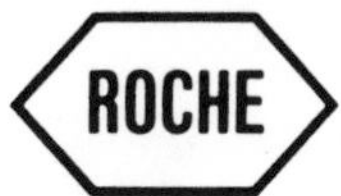

PRESENTED WITH

THE COMPLIMENTS OF

ROCHE LABORATORIES

DIVISION OF

HOFFMANN - LA ROCHE INC.

NUTLEY, N. J.

Emergency Care
as Practiced
at the
Massachusetts
General Hospital,
Boston

emergency medicine

Scientific Foundations and Current Practice

THIRD EDITION

Emergency Care as Practiced at the Massachusetts General Hospital, Boston

emergency medicine

Scientific Foundations and Current Practice

THIRD EDITION

EDITOR

EARLE W. WILKINS, JR., M.D.
Chief, Emergency Services, 1961–1988

ASSOCIATE EDITORS

JAMES J. DINEEN, M.D.
Associate Physician

PETER L. GROSS, M.D., F.A.C.E.P.
Associate Chief, Emergency Services

CHARLES J. McCABE, M.D.
Associate Chief, Emergency Services

ASHBY C. MONCURE, M.D.
Visiting Surgeon

PATRICIA J. O'MALLEY, M.D.
Assistant Chief, Emergency Services

Editor: Timothy H. Grayson
Associate Editor: Carol Eckhart
Copy Editors: Klemie Bryte, Judith F. Minkove
Design: Norman W. Och
Illustration Planning: Lorraine Wrzosek
Production: Raymond E. Reter

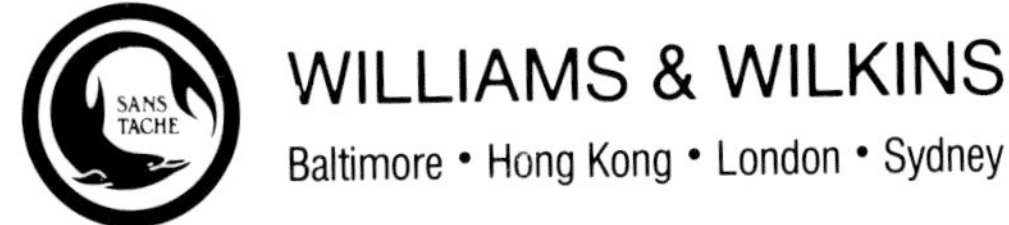

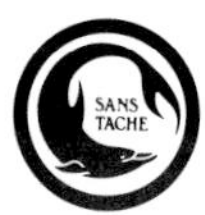

Editor: Timothy H. Grayson
Associate Editor: Carol Eckhart
Copy Editors: Klemie Bryte, Judith F. Minkove
Design: Norman W. Och
Illustration Planning: Lorraine Wrzosek
Production: Raymond E. Reter

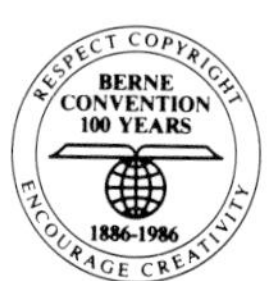

Accurate indications, adverse reactions, and dosage schedules for drugs are provided in this book, but it is possible that they may change. The reader is urged to review the package information data of the manufacturers of the medications mentioned.

Printed in the United States of America

Previously published as *MGH Textbook of Emergency Medicine*
First Edition, 1978
Second Edition, 1983

Library of Congress Cataloging-in-Publication Data

Emergency medicine.
Rev. ed. of: MGH textbook of emergency medicine.
2nd ed. c1983.
Includes bibliographies and indexes.
1. Emergency medicine.
2. Wilkins, Earle W., 1919- II. Dineen,
James J., 1938- . III. MGH textbook of emergency
medicine. [DNLM: 1. Emergency Medicine. WB 105 E559]
RC86.7.E5785 1988 616′.025 87-25320
ISBN 0-683-09085-2

89 90 91 92 10 9 8 7 6 5 4 3

To Emergency Physicians everywhere

Foreword

Emergency medicine has emerged not only as a specialty but, indeed, as a true science, as well. The purpose of this textbook is, as its name implies, to provide a scientific foundation for the therapeutic practices that are currently used in the emergency department. As we address further scientific investigation in this arena, we can explore a hitherto unknown facet of disease—one that begins in the field, continues in transport (by air or ground), centers in the emergency department, and ultimately integrates with established research in the operating rooms, intensive care units and the research laboratories of our hospitals. Hopefully, this investigation will lead to more effective patient management not only in the field but throughout a patient's acute care and rehabilitation process.

It has been my privilege this year to take over the duties as Chief of Emergency Services at the Massachusetts General Hospital succeeding the Senior Editor of this text. Dr. Wilkins' tenure extended back to 1961 and so covered the entire temporal frame in the development of emergency medicine. It culminated in chairmanship of the board of Boston Med Flight, the unique consortium of teaching hospitals that sponsor aeromedical transport in northern and eastern New England. As Medical Director of that most successful operation and as a surgeon, I welcomed association with him in that project and now in his book.

Alasdair K. Conn, M.D.
Boston, Massachusetts

Preface to the Third Edition

It has been 10 years since the debut of this textbook in its first edition. The decade has been full, from the birth of the American Board of Emergency Medicine in 1979 to the organization of complex systems of emergency medical services nationwide. The body of knowledge required of the emergency physician has continued to expand. A flurry of emergency medicine textbooks has appeared, one indicator of the acceptance and growth of the specialty. It is time then for a renewal of this particular effort.

The renewal begins with a renaming. The new title *Emergency Medicine: Scientific Foundations and Current Practice* more accurately reflects both its purpose and content. This book continues to call upon experts in each specialty from the Massachusetts General Hospital under the premise that the in-depth experience of each is the best foundation for presentation of any given subject. Although the practice of emergency medicine is not limited to the emergency department—the intensive care unit and the surgical recovery room are hospital areas requiring the same body of knowledge—an attempt has been made to orient content to the emergency physician. Associate Editor Peter L. Gross is boarded in Emergency Medicine and a Fellow of the American College of Emergency Physicians.

The format continues to emphasize medical and surgical subspecialties, but new sections have been added for pediatrics and radiology. These two fields, like emergency medicine, are horizontally structured across the medical fields and anatomic systems that constitute traditional specialization. The Pediatrics section was added because of the frequent comment that giving care to the neonate and young pediatric patient aroused the greatest insecurity. The Radiology section was added to reflect its diagnostic role in trauma, to emphasize pertinent and new imaging techniques, to expand on angiographic methodology and, again, to underscore particular concerns in pediatrics.

In addition, the Illustrated Techniques section has been expanded by 10 procedures commonly encountered in the emergency department. An Appendix has been included: a useful drug reference guide calling attention to important matters of dosage, side effects, and contraindications. An expanded Index has been bolstered by outlines at the beginning of each chapter indicating location of particular subject content and by the addition of major topics in the Contents.

A chapter on emergency medical services systems has been dropped to conserve space. Its content would have been unchanged, except for modernization with coverage of aeromedical evacuation and transport systems. The Boston system, which the chapter reflected, can still be researched in the second edition, which is available in most libraries.

This third edition presents the scientific basis for emergency medicine, providing an essential foundation for all residents working in emergency departments. This book will be a ready reference for the continuing education of the emergency physician and a useful resource for all physicians encountering emergency situations in hospital settings.

EARLE W. WILKINS, JR., M.D.

Preface to Second Edition

The first national medical specialty board was recognized in 1917. In September 1979, 62 years later, the American Board of Emergency Medicine (ABEM) became the 23rd specialty board. A resolution adopted by the American Board of Medical Specialties recognized the ABEM as a conjoint board of the American Board of Family Practice, the American Board of Internal Medicine, the American Board of Obstetrics and Gynecology, the American Board of Otolaryngology, the American Board of Pediatrics, the American Board of Psychiatry and Neurology, the American Board of Surgery, the American College of Emergency Physicians, the American Medical Association's Section on Emergency Medicine, and the University Association for Emergency Medicine. Like the American Board of Family Practice, the ABEM is structured by means of "horizontal categorization" rather than the conventional "vertical categorization." Because of this cross-disciplinary framework, Emergency Medicine must be prepared to provide diagnosis and treatment for the entire spectrum of problems cared for by the sponsoring boards. This is a mighty challenge!

The coming-of-age of the specialty of Emergency Medicine has brought added responsibilities. Foremost among these are medical education, the development of standards of care for emergency departments as well as patterns of follow-up care that compensate for the episodic nature of the doctor-patient relationship, the formulation of mutually acceptable working arrangements with other specialties, and research into the common problems that are encountered in this broad field.

This textbook is directed toward the difficult task of education in perhaps the broadest specialty of all. Its contents originally stemmed from lectures presented to participants in the 2-week practical course sponsored by the Department of Continuing Education at the Harvard Medical School and the Massachusetts General Hospital (Emergency Care: An Extended Workshop). This course is now in its 14th year, and the present course director, Dr. Peter L. Gross, has been added as associate editor of this second edition.

Textbook preparation has been an immense task. An attempt has been made to avoid an encyclopedic treatise and to maintain a physically manageable size, while providing an in-depth approach to specific patient problems. The purpose has been to include material covering all aspects of medical care in the emergency department, to help bridge the sometimes difficult transition from emergency department to hospital specialty care, and to provide insights into subsequent diagnosis and therapy that may be affected by decisions made in the first moments of care. A criticism of the first edition was that it was largely written by traditional specialists and not by emergency physicians. Although this is still the case, every effort has been made in the second edition to heed specific suggestions of earlier critics.

The basic format of five sections has been maintained. In section 1, Life Support, a chapter on the treatment of the patient with multisystem trauma has been added, and in section 2, Medicine, chapters have been added on environmental hazards (including hyperthermia, radiation, barotrauma, and bites and stings) and on states of altered consciousness. In addition, Chapter 14 (new Chapter 17), Toxicologic Emergencies, has been reorganized. In section 4, Administration, the two chapters on the Massachusetts General Hospital Emergency Ward have been deleted; teaching hospitals that found this information useful can still refer to the first edition. Chapter 36, Emergency Medical Services Systems, is new, and describes the development and management of the excellent prehospital system of patient care in the city of Boston; this chapter was written by two authorities from the Boston City Hospital, which is the resource hospital for Medic IV, the regional emergency medical services system project. Finally, section 5, Illustrated Techniques, has been expanded, with the continued excellence of principal artist Mrs. Edith Tagrin.

The editors wish to express special gratitude to Ms. Catherine P. Fitzgerald, Editorial Associate, and to Mrs. Jane S. McDermott, who has skillfully handled the entire task—familiar to all editors—of coaxing authors, correlating material, and meeting deadlines.

Earle W. Wilkins, Jr., M.D.

Contributors

Ran D. Anbar, M.D.
(Chapter 25) Clinical Fellow in Pediatrics, Massachusetts General Hospital; Research Fellow in Pediatrics, Harvard Medical School, Boston, Massachusetts

William H. Anderson, M.D.
(Chapter 18) Associate Psychiatrist, Massachusetts General Hospital; Chairman, Department of Psychiatry, St. Elizabeth's Hospital; Lecturer in Psychiatry, Harvard Medical School, Boston, Massachusetts

Christos A. Athanasoulis, M.D.
(Chapter 46) Radiologist and Head, Vascular Radiology, Massachusetts General Hospital; Professor of Radiology, Harvard Medical School, Boston, Massachusetts

Ann S. Baker, M.D.
(Chapter 10) Associate Physician and Member, Infectious Disease Unit, Massachusetts General Hospital; Assistant Professor of Medicine, Harvard Medical School, Boston, Massachusetts

Peter C. Block, M.D.
(Illustrated Technique 8) Physician and Director, Cardiac Catheterization Laboratory, Massachusetts General Hospital; Associate Professor of Medicine, Harvard Medical School, Boston, Massachusetts

Lawrence F. Borges, M.D.
(Chapter 37) Assistant Visiting Neurosurgeon, Massachusetts General Hospital; Assistant Professor of Surgery (Neurosurgery), Harvard Medical School, Boston, Massachusetts

Michael Broad, Esq.
(Chapter 49) Deputy General Counsel, Massachusetts General Hospital, Boston, Massachusetts

Frank P. Castronovo, Jr., Ph.D.
(Chapter 10) Associate Radiopharmacologist and Radiation Safety Officer, Massachusetts General Hospital; Associate Professor of Radiology, Harvard Medical School, Boston, Massachusetts

Elizabeth A. Catlin, M.D.
(Chapter 22) Assistant Pediatrician, Massachusetts General Hospital; Instructor in Pediatrics, Harvard Medical School, Boston, Massachusetts

David S. Chapin, M.D.
(Chapter 34; Illustrated Technique 17) Clinical Associate in Gynecology, Massachusetts General Hospital; Director of Gynecology, Beth Israel Hospital; Instructor in Obstetrics and Gynecology, Harvard Medical School, Boston, Massachusetts

Robert H. Cleveland, M.D.
(Chapter 47) Associate Radiologist, Massachusetts General Hospital; Associate Professor of Radiology, Harvard Medical School, Boston, Massachusetts

Cecil H. Coggins, M.D.
(Chapter 8) Physician and Clinical Director, Renal Unit, Massachusetts General Hospital; Associate Professor of Medicine, Harvard Medical School, Boston, Massachusetts

Rita Colley, R.N.
(Illustrated Technique 5) *Formerly* Nurse Clinician, Hyperalimentation Unit, Massachusetts General Hospital, Boston, Massachusetts

David J. Cullen, M.D.
(Illustrated Techniques 1 and 2) Anesthetist and Director of the Recovery Room, Massachusetts General Hospital; Professor of Anesthesia, Harvard Medical School, Boston, Massachusetts

Gilbert H. Daniels, M.D.
(Chapter 14) Associate Physician and Co-Director, Thyroid Associates, Massachusetts General Hospital; Associate Professor of Medicine, Harvard Medical School, Boston, Massachusetts

G. William Dec, M.D.
(Chapter 6) Assistant in Medicine and Director, Medical Intensive Care Unit, Massachusetts General Hospital; Instructor in Medicine, Harvard Medical School, Boston, Massachusetts

Harold J. Demonaco, M.S.
(Drug Index) Director, Pharmacy, Massachusetts General Hospital, Boston, Massachusetts

Roman W. DeSanctis, M.D.
(Chapter 5) Physician and Director, Clinical Cardiology, Massachusetts General Hospital; Professor of Medicine, Harvard Medical School, Boston, Massachusetts

James J. Dineen, M.D.
(Associate Editor) Associate Physician, Massachusetts General Hospital; Assistant Professor of Medicine, Harvard Medical School, Boston, Massachusetts

R. Bruce Donoff, D.M.D., M.D.
(Chapter 40) Chief, Oral and Maxillofacial Surgery Service, Massachusetts General Hospital; Professor and Chairman, Oral and Maxillofacial Surgery Department, Harvard School of Dental Medicine, Boston, Massachusetts

Elizabeth C. Dooling, M.D.
(Chapter 28) Associate Neurologist and Associate Pediatrician, Massachusetts General Hospital; Associate Professor of Neurology, Harvard Medical School, Boston, Massachusetts

Stephen P. Dretler, M.D.
(Chapter 35) Associate Urologist and Director of Lithotriptor Unit, Massachusetts General Hospital; Associate Professor of Urology, Harvard Medical School, Boston, Massachusetts

Roland D. Eavey, M.D.
(Chapter 23) Director, Ear, Nose and Throat Pediatric Service, Massachusetts Eye and Ear Infirmary; Assistant Professor of Otolaryngology, Harvard Medical School, Boston, Massachusetts

Leonard Ellman, M.D.
(Chapter 13) Physician and Director, Hematology Laboratories, Massachusetts General Hospital; Associate Professor of Medicine, Harvard Medical School, Boston, Massachusetts

A. John Erdman III, M.D.
(Illustrated Technique 10) *Deceased*

Michael A. Fifer, M.D.
(Chapter 7) Assistant in Medicine, Massachusetts General Hospital; Assistant Professor of Medicine, Harvard Medical School, Boston, Massachusetts

Josef E. Fischer, M.D.
(Illustrated Technique 5) Surgeon-in-Chief, University Hospital; Christian R. Holmes Professor and Chairman, Department of Surgery, University of Cincinnati College of Medicine, Cincinnati, Ohio

Thomas B. Fitzpatrick, M.D., Ph.D.
(Chapter 19) Dermatologist (*formerly* Chief), Dermatology Service, Massachusetts General Hospital; Edward Wigglesworth Professor of Dermatology, Harvard Medical School, Boston, Massachusetts

Albert R. Frederick, Jr., M.D.
(Chapter 43) Associate Surgeon in Ophthalmology, Massachusetts Eye and Ear Infirmary; Clinical Instructor in Ophthalmology, Harvard Medical School, Boston, Massachusetts

Herbert Freund, M.D.
(Illustrated Technique 5) Senior Lecturer in Surgery, Hadassah Hebrew University, Jerusalem, Israel

Stuart C. Geller, M.D.
(Chapter 46) Assistant Radiologist, Massachusetts General Hospital; Instructor in Radiology, Harvard Medical School, Boston, Massachusetts

Peter L. Gross, M.D., F.A.C.E.P.
(Associate Editor; Chapters 10 and 17) Associate Physician and Associate Chief, Emergency Services, Massachusetts General Hospital, Boston, Massachusetts

Walter Guralnick, D.M.D.
(Chapter 40) Visiting Oral and Maxillofacial Surgeon, Massachusetts General Hospital; Emeritus Professor of Oral and Maxillofacial Surgery, Harvard School of Dental Medicine, Boston, Massachusetts

Ernest M. Haddad, Esq.
(Chapter 49) Secretary and General Counsel, Massachusetts General Hospital, Boston, Massachusetts

Charles A. Hales, M.D.
(Chapter 9) Associate Physician, Pulmonary Unit, Massachusetts General Hospital; Associate Professor of Medicine, Harvard Medical School, Boston, Massachusetts

Hamilton R. Hayes, M.D., F.A.C.E.P.
(Chapter 2) Emergency Physician, Anna Jaques Hospital, Newburyport, Massachusetts

John M. Head, M.D.
(Chapter 32) Chief, Surgical Service, and Associate Chief of Staff, Veterans Administration Hospital, White River Junction, Vermont; Professor of Clinical Surgery and Vice Chairman, Department of Surgery, Dartmouth Medical School, Hanover, New Hampshire

Daniel G. Heller, M.D.
(Chapter 27) Associate Pediatrician, Massachusetts General Hospital; Instructor in Pediatrics, Harvard Medical School, Boston, Massachusetts

Thomas E. Herman, M.D.
(Chapter 47) Assistant Radiologist, Massachusetts General Hospital; Assistant Professor of Radiology, Harvard Medical School, Boston, Massachusetts

John T. Herrin, M.B.B.S.
(Chapter 27) Chief, Pediatric Nephrology, and Pediatrician, Massachusetts General Hospital; Chief, Pediatrics, Shriners Burns Institute; Associate Clinical Professor of Pediatrics, Harvard Medical School, Boston, Massachusetts

Alan D. Hilgenberg, M.D.
(Chapter 31) Associate Visiting Surgeon, Massachusetts General Hospital, Boston; Chief of Thoracic and Cardiovascular Surgery, Mt. Auburn Hospital, Cambridge; Assistant Professor of Surgery, Harvard Medical School, Boston, Massachusetts

B. Thomas Hutchinson, M.D.
(Chapter 43) Associate Chief of Ophthalmology, Massachusetts Eye and Ear Infirmary; Associate Clinical Professor of Ophthalmology, Harvard Medical School, Boston, Massachusetts

Adolph M. Hutter, Jr., M.D.
(Chapter 6) Physician and Chairman, Medical Intensive Care Coordinating Committee, Massachusetts General Hospital; Associate Professor of Medicine, Harvard Medical School, Boston, Massachusetts

Richard A. Johnson, M.D.
(Chapter 19) Clinical Associate in Dermatology, Massachusetts General Hospital; Clinical Instructor in Dermatology, Harvard Medical School, Boston, Massachusetts

Robert A. Johnson, M.D.
(Chapter 7) Walla Walla, Washington; *formerly* Assistant Physician, Massachusetts General Hospital; Assistant Professor of Medicine, Harvard Medical School, Boston, Massachusetts

Dorothy H. Kelly, M.D.
(Chapter 24) Associate Pediatrician and Co-Director, Pediatric Pulmonary Laboratory, Massachusetts General Hospital; Assistant Professor of Pediatrics, Harvard Medical School, Boston, Massachusetts

John P. Kelly, D.M.D., M.D.
(Chapter 40) Visiting Oral and Maxillofacial Surgeon, Massachusetts General Hospital; Assistant Professor, Harvard School of Dental Medicine, Boston, Massachusetts

Sean Kennedy, M.D.
(Chapter 3) Associate Anesthetist and Co-Director, Neurological-Neurosurgical Intensive Care Unit, Massachusetts General Hospital; Assistant Professor of Anesthesia, Harvard Medical School, Boston, Massachusetts

Samuel H. Kim, M.D.
(Chapter 30) Visiting Surgeon, Division of Pediatric Surgery, Massachusetts General Hospital; Associate Clinical Professor of Surgery, Harvard Medical School, Boston, Massachusetts

Glenn M. LaMuraglia, M.D.
(Chapter 30) Assistant in Surgery, Massachusetts General Hospital; Instructor in Surgery, Harvard Medical School, Boston, Massachusetts

Daniel Chia-Sen Lee, M.D.
(Chapter 7) Dedham Medical Associates, Dedham, Massachusetts

Michael B. Lewis, M.D.
(Chapters 38 and 39) Assistant in Surgery, Massachusetts General Hospital; Surgeon and Chief, Division of Plastic Surgery, New England Medical Center Hospital; Associate Professor in Surgery, Tufts University Medical School; Instructor in Surgery, Harvard Medical School, Boston, Massachusetts

David A. Link, M.D.
(Chapter 27) Pediatrician, Massachusetts General Hospital; Instructor in Pediatrics, Harvard Medical School, Boston, Massachusetts

David B. Lovejoy, M.D.
(Chapter 36) Assistant Orthopaedic Surgeon, Massachusetts General Hospital; Chief of Orthopaedics, The Cambridge Hospital, Cambridge, Massachusetts; Clinical Instructor in Orthopaedic Surgery, Harvard Medical School, Boston, Massachusetts

Dennis P. Lund, M.D.
(Chapter 30) Assistant in Surgery, Massachusetts General Hospital; Clinical Fellow in Surgery, Harvard Medical School, Boston, Massachusetts

Douglas J. Mathisen, M.D.
(Chapter 32) Assistant Surgeon, Massachusetts General Hospital; Assistant Professor of Surgery, Harvard Medical School, Boston, Massachusetts

Charles J. McCabe, M.D.
(Associate Editor; Chapters 1, 4, and 33; Illustrated Techniques 4, 6, 7, 9, 11, 13, 18–22, 26, and 27) Associate Visiting Surgeon and Associate Chief, Emergency Services, Massachusetts General Hospital; Assistant Professor of Surgery, Harvard Medical School, Boston, Massachusetts

Ashby C. Moncure, M.D.
(Associate Editor; Chapters 31 and 33; Illustrated Techniques 3 and 15) Visiting Surgeon, Massachusetts General Hospital; Associate Clinical Professor of Surgery, Harvard Medical School, Boston, Massachusetts

Thomas J. Mulvaney, M.D.
(Chapter 42) Medical Director, Ear, Nose and Throat Ambulatory Services, Massachusetts Eye and Ear Infirmary; Clinical Instructor in Otolaryngology, Harvard Medical School, Boston, Massachusetts

Edward A. Nardell, M.D.
(Chapter 9) Department of Medicine, Cambridge Hospital, Cambridge, Massachusetts; Assistant Professor of Medicine, Harvard Medical School, Boston, Massachusetts

Robert A. Novelline, M.D.
(Chapters 44 and 45) Radiologist and Director of Emergency Radiology, Massachusetts General Hospital; Associate Professor of Radiology, Harvard Medical School, Boston, Massachusetts

Nicholas E. O'Connor, M.D.
(Chapter 38) Department of Plastic Surgery, Brigham and Women's Hospital; Instructor in Surgery, Harvard Medical School, Boston, Massachusetts

Patricia J. O'Malley, M.D.
(Associate Editor; Chapters 20, 21, 26, and 29) Associate Pediatrician and Director, Pediatric Emergency Unit, Massachusetts General Hospital; Instructor in Pediatrics, Harvard Medical School, Boston, Massachusetts

Leslie W. Ottinger, M.D.
(Chapter 33) Visiting Surgeon, Massachusetts General Hospital; Associate Professor of Surgery, Harvard Medical School, Boston, Massachusetts

Rufus C. Partlow, Jr., M.D.
(Chapter 42) Tuscaloosa, Alabama; *formerly* Associate Surgeon, Massachusetts Eye and Ear Infirmary; Clinical Instructor in Otolaryngology, Harvard Medical School, Boston, Massachusetts

Donald C. Patterson, M.D.
(Chapter 34) Department of Obstetrics and Gynecology, Columbia Regional Hospital, Boone Health Center, University of Missouri Medical Center, Columbia, Missouri

Amy A. Pruitt, M.D.
(Chapters 15 and 16; Illustrated Technique 14) Associate Neurologist, Massachusetts General Hospital; Assistant Professor of Neurology, Harvard Medical School, Boston, Massachusetts

James M. Richter, M.D.
(Chapter 12) Assistant Physician, Massachusetts General Hospital; Assistant Professor of Medicine, Harvard Medical School, Boston, Massachusetts

Carter R. Rowe, M.D.
(Illustrated Technique 23) Senior Orthopaedic Surgeon, Massachusetts General Hospital; Emeritus Associate Clinical Professor of Orthopaedic Surgery, Harvard Medical School, Boston, Massachusetts

Eric. J. Sacknoff, M.D.
(Illustrated Technique 16) Attending Urologist, Mt. Auburn Hospital, Cambridge, Massachusetts; Clinical Instructor in Urology, Harvard Medical School, Boston, Massachusetts

Richard Sacknoff, M.D.
(Chapters 44 and 45) Assistant Radiologist, Massachusetts General Hospital; Instructor in Radiology, Harvard Medical School, Boston, Massachusetts

Stephen F. Schiff, M.D.
(Chapter 35) Assistant Professor of Surgery (Urology), Section of Urology, Yale University School of Medicine, New Haven, Connecticut

Daniel C. Shannon, M.D.
(Chapter 24) Pediatrician, Massachusetts General Hospital; Associate Professor of Pediatrics, Harvard Medical School, Boston, Massachusetts

Bradford J. Shingleton, M.D.
(Chapter 43) Director, Eye Emergency Service and Associate Surgeon in Ophthalmology, Massachusetts Eye and Ear Infirmary; Clinical Instructor in Ophthalmology, Harvard Medical School, Boston, Massachusetts

Harvey B. Simon, M.D.
(Chapter 11) Associate Physician, Infectious Disease Unit, Massachusetts General Hospital; Assistant Professor of Medicine, Harvard Medical School, Boston, Massachusetts

Richard J. Smith, M.D.
(Chapter 41) Deceased; *formerly* Chief, Hand Surgery Service, Department of Orthopaedic Surgery, Massachusetts General Hospital; Clinical Professor of Orthopaedic Surgery, Harvard Medical School, Boston, Massachusetts

Theodore A. Stern, M.D.
(Chapter 18) Assistant Psychiatrist, Massachusetts General Hospital; Assistant Professor of Psychiatry, Harvard Medical School, Boston, Massachusetts

Denise J. Strieder, M.D.
(Chapter 25) Associate Pediatrician, Massachusetts General Hospital; Associate Professor of Pediatrics, Harvard Medical School, Boston, Massachusetts

David M. Systrom, M.D.
(Chapter 9) Clinical Assistant in Medicine, Pulmonary Unit, Massachusetts General Hospital; Instructor in Medicine, Harvard Medical School, Boston, Massachusetts

George E. Thibault, M.D.
(Chapter 5) Physician and Associate Chief, Medical Services, Massachusetts General Hospital; Associate Professor of Medicine, Harvard Medical School, Boston, Massachusetts

B. Taylor Thompson, M.D.
(Chapter 9) Assistant in Medicine, Pulmonary Unit, Massachusetts General Hospital; Instructor in Medicine, Harvard Medical School, Boston, Massachusetts

I. David Todres, M.D.
(Chapters 21 and 23) Pediatrician and Anesthesiologist, Director of Pediatric Intensive Care and Neonatal Units, Massachusetts General Hospital; Associate Professor of Anesthesia (Pediatrics), Harvard Medical School, Boston, Massachusetts

Katherine K. Treadway, M.D.
(Chapter 8) Assistant Physician, Massachusetts General Hospital; Instructor in Medicine, Harvard Medical School, Boston, Massachusetts

Virginia Tritschler, R.N., B.S.
(Chapter 48) *Formerly* Clinical Nurse Leader, Emergency Services, Massachusetts General Hospital, Boston, Massachusetts

Arthur C. Waltman, M.D.
(Chapter 46) Radiologist, Massachusetts General Hospital; Professor of Radiology, Harvard Medical School, Boston, Massachusetts

Nancy Weber-Bornstein, M.D.
(Chapter 10) Emergency Physician, Boston City Hospital; Boston University, Boston, Massachusetts

James G. Wepsic, M.D.
(Chapter 37) Assistant Visiting Neurosurgeon, Massachusetts General Hospital; Neurosurgeon, New England Baptist Hospital, Boston, Massachusetts

Ernest A. Weymuller, Jr., M.D.
(Chapter 42) Otolaryngologist-in-Chief, Harborview Medical Center; Associate Professor of Otolaryngology, University of Washington, Seattle, Washington

Earle W. Wilkins, Jr., M.D.
(Editor; Illustrated Technique 12) Chief, Emergency Services (Retired), Visiting Surgeon, Massachusetts General Hospital; Clinical Professor of Surgery, Harvard Medical School, Boston, Massachusetts

Edwin T. Wyman, Jr., M.D.
(Chapter 36) Chief of Fracture Service and Visiting Orthopaedic Surgeon, Massachusetts General Hospital; Assistant Clinical Professor of Orthopaedic Surgery, Harvard Medical School, Boston, Massachusetts

Bertram Zarins, M.D.
(Illustrated Techniques 23, 24, and 25) Associate Orthopaedic Surgeon, Massachusetts General Hospital; Assistant Clinical Professor of Orthopaedic Surgery, Harvard Medical School, Boston, Massachusetts

Contents

SECTION 3

Pediatrics

Associate Editor, Patricia J. O'Malley, M.D.

SECTION 4

Surgery

Associate Editor, Ashby C. Moncure, M.D.

SECTION 5

Radiology

Editor, Earle W. Wilkins, Jr., M.D.

SECTION 6

Supporting Services

Associate Editor, Peter L. Gross, M.D., F.A.C.E.P.

SECTION 7

Illustrated Techniques

Medical Artist, Edith Tagrin
Associate Editor, Charles J. McCabe, M.D.

SECTION 1

Life Support

CHARLES J. McCABE, M.D.
Associate Editor

CHAPTER 1

Prehospital Medical Care

CHARLES J. McCABE, M.D.

The prehospital management of the acutely ill or injured and the emergency department management of these same patients form a natural continuum. As a result, the emergency physician has an obligation to participate in the field management by both on-line and off-line medical direction, as well as by quality assurance monitoring of the care provided. In order for the prehospital emergency medical technician and paramedic to become the "physician extenders," the physician must play an active role in their continuing education and the development of their knowledge base and skills.

THE EMERGENCY MEDICAL SERVICES SYSTEM

There are 10 components to a well-developed emergency medical services (EMS) system, (Table 1.1). Each is critically dependent upon the other, and the statement that the system is only as strong as its "weakest link" is applicable to EMS. An injury or acute illness must be recognized, immediate care provided, and a call for help initiated. In well-developed EMS systems, the universal emergency number 911 is available. It is surprising how many areas of the country do not have this access number to an EMS system, and often the phone book must be consulted before help can be summoned. Commonly, the operator or the police are called, which results in additional response delay. Ideally, an ambulance company should respond to an emergency call within 5 minutes, and decreasing the response time is an area that needs concerted effort. Voluntary ambulance services supply the emergency care in many areas and states of this country. They may be unavailable or response times may be in excess of what is required.

Table 1.1.
Components of an Emergency Medical Services (EMS) System

1. Recognition of the emergency or the initiation of first aid
2. Activation of the EMS system (911)
3. Initiation of treatment at the scene by first responders, EMS personnel
4. Transport by EMS personnel (EMT/paramedic)
5. Treatment in emergency department
6. Treatment in operating room
7. Treatment in intensive care unit (ICU)
8. Organization/communication
9. Planning, education, evaluation
10. Research

The ambulance personnel have an obligation to initiate care and transport the patient safely to an appropriate facility. The hospital and the emergency department often provide direction by radio to the personnel in the street, and the patient's arrival in the emergency department may be anticipated and the care already delivered understood. The hospital is then responsible for providing care in the emergency department, the operating room (if necessary), and the regular or intensive care units. The remaining elements of the EMS system are case review, quality assurance, and research into methods of improving the delivery of care.

The provision of this care is not inexpensive. It has been estimated that to provide a single paramedic-staffed vehicle may cost in excess of $350,000/year. The communication system is also costly. Obviously, not all communities can bear this expense, and many innovative techniques have been facilitated in order to provide advanced life support care. Many of these use hospital-based advanced life support personnel in nontransport vehicles to respond to advanced life support calls as a backup to basic life support ambulances. This has worked reasonably well and may provide care to multiple communities, thereby defraying the expense.

PERSONNEL AND EQUIPMENT

The ambulance and its operator have changed dramatically since 1965. Prior to that time, the vehicles available to transport patients in the supine position were often hearses, driven by morticians. The care that patients received prior to arrival in the emergency department was limited. In 1966, the National Academy of Science published the National Research Council's report, "Accidental Death and Disability, The Neglected Disease of Modern Society." This publication exposed the inadequacies of emergency care for the acutely ill and injured, and the Department of Transportation was given the task of developing a training program for providers of prehospital care. A modular system of training and skill development was instituted and has since become the standard of training for the new paraprofessional—the emergency medical technician (EMT). Similarly, ambulances and their equipment were standardized.

The goals of prehospital care are to assess the emergency problem, to provide immediate support for life-threatening emergencies, and to transport the patient safely and rapidly to an appropriate care facility. The care is delivered at either a basic or an advanced level. Basic EMTs are trained in a 110-hour, Department of Transportation-approved program that educates them in cardiopulmonary resuscitation, management of the obstructed airway, methods of immobilization, care of wounds, and control of external hemorrhage. The use of the military antishock trousers (MAST) has recently also become part of standard education. All of this care is provided by noninvasive techniques and does not necessarily require on-line medical communication.

In some states the basic EMT has been trained and is allowed to defibrillate patients who have suffered out-of-hospital cardiorespiratory arrest. This movement has been spearheaded by Eisenberg and Stults, and in their well-developed EMS system with short response times, the improvement in survival

Table 1.2.
Components of the Original Paramedic Didactic Course

	Module	
*	I	The emergency medical technician
*	II	Human systems and patient assessment
*	III	Shock and fluid therapy
	IV	General pharmacology
*	V	Respiratory system
	VI	Cardiovascular system
	VII	Central nervous system
	VIII	Soft tissue injuries
	IX	Musculoskeletal system
	X	Medical emergencies
	XI	Obstetric/gynecologic emergencies
	XII	Pediatrics and neonatal transport
	XIII	Emergency care of the emotionally disturbed
	XIV	Extrication/rescue techniques
*	XV	Telemetry and communications

* = EMT-I.

with basic EMT defibrillation (EMT-D) has been up to 40% versus 2–3%. Eisenberg has emphasized that time is the important element in predicting survival from out-of-hospital cardiac arrest. The important time factors include a witnessed arrest and the initiation of cardiopulmonary resuscitation (CPR) within 4 minutes. Definitive care, that is, defibrillation, must be provided within 8 to 10 minutes in order for improved outcomes to be realized. Many systems have attempted to duplicate Eisenberg and Stults' results without first developing the framework of quick response times and early CPR.

Advanced life support is provided in several categories (intermediate, paramedic). At this level the basic EMT is upgraded in education and in skill capabilities. Normally, a paramedic has 500–1500 hours of didactic, clinical, and field experience and develops many advanced capabilities in caring for acutely ill or injured patients. The education includes normal anatomy and physiology and the alterations induced by illness or injury (Table 1.2). Technical skills are developed, including the insertion of intravenous lines and the administration of fluids, the use of intravenous medications and the defibrillator, and—probably the most important skill—the invasive management of the airway with an endotracheal tube. These skills are initially learned on manikins, then developed in the clinical hospital setting under supervision, and finally performed in the field.

The EMT Intermediate (EMT-I) has been trained specifically to care for the trauma patient. The training is less intense and covers five of the 15 paramedic modules (Table 1.2): patient assessment, anatomy, physiology, shock, and the respiratory system. The technical skills of the EMT-I include advanced airway management (endotracheal tube, esophageal obturator airway), intravenous administration of fluids (but not medications), and use of the military antishock trousers. Unfortunately, for the majority of calls to which an ambulance service responds (medical emergencies), the EMT-I is not able to provide the necessary emergency care. If equipped with a defibrillator and a few medications, their skills would be put to greater use.

One of the most important aspects of training prehospital personnel is assessment of patients' complaints and, by physical examination, determination of the etiology. Communication then can be established between the EMT-I/paramedic and the hospital-based physician so that appropriate therapy can be instituted in the field. The EMT-I/paramedic acts as the eyes and hands of the on-line medical control physician, and a reliance and confidence must be established between the two.

PREHOSPITAL CARE

The EMS system must deal with seven major areas of acute illness or injury: (*a*) spinal cord injuries, (*b*) trauma, (*c*) psychiatric disturbances, (*d*) pediatric problems, (*e*) cardiac disease, (*f*) burns, and (*g*) poisoning/drug abuse. Of these, trauma and cardiac disease account for the vast majority of cases. Trauma causes approximately 10 million disabling injuries and 165,000 deaths/year. Accidents have become the leading cause of death in children over age 1. In the nontraumatic category, approximately 1 million people die each year of cardiac disorders.

The field treatment of medical patients versus trauma patients is very different. For the trauma patient, the goals are simple and based on the premise that *stabilization and definitive care cannot be provided in the field.* They consist of patient extrication, rapid assessment, immediate lifesaving maneuvers, and rapid transport to an appropriate hospital. The amount of time spent in the prehospital management of the trauma patient has been described as the "golden 10 minutes" and sets the time frame for treatment. Unfortunately, with the development of advanced life support in the pre-

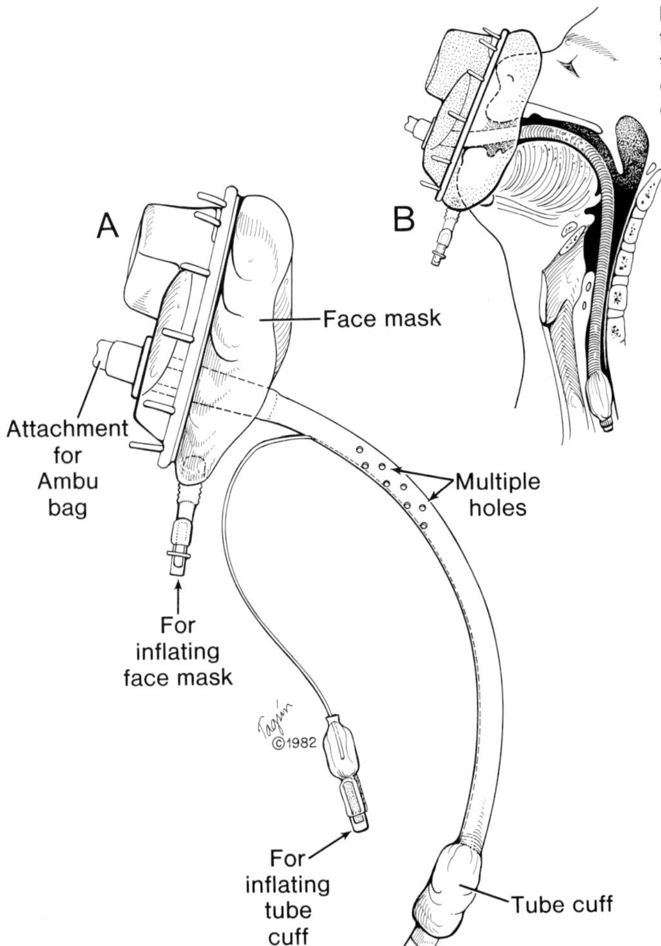

Figure 1.1. The esophageal obturator airway (EOA). *A,* The structure of the device. *B,* Correctly placed in the esophagus with cuff inflated and mask creating a seal.

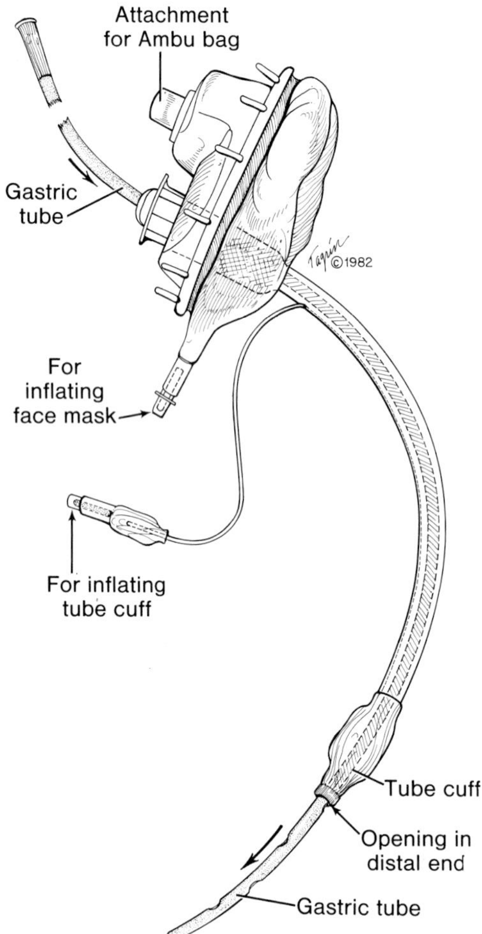

Figure 1.2. The esophageal-gastric tube airway (EGTA) has a port permitting insertion of a tube and removal of gastric contents.

hospital arena, an all too frequent problem has developed: delaying transport of the trauma patient while advanced procedures are performed in an attempt to stabilize the patient in the field. This attempt at stabilization has no place in trauma management.

There should be little time wasted treating the trauma patient in the prehospital arena. An absolute requirement is the provision of a patent airway and adequate ventilation. The appropriate airway used in the trauma patient, when necessary, is the endotracheal tube. The esophageal obturator airway (EOA) (Fig. 1.1) and the esophagogastric tube airway (EGTA) (Fig. 1.2) have been popular in some systems. Unfortunately, they were utilized before their efficacy had been established in the prehospital arena. Studies indicate that they are often ineffective in providing ventilation and oxygenation in the prehospital setting. Recently, the pharyngeal-tracheal lumen airway (PTLA) (Fig. 1.3) has been marketed for use in the field. This device is similar in many respects to the EOA/EGTA. It has not yet proven beneficial when used in the prehospital arena and must be field-tested before it can be widely used.

The resuscitation of the trauma patient in the field is often attempted with the utilization of the MAST (Fig. 1.4) and intravenous volume support. The MAST splints fractures, tamponades external hemorrhage and potential internal hemorrhage, and autotransfuses a small amount of blood. Its predominant effect on the cardiovascular system is to increase afterload. Obviously, in patients with thoracic trauma resulting in a torn thoracic aorta or bleeding from the thoracic aorta for any reason, this increase in afterload may intensify the problem. It has not been demonstrated to increase survival among patients on whom it has been used.

The utilization of intravenous fluids in the prehospital arena is often a waste of valuable time. If it should take the paramedic 10 minutes to start an intravenous line with the patient in hemorrhagic shock, 1000 to 1500 ml of blood may be lost while the intravenous line is inserted. Often, only 500 to 1000 ml of asanguinous crystalloid solution can be administered during the transport of the patient. The result is often a net loss of volume. It is now clear that transport of the patient a short distance should not be delayed in order to start an intravenous line, and ideally, it can be started in the ambulance while

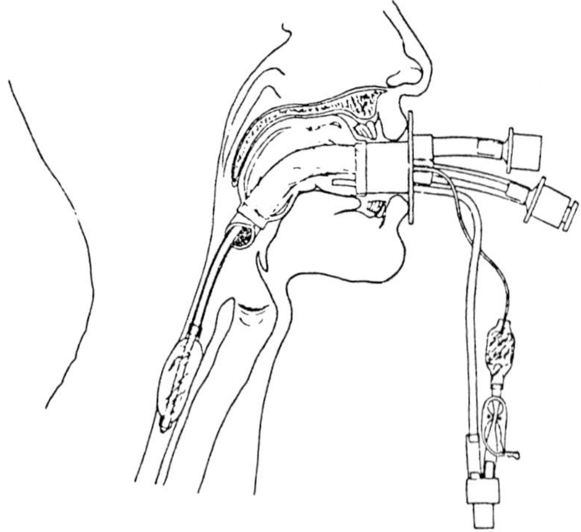

Figure 1.3. The pharyngeal-tracheal lumen airway (PTLA). The tube has two proximal lumens and two distal balloons. With the balloons inflated and the esophagus intubated, ventilation will occur in a fashion similar to that with the esophageal obturation airway. If the trachea should be intubated and it is recognized, a stylet can be removed and the appropriate lumen used as if it were an endotracheal tube.

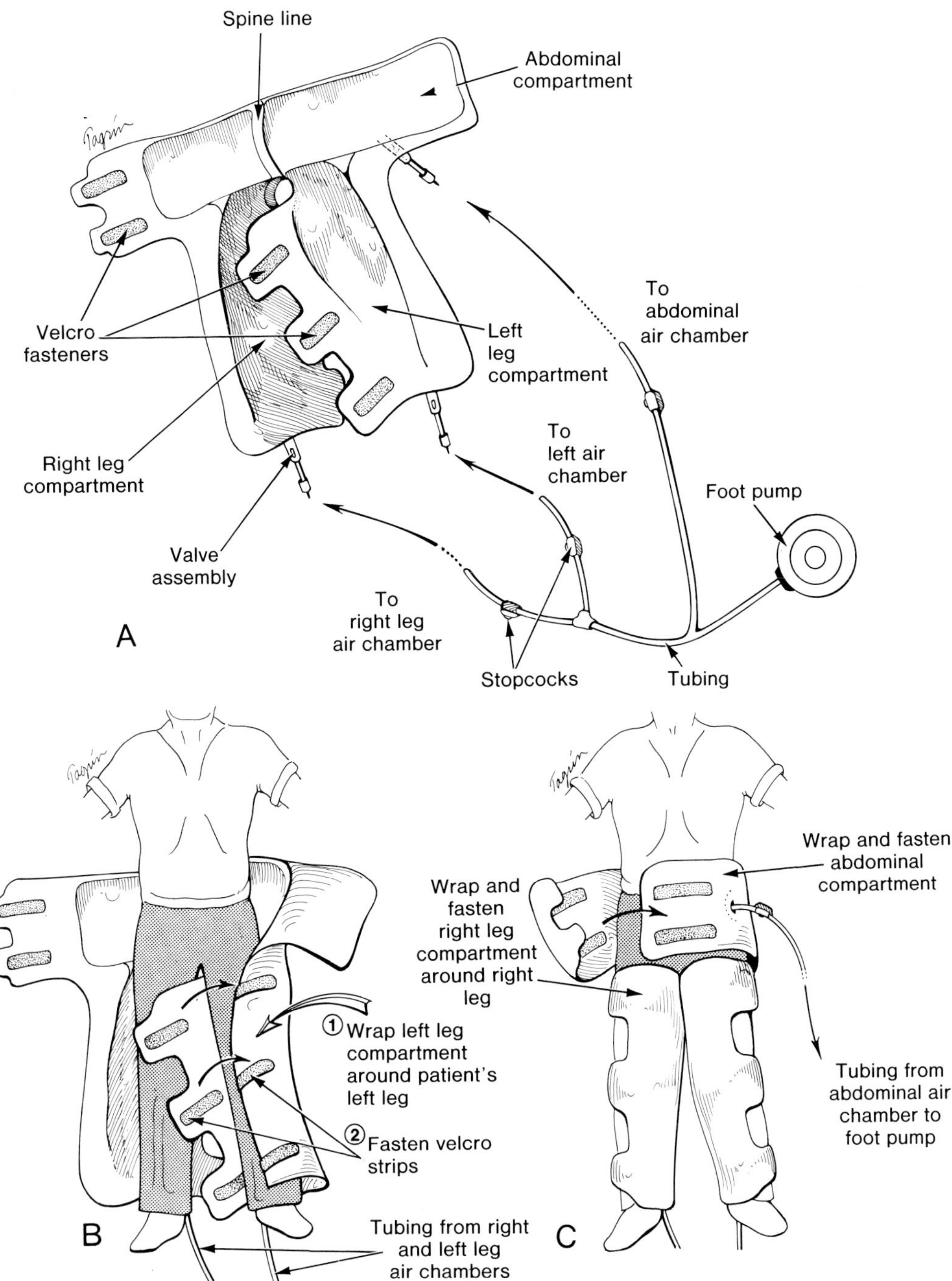

Figure 1.4. Application of the military antishock trousers (MAST). *A,* The garment is opened and spread with the left leg overlying the right, ready to receive the patient. Place patient on garment, supine, with top of abdominal section resting just below the lowest rib. *B,* Individual compartments are wrapped and secured with Velcro strips, beginning with the left leg, and the tubing is connected to the foot pump. *C,* After all indicated compartments are closed, the valves are opened and the garment inflated, again beginning with the legs. A pop-off valve or needle gauge regulates the final pressure attained.

Table 1.3.
Trauma Score[a]

Glasgow Coma Scale (GCS) (see below)	14–15	5
	11–13	4
	8–10	3
	5–7	2
	3–4	1
Respiratory rate	10–24/min	4
	25–36/min	3
	36/min or greater	2
	1–9/min	1
	None	0
Respiratory expansion	Normal	1
	Retractive/none	0
Systolic blood pressure	90 mm Hg or greater	4
	70–89 mm Hg	3
	50–69 mm Hg	2
	0–49 mm Hg	1
	No pulse	0
Capillary refill	Normal	2
	Delayed	1
	None	0
Total trauma score (maximal)		16

Glasgow Coma Scale (GCS)

Eye opening response	Spontaneous	4
	To voice	3
	To pain	2
	None	1
Best verbal response	Oriented	5
	Confused	4
	Inappropriate words	3
	Incomprehensible sounds	2
	None	1
Best motor response	Obeys command	6
	Localizes pain	5
	Withdraws (pain)	4
	Flexion (pain)	3
	Extension (pain)	2
	None	1
Total (Apply this score to GCS portion of Trauma Score left.)		3–15

Trauma score operational definitions

Respiratory rate	Number of respirations in 15 seconds; multiply by 4.
Respiratory expansion	Retractive: use of accessory muscles or intercostal muscle retraction.
Systolic blood pressure	Systolic cuff pressure; either arm—auscultate or palpate. No pulse: no carotid pulse.
Capillary refill	Normal: nail bed, forehead, or lip mucosa color refills in 2 seconds. None: no capillary refill.
Best verbal response	Arouse patient with voice or painful stimulus.
Best motor response	Response to command or painful stimulus.

[a] The Trauma Score is a numeric grading system for estimating the severity of injury. The score is composed of the Glasgow Coma Scale (reduced to approximately one-third value) and measurements of cardiopulmonary function. Each parameter is given a number (high for normal and low for impaired function). Severity of injury is estimated by summing the numbers. The lowest score is 1, and the highest score is 16.

the patient is being transported. Extremity fractures and the cervical spine should be immobilized to prevent further injury during transport. The emphasis in the trauma patient is to transport early and quickly and not to waste time in the field.

In the medical patient, on the other hand, many of the conditions causing the acute problem can be treated with prehospital therapy that not only *might* be definitive but also *must* be applied in the prehospital arena to be effective (defibrillation, treatment of anaphylaxis). In general, in the medical patient, every attempt is made to reverse and control the problem before the patient is transported. Many of the conditions can be satisfactorily treated in the prehospital arena by the paramedic (more so than by the EMT-I). Patients in cardiac arrest can be quickly defibrillated, and it has been shown that in well-developed systems early defibrillation in patients with ventricular fibrillation can result in up to a 40% rate of patient discharge from the hospital. A narcotic overdose can be reversed with the intravenous use of Narcan, the hypoglycemic patient can be treated with 50% dextrose, and anaphylaxis can be treated with subcutaneous epinephrine immediately at the scene. The important element is well-developed paramedic assessment skills so that the EMT can diagnose the problem and communicate it to the physician in the emergency department. The prehospital system must develop protocols for the management of each problem with which the prehospital paraprofessional is faced. In this way, the medical control physician and the paramedic have predetermined actions which both the physician and the paramedic understand and upon which they have agreed. Rarely do they vary from these protocols.

THE HOSPITAL

The object of an emergency medical system is to transport the *right* patient to the *right* hospital at the *right* time. The American Medical Association stated the purpose of hospital categorization:

to identify the readiness and capability of the hospital and to receive and treat correctly and expeditiously emergency patients. Ambulance personnel

Table 1.4.
Historical and Anatomical Data[a]

1. Accidents involving great force (e.g., explosions, falls from greater than 20 feet)
2. Patient's age less than 14 with major system injury
3. Patient thrown from a high-speed *moving* vehicle
4. Death of another passenger resulting from a *high-speed* accident
5. Significant combined system injury
6. Penetrating injury of the groin, neck, or chest
7. Avulsion amputation other than digits
8. CNS injury producing prolonged loss of consciousness, posturing, or paralysis
9. Spinal cord injury with neurologic deficit
10. Unstable chest
11. Blunt and/or penetrating abdominal trauma with shock
12. Burns: partial thickness or full-thickness involving 25% of body surface area

[a] Historic and anatomic data are helpful in triaging patients. The Trauma Score underestimates serious trauma, i.e., has significant numbers of false negatives. Therefore, additional criteria are necessary to triage trauma victims to trauma centers appropriately.

. . . having advanced knowledge of the designated categories of emergency capabilities of the various hospitals in the area, may thus select the proper institution to which patients should be taken.

The AMA also noted that this applied to both medical and surgical emergencies.

The emergency department caring for patients with medical/surgical emergencies must be staffed with physicians, nurses, and administration personnel and be equipped to care for emergency problems. The Joint Commission on the Accreditation of Hospitals has an item-by-item list of the necessary and essential personnel and equipment requirements. In a similar fashion, designated trauma centers with immediately available diagnostic and therapeutic capabilities to manage all potential injuries are the appropriate hospitals to which severely traumatized patients are triaged. The goal of an EMS system requires that the emergency medical technician recognize the capabilities of the surrounding hospitals so that patients can be appropriately triaged from the scene of the acute illness or injury. Tables 1.3–1.6 describe several categorization schemes and scoring systems for assisting in appropriate triage of the trauma patient. Ideally, EMS personnel are able to assess the patient at the scene and appropriately triage the patient to the facility capable of caring for the problem. Unfortunately, many obstacles result in imperfect implementation of this triage system. Besides ground transportation, helicopter transport of the acutely ill or injured patient has recently become available. With many up and running helicopter programs, most states have the ability to transport patients rapidly to an appropriate care facility.

Table 1.5.
Hospital Categorization: Trauma Centers

Level I
1. More than 500 beds
2. Metropolitan area
3. Sees 600–1000 trauma cases/year
4. Trauma training program and research
5. Trauma service
6. Full-time supportive service and staff

Level II
1. Commitment to quality care is the same as in a Level I
2. Sees 350–600 trauma cases/year
3. Does not provide training or do research

Level III
1. 100–200 beds
2. Community area
3. Lack of full-time staff specialists

Table 1.6.
Trauma Patient Categorization

Category I Patients
1. Combined system injury
2. Bleeding open fractures
3. Uncontrolled hemorrhage
4. Severe maxillofacial injuries
5. Severe head, neck, and upper respiratory injuries
6. Unstable chest injuries
7. Pelvic fractures
8. Blunt abdominal trauma with hypotension and/or penetrating abdominal injuries
9. Severe neurologic injuries

Category II Patients
1. Open or closed fractures
2. Soft tissue injuries, stabilized bleeding
3. Multiple rib fractures with flail
4. Blunt abdominal trauma without hypotension
5. Transient loss of consciousness

Category III Patients
1. Uncomplicated fractures
2. No hypovolemia or hypotension
3. No neurologic injury
4. No abdominal injury
5. Moderate soft tissue injuries
6. Chest injuries without respiratory distress

THE FUTURE

Prehospital care is in many respects in its infancy. Improvements in care are being developed. Much of this progress will result from improved technology. The basic EMT is now able to provide immediate defibrillation to a cardiac arrest patient. Combined with advanced life support, this has improved out-of-hospital cardiac arrest survival rates to approximately 40% in fully developed systems.

Unfortunately, public knowledge of what prehospital services are available to them is imperfect, and as a result, the amount of money spent to support the prehospital arena is insufficient. One of the obligations of emergency department physicians is to educate the community that is served by their hospital and emergency system. Hopefully, an increase in awareness of the prehospital arena will improve public support. The public must know what EMS systems are available within their community and must support their development.

SUGGESTED READINGS

Trauma

Abraham E, Cobo JC, Bland RD. Cardio-respiratory effects of the pneumatic trousers in critically ill patients. *Arch of Surg,* 1984;119:912–915.

Aprahamian C, Thompson BM, Towne JB, et al. The effect of a paramedic system on mortality of major open intra-abdominal vascular injuries. *J Trauma,* 1983;23:687–690.

Auerbach PS, Geehr EC. Inadequate oxygenation and ventilation using the esophageal gastric tube airway in the prehospital setting. *JAMA,* 1983;250:3067–3071.

Border JR. Panel discussion. Prehospital trauma care—Stabilize or scoop and run. *J Trauma,* 1983;23:708–711.

Champion HR, Sacco WJ, Hannar DS, et al. Assessment of injury severity: The triage index of critical care medicine. *Crit Care Med,* 1980;8:201–208.

Commission on Emergency Medical Services. *Categorization of Hospital Emergency Capabilities.* Chicago, American Medical Association, 1971.

Copass MR, Oreskobich MR, Bladergroen MR. Prehospital cardiopulmonary resuscitation of the critically injured patient. *Am J Surg,* 1984;148:20–26.

Eggold R. Trauma care regionalization—A necessity. *J Trauma,* 1983;23:260–262.

Fisher RP, Flynn TC, Miller PW, et al. The economics of fatal injury, dollars and cents. *J Trauma,* 1985;25:746–750.

Freeark RJ. The 1982 AAST presidential address. The trauma center, its hospitals, head injuries, helicopters, and heroes. *J Trauma,* 1983;23:173–178.

Godbout B, Burchard KW, Slotman GJ, et al. Crush syndrome with death following pneumatic antishock garment application. *J Trauma,* 1984;24:1052–1056.

Hospital resources for optimal care of the injured patient. *Bulletin of the American College of Surgeons,* August 1979, October 1983, and October 1986.

Jacobs LM, Bennett BP. Emergency patient care. Prehospital ground and air procedures. MacMillan, New York, 1983.

Jacobs LM, Berrizbeitia LD, Bennett B, et al. Endotracheal intubation in the prehospital phase of emergency medical care. *JAMA,* 1983;250:2175–2177.

Jurkovich GJ, Campbell B, Padrta J, et al. Paramedic perception of elapsed field time. *J Trauma,* 1987;27:892–897.

Kerr HD. Prehospital emergency services and health maintenance organizations. *Ann Emerg Med,* 1986;15:727–729.

Lowe DK, Ott GR, Neely KW, et al. Evaluation of injury mechanism as a criterion in trauma triage. *Am J Surg,* 1986;152:6–10.

Mackensie RC, Christense JM, Lewis FR. The prehospital use of external counterpressure—Does MAST make a difference? *J Trauma,* 1984;14:882–883.

Mattox KL, Feliciano DV. Role of external cardiac compression in truncal trauma. *J Trauma,* 1982;22:934–936.

Mattox KL, Pepe PE, Bickell W, et al. Prospective randomized evaluation of the "MAST" garment in hemorrhagic shock. *J Trauma,* 1986;26:779–786.

Morris JA, Averbach PS, Marshall GA, et al. The trauma score as a triage tool in the prehospital setting. *JAMA,* 1986;256:1319–1325.

National Academy of Sciences, National Research Council. Accidental death and disability—The neglected disease of modern society. National Academy of Sciences, 1966.

Niemann JT, Rosborough JP, Myers R, et al. The pharyngeal-tracheal lumen airway, preliminary investigation of a new adjunct. *Ann Emerg Med,* 1984;13:591–596.

Oakes DD, Holcromb SF, Sherck JP. Patterns of trauma care costs and reimbursements, the burden of uninsured motorists. *J Trauma,* 1985;25:740–745.

Podolsky S, Baroff LF, Simon RR, et al. Efficacy of cervical spine immobilization. *J Trauma,* 1983;23:461–465.

Pons PT, Honigman B, Moore EE, et al. Prehospital advanced trauma life support for critical penetrating wounds to the thorax and abdomen. *J Trauma,* 1985; 25:828–832.

Prehospital trauma life support. Butman AM, Paturas JL, McSwain NE, Dineen JP, eds. *Emergency Training,* 1986, Akron, Ohio.

Rhee KJ, Strozeski M, Burney RE, et al. Is the flight physician needed for helicopter emergency medical services? *Ann Emerg Med,* 1986;15:174–177.

Sacco WV, Champion HR, Carnozzo AJ. Trauma score. *Curr Concepts Trauma Care,* Spring 1981:9–11.

Smith JP, Bodai BI, Aubourg R, et al. A field evaluation of the esophageal obturator airway. *J Trauma,* 1983; 23:317–321.

Smith JP, Bodai BI, Hill AS, et al. Prehospital stabilization of critically injured patients: A failed concept. *J Trauma,* 1985;25:65–70.

Smith JP, Bodai BI, Seifkin A, et al. The esophageal obturator airway—A review. *JAMA,* 1983;250:1081–1084.

Stewart RD, Paris PM, Winter PM, et al. Field endotracheal intubation by paramedical personnel. *Chest,* 1984;85:341–345.

Tempelman D, Lange R, Harris B. Lower extremity compartment syndrome associated with the use of pneumatic antishock garments. *J Trauma,* 1987;27:779–781.

The law of the ninety-third congress—Emergency medical services systems acts of 1973. Public law 93–154, Washington, DC, 1976.

Vollmer TP, Stewart RD, Paris PM, et al. Use of a lighted stylet for guided orotracheal intubation in the prehospital setting. *Ann Emerg Med,* 1985;14:324–328.

West JG, Cales RH, Gazzanega AR. Impact of regionalization, the Orange County experience. *Arch Surg,* 1983;118:740–744.

West JG, Trunkey DD, Lim RC. Systems of trauma care. *Ann Surg,* 1979;114:455-460.

Medical

Bachman JW, McDonald GS, O'Brien PC. A study of out-of-hospital cardiac arrests in northeastern Minnesota. *JAMA,* 1986;256:477–483.

Cummins RO, Eisenberg MS, Moore JE, et al. Automatic external defibrillators: Clinical, training, psychological, and public health issues. *Ann Emerg Med,* 1985;14:755–760.

Diamond NJ, Schofferman J, Elliot JW. Factors in successful resuscitation by paramedics. *J Am Coll Emerg Physicians,* 1977;6:42–46.

Eisenberg MS, Copass MK, Hallstrom AP, et al. Treatment of out-of-hospital cardiac arrests with rapid defibrillation by emergency medical technicians. *N Engl J Med,* 1980;302:1379–1383.

Eisenberg MS, Bergner L, Hallstrom A. Cardiac resuscitation in the community. Importance of rapid provision and implications for program planning. *JAMA,* 1979;241:1905–1907.

Eisenberg MS, Bergner L, Hallstrom A. Paramedic programs and out-of-hospital cardiac arrest. I. Factors associated with successful resuscitation. *Am J Public Health,* 1979;69:30–38.

Eisenberg MS, Bergner L. Hallstrom A. Paramedic programs and out-of-hospital cardiac arrest. II. Impact on community mortality. *Am J Public Health,* 1979;69:39–42.

Eisenberg MS, Hallstrom A, Bergner L. Long-term survival after out-of-hospital cardiac arrest. *N Engl J Med,* 1982;306:1340–1343.

Gillium RF, Folsom A, Luepker RV, et al. Sudden death and acute myocardial infarction in a metropolitan area, 1970–1980. *N Engl J Med,* 1983;309:1353–1358.

Holroyd BR, Knopp R, Kallsen G. Concepts in emergency and critical care. *JAMA,* 1986;256:1027–1031.

Jaggarao NSV, Grainger R, Heber M. Use of an automated external defibrillator-pacemaker by ambulance staff. *Lancet,* 1982;2:73–75.

Lund I, Skulberg A. Cardiopulmonary resuscitation by lay people. *Lancet,* 1976;2:702–704.

Luterman A. Ramenofsky M, Berryman C. Evaluation of prehospital emergency medical service (EMS): Defining areas of improvement. *J Trauma,* 1983;23:702–707.

Newman M. Twenty-five years of CPR. *J Emerg Med Services,* 1985;13:26–30.

Ornato JP, McNeill SE, Craren EJ, et al. Limitation on effectiveness of rapid defibrillation by emergency medical technicians in a rural setting. *Ann Emerg Med,* 1984; 13:1096–1099.

Rinke CM. Concepts in emergency and critical care. *JAMA,* 1985;253:544–548.

Standards and guidelines for cardiopulmonary resuscitation (CPR) and emergency cardiac care (ECC). *JAMA,* 1986;255:2905–2989.

Stults KR, Brown DD, Schug VL, et al. Prehospital defibrillation performed by emergency medical technicians in rural communities. *N Engl J Med,* 1984;310:219–223.

Thompson RG, Hallstrom AP, Cobb LA. Bystander-initiated cardiopulmonary resuscitation in the management of ventricular fibrillation. *Ann Intern Med,* 1979;90:737–740.

Tweed WA, Bristow G, Donen N. Resuscitation from cardiac arrest: Assessment of a system providing only basic life support outside of hospital. *Can Med Assoc J,* 1980;122:297–300.

White RD. Making EMT-D work. *J Emerg Med Services,* 1986:February 14:26–30.

CHAPTER 2

Cardiopulmonary Resuscitation

HAMILTON R. HAYES

Editor's note: In this third edition a pediatrics section has been introduced. Thus, cardiopulmonary resuscitation for the pediatric patient is discussed in Chapter 21.

INTRODUCTION

Resuscitation is in a field in flux. A decade of intensive investigation has exposed weakness in the scientific underpinnings of the discipline, and analysis of resuscitation outcomes from numerous localities has been sobering. Truly successful resuscitations—returning neurologically functional individuals to their premorbid social settings—have been in the minority in reported series. In particular subsets—the pediatric age group, bradycardic and asystolic arrests at any age, trauma-related cardiac arrests—the record has been dismal. Brain protection has been ineffectual. Critical review has shown some drugs to be ineffective, even detrimental, and the efficacy of certain advanced life support adjuncts has increasingly been debated.

Because the field is undergoing major upheavels, textbook chapters and American Heart Association standards must be appreciated for what they are: efforts at consensus and attempts to summarize work in progress.

BASIC CARDIOPULMONARY RESUSCITATION (CPR)

The purpose of basic CPR is to buy time by adequately perfusing the heart and brain with partially oxygenated blood, thereby maintaining viability until definitive therapy can restore spontaneous circulation and ventilation. It is clear that basic CPR is a technique that can be codified, taught, widely disseminated, and incorporated into emergency medical service systems. It is less obvious how effective it is at achieving its purpose. Clinical experience and more sophisticated research techniques have shown us that basic CPR is a weaker tool than once thought (Table 2.1). Where we once took satisfaction in saying that well-performed CPR could generate up to 30% of the baseline cardiac output, we now realize that it is the end-organ distribution of this output that is critical. Even when optimally performed, basic CPR produces myocardial and cerebral blood flow that is well below the levels considered thresholds for viability. Even when begun promptly, basic CPR provides a shorter window of viability than had been thought.

Reported statistics on success of basic CPR vary greatly. These variations reflect the different standards employed in particular series for such critical parameters as criteria for exclusion, advanced life support response time, and definitions of a "save." Indeed, some of the successes attributed to the technique of CPR may, in fact, be due to such simple techniques as opening the airway. Representative samples of the reported experience are presented in Tables 2.1 and 2.2.

These observations notwithstanding, it does appear that for a percentage of victims of cardiopulmonary arrest basic standard CPR, skillfully

Table 2.1.
Summary of CPR Success Rates in Several Representative Series[a]

Location/System[b]	Witnessed	Rhythm[c]	Response Time	No.[d]	% (No.) Discharged from Hospital Alive
Oslo, EMTs only	Not reported	Not reported	Median "driving time" = 8 min	BYS CPR = 75 Delayed CPR = 556	36% (27) 8% (43)
Birmingham, AL, paramedics only	Implied yes	VF or VT	>5 min from call to arrival	BYS CPR = 7 Medic CPR = 12	86% (6) 50% (6)
Seattle, EMTs and paramedics	76% overall were witnessed	VF only	mean = 3 min from dispatch to arrival	BYS CPR = 109 EMT CPR = 207	43% (47) 21% (43)
Winnipeg, Manitoba, EMTs only	Not reported	VF or VT	<10 min from call to arrival for only 12% of cases	BYS CPR = 65 EMT CPR = 161	25% (16) 5% (8)
Iceland, EMTs only	Not reported	All rhythms (42% = VF)	Mean = 7.3 min from call to arrival	BYS CPR = 38 EMT CPR = 84	42% (16) 6% (5)
Vancouver, EMTs and paramedics	77% overall were witnessed	All rhythms	Not reported	BYS CPR = 43 Delayed CPR = 272	21% (9) 6% (17)
Los Angeles, paramedics	41% overall were witnessed	All rhythms	Mean = 5.0 min from call to arrival	BYS CPR = 93 Medic CPR = 150	22% (20) 5% (7)
		VF only		BYS CPR = 45 Medic CPR = 70	27% (12) 6% (4)
King County WA, EMTs and paramedics	Not reported	All rhythms	Mean = 6 min from collapse to EMT arrival	BYS CPR = 108 EMT CPR = 379	23% (25) 12% (45)
Pittsburgh, paramedics	Not reported	VF/VT only	Mean = 6.0 min dispatch to arrival	BYS CPR = 25 Medic CPR = 59	24% (6) 7% (4)

[a] From Cummins RO, Eisenberg MS. Prehospital cardiopulmonary resuscitation. Is it effective? *JAMA*, 1985; 253:2408-2412
[b] EMTs, emergency medical technicians, or trained first responders.
[c] VF, ventricular fibrillation; VT, ventricular tachycardia.
[d] BYS, bystander.

applied, will maintain the myocardium in a state receptive to being restarted and the brain in a condition permitting it to regain near normal functioning. Basic CPR is of particular value in localities having limited advanced life support capability and has application in numerous noncardiac arrest situations, as well.

In the field, CPR should be begun on any individual seen to arrest, or found in arrest, unless there is gross evidence of irreversible death (decapitation, rigor mortis, severe dependent livedo). In the emergency department, CPR should be continued until there is indication of cardiovascular unresponsiveness or additional information (preexisting medical condition, living will, "do not resuscitate status") becomes available.

Parameters of CPR

To have a chance for effectiveness, CPR must be started within 4 minutes of arrest in a normothermic individual (Table 2.2). Direct measurement of flow rates through the coronary arteries during CPR have shown values ranging from 5–10% of normal to coronary perfusion pressures that were actually negative. Internal carotid artery flow rates in the 5–10% of normal range may be generated

Table 2.2.
The Importance of Prompt Institution of CPR[a]

	Witnessed Arrests	Unwitnessed Arrests	Totals
Bystander cardiopulmonary resuscitation	32% (189/598)	7% (10/147)	27% (199/745)
Delayed cardiopulmonary resuscitation	21% (162/766)	3% (19/599)	13% (181/1365)
Totals	26% (351/1364)	4% (29/746)	18% (380/2110)

[a] Data from King County, WA, between 1976 and 1982 for patients in cardiac arrest, all rhythms, given care by paramedics. From Cummins RO, Eisenberg MS. Prehospital cardiopulmonary resuscitation. Is it effective? *JAMA*, 1985;253:2408-2412. Copyright 1985, American Medical Association.

early, but drop off to near zero after 5 minutes of standard CPR. It is not clear how these seemingly inadequate perfusion pressures allow the myocardium of some arrest victims to sustain ventricular tachycardia fibrillation for several minutes.

Conceptual Changes: The Physiology of Closed Chest CPR

It was previously assumed that closed chest compressions generated cardiac output literally by cardiac massage, that is, by physically compressing the heart between the sternum and the vertebral column. However, this "cardiac pump" theory has been challenged by many studies, including those demonstrating that the atrioventricular valves remain open and that the heart simply functions as a passive conduit during CPR. It has also been shown that the act of coughing (which transiently elevates general intrathoracic pressure) can generate forward blood flow, much like closed chest CPR. These and other observations have led to the concept of the "thoracic pump" to account for the propulsion of blood by closed chest CPR. This latter theory attributes the production of cardiac output to rhythmic elevations in the general intrathoracic pressure, not to massage of the heart, the unidirectional flow being achieved by a valve-like collapsing of the major veins at the thoracic inlet during the downstroke of compression.

"New CPR"

As it has become apparent that both the underlying theory and the demonstrated effectiveness of basic life support techniques were open to question, various investigators have attempted to modify CPR in an effort to improve organ perfusion. These technical modifications have endeavored to raise intrathoracic pressure by such measures as simultaneously ventilating the patient while compressing the chest, or by interposing abdominal compression between chest compressions. In addition, the application of various types of abdominal binders—including the military antishock trousers (MAST) garment—has been investigated in an effort to increase abdominal and, thereby, intrathoracic pressure in continuous fashion.

Unfortunately, none of these new CPR techniques has been shown to increase critical organ perfusion by an increment large enough to be clinically meaningful; moreover, the modified techniques are more complex, some requiring more than two rescuers, some needing specialized equipment. They have, in addition, potential complications of their own, including damage to the abdominal viscera and increased intracranial pressure causing reduced cerebral blood flow. Likewise, abdominal binding, by increasing return to the right side of the heart, raises right arterial pressure and thereby reduces the coronary perfusion gradient. Given these considerations, the new CPR techniques must at this stage be considered to be experimental.

Technique of Basic Life Support

The third edition of "Standards and Guidelines for Cardiopulmonary Resuscitation (CPR) and Emergency Cardiac Care (ECC)" details the consensus of the national conference on this subject in 1986. This publication represents a reasonable summary of the state of the art; however, the standards should be viewed as guidelines, not rigid dogma, and the clinician is certainly justified in deviating from their recommendations, if such deviations are based on thoughtful reading of the medical literature, the incorporation of new advances, and special considerations in a given patient.

The new standards attempt to simplify protocols, thereby facilitating teaching and retention of details. Where previously taught parallel techniques were considered to be equivalent, only one is now to be presented (e.g., the chin-lift, head-tilt as the only way to open the airway (Fig. 2.1)). Some procedures, such as two-person CPR, are no longer to be taught to lay persons.

Technically, rescue breathing has been modified in recognition of the dangers of gastric distention and regurgitation. The new standards advocate

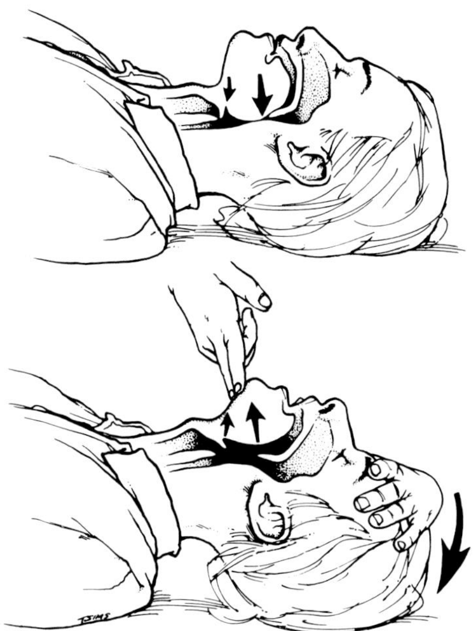

Figure 2.1. American Heart Association Guidelines' recommended airway maneuver for basic CPR. Opening the airway. Top, Airway obstruction produced by tongue and epiglottis; *bottom*, relief by head-tilt, chin-lift. (From American Heart Association. Standards and guidelines for cardiopulmonary resuscitation (CPR) and emergency cardiac care (ECC). *JAMA,* 1986;255:2905–2989. Copyright 1986, American Medical Association.)

slower patient lung inflation rates and more modest delivered volumes. For the same reason, the "staircase" initial breaths are no longer advised. In recognition of the importance of cerebral perfusion, the standards caution against elevating the head during CPR and suggest that elevating the lower extremities might be beneficial. With regard to chest compressions, emphasis has been focused on correct hand position, the appropriate depth of sternal compression, and, most importantly, the duration of the compression cycle. In order to maximize perfusion, 50% or more of the cycle should be spent in the compression phase. For the same reason, it is recommended that the compression rate be increased from the presently advocated 60 compressions/minute to 80 to 100, when possible. Recognizing that primary upper airway obstruction is a significant cause of mortality, considerable attention in this edition of the Standards is devoted to techniques for clearing the airway. Emphasis is placed on the importance of clearing the airway in a child or infant. The nomenclature and description of the Heimlich maneuver have been standardized. Back blows are no longer endorsed in the adult or older child.

The reader is referred to the Standards for a comprehensive presentation of basic CPR.

ADULT ADVANCED CARDIAC LIFE SUPPORT (ACLS)

Ten years of CPR have taught that the early restoration of spontaneous cardiac action/tissue perfusion is critical. With currently available methodology, only victims of ventricular tachycardia, ventricular fibrillation, and primary respiratory arrests have any meaningful survival and recovery potential. Time is of the essence if brain function is to be preserved. Concepts once considered axiomatic ("coarse fibrillation is more easily defibrillated") have been found to have no basis in science and have been discarded, and certain drugs recommended for advanced cardiac life support in previous editions of the AHA Standards and this textbook are now considered to be ineffective or harmful. Priorities in administering ACLS have been reordered.

Defibrillation

Approximately 70% of adult patients suffering extrahospital cardiac arrest do so with a rhythm that is initially amenable to defibrillation (ventricular fibrillation or ventricular tachycardia). Patients with these rhythms need immediate defibrillation. Since the overriding imperative is the restoration of spontaneous circulation, this should be done before time is taken for intubation, intravenous line placement, or drug administration. Contrary to previous thinking, it has been shown that the heart *can* be defibrillated in an acid environment and that "coarsening" ventricular fibrillation with epinephrine not only fails to make the heart more easily defibrillated, but actually increases the work done by the inadequately perfused heart, increases its oxygen consumption, and deflects perfusing blood away from the subendocardium.

The principal predictors of success in defibrillation seem to be the duration of the episode of fibrillation and coronary artery perfusion (which maintains the myocardium in a receptive state). The first approach to the arrested patient in the field (if local advanced life support has the capability) or in the emergency department, then, should be to apply the defibrillator paddles to the chest wall in the quick-visualization mode. If ventricular tachycardia or ventricular fibrillation is present, the patient should be defibrillated immediately. If the defibrillator does not have monitoring capability, blind defibrillation is in order. The energy selected for the first defibrillation should be the lowest that is likely to be effective. High energy levels may cause myocardial necrosis and later adverse electrophysiologic effects (recurrent ventricular fibrillation/atrioventricular blocks). The objective is to depolarize a critical mass of myocardium, not to injure

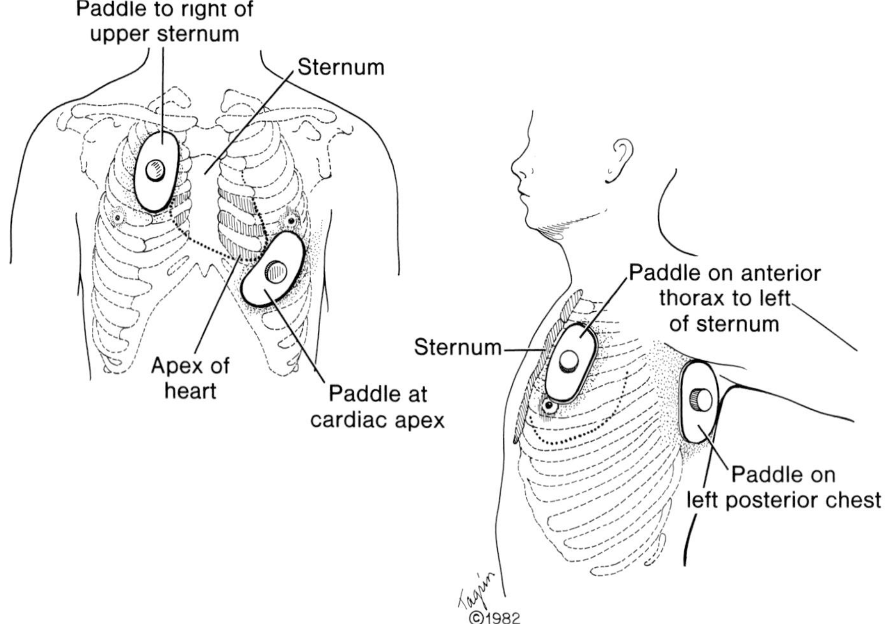

Figure 2.2. Acceptable defibrillation paddle placement. *A*, Both paddles are applied to the anterior chest wall. *B*, Paddles are applied anteriorly and posteriorly to the left thorax.

it. The current actually flowing through the heart is determined by the energy delivered to the chest wall, minus the transthoracic impedance. Impedance is a function of numerous factors, including paddle size, placement, pressure, the conductance of the interface material between paddle and skin, and the number and timing of previous discharges. Defibrillation temporarily reduces the impendance of the thorax for a following repeat shock, so tandem defibrillation is a recommended technique. The commonest choice for electrode placement is on the right anterior chest wall just beneath the clavicle adjacent to the sternum and over the apex of the heart (Fig. 2.2). The anterior/posterior placement of the paddles offers no advantage in emergency defibrillation and is somewhat time consuming and disruptive of CPR.

Good electrode-skin contact is essential, and firm pressure (approximately 25 pounds) has the dual advantage of maintaining such pressure and also forcing some of the air out of the lungs, potentially reducing impedance. Larger paddle size also decreases transthoracic resistance. However, if the paddle surface area is excessive, the density of the current passing through heart muscle will also be reduced, so a technical compromise must be reached in paddle design. Current recommendations are for a 10-cm diameter electrode in adults.

The latest Standards for CPR and ECC recommend a triplet of defibrillation shocks, administered rapidly and sequentially, delaying only to recharge the defibrillator and to assess the results. For ventricular fibrillation in the adult, the initial discharge should be 200 joules, the second in the 200–300 joule range, and the third up to 360 joules. For ventricular tachycardia, much lower levels of energy are required. The patient who is tolerating ventricular tachycardia well may be sedated and cardioverted with 50–100 joules. If the patient with ventricular tachycardia is, however, pulseless and/or unconscious, immediate cardioversion with an initial energy level between 100 and 150 joules is appropriate.

Failure to cardiovert with three such shocks is an indication to proceed with intubation, drug therapy, and repeated defibrillation attempts. Specific pharmacologic agents are discussed below. Failure to achieve defibrillation should also raise the question of an underlying correctable cause, such as the presence of pneumothorax.

Two lines of reasoning have been advanced that advise defibrillation in patients with a straight-line monitor pattern. The first of these is an imprecise concept, suggesting that an asystolic heart can be "jump-started" with an electric shock. This is an unsubstantiated theory and may well be erroneous. Defibrillating a truly arrested heart is likely to damage the myocardium and nothing more, so it is not recommended. However, some cases of apparent asystole may represent "occult" ventricular fibrillation because of an artifact of lead placement. Ventricular fibrillation has an electrical vector, and if that vector happens to be at right angles to the axis of the defibrillator electrodes during the "quick look," it would appear as a straight line. However, given this circumstance (a straight-line monitor pattern), the appropriate response is to reposition the paddles at 90° to the original axis to seek the pattern of fibrillation, not simply to deliver an electroshock to the heart.

Since the majority of extrahospital arrests are due to rhythms that are susceptible to defibrillation and since time is critical, it seems appropriate to press for defibrillation by emergency medical technicians (EMTs) in the field. Indeed, it seems much more logical than teaching skills of limited lifesaving potential (such as intravenous line insertion) to EMTs with basic or intermediate training. Newer automatic defibrillators, which both detect the rhythm and defibrillate through the same electrodes, should go far toward overcoming objections to EMT defibrillation on the grounds of skill level and skill decay and may be appropriate for home use. Statistically, the incidence of significant complications following unsynchronized cardioversion of supraventricular tachyarrhythmias is low.

A chest thump can deliver approximately 5 joules of energy to the heart. On occasion, that can be enough to convert an arrhythmia (especially ventricular tachycardia, but less commonly ventricular fibrillation) into an organized, pulse-producing rhythm. It is therefore probably reasonable to administer a single precordial blow to a patient who is monitored and who slips into ventricular tachycardia or ventricular fibrillation if no defibrillator is immediately available. However, there is a significant potential for the chest thump to convert ventricular tachycardia or ventricular fibrillation to asystole, so the ability to respond rapidly with ACLS must be near at hand when the thump is employed.

Airway Management

Clearly, the priority in any cardiac arrest situation must be the establishment of an open airway. The resuscitator needs a patent and secure airway passage to permit oxygenation of the victim, to allow hyperventilation to relieve respiratory acidosis, to provide access for the transtracheal administration of drugs, and to protect the lungs against regurgitation/aspiration. Accordingly, the physician must possess several airway skills: oral endotracheal intubation, nasotracheal intubation (for use in the presence of trismus or facial injuries), and some alternative technique, such as cricothyrotomy, to be employed if the upper airway is totally occluded. Although it does not fulfill the criteria of an airway secure from aspiration, the technique of bag-mask ventilation with an oropharyngeal airway is a vital one, and this modality should be employed prior to attempting endotracheal intubation (Figs. 2.3 and 2.4).

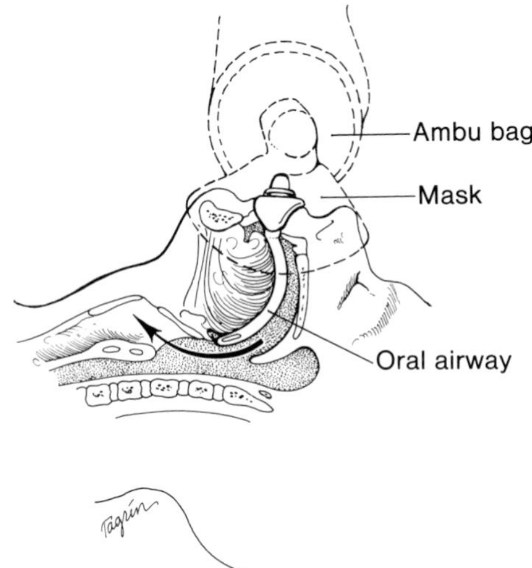

Figure 2.3. Oropharyngeal airway is correctly positioned to permit ventilation.

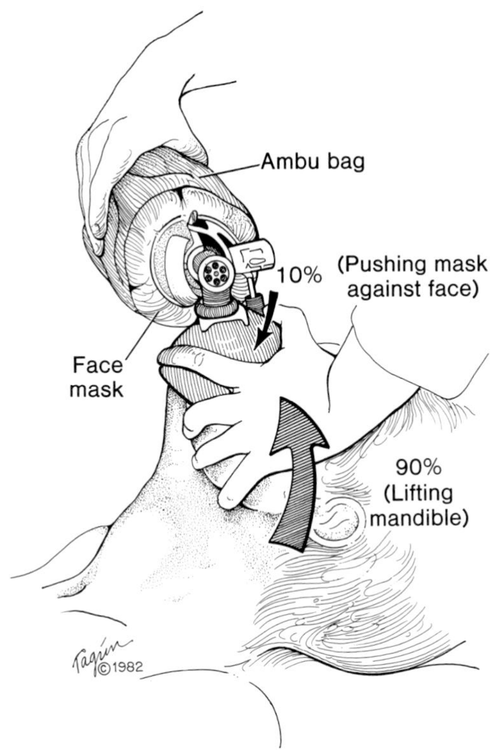

Figure 2.4. Technique of bag-mask ventilation indicates the importance of lifting the mandible to create a seal without occluding the airway.

Endotracheal Intubation

Many refinements in equipment and in technique for endotracheal intubation have been suggested; these range from the use of stylets within the lumen of the tube to the employment of the newer lighted flexible laryngoscopes, from cricoid pressure to digital blind intubation. However, the basic procedure is straightforward. The patient is first ventilated with 100% oxygen with a bag-mask respirator and an oral pharyngeal airway. A suction apparatus equipped with a tonsil tip must be available. The patient's head is supported in the sniffing position (see Illustrated Technique 1) brought forward, and extended on the neck to align the oral and pharayngeal-laryngeal axes. With the laryngoscope most familiar to the physician, curved or straight, the tongue is moved to the left and the mandible is lifted upward along the vector parallel to the handle of the laryngoscope (care being taken not to use the upper teeth as a fulcrum) (see also Illustrated Technique 1). Under direct visualization the endotracheal tube is inserted into the glottic opening, positioning the cuff just below the vocal cords. The epigastrium and both axillae should be promptly auscultated to rule out inadvertent esophageal or mainstem bronchus intubation. In a child, breath sounds are well-transmitted widely throughout the thorax, so it is preferable to verify the tube position by *inspecting* the chest for symmetric expansion rather than by auscultation.

If the oral route is not available (due to facial trauma or oral burns, for example) and the patient is breathing on his/her own, nasotracheal intubation can provide a secure airway. Nasotracheal intubation is a blind procedure (see Illustrated Technique 2) that is carried out by advancing the tube gradually with the physician's ear close to its proximal opening. This permits the physician to listen for breath sounds and to feel expired air while guiding the tube into the glottic opening. The respiratory efforts in a spontaneously breathing patient will often actually cause the tip of the advancing nasotracheal tube to be inhaled into the larynx.

If the upper airway is completely obstructed (due to retropharyngeal swelling, trauma, the presence of a foreign body, or other mechanical factor (cricothyrotomy (needle or surgical) is a technique that may provide a lifesaving airway (see Illustrated Techniques 3 and 4). A cricothyrotomy is more rapidly accomplished and less likely to produce hemorrhage than is a traditional tracheotomy. Surgical cricothyrotomy is not recommended in children under the age of 12 years, since the cricoid cartilage may be damaged, but needle cricothyrotomy may be attempted if there is facial trauma or airway obstruction, unrelieved by the usual initial measures.

Other Airway Adjuncts

The esophageal obturator airway (EOA) (see Fig. 1.1) and its variant, the esophageal-gastric tube airway (EGTA) (see Fig. 1.2), are currently in use in some advanced prehospital systems. The EOA consists of a face mask with an attached 37-cm long cuffed tube having its distal end blocked with an obturator. There are numerous fenestrations in the proximal portion of the tube. In use, it is passed blindly by mouth into the esophagus, the cuff is inflated to seal the esophagus, the mask is seated against the face, and the patient is ventilated with a bag ventilator through a fitting in the end of the tube. The principal advantages of the EOA are the reported ease of insertion, simplicity of training, and relatively lesser skill decay. The problems and complications of the EOA include upper airway and esophageal trauma, inadvertent tracheal intubation (a lethal complication, if not promptly detected), and postremoval regurgitation with potential aspiration, a common problem. The greatest difficulty with the EOA is inability to maintain a tight mask seal. This is equivalent in degree of difficulty to a bag mask ventilator and accordingly presents problems in training and use in this field.

The EGTA variation has a no. 16 gastric tube that passes through the obturator into the stomach and has a second port in the mask for ventilation. The gastric tube allows the stomach to be decompressed prior to extubation and offers some protection against gastric distention, regurgitation, and aspiration while in place.

A new device, the pharyngeal-tracheal lumen airway (PTLA) (see Fig. 1.3), which seals the pharynx and obviates the need for a mask, is in a stage of experimental development. Neither the EOA nor the EGTA is suitable for children younger than 16.

Because of the danger of regurgitation on removal, it is standard practice to intubate the trachea with an endotracheal tube while the esophageal obturator airway is still in place, then to withdraw the EOA. In practice, the EOA and EGTA are inferior to endotracheal intubation. Where the latter technique can be taught and its skill maintained, it is the preferable airway. On rare occasions the EOA or one of its refinements may be an acceptable device. Modifications of the technique—for instance, use of an oxygen-powered device—may improve the performance of the EOA.

Transtracheal jet ventilation (see Illustrated Technique 4) involves the use of a 14-gauge catheter inserted through the cricothyroid membrane which allows intermittent jets of pressurized oxygen to be injected at high flow rates, resulting in chest expansion. Expiration is passive via the normal anatomic route. The transtracheal jet technique has the advantage of rapid oxygenation but it is at best a stopgap technique because it does not adequately protect against aspiration or permit suctioning. It is not effective in the presence of complete upper airway obstruction because of inadequate exhalation.

The issue of pharmacologic muscle relaxation for intubation resolves into indication, skill levels, and the availability of assistance. It may be indicated when a patient with trismus needs intubation. Rather than wait for the patient to deteriorate into flaccidity, a muscle relaxant such as succinylcholine may be employed, allowing intubation. However, the use of muscle relaxants in the emergency department should be undertaken only by a physician fully trained in the use of such drugs and skilled in intubation procedure, who has a second physician standing by, gloved and ready to carry out a surgical approach to the airway if intubation is not achieved promptly after paralyzing the patient.

Intravenous Access

Access to the circulation is required for administration of medication, volume expanders, and blood. Considerable discussion has occurred in the literature regarding the relative desirability of various intravenous access points. During states of normal cardiac action and circulatory flow, there is probably little difference in effectiveness of drugs administered peripherally or centrally. The route chosen for the injection of medications and fluids may be of significant consequence in the cardiac arrest circumstance, however, because the cardiac output is redistributed and circulation time is prolonged. There may be a 2-minute or more delay between the administration of a drug peripherally (during cardiac arrest) and the onset of its central effect. Access to the central circulation is desirable, but the subclavian and internal jugular routes should probably be avoided during initial resuscitation efforts. Of the several other available avenues to the circulation, the first choice for drug administration is a large vein in the antecubital fossa, perhaps using a long central catheter. This approach permits central delivery of medications but does not require the cessation of CPR while the line is being inserted. Less desirable options include the subclavian vein and the external jugular vein (both require cessation of CPR) or the femoral vein with an intravenous catheter long enough to reach above the diaphragm. Each of these three latter possible sites carries a greater risk of complications.

Long venous catheters are not, however, appropriate for the rapid infusion of volume expanders or blood. Volume expansion is much more readily achieved through a short, large-bore (14- or 16-gauge) peripheral catheter. The act of placing an intravenous line should not be allowed to delay defibrillation. Intracardiac injection is generally unwise because of the possibilities of inducing pneumothorax or hemopericardium, inadvertent injection directly into the myocardium, and/or laceration of a coronary artery.

Endotracheal Drug Administration

The transtracheal route of drug administration is appropriate and useful. Certain agents—notably epinephrine, lidocaine, and atropine—are well-absorbed across the respiratory epithelium and may, therefore, be administered via the endotracheal tube before central venous access is achieved. The technique is to inject the drug as a bolus using a long needle, then to ventilate the patient vigorously. In general, the onset of drug effect is rapid. The peak level is somewhat less than via the intravenous route and the duration of action is prolonged. Lipophobic drugs such as bretylium tosylate should not be thus administered.

Open Chest Cardiac Massage

Recent resuscitative research using state-of-the-art technology has raised questions about the adequacy of closed chest cardiac massage (even when augmented with pressors and when employing the so-called new CPR techniques). This has prompted a reevaluation of open cardiac massage. Repeatedly, studies have demonstrated that the open chest procedure can generate nearly normal cardiac output and tissue perfusion and can actually shunt cranial blood flow from the face to the brain, in direct contrast to the effect of the closed chest technique. Open chest massage can achieve a cerebral blood flow level well above the 20–30% of normal that is considered critical for survival of the brain.

Several indications for open chest cardiac massage are listed in the Standards for CPR and EEC (Table 2.3). However, few practitioners are pre-

Table 2.3.
Indications for Open Chest Cardiac Massage

Cardiac arrest associated with penetrating chest trauma
Anatomic deformity of the chest or severe emphysema
Cardiac arrest secondary to severe hypothermia
Cardiac arrest secondary to ruptured aortic aneurysm (when bypass facilities are available)
Intraoperative cardiac arrest when the chest is already open
Crushed chest injury with lateral instability
Failure of closed chest compression in ventricular fibrillation refractory to external defibrillation

pared technically to carry out the open procedure in the emergency department, despite its potential efficacy in certain circumstances. Continued experience and research will likely define the role of this modality for the emergency physician.

Pharmacology of ACLS

In no other area of resuscitation have changes been so sweeping. Drugs that were considered mainstays of therapy, such as sodium bicarbonate, calcium chloride, and isoproterenol, are less effective than previously thought and may actually be harmful. Earlier recommendations were often based on anecdotes, misconstrued studies, or vague theoretical impressions. The indications for some drugs have been markedly limited or the drugs have been flatly contraindicated. Controversy still abounds; the recommendations herein represent an attempt at a workable consensus. It is fully recognized that this is an area in flux and that both recommendations and indications will change as future investigations are reported.

Oxygen

Oxygen is perhaps the only agent that has emerged unscathed from this period of reassessment. One hundred percent oxygen should be administered early in any resuscitative procedure by whatever route is available—bag mask, EOA, endotracheal tube, cricothyrotomy. Cell viability is ultimately dependent on the delivery of oxygen and substrate so that energy-requiring cell mechanisms can be maintained. When the patient is intubated and being mechanically hyperventilated, 100% oxygen may be administered since there is no need for concern over the CO_2 retention in that circumstance.

Epinephrine

Epinephrine has been shown to improve resuscitation rates from cardiac arrest in experimental and clinical studies from the turn of the century to the present. It has now been persuasively demonstrated that it is epinephrine's potent α-adrenergic agonist effect that is critical in improving salvage. The beneficial role, if any, played by epinephrine's β-receptor stimulating properties in the arrest situation is not well-understood.

By stimulating α-receptors in muscle, skin, and visceral beds, epinephrine increases the total peripheral resistance, thereby raising aortic diastolic blood pressure above 40 mm Hg, which seems to represent a critical threshold value. This aortic diastolic pressure (ADP) is the driving force behind coronary perfusion (the perfusion gradiant being ADP less right atrial pressure) so this α effect of epinephrine maintains coronary arterial flow, myocardial oxygenation, and myocardial viability.

Epinephrine may also be brain protective because it potentially redistributes the limited cardiac output from CPR to the cerebral vasculature. The improved cerebral flow may outweigh any potential increase in central nervous system (CNS) metabolic activity induced by epinephrine. Animal studies confirm that epinephrine is inactivated in alkaline media, but suggest that it is more effective in an acidic environment than was previously thought, and its administration need not be delayed in the arrest situation. A previous tenet of epinephrine use was that it coarsened fine ventricular fibrillation, thereby facilitating subsequent defibrillation. This allegedly improved ease of defibrillation is not substantiated by animal or human data, and it now appears that there is no difference in the ability to defibrillate coarse versus fine fibrillation. Moreover, the coarsening of fibrillation by epinephrine's positive inotropic effect (β) increases myocardial work, increases intramyocardial resistance to blood flow, and selectively shunts blood away from the endocardium. Obviously, these effects are undesirable and to some degree offset epinephrine's beneficial effect on coronary perfusion.

Accordingly, in cardiac arrest, a case can be made for using a pure α agent to avoid epinephrine's potentially detrimental β effects. Methoxamine has been suggested for this indication. While it is clear that pure β agents are detrimental and it has been demonstrated that pure α agents can enhance restoration of circulation, questions remain. Do the pure α agents selectively redistribute blood to brain and heart as well as epinephrine does? Do they cause sustained peripheral vasoconstriction that can produce lactic acidosis and impair long-term survival postresuscitation? Would a potent α agent raise right atrial pressure and ultimately diminish the gradient driving coronary artery perfusion? Until such doubts are resolved, epinephrine will remain the drug of choice in managing cardiac arrest. The recommended dose in the guidelines is 5–10 ml of a 1:10,000 solution (0.5–1.0 mg) given intravenously every 5 minutes during the resuscitation effort. However, studies indicate that a more frequent administration (every 2 minutes) may be necessary to sustain epinephrine's therapeutic levels and, consequently, the diastolic blood pressure.

Epinephrine may be given by the endotracheal route as well, but the optimal dose for such administration has yet to be determined. The guidelines recommend 10 ml of a 1:10,000 solution instilled as a single bolus. It is clear that the drug instilled by the endotracheal route has a prolonged depot effect relative to an intravenous injection, but equally high peak levels are not achieved. The possibility of a postresuscitative hypertensive effect of depot epinephrine exists.

Atropine

Atropine sulfate is a vagolytic agent used to accelerate the spontaneous firing rate of the sinoatrial node and to speed conduction through the atrioventricular (A-V) node. Accordingly, it is of use in managing hemodynamically significant sinus bradycardia (evidenced by inadequate cerebral perfusion, hypotension, and/or frequent ventricular escape beats). Some cases of A-V nodal blockade respond to atropine, and there are advocates of its use in asystole (reasoning that sustained elevation of parasympathetic tone may produce cardiac standstill by supressing supraventricular and ventricular pacemakers).

The recommended dose varies by indication: for symptomatic bradycardia, 0.5 mg intravenously as a bolus administered every 5 minutes to a maximum of 2.0 mg (at this level the vagal effect is fully blocked). For asystole, the suggested dose is twice that, 1.0 mg every 5 minutes. Like epinephrine and lidocaine, atropine may be administered by the endotracheal route. Tachycardia increases myocardial work and can extend an area of infarction, so atropine should be used with caution in the setting of acute myocardial ischemia.

Lidocaine

Lidocaine has the ability to suppress ventricular ectopy when administered prophylactically and/or therapeutically. It has also been shown experimentally to raise the fibrillatory threshold. Lidocaine has been employed extensively and successfully in the prevention of primary and recurrent ventricular ectopy and fibrillation in the patient with acute myocardial infarction, making it the drug of choice for this indication. Like bretylium tosylate, it has been an effective adjunct to electrical defibrillation of refractory ventricular fibrillation.

Since many episodes of ventricular fibrillation begin unheralded by the "classic" premonitory signals (coupled premature ventricular contractions (PVCs), multifocal PVCs, etc.) and since lidocaine is neither a myocardial nor a cardiac conduction system depressant, it should be routinely administered prophylactically in the patient with a suspected myocardial infarct. Lidocaine administered prophylactically in the field by paramedics and/or self-administered intramuscularly by patients themselves is under active investigation and has shown promising results. When used prophylactically in the emergency department, a loading bolus of 0.5–1.0 mg/kg should be administered intravenously and a drip started at 2 mg/minute. The bolus dose should be repeated in 5 minutes to achieve prophylactic blood levels.

For the management of refractory ventricular fibrillation, lidocaine and bretylium tosylate have demonstrated essentially a comparable efficacy, at facilitating electrical defibrillation, in randomized clinical trials. For simplicity, the American Heart Association (AHA) Guidelines have arbitrarily designated lidocaine as the drug of choice for this indication, but research is ongoing in this field. If the triplet of countershocks described above (p 14) has not been successful in terminating ventricular fibrillation, lidocaine should be given in a 1 mg/kg bolus intravenously, repeated every 5–8 minutes, to a maximum of 3 mg/kg. After a regular rhythm has been restored, the blood level of lidocaine should be sustained with a drip infusion at 4 mg/minute. Lidocaine can also be administered by endotracheal tube, and the recommended dose is 1 mg/kg. Future studies may recommend a different dosage for the endotracheal route.

A population of patients in refractory ventricular fibrillation seem to respond to multiple agents. Accordingly, if the combination of lidocaine and defibrillation is not effective, bretylium tosylate should be added to the regimen (Fig. 2.5).

Lidocaine manifests toxicity primarily through CNS changes ranging from muscle twitching and slurred speech to simulated cerebrovascular accidents and seizures.

Bretylium Tosylate

Bretylium tosylate (BT) is an antiarrhythmic agent that lowers the defibrillation threshold in experimental animals and has been reported to achieve chemical defibrillation in some clinical settings. Most authors designate BT as a second line drug (after lidocaine or procainamide), advising that it be employed for the treatment of "refractory" ventricular fibrillation. But this relegation to secondary status may be rooted more in tradition than logic. To date, comparative clinical studies have not demonstrated that either BT or lidocaine is clearly superior. BT does have its staunch advocates as the drug of choice for managing ventricular fibrillation refractory to electrical defibrillation. They maintain that it should be employed early rather than withheld until all else has failed.

The effect of bretylium tosylate is principally the result of its ability to release neuromediators from adrenergic nerve terminals. This produces a transient hypertensive phase with some increase in ectopy in patients with normal cardiac action. The release phase is followed by a period of depletion of the mediator that is characterized in the ambulatory patient by orthostatic hypotension. Bretylium tosylate does not impair cardiac conduction velocity or automaticity. It has a positive inotropic effect. BT is effective in the treatment of both ventricular tachycardia and ventricular fibrillation. It may be administered intravenously in a dosage of 5–10 mg/

Figure 2.5. Ventricular fibrillation (and pulseless ventricular tachycardia). This sequence was developed to assist in teaching how to treat a broad range of patients with ventricular fibrillation (*VF*) or pulseless ventricular tachycardia (*VT*). Some patients may require care not specified herein. This algorithm should not be construed as prohibiting such flexibility. Flow of algorithm presumes that VF is continuing. *CPR,* cardiopulmonary resuscitation.
[a]Pulseless VT should be treated identically to VF.
[b]Check pulse and rhythm after each shock. If VF recurs after transiently converting (rather than persists without ever converting), use whatever energy level has previously been successful for defibrillation.
[c]Epinephrine should be repeated every 5 minutes.
[d]Intubation is preferable. If it can be accomplished simultaneously with other techniques, then the earlier the better. However, defibrillation and epinephrine are more important initially if the patient can be ventilated without intubation.
[e]Some may prefer repeated doses of lidocaine, which may be given in 0.5 mg/kg boluses every 8 minutes to a total dose of 3 mg/kg.
[f]Value of sodium bicarbonate is questionable during cardiac arrest, and it is not recommended for routine cardiac arrest sequence. Consideration of its use in a dose of 1 mEq/kg is appropriate at this point. Half of original dose may be repeated every 10 minutes if it is used. (From American Heart Association: Standards and guidelines for cardiopulmonary resuscitation (CPR) and emergency cardiac care (ECC). *JAMA*, 1986;255:2905–2989. Copyright 1986, American Medical Association.)

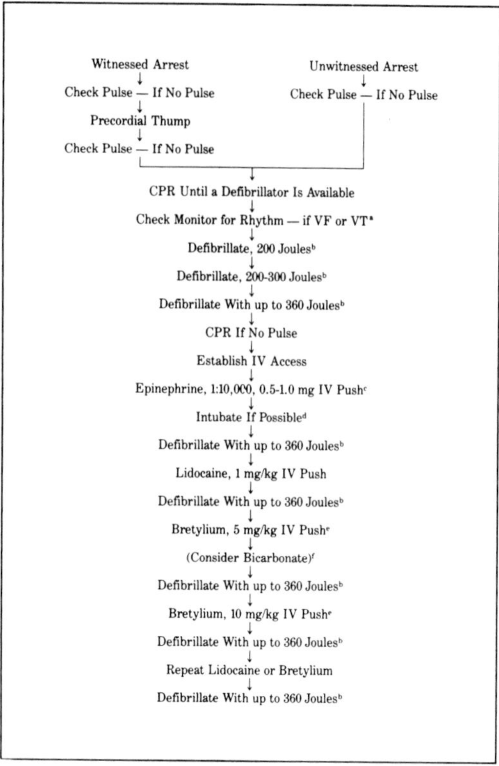

kg as a slow intravenous bolus for ventricular tachycardia. There follows an approximately 2-minute interval before effects are noted. The intravenous bolus dose may be repeated every 15–30 minutes to a maximum of 30 mg/kg. Like lidocaine, its bolus administration may be followed by a drip at 1–2 mg/minute. For ventricular fibrillation, the bolus may be given more rapidly as a push dose.

Sodium Bicarbonate

The most radical change in advanced cardiac life support protocol recommendations centers on the use of sodium bicarbonate. This drug was once the centerpiece of therapy—the first to be administered in the arrest situation—but it is now deemed unnecessary in most resuscitation efforts and may have harmful effects if given in previously recommended dosages. Animal data indicate that sodium bicarbonate neither facilitates defibrillation nor improves the rate of survival. Acidosis attenuates myocardial response to catecholamines and depresses myocardial contractility, but alkalosis is also detrimental. The main cause of initial acidemia during cardiac arrest is respiratory failure. Accordingly, the appropriate response is intubation and hyperventilation, not the administration of sodium bicarbonate.

The adverse effects of bicarbonate are many: hyperosmolality, increased arterial P_{CO_2}, intracellular acidosis, myocardial depression, CNS acidosis, impaired delivery of oxygen from hemoglobin molecule to tissue, and sodium overload. Bicarbonate should, then, be withheld early in the resuscitation procedure. Interventions of proven benefit (defibrillation, intubation and ventilation, administration of epinephrine) have priority. The principal indication for administering bicarbonate is profound acidosis (pH less than 7.0 despite effective ventilation).

The recommended dosage of bicarbonate in this situation is 1 mEq/kg as an initial bolus, followed by 0.5 mEq/kg at 10-minute intervals if blood gas determinations indicate persistent severe acidosis.

Calcium Chloride

As with sodium bicarbonate, recent experimental studies, a critical survey of the literature, and assessment of clinical outcomes have narrowed the indications for the administration of calcium chloride in cardiac arrest. Calcium is a vital ion, essential for the process of muscle contraction. However, hypocalcemia is not found in the typical cardiac arrest, and there is no evidence that raising the serum calcium concentration above normal is beneficial. Indeed, the elevated level of calcium ion produced by previously recommended doses may be injurious to both the myocardium (decreased contractility) and the cerebral perfusion (through increased microvascular resistance). It has been shown that, in some cases, calcium chloride administration causes intractable ventricular fibrillation and sudden death. Given these facts, the recommendation that calcium chloride be administered in refractory asystole has been withdrawn.

However, there continue to be reports of slight increase in short-term salvage from electromechanical dissociation (EMD) associated with the use of calcium. The benefit seems to be restricted to cases of refractory EMD in which the QRS segment duration is greater than 0.12 second. Calcium *is* indicated in cardiac arrest with hyperkalemia, profound hypocalcemia, and poisoning with calcium channel blockers. The recommended dosage for these indications is 2–5 ml or a 10% solution of calcium chloride as an intravenous bolus.

Isoproterenol Hydrochloride

Isoproterenol, true to its history as a drug subject to wide swings in acceptability, is now out of favor in ACLS. This is because myocardial perfusion—not cardiac output—is the single most important determinant of resuscitative success. Isoproterenol, a pure β agent, stimulates the heart and increases cardiac output and its myocardial oxygen demands, while at the same time reducing peripheral resistance, diastolic blood pressure, and coronary perfusion pressure. Worse, despite raising overall cardiac output, isoproterenol shunts blood away from the heart and brain. Consequently it is not indicated in patients in cardiac arrest. These same comments apply to the β agent dobutamine hydrochloride and to dopamine hydrochloride, when given in low doses.

The only remaining indication for isoproterenol

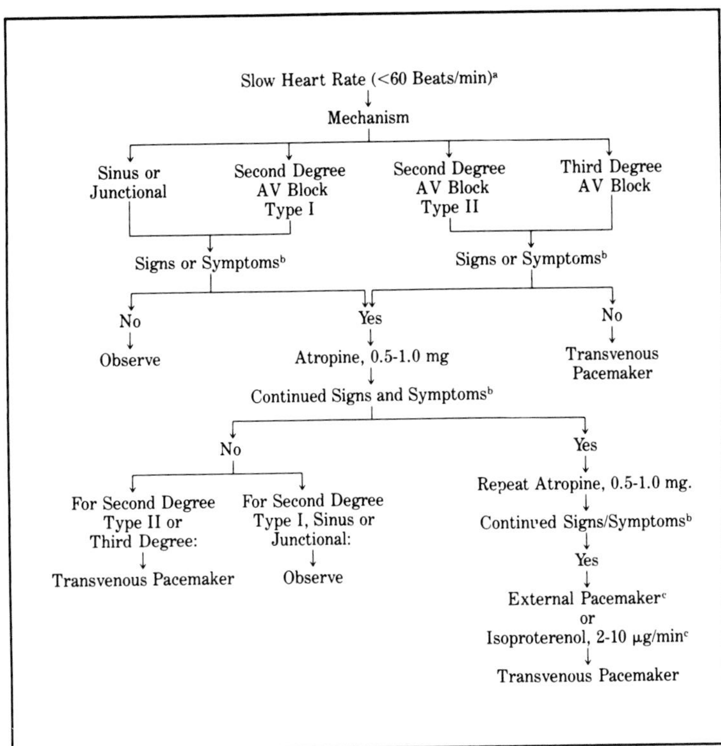

Figure 2.6. Bradycardia. This sequence was developed to assist in teaching how to treat a broad range of patients with bradycardia. Some patients may require care not specified herein. This algorithm should not be construed to prohibit such flexibility. *AV,* atrioventricular.

[a]A solitary chest thump or cough may stimulate cardiac electrical activity and result in improved cardiac output and may be used at this point.

[b]Hypotension (blood pressure <90 mm Hg), premature ventricular contractions, altered mental status or symptoms (eg, chest pain or dyspnea), ischemia, or infarction.

[c]Temporizing therapy. (From American Heart Association: Standards and guidelines for cardiopulmonary resuscitation (CPR) and emergency cardiac care (ECC). *JAMA,* 1986;255:2905–2989. Copyright 1986, American Medical Association.)

If Rhythm Is Unclear and Possibly Ventricular Fibrillation, Defibrillate as for VF. If Asystole is Present[a]
↓
Continue CPR
↓
Establish IV Access
↓
Epinephrine, 1:10,000, 0.5 - 1.0 mg IV Push[b]
↓
Intubate When Possible[c]
↓
Atropine, 1.0 mg IV Push (Repeated in 5 min)
↓
(Consider Bicarbonate)[d]
↓
Consider Pacing

Figure 2.7. Asystole (cardiac standstill). This sequence was developed to assist in teaching how to treat a broad range of patients with asystole. Some patients may require care not specified herein. This algorithm should not be construed to prohibit such flexibility. Flow of algorithm presumes asystole is continuing. *VF,* ventricular fibrillation; *IV,* intravenous.
[a]Asystole should be confirmed in two leads.
[b]Epinephrine should be repeated every 5 minutes.
[c]Intubation is preferable; if it can be accomplished simultaneously with other techniques, then the earlier the better. However, cardiopulmonary resuscitation (CPR) and use of epinephrine are more important initially if patient can be ventilated without intubation. (Endotracheal epinephrine may be used.)
[d]Value of sodium bicarbonate is questionable during cardiac arrest, and it is not recommended for the routine cardiac arrest sequence. Consideration of its use in a dose of 1 mEq/kg is appropriate at this point. Half of original dose may be repeated every 10 minutes if it is used. (From American Heart Association. Standards and guidelines for cardiopulmonary resuscitation (CPR) and emergency cardiac care (ECC). *JAMA,* 1986;255:2905–2989. Copyright 1986, American Medical Association.)

in ACLS is to accelerate the heart rate in a patient with symptomatic bradycardia and a palpable pulse who is unresponsive to atropine. In this indication, isoproterenol is considered to be a temporizing measure employed until a pacemaker can be inserted. The dose is 2–10 μg/minute as an intravenous infusion.

Bradyasystolic and Pulseless Idioventricular Arrests

This group of entities carries a uniformly dismal prognosis with a mortality rate approaching 100%. Several avenues of research are being pursued, including immediate countershock for asystole, drug regimens, and early transcutaneous pacing. These have shown only limited promise. As noted above, calcium chloride seems to be of short-term benefit in selected cases of wide complex electromechanical dissociation, but otherwise it is not indicated in these conditions. The administration of atropine in asystole may be of value in some cases. Defibrillator sensing paddles should be repositioned in the case of an initial straight line to rule out occult ventricular fibrillation. Lacking any better agent, epinephrine remains the drug of choice for these lethal situations. The AHA protocols for these specific indications are presented in Figures 2.6–2.8.

Brain Resuscitation

A resuscitation that yields a brain-damaged or brain-dead "survivor" is a Pyrrhic victory. With

Continue CPR
↓
Establish IV Access
↓
Epinephrine, 1:10,000, 0.5 - 1.0 mg IV Push[a]
↓
Intubate When Possible[b]
↓
(Consider Bicarbonate)[c]
↓
Consider Hypovolemia,
Cardiac Tamponade,
Tension Pneumothorax,
Hypoxemia,
Acidosis,
Pulmonary Embolism

Figure 2.8. Electromechanical dissociation. This sequence was developed to assist in teaching how to treat a broad range of patients with electromechanical dissociation. Some patients may require care not specified herein. This algorithm should not be construed to prohibit such flexibility. Flow of algorithm presumes that electromechanical dissociation is continuing. *CPR,* cardiopulmonary resuscitation; *IV,* intravenous.
[a]Epinephrine should be repeated every 5 minutes.
[b]Intubation is preferable. If it can be accomplished simultaneously with other techniques, then the earlier the better. However, epinephrine is more important initially if the patient can be ventilated without intubation.
[c]Value of sodium bicarbonate is questionable during cardiac arrest, and it is not recommended for routine cardiac arrest sequence. Consideration of its use in a dose of 1 mEq/kg is appropriate at this point. Half of original dose may be repeated every 10 minutes if it is used. (From American Heart Association. Standards and guidelines for cardiopulmonary resuscitation (CPR) and emergency cardiac care (ECC). *JAMA,* 1986;255:2905–2989.)

current techniques, 50% of initial survivors will ultimately die of CNS-related causes and 20% of those who become long-term survivors will evidence some degree of brain damage. The processes that are injurious to the CNS are initiated during the arrest and resuscitation and mature in the postarrest ("reperfusion") period. Consequently, rescuers must think in terms of cerebral preservation early in basic CPR and continue such concern into ACLS and after circulation is restored. At present, research into brain resuscitation is in its infancy.

Pathophysiology

The injuries to the cerebrum occur during two phases: the period of cessation of blood flow and the postreperfusion phase. During the primary event of global ischemia, cerebral oxygen stores are rapidly depleted (within 10–30 seconds) and CNS glucose and glycogen stores are expended over 4–5 minutes (Fig. 2.9). Energy-requiring cell protective functions soon fail. Ion shifts occur and intracellular edema develops. Changing to anaerobic metabolism results in the production of toxic lactic acid with cell membrane disruption and neuronal death. The blood-brain barrier is disrupted and brain swelling occurs as a consequence of the loss of vascular integrity.

In the second phase (after the reestablishment of the cerebral circulation), ongoing injury proceeds (Fig. 2.10). Blood flow to the brain may transiently increase immediately postresuscitation, but then the combination of tissue edema, vasospasm, sludging of aggregates, and endothelial swelling terminates this hyperemic phase and leads to regional hypoperfusion in the central nervous system. This secondary reaction is referred to as the no-reflow phenomenon. Cascades of chemical reactions catalyzed in part by iron molecules lead to the production of superoxide free radicals that, in turn, attack cell organelles and membranes, killing additional cells.

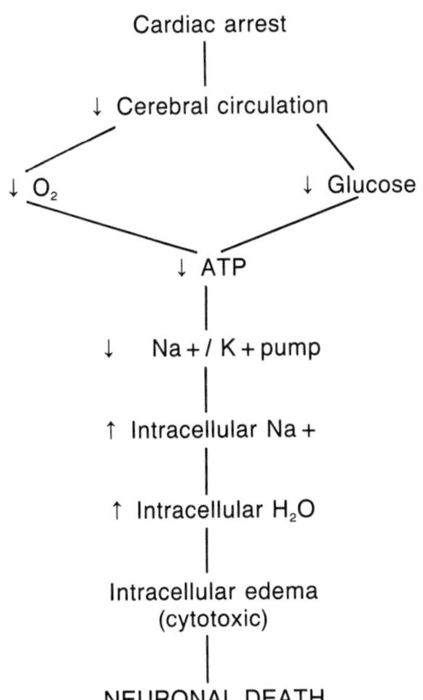

Figure 2.9. Pathophysiologic processes occurring during the initial ischematic event. (From Henneman EA. Brain Resuscitation. *Heart Lung,* 1986;15:3–13.

↓ Vessel size

Cardiac arrest

↑ Blood viscosity

\+ NEURONAL DEATH

→ →

↑ Hypermetabolism

Reperfusion

↑ Intracellular Ca^{++}

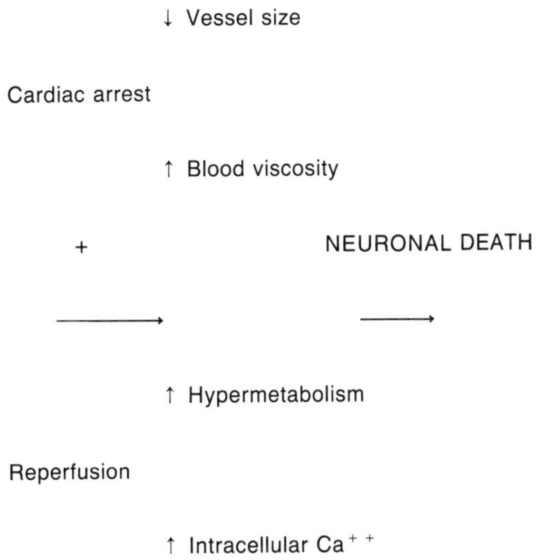

Figure 2.10. Pathophysiologic processes occurring after the reestablishment of circulation. (From Henneman EA: Brain Resuscitation. *Heart Lung,* 1986;15:3–13.

Research into brain resuscitation has raised a profoundly disturbing question: Is standard CPR worse than no therapy at all? Animal studies have shown that even normothermic neurons can survive 20–60 minutes of total anoxia. After having used up available oxygen and glucose, brain cells appear to enter a stage with no progression of the insult ("ischemic freeze"). However, if the neurons are provided with a source of glucose while they are anoxic, anaerobic glycolysis proceeds, leading to the production of lactic acid. This state, with the brain receiving insufficient oxygen but some glucose for a substrate, occurs during standard CPR and is referred to as the "trickle flow" phenomenon. The lactate produced during this phase will ultimately lead to irreversible morphologic changes, which would not have occurred without the trickle flow. This theoretical objection to basic CPR has not been resolved as of this writing.

Protective Measures

The approach should be to maximize cerebral blood flow and tissue oxygenation during CPR. At present this can be done only by keeping the head of the stretcher flat, employing excellent technique for chest compressions, intubating and ventilating the patient with 100% oxygen, and administering epinephrine early and repeatedly. The objective is to produce a cerebral blood flow greater than 20–30% of normal, thereby maintaining neuronal viability, but this is rarely, if ever, achieved by basic CPR. The key to cerebral protection, then, is the early restoration of spontaneous circulation. All efforts should be directed toward this goal.

If spontaneous circulation can be restored, the next objective is to maintain cerebral perfusion and oxygenation in the face of the ongoing pathologic changes detailed above. At present there is no single protocol that is unequivocally successful in accomplishing this, but several approaches have been explored in animal models. These data indicate that the administration of a loop diuretic may reduce cerebral edema by selectively dehydrating edematous tissues (in contrast to osmotic diuretics, which withdraw fluid from the normal brain and which are subject to the phenomenon of rebound swelling). Some investigators have attempted hemodilution and the induction of a brief episode of hypertension to "flush out the sludge" in the brain's microvasculature during the reperfusion stage. A trial of barbiturate loading has been found to be ineffective in modifying outcome in a large cooperative study. Calcium channel blockers have been used to prevent delayed vasospasm. Moreover, the fact that high intracellular calcium concentrations were found in the damaged brain tissue suggested that calcium channel blockers might be used beneficially to prevent the influx of damaging calcium ions. However, the calcium channel blockers have not been effective in doing so because the calcium appears to enter through the damaged cell membranes and not the calcium channels. That is, the influx of calcium seems to be a result, not a cause, of the injury. Research is proceeding on the use of iron chelating agents to protect against the formation of superoxide radicals, but this investigation is in its early stages. At this time, brain resuscitation remains an objective, not an achievement.

CESSATION OF CPR

Analysis of experience has permitted a somewhat more defined approach to the decision to terminate efforts. The reality is as follows. Most successful resuscitations occur in the field. Patients arriving in the emergency department in asystole or pulseless bradycardia currently have virtually no chance of successful resuscitation. Resuscitation efforts in the normothermic and nondrug-intoxicated patient going beyond 35 minutes have virtually no probability of success. In the case of hypothermia, immersion, and drug-induced comas in young patients, prolonged vigorous efforts are justified.

Bystander estimates of down time are notoriously inaccurate. Such neurologic signs as fixed, dilated pupils are unreliable. Therefore, the appropriate endpoint for resuscitation is cardiovascular unresponsiveness.

SUGGESTED READINGS

American Heart Association. Standards and guidelines for cardiopulmonary resuscitation (CPR) and emergency cardiac care (ECC). *JAMA,* 1986;255:2905–2989.

Babbs CF. Role of iron ions in the genesis of reperfusion injury following successful cardiopulmonary resuscitation: Preliminary data and a biochemical hypothesis. *Ann Emerg Med,* 1985;14:777–783.

Cardiopulmonary-cerebral resuscitation: State of the art. *Ann Emerg Med,* 1984;13:755–875.

Cummins RO, Eisenburg MS, Stults KR. Automatic external defibrillators: Clinical issues for cardiology. *Circulation,* 1986;73:381–385.

Hammargren Y, Clinton JE, Ruiz E. A standard comparison of esophageal obturator airway and endotracheal tube ventilation in cardiac arrest. *Ann Emerg Med,* 1985;14:953–958.

Kosnik JW, Jackson RE, Keats S, et al. Dose-related response of centrally administered epinephrine on the change in aortic diastolic pressure during closed-chest massage in dogs. *Ann Emerg Med,* 1984;14:204–208.

Proceedings of the 1985 UAEM/IRIEM research symposium on resuscitation. *Ann Emerg Med,* 1985;14:712–823.

Ralston SA, Voorhees WD, Babbs CF. Intrapulmonary epinephrine during prolonged cardiopulmonary resuscitation: Improved regional blood flow and resuscitation in dogs. *Ann Emerg Med,* 1984;13:79–86.

Sanders AB, Kern KB, Ewy GA, et al. Improved resuscitation from cardiac arrest with open-chest massage. *Ann Emerg Med,* 1984;13:672–675.

Shea SR, MacDonald JR, Gruzinski G. Prehospital endotracheal tube airway or esophageal gastric tube: A critical comparison. *Ann Emerg Med,* 1985;14:102–112.

Smith JP, Bodai BI. Guidelines for discontinuing prehospital CPR in the emergency department—A review. *Ann Emerg Med,* 1985;14:1093–1098.

Spivey WH, Lathers CM, Malone DR, et al. Comparison of intraosseous, central, and peripheral routes of sodium bicarbonate administration during CPR in pigs. *Ann Emerg Med,* 1984;14:1135–1140.

Stueven HA, Thompson B, Aprahamian C, et al. The effectiveness of calcium chloride in refractory electromechanical dissociation. *Ann Emerg Med,* 1985;14:626–629.

Stueven HA, Thompson B, Aprahamian C, et al. Lack of effectiveness of calcium chloride in refractory asystole. *Ann Emerg Med,* 1985;14:630–632.

Syverud SA, Dalsey WC, Hedges Jr. Transcutaneous and transvenous cardiac pacing for early bradysystolic arrest. *Ann Emerg Med,* 1986;15:121–124.

Chapter **3**

Shock

Glenn LaMuraglia, M.D.
Sean Kennedy, M.D.

Shock is best defined as a state of inadequate tissue perfusion that may develop secondary to diverse etiologies. Although shock is classified in many ways, it will be here categorized into: (*a*) hypovolemic, (*b*) cardiogenic, (*c*) obstructive, and (*d*) peripheral (Table 3.1). Figure 3.1 presents a diagrammatic representation of the several shock states according to the underlying pathophysiologic derangement.

The clinical presentation of the patient with established shock reflects the lack of perfusion and is characterized by alteration in the sensorium, ranging from anxiety to obtundation, weakness or prostration, pallor, diaphoresis, clamminess, tachycardia, thready pulse, hypotension, and tachypnea. The most notable variation is "warm shock" presenting with peripheral vasodilatation that is associated with early sepsis, spinal cord injury, or anaphylaxis.

Hemorrhage, myocardial infarction, sepsis, anaphylaxis, and spinal cord injury are the predominant causes of the shock syndrome. Although seemingly unrelated, these processes all affect the microcirculation and the cells lining the capillary beds. Their common impact is to produce diminished perfusion in the capillaries, which deprives the cells of needed oxygen and nutrients, allowing accumulation of waste products and leading to lactic acidosis.

PHYSIOLOGIC RESPONSES

To defend against this life-threatening sequence, the body employs several compensatory mechanisms, designed to maintain perfusion pressure in tissues. The initial response is a sympathetic discharge, an outflow of catecholamines that stimulates the heart, increasing the rate and force of contraction. The afferent arterioles of nonessential vascular beds are simultaneously constricted, raising peripheral resistance in an attempt to increase intraarterial pressure. These neurohumoral responses produce the pale, cool, clammy skin and rapid, thready pulse characteristic of the shock state. Their principal goal is to increase circulating blood volume and, thereby, to maintain blood flow through the coronary and carotid arteries. If sustained, however, this vasoconstricted state itself becomes harmful, leading to sludging of the blood trapped in the capillaries, disseminated intravascular coagulation, and profound acidosis. Ultimately, tissue hypoxia results in loss of cell function and membrane integrity, followed by cell death and organ failure. In addition, the venous capacitance vessels are constricted, reducing the size of the intravascular compartment and transiently increasing right heart venous return. In the subacute state, diminution of intravascular hydrostatic pressure allows interstitial fluid to return to the intravascular compartment. This shift, of cell-

Table 3.1.
Categories of Shock

Shock State	Symptoms and/or Causes
Hypovolemic	
Hemorrhage	External
	Internal
Gastrointestinal	Poor intake
	Vomiting
	Diarrhea
Fluid losses	Diaphoresis (heat stroke)
	Burn
Cardiogenic	
Mechanical	Valvular disease
	Acute: myocardial infarction, aortic dissection
	Chronic: regurgitation or stenosis
	Myxoma
	Thrombus
	Idiopathic hypertrophic subaortic stenosis
Myocardial	Impaired contractility
	Right myocardial infarct
	Left myocardial infarct
	Impaired compliance
	Amyloidosis
	Sclerosis
Arrhythmia	
Obstructive	
Pulmonary embolus	
Tension pneumothorax	
Cardiac tamponade	Effusion
	Constriction
Peripheral	
Septic	
Neurogenic	Brain injury
	Spinal cord injury
Vasogenic	Anaphylactic
	Anesthetic
	Overdose

free and protein-free solution occurs at rates up to 1 liter/hr. The clinician can attempt to augment this physiologic shift by elevating the patient's legs or applying military anti-shock trousers (MAST), which may contribute an autotransfusion of intravascular volume.

Thus, the body constricts both arterioles and venules to increase the central blood volume, increases the cardiac output to circulate the available blood more rapidly, and draws on interstitial fluid reserves to supplement the total intravascular fluid volume. Through these mechanisms, loss of up to 30% of intravascular fluid can be compensated; however, additional losses or continuing stress at this level for extended periods can lead to rapid deterioration of the clinical status.

HYPOVOLEMIC SHOCK

The classic example of the pattern of derangement and response just described is exemplified by hypovolemic shock. The fluid loss can be water, plasma, or whole blood with the same effect on circulatory dynamics. Dehydration through inadequate fluid intake, excessive sweating, or loss from the gastrointestinal tract (vomiting or diarrhea) can produce spontaneous hypovolemia. Blood loss from trauma or bleeding into body cavities or the intestine can lead to shock without overt hemorrhage. Two important clinical objectives are early recognition of the hypovolemic patient and detection of occult blood loss (Table 3.2). This may be recognized by orthostatic vital signs and a narrow pulse pressure. Decrease of more than 10 mm Hg systolic pressure or an increase in heart rate of more than 10 beats/minute in assuming the upright position indicates hypovolemia.

In hemorrhagic shock a bleeding source must be aggressively sought. A careful, thorough history and

Table 3.2.
Correlation of Magnitude of Volume Deficit and Clinical Presentation (70-kg Patient); (Intravascular Volume = 7% Body Weight)

Approximate Deficit	Decrease in Blood Volume	Shock	
		Degree	Signs
ml	%		
500–750	10–15	None	None
800–1500	15–30	Mild (compensated)	Tachycardia (>100); postural blood pressure changes; mild peripheral vasoconstriction
1500–2000	30–40	Moderate	Thready pulse 100–120 beats/min; blood pressure 90–100 mm Hg systolic; marked vasoconstriction; diaphoresis; anxiety, restlessness; decreased urinary output
>2000	>40	Severe	Thready pulse >120 beats/min; blood pressure <60 mm Hg systolic; marked vasoconstriction; marked diaphoresis; obtundation; no urinary output

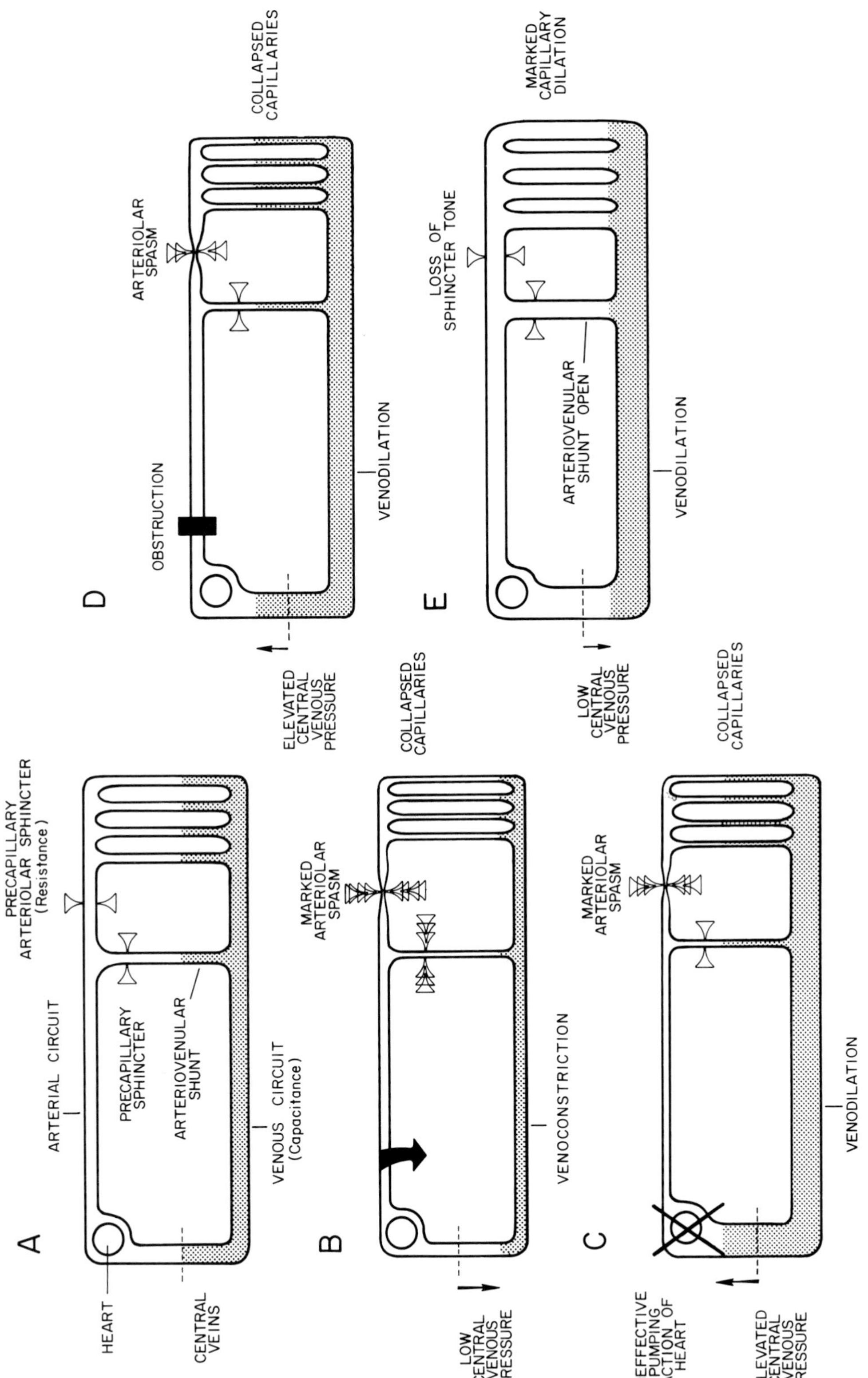

FIGURE 3.1. Schema of circulatory system: mechanisms of production of shock. *A*, Normal circulatory system. *B*, Shock due to loss of intravascular volume from hemorrhage, extravasation, dehydration, or burn. *C*, Cardiogenic shock from myocardial infarction or arrhythmia. *D*, Obstructive shock from pulmonary embolus or pericardial tamponade. *E*, Peripheral shock of septic, anesthetic, or neurogenic origin, or anaphylaxis.

physical examination are essential. Percussion of the chest for dullness, palpation of the abdomen for rigidity, careful measurement of thigh girths, and digital examination of the rectum are included in the examination. Nasogastric aspiration with guaiac testing, and peritoneal lavage may be indicated in individual instances.

The clinical laboratory plays a limited but important role in the assessment of the patient with shock. Initial hemoglobin and hematocrit determinations offer no clues to the magnitude of acute blood loss, since hemodilution by interstitial fluid requires time. These values, however, serve as important baseline information. Arterial blood gas studies indicate the severity of any acid-base imbalance, and indicate whether the patient has adequate ventilation. Serum electrolyte and renal function tests provide additional baseline data. In situations where blood loss is suspected as a contributing factor in hypovolemic shock, blood for transfusion should be made immediately available. Table 3.2 correlates the magnitude of fluid deficit with the clinical status and, along with estimated ongoing loss, may assist in determining the initial quantity of blood to be ordered.

A major aspect of the care of patients with shock of any cause is the reevaluation and ongoing monitoring of vital parameters. This is best done in an intensive care unit (ICU). These observations include vital signs determinations, repeated physical examinations and assessment of mental status, hourly monitoring of the urine output by an indwelling catheter, evaluation of the pulmonary status by portable chest x-ray, and continuous electrocardiographic monitoring. The mental status and urinary output reflect perfusion of the cerebral cortex and kidney. In selected patients, the central venous, pulmonary arterial wedge, and radial artery pressures should be measured since they serve as determinants of fluid status and cardiac function. Adequacy of ventilation is assessed with arterial blood gas measurements. Patients in shock should *not* remain in the emergency department. The ICU or operating room is the appropriate care area.

Therapy

Patients in shock should undergo evaluation and immediate resuscitation simultaneously. The measures involved in treating patients with hypovolemic shock include controlling hemorrhage (e.g., by direct pressure, tourniquet, MAST, Sengstaken-Blakemore tube, or ligation of bleeders), establishing and maintaining an airway, assisting ventilation if necessary, supplying oxygen, replacing lost volume and red blood cell mass, and correcting acid-base or electrolyte disturbances. Fluid administration is the essential early therapy for hypovolemic shock. Vasoactive drugs are never primary therapy.

Table 3.3.
Use of MAST

- Indications for use
  - Hypovolemic shock ("autotransfusion")
    - Blood loss (e.g., trauma, gastrointestinal bleeding, leaking abdominal aortic aneurysm, ruptured ectopic pregnancy)
  - Relative hypovolemia
    - Compression of vascular space (e.g., neurogenic shock, anaphylaxis, drug overdose)
  - Skeletal stabilization
    - (e.g., pelvic or lower extremity fracture)
  - Control of hemorrhage in lower extremities
- Contraindications to use
  - Absolute
    - Pulmonary edema (MAST increases afterload)
  - Relative
    - Pregnancy
    - Dyspnea/thoracic injury
    - Head injury

MAST

An early step in treating hypovolemic shock, secondary to trauma, has been the application of MAST (Table 3.3). MAST has been increasingly utilized in the field and in emergency departments, but does have certain limitations. MAST is available in several configurations commercially but is, in essence, a compartmented pneumatic garment designed to be applied to the lower extremities and abdomen (see Chapter 1, p 5). When inflated, the suit applies external compression to the anatomic parts it encircles. In doing so, it produces several effects: (*a*) a redistribution of an estimated 300–1200 ml of blood from the legs to the central circulation, (*b*) a reduction in the size of the vascular compartments by compression of vessels within the trousers (causing increased afterload), (*c*) a tamponading of ongoing bleeding in the parts enclosed, and (*d*) stabilization of fractures of the pelvis or lower extremities.

There are disadvantages to the use of MAST: (*a*) inaccessibility of the covered areas to repeated examination, (*b*) restriction of diaphragmatic excursion and lung expansion, (*c*) distal leg ischemia, and (*d*) potential increased thoracic bleeding.

Of critical importance is careful deflation of the MAST. It should never be removed abruptly and, in particular, it should never be cut off, because a precipitous fall in blood pressure can occur. Rather, it should be removed in stepwise fashion, compartment by compartment, in the reverse order in which it was inflated. MAST is only to be removed in two circumstances: (*a*) in the operating room where all is in readiness for definitive surgical intervention, or (*b*) in the emergency department after bleeding has been controlled and intravascular volume has been repleted. In this situation, the deflation is done in a sequential manner with vital signs measured as each chamber is deflated. If the systolic pressure falls by 5–10 mm Hg at any stage, that compartment is reinflated and additional fluid volume administered. Although frequently used, there has still been no study proving that the MAST enhances outcome in patients with hypovolemic shock after trauma.

Fluid Administration

The objective of volume expansion is to refill the vascular compartment. This allows the heart to generate adequate cardiac output and to produce enough hydrostatic pressure to perfuse the tissue. There are many types of solutions for fluid therapy, some containing electrolytes only (crystalloids), some containing large molecular weight molecules (colloids), and some containing red blood cells (whole blood or packed cells). The reasons for choosing each fluid are important, and the choice is governed by the clinical situation.

Two generalizations can be made about fluid replacement therapy. First, any fluid will improve perfusion, at least transiently. Second, only red blood cells carry significant amounts of oxygen. Fluid for rapid volume replacement should be administered via short, large-bore, indwelling venous cannulas. The amount administered depends on the clinical presentation of the patient. If the deficit has been present for some time, it is necessary to replenish both the intravascular fluid and some of the interstitial fluid. The rate of administration is governed by the rapidity of the ongoing bleeding and the magnitude of the preexisting loss.

Central venous pressure lines should not be routinely used for the rapid administration of fluid. They can be useful, however, as a guide to fluid administration and are most dependable in patients with hypovolemic shock without complications. If primary myocardial dysfunction or respiratory disease is suspected, central venous pressure reading may be deceptive and pulmonary artery wedge pressure measurements may be necessary. In all patients, the central venous pressure measurement should be supplemented with repeated auscultation of the chest and, when indicated, arterial blood gas measurement and chest x-ray films during vigorous fluid replacement.

Selection of Replacement Fluids

Not only is the selection of a solution for correcting hypovolemia important, it is also the subject of controversy. Logically, blood lost should be replaced with blood. In practice, however, there are safer and less expensive solutions available that can be used to correct mild to moderate deficits. Asanguinous replacement solutions, crystalloids and colloids, both have had extensive clinical use, but there, too, controversy surrounds their selection.

The debate hinges on which fluid is more likely to produce interstitial pulmonary edema when administered in quantity. Crystalloid solutions contain small molecules and rapidly escape from the vascular space into the interstitium to produce peripheral and pulmonary edema. Consequently, their volume expansion effects are short-lived. Colloid solutions, in contrast, contain large macromolecular polymers and leave the circulation less easily when capillary endothelial integrity is present. They increase the plasma oncotic pressure, allowing attraction of water from the interstitium, actually producing intravascular volume expansion in an increment above that which is administered.

The rebuttal argument is that colloids ultimately escape the circulation when capillary damage exists. They raise interstitial oncotic pressure in a similar fashion and draw water back into the perivascular spaces. Obviously, if the lung interstitium is damaged, this can lead to a particularly resistant form of pulmonary edema. There is currently no conclusive evidence that the type of fluid used in volume resuscitation influences the development of pulmonary complications.

Crystalloids. For these reasons, crystalloids are the mainstay of asanguinous fluid replacement therapy. Those commonly employed are normal saline and lactated Ringer's solution. Both are "balanced" (isotonic with the extracellular fluid). There is no compelling reason to choose one over the other. Unless the patient is at risk of developing hyperkalemia, in which case lactated Ringer's should be avoided, the sodium lactate in lactated Ringer's solution does not contribute to lactic acidosis and is metabolized in the liver to bicarbonate. Crystalloids are nonallergenic, have no potential to produce a hypotensive reaction, and are virus-free. They are much less expensive than colloidal solutions. Glucose-containing solutions are avoided if concurrent blood transfusions are anticipated.

Colloids. There are currently three colloidal solutions available for clinical use: dextran, hetastarch, and preparations of serum albumin.

Dextran. This solution is a polysaccaride, a polymer of glucose, available in two forms—high molecular weight (dextran 70, a 6% solution with an average molecular weight in the 70,000–75,000 range) and low molecular weight (dextran 40, a 10% solution averaging 40,000). Both dextran preparations offer low cost and effective volume expansion. Dextran 70 remains in the vascular bed 2–3 days, and dextran 40 lasts for 12–18 hours. Red cell and platelet-coating effects occur; this is advocated as a beneficial antisludging factor.

However, serious difficulties limit the usefulness of dextran. Dextran can cause anaphylactic reactions and should be administered only after Promit. Promit is a glucose polymer that forms monovalent haptens with any antibodies that could combine with dextran. This inhibits formation of immune complexes and anaphylactic reactions. Dextran 70 impairs platelet and fibrinogen function and can cause a bleeding diathesis, limiting its use as a replacement fluid. Even more important, dextran can agglutinate red blood cells, making subsequent cross-matching difficult or even impossible.

Hetastarch. A colloidal plasma volume expander more recently introduced into clinical practice, hetastarch (Hespan) is an artificial polymer derived from the waxy starch amylopectin that closely resembles glycogen. It has a molecular weight averaging 450,000 and, consequently, provides a long-lasting volume expansion effect. It is detectable in the circulation 24–36 hours after administration. It is supplied as a 6% solution in normal saline.

Hetastarch alters coagulation but does not interfere with subsequent blood typing and cross-matching. This colloid is relatively nonallergenic, having a reaction rate similar to that for albumin. It is less expensive than albumin; however, no additional benefit has been demonstrated for hetastarch over crystalloid in the treatment of acute hypovolemic shock.

Serum Albumin. This is available in 5 and 25% solutions. The former is an effective plasma volume expander; the latter, a more potent elevator of plasma oncotic pressure. Both are stabilized and heat-treated to kill hepatitis virus. Albumin has a lower incidence of serious allergic reactions than other colloid preparations, has no deleterious effect upon hemostasis, and does not produce a paradoxical idiosyncratic hypotensive effect. Therefore, unlike dextran, the volume of albumin that may be transfused is not restricted. Albumin preparations are expensive.

Beyond expense, however, several recent studies have questioned the use of albumin. There is evidence that albumin has a negative inotropic effect and causes excessive salt retention. In addition, coagulation deficits and typing and cross-matching difficulties have been reported. Nevertheless, albumin has a long track record of favorable clinical use.

Guidelines

Given these controversies, the following guidelines provide a practical approach to the treatment of hypovolemic shock: (*a*) establish at least two short, large-bore intravenous lines; (*b*) obtain blood for typing and cross-matching, for an appropriate number of units for the clinical situation; (*c*) regard crystalloid as the keystone of therapy and begin an infusion of saline or lactated Ringer's, giving two to three times the estimated blood loss as a bolus (for pediatric patients, approximately 20 ml/kg); and (*d*) carefully monitor vital signs and pulmonary status after each 500 ml are infused. Urine output is a good monitor for adequacy of volume replacement with blood pressure and pulse rate. The clinical objective is a systolic blood pressure over 90. If there is an inadequate clinical response to 2–3 liters of crystalloid, whole blood or packed red blood cells are administered.

Blood Transfusion. Currently, blood is the only solution that permits oxygen transport, and therefore it is ultimately required in profound blood loss. Whole blood has historically been advocated for the treatment of patients with hemorrhagic shock with the compelling logic of matching fluid administered to fluid lost. Current practice, however, favors administration of packed red blood cells suspended in a crystalloid solution. This practice reflects standard blood bank procedure in which drawn blood is immediately fractionated into platelets, plasma, and packed red cells.

Ideally, adequate time exists or can be gained to permit typing and complete cross-matching of the patient's blood. However, if exsanguination or irreversible shock is imminent, complete matching cannot be accomplished and compromises must be made. The best choice in the urgent situation is type-specific blood, which is available in minutes and which avoids the incompatibility reaction of the ABO blood group. Type-specific blood is preferable to O-negative (universal donor) blood for several reasons: type O Rh-negative blood is not available in many blood banks; there is an increasing incidence of anti-A and anti-B antibody titers in O-negative donors, and transfusion of large amounts of type O blood can make subsequent typing and cross-matching of the patient's blood difficult. If type O-negative blood is used, only blood from donors with low titers of anti-A and anti-B antibodies or O-negative packed red blood cells suspended in AB plasma or saline should be transfused.

If an additional 15 minutes are available, saline cross-matching can be carried out in addition to typing. This permits determination of the Rh factor and detects strong antibodies of the minor blood groups (e.g., anti-Kell), avoiding severe reactions.

It is preferable to use the freshest blood available because stored blood undergoes undesirable changes (Table 3.4), becomes acidic, and 2,3-diphospho-

Table 3.4.
Some Potentially Deleterious Effects of Massive Transfusion of Stored Blood[a]

Volume-related
Transmission of disease
Immunologic mismatch
Immunization of recipient
Rate- and volume-related
Altered hemoglobin affinity for oxygen
Coagulation abnormalities
Acid-base imbalance
Citrate toxicity
Hypothermia
Microembolization
Impaired red blood cells deformability
Infusion of plasticizers
Infusion of denatured proteins
Infusion of vasoactive substances
Elevated potassium, phosphate, ammonia levels
Hemolyzed blood products
Impaired antibacterial defenses
Graft-vs.-host reactions
Toxicity of new additives

[a] From Collins JA. Problems associated with the massive transfusion of stored blood. *Surgery*, 1974;75:274–295.

glycerate levels decrease in the red blood cells. Much like lactate, the high citrate content of preserved blood is metabolized by the liver to bicarbonate once circulation is restored. This can produce metabolic alkalosis after resuscitation. Banked blood is also hypocalcemic, since citrate binds calcium.

In the case of massive transfusion, a blood warmer is helpful to protect the core temperature of the patient and the heat-sensitive coagulation mechanism. Fresh frozen plasma, containing clotting factors, should be administered in the ratio of 2 units for every 8 units of packed cells. Calcium gluconate is rarely needed unless the infusion rate of blood is more than 75–100 ml/min for more than several units.

In summary, specific therapy for hypovolemic shock involves control of hemorrhage, administration of appropriate intravenous fluids, and maintaining body temperature. The application of external pneumatic compression devices may be of value while volume is being replaced or while the patient is being transported to a tertiary care facility or to the operating room. Pressor agents are rarely, if ever, indicated in treating hypovolemic shock.

All fluids used should be warmed to body temperature. A microwave oven or incubator can be utilized for this purpose with crystalloids (Ringer's lactate can be maintained at 40°C in the emergency department). Blood, however, must be warmed using blood warmers. Some patients may require immediate or urgent operative intervention to control hemorrhage.

CARDIOGENIC SHOCK

The second major category of the shock state is cardiogenic, in which failure to perfuse tissues adequately is a consequence of impaired cardiac function. This results most commonly from destruction of contractile muscle secondary to myocardial infarction. Disruption of the normal conduction sequence, as in heart block or arrhythmia, and mechanical factors resulting from valvular disease, intramyocardial masses (thrombus, myxoma), or idiopathic hypertrophic subaortic stenosis are other important etiologies. The result of these pathologic mechanisms is decreased cardiac output, the fundamental physiologic defect in cardiogenic shock. Thus, in contrast to hypovolemic shock, central venous pressure and pulmonary capillary wedge pressure are elevated in typical cardiogenic shock.

Attention is directed to the most common situation, cardiogenic shock after myocardial infarction (Chapter 6). Management of arrythmias is discussed in Chapter 5.

Cardiogenic shock has been defined by a set of clinical criteria, useful in facilitating a comparison of results of therapy. These diagnostic criteria include systolic pressure less than 80 mm Hg, cardiac index less than 2.1 liters/min/m^2, urinary output less than 20 ml/hr, diminished cerebral perfusion with confusion or obtundation, and cool, clammy, mottled skin characteristic of the low output state. Cardiogenic shock is the most lethal variety of shock. It occurs in 15% of patients with myocardial infarcts; the resulting mortality in these 15% ranges from 70 to 90%. Among patients who fail to respond to the initial conventional measures of treatment and who have no surgically correctable lesion, the mortality approaches 100%. This grim prognosis has spawned the development of specialized therapy. Approaches include intraaortic balloon counterpulsation, coronary recanalization and bypass procedures, and heart transplantation. The role of the emergency physician is to recognize the situation, to institute stabilization measures, and to ensure transport of the patient to the appropriate treatment facility in the hospital or geographic area.

Barring the appearance of arrhythmias or conduction blocks, the development of cardiogenic shock is a function of the location and size of the infarct. Typically, shock occurs when more than 40% of the left ventricular myocardium is involved. However, it can present as acute right heart failure as well. The onset of the shock syndrome occurs within the first 24 hours after infarction in 70% of patients and by 72 hours in 90%.

Table 3.5.
Drugs to Improve Inotropic State of the Myocardium

Drug	Dose[a]	Action	Arrythmogenicity	Comments
Amrinone (Inocor)	i.v.: loading dose 0.75 mg/kg,5–10 μg/kg/min STD MIX 200 mg in 250 ml (1 mg/ml) nondextrose solution	Non-β receptor inotropic agent	Minimal	Useful in treatment of congestive heart failure, smooth muscle relaxant, dose-dependent thrombocytopenia, and gastrointestinal toxcity
Dobutamine (Dobutrex)	i.v.: 2.5-10 μg/kg/min STD MIX 250 mg in 250 ml	Inotropic agent major β_1-adrenergic agonist with minor β_2- and α-adrenergic agonist	Minimal	Useful for cardiogenic shock and ischemia
Dopamine (Intropin)	i.v.: 0.5-2 μg/kg/min	Mainly dopaminergic splanchnic dilatation	Moderate	Good agent to increase cardiac output, blood pressure, and urine output
	i.v.: 2-10 μg/kg/min STD MIX 400 mg in 250 ml	Includes β_1- and α-adrenergic agonist		
Ephedrine	i.v.: 10-25 mg i.v. bolus slowly, may repeat every 5-10 min max 150 mg/24 hr,	β_1 and α agonist	Moderate	Increases autorhythmicity of idioventricular or nodal pacemaker and can be useful during temporary pacemaker placement
Epinephrine (Adrenalin)	i.v.; 0.5-1 mg i.v. bolus or 0.5-5 μg/min STD MIX 1 mg in 250 ml	Mostly β_1, β_2 agonist, also α agonist at higher doses	Marked	In asystole may activate sinus node; increases myocardial oxygen consumption; can be administered through an endotracheal tube if no i.v. access available
Isoproterenol (Isuprel)	i.v.: 0.5-5 μg/min STD MIX 1 mg in 250 ml	β agonist	Marked	Increases myocardial oxygen consumption; causes marked tachycardia, useful for bradycardia
Metaraminol (Aramine)	i.v.: 0.5-5 mg i.v. bolus, 5-15 μg/kg/min STD MIX 100 mg in 250 ml	Primary α agonist, also minor β_1 agonist	None	Releases endogenous norepinephrine; increases myocardial oxygen consumption
Norepinephrine (Levophed)	i.v.: 2-12 μg/min STD MIX 40 mg in 250 ml; mixture must contain D_5W to avoid oxidation	α agonist, may be β agonist at higher doses	Moderate	Causes indiscriminate peripheral vascular constriction; should be administered in central vein
Phenylephrine	i.m.: 2-5 mg i.v.: initial dose: 0.1–0.5 mg, slowly maintain 0.05–0.2 mg/min STD MIX 10 mg in 250 ml	Predominantly α agonist	None	Primarily constricts resistance blood vessels; useful in spinal anesthesia

[a] STD MIX, standard mixture; D_5W, 5% dextrose in water. Modified by permission, from DeSanctis RW, Zusman RW. In: Rubinstein E, Federman DD (eds): Scientific American *Medicine*. Section 1, Subsection III.

Principles of Therapy

Basic therapy is the same as for other forms of shock: establishment of an adequate airway, ventilation, oxygenation, relief of pain, and correction of acidosis. Derangement of ventilation-perfusion ratios may be exaggerated because of pulmonary edema and microembolization. Scrupulous attention to pulmonary status is most important in this variety of shock.

The cardiac rhythm must be monitored because poor coronary artery perfusion, hypoxia, and acidosis all depress the myocardium and favor the development of arrhythmias. In a patient with cardiogenic shock, the objective is to determine and reverse the primary etiology (myocardial, mechanical, and/or arrhythmic) and any contributing factor so that cardiac output can be optimized. Besides attempting to reverse specific derangements, there are three possible ways to improve cardiac output in the emergency department. First, if the patient is not in congestive heart failure, intravascular volume can be increased modestly to elevate the cardiac preload. This stretches the myocardial fibers at the end of diastole, amplifying left ventricular stroke work. Second, the force of the myocardial contraction (inotropy) can be increased with pharmacologic agents. Third, the afterload against which the heart must pump can be decreased by lowering the peripheral resistance. Special care must be used when applying this modality in hypotensive patients. In practice, these techniques may be applied in various combinations either simultaneously or sequentially. Ideally, this care is best delivered in an intensive care unit where proper monitoring is possible with peripheral and pulmonary artery lines and measurements of cardiac output (CO).

Optimizing the Preload

Patients in cardiogenic shock are often hypovolemic because of reflex vasodilation, reduced oral intake, vomiting, sweating, or drug therapy with nitrates or morphine. In addition, the damaged left ventricle is shifted to a Starling's curve position, which functions better at filling pressures above normal. Thus, if an adequate stroke volume is to be produced, a fluid push is needed to achieve a pulmonary capillary wedge pressure in the 16–20 mm Hg range. This is especially true in the normally hypertensive patient with left ventricular hypertrophy and a small noncompliant ventricular lumen. As drug treatment is undertaken to reverse myocardial ischemia and patient anxiety, the volume status may change frequently and requires continual reassessment.

The same myocardial dysfunction that puts patients into shock renders them extremely sensitive to volume overload and makes them prone to pulmonary vascular congestion. Again, close monitoring of this phase of volume expansion is essential. As noted, this is a situation in which central venous pressure measurement is unreliable; therefore, repeated physical examination, serial chest x-rays, and data gained from a Swan-Ganz pulmonary artery catheter and a peripheral arterial line are most valuable.

Improving the Inotropic State of the Myocardium

If the response to volume expansion is inadequate, pharmacologic agents are employed. Several categories of drugs (Table 3.5) have been advocated, including vasopressors, digitalis glycosides, sympathomimetic cardiac stimulants, adrenergic blocking agents, and corticosteroids. Many protocols have been tried using various drugs, but the issue of the best program remains controversial.

Catecholamines are the drugs most commonly utilized in the treatment of cardiogenic shock. They act by stimulating myocardial and vascular smooth muscle receptors. Catecholamines are categorized by the specific receptors they stimulate. These receptor sites are designated α (causing peripheral vasoconstriction when stimulated), β_1 (cardiac stimulation), and β_2 (peripheral vasodilation). These amines have the ability to stimulate receptors with varying degrees of specificity. Methoxamine, for example, is a pure α stimulant, whereas isoproterenol is strictly a β agent. Most of these agents have some effect on both central and peripheral receptors so that they are not "pure" agents, and the particular response is often dose-dependent. Dopamine is exceptional in its ability to stimulate unique δ (dopaminergic) splanchnic and renal vasodilating receptors.

It is important to understand that the use of sympathetic amines in the immediate postinfarct period is a double-edged sword: the drugs may be beneficial in maintaining blood pressure at a level adequate to perfuse the coronary arteries, but this benefit may be obtained at the expense of increased myocardial oxygen consumption and possible extension of the infarct. The potent cardiac stimulants are also potent arrhythmogenic agents.

α Agents. Pure or predominantly α drugs, such as methoxamine, metaraminol, and phenylephrine, once the keystones of shock therapy, are rarely used to treat cardiogenic shock. The peripheral vasoconstriction they produce may elevate blood pressure, but it does so at the expense of increased cardiac work, and actually decreases cardiac output, impairing tissue perfusion. These pressors may have limited utility as stopgap measures to maintain coronary artery circulation while other modalities are readied (e.g., the intraaortic balloon pump). They may be indicated for the treatment of peripheral shock. In general, however, the agents listed in the following sections are more appropriate in this setting.

Mixed α, β Agents. Drugs with both α and β stimulating properties have been used widely in the therapy of cardiogenic shock. Included in this group are epinephrine, norepinephrine, and dopamine.

Norepinephrine is a potent α and weaker β_1 stimulant that constricts both venous capacitance vessels and arteriolar resistance vessels and also stimulates the heart. Initially, the cardiac output either remains the same or is decreased slightly, but arterial blood pressure is increased. By stimulating the heart and supporting diastolic blood pressure, norepinephrine enhances coronary artery perfusion, resulting in improved cardiac output. Thus, it differs from the pure α agents by improving coronary blood flow as well as increasing cardiac work. Administration of norepinephrine leads to a decrease in myocardial lactate production, reflecting the improved perfusion. Renal, splanchnic, skeletomuscular, and cutaneous blood flows are all decreased, but cerebral perfusion is augmented. Norepinephrine is indicated in cardiogenic shock characterized by profound hypotension. The therapeutic objective is to produce a systolic blood pressure in the 80–100 mm Hg range to alleviate the shock state, not to restore the pressure to its preinfarction level. Better understanding of the underlying pathophysiology of cardiogenic shock has resulted in decreasing reliance on norepinephrine in favor of vasodilating drugs to reduce afterload.

Epinephrine is one of the most powerful vasopressor drugs known; it is primarily a β- but also a potent α-adrenergic agonist. It differs from norepinephrine by exerting its effect more on the heart than on the vascular tree. The positive chronotropic effect on the sinoatrial node and the positive inotropic effect on the myocardium contribute to the increased cardiac output and oxygen consumption of the heart. The direct constricting effect on all blood vessels excluding the cerebral circulation is more pronounced at higher doses of administration. With increase in blood pressure from both α and β stimulation, the heart rate generally increases, but this may vary secondary to vagal stimulation with higher arterial pressure. Epinephrine increases ventricular irritability, especially when cardiac ischemia or drugs such as digitalis and certain anesthetics have sensitized the heart. Enhanced cardiac electrical activity makes epinephrine the drug of choice in asystolic cardiac arrest. However, because it causes marked increase in myocardial oxygen consumption, it is not the drug of choice in cardiogenic shock. Epinephrine is inactivated by alkali and it should never be administered in the same intravenous line with sodium bicarbonate.

Dopamine is another mixed α and β agonist that has the unique property, mentioned previously, of dilating mesenteric and renal vascular beds. Protecting the kidneys from vasoconstriction and hypoperfusion has increased its utility. Dopamine is remarkably dose-dependent in its effects. At low dose ranges, (1–2 μg/kg/min), the δ (dopaminergic renal and mesenteric) dilatation effect is seen with little cardiac stimulation or pressor response. At intermediate dose ranges (2–10 μg/kg/min), the β (cardiac stimulant) effect of dopamine predominates. In this regard, dopamine is less potent than isoproterenol and dobutamine, but it does increase cardiac output. At progressively higher infusion rates (10–20 μ/kg/min), the α stimulating effect of dopamine becomes more prominent, producing peripheral vasoconstriction that overrides the dopaminergic effect when it reaches rates above 20 μg/kg/min. At these high levels, there is also a corresponding increase in the cardiac stimulating effect.

In practice, the infusion is begun in the 2–5 μg/kg/min range and is increased carefully, noting response of blood pressure and urine output. The principal limitation to the use of dopamine is its tendency to produce undesirable tachycardia and excessive vasoconstriction at high dosage levels. Dopamine is also inactivated in alkaline solutions and should not be administered in the same line as sodium bicarbonate. Dopamine works partly by the release of endogenous catecholamines and may be less reliable in patients whose stores have been depleted (as in patients previously treated with reserpine).

Pure β Agents. *Isoproterenol* is a pure β agent that increases both the heart rate (chronotropy) and myocardial contraction (inotropy) while producing considerable peripheral vasodilation. This seemingly desirable combination produces some undesirable side effects. The peripheral vasodilatation is nonselective with increasing blood flow to nonessential organs, such as the skin and skeletal muscles. This occurs partly at the expense of the renal circulation; the proportion of cardiac output that reaches the kidney decreases. Moreover, as vasodilation lowers the diastolic pressure, coronary artery perfusion suffers, and myocardial lactate production increases. In effect, isoproterenol stimulates the heart while simultaneously diminishing the myocardial blood supply. The main indication for its use is shock with only mild hypotension. In this situation, it can be administered alone or with another pressor agent to increase cardiac output. All β drugs have a strong potential to produce arrhythmias and to extend infarct size due to increasing myocardial oxygen consumption.

Dobutamine is primarily a potent β_1 (inotropic) stimulant, on a par with isoproterenol in this regard. However, it has much less tendency to dilate the peripheral vessels; hence there is virtually no reflex tachycardia with its use (when administered in a 2.5–10 μg/kg/min range). Furthermore, dobutamine has essentially no *a* (peripheral vasoconstrictive) effect and has a low potential for arrhythmia production. Thus, as a selective inotropic agent capable of raising cardiac output and blood pressure without real increase in heart rate, it seems to be a good drug for treating cardiogenic shock.

Other Agents. Amrinone and digitalis glycosides also improve the inotropic state of the myocardium.

Amrinone lactate, a bipyridine derivative unrelated to sympathomimetic agents or digitalis glycosides, is an inotropic drug with vasodilating properties. Its action is not well-understood, but it is thought to inhibit intracellular phosphodiesterase and increase the concentrations of cyclic adenosine monophosphate (cAMP). Primarily indicated in patients with congestive heart failure, it has been shown to increase the cardiac index by 40–80% and to decrease systemic and pulmonary vascular resistance. There is no appreciable increase in heart rate, decrease in blood pressure, or arrhythmia with conventional doses. Amrinone should not be administered concurrently with disopyramide (Norpace) because severe hypotension has been reported. A new, more potent derivative, milrione, reportedly has fewer adverse effects and is being tested in clinical trials.

Digitalis glycosides have been demonstrated to have little utility in the acute phase of cardiogenic shock. Indeed, awareness of the potential for digitalis toxicity is an important factor. However, survivors of the cardiogenic shock state are likely to require digitalization in subacute or chronic phases.

Reducing the Afterload

The cardiac output is in large measure dependent on the afterload of the heart when the heart has sustained injury. Consequently, after the preload has been optimized and efforts have been made to improve the inotropic status of the heart, the remaining variable that can be manipulated is afterload. The damaged heart appears to be exquisitely sensitive to alterations in afterload. Consequently, various vasodilators, alone or in combination with sympathetic amines, have been employed in treating patients with myocardial damage. This is done in an effort to decrease vascular impedance, promote ventricular emptying, and thereby lower filling pressure of the heart. Hypotension must be controlled before this modality for increasing cardiac output is employed.

Nitroglycerin. Nitroglycerin is a potent smooth muscle relaxant and vasodilator that has been the mainstay of cardiac ischemia therapy for many years. Its primary action is the dilatation of the coronary arteries, systemic venous dilatation, and to a lesser extent, arteriolar dilatation. Although blood pressure is decreased, it is primarily systolic rather than diastolic. In fact, the latter may remain the same. This puts less strain on the heart by decreasing myocardial oxygen consumption while maintaining coronary artery perfusion. When using nitroglycerin, careful attention must be given to the volume status of the patient because of its venodilatation.

Sodium Nitroprusside. The benefits of using nitroprusside are rapid onset of action and rapid inactivation, making it a useful vasodilator in cardiogenic shock. If doses are titrated properly, it is often possible to improve tissue perfusion, enhance cardiac output enough to offset the reduction in total peripheral resistance, and maintain systemic blood pressure without triggering reflex tachycardia. However, nitroprusside is cumbersome to use because of its photoinactivation and higher incidence of reflex tachycardia than nitrogycerin.

Vasodilator therapy is particularly effective in treating cardiogenic shock with an element of congestive failure. In this situation, venodilatation reduces right heart return and enhances ventricular emptying. In so doing, it drops the left ventricular end-diastolic pressure and helps to alleviate pulmonary congestion. In the difficult clinical situation of simultaneously developing hypotension and congestive failure in the postinfarct state, the combination of an inotropic agent and a vasodilator offers a logical and sometimes effective approach.

Other Modalities

Invasive approaches available for treating cardiogenic shock include the intraaortic balloon pump, used primarily in supporting a patient with a surgically reparable cause of shock, such as ruptured chordae tendineae or intraventricular septal defects, in the preoperative period. Efforts can be made to reopen occluded coronary arteries mechanically or with drugs such as streptokinase or tissue plasminogen activator (TPA). Advocates of coronary artery bypass grafts or coronary angioplasty in the acute postinfarct stage have demonstrated improvement in survival statistics in selected cases. Temporary pacing can be a valuable adjunct in patients with bradycardia or heart block and cardiogenic shock. Although new drugs are being tested and hold some promise, cardiogenic shock is still frequently a lethal condition.

OBSTRUCTIVE SHOCK

The third major category is "obstructive shock," a state in which failure of tissue perfusion results from vascular obstruction or mechanical impairment of cardiac filling. The causes of this state are listed in Table 3.1 and include: (*a*) pulmonary embolus, (*b*) cardiac tamponade, and (*c*) tension pneumothorax.

Pulmonary Embolus

Pulmonary embolus is usually characterized by the sudden onset of chest pain, tachypnea, tachycardia, elevated jugular venous pressure, hypoxia, and at times hemoptysis. Right-sided cardiac pressures are elevated with normal or low pulmonary capillary wedge pressures. In severe cases, the pulmonary artery obstruction results in pulmonary hypertension and even acute right heart failure. This form of obstructive shock differs from cardiac tamponade and tension pneumothorax, the two other causes, in that both of these result from inadequate cardiac filling.

Cardiac Tamponade

Cardiac tamponade can occur acutely as a result of blunt or penetrating trauma or can develop chronically, in a more subtle fashion, as the result of constrictive pericarditis, renal failure, or a malignant pericardial effusion. Symptoms depend largely on the primary disease process. Acute cardiac tamponade is suspected in any patient in shock who suffers chest trauma. These patients present with Beck's triad: elevated neck veins, shock, and muffled or distant heart sounds. An important sign is pulsus paradoxus. This is the phenomenon of a decrease in systolic arterial pressure greater than 10 mm Hg during spontaneous inspiration. In the more chronic evolution of cardiac tamponade, the patient develops symptoms of right heart failure with peripheral edema, dyspnea, venous congestion, and tachycardia. The chest x-ray demonstrates cardiomegaly with a widened transverse diameter and a globular appearance of the cardiac silhouette. An echocardiogram confirms the diagnosis.

Tension Pneumothorax

Tension pneumothorax must be differentiated from pericardial tamponade. Both can cause the shock state with distended neck veins. In tension pneumothorax, however, there are no breath sounds on the affected side and the mediastinum is shifted, with displacement of the trachea away from that side. The patient also has a hyperresonant hemithorax to percussion. If the patient is in shock, tension pneumothorax should be ruled out quickly because its therapy will reverse not only the respiratory dysfunction but also the shock-like state. Tension pneumothorax is a cause of obstructive shock since, with a shift of the mediastinum, it results in obstruction of blood return to the right side of the heart.

Therapy

The initial treatment of these causes of obstructive shock follows treatment plans listed previously. A patent airway must be maintained and the cardiovascular system supported with volume and appropriate pharmacologic agents. In patients with pulmonary embolus, heparinization is often effective. Alternative methods include the use of fibrinolytic agents, transjugular suction-catheter embolectomy, and surgical embolectomy of the pulmonary artery. Tension pneumothorax requires early diagnosis and rapid needle decompression of the tension, followed by the appropriate placement of a chest tube (see Illustrated Technique 13). Acute traumatic cardiac tamponade, on the other hand, is best treated in the operating room. In many situations, temporary decompression of the pericardium can be obtained by pericardiocentesis in the emergency department (see Illustrated Technique 10). In patients with chronic pericarditis or chronic pericardial effusions, the immediate therapy includes volume support with pericardiocentesis. Patients with constrictive pericarditis may require pericardiectomy but usually respond to volume support until such surgical intervention is possible.

PERIPHERAL SHOCK

The fourth major category of the shock state is collapse of peripheral vasomotor tone, resulting in the failure of adequate tissue perfusion. There are three major subdivisions (Table 3.1): (*a*) neurogenic, (*b*) vasogenic, and (*c*) septic.

Neurogenic

Neurogenic shock results from a severe midbrain or spinal cord injury. Besides checking for associated injury, care must be directed at delineating the extent of neurologic damage. Maintenance of an airway and checking for adequate ventilation are important, especially if the patient is unconscious. While physical examination, spine x-rays, and computed tomography are undertaken for evaluation of the patient, vital signs must be closely monitored. Shock occurs by the loss of vasomotor tone through the relaxation of the vascular smooth muscle. The heart rate is often normal and the periphery warm and perfused. The drugs of choice for blood pressure support in this setting are the α-adrenergic drugs: phenylephrine, methoxamine, and metaraminol.

Vasogenic

Vasogenic shock is similar to neurogenic shock in its pathophysiology. Treatment is the same although fluid replacement can be given more liberally. In anaphylactic reactions, 0.5 ml of epinephrine 1:1000 is administered subcutaneously to alleviate bronchospasm. In cases of greater respiratory or vascular compromise, epinephrine is given intravenously. To counteract the effect of histamine, an H_2-blocker, cimetidine (600 mg) or ranitidine (300 mg), and an H_1-blocker, preferably chlorpheniramine (Chlor-Trimeton, 2–4 mg), are given intravenously. Chlorpheniramine is preferable to other antihistamines because it causes the least vasodilatation when given intravenously. Corticosteroids, such as hydrocortisone 500 mg or dexamethasone 4 mg, are administered intravenously to help prevent subsequent return of the syndrome.

Septic

Septic shock is defined as hypoperfusion of tissues that results from the action of bacterial toxins on the circulatory system. Until recently, bacteremic shock was virtually synonymous with Gram-negative sepsis and was seen principally in newborns, the elderly, and the debilitated. Two factors have modified this epidemiologic pattern: an increase in intravenous drug abuse and an increase in the number of compromised hosts in the general population. Compromised hosts include patients receiving cancer chemotherapy, corticosteroids, and immunosuppressive drugs, patients who have had splenectomy, and patients with advanced or debilitating disease, such as cirrhosis, acquired immune deficiency syndrome (AIDS), nephrosis, diabetes, and severe burns. In persons with impaired defenses, usually innocuous agents, such as *Candida albicans*, can become deadly pathogens. The overuse of potent antibiotics in clinical care has resulted in the development of drug-resistant bacterial strains, particularly in the hospital setting.

Although the epidemiologic and microbiologic aspects of septic shock have changed, the mortality remains high, ranging from 50 to 80% in reported series. In part, this reflects the nature of the population at risk and, in part, the refractory character of the disease process itself.

The pathophysiologic development of bacteremic shock is complex and incompletely elucidated. Two hemodynamic phases occur. Initially, peripheral resistance falls with the opening of arteriovenous shunts; heart rate and cardiac output rise, though not enough to offset the drop in total peripheral resistance; and the blood pressure is maintained only with difficulty. In this hyperdynamic or warm stage, the skin is pink and dry, and the patient is likely to be alkalotic secondary to the hyperventilation. Later, peripheral vasoconstriction develops and cardiac output falls. The patient then assumes the classic picture of shock with cool clammy skin, cyanosis, and the development of lactic acidosis. The tendency toward hypotension is further exacerbated by impaired capillary integrity and the loss of fluid from the vascular compartment to the interstitium. The mechanism appears to be the following. A septic focus or blood-borne bacterial infection releases lipopolysaccharide endotoxins into the circulation. These activate factors in the coagulation and complement sequences that generate vasoactive kinins and trigger the intrinsic coagulation system. Consequently, the clinical picture of decreased total peripheral resistance, increased capillary permeability, and disseminated intravascular coagulation occurs. This activation of the complement cascade further increases capillary permeability and impairs antibody function. The switch from vasodilatation to vasoconstriction may correspond to an early rise in the vasodilating prostaglandin E_2 and a subsequent appearance of the vasoconstricting prostaglandin F_2. As a further insult, myocardial function falters with a rising left ventricular end-diastolic pressure. This deterioration occurs in association with shifts in calcium ion, but the bacterial endotoxins responsible for the development of septic shock may themselves be injurious to the myocardium.

The general therapeutic measures discussed for hypovolemic and cardiogenic shock (establishment of an airway, oxygenation, ventilation, monitoring, correction of acidosis, volume expansion, and administration of vasoactive agents as needed to maintain coronary and cerebral perfusion) apply to septic shock as well. The efficacy of corticosteroids remains controversial. The studies that recommend treatment (methylprednisolone, 30 mg/kg) indicate that only one or two early doses are efficacious. Specific therapy for bacteremic shock involves antibiotic administration, surgical intervention when indicated, such as drainage of an abscess or removal of an obstruction, and correction of the nutritional deficit. Recently, investigation has been undertaken in the role of endorphins and opiate receptors in shock, particularly in septic shock. Experimental models have demonstrated improvement in cardiac function and in survival with the administration of naloxone, an opiate receptor agonist-antagonist. However, clinical trials using 0.01–0.1 mg/kg of naloxone intravenously have not consistently demonstrated the same hemodynamic improvement. Thyroid-releasing hormone (TRH) has been noted to have a pressor effect in higher than usual physiologic doses in shock models. The mechanism is not clearly defined, but it is known not to occur via the opiate receptor pathway. Further investigation needs to be undertaken with these agents before insight into their usefulness is apparent.

Pretreatment Assessment

The classic history in patients with septic shock includes a shaking chill leading to prostration. To aid in identifying the organism, the physician seeks a description of antecedent symptoms including cough, dysuria, or a history of underlying disease, drug abuse, alcohol consumption, medications, or recent medical instrumentation or dental or surgical procedure.

Table 3.6.
Bacteremia: Common Initiating Infections and Probable Pathogens

Anatomic Site and Condition	Pathogens Likely in Unmodified Host	Possible Complicating Factors	Additional Organisms to Be Considered in Compromised Host
Respiratory tract			
Pneumonia	*Haemophilus influenzae* (children <6 years; adults with chronic obstructive pulmonary disease)	*Streptococcus pneumoniae* Aspiration, alcoholism	*Escherichia coli, Bacteroides, Klebsiella-Enterobacter-Serratia,* oral flora
	Staphylococcus aureus (especially after influenza) Group A streptococci	Nosocomial infection (tracheostomy, ventilatory assistance)	*Pseudomonas aeruginosa, Klebsiella-Enterobacter-Serratia, Acinetobacter (Herellea)* species, *E. coli*
Pulmonary abscess	*Bacteroides* Fusospirochetes Anaerobic streptococci	after aspiration	
	Klebsiella *S. aureus*	progression from necrotizing pneumonia	
Empyema	*Bacteroides* Fusospirochetes Anaerobic streptococci	after aspiration	
	Intestinal flora (progression from subdiaphragmatic process)		
Central nervous system			
Meningitis	*S. pneumoniae* (direct extension from otitis or sinusitis; bacteremia from lung) Meningococcus *H. influenzae* (2 months to 6 years) *E. coli* and other enteric Gram-negative organisms (newborns)	Immunosuppression, debilitation, neurosurgical procedure, head trauma	Gram-negative bacilli, *Staphylococcus, Streptococcus*
Peritoneal cavity			
Peritonitis of intestinal origin (appendicitis, diverticulitis)	*Bacteroides fragilis* *E. coli*		
Intraperitoneal abscess	*Proteus* species Other Gram-negative bacilli Enterococcus (aerobic group D streptococcus)		
Biliary tree and liver			
Cholangitis Cholecystitis	*E. coli* *Proteus* species *Klebsiella-Enterobacter-Serratia* Enterococcus		

Table 3.6—*continued*

Anatomic Site and Condition	Pathogens Likely in Unmodified Host	Possible Complicating Factors	Additional Organisms to Be Considered in Compromised Host
Urinary tract			
Acute pyelonephritis	*E. coli* Enterococcus *Proteus mirabilis* *Morganella morganii* Other Gram-negative organisms (*Citrobacter, Enterobacter, Klebsiella*)	Recurrent, treated urinary tract infection, instrumentation	*E. coli, Klebsiella-Enterobacter-Serratia, Proteus* species, *P. aeruginosa*, enterococcus
Genitalia			
Pelvic inflammatory disease	*Neisseria gonorrhoeae* Intestinal flora (*Bacteroides, E. coli*, groups A, B, and C streptococci)	Instrumentation, abortion, postpartum sepsis	*Bacteroides* species, clostridia, anaerobic streptococci
Urethritis	*N. gonorrhoeae*		
Toxic shock syndrome	*S. aureus*	Prolonged use of superabsorbent tampon	
Bones and joints			
Septic arthritis	*N. gonorrhoeae* Meningococcus	Pediatric age group	*H. influenzae*
	S. aureus *S. pneumoniae* *Streptococcus*	Debilitation, drug addiction	Gram-negative bacilli
Osteomyelitis	*S. aureus*	Drug addiction	*Pseudomonas*
Skin and subcutaneous tissues	*S. aureus* Group A steptococci	Traumatic and surgical wounds	Gram-negative bacilli, clostridia, anaerobic streptococci
		Immunosuppression, burns	Gram-negative bacilli, *P. aeruginosa, Acinetobacter (Herellea)* species, *Serratia*
Cardiovascular system			
Acute bacterial endocarditis	*S. aureus* Enterococcus	Drug addiction	Gram-negative bacilli
Other	*Salmonella* species	Venous cutdown, indwelling catheter, intracardiac pacemaker	*S. aureus, Staphylococcus epidermidis, P. Aeruginosa, Acinetobacter (Herellea)* species, *Serratia*

Physical examination is detailed. Inspection of the skin may reveal needle tracks, septic emboli, abscesses, or characteristic eruptions such as those seen in ecthyma gangrenosum caused by *Pseudomonas*. Nuchal rigidity, tenderness of the costovertebral angle, lymphadenopathy, auscultatory evidence of pneumonia or pleural effusion, localized abdominal tenderness, guarding or masses, perirectal abscess, and prostate swelling and tenderness are some of the critical observations possible on physical examination. Examination of each area is important.

Laboratory studies include a complete blood count, coagulation studies, urinalysis, and Gram's stain of the unspun urine sediment. Cerebrospinal fluid (if indicated), sputum, and purulent discharges are examined. Chest x-ray films, abdominal x-ray films, or other specialized radiologic studies may aid in localizing the infectious process. One must ensure that all appropriate specimens are expeditiously and correctly obtained before antibiotics are administered. Typical specimens for culture include blood samples, urine, sputum, cerebrospinal fluid, and purulent aspirates or drainage. Of particular importance is the Gram's stain because it offers the opportunity to identify specific organisms before receiving culture results, thus saving 24 hours or more time.

While it is true that urgent institution of antibiotic therapy is necessary, it is also true that the interval between presentation and institution of treatment may represent the *only* chance to obtain meaningful bacteriologic specimens. The choice of antibiotic presents difficult decisions since the urgency of the patient's condition frequently demands institution of therapy before the causative organism can be identified with certainty by culture. The correctness of the initial choice of antibiotic may determine the chance of survival. The problem for the emergency physician in selecting initial therapy may be less difficult than for the physician dealing with hospitalized patients. The latter is likely to encounter the unusual or antibiotic-resistant organisms common in the hospital setting. However, there are drug addicts and compromised hosts in the population who may be seen in the emergency department with infections caused by atypical organisms.

With improved culture techniques, it has become apparent that anaerobic organisms, which are normal inhabitants of the mouth and pharynx, the intestine, and the female reproductive system, can be recovered from patients with septic shock. With proper technique, anaerobic bacteria can be cultured from the "sterile" collection often recovered from intraabdominal, tuboovarian, and pulmonary abscesses. Studies have shown that infections associated with contamination by the fecal, oral, or vaginal flora are likely to be the result of both aerobes and anaerobes. Therefore, in the treatment of potentially life-threatening infections derived from contamination from these routes, it is prudent to assume that anaerobes are involved and to administer the proper full antibiotic coverage.

With this admonition and the knowledge of local patterns of infection, the emergency physician should be able to categorize the septic patient into one of three groups: those in whom no specific organ or organ system can be implicated as the likely source of sepsis; those in whom involvement of a specific organ or organ system (for example, the urinary tract) is likely, but no causative pathogen can be identified; and those in whom a particular bacterium can be identified with some degree of certainty, usually by means of a Gram's stain. Patients in the first group, which fortunately is small, are treated with antibiotics chosen to cover a wide spectrum. For patients in the third group, a specific antibiotic can be matched to the suspected pathogen. It is the large middle group that poses the greatest judgmental challenge. Knowing the likely source allows the spectrum of possible antibiotics to be narrowed, but the physician must choose carefully to cover both the most common causative pathogens and the important unusual organisms.

The prognosis for the patient correlates with his/her cardiac output. If the cardiac output is greater than 3.5 liters/min, survival rates are greater than 60%. If the cardiac output is less than 3.0 liters/min, mortality approaches 100%.

Choice of Antibiotic

Several general statements can be made regarding the choice of an antibiotic in septic shock. The antibiotic should be bactericidal when possible; it should be administered intravenously; due regard must be given to allergies of the patient and to the specific toxicities of the drugs used; and the maintenance dose must be tailored to renal and hepatic function, depending on the method of excretion of the drug. Specific recommendations regarding choice of antibiotic therapy are based on two factors: knowledge of the pathogens likely to invade a specific site (Table 3.6) and knowledge of the typical patterns of antibiotic sensitivities of those pathogens. When no insight into the likely pathogen can be gained, a broad spectrum regimen, such as a semisynthetic penicillin plus an aminoglycoside in full dosage, should be given (see Chapter 11).

Role of Surgery

Septic shock is usually associated with a high degree of septicemia, which is frequently produced by undrained septic collection often under pressure. Early surgical consultation and intervention are mandatory if such a situation is suggested. For example, drainage of an obstructed, infected gallbladder is the definitive therapeutic measure and will do more for the well-being of the patient than administration of antibiotics.

Shock Lung

As more patients were resuscitated successfully from the acute phase of various shock states, it became apparent that many had several and often fatal pulmonary complications. Known as shock lung, the adult respiratory distress syndrome (ARDS), postperfusion lung, and other descriptive phrases, this syndrome of pulmonary involvement is seen in many clinical situations. It has reportedly been associated with hypovolemic or septic shock, but an identical syndrome has been associated with nonthoracic trauma, particularly cranial, cardiopulmonary bypass procedures, massive blood transfusions, respirator-assisted ventilation, aspiration pneumonia and pancreatitis.

The onset of shock lung is heralded by increased tracheobronchial secretions, tachypnea, and cyanosis. Laboratory investigations reveal a decreased arterial partial pressure of oxygen (Pa_{O_2}); an arterial partial pressure of carbon dioxide (Pa_{CO_2}), initially low, rises as the condition of the patient decompensates. Metabolic acidosis is frequently followed by a respiratory acidosis. Bedside pulmonary function studies demonstrate decreased tidal volume and reduced pulmonary compliance. This requires increased inspiratory pressure during ventilation to maintain a given tidal volume.

No single cause of shock lung has been identified. Numerous factors have been implicated, and it is likely that the syndrome represents a final convergent pathway of several insults, including injury to the central nervous system, aspiration, disseminated intravascular coagulation, microembolization, fat embolization, and infection.

The pathophysiologic sequence leading to shock lung has not been clearly delineated, in part because of the paucity of observations regarding the early phases. Loss of integrity of the pulmonary-vascular endothelium, diminished plasma oncotic pressure, increased hydrostatic pressure with escape of protein into the alveolar spaces, and decreased surfactant activity have been observed. Increased affinity of the interstitial collagen for sodium apparently occurs, contributing to interstitial edema. A consistent finding quite early in the process is an increase in pulmonary vascular resistance occurring at the distal end of the pulmonary capillaries or in the pulmonary veins. Pathologic findings vary with the stage of the process. Shock lung is characterized by interstitial edema followed by alveolar edema, atelectasis, microthrombosis, hemorrhage, and consolidation.

Recommendations for prevention and therapy are not specific at present. Careful infusion to avoid overhydration, filtration of blood products to prevent microembolization, maintenance of oxygen administration at the minimal effective concentration (FIO_2 less than 0.5 if possible), and good pulmonary toilet are all reasonable suggestions. Intubation and assisted ventilation utilizing intermittent positive-pressure breathing and positive end-expiratory pressure are indicated. The judicious administration of fluids and nutrition are beneficial. More definitive therapy awaits improved knowledge of the underlying pathophysiologic mechanisms.

Summary

Untreated shock is fatal. Its management, whatever its etiology, requires the full, imaginative concentration of the treating physician, whose attention must be undivided. Advisory consultation is wise. The emergency physician is in good position to contact the intensive care unit physician early.

SUGGESTED READINGS

Baim DS, McDowell AV, Cherniles J, et al. Evaluation of a new bipyridine inotropic agent—milrione—in patients with severe congestive heart failure. *N Engl J Med,* 1983;309:748–756.

Benotti JR, Grossman W, Braunwald E, et al. Hemodynamic assessment of amrinone. A new inotropic agent. *N Engl J Med,* 1978; 25:1373–1377.

Bernton EW. Naloxone and TRH in the treatment of shock and trauma. What future roles? *Ann Emerg Med,* 1985;14:229–235.

Billhardt RA, Rosenbush SW. Cardiogenic and hypovolemic shock. *Med Clin North Am,* 1986;70:854–876.

Bonnet F, Bilaine J, Lhoste F, et al. Naloxone therapy of human septic shock. *Crit Care Med,* 1985;13:972–975.

Braunwald E. Vasodilator therapy—A physiologic approach to the treatment of heart failure (editorial). *N Engl J Med,* 1977, 297:331–332.

Collins JA. Problems associated with the massive transfusion of stored blood. *Surgery,* 1974;75:274–295.

Collins JA. The pathophysiology of hemorrhagic shock. *Prog Clin Biol Res,* 1982;108:5–29.

Czer LS, Appel P, Shoemaker WC. Pathogenesis of respiratory failure (ARDS) after hemorrhage and trauma. II. Cardiorespiratory patterns after the development of ARDS. *Crit Care Med,* 1980;8:513–518.

Goldberg LI. Dopamine—Clinical uses of an endogenous catecholamine. *N Engl J Med,* 1974;291:707–710.

Gorbach SL, Bartlett JG. Anaerobic infections. *N Engl J Med,* 1979; 290:1177–1184, 1237–1245, 1289–1294.

Gould SA, Sehgal LR, Rosen M, et al. Red cell substitutes: An update. *Ann Emerg Med,* 1985;14:798–803.

Huss P, Miller J. Unverferth DV, et al. The new inotropic drug, dobutamine. *Heart Lung,* 1981;10:121–126.

Karakusis PH. Considerations in therapy of septic shock. *Med Clin North Am,* 1986;70:933–944.

Kones RJ. The catecholamines: Reappraisal of their use for acute myocardial infarction and the low cardiac output syndromes. *Crit Care Med,* 1973;1:203–220.

Lew AS, Weiss AT, Shah PK, et al. Extensive myocardial salvage and reversal of cardiogenic shock after reperfusion of the left main coronary artery by intravenous streptokinase. *Am J Cardiol,* 1984;54:450–452.

Moss GS. Plasma expanders: an update. *Am J Surg,* 1988;155:425–434.

Moss GS, Lowe RJ, Jilek J, et al. Colloid or crystalloid in the resuscitation of hemorrhagic shock; a controlled clinical trial. *Surgery,* 1981;89:434–438.

Mueller HS. Inotropic agents for the treatment of cardiogenic shock. *World J Surg,* 1985;9:3–10.

Resnekov L. Cardiogenic shock. *Chest,* 1983;83:893–898.

Rude KE. Pharmacologic support in cardiogenic shock. *Adv Shock Res,* 1983;10:35–49.

Schumer W. Pathophysiology and treatment of septic shock. *Am J Emerg Med,* 1984;2:74–77.

Shatney CH, Cohen RM, Cohen MR, et al. Endogenous opioid activity in clinical hemorrhagic shock. *Surg Gynecol Obstet,* 1985;160:547–551.

Shoemaker WC, Appel P, Czer LS, et al. Pathogenesis of respiratory failure (ARDS) after hemorrhage and trauma. I. Cardiorespiratory patterns preceding the development of ARDS. *Crit Care Med,* 1980;8:504–512.

Smith CB, Jacobsen JA. Toxic shock syndrome. *Disease a Month,* 1986;32:77–118.

Sprung CL, Coralis PV, Marcial EG, et al. The effects of high-dose corticosteroids in patients with septic shock. A prospective, controlled study. *N Engl J Med,* 1984;311:1137–1143.

Tarazi RC. Sympathomimetic agents in the treatment of shock. *Ann Intern Med,* 1984;81:364–371.

Trambaugh RF, Lewis FR. Crystalloid versus colloid for fluid resuscitation of hypovolemic patients. *Adv Shock Res,* 1983;9:203–216.

Wayne MA, MacDonald SC. Clinical evaluation of the antishock trouser: retrospective analysis of five years of experience. *Ann Emerg Med,* 1983;12:342–347.

CHAPTER **4**

Emergency Department Management of Trauma

CHARLES J. McCABE, M.D.

INTRODUCTION

The litany of yearly trauma statistics is well known. The National Academy of Science first exposed trauma as the "Neglected Disease of Modern Society" in 1965. The reported statistics at that time revealed that trauma was the leading cause of death in patients under 40 years of age and accounted for 10 million disabling injuries and more than 100,000 deaths/year at a cost of $18 billion in lost wages, hospitalization costs and disability benefits. Many recommendations were made in an attempt to alter this epidemic. These were incompletely implemented and, unfortunately, subsequent improvements have not been realized. In fact, the death toll has continued to increase by 1%/year since 1977. The majority of these deaths has resulted from motor vehicle accidents (approximately 50,000 cases). The principal other causes were falls, homicides, suicides, burns, and drownings. Trauma has become the leading cause of death in children over age 1.

The cost in human lives is enormous, as is the financial expense of medical care and rehabilitation of the survivors. Hospital expenses, lost wages, and disability benefits have been estimated at $60 to $80 billion/year. The best solution to this very real problem is prevention, but necessary methods are difficult to implement. They include enforced speed limits, motor vehicle safety regulations that include mandating the use of seatbelts and motorcycle helmets, as well as strong legislation to combat drunk driving. Narcotic and handgun regulations are also necessary. These are sensitive issues and would take enormous effort to implement. In present day trauma management, the major focus has been on providing improved care once the accident has occurred rather than preventing accidents.

The principal causes of death after trauma are: (*a*) neurologic injury, (*b*) hemorrhage, and (*c*) post-injury sepsis and multiorgan failure. Deaths occur in groups identifiable by time intervals from time of injury. Within the first few minutes, deaths result from massive brain and spinal cord injury, from airway obstruction, or from exsanguinating hemorrhage. Little can be done to alter the outcome of these patients. The second group of deaths occurs secondary to epidural or subdural hematomas or due to hemorrhage in the first 2–6 hours after the traumatic episode. These patients will normally survive to reach the hospital where therapy, including operation, may alter the outcome. The last group of deaths occurs secondary to sepsis and multiorgan failure (MOF) in the post-injury period, and commonly occurs following surgical intervention.

Proper emergency department management will have its greatest impact in preventing death in the second group of patients. Prompt injury recognition and appropriate intervention should lead to improved survival. This chapter deals with the means of providing improved care in the setting of the emergency department.

EMERGENCY DEPARTMENT SETTING

Each emergency department (ED) is different with respect to staffing patterns and care capabilities. This chapter approaches the trauma victim's care under "ideal" conditions. Some recommendations and suggestions do not apply to all emergency services. In many respects the trauma victim is simple to care for, but therapy requires a sense of calm, and the trauma team, regardless of size and makeup, must be organized, well-practiced, and have a designated leader. The goal is to establish order from chaos. Each member of the team should have a predetermined responsibility, and the only needed element for the team to be activated is the presence of a patient. In a similar fashion, necessary action should be automatic such that once the specific injury is recognized, the therapy is clear to the entire team and easily implemented.

Trauma teams vary from hospital to hospital, from suburban to urban areas, and from community hospital to teaching hospital. The average non-trauma center emergency department will be staffed by an emergency physician alone. The operating room will not be open 24 hours a day, and the operating room team, including the surgeon and anesthesiologist, may not always be in-house. In this situation it is even more important for the available personnel to be organized. In major trauma centers, an organized in-house trauma team is a necessary requirement for designation.

The relationship between the emergency department staff and the trauma surgeons involved with the care should be well-developed. In general, trauma creates "surgical" problems, and operative intervention is often necessary. Even if a general surgical operation is not necessary, the combined experience of the general surgeon and the ED physician will provide the necessary tools for appropriate triage of the patient with multiple injuries. The individual roles of the emergency physician and the surgeon should be mutually understood, and agreed upon and respected. Both professional groups can help each other and, more importantly, the patient.

There should be a designated admitting and resuscitation area equipped with all necessary technical equipment and large enough to permit access to the patient by the trauma team. This area should be in proximity to the operating room. The availability and access to computed tomographic (CT) scanning is also ideal.

PATIENT ASSESSMENT

An aggressive intervention-directed approach to the patient is encouraged, and actions often must precede accurate diagnosis. It is wise to assume that the patient is more ill than is initially apparent. A quick overview is obtained by assessing mental status, capillary refill, skin color, and temperature. The patient with cool, poorly perfused extremities and altered mental status requires rapid intervention. The physician in the ED should assess the trauma patient early and call for appropriate help when indicated (surgeon, anesthesiologist, or other expert). Similarly, the physician should rationally assess the hospital care capabilities and arrange for *early* transfer of the patient if clearly required. Appropriate field triage and transport can often avoid this necessity. If transfer is necessary, it may require advanced life support monitoring en route, creating staffing difficulties.

Proper management of the trauma patient is divided into three phases:

Phase 1: Primary survey and resuscitation;
Phase 2: Secondary survey;
Phase 3: Definitive care.

Phase 1: Primary Survey and Resuscitation

The goal in phase 1 is to determine and correct conditions that would be lethal if not recognized and reversed immediately. Phase 1 consists of evaluation of the airway, breathing, and circulatory status and correction of any problems. The physician in charge should go to the patient's head. This initiates the proper sequence of assessment and therapy. The following divisions are arbitrary; much of what follows occurs simultaneously.

The Airway and Breathing

The causes of inadequate ventilation are divided into (*a*) airway obstruction, (*b*) altered chest wall mechanics, and (*c*) neurologic injury. The airway is first assessed for patency.The mouth is opened and any foreign body, food, vomitus, blood, or obstructing dentures are removed. A tonsil tip suction device is very useful to clean the oropharynx mechanically. The most common cause of airway obstruction is the tongue; this situation can easily be relieved by proper positioning of the jaw anteriorly (jaw lift or thrust). An oropharyngeal airway may be useful if the patient tolerates it. If there is respiratory impairment secondary to upper airway obstruction that cannot be resolved by these measures, an oral or nasal endotracheal tube, or rarely a cricothyrotomy or tracheostomy, is necessary.

The trauma patient, particularly if unconscious or with injuries above the clavicle, must be suspected of a cervical spine (C-spine) injury. If conditions permit, the cervical spine should be assessed by a lateral x-ray, visualizing all seven cervical vertebrae before moving the neck from the neutral position (Fig. 4.1). It must be remembered that the first priority is ventilation; however, possible spinal cord injury, although a "secondary" consideration, must be kept in mind. The nasotracheal approach to intubation (see Illustrated Technique 2) is a good method in the breathing patient with injuries that

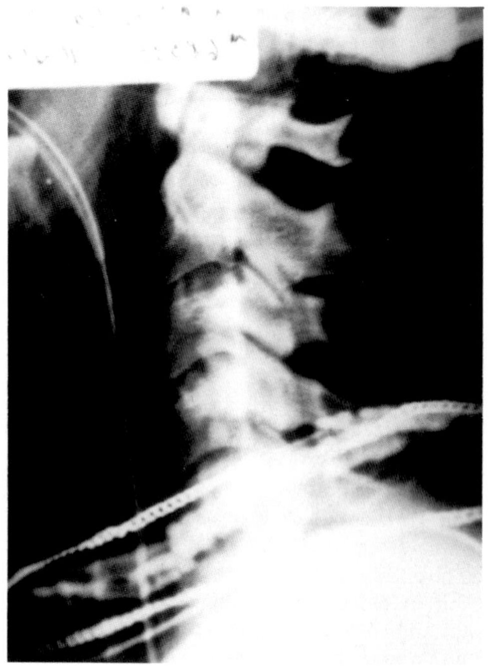

Figure 4.1. This lateral cervical spine x-ray does not adequately visualize all seven cervical vertebrae. This patient had a C-4-5 fracture-dislocation.

require intubation, since it can be performed without laryngoscopy and neck extension.

If this is unsuccessful, manual immobilization of the head, in-line to prevent flexion or extension, is maintained while oral intubation is attempted. If this is not possible, or if anatomic injuries preclude these methods, an emergency airway is best obtained by performing a cricothyrotomy. A needle cricothyrotomy has been successful and is a technique with which most physicians are comfortable (see Illustrated Technique 4). A 14-gauge angiocatheter with needle is inserted into the trachea through the easily palpable cricothyroid membrane. A syringe, attached to the catheter as it is inserted, permits aspiration of air as the trachea is entered. The position of the needle is then readily apparent. The catheter is advanced over the needle into the trachea and the needle is removed. The catheter is attached at its hub through a no. 3 pediatric endotracheal tube adapter, and this adapter is then connected to two pieces of oxygen extension tubing, separated by a Y-piece. This equipment should be set up and always be available. The end of the oxygen tubing is connected to 100% oxygen to provide 50 pounds/inch^2 of pressure. Oxygenation is performed by occluding the Y-piece for 1 second, which allows rapid insufflation of oxygen into the lungs. The finger is removed from the Y-piece and exhalation occurs through the normal anatomic route. Four seconds are allowed for this phenomenon. If the airway is *totally* occluded proximal to the catheter, this jet insufflation of oxygen will lead to a tension pneumothorax because the catheter is too small to permit proper exhalation. A surgical cricothyrotomy (Illustrated Technique 3) or tracheostomy is then necessary. Cricothyrotomy will not provide a successful airway in patients with injuries below the cricothyroid membrane, and a direct tracheostomy is necessary. The need for a surgeon should be apparent well before this procedure is necessary.

The airway and breathing are assessed simultaneously. The entire chest must be exposed. Aside from airway obstruction, the causes of inadequate ventilation in a trauma victim result from altered chest wall mechanics and consist of (*a*) open pneumothorax, (*b*) tension pneumothorax, (*c*) hemothorax, and (*d*) flail chest. These problems should be readily identified and therapy instituted. While identification of these physiologic problems is under way, oxygen is usually supplied by nasal prongs or face mask.

The *open pneumothorax* is recognized by the noisy respiration and appearance of air and blood bubbling from the wound. The wound should be covered with a Vaseline gauze pack and a chest tube inserted at a separate location, connected to underwater drainage.

A *tension pneumothorax* (Fig. 4.2) must be identified early in patients who present with the combination of shock and respiratory embarrassment

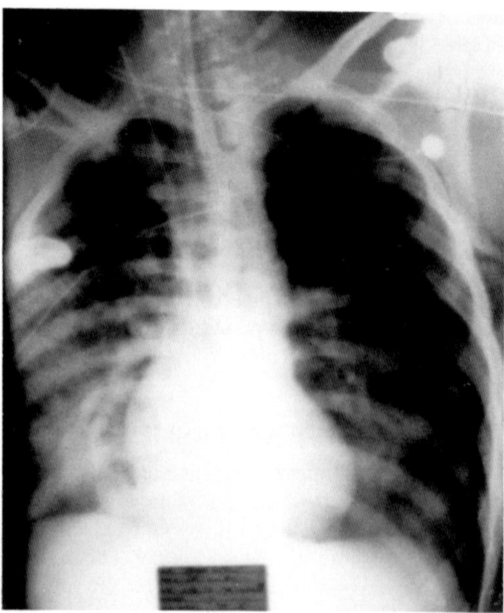

Figure 4.2. The mediastinum is shifted to the right with a left-sided tension pneumothorax. There is also a right basilar contusion.

since appropriate treatment is necessary to reverse both problems. In all patients who present in shock, a tension pneumothorax should be considered, and excluded early in the assessment. The mediastinum is shifted to the side opposite the tension pneumothorax, the affected side is hyperresonant to percussion, and breath sounds are absent. Deviation of the trachea may be recognized. If the patient has severe cardiovascular compromise, a 12-gauge needle is immediately placed into the chest in the second anterior intercostal space at the midclavicular line to relieve the pressure, converting the tension pneumothorax to an open pneumothorax. A chest tube can then be placed, usually laterally behind the pectoral muscles. If, on the other hand, the patient is not severely compromised, a chest tube may be the initial therapy (see Illustrated Technique 13). An experienced emergency department physician is capable of inserting the chest tube, but a good working relationship with the general surgical staff, as well as supervision by the surgical staff, is essential in the multiinjured patient.

Hemothorax is a common event after chest trauma and may result from either blunt or penetrating injuries. The bleeding is usually not massive. Although optimal, it is unlikely that an upright chest x-ray can be obtained on an unstable patient. A chest x-ray taken on such patients in the supine position reveals haziness on the affected side but not a clear fluid line. The treatment of hemothorax requires insertion of intravenous catheters and then the placement of a size 32–36 chest tube connected to suction. The blood is optimally collected in an autotransfusion device so that it can be returned to the patient and used as part of the resuscitation fluid. Massive hemorrhage results from intercostal, internal mammary, major hilar or great vessel disruption. Patients with these injuries require immediate operation to control bleeding. Usually 500–1000 ml of blood will drain from the chest. In most circumstances bleeding will then slow to approximately 200–300 ml/hour for 1 or 2 hours and then decrease from that. If drainage continues at a rate of 300–500 ml/hour for several hours, operative intervention is necessary. Each thoracic or general surgeon has his or her own protocol for determining whether an operation is necessary.

The *flail chest* is identified by paradoxical motion of the chest wall with spontaneous respiration. If the paradox is substantial, and the patient is suffering respiratory embarrassment, intubation and volume ventilation may be immediately necessary. Attempts at stabilizing the chest wall with sandbags or by turning the patient onto the affected side are only temporizing.

The last cause of inadequate ventilation is severe neurologic injury; the airway must be protected by intubation and ventilation must be provided. C-spine precautions are necessary.

Table 4.1.
Causes of Traumatic Shock

Hemorrhage
External
Internal
Chest
Abdomen
Extremities
Retroperitoneum
Cardiac dysfunction
Pericardial tamponade
Myocardial contusion
Infarction
Air embolus
Tension pneumothorax[a]
Spinal cord injury

[a] This primary diagnosis requires early treatment or exclusion.

Circulation

The *circulatory system* is evaluated next. An assessment of perfusion must be made, and if the patient is in shock, treatment and diagnosis proceed simultaneously. The causes of traumatic shock are listed in Table 4.1.

The neck veins are a useful source of information in determining etiology. Flat neck veins imply hypovolemia which is most commonly due to hemorrhage. Bleeding occurs either externally or internally. The external hemorrhage may be ongoing in the emergency department and is controlled by pressure, or it may have stopped after a large amount of blood loss at the accident scene. Any external source of hemorrhage is controlled by direct pressure; tourniquets and clamps are to be avoided. The potential internal sites of hemorrhage in the adult are only four and can be rapidly identified: (*a*) the chest, (*b*) the abdomen, (*c*) the retroperitoneum, and (*d*) the extremities. A chest x-ray (CXR) identifies chest blood losses, which can be as much as 3000 ml in one hemithorax. A physical examination reveals any losses into the extremity (usually underestimated). A peritoneal lavage reveals intraperitoneal hemorrhage. The only location not immediately accessible is the retroperitoneum. It can be a major site of blood loss, which should be suspected in patients with pelvic fractures.

Distended neck veins, on the other hand, suggest either tension pneumothorax or cardiac dysfunction. An examination of the chest may reveal absent breath sounds and a hyperresonant chest characteristic of a tension pneumothorax. Additional evidence includes a tracheal shift. If there is any doubt, treatment of the presumed diagnosis should precede any further diagnostic efforts, such as x-rays. Cardiac dysfunction results from cardiac tamponade, from myocardial contusion or infarction, or from air embolus. Both blunt and penetrating injuries to the chest may cause pericardial tamponade. With improved transportation and emergency medical service response times, patients suffering blunt trauma to the heart with tamponade are now reaching emergency facilities alive. Therefore, this diagnosis must be entertained. Likewise, penetrating injury to the chest at any entry site may cause tamponade. The classic Beck's triad of distended neck veins, shock, and distant heart sounds is not always clear in an emergency situation.

Once tamponade is suspected, the patient should be placed in the operating room. Aspirating the pericardium is often unsuccessful in the acute trauma victim and wastes valuable time. If the hospital is unable to provide definitive care for pericardial tamponade in the operating room, transfer of the patient is necessary. In this situation, the pericardium should be aspirated and perhaps a catheter left in the pericardial space to allow for repeated aspiration and drainage. This may be successful in patients with stab wounds to the heart, but it is unlikely to be beneficial in patients with gunshot wounds or blunt rupture of the heart. An aggressive operative approach is necessary. The subxiphoid operative approach to the pericardium is not recommended in the emergency department.

The other causes of myocardial dysfunction are myocardial contusion, myocardial infarction, and coronary artery air embolus. Myocardial contusions are common but usually do not cause significant myocardial dysfunction. However, they may behave exactly like an acute infarction. If the emergency medical technician reports that the steering wheel was broken or if the patient has a contusion on the chest anterior to the sternum, this injury should be suspected. Myocardial infarction and arrhythmias may precede or follow trauma. An electrocardiogram reveals the rhythm disturbance of ischemia. A rare but potential cause of myocardial dysfunction and distended neck veins is an air embolus to the coronary arteries. This is usually the result of a combination of parenchymal lung disruption in a patient requiring positive pressure ventilation. The positive pressure ventilation forces air into the disrupted pulmonary venous circuit, through the left heart to the systemic circulation. Air in the coronary arteries causes severe myocardial dysfunction. Mental aberrations may also occur from cerebral air emboli.

Finally, spinal cord injuries may result in hypotension as a result of vasomotor dysfunction. The blood pressure rarely falls below 80 mm Hg. Aids in making this diagnosis are the absence of tachycardia and the presence of warm, perfused, insensate, and paralyzed extremities associated with the hypotension. This diagnosis should be considered last since its therapy is different from that of the other etiologies of shock and may require vasopressors in addition to volume replacement.

Associated trauma to the head is common in the multitrauma patient but is the cause of hypotension only as a preterminal event. Normally, head trauma with increased intracranial pressure will result in the "Cushing response," with bradycardia and hypertension. The patient with a head injury and hypotension usually has a secondary cause for the hypotension. It is a wise rule, in general, not to implicate head trauma as the cause of hypotension.

Volume Resuscitation

Resuscitation of the traumatized victim almost always requires volume replacement. The location of insertion and the size and type of catheter utilized are as important as the fluid used. With chest injuries, if the superior vena cava is injured, infusions into the upper extremities may extravasate. Pelvic fractures or abdominal injuries may interfere with fluids administered into the lower extremities. Lines placed both above and below the diaphragm will circumvent this problem. Two to four lines may be necessary. The massively hypovolemic and vasoconstricted patient will have poor peripheral hand access sites; therefore, the basilic or cephalic veins in the antecubital space are a better choice. Cutdowns at the ankle are useful for the short term, as are femoral vein lines placed percutaneously. The catheter should be a short 14- or 16-gauge to optimize flow. Direct insertion of sterile intravenous tubing by cutdown is also a good method. The standard 16-gauge central venous pressure (CVP) line placed by the subclavian or internal jugular route does not have good flow characteristics for rapid volume infusion and may cause complications, such as pneumothorax, hydrothorax, or bleeding, on insertion. The introducer used for pulmonary artery line insertion is a better alternative but has the same potential risks. The initial solution used in resuscitation is lactated Ringer's. Five percent albumin, although popular in some centers, is expensive and may cause coagulation abnormalities. It has no proven benefit over Ringer's lactate. If the patient remains unstable after 2–3 liters of Ringer's lactate have been infused, blood should be added to the resuscitation fluids. Type 0-negative is used if blood is immediately necessary; if time permits, type-specific blood can be available in 15 minutes. Fresh frozen plasma and fresh platelets are commonly necessary as the number of blood transfusions increases in order to prevent the development of a coagulopathy. To prevent hypothermia, both the Ringer's lactate and the blood should be warmed at least to body temperature (37°C) before infusion. This may be difficult with blood but is easily accomplished by making prewarmed Ringer's lactate available (heated in plastic bags in a microwave oven).

It must be recognized that in some situations adequate resuscitation of the traumatized victim requires immediate surgical intervention, and the resuscitation can be done only in the operating room when the bleeding is surgically controlled. These patients are recognized by their failure to respond to the initial 2–3 liters of Ringer's lactate resuscitation. If a patient does initially respond but then very quickly becomes hypotensive again, it is likely that this is a manifestation of continued hemorrhage and that surgical intervention is quickly necessary.

Although its exact physiologic effect has not been defined, the pneumatic antishock garment has at times been useful in patients refractory to volume replacement. Its effects include: (*a*) tamponade of external and internal hemorrhage, (*b*) splinting of fractures, (*c*) autotransfusion of an estimated 300–1200 ml of blood, and (*d*) increase in cardiac afterload. The garment may be placed on the trauma stretcher beneath the patient and be available for immediate inflation if it becomes necessary. Patients will often have had the garment applied in the prehospital setting, and it may or may not have been inflated. This occasionally obscures peripheral examinations and certainly makes examination of the abdomen difficult.

Emergency Department Thoracotomy

A left anterolateral thoracotomy is sometimes necessary in the emergency department. Its objectives are to relieve pericardial tamponade, to control hemorrhage, and to prevent air emboli. The indications for thoracotomy vary from center to center. The decision to perform an ED thoracotomy should be made early with clear specific objectives (control hemorrhage, open pericardium, clamp aorta). The arrested, hypovolemic patient cannot be resuscitated with closed chest cardiopulmonary resuscitation (CPR), and an early decision to open the chest offers the only chance for survival. This creates a difficult situation for the nonsurgeon emergency department physician. This is another situation in which the emergency physician must have developed a good working relationship with the surgical staff of the hospital. In the majority of emergency physician training programs, an opportunity to perform emergency room thoracotomy is not available. This training might be obtained "on the scene" by participating in thoracotomies done by the surgical staff either in the emergency department or in the operating room. This is not a procedure to be utilized unless prompt surgical backup and intervention are possible.

In general, the patient who presents with any type of chest wound without blood pressure or pulse should undergo a left thoracotomy in order to evaluate the pericardium for cardiac tamponade and to control any sources of exsanguinating hemorrhage. A right chest tube is also inserted. Under normal circumstances, control of the descending thoracic aorta is obtained with compression or clamping. Open cardiopulmonary resuscitation is performed and vigorous volume replacement is carried out. Any wounds to the heart are obturated with insertion of the index finger. Suturing may be attempted or delayed until the patient is in the operating room. A Foley catheter can be inserted through the hole and the balloon inflated and pulled taut to seal the hole from inside the heart. In some series, emergency department thoractomy is shown to be effective in approximately 25% of patients (if some neurologic function is present on admission). Stab wounds to the chest that result in acute pericardial tamponade or hemorrhage have a better outcome than do gunshot wounds. Gunshot wounds to the chest usually have an unfortunate outcome due to the massive destruction of the heart wall. Likewise the success rate is poor when emergency thoractomy is used in arrested patients to control intraabdominal hemorrhage. Clearly, if emergency department thoractomy is successful, the patient must be rapidly transported to the operating room for more definitive care.

Diagnostic Studies

Blood is drawn immediately for hematocrit, prothrombin time, partial thromboplastin time, blood bank sample, blood urea nitrogen, blood sugar, and arterial blood gases. Occasionally, an early amylase level will be helpful; no other studies are immediately necessary. A lateral C-spine x-ray is obtained quickly in patients suspected of neck injury, as are a chest x-ray and plain film of the pelvis. Other diagnostic films can await stabilization. (Note: A normal lateral C-spine is *not* conclusive evidence that the cervical spine is uninjured.) Often an adequate C-spine study is not possible (all seven vertebrae must be visualized). In that situation C-spine immobilization should be maintained until a full cervical series is possible (anteroposterior, lateral, oblique, odontoid views).

The remaining workup and therapy depend on the injury and the patient's status. Abdominal lavage, placement of chest tubes, CT scanning, and arteriography may be necessary. It is often useful to perform a "one shot" intravenous pyelogram to define the presence of two kidneys. A nasogastric tube and Foley catheter should be placed if there are no contraindications (cribriform plate fracture, suspected urethral tear). Antibiotics and tetanus toxoid should be administered.

Phase 2: Secondary Survey

Once the life-threatening problems have been reversed and the situation is stabilized, a full secondary survey of the patient must be performed. The entire body is examined from head to foot and from front to back in order to deterine what other injuries the patient may have suffered. The simplest method of performing this survey is to begin with the cranium and work down to the lower extremities. The back is often missed and is optimally visualized when the patient first arrives. This is particularly important in penetrating injuries. The level of consciousness, respiratory status, and airway are continuously assessed as the secondary survey is performed. A brief history is usually obtainable at this time. The AMPLE mnemonic provides all the necessary historical information (Table 4.2). It is particularly important to obtain the details surrounding the accident: Was anyone killed? How damaged was the car? Was the steering wheel or windshield damaged? Was the patient thrown from the vehicle or wearing a seatbelt? How far was the fall? What kind of knife or gun? All of these pieces of information imply the "force" of the injury. The emergency medical technician can be the source of these data.

Head

The cranial vault is examined for any signs of depressed fracture, brain evisceration, cerebrospinal fluid (CSF) leaks, and facial bone injuries. All open scalp wounds are sterilely palpated for bony deficits. Eviscerated brain substance will be obvious and is a particularly grave sign. The so-called "Battle's sign" or "raccoon eyes," indicative of basilar skull fracture is a late finding and is not seen acutely. The facial bones are palpated systematically. In the conscious patient, pain will be elicited if fractures are present. Deformity will also be obvious, and inspection of the face from the side reveals most zygomatic and midface fractures. The mouth is opened, and with the thumb on the maxilla and the forefinger on the palate, the stability of the foreface is assessed. Any fracture of the body of the mandible can lead to airway obstruction from the tongue. Proper support of the mandible prevents this. Blood accumulation in the oropharynx must be prevented by suctioning.

Table 4.2.
The AMPLE Mnemonic

A –	**A**llergies
M –	**M**edicines
P –	**P**ast medical history
L –	**L**ast meal
E –	**E**vents leading to the accident (kinematics)

Head trauma is the cause of more than 50% of trauma deaths, and aggressive and expeditious diagnosis and intervention are required for any chance for survival. The common, serious problems include skull fracture, brain contusion, and subdural and epidural hematomas. All skull fractures require hospital admission for a period of observation. The CT scan has become an invaluable diagnostic tool in the differential diagnosis of brain contusion and intracranial blood collections, and it allows for definitive, accurate intervention. The initial goals of management are to protect the airway and assess the severity of damage. A brief neurologic examination establishes a baseline, and reassessment is essential. A CT scan is absolutely required for full and accurate evaluation of the extent of brain trauma. With severe injuries, hyperventilation and mannitol (see Chapter 37), when employed early, may decrease intracranial pressure. A neurosurgical consultation is necessary. All time delays must be avoided.

Neck

The neck is examined for jugular venous distention, tracheal position, and evidence of subcutaneous air, penetrating injuries, and hematoma formation. Penetrating injuries may injure major vascular structures as well as the trachea and the esophagus. Any injury to the trachea may result in massive subcutaneous emphysema, and the airway is always tenuous. Penetrating injuries have become an area for major clinical research. Formerly, any neck wound that penetrated the platysma was explored surgically. In follow-up of these patients, a high incidence of nontherapeutic neck explorations was obvious. It has now become apparent that penetrating injuries of the platysma do not necessarily require surgical exploration. The neck is divided into three zones. Zone 1 includes the area of the neck from the suprasternal notch to the cricoid cartilage. Zone 2 extends from the cricoid cartilage to the angle of the mandible. Zone 3 extends from the angle of the mandible to the base of the skull. Penetrating injuries in zones 1 and 3 require arteriography for full evaluation. Numerous clinical studies indicate that patients with stab wounds of the neck may successfully be managed by clinical observation and reevaluation. Clinical indications for operative intervention then include an expanding hematoma, subcutaneous air, frank pain on swallowing, and/or any neurologic deficit. Studies that may be beneficial in evaluating penetrating injuries to the neck include a Gastrografin swallow and endoscopy of both the trachea and the esophagus. Arteriography is helpful in defining arterial injuries. This should be performed in stable patients with penetrating injuries at the base of the neck or those near the cranial vault. In any blunt injury above the clavicle, auscultation of the carotid arteries is essential. Bruits indicate possible intimal damage from stretching of the artery across the transverse process of the adjacent vertebral body.

Chest

Chest trauma should always be considered potentially lethal. With essential life support structures in the chest, trauma to this area is responsible for about 25% of traumatic deaths. This statistic is disturbing in that only approximately 15% of chest trauma requires operative intervention or the skills of a trained thoracic surgeon. This implies that the physician in the emergency department may have a most important role in the outcome of these patients. The first physician who sees a patient with chest trauma has the best opportunity to affect outcome. Injuries involving the chest are most easily divided into two groups: those that are immediately life-threatening and those that are not. The causes are blunt or penetrating trauma. The first group consists of injuries that have already been discussed: airway obstruction, cardiac tamponade, and the mechanical chest wall difficulties, including open pneumothorax, tension pneumothorax, hemothorax, and flail chest. The second group consists of six entities that are most easily remembered by dividing them into "the contusions" and "the tears." The contusions consist of injuries to the two parenchymal organs in the chest, the heart and lungs, and the tears consist of disruption of the other structures in the chest: the aorta, the tracheobronchial tree, the esophagus, and the diaphragm.

Contusions of the heart are common; approximately 70% of patients who suffer chest trauma have myocardial contusions identified by radioisotopic scanning. Clinically, these injuries are identified or at least suspected by physical examination of the precordial area. Often the patient has an imprint of the steering wheel, or the electrocardiogram may show evidence of injury. In examining the sternum, a sternal click may be palpable. In general, admission to the hospital is recommended, and the patient should be carefully monitored for the development of arrhythmias. Current data suggest that prophylactic lidocaine is probably unnecessary. Cardiac enzymes (creatine phosphokinase-MB) are elevated and a radioisotopic scan reveals a lack of perfusion to the contused segment of the myocardium. Bed rest, electrocardiographic monitoring, oxygen therapy, and occasionally antiarrhythmic drugs will be necessary. These injuries usually do not cause true cardiovascular abnormalities but may result in ventricular arrhythmias; in severe cases, coronary occlusion can occur with myocardial dysfunction and congestive heart failure. Left ventricular aneurysms have been reported as a consequence of myocardial contusion (Figs. 4.3 and 4.4).

Pulmonary contusions are also common in chest trauma but normally do not cause symptomatic respiratory dysfunction or hypoxia. If a patient has a pulmonary contusion without other major trauma, fluid restriction is essential to avert accumulation of lung fluid and pulmonary insufficiency. If volume resuscitation is necessary, the pulmonary contusion may be magnified. Pulmonary compromise may require intubation with volume ventilation and positive end-expiratory pressure (PEEP). Steroids have not been beneficial in these patients.

The second group of injuries, the tears, usually results in surgical pathology. The aortic tear is one of the major problems identified in the emergency department after a motor vehicle accident. The common finding is an abnormal chest x-ray with widening of the mediastinum and obscuring of the aortic knob (Fig. 4.5). Other possible x-ray findings include an apical pleural cap, first rib fracture, hemothorax on the affected side, a shift of medi-

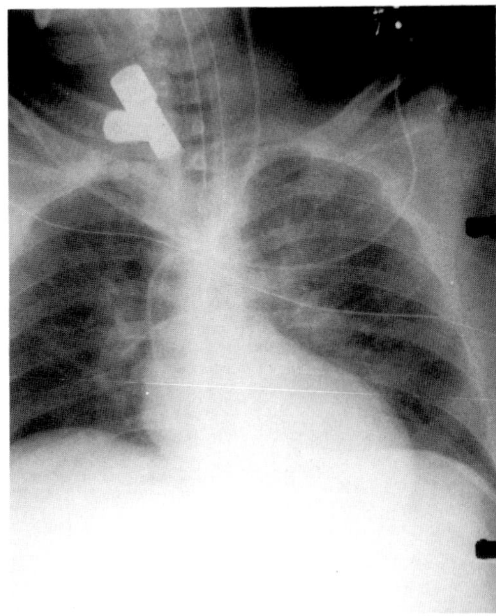

Figure 4.3. Chest x-ray of a patient admitted after blunt trauma to the sternum. The imprint of the steering wheel was present over the sternal skin.

astinal structures to the right, and depression of the left mainstem bronchus. Once this diagnosis is suspected, aortography should be performed expeditiously to document and identify the location of the aortic injury (Fig. 4.6). During this evaluation, arterial blood pressure should be continuously monitored with a radial arterial line and hypertension controlled using propranolol and nitroprusside. The aortogram should be performed in a hospital with capability of repairing the injury. Emergency repair of aortic disruptions, except in rare situations, is essential. These patients commonly have multiple injuries, and triage for the sequence of appropriate surgical procedures is necessary. The unstable patient should undergo peritoneal lavage and, if positive, abdominal exploration. Aortography should immediately follow laparotomy with aortic repair if positive. In the stable patient, peritoneal lavage may be done, followed by aortography. Operation then depends on the results.

Tracheal trauma occurs with both blunt and penetrating injuries to the neck. Penetrating wounds cause partial or complete disruption of the trachea. These patients present with air bubbling from the wound and with subcutaneous emphysema. Blunt injuries may cause laryngeal fracture, compression, and the development of mucosal flaps.

The airway must be cleared of blood and securely maintained until the injury is repaired. Consultation with an otolaryngologist or thoracic surgeon is judicious. Tracheostomy may be necessary for proximal injuries. Injuries to the distal trachea and bronchi are possible and may result from any penetrating injury that passes through the mediastinum. Blunt trauma is usually secondary to motor vehicle accidents with acceleration/deceleration types of force, the injury commonly occurring just beyond the carina. The patient usually presents with subcutaneous emphysema and a tension pneumothorax that does not resolve with placement of a chest tube. Continuous bubbling from the Pleur-Evac chest suction indicates the diagnosis. Bronchoscopy permits visualization of the tear. Surgical repair is necessary.

The esophagus is uncommonly injured secondary to blunt trauma. Blunt trauma to the abdomen in a patient with a full stomach causes an increase in intragastric pressure. A traumatic "Boerhaave's" esophageal rupture may then result. The esophagus can be injured by any type of penetrating injury that traverses the neck, chest, or mediastinum. The injury is suspected with any direct posterior penetration of the chest. Evaluation commonly requires esophagoscopy and a Gastrografin esophagogram in order to define the presence and level of the injury. Should Gastrografin not identify an esophageal leak, the use of a barium swallow is permissible.

The diaphragm may be disrupted secondary to high abdominal or low chest penetrating wounds. An increase in intraabdominal pressure secondary to blunt trauma to the abdomen can cause a diaphragmatic tear. These injuries are most commonly recognized on the left and usually present with a chest x-ray often misread as "an elevated left hemidiaphragm" or "a loculated pneumothorax" (Fig. 4.7). In these patients a nasogastric tube may not

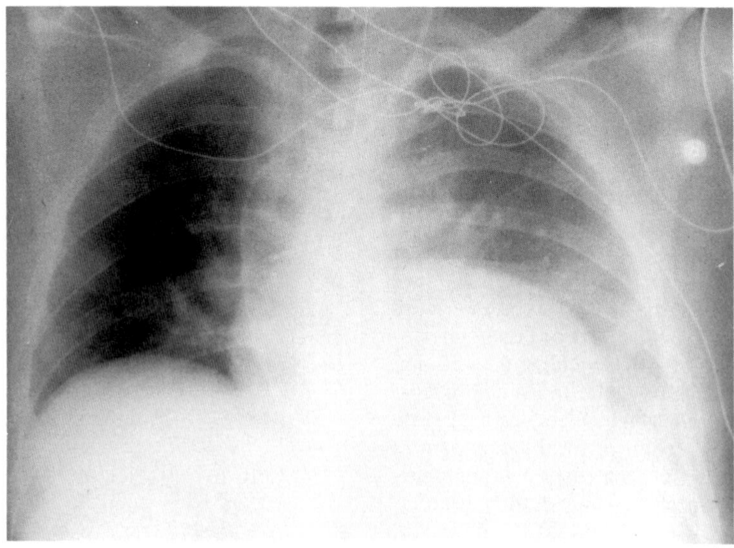

Figure 4.4. Chest x-ray of the same patient shown in Figure 4.3 after 1 week, revealing a large left ventricular aneurysm.

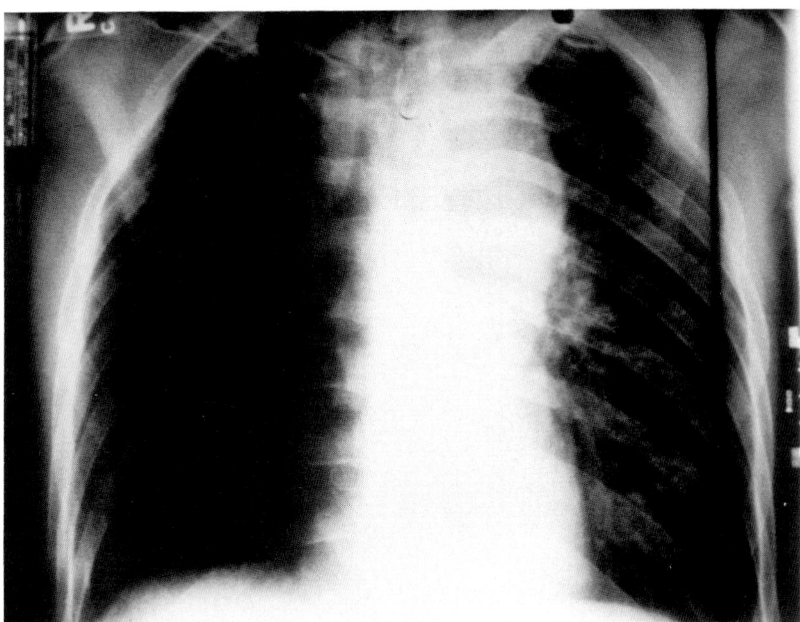

Figure 4.5. This chest x-ray reveals the classic findings of a widened mediastinum with an obscured aortic knob.

pass into the stomach. A barium swallow may be necessary to make the diagnosis. If a chest tube is placed because of the erroneous interpretation of the chest x-ray, injury to the herniated organ can result. Abdominal exploration is necessary to repair this injury and any associated intraabdominal damage. Right-sided diaphragmatic hernias do occur, but they are not easily recognized since the liver prevents herniation of any intraabdominal viscus. If the tear is large, the right hemidiaphragm will be obscure on chest x-ray and should suggest the diagnosis (Figs. 4.8 and 4.9).

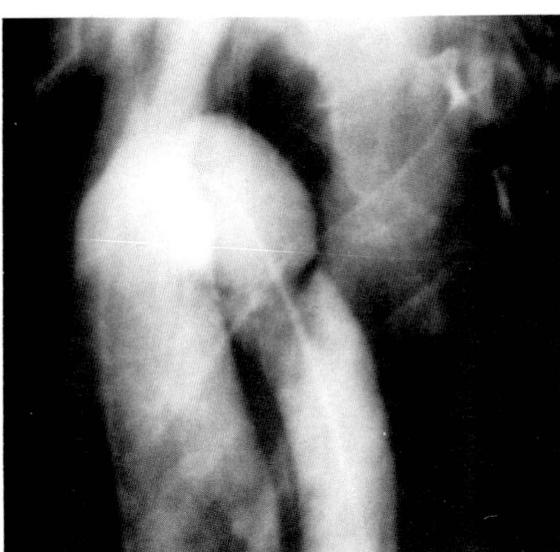

Figure 4.6. This transfemoral aortogram reveals an aortic tear at the common location, just distal to the take-off of the left subclavian artery.

It is wise to be aware that any low injury to the chest or high abdominal wound may have traversed the diaphragm, causing injury away from the cavity penetrated. Chest tubes should be inserted on minimal indications, particularly in patients with penetrating chest wounds or rib fractures that require intubation, anesthesia, or transfer to other hospitals. It is not uncommon for a large hemothorax or a tension pneumothorax to develop occultly, and prophylactic chest tube insertion, under these circumstances will avoid this. Similarly, chest tubes should be placed in these patients before air transport.

Abdomen

As with chest trauma, trauma to the abdomen is divided into blunt and penetrating. Gunshot wounds and stabbings are the most common penetrating injuries. Patients may present with multiple stab or gunshot wounds. It must be kept in mind that any penetrating injury may have transgressed the diaphragm and caused injury remote from the point of entrance. Penetrating wounds of the chest below the nipple or scapula will more commonly cause abdominal trauma than chest trauma, and peritoneal lavage may be necessary to evaluate the abdomen. Again, the use of chest tubes is encouraged in any patient with penetrating chest wounds or rib frac-

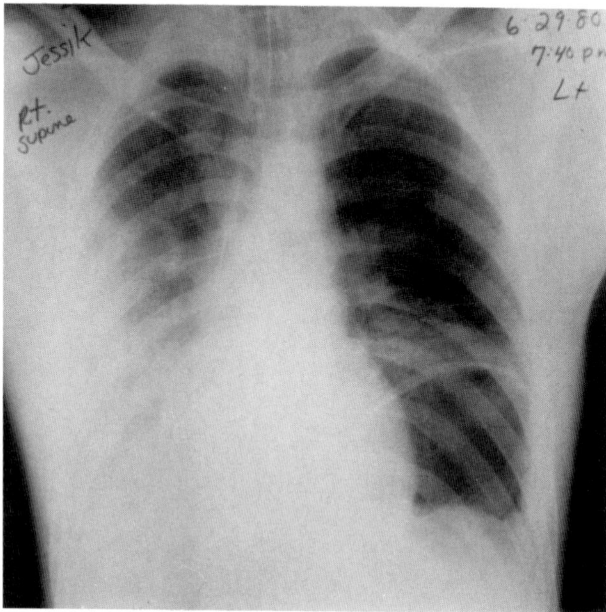

Figure 4.7. Chest x-ray of a patient who suffered blunt abdominal trauma. The ruptured left hemidiaphragm is often misinterpreted as a loculated left pneumothorax or as an elevated hemidiaphragm. This is actually the herniated stomach in the left chest.

tures who is to undergo nonthoracic surgical procedures.

Blunt trauma results from falls, seatbelts in decelerating auto accidents, blast injuries, and crushing forces. These are difficult to evaluate, particularly when the abdominal examination is obscured by spinal cord injuries or by the effects of drugs or alcohol. One method of assessing blunt abdominal trauma is serial clinical examination of the patient. Unfortunately, in patients with altered mental status, this is inaccurate and may result in unnecessary time delay and blood loss. If injury is suspected, a peritoneal lavage or a CT scan is performed. If CT scanning and its interpretation of a stable patient are immediately available, this is probably the optimal method of evaluating the abdomen for visceral injuries and the presence of intraabdominal blood. If CT is not available, peritoneal lavage should be performed on a patient suspected of having intraabdominal trauma (Table 4.3).

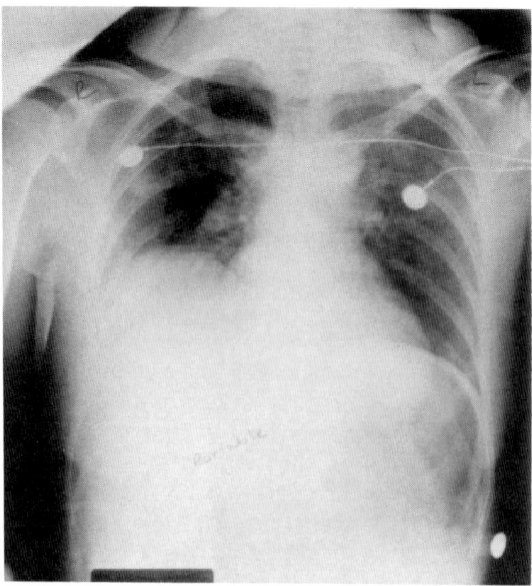

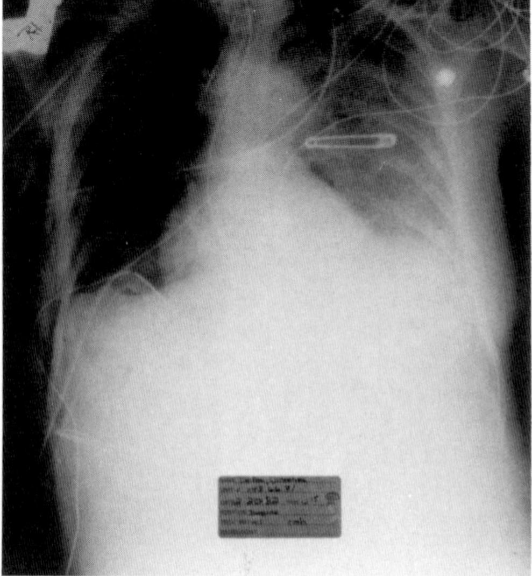

Figure 4.8. This pedestrian was struck by a car and suffered blunt abdominal trauma. The x-ray on the left reveals an abnormal right hemidiaphragm. The x-ray on the right shows the postoperative x-ray.

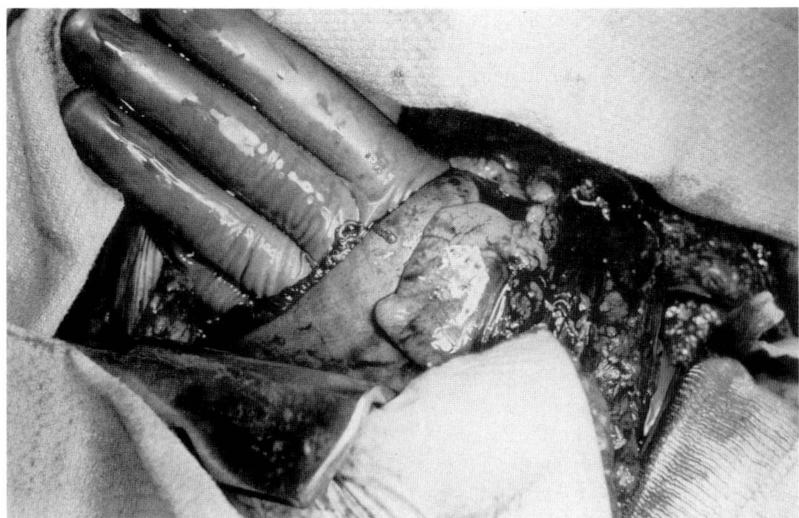

Figure 4.9. Intraoperative findings of a right-sided hemidiaphragmatic rupture (same patient as shown in Figure 4.8). The surgeon's hand is placed through the tear in the right hemidiaphragm.

The accuracy of peritoneal lavage is approximately 98% and with experience is very safe. However, false-negative lavages do occur! Immediate operation is required on patients who have clear physical signs of injury.

Peritoneal lavage is performed using an infraumbilical approach (see Illustrated Technique 15), except in a patient with pelvic fracture, when a supraumbilical incision is used. The incision is made under local anesthesia using 1% lidocaine with epinephrine, and the linea alba is identified. The cannula is inserted with a trocar after making a small incision in the linea alba. In thin patients, direct exposure and opening of the peritoneum and insertion of the cannula alone can be carried out (so-called "minilap"). Fluid is aspirated and, if 10 ml of blood are present, the examination is considered positive and no lavage is performed. Otherwise, saline or Ringer's lactate is instilled into the peritoneal space, allowed to equilibrate, and then drained. If the red blood cell count is greater than $100{,}000/mm^3$ or the white blood cell count is greater than $500/mm^3$ in the effluent, the lavage is considered positive. The presence of bile, bacteria, or particulate matter is also considered a positive test. Drainage of the lavage fluid through a chest tube or Foley catheter likewise indicates a positive lavage (Table 4.4).

The performance of peritoneal lavage is not difficult. With proper training and experience, the physician in the emergency department may perform this procedure. An agreement and understanding must be developed between the operating surgeon and the physician in the emergency department so that performance of this technique is standardized and noncontroversial. Many surgeons prefer to perform this procedure personally, a not unreasonable surgical preference. It should be established in each emergency department who performs peritoneal lavage and how it should be performed.

With any penetrating sharp object or bullet injury to the abdomen, if the patient presents in shock, the cause of the shock must be considered intraabdom-

Table 4.3.
Indications and Contraindications for Peritoneal Lavage

Abdominal trauma plus
1. Altered mental status
   a. Drugs
   b. Alcohol
   c. Head injury
   d. Anesthesia required for nonabdominal injury
2. Spinal cord injury

Contraindications
1. Clear-cut indications for laparotomy
2. Multiple previous abdominal procedures
3. Pregnancy

Table 4.4.
Criteria for Positive Peritoneal Lavage

1. Aspiration of 10 ml of free, nonclotting blood.
2. Red blood cell count > $100{,}000/mm^3$[a]
3. White blood cell count > $500/mm^3$
4. Bile, bacteria, food, feces in effluent
5. Dialysate draining through chest tubes or Foley catheter

NOTE: [a] Red blood cell counts of 50,000–100,000 are *not* negative. Further diagnostic workup or observation is necessary.

inal hemorrhage. That patient needs to be sent expeditiously to the operating room. Bullet wounds of the abdomen, with rare exception, all require abdominal exploration; and this makes their evaluation in the emergency department straightforward. A plain film of the abdomen and chest x-rays to determine location of the bullet and an intravenous pyelogram may be helpful.

Stab wounds of the abdomen are often difficult to evaluate. In the presence of shock, evisceration, or signs of peritonitis, the patient requires abdominal exploration. On the other hand, if none of these critical signs is present, the methods of evaluation are either selective observation of the patient with serial clinical examination, or attempts to prove intraperitoneal penetration. It has been demonstrated that not all stab wounds of the abdomen that penetrate the peritoneum require abdominal exploration. The proponents of selective observation have shown that, with careful recurrent patient assessment, the incidence of unnecessary laparotomy is decreased and the risk of delayed operation is very low. This requires meticulous attention on the part of one observer over a period of time. If, on the other hand, the surgeon believes that peritoneal penetration requires abdominal exploration, then assessment of the stab wound tract is essential to determine if the peritoneum has been penetrated. A sinogram is not used to prove penetration. A Kelly clamp may drop easily into the peritoneum. The optimal method is to anesthetize the area of the stab wound and then to enlarge the injury site. In so doing, the tract of the knife is explored and the fascia is identified. If fascial penetration is proven, then it is presumed that the peritoneum is penetrated as well. In some centers exploratory laparotomy is performed on these patients. In others, peritoneal lavage may be added to the evaluation in an attempt to decrease the incidence of unnecessary laparotomy.

Pelvic Fractures

Pelvic fractures continue to present major difficulties in management. These injuries are not easily identified by physical examination, and the plain x-ray film of the pelvis is often the only method of making the diagnosis. In addition to skeletal fractures, problems may involve injuries to the rectum and perineum, the urethra and bladder, and disruption of pelvic arterial and venous blood vessels.

In all patients with pelvic fracture, the perineum and pelvic organs must be evaluated. In a female, vaginal bleeding implies laceration of this structure. A rectal examination is essential to look for blood. Lacerations of the rectum, vagina, and perineum must be identified early. If blood is present in any of these locations, anoscopy, sigmoidoscopy, vaginal examination, and even Gastrografin enema may be necessary. Urethral injuries in a female are associated with anterior vaginal tears. The signs of a urethral tear in a male consist of blood at the meatus, either spontaneously or after milking the urethra, and the presence of a "floating prostate." In a male patient with a major pelvic fracture, prior to insertion of a Foley catheter, a rectal examination should always be performed. The examiner is searching for the presence or absence of the prostate in its normal position. Other signs of a urethral tear, the inability to void and a distended bladder, are often not easily assessed in the traumatized patient. If a urethral or bladder injury is suspected, a retrograde urethrogram and cystogram should be performed (Figs. 4.10 and 4.11). A cystogram that fails to reveal extravasation should be followed by a plain x-ray film of the pelvis once the dye has been emptied from the bladder. This demonstrates any posterior leak obscured by the dye-filled bladder. If a urethral tear is identified, a Foley catheter should not be inserted and a suprapubic cystocatheter placed (see Illustrated Technique 16). Ruptures of the bladder can occur either extraperitoneally or intraperitoneally. The extraperitoneal tears may occasionally be satisfactorily cared for with catheter drainage alone. The intraperitoneal injuries, on the other hand, require operative intervention.

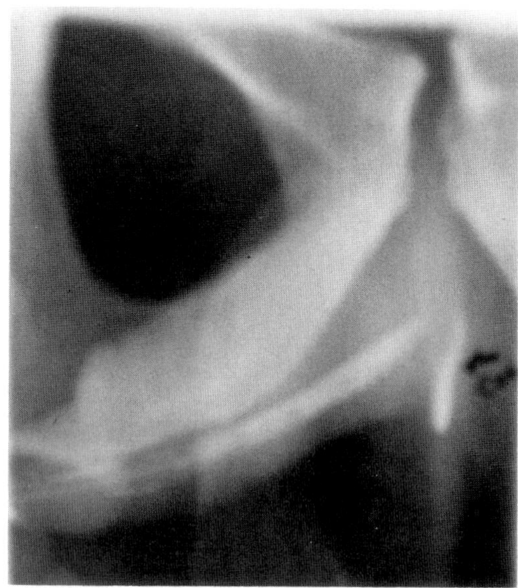

Figure 4.10. This retrograde urethrogram reveals extravasation of dye from the urethra.

The other major problem with pelvic fractures is massive hemorrhage into the retroperitoneum from a disruption of either arterial or venous channels in the pelvis. The management of these patients in the

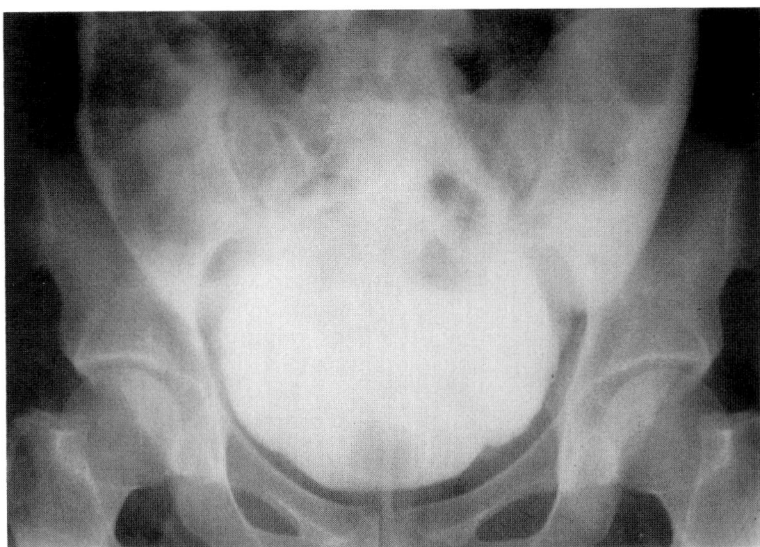

Figure 4.11. A cystogram revealing free extravasation of dye from a ruptured bladder into the peritoneal cavity.

emergency department consists of volume resuscitation and the application of a tamponading device (G-suit, MAST, pneumatic antishock garment (PASG)). The patient must be managed aggressively and massive blood loss must be anticipated. Further intervention may include angiography with identification of arterial bleeding and embolization of the vessel. Rarely, the iliac arteries may be torn; these require surgical repair. The external fixiter, a mechanical orthopaedic fracture device (see Chapter 36), has been used to reoppose the bones of the pelvis but may not be successful in controlling arterial hemorrhage secondary to pelvic fractures. There is no evidence that bilateral ligation of the hypogastric arteries is effective for these patients. If the perineum is lacerated, the injury is even more complex (compound pelvic fracture). Fecal diversion by colostomy is necessary in these patients.

Vascular and Extremity Injuries

The bony skeleton is quickly assessed for deformity, swelling, and tenderness. The orthopaedic injury will not usually cause life-threatening problems, but the blood loss may be substantial. Fractures are probably the most common cause of blood loss in traumatized patients, owing to the frequency of this injury. All fractures require x-ray definition. The circulation, sensory, and motor function must be assessed distal to every fracture. The signs of vascular injury consist of distal ischemia, loss of distal pulses, presence of a wound or bruit over a major vascular structure, an expanding hematoma, and obvious external arterial hemorrhage. The presence of pulses distal to a fracture site does not necessarily exclude an arterial injury. If there is any suspicion that a patient has suffered an arterial disruption, the arterial anatomy must be identified either angiographically or by direct surgical exploration. Injury to the popliteal artery secondary to distal femur injuries, proximal tibia and fibula injuries, and also secondary to a posteriorly dislocated knee must be recognized early. (Fig. 4.12).

Other sites commonly injured include the subclavian artery with a clavicular fracture and the brachial artery in severe humeral fractures or with elbow dislocations. Any penetrating injury to the neck may injure both the arterial and venous systems. Injuries to the carotid artery are not uncommon after blunt trauma to the head. It is important to listen over the carotid arteries for the presence of a bruit after a patient has suffered injury above the clavicle. The presence of a bruit leads to the suspicion of a carotid artery injury and the need for angiographic evaluation.

Burns

A patient who suffers major thermal injury presents two problems that must be cared for rapidly: (*a*) airway and ventilatory compromise and (*b*) volume depletion. These injuries often occur in a closed space, and inhalation of carbonaceous fumes is common. The patients present with singed hair, carbonaceous material in the oropharynx, and respiratory distress. Early control of the airway and ventilation offers the best and safest management.

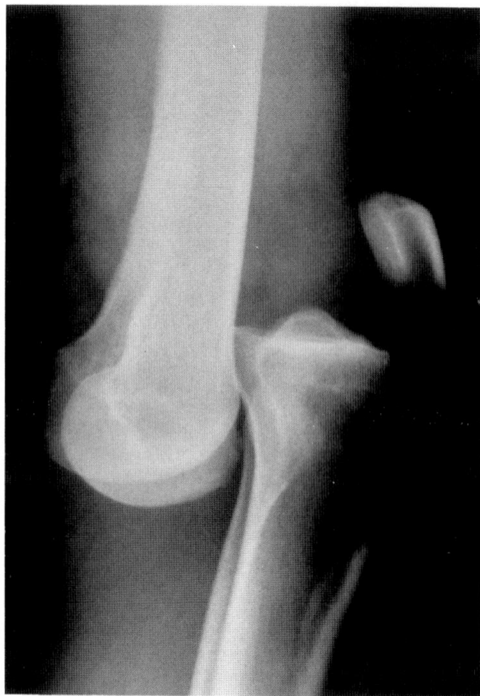

Figure 4.12. An obvious dislocation of the knee. An arterial disruption is always suspect; after relocating the knee, an arteriogram or direct arterial exploration is indicated.

The patient requires early and aggressive volume replacement. Fluids and formulas for resuscitation are variable (see Chapter 38), but the important component of any plan is that the patient produces urine. Ringer's lactate is the ideal solution for early use.

The burn is handled in standard fashion. All clothing is removed and the extremities examined for circumferential burns that require escharotomy. All jewelry is removed. Once cleansing of the burn is performed, the wounds are dressed with silver nitrate, Sulfamylon, or Silvadene. The latter two are preferred for the facial area.

If circumferential injuries compromise perfusion, such as with deep second- and third-degree burns, escharotomies are performed. The eschar is anesthetic, and the blood vessels are thrombosed so that the procedure is bloodless and painless. Rarely, if the third-degree burn involves the chest, an escharotomy of the chest wall may be necessary to permit normal respiratory mechanics.

Phase 3: Definitive Care

Once the emergency evaluation is complete, the last phase of care may require operative intervention. As a final check prior to this, the physician should ask the question, "Has every orifice been intubated?" It is at this time that the failure to insert the Foley catheter and nasogastric tube or perform a rectal examination becomes obvious. Definitive care will be discussed throughout the text.

SUMMARY

A thorough, aggressive, and well-planned approach to the trauma victim is essential. Proper implementation requires frequent usage. Proper emergency department care can favorably affect outcome and present to the operating team a patient fully prepared for the necessary surgical procedures.

SUGGESTED READINGS

General Information

Accidental Death and Disability, The Neglected Disease of Modern Society. Washington, DC: Division of Medical Sciences, The National Academy of Sciences, The National Research Council, 1965.

Baker CC, Oppenheimer L, Stephens B, et al. The epidemiology of trauma deaths. *Am J Surg*, 1980;140:144–150.

Baker SP, *Injuries*: The neglected epidemic (Stone Lecture, 1985), *J Trauma*, 1987;23:343–348.

Blaisdell FW. Trauma myths and magic: 1984 FITTS lecture. *J Trauma*, 1985;25:856–863.

Cales RA, Trunkey DD. Preventable trauma deaths—A review of trauma care systems development. *JAMA*, 1985;254:1059–1063.

Definition of impairment essential for prosecuting "drunken drivers." *JAMA*, 1985;258:3509–3517.

Freeark RJ. The 1982 AAST presidential address: The trauma center, its hospitals, head injuries, helicopters, and heroes. *J Trauma*, 1983;23:173–178.

Gann DS. Injury in America. *Bull Am Coll Surg*, 1987;72:12–15.

Improving trauma care. *Bull Am Coll Surg*, 1984:69:1–36.

Injury in America. The Committee on Trauma Research, Commission on Life Sciences. The National Research Council and the Institute of Medicine. Washington, DC: National Academy Press, 1985.

Long WB, Bachulis BL, Hines GD. Accuracy and relationship of mechanisms of injury, trauma score, and injury severity score in identifying major trauma. *Am J Surg*, 1986;151:581–584.

Luna GK, Maier RV, Sowder L, et al. The influence of ethanol intoxication and outcome of injured motorcyclists. *J Trauma*, 1984;24:695–700.

Munoz E. Economic costs of trauma in the United States (1982). *J Trauma*, 1984;24:237–244.

Oakes DD, Holcomb SF, Sherck JP. Patterns of trauma care costs and reimbursements—the burden of uninsured motorists. *J Trauma,* 1985;25:740–745.

Rhee KJ, Burney RE, Mackenzie JR, et al. Therapeutic intervention scoring as a measure of performance in a helicopter emergency medical services program. *Ann Emerg Med*, 1986;15:79–82.

Rhee KJ, Strozeski M, Burney RE, et al. Is the flight physician needed for helicopter emergency medical services? *Ann Emerg Med*, 1986;15:174–177.

Slagel SA, Skiendzielewski JJ, Martyak GG, et al. Emergency medicine and surgery resident roles on the trauma team: a difference of opinion. *Ann Emerg Med*, 1986;15:28–32.

Trunkey DD. Trauma. *Sci Am*, 1983;249:28–35.

Trunkey DD. The Presidential Address; On the nature of things that go bang in the night. *Surgery*, 1983;92:125–132.

Wintemute GJ, Firearms as a cause of death in the United States 1920–1982. *J Trauma*, 1987;27:532–536.

Resuscitation

Baker CC, Thomas NA, Trunkey DD. Role of emergency room thoracotomy in trauma. *J Trauma*, 1980;20:848–855.

Carrico CJ, Canizaro PC, Shives T. Fluid resuscitation following injury, rationale for the use of balanced salt solution. *Crit Care Med*, 1976;4:46–54.

Cogvill TH, Moore EE, Millikan JS. Rationale for selective application of emergency department thoracotomy in trauma. *J Trauma*, 1983;23:453–460.

Gervin AS, Fisher RP. Resuscitation of trauma patients with type-specific uncrossed matched blood. *J Trauma*, 1983;24:327–331.

Harnar TJ, Oreskovich MP, Copass MK, et al. Role of emergency thoracotomy in the resuscitation of moribund trauma victims. *Am J Surg*, 1981;142:96–99.

Hoffman JR. Emergency department thoracotomy. *Ann Emerg Med*, 1981;10:275–278.

Horton J, Landreneau R, Tuggie D. Cardiac response to fluid resuscitation from hemorrhagic shock. *Surg Gynecol Obstet*, 1985;160:442–452.

Jordan RC, Moore EE, Marx JA, et al. A comparison of PTV and endotracheal ventilation in an acute trauma model. *J Trauma*, 1985;25:978–983.

Leipold WC, Lucas CE, Ledgerwood AM, et al. The effect of albumin and resuscitation on canine coagulation activity and content. *Ann Surg*, 1983;198:630–633.

Lucas CE, Ledgerwood AM, Higgins RF, et al. Impaired pulmonary function after albumin resuscitation from shock. *J Trauma*, 1980;20:446–451.

Luna GK, Maier RV, Paulin EG, et al. Incidence and effect of hypothermia in seriously injured patients. *J Trauma*, 1987;27:1014–1018.

Millikan JSA, Cain TL, Hansborough J. Rapid volume replacement for hypovolemic shock—A comparison of techniques and equipment. *J Trauma*, 1984;24:428–431.

Neff CC, Pfister RC, Van Sonnenberg E. Percutaneous transtracheal ventilation, experimental and practical aspects. *J Trauma*, 1983;23:84–90.

Reed RL, Heimbach DM, Counts RB, et al. Prophylactic platelet administration during massive transfusion. *Ann Surg*, 1986;203:40–48.

Rohman M, Ivatory RR, Steichen FM. Emergency room thoracotomy for penetrating cardiac injuries. *J Trauma*, 1983;23:570–576.

Shaver J, Camarata G, Taleisnik A, et al. Changes in epicardial and core temperature during resuscitation of hemorrhagic shock. *J Trauma*, 1984;24:957–963.

Shimozu S, Shatney CH. Outcome of trauma patients with no vital signs on hospital admission. *J Trauma*, 1983;23:213–216.

Silva R, Moore EE, Bar-Or D. The risk benefits of autotransfusion—comparison to banked blood in a canine model. *J Trauma*, 1984;24:557–564.

Swanson RS, Uhlig PN, Gross PL, et al. Emergency intravenous access through the femoral vein. *Ann Emerg Med*, 1984;4:244–247.

Phillips TF, Soutier G, Wilson RF. Outcome of massive transfusion exceeding two blood volumes in trauma and emergency surgery. *J Trauma*, 1987;27:903–909.

Vij R, Simoni E, Smith RF, et al. Resuscitation thoracotomy for patients with traumatic injury. *Surgery*, 1983;94:554–561.

Yamada Y, Yasoshima A. Rapid warming of infusion solution. *Surg Gynecol Obstet*, 1985;160:400–402.

Chest

Bauchamp J, Khalfallah A, Gerard R, et al. Blunt diaphragmatic rupture. *Am J Surg*, 1984;148:292–295.

Calhoon JH, Hoffman TH, Trinkle JK, et al. Management of blunt rupture of the heart. *J Trauma*, 1986;26:495–502.

Chrestophi C. Diagnosis of traumatic diaphragmatic hernia, analysis of 63 cases. *World J Surg*, 1983;7:277–280.

Demetriades S, Rabinowitz B, Sofianos C. Emergency room thoracotomy for stab wounds of the chest. *J Trauma*, 1987;27:483–485.

Gundry SR, Burney RE, Mackenzie JR, et al. Assessment of mediastinal widening associated with traumatic rupture of the aorta. *J Trauma*, 1983;23:293–299.

Harley DP, Mena I. Cardiac and vascular sequelae of sternal fractures. *J Trauma*, 1986;26:553–555.

Jones SW, Mavroudis C, Richardson JD, et al. Management of tracheal-bronchial disruption resulting from blunt trauma. *Surgery*, 1984;95:319–322.

Marshall WS, Bell JL, Kouchoukos NT. Penetrating cardiac trauma. *J Trauma*, 1984;24:147–149.

Martin TD, Flynn TC, Rowlands RJ, et al. Blunt cardiac rupture. *J Trauma*, 1984;24:287–290.

Mattox KL, Limacher MC, Feliciano DV, et al. Cardiac evaluation following heart injury. *J Trauma*, 1985;25:758–765.

Tate JS, Horan DP. Penetrating injuries of the heart. *Surg Gynecol Obstet*, 1983;157:57–63.

Tenzer ML. The spectrum of myocardial contusion—A review. *J Trauma*, 1985;25:620–627.

Abdominal

Coppa GF, Davalle M, Pachter A, et al. Management of penetrating wounds of the back and flank. *Surg Gynecol Obstet*, 1984;159:514–518.

Cox EE. Blunt abdominal trauma, a five-year analysis of 870 patients requiring celiotomy. *Ann Surg*, 1984;199:467–474.

Davis RA, Shayne JP, Max MH, et al. The use of computerized axial tomography versus peritoneal lavage in the evaluation of blunt abdominal trauma: a prospective study. *Surgery*, 1985;98:845–849.

Federle MP, Brant-Zawadzki MB. Computed tomography in the evaluation of trauma. 2nd ed. Baltimore: Williams & Wilkins, 1986.

Feliciano DV, Bitondo CG, Steed G, et al. Five hundred open taps or lavages in patients with abdominal stab wounds. *Am J Surg*, 1984;148:772–777.

Flint LM, Brown A, Richardson D, et al. Definitive care of bleeding from severe pelvic fractures. *Ann Surg*, 1979;189:709–716.

Galbraith TA, Oreskovich MR, Heimbach DM, et al. The role of peritoneal lavage in the management of stab wounds of the abdomen. *Am J Surg*, 1980;140:60–64.

Goldstein AS, Sclafani SJ, Kupferstein NH, et al. The diagnostic superiority of computed tomography. *J Trauma*, 1985;25:938–946.

Gomez GA, Alvarez R, Plasencia G, et al. Diagnostic peritoneal lavage in the management of blunt abdominal trauma & reassessment. *J Trauma*, 1987;27:1–5.

Hauser GJ, Huprich JE, Bosec P, et al. Triple contrast computed tomography in the evaluation of posterior penetrating abdominal injuries. *Arch Surg*, 1987;122:1112–1115.

Jones RC, Thal ER, Johnson NA, et al. Evaluation of antibiotic therapy following penetrating abdominal trauma. *Ann Surg*, 1985;201:576–585.

Jorgens ME. Peritoneal lavage. *Am J Surg*, 1977;133:365–369.

Lee WC, Uddo JK, Nance FC. Surgical judgment in the management of abdominal stab wounds. *Ann Surg*, 1984;199:549–554.

Mahon PA, Sutton JE. Non-operative management of adult splenic injury due to blunt trauma: a warning. *Am J Surg*, 1985;149:716–721.

Marx JA, Moore EE, Jordan RC, et al. Limitations of computed tomography in the evaluation of acute abdominal trauma: a prospective comparison with diagnostic peritoneal lavage. *J Trauma*, 1985;25:933–937.

Merlotti GJ, Marcet E, Sheaff CM, et al. Use of peritoneal

lavage to evaluate abdominal penetration. *J Trauma*, 1985;25:228–231.

Moore EE, Marx JA. Penetrating abdominal wounds: rationale for exploratory laparotomy. *JAMA*, 1985;25:2705–2708.

Mucha P, Farnell MD. Analysis of pelvic fracture management. *J Trauma*, 1984;24:379–386.

Nance FC, Wennar M, Johnson LW, et al. Surgical judgment in the management of penetrating wounds of the abdomen. *Ann Surg*, 1974;179:639–646.

Obeid FN, Sorensen V, Vincent G, et al. Inaccuracy of diagnostic peritoneal lavage in penetrating colonic trauma. *Arch Surg*, 1984;119:906–908.

Oreskovich MR, Carrico CJ. Stab wounds of the anterior abdomen. *Ann Surg*, 1983;198:411–419.

Urologic

Cass AS. The multiple injured patient with bladder trauma. *J Trauma*, 1984;24:731–734.

Cass AS. Urethral injury in the multiple-injured patient. *J Trauma*, 1984;24:901–906.

Weems WL. Management of genito-urinary injuries in patients with pelvic fractures. *Ann Surg*, 1979;189:717–722.

Neurosurgical

Seelig JM, Becker DP, Miller JD, et al. Traumatic acute subdural hematomas, major mortality reduction in comatose patients treated within four hours. *N Engl J Medi*, 1981;304:1511–1518.

Stone JL, Lowe RJ, Jonasson O, et al. Acute subdural hematoma: direct admission to a trauma center yields improved results. *J Trauma*, 1986;26:445–449.

Neck

Bachulis BL, Long WD, Hynes GT, et al. Clinical indications for cervical spine radiographs in the traumatized patient. *Am J Surg*, 1987;153:473–478.

Golueke PJ, Goldstein AS, Salvatore JA, et al. Routine versus selective exploration of penetrating neck injuries: a randomized prospective study. *J Trauma*, 1986;26:1010–1014.

Jurkovich GJ, Zingarelli W, Wallace J, et al. Penetrating neck trauma: diagnostic studies in the asymptomatic patient. *J Trauma*, 1986;26:819–822.

Noyes LD, McSwain NE Jr, Markowitz IP, et al. Panendoscopy with arteriography versus mandatory exploration of penetrating wounds of the neck. *Ann Surg*, 1986;204:21–31.

Obeid FN, Haddad GS, Horse HM, et al. A critical reappraisal of a mandatory exploration policy for penetrating wounds of the neck. *Surg Gynecol Obstet*, 1985;160:517–522.

Ross SE, Schwab W, David ET, et al. Clearing the cervical spine: initial radiologic evaluation. *J Trauma*, 1987;27:1055–1060.

Sclafani SJ, Panetta T, Goldstein AS, et al. The management of arterial injuries caused by penetration of zone III of the neck. *J Trauma*, 1986;26:871–881.

Walter J, Doris PE, Shaffer MA, et al. Clinical presentation of patients with acute cervical spine injury. *Ann Emerg Med*, 1984;13:512–515.

SECTION 2

Medicine

PETER L. GROSS, M.D., F.A.C.E.P.
JAMES J. DINEEN, M.D.
Associate Editors

CHAPTER 5

Cardiology: Arrhythmias

GEORGE E. THIBAULT, M.D.
ROMAN W. DESANCTIS, M.D.

Editor's note: In contradistinction to other topics, cardiology is arbitrarily divided into three sections—Chapters 5, 6, and 7—stressing three distinct aspects of the subject. It would be wise for an emergency physician to review this entire subject of arrhythmia before utilization in the emergency department.

It is essential to remember that cardiac rhythm disturbances do not occur in isolation—they occur in a particular patient whose age, previous therapy, and coexisting cardiac and noncardiac diseases are important determinants of how well the arrhythmia is tolerated and of the urgency and appropriateness of treatment. The diagnosis and the treatment of an arrhythmia, which are only the first steps in the total evaluation of the patient's condition, should raise several important questions: Why did the arrhythmia occur? Does the patient have heart disease, and if so, what kind? What other diagnoses may be suggested or modified by the rhythm disturbance? What additional diagnostic or therapeutic measures should be instituted to elucidate causes further and to prevent recurrences?

To treat cardiac arrhythmias successfully in the emergency department, the physician must understand the normal anatomy and physiology of the cardiac pacemaking and conducting systems and the ways in which they can be deranged, must know what methods are available for accurate diagnosis of the rhythm disturbance, and finally, must select the correct therapy for restoring normal rhythm.

ANATOMY AND PHYSIOLOGY

Automaticity

Any cardiac cell that can spontaneously depolarize, reach its threshold potential, and discharge without the aid of another stimulus is capable of acting as a cardiac pacemaker cell. This property is known as *automaticity* and is possessed by specialized cells in several locations in the heart, such as the sinus (sinoatrial) node, the atrioventricular (A-V) node and junction, and the His-Purkinje system. At any given time, the cells with the fastest rate of spontaneous diastolic depolarization constitute the dominant pacemaker and suppress the formation of impulses in cells with slower discharge rates.

Sinus Node

This dominant-pacemaker function is usually served by the sinus node, a collection of cells and fibrous tissue located at the junction of the superior vena cava and the right atrium. Since it is a superficial structure, it is easily affected by pericardial inflammation, resulting in the atrial arrhythmias common in patients with pericarditis. The artery to the sinus node courses directly through it, and pressure within the artery may help regulate the discharge rate of the pacemaker cells; this artery is a proximal branch of the right coronary artery in 55% of patients and of the left circumflex coronary artery in the remainder. The impulse generated in the sinus node is propagated through the atria along at least three loosely organized internodal bundles that terminate in the node.

A-V Node

The A-V node is located near the junction of the interatrial and interventricular septa; its slow conduction time limits the number of impulses that can reach the ventricle and provides a delay between atrial systole and ventricular systole that facilitates proper ventricular filling. The artery to the A-V node comes from the right coronary artery in 90%

of patients and from the left circumflex coronary artery in the remainder.

His Bundle and Bundle Branches

From the A-V node, the impulse is conducted down the bundle of His, which soon divides into a thin right branch coursing into the right ventricle and a thicker left branch entering the left ventricle. The left bundle branch divides into anterior and posterior segments. Hence, there are three major divisions or fascicles—the right bundle branch and the anterior and posterior divisions of the left bundle branch. The blood supply to the bundle branches is primarily from septal branches of the left anterior descending coronary artery.

Depolarization Physiology

Throughout its course, the propagation of the impulse depends on its reaching cells that are *excitable*, that is, capable of being depolarized. A cell that is not excitable is *refractory*. The *refractory period* is the time needed for a depolarized cell to recover so that it can discharge again in response to a stimulus. The normal electrical sequence, therefore, depends on coordination of automaticity, conduction velocities, excitability, and refractoriness. Disorders of cardiac rhythm result from abnormalities in these functions that occur individually or in combination. For example, atrial tachycardia with block represents a combination of enhanced atrial automaticity and depressed A-V conduction. Furthermore, each of these properties may be altered by physiologic events (for example, electrolyte changes or alteration in sympathetic or parasympathetic tone), pathologic processes (for example, ischemia, infarction, fibrosis, or inflammation), or drugs.

CONSEQUENCES OF ARRHYTHMIAS

The ability of a patient to tolerate an arrhythmia depends on the nature of the arrhythmia, its duration, the vigor of the heart, and the patient's general health. Certain principles may be applied in understanding the consequences of arrhythmias.

Rate Tolerance

The normal heart tolerates a wide range of rates without decompensation. In healthy persons, a satisfactory cardiac output can be maintained with heart rates in excess of 170 beats/min or as low as 40 beats/min.

Tachycardia, however, shortens diastole, and also increases myocardial oxygen consumption considerably. Two important events occur during diastole—ventricular filling and coronary artery perfusion. For these reasons, sustained tachycardia is tolerated poorly by patients dependent on long diastolic periods for ventricular filling, such as those with mitral stenosis, and by patients who cannot tolerate increased myocardial oxygen consumption and decreased coronary artery perfusion, such as those with angina pectoris or acute myocardial infarction.

Bradycardia is tolerated poorly by patients with relatively fixed stroke volumes, such as those with aortic valvular disease or a failing left ventricle. A bradycardic rhythm may cause no problems until a stress such as fever or increased activity requires increased cardiac output. The ability to tolerate either tachycardia or bradycardia is directly related to the functional state of the heart, primarily the left ventricle; this point is fundamental in deciding on the urgency with which an arrhythmia should be terminated in any given patient.

Atrial Transport

Atrial contraction at the end of diastole completes ventricular filling before the ventricle contracts and may be responsible for 10–30% of the cardiac output. This atrial transport function is more important in diseased hearts than it is in healthy hearts and is particularly needed in patients with hypertrophic or noncompliant left ventricles, such as patients with aortic stenosis, idiopathic hypertrophic subaortic stenosis, and hypertensive heart disease, and some patients with coronary artery disease. Loss of this atrial "kick" may be important in the deterioration of hemodynamic status that can result from atrial fibrillation, ventricular tachycardia, or complete heart block.

Rhythm Deterioration

Because of hemodynamic deterioration and underlying heart disease—particularly ischemic heart disease—it is common for one arrhythmia to give way to another, which further jeopardizes the patient's condition. For example, the rapid heart rate of paroxysmal atrial tachycardia may cause coronary ischemia which, in turn, can precipitate ventricular tachycardia or ventricular fibrillation. Bradyarrhythmias such as complete heart block may result in either asystole or ventricular fibrillation. The prevention of such a sequence is one of the strongest reasons for the prompt treatment of arrhythmias, particularly in elderly patients and in those with coronary artery disease.

GENERAL PRINCIPLES IN DIAGNOSIS OF ARRHYTHMIAS

Three sources of information are available to the physician in diagnosing an arrhythmia: the history, physical examination, and electrocardiogram.

History

As much information as possible should be gathered regarding the patient's drug history, known cardiac diagnoses, and any previous arrhythmias and response to therapy. Being alert to the possibility of digitalis toxicity, electrolyte disorders (particularly hypokalemia in patients receiving diuretics), and previous adverse drug reactions may help in both diagnosis and choice of therapy. In a patient who has had recurrent arrhythmias, such as paroxysmal supraventricular tachycardia, it is useful to know which therapeutic maneuvers or drugs have or have not been effective. The duration of the rhythm disturbance, possible precipitating events, and the patient's report of symptoms such as angina, dyspnea, or syncope are all important in guiding therapy.

Physical Examination

Awareness of the patient's state of perfusion as indicated by blood pressure, skin color and temperature, mental status, and urinary output is essential to establish how well the arrhythmia is being tolerated and how urgently intervention is required. If the patient has no pulse and is unconscious, a "blind" defibrillation is indicated. If the patient has a rapid heart rate (150 beats/min or more) and evidence of severely decreased perfusion, immediate cardioversion also may be required even before establishing a definitive diagnosis. If the patient is not in such a state of hemodynamic collapse, more time can be taken for a careful physical examination before therapy.

Inspection of the jugular veins can yield information about atrial activity and the presence or absence of A-V dissociation. With practice, the physician can recognize the normal "a" waves (P waves on the electrocardiogram) caused by atrial contraction and their relation to the normal "v" waves of ventricular contraction (QRS interval). Two "a" waves per ventricular systole suggest 2:1 heart block. Large intermittent cannon "a" waves are diagnostic of A-V dissociation, which suggest either complete heart block or ventricular tachycardia with an independent atrial rhythm. Cannon waves result from the backward pressure generated by the atrium contracting against a tricuspid valve closed by simultaneous ventricular contraction. Occasionally, the rapid flutter waves (300 waves/min) of atrial flutter can be seen in the neck. An "irregularly irregular" pulse and absence of "a" waves suggest atrial fibrillation.

Cardiac auscultation may provide additional diagnostic information. Variability of the first heart sound suggests either atrial fibrillation, a changing P-R interval, or some type of A-V dissociation. Wide splitting of both the first and second sounds and gallop sounds, which may be variable in intensity and timing, strongly suggests ventricular tachyarrhythmia. Auscultation is also important for the identification of murmurs, gallops, or rubs that may enable more accurate diagnosis of the underlying heart disease. Knowing that the patient has mitral or aortic valvular disease or a dilated, failing heart is important in predicting how well a rhythm disturbance is likely to be tolerated.

A-V dissociation, which usually occurs in ventricular tachycardia, often can be recognized more readily from physical examination than from the electrocardiogram. When the atria and ventricles beat asynchronously, there is a veritable cacophony on auscultation, with variation in the intensity and splitting of the heart sounds and intermittent gallop sounds. Inconstant cannon waves are seen in the jugular veins, and there is beat-to-beat variation in the systolic blood pressure. All these findings are due to the random relation of the atrial and ventricular contractions. In contrast, the heart sounds in arrhythmias in which the atria and ventricles beat synchronously—as in paroxysmal atrial tachycardia—are similar to each other, and there are no beat-to-beat variations in heart sounds, the jugular veins, or systemic blood pressure.

In the remainder of the physical examination, the physician should establish whether there is evidence of left or right ventricular failure (rales, jugular venous distention, hepatomegaly, or peripheral edema), and should look for coexisting diseases that may have precipitated the arrhythmia, such as pneumonia, pulmonary embolic disease, or thyrotoxicosis.

Electrocardiogram

Electrocardiographic examination is crucial in the diagnosis of an arrhythmia, and it must be approached systematically. The physician should ask four key questions:

1. Is there evidence of atrial activity represented by P waves or flutter waves?
2. Is the QRS complex, representing ventricular depolarization, normal or wide (more than 0.12 second), fast or slow, regular or irregular?
3. Is there any relation between the P waves and the QRS complex?
4. Are there premature beats or pauses that need to be explained?

Atrial Activity

In the standard electrocardiogram, atrial activity is represented by the P waves, usually best seen in the inferior leads (II, III, and AVF) or right precordial leads (V_1 and V_2). Additional right precordial leads such as V_3R and V_4R may be helpful.

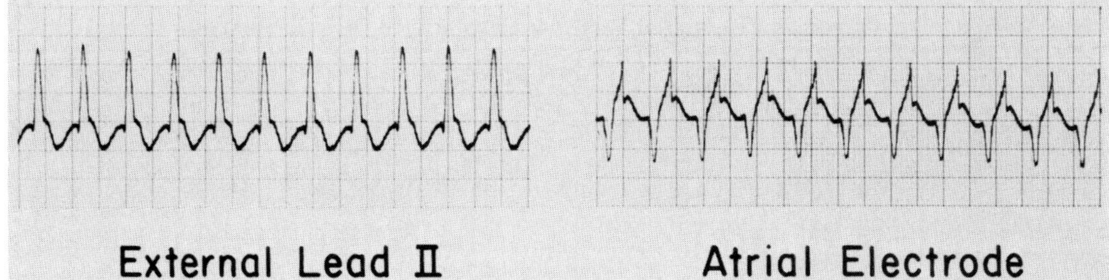

Figure 5.1. Use of atrial electrode to diagnose arrhythmia. External electrocardiogram reveals a regular tachycardia at 160 beats/min with narrow QRS complexes and no discernible atrial activity. The atrial electrode reveals regular atrial activity with 1:1 relation between P waves and QRS complexes. The diagnosis of paroxysmal atrial tachycardia can now be made and appropriate therapy instituted. (Reproduced by permission of the American Heart Association, Inc., from De Sanctis, RW. Diagnostic and Therapeutic Uses of Atrial Pacing. *Circulation,* 43:745–761. © 1971.)

Modification of the lead system sometimes may reveal atrial activity not seen with the standard leads. One such modification is the CR system, in which the right arm electrode is used as the indifferent electrode and the left arm electrode is used as an exploring precordial electrode while the electrocardiogram is recorded from lead I.

If these leads are not sufficient to define atrial activity, other means must be used. An esophageal electrode may be placed behind the left atrium by passing it down the esophagus a distance of 32–36 cm from the nares. This then can be connected to the exploring V electrode by an insulated wire with an alligator clamp at each end, the electrocardiogram being recorded from the V lead. Because this procedure is often uncomfortable for the patient, it may be difficult to perform.

A right atrial electrocardiogram can be recorded directly by means of a central venous pressure line, the tip of which is positioned in the right atrium. The line is filled with a 10% solution of sodium bicarbonate, and an external metal needle is connected by alligator clips to the V electrode. In many instances, this salt bridge will provide an interpretable atrial electrocardiogram recorded from the V lead. Finally, a definitive atrial electrocardiogram can usually be obtained by passing a pacemaker electrode transvenously into the right atrium and connecting the external tip of the wire to the V lead with alligator clips (Fig. 5.1). This can be done at the bedside with virtually no risk to the patient.

QRS Complex

The width of the QRS complex represents the amount of time required for the depolarizing electrical impulse to travel from the A-V node throughout the ventricle. Normally, the QRS width is less than 0.12 second because the impulse travels along the left and right bundles, which are high-speed conduction tissue. A QRS width less than 0.12 second represents a rhythm starting above the ventricle and having access to a normal conduction system via the A-V node, that is, a supraventricular rhythm. If the QRS complex is wider than normal, three possibilities exist: (*a*) the impulse may start within the ventricle, and thus not have access to the conduction system; (*b*) the conduction system may be permanently interrupted, that is, the patient may have left or right bundle-branch block; or (*c*) there may be a temporary dysfunction of the conduction system resulting in aberrant conduction. Such aberrant conduction may occur if a demand is made on the system to conduct too many beats per minute (rate-related) or to handle a premature beat before it has recovered from the previous beat. The distinction between supraventricular tachycardia with aberrant conduction and ventricular tachycardia can be difficult. The following considerations are helpful (Table 5.1).

A-V Dissociation. A-V dissociation refers to that situation in which atrial and ventricular complexes are independent of each other. If a tachycardia originates in the atrium, the ventricular response bears a constant relation to atrial activity. However, if the tachycardia is ventricular, the atria often but not always depolarize independently at an entirely different and usually slower rate; the exception to this is the occasional case of ventricular tachycardia with constant retrograde atrial activation. Electrocardiographic evidence of A-V dissociation is the strongest indication of a ventricular tachycardia (Fig. 5.2). As previously mentioned, physical findings of A-V dissociation, such as cannon waves in the jugular veins and variable heart sounds, may provide additional clues.

Capture or Fusion Beats. If the atria are beating independently of the ventricles and there is normal A-V nodal function, occasionally a supraventricular impulse may be timed such that it finds the ventricle vulnerable. This results in an entirely normal and usually premature QRS complex in the midst of the widened complexes (a capture beat) or

Table 5.1.
Differential Electrocardiographic Features of Tachycardia with Wide QRS Complexes

Differential Feature	SVT with Aberrant Conduction	Ventricular Tachycardia
Atrioventricular dissociation on electrocardiogram and physical examination	No	Often (diagnostic if present) (about 20% have retrograde atrial activity and therefore do not show A-V dissociation)
Capture or fusion beats or both	No	Often (diagnostic if present)
QRS structure	Commonly right bundle-branch block, especially with RSR′ in V_1 (R′ usually > R)	Less often right bundle-branch block, rarely with RSR′ in V_1 (R > R′), more commonly R or QR in V_1
Initial 0.04-sec vector of QRS complex	Identical with normally conducted beats	Different from normally conducted beats
Rate	150–240 beats/min	120–250 beats/min
Regularity	Usually regular (unless atrial fibrillation or supraventricular tachycardia with variable block)	May have slight variation in cycle length (0.02–0.03 sec)
Response to carotid sinus pressure	May slow or revert to normal sinus rhythm	No response
Relation to prior electrocardiographic events	Structure may resemble preexisting bundle-branch block or previous aberrantly conducted premature beats	Structure may resemble previous ventricular premature beats

in a complex intermediate in width and configuration between the normal and abnormal complexes (a fusion beat or Dressler beat). Capture or fusion beats are further evidence that a tachycardia is ventricular. They usually occur when the ventricular ectopic rate is relatively slow, thus allowing enough time for the A-V node to recover sufficiently to conduct a sinus impulse.

Structure of the QRS Complex. Since the refractory period of the right bundle is normally longer than that of the left, aberrant ventricular conduction usually assumes the pattern of right bundle-branch block. Unfortunately, rhythms arising in the left ventricle also have a right bundle-branch block configuration. A right bundle-branch block pattern due to ventricular origin of the tachycardia is more likely to be monophasic or, if bi- or tri-phasic (RR′ or RSR′), the R wave is of greater amplitude than the R′. With aberrant conduction, an RSR′ pattern is more common and the R′ wave is usually of greater amplitude than the R.

Additional information may be obtained from analysis of the first 0.04-second vector of the QRS complex. This portion is usually unaffected by aberration, that is, it is in the same direction as it is in the patient's normally conducted beats. If it is different from that of the normal beats, the tachycardia is likely to be ventricular. To determine the direction of this vector accurately, it is necessary to examine the QRS complex in all the standard leads.

Rate, Regularity, and Response to Carotid Sinus Pressure. There is considerable overlap in rate between ventricular and supraventricular rhythms, but ventricular tachycardia rarely exceeds

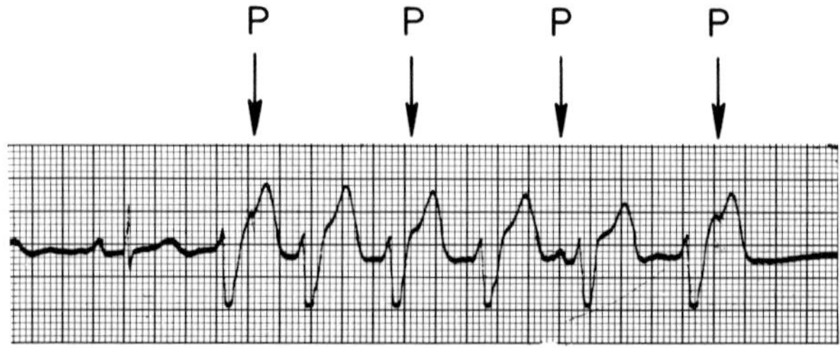

Figure 5.2. Ventricular tachycardia. This 6-beat aberrant tachycardia can be diagnosed as ventricular in origin because of electrocardiographic evidence of A-V dissociation. Sinus P waves that continue through the tachycardia indicate that the atrium is beating independently of the ventricle.

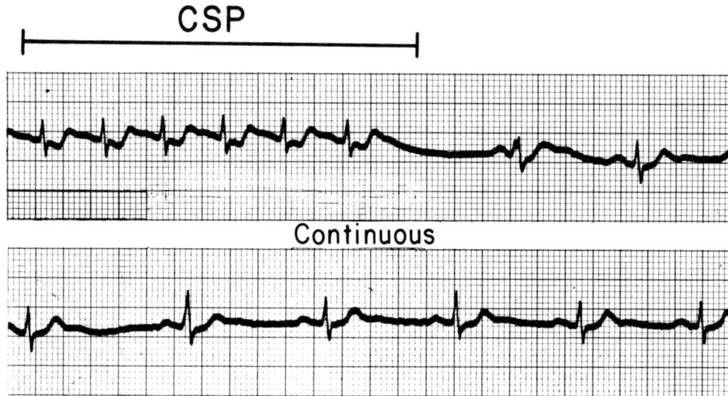

Figure 5.3. Paroxysmal atrial tachycardia converting to normal sinus rhythm with carotid sinus pressure. Initially there is a regular tachycardia at 140 beats/min with narrow QRS complexes and no clear atrial activity. With carotid sinus pressure, the rhythm changes abruptly—initially a pause, then a junctional escape beat, then return of normal sinus rhythm with gradual increase in rate as sinus node "warms up"

200 beats/min. There is more likely to be slight variation in the R-R interval (0.02–0.03 second) with ventricular tachycardia, whereas supraventricular tachycardia is more likely to be absolutely regular, with the exception of atrial fibrillation, which is characterized by total irregularity. A decrease in rate or conversion to sinus rhythm with carotid sinus pressure is diagnostic of a supraventricular origin (Fig. 5.3). (Technique is described on p 90).

Relation to Previous Electrocardiographic Events. Review of the patient's past electrocardiograms may provide diagnostic information. If the patient has had previous ventricular premature beats of identical configuration or has had similar aberrantly conducted supraventricular beats, the arrhythmia is likely to be related to these events.

Premature Beats and Pauses

The electrocardiogram must be analyzed for premature beats and pauses. Once the regular pattern of atrial and ventricular activation has been identified, it is possible to recognize beats that occur earlier than expected; these usually indicate increased automaticity of another pacemaker focus. It is also important to appreciate the failure of a beat to occur on time, which usually indicates delay within the conduction system or a disturbance of impulse formation within the dominant pacemaker. Premature beats and pauses often accompany each other, as is the case with either a ventricular premature beat followed by a compensatory pause or a nonconducted atrial premature beat.

DIAGNOSIS AND TREATMENT OF SPECIFIC ARRHYTHMIAS

We prefer to consider the recognition and treatment of cardiac rhythm disturbances according to features that are easily distinguished on the electrocardiogram. Three fundamental electrocardiographic characteristics form the basis of this approach: the heart rate, the regularity of the QRS complexes, and the width of the QRS complexes. This approach is schematically represented in Figure 5.4.

Tachycardias

Tachycardias are rhythms with rates more than 100 beats/min.

Regular Tachycardias with Narrow QRS Complexes

These constitute the most common group of rhythm disturbances. The narrow QRS complex indicates that the arrhythmia originated above the bifurcation of the bundle of His; hence, these are all supraventricular. The differential diagnosis is among *sinus tachycardia, paroxysmal supraventricular (atrial* or *junctional) tachycardia, atrial flutter,* and *nonparoxysmal junctional tachycardia.* Although junctional rhythms have been referred to as nodal rhythms, recent studies indicate that the A-V node has little spontaneous automaticity and that most such rhythms arise in sites distal to the A-V node but proximal to the bifurcation of the bundle of His—hence the term "junctional."

Sinus Tachycardia. This is not a true cardiac arrhythmia, but is merely an acceleration of the normal discharge rate of the sinus node. Sinus tachycardia is invariably secondary to a condition that is driving the heart at a faster rate.

In patients with sinus tachycardia, the heart rate rarely exceeds 150 beats/min, except in infants and children and in adults engaging in maximal physical exertion. There may be slight irregularity due to

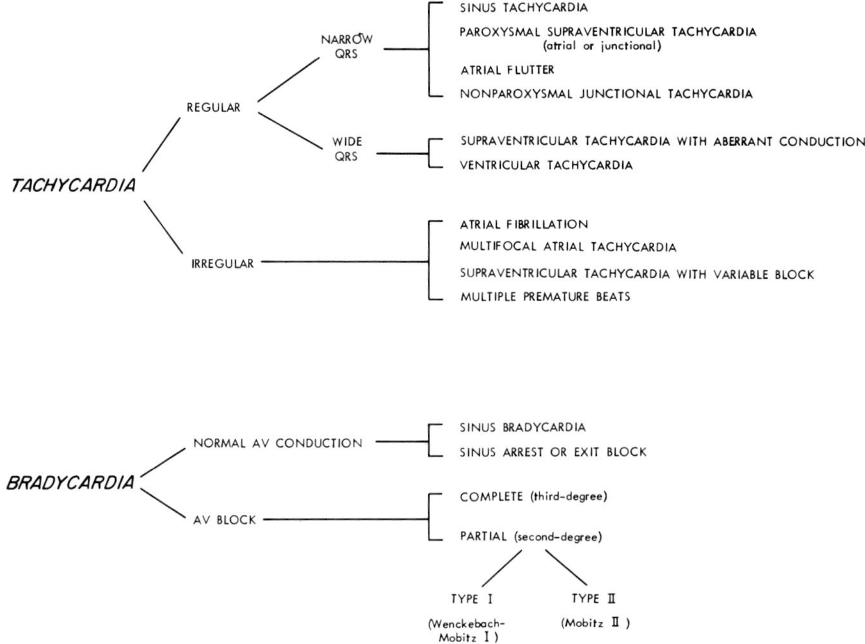

Figure 5.4. Arrhythmia flow sheet based on electrocardiographic features.

sinus arrhythmia, although at rapid heart rates, sinus arrhythmia is usually not present.

Diagnosis. One of the problems in diagnosing sinus tachycardia lies in the fact that the P wave may be incorporated into the T wave of the preceding beat. A constant hump often subtly inscribed in the T wave may indicate the P wave. Also, comparison of prior electrocardiograms at slower rates may reveal more peaked T waves resulting from a combination of P and T waves. Carotid sinus pressure may produce enough slowing to dissociate the P wave from the T wave. Slowing is always gradual, and the heart usually resumes its prior rate on release of carotid sinus pressure. If premature beats are present, the sinus P wave may appear in the beat after the compensatory pause. If the P wave can be dissociated from the previous T wave, its axis will be normal—approximately +60 degrees.

Treatment. With rare exceptions, treatment of sinus tachycardia is not directed at the rhythm itself. Rather, a careful search should be made for the underlying cause, and this should be appropriately managed. Common causes include fever, sepsis, congestive heart failure, hypovolemia, hypoxemia, anemia, pulmonary embolism, thyrotoxicosis, anxiety, and drugs that accelerate the heart rate. Digitalis glycosides are indicated *only* if the sinus tachycardia is secondary to congestive heart failure.

One exception regarding therapy is sinus tachycardia in the presence of angina pectoris or acute myocardial infarction. Since the heart rate is a major determinant of myocardial oxygen consumption, slowing it may be important in the patient with myocardial ischemia. Angina may be relieved by slowing the heart rate with carotid sinus pressure. Slowing of sinus tachycardia may also abolish the ischemic pain of myocardial infarction and may even limit the size of the infarct area. Propranolol (Inderal), 1–5 mg intravenously to a maximum of 0.1 mg/kg of body weight, may be administered for this purpose if the sinus tachycardia is not associated with congestive heart failure. *Propranolol is contraindicated when congestive heart failure is present.* Caution should be exercised in administering intravenous propranolol to any patient with electrocardiograhic evidence of an acute myocardial infarction. In general, we prefer to have a pulmonary artery line in place to monitor the pulmonary capillary wedge pressure and cardiac output before administering intravenous propranolol to patients with an acute myocardial infarction.

Paroxysmal Supraventricular Tachycardia. **Diagnosis.** The term paroxysmal supraventicular tachycardia (SVT) includes paroxysmal tachycardia of both atrial and junctional origin, since in practice these are indistinguishable. The heart rate is usually between 150 and 200 beats/min, but it occasionally may be faster, especially in infants and patients with Wolff-Parkinson-White syndrome.

These tachyarrhythmias are usually characterized by abrupt onset and termination, and the history

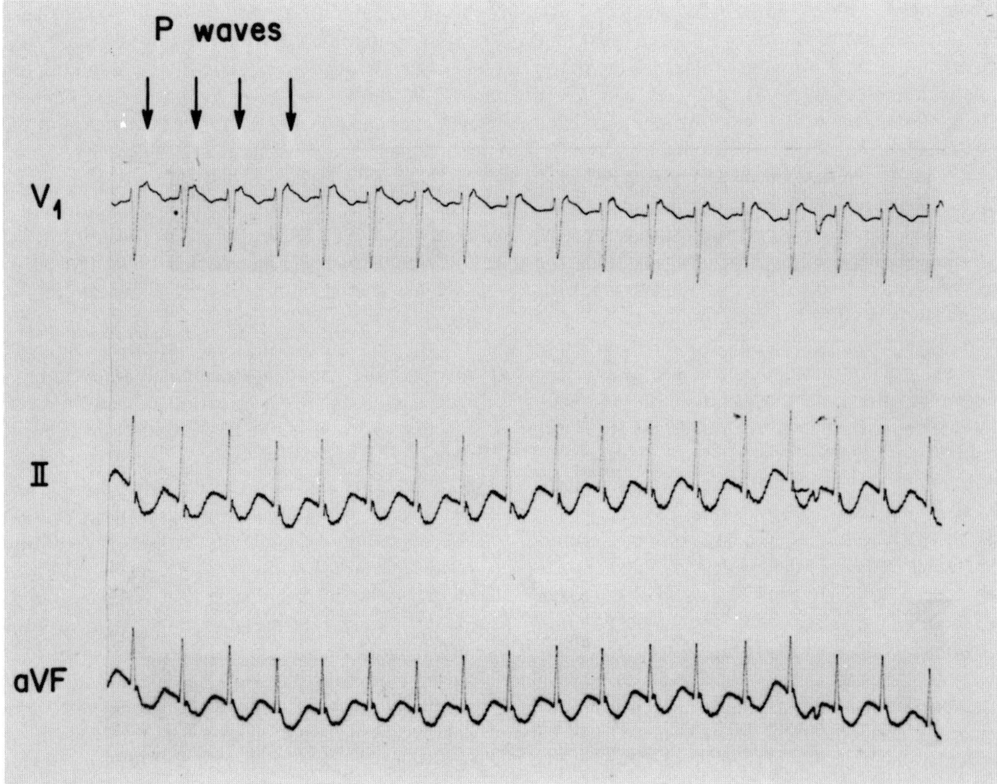

Figure 5.5. Paroxysmal atrial tachycardia. This is a regular tachycardia at 180 beats/min with narrow QRS complexes. P waves at rate of 180 waves/min can be seen in lead V_1.

often suggests the diagnosis. They tend to recur and may occur in young persons without heart disease. Some patients experience polyuria concomitantly.

Pathophysiology. There are at least four types of paroxysmal supraventricular tachycardia and sometimes distinctions can be made based on the location and morphology of the P wave. The most common mechanism is a reentry mechanism involving the A-V node. In these cases, the P wave is usually invisible as it is buried in the QRS complex. If the P wave is visible, it is inverted in leads II, III, and F and is seen immediately after the QRS complex (Fig. 5.5). If the tachycardia is due to a reentry mechanism involving an accessory pathway (see below), the P wave always follows the QRS complex and is retrograde. If the tachycardia is due to sinus node or atrial reentry, the P wave will precede the QRS complex and usually will be of normal or nearly normal configuration. Finally, the tachycardia may be due to enhanced automaticity of an ectopic pacemaker. In these cases, the P wave precedes the QRS complex and its morphology is variable depending on the site of the ectopic focus. SVTs due to this last mechanism may not have the abrupt onset or termination that is characteristic of those that occur by any of the reentry mechanisms. In addition, they may be more resistant to therapy.

Physical Examination. On physical examination, the heart sounds are uniform. In some cases, the atria and ventricles may contract simultaneously, causing constant cannon waves in the jugular veins. The response to carotid sinus pressure is often diagnostic, since abrupt cessation of the rhythm may be seen. Sinus rhythm returns after a pause, which sometimes is interrupted by junctional escape beats while the sinus "warms up" (Fig. 5.3). The tachycardia is characteristically regular, although it may be irregular for the first few beats. If the beginning of the arrhythmia is recorded, an atrial or junctional premature beat will be seen initiating the tachycardia. Once sinus rhythm is restored, sporadic atrial or junctional premature beats may provide further diagnostic clues. On application of carotid sinus pressure, a small number of patients have some degree of A-V block rather than reversion to normal sinus rhythm. This should arouse suspicion of digitalis toxicity, which is present in about 75% of such patients.

Treatment. *Vagal Tone Measures.* Initial treatment includes measures to increase vagal tone, such as carotid sinus pressure, Valsalva's maneuver, or induction of gagging. Vagal tone can be increased pharmacologically with edrophonium chloride (Tensilon), 5–10 mg intravenously. Its effect peaks in 1–3 minutes and is dissipated in 10–15 minutes. Some patients experience nausea, cramps, or increased salivation. Administration of this drug to digitalized patients must be very cautious, because of an increased risk of profound bradycardia. Atropine sulfate, 0.5–1.0 mg, should be ready for immediate intravenous administration if an excessive vagal reaction develops. If conversion has not occurred by the time the effect of edrophonium chloride peaks, the maneuvers to increase vagal tone should be repeated.

Verapamil. If vagal maneuvers are unsuccessful, verapamil is the drug of choice. It is particularly effective for the cessation of reentry arrhythmias involving the A-V node. The intravenous dose is 0.075 to 0.15 mg/kg (5–10 mg total dose in an average-sized adult) given over 2–3 minutes. It has its peak effect within 10 minutes, and a repeat dose may be given if necessary in 30 minutes. Verapamil should be used with caution in the presence of hypotension, severely depressed left ventricular function, or known conduction system disease. Elderly patients may be more prone to its adverse effects, particularly its bradycardic response.

Propranolol. Propranolol is another useful drug for the treatment of paroxysmal SVTs, provided that the patient has neither severe hypotension nor a history of severe congestive heart failure or bronchospastic pulmonary disease. Propranolol may be administered intravenously in 1-mg increments every 5 minutes until either conversion is achieved or a total dose of 0.1 mg/kg (5–10 mg) is administered. Electrocardiographic monitoring and frequent determinations of blood pressure must accompany administration of propranolol, since profound bradycardia and hypotension may develop. Intravenous propranolol should never be given in close proximity to intravenous verapamil because of the risk of profound bradycardia and/or profound dysgenesis of ventricular function.

Digitalis Glycosides. If all of these measures are unsuccessful, a rapid-acting intravenous digitalis glycoside should be administered. We prefer digoxin (Lanoxin) 0.5 mg, initially in the patient known not to be on digitalis glycosides. Digoxin begins to exert its effect in 15–30 minutes. Vagal stimulation should be repeated if conversion has not occurred by this time, since the digitalis glycosides further enhance vagal tone and increase responsiveness to these maneuvers. Digoxin may be given in additional 0.25 mg increments every 30 to 60 minutes until the rhythm responds, there is evidence of toxicity, or a total digitalizing dose of 0.02 mg/kg has been given. If the patient has already been given verapamil or propranolol, there is a higher risk of inducing high degree A-V block, and therefore lower doses separated by longer intervals should be employed. If the patient is already taking a digitalis preparation, dose increments of 0.125 mg should be employed with a heightened sensitivity to the appearance of any signs of digitalis toxicity.

Vasopressors. If the arrhythmia is still refractory, vasopressor agents may be administered to selected patients. Because of the risk of an adverse reaction to an excessive rise in blood pressure, this therapy should be reserved for young patients with healthy hearts and with relative hypotension accompanying the arrhythmia. The agent may be administered as an intravenous bolus [for example, phenylephrine (Neo-Synephrine), 0.5–1.5 mg, or methoxamine hydrochloride (Vasoxyl), 5-10 mg] or as a continuous intravenous infusion [for example, metaraminol (Aramine), 100 mg in 500 ml of 5% dextrose in water], titrating the infusion rate against the blood pressure. The goal is to return the blood pressure to a normal range or to slightly above normal, for example, approximately 150/90 mm Hg or 150/100 mm Hg. Drug administration must be stopped immediately on conversion or if blood pressure becomes excessively elevated. Blood pressure must be monitored carefully, and an intravenous α-adrenergic antagonist such as phentolamine (Regitine), 1-3 mg, must be available to counteract a potentially dangerous blood pressure elevation. A common consequence of excessive blood pressure response is severe occipital headache. Fatal intracerebral hemorrhage has resulted from the overzealous use of vasopressor agents.

Other Agents. In addition to the aforementioned drugs, intravenous lidocaine (Xylocaine) has been successful in a small number of patients. Intravenous phenytoin (Dilantin) may also be administered, but its effectiveness may be restricted to patients with digitalis toxicity, who have ectopic atrial tachycardia accompanied by A-V block. Rarely either quinidine sulfate or procainamide may be useful in treating these arrhythmias, particularly if they are associated with a preexcitation syndrome or if the SVT is ectopic in origin.

If these interventions have failed, and the patient is not tolerating the arrhythmia, either synchronized direct-current countershock or rapid atrial stimulation (see pp 69–70) is likely to be successful. It is unusual, however, to have to apply either of these measures.

Further Treatment. Once conversion to sinus

rhythm has been achieved, consideration must be given to prescribing an antiarrhythmic agent to prevent recurrences. The decision should be based on the frequency of the attacks and the severity of associated symptoms. The agents most likely to be successful in long-term prophylaxis are digoxin, 0.25 mg daily, or propranolol, 20–30 mg four times a day, or both. Quinidine, 200-300 mg four times a day, may also be effective as may procainamide or disopyramide. It is important to caution the patient about the possible role that caffeine, nicotine, sympathomimetic drugs, and other stimulants may play in the initiation of paroxysmal SVT.

Atrial Flutter. Diagnosis. This arrhythmia, which tends to occur in patients with heart disease, is usually episodic. Atrial flutter is due to regular atrial depolarization at a rate of 250-300 beats/min. Since in most situations the A-V node cannot conduct impulses at this rate, a physiologic 2:1 A-V block results, in which the ventricular response is approximately 150 beats/min (Fig 5.6*A*). In infants, 1:1 conduction can occur. *Any absolutely regular SVT at a rate of 150 beats/min should raise the suspicion of atrial flutter.* The response to carotid sinus pressure may be characteristic in that it results in a stepwise decrease in rate caused by increasing degrees of A-V block (usually from 2:1 to 4:1) without a change in the underlying atrial mechanism. Atrial activity can be seen on the electrocardiogram at a rate of approximately 300 beats/min appearing as ''sawtooth'' deflections in the inferior leads or as positive deflections in the inferior leads or as positive deflections in the right precordial leads (Fig. 5.6*B*). When atrial activity cannot be clearly distinguished in the baseline electrocardiogram or after carotid sinus pressure, edrophonium chloride, 5-10 mg intravenously, may cause transient A-V block and allow identification of flutter waves. If this fails, a right atrial electrocardiogram usually permits clear definition of atrial activity.

Treatment. *Drug Therapy.* The drugs of choice for conversion or control of heart rate or both in patients with atrial flutter are the digitalis glycosides, verapamil, or propranolol alone or in combination. Digoxin can be administered in an initial bolus of 0.5 mg intravenously. Digoxin may result either in the establishment of a higher degree of A-V block or may cause conversion to sinus rhythm. Verapamil (5-10 mg intravenously) has its primary effect on A-V conduction, so it may result in a beneficial slowing of the ventricular response. In a small percentage of cases (20–30%) it will convert atrial flutter to sinus rhythm or atrial fibrillation. Propranolol can be administered intravenously at the rate of 1 mg/min every 3–5 minutes until conversion has been achieved, the heart rate has been slowed, or a total dose of 0.1 mg/kg has been given. As noted above, intravenous propranolol should not be given in close proximity to intravenous verapamil.

Cardioversion. If conversion to sinus rhythm does not occur with initial drug administration, we prefer to convert the arrhythmia electrically. Atrial flutter is extraordinarily responsive to electrical cardioversion and can usually be terminated with low energy levels, for example, 20–50 joules. Cardioversion is safe with the small amounts of digitalis

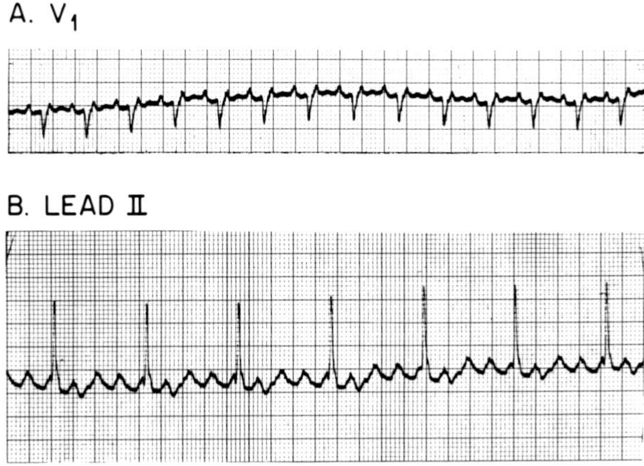

Figure 5.6. Atrial flutter. *A,* Atrial rate is 300 beats/min and ventricular rate is 150 beats/min; there is a physiologic 2:1 A-V block. This is the most common presentation of atrial flutter: a regular tachycardia at 150 beats/min with narrow QRS complexes. Note that flutter waves are positive in lead V_1. *B,* Electrocardiogram from different patient, which illustrates atrial flutter with 4:1 A-V block. This occurred in a fully digitalized patient in whom digitalis caused a higher degree of A-V block. Atrial rate is 280 beats/min, and ventricular rate is 70 beats/min with narrow QRS complexes. Note that flutter waves are negative sawtooth deflections in lead II.

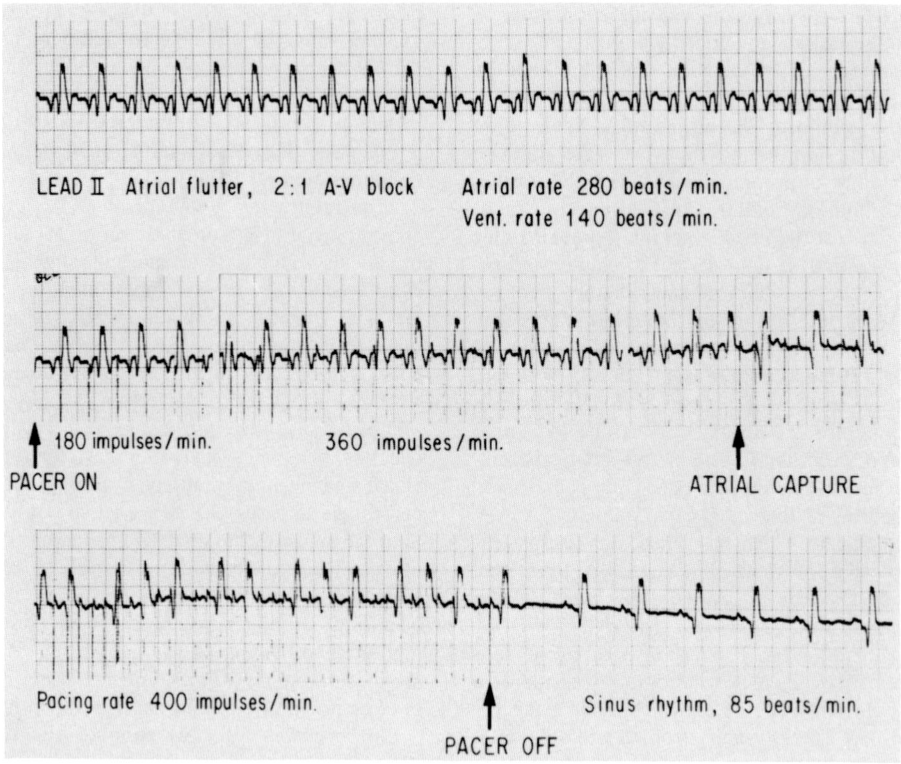

Figure 5.7. Rapid atrial pacing to convert atrial flutter. *Top panel* shows classic atrial flutter with negative atrial depolarization at rate of 280 beats/min (flutter waves) in lead II and with regular ventricular response of 140 beats/min. Rate of atrial pacemaker was increased progressively until atrium was captured, and sinus rhythm returned with cessation of pacing. (Reproduced by permission of the American Heart Association, Inc., from De Sanctis, RW. Diagnostic and Therapeutic Uses of Atrial Pacing. *Circulation,* 43:745–761. © 1971.)

glycosides that have been recommended, but it becomes risky if larger quantities have been given as is often necessary to control the ventricular response. Hence, we prefer to cardiovert early in the course of atrial flutter.

Rapid Atrial Pacing. In refractory cases and when digitalis excess is suspected, rapid atrial stimulation may be successful in converting the rhythm (Fig. 5.7). A transvenous electrode is placed in the right atrium, and the position is confirmed electrocardiographically and radiographically. The atrium is stimulated initially at a rate of 150 impulses/min with sufficient current (usually about 5 milliamperes) to capture it or to interrupt the flutter waves. The rate and amperage may be progressively increased to 1200 impulses/min and 25 milliamperes, respectively, if necessary. The pacemaker must be turned off after several seconds of pacing at each increment to determine whether the rhythm has been altered. In 40-50% of patients, sinus rhythm is restored. In 25%, atrial flutter is converted to atrial fibrillation, which may then spontaneously revert to sinus rhythm; even if it does not, however, the heart rate can be controlled more easily with digitalis glycosides, verapamil, or propranolol than is the case with atrial flutter. Atrial fibrillation cannot be converted by rapid atrial stimulation.

Once conversion has occurred, it is wise to leave the pacing electrode in the atrium for a period of observation so that it is available for the diagnosis or treatment of any subsequent arrhythmias.

Quinidine Conversion. Occasionally a patient is tolerating atrial flutter sufficiently well to allow a more leisurely approach, in which case one can slowly digitalize the patient over 24 or 48 hours (with or without adjunctive therapy with propranolol or verapamil). If control of the ventricular response is achieved in this way, but the patient remains in atrial flutter, then an attempt can be made to convert the patient pharmacologically with an agent such as quinidine sulfate. There is a small risk of acceleration of the ventricular response with the addition of quinidine and patients need to be hospitalized and closely monitored if this approach is taken.

Long-term oral administration of digoxin and an agent such as quinidine sulfate, 200–300 mg every 6 hours, may be helpful in preventing recurrences.

Nonparoxysmal Junctional Tachycardia. Diagnosis and Pathophysiology. This arrhythmia is due to gradual acceleration of the junctional pacemaker and is distinguished from the paroxysmal SVTs by its gradual onset and termination and its slower rate, which rarely exceeds 140–150 beats/min. It occurs most commonly in patients with digitalis toxicity or acute inferior myocardial infarction and may also be seen after cardiac operations (particularly mitral valve replacement) and in patients with inflammation in the region of the A-V node due to acute rheumatic or viral myocarditis or bacterial endocarditis. The electrocardiogram reveals regular QRS complexes of normal width with absent or retrograde atrial activity. Carotid sinus pressure usually evokes no response. Constant cannon waves may be seen in the jugular veins.

Treatment. Nonparoxysmal junctional tachycardia is usually well-tolerated and rarely requires therapy other than withholding digitalis if digitalis excess is the cause. Correction of hypokalemia is also important. This arrhythmia is usually unresponsive to conventional antiarrhythmic drugs, and its presence should stimulate a search for a possible underlying cause. Occasionally a patient with severely impaired ventricular function may not tolerate this rhythm because of a fall in cardiac output due to the loss of atrial systole. In these cases, overdrive atrial pacing may be necessary to restore physiologic atrial and ventricular synchrony.

Regular Tachycardias with Wide QRS Complexes

These are among the most challenging of all the arrhythmias because the differential diagnosis lies between a *SVT with aberrant conduction and ventricular tachycardia.* The principles followed in making this differentiation have already been detailed (Table 5.1). It should be stressed that, if the condition of a patient with such an arrhythmia is hemodynamically compromised, the treatment of choice is cardioversion, whether the arrhythmia is ventricular or supraventricular. The only possible exception is the patient in whom digitalis toxicity is suspected.

SVT with Aberrant Conduction. Treatment is that of the particular supraventricular rhythm disturbance. The presence of aberrantly conducted ventricular complexes does not influence the choice of therapy. The hemodynamic status of these patients is usually more stable than that of a patient with ventricular tachycardia at a similar rate and, thus, there usually is time to employ drug therapy safely.

Ventricular Tachycardia. Diagnosis. This type of tachycardia is diagnosed by electrocardiographic evidence of A-V dissociation (Fig. 5.2) and by findings on physical examination such as cannon waves and variable heart sounds and blood pressure. Physical findings of A-V dissociation are absent in ventricular tachycardia if either atrial fibrillation or 1:1 retrograde activation of the atria by the ventricles is present. Ventricular tachycardia almost always is associated with underlying heart disease, which is often ischemic; a small number of patients, however, may have isolated or recurrent ventricular tachycardia without any other evidence of heart disease.

Treatment. *Cardioversion.* Cardioversion is the treatment of choice in the presence of significant hemodynamic compromise, and the decision whether to perform cardioversion must be made quickly at the bedside. Some patients are obviously moribund when first seen, in which case cardioversion should be performed immediately. Others tolerate the arrhythmia reasonably well. Cardioversion should usually be undertaken if any of the following complications are present: (*a*) a systolic blood pressure of 90 mm Hg or less; (*b*) poor peripheral perfusion indicated by cool, clammy, mottled extremities, mental obtundation, and oliguria; (*c*) congestive heart failure manifested by dyspnea, orthopnea, pulmonary edema, or a considerably elevated systemic venous pressure; and (*d*) ischemic myocardial pain. Once again, the only relative contraindication to cardioversion in patients with ventricular tachycardiais is digitalis toxicity (see pp 84–85).

Cardioversion is successful in more than 90% of patients and can usually be accomplished with a low energy level from 50–100 joules. A firm thump delivered to the precordium with a clenched fist may deliver enough energy to cardiovert this rhythm in some instances. This technique (thump version) should be tried once the diagnosis has been made and while preparing for cardioversion, but one should not persist with repeated attempts once ready to cardiovert electrically.

Lidocaine. In less urgent situations and when ventricular tachycardia recurs after initial conversion, pharmacologic therapy is indicated. Lidocaine is the first agent of choice because of its efficacy and relative safety. An initial intravenous bolus, 1–2 mg/kg, should be administered to achieve a therapeutic level in the blood rapidly (2-5 μg/ml). Additional boluses of 1 mg/kg can be administered every 5-10 minutes until either conversion has occurred or a maximum of 5 mg/kg has been administered. The most common toxic effects are central nervous system reactions such as drowsiness, dysarthria, tinnitus, bizarre behavior, and seizures. After conversion, further ventricular ectopy can usually be suppressed by a constant intravenous infusion of lidocaine, 20-55 μg/kg/min, which is about 1-4 mg/min in an average-sized adult. Lidocaine has little depressant effect on myocardial contractility and on conduction time, although isolated cases of sinoatrial and A-V block have been reported after lidocaine therapy. The drug is quickly metabolized, primarily in the liver, and toxic levels may be more rapidly achieved in the presence of severe hepatic disease or congestive heart failure.

Procainamide. Lidocaine may be ineffective in 10-20% of patients, and procainamide (Pronestyl) is the next drug of choice. Although there is slightly greater risk of hypotension with intravenous use of this drug, it usually can be administered safely in 100-mg increments every 5 minutes to a total dose of 1 gm or until a toxic reaction or abolition of the arrhythmia occurs. Blood pressure must be carefully monitored during intravenous administration of procainamide, and the electrocardiogram must be watched closely for evidence of A-V or intraventricular block, since procainamide can prolong conduction times. Therapeutic levels of the drug are between 4 and 8 μg/ml; above these levels, significant prolongation of QRS complexes and of QT intervals is likely. Since the drug is rapidly metabolized and excreted by the kidney, oral or intramuscular doses should be repeated at 3-hour intervals to maintain a therapeutic level. Usually, 250-500 mg every 3-4 hours provides adequate suppression of further ventricular ectopic activity.

In cases of stubborn ventricular irritability unresponsive to intravenous lidocaine, an intravenous infusion of procainamide, 20-40 μg/kg/min (1-4 mg/min), may be effective in suppressing the ectopy. When given in this manner, procainamide should be administered by means of a constant infusion pump.

Bretylium. A third drug for the treatment of recurrent or resistant ventricular tachycardia is bretylium tosylate. It may be given as a single intravenous dose of 5 mg/kg over 10 minutes. Since bretylium initially causes release of stored catecholamines from nerve terminals, there may be an initial hypertensive response, and it also has been reported to cause an initial exacerbation of ventricular ectopy in some patients. Though the drug may immediately lower the ventricular fibrillation threshold, its effect in suppressing ventricular ectopy may not be seen for 20 minutes to 2 hours. The major side effect of the drug is hypotension due to peripheral vasodilatation. In some cases, this may be profound and may require rapid volume infusion or administration of α-adrenergic agents. For this reason, patients should always be in the supine position when given the drug. There also may be an increased risk of exacerbating ventricular ectopy if bretylium is administered to patients with digitalis intoxication. In some cases of refractory ventricular tachycardia, continuous infusion with bretylium (1-2 mg/min) is necessary for control of these arrhythmias.

Phenytoin. Another drug which is sometimes effective in the treatment of venticular tachycardia is phenytoin. This is more likely to be successful—and may be the drug of choice—if the arrhythmia is induced by digitalis. It is not very effective in terminating ventricular tachycardia that is not due to digitalis excess. Phenytoin may safely be administered intravenously in 100-mg increments every 5 minutes until a total of 1 gm has been given, the arrhythmia has been controlled, or side effects have developed. It has little myocardial depressant effect and causes little or no depression of conduction times, although hypotension, bradyarrhythmias, and respiratory arrest have been reported during rapid intravenous administration. The therapeutic level in the blood is 10-18 μg/ml; above this level, neurologic toxic reactions develop, such as nystagmus, ataxia, and somnolence. Phenytoin is caustic, and when administered intravenously, it should be delivered through a central line or into a peripheral line with a rapidly running solution of 5% dextrose in water. It should not be administered intramuscularly because of erratic absorption. Once a therapeutic blood level has been achieved, it usually can be maintained with oral doses of 300-400 mg daily.

Propranolol. Intravenous propranolol also may be administered, either alone or in conjunction with one or more of the aforementioned agents. Like phenytoin, it appears to be more effective if the ventricular tachycardia is digitalis-induced. The intravenous dose is 1 mg every 5 minutes up to either 0.1 mg/kg, cessation of the arrhythmia, or tolerance. Major limitations are its considerable myocardial depressant effect and its potential for inducing bronchospasm. Antiarrhythmic blood levels usually can be maintained with a total dose of 80-240 mg daily in four to six divided doses.

Quinidine. Quinidine may also be useful in suppressing recurrent ventricular arrhythmias, but because its intravenous administration has been associated with severe hypotensive reactions, it plays little role in the management of the acute arrhythmia. Therapeutic blood levels can usually be maintained with doses of 300–600 mg orally or intramuscularly every 6 hours. It has now been well shown that in some cases, quinidine actually may exacerbate ventricular ectopy. This phenomenon in part may be mediated by quinidine's capacity for prolonging the QT interval, though its does not correlate entirely with that phenomenon. It is likely that this potential for exacerbating ventricular ectopy is also true of other antiarrhythmic agents, and it should be considered as a possible cause for refractory or worsening ventricular ectopy in the face

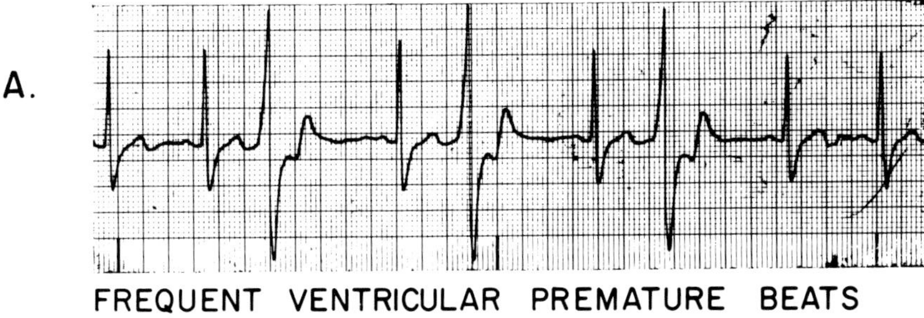

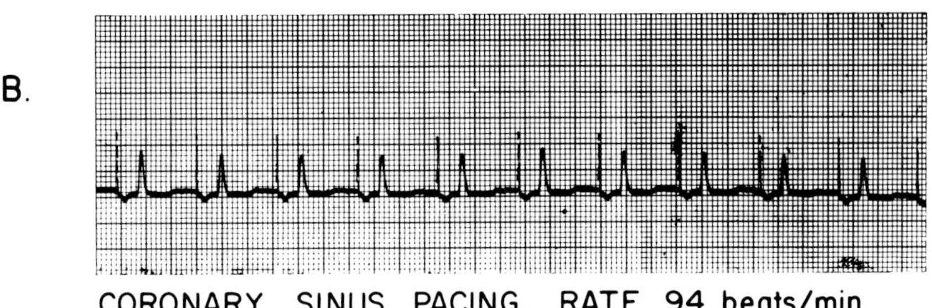

Figure 5.8. Overdrive pacing for suppression of ventricular ectopic beats. *A*, Ventricular bigeminy in patient with history of recurrent ventricular tachycardia resistant to pharmacologic suppression. *B*, Ventricular ectopic activity has been eliminated by instituting coronary sinus (atrial) pacing at 94 impulses/min. (Reproduced by permission of the American Heart Association, Inc., from De Sanctis, RW. Diagnostic and Therapeutic Uses of Atrial Pacing. *Circulation,* 43:745–761. © 1971.)

of escalating numbers and doses of antiarrhythmic therapy.

Other Agents: Disopyramide, Tocainide, and Mexiletine. In addition to quinidine, one other oral agent with similar electrophysiologic properties that may be useful as maintenance therapy to prevent recurrence of ventricular tachycardia is disopyramide (100–300 mg q6h). Disopyramide may also prolong the QT interval and is a potent myocardial depressant, so is contraindicated in the presence of severe heart failure. Two new lidocaine analogues are also now available for oral maintenance therapy. These are tocainide (400–800 mg q8h) and mexiletine (200–300 mg q8h). These have the advantage that they do not prolong the QT interval and they are not myocardial suppressants. They may be particularly useful if the acute arrhythmia has been responsive to lidocaine, although this has not always predicted response to these drugs.

Overdrive Pacing. If drug therapy fails to prevent recurrence of ventricular tachycardia, *overdrive pacing* of either the right atrium or the right ventricle may be successful in suppressing an ectopic pacemaker (Fig. 5.8). Pacing is more likely to be successful if the patient's normal heart rate is slow. Suppression is usually achieved with pacing rates between 90 and 120 impulses/min. In patients with coronary artery disease, pacing at such rates may be tolerated poorly because of the concomitant increase in oxygen consumption, and ischemic pain or a paradoxical increase in ventricular irritability may result.

Other Factors. Every effort must be made to identify and to treat the factors contributing to the genesis and propagation of ventricular tachycardia.The importance of recognizing digitalis excess has already been mentioned. The serum potassium level should be brought to the upper range of normal (4.5-5.0 mEq/liter) by an intravenous infusion of potassium chloride, 10-20 mEq/hr. Hypoxemia should be corrected, and any exogenous source of β-adrenergic stimulation should be withdrawn. The possible role of intracardiac mechanical factors should also be kept in mind. A central venous pressure catheter that has migrated into the right ventricle or a pacing electrode or Swan-Ganz pulmonary artery catheter in the right ventricle may be responsible for persistent or recurrent ventricular tachycardia that is particularly resistant to therapy.

Torsade de Pointe. A particularly malignant form of ventricular tachycardia with a characteristic morphology has been named "Torsade de pointe," a name chosen to reflect the turning of the QRS axis during the tachycardia. This form of ventricular tachycardia has been particularly associated with situations that prolong the QT interval (such as

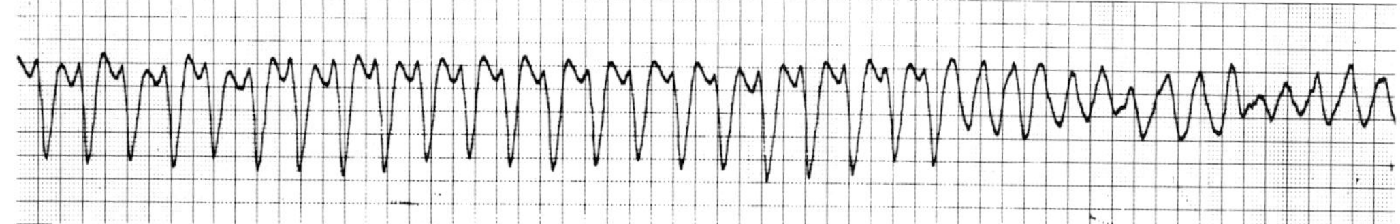

Figure 5.9. Ventricular fibrillation. Ventricular tachycardia at 155 beats/min degenerates into ventricular fibrillation with chaotic, disorganized ventricular rhythm.

quinidine, procainamide, or disopyramide therapy), underlying bradyarrhythmias, acute ischemia or inflammation, hypokalemia, or hypomagnesemia. Frequently more than one predisposing factor may be present. This arrhythmia has a high risk of degenerating into ventricular fibrillation. Antiarrhythmic agents which prolong the QT interval are contraindicated. Cardioversion is often necessary, but the arrhythmia is likely to recur unless the underlying predisposing factors are corrected. Overdrive pacing may be necessary to prevent recurrences, and in some instances an isoproterenol infusion (2–8 μg/min) to shorten the QT interval has proven to be successful.

To suppress refractory ventricular irritability the aforementioned drugs (see pp 71–73) may be administered in combination; at present such therapy in the acute situation is largely empirical.

Ventricular Flutter and Fibrillation. Ventricular flutter is a prefibrillatory rhythm in which there is still regular ventricular electrical activity at rates of 200-300 beats/min, but there is little or no effective mechanical activity. Ventricular fibrillation represents totally chaotic ventricular electrical activity with no cardiac output (Fig. 5.9). Both of these rhythms are medical emergencies requiring immediate electrical conversion. Ventricular fibrillation is likely to recur, particularly in the patient with ischemic heart disease. Therefore, once the heart is successfully defibrillated, immediate attention must be given to correction of underlying causes and to institution of prophylactic antiarrhythmic therapy with lidocaine or procainamide or both.

Irregular Tachycardias with Narrow or Wide QRS Complexes

Only rarely is a very irregular tachycardia exclusively ventricular. With an irregular tachycardia, widening of the QRS complex is due to either aberrant conduction or ventricular ectopic beats in the presence of another rhythm. Whether the QRS complexes are wide or narrow, the differential diagnosis of an irregular tachycardia is among *atrial fibrillation, multifocal atrial tachycardia, SVT with varying degrees of A-V block,* and *multiple premature beats of atrial, junctional,* or *ventricular origin.*

Atrial Fibrillation. Diagnosis. This is usually easily recognized by its irregularly irregular ventricular response and the undulating baseline between QRS complexes (Fig. 5.10). There is no organized atrial activity. At very fast rates, the ventricular response is less irregular than at slow rates. The fibrillatory waves in the baseline may be almost inapparent ("fine" atrial fibrillation) or may be several millimeters in amplitude ("coarse" atrial fibrillation). Fine fibrillatory waves are seen more commonly in ischemic or hypertensive heart disease, and coarse waves are more common in rheumatic mitral valvular disease. Carotid sinus pressure characteristically results in gradual slowing of the ventricular response without affecting the atrial mechanism or degree of irregularity.

Ashman Phenomenon. Atrial fibrillation may occur with either narrow or wide QRS complexes. Wide complexes are uniformly present if right or left bundle-branch block accompanies the atrial fibrillation. When wide complexes are present intermittently, the distinction must be made between an occasional aberrantly conducted beat and coexisting ventricular premature beats. This can be done by recognizing the *Ashman phenomenon*, that is, that an aberrantly conducted beat often ends a short cycle (R-R interval) that has followed a long cycle (Fig. 5.11). These aberrantly conducted beats almost invariably exhibit a right bundle-branch block pattern. The ventricular origin of wide beats is favored by the absence of the Ashman phenomenon, the presence of a left bundle-branch block pattern, or a difference between the initial 0.04-second vector of the normal and abnormal beats. In addition, ventricular premature beats are likely to have a nearly constant coupling interval with the preceding normal beats and are likely to be followed by a pause. The distinction between aberrancy and ventricular ectopy may be important in deciding whether a patient with atrial fibrillation requires more digitalis or is already showing signs of digitalis excess.

Pathophysiology. Atrial fibrillation usually occurs in patients with heart disease, and it should stimulate attempts to determine the underlying condition. Arteriosclerotic and hypertensive heart dis-

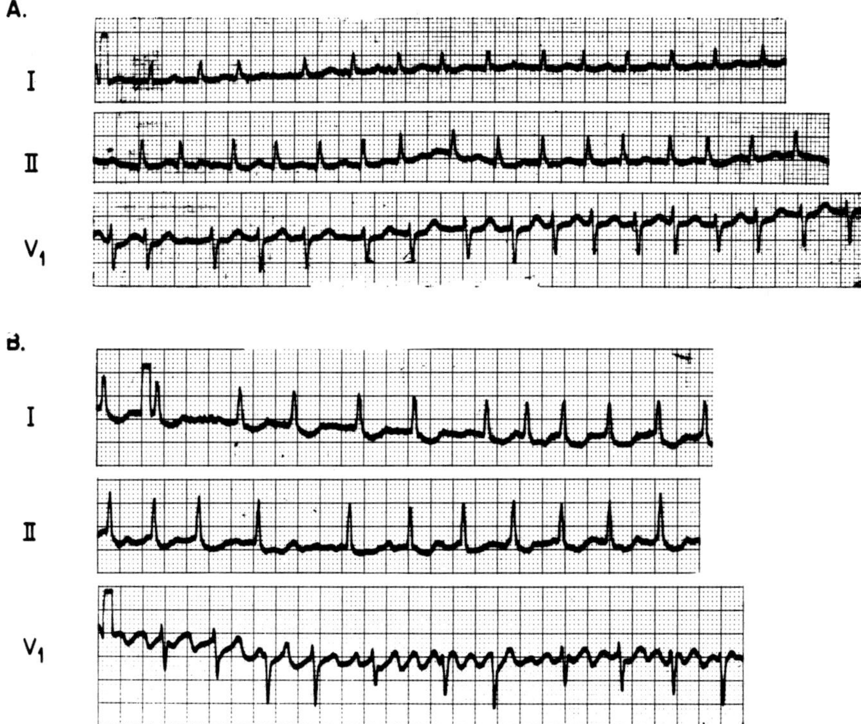

Figure 5.10. Atrial fibrillation. *A,* Irregularly irregular ventricular response with narrow QRS complexes and no clearly definable atrial activity. This is a fine atrial fibrillation with rapid ventricular response. *B,* QRS complexes are narrow and are irregularly irregular. Atrial activity is seen in lead V, as irregular fibrillatory waves bearing no constant relation to QRS complexes. This is coarse atrial fibrillation with rapid ventricular response.

eases are the most common causes, but rheumatic heart disease always must be considered, particularly with mitral stenosis or regurgitation or both. Cardiomyopathy, pericarditis, and certain noncardiac diseases, such as pulmonary embolism, pneumonia, chronic obstructive pulmonary disease, and thyrotoxicosis, are also possible underlying causes.

A small number of patients have *paroxysmal* atrial fibrillation without other evidence of heart disease. These patients are often young, and the onset of fibrillation may be correlated with stress or the use of alcohol or other stimulants. A smaller group of patients may have chronic atrial fibrillation in the absence of any obvious heart disease; this is "lone"

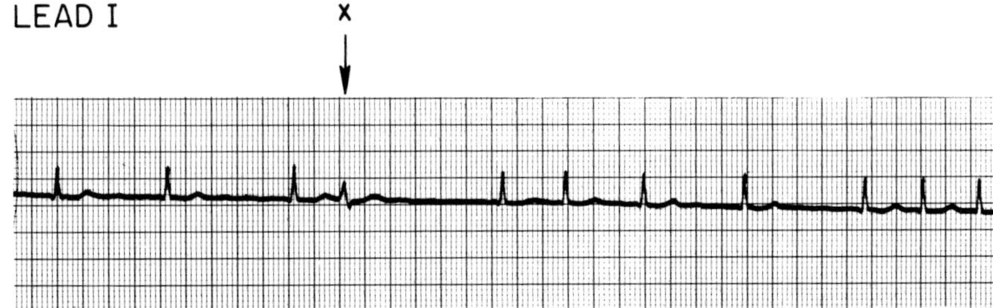

Figure 5.11. Atrial fibrillation with Ashman phenomenon. The ventricular activity is irregularly irregular with no discernible atrial activity. One beat (marked X) is broader than other complexes and has terminal S wave. This beat concludes shortest R-R interval on strip and follows one of longest intervals. This sequence of long interval followed by short interval favors aberrant conduction (often with right bundle-branch block pattern) as shown here. This type of aberrant conduction seen in atrial fibrillation is known as the Ashman phenomenon.

atrial fibrillation and is probably a form of sick sinus syndrome (see pp 89–90).

Treatment. *Digitalis Glycosides.* Digitalis glycosides are the drugs of choice for rate control. Large amounts may be needed, particularly in patients who have atrial fibrillation of recent onset, who previously have not been receiving digitalis, or who are acutely ill. The shorter-acting digitalis preparations offer little advantage over digoxin, and the physician should be familiar with this preparation, which can be used in both acute and chronic situations. In the patient who has not been receiving a digitalis preparation, initial doses of 0.5–0.75 mg of digoxin may be administered intravenously; in the patient who has previously received digitalis, 0.125 or 0.25 mg is the proper dose if the ventricular rate is rapid. Intravenous digoxin begins to exert its effect in 15-30 minutes, and its peak effect occurs in 1½-4 hours. Additional digoxin may be administered every 2-4 hours in increments of 0.125 or 0.25 mg as needed for rate control. Sometimes up to 2 mg is necessary in the first 24 hours. If the heart rate is refractory to digitalis, intravenous propranolol in 1-mg increments may be administered if no contraindications are present; the total dose must not exceed 0.1 mg/kg.

Verapamil. The calcium channel blocking agent verapamil is very effective for control of the ventricular response to atrial fibrillation and is the drug of choice if rapid control of the ventricular response is necessary. It exerts its electrophysiologic effects solely on the A-V node. It may be administered in an intravenous dose of 5-10 mg and it usually will exert its slowing effect in 10 minutes. Its main side effects are hypotension and depression of ventricular function. In some instances, it may cause profound bradycardia, particularly in elderly patients with underlying conduction system disease or prior administration of β-adrenergic blocking drugs. Though it has the advantage over digoxin of being more rapidly acting and more specific in its site of action, its duration of action is shorter (30-60 min) and it usually will not obviate the need to give digitalis glycosides.

"Adequate" control of heart rate usually means a ventricular response of 70-90 beats/min. However, a rapid ventricular response in a patient with atrial fibrillation may be partly a physiologic response to hypoxemia, fever, hypovolemia, congestive heart failure, or other stimuli. Thus, measures to correct these problems should be instituted while administering drugs to slow the ventricular response.

Cardioversion. In most patients with rapid atrial fibrillation, the heart rate is slowed with the measures just mentioned, but atrial fibrillation continues. In about 15-20% of patients with new onset of atrial fibrillation, conversion to sinus rhythm occurs with digitalis, verapamil, propranolol, or simply the passage of time. In another small percentage, the hemodynamic status may deteriorate because of the rapid rate and loss of atrial transport, and these patients should be considered for early emergency synchronized cardioversion. If the patient is unresponsive to therapy, it is best to perform cardioversion early, since the risk of this procedure is substantially increased if it is performed after large doses of digitalis have been administered. Cardioversion has been successful in restoring sinus rhythm at least transiently in about 90% of patients with atrial fibrillation.

Some patients with atrial fibrillation have bradycardia rather than tachycardia. In this situation, digitalis toxicity or intrinsic conduction system disease should be suspected, and digitalis and other drugs that further depress A-V conduction should be administered very cautiously, if at all. Digitalis toxicity is particularly likely if the patient has either a slow but regular ventricular rate (indictating a junctional rhythm, Fig. 5.12) or frequent ventricular premature beats or both. Rarely, pervenous ventricular pacing is required to accelerate the heart rate.

Multifocal Atrial Tachycardia. Diagnosis. This condition is easily confused with atrial fibrillation. It is similar in rate and irregularity, but is distinguished by the presence of organized atrial activity. Characteristically, P waves of three or more configurations occur at varying P-P intervals with variation in P-R intervals as well (Fig. 5.13). The arrhythmia is usually unresponsive to carotid sinus pressure, although some degree of A-V block may be induced. It occurs most commonly in elderly patients with acute or chronic respiratory disease.

Treatment. Treatment is primarily that of the underlying causative respiratory and metabolic abnormalities. The most serious error in the management of this arrhythmia is administration of increasing doses of digitalis glycosides for rate control in the belief that the rhythm is atrial fibrillation. Although it does not appear that the rhythm itself is often due to digitalis toxicity, it does not respond to digitalis, and digitalis toxicity may readily result. If congestive heart failure is present, however, digitalis may be indicated. Antiarrhythmic agents usually do not suppress multifocal atrial tachycardia satisfactorily, though verapamil may occasionally be successful. Efforts must be directed at correcting hypoxemia, hypokalemia, and acid-base disorders. The arrhythmia is associated with a high mortality of 40-50%, primarily because of the critical condition of the patients in whom it is seen.

Wandering atrial pacemaker is a variant of the same rhythm disturbance in that varying P-wave structures are seen, but at a slower rate. Unlike

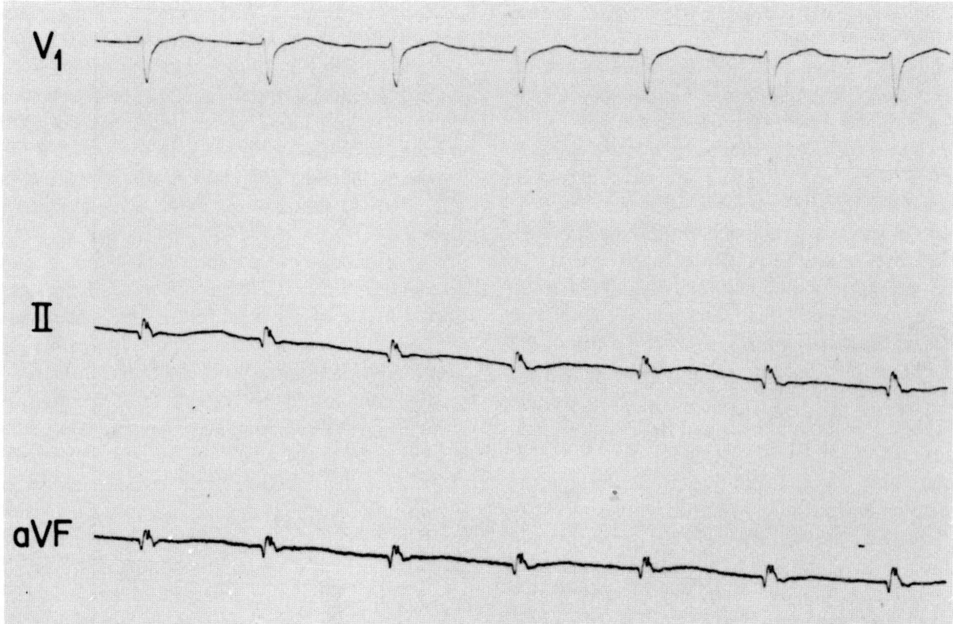

Figure 5.12. Accelerated junctional rhythm due to digitalis toxicity. There is no discernible atrial activity and there is a regular ventricular rate of 70 beats/min with narrow QRS complexes. The patient has been in atrial fibrillation, and increasing doses of digitalis had been given to control ventricular response. This "regularized" rhythm resulted and is due to acceleration of the junctional pacemaker. Atrial mechanism is still atrial fibrillation, and an irregularly irregular ventricular response returned when digitalis was withheld.

multifocal atrial tachycardia, this rhythm may occur in the absence of cardiac or systemic disease and is usually benign.

SVT with Varying Degrees of A-V Block. **Diagnosis.** If the A-V node permits every second, third, or fourth beat to be transmitted from the atrium to the ventricle at different times, an arrhythmia that ordinarily might be a regular SVT, such as atrial flutter, paroxysmal SVT, or ectopic SVT becomes manifested as an irregular ventricular response. The diagnosis depends on identification of atrial activity, as well as appreciation of a recurrent pattern to the irregularity rather than the irregular irregularity of atrial fibrillation or multifocal atrial tachycardia.

Treatment. Treatment is that of the particular supraventricular arrhythmia; however, either digitalis toxicity or intrinsic A-V nodal disease may be present in patients with SVT and variable A-V block. Atrial tachycardia with A-V block must be presumed to be due to digitalis toxicity whenever it occurs in a patient known to be receiving a digitalis preparation.

Atrial or Junctional Premature Beats. Multiple premature beats may simulate a tachyarrhythmia and may produce similar hemodynamic

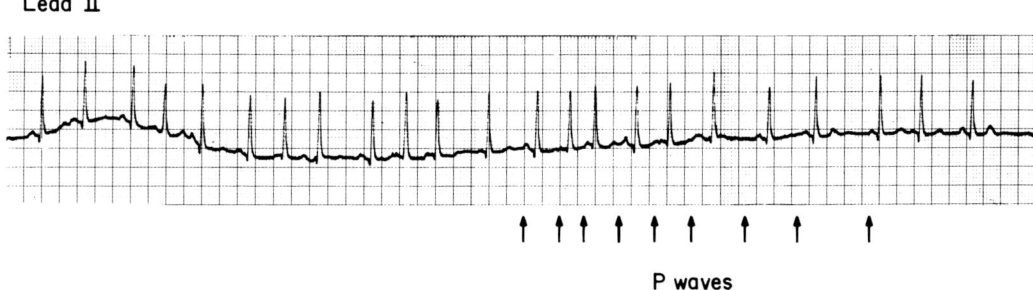

Figure 5.13. Multifocal atrial tachycardia. This is an irregular rhythm with narrow QRS complexes in which every QRS complex is preceded by a P wave. There are, however, several different P-wave morphologies and P-R intervals; this indicates that impulses arise from several different foci in atrium.

consequences if they diminish the number of mechanically effective beats.

Diagnosis. Atrial or junctional premature beats usually have QRS complexes similar to or only slightly different from the QRS complexes of the sinus beats. If they are preceded by upright P waves in leads II, III, and AVF, they are presumed to be atrial; if there is no identifiable atrial activity or if there are P waves preceding or following the QRS complex that are inverted in leads II, III, and AVF, they are presumed to be junctional. Atrial and junctional premature beats that retrogradely depolarize the atrium characteristically reset the sinus pacemaker. Therefore, the interval from the premature beat to the next normally conducted beat is usually approximately equal to the normal R-R interval, that is, there is no compensatory pause.

Treatment. Atrial and junctional premature beats are benign and rarely require treatment. They may, however, indicate the potential development of a more serious supraventricular arrhythmia, such as atrial fibrillation, atrial flutter, or paroxysmal SVT. When multiple atrial or junctional premature beats occur in a patient with a history of sustained or recurrent supraventricular arrhythmia, prophylactic suppression with drugs such as quinidine or propranolol may be indicated.

Ventricular Premature Beats. Diagnosis. These beats, which have wide, sometimes bizarre QRS complexes, must be distinguished from supraventricular premature beats with aberrant conduction. In addition to the absence of preceding atrial activity and the presence of the morphologic features of the QRS complex listed in Table 5.1, ventricular premature beats usually are followed by a compensatory pause, and the resultant interval from the premature beat to the subsequent conducted beat exceeds the normal R-R interval (Fig. 5.14). The interval from the preceding conducted beat to the subsequent conducted beat equals *two* normal R-R intervals. Occasionally, a ventricular premature beat is timed in such a way that the next conducted beat occurs exactly when it should, without a pause. Such a premature beat is said to be *interpolated*, occurring between two normally conducted beats.

Reentrant Beats. Ventricular premature beats are of two types: reentrant and parasystolic. Reentry results from delay in the passage of a normally conducted impulse through an area of the ventricle; delay may be caused by ischemia, fibrosis, inflammation, or other factors. When the impulse finally traverses the area of retarded conduction, it finds the ventricle repolarized and it is discharged prematurely.

Parasystole. In contrast, parasystole is caused by the repetitive discharge of a so-called protected focus in one of the ventricles, which captures the ventricles whenever it finds them susceptible. Most ventricular premature beats are due to reentry.

The coupling interval between a reentrant ventricular premature beat and the preceding normal beat is usually constant, and intervals that vary up to 0.06–0.08 second are still considered ''fixed.'' When no constant coupling intervals occur and the beats are clearly ventricular, parasystole should be suspected. This diagnosis is confirmed by examining a long rhythm strip and finding that the intervals between ectopic beats are whole-number multiples of a common interval. An additional feature of parasystole is that fusion beats are common. Fusion beats have a configuration intermediate between that of ectopic beats and normally conducted beats.

Treatment. Ventricular premature beats originating in the left ventricle usually display a pattern of right bundle-branch block, and those originating in the right ventricle usually exhibit a left bundle-branch block configuration. They are the most common form of cardiac rhythm disturbance, and although they do not necessarily indicate heart disease, they are more common in such patients, particularly those with coronary artery disease. The decision as to whether treatment is required depends on the presence or absence of symptoms, the setting in which they occur, and the presence or absence of certain features that suggest the possibility of a more serious condition.

In general, ventricular premature beats should be suppressed if any of the following is fulfilled, alone or in combination: (*a*) the patient is symptomatic, with palpitations, light-headedness, or syncope presumably related to more serious ventricular arrhyth-

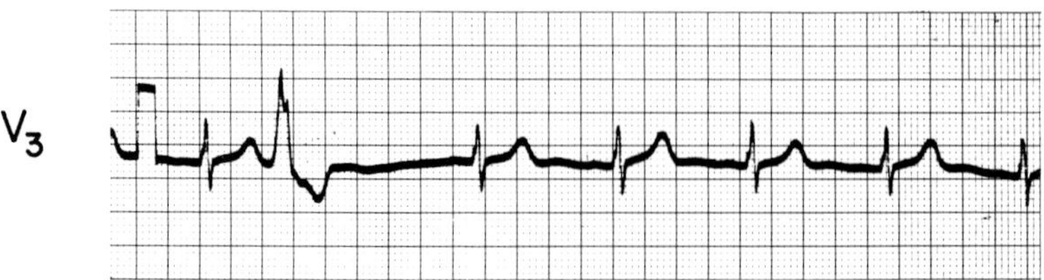

Figure 5.14. Ventricular premature beat. An isolated ventricular premature beat is recorded. There is a full compensatory pause. QRS complex of premature beat has left bundle-branch block pattern.

mias triggered by the premature beats; (*b*) there is evidence of active myocardial ischemia or infarction as indicated by ischemic chest pain or electrocardiographic changes or both; (*c*) digitalis toxicity is suspected; or (*d*) the premature beats occur sequentially, arise from more than one focus, fall close to or on the T wave of the preceding beat, or are very frequent (usually more than 5–10 beats/min).

The drugs used to suppress ventricular premature beats are the same as those discussed for ventricular tachycardia—lidocaine, procainamide, bretylium, phenytoin, propranolol, and quinidine—and attention must be given to the possible role of hypokalemia, hypoxemia, drugs, or mechanical factors in predisposing the heart to ventricular irritability.

Bradycardias

Rhythms with rates less than 60 beats/min are classified as bradycardias. The differential diagnosis is less complex than with the tachyarrhythmias, but the same principles are followed—identification of atrial and ventricular activity and determination of their relation. These rhythm disturbances involve *dysfunction of the sinus or A-V nodes*.

Sinus Bradycardia

Diagnosis. In sinus bradycardia, there is a normal 1:1 relation between P waves and QRS complexes; only the rate is slow. Sinus bradycardia may indicate dysfunction of the sinus node, or it may be a normal, physiologic arrhythmia, especially in well-trained athletes. It also may be drug-induced, particularly by propranolol or other β-adrenergic blockers, and it may be seen in states of heightened vagal tone and in patients with hypothyroidism.

Treatment. Sinus bradycardia usually does not require treatment, unless the slow rate is associated with hypotension, congestive heart failure, or symptoms. If treatment is required, atropine sulfate, 0.5–1.0 mg intravenously, or isoproterenol (Isuprel), 1–2 μg/min intravenously, is the agent of choice. Rarely, transvenous pacing may be required if the bradycardia is profound or refractory to these medications.

Sinus Arrest or Exit Block

Diagnosis. In sinus arrest or exit block, P waves are either absent or only intermittent. If present, each P wave is followed by a QRS complex, but long pauses may be ended by QRS complexes without P waves (*junctional escape beats,* Fig. 5.15). Isolated pauses simulating sinus arrest may be caused by *nonconducted atrial premature beats.* These can be diagnosed by appreciating some deformity in the T wave preceding the pause. This deformity results from superimposition of a premature P wave on a normal T wave.

Treatment. The indication for treating sinus arrest or exit block is the same as that for treating sinus bradycardia. Likewise, treatment is the same, except that sinus arrest or exit block is more often resistant to drug therapy, and if the patient is symptomatic, transvenous pacing is more likely to be required.

A-V Block

Diagnosis. First-degree A-V Block. First-degree A-V block is present if the P-R interval is prolonged beyond 0.20 second but all P waves are followed by a QRS complex.

Second-degree A-V Block. In second- and third-degree A-V block, there are more P waves than QRS complexes. In second-degree block, some P waves are conducted to the ventricles and some are not. This degree of heart block, which is described by the ratio of P waves to QRS complexes (for example, 2:1, 3:2, or 4:3), can be divided into type I (Wenckebach-Mobitz I) and type II (Mobitz II). In type I, the P-R intervals of the conducted beats become progressively longer until a P wave is

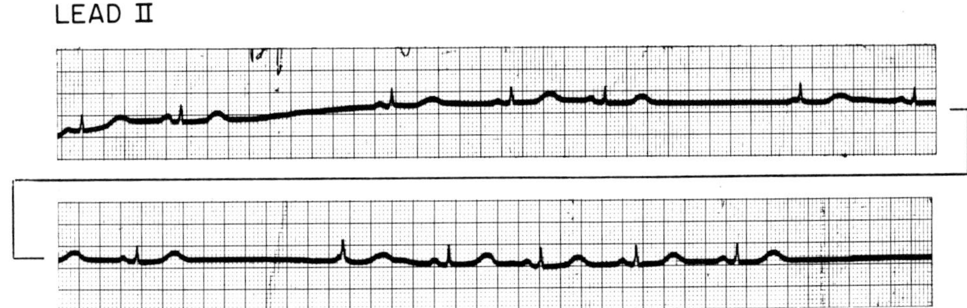

Figure 5.15. Sinus arrest. Sinus rhythm is present with slight sinus arrhythmia. There are several pauses lasting approximately 2 seconds in which no P waves are seen. Two pauses are ended by narrow (supraventricular) complexes that are not preceded by P waves, and then a sinus beat follows. Pauses are due to sinus arrest, and some pauses are terminated by junctional escape beats. If patient's condition is symptomatic during pauses, a pacemaker is indicated.

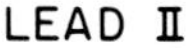

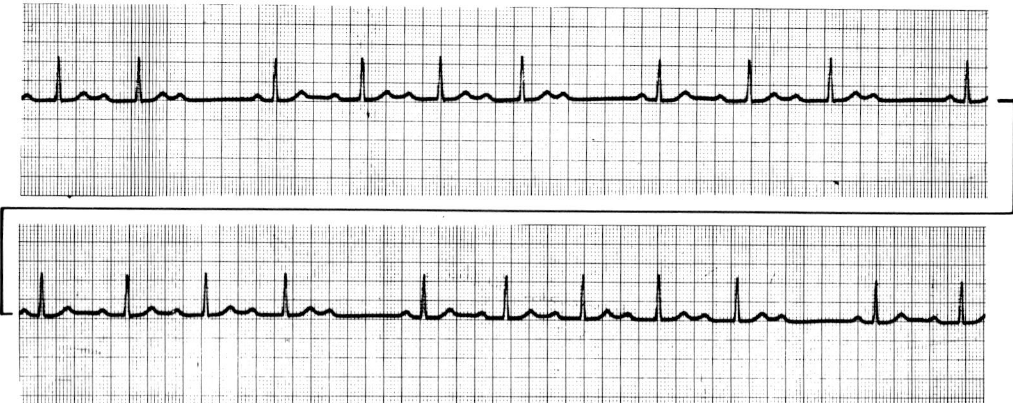

Figure 5.16. Type I (Wenckebach-Mobitz I) second-degree A-V block. There is a regular atrial activity at 72 beats/min. P-R interval becomes progressively prolonged, and every fourth, fifth, or sixth P wave is not conducted to ventricle. QRS complexes are narrow, and R-R interval becomes progressively shorter before each pause.

not conducted (Fig. 5.16). In type II, the P-R intervals of the conducted beats are constant; blocked beats occur without progressive prolongation of the P-R interval (Fig. 5.17). To some extent, these two types of block correspond to disorders at different levels of the conducting system. Type I block usually occurs in the A-V node and type II in the more distal His-Purkinje system. The features of these two types of block are summarized in Table 5.2.

Third-degree A-V Block. In contrast with second-degree block, third-degree block is characterized by total absence of any relation between P waves and QRS complexes (Fig. 5.18). P waves are seen to march through the QRS complexes—sometimes in front of, sometimes buried in, and sometimes following them. The QRS complexes, which are usually regularly spaced, may be relatively narrow, indicating a junctional origin of the subsidiary escape pacemaker, or they may be very wide and clearly ventricular. If the pacemaker is junctional, the ventricular rate may be 40–60 beats/min, a rate that is tolerated well. In contrast, a ventricular escape focus usually has a slower rate (20–40 beats/min) and is more likely to result in symptoms that are due to decreased cardiac output.

In third-degree block, physical findings of A-V dissociation are present. Intermittent cannon waves are seen in the jugular veins, and there is variability

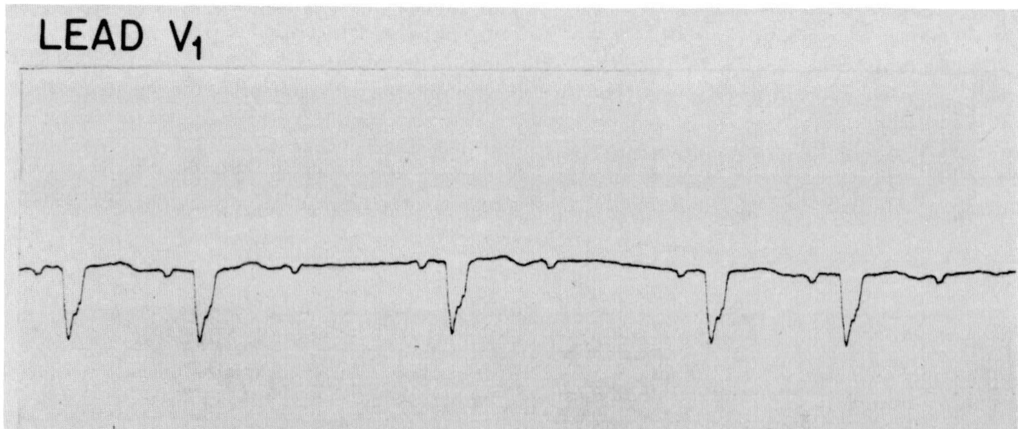

Figure 5.17. Type II (Mobitz II) second-degree A-V block. P-R interval is constant at 0.18 second, and every second or third P wave is not conducted, which results in periods of 3:2 and 2:1 A-V block. QRS complex has left bundle-branch block pattern, indicating disease of His-Purkinje system. Atrial rate is regular at 80 beats/min.

Table 5.2.
Differential Electrocardiographic Features of Atrioventricular Block

Differential Feature	Type I (Wenckebach-Mobitz I)	Type II (Mobitz II)
P-R interval	Progressively prolonged in conducted beats, never normal	Constant in conducted beats, may be normal
QRS complex of conducted beats	Usually normal	Often prolonged, bundle-branch block or hemiblock frequent
Time course	Often transient, sudden asystole rare	More likely chronic, definite risk of sudden asystole
Ventricular rate if complete heart block occurs	Usually 40–50 beats/min because of effective junctional pacemaker	Very slow (ventricular pacemaker) or asystole
Response to drug therapy	Conduction usually improves with atropine or isoproterenol	Poor response
Associated conditions	Digitalis toxicity, inferior myocardial infarction, inflammatory condition involving the atrioventricular node	Anterior myocardial infarction, chronic conduction system disease
Level of conduction abnormality	Atrioventricular node	His-Purkinje system

of the first heart sound and of the systemic blood pressure corresponding to the beat-to-beat changes in the relation of atrial and ventricular systole.

Fascicular Block. Complete heart block is often preceded by block in two of the three fascicles of the bundle branches. Bifascicular block may be manifested by any of the following patterns: (*a*) complete left bundle-branch block; (*b*) right bundle-branch block with block of the left anterior fascicle of the left bundle, giving an electrocardiographic pattern of right bundle-branch block with left axis deviation; or (*c*) right bundle-branch block with block of the left posterior division of the left bundle, giving a pattern of right bundle-branch block with considerable right axis deviation. Right bundle-branch block with left anterior fascicular hemiblock is 10–20 times more common than right bundle-branch block with left posterior hemiblock.

Syncope (Adams-Stokes attacks) in patients with heart block usually is due to profound bradycardia or asystole, but can also be secondary to recurrent ventricular tachycardia or ventricular fibrillation (Fig. 5.19). At slow heart rates, the ventricles tend to repolarize less uniformly, and ventricular tachycardia or fibrillation may result. *Whether symptoms are due to asystole or recurrent ventricular arrhythmias, the treatment of choice is acceleration of the heart rate by transvenous ventricular pacing.* This intervention in the emergency department may be lifesaving.

When Adams-Stokes attacks are caused by recurrent ventricular arrhythmias, the tendency is to administer antiarrhythmic drugs. These may aggravate rather than improve the situation, however, since they suppress the automaticity of the lower escape foci, and they are contraindicated in therapy for complete heart block *unless* the ventricles are electrically paced.

Lesser degrees of heart block do not necessarily require emergency therapy; treatment is dictated by the patient's symptoms and by the setting in which heart block occurs (see p 84 for discussion of heart block in the presence of myocardial infarction).

Treatment. Type I second-degree A-V block is more likely to be transient and to respond to pharmacologic therapy (atropine sulfate or isopro-

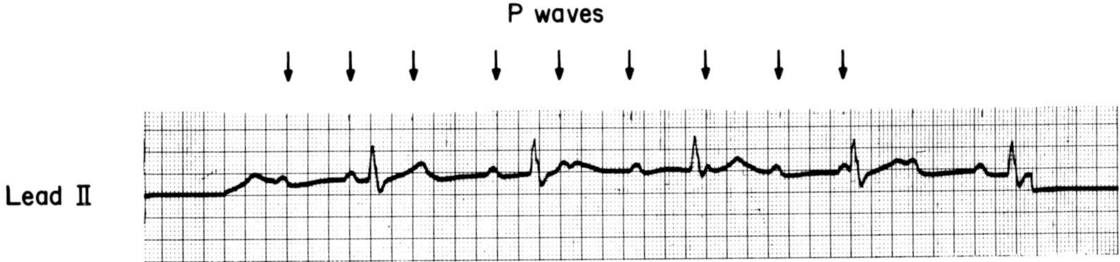

Figure 5.18. Complete heart block. There is no constant relation between P waves and QRS complexes. Atrial rate is 88 beats/min and ventricular escape rate is 39 beats/min. Nonconducted P waves distort T waves as they march through QRS complexes. This rhythm is an indication for a temporary pacemaker.

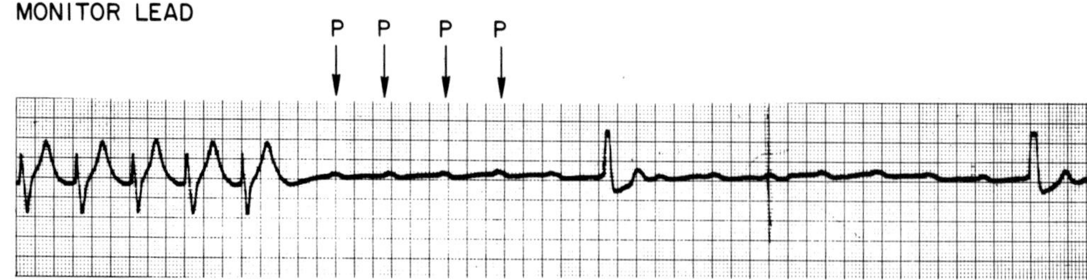

Figure 5.19. Complete heart block. Initially there is a regular tachycardia at 105 beats/min, and then there is sudden loss of ventricular activity with continuation of atrial activity at 105 beats/min. There is a slow, irregular ventricular escape pacemaker at about 15 beats/min. This sudden development of complete heart block was associated with syncope (Adams-Stokes attack).

terenol) than is type II. In any patient with type I block known to be receiving a digitalis preparation, digitalis toxicity should be suspected. Temporary pacing is indicated for type I block only in the presence of hypotension, congestive heart failure, or severe ventricular irritability. Prophylactic pacing is not indicated.

In contrast, patients with type II second-degree A-V block are much more likely to have a chronic disorder of A-V conduction and at some time to have symptomatic bradycardia. Many also have coexisting bundle-branch block. All patients with type II block should receive a temporary transvenous pacemaker, and most require permanent pacing.

An additional therapeutic dilemma is posed by the patient with chronic bifascicular disease without A-V block. It has been our practice to place temporary pacemakers in these patients only if they have had symptoms (syncope or presyncope) or if monitoring reveals intermittent second- or third-degree A-V block. In an acute medical or surgical emergency, patients with first-degree A-V block and bifascicular block of unknown duration should probably also receive a temporary pacemaker; subsequent monitoring or further studies of the A-V conduction may then help determine whether permanent pacing is indicated.

ARRHYTHMIAS IN SPECIAL SITUATIONS

Myocardial Infarction

At least 90% of patients with acute myocardial infarction seen in the hospital experience some disturbance of cardiac rhythm, which usually occurs soon after infarction. For example, the likelihood of ventricular fibrillation is estimated to be 15 times greater in the first 4 hours after the onset of infarction than in the next 8, and 25 times greater than in the 12–24 hours after infarction. Arrhythmias are also more likely to occur in patients with severe left ventricular dysfunction due to the infarct.

Table 5.3 summarizes the incidence of arrhythmias in four series of hospitalized patients with acute myocardial infarction. These arrhythmias are managed in generally the same way as in patients without infarction. However, it is even more important to treat tachyarrhythmias and ventricular ectopy promptly, because the increased oxygen consumption caused by the tachycardia may increase the size of the infarct, and ischemic myocardium is more unstable electrically and more susceptible to the development of life-threatening arrhythmias.

Several specific circumstances should be considered.

Table 5.3.
Arrhythmias in Patients with Acute Myocardial Infarction[a]

Rhythm[b]	Average Incidence	Range
	%	
Ventricular		
Extrasystoles	90	45–100
Tachycardia	23	6–30[c]
Fibrillation	5	2–10
Supraventricular		
Sinus tachycardia	35	30-43
Atrial and nodal tachycardia	8	4-11
Atrial fibrillation	11	7-16
Atrial flutter	4	2-5
Sinus bradycardia	18	11-26
Atrioventricular block		
Second degree	7	4-10
Third degree	7	4-10

[a] Based on four series totaling 791 patients (Julian et al., Kimball and Killip, Lown et al., and Meltzer and Kitchell).
[b] Many patients have more than one rhythm disturbance.
[c] Many series do not distinguish between ventricular tachycardia (rate > 100 beats/min) and accelerated idioventricular rhythm (rate < 100 beats/min). In our experience, about 8–10% of patients have ventricular tachycardia and 10–15% have accelerated idioventricular rhythm.

Bradycardia with Inferior Myocardial Infarction

Pathophysiology. Bradycardia is likely to develop in patients with inferior myocardial infarction because of compromise of circulation to A-V nodal arteries and because of increased vagal tone. Recent studies have questioned whether such bradycardia should be treated to prevent electrical and hemodynamic deterioration and have suggested that bradycardia is not itself dangerous and even may be desirable. When bradycardia occurs with hypotension, however, as it frequently does in the early phase of infarction, the heart rate should be accelerated. Bradycardia should also be treated when congestive heart failure or significant ventricular irritability is present.

Treatment. Atropine. When heightened vagal tone is the apparent cause (as suggested by hypotension coexisting with diaphoresis, cool and mottled extremities, nausea, vomiting, tenesmus, or tracheal burning) and the situation is not urgent, atropine sulfate is the drug of choice, 0.4–0.6 mg intravenously every 10–15 minutes until vagal manifestations have been reversed or a total of 2 mg has been administered. The most serious complication of atropine therapy is potentially hazardous tachycardia from an excessive dose. Atropine sulfate also may cause urinary retention, and it may cause a toxic reaction of the central nervous system manifested in its most severe form as an agitated, hallucinatory psychosis that may last for days. Because these complications are more common in elderly patients, the emergency physician should rarely administer more than 1 mg to patients over 65 years old.

Isoproterenol. In more urgent situations, isoproterenol or epinephrine, 1–3 μg/min, can be administered as a continuous intravenous infusion. These drugs must be used with caution because they increase myocardial oxygen demands considerably and may extend the area of myocardial ischemia or infarction. They should be used only until a temporary pacemaker can be placed.

Temporary Pacing. The most reliable means of accelerating the heart rate is temporary transvenous pacing, which should be undertaken if the bradycardia is not quickly responsive to pharmacologic therapy or if complications of drug therapy occur. Pacing may be done from the right atrium if A-V nodal function is normal—thus preserving the benefit of atrial transport—or from the right ventricle if A-V block is present. The latter is generally preferred in emergency situations because of the greater ease in positioning a temporary pacing wire in the ventricle to achieve reliable pacing.

Ventricular Premature Beats

Prophylactic Lidocaine. In patients with acute myocardial infarction, all ventricular premature beats should be suppressed because of the risk of ventricular fibrillation. Since up to 50% of instances of ventricular fibrillation in acute infarction occur without premonitory ventricular ectopy, it has been argued that prophylactic antiarrhythmic agents should be used. In several studies testing this hypothesis with procainamide, quinidine, or lidocaine, a decrease in serious ventricular arrhythmias has been seen, but with no change in survival in the setting of a coronary unit.

Nonetheless, it has been our practice routinely to administer intravenous lidocaine prophylactically (50- to 100-mg bolus followed by a continuing 1–3 mg/min) in all patients in whom an acute myocardial infarction is definitely present or in whom the suspicion is high. The rationale for this is that even though the patient is likely to be resuscitated successfully from ventricular tachycardia or fibrillation, the occurrence of such an arrhythmia is likely to have an adverse effect in a number of other ways such as the size of the infarct, the perfusion of other organs, and the patient's psyche. It, therefore, seems the most prudent course to prevent these arrhythmias if at all possible. Prophylactic drugs should not be administered to patients with second- or third-degree A-V block unless a pacemaker is in place.

If patients have ventricular ectopy after initiation of lidocaine therapy, the first step would be to give another bolus of 50-75 mg of lidocaine and increase the infusion rate by 1 mg/min (provided there are no signs of lidocaine toxicity). If there is still ventricular ectopy present after realizing an infusion rate of 4 mg/min (or signs of lidocaine toxicity), then either procainamide or bretylium should be added, as outlined in the previous section on the treatment of ventricular arrhythmias.

A-V Conduction Abnormalities

Inferior Myocardial Infarction. Inferior myocardial infarction may be associated with transient abnormalities of A-V conduction, such as first-degree block, type I second-degree block, and rarely, third-degree block. These abnormalities, which are due to either increased vagal tone or reversible ischemia of the A-V node, are usually transient and do not appear to alter prognosis. Atropine sulfate may reverse the component of A-V block that is due to vagotonia. Ventricular pacing is not recommended unless hypotension, congestive heart failure, or ventricular irritability exist in the presence of bradycardia. Even third-degree block may be well-tolerated, since the junctional pacemaker usually provides an adequate heart rate, but pacing is indicated if the escape rate is inadequate.

Anterior Myocardial Infarction. Anterior infarction, on the other hand, may be associated

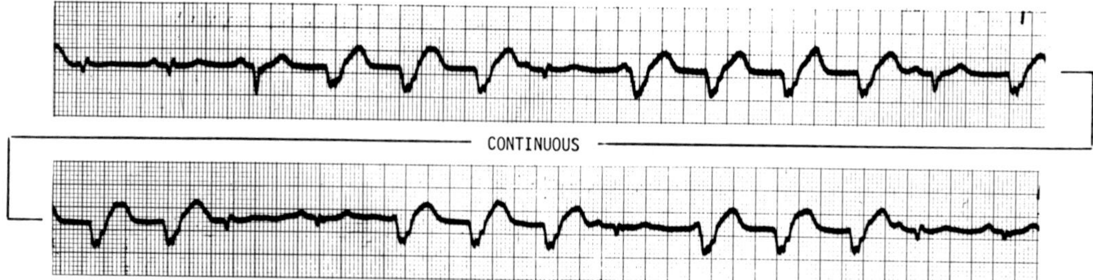

Figure 5.20. Idioventricular rhythm. This patient had recent inferior-wall myocardial infarction. There is an accelerated ventricular pacemaker with rate of 85 beats/min, which is slightly faster than sinus rate. The two pacemakers are competing, and the patient alternates between sinus rhythm and idioventricular rhythm. Ventricular origin of rhythm is confirmed by the fusion beat, which initiates first period of idioventricular rhythm. This rhythm is usually benign and does not require treatment unless patient's hemodynamic status is compromised or unless rhythm accelerates to ventricular tachycardia.

with bundle-branch block and higher degrees of A-V block that carry a grave prognosis. This prognosis is dictated by the fact that conduction abnormalities in anterior infarction usually indicate a large area of myocardial damage, and consequently, coincident severe ventricular failure is common. Some deaths, however, are related to sudden asystole due to the failure of an escape junctional or ventricular pacemaker to emerge when heart block develops. For this reason, temporary ventricular pacing is indicated in any patient with anterior infarction and complete heart block.

Indications for Emergency Pacing. The emergency physician should arrange for a prophylactic transvenous pacemaker in any patient with anterior infarction and evidence of *new* bifascicular block or with type II second-degree A-V block. Although prophylactic pacing has not yet been shown to alter survival in these patients, it can be accomplished at low risk, and it may avoid the need for emergency pacemaker placement. It also may provide a smoother hemodynamic transition with the onset of heart block. Because of the risk of competition with conducted or premature beats, ventricular pacing in patients with myocardial infarction should always be of the demand type.

Accelerated Idioventricular Rhythm

This is a slow ventricular rhythm with a rate between 60 and 100 beats/min, which results from a combination of acceleration of an ectopic ventricular pacemaker and slowing of the rate of the sinus node (Fig. 5.20). It occurs most commonly in inferior myocardial infarction and usually appears as an end-diastolic rhythm lasting from 4 to 30 beats. It is generally well-tolerated and appears to be benign. Occasionally, it may herald or be accompanied by other more serious ventricular arrhythmias requiring treatment. If the rhythm is well-tolerated and is unaccompanied by other more serious ventricular ectopy, therapy is not needed. If suppression is required, increasing the sinus rate with atropine sulfate or pacing may be successful, but frequently, active suppression with the drugs used to treat ventricular ectopy may be necessary.

Digitalis Toxicity

Between 20 and 30% of hospitalized patients who have been receiving digitalis may have digitalis toxicity. Virtually every known rhythm disturbance can result from this complication; Table 5.4 lists the incidence of various arrhythmias in four series of patients. These arrhythmias are a manifestation of the ability of digitalis to increase automaticity and to decrease conduction.

Table 5.4.
Arrhythmias as Manifestations of Digitalis Toxicity[a]

Rhythm[b]	Average Incidence	Range
	%	
Ventricular premature beats (often multifocal)	63	47–85
Second- or third-degree atrioventricular block	21	11-40
Nonparoxysmal junctional tachycardia	17	6-30
Junctional escape rhythm (usually with atrial fibrillation)	16	5-35
Atrial tachycardia (with or without block)	10	6-12
Ventricular tachycardia	10	4-18
Atrial flutter or fibrillation	7	6-13
Sinus arrest or exit block	4	3-5

[a] Based on four series totaling 392 patients (Beller et al., Chung, Resnekov, and Rios et al.).
[b] Many patients have more than one rhythm disturbance.

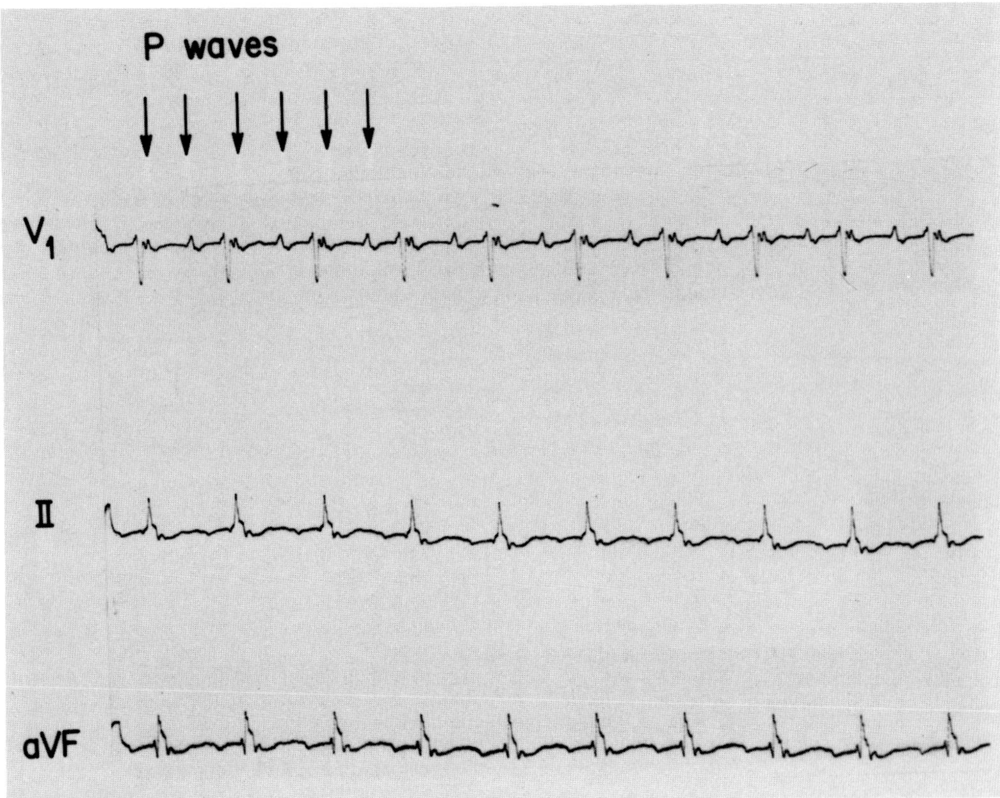

Figure 5.21. Atrial tachycardia with 2:1 A-V block. Atrial rate is 200 beats/min and ventricular rate is 100 beats/min. Nonconducted P wave is apparent in initial portion of each ST segment. This rhythm should be presumed to be due to digitalis toxicity.

Treatment

Digitalis Adjustment. Treatment of these arrhythmias is similar to that when they occur in the absence of digitalis toxicity, with a few notable exceptions. Administration of digitalis glycosides should be stopped immediately. In some instances, it may be difficult to be sure of the role of digitalis, but if there is any suspicion at all, digitalis should be withheld. Atrial tachycardia with block (Fig. 5.21) is perhaps the most difficult rhythm to judge in this regard; it is often secondary to digitalis intoxication, but if it is not due to digitalis excess it may respond to digitalis therapy.

Potassium. Potassium deficiency commonly precipitates or aggravates the arrhythmic manifestations of digitalis toxicity, and potassium replacement is of prime importance in therapy. If the serum potassium level is low, potassium should be infused intravenously at a rate of 10–20 mEq/hr to raise the serum level to 4.5–5.0 mEq/liter. The one toxic manifestation of digitalis that should not be treated aggressively with potassium is A-V block (except paroxysmal atrial tachycardia with block), since it may be aggravated by elevating potassium levels to above normal. Even in this case, however, potassium replacement is indicated if the serum potassium is low.

Phenytoin and Lidocaine. In the presence of digitalis toxicity, ventricular premature beats and ventricular tachycardia are ominous and must be treated promptly. Phenytoin is the drug of choice (Table 5.5). Lidocaine is also effective, and propranolol may be successful in the absence of overt congestive heart failure. Procainamide also may be effective if the other agents fail, though rarely is this necessary unless the patient has a preexisting tendency to ventricular arrhythmias. Quinidine should be used with great caution (if at all) in this situation because of its well-documented capacity for elevating the serum digoxin level. Worsening of ventricular ectopy in the presence of digitalis toxicity also has been reported following the administration of bretylium.

Cardioversion. Cardioversion usually is contraindicated in the presence of digitalis toxicity because of the risk of precipitating an even more serious arrhythmia. In rare instances, cardioversion

Table 5.5.
Agents Commonly Administered Intravenously for Emergency Treatment of Arrhythmias

Drug	Dosage	Indications	Complications
Atropine sulfate	0.5–1.0 mg initially, not to exceed 2.0 mg total	Symptomatic sinus bradycardia or atrioventricular block	Tachycardia Central nervous system toxicity Urinary retention
Digoxin	0.25–0.50 mg initially, with 0.125–0.25 mg increments to total of 1.0–2.0 mg	Rate control in rapid atrial fibrillation Rate control in atrial flutter (do not exceed 0.75 mg if cardioversion indicated) Conversion of paroxysmal SVT (in absence of atrioventricular block)	Ventricular arrhythmias Atrioventricular block
Phenytoin sodium (Dilantin)	100 mg every 5 min, not to exceed 1 gm total	Ventricular arrhythmias in presence of digitalis toxicity Refractory ventricular arrhythmias when lidocaine and procainamide ineffective SVT due to digitalis toxicity	Hypotension Bradycardia Central nervous system toxicity
Lidocaine (Xylocaine)	50 to 100-mg bolus followed by 1–4 mg/min continuous infusion	Ventricular arrhythmias (treatment of choice) Refractory paroxysmal SVT (occasionally successful)	Central nervous system toxicity Heart block or sinus arrest (rare)
Procainamide	100 mg every 5 min, not to exceed 1 gm total; 1-4 μg/min continuous infusion	Ventricular arrhythmias refractory to lidocaine Refractory SVT (rarely)	Hypotension Congestive heart failure Heart block
Propranolol	1 mg every 5 min, not to exceed 10 mg total	Rate control in atrial fibrillation or atrial flutter refractory to digitalis Conversion of paroxysmal SVT or atrial flutter Ventricular arrhythmias refractory to other agents	Congestive heart failure Hypotension Bradycardia Bronchospasm
Verapamil	5-10 mg i.v. over 3 min, may repeat in 30 min	Conversion of paroxysmal SVT Rate control in AF and atrial flutter	Hypotension Congestive heart failure Bradycardia
Bretylium	300 mg i.v. over 5-10 min, rarely continuous infusion 1–2 mg/min	Refractory ventricular arrhythmias	Hypotension Rarely worsening of ventricular ectopy

may be necessary to convert a tachycardia, in which case the risk can be lessened by prior administration of phenytoin or lidocaine.

Digoxin Antibodies and Other Agents. Other agents, such as magnesium and ethylenediaminetetraacetic acid (EDTA), have also been used to treat digitalis toxicity, but conventional antiarrhythmic therapy and correction of metabolic abnormalities usually suffice. The administration of digoxin-specific antibodies to reverse the effects of digitalis directly appears promising, particularly in instances of massive overdose.

Pacemaker-related Arrhythmias

Fixed Rate Pacemakers

In patients with fixed-rate ventricular pacemakers and preservation of normal sinus and A-V nodal function, there is a potential for competition between the intrinsic pacemaker and the artificial pacemaker. Although such competition rarely provokes serious ventricular arrhythmias, it may do so in the presence of ischemia or ectopic beats. With the increasing use of demand pacemakers, this is now seldom a problem.

Ventricular Demand Pacemakers

Ventricular demand pacemakers are of two types: "R wave inhibited" in which no pacemaker spike is seen if the ventricle is spontaneously depolarizing at a rate faster than the preset rate of the pacemaker, and "R wave synchronous," in which each spontaneously occurring QRS complex discharges the pacemaker and is deformed by a pacemaker spike. Both types pace the heart when the heart rate falls below the present rate of the unit.

R-Wave Inhibited Pacemakers. The R-wave inhibited pacemaker has the advantage that it permits interpretation of structural changes in the QRS complex, ST segment, and T wave in normally conducted beats, as in cases of suspected myocardial infarction. Its disadvantage is that it may be difficult to differentiate between a nonfunctioning pacemaker and one that is appropriately suppressed by a faster intrinsic heart rate. Slowing the heart rate with carotid sinus pressure may enable paced beats to emerge, and many recent models can be converted temporarily to a fixed rate by applying a magnet directly over the unit.

R-Wave Synchronous Pacemakers. Since the R-wave synchronous pacemaker shows a pacemaker spike in each QRS complex, its function can be assessed easily. Its major disadvantage is that the QRS complex is deformed by the pacemaker artifact, making it difficult to detect any change in the QRS complex, ST segment, or T wave. The location of the pacemaker spike must be scrutinized to determine whether it initiates or follows the beginning of the QRS complex, thus indicating if the beat is paced or spontaneous. If the patient has spontaneous tachycardia, it may appear to be pacemaker-induced unless this fact is appreciated.

Additionally, all demand pacemakers have a refractory period that is usually about 400 msec, during which they will not sense a beat and will not discharge. In the presence of a spontaneous tachyarrhythmia, this can create a confusing electrocardiographic tracing in which there are conducted beats with pacemaker spikes, normally conducted beats without a pacemaker artifact, and perhaps paced beats as well. These must be analyzed carefully, and they do not necessarily indicate pacemaker failure.

Pacemaker Failure

Pacemaker failure is usually manifested by slowing of the paced rate, failure to sense spontaneous beats (hence converting a demand pacemaker to a fixed mode), or failure to capture the ventricle (Fig. 5.22). Older models may accelerate when failure occurs, causing ventricular tachycardia. Atrial pacing, either alone or as part of a dual chamber system, is becoming more widely employed. The atrial electrode may either sense or pace. It is always wise to get an x-ray of a patient with a pacemaker if you suspect pacemaker malfunction. This will give valuable information regarding electrode site, position, possible wire fractures and also the type of pacing unit. It may also be possible to identify the type of pacemaker from the patient's identification card in addition to the radiographic appearance of the unit and to obtain detailed information from the manufacturer regarding the features of the particular device.

Wolff-Parkinson-White Syndrome and Other Preexcitation Syndromes

Types

Patients with this syndrome or a variant have one or more anomalous conduction pathways that bypass all or a portion of the normal A-V junctional system. When conduction occurs through the bypass tract, the electrocardiogram has the characteristic features of a *short P-R interval*, a *Δ-wave*, and a *wide QRS complex* (Fig. 5.23). Three types are distinguished on the basis of the orientation of the Δ-wave: (*a*) type A, in which the Δ-wave is anteriorly directed and is positive in leads V_1 and V_6, creating a pattern that resembles right bundle-branch block; (*b*) type B, in which the Δ-wave is posteriorly directed and is negative in lead V_1 and positive in Lead V_6, creating a pattern that resembles left bundle-branch block; and (*c*) type C, which includes patients who are not easily classified as having type A or type B. In other forms of preexcitation syndrome due to other types of bypass pathways, the P-R interval may be shortened without change in the QRS complex or there may be a wide QRS complex with Δ-wave without P-R interval shortening.

Patients with Wolff-Parkinson-White syndrome may have normal conduction patterns at some times and abnormal patterns at other times. During abnormal conduction, QRS patterns may simulate those in myocardial infarction. There may also be repolarization abnormalities simulating ischemia.

A. Lead II

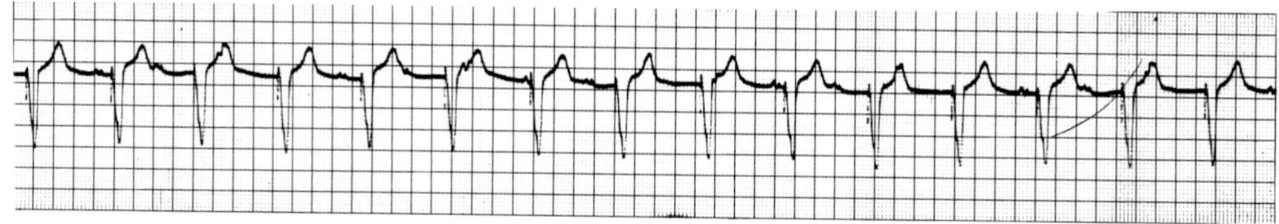

B. Lead II

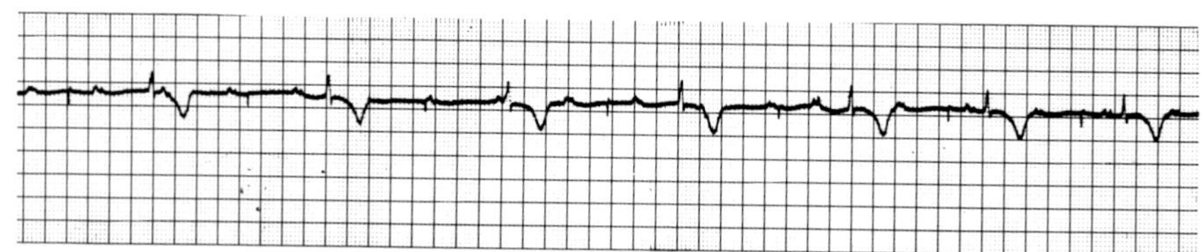

Figure 5.22. Ventricular pacemaker with pacemaker failure. *A,* A demand ventricular pacemaker is firing at 72 beats/min with 1:1 capture of ventricle. Atrial rate is 95 beats/min and P waves march through QRS complexes without being conducted to ventricle (complete heart block is present). This is a right ventricular endocardial pacemaker, and paced beats have left bundle-branch block pattern. *B,* In same patient, pacemaker rate is still 72 beats/min, but none of paced beats now results in ventricular depolarization. Atrial rate is still 95 beats/min, and there is junctional escape rhythm at about 40 beats/min. This is pacemaker failure, which was due to perforation of right ventricle by pacemaker wire.

Treatment of Arrhythmias

Paroxysmal SVT. The availability of two or more pathways for conduction from the atria to the ventricles creates a situation in which a *reentry* or *reciprocating tachycardia* may occur. The most common manifestation of this is paroxysmal SVT. The QRS complexes are usually normal during such a tachycardia, indicating antegrade conduction through normal pathways and retrograde conduction through the anomalous pathway. If P waves are visible, they will follow the QRS complex and be of retrograde fashion (i.e., inverted in leads II, III, and F). Treatment of this arrhythmia is similar to that described previously, with the exception that the rate may be more rapid in patients with Wolff-Parkinson-White syndrome, and the tachycardia may be more resistant to therapy. Digoxin is often effective because of its effect on A-V conduction, but it does not affect conduction in the bypass pathway. The use of digoxin may, however, be hazardous if the patient also is prone to atrial fibrillation with a rapid ventricular response (see below). Propranolol, other β-adrenergic blocking drugs, and verapamil also have been found effective. Quinidine and procainamide have been particularly effective in many difficult cases because they have been shown to affect conduction in the bypass tract. Because of symptomatic recurrences, many of these patients require long-term antiarrhythmic prophylaxis, at times with several agents. A small number may require either permanent pacing or resection of the anomalous pathway. Patients with difficult-to-control or life-threatening arrhythmias are candidates for electrophysiologic studies for select appropriate therapy.

Atrial Fibrillation. Atrial fibrillation also is seen in patients with Wolff-Parkinson-White syndrome. It is particularly dangerous in these patients because conduction of impulses to the ventricle may be by means of the rapidly conducting bypass pathway rather than through the A-V node. Ventricular rates up to 300 beats/min may occur, and may precipitate hemodynamic collapse, although young patients may tolerate such rates remarkably well. The QRS complexes are aberrant because of antegrade conduction in the anomalous pathway. Digitalis and verapamil are often unsuccessful in slowing the ventricular response and may in fact result in a faster ventricular rate. This is the one situation in which both digitalis and verapamil are *contraindicated* for the control of the ventricular response in atrial fibrillation. Lidocaine, procainamide, quinidine, and cardioversion are the treatments of choice.

Sick Sinus Syndrome

This is not a single arrhythmia, but a group of arrhythmias. It deserves special mention because the treatment of a given arrhythmia in this context may be slightly different from its treatment if it occurred alone. The sick sinus syndrome usually occurs in elderly patients, who often have no other evidence of heart disease. These patients may have periods of sinus bradycardia or sinus arrest that frequently

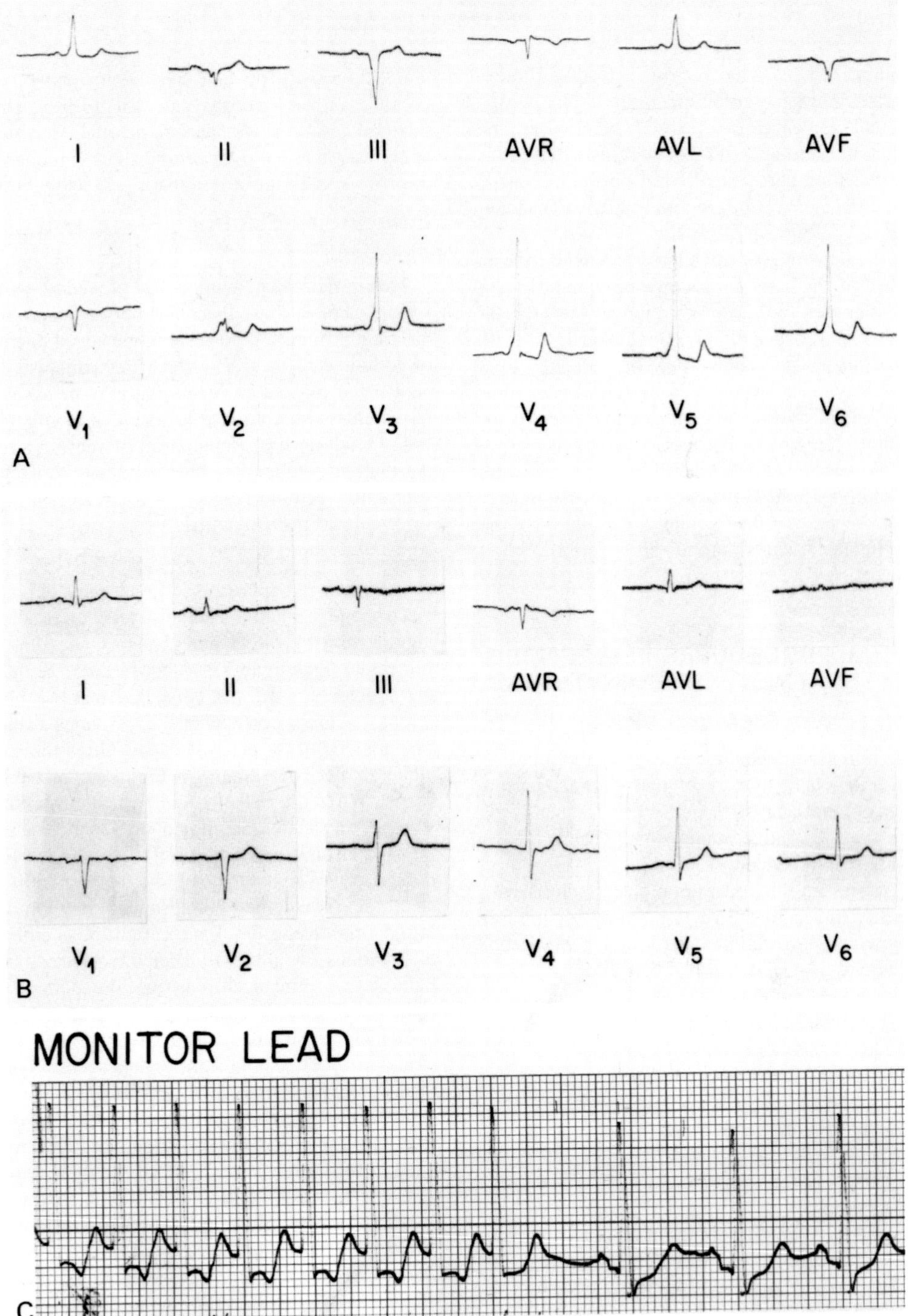

Figure 5.23. Type A Wolff-Parkinson-White syndrome. *A,* Classic findings of Wolff-Parkinson-White syndrome are illustrated in this electrocardiogram from patient with recurrent paroxysmal atrial tachycardia. P-R interval is 0.12 second and there is a Δ-wave that is anteriorly and superiorly directed. QRS complex in leads II, III, and aVF has "pseudoinfarct" pattern. Abnormal conduction pattern was intermittent, and there were no inferior Q waves when conduction pattern was normal. *B,* Electrocardiogram from same patient. Conduction pattern is now normal and Wolff-Parkinson-White syndrome cannot be diagnosed. *C,* Monitor lead from same patient showing brief run of paroxysmal atrial tachycardia at 180 beats/min. Note narrow QRS complex and normal conduction pattern during this episode. This is true in about 85% of cases of SVT with Wolff-Parkinson-White syndrome and indicates that antegrade conduction is through the A-V node (normal pathway) and that retrograde conduction uses the anomalous pathway, thus completing the reentry cycle.

are punctuated by atrial tachyarrhythmias (bradycardia-tachycardia syndrome). There is also a high associated incidence of A-V nodal and His-Purkinje dysfunction. The spectrum of tachyarrhythmias is wide, including paroxysmal atrial fibrillation, atrial flutter, atrial tachycardia, and multifocal atrial tachycardia.

In patients with sick sinus syndrome who have an atrial tachyarrhythmia, profound symptomatic bradycardia may develop on termination of the arrhythmia; this may occur either spontaneously or with therapy. Such a possibility may be indicated by a history of syncopal episodes or by evidence of sinus or A-V nodal dysfunction on previous electrocardiograms. Negatively chronotropic agents, especially propranolol and verapamil, must be used with great caution in these patients. Cardioversion may be risky because of the likelihood that there will be no spontaneous sinus activity after conversion. If cardioversion is required, a prophylactic temporary pacing catheter should be used.

SPECIAL PROCEDURES IN DIAGNOSIS AND TREATMENT OF ARRHYTHMIAS

Carotid Sinus Pressure

This important technique is used in the differential diagnosis and therapy of many atrial tachyarrhythmias, and lack of response can frequently be ascribed to its faulty application. The following steps are recommended.

1. Attach an electrocardiographic monitor with the ability to record the rhythm. Insert an intravenous line and have equipment for emergency defibrillation and pacing at hand.
2. In elderly patients, auscultate the carotid arteries for evidence of a stenotic bruit. If one is heard, do not apply carotid sinus pressure.
3. Extend the patient's neck as much as possible, using a small pillow or some folded towels placed behind the base of the neck and shoulders. Rotate the patient's head slightly away from the side to be compressed. These maneuvers expose the carotid sinus maximally.
4. Locate the area of the carotid sinus, which is at the carotid bifurcation just below the angle of the jaw. The carotid sinus is usually at the point of maximal palpable carotid pulsation.
5. Apply light pressure first. If there is no response or no adverse effect, more pressure—enough to cause the patient slight discomfort—may be applied. Firm pressure should be exerted for 5–10 seconds and released immediately on evidence of a change in rhythm. If there is no effect, pressure may be reapplied, especially after edrophonium chloride or digitalis had been administered to increase vagal tone.
6. If pressure on one side is ineffective, exert pressure on the opposite side. At no time should bilateral carotid sinus pressure be applied. Usually, compression of the right carotid sinus is more likely to prove successful in terminating an arrhythmia.

Intracardiac Electrode Placement

Indication

This is an extremely important procedure that has several applications. Placement of an electrode in the right atrium to record activity enables diagnosis of complicated or obscure tachyarrhythmias. Right ventricular placement for pacing may be lifesaving in patients with complete heart block or other profound bradycardias. Rapid atrial or ventricular pacing may also be applied therapeutically to suppress ventricular ectopic activity or to convert a supraventricular tachyarrhythmia.

Technique

The preferred approach for temporary pervenous electrode placement is via the subclavian or internal jugular vein by direct percutaneous puncture (see Illustrated Technique 8). Many flexible, semifloating pacemakers are available that may be passed through a large polyethylene intravenous catheter. The position of the electrode can be monitored with either an electrocardiograph (Fig. 5.24) or a fluoroscope. When only electrocardiographic monitoring is used, the electrode should be advanced slowly into the atrium, and the point at which ventricular potentials are first recorded should be noted. The electrode should then be advanced 2–4 cm more into the right ventricle. Except in the most emergent of situations, we prefer to place the electrode under fluoroscopic guidance to assure the optimal and most stable pacing position.

The electrode usually can be positioned in the atrium from either the right or left venous system. Stable ventricular positioning, however, is often better achieved from the left side. The tip of the electrode should be directed slightly downward and fixed in the trabeculae carneae of the right ventricle so that it does not float freely with each contraction. It usually is possible to find an area with a pacing threshold of 1–2 milliamperes that will accurately sense spontaneous ventricular depolarization. The optimal pacing rate for each patient must be determined individually. Rates of 90–100 impulses/min usually maximize cardiac output if congestive heart failure or hypotension is the indication for pacemaker placement, although lower rates often are desirable in patients with ischemia or if the electrode has been placed for prophylactic purposes.

Complications

The diaphragm may be paced with right atrial pacing; pacing of the diaphragm or of the intercos-

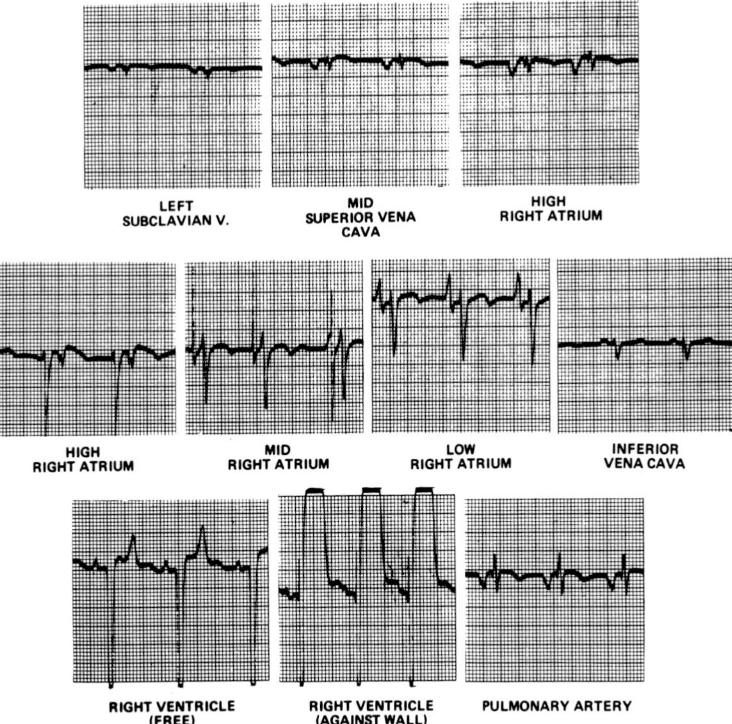

Figure 5.24. Electrocardiographic monitoring of electrode placement. With external end of pacemaker attached to lead V of electrocardiograph by means of alligator clip, tracings can be recorded for various locations to guide in bedside pacemaker placement. Of particular importance are large atrial deflections obtained with electrode in atrium and large intracavitary QRS complex (similar to aVR) with electrode in ventricle. Injury current is obtained with electrode against right ventricular wall (optimal position for ventricular pacing). (Reproduced by permission, from Bing HL, McDowell JW, Hantman J, et al. *N Engl J Med,* 1972;287:651.)

tal muscles with ventricular pacing may indicate perforation of the ventricular wall or may result from excessive current. If the pacemaker wire has perforated the ventricle, it usually malfunctions, that is, it fails to capture or sense or both. This is successfully managed by withdrawing the pacemaker until pacing is restored, and there is rarely sufficient bleeding to cause cardiac tamponade. Rarely, perforation of the ventricular septum also may occur. This results in pacing of the left ventricle, which is indicated by a right bundle-branch block pattern on the electrocardiogram and a widely but physiologically split second sound. Right ventricular pacing results in a left bundle-branch block pattern and single or paradoxically split second sound.

Electrode placement may also be achieved via the femoral veins or brachiocephalic system. In extreme emergencies, transthoracic pacing may be achieved by direct cardiac puncture and insertion of a pacing needle or a special electrode. This maneuver may be lifesaving in some situations and may provide time to institute more stable measures in others.

Cardioversion

A distinction must be made between emergency cardioversion in the case of circulatory arrest and semielective or elective cardioversion of an arrhythmia that has been resistant to therapy but that the patient is tolerating reasonably well. In treating circulatory arrest, the physician is treating either ventricular fibrillation or an unknown rhythm disturbance in a pulseless patient. Cardioversion should be applied at maximal energy (400 joules), without premedication or synchronization. In the case of an elective conversion, there is usually time to premedicate the patient. Intravenous diazepam (Valium), 5–10 mg, is both effective and safe. We also frequently use sodium methohexital (Brevital), a short-acting barbiturate administered by an anesthetist in doses up to 1 mg/kg. Equipment must be available for tracheal intubation, and an anesthesiologist should be present. Synchronized direct-current cardioversion is preferred to minimize the risk of serious ventricular arrhythmias. Cardioversion should initially be attempted with an energy level of 25–50 joules, and increments of 50–100 joules should be employed until cardioversion has been achieved or a level of 300–400 joules has been reached. Some arrhythmias, such as atrial flutter, are more likely to be converted at low energy levels. If digitalis toxicity is suspected as causing the arrhythmia, it is particularly important to begin with extremely low energy levels (5–10 joules), and lidocaine, 2–4 mg/min, should be infused prophylactically. The same precautions apply if the patient has had an acute myocardial infarction. Since serum enzyme levels may be elevated after cardioversion, their subsequent interpretation in diagnosing acute myocardial infarction may be difficult.

SUGGESTED READINGS

Arrhythmias: General

Cranefield PF, Wit AL, Hoffman BF. Genesis of cardiac arrhythmias. *Circulation,* 1973, 47:190–204.

Harvey WP, Ronan JA, Jr. Bedside diagnosis of arrhythmias. *Prog Cardiovasc Dis,* 1966;8:419–445.

Marriott HJL, Sandler IA. Criteria, old and new, for differentiating between ectopic ventricular beats and aberrant ventricular conduction in the presence of atrial fibrillation. *Prog Cardiovasc Dis,* 1966;9:18–28.

Schamroth L. How to approach an arrhythmia. *Circulation,* 1973; 47:420–426.

Tachyarrhythmias

Supraventricular

Antman EM, Stone PH, Muller JE, et al. Calcium channel blocking agents in the treatment of cardiovascular disorder. Part I. Basic and clinical electrophysiologic effects. *Ann Intern Med,* 1981;93:875–885.

Josephson ME. Paroxysmal SVT: An electrophysiologic approach. *Am J Cardiol,* 1978;41:1123–1126.

Klein GJ, Sharma AD, Yee R. An approach to therapy for paroxysmal supraventricular tachycardia. *Am J Cardiol,* 1988;61:77A–82A. (Review).

Pittman DE, Makar JS, Kooros KS, et al. Rapid atrial stimulation: Successful method of conversion of atrial flutter and atrial tachycardia. *Am J Cardiol,* 1973;32:700–706.

Rosen KM. Junctional tachycardias: Mechanisms, diagnosis, differential diagnosis and management. *Circulation,* 1973;47:654–664.

Shine KL, Kastor JA, Yurchak PM. Multifocal atrial tachycardia: Clinical and electrocardiographic features in 32 patients. *N Engl J Med,* 1968; 279:344–349.

Ticzon AR, Whalen RW. Refractory supraventricular tachycardias. *Circulation,* 1973;47:642–653.

Yee R, Gulamhusein SS, Klein GJ. Combined verapamil and propanolol for supraventricular tachycardia. *Am J Cardiol,* 1984;53:757–763.

Ventricular

Austin JL, Preis LK, Crampton RS. et al. Analysis of pacemaker malfunction and complications of temporary pacing in the coronary care unit. *Am J Cardiol,* 1982;49: 301–306.

Bauman JL, Bauernfeind RA, Hoff JV, et al. Torsade de Pointes due to quinidine: observation in 31 patients. *Am Heart J,* 1984;107:425–430.

Bigger JT, Schmidt DH, Kutt H. Relationship between the plasma level of diphenylhydantoin sodium and its cardiac antiarrhythmic effects. *Circulation,* 1968;38:363–374.

Campbell RW. Mexiletine. *N Eng J Med,* 1987;316:29–34. (Review).

Collinsworth KA, Kalman SM, Harrison DC. The clinical pharmacology of lidocaine as an antiarrhythmic drug. *Circulation,* 1974;50:1217–1230.

DeSanctis RW, Kastor JA. Rapid intracardiac pacing for treatment of recurrent ventricular tachyarrhythmias in the absence of heart block. *Am Heart J* 1968;76:168–172.

Giardina EV, Heissenbuttel RH, Bigger JT. Intermittent intravenous procainamide to treat ventricular arrhythmias: Correlation of plasma concentration with effect on arrhythmia, electrocardiogram, and blood pressure. *Ann Intern Med,* 1973;78:183–193.

Hohnloser SH, Lanse HW, Raeder EA, et al. Short- and long-term therapy with tocainide for malignant ventricular tachyarrhythmias. *Circul.* 1986;73:143–149.

Koch-Weser J: Drug therapy: Bretylium. *N Engl J Med,* 1979;300:473–477.

Morsanroth J, Nestico PF, Horowitz LN. A review of the uses and limitations of tocainide—a Class IB antiarrhythmic agent. *Am Heart J,* 1985;110:856–863. (Review).

Pick A, Langendorf R. Parasystole and its variants. *Med Clin North Am,* 1976;60:125–147.

Pottase A. Clinical profiles of newer Class I antiarrhythmic agents-tocainide, mexiletine, encainide, flecainide, and lorcainide. *Am J Cardiol,* 1983;52:24C–31C. (Review).

Roden DM, Woosley RL. Drug therapy Tocainide. *N Eng J Med,* 1986;315:41–45. (Review).

Rothfeld EL, Zucker IR, Parsonnet V, et all. Idioventricular rhythm in acute myocardial infarction. *Circulation,* 1968;37:203–209.

Smith WM, Gallagher JJ: "Les Torsades de pointes": An unusual ventricular antirhythm. *Ann Intern Med,* 1980;93:578–584.

Willerson JT, Yurchak PM, DeSanctis RW. Ventricular tachycardia. *Cardiovasc Clin,* 1970;2:69–86.

Woosley RL, Wans T, Stone W, et al. Pharmacology, electrophysiology, and pharmacokinetics of mexiletine. *Am Heart J,* 1984;107:1058–1065.

Yee R, Gulamhusein SS, Klein GJ, et al. Electropharmacology of antiarrhythmic drugs. *Am Heart J,* 1983;106:829–839. (Review).

Bradyarrhythmias

Kastor JA. Atrioventricular block. *N Engl J Med,* 1975;292:462–465, 572–574.

Rosenbaum MB, Elizari MV, Lazzari JO. The Hemiblocks: New Concepts of Intraventricular Conduction Based on Human Anatomical Physiological and Clinical Studies. Oldsmar, FL: Tampa Tracings, 1970

Arrhythmias in Special Situations

Myocardial Infarction

Campbell RW. Treatment and prophylaxis of ventricular arrhythmias in acute myocardial infarction. *Am J Cardiol,* 1983;52:55C–59C.

Dhurandhar RW, Macmillan RL, Brown KW. Primary ventricular fibrillation complicating acute myocardial infarction. *Am J Cardiol,* 1971;27:347–351.

Julian DG, Valentine PA, Miller GG. Disturbances of rate, rhythm, and conduction in acute myocardial infarction: A prospective study of 100 consecutive unselected patients with the aid of electrocardiographic monitoring. *Am J Med,* 1964;37:915–927.

Kimball JT, Killip T. Aggressive treatment of arrhythmias in acute myocardial infarction: Procedures and results. *Prog Cardiovasc Dis,* 1968;10:483–504.

Koch-Weser J, Klein SW, Foo-Canto LL, et al. Antiarrhythmic prophylaxis with procainamide in acute myocardial infarction. *N Engl J Med,* 1969;281:1253–1260.

Lown B, Klein MD, Hershberg PL. Coronary and precoronary care. *Am J Med,* 1969;46:705–724.

Lucchesi, BR. Rationale of therapy in the patient with acute myocardial infarction and life-threatening arrhythmias: a focus on bretylium. *Am J Cardiol,* 1984;54:14A–19A.

Meltzer LE, Kitchell JB. The incidence of arrhythmias associated with acute myocardial infarction. *Prog Cardiovasc Dis,* 1966;9:50–63.

Nimetz AA, Shubrooks SJ, Jr, Hutter AM, Jr, et al. The significance of bundle-branch block during acute myocardial infarction. *Am Heart J,* 1975;90:439–444.

Norris RM. Heart block in posterior and anterior myocardial infarction. *Br Heart J,* 1969;31:352–356.

Susiura T, Iwasaka T, Osawa A, et al. Atrial fibrillation in acute myocardial infarction. *Am J Cardiol,* 1985;56:27–29.

Digitalis Toxicity

Beller GA, Smith TW, Abelmann WH, et al. Digitalis intoxication, a prospective clinical study with serum level correlations. *N Engl J Med,* 1971;284:989–997.

Chung EK. Digitalis Intoxication. Baltimore: Williams & Wilkins, 1969.

Resnekov L. Prevalence diagnosis and treatment of digitalis-induced dysrhythmias. In: Sandoe E. Flensted-Jensen E, Olesen KH, Eds. Symposium on Cardiac Arrhythmias. Sodertalje, Sweden: AB Astra, 1970.

Rios JC, Dziok CA, Ali NA: Digitalis-induced arrhythmias: Recognition and management. *Cardiovasc Clin,* 1970;2:261–279.

Pacemaker-Related Arrhythmias

Castellanos A, Jr, Lemberg L. Pacemaker arrhythmias and electrocardiographic recognition of pacemaker. *Circulation,* 1973;47:1382–1391.

Littleford PO, Curry RC, Jr, Schwartz KM, et al. Pacemaker-medicated tachycardias: a rapid bedside technique for induction and observation. *Am J Cardiol,* 1983;52:287–291.

Luceri RM, Castellanos A, Zaman L, et al. The arrhythmias of dual-chamber cardiac pacemakers and their management. *Ann Intern Med,* 1983;99:354–9.

Walter WH, III, Wenger NK. Radiographic identification of commonly used implanted pacemakers. *N Engl J Med,* 1969;281:1230–1231.

Wolff-Parkinson-White Syndrome

Klein GJ, Gulamhusein SS. Intermittent preexcitation in the Wolff-Parkinson-White syndrome. *Am J Cardiol,* 1983;52:292–296.

Narula OS: Wolff-Parkinson-White syndrome: A review. *Circulation,* 1973;47:872–887.

Rinne C, Klein GJ, Sharma AD, el al. Relation between clinical presentation and induced arrhythmias in the Wolff-Parkinson-White syndrome. *Am J Cardiol,* 1987;60:576–579.

Sick Sinus Syndrome

Rosenqvist M, Vallin H, Edhas O. Clinical and electrophysiologic course of sinus node disease: five year follow-up study. *Am Heart J,* 1985;109:513–522.

Rubenstein JJ, Schulman CL, Yurchak PM, et al. Clinical spectrum of the sick sinus syndrome. *Circulation,* 1972;46:5–13.

Special Procedures

DeSanctis RW. Diagnostic and therapeutic uses of atrial pacing. *Circulation,* 1971;43:745–761.

Lown B. Electrical reversion of cardiac arrhythmias. *Br Heart J,* 1967;29:469–489.

Phibbs B, Marriott HJ. Complications of permanent transvenous pacing. *N Eng J Med,* 1985;312:1428–1432. (Review).

Resnekov L. Present status of electroversion in management of cardiac dysrhythmias. *Circulation,* 1973;47:1356–1363.

CHAPTER **6**

Cardiology: Unstable Angina and Acute Myocardial Infarction

ADOLPH M. HUTTER, JR., M.D.
G. WILLIAM DEC, M.D.

DIAGNOSIS OF ISCHEMIC CARDIAC PAIN

The accurate and expeditious evaluation of chest pain is one of the most important responsibilities of the physician in the emergency department. Many patients whose chest pain ultimately proves to have been noncardiac are mislabeled as suffering from angina. Too frequently, the misdiagnosis is the result of an inadequate history or physical examination.

Differential Diagnosis

A number of conditions are commonly confused with angina. Pulmonary embolism, aortic dissection, and chest trauma are fully discussed elsewhere (see Chapters 9, 31, and 32).

Esophageal Spasm

Esophageal spasm may cause substernal, squeezing pain closely resembling angina pectoris. Pain from this source tends to occur in the supine position, especially after a big meal, and it may be relieved by antacids. The fact that the pain may also be relieved by nitroglycerin (Orlando and Bozymski, 1973) or calcium channel blockers (Castell, 1985) increases the confusion with coronary ischemia.

Chest Wall Pain

Chest wall pain due to costochondritis is classically exacerbated by chest movement, especially deep breathing, coughing, and forward bending. It is associated with tenderness over the costochondral joints along the sternal border or the inferior edges of the rib cage. This condition, however, is frequently overlooked because the examining physician fails to ask the proper questions or to palpate each costochondral junction, looking specifically for tenderness.

Pericarditis

Pericarditis (see also Chapter 11) may be confusing since it is commonly associated with sternal or parasternal chest pain that can extend to the neck or shoulder, but rarely down the arm. Careful questioning usually elucidates the sharpness of the pain intensified by deep inspiration, the recumbent position (especially left lateral decubitus), coughing, deep breathing, and even swallowing. Relief of pain is noted on sitting up, bending forward, or holding the breath. A pericardial friction rub confirms the diagnosis; this is a scratchy, superficial sound that occasionally has a coarse, leathery quality. There may be one to three components (ventricular systole and diastole and atrial systole). The pericardial rub usually is best heard to the left of the lower part of the sternum with the patient leaning forward, but sometimes is heard only in the supine position. During auscultation, the patient should hold his breath in various phases of respiration, since the rub sometimes is best heard in expiration and sometimes in inspiration. The rub may be evanescent and may not be audible a few hours later. The electrocardiogram may reveal diffuse elevation of the ST segments with upright T waves early in the course of pericarditis. Later, the T waves invert after the ST segments return to baseline. This contrasts with ST segment elevations due to coronary ischemia, which frequently have concurrent T wave inversion. However, differentiation between the ST segment and T wave changes of pericarditis and those of ischemia, particularly "hyperacute" ischemic changes with upright T waves, can be difficult. A clue to the diagnosis of pericarditis is a depressed P-R interval, which is often overlooked because of its association with elevated ST segments (Spodick, 1974). This phenomenon (Fig. 6.1) is best seen in the inferior leads (II, III, and AVF) and occasionally in the apical leads (V_5 and V_6) and is not a feature of coronary ischemia. Reciprocal P-R segment elevation may be seen in AVR. Since late pericarditis may occur after myocardial infarction (Dressler's syndrome) or cardiac surgery (postpericardiotomy syndrome), this possibility should be considered in patients with return of chest pain after either of these events.

Even a careful history and physical examination may not result in accurate differentiation among the various possible causes of chest pain, particularly in patients who complain of more than one type of pain or who have multiple potential sources. Correct determination that the pain is of ischemic cardiac origin is crucial to the subsequent diagnostic and therapeutic plan. The misdiagnosis of severe or unstable angina pectoris made on the basis of an inadequate history may lead to unnecessary coronary angiography, which may nevertheless demonstrate obstructive coronary lesions. The resultant choices between medical and surgical therapy and decisions to restrict patient activity will be inappropriate for the patient who has costochondritis or esophageal spasm and in whom the finding of coronary artery disease is, in fact, coincidental.

Physical Examination

Proof that chest pain is due to myocardial ischemia can be established by recording an electrocardiogram, examining the patient, and monitoring hemodynamic parameters *during* pain. Physical examination during such episodes may reveal tachycardia, elevated systemic blood pressure, transient paradoxical splitting of the second heart sound, the appearance or intensification of a fourth heart sound, and occasionally, a third heart sound (S_3 gallop) or a systolic murmur indicating mitral regurgitation due to papillary muscle dysfunction. Hemodynamic findings may include a rise in left ventricular filling pressure consequent to decreased ventricular com-

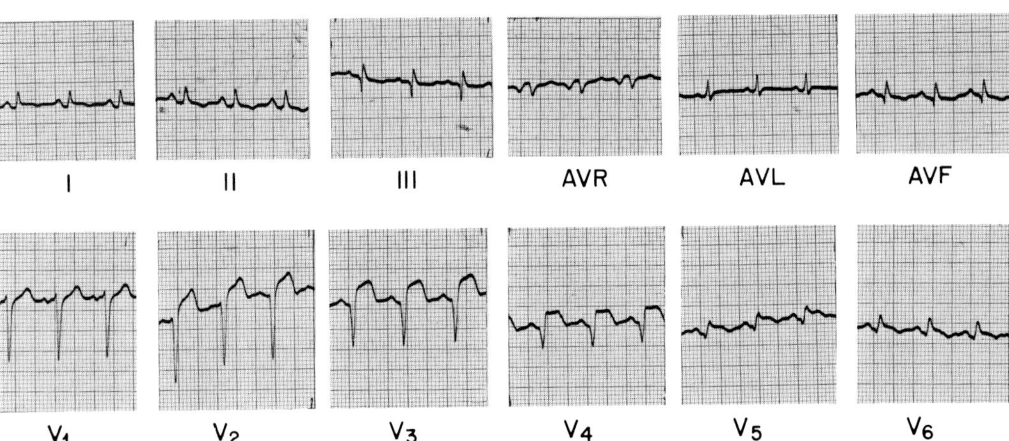

Figure 6.1. Pericarditis. Electrocardiogram of patient with acute anterior myocardial infarction. P-R interval is depressed relative to T-P interval in leads I, II, V_5, and V_6 with reciprocal P-R elevation in AVR. This finding suggests pericarditis, but is often overlooked because of the ST segment elevation.

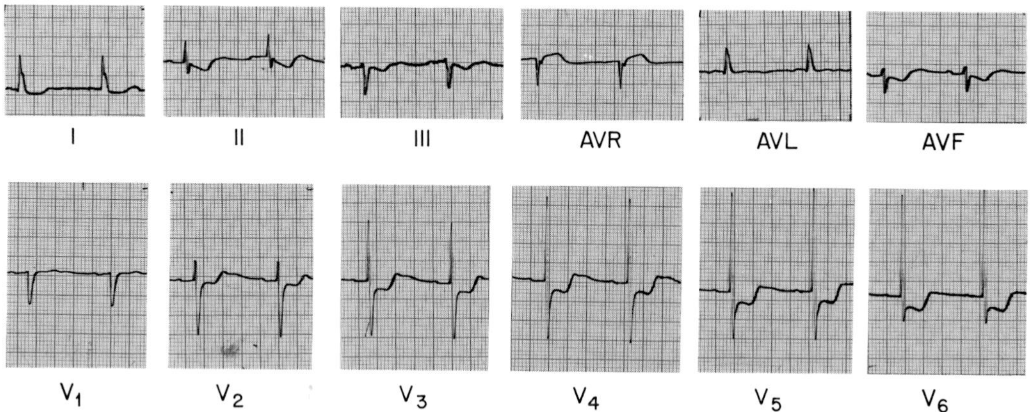

Figure 6.2. Subendocardial ischemia during chest pain. ST segment depression in leads V_2 through V_5 begins with marked J point depression and ends with sharp "squaring" of the ST-T junction, giving a horizontal ST segment depression characteristic of subendocardial ischemia. Lesser but similar changes are seen in leads II, III, and AVF. This electrocardiogram indicates ischemia of the anteroseptal, anterior, apical, and inferior surfaces of the heart.

pliance and reflected by the pulmonary capillary wedge pressure measured with a Swan-Ganz catheter. Although hemodynamic monitoring is not routine, especially in the emergency department, the emergency physician should make every attempt to record an electrocardiogram and to examine the patient during pain to establish with certainty that the pain in question is angina.

Electrocardiogram Interpretation

A repeat electrocardiogram may provide valuable information, showing electrocardiographic abnormalities that occur during anginal pain usually returning to baseline when the pain abates. The most common electrocardiographic abnormality during pain is transient ST segment depression (Fig. 6.2), although ST segment elevation may occur in vasospastic (variant) angina. Sometimes only T wave inversions appear, and occasionally, previously inverted T waves become upright during pain ("pseudonormalization" of T waves), as seen in Figure 6.3.

Anatomical Correlations

In addition to helping establish the cardiac origin of pain, the fluctuating electrocardiographic abnormalities indicate the area of heart involved and, to some degree, the extent of myocardium jeopardized. Table 6.1 correlates the area of myocardium and the coronary artery usually involved with the electrocardiographic leads showing ischemic changes. For example, transient marked depression of ST segments over the entire anterior precordium (leads V_2 to V_6) as well as over the inferior surface (leads II, III, and AVF) usually indicates that a large area of myocardium is at risk from the ischemic episode. Another example is that of ST segment depression over the anterior surface in a patient with recurrent pain after an old inferior myocardial infarction, indicating that a second coronary artery is involved.

The prognosis for patients with coronary artery disease and the decisions for medical or surgical therapy are best correlated with the amount of myocardium put at ischemic risk by coronary obstructive lesions and the state of left ventricular function (CASS Investigators, 1983; European Coronary Surgical Group, 1980; Hutter, 1980; Takaro et al., 1976). Documentation of transient ST segment and T wave changes during pain is important not only to establish the ischemic nature of the pain, but also to identify patients with a large amount of viable myocardium at ischemic risk. If such patients are otherwise suitable candidates, they should be considered for coronary angiography.

Vasospastic (Variant) Angina

In vasospastic (variant) angina, ST segment elevation rather than ST segment depression is seen during pain, with resolution to baseline after relief of pain (Prinzmetal et al., 1959; Pasternak et al., 1979; National Cooperative Study Group, 1980) (Fig. 6.4). Ischemic pain is due to intermittent coronary artery spasm often superimposed on fixed atherosclerotic lesions. The diagnosis cannot be made until subsequent electrocardiograms prove that the ST segments have returned to baseline *without* evolution of a myocardial infarction. Characteristically, the pain occurs at rest, often at similar times during the day. Some patients may also have exertional pain. Arrhythmias are common during pain: ventricular premature beats, ventricular tachycar-

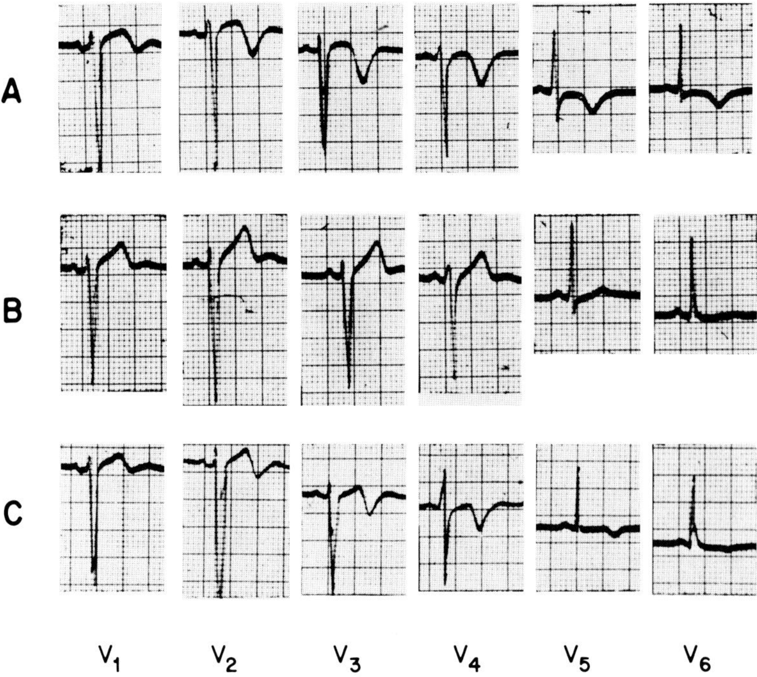

Figure 6.3. "Pseudonormalization" of abnormal T waves during angina. *A*, Baseline electrocardiogram shows recent anteroseptal infarction. *B*, during angina, T waves become upright and appear more "normal." *C*, After pain, T waves revert to baseline. These changes indicate that the anterior wall is the location of the ischemia and that, therefore, there must still be live muscle in the area of the recent anteroseptal infarction.

dia, ventricular fibrillation, atrioventricular block, sinus bradycardia, sinoatrial exit block, and supraventricular tachyarrhythmia.

UNSTABLE ANGINA PECTORIS

Diagnosis

The syndrome of unstable angina pectoris is in the "gray zone" between stable angina on the one hand and acute myocardial infarction and perhaps sudden death on the other. It is best divided into three main groups. First, in patients with previously stable angina, the frequency, severity, or duration of pain may increase considerably. Pain is brought on with less and less activity, occurring even at rest, and becomes more and more resistant to relief from nitrates. This crescendo pattern occurs in the absence of precipitating factors such as anemia, arrhythmias, or thyrotoxicosis. Second, in patients without previous angina, pain begins abruptly and demonstrates the same rapidly progressive pattern usually in the course of days or weeks. Third, in some patients, a prolonged episode of coronary pain developes that suggests myocardial infarction but without electrocardiographic or enzymatic evidence of infarction.

Table 6.1.
Correlation Between Location of Ischemic Changes on Electrocardiogram and Involved Myocardial Region

Electrocardiographic Leads	Myocardial Region	Coronary Artery[a]
II, III, AVF	Inferior	RCA
V_1, V_2 (reciprocal changes)	Posterior	RCA
V_2–V_4	Anteroseptal	Left anterior descending branch of LCA
V_3–V_5	Anterior	Left anterior descending branch of LCA
I, AVL	High lateral	Circumflex marginal or diagonal branch of LCA
V_5–V_6	Apical	Usually left anterior descending branch of LCA; can be posterior descending branch of RCA

[a] RCA, right coronary artery; LCA, left coronary artery.

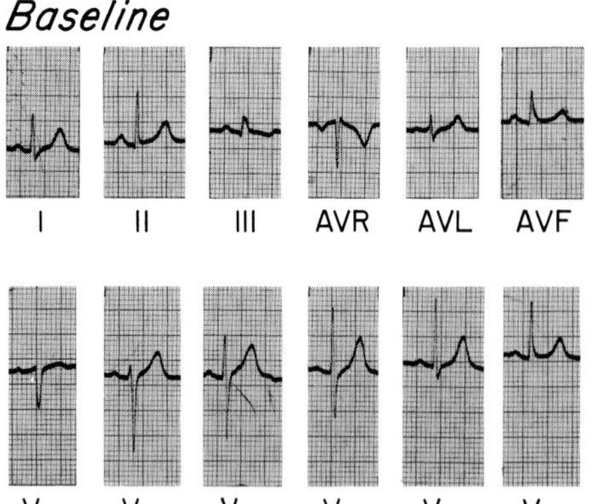

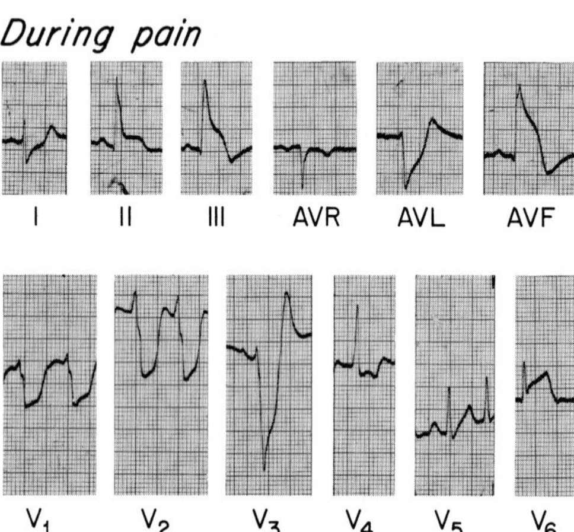

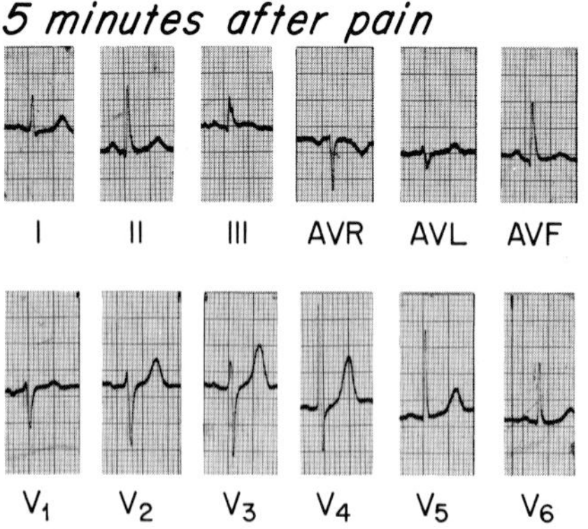

Figure 6.4. Prinzmetal's angina. During pain, marked ST segment elevation is seen in leads II, III, AVF, and V_6 with reciprocal ST segment depression in leads AVL, V_1, V_2, and V_3 indicating inferoposteroapical epicardial injury current. After pain, ST segments return to baseline without subsequent evolution to myocardial infarction.

Once unstable angina is diagnosed, the emergency physician should hospitalize the patient, preferably in a coronary care unit. Hospitalization is necessary to stabilize the patient's condition, to exclude the diagnosis of myocardial infarction, to institute prompt medical therapy, and to consider further diagnostic studies, including coronary angiography, in order to decide between continued medical treatment, coronary revascularization, or coronary angioplasty. Once myocardial infarction has been ruled out and the patient's condition is stabilized on medical therapy, coronary angiography can be carried out as safely as in patients with stable angina (National Cooperative Study Group, 1976).

Treatment

In the emergency department the medical treatment of angina pectoris should be instituted promptly and aggressively. When pain cannot be controlled with other measures, morphine sulfate, 2–5 mg intravenously, is preferable to other analgesics. Adequate sedation can usually be achieved with oxazepam (Serax), diazepam (Valium), lorazepam (Ativan), or chlordiazepoxide hydrochloride (Librium).

Nitrates, β-adrenergic blocking agents, and calcium antagonists are the mainstays of medical therapy. The general aim of these is to improve the relationship between myocardial oxygen demand and its supply.

Nitrates

Nitrates, which may cause reflex tachycardia when administered alone, are used effectively in conjunction with β-adrenergic blocking agents. When the drugs are given concurrently, control of both heart rate (50–60 beats/min) and blood pressure (100–120 mm Hg systolic, depending on the individual) can usually be achieved. The primary systemic effect of the nitrates is venodilatation, which results in diminished venous return to the heart and, thus, in a decreased preload. Nitrates also cause some dilatation of the arterioles, resulting in lower blood pressure. They also dilate coronary arteries (Badger et al., 1985) and increase circulation through collaterals between major coronary arteries (Goldstein et al., 1974). The patient with active unstable angina and adequate blood pressure should be treated in the emergency department with nitroglycerin, 0.3 or 0.4 mg sublingually. If the blood pressure is well-maintained, the dose can be repeated every 5 minutes. If pain persists after three doses, however, morphine sulfate should be given. Once pain is controlled, longer-term treatment may be started with isosorbide dinitrate, 5–20 mg every 2–3 hours sublingually, as permitted by blood pressure (Thadani et al., 1980). If pain is not relieved, intravenous nitroglycerin can be administered as a constant infusion, starting with 15–20 μg/min and increasing to as high as 400 μg/min (Armstrong et al., 1980). Because of the potential for hypotension, patients receiving intravenous nitroglycerin should be followed with continuous intraarterial pressure monitoring or an automated cuff sphygmomanometer and, in most cases, a pulmonary arterial line to measure left ventricular filling pressure. Because of these requirements, intravenous nitrate administration usually is deferred until the patient has arrived in the intensive care unit.

The less acutely ill patient may be treated with isosorbide dinitrate, 10–80 mg every 4 hours orally (Thadani et al., 1980). Nitroglycerin ointment, when applied to the skin in 1- to 3-inch ribbons of extruded paste, has a duration of action up to 6 hours and can be used effectively, particularly for extended nighttime protection (Reichek et al., 1974). Headache, the most frequent limiting side effect of nitrate therapy, may be ameliorated in patients by switching from oral to cutaneous administration. Isosorbide dinitrate capsules (Isordil Tembids) have an extended antianginal effect and result in improved exercise tolerance for as long as 6 hours (Lee et al., 1976), but they have variable absorption and should not be used in an unstable situation in the emergency department. In addition to headache, hypotension may be a limiting factor in administration of nitrates. This is particularly true in elderly patients with attenuated autonomic nervous system responses and in patients who are depleted of volume because of concurrent administration of diuretics or inappropriate vasodilatation related to a recent myocardial infarction, particularly inferior infarction. Thus, fluids may have to be administered to patients with large nitrate requirements who are hypotensive with a low left ventricular filling pressure.

β-*Blocking Agents*

β-Blocking agents diminish myocardial oxygen demand by reducing heart rate, blood pressure, and cardiac inotropy. In the absence of contraindications, such as evident congestive heart failure, marked bradycardia, or history of bronchospasm, they should be started immediately and increased until adequate physiologic levels are reached, as indicated by a resting heart rate of 50–60 beats/min (Nies and Shand, 1975). Propranolol hydrochloride (Inderal) is the most commonly used β-adrenergic blocking agent in the United States. Oral dosage ranges from 40 mg/day to 800 mg/day in two to four divided doses. A long-acting preparation is also available. When the oral route is unavailable or when more immediate onset of action is desired, propranolol can be given intravenously. Increments of 0.5 to 1.0 mg can be given every 5 minutes until an appropriate physiologic effect is achieved. Usually, 0.05 mg/kg is a reasonable total initial dose, although some patients require more. A maintenance dose, usually equal to the initial dose, can be administered as an intravenous drip. Intravenous doses are usually 5–10% of the oral dose.

Propranolol is generally contraindicated in patients with left ventricular failure, high-grade atrioventricular block, or hypotension. In addition, by blocking β-adrenergic receptors in the bronchial tree, propranolol can precipitate bronchial spasm. Patients who have resting bradycardia must be carefully monitored for additional slowing after administration of propranolol and may benefit from a β-blocker with intrinsic sympathomimetic activity such as pindolol (Visken). Other β-adrenergic blocking agents currently approved in the United States for oral use include: metoprolol tartrate (Lopressor), which is relatively cardioselective and therefore less likely to induce bronchospasm; nadolol (Corgard), a nonselective β-adrenergic blocking agent that requires administration only once a day because of longer duration of action; timolol maleate (Blocadren), a nonselective agent; atenolol (Tenormin), a cardioselective agent that also can be given once a day; acebutolol hydrochloride (Sectral), a selective agent with mild intrinsic sympathomimetic activity; and labetalol hydrochloride (Normodyne), a combined A and nonselective β-blocker. Atenolol, nadolol, timolol, and acebutolol are less lipophilic than propranolol and metoprolol and therefore may be associated with fewer central nervous system side effects (Frishman, 1981). In addition to propranolol, both metoprolol and labetalol can be administered intravenously when rapid onset of action is required.

Calcium Antagonists

Calcium antagonists have rapidly become of major importance in the treatment of ischemic heart disease (Zelis and Flaim, 1981; Ellrodt et al., 1980). Nifedipine (Procardia) is effective in the treatment of coronary spasm (Antman et al., 1980; Hill et al., 1982) and in the treatment of angina pectoris resulting from fixed coronary artery obstruction (Liang et al., 1985; White et al., 1985; Gerstenblith et al., 1982). It dilates coronary and peripheral arterioles and enhances collateral circulation. Oral dosage of nifedipine is 10–40 mg three to four times a day. Nifedipine is also effective when given sublingually. Verapamil hydrochloride (Isoptin, Calan) has antianginal effects similar to those of nifedipine and is, in addition, highly effective in the treatment of supraventricular tachyarrhythmias which involve the A-V node. It is available for both intravenous and oral use, with oral doses ranging from 240 to 480 mg/day. Diltiazem is as effective as nifedipine in the treatment of exertional and vasospastic angina, yet has fewer side effects (Prida et al., 1985; Broden et al., 1985). It is currently available for oral use with a dosage range of 90–360 mg/day. Frequently, the management of acute unstable ischemic states requires that all three types of anti-ischemic agents (nitrates, β-blocking agents, and calcium channel blockers) be used in appropriate combination.

Afterload Reduction

Patients with continuing pain in the setting of persistent hypertension may benefit from blood pressure (afterload) reduction. Although all of the antianginal treatments previously described have hypotension-producing potential, hypertension persisting even in the face of treatment with anti-ischemic medications should be aggressively managed. In most cases, treatment with diuretics or other specific antihypertensive agents will suffice. For those patients requiring immediate blood pressure reduction for ongoing ischemia, intravenous infusion of a hypotensive agent closely titrated to blood pressure is preferable to a "bolus" that may result in uncontrolled hypotension and exacerbation of the ischemia. If sublingual or intravenous nitroglycerin is insufficient to control blood pressure, sodium nitroprusside may be added, 20–50 μg/min intravenously (Miller et al., 1975; Palmer and Lasseter, 1975). Except in the most serious emergency during which pressure may be continuously monitored manually, intraarterial pressure monitoring should be a prerequisite to the administration of this medication. This should be carried out in the intensive care unit, not the emergency department. In addition, since sodium nitroprusside may unfavorably affect the coronary circulation in the ischemic heart (Chiariello et al., 1976), it should be added to a nitrate regimen already increased to a high level.

Anticoagulation

A variety of pathophysiologic mechanisms have been proposed to explain the development of unstable angina, including: progressive coronary arterial narrowing, plaque hemorrhage, arterial spasm, and platelet aggregation at the site of coronary stenosis (Willerson et al., 1984). Recent attention has focused upon the role of platelet aggregation in the alteration of coronary blood flow. At least one large, randomized, placebo-controlled clinical trial has demonstrated the protective effect of aspirin against acute myocardial infarction in men with unstable angina (Lewis et al., 1983). The dosage was 325 mg of buffered aspirin per day. A large Canadian study confirmed the protective action of aspirin in unstable angina patients using 325 mg four times daily (Cairns et al., 1985). Many cardiologists are routinely prescribing one aspirin tablet daily to all patients with known coronary artery disease in an attempt to inhibit platelet cyclooxygenase action and prevent the development of unstable angina or myocardial infarction. Systemic anticoagulation with intravenous heparin has been studied in patients with unstable angina and has also been shown in one small controlled clinical trial to decrease the likelihood of myocardial infarction (Telford and Wilson, 1981). Since this study has not yet been reproduced by other investigators, the exact role for systemic heparin therapy in unstable angina should be considered unsettled. Nevertheless, current treatment of unstable angina may include the addition of aspirin or heparin for those patients who fail to respond to anti-ischemic therapy.

Treatment of Left Ventricular Failure

When left ventricular failure is evident and seems to contribute to unstable angina, digitalis glycosides and diuretics may relieve pain by reducing left ventricular volume, transmural pressure, and therefore, myocardial oxygen consumption. Except in this setting, digitalis has no role in the therapy for unstable angina, since it may increase peripheral vascular resistance, myocardial oxygen consumption, and ischemia.

Management of Arrhythmia

The treatment of arrhythmias is discussed in Chapter 5, but it should be emphasized here that achievement of normal sinus rhythm is urgent in patients with ongoing coronary ischemic pain, whether due to unstable angina or acute myocardial infarction. By increasing myocardial oxygen consumption, persistent rapid atrial fibrillation or paroxysmal atrial tachycardia may result in progression of unstable angina to myocardial infarction or extension of an existing myocardial infarct. Thus, prompt cardioversion to normal sinus rhythm in such patients is recommended. Similarly, use of a temporary pacemaker or appropriate pharmacologic therapy for bradyarrhythmias is more urgent in the patient with ongoing ischemia in whom a normal heart rate is essential for maintenance of adequate cardiac output and coronary perfusion.

Intraaortic Balloon Counterpulsation

Ongoing coronary pain, despite a maximal medical program, can often be managed with intraaortic balloon counterpulsation (Gold et al., 1973; Levine et al., 1978). With deflation just before systole, the balloon reduces the pressure against which the left ventricle must empty (afterload). In addition, it reduces left ventricular end-diastolic pressure (preload) and, therefore, left ventricular size and wall tension. Both of these effects reduce myocardial oxygen consumption. With inflation in diastole, the balloon transiently increases diastolic pressure and improves coronary artery blood flow. In patients whose condition is very unstable, the intraaortic balloon is useful not only in relieving pain but also in enhancing the safety of coronary angiographc examinations and revascularizing surgery (Levine et al., 1978). Although intraaortic balloon counterpulsation is not used in the emergency department and is not available in all hospitals, knowledge of its indications and effectiveness is necessary so that the emergency physician can either mobilize the appropriate resources within the hospital or transfer the patient to an institution with such equipment.

ACUTE MYOCARDIAL INFARCTION

In the emergency department, careful history, thorough physical examination, and evaluation of the electrocardiogram form the basis for diagnosing acute myocardial infarction.

History

The usual complaint is chest pain, often with extension to the neck or arm, commonly accompanied by sweating, nausea, shortness of breath, and pallor. If the patient has preexisting angina, the pain is frequently reminiscent of this pain, but is more intense and unremitting. Many patients have symptoms that are not typical. Elderly patients, in particular, are frequently seen without pain after the sudden onset of dyspnea or worsening of congestive heart failure (Pathy, 1967). If the history continues to suggest ischemia or infarction without evidence of other possible causes of chest pain, the patient should be admitted and myocardial infarction ruled out, even in the presence of an initial normal electrocardiogram.

Electrocardiographic Changes

Figure 6.5 depicts the electrocardiographic evolution of acute myocardial infarction. The electrocardiogram may be diagnostic in the emergency department if pathologic Q waves are seen with ST segment elevation and T wave inversion. These findings may also indicate an old myocardial infarct with ventricular aneurysm, but the burden of proof is on the person who claims the changes are old. The location of Q waves indicates the location of the infarct, the coronary artery involved, and, to some degree, the extent of damage (Table 6.1). In a true posterior infarction, Q waves are not seen on the standard electrocardiogram; rather, reciprocal changes occur in leads V_1 and V_2 with tall, broad R waves (more than 0.04 second), depressed ST segments, and upright T waves. The Q waves would be seen in lead V_{10} placed behind the heart on the left posterior region of the chest.

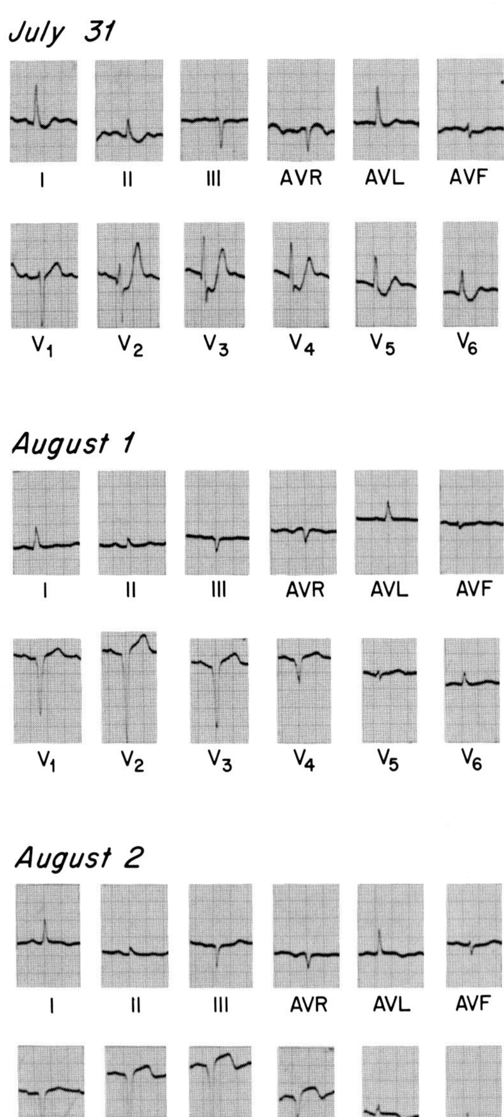

Figure 6.5. Evolution of anteroseptal myocardial infarction. Hyperacute tall T waves associated with depressed ST segments may be seen in the first few hours (*July 31*). Later, T-wave inversion and ST-segment elevation occur in association with loss of R wave and development of Q waves in leads V_1 through V_4 (*August 1* and *2*).

Since the amount of muscle still in jeopardy as well as the amount already infarcted is extremely important in determining the patient's ultimate course, other leads should be studied for evidence of additional areas of compromise. For example, a

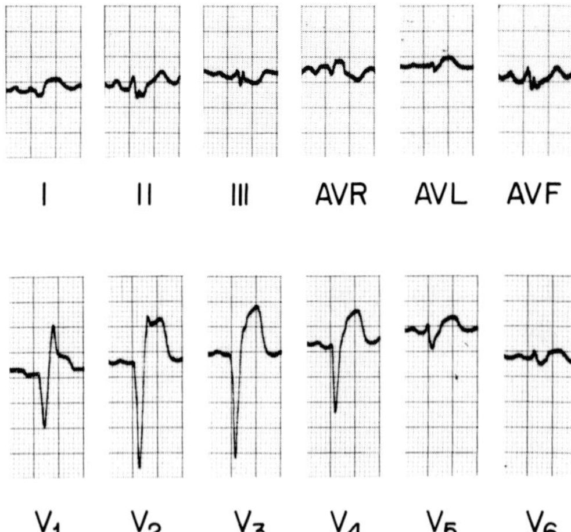

Figure 6.6. Acute anteroseptal myocardial infarction and right bundle-branch block (RBBB). Q-wave and ST-segment elevation is clearly seen in leads V_1 through V_3 in presence of complete RBBB. The latter is indicated by the tall terminal R′ in lead V_1 and 0.16-second duration of QRS complex.

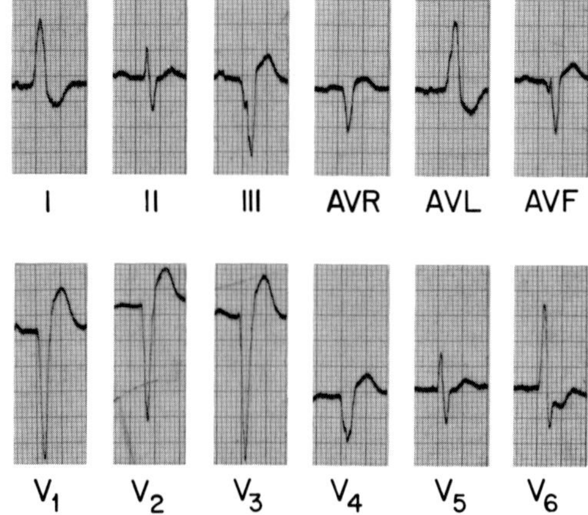

Figure 6.7. Old inferior myocardial infarction in presence of left bundle-branch block (LBBB). QRS-complex duration of 0.12-second, initial positive deflection of QRS in leads I and AVL, and poor R-wave progression in leads V_1 through V_4 are all features of LBBB. Q waves in leads III and AVF indicate inferior myocardial infarction since an R wave is normally present in leads II, III, and AVF in LBBB, even if there is marked left axis deviation. (Lead V_2 was taken at one-half standarization.)

patient with classic inferior myocardial infarction with Q waves and elevated ST segments in leads II, III, and AVF may also have ST segment depression in leads V_3 and V_4, indicating anterior subendocardial ischemia. A second electrocardiogram recorded only a few hours later may show the evolving inferior myocardial infarction, but no longer may show any anterior changes. Nevertheless, the patient probably has two-vessel disease (right coronary artery and left anterior descending branch of the left coronary artery) rather than single-vessel, right coronary artery disease. This observation is important and should be documented, since it may indicate a need for subsequent coronary angiographic examination.

Ischemia in Bundle-Branch Block

The diagnosis of acute ischemia and myocardial infarction can be made in the presence of right bundle-branch block (RBBB) since only the terminal part of the QRS complex is involved with this conduction defect, causing an R′ in lead V_1 and a broad, slurred S wave in lead I. Thus, pathologic Q waves (more than 0.04 second) can still be read in any lead (Fig. 6.6).

In left bundle-branch block (LBBB), on the other hand, the initial as well as the terminal portions of the QRS complex are abnormal, and therefore it is often taught that infarction cannot be read in the presence of LBBB. There are two important exceptions to this rule. First, in LBBB an R wave is normally present in leads II, III, and AVF even in the presence of considerable left axis deviation, in which case lead II has an RS configuration. The occurrence of Q waves in leads II, III, and AVF, therefore, permits diagnosis of inferior myocardial infarction in the presence of LBBB (Fig. 6.7). Second, anteroseptal infarction can also be determined in the presence of LBBB, although not by the usual poor anterior R wave progression since this is a normal feature in LBBB. In LBBB, the ventricular septum, which normally depolarizes from left to right, depolarizes from right to left. This results in an initial positive deflection of the QRS complex in leads I and AVL, which "look at" the free left ventricular wall from the left shoulder. In an anteroseptal infarct, the initial septal forces are lost, and the second forces, which are right ventricular and therefore directed to the right, initiate the QRS complex, resulting in Q waves in leads I and AVL. Thus, new Q waves in leads I and AVL in a patient with LBBB indicate a septal infarct (Fig. 6.8).

Acute injury currents can also be read in the presence of LBBB. The repolarization changes of uncomplicated LBBB consist of downsloping ST segments and asymmetric T wave inversion in those leads with a positive QRS complex (leads I, AVL, V_5, and V_6). Reciprocal changes of upsloping ST segments and upright T waves are seen in those leads with a negative QRS complex (leads V_1 to V_3). Therefore, elevation of ST segments in a lead with an upright QRS complex may indicate epicardial injury (Fig. 6.9), and depression of ST segments in

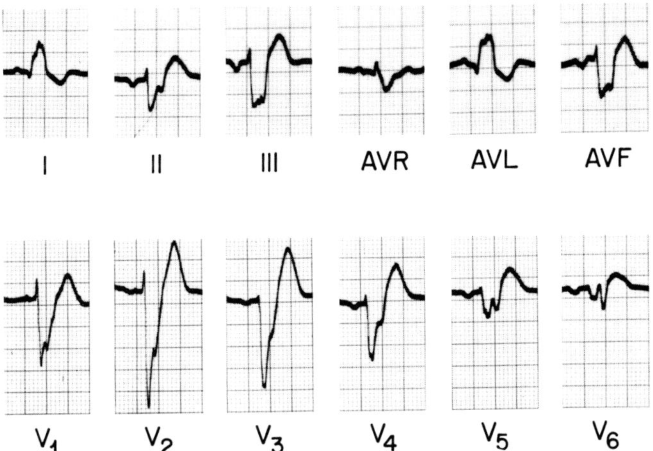

Figure 6.8. Septal myocardial infarction in LBBB. Q waves in leads I and AVL indicate septal (and, therefore, anteroseptal) infarction in presence of LBBB.

a lead with a negative QRS complex may indicate subendocardial injury.

Cardiac Enzymes

Another important aspect in diagnosing myocardial infarction is knowledge of serial myocardial enzyme levels. In patients without classically evolving Q waves, the differentiation between unstable angina and myocardial infarction depends greatly on valid interpretation of enzyme levels. In such patients, three sets of enzyme determinations should be performed within the first 24 hours, since levels can peak and then decrease to normal within this time. It is precisely for those patients with only ST segment and T wave changes that this more subtle knowledge of the enzyme curve is needed. An assay for creatinine phosphokinase-MB, the myocardium-specific subtype of creatinine phosphokinase, should be performed with each set of cardiac enzyme determinations (Roberts and Sobel, 1978). Since the creatinine phosphokinase level or serum glutamic oxaloacetic transaminase level or both can be elevated just with intramuscular injections, it is important to avoid this method of drug administration and to use subcutaneous or intravenous routes in such patients.

Physical Examination

Physical examination during acute myocardial infarction may reveal those phenomena associated with angina pectoris, namely, tachycardia, elevated systemic blood pressure, transient paradoxical splitting of the second heard sound, and appearance or exacerbation of a fourth heart sound. More significant left ventricular failure may be indicated by a third heart sound (S_3 gallop), congestive rales, or hypotension.

Papillary Muscle Dysfunction

Murmurs indicating mitral regurgitation due to papillary muscle dysfunction are relatively frequent, occurring in more than 70% of patients with inferior myocardial infarction and in more than 50% with anterior myocardial infarction under ideal conditions for auscultation (Heikkila, 1967). The murmur frequently is missed unless the patient is examined in the left lateral decubitus position with full expiration in a quiet room and with the diaphragm of the stethoscope placed directly over the apex. This murmur is usually of auscultatory interest only, and the mitral regurgitation is of no hemodynamic significance.

Acute Mitral Regurgitation

Occasionally, regurgitation may be severe, requiring aggressive therapy. Papillary muscle rupture occurs in only about 1% of patients with acute myocardial infarction and usually is indicated by abrupt onset of a harsh systolic murmur at the apex, with extension to the axilla or to the left sternal border. These patients are almost always critically ill with severe pulmonary edema or cardiogenic shock, or both. The acute congestive heart failure is left-sided and is manifested by pulmonary edema and a loud S_3 gallop in both severe papillary muscle dysfunction and papillary muscle rupture. The murmur may be absent in the presence of profound hypotension. Right-heart catheterization with a Swan-Ganz catheter reveals a high pulmonary capillary wedge pressure with tall V waves.

Septal Rupture

Rupture of the ventricular septum is another mechanical complication of myocardial infarction as-

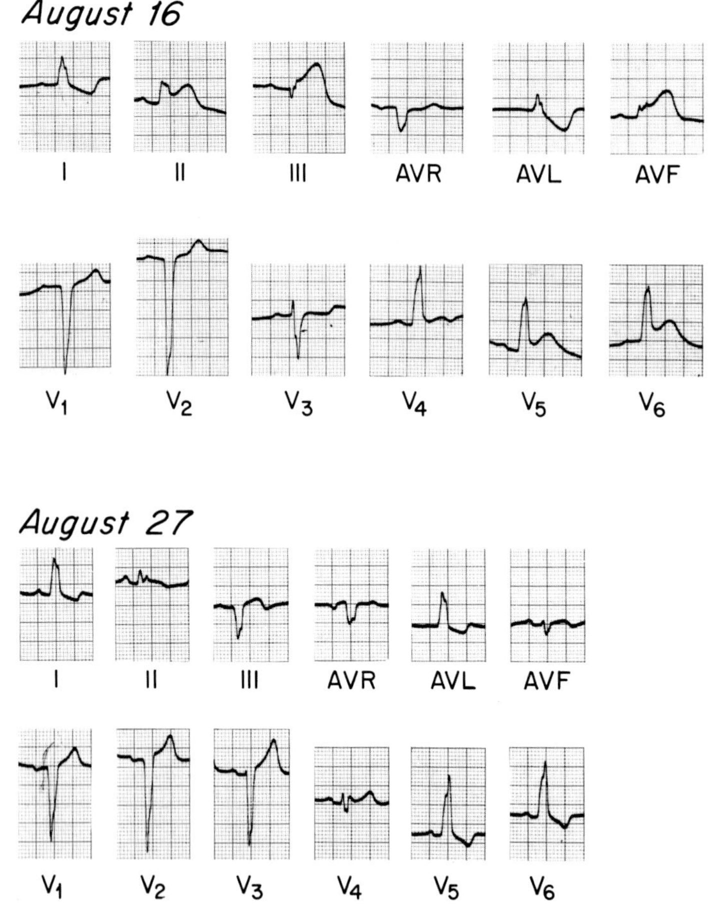

Figure 6.9. Acute inferoapical injury in LBBB. ST-segment elevation in leads II, III, AVF, V_5, and V_6, indicates epicardial injury current (*August 16*) since ST segments should be downsloping in leads with a positive QRS complex in LBBB. ST segments return to baseline on *August 27*.

sociated with a systolic murmur. The murmur is usually loud, diamond-shaped, and holosystolic, beginning just before the first heart sound and best heard at the left sternal border. A systolic thrill is often palpable. In contrast with the clinical appearance of pulmonary edema associated with acute mitral regurgitation, rupture of the ventricular septum overloads the right ventricle, causing the clinical findings of severe right-sided congestive heart failure with less pulmonary congestion. Since some patients may have both papillary muscle dysfunction and a ruptured ventricular septum, any patient with acute myocardial infarction who has a new systolic murmur and whose hemodynamic status is unstable should undergo right-heart catheterization. Blood samples should be obtained from the right atrium, right ventricle, and pulmonary arteries to determine the presence of an oxygen step-up. The pulmonary capillary wedge pressure should be determined with a Swan-Ganz catheter, and the tracing should be inspected for tall V waves.

Pericarditis

Pericarditis may occur early in the course of transmural acute myocardial infarction, resulting in pain that can be misinterpreted as ongoing ischemic pain. Since the implications of the two entities differ greatly, careful examination for a pericardial friction rub and determination of pain changes with change in position are important. If the pain is exacerbated by a deep breath and is either relieved or made worse by sitting up, it is more likely to be pericarditis, even in the absence of a pericardial friction rub. In questionable cases, a short-term trial with an effective anti-inflammatory agent such as indomethacin, 25 mg every 6 hours for 2 or 3 days, is sometimes helpful (see Chapter 11).

Treatment

The treatment of acute myocardial infarction has changed markedly in the past decade. Many studies have indicated that the size of infarction may be reduced by techniques designed either to lessen myocardial oxygen consumption, such as the use of β-blockers or nitrates (Maroko and Braunwald, 1973; Maroko et al., 1971), or to increase coronary perfusion with angioplasty or thrombolytic therapy (Laffel et al., 1984).

Nitrates

Sublingual nitroglycerin acts primarily as a venodilator reducing preload (left ventricular filling pressure) (Gold et al., 1972; Williams et al., 1975). Intravenous nitroglycerin has a greater effect on arteriolar dilatation, decreasing afterload (peripheral resistance) (Epstein et al., 1975; Flaherty et al., 1983; Williams et al., 1975). It reduces the area of ST segment elevation and presumably myocardial injury after coronary artery ligation in dogs (Epstein et al., 1975) and after myocardial infarction in human beings (Borer et al., 1975; Come et al., 1975; Jaffe et al., 1983; Flaherty et al., 1983). In the emergency department, however, sublingual nitroglycerin or sublingual isosorbide dinitrate, or both, should be administered with careful measurement of blood pressure before and after administration. Since an adequate nitrate effect can be achieved via this route, there is, in general, no indication for intravenous nitrates in the emergency department.

β-Blockers

Intravenous administration of a β-blocker has also been shown to limit eventual myocardial infarct size (Mueller and Ayers, 1977). Propranolol hydrochloride (Peter et al., 1978; Norris et al., 1981; Roberts et al., 1984), metoprolol (Goteborg Metroprolol Trial, 1984; Boyle et al., 1983), timolol (International Collaborative Study Group, 1984), and atenolol (Yusuf et al., 1983) have all been shown in acute randomized intervention trials to reduce infarct size when given within 6 hours of onset of symptoms. All trials began with β-blocker administration by the intravenous route; some continued intravenous administration while others used oral dosage. The beneficial effects of β-blockers are felt to derive from reduced myocardial oxygen consumption due to decreased heart rate, myocardial contractility, and systemic blood pressure. Propranolol and metoprolol are currently the most commonly utilized β-blockers following acute myocardial infarction. In patients with adequate blood pressure and no evidence of congestive heart failure, the initial intravenous dose of propranolol is 0.05 mg/kg given in increments of 0.5 mg every 5–10 minutes. The maintenance intravenous dose ranges from 1 to 3 mg every 4–6 hours, but most patients should be converted to oral dosage once their condition stabilizes. Metoprolol is generally given in three divided doses of 5 mg each over 5–10 minutes. If the initial doses have been well-tolerated, oral therapy is then begun at 50 mg every 6 hours for the next 48 hours. The patient should be closely observed for evidence of congestive heart failure, an unacceptably slow heart rate, or hypotension. As a general rule, patients with evidence of real anterior wall injury should be monitored with a Swan-Ganz pulmonary artery line during institution of β-blockade to ensure that the additive myocardial depressant effects of the evolving infarction and the medication do not combine to precipitate frank congestive heart failure.

Lidocaine

Because "warning arrhythmias" are an unpredictable precursor of disastrous ventricular arrhythmias, and because prophylactic administration of lidocaine hydrochloride (Xylocaine) has been shown to diminish the frequency of primary ventricular fibrillation (Lie et al., 1974; Wyman and Hammersmith, 1974), lidocaine is routinely infused prophylactically for the first 24–48 hours after acute myocardial infarction. An effective regimen requires a loading dose of 50–75 mg as an intravenous bolus, followed by an infusion of 1–4 mg/min. Administration of a second bolus of 50 mg approximately 20 minutes after the first dose may be required to maintain adequate levels (Greenblatt et al., 1976). Doses should be reduced in the elderly, in patients with hepatic dysfunction, and in patients with incipient circulatory collapse.

Intraaortic Balloon Counterpulsation

Intraaortic balloon counterpulsation reduces both afterload and preload, and at the same time, increases coronary artery perfusion pressure by augmenting diastolic blood pressure. The device can now be inserted percutaneously (Subramanian et al., 1980), and thus, it may in rare cases be considered part of the emergency department armamentarium. Indeed, such patients now arrive at tertiary center emergency departments by advanced life support ground or air ambulance transport with balloon counterpulsation support. Although balloon counterpulsation can relieve pain and stabilize hemodynamics, studies performed on patients with or without congestive heart failure soon after myocardial infarction have thus far failed to demonstrate long-term benefit (Leinbach et al., 1978; O'Rourke et al., 1981). Thus, with rare exception, this mode of early intervention is reserved for patients who may be expected to benefit from nearly immediate operative intervention, but who require short-term stabilization before operation.

Vasodilators

Nitroprusside has both strong venodilating (preload) and arteriolar dilating (afterload) actions and can be administered effectively to patients with persistent elevation of blood pressure, especially when it is associated with a high left ventricular filling pressure. For the reasons previously noted, when nitroprusside is administered in the presence of acute ischemia or infarction, concurrent treatment with nitroglycerin is preferred, in the hope of maintaining coronary circulation through the collateral channels.

Acute Interventional Therapy

In addition to attempts to limit infarct size with agents which decrease myocardial oxygen demand, recent efforts have focused upon restoring coronary artery perfusion during the acute myocardial infarction. At present, reperfusion can be achieved by: (*a*) the administration of thrombolytic agents, such as streptokinase or tissue plasminogen activator (TPA); (*b*) percutaneous coronary artery angioplasty; or (*c*) surgical revascularization.

Thrombolytic Agents

Intracoronary streptokinase has been shown to establish reperfusion in approximately 75% of patients with acute myocardial infarction (Cowley, 1983). Comparison of regional and overall left ventricular function strongly suggests that effective thrombolysis with intracoronary streptokinase results in a higher ejection fraction, improvement in regional wall motion, and reduction in enzymatic infarct size, particularly in patients who undergo reperfusion within 4 hours of onset of symptoms (Anderson et al., 1983). Following demonstration of total or subtotal occlusion of the infarct-related coronary artery by coronary angiography, intracoronary streptokinase is administered as a bolus of 10,000–30,000 units. This is followed by a continuous infusion of 2,000–4,000 units/min. The infusion is maintained until thrombolysis has occurred, or until the preset maximum dose (150,000–500,000 units) has been administered. The response to therapy is monitored both clinically and angiographically. The sudden relief of chest pain, the new onset of ventricular arrhythmias, or the resolution of ST segment elevation usually signifies successful reperfusion (Mathey et al., 1981; Rentrop et al., 1979). The streptokinase infusion is generally administered for an additional hour and then anticoagulation with intravenous heparin is begun. Antiplatelet therapy with aspirin and dipyridamole (Persantine) is usually begun prior to discharge. Additional studies suggest that intravenous administration of streptokinase may also be effective in reestablishing antegrade coronary blood flow; however, high rates of arterial reocclusion have so far prevented the widespread use of this technique (ISAM Study Group, 1986).

More recently, TPA has been shown to be effective in lysing coronary thrombi during acute myocardial infarction (VanDeWerf et al., 1984). Preliminary results of a multicenter trial suggest that intravenous TPA may be more effective than intravenous streptokinase during acute infarction (TIMI Study Group, 1985). If results of ongoing clinical trials demonstrate either intravenous streptokinase or TPA to be highly effective in limiting myocardial infarction size, the emergency department approach to acute infarction will undergo major reevaluation.

Angioplasty

Percutaneous transluminal coronary angioplasty (PTCA) is also being utilized in acute myocardial infarction, either alone or following thrombolytic therapy. This technique appears especially useful in three clinical settings: (*a*) failure of thrombolytic agents to establish reperfusion; (*b*) with effective clot lysis, but a residual severe stenosis due to fixed atherosclerosis; and (*c*) with "partial" reperfusion demonstrated by slow antegrade flow, yet persistent chest pain and ST segment elevation, suggesting ongoing myocardial ischemia. Emergency angioplasty may also be helpful in patients in whom there are contraindications to thrombolytic therapy (such as recent surgery, cardiopulmonary resuscitation, or recent stroke (O'Neill et al., 1986)).

Selection of Patients

Patients with a history of typical ischemic chest pain of short duration (usually less than 4 hours) who demonstrate ST segment elevation greater than 1 mm that persists after sublingual nitroglycerin and who are hemodynamically stable should be considered for acute interventional therapy. Those individuals with pathologic Q wave development in the leads in which ST segment elevations are seen are usually excluded, since most have already had complete, or virtually complete, infarction. Likewise, patients with prolonged chest pain who demonstrate only ST segment depression or T wave inversion are usually excluded, since the incidence of occlusive thrombi is relatively low (Laffel and Braunwald, 1984). Patients with multiple prior infarctions, cardiogenic shock, advanced age, recent surgery, or cerebral vascular accident are poor candidates for acute interventional therapy and are usually best managed with conventional techniques and medications. Since the duration of myocardial ischemia is a major determinant of successful infarct limitation, the emergency physician must be familiar with the current indications for acute interventional therapy and seek to expedite the transfer of suitable patients from the emergency department to more appropriate facilities.

Such aggressive forms of therapy designed to limit infarct size are clearly unnecessary and inappropriate in patients with an uncomplicated infarction and adequate blood pressure and heart rate. Such patients should be treated in the emergency department with the classic regimen consisting of pain relief and sedation. Usually this is best accomplished with morphine sulfate, oxygen delivered through a nasal cannula, close monitoring of the heart rate, rhythm, and blood pressure, and expeditious transportation to the coronary care unit.

For patients with continuing ischemic pain or congestive heart failure in whom aggressive therapy is appropriate, the emergency physician should make immediate arrangements either for insertion of an intraarterial cannula for constant monitoring of the arterial blood pressure or of a Swan-Ganz pulmonary arterial catheter for measurement of left ventricular filling pressure, on prompt transfer to the appropriate intensive care unit. In the emergency situation, when medications such as nitroprusside, nitroglycerin, and propranolol are administered without monitoring devices, counteracting agents should always be available. Those would include an intravenous solution of isoproterenol or epinephrine to combat the effect of propranolol and a pure α-adrenergic agonist such as phenylephrine hydrochloride to negate the nitroprusside or nitroglycerin effects on blood pressure.

Hypotension in Acute Myocardial Infarction

Rhythm Disturbances

Hypotension complicating acute myocardial infarction may be related to easily reversible causes or may presage a truly ominous syndrome of cardiogenic shock. Easily reversible causes include considerable sinus bradycardia in a patient with inferior myocardial infarction, treatable with atropine, isoproterenol, or a temporary pacing wire, and rapid paroxysmal atrial tachycardia, treatable with cardioversion and appropriate antiarrhythmic drugs. The treatment of bradycardia in the absence of symptoms, ventricular premature beats, or hypotension remains controversial. Treatment in this setting is usually withheld to avoid unnecessary and perhaps dangerous stimulation (Epstein et al., 1975). When atropine is given, the minimum dose should be 0.4 mg intravenously to avoid the paradoxical slowing that has been reported with lower doses. The maximum dose should be 1.0 mg to avoid the sinus tachycardia occasionally seen with high doses. Loss of a properly timed atrial contraction may cause diminution in cardiac output in patients with impaired myocardial function, and restoration of atrioventricular synchrony by cardioversion, atrial pacing, or atrioventricular sequential pacing may improve both cardiac output and blood pressure.

The appearance of a bifascicular conduction system disturbance, including LBBB or RBBB with either left anterior or posterior hemiblock, may herald imminent progression to complete atrioventricular block. Most patients who die with this complication have extensive anterior infarction and ventricular failure. A small number of patients have relatively well-preserved left ventricular function and thus will benefit from the prompt prophylactic insertion of a temporary transvenous right ventricular pacing wire at the time of the appearance of the bifascicular block (Hindman et al., 1978).

Hypovolemia

Another promptly reversible but often unrecognized cause of hypotension in myocardial infarction is relative hypovolemia due to excessive diuresis or inappropriate peripheral vasodilatation. The classic example is the patient with pulmonary edema who has received a potent diuretic such as furosemide that has prompted considerable diuresis with subsequent hypotension. Such a patient may have a low intravascular volume at a time (even up to 24 hours) when interstitial edema is still present, either seen on the chest x-ray film or clinically manifested as congestive rales.

Right Ventricular Infarction

Right ventricular infarction, usually associated with infarction of the inferior left ventricular wall, may result in systemic hypotension in the absence of severe left ventricular dysfunction. The failure of the right ventricle in this setting results in insufficient left-sided filling pressure and, thus, reduced cardiac output (Isner and Roberts, 1978; Lorell et al., 1979). Unlike left ventricular failure, hypotension from this cause responds to volume expansion.

Knowledge of the left ventricular filling pressure obtained with a Swan-Ganz catheter allows appropriate volume replacement, employing either normal saline or lactated Ringer's solution. If knowledge of the left ventricular filling pressure is not readily obtainable, rapid administration, within 10 minutes, of 200 ml of 5% dextrose in water may be helpful. The pulse and blood pressure should be measured every 3 or 4 minutes. If the pulse rate slows and the blood pressure rises with the fluid challenge, good evidence of hypovolemia is obtained and longer-term replacement therapy can be instituted. If no beneficial effect is seen, even with a repeated challenge, the need for volume replacement must be questioned. Rapid administration of 5% dextrose in water is recommended because it moves into the intracellular space quickly, thus challenging the intravascular compartment briefly and safely.

Another cause of hypovolemia, recognized more often, is inappropriate peripheral vasodilatation in patients with acute infarction. Although this is noted more frequently in inferior and posterior myocardial infarction, perhaps related to stimulation of the vagal afferent or efferent nerves, it also occurs in anterior myocardial infarction. Here again, knowledge of the left ventricular filling pressure or a challenge with 5% dextrose in water will allow appropriate decisions concerning volume replacement. In most patients, inappropriate peripheral vasodilatation resolves after 24–72 hours.

Cardiogenic Shock

Severe hypotension not due to arrhythmias or hypovolemia may indicate cardiogenic shock with its ominous prognosis. In patients with cardiogenic shock, systolic blood pressure is usually less than 90 mm Hg or is 50 mm Hg lower than normal levels for the patient and is accompanied by signs of peripheral vasoconstriction, a urinary output less than 20 ml/hr, and mental obtundation. Pulmonary congestion may or may not occur. The characteristic hemodynamic findings are a cardiac index less than 2 liters/min/m^2, a mean arterial pressure less than 60 mm Hg, and a pulmonary capillary wedge pressure more than 20 mm Hg. A vicious cycle ensues, with low cardiac output causing low arterial blood pressure leading to reduced coronary artery perfusion, resulting in further reduction of cardiac output, and so on.

The goal of therapy is to support the blood pressure at a level sufficient to maintain both peripheral circulation and coronary artery perfusion pressure, aiming at a mean arterial pressure of 70 mm Hg, in such a way that myocardial oxygen consumption does not increase. This poses a problem since agents such as epinephrine, isoproterenol, and norepinephrine increase myocardial oxygen consumption by their central β-adrenergic action, and yet this direct stimulation of the heart is usually essential to maintain overall circulation. Pure α-adrenergic agents, such as phenylephrine hydrochloride and methoxamine hydrochloride, are usually ineffective in patients with cardiogenic shock.

Probably the best supporting pharmacologic agent currently in clinical use is norepinephrine, 2–30 μg/min intravenously. This agent has both an α action (peripheral vasoconstriction) and central β action (increased cardiac contractility), but the former action is stronger. An acceptable compromise results in which the peripheral circulation, the central coronary artery perfusion pressure, and the myocardium are supported. Dobutamine, a synthetic catecholamine, improves cardiac output and lowers left ventricular filling pressure in patients with evolving myocardial infarction without significantly accelerating heart rate or precipitating arrhythmias (Gillespie et al., 1975; Goldstein et al., 1980). Except in the treatment of atrial tachyarrhythmias, digitalis has no role in the emergency department therapy of heart failure from acute myocardial infarction.

The most effective therapeutic device in the management of cardiogenic shock is intraaortic balloon counterpulsation (Corral and Vaughn, 1986; Dunkman et al., 1972). As mentioned previously, by deflating in systole, the balloon reduces the afterload and preload, decreasing myocardial oxygen consumption; and by filling in diastole, it augments the central diastolic aortic pressure, increasing coronary artery perfusion pressure. The intraaortic balloon is now established as an effective device that allows subsequent coronary angiographic examination and operation in suitable candidates. The ideal patient is a young person with no previous infarct and with a normal-sized heart in whom balloon support is initiated within 24 hours of acute infarction. Other favorable indicators include a murmur signaling a possibly treatable mechanical complication or angina indicating viable but ischemic myocardium. The poorest candidate is the older patient with multiple previous infarcts and a large heart with no evidence of a surgically correctable mechanical lesion, such as a ventricular septal defect, severe mitral regurgitation, or a large discrete aneurysm. It is useful to keep these guidelines in mind, because the best results in cardiogenic shock are obtained with early use of the balloon, and the decision for or against such therapy must often be made in the emergency department.

REFERENCES

Anderson JL, Marshall HW, Bray BE, et al. A randomized trial of intracoronary streptokinase in the treatment of acute myocardial infarction. *N Engl J Med*, 1983;308: 1312–1318.

Antman E, Muller J, Goldberg S, et al. Nifedipine therapy for coronary-artery spasm. *N Engl J Med*, 1980;302: 1269–1273.

Armstrong PW, Armstrong JA, Marks GS. Pharmacokinetic-hemodynamic studies of intravenous nitroglycerin in congestive heart failure. *Circulation*, 1980;62:160–166.

Badger RS, Brown BG, Gallery CA, et al. Coronary artery dilation and hemodynamic responses after isosorbide dinitrate therapy in patients with coronary artery disease. *Am J Cardiol*, 1985;56:390–395.

Borer JS, Redwood DR, Levitt B, et al. Reduction in myocardial ischemia with nitroglycerin or nitroglycerin plus phenylephrine administered during acute myocardial infarction. *N Engl J Med*, 1975;293:1008–1012.

Boyle DC, Barber JM, McIlmoyle EL, et al. Effect of very early intervention with metoprolol on myocardial infarct size. *Br Heart J*, , 1983;49:229–233.

Broden WE, Bough EW, Reichman MJ, et al. Beneficial effects of high-dose diltiazem in patients with persistent effort angina on beta-blockers and nitrates: a randomized, double-blind, placebo-controlled cross-over study. *Circulation*, 1985;71:1197–1205.

Cairns, JA, Gent M, Singer J, et al. Aspirin, sulfinpyrazone, or both in unstable angina: Results of a Canadian multicenter trial. *N Engl J Med*, 1985;313:1369–1375.

CASS Investigators. Coronary artery surgery study (CASS): A randomized trial of coronary artery bypass surgery survival data. *Circulation*, 1983;68:939–950.

Castell DO. Calcium channel blocking agents for gastrointestinal disorders. *Am J Cardiol,* 1985;55:210B–213B.

Chiariello M, Gold HK, Leinbach RC, et al. Comparison between the effects of nitroprusside and nitroglycerin on ischemic injury during acute myocardial infarction. *Circulation*, 1976;54:766–773.

Come PC, Flaherty JT, Baird MG, et al. Reversal by phenylephrine of the beneficial effects of intravenous nitroglycerin in patients with acute myocardial infarction. *N Engl J Med*, 1975;293:1003–1007.

Corral, CM, Vaughn CC. Intraaortic balloon counterpulsation: An eleven year review and analysis of determinants of survival. *Tex Heart Inst J*, 1986;13:39–44.

Cowley, MJ. Methodologic aspects of intracoronary thrombolysis: Drugs, dosage and duration. *Circulation,* 1983;68 (suppl):90–95.

Dunkman WB, Leinbach RC, Buckley MJ, et al: Clinical and hemodynamic results of intraaortic balloon pumping and surgery for cardiogenic shock. *Circulation*, 1972;46:465–477.

Ellrodt G, Chew CYC, Singh BN: Therapeutic implications of slow-channel blockade in cardiocirculatory disorders. *Circulation*, 1980;62:669–679.

Epstein SE, Kent KM, Goldstein RE, et al: Reduction of ischemic injury by nitroglycerin during acute myocardial infarction. *N Engl J Med*, 1975;292:29–35.

European Coronary Surgical Group: Prospective randomized study of coronary artery bypass surgery in stable angina pectoris. *Lancet*, 1980;2:491–495.

Flaherty JT, Becker LC, Buckley BH, et al: A randomized prospective trial of intravenous nitroglycerin in patients with acute myocardial infarction. *Circulation*, 1983;68:576–588.

Frishman WH: Drug therapy: Beta-adrenoceptor antagonists: New drugs and new indications. *N Engl J Med*, 1981;305:500–506.

Gerstenblith G, Ouyang P, Achuff SC, et al: Nifedipine in unstable angina: A double-blind, randomized trial. *N Engl J Med*, 1982;306:885–889.

Gillespie TA, Ambos HD, Sobel BE, et al: Effects of dobutamine in patients with acute myocardial infarction. *Am J Cardiol*, 1975;39:588–594.

Gold HK, Leinbach RC, Sanders CA: Use of sublingual nitroglycerin in congestive failure during acute myocardial infarction. *Circulation*, 1972;46:839–845.

Gold HK, Leinbach RC, Sanders CA, et al: Intraaortic balloon pumping for control of recurrent myocardial ischemia. *Circulation*, 1973;47:1197–1203.

Goldstein RE, Stinson EB, Scherer JL, et al: Intraoperative coronary collateral function in patients with coronary occlusive disease: Nitroglycerine responsiveness and angiographic correlations. *Circulation*, 1974;49:298–308.

Goldstein RA, Passamani ER, Roberts R: A comparison of digoxin and dobutamine in patients with acute infarction and cardiac failure. *N Engl J Med*, 1980;303:846–850.

Goteborg Metoprolol Trial in Acute Myocardial Infarction: *Am J Cardiol*, 1984;53:10D–50D.

Greenblatt DJ, Bolognini V, Koch-Weser, J, et al: Pharmacokinetic approach to the clinical use of lidocaine intravenously. *JAMA*, 1976;236:273–277.

Heikkila J: Mitral incompetence complicating acute myocardial infarction. *Br Heart J*, 1967;29:162–169.

Hill JA, Feldman RL, Pepine CJ, et al: Randomized double-blind comparison of nifedipine and isosorbide dinitrate in patients with coronary arterial spasm. *Am J Cardiol*, 1982;49:431–438.

Hindman MC, Wagner GS, JaRo M, et al: The clinical significance of bundle branch block complicating acute myocardial infarction. 1. Clinical characteristics, hospital mortality, and one-year follow-up. *Circulation*, 1978;58: 679–688.

Hutter AM, Jr: Is there a main left equivalent? *Circulation*, 1980;62:207–211.

International Collaborative Study Group: Reduction of infarct size with the early use of timolol in acute myocardial infarction. *N Engl J Med*, 1984;310:9–15.

ISAM Study Group: A prospective trial of intravenous streptokinase in acute myocardial infarction: Mortality, morbidity, and infarct size at 21 days. *N Engl J Med*, 1986;314:1465–1471.

Isner JM, Roberts WC: Right ventricular infarction complicating left ventricular infarction secondary to coronary heart disease. *Am J Cardiol*, 1978;42:885–894.

Jaffe AS, Geltman EM, Tiefenbrunn AJ, et al: Reduction of infarct site in patients with inferior infarction with intravenous glyceryl trinitrate: A randomized study. *Br Heart J,* 1983;49:452–460.

Laffel GL, Braunwald E: Thrombolytic therapy. A new strategy for the treatment of acute myocardial infarction. *N Engl J Med*, 1984;311:710–717, 770–776.

Lee G, Mason DT, Amsterdam EA, et al: Improved exercise tolerance for six hours following isosorbide dinitrate capsules in patients with ischemic heart disease (Abstract). *Am J Cardiol*, 1976;37:150.

Leinbach RC, Gold HK, Harper RW, et al: Early intraaortic balloon pumping for anterior myocardial infarction without shock. *Circulation*, 1978;58:204–210.

Levine FH, Gold HK, Leinbach RC, et al: Management of acute myocardial ischemia with intraaortic balloon pumping and coronary artery bypass surgery. *Circulation*, 1978;58 (suppl):69–72.

Lewis HD Jr, Davis JW, Archibald DG, et al: Protective effects of aspirin against acute myocardial infarction and death in men with unstable angina. Results of a Veterans Administration Cooperative Study. *N Engl J Med* 1983;309:396–403.

Liang C-S, Coplin B, Wellington K: Comparison of antianginal efficacy of nifedipine and isosorbide dinitrate in chronic stable angina: A long-term, randomized, double-blind, crossover study. *Am J Cardiol*, 1985;55:9E–14E.

Lie KI, Wellens HJ, Van Capelle FJ, et al: Lidocaine in the prevention of primary ventricular fibrillation: A double-blind randomized study of 212 consecutive patients. *N Engl J Med*, 1974;291:1324–1326.

Lorell B, Leinbach RC, Pohost GM, et al: Right ventricular infarction. *Am J Cardiol*, 1979;43:465–471.

Maroko PR, Braunwald E: Modification of myocardial infarction size after coronary occlusion. *Ann Intern Med*, 1973;79:720–733.

Maroko PR, Kjekshus JK, Sobel BE, et al: Factors influencing infarct size following experimental coronary artery occlusions. *Circulation*, 1971;43:67–82.

Mathey, DC, Kuck K-K, Tilsner V, et al. Nonsurgical coronary artery revascularization in acute transmural myocardial infarction. *Circulation*, 1981;63:489–497.

Miller RR, Vismara LA, Zelis R, et al: Clinical use of sodium nitroprusside in chronic ischemic heart disease: Effects on peripheral vascular resistance and venous tone and on ventricular volume, pump and mechanical performance. *Circulation*, 1975;51:328–336.

Mueller HS, Ayers SM: The role of propranolol in the treatment of acute myocardial infarction. *Prog Cardiovasc Dis,* 1977;19:405–412.

National Cooperative Study Group to Compare Medical and Surgical Therapy: Unstable angina pectoris: I. Report of protocol and patient population. *Am J Cardiol*, 1976;37:896–902.

National Cooperative Study Group to Compare Surgical and Medical Therapy: Unstable angina pectoris: III. Results in patients with ST segment elevation during pain. *Am J Cardiol*, 1980;45:819.

Nies AS, Shand DG: Clinical pharmacology of propranolol. *Circulation*, 1975;52:6–15.

Norris RM, Sammel NL, Clarke ED, et al. Treatment of acute myocardial infarction with propranolol. *Br Heart J,* 1981;43:617–622.

O'Neill W, Timmis GC, Bourdillon PD, et al: A prospective randomized clinical trial of intracoronary streptokinase versus coronary angioplasty for acute myocardial infarction. *N Engl J Med*, 1986;314:812–818.

Orlando RC, Bozymski EM: Clinical and manometric effects of nitroglycerin in diffuse esophageal spasm. *N Engl J Med*, 1973;289:23–25.

O'Rourke MF, Norris RM, Campbell TJ, et al: Randomized controlled trial of intraaortic balloon counterpulsation in early myocardial infarction with acute heart failure. *Am J Cardiol*, 1981;47:815–820.

Palmer RF, Lasseter KC. Drug therapy: Sodium nitroprusside. *N Engl J Med*, 1975;292:294–297.

Pasternak RC, Hutter AM Jr, DeSanctis RW, et al. Variant angina: Clinical spectrum and results of medical and surgical therapy. *J Thorac Cardiovasc Surg*, 1979;78:614–622.

Pathy MS: Clinical presentation of myocardial infarction in the elderly. *Br Heart J*, 1967;29:190–199.

Peter T, Norris RM, Clarke ED, et al. Reduction of enzyme levels by propranolol after acute myocardial infarction. *Circulation*, 1978;57:1091–1095.

Prida XE, Feldman RL, Hill JA, et al. Comparison of diltiazem and nifedipine in patients with coronary artery spasm. *Circulation*, 1985;72(suppl III):276.

Prinzmetal M, Kennamer R, Merliss R, et al: Angina pectoris. 1. A variant form of angina pectoris: Preliminary report. *Am J Med*, 1959;27:375–388.

Reichek N, Goldstein RE, Redwood Dr, et al: Sustained effects of nitroglycerin ointment in patients with angina pectoris. *Circulation*, 1974;50:348–352.

Rentrop KP, Blanze H, Karsh FR, et al. Initial experience with transluminal recannulization of the recently occluded infarct-related coronary artery in acute myocardial infarction: Comparison of conventionally treated patients. *Clin Cardiol*, 1979;2:92–105.

Roberts R, Sobel BE: Creatinine kinase isoenzymes in the assessment of heart disease. *Am Heart J,* 1978;95:521–528.

Roberts R, Croft C, Gold HK, et al. Effect of propranolol on myocardial infarct size in a randomized blinded multicenter trial. *N Engl J Med*, 1984;311:218–225.

Spodick DH: Electrocardiogram in acute pericarditis: Distributions of morphologic and axial changes by stages. *Am J Cardiol*, 1974;33:470–474.

Subramanian VA, Goldstein JJ, Sos TA, et al. Preliminary clinical experience with percutaneous intraaortic balloon pumping. *Circulation,* 1980;62(suppl 1):123–129.

Takaro T, Hultgren HN, Lipton MJ, et al: The Virginia Cooperative Randomized Study of Surgery for Coronary Arterial Occlusive Disease. II. Subgroup with significant left main lesions. *Circulation,* 1976;54(suppl III):107–117.

Telford AM, Wilson C: Trial of heparin versus atenolol in treatment of myocardial infarction in intermediate coronary syndrome. *Lancet*, 1981;1225–1228.

Thadani U, Fung HL, Darke AC, et al: Oral isosorbide dinitrate in the treatment of angina pectoris: Dose response relationship and duration of action during acute therapy. *Circulation*, 1980;62:491–502.

TIMI Study Group: The thrombolysis in myocardial infarction (TIMI) trial. *N Engl J Med*, 1985;312:932–936.

VanDeWerf F, Ludbrook PA, Bergmann SR, et al: Coronary thrombolysis with tissue-type plasminogen activator in patients with evolving myocardial infarction. *N Engl J Med*, 1984;310:609–613.

White HD, Polak JF, Wynne J. et al. Addition of nifedipine to maximal nitrate and beta-adrenoreceptor blocker therapy in coronary artery disease. *Am J Cardiol*, 1985;55:1303–1307.

Willerson JT, Campbell WB, Winniford MD, et al. Conversion from chronic to acute coronary disease: Speculation regarding mechanisms. *Am J Cardiol*, 1984;54:1349–1354.

Williams DO, Amsterdam EA, Mason DT: Hemodynamic effects of nitroglycerin in acute myocardial infarction: Decrease in ventricular preload at the expense of cardiac output. *Circulation*, 1975;51:421–427.

Wyman MG, Hammersmith L: Comprehensive treatment plan for the prevention of primary ventricular fibrillation in acute myocardial infarction. *Am J Cardiol*, 1974;33:661–667.

Yusuf S, Sleight P, Rossi P, et al. Reduction in infarct size, arrhythmias and chest pain by early intravenous betablockade in suspected acute myocardial infarction. *Circulation*, 1983;67:32–41.

Zelis R, Flaim SF: "Calcium influx blockers" and vascular smooth muscle: Do we really understand the mechanism? [Editorial]. *Ann Intern Med*, 1981;94:124.

CHAPTER 7

Cardiology: Heart Failure

MICHAEL A. FIFER, M.D.
ROBERT ARNOLD JOHNSON, M.D.
DANIEL CHIA-SEN LEE, M.D.

DEFINITION AND CAUSES OF HEART FAILURE

Confusion regarding use of the term "heart failure" is a persistent problem in medical practice. The following definition is often offered: heart failure is the inability of the heart to supply blood in an amount adequate for the metabolic needs of the tissues. In practice, it is usually very difficult for the emergency physician to determine whether such a disparity between blood supply and metabolic needs exists in an individual patient. Furthermore, the term heart failure is generally applied by emergency physicians when there is an elevation of left and/or right heart filling pressure, irrespective of whether the metabolic needs of the tissues are satisfied. This latter definition of heart failure is attractive in that it is simple and clinically useful. Thus, *left heart failure* (LHF) may be defined as an increase in mean left atrial pressure (as commonly approximated by the pulmonary capillary "wedge" pressure) above 12 mm Hg; *right heart failure* (RHF) as an increase in mean right atrial pressure (as commonly estimated by the central venous pressure) above 6 mm Hg (or 8 cm H_2O); and *bisided heart failure,* as abnormal elevation of both atrial pressures. The manifestations of LHF are those of pulmonary venous congestion, and the manifestations of RHF are those of systemic venous congestion.

Several aspects of these definitions are noteworthy. First, the term heart failure does not imply impairment of either systolic or diastolic function of the ventricular myocardium. Having made a diagnosis of heart failure, the physician must determine the contributions of both myocardial and nonmyocardial factors to the elevation of atrial pressure. For example, in patients with mitral stenosis, obstruction of the mitral valve results in elevation of left atrial pressure; this may be appropriately termed heart failure, yet left ventricular (LV) function is usually normal. Second, no statement is made regarding the cardiac output, which may be high, normal, or low, depending on the cause of heart failure.

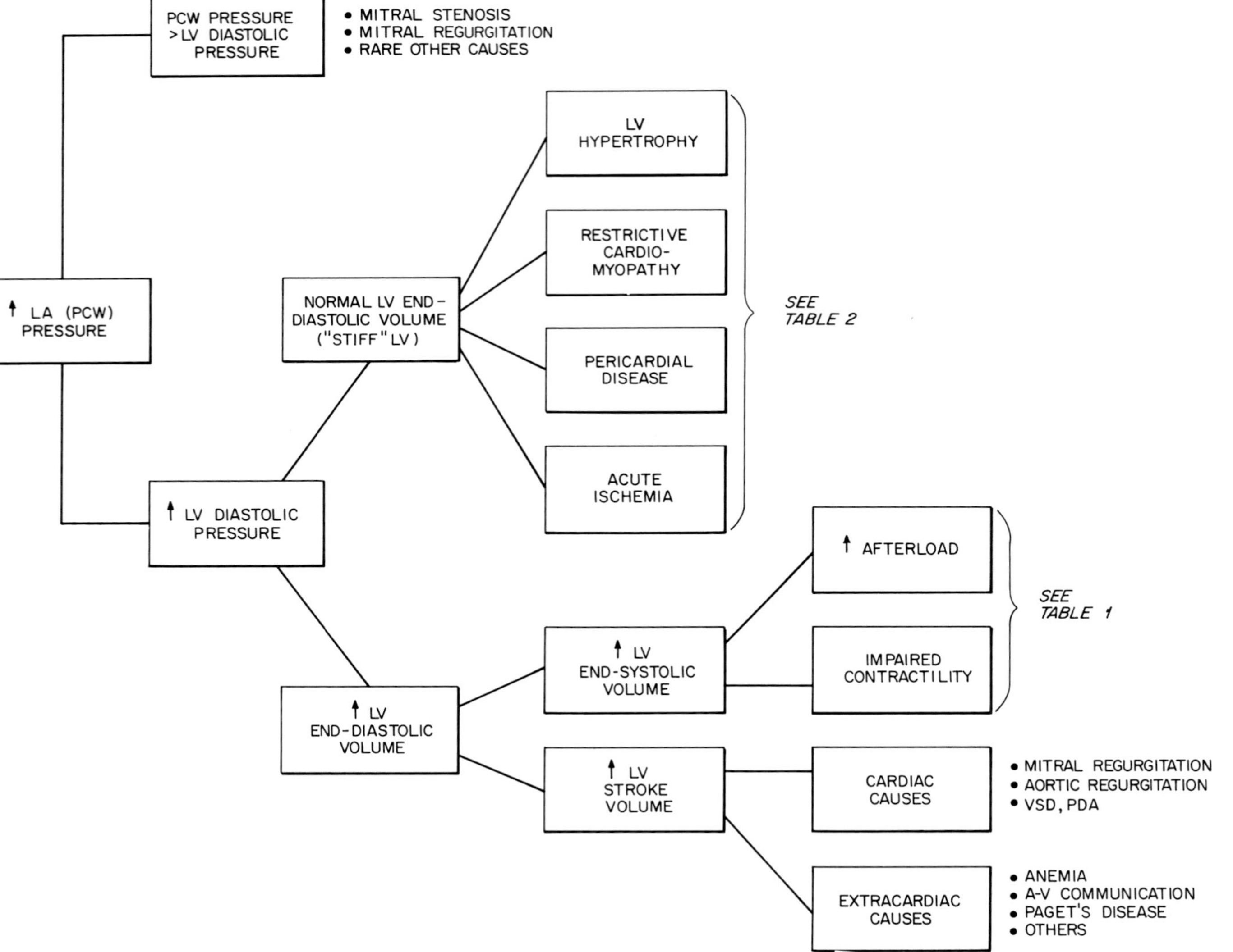

Figure 7.1. Schematic outline of differential diagnosis of left heart failure. *PCW pressure*, pulmonary capillary wedge pressure; *VSD*, ventricular septal defect; *PDA*, patent ductus arteriosus; *A-V communication*, arteriovenous communication.

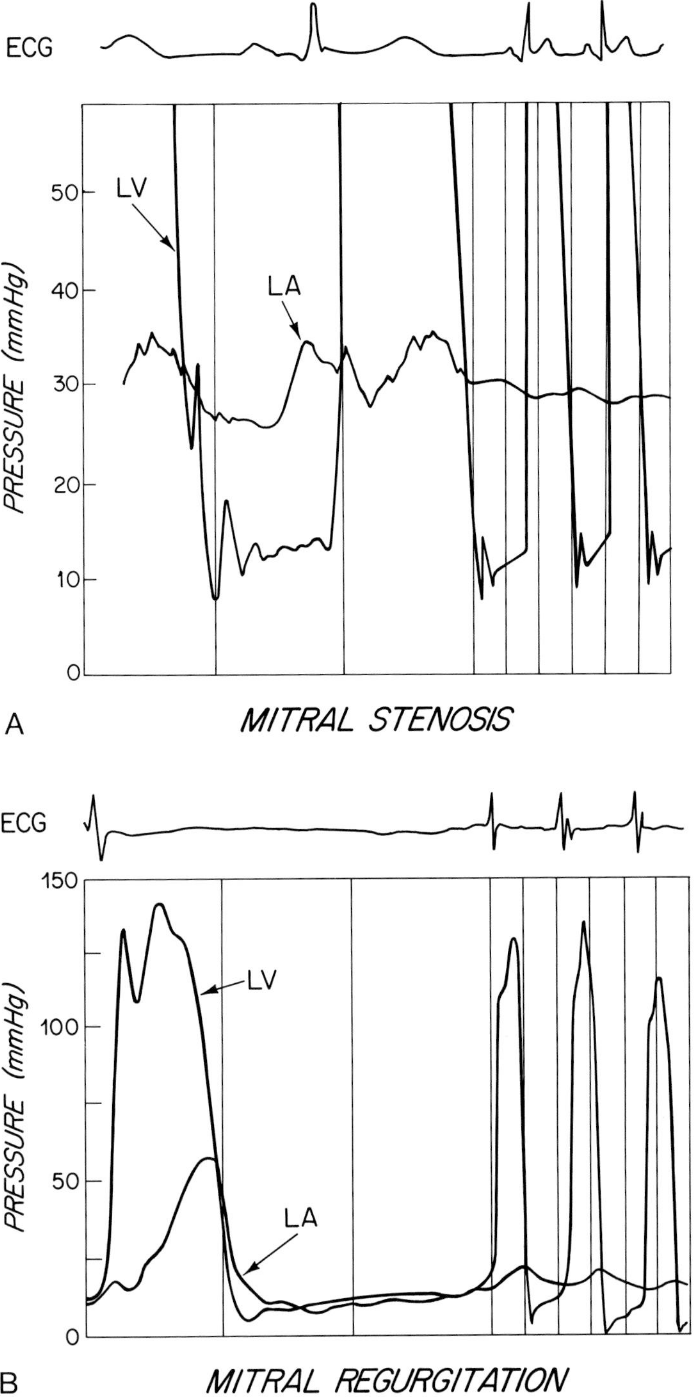

Figure 7.2. Elevation of mean left atrial *(LA)* pressure despite normal or near-normal left ventricular *(LV)* diastolic pressure. *A*, mitral stenosis: mean LA pressure exceeds LV diastolic pressure because of gradient across stenotic mitral valve in diastole. *B*, mitral regurgitation: mean LA pressure incorporates (systolic) regurgitant or "v" waves and is therefore higher than LV diastolic pressure.

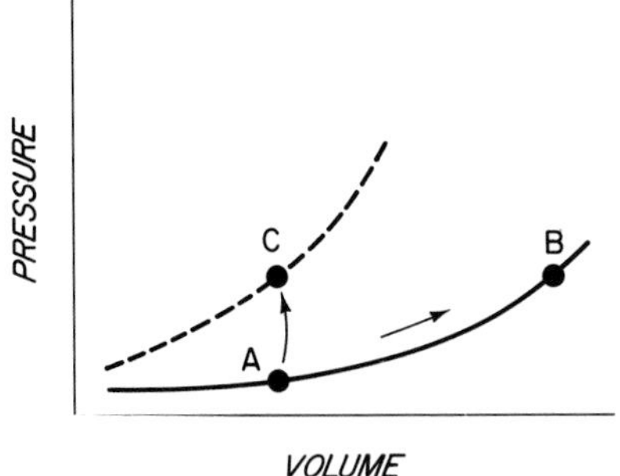

Figure 7.3. Mechanisms of elevation of left ventricular end-diastolic pressure. With left ventricular dilatation (due to volume overload or systolic dysfunction), end-diastolic volume and pressure increase (from *point A* to *point B*) along the normal passive diastolic pressure-volume curve *(solid line).* In diastolic dysfunction (stiff left ventricle), there is an upward shift of the pressure-volume relation *(dashed line),* such that end-diastolic pressure is elevated *(point C)* despite normal end-diastolic volume.

Table 7.1.
Causes of LV Systolic Dysfunction (Low LV Ejection Fraction)

Extreme elevation of LV afterload
Aortic stenosis
Severe, acute hypertension
Coarctation of the aorta (in infancy)
Impaired Contractility
Multiple myocardial infarctions
Large, single myocardial infarction
Acute
Remote (often with LV aneurysm)
Widespread acute myocardial ischemia
Idiopathic dilated cardiomyopathy
Myocarditis
Chronic mitral or aortic regurgitation
Alcoholic cardiomyopathy
Peripartum cardiomyopathy
Doxorubicin (Adriamycin) cardiotoxicity
Hemochromatosis
Hypophosphatemia
Many other rare causes

Third, this view of heart failure encourages the physician from the outset to consider separately those therapeutic maneuvers aimed at treating the consequences of elevated atrial pressure and those aimed at treating the underlying cause.

Causes of Left Heart Failure

A schematic flow chart outlining the causes of left heart failure is shown in Figure 7.1. Elevation of left atrial (or pulmonary capillary wedge) pressure generally reflects elevation of the left ventricular diastolic pressure (LVDP). Two exceptions to this rule are mitral stenosis and mitral regurgitation. In mitral stenosis, the pressure gradient across the narrowed mitral valve results in elevation of the left atrial pressure (LAP) even in the presence of normal LVDP (Fig. 7.2*A*). It is perhaps less well-appreciated that, in mitral regurgitation as well, the mean LAP is often elevated even when LVDP is not. This is so because the *mean* LAP incorporates the large regurgitant or "v" wave generally seen in mitral regurgitation (Fig. 7.2*B*); because the v wave reflects blood regurgitated during *systole*, it results in elevation of the mean left atrial pressure out of proportion to that of LVDP, which may, in fact, be normal. Other causes of elevation of LAP despite normal LVDP, such as left atrial myxoma, are rare.

In the absence of mitral valve disease, elevation of LAP generally reflects abnormally high LVDP. LVDP may be elevated by either of two mechanisms (Fig. 7.3). If the LV is dilated, i.e., if LV end-diastolic volume is elevated, then LV end-diastolic pressure will be passively increased because of movement along the normal compliance curve of the LV (*point B*). Alternatively, LV end-diastolic pressure may be elevated in the presence of normal LV end-diastolic volume if the ventricle is abnormally stiff, or noncompliant (*point C*).

High LV End-diastolic Volume

Since LV end-diastolic volume is the sum of end-systolic volume and stroke volume, elevation of end-diastolic volume may reflect either high end-systolic volume (i.e., systolic dysfunction, with low ejection fraction) or high stroke volume (i.e., volume overload). As outlined in Figure 7.1, systolic dysfunction is usually due to impaired myocardial contractility, but, in some cases, results from excessively high afterload, as in aortic stenosis or severe, acute hypertension. Some causes of systolic dysfunction are listed in Table 7.1. Volume overload may be due to mitral or aortic regurgitation, or to extracardiac conditions such as anemia.

Abnormal LV Stiffness

The LV may be abnormally noncompliant because there is too much myocardium (LV hypertrophy), because there is an infiltrative disorder of the myocardium (restrictive cardiomyopathy), because the myocardium is abnormally constrained from without (pericardial disease), or because the myocardium is acutely ischemic. Specific causes of abnormal LV stiffness are listed in Table 7.2. Pericardial disease and some types of restrictive cardiomyopathy typically produce bisided heart failure.

Two or more mechanisms of LAP elevation may be operative in a single cardiac disorder. For example, a patient with aortic stenosis may exhibit abnormal LV stiffness (i.e., *diastolic* dysfunction)

Table 7.2.
Causes of LV Diastolic Dysfunction (Abnormal LV Stiffness)

LV hypertrophy
- Aortic stenosis
- Chronic hypertension
- Hypertrophic cardiomyopathy (including idiopathic hypertrophic subaortic stenosis)

Restrictive cardiomyopathy
- Amyloid heart disease
- Idiopathic restrictive cardiomyopathy
- Endomyocardial disease

Pericardial disease
- Pericardial constriction
- Pericardial tamponade
- Effusive-constrictive pericarditis

Acute myocardial ischemia

due to LV hypertrophy, *and* impaired LV emptying (i.e., *systolic* dysfunction) due to excessive afterload.

Left Heart Failure in Coronary Artery Disease

Coronary artery disease may bring about LHF by a number of mechanisms. Papillary muscle dysfunction, infarction, or, in the extreme case, rupture may cause elevation of the pulmonary wedge pressure with normal or near-normal LV function. Alternatively, LV systolic dysfunction may result from multiple previous infarctions, one large past infarction (sometimes with formation of a LV aneurysm), acute infarction, or widespread acute ischemia. It is common for heart failure to complicate an acute anterior myocardial infarction, but uncommon for heart failure to complicate an inferior myocardial infarction unless there are associated mechanical complications (infarction or rupture of a papillary muscle, rupture of the interventricular septum), unrecognized old infarctions, concomitant areas of ischemia, or right ventricular infarction. Finally, acute ischemia often causes abnormal LV stiffness, which may result in heart failure in the presence of normal LV systolic function.

Causes of Right Heart Failure

Causes of right heart failure are listed in Table 7.3. Tricuspid stenosis or primary tricuspid regurgitation may result in elevation of right atrial pressure. Right ventricular (RV) diastolic pressure may be elevated due to high RV end-diastolic volume associated with volume overload (tricuspid or pulmonic regurgitation, atrial septal defect), or, more commonly, with RV systolic dysfunction. RV systolic dysfunction (low RV ejection fraction) may be due to RV pressure overload, i.e., pulmonary hypertension due to LHF, lung disease (cor pulmonale), massive acute pulmonary embolism, or

Table 7.3.
Causes of Right Heart Failure

Tricuspid valve disease
- Tricuspid stenosis
- Tricuspid regurgitation

Right ventricular volume overload
- Cardiac cause
  - Atrial septal defect
  - Tricuspid regurgitation
  - Pulmonic regurgitation
- Extracardiac cause
  - Anemia
  - Arteriovenous communication
  - Paget's disease

Right ventricular systolic dysfunction (low RV ejection fraction)
- Elevation of RV afterload
  - Pulmonic stenosis
  - Pulmonary hypertension
    - Due to left heart failure
    - Due to lung disease (cor pulmonale)
    - Pulmonary embolism
    - Primary pulmonary vascular disease
- Impaired contractility
  - Cardiomyopathy
  - Acute RV infarction
  - Chronic volume overload

Right ventricular diastolic dysfunction (abnormal RV stiffness)
- RV hypertrophy
  - Pulmonic stenosis
  - Pulmonary hypertension
  - Hypertrophic cardiomyopathy with RV involvement
- Restrictive cardiomyopathy
- Pericardial disease
  - Pericardial tamponade
  - Pericardial constriction
  - Effusive-constrictive pericarditis

primary pulmonary vascular disease. Of these, the most common is LHF—thus, the clinical maxim, "the most common cause of right heart failure is left heart failure." Alternatively, low RV ejection fraction may be due to depressed contractility of the RV myocardium. Impaired RV myocardial contractility may result from cardiomyopathy of any cause, acute RV infarction, or chronic volume or pressure overload. Finally, RHF may be due to abnormal RV stiffness resulting from RV hypertrophy (as in pulmonic stenosis), restrictive cardiomyopathy, or pericardial constriction or tamponade.

Like LHF, RHF may result from two or more mechanisms. For example, some patients with rheumatic heart disease may have intrinsic tricuspid valve disease causing regugitation, as well as RV pressure overload due to concomitant mitral stenosis with LHF and pulmonary hypertension.

Precipitating Factors

In many of the diseases causing LHF or RHF or both, the condition of the patient is often "compen-

Table 7.4.
Precipitating Factors of Heart Failure

States resulting in increased cardiac output
- Infection
- Anemia
- Dietary salt excess
- Fluid overload
- Fever
- Renal failure
- Pregnancy
- Hypoxia
- Heat
- Hyperthyroidism
- Emotional stress
- Obesity
- Hepatic disease
- Acute minor pulmonary embolism
- Acute abdominal disease (e.g., intestinal infarction, pancreatitis)

Fluid retention due to nonsteroidal anti-inflammatory drugs
Negative inotropic agents (β-blockers, calcium channel blockers, disopyramide)
Tachy- or bradyarrhythmia
Poorly controlled hypertension
Poor compliance with medical regimen

sated,'' i.e., atrial pressures are normal or only mildly elevated, until a precipitating event results in an increase in one or both atrial pressures. These factors (Table 7.4) do not in themselves usually cause heart failure, but, when superimposed on underlying heart disease, may ''tip the scales.'' Special mention should be made of pulmonary emboli, which, in addition to being a cause of isolated RHF when massive or multiple, may precipitate LHF in patients who have underlying left heart disease. The mechanism is uncertain, but possibly involves the increased cardiac output due to hypoxemia caused by pulmonary embolism.

MANIFESTATIONS AND DIAGNOSIS OF HEART FAILURE

History

Both LHF and RHF may produce *dyspnea* on exertion and fatigue because of associated limitation of forward cardiac output. Paroxysmal nocturnal dyspnea, orthopnea, and nonproductive cough are symptoms of elevated left atrial pressure in LHF, while right upper quadrant discomfort is a particular symptom of elevated right atrial pressure in RHF.

Peripheral *edema* may be caused by RHF, by impaired renal perfusion due to LHF alone, or by a combination of these; severe fluid retention, with ascites and anasarca, generally reflects some degree of RHF. Ankle edema is correctly attributed to RHF only if the jugular venous pressure is elevated. Most patients with ankle edema do not have heart failure at all. More common causes are bilateral chronic venous insufficiency of the lower extremities and prolonged dependency of the legs in obese or disabled persons. Edema is also a common side effect of the calcium channel blocker nifedipine. Less commonly, edema is due to hepatic disease, renal disease, or another systemic cause. In some cases, an explanation cannot be found.

While even moderate elevation of left atrial pressure produces severe symptoms in patients with previously normal hemodynamics (as in ruptured mitral chordae tendineae), patients with chronic elevation of left atrial pressure, even to levels as high as 30 mm Hg, may tolerate this remarkably well, probably due to an increase in pulmonary lymphatic drainage. High right atrial pressures, on the other hand, are not well-tolerated, because of the lack of a compensatory mechanism. For these reasons, the clinical presentation of RHF ''out of proportion'' to LHF may be misleading; in such cases, left atrial pressure is often equal to or greater than right atrial pressure.

The history may provide clues as to the underlying cause of or factors precipitating heart failure (Table 7.5). In cases of pulmonary edema, the patient may be physically unable to give a history, which must then be obtained if possible from family members or neighbors. In elderly patients in particular, the classic symptoms of heart failure may be

Table 7.5.
Initial Evaluation of the Patient with Heart Failure: Clues to the Causative Mechanism

History
- Chronic symptoms (previous myocardial infarction, rheumatic mitral regurgitation, idiopathic dilated cardiomyopathy) vs. sudden symptoms (acute myocardial infarction, ruptured chordae tendineae)
- Chest pain (coronary artery disease)
- Infection, poor compliance with diet or medication (precipitating causes)

Physical examination
- Pulsus paradoxus (pericardial tamponade)
- Kussmaul's sign (pericardial constriction)
- Weak and delayed carotid pulsation (aortic stenosis)
- Lateral displacement of LV apical impulse (LV enlargement)
- S_3 (LV systolic dysfunction)
- Opening snap or loud S_1 (mitral stenosis)

Electrocardiogram
- Left ventricular hypertrophy (aortic stenosis, chronic hypertension, hypertrophic cardiomyopathy)
- Previous transmural infarction (chronic LV systolic dysfunction)
- Acute ischemia (LV systolic and/or diastolic and/or papillary muscle dysfunction)

obscure, and it may be reported by others that the patient "just hasn't been doing well" recently, as evidenced by change in mental status, anorexia, insomnia, or decreased activity.

Overemphasis on the role of dietary salt "indiscretion" in precipitating pulmonary edema should be avoided. While excessive sodium ingestion may lead to heart failure in a patient with underlying heart disease, it is often incorrectly assigned a role in the absence of these conditions. As a consequence, more significant causative factors may be overlooked.

The physician should not assume that a history generally consistent with coronary artery disease is an adequate explanation for heart failure. As discussed previously, LHF may complicate coronary artery disease by a number of mechanisms; since therapy is often directed at the causative mechanism(s), it is important to determine which of these is most likely in a given patient.

Physical Examination

General Appearance

The physical examination in acute pulmonary edema is usually dominated by the general appearance of an extremely dyspneic, profusely diaphoretic patient with rapid, shallow respirations and a variable degree of cyanosis. Pink, frothy sputum may be evident. Exceptions are elderly patients or those with cardiogenic shock, who may not appear typically dyspneic because of obtundation. Patients with less severe heart failure have correspondingly less dramatic physical findings.

Vital Signs

Sinus tachycardia is usually present, although frequent exceptions occur. For example, atrial fibrillation is common in chronic mitral valve disease and in cardiomyopathy. In addition, a primary rhythm disturbance superimposed on underlying heart disease may have been the precipitating factor for heart failure; such rhythm disturbances include supraventricular tachyarrythmias, ventricular tachycardia, marked sinus bradycardia with inadequate escape rhythm, and high-grade atrioventricular block. Finally, treatment with β-blockers or calcium channel blockers may blunt the compensatory tachycardia that usually accompanies heart failure or contribute to the arrhythmia that precipitates it.

Elevated blood pressure is common in patients with pulmonary edema, probably because of outpouring of endogenous catecholamines; this does not imply an independent hypertensive state, even when the degree of elevation is considerable. On the other hand, when hypertension is severe (diastolic pressure more than 120 mm Hg), it is sometimes difficult to know whether the situation represents malignant hypertension complicated by pulmonary edema or pulmonary edema that has led to hypertension. Examination of the ocular fundi is important in this situation, since the absence of typical funduscopic findings argues strongly against malignant hypertension. The absence of electrocardiographic indications of left ventricular hypertrophy also argues against a primary hypertensive state.

The physician should personally check the blood pressure, and, in doing so, carefully monitor for *pulsus paradoxus,* i.e., an inspiratory fall in the systolic blood pressure in excess of 10 mm Hg. This and other physical signs particularly important for determining the mechanism of heart failure are outlined in Table 7.5. Except in extreme cases, in which respiratory variation in systolic blood pressure may even be palpable in peripheral pulses, detection of pulsus paradoxus demands careful attention on the part of the physician. After the approximate blood pressure is determined, the physician should inflate the cuff to the highest level at which the blood pressure can be auscultated during expiration and then determine the highest pressure at which sounds are heard throughout the respiratory cycle. If the difference between those two readings is greater than 10 mm Hg, pulsus paradoxus is present. In a patient with mild to moderate heart failure, the presence of pulsus paradoxus suggests pericardial tamponade. In a patient with severe pulmonary edema, tachypnea may prevent accurate determination of whether pulsus paradoxus is present; if it is found, it is more likely due to the respiratory distress itself than to pericardial tamponade. Detection of pulsus paradoxus is difficult or impossible in the presence of atrial fibrillation. Pulsus paradoxus is *not* typically found in pericardial constriction.

Jugular Venous Pressure

The height of the top of the venous column, which may be seen in the internal or external jugular veins, reflects right atrial pressure and is central to the diagnosis of RHF. The position of the head and torso must be adjusted so that the top of the venous column is visible. The central venous pressure is then estimated by assuming the sternal angle to lie 5 cm above the right atrium, so that 5 cm H_2O is added to the height of the column above this landmark. Central venous pressures above 8 cm H_2O are abnormal. Obstruction of the superior vena cava, as by tumor or aortic aneurysm, rarely produces elevation of the jugular venous pressure in the absence of RHF. In some patients, obesity or an unusual neck anatomy makes identification of the jugular veins impossible. In such instances, direct measurement of the right atrial or central venous pressure may be necessary before a diagnosis of RHF is confirmed or excluded.

The height of the venous column normally falls during inspiration, due to the accompanying decrease in intrathoracic pressure. When the height of the column *rises* during inspiration, then *Kussmaul's sign* is present. This sign is highly suggestive of pericardial constriction; it is usually absent in pericardial tamponade.

Carotid Pulse

Since critical *aortic stenosis* is a correctible cause of heart failure, the typical weak and delayed carotid upstroke should be sought in each patient, particularly if a systolic ejection murmur is present. A transmitted murmur, and often a thrill, are generally evident in the neck. Any cause of heart failure may produce a "low volume" carotid impulse, making assessment of the speed of the upstroke difficult or impossible. In addition, carotid artery disease may produce not only weak and delayed pulsations, but bruits that mimic the transmitted murmur of aortic stenosis as well.

Most patients with LHF due to aortic stenosis improve with therapy and may subsequently undergo cardiac catheterization and aortic valve replacement. Occasionally, however, patients with critical aortic stenosis have pulmonary edema or cardiogenic shock that is unresponsive to therapy. These patients are at great risk for sudden cardiac arrest and often cannot be resuscitated. It is important that they be recognized early, since emergency aortic valve replacement may be lifesaving. The physician should consider the diagnosis of aortic stenosis in all patients with LHF of inapparent cause, especially in the elderly. Carotid pulses must be carefully examined for even a hint of an upstroke plateau or thrill. The characteristic harsh, grunting systolic murmur may be heard best in the subclavicular area, in the neck, or at the cardiac apex. Evidence of left ventricular hypertrophy is sought on examination of the apical impulse (sustained) and on the electrocardiogram. High-quality chest films, including a lateral view, are obtained as soon as possible, so that the presence of aortic valve calcification may be evaluated; the absence of calcium, however, does not exclude the diagnosis. If aortic stenosis cannot be excluded by routine clinical examination, then further diagnostic measures (echocardiography, cardiac catheterization) are required.

Lungs

In mild LHF, examination of the chest may reveal fine, moist, crackling inspiratory *rales* extending part way up from the bases. In overt pulmonary edema, loud rales extending from lung bases to apices may completely obscure the heart sounds. Rales may be accompanied by expiratory *wheezes*. In some cases, wheezing may be prominent, even in the absence of rales; in such cases, the distinction between heart failure and primary bronchial disease may be difficult. Conversely, pulmonary disease may produce rales indistinguishable from those of cardiac pulmonary edema. Unwarranted emphasis on either the presence or absence of rales constitutes one of the more common reasons for misdiagnosis of LHF. The presence of a pleural effusion, with dullness, diminished breath sounds, and egophony, often reflects the presence of bisided heart failure.

Heart

On initial examination, cardiac findings may be completely obscured by the manifestations of respiratory distress. It is important in these cases to reexamine the patient frequently as he or she begins to improve following the institution of therapy.

The location of the *LV apical impulse* provides important information regarding the mechanism of LHF. Displacement away from the midclavicular line toward the anterior axillary line indicates that LV enlargement is the cause of elevated left atrial pressure. An impulse that is palpable with the palm of the hand placed on the sternum as a RV tap or heave indicates RV pressure and/or volume overload. A loud S_1 or an opening snap may be the first clue to the presence of mitral stenosis; the associated rumble may be soft or inaudible. The presence of an S_3 indicates LV systolic dysfunction as the mechanism of heart failure. Both the S_3 and the rumble of mitral stenosis are sought with the patient in the left lateral decubitus position.

If heart failure is due to mitral regurgitation, a loud holosystolic murmur is present. In critical aortic stenosis, cardiac output may be severely depressed, so that the aortic valve gradient is low and the corresponding murmur misleadingly soft. The murmur of aortic insufficiency is often best heard at the lower left sternal border in sustained expiration with the patient sitting forward.

Electrocardiogram

The electrocardiogram (ECG) may reveal heart rhythm abnormalities associated with the underlying condition, or in themselves contributing to the pathophysiology of heart failure. Left atrial enlargement is common in patients with elevated left atrial pressure of any cause. Electrocardiographic left ventricular hypertrophy is a specific but insensitive indicator of actual wall thickening and/or chamber enlargement; in the absence of chronic hypertension, it should prompt a particularly diligent effort to exclude aortic stenosis. Electrocardiographic signs of acute myocardial infarction or ischemia are sought. Chronic heart failure due to coronary artery disease generally results from previous myocardial infarction but the absence of ECG abnormalities diagnostic of previous transmural infarction call this diagnosis into question.

Chest X-ray

The chest x-ray is the most important tool in the diagnosis of LHF. Normally, in the upright position, pulmonary blood flow is greater to the lung bases than to the apices. This is apparent on the plain chest film in comparing the caliber of the vessels, particularly the veins, of the lower lung zones with that of the upper lung zones. Patients with LHF have a *redistribution* of pulmonary blood flow to the upper zones, so that the caliber of upper zone vessels becomes equal to or greater than the caliber of lower zone vessels. Redistribution occurs because interstitial edema is more severe in lower lung fields as a result of gravity. The microvasculature is consequently compressed, and blood flow is shunted upward. Radiologic interstitial and alveolar edema are nonspecific in that they occur in a wide variety of circumstances. The specific hallmark of LHF is upper zone redistribution.

There are at least three situations in which caution need be exercised in interpreting upper zone redistribution. First, some patients with emphysema have pulmonary parenchymal loss that is much greater in the lower zones. Consequently, the pulmonary vascular resistance is higher in the lower zones, and blood flow to the apices increases, simulating the pattern of LHF. The clue that emphysema, rather than LHF, is the cause of flow redistribution consists of the concomitant presence of hyperinflation, especially depressed diaphragms, and basilar rarefaction. In the absence of these stigmata, upper zone redistribution may usually be attributed to LHF, even if the patient also has chronic obstructive lung disease. Second, chest films taken with the patient supine may not reveal flow redistribution, since its occurrence depends on the effect of gravity on the upright lung. Third, there may be chronic loss of vascular definition by interstitial scarring, making it difficult to interpret vessel size. This is particularly likely in elderly patients, and also in patients with diseases producing interstitial pulmonary fibrosis.

Interstitial Pulmonary Edema

Interstitial pulmonary edema occurs when LAP is elevated above 20 mm Hg. The radiologic pattern of interstitial edema consists of varying combinations of septal, perivascular, and subpleural edema. Septal edema is manifested by Kerley B lines, i.e., short, nonbranching lines seen at the periphery of the lower lung fields, extending to and perpendicular to the pleural surface (Fig. 7.4). Perivascular

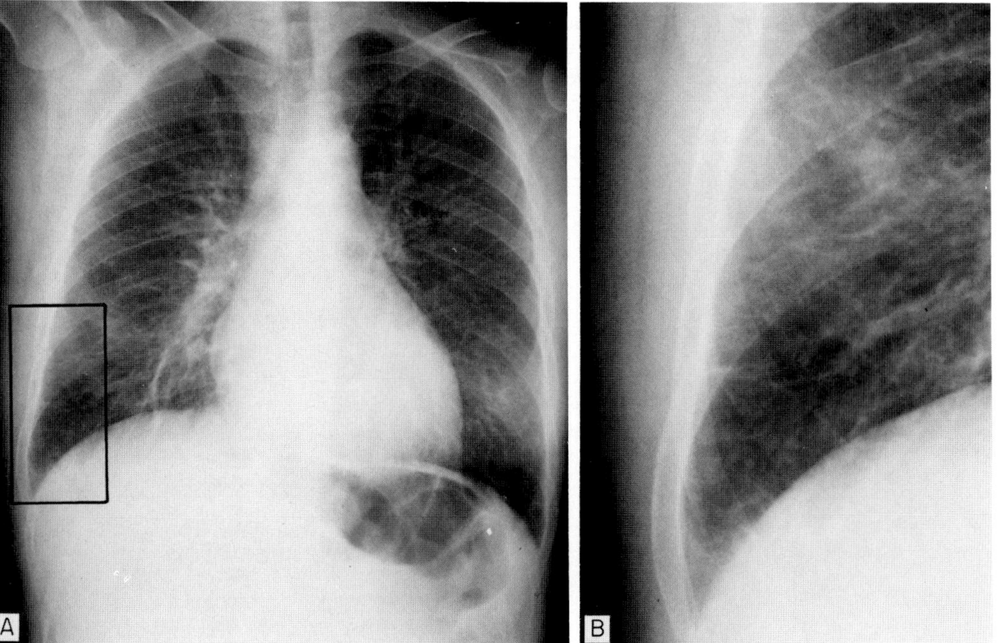

Figure 7.4. *A*, Prominence of upper zone vessels and loss of vascular definition in lower zone vessels (flow redistribution) in 51-year-old patient with myocardial infarction. There are also Kerley B lines at periphery of bases. *B*, Enlargement of area outlined in *A*.

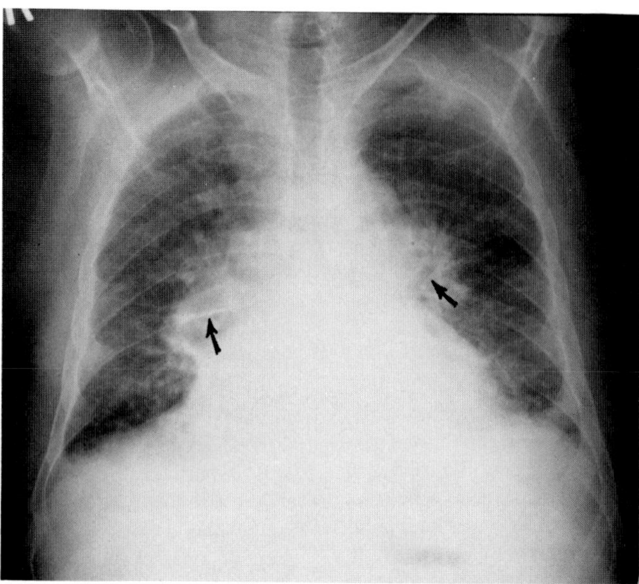

Figure 7.5. Upper zone blood flow redistribution and marked interstitial edema. Note complete loss of vascular definition in lower zones. Blurring of central vascular definition gives impression of hilar enlargement. Kerley A lines are present *(arrows).* There is peripheral haze in lower and midpulmonary zones.

edema is manifested both as a central (hilar) haze and as loss of definition of lower zone vessels (Figs. 7.4 and 7.5). Hilar haze (loss of definition of central vessels) often results in a general impression of hilar enlargement (Fig. 7.5). Subpleural edema is indicated by a sharp pleural margin associated with a poorly defined density extending into the underlying lung. Interstitial edema is also seen as peribronchial "cuffing" when airways are viewed in cross-section (Fig. 7.6).

Alveolar Edema

Alveolar edema occurs when LAP is elevated above 30 mm Hg and is manifest by frank pulmonary opacification. The distribution of alveolar edema may be the typical central "batwing" pattern (Fig. 7.6), may be diffuse (Fig. 7.7), or may be asymmetric, even unilateral. Opacification is usually homogeneous, but occasionally resembles miliary densities, nodules, or patchy pneumonia.

Figure 7.6. Upper zone flow redistribution and alveolar edema in central batwing distribution. Note peribronchial cuffing *(arrow).*

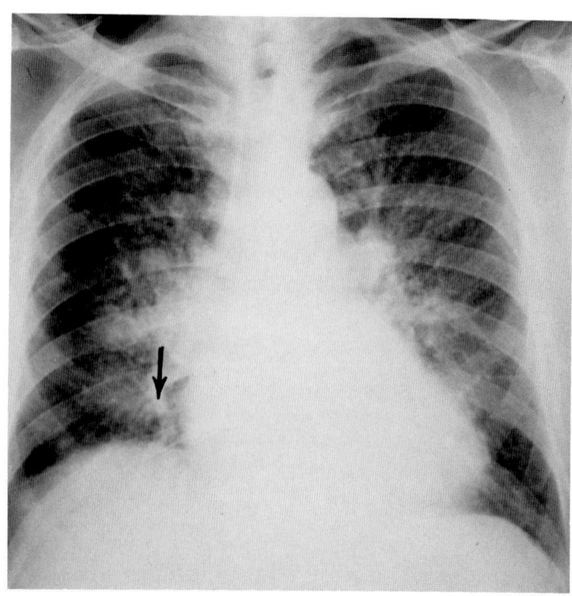

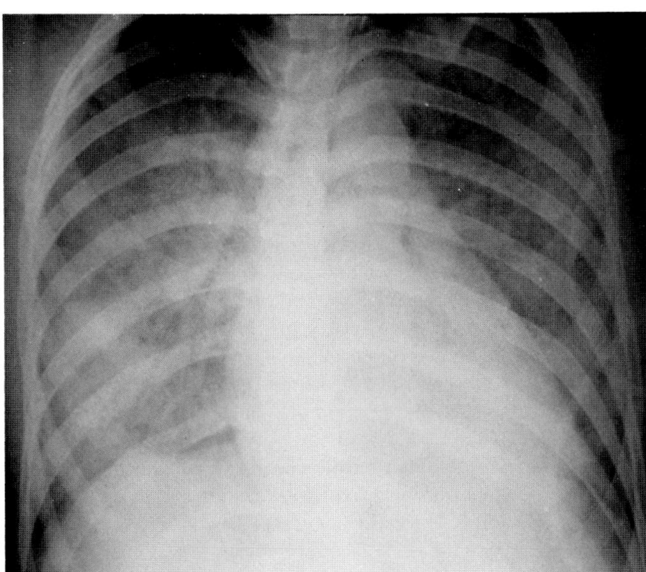

Figure 7.7. Diffuse alveolar edema in patient with mean pulmonary capillary wedge pressure of 40 mm Hg because of ruptured papillary muscle leading to acute mitral regurgitation.

The relationship between interstitial and alveolar edema and LAP may be modified by several factors. First, it may be affected by alterations in serum oncotic pressure. At a low serum albumin level, radiologic edema may occur at a relatively low atrial pressure; in the extreme, a very low serum albumin level may cause pulmonary edema when the LAP is normal. Second, a LAP exceeding 35 mm Hg may be manifest only by interstitial edema if the elevation of LAP has been long-standing, because of an expanded capacity of the interstitial lymphatic system. Third, there may be a lag of several hours before the appearance of radiologic pulmonary edema when the elevation of LAP occurs acutely, as in myocardial infarction. Conversely, when LAP is rapidly lowered with therapy, the chest x-ray may continue to show edema for several hours.

Despite these considerations, respiratory distress due to LHF is generally associated with typical radiologic features. If a patient with respiratory distress does not manifest upper zone distribution and interstitial or alveolar edema, the diagnosis of LHF as the cause of the respiratory distress should be suspect, and another cause of respiratory distress should be sought.

Pleural Effusions

Small pleural effusions may be due to isolated LHF, but large pleural effusions due to heart failure are almost always associated with bisided heart failure. Thus, when a large effusion occurs in the presence of a normal right atrial or central venous pressure, a cause other than LHF is sought. Isolated RHF is seldom a cause of pleural effusion. Pleural effusion due to heart failure is often bilateral; when unilateral, it usually occurs on the right. When isolated left-sided pleural effusion is present, a cause other than heart failure is sought.

Blood Tests

Arterial hypoxemia, as measured by *arterial blood gas* samples, is present in interstitial pulmonary edema because of ventilation-perfusion mismatching. Arterial PCO_2 is usually modestly decreased because of associated hyperventilation. In alveolar edema, arterial PO_2 is depressed both by ventilation-perfusion mismatching and by intrapulmonary right-to-left shunting; arterial PCO_2 may be mildly decreased or normal. In extremely severe pulmonary edema, particularly in the elderly, fatigued, or obtunded patient, arterial PCO_2 may be elevated. If the cause of pulmonary edema is also a cause of critically low cardiac output, metabolic (lactic) acidosis may be present. *Liver function tests* (serum glutamic oxaloacetic transaminase, alkaline phosphatase, or bilirubin) may be elevated in the presence of RHF or low cardiac output. The *white blood cell count* is often elevated because of demargination of leukocytes; this does not in itself constitute evidence of infection.

Echocardiography

When available on an emergency basis, echocardiography may be extremely useful in the search for correctible causes of heart failure, such as pericardial tamponade and aortic stenosis. Small, moderate, and occasionally large pericardial effusions often occur in the absence of actual tamponade; if an effusion is present, but pulsus paradoxus absent, then another cause of heart failure must be sought.

MANAGEMENT OF ACUTE PULMONARY EDEMA

In the emergency department, the patient often presents with heart failure in its most dramatic form, acute pulmonary edema. In this setting, the emergency physician immediately assesses the severity of respiratory distress. In the extreme case, immediate endotracheal intubation is required. The presence of hypotension generally indicates severe illness. It should be noted, however, that hypotension may be due to respiratory failure and associated acidosis and may normalize promptly after their correction. The severity of pulmonary edema dictates the priority of diagnostic and therapeutic steps. What follows is an outline of an approximate sequence for the evaluation and management of acute pulmonary edema.

Initial Measures

The goal of initial assessment is recognition of specific mechanisms that cause or precipitate heart failure, such as acute myocardial infarction, pericardial tamponade, or arrhythmia. Many of the measures utilized in the treatment of pulmonary edema, however, are applicable regardless of cause. Initial therapy (Table 7.6) is directed at improving oxygenation, lowering left atrial pressure, and allaying the anxiety of the patient.

Table 7.6.
Therapy for Cardiogenic Pulmonary Edema

Useful in Emergency Department	Useful in Intensive Care Unit or in Special Circumstances
Improve oxygenation	
Increase FiO_2 by face mask	Positive end-expiratory pressure
Aminophylline for bronchospasm	
Endotracheal intubation and controlled ventilation	
Treat anxiety	
Morphine	
Lower left atrial pressure	
Morphine	Intravenous vasodilators:
Diuretics	Nitroprusside
Sublingual nitroglycerin	Nitroglycerin
? Rotating tourniquets	Amrinone
Phlebotomy	Dialysis
	Pericardiocentesis
Provide inotropic and/or blood pressure support	
	Inotropic agents
	Dobutamine
	Amrinone
	Dopamine (medium doses)
	Pressors
	Norepinephrine
	Dopamine (high doses)
	Intraaortic balloon counterpulsation

Oxygen

The emergency department stretcher is adjusted so that the patient is sitting at approximately 80°; in fact, the patient usually insists on sitting upright. Oxygen is administered immediately by face mask at a high flow rate. A positive-pressure mask may further improve oxygenation by preventing alveolar collapse. Some patients, however, do not tolerate this close-fitting device. Nasal prongs are usually inadequate because the patient breathes through the mouth. If there is a possibility that the patient has chronic carbon dioxide retention due to concomitant chronic obstructive pulmonary disease, a face mask delivering oxygen at a controlled concentration of 24% should be used, and the physician should be prepared to intubate the patient should obtundation occur.

Intravenous Line

An adequate intravenous cannula is secured; a scalp-vein needle is not sufficient. If hypotension is present or anticipated, an attempt should be made to place a central venous "long line" from the antecubital fossa. Placement of a subclavian or internal jugular line, which requires that the patient be supine, is generally not possible unless endotracheal intubation has already been performed. When the intravenous cannula is placed, blood samples are sent for electrolytes, blood urea nitrogen, creatinine, and complete blood cell count.

Rapid Clinical Assessment

The severity of pulmonary edema dictates the thoroughness of the initial assessment. A brief history is obtained from the patient or accompanying persons, with particular attention to the items listed in Table 7.5. It is important, in addition, to ascertain the medications taken by the patient. Vital signs, jugular venous pulse, and carotid pulse are recorded, and the lungs and heart are examined. The presence of peripheral edema is sought. The initial cardiac examination may be at least partially obscured by respiratory noise, so that cardiac auscultation must be repeated as respiratory distress lessens. A 12-lead electrocardiogram is obtained, and continuous electrocardiographic monitoring initiated.

Treatment of Arrhythmias

Ventricular premature beats are treated with lidocaine, 75 mg given as an intravenous bolus over 1 minute, followed by an infusion at 1 mg/min. In this setting, infusions of 2 mg/min sometimes, 3 mg/n in often, and 4 mg/min almost always result in manifestations of toxicity. Ventricular tachycardia must be quickly converted with synchronized electrical cardioversion (Chapter 5). Occasionally, a bolus of 75–100 mg of lidocaine, given while preparation for cardioversion is taking place, will terminate the arrhythmia.

Patients with rapid supraventricular tachyarrhythmias (atrial fibrillation or flutter or paroxysmal supraventricular tachycardia) may be treated with intravenous verapamil only if hypotension is not present and the cause of pulmonary edema is not impaired LV contractility. If the arrhythmia is known or suspected to be of recent onset, and significant hypotension is present, electrical cardioversion should be carried out. Electrical cardioversion is hazardous in the presence of excessive digoxin levels, but not in the presence of "therapeutic" levels. If atrial fibrillation is chronic, then sinus rhythm is not likely to be maintained after cardioversion. The rapid rate is likely secondary to noncompliance with medications or to the sympathetic stimulation associated with hemodynamic compromise.

If atrial fibrillation is chronic, if the patient is not severely ill, and if impaired contractility is present or cannot be excluded, then an attempt should be made to control the ventricular response with digoxin. The onset of action following intravenous administration occurs at 15–30 minutes, and the peak effect at 1½–5 hours. In a patient not previously taking digoxin, the initial dose is 0.5–0.75 mg; if the patient has been treated chronically with digoxin, the initial dose is 0.125–0.25 mg. In the setting of hemodynamic compromise, the ventricular response rate is only a rough guide to the adequacy of digitalization; an increase in sympathetic stimulation may make the A-V node insensitive to digoxin, and digitalis arrhythmias may occur before the ventricular response rate is controlled. Small doses of verapamil are often helpful in this setting, although hypotension or worsening of ventricular systolic function may complicate treatment with this drug.

Morphine

If the diagnosis of cardiogenic pulmonary edema is secure, morphine sulfate is administered. Morphine acts by venous and arterial vasodilatation and reduction of anxiety. Contraindications to the use of morphine include respiratory depression and hypotension. The drug is adminstered intravenously, since the rate of absorption from subcutaneous and intramuscular sites is unpredictable in the presence of peripheral vasoconstriction. Initial dosage is 2–5 mg intravenously, given slowly; the drug may be given at 5–15-minute intervals, with the dosage carefully titrated to clinical effects.

Patients who are not significantly obtunded or hypotensive require morphine for severe respiratory distress due to pulmonary edema. It should not be withheld, or postponed until arterial blood gas results are available, for fear of inducing hypoventilation. If severe hypoventilation occurs following administration of morphine—and it occasionally does—endotracheal intubation is required for controlled ventilation; Narcan can be used adjunctively, as well.

The effectiveness of morphine in allaying the anxiety of the patient is enhanced by calm reassurance from the physician. This may be difficult, especially for the inexperienced physician, since the awesome anxiety of the patient with acute pulmonary edema is frequently contagious to medical personnel. The physician may find it helpful to keep in mind that while, in most cases, the initial therapy of pulmonary edema is designed to avoid endotracheal intubation, this procedure can be performed if necessary at any time. Once controlled ventilation is instituted, the care of the patient is considerably easier and less anxiety is provoked in the attendant staff.

Diuretics

Furosemide is administered intravenously. In the patient who has not been treated chronically with the oral furosemide (the so-called "Lasix virgin"), the initial dose is 20–40 mg intravenously; in the patient on chronic oral therapy, the initial intravenous dose is equal to or greater than his or her usual oral dose. In moderately or severly ill patients, a catheter is placed into the bladder. Urinary flow begins to increase 10–30 minutes after intravenous administration of furosemide. If the expected response is not seen, the dose is doubled. Thus, the patient accustomed to a daily furosemide dose of 80 mg orally receives 80 mg intravenously as the initial dose; if diuresis were not evident 20–30 minutes later, the patient receives an additional 160 mg intravenously. The effect of furosemide on vascular tone has recently been reevaluated. While administration of the drug to patients with acute myocardial infarction was previously found to produce venodilatation preceding the diuretic effect (see Dikshit et al., Suggested Readings), a more recent study has demonstrated an acute vasoconstrictor response in patients with chronic heart failure (see Francis et al., Suggested Readings).

Other powerful, rapidly acting diuretics, such as ethacrynic acid, 50 mg intravenously, or bumetanide, 1 mg intravenously, may be substituted for furosemide. The addition of chlorthiazide, 500 mg intravenously may facilitate diuresis in patients who do not respond to single-agent therapy.

Furosemide and other diuretics should be administered with caution to patients with impaired LV compliance (''stiff'' ventricle), as in aortic stenosis, left ventricular hypertrophy due to chronic hypertension, hypertrophic cardiomyopathy, and pericardial tamponade or constriction. In these patients, excessive reduction of LV filling pressure may result in hypotension.

The diuretic response is accompanied by an increase in potassium excretion. Potassium levels are checked at frequent intervals, and replacement instituted promptly, particularly for total-body potassium depletion due to chronic diuretic therapy. Hypokalemia may induce ventricular tachyarrhythmias and occasionally atrioventricular block. The likelihood of these rhythm disturbances is increased in the coexistence of digoxin administration and hypokalemia. It is emphasized that hypokalemia may cause arrhythmias even in the absence of digoxin.

Sublingual Nitroglycerin

The administration of sublingual nitroglycerin brings about venodilatation, which lowers left atrial pressure. Since nitroglycerin is also a coronary and systemic arterial dilator, it may produce further benefit in relief of myocardial ischemia and in reduction of afterload. In pulmonary edema, higher doses are required than those effective in the treatment of angina. A preferred plan is as follows: administer 0.3 mg, measure blood pressure 5 minutes later, administer 0.6 mg, recheck blood pressure 5 minutes later, and repeat doses of 0.6 mg every 10 minutes until improvement occurs or the systolic blood pressure falls to 100–110 mm Hg. Nitroglycerin is not administered if the initial blood pressure is below this level.

Arterial Blood Gases

A sample of arterial blood is sent to monitor the effectiveness of oxygenation, to check for carbon dioxide retention, and to assess acid-base status. Acute carbon dioxide retention due to pulmonary edema does not contraindicate high-flow oxygen therapy so long as the patient is observed carefully for increasing obtundation.

Acidemia (blood pH less than 7.36) is common in acute pulmonary edema and may be due to respiratory acidosis, metabolic acidosis, or both. Severe respiratory acidosis (pH less than 7.15–7.20, Pco_2 greater than 65–75 mm Hg) necessitates institution of controlled ventilation. Mild or moderate metabolic (lactic) acidosis does not require specific therapy. When metabolic acidosis is severe (pH less than 7.15–7.20), sodium bicarbonate is administered. While the associated sodium load may temporarily exacerbate pulmonary edema, such patients generally require controlled ventilation.

Arterial blood gases must be repeated as the clinical condition changes and new therapies, particularly controlled ventilation, are introduced.

Chest X-ray

A chest x-ray, usually portable, is obtained at this time to confirm the diagnosis of pulmonary edema, to ascertain the presence of other conditions, and to assess heart size, allowing for the anteroposterior technique. Physicians sometimes think that LHF and cardiomegaly are inseparable except in mitral stenosis. This is not the case. Causes of LHF with normal heart size include some cases of aortic stenosis, LV hypertrophy due to long-standing hypertension, acute myocardial infarction, acute mitral regurgitation, and pericardial constriction.

Aminophylline

Aminophylline, a phosphodiesterase inhibitor, is primarily a bronchodilator, but is also, to a lesser extent, a diuretic, vasodilator, and positive inotropic agent. Its bronchodilator effect is useful in treating the wheezing (''cardiac asthma'') associated with pulmonary edema. Its other actions may also be of benefit in heart failure, although the positive inotropic effect may not be desirable in a patient with acute myocardial infarction or ischemia. Aminophylline is always used with caution. An initial intravenous dose of 4–6 mg/kg over 20–30 minutes, followed by a continuous infusion of 0.2–0.5 mg/kg/min, yields a therapeutic serum theophylline level of 10–20 μg/ml. In patients with pulmonary edema, the lower doses may be sufficient. Toxic effects include nausea, vomiting, tachyarrhythmias, and seizures.

Aminophylline is extremely useful in the occasional patient in whom it is difficult to determine whether respiratory distress is due to pulmonary edema or to an exacerbation of chronic pulmonary obstructive disease by acute bronchitis. Early use of this medication may buy time while diagnostic measures, such as a chest x-ray, are carried out to aid in the differential diagnosis.

Further Measures

Most patients with pulmonary edema improve dramatically with the measures outlined above. In some patients, further steps, as described below, are necessary (Table 7.6). Some of these require invasive monitoring with arterial and pulmonary artery catheters, in which case they are generally instituted after the patient is transferred from the emergency department to the intensive care unit. The goals of therapy are improvement of oxygenation, lowering left atrial pressure, decreasing afterload (when appropriate), and improving contractility and/or supporting blood pressure (when appropriate).

Rotation of Tourniquets

Tourniquets placed on three extremities at a time and rotated every 15–20 minutes, tightened sufficiently to occlude venous but not arterial flow, constitute a traditional adjunct to the treatment of pulmonary edema. Devices that automatically inflate and deflate blood pressure cuffs are now widely employed instead of tourniquets. Cuffs should be inflated to a level lower than arterial pressure but higher than venous pressure. This therapy has limited effectiveness, and its use has been called into question. Inflated cuffs or tourniquets are not used in patients with hypotension or severe peripheral vascular disease.

Phlebotomy

A favorable, occasionally dramatic response, is sometimes produced by the withdrawal of 100–500 ml of blood by phlebotomy. As with diuretic therapy, phlebotomy is used cautiously when pulmonary edema has developed in the presence of a normal blood volume. This is most common in patients with acute myocardial infarction and in some patients with aortic stenosis. If collected by properly sterile technique, the blood may later be given back as packed red blood cells.

Controlled Ventilation

If the patient is severely dyspneic, tiring, or obtunded, if respiratory acidosis is severe (pH less than 7.15) and does not rapidly improve, or if arterial Po_2 is lower than 50 mm Hg with initial therapy, endotracheal intubation is then performed and controlled positive-pressure ventilation instituted. The decision whether to institute controlled ventilation is often difficult. While endotracheal intubation is not without its hazards, it should be performed before severe respiratory acidosis or hypoxemia leads to severe hypotension, ventricular fibrillation, or asystole. It is preferable to perform intubation too early in a patient in whom it might have been avoided, than to proceed to intubation too late, such as for cardiopulmonary arrest.

Nasotracheal intubation (see Illustrated Technique 2) is the method of choice, in the absence of systemic anticoagulation with heparin or warfarin, for the patient with pulmonary edema, since it may be performed with the patient sitting upright, and results in less vocal cord trauma. Once cardiopulmonary arrest has occurred, orotracheal tracheal intubation (Illustrated Technique 1) is necessary.

Controlled ventilation is initially applied with a pressure-cycled respirator. Since patients with pulmonary edema often have erratic, unpredictable tidal volumes on pressure-cycled respirators, however, a volume-cycled respirator is substituted as soon as it is practicable, usually in the intensive care unit. It is important that a large tidal volume (600–1000 ml) be ensured, to prevent subsegmental atelectasis, which further worsens gas exchange. Positive-pressure ventilation reduces venous return. As with other measures that reduce venous return, care is taken that hypotension does not ensue.

Occasionally, gas exchange remains critically impaired even after controlled ventilation is instituted with a volume-cycled respirator. Oxygenation may then be improved by employing positive end-expiratory pressure ("PEEP") of 5–10 cm H_2O to prevent or treat alveolar collapse. This technique may further compromise venous return.

Vasodilators

Reduction of preload and afterload with vasodilators has assumed an important role in both the acute and chronic management of heart failure. The effects of the available vasodilator drugs are summarized in Table 7.7. In the patient with pulmonary edema without evidence of myocardial ischemia or infarction, *nitroprusside* is the drug of choice. Nitroprusside is both a venous and arterial vasodilator and thus has balanced effects on preload and afterload. Treatment with this agent requires monitoring of arterial blood pressure with an intraarterial line or an automated blood pressure cuff, and, in most cases, monitoring of pulmonary capillary wedge pressure with a right heart catheter. These are generally initiated after transfer of the patient from the emergency department to the intensive care unit. Therapy is initiated at a dose of 15–25 μg/min and titrated upward to a maximum dose of 300–400 μg/min to obtain the desired effects on pulmonary capillary wedge pressure and cardiac output without causing undue reduction in systemic arterial pressure. Systemic arterial Po_2 may fall on nitroprusside, due to worsening of ventilation-perfusion mismatch. This effect is usually mild and is counterbalanced by an increase in cardiac output, so that tissue oxygenation is rarely compromised. Side effects include nausea, vomiting, sweating, restlessness, and headache. Prolonged infusions at high doses may result in frank thiocyanate toxicity, manifest as delirium or coma. Afterload reduction with nitroprusside may be particularly effective in patients with acute hypertension and in those with mitral or aortic regurgitation, in whom the fall in systemic vascular resistance permits forward, rather than regurgitant blood flow.

In patients with pulmonary edema complicating myocardial ischemia or infarction, intravenous *nitroglycerin* is preferred over nitroprusside, since this

Table 7.7.
Intravenous and Oral Vasodilators

Agent	Hemodynamic Effescts			Dosage
	Preload	Afterload	Contractility	
Intravenous				
Nitroprusside	↓	↓	0	15–400 μg/min
Nitroglycerin	↓	↓	0	10–500 μg/min
Amrinone	↓	↓	↑	0.75 μg/kg bolus 5–10 μg/kg/min
Oral				
Isosorbide dinitrate	↓	↓	0	10–80 mg QID
Hydralazine	0	↓	0	10–200 mg QID
Prazosin	↓	↓	0	1–5 mg TID
Converting enzyme inhibitors				
Captopril	↓	↓	0	6.25–50 mg TID
Enalapril	↓	↓	0	2.5–10 mg BID
Calcium channel blockers				
Nifedipine	0	↓	0 or ↓	10–30 mg QID
Diltiazem	0	↓	0 or ↓	30–90 QID

agent may have more salutary effects on the blood flow to the ischemic myocardium. The initial dose is 10–20 μg/min. It may be titrated to a maximum dose of 400–500 μg/min.

Amrinone, like aminophylline, is a phosphodiesterase inhibitor. Unlike aminophylline, it is relatively specific for the type of phosphodiesterase in cardiac muscle. It has positive inotropic properties and is also a very powerful vasodilator, with balanced effects on preload and afterload. It is discussed in more detail in the next section.

After acute pulmonary edema has been effectively treated, it may be desirable to replace intravenous vasodilators with oral agents, which are listed in Table 7.7. While *isosorbide dinitrate,* like other nitrate preparations including transdermal nitroglycerin, is predominately a venodilator and *hydralazine* is an arterial vasodilator, the combination of the two provides balanced vasodilatation and is often effective in the management of heart failure. While *prazosin* may be effective in some patients, experience has shown that only a minority enjoy sustained benefit from this drug. The converting enzyme inhibitors *captopril* and *enalapril* provide balanced vasodilatation and generally provide sustained benefit. Side effects, including hypotension, hyperkalemia, and renal dysfunction, are most likely to occur in patients with hyponatremia. In such patients, therapy is initiated with a test dose of 6.25 mg of captopril or 2.5 mg of enalapril, proceeding cautiously to higher doses.

In patients with heart failure and intermittent ischemia, isosorbide dinitrate is the drug of choice. If a second agent is needed, a calcium channel blocker, *nifedipine* or *diltiazem,* may be added, although it is noted that these agents have modest negative inotropic effects, which may be clinically evident in an occasional patient. Verapamil is a less effective vasodilator than nifedipine or diltiazem. Thus, verapamil is not prescribed for afterload reduction in patients with heart failure. There is little reason to choose any calcium channel blocker in patients with heart failure without ischemia, since vasodilators without negative inotropic effect are available.

Inotropic Agents

When intravenous vasodilators are ineffective in treating refractory pulmonary edema, or when borderline blood pressure prevents or limits their use, positive inotropic agents may be beneficial. Amrinone, dobutamine, and dopamine are all powerful inotropic agents. They differ markedly, however, in their associated vascular effects (Table 7.8).

Table 7.8.
Inotropic Agents: Associated Vascular Effects

Agent	Preload	Afterload	Specific Renal Effect
Amrinone	↓	↓	0
Dobutamine	0 or ↓	↓	0
Dopamine	0 or ↓	0, ↓, or ↑	+ (low doses)

Amrinone is a powerful balanced venous and arterial vasodilator with a concomitant positive inotropic effect. It provides appropriate therapy for patients with severe systolic dysfunction causing pulmonary edema. It is administered in the intensive care unit with systemic arterial and pulmonary arterial pressure monitoring. Therapy is initiated with a bolus of 0.75 mg/kg, followed by an infusion of 5–10 μg/kg/min. Amrinone is not a pressor; blood pressure usually remains constant or falls. In patients in whom preload falls markedly on amrinone, frank hypotension may occur. This may be prevented by lower doses. Heart rate typically increases by 5–10%. In occasional patients, atrial and ventricular irritability may be encountered. Because of the pronounced vasodilator effects, myocardial oxygen demand does not usually increase, and clinical myocardial ischemia is rare. Thrombocytopenia may occur, so that platelet count must be monitored.

Dobutamine, a synthetic catecholamine β_1 agonist, is the "purest" positive inotropic agent available. It has few vascular effects, although arterial vasodilatation may occur, in part due to withdrawal of intrinsic sympathetic tone. The usual dose is 2–15 μg/kg/min. Tachyarrhythmias and myocardial ischemia may occur, although these are fairly unusual.

Dopamine has diverse effects that depend on the dose administered. The lowest doses (approximately 1–3 μg/kg/min) have a selective, so-called dopaminergic effect on dilating the renal vasculature, which may improve renal function. At intermediate doses (approximately 3–8 μg/kg/min), β-adrenergic effects, i.e., inotropic support and systemic vasodilatation, predominate. Finally, at higher doses (up to 20 μg/kg/min), α-adrenergic stimulation comes into play; systemic vasoconstriction occurs, and cardiac output may fall in response to the increase in afterload. At these doses, renal blood flow may decline from its maximal level. Thus, low doses may be used to improve renal function, middle doses to increase cardiac output, and high doses to support blood pressure. There is however, considerable patient variation in the response to a given dose of dopamine, so that dosage must be titrated carefully in the individual patient. Side effects include sinus tachycardia, other tachyarrhythmias, and myocardial ischemia.

Of amrinone, dobutamine, and dopamine, amrinone has by far the greatest effect on lowering the pulmonary capillary wedge pressure. Since this drug is a powerful vasodilator, it is useful to think of amrinone as intermediate in its effects between nitroprusside and dobutamine. Of dobutamine and dopamine, dobutamine is the agent of choice for heart failure. The combination of dobutamine and dopamine, in the low renal dose range, is beneficial in some cases. In patients with acute ischemia, any inotropic agent may worsen the balance between myocardial oxygen supply and demand. When available, intraaortic balloon counterpulsation is preferable.

In patients without supraventricular tachyarrhythmias, digoxin has little or no place in the emergency management of left heart failure because its inotropic effect is modest and the incidence of arrhythmias due to digitalis toxicity is higher than in chronic medication. Digitalis toxicity is discussed in Chapter 5. In the absence of hypocalcemia, intravenous preparations of calcium have no demonstrated benefit in the treatment of left failure. They should be withheld. When emergency inotropic support is required, one of the agents listed in Table 7.8 or intraaortic balloon counterpulsation should be employed.

Pressors

When hypotension coexists with pulmonary edema despite endotracheal intubation and controlled ventilation, then the patient is in cardiogenic shock. Treatment with norepinephrine (Levophed) or *high*-dose dopamine provides blood pressure support, but is likely to compromise cardiac output. When the cause of heart failure, such as acute myocarditis, is reversible, these drugs are used to buy time. When no reversible cause of heart failure is evident, pressor requirement is a very poor prognostic sign.

Special Measures

When preexisting or acute oliguric renal failure is present, hemodialysis may be required for fluid removal. In some cases, echocardiography, if available, should be performed on an emergency basis to evaluate the presence of pericardial tamponade or critical aortic stenosis. Heart failure resulting from pericardial tamponade should be treated with pericardiocentesis (see Illustrated Technique 10). When the clinical condition of the patient allows and facilities are available, this procedure is combined with right-heart catherization in the cardiac catheterization laboratory. This permits confirmation of the diagnosis of tamponade and the detection of concomitant pericardial constriction (so-called effusive-constrictive pericarditis). Patients with aortic stenosis may require emergency cardiac catheterization and even aortic valve replacement. In patients with heart failure complicating myocardial ischemia or acute infarction, intraaortic balloon counterpulsation, emergency cardiac catheterization, and thrombolytic therapy, and/or coronary angioplasty may be appropriate, if available.

Precipitating Factors

Once the patient has been stabilized, attention should be directed at potentially reversible precipitating factors, such as infection and anemia. Fever is aggressively treated with aspirin, acetaminophen, and cooling blankets.

Effects of Diuretics

The effects of intravenous diuretics must be continually monitored. In particular, serum potassium levels must be checked frequently. If an initially favorable diuretic response is followed by a fall-off in urine output, and heart failure persists, diuretic doses should be repeated. The most common cause of recurrent pulmonary edema after transfer to the intensive care unit is inadequate initial diuresis.

DIFFERENTIAL DIAGNOSIS OF ACUTE CARDIOGENIC PULMONARY EDEMA

The causes of acute respiratory distress are listed in Table 7.9.

Acute Bronchitis with Bronchospasm

Acute bronchitis with bronchospasm is not usually a diagnostic problem in younger patients with atopic asthma and in patients with obvious exposure to noxious fumes, including smoke (see Chapter 10). In the elderly patient with or without chronic lung disease, however, distinguishing bronchitis with bronchospasm from acute pulmonary edema is a common and difficult problem. Oxygen is administered at an Fio_2 of 24% until blood gas determination excludes carbon dioxide retention. Until a diagnosis is made, morphine should be withheld, but aminophylline may be very helpful.

Pulmonary Emboli

Pulmonary emboli are a common source of diagnostic confusion, both as a direct cause of respiratory distress and as a precipitant of pulmonary edema in patients with underlying left heart disease. In the former, the chest x-ray does not show pulmonary edema. In the latter, treatment for pulmonary edema proceeds, and the diagnosis of pulmonary emboli is made subsequently by appropriate means (see Chapter 9).

Pneumonitis

Widespread pneumonitis (viral, bacterial, or a noninfectious inflammatory state) and pneumonia superimposed on chronic pulmonary disease are also causes of acute respiratory distress (see Chapter 11). Bronchospasm may develop in these patients. The approach to treatment is similar to that described for acute bronchitis. It is particularly important to withhold morphine and to avoid the development of hypovolemia with diuretics.

Patients with bronchitis, pulmonary emboli, and pneumonia may have chest x-ray findings that do not allow confident exclusion of cardiogenic pulmonary edema. Conversely, the radiographic findings in cardiogenic pulmonary edema are sometimes not distinctive enough to allow confident confirmation of the diagnosis. In these patients, specific treatment for cardiogenic pulmonary edema, especially administration of morphine and diuretics, may have to be deferred in the emergency department and await measurement of the pulmonary capillary wedge pressure in the intensive care unit.

With widespread application of the bedside technique for measurement of pulmonary capillary wedge pressure, it has become apparent that there are many causes of radiologic pulmonary edema other than heart failure. These are listed in Table 7.9 as causes of *noncardiogenic pulmonary edema.* Opium alkaloid overdose has been recognized for many years as a cause of pulmonary edema, and is a common emergency department problem (see Chapter 17). The treatment of these patients is mentioned here only to emphasize that general measures for treating impaired gas exchange are the cornerstone of therapy. Except when the cause is obvious, as in opium alkaloid overdose, the diagnosis of noncardiogenic pulmonary edema is usually made outside the emergency department after measurement of the pulmonary capillary wedge pressure.

Table 7.9.
Causes of Acute Respiratory Distress

Cardiogenic pulmonary edema (resulting from elevation of left atrial pressure; see Figure 7.1 and Tables 7.1 and 7.2)

Noncardiogenic pulmonary edema
- Increased negativity of intrathoracic pressure
  - Upper airway obstruction
    - Larynogospasm after attempted intubation
    - Epiglottitis/croup
    - Suffocation
    - Hanging
  - Unilateral pulmonary edema after reexpansion of collapsed lung
- Increased alveolocapillary membrane permeability
  - Infectious pneumonia—viral, bacterial, parasitic
  - Inhaled toxins

Beryllium salts	Oxygen in high concentration
Boron	Ozone
Cadmium salts	Phosgene
Carbon monoxide	Polyvinyl derivatives
Chlorine	Rocket propellants
Diethyl sulfate	Smoke
Hydrogen fluoride	Teflon fumes
Hydrogen sulfide	Toluene
Metallic chloride salts	Toluidine

Table 7.9—*continued*

- Methyl bromide
- Nitrogen dioxide
- compounds
- Turpentine
- Xylene

- Circulating foreign substances
  - Snake venon
  - Bacterial endotoxins (in bacteremia)
- Aspiration of gastric contents
- Aspiration of baby powder
- Acute radiation pneumonitis
- Drowning
- Disseminated intravascular coagulation
- Hereditary angioneurotic edema
- Idiopathic capillary leak syndrome
- Immunologic or idiosyncratic
  - Hypersensitivity pneumonitis
  - Leukoagglutinin (transfusion reaction)
  - Systemic lupus erythematosis and other vasculitides
- Drug-induced
  - Busulfan
  - Colchicine
  - Cyclophosphamide
  - Dextran 40
  - Diphenhydramine hydrochloride
  - Hydralazine
  - Hydrochlorothiazide
  - Methotrexate
  - Nitrofurantoin
  - Radiographic contrast material

Lymphatic insufficiency
- After lung transplantation
- Lymphangitic carcinomatosis
- Fibrosing lymphangitis (e.g., silicosis)

Unknown or incompletely understood
- High altitude
- Uremia
- Neurogenic (intracranial hypertension or postictal)
- Pulmonary embolism (fat, air, amniotic fluid, or thrombus)
- Overdose
  - Opium alkaloids, including meperidine (Demerol)
  - Methadone
  - Propoxyphene hydrochloride (Darvon)
  - Pentobarbital
  - Chloral hydrate
  - Methaqualone
- Postcardioversion
- Postanesthesia
- Postcardiopulmonary bypass
- Recovery from diabetic ketoacidosis
- Hepatic failure
- Pancreatitis
- Closed chest trauma
- Nonthoracic trauma

Causes not associated with pulmonary edema
- Acute massive pulmonary thromboembolism
- Atopic asthmatic bronchitis
- Asthmatic bronchitis superimposed on chronic lung disease
- Upper airway obstruction (laryngeal or tracheal)
- Pneumothorax
- Hypovolemic or septic shock
- Transient reversible restrictive pulmonary disease
- Dyskinetic respiratory muscles

The differential diagnosis of acute cardiogenic pulmonary edema constitutes one of the most difficult problems in clinical medicine. There are helpful guidelines.

1. Do not be intimidated into making a specific diagnosis. It is better to proceed initially with a diagnosis of acute respiratory distress of uncertain cause than to start therapy for a specific cause that later turns out to be nonexistent.

2. The end result of all causes of respiratory distress is impaired gas exchange. Give oxygen by face mask. If there is concern that the patient may have chronic hypercapnia due to pulmonary disease, give low-flow oxygen by a mask delivering a controlled Fio_2 of 24%. If the patient has bronchospasm, give aminophylline. If severe hypoxemia persists despite face mask oxygen therapy, if severe respiratory acidosis exists, or if the patient is obtunded, initiate controlled ventilation.

3. If the diagnosis of cardiogenic pulmonary edema is uncertain, withhold morphine unless it has been decided that endotracheal intubation is imminent regardless.

4. Do not equate the presence of diffuse rales with the diagnosis of cardiogenic pulmonary edema. The most powerful diagnostic evidence of cardiogenic pulmonary edema, other than an elevated pulmonary capillary wedge pressure, is provided by the chest x-ray.

5. Almost all patients with cardiogenic pulmonary edema have some clue that implicates the heart, although the nature of the clue depends on the type of heart disease present. Such clues include: angina, cardiac enlargement shown by examination or chest x-ray, gallop rhythms, murmurs, and myocardial infarction shown on the electrocardiogram. Electrocardiographic evidence of left atrial enlargement is a common, although not invariable, manifestation of almost all forms of left heart disease severe enough to be associated with elevated LAP.

Be reluctant to diagnose cardiogenic pulmonary edema in the absence of at least one of these clues. Old age by itself does not constitute such a clue. Neither does the presence of atrial fibrillation, which may be associated with chronic lung, rather than heart, disease. This rule cannot be inverted; patients with heart disease may suffer from causes of acute respiratory distress other than pulmonary edema.

ACUTE RIGHT HEART FAILURE WITH HYPOTENSION

As discussed previously, RHF may be more evident than LHF despite the presence of LAP greater than or equal to right atrial pressure (RAP). Thus, many patients presenting with RHF clinically out of proportion to LHF have, in fact, bisided heart failure. Patients presenting with acute RHF and hypotension may, therefore, have disease affecting predominantly the right side of the heart (massive pulmonary embolism, right ventricular infarction), or affecting both sides symmetrically (pericardial tamponade).

Massive Pulmonary Embolism

Massive pulmonary embolism may present as acute cor pulmonale. Its clinical features consist of the abrupt onset of intense dyspnea, cyanosis varying from mild to profound, elevation of the jugular venous pressure, and, in some cases, extreme agitation. Syncope is a frequent initial manifestation. A right ventricular impulse may be palpable. An increase in the intensity of pulmonic second sound may not be initially apparent. Electrocardiographic abnormalities are common. This disorder is discussed in detail in Chapter 9.

Right Ventricular Infarction

Clinical right ventricular infarction sometimes complicates inferior infarction of the left ventricle. While a variable degree of LHF may therefore be present, RAP is generally equal to or greater than LAP. The initial treatment of hypotension in this setting consists of rapid volume infusion (see Chapter 6).

Pericardial Tamponade

The recognition of pericardial tamponade as a cause of hypotension is extremely important since pericardiocentesis is often lifesaving. The key clinical feature of pericardial tamponade, as discussed previously, is pulsus paradoxus, which is almost always present in the patient with hypotension in sinus rhythm. Fluids, and, if necessary, pressors may be administered until pericardiocentesis is performed (see Illustrated Technique 10).

Table 7.10.
Criteria of Left Heart Failure[a]

Event [b]	Points for Diagnosis [c]
Chest x-ray film	
Alveolar edema	4
Interstitial edema	3
Upper zone flow redistribution	2
Causal relationship	
Third heart sound	3
Presence of known potential cause of heart failure	2
Cardiothoracic ratio > 0.50	2
Dyspnea	
Rest dyspnea on orthopnea	2
Paroxysmal nocturnal dyspnea	2
Dyspnea on exertion	1
Evidence that heart failure is bisided (JVP > 7 cm H_2O)	2
Other	
Pulmonary crackles (posttussive)	1
P-wave negativity in V_1 > 0.03 mm/sec	1
Heart rate (sinus)	
> 90	1
> 100	2

[a] Reproduced by permission from Johnson RA. Heart failure. In: Johnson RA, Haber E, Austen WG, eds. The Practice of Cardiology. Boston: Little, Brown & Co., 1980: 31–95.
[b] JVP, mean jugular venous pressure.
[c] Six points or more are required for diagnosis. Only one event each can be counted from the chest x-ray film, causal relationship, dyspnea, or "other" categories.

SUBACUTE AND CHRONIC HEART FAILURE: DECISIONS IN THE EMERGENCY DEPARTMENT

Diagnosis

The most obvious need for patients with heart failure in the emergency department is treatment of acute pulmonary edema. The emergency department is used increasingly, however, as a source of primary medical care. Physicians in the emergency department must frequently make decisions with respect to the diagnosis and management of heart failure that is manifest in forms milder than acute pulmonary edema that are not true medical emergencies. When the condition is severe, the diagnosis of heart failure is usually not difficult. When heart failure is mild, however, the diagnosis may be elusive. Formalization of the process by which physicians establish the presence of LHF may help to avoid both underdiagnosis and overdiagnosis of the condition. Table 7.10 shows one set of criteria for the diagnosis of LHF. When these criteria are not met, but LHF is nevertheless suspected, the physician considers measuring, in an intensive care unit, the pulmonary capillary wedge pressure or, in other circumstances, instituting a therapeutic trial for heart failure. If the latter route is chosen, the therapy should be appropriate to the suspected mechanism of heart failure. The physician should have clear endpoints for declaring the trial a success or a failure. Otherwise, the patient is committed to a protracted course of therapy, the risk of which may exceed its benefit.

Therapeutic Decisions

Patients with heart failure of any stage of severity require ongoing primary medical care. Follow-up referral is essential. Heart failure always implies cardiac impairment. "A little heart failure" is a euphemism. Patients must be carefully evaluated to establish a cause, even when the symptoms are mild, because the natural history of some forms of heart disease is not clearly related to the severity of accompanying left atrial hypertension, for example, the high incidence of sudden death in aortic stenosis once symptoms develop. In addition, therapy for some causes of heart failure must be specific, such as valve replacement in valvular disease and β-adrenergic or calcium channel blockade in hypertrophic cardiomyopathy. These causes of heart failure are often unrecognized on initial evaluation in the emergency department. They may be suspected only during follow-up primary care evaluation, at which time cardiologic consultation may be obtained.

Digoxin is appropriate in most cases in which left ventricular enlargement is present, but care is taken to avoid digitalis toxicity. Outpatient diuretic therapy is carefully monitored, and serum potassium concentration checked. Some causes of left heart failure are associated with a high risk of thromboembolism, so that certain patients should be treated with warfarin. Vasodilator therapy (Table 7.7) benefits many patients with heart failure. When "balanced" arterial and venous vasodilatation is desired, as in the patient with idiopathic dilated cardiomyopathy, the combination of hydralazine and isosorbide dinitrate, or, alternatively, single-agent therapy with a converting enzyme inhibitor (captopril or enalapril), may be helpful. Patients with mitral or aortic regurgitation may benefit in particular from afterload reduction with hydralazine. When intermittent ischemia coexists with chronic heart failure, isosorbide dinitrate and calcium channel blockers (nifedipine or diltiazem) are the drugs of choice. Vasodilator therapy is associated with potentially adverse effects (Table 7.7). Once therapy of heart failure is initiated, close output follow-up is required.

Neither systematic evaluation nor systematic management can be provided by erratic visits to an emergency department. When patients who have not had the care of a primary physician come to an emergency department with mild or chronic heart failure, they must be referred to a primary care physician for subsequent care.

Admission Criteria

A corollary of this problem involves decisions regarding hospital admission for patients not previously followed by a physician. Patients with dyspnea at rest, even without frank pulmonary edema, should be admitted to the hospital for evaluation and initiation of therapy. In addition, the following criteria for admission are useful.

1. When symptoms have progressed in the course of several days or when their progression is uncertain.
2. When the cause or suspected cause is in itself grounds for admission. An example is heart failure due to coronary artery disease when it is accompanied by unstable angina. Another example is heart failure due to aortic stenosis, which always prompts admission because management is difficult and early evaluation for surgery may be required.
3. When there is a suspected precipitating factor such as arrhythmia, pneumonia, or urinary tract infection. The course of heart failure in these patients is usually too uncertain to allow outpatient management, even if the precipitating factor itself does not necessitate hospital admission.
4. When there is RHF, as indicated by neck vein distention, of any cause in a patient not previously evaluated. RHF always has serious implications. It is not a complication of left heart disease unless LHF is severe. The other causes of RHF are serious in themselves (Table 7.3) and necessitate careful evaluation because treatment must often be directed specifically toward the cause and not limited to management of the symptomatic consequences of elevated RAP.

Having made the decision to admit a patient with heart failure, but who does not have pulmonary edema, the physician in the emergency department must decide whether intensive or routine care is necessary. In general, intensive care should be provided whenever hemodynamic or electrical instability is present, or is anticipated as a result of the underlying disease or its treatment, or whenever the progression of heart failure appears unrelenting despite initiation of treatment in the emergency department.

Indications for Pulmonary Artery Lines

Pulmonary arterial catheterization should be considered in the following situations:

1. When the diagnosis of heart failure remains in doubt and the choice of several divergent therapeutic courses hinges on establishing an accurate diagnosis;
2. When the regulation of treatment is difficult without the aid of precise and easily accessible hemodynamic measurements;
3. When hemodynamic studies may help establish the cause of heart failure, for example, acute mitral regurgitation or ventricular septal rupture.

SUGGESTED READINGS

Bencowitz HZ, LeWinter MM, Wagner, PD. Effect of sodium nitroprusside on ventilation-perfusion mismatching in heart failure. *J Am Coll Cardiol,* 1984;4:918–922.

Bussmann W, Schupp D. Effect of sublingual nitroglycerin in emergency treatment of severe pulmonary edema. *Am J Cardiol,* 1978;41:931–936.

Colucci WS, Fifer MA, Lorell BH, et al. Calcium channel blockers in congestive heart failure: Theoretic considerations and clinical experience. *Am J Med,* 1985;78 (suppl 2B):9–17.

Colucci WS, Wright RF, Braunwald E: New positive inotropic agents in the treatment of heart failure. *N Engl J Med,* 1986;314:290–299, 349–358.

Dikshit K, Vyden JK, Forrester JS, et al. Renal and extrarenal hemodynamic effects of furosemide in congestive heart failure after acute myocardial infarction. *N Engl J Med,* 1973;288:1087–1090.

Dougherty AH, Nacarelli GV, Gray EL, et al. Congestive heart failure with normal systolic function. *Am J Cardiol,* 1984;54:778–782.

Franciosa JA, Wilen MM, Jordan RA: Effects of enalapril, a new angiotensin-converting enzyme inhibitor, in a controlled trial in heart failure. *J Am Coll Cardiol,* 1985;5:101–107.

Francis GS, Siegel RM, Goldsmith SR, et al. Acute vasoconstrictor response to intravenous furosemide in patients with chronic congestive heart failure. Activation of the neurohumoral axis. *Ann Int Med,* 1985;103:1–6.

Goldberg LI, Hsieh Y, Resnekov L: Newer catecholamines for treatment of heart failure and shock: An update on dopamine and a first look at dobutamine. *Prog Cardiovasc Dis,* 1977;19:327–340.

Habak PA, Mark AL, Kioschos JM, et al. Effectiveness of congesting cuffs ("rotating tourniquets") in patients with left heart failure. *Circulation,* 1974;50:366–371.

Johnson RA: Heart failure. In: Johnson RA, Haber E, Austen WG, eds. The Practice of Cardiology. Boston: *Little, Brown & Co.,* 1980:31–95.

Johnson RA, Palacios I: Dilated cardiomyopathies of the adult. *N Engl J Med,* 1982;307:1051–1058, 1119–1126.

Johnson MW, Mitch WE, Wilcox CS: The cardiovascular actions of morphine and the endogenous opioid peptides. *Prog Cardiovasc Dis,* 1985;27:435–450.

Lee DCS, Johnson RA, Bingham JB, et al. Heart failure in outpatients: A randomized trial of digoxin vs. placebo. *N Engl J Med,* 1982;306:669–705.

Leier CV, Unverfeth DV: Dobutamine. *Ann Int Med,* 1983;99:490–496.

Meszaros WT: Lung changes in left heart failure. *Circulation,* 1973;47:859–871.

Packer M: Is the renin-angiotensin system really unnecessary in patients with severe chronic heart failure? The price we pay for interfering with evolution. *J Am Coll Cardiol,* 1985;6:171–174.

Palmer RF, Lasseter KC: Nitroprusside. *N Engl J Med,* 1975;292:294–297.

Robin ED, Cross CE, Zelis R: Pulmonary edema. *N Engl J Med,* 1973;288:239–246, 292–304.

Simon M: The pulmonary vessels: Their hemodynamic evaluation using routine radiographs. *Radiol Clin North Am,* 1963;1:363–376.

Slutsky RA, Brown JJ: Chest radiographs in congestive heart failure: Response to therapy in acute and chronic disease. *Radiology,* 1985;154:577–580.

CHAPTER 8

Management of Hypertensive Emergencies

CECIL H. COGGINS, M.D.
KATHARINE K. TREADWAY, M.D.

Hypertension is epidemic, with elevated blood pressure existing in more than 15% of the adult population of the United States. The percentage is higher among blacks and in the older age groups, and it is still higher if borderline hypertension is included.

Even mild degrees of blood pressure elevation increase the risk of cardiovascular disease and death from cerebral thrombosis or hemorrhage, heart failure, myocardical infarction, and renal failure. Effective treatment decreases the death rate toward normal; however, only about one-half of the hypertensive patients in the population have been discovered, and in only a small minority of these is hypertension satisfactorily controlled.

It is therefore not surprising that the emergency physician is often challenged with hypertensive crises. These crises may be the malignant culmination of prolonged essential hypertension or of hypertension secondary to other disease (Table 8.1), or they may represent the major manifestation of a new illness. Even moderate hypertension may constitute an emergency when it is superimposed on arterial bleeding, aortic dissection, or severe heart failure. This chapter will discuss the diagnosis and management of the hypertensive crisis.

HYPERTENSIVE EMERGENCIES

The key to successful management of a hypertensive emergency is prompt recognition and initiation of treatment, the goal being rapid reduction of blood pressure within minutes to hours. Usually this requires that treatment be started after only a brief evaluation. Table 8.2 lists the situations considered to represent hypertensive emergencies. These conditions are discussed below.

Malignant Hypertension

Malignant hypertension is defined as severe hypertension with diastolic blood pressure usually greater than 130–140 mm Hg and with grade IV Keith-Wagner retinopathy (papilledema, hemorrhages, and exudates). Patients with a similar elevation of blood pressure and grade III retinopathy (hemorrhages and exudates without papilledema) are considered to have accelerated hypertension. These conditions represent a continuum, and both are associated with diffuse arteriolitis and fibrinoid necrosis.

Malignant hypertension usually occurs in the setting of poorly controlled essential hypertension, although it may occur in young patients, particularly black males, without a known history of hypertension. It also may occur with some forms of secondary hypertension, namely, pheochromocytoma and renovascular hypertension, as well as in association with acute or chronic renal failure. Patients most commonly have headache and visual complaints. They may or may not have encephalopathy, and they also may have signs of chronic hypertension such

Table 8.1.
Hypertension Classified by Cause

Essential hypertension—not associated with defined disease; more than 90% of hypertensive patients

Secondary hypertension—less than 10% of hypertensive patients
- Coarctation of aorta
- Renal disease
  - Parenchymal
  - Vascular
- Adrenal disease
  - Medulla or chromaffin cells—pheochromocytoma
  - Cortex
    - Cushing's syndrome
    - Primary hyperaldosteronism
    - Other mineralocorticoid excess
- Toxemia of pregnancy
- Central nervous system disease
- Hypertension associated with contraceptive pills

as left ventricular hypertrophy, congestive heart failure, or other atherosclerotic disease. Less commonly, patients are entirely asymptomatic. Prompt treatment is mandatory. Untreated, the patient's condition may progress rapidly to coma, convulsions, and death, with survival of less than 1% at the end of 1 year. Recent statistics suggest that with proper treatment more than 75% are alive at 1 year.

Hypertensive Encephalopathy

Encephalopathy usually occurs as an acute or subacute depression of central nervous system function in the setting of severely elevated blood pressure. Patients usually have symptoms ranging from confusion to coma, with or without associated headache and nausea. It is important to note that in patients without a history of hypertension (as in patients with acute renal failure or eclampsia) encephalopathy may occur with diastolic blood pressure from 95 to 120 mm Hg. Hypertensive encephalopathy must be distinguished from other central nervous system catastrophes (Table 8.3). Although focal neurologic deficits are not common in patients with hypertensive encephalopathy, they can occur. When present, they are often migratory and transient, and resolve rapidly after blood pressure is controlled. Significantly elevated diastolic blood pressure, evidence of chronic hypertension, hypertensive retinopathy, with a gradual onset, over 24–48 hours, of headache and lethargy with or without focal signs, as well as prompt clearing of central nervous system symptoms with effective therapy (often within several minutes) usually will establish the diagnosis.

Table 8.2.
Hypertensive Emergencies

- Malignant hypertension
- Hypertensive encephalopathy
- Eclampsia
- Catecholamine excess secondary to
  - Pheochromocytoma
  - Monoamine oxidase inhibitors
  - Clonidine hydrochloride withdrawal
- Severe hypertension associated with
  - Acute left ventricular failure
  - Myocardial infarction
  - Acute aortic dissection
  - Intracranial hemorrhage
  - Acute glomerulonephritis

Table 8.3.
Differential Diagnosis of Hypertensive Encephalopathy

- Uremic encephalopathy
- Encephalopathy secondary to metabolic derangements
- Subarachnoid hemorrhage
- Intracerebral hemorrhage
- Cerebrovascular accident
- Subdural hemorrhage
- Head injury
- Intracranial mass
- Postictal state
- Encephalitis
- Cerebral vasculitis

Eclampsia

Preeclampsia is characterized by acute vasospasm and sodium retention in a previously healthy woman during the third trimester of pregnancy. Manifested by hypertension, edema, and proteinuria, preeclampsia puts the patient at great risk for progression to *eclampsia,* with convulsions, coma, and frequently, renal failure. It is most likely to occur in women who have never borne children before, women over 35 years old, patients carrying multiple fetuses, and patients with hydatidiform moles. It should be remembered that blood pressure is normally somewhat lower than usual during the second and third trimesters of pregnancy (often averaging 100–90/50–60 mm Hg) and that a rapid rise in blood pressure to 160/100mm Hg may be severe enough to cause encephalopathy. These patients also must be distinguished from those who have a history of hypertension. The latter patients usually have hypertension before the third trimester and do not have accompanying edema or proteinuria. Eclampsia is ordinarily an indication to terminate the pregnancy, but extreme elevations of blood pressure require immediate pharmacologic control.

Catecholamine Crisis

Catecholamine crisis may occur associated with tumor, drug use, or withdrawal of antihypertensive medication. In a patient with pheochromocytoma, extreme hypertension may accompany the release of catecholamines from epinephrine- or norepinephrine-secreting chromaffin tumors in the adrenal medulla or elsewhere in the abdomen. The diagnosis should be suspected in any patient with a history of episodic headache, palpitation, tremors, sweating and tachycardia associated with elevated blood pressure; the condition should not be mistakenly diagnosed as an anxiety attack.

In these patients, hypertension may be either labile or sustained. Patients with pheochromocytoma are usually thin and frequently exhibit a decrease in blood pressure when standing, unlike most patients with essential hypertension. Patients who have pheochromocytoma and episodic blood pressure elevation often do not have the cardiac enlargement and retinopathy that would be expected with sustained hypertension of a similar degree. Signs of chronic hypertension may be present, however, in those patients with sustained hypertension.

A catecholamine crisis may also result from intake of catecholamine precursors or analogues by a person whose ability to metabolize such compounds is impaired. Such impairment results from the use of antidepressant monoamine oxidase inhibitors (Table 8.4). Catecholamine precursors include tyramine, which is naturally found in foods such as aged cheese and Chianti wine, and amphetamine or ephedrine, which may be found in cold preparations and cough medicines. In addition, the extreme elevations of blood pressure that have been reported to occur after abrupt withdrawal of the antihypertensive drug clonidine hydrochloride in many respects resemble a catecholamine crisis.

Table 8.4.
Significant Nonproprietary and Proprietary Names

Nonproprietary Name	Proprietary Name
Monoamine oxidase inhibitors	
Isocarboxazid	Marplan
Nialamide	Niamid
Pargyline hydrochloride	Eutonyl
Phenelzine sulfate	Nardil
Tranylcypromine sulfate	Parnate
Other	
Captopril	Capoten
Clonidine hydrochloride	Catapres
Diazoxide	Hyperstat
Furosemide	Lasix
Hydralazine hydrochloride	Apresoline
Labetalol	Normodyne, Trandate
Nifedipine	Procardia
Sodium nitroprusside	Nipride
Phenoxybenzamine hydrochloride	Dibenzyline
Phentolamine	Regitine
Propranolol hydrochloride	Inderal
Trimethaphan camsylate	Arfonad

Complicated Hypertension

Even when hypertension is not itself an immediate threat to life, it may demand emergency treatment when combined with another illness such as acute left ventricular failure, myocardial ischemia or infarction, acute aortic dissection, or intracranial hemorrhage. In these settings, severe hypertension usually exacerbates the underlying condition, and in the case of aortic dissection or intracranial hemorrhage, even modest degrees of hypertension may become life-threatening. These conditions require special treatment considerations, which are discussed on page 139; their clinical appearance and approaches to diagnosis are described in Chapters 6, 7, 15, and 31.

PHARMACOLOGIC AGENTS

Although several potent, rapidly acting antihypertensive drugs are now available, the physician will treat hypertensive emergencies most effectively by becoming expert in the use of a few agents. Almost all hypertensive emergencies can be managed with one of two primary drugs (diazoxide and nitroprusside), two ancillary drugs (propranolol hydrochloride and furosemide), and special purpose drugs for pheochromocytoma and aortic dissection.

Diazoxide

Diazoxide is a benzothiadiazide compound structurally related to the thiazide diuretics, but with a sodium-retaining effect rather than a diuretic effect.

Action

The primary action of diazoxide is to relax arteriolar smooth muscle, thus reducing peripheral resistance. It has little effect on capacitance vessels (veins) and no direct cardiac effect. The onset of action is within 1 minute. Peak action is in 5–10 minutes and the duration is 3–18 hours. A sympathetic reflex response to the lower blood pressure produces increased heart rate, cardiac index, and cardiac work. Sympathetic or ganglionic blocking agents such as propranolol or guanethidine may therefore have a synergistic effect by blocking this reflex response. Diazoxide is highly bound to plasma proteins. The antihypertensive effect results from the unbound fraction and hence is poorly correlated with total serum levels. In patients with uremia, the drug is less completely bound and more slowly excreted, so required doses may be reduced. In the pregnant patient, the relaxant effect on smooth muscle may arrest labor, and the patient may require oxytocin to resume uterine contractions.

Administration

An average dose of diazoxide is 300 mg (5 mg/kg) injected over 10 or 15 seconds through an already established large-bore intravenous line. Pressure will begin to decrease within 2–5 minutes. Although it is generally believed that rapid injection is essential to ensure that some of the drug will not be bound to the circulating albumin, recent studies have demonstrated efficacy with 100–150 mg repeated after 5 minutes if response is inadequate. Slow intravenous infusion at 20 mg/min is also effective, producing a response within 20 minutes. Blood pressure should be measured every 5 minutes for the first 30 minutes and less frequently thereafter. If the effect in 30 minutes is insufficient, the dose may be repeated. Smaller amounts may be given with proportionately smaller effects. Caution should be used if another antihypertensive drug has already been administered, because in this circumstance blood pressure may decrease to subnormal levels after administration of a standard dose of diazoxide. Volume depletion or β-blockade will also enhance the effect of diazoxide.

Side Effects

Salt and water retention regularly occur after use of diazoxide. Furosemide, 40 mg intravenously, may be given either initially or with each successive dose, unless volume depletion is present. Hyperglycemia occurs, but rarely requires treatment unless diazoxide is given repeatedly over 2–3 days. Hyperuricemia and hyperlipidemia also may occur. If blood pressure decreases to undesirable levels, the patient's head should be lowered and the legs may be raised.

Sodium Nitroprusside

The action of sodium nitroprusside in reducing blood pressure has been apparent since 1929, but no stable commercial preparation became available until recently.

Action

Sodium nitroprusside acts by direct dilatation of vascular smooth muscle. This not only reduces peripheral resistance but, by diminishing venous tone (increasing capacitance), it also reduces cardiac filling pressure. Therefore, blood pressure decreases with little change in cardiac output. In addition, reflex tachycardia does not occur. There is little direct effect on the heart itself. Sodium nitroprusside is in large part metabolized to cyanide in the red blood cells; the cyanide reacts with thiosulfate in the liver to form thiocyanate. Thiocyanate, in turn, is excreted by the kidneys. In hepatic failure, therefore, cyanide may accumulate, and in renal failure or with infusions lasting 2 or more days, toxic levels of thiocyanate may occur.

Administration

Administered by constant intravenous infusion, sodium nitroprusside has an immediate effect proportionate to the infusion rate and lasting only as long as the infusion continues. It therefore requires minute-to-minute titration and constant attention in the emergency department or intensive care unit. When available, constant infusion pumps aid in precise regulation of administration, and arterial lines aid in monitoring pressure. One vial (50 mg) is dissolved in 500 ml of 5% dextrose in water, and the bottle is covered with aluminum foil or a paper bag because of sensitivity to light. An initial infusion of 0.5 μg/kg/min (35 μg/min or 0.35 ml/min for a 70-kg patient) should be given and the rate adjusted for adequate control. Different individuals may require from 0.5 to 8.0 μg/kg/min, with an average dose of 3 μg/kg/min.

Side Effects

Nausea, sweating, or apprehension initially may be noted, but usually diminishes with time. The main disadvantage is not the presence of side effects, but rather the extreme potency of the drug, which requires very close attention to blood pressure and infusion rate. If thiocyanate in the blood rises to toxic levels, muscular weakness, delirium, or coma may develop. In patients at risk, thiocyanate levels should be monitored and infusion discontinued if possible when levels exceed 10 mg/100 ml. If necessary, thiocyanate may be removed by dialysis. One instance of methemoglobinemia occurring on the fourth day of infusion has been reported.

Nifedipine

Action

Nifedipine, one of the class of calcium channel blocking drugs, has become increasingly used in the treatment of hypertensive emergencies. (Although nifedipine has not been officially approved for this purpose at the time of writing, it seems likely that approval will soon be forthcoming.) It causes direct vasodilatation of arterioles, reducing peripheral vascular resistance promptly, smoothly, and with relatively few side effects. Its action begins within 15 minutes of sublingual administration, peaks at 30 to 60 minutes, and lasts 4–6 hours. Swallowed, its onset is a bit slower. It is metabolized by the liver and, because of "first pass" metabolism, has somewhat limited gastrointestonal absorption. Mean arterial pressure can be expected to fall by 20–30% following the administration of 10–20 mg. Excessive hypotension has been reported but is rare. Renal and cerebral blood flow are well-preserved when the drug is administered to hypertensive patients (although some fall in glomerular fittration rate may be observed with chronic administration to patients with renal disease.) A mild increase in heart rate may be seen.

Administration

A simple means of administration is to chew a 10-mg capsule for 2 or 3 minutes, allowing for oral as well as gastric absorption. This may be repeated in 20 minutes, if necessary, to control the blood pressure.

Labetalol

Action

Labetalol is a combined blocker of α- and β-adrenergic receptors. When given intravenously, it has a predominently β-blocking effect with a β-to-α ratio of about 7:1. An intravenous dose has a hypotensive effect, beginning in 5 minutes and lasting for at least 4–6 hours. The fall in blood pressure results from a decrease in peripheral vascular resistance accompanied by a slight fall in cardiac output. When pulmonary artery wedge pressure is initially elevated, labetalol can lower it. It has been used successfully in the emergency treatment of malignant hypertension, catecholamine crisis, and hypertension of late pregnancy. Since the drug is also effective as an oral antihypertensive agent, the initial parenteral treatment can be smoothly followed with oral administration.

Administration

Continuous intravenous infusion, bolus doses, or repeated "miniboluses" have been successfully used. A reasonable protocol is to give an initial intravenous bolus dose of 0.25 mg/kg, followed each 15 minutes as necessary with somewhat larger boluses of 0.5 mg/kg until blood pressure is controlled or a total dose of 3.25 mg/kg has been given.

Side Effects

Side effects are few but include nausea, sedation, diaphoresis, and rarely marked hypotension.

Trimethaphan Camsylate

Trimethaphan camsylate is a ganglionic blocking agents that causes inhibition of both adrenergic and cholinergic ganglia. This accounts for both its efficacy and its numerous side effects. Adrenergic blockade causes vasodilatation and subsequent reduction in blood pressure; it also reduces systolic ejection velocity and cardiac output. Anticholinergic action may cause urinary retention, hypomotility of the intestine with development of ileus or gastric retention, and blurred vision. Respiratory paralysis has been reported.

Administration is by constant intravenous infusion; 500 mg is mixed in 500 ml of 5% dextrose in water and given as an initial dose of 0.5–1.0 mg/min. The dose is then titrated to achieve desired pressure. Elevation of the head at 45° will enhance the antihypertensive effect.

Because trimethaphan camsylate is extremely potent, its use requires constant monitoring, preferably with an arterial line. Tachyphylaxis is common and usually occurs within 48–72 hours.

Phentolamine

Phentolamine is a pure α-adrenergic blocking agent used specifically for treatment of catecholamine crisis. It is given as a 5–10-mg intravenous bolus. The effect is immediate and lasts approximately 15 minutes, so constant intravenous infusion is used to continue the effect. Phentolamine may cause tachyarrhythmias or angina. Phenoxybenzamine, a long-acting α-adrenergic blocking agent may be given orally after initial treatment with phentolamine.

Captopril

Action

Captopril is a rapidly acting and powerful oral inhibitor of the angiotensin converting enzyme. Although its action is not rapid enough to be considered in the first line of drugs for the treatment of true emergency hypertension, it can provide a means to reduce severe hypertension within 30–60 minutes without the need for constant or elaborate blood pressure monitoring. It is particularly effective when combined with a rapidly acting diuretic such as furosemide. One can give captopril, 25 mg orally, accompanied by furosemide, 40 mg orally. If insufficient response is noted at 30 minutes, the captopril dose may be repeated one or two times. If blood pressure remains severely elevated, then parenteral agents should probably be used. The drug appears to be well-tolerated in elderly patients (perhaps because cerebral blood flow is maintained while arterial pressure falls) and may be particularly effective when heart failure complicates the severe hypertension.

MANAGEMENT

Does An Emergency Exist?

When the patient is not outwardly critically ill or in extreme distress, the most difficult decision is whether to use potent rapidly acting intravenous hypertensive drugs or to use slower drugs that can be incorporated later into the chronic treatment program. The physician must estimate the threat to the patient posed by several hours or a day of continued, severe hypertension. In general, severe hypertension associated with any of the following requires rapid (within minutes) lowering of blood pressure: grade III or IV retinopathy with or without symptoms of encephalopathy, eclampsia, aortic dissection, acute myocardial ischemia or infarction, or intracranial hemorrhage. Asymptomatic hypertension without papilledema or complications usually does not require parenteral drug treatment.

Evaluation of the Patient

Although severe hypertension requires consideration of correctable secondary causes and often a series of laboratory studies, initial therapy in a hypertensive emergency must begin after the briefest evaluation. The only benign conditions in the differential diagnosis of severe hypertension are anxiety attacks and defective blood pressure measuring equipment, including undersized cuffs applied to obese patients.

History

The physician should determine the following: Is there a history of hypertension? Is the patient taking any medication, including diuretics, antihypertensive drugs, monoamine oxidase inhibitors, or birth control pills? Have there been episodes of palpitation, pallor, sweating, and headache that would suggest pheochromocytoma? Has dyspnea, orthopnea, angina pectoris, or papilledema been noted? In a patient suspected of having hypertensive encephalopathy, a careful history of the symptoms and the course of onset is especially important.

Physical Examination

Immediate examination should include determination of blood pressure in both arms and evaluation of the heart, lungs, and neck veins for evidence of congestive failure, examination of the optic fundi for retinopathy or papilledema, and determination of all pulses, especially if aortic dissection is suspended. The examiner also should look briefly for café au lait spots and neurofibromas that many accompany pheochromocytoma and should perfom a rapid neurologic examination, including determination of mental status.

An electrocadiogram should be obtained, an intravenous line of at least 18-gauge tubing established, the patient's head elevated at a 45° angle, and arrangements made for admission to the hospital. A chest x-ray film is usually obtained, but treatment should not be delayed by a slow trip through the radiology department.

Treatment

General Considerations

The selection of appropriate therapy will be simplified by taking the following into consideration.

1. Urgency—patients with malignant hypertension, encephalopathy, or complicated hypertension require immediate control with rapidly acting antihypertensive agents. In the asymptomatic patient with accelerated hypertension, the condition may be controlled in the course of hours.

2. Blood pressure goal—Except in patients previously normotensive (such as children or patients with eclampsia or acute renal failure) and patients with aortic dissection, the initial goal of treatment is not to achieve completely normal blood pressure. Patients with chronic hypertension often have thickened arterial walls and atherosclerosis, so perfusion to vital organs may be compromised by normal pressures. In general, in the previously hypertensive patient the immediate blood pressure goal is 180–160/110–100 mm Hg. In the patient who was previously normotensive, the goal is 140/90 mm Hg or lower. In the presence of aortic dissection, despite a history of hypertension, the blood pressure goal is usually approximately 100–110/60 mm Hg to prevent further dissection. In the patient with myocardial ischemia or infarction, the physician must weigh the need to lower the blood pressure for reduction of myocardial work against the need to maintain adequate coronary perfusion.

3. Hemodynamic stability—Because of its relatively long duration of action, diazoxide is ideal for patients with uncomplicated hypertensive emergencies. In situations that may become potentially unstable, such as myocardial infarction, pulmonary edema, or intracranial hemorrhage, more precise control is necessary, and sodium nitroprusside is preferred.

Uncomplicated Hypertension—Specific Recommendations

In uncomplicated hypertensive emergencies, the primary circulatory abnormality is increased peripheral resistance. In this circumstance, the ideal emergency drug would be one with a predominant action of reducing resistance, rapid onset of action, and relatively few side effects. Diazoxide and sodium nitroprusside approach this ideal, although neither is perfect.

In general, except in catecholamine crisis, uncomplicated hypertensive emergencies are best treated with diazoxide because of its ease of administration and proven efficacy. In complicated hypertensive emergencies, sodium nitroprusside is preferred because of its lack of reflex cardiac stimulation and its potency and short duration of action, which allow precise control in hemodynamically unstable situations. Nifedipine also appears to be an excellent drug for the emergency treatment of uncomplicated hypertension. Its oral administration and prompt, safe action are major advantages. It has not been adequately compared with nitroprusside and diazoxide in the treatment of malignant hypertension and hypertensive encephalopathy and should not be considered the drug of choice for these conditions. It appears to be a good choice for patients without encephalopathy and for those in whom severe hypertension is combined with cardiac ischemia or heart failure. Recommendations for treatment of hypertensive emergencies are summarized in Tables 8.5 and 8.6.

Complicated Hypertension—Specific Recommendations

Pulmonary Edema. Patients with pulmonary edema frequently have extreme hypertension. Initial management should be directed at specific treatment of the pulmonary edema including diuretics, morphine, and oxygen. Occasionally, pulmonary congestion does not resolve with standard measures and blood pressure remains elevated. In such cases, sodium nitroprusside is the drug of choice. Nifedipine may be of benefit as well.

Acute Myocardial Ischemia. Similarly, sodium nitroprusside is the drug of choice in acute myocardial ischemia complicated by severe hypertension. It allows gradual, precise reduction of blood pressure without increasing ischemia. Intravenous nitroglycerin also may be useful in the patient with hypertension and ongoing ischemia. Used alone, it is inadequate to control severe hypertension. If hypertension is less severe and the patient's condition is hemodynamically stable, nitrates and propranolol hydrochloride may be tried initially. The two newer agents, labetalol and, in particular, nifedipine, may be particularly useful in this condition.

Aortic Dissection. The treatment of aortic dissection is aimed at reducing the forces that propagate the dissection—elevated pressure and velocity of systolic ejection. This is achieved by a combination of propranolol hydrochloride and sodium nitroprusside. Propranolol is given first as a 0.5-mg intravenous test dose, followed in 5 minutes by 1 mg intravenously which is repeated every 5 minutes until the heart rate is between 60 and 70 beats/min or until a total dose of 0.15 mg/kg has been attained. Nitroprusside is then given to lower pressure to approximately 100/60 mm Hg. During this time, arrangements should be made either to have the patient evaluated by a cardiologist and a cardiac surgeon or to transfer the patient immediately to a facility in which aortic angiography and cardiac surgery can be performed. If the patient has congestive heart failure or a history of significant pulmonary disease or asthma, propranolol is hazardous and the drug of next choice is trimethaphan camsylate. Trimethaphan may be given by intravenous infusion, 0.5–1.0 mg/min, and titrated until the desired pressure is reached. As a ganglionic blocking agent, it both lowers blood pressure through vasodilatation and reduces systolic ejection velocity and cardiac output. Therefore, it may be used alone. In the patient with aortic dissection, its effect is enhanced by elevating the upper portion of the patient 45°. Like sodium nitroprusside, it is an extremely potent antihypertensive agent and requires constant monitoring to avoid profound hypotension.

Intracranial Hemorrhage. While severe hypertension may precede intracranial hemorrhage, it may also be secondary to increased intracranial pressure, and thus it may fluctuate in response to measures that reduce intracranial pressure. In such a situation, sodium nitroprusside is the drug of choice if monitoring is available. Intracranial hemorrhage has not been shown to benefit from blood pressure control; thus, pressure should be lowered carefully to about 20–30% below the original systolic pressure. Any drug that may depress central nervous system function such as reserpine or methyldopa should be avoided.

Catecholamine Crisis. Because catecholamine crisis occurs secondary to a sudden excess of catecholamines, whether endogenous or exogenous, treatment is aimed at blocking both α- and β-adrenergic effects. To avoid an increase in peripheral resistance and thus further pressure elevation, the physician must achieve α-blockade first. This is accomplished with the α-blocking agent, phentolamine, 1–10 mg as an intravenous bolus every 5 minutes until pressure is lowered. This then may be followed by intravenous propranolol hydrochloride as previously described. Sodium nitroprusside is also effective, and if there is any doubt about the diagnosis, it is the preferred agent.

Eclampsia. It has been recently suggested that, when the diastolic blood pressure exceeds 105 mm Hg, intravenous hydralazine should be given in repeated doses of 5 or 10 mg until the diastolic pressure remains below 105 mm Hg. Diazoxide may be given in small repeated doses of 30 mg intravenously for resistant cases.

Table 8.5.
Drug Considerations in the Treatment of Hypertensive Emergencies

	Route and Dosage[a]	Time Course			Mechanism of Action	Side Effects	Disadvantages	Advantages
		Onset	Peak	Duration				
General								
Diazoxide	i.v. push: 300 mg (5 mg/kg), 150 mg, or infusion	1–2 min	2–4 min	4–12 hr	Direct arterial vasodilatation	Reflex tachycardia, sodium retention, hyperglycemia, vomiting, uterine atony	Hypotension, painful extravasation	Prompt effect, potent, continuous infusion not required, constant monitoring not required
Sodium nitroprusside	i.v. infusion: 50 mg in 500 ml D_5W—begin at 25–50 μ/min and titrate ↑	<1 min	1–2 min	2–5 min	Direct smooth muscle relaxation (arterial and venous)	Nausea, restlessness, hypotension, thiocyanate toxicity after prolonged use	Constant monitoring required, extreme photosensitivity	Precise control, ↓ both preload and afterload
Nifedipine[b]	Oral, sublingual. Chew and swallow	10 min	30 min	1–6 hr	Smooth muscle relaxation	Nausea, flushing	Hypotension (rare)	Oral, sublingual
Labetalol	repeated i.v. pushes of 0.5 mg/kg doses	5 min	60 min	4–6 hr	β- and α-blocker	Nausea, sedation	Avoid in asthma	Constant monitor not required
Hydralazine	10–50 mg given i.v.	15 min	60 min	1–6 hr	Direct arteriolar vasodilatation	Reflex tachycardia, increased pulse pressure	Avoid in cardiac ischemia, aneurysm, or bleeding	Maintains renal blood flow. Good for pregnancy use.
Special purpose								
Trimethaphan camsylate	i.v. infusion; 500 mg in 500 ml D_5W—begin at 0.5–1.0 mg/min and titrate ↑	1–2 min	2–5 min	10 min	Ganglionic blockade	Ganglionic blockade, urinary retention, ileus, cycloplegia, respiratory arrest	Tachyphylaxis, constant monitoring required	Potent, precise control

Propranolol hydrochloride	0.5 mg i.v. test dose, then 1 mg i.v. q 5 min until pulse <70 or total 0.15 mg/kg	<1 min	1–2 min	2–6 hr	α-Blockade	Bradycardia, ↓ atrioventricular conduction, bronchospasm, myocardial depression		
Phentolamine	i.v. bolus 5–10 mg followed by i.v. infusion of 1.5–2 μgm/kg/min	<1 min		5–30 min	α-Adrenergic blockade	Tachyarrhythmias, angina, palpitation		Use only in circumstances of catecholamine excess
Severe hypertension, but not an acute emergency (see text)								
Captopril	25 mg orally accompanied by 40 mg furosemide	30 min	2 hr	8–12 hr	Inhibitor of angiotensin converting enzyme	Dysgeusia	Hypotension	Oral, no intensive monitoring. Cerebral blood flow maintained. Good in heart failure.

[a] i.v., intravenous; D_5W, 5% dextrose in water.
[b] Nifedipine is not yet official for this use.

Table 8.6.
Specific Pharmacologic Recommendations[a]

Syndrome	Drugs of Choice	Drugs to Be Avoided
Malignant hypertension	Diazoxide or sodium nitroprusside	
Hypertensive encephalopathy	Diazoxide or sodium nitroprusside	Reserpine, methyldopa
Eclampsia	Hydralazine, diazoxide, labetalol	
Excess catecholamines	Phentolamine followed by propranolol hydrochloride or sodium nitroprusside	Propranolol hydrochloride in the absence of α-blockade
Hypertension complicated by		
Acute left ventricular failure	Sodium nitroprusside, nifedipine	
Intracranial hemorrhage	Sodium nitroprusside	Reserpine, methyldopa, diazoxide
Aortic dissection	Sodium nitroprusside and propranolol hydrochloride or trimethaphan camsylate	Diazoxide, hydralazine
Aortic ischemia or infarction	Sodium nitroprusside, nifedipine	Diazoxide, hydralazine

[a] These recommendations are based on known benefits and hazards and may not be universally applicable.

Magnesium sulfate remains the drug of choice to treat impending seizures, but should not be considered a very effective agent for the management of severe hypertension. Nitroprusside and diuretics are less desirable than hydralazine or diazoxide. Special care must be taken to avoid intravascular volume depletion since eclamptic patients are frequently hypovolemic despite peripheral edema. A central venous pressure line usually is recommended. Stabilization of the patient's condition with subsequent rapid delivery is the treatment of choice.

Other Drug Therapy

We have emphasized the usefulness of diazoxide and sodium nitroprusside in most hypertensive emergencies. This should not imply that these are the *only* drugs useful in such emergencies. It is likely, however, that the emergency physician who is thoroughly experienced with the actions of two drugs will treat hypertensive crises more effectively than one who has passing familiarity with a large number.

Once blood pressure is under control, treatment has only begun. An oral regimen of therapy should be started if possible, even as the emergency program is in progress. A search for correctible causes of secondary hypertension should be instituted—the extent of the search depending on the age and clinical characteristics of the patient.

SUGGESTED READINGS

Chiariello M, Gold HK, Leinbach RC, et al. Comparison between the effects of nitroprusside and nitroglycerin on ischemic injury during acute myocardial infarction. *Circulation,* 1976;54-766–773.

Cohn JN, Burke LP. Nitroprusside. *Ann Intern Med,* 1979;91:752–757.

Ellrodt AG, Adult MG, Riedinger, MS, et al. Efficacy and safety of sublingual nifedipine in hypertensive emergencies. *Am J Med,* 1985;79:19–25.

Ferguson, RK, Vlasses, PH. Hypertensive emergencies and urgencies. *JAMA,* 1986;255:1607–1613.

Finnerty FA: Treatment of hypertensive emergencies. *Heart Lung,* 1981;10:275–284.

Grossman SH, Gunnels JC: Recognition and treatment of hypertensive emergencies. *Cardiovasc Clin,* 1981;12, No 3:47–54.

Guiha NH, Cohn JN, Mikulic E, et al: Treatment of refractory heart failure with infusion of nitroprusside. *N Engl J Med,* 1974;291:587–592.

Houston, MC. Treatment of hypertensive urgencies and emergencies with nifedipine. *Am Heart J,* 1986;111:963–969.

Koch-Weser J: Drug therapy: Diazoxide. *N Engl J Med,* 1976;294:1271–1274.

Lebel M, Langlois S, Belleau, LJ, et al. Labetalol infusion in hypertensive emergencies. *Clin Pharmacol Ther,* 1985;37:615–618.

Lindheimer MD, Katz AL. Hypertension in pregnancy. *New Engl J Med,* 1985;313:675–680.

Mukherjee D, Feldman MS, Helfant RH: Nitroprusside therapy: Treatment of hypertensive patients with recurrent resting chest pain, ST-segment elevation, and ventricular arrhythmias. *JAMA,* 1976;235:2406–2409.

Palmer RF, Lasseter KC: Drug therapy: Sodium nitroprusside. *N Engl J Med,* 1975;292:294–297.

Ram CVS, Kaplan N: Individual titration of diazoxide dosage in the treatment of severe hypertension. *Am J Cardiol* 1979;43:627.

Slater EE, DeSanctis RW: The clinical recognition of dissecting aortic aneurysm. *Am J Med,* 1976;60:625.

Wheat MR Jr, Palmer RF: Dissecting aneurysms of the aorta. In: Sabiston DC Jr, Spencer FC, eds. Gibbon's Surgery of the Chest. ed 3. Philadelphia: WB Saunders, 1976;913–933.

Wilson, DJ, Wallin JD, Vlachakis, ND, et al. Intravenous labetalol in the treatment of severe hypertension and hypertensive emergencies. *Am J Med,* 1983;75:95–102.

CHAPTER **9**

Pulmonary Emergencies

B. TAYLOR THOMPSON, M.D.
DAVID M. SYSTROM, M.D.
EDWARD A. NARDELL, M.D.
CHARLES A. HALES, M.D.

PULMONARY EMBOLISM

A frequently unrecognized emergency medical problem, pulmonary embolism is the result of clot or other particulate matter lodging in the pulmonary vascular bed. Annual incidence of symptomatic pulmonary emboli in the United States probably exceeds 500,000 but as many as two-thirds go undiagnosed. Ten percent are fatal within one hour of onset of symptoms. If the patient survives the initial embolic event, subsequent mortality is 30–40%, primarily the result of recurrent embolism. However, when the diagnosis is established and anticoagulant therapy is administered, the mortality is reduced to 8–9%.

Natural History

Pulmonary embolism is usually the consequence of clot from the deep venous system, known as deep venous thrombosis (DVT). DVT usually begins in the lower extremities although occasionally clots form in pelvic veins and rarely in renal veins or veins of the upper extremities. Most thrombi originate in the soleus veins of the calf, often at sites of decreased flow such as valve cusps or bifurcations. The majority of calf thrombi resolve spontaneously; if embolization to the lung occurs, clinical manifestations may be absent. About 20–30% of clots propagate to the iliofemoral system, and an additional 10–20% of all DVT begin in proximal veins without prior calf involvement. Iliofemoral thromboses appear to be the source of most clinically significant pulmonary emboli.

Once in the pulmonary circulation, large clots lodge at the bifurcation of the pulmonary and lobar arteries and may cause hemodynamic compromise. Smaller clots continue distally to arterioles or capillaries. Lower lobes are more often involved than upper lobes, and emboli are usually multiple. Only about 10% of emboli cause infarction, probably because of collateral flow between the bronchial and pulmonary circulations. Infarction is more common in patients with preexistent cardiopulmonary disease.

Factors predisposing to pulmonary emboli include: 1) history of prior embolism; 2) factors promoting stasis, including bed rest, inactivity, or congestive heart failure; 3) endothelial damage following surgery or trauma to the lower extremity; 4) primary hypercoagulable states, such as a deficiency of antithrombin III, protein C, or protein S; and 5) secondary hypercoagulable states, such as malignancy, use of oral contraceptives, and pregnancy, particularly in the postpartum period.

Clinical Manifestations

Autopsy series show a prevalence of pulmonary embolism as high as 64% and suggest that many emboli are silent. The clinical presentation most suggestive of the diagnosis is that of the acute and unexplained onset of dyspnea. Other symptoms depend primarily on the size of the emboli. Small to medium emboli lodge in segmental or more distal branches of the pulmonary artery. Symptoms of these smaller emboli are usually pulmonary, including dyspnea, chest pain, and cough (Table 9.1). Tachycapnea and tachycardia are present in most patients. Mild fever below 102.2°F (39°C) is common and wheezing occurs in less than 5% of patients, often those with underlying lung disease. If infarction occurs, hemoptysis, pleuritic pain, and a pleural rub may be present (Table 9.2).

Massive pulmonary emboli occur in lobar arteries or the main pulmonary arteries with predominantly cardiovascular findings. Symptoms include syncope, chest pain, and dyspnea. The following signs of right ventricular dysfunction may be present: right ventricular heave, increased pulmonary component of the second heart sound, right ventricular S_3 gallop, jugular venous distention, and tricuspid regurgitant murmur. Systemic hypotension in a previously normotensive patient almost always signifies elevated right ventricular pressures. However, some patients may have normal pulmonary artery pressures and no evidence of right ventricular dysfunction despite massive embolization.

In patients in whom pulmonary embolism is suspected, the emergency physician should seek a history or findings of deep venous thrombosis. A history of calf or leg pain, signs of unilateral edema, and increased calf warmth or tenderness combined with the respiratory symptoms should heighten the suspicion of pulmonary embolism and focus the diagnostic approach. However, less than half of patients with pulmonary emboli have clinically evident DVT, in part, because DVT is often silent. Thus, the absence of clinically apparent DVT does not lessen the likelihood of pulmonary embolism. Factors predisposing to DVT, however, are almost invariably present.

Noninvasive studies of the legs with impedance plethysmography aid greatly in documenting proximal DVT but are less useful in documenting DVT of the calf veins. Calf veins, however, are rarely the source of symptomatic pulmonary emboli. Venography provides the definitive diagnosis of DVT, although it is more uncomfortable for the patient and carries a low risk of resultant phlebitis. Positive lower extremity noninvasive studies, confirmed with venography, establish with certainty the diagnosis of DVT in patients with pulmonary emboli and thus establish the need for anticoagulation. However, negative noninvasive studies and negative bilateral lower extremity venography in patients suspected of having pulmonary emboli do not exclude the diagnosis as these tests may be negative in one-third to

Table 9.1.
Frequency of Symptoms of Pulmonary Embolism in 160 Patients[a]

Symptom	Percent
Dyspnea	81
Pleuritic pain	72
Apprehension	59
Cough	54
Hemoptysis	34
Sweats	26
Syncope	14

[a] Modified by permission, from Sasahara AA. The urokinase pulmonary embolism trial: A national cooperative study. *Circulation,* 1973; *47* and *48* (suppl II):1–108, © The American Heart Association, Inc.

Table 9.2.
Frequency of Physical Signs of Pulmonary Embolism in 160 Patients[a]

Sign	Percent
Respiration rate > 16/min	88
Rales	53
Elevated S_2P	53
Pulse rate > 100/min	43
S_3-S_4 gallop	34
Diaphoresis	34
Thrombophlebitis	33
Edema	23
Murmur	23
Cyanosis	18

[a] Modified by permission, from Sasahara AA. The urokinase pulmonary embolism trial: A national cooperative study. *Circulation,* 1973; *47* and *48* (suppl II):1–108, © The American Heart Association, Inc.

one-half of patients with angiographically documented pulmonary emboli.

In patients with smaller pulmonary emboli, the differential diagnosis includes hyperventilation, asthma, congestive heart failure, pleurodynia, and serositis. If infarction is present, clinical findings may resemble pneumonia, bronchial obstruction by mucus or tumor, or pleural effusion of various causes.

In summary, signs and symptoms of pulmonary embolism are often nonspecific. Vigilance is required to suspect the diagnosis and to initiate further evaluation. The emergency physician is thus frequently in the position to make an important, potentially lifesaving diagnosis.

Laboratory Evaluation

General Studies

Noninvasive laboratory findings may further suggest, but rarely confirm, the diagnosis of pulmonary embolism. Nonspecific findings include leukocytosis, elevated erythrocyte sedimentation rate, and abnormal serum lactate dehydrogenase (LDH) or serum glutamic oxaloacetic transaminase (SGOT) level with normal bilirubin level. Fibrin degradation products are more common in the serum of patients with pulmonary emboli, but are nondiagnostic. However, the absence of these products and soluble fibrin complexes makes the diagnosis less likely.

Arterial Blood Gases

Arterial blood gas studies usually reveal hypoxemia, hypocapnia, and respiratory alkalosis. Massive pulmonary embolism with hypotension and respiratory collapse may lead to hypercapnia and combined respiratory and metabolic acidosis.

The arterial oxygen tension (Pao_2) is less than 90 mm Hg in almost all patients with pulmonary embolism and less than 80 mm Hg in 90% of these patients; the average is 60–65 mm Hg. However, the Pao_2 must be interpreted with caution since the normal level varies with age and position of the patient.

Formulas for estimating Pao_2 are:

$$Pao_2\ (\text{seated}) = 104.2 - (0.27 \times \text{age in years})$$
$$Pao_2\ (\text{supine}) = 103.5 - (0.42 \times \text{age in years})$$

Further, measured Pao_2 must be corrected for $Paco_2$ since the two coexist in alveolar gas: for every millimeter of mercury increase in $Paco_2$, Pao_2 decreases in roughly the same amount (assuming a respiratory quotient of 1). Therefore, a patient with a Pao_2 of 100 mm Hg and a $Paco_2$ of 20 mm Hg may be relatively hypoxemic, since correction to a $Paco_2$ of 40 mm Hg yields a Pao_2 of 80 mm Hg.

Table 9.3.
Frequency of Chest Radiologic Abnormalities before Heparin Infusion in 128 Patients

Finding	Patients No.	Patients %
Lung parenchyma	60[a]	47
Consolidation	53	41
Atelectasis	26	20
Other	2	2
Pleural effusion	36	28
Diaphragmatic elevation	52	41
Pulmonary vessels	50	39
Distention of proximal pulmonary arteries	30	23
Focal oligemia	19	15
Pulmonary arterial hypertension	4	3
Pulmonary venous hypertension	4	3
Other	3	2

[a] Number of patients with at least one radiologic finding of that subgroup. Modified by permission, from Sasahara AA. The urokinase pulmonary embolism trial: A national cooperative study. *Circulation,* 1973; *47* and *48* (suppl II):1–108, © The American Heart Association, Inc.

This is especially important, given the frequency of hypocapnia in pulmonary embolism. However, a rare patient with pulmonary embolism may have a completely normal Pao_2 for age and a normal $Paco_2$.

Hypoxemia may be detected up to 14 days after embolism and is due mainly to ventilation-perfusion inequalities with a small proportion due to shunt. Since hypoxemia is common in other diseases, it remains suggestive but nonspecific for pulmonary embolism.

Electrocardiogram

The electrocardiogram is often abnormal in patients with small to medium pulmonary emboli, but findings are nonspecific including ST-segment and T-wave changes. In the presence of massive pulmonary embolism, findings of right ventricular dysfunction are more common, including right axis deviation, right bundle-branch block, and the classic $S_1\ Q_3\ T_3$ pattern.

Chest X-ray

Even without infarction, radiographic abnormalities occur in many patients with pulmonary emboli (Table 9.3). These include elevation of a hemidiaphragm, atelectasis (Fig. 9.1), and effusion. An infarct classically appears as a pleural-based infiltrate with a convex margin directed toward the heart. Effusions are usually small, unilateral, and either exudative or transudative. Blood is present in over half, and white blood cell count and differential vary widely.

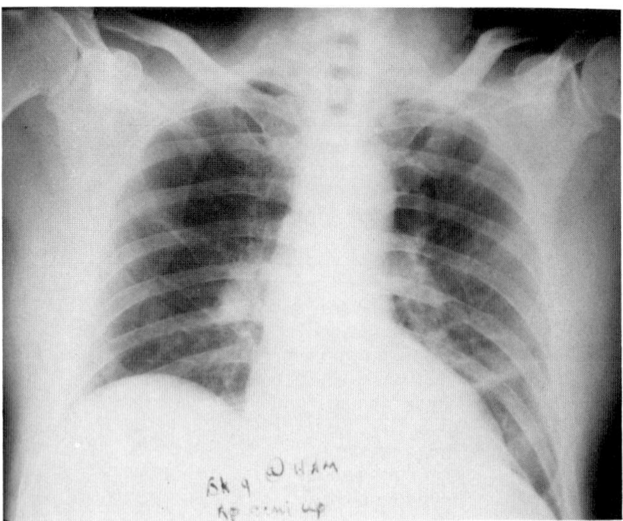

Figure 9.1. Posteroanterior chest x-ray film shows bilateral atelectasis, elevated right diaphragmatic leaf, and diminution of lung markings on right.

Perfusion Scanning

Perfusion lung scanning is performed by injection of radioisotope-labeled albumin macroaggregates or microspheres. Scanning is sensitive; negative findings virtually exclude pulmonary embolism. Positive results, however, are nonspecific. Since pulmonary arterioles constrict in response to hypoxia, pulmonary defects, especially if nonsegmental, may be secondary to a ventilation abnormality and not to obstruction of flow caused by an embolism. Findings may also be abnormal in patients with atelectasis, asthma, chronic airways obstruction and emphysema, pneumonia, or other causes of regional hypoventilation or destruction of the pulmonary vascular bed.

Ventilation scans may be used to increase the specificity of perfusion scans although sensitivity is not altered. Ventilation scans are particularly useful when there is no infiltrate on the chest x-ray and when segmental or larger perfusion scan defects are present (Figs. 9.2 and 9.3).

Lung scans are extremely helpful if the perfusion image is completely normal, thus excluding clini-

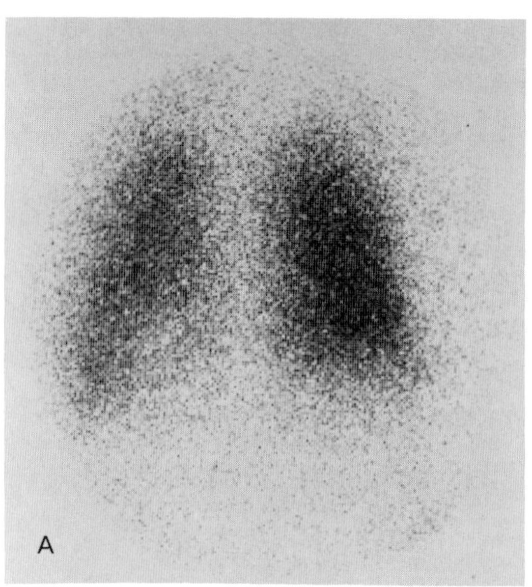

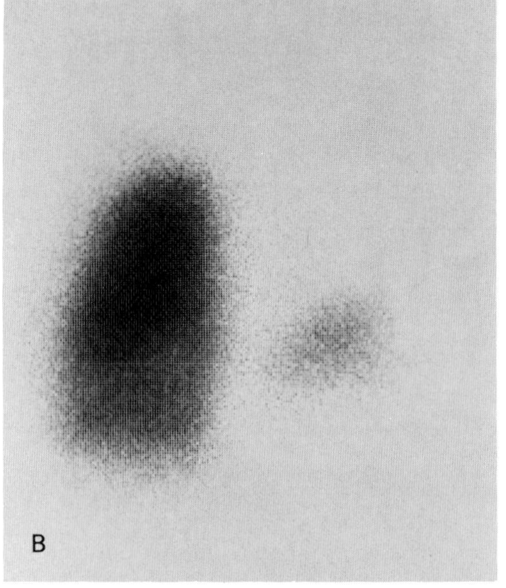

Figure 9.2. Ventilation *(A)* and perfusion *(B)* combined lung scan (posterior view, same patient as in Fig. 9.1) shows normal ventilation in right lung but almost complete absence of blood flow, except for minimal perfusion in middle lobe.

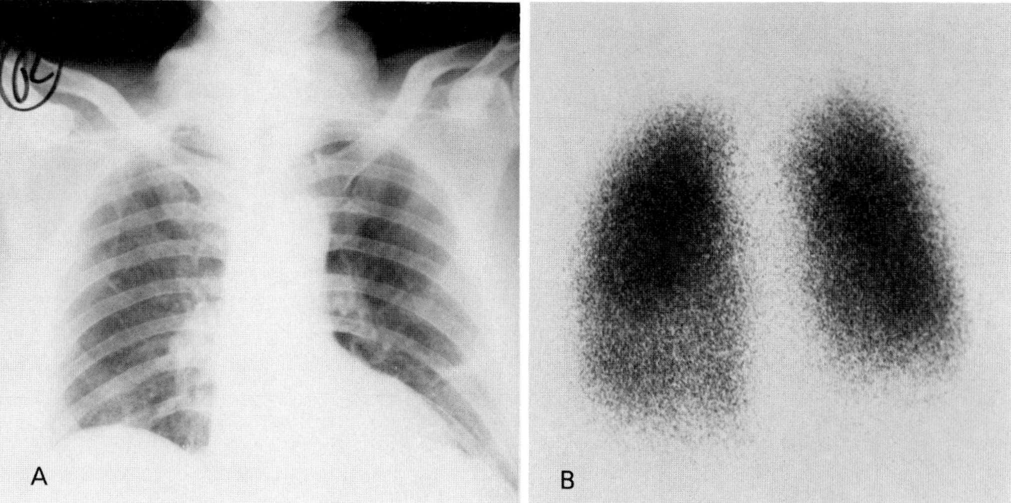

Figure 9.3. *A,* Posteroanterior chest x-ray film 2 weeks later reveals minimal atelectasis in left lower lobe. *B,* Posterior perfusion scan shows return of right lung perfusion.

cally significant pulmonary emboli. Scans are also helpful when multiple large (segmental or greater) perfusion defects are present that ventilate normally. This scan pattern suggests pulmonary vascular occlusion and is highly suggestive for pulmonary emboli (>90%). When highly suggestive or high probability scans are coupled with a characteristic clinical picture for pulmonary embolism or documentation of DVT in the lower extremities, further studies may be avoided. However, other scan patterns must be interpreted with caution. Multiple subsegmental and nonsegmental defects, with or without associated ventilation abnormalities, have been traditionally considered of low probability for pulmonary emboli. However, a recent prospective study of patients suspected of having pulmonary emboli found pulmonary emboli at angiography in 25–40% of patients with these "low probability" scan defects.

Pulmonary Angiography

Many patients have uncharacteristic clinical presentations or nonspecific lung scan abnormalities and require the use of pulmonary angiography to diagnose pulmonary embolism. Angiography, the definitive diagnostic technique in this disease, is performed by injecting radiographic contrast dye into a branch of the pulmonary artery after percutaneous, usually transfemoral, catheterization. The catheter is advanced at least to the main pulmonary artery and preferably selectively to the left or right pulmonary artery to achieve good dye concentration in the pulmonary vessels. A positive result consists of a filling defect or sharp cutoff of small vessels (Fig. 9.4). Selective injection with magnification views increases sensitivity. Negative findings appear to exclude pulmonary embolism, and one follow-up study has shown the risk of embolization in patients with negative selective pulmonary angiograms to be extremely low. Mortality from the procedure is less than 0.4%; deaths that occur are usually in patients with markedly elevated pulmonary artery pressure. Complications related to catheter insertion occur in about 4% of studies.

Treatment

Treatment of pulmonary embolism requires the prompt use of either anticoagulants or thrombolytic agents.

Heparin Therapy

The objective of heparin therapy is to prevent further thrombosis in the lower extremities and recurrent embolism, allowing endogenous fibrinolytic mechanisms to dissolve existing thrombi. Heparin combines with antithrombin III, leading to rapid inactivation of thrombin. Constant intravenous infusion of heparin appears to cause fewer hemorrhagic complications than intermittent infusion. A bolus of 5000 units is followed by approximately 1000 units/hr in most patients; doses are decreased if a bleeding tendency or renal or hepatic disease is present. An activated partial thromboplastin time of 1½ to 2½ times the control value should be maintained. Lower levels may allow recurrent thromboembolism; higher levels increase the risk of bleeding.

Hemorrhage is the major complication of heparin therapy, occurring in about 5% of patients. Heparin may also cause thrombocytopenia, especially with

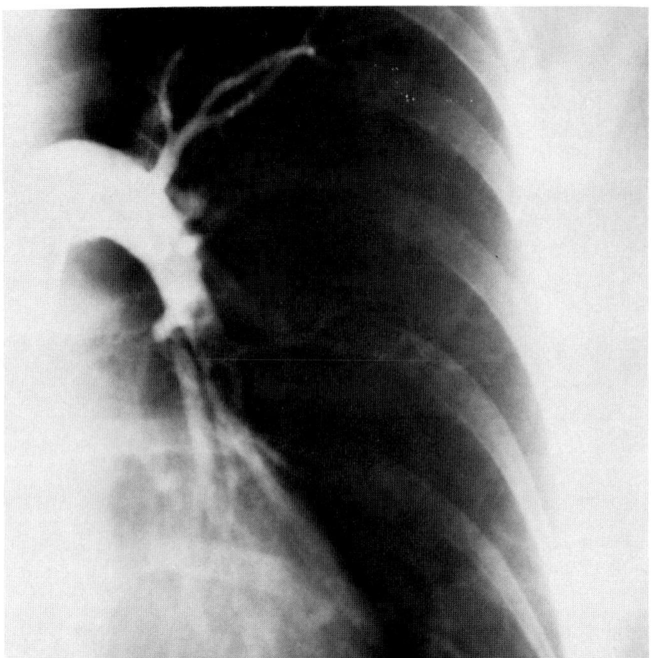

Figure 9.4. Pulmonary angiogram of left lung shows occlusion of artery to left lower lobe.

bovine preparation but this is rarely clinically significant. Contraindications to heparin administration include intracranial hemorrhage and active bleeding. A known bleeding diathesis and recent operation are relative contraindications. Sodium warfarin alone should not be given in the acute situation because of its delayed onset of action and because depletion of protein C, a vitamin K-dependent anticoagulant protein, may aggravate thrombosis initially.

Thrombolytic Therapy

Thrombolytic therapy is approved for massive pulmonary emboli. On angiographic examination, these are seen as filling defects in two or more lobar vessels. In the clinical setting, they are defined as emboli causing hemodynamic instability. The objective of thrombolytic agents is to accelerate clot lysis, as well as to prevent further thrombosis. Although no clear reduction in mortality has been shown in comparison with heparin, thrombolytic therapy allows more rapid dissolution of clot and reduction of pulmonary artery pressures and may improve pulmonary function after recovery. If thrombolytic therapy is administered carefully, the risk of bleeding may be no greater than with heparin. Contraindications include intracranial bleeding (or its strong possibility) or active bleeding. Relative contraindications are recent operation or trauma.

Thrombolytic therapy seems most justified for acute massive pulmonary embolism in the patient who is hemodynamically compromised. There the reduction in pulmonary artery pressure and resistance can be impressive. The issue of treating smaller emboli in patients who are not clinically compromised becomes more debatable. While mortality may not be decreased, there is evidence that the pulmonary microvasculature is somewhat better preserved by thrombolytic therapy. Resolution of DVT may be better with 24 hours of thrombolytic therapy, although this is controversial. Seventy-two hours of thrombolytic therapy seems necessary to provide consistent lessening of the postphlebitic leg syndrome. The issue of thus exposing patients to added risk must be weighed against the clinical status and with the small, and somewhat controversial, improvement that thrombolytic therapy can provide.

Two thrombolytic agents are currently available: urokinase and streptokinase. Tissue plasminogen activator is currently in the evaluation stage. Urokinase is extremely expensive and is seldom used. Streptokinase increases conversion of plasminogen to plasmin. It is antigenic in humans, cross-reacting with anti-streptococcal antibodies. Therefore, a loading dose must be given to bind these antibodies, 250,000 units over 30 minutes in most patients. This is followed by infusion of 100,000 units/hr for 24 hours. No test of the clotting system correlates with thrombolytic effect. Nonetheless, thrombin time or activated partial thromboplastin time is determined after about 4 hours to ensure the presence of a thrombolytic state. If either test is prolonged, the fixed dose should be continued. If results are normal, the presence of excess antibodies should be determined and the dose adjusted.

Bleeding complications do not correlate with clotting parameters, but rather with invasive procedures. Patients in whom thrombolytic therapy is considered should have procedures performed in distal vessels if possible. If significant bleeding occurs, streptokinase administration should be stopped and whole blood given. Rarely, ϵ-aminocaproic acid is required to reverse the thrombolytic state. As many as one-third of patients treated with streptokinase have mild fever as a result, and a smaller number have allergic reactions, usually manifested by urticaria, itching, or flushing. Many physicians elect to administer steroids concomitantly with streptokinase to reduce the likelihood of such reactions. A course of streptokinase may induce an antibody response and increase the likelihood of allergic reactions during retreatment. Accordingly, if thrombolytic therapy is necessary within a 6–12-month period following streptokinase treatment, urokinase is recommended.

Vena Caval Clipping

If anticoagulant therapy is strongly contraindicated, if septic pulmonary emboli occur, or if emboli recur despite adequate anticoagulant therapy, an inferior vena cava interruption procedure should be performed to prevent further embolization from leg or pelvic veins. Ligation of the inferior vena cava may result in serious lower extremity morbidity and even mortality and should be reserved for septic emboli. Clipping the inferior vena cava is tolerated better by the patient with less leg edema but recent advances in transvenously placed filters will likely supplant their use. Transvenously placed filters avoid a direct operative procedure and serve the same function as inferior vena caval clipping. The Kimray-Greenfield filter is the most widely used and is customarily placed via a surgical cutdown in the jugular vein, although percutaneous placement is performed in some centers. A number of other percutaneously placed filters are presently being evaluated.

Embolectomy

The usefulness of embolectomy for acute massive pulmonary embolus is uncertain and, in part, depends on the immediate availability of a cardiopulmonary bypass pump team. Mortality is extremely high, 57% in emergency procedures and 25% in moderately urgent procedures. These mortality figures must also be placed in the perspective that most patients who die from massive pulmonary emboli do so in the first hour, often before a pump team can be gathered. Randomized comparison with thrombolytic therapy has not been performed.

Other Types of Embolic Disease

Upper Extremity Thrombosis

Upper extremity thrombosis is uncommon and may occur spontaneously or following upper extremity trauma or after cannulation of the subclavian veins. Whether pulmonary emboli occur is uncertain. Postphlebitic complications are common following upper extremity DVT treated only with heparin, and thrombolytic therapy should be strongly considered, although prospective trials have not been performed.

Septic Emboli

Septic emboli usually occur in patients with bacterial endocarditis (for example, tricuspid or left-sided bacterial endocarditis with ventricular septal defect) or septic thrombophlebitis. Diagnosis is based on a chest film showing multiple migratory infiltrates, and therapy consists of antibiotics and excision of the septic vein source.

Fat Emboli

The fat embolism syndrome is most often seen after trauma with fracture of the pelvis or long bones of the lower extremity. Clinical findings occur hours to several days after trauma and include changes in mental status, petechiae, and hypoxemia, with diffuse infiltrates on chest x-ray that may progress to the adult respiratory distress syndrome. Therapy may include corticosteroids early but not anticoagulants.

Amniotic Fluid Embolism

Amniotic fluid embolism occurs after childbirth as a result of infusion of amniotic fluid into endocervical veins. It is more common in older, multiparous patients and after complicated labor. Findings are similar to those seen with other types of pulmonary embolism except that hypotension is common and prognosis is poor. Therapy is supportive.

ASTHMA

Asthma is defined by the American Thoracic Society as increased responsiveness of the tracheobronchial tree to various stimuli, manifested by reversible widespread narrowing of the airways. It is a common disease, affecting approximately 7% of the population of the United States. In its severe form, it is also a dangerous disease, directly responsible for the death of up to 7% of asthmatics.

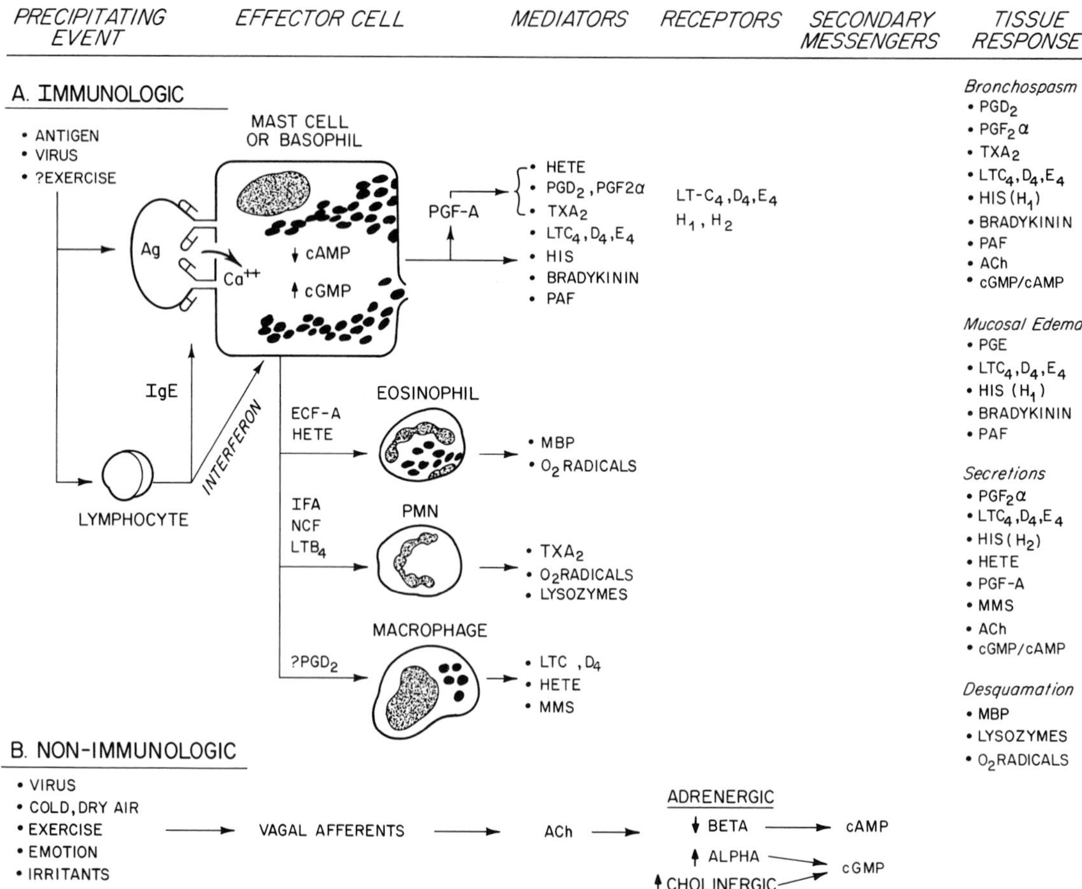

Figure 9.5. Overlapping pathophysiologic pathways leading to airways obstruction in asthma. Extrinsic asthma may result from mast cell degranulation, release of mediators, and recruitment of other effector cells. Intrinsic asthma may depend more on neural pathways. Airways obstruction is due to a combination of bronchospasm, mucosal edema, and bronchial lumen plugging with secretions and desquamated cells. Ag, antigen; cAMP, cyclic 3′, 5′—adenosine monophosphate; cGMP, cyclic 3′, 5′—guanosine monophosphate; ECF—A, eosinophil chemotactic factor of anaphylaxis; HETE, monohydroxyeicosatetraenoic acid; NCF, neutrophil chemotactic factor; PGD_2, E, F_2, prostaglandin D_2, E, F_2; TXA_2, thromboxane A_2; LTC_4, D_4, E_4, leukotriene C_4, D_4, E_4; HIS, histamine; PAF, platelet-activating factor; PGF-A, prostaglandin-generating factor of anaphylaxis; IFA, inflammatory factor of anaphylaxis; MBP, major basic protein; MMS, macrophage mucus secretagogue; ACh, acetylcholine.

Pathophysiology

Extrinsic Asthma

Immunologic and nonimmunologic mechanisms play roles of varying degrees of importance in initiating and perpetuating as asthmatic attack (Fig. 9.5). The atopic patient, for instance, may note an exacerbation after exposure to certain antigens. Cross-bridging of two specific IgE molecules attached to the cell membrane of mast cells or basophils leads to calcium ion (Ca^{++}) influx and the release into surrounding tissue of a variety of preformed and newly generated chemical mediators. Substances such as histamine, bradykinin, leukotrienes, and prostaglandins cause bronchospasm directly or through interaction with receptors on bronchial smooth muscle cells. Bronchial wall edema due to increased capillary and venule permeability, as well as increased mucous gland secretion, worsen bronchial obstruction. With time, chemoattractants, such as eosinophil chemotactic factors of anaphylaxis (ECF-A), neutrophil chemotactic factor (NCF), and leukotriene B_4 (LTB_4) recruit neutrophils, eosinophils, and macrophages. These cells, through the release of lysozymes, O_2 radicals, and major basic protein, cause epithelial cell damage and desquamation which further compromise bronchial lumen patency.

Intrinsic Asthma

The "intrinsic" asthmatic, on the other hand, often associates exacerbations with nonspecific irritants, cold air, exercise, and emotion. The fundamental defect underlying this type of asthma is unknown but it may be that these stimuli increase vagal tone which causes a secondary elevation of intracellular cyclic guanosine 3′,5′—monophosphate (cGMP). An increased concentration of cGMP relative to cyclic adenosine monophosphate (cAMP) is associated with bronchospasm and increased bronchial secretions.

The immunologic and reflex pathways are by no means mutually exclusive. Histamine, for instance, released from mast cells by an IgE-dependent mechanism, may stimulate vagal afferents. Conversely, increased vagal tone is associated with elevated mast cell cGMP levels and enhanced mediator release.

Physiologic Effects

The net physiologic result of the intracellular events described above is a combination of large and small airway obstruction. An increased *demand* is then placed on the ventilatory pump in several ways. Ventilation-perfusion ($\dot{V}/\dot{Q}$) mismatching, both from obstruction and treatment, results in wasted ventilation and hypoxemia. Obstruction increases resistive work of breathing directly and elastic work of breathing indirectly, through air trapping and hyperinflation.

Table 9.4.
Differential Diagnosis of Acute Dyspnea and Wheezing

Diagnosis	Symptoms
Upper airway obstruction	Hoarseness, inspiratory stridor, normal alveolar-arterial O_2 gradient, peak flow (liters/sec) < 1.7 × FEV_1 (liters)
Fixed lower airway obstruction due to tumor or foreign body	History of aspiration, hemoptysis, localized wheeze, volume loss on chest x-ray
Left ventricular failure[a]	Symptoms of congestive heart failure, jugular venous distention, S_3 gallop, rales, chest x-ray
Pulmonary embolism[a]	Risk factors, sudden onset of symptoms, chest pain, hemoptysis, leg pain or swelling, chest x-ray (all notoriously insensitive and nonspecific)

[a] Uncommon causes of wheezing in absence of coexistent lung disease.

Conversely, the ability of the respiratory system to *respond* to the increased ventilatory demands of an asthmatic exacerbation is limited. Hypoxemia and respiratory acidosis impair respiratory muscle contractility. Alveolar hypoxia, acidemia, and hyperinflation increase pulmonary vascular resistance. The left heart may become underfilled. This, combined with increased left ventricular afterload due to markedly negative intrapleural pressure, may impair cardiac output and thereby respiratory muscle blood flow. Finally, hyperinflation puts the respiratory muscles at a disadvantageous length-tension relationship, further compromising contraction.

Clinical Presentation

When confronted with a tachypneic, wheezing patient, the emergency physician must in rapid succession make a diagnosis, assess the severity of disease, and institute appropriate therapy. It is of utmost importance to remember "all that wheezes is not asthma." History, physical examination, and laboratory studies will suggest diagnoses other than asthma (Table 9.4).

History

The true asthmatic gives a long history of episodic wheezing and shortness of breath. Up to 15% of asthmatics, however, suffer their first asthmatic attack after the age of 50. Older age and intrinsic disease predict slow response to therapy. Prior in-

Table 9.5.
Indications of Severe Asthma

History
Previous ICU treatment, especially with intubation[a]
Steroid dependence
Diurnal variation of peak flow > 50%
Physical examination
Central cyanosis
Accessory respiratory muscle use
Pulsus paradoxus > 15
Respiratory rate > 35
Pulse > 130
Respiratory alternans
Abdominal paradox
Absence of wheezes
Asterixis
Mental status change
Laboratory
FEV_1 < 750 ml or peak flow < 100 liters/min
Pao_2 < 50 mm Hg on room air
$Paco_2$ normal or increased
Metabolic acidosis

[a] ICU, intensive care unit.

tubation, steroid dependence, or greater than 50% diurnal variation of flow rates indicate severe disease and the need for close monitoring (Table 9.5).

The current episode may have developed over hours to weeks. An exacerbation beginning more than a week before the emergency department visit in a patient taking full doses of bronchodilators suggests the response to therapy will be slow. A thorough historical search should be made for a precipitating factor including allergy, nonspecific inhaled irritant, and infection. Purulent sputum production, however, seldom suggests a bacterial infection in the asthmatic, as most exacerbations are viral or nonspecific. Significant weight should be given to the patient's own assessment of the severity of an attack, as this correlates with objective measurements of airflow obstruction better than physical examination.

Physical Examination

Certain signs alert the physician to the presence of severe disease (Table 9.5). These findings, while quite specific for severe disease, are relatively insensitive and their absence, therefore, should not be used to exclude serious illness. Central cyanosis, use of accessory respiratory muscles, pulsus paradoxus greater than 15 mm Hg, respiratory rate greater than 35 breaths/min, and heart rate greater than 130 beats/min have all been correlated with a forced expiratory volume in 1 second (FEV_1) of less than 1.0 liter and therefore severe airways obstruction. Increasing tachypnea, respiratory alternans (alternating thoracic and abdominal breathing), and abdominal paradox (inspiratory descent of abdomen) may occur in sequence and herald the onset of respiratory failure and the need for intubation. Fever suggests a bacterial complication, such as pneumonia. Diffuse polyphonic expiratory wheezes are commonly heard, but may be absent when obstruction is severe and airflow greatly diminished. Unilateral diminution of breath sounds, tracheal deviation, or subcutaneous crepitus suggest pneumothorax and/or pneumomediastinum. A careful search should be made for inspiratory stridor, signs of right and left heart failure, and lower extremity warmth, erythema, tenderness, edema, and palpable venous cords. Mental status changes and asterixis suggest CO_2 retention and the need for assisted ventilation.

Laboratory

Routine Studies. Routine laboratory studies for the acute asthmatic include a complete blood count, electrolyte and plasma theophylline levels, and microscopic examination of the sputum. Leukocytosis with a left shift and Gram's stain of the sputum may suggest a bacterial infection, while blood or sputum eosinophilia by Wright's stain indicate steroid responsiveness. Potentially fatal hypokalemia may result from dehydration and contraction alkalosis, respiratory alkalosis, as well as treatment with theophylline, sympathomimetics, and steroids. The plasma theophylline level confirms compliance with treatment and provides a rational basis for further therapy.

Airflow Measurements. The single most useful diagnostic test in the emergency department treatment of asthma is a direct measurement of airflow obstruction. The peak expiratory flow rate (PEFR) and FEV_1 are easily measured at the bedside in all but the most critically ill patient. A PEFR < 100 liters/min or an FEV_1 < 750 ml indicates very severe disease.

Arterial Blood Gases. Blood for arterial blood gases should be drawn if physical examination or spirometry suggest a serious asthmatic exacerbation or if another diagnosis is being entertained. Classical teaching holds that mild asthma causes hypocapnia alone and that with increasingly severe obstruction, hypoxemia, normocapnia, and finally hypercapnia are seen in sequence. As with the physical examination, however, arterial blood gas (ABG) abnormalities are specific for, but quite insensitive to, serious disease. Thus, a room air Pao_2 less than 50 mm Hg and hypercapnia (Table 9.5) do correlate with a PEFR or FEV_1 less than 25% predicted, but their absence does not preclude life-threatening illness. One study has associated metabolic acidosis, presumably due to ventilatory muscle-generated lactate, with impending respiratory failure.

Electrocardiogram. The electrocardiogram

Table 9.6.
Treatment of Acute Asthma

Drug	Dose and Route	Toxicity
Sympathomimetics		*All sympathomimetics*
Metaproterenol	0.1–0.3 ml of 5% solution (5–15 mg) in 3 ml normal saline via aerosol q15 min × 4 then q1–4 hr	*CNS*[a]*:* anxiety, headache, tremor *Cardiac:* tachycardia, tachyarrhythmia
Isoetharine 1% and phenylephrine 0.25% (Bronkosol)	0.5 ml in 1.5 ml saline via aerosol q4–6 hr	
Terbutaline	1.5–2.5 mg in 3 ml saline, as above	
Albuterol[b]	0.3 ml in 2.5 ml saline as above	
Epinephrine	0.01 ml/kg (maximum 0.3 ml) of 1:1000 solution subcutaneously × 1 or 2 doses q20 min followed by Sus-Phrine	
Sus-Phrine	0.005 ml/kg (0.025 mg/kg) of 1:200 solution (maximum 0.15 ml) subcutaneously alone or 20 min after epinephrine as above, × 1.	
Isoproterenol	0.5–5 μg/min i.v.	
Theophylline		
Aminophylline	5–6 mg/kg *actual* weight in 100 ml D_5W i.v. over 20 min. If patient has been taking aminophylline, 3 μg/kg load will increase theophylline level by 5 μg/ml. Maintenance dose for first 12 hr = 0.7 mg/kg/hr *ideal* body weight for adults, 0.6 mg/kg/hr for older patients, and 0.5 mg/kg/hr for patients with congestive heart failure and liver disease. Adjust for serum level = 10–20 μg/ml.	*CNS:* anxiety, headache, tremor, seizures *Cardiac:* tachycardia, tachyarrhythmias *GI:* nausea and vomiting
Corticosteroids		
Methylprednisolone	40–125 mg i.v. q6 hr	*CNS:* anxiety, psychosis, seizures *Metabolic:* hypokalemia, hyperglycemia *GI:* nausea *Bones:* osteoporosis, avascular necrosis of femoral head

[a] CNS, central nervous system; GI, gastrointestinal; D_5W, 5% dextrose in water.
[b] Has not yet received final Food and Drug Administration approval.

in acute asthma may show reversible right axis deviation, P-pulmonale, right ventricular hypertrophy with strain, and right bundle-branch block. The chest x-ray is useful in ruling out pneumomediastium, pneumothorax, atelectasis due to mucous plugging, and pneumonia.

Treatment (Table 9.6)

β-Adrenergic Agents. These agents bind to *β*-adrenergic receptors on the cell membrane, increase intracellular cAMP through activation of adenylate cyclase, and enhance binding of intracellular calcium to cell membrane and endoplasmic reticulum. These events are associated with bronchial smooth muscle relaxation, inhibition of mast cell mediator release, decrease in mucous gland secretion, and enhanced mucociliary clearance.

Epinephrine. First line therapy for acute asthma in the emergency department should include the sympathomimetics. As single agents, they offer more prompt relief, are more effective, and are associated with less toxicity than intravenous theophylline. They may be given parenterally or via aerosol. Classic therapy has consisted of epinephrine subcutaneously every 20 minutes for three doses. Recent studies have shown the greatest bronchodilation occurs after the first dose and little is added by the second two. Furthermore, an increased relapse rate was associated with failure to add a long-acting epinephrine to the treatment regimen. There is little advantage in using subcutaneous terbutaline because β_2 specificity is lost when the drug is given parenterally and blood pressure and pulse usually fall with relief of airway obstruction after epinephrine.

Other Sympathomimetics. The newer inhaled sympathomimetics (see Table 9.6) may have several advantages over subcutaneous epinephrine. Chemical substitution of the catecholamines has led to increased β_2 specificity, theoretically with less cardiac toxicity, and a prolonged duration of action. In contrast to subcutaneous epinephrine, significant increments in flow rates are seen with sequential doses. Prior fears of tachyphylaxis in patients using outpatient β_2 inhalers, increased cardiac toxicity after sequential doses, and ineffective drug deposition in the setting of severe bronchospasm have not been borne out by recent clinical trials. These agents should be given via a loose-fitting face mask or hand-held nebulizer. The gas supply to the mask should be 40–60% O_2 and not room air (see "Oxygen"). Intermittent positive pressure breathing (IPPB) therapy has been associated with increased morbidity and mortality and should not be used.

Rarely, in refractory children or young adults free of cardiovascular disease, intravenous isoproterenol may be used, while closely monitoring heart rate.

Theophylline. Past teaching has been that these agents act through phosphodiesterase inhibition and elevation of cAMP. Tissue theophylline levels that produce effective bronchodilation, however, have little effect on phosphodiesterase activity. In addition, potent inhibitors of the enzyme, such as dipyridamole, are not bronchodilators. Postulated mechanisms of action include changes in calcium ion flux, increased levels of endogenous catecholamines or β-adrenergic receptor function, and inhibition of prostaglandins or adenosine. Physiologic effects include bronchodilation, decrease in bronchial mucosa edema, increased mucociliary clearance, and improved diaphragmatic contractility.

Intravenous aminophylline has been used for years in the emergency department treatment of asthma. Recent double-blind, controlled trials have suggested that, in the emergency department setting, theophylline adds little but increased toxicity to sequential β-adrenergic therapy. These studies have not, however, examined combination therapy during hospitalization. It therefore seems prudent to begin an aminophylline drip in the emergency department when it becomes clear that the patient will require hospitalization. Doses and toxic effects are detailed in Table 9.6.

Corticosteriods. These agents affect virtually every immunologic and inflammatory pathway thought to be important in the pathogenesis of asthma. They inhibit mediator synthesis and release, as well as effector cell migration. The secondary messenger cAMP is increased through steroid-induced synthesis of β-adrenergic receptors while cholinergic-mediated cGMP is decreased. Net physiologic effects include bronchodilation, decreased mucous gland secretion, bronchial wall edema, and increased mucociliary clearance.

Steroids should be considered in patients with eosinophilia or a past history of steroid responsiveness. Patients on a recent course may need steroids both for their asthma and relative adrenal insufficiency.

The beneficial effects of corticosteroids are not apparent for 6–24 hours following administration. They should, therefore, be given early in the treatment of acute severe asthma and the need for its continuation assessed later. One study (see Haskell et al., Suggested Readings) suggests dose dependence of bronchodilation when methylprednisolone was increased from 15–40 to 125 mg intravenously every 6 hours for 3 days. The two higher doses were associated with more rapid resolution of bronchospasm in a small series. It is therefore reasonable in most cases of acute asthma to give at least the equivalent of methylprednisolone, 15 mg intravenously every 6 hours for 3 days; higher doses should be considered but their choice remains controversial pending accumulation of more data. Acute toxicity includes central nervous system effects, hypokalemia, hyperglycemia, nausea, and rarely avascular necrosis of the femoral heads. The latter may not be dose-related. Short courses of steroids are not likely to exacerbate peptic ulcer disease, quiescent tuberculosis, hypertension, or cause adrenal suppression.

Other Agents. Current calcium channel blockers, anticholinergics, antihistamines, and α-adrenergic antagonists have limited usefulness in the treatment of *chronic* asthma. Furthermore, the weight of current evidence suggest that these agents have no place in the treatment of status asthmaticus. Similarly, cromolyn sodium and inhaled steroid preparations are useful for asthma prophylaxis, but may cause paradoxical aggravation of existing bronchospasm and should not be used in the acute situation.

Supportive Therapy

Rehydration. During an asthmatic attack, a combination of decreased oral intake and increased water loss often leads to dehydration. This, in turn, may be responsible for inspissation of bronchial secretions and worsening obstruction. Rehydration should therefore be vigorous, with careful clinical monitoring including the blood urea nitrogen and hematocrit.

Oxygen. During status asthmaticus, airways obstruction and bronchodilator inhibition of hypoxic pulmonary vasoconstriction cause significant $\dot{V}/\dot{Q}$ mismatching and hypoxemia. Low flow O_2 should therefore be given for all but the mildest exacerbations of asthma. Contrary to the situation in chronic obstructive pulmonary disease (COPD), chronic CO_2 retention and suppression of the CO_2 ventilatory drive seem not to be significant. O_2 may therefore be given without fear of causing CO_2 retention.

Antibiotics. These should not be given routinely for acute asthma. As noted, most infectious exacerbations are viral. Antibiotics are reserved for the patient with fever, leukocytosis, or an infiltrate on chest x-ray.

Mechanical Ventilation. Rarely, despite all these measures, a patient may exhibit progressive respiratory acidosis and require endotracheal intubation. If possible the patient should be premedicated with atropine, 0.4–0.6 mg subcutaneously, to avoid increased reflex bronchospasm due to vagal stimulation by the endotracheal tube. During ventilation, the inspiratory time setting should be shortened to allow sufficient time for expiration and avoid further air trapping. Increased inspiratory flow rates should not, however, be permitted to increase peak airway pressures and increase the risk of barotrauma. Restoration of a normal P_{CO_2} and pH will improve both the effectiveness of β-adrenergic agents and of the contractility of respiratory muscle. Sedation, without fear of respiratory depression, but with decreased work of breathing on the ventilator, decreases P_{CO_2} and P_{O_2} and, therefore, the demands on a failing ventilatory pump. Paralysing with pancuronium bromide is often necessary to prevent high airways pressures due to dysynchronous breathing ("fighting") against the respirators and to achieve adequate ventilation. If the pH cannot be raised above 7.30 with these steps, $NaHCO_3$, 1–2 mEq/kg, should be given intravenously.

General Anesthesia. As a measure of last resort, general anesthesia with halothane or enflurane may be induced after intubation. These agents may work on bronchial smooth muscle by inhibiting reflex bronchospasm. They may increase cardiotoxicity from theophylline, sympathomimetics, hypoxia, and acidosis.

Lavage. Mucous plugging of large or small airways may prevent adequate oxygenation or ventilation, even after intubation. Although reports are anecdotal, bronchial lavage can be considered in this setting. When segmental or lobar atelectasis is demonstrated on chest x-ray, lavage may be done in a limited fashion using 3–5 ml of 10% *N*-acetylcysteine, watching closely for increased bronchospasm. Alternatively, for more diffuse bronchial plugging, bronchoscopic lavage may be carried out with normal saline, particularly of subsegmental bronchioles distal to the wedged bronchoscope. Monitoring is essential to watch for worsening hypoxemia.

Hospitalization or Outpatient Care

The pathophysiologic process during recovery from an asthmatic attack must be understood if the patient is to be appropriately admitted or discharged from the emergency department. With treatment, small improvements in FEV_1 are first associated with disappearance of the physical signs of severe disease listed in Table 9.4. By the time the patient considers the attacks over, flow rates may remain less than 50% of normal and still require aggressive treatment. Wheezes disappear after symptoms, followed, in turn, by return of spirometric measurements to normal. Hyperinflation and mild hypoxemia may persist for 2 weeks after the initial attack. Laboratory studies suggest that the reversible changes noted are related to medium and large airways bronchospasm. Changes persisting for days to weeks, on the other hand, are related to small airways obstruction secondary to retention of secretions and desquamated epithelium. The latter are sometimes related to the IgE-dependent reaction and may be steroid-responsive.

One might predict that successful discharge of the asthmatic patient from the emergency department depends on both the nature and severity, i.e. reversibility, of obstruction and the effectiveness of emergency department treatment. Indeed, retrospective clinical trials have shown that patients with an initial FEV_1 < 700 ml (PEFR < 100 liters/min) failing to improve to > 2.1 liters (PEFR > 300 liters/min) needed hospitalization. A multifactorial index based on presenting clinical signs, applied prospectively, did not reliably predict successful discharge.

Pathophysiology suggests that the outpatient medical regimen following emergency treatment is an important determinant of successful discharge. One prospective study has demonstrated a lower relapse rate in acute asthmatic patients given methylprednisolone, 4 mg/kg intravenously, in the emergency department followed by a dose of oral methylprednisolone, tapering from 32 mg/day to 0, over 8 days.

ACUTE DECOMPENSATION OF CHRONIC RESPIRATORY FAILURE

As long as cigarette smoking and air pollution persist, chronic bronchitis and emphysema will continue to cause illness and death. Although it is often useful to separate these diseases because of their distinct pathologies and for the purpose of therapy and prognosis, they often occur together, and in the end stage—when respiratory failure occurs—their differences are less apparent and their treatment usually similar. Thus, they are considered in this section as one syndrome best described by their common physiologic defect, chronic airways obstruction (CAO).

Whereas the complications of chronic bronchitis and emphysema are many, their common natural course is the progressive loss of pulmonary function punctuated by episodes of acute respiratory failure. Despite an apparent inability to prevent or to cure the underlying disease processes, advances have been made in the outpatient management of CAO. Early empirical antibiotic treatment of bronchitis flare-ups and immunizations against influenza and pneumococci may prevent decompensation. They are standard procedures in most chest clinics. Use of home and portable equipment for the delivery of low-flow oxygen clearly diminishes the discomfort of daily activities for many hypoxemic patients (Pa_{O_2} less than 55 mm Hg) and its continuous use has been shown to increase life expectancy and decrease the frequency of hospitalization. Multidisciplinary pulmonary rehabilitation programs, including inspiratory muscle training, reduce hospitalization time and improve life quality, if not its duration. In the treatment of patients with prominent bronchospasm, new and improved bronchodilator drugs have made a major impact.

Despite the best in outpatient management, acute decompensation of chronic respiratory failure still occurs. This section reviews the pathophysiology and treatment of acute or chronic respiratory failure and emphasizes its differences from the treatment of acute respiratory failure uncomplicated by underlying obstructive lung disease. Although intubation and mechanical ventilation are sometimes required in the management of decompensated chronic respiratory failure, such interventions are associated with poorer results and greater morbidity than in uncomplicated respiratory failure. The explanation for this distinction lies in the pathophysiology of chronic hypercapnia, an understanding of which has led to reliance on continuous low-flow oxygen as the mainstay of therapy for acute decompensation. However, as the role of inspiratory muscle fatigue in respiratory decompensation becomes better understood, the potential benefit of resting the respiratory muscles through mechanical ventilation is under investigation. Before therapeutic guidelines are detailed, it is important to review the pathophysiology of inspiratory muscle fatigue, carbon dioxide retention, acid-base regulation, respiratory control, and oxygen transport, as they apply to acute or chronic respiratory failure.

Pathophysiology

Inspiratory Muscle Fatigue

Severe CAO increases the work of breathing by increasing airway resistance, functional residual capacity, and respiratory rate. Moreover, the mechanical derangements consequent to long-standing CAO, such as diaphragmatic flattening, reduce the capacity of the inspiratory muscles to sustain the increased ventilatory workload. Undernutrition, present in about 20% of cases, further impairs ventilatory function by reducing respiratory muscle mass. Decreases in local or systemic blood supply to the diaphragm are another potential mechanism tipping the energy supply-and-demand balance toward failure. While transient inspiratory muscle fatigue is a feature of acute respiratory failure due to many causes, more sustained fatigue often accompanies chronic CAO.

The diagnosis of inspiratory muscle fatigue is made on clinical grounds. Dyspnea and tachypnea are early, nonspecific signs. The combination of rapid, shallow breathing, abdominal paradoxical motion, and alteration between rib cage and abdominal breathing is thought, with reasonable certainty, to correlate with inspiratory muscle fatigue. While a number of research techniques are used to describe and measure fatigue, none is applicable to clinical practice.

The goal of therapy for inspiratory muscle fatigue is restoration of the balance of energy supply and demand. Bronchodilatation, control of secretion through antibiotic and physical therapy, and the treatment of heart failure all reduce the work of breathing, while oxygen, nutrition, aminophylline, and β-adrenergic drugs may enhance muscle contractility. The specific treatment of muscle fatigue, however, is rest. For the muscles of inspiration, rest may be achieved by mechanical ventilation, partial or complete, whether by positive or negative pressure. For the "low frequency" fatigue associated with chronic respiratory failure, 12 or more hours of rest are required for recovery. Hence, a potential dilemma arises in managing decompensated chronic respiratory failure. Rest clearly offers potential benefits, but intubation and positive pressure ventilation for all cases clearly increases the risk of unnecessary mechanical ventilation, an unpleasant experience with its own morbidity. The benefits of early ventilation over conservative management have yet to be proved. A possible negative consequence of this change in strategy (intubating all patients) is an increase in the number of end-stage patients, for whom there is no hope of weaning, who may spend their last days on ventilators. A way of predicting which patients will benefit from ventilatory rest is needed before the data on respiratory muscle fatigue can be fully incorporated into clinical practice. It is clear, however, that once a fatigued patient is placed on a respirator, full rest must be allowed for 12–24 hours before an attempt at weaning.

Carbon Dioxide Retention

Carbon dioxide is both a waste product of aerobic metabolism and a vital participant in acid-base homeostasis. Although it is artificial to separate these interrelated roles, carbon dioxide is considered here as a potentially toxic by-product, the elimination of which is a major function of the respiratory system. Whenever an excretory organ is obstructed, the result is retention of the product to be excreted. Thus, it is not surprising that carbon dioxide retention can result from chronic bronchitis and emphysema, since airways obstruction is their fundamental physiologic aberration. The unanswered question is why some patients with comparably obstructed airways retain carbon dioxide while others do not. Several theories have been advanced, but none is totally satisfactory.

One factor agreed to be important to the development and treatment of carbon dioxide retention is the work of breathing. Although expiration is normally a passive process, breathing against obstructed airways requires energy and can account for a large part of resting oxygen consumption and carbon dioxide production in the severely obstructed patient.

The $Paco_2$ is determined not only by the volume of air moving in and out of the alveoli each minute but also by the amount of carbon dioxide produced and, in the steady state, excreted each minute, as expressed by the following equation in which 0.863 is a constant:

$$Paco_2 = \frac{CO_2 \text{ production (or excretion)}}{\text{alveolar ventilation}} \times 0.863$$

Normally, carbon dioxide production is relatively constant and $Paco_2$ is a reciprocal function of alveolar ventilation. As alveolar ventilation increases, $Paco_2$ decreases. With severe airways obstruction, however, the work required to increase ventilation results in an increase in carbon dioxide production and renders the added ventilation less effective in lowering $Paco_2$. The oxygen required to increase ventilation, moreover, is no longer available for use by other tissues. Chronic hypercapnia therefore may be thought of as a physiologic compromise that conserves oxygen for nonventilatory use and that at the same time minimizes carbon dioxide production. In the steady state, carbon dioxide excretion again equals carbon dioxide production, but at a higher total body content of carbon dioxide. Higher tissue, venous, and alveolar Pco_2 allows more carbon dioxide to be eliminated per breath and, thus, fewer breaths per minute to maintain the balance of production and excretion. Patients with chronic respiratory failure live for long periods in this compensated state until factors such as excessive bronchial secretions and bronchospasm further increase the work of breathing, upset the equilibrated state, and cause acute carbon dioxide retention. Most effective therapeutic modalities such as bronchodilators, antibiotics, and chest physical therapy work by decreasing airway resistance, lowering the work of breathing, and restoring equilibrium. Mechanical ventilation also helps relieve the work of breathing, although it acts primarily in the inspiratory phase, leaving expiratory work for the patient.

If carbon dioxide is a potentially noxious by-product, how do patients with chronic respiratory failure tolerate such excessive amounts? The answer is the slow rate with which chronic hypercapnia develops. The toxicity of rapidly developing or extremely high levels of carbon dioxide can be thought of as both pharmacologic and physical.

Pharmacologic Effects. The pharmacologic effects of carbon dioxide retention are closely related to its role in acid-base chemistry. Carbon dioxide is normally transported from tissues to the lungs largely as bicarbonate ion formed by the reaction of dissolved carbon dioxide with water:

$$\underset{\text{dissolved}}{CO_2} + H_2O \underset{\text{carbonic anhydrase}}{\rightleftharpoons} H_2CO_3 \rightleftharpoons H^+ + HCO_3^-$$

The reaction occurs extremely rapidly in the presence of carbonic anhydrase found in red blood cells; it also occurs more slowly in the absence of this enzyme. Since hydrogen ions are formed in the process, carbon dioxide is potentially a weak acid. Normally the hydrogen ions are buffered by hemoglobin and plasma proteins, which allows the reaction to go to the right. When bicarbonate reaches the pulmonary capillary bed, the process is reversed and carbon dioxide is eliminated as a gas. Smaller amounts of carbon dioxide are transported as carbamino compounds, carbonic acid, and dissolved carbon dioxide.

With acute carbon dioxide retention, hydrogen ions are produced in excess of blood buffering capacity and acidemia results. The mechanisms that exist to minimize pH change in acute and chronic hypercapnia are discussed on pp 159–161.

The signs and symptoms of carbon dioxide toxicity due to acidosis or due to direct effects of carbon dioxide so overlap with the manifestations of hypoxemia that it is unrealistic to separate them. Restlessness, tachycardia, confusion, diaphoresis, jerking tremor, headache, and various degrees of stupor are nonspecific and may not even be present despite severe hypoxemia and hypercapnia. The diagnosis of acute respiratory failure must be based on arterial blood gas determinations.

Physical Effects. Dalton's law states that the pressure exerted by each component of a gas mixture is independent of the other gases in the mixture and that the total pressure exerted is the sum of the individual gas pressures. Because alveoli are in contact with atmospheric pressure via the airways, total alveolar gas pressure is considered atmospheric. Since water vapor and nitrogen pressures vary relatively little, carbon dioxide shares the alveolar space with only one other variable gas, oxygen, as expressed in the simplified alveolar gas equation. For convenience the readily obtained $Paco_2$ (a = arterial) is substituted for $PAco_2$ (A = alveolar) since the two values are usually almost identical:

$$PAo_2 = \text{inspired } Po_2 - \frac{Paco_2}{R}$$

If equal amounts of oxygen and carbon dioxide are exchanged, R, the respiratory quotient, equals 1 and the relationship is reciprocal; that is, PAo_2 must decrease 1 mm Hg for each 1 mm Hg rise in $Paco_2$ since total gas pressure does not change. When R is the usual 0.8, as it is when 200 ml of carbon dioxide is produced for each 250 ml of oxygen taken up per minute, the decrease in PAo_2 for a given increase in $Paco_2$ is even greater. Unlike the case with Pco_2, a gradient always exists between alveolar and arterial Po_2. The Pao_2 will therefore follow the change in PAo_2, but will be lower.

Using these facts, McNicol and Campbell (see Suggested Readings) theorized that in untreated patients with respiratory failure the rise in $PAco_2$ would displace enough oxygen from the alveoli that life-threatening hypoxemia (Pao_2 less than 25 mm Hg) would result before the $Paco_2$ would reach dangerous levels ($Paco_2$ greater than 80 mm Hg, pH less than 7.20). Patients with a $Paco_2$ much higher than 80 mm Hg, therefore, must have been supported by prior oxygen therapy to allow the $Paco_2$ to rise to that level without lethal hypoxemia.

The prediction of McNicol and Campbell proved true in a large series of previously untreated patients with decompensation of known chronic respiratory failure. They found that, whereas most patients had a $Paco_2$ between 60 and 80 mm Hg and a pH between 7.22 and 7.44, the majority had a Pao_2 between 25 and 40 mm Hg. The body normally has large carbon dioxide stores and appears to tolerate $Paco_2$ increases of this magnitude relatively well, especially when they develop slowly, allowing the body's buffer systems to minimize pH shifts. Oxygen stores, however, are small, and severe hypoxemia like that observed by McNicol and Campbell can rapidly lead to tissue injury. These data, therefore, not only illustrate the physical consequences of carbon dioxide retention but also emphasize that it is usually hypoxemia, not hypercapnia in itself, that is life-threatening to the CAO patients with acute respiratory failure who are seen in the emergency department. Oxygen therapy in this setting, therefore, is paramount.

Acid-Base Regulation in Acute and Chronic Hypercapnia

Carbon dioxide retention results in $[H^+]$ increase through the hydration reaction. Multiple buffer systems interact, however, to minimize pH changes due to respiratory or metabolic causes. The understanding of these complex acid-base interactions is greatly simplified by the belief that changes in one buffer pair—carbonic acid and its conjugate base, bicarbonate—are representative of changes in all other buffer systems with which the pair are in equilibrium. The physiocochemical relationship of the three variable components of the carbonic acid system, pH, $Paco_2$, and $[HCO_3^-]$, is given by the Henderson-Hasselbalch equation, in which α is the solubility coefficient for carbon dioxide and pK is a constant:

$$pH = pK + \log \frac{[HCO_3^-]}{\alpha \cdot Paco_2}$$

The equation states that, when $Paco_2$ is elevated, pH will decrease unless $[HCO_3^-]$ rises by an amount proportional to the rise in $Paco_2$. When hypercapnia is acute, the readily available sources for buffering hydrogen ions and for elevating $[HCO_3^-]$ are easily depleted and pH falls. In the first 24 hours after the onset of hypercapnia, buffering of excess hydrogen ions is almost entirely due to cellular proteins. The hydrogen ions enter the blood and tissue cells in exchange for potassium and sodium ions, and chloride enters in exchange for bicarbonate:

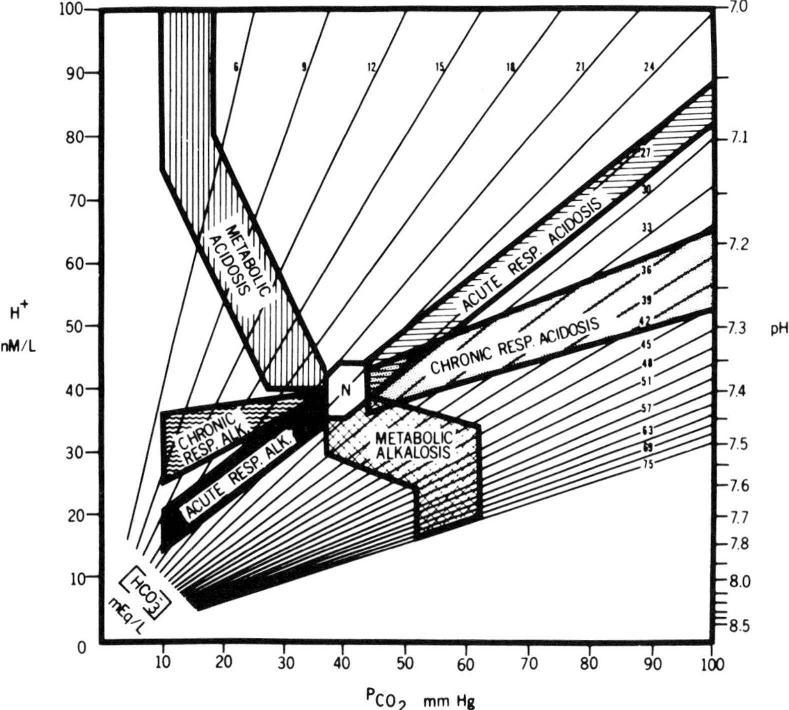

Figure 9.6. Acid-base diagram. *Shaded areas* represent the normal response anticipated for P_{CO_2}, $[HCO_3^-]$, and pH or $[H^+]$ for each of the six simple acid-base disturbances. *Numbered lines* are bicarbonate isopleths in milliequivalents/liter. (Reproduced by permission, from Goldberg M, Green SB, Moss ML, et al. Computer-based instruction and diagnoses of acid-base disorders: A systematic approach. *JAMA,* 223:269–275 ©1973, by The American Medical Association.)

dissolved

$$CO_2 + H_2O \rightleftharpoons H_2CO_3 \rightleftharpoons H^+ + HCO_3^-$$

$$\begin{array}{rcl} HCO_3^- \leftarrow & \boxed{\begin{array}{c}\text{cellular}\\ \text{protein}\\ \text{buffers}\end{array}} & \rightarrow K^+ \\ Cl^- \rightarrow & & \rightarrow Na^+ \end{array}$$

The net result of the limited cellular buffering of acute hypercapnia is only a small increase in the calculated $[HCO_3^-]$ and a relatively large decrease in pH.

When hypercapnia is prolonged, $[HCO_3^-]$ increases to levels well above that achievable in the first 24 hours, raising pH toward normal and replenishing cellular buffers depleted during the acute period. Increased renal retention of bicarbonate accounts for most of the improved pH regulation, although hydrogen is also eliminated in the urine as ammonium and other titratable acids. For electrochemical balance, chloride is excreted as bicarbonate is retained.

Because acute and chronic respiratory acidosis usually requires distinct therapies, their differentiation is important. Acid-base diagrams like that proposed by Goldberg et al. (see Suggested Readings and Fig. 9.6) are helpful in the rapid interpretation of arterial blood gas findings. According to the diagram, a patient with a Pa_{CO_2} of 80 mm Hg has acute respiratory acidosis if the pH is between 7.14 and 7.18, chronic respiratory acidosis if the pH is between 7.24 and 7.32, and acute decompensation of a chronic respiratory acidosis if the pH is between the bands, that is, 7.18–7.24.

At the bedside it is helpful to estimate the change in hydrogen ion concentration ($\Delta[H^+]$) expected for a change in Pa_{CO_2} (ΔPa_{CO_2}) by use of the following two relationships:

Acute respiratory acidosis:

$$\Delta[H^+] = 0.8 \times \Delta Pa_{CO_2}$$

Chronic respiratory acidosis:

$$\Delta[H^+] = 0.3 \times \Delta Pa_{CO_2}$$

The substitution of $[H^+]$ for pH eliminates the logarithm and allows use of a linear relationship. Hydrogen ion concentration can be estimated by its coincidental relationship with pH whereby the two decimal digits of the pH are numerically similar to and vary reciprocally with the $[H^+]$ expressed in nanomoles/liter within the clinically important pH range of 7.10–7.50:

pH		[H+]
7.10	=	70 nmol/liter
7.20	=	60 nmol/liter
7.30	=	50 nmol/liter
7.40	=	40 nmol/liter
7.50	=	30 nmol/liter

Problem: Do the following arterial blood gas data—pH 7.35; Pco_2, 60 mm Hg; Po_2, 40 mm Hg—represent acute or chronic respiratory acidosis?

Solution: Consult an acid-base diagram (Fig. 9.6) or use the bedside estimate as just outlined:

$$\Delta Paco_2 = 60 \text{ mm Hg} - 40 \text{ mm Hg (normal)} = 20 \text{ mm Hg}$$

If this is a chronic condition, the $[H^+]$ increase is predicted by

$$\Delta[H^+] = 0.3 \times \Delta Paco_2 = 0.3 \times 20 = 6 \text{ nmol/liter}$$

Predicted $[H^+]$ = 40 nmol/liter (normal) + 6 nmol/liter = 46 nmol/liter. Using the reciprocal $[H^+]$−pH relationship:

[H+]		pH
40 nmol/liter	=	7.40
46 nmol/liter	=	7.34

An increase in $[H^+]$ of 6 nmol/liter equals a decrease in pH of 0.06 unit.

The measured pH, 7.35, is close to the 7.34 predicted for chronic respiratory acidosis. If hypercapnia were acute, a much greater decrease in pH would be predicted:

$$\Delta[H^+] = 0.8 \times \Delta Paco_2 = 0.8 \times 20 = 16 \text{ nmol/liter}$$

Predicted $[H^+]$ = 40 nmol/liter + 16 nmol/liter = 56 nmol/liter. Using the reciprocal $[H^+]$−pH relationship:

[H+]		pH
56 nmol/liter	=	7.24

The measured pH 7.35 was not nearly so low as would be predicted in acute respiratory acidosis. In this example, there has evidently been time for both cellular and renal mechanisms to modify the change in pH.

A pH of 7.30 in the same example would be compatible with either decompensated chronic respiratory acidosis or acute respiratory acidosis prior to maximal renal compensation.

This problem illustrates the use of acid-base diagrams and bedside formulas in the diagnosis of hypercapnia as acute, chronic, or acute superimposed on chronic. Aside from ease, the advantage of using an acid-base diagram over using the beside approximations is that the diagrams provide a range of biologic variation whereas the regression equations do not. Without some guide to normal variance, there is no way at the bedside to predict whether a given acid-base permutation is explainable by a single disturbance or whether multiple disturbances are more likely. It must be remembered that patients with acute respiratory distress, especially the elderly and those with multisystem disease, frequently have more than one acid-base disturbance. The diagnoses suggested by the acid-base diagram are meaningful only in the context of a careful history and physical examination in which causes of nonrespiratory acidosis and alkalosis are sought. Diuretic therapy resulting in hypochloremic-hypokalemic metabolic alkalosis is probably the most common concomitant disturbance. Lactic acidosis is much less common in patients with respiratory failure, occurring in the setting of severe hypoxemia combined with impaired circulation due to peripheral vascular disease or congestive heart failure. Serum electrolyte determinations are therefore a vital part of acid-base assessment. Not only do they reveal the presence of hypokalemia or hypochloremia but also the calculation of an elevated unmeasured anion may provide the only readily available clue to lactic acidosis. A serum lactic acid determination is confirmatory.

In the clinical setting, Kettel et al. (see Suggested Readings) plotted the pH and $Paco_2$ values obtained before, during, and after 87 consecutive episodes of acute ventilatory failure in patients with CAO. The confidence bands in Figure 9.7 are similar to those in the complete acid-base diagram (Fig. 9.6). As expected, most values 24 or more hours before acute decompensation (Fig. 9.7*A*) fell within the chronic hypercapnia band and returned there after successful treatment (Fig. 9.7*C*). A $Paco_2$ of 65 mm Hg or more was usually associated with an abnormal pH even in the chronic state. During the acute episodes, most values were between the acute and chronic bands (Fig. 9.7*B*). The extremely high $Paco_2$ values achieved by some patients indicate that they had been supported with prior oxygen therapy.

In addition to confirming the usefulness of the acid-base diagram, the above data suggest rational goals in the treatment of patients with CAO. The findings before and after the acute episodes indicate that no purpose is served by correcting pH or $Paco_2$ in acute respiratory decompensation beyond what the patient can achieve in the chronic well-compensated state.

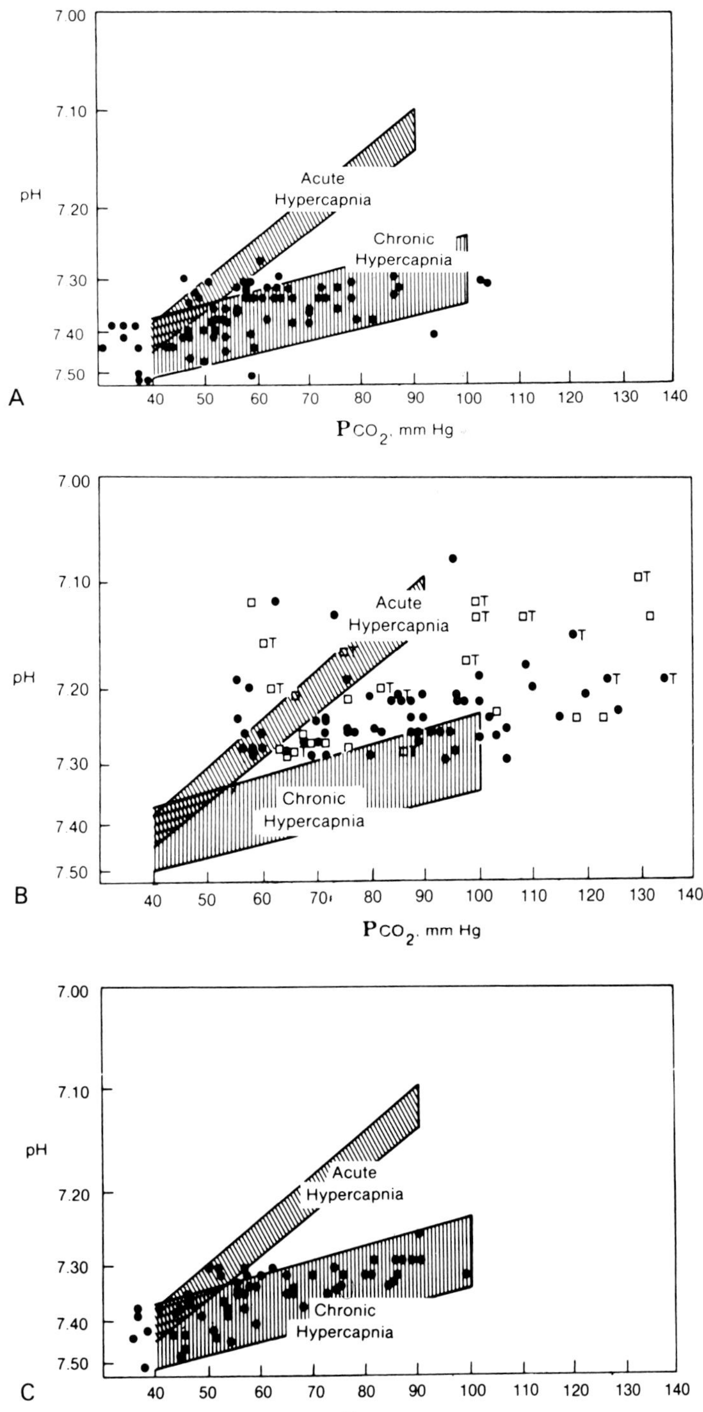

Figure 9.7. Acid-base values observed in CAO patients before, during, and after acute respiratory decompensation. Shaded areas are similar to those in right upper quadrant of Figure 9.6. *A,* Arterial blood-gas values 24 hours or more before 87 episodes of acute respiratory decompensation. *B,* Arterial blood-gas values during acute respiratory decompensation at time of lowest observed pH. Episodes of acute respiratory acidosis from which patient survived (●) and episodes that resulted in death (□) are shown. *T* identifies episodes in which tracheal intubation was used with mechanically assisted ventilation. *C,* Arterial blood-gas values after acute respiratory decompensation. Values shown are those observed closest to normal pH. (Reproduced by permission, from Kettel LJ, Diener CF, Morse JO, et al. Treatment of acute respiratory acidosis in chronic obstructive lung disease. *JAMA* 217:1503–1508, ©1971, by The American Medical Association.)

Chronic Hypercapnia and Control of Respiration

The pH of the blood is regulated less well in response to an acute change in $Paco_2$ and relatively better when hypercapnia is sustained. The pH of the brain interstitial fluid as reflected in the cerebrospinal fluid is normally slightly lower than that of blood and ever better protected against chronic $Paco_2$ elevation, which suggests that pH may be critical to the brain's complex functions. Carbon dioxide retained in respiratory failure crosses the blood-brain barrier readily and produces acidosis. As in the blood, pH regulation in the brain appears to be due to bicarbonate accumulation. Although initial cellular buffering is ineffective in preventing brain acidosis in acute hypercapnia, within hours of the onset of an elevated $Paco_2$ the bicarbonate level in the cerebrospinal fluid begins to increase, which results in a pH closer to normal than that of the blood in chronic hypercapnia. Some of the bicarbonate increase appears to be due to endogenous production, while another portion enters the cerebrospinal fluid from the circulation.

These findings would be no more than physiologic curiosities to all but the neuroscientist were it not for the presence of the $[H^+]$-sensitive respiratory center within the brain substance. The elevated brain bicarbonate level in chronic hypercapnia minimizes the $[H^+]$ change resulting from futher increases in $Paco_2$ and therefore lessens the respiratory center output for a given $Paco_2$ stimulus. In the clinical setting this is seen as a flattened carbon dioxide ventilatory response curve when such patients are tested.

The carotid bodies sense the oxygen tension of the arterial blood and ordinarily begin to respond with a strong ventilatory stimulus when a Pao_2 of 50 mm Hg or less occurs. Although this response to hypoxia usually plays a minor role in respiratory control in healthy persons, because of diminished $Paco_2$ responsiveness, patients with chronic hypercapnia often rely on the hypoxic drive to ventilate. Relief of the hypoxic drive by uncontrolled oxygen therapy may lead to acute ventilatory depression with marked carbon dioxide retention and acidosis. Use of controlled oxygen therapy, however, can provide adequate oxygen delivery to tissues with only insignificant increases in $Paco_2$.

Controlled Oxygen Therapy

Patients with chronic respiratory failure often live productive lives with moderate degrees of hypoxemia without need of oxygen therapy. When hypoxemia becomes severe either acutely or gradually, symptoms may develop and supplemental oxygen is indicated. As in hypercapnia, the symptoms and signs of hypoxemia are nonspecific, and its accurate assessment depends on measurement of arterial ox-

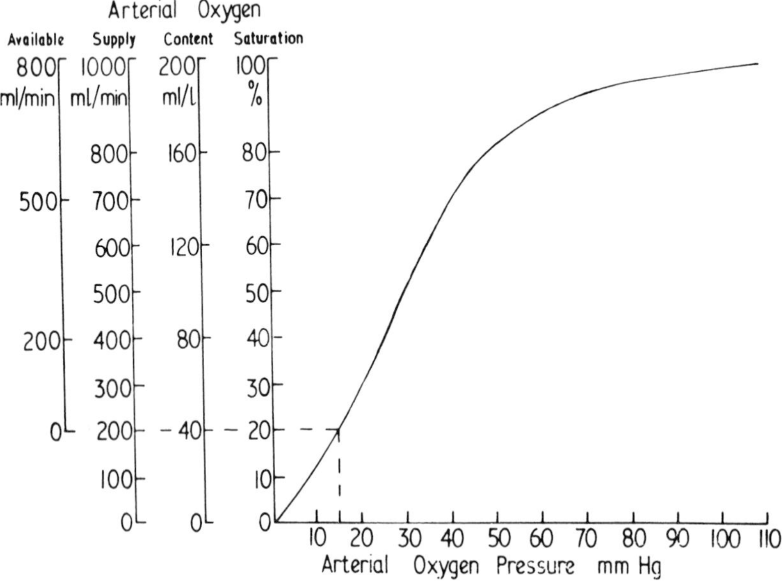

Figure 9.8. Oxygen-hemoglobin dissociation curve and oxygen supply. Vertical scale labeled *Content* assumes a normal hemoglobin level of 15 gm/100 ml. Oxygen *supply* to tissues is calculated on the basis of a normal cardiac output of 5 liters/min. *Available* oxygen assumes that tissues are unable to extract the last 20% of oxygen from hemoglobin. (Reproduced by permission, from Campbell EJM. The J Burns Amberson Lecture: The management of acute respiratory failure in chronic bronchitis and emphysema. *Am Rev Respir Dis,* 1967;96:626–639.)

ygen tension. Cyanosis, which is thought to require 5 gm of reduced hemoglobin/100 ml, is particularly unreliable as an index of hypoxemia, occurring at lower oxygen tensions in severe anemia and at higher oxygen tensions when peripheral blood flow is impaired, which allows greater oxygen extraction.

An adequate oxygen supply to tissues depends not only on the Pao_2 but also on adequate amounts of hemoglobin capable of carrying oxygen and on sufficient cardiac output and local circulation to deliver it to the tissues.

Figure 9.8 depicts the oxygen-hemoglobin dissociation curve. The x axis expresses hemoglobin saturation. The next scale to the left, which assumes a normal hemoglobin concentration of 15 gm/100 ml, gives the oxygen content of the blood. Based on a normal cardiac output of 5 liters/min, the next scale estimates oxygen supply to tissues. Finally, since tissues cannot extract the last 20% of oxygen from the blood, the scale furthest to the left predicts the oxygen actually available to tissues at a given Pao_2. Since the healthy person at rest requires at least 200 ml of oxygen/minute, the lowest tolerable level of hemoglobin saturation is estimated at 40% (Po_2, 25 mm Hg). This would prove inadequate, however, in the presence of increased metabolic demands, severe anemia, congestive heart failure, or impaired peripheral circulation.

Fortunately, the remarkable properties of the hemoglobin molecule make therapy for hypoxemia relatively easy. The oxygen-hemoglobin dissociation curve is steep in its unsaturated portion, so small increases in Pao_2 result in relatively large increases in saturation and, therefore, in oxygen content and supply to the tissues. A 15 mm Hg increase in Pao_2—from 25 to 40 mm Hg, for example—results in almost a 2½-fold increase in available oxygen. This can often be achieved with only a small increase in inspired oxygen from 21% (ambient air) to 28%. Since the flat (saturated) portion of the curve is reached at about a Pao_2 of 50 mm Hg, further increases in Pao_2 result in relatively small increases in hemoglobin saturation. Oxygen tensions higher than 50 or 60 mm Hg, therefore, result in little benefit and risk dampening the hypoxic stimulus to ventilate on which patients with CAO often depend. In clinical practice, the point at which severe hypoventilation limits oxygen therapy is highly variable and requires a cautious trial and error approach monitored by arterial blood gas determinations 15–20 minutes after each adjustment in oxygen flow. Because of the physiologic considerations just discussed, oxygen therapy should always begin with the lowest controllable concentration and should progress in small increments to higher concentrations. A satisfactory goal is a Pao_2 between 50 and 60 mm Hg, which should be adequate for tissues as estimated by the patient's cerebral function, for example, and which should also result in little increase in $Paco_2$ or in a stable, tolerable increase as monitored by serial arterial blood gas determinations.

Adequate oxygen administration is important for yet another reason. Unlike systemic arterioles, which dilate in the presence of tissue hypoxia to permit increased blood flow, the arterioles of the pulmonary vascular tree constrict with alveolar hypoxia, allowing the normal lung to regulate its regional balance of perfusion and ventilation. Were blood flow to continue to a region of the lung where alveoli are underventilated and therefore hypoxic, a low ventilation-perfusion ($\dot{V}/\dot{Q}$) area would exist and contribute to systemic hypoxemia. Local pulmonary vasoconstriction tends to restore the balance between perfusion and ventilation, thus reducing hypoxemia. The design of the pulmonary circulation is such that constriction of as much as half of the pulmonary vasculature normally does not result in a significant increase in pulmonary arterial pressure since the remaining pulmonary vessels may dilate and closed vessels may open. When alveolar hypoxia is generalized, however, most of the pulmonary vasculature is constricted and pulmonary arterial pressure rises. This results in increased work for the right side of the heart, which is normally thin walled and ill equipped to handle a pressure load. Prolonged widespread alveolar hypoxia, such as in severe chronic bronchitis, can lead to right heart failure (cor pulmonale). Consequently, the treatment of heart failure of this type should be directed primarily not at the heart itself but at the elevated pulmonary arterial pressure and the responsible alveolar hypoxia.

Providing a PAo_2 of 60 mm Hg or more assures minimal pulmonary vasoconstriction. In practice, since alveolar gas tensions are not readily obtainable and since a large alveolar-arterial gradient is known to exist in patients with CAO, a Pao_2 of 50 mm Hg is considered a reasonable goal in preventing reactive pulmonary hypertension. Again the clinician may be faced with the delicate balance between providing enough oxygen to prevent tissue hypoxia and pulmonary vasoconstriction while not suppressing ventilation. Unless the patient is ill enough to require a pulmonary artery catheter to measure right-sided pressure, the clinician must rely on empirical guidelines such as those just presented and, in the long term, on the signs and symptoms of right-sided heart failure.

Careful control of oxygen administration is difficult to achieve with nasal prongs or with face masks whose oxygen delivery rates vary with the patient's ventilation. Development of the Venturi mask, which delivers a predetermined mixture of oxygen and room air regardless of the patient's ventilation, has made controlled oxygen therapy much safer. It must be properly worn, of course, and has the disadvantage of not permitting eating or talking when in place. Such masks are available to deliver 24, 28, 35, and 40% oxygen.

Treatment

The previous discussion provides background for the recommendations that follow.

Intubation

When the patient is apneic or nearly apneic, immediate intubation and mechanical ventilation are indicated and should be performed when: (*a*) adequate oxygenation cannot be provided without severe carbon dioxide retention and acidosis; and/or (*b*) there is pharmacologic ventilatory depression or mechanical interference with chest wall function. The role of elective mechanical ventilation to rest respiratory muscles, by positive or negative pressure, is not established at this time. Negative pressure ventilators such as the cuirass ventilator or the iron lung are effective adjuncts in some patients, although in many the machine-engendered pressure is not adequate and secretion clearance remains a major problem. Intubation for positive pressure ventilation is a more serious step, both medically and ethically. Use of this procedure must be individualized.

Intubation should take into consideration the patient's expressed wishes, current status, and medical history. End-stage associated illness or recurrent intractable respiratory failure raises difficult ethical questions as to the appropriateness of this procedure that are best addressed by the primary physician and patient before the final acute emergency exists.

Low Flow Oxygen Therapy

When spontaneous ventilation is present, arterial blood gas levels should be determined and oxygen therapy begun with a 24% Venturi mask.

The patient's response to therapy must be monitored with serial arterial blood gas determinations, especially 15–20 minutes after each change in oxygenation or ventilation. Since the time required to obtain results from the blood gas laboratory may be substantial, it is good practice to return the patient to previously established safe levels of oxygenation or ventilation after arterial blood samples are taken at the new settings. If the values are satisfactory, the new settings can be re-established.

If the patient has a history or physical signs of long-standing obstructive airways disease or if initial arterial blood gas levels suggest chronic or acute-on-chronic respiratory acidosis, a Pao_2 of 50 to 60 mm Hg should be the goal. A mild increase in $Paco_2$ is acceptable if it does not produce severe acidosis or clinical signs of carbon dioxide toxicity. The acid-base diagram (Fig. 9.6) or the bedside approximations are recommended to help interpret the pH and $Paco_2$.

Bicarbonate Therapy

Bicarbonate therapy is not indicated for respiratory acidosis. Bicarbonate was once recommended for hypoxic lactic acidosis, but is now thought to be detrimental in that setting. Treatment of hypoventilation, oxygenation, and perfusion are the mainstays of acidosis management for most cases of respiratory failure.

Etiology of Decompensation and Specific Treatment

The cause of decompensation must be sought and treated. A history of gradual decline with increasing sputum and dyspnea is most common and suggests infection as the cause. More acute failure may also be due to infection, but acute pulmonary embolism, heart failure, and pneumothorax are also considerations.

Antibiotics

Unless a Gram's stain of sputum reveals a predominance of a single organism, a broad-spectrum antibiotic such as ampicillin or tetracycline should be given since *Hemophilus influenzae* is commonly recovered from the sputum of patients wth CAO.

Bronchodilators

Bronchodilators may improve ventilation and reduce the work of breathing. Intravenous aminophylline has the advantage of rapid control, and it can be monitored by serum theophylline levels. It may also provide central respiratory stimulation that may help counteract the ventilatory depression due to oxygen therapy. The intravenous dosage recommended for asthmatic patients (Table 9.6) may require modification for patients with CAO, who are often older and more subject to central nervous system complications and cardiac arrhythmias resulting from aminophylline therapy.

Systemic and topical β-adrenergic drugs act synergistically with aminophylline and should be given to patients in whom an added bronchodilator effect is needed. Inhaled β_2 selective sympathomimetic agents such as albuterol and metaproterenol are extremely useful in patients with CAO who are subject to atrial arrhythmias since the effective dose by aerosol is much less than that required by the oral route. More details on bronchodilators and on corticosteroids that are occasionally required for resistant bronchospasm in patients with CAO may be found in Table 9.6.

Chest Physiotherapy

Frequent chest physical therapy plays an important role in helping CAO patients clear secretions. Neither physical therapy nor regular side-to-side repositioning of patients should be neglected because of mechanical ventilation, intravenous catheters, or cardiac monitors. Oxygen therapy should not be discontinued during physical therapy or tracheal suction.

Corticosteroids

Corticosteroids administered intravenously in divided doses over the course of the day have also been shown to hasten recovery of flow rates in decompensation of CAO not due to asthma.

Complications and Special Considerations

Mask Choices

Once oxygen therapy is begun, it should be continuous. Because carbon dioxide stores are much greater than oxygen stores in the body, an elevated $Paco_2$ due to oxygen therapy stays elevated for several minutes after decrease in alveolar, arterial, and tissue Po_2 on discontinuance of supplemental oxygen. The elevated $Paco_2$ continues to displace oxygen from the alveolus after the inspired oxygen fraction is lowered and may result in hypoxemia more severe than before treatment.

Whereas Venturi masks provide better oxygen control during the initial treatment period, when the patient's condition becomes stablized, low-flow oxygen by nasal prongs has the advantage of allowing unimpaired eating and speech without interruption of oxygen therapy. Since there is no way of knowing the exact fraction of inspired oxygen delivered with nasal prongs, safe flow must be established by trial and error, with administration of 1 liter/min initially.

Dehydration

Dehydration and overhydration are important considerations. Dehydration causes thick tenacious sputum, whereas overhydration or left ventricular heart failure can interfere with oxygen transport, decrease lung compliance, and increase the work of breathing.

While humidification of inspired gases appears essential to normal mucociliary clearance when the nasopharynx is bypassed by intubation or tracheotomy, the role of high humidity and ultrasonic nebulization of water outside these limited circumstances is controversial. Ultrasonic nebulizers carry large quantities of moisture to the nasopharynx, although only a small amount reaches the bronchial tree. What beneficial or harmful effects increased inspired moisture has in patients with CAO is uncertain. Some authorities believe that mucus consistency depends more on systemic hydration than on moisture added via the bronchus. Breathing humidified gases does minimize insensible fluid losses through the respiratory tract. Replacement fluids therefore must be appropriately reduced when fluid balance is critical.

The roles of diuretics and digoxin in treating respiratory failure complicated by left heart failure are discussed in Chapter 7.

Hypokalemia-Hypochloremia

Hypokalemia and hypochloremia secondary to chronic acidosis or diuretic therapy should be treated by parenteral or intravenous administration of potassium chloride. The hypokalemic hypochloremic metabolic alkalosis so often seen in patients with CAO further diminishes the central drive to ventilate and can result in fatal alkalosis if mechanical hyperventilation with subsequent acute respiratory alkalosis is superimposed.

Pulmonary Emboli

CAO patients at high risk from pulmonary embolus—especially those with polycythemia, congestive heart failure, or peripheral venous disease—are candidates for prophylactic anticoagulation.

Central Nervous System Alkalosis

When patients with severe *hypercapnia* require mechanical ventilation, care must be taken not to lower $Paco_2$ too quickly, causing systemic and central nervous system alkalosis. The bicarbonate accumulation resulting from chronic hypercapnia requires adequate chloride and sufficient time (hours to days) to be eliminated by the kidneys. During that period, arterial pH may not represent central nervous system pH since the blood-brain barrier blocks bicarbonate flux. Importantly, cerebral perfusion is considerably reduced in response to central nervous system alkalosis induced by overventilation. Hypoxic brain damage has resulted from overventilation under these circumstances.

Prognosis

Bates (see Suggested Readings) suggested that the progression of obstructive airways disease, as determined by pulmonary function tests, occurs rather independently of acute exacerbations of bronchitis. For the individual CAO patient, however, each episode of acute respiratory failure represents a potential life-threatening situation. The data of Kettel et al. (see Suggested Readings and Figure 9.7*B*) correlate patients surviving the acute episode (*black circles*) with type of therapy and degree of acidosis. Among the patients who responded to conservative management or who were not intubated for medical or humanitarian reasons, the survival rate was 87.5%. Only a small number of patients were intubated—presumably, the sickest who were still treatable with expectation of survival. Their survival rate was 20%. Thus, although this type of investigation cannot be done as a controlled study, the results suggest that, when patients with CAO do not respond to conservative management, the prognosis with intubation and assisted ventilation is grim. It is possible that earlier, elective mechanical ventilation of selected patients will improve results through recovery of inspiratory muscle fatigue. However, the selection criteria, methods of ventilation, and results, compared to conservative approaches, have yet to be established.

Conclusion

Acute respiratory failure in patients with chronic hypercapnia differs in several respects from acute respiratory failure in the absence of chronic pulmonary disease. Obstructed airways increase the work of breathing and, in some patients, leads to inspiratory muscle fatigue and carbon dioxide retention. Carbon dioxide is well-tolerated when it accumulates slowly, but causes acidosis when the increase is rapid or in excess of cellular buffering. Carbon dioxide increase also worsens hypoxemia by displacing oxygen from the alveolus. Chronic hypercapnia blunts the normal ventilatory carbon dioxide response and leads to dependence on the hypoxic response mediated by the carotid bodies. Low-flow oxygen therapy is the basis of conservative management of acute respiratory decompensation, together with methods reducing the work of breathing. At this time, intubation and mechanical ventilation should be reserved for patients whose medical history and current status suggest a reasonable chance for survival and who fail to respond to conservative management. The role of elective ventilation to reverse inspiratory muscle fatigue is not established at this time.

Suggested Readings

Pulmonary Embolism

Cheely R. The role of noninvasive tests versus pulmonary angiography in the diagnosis of pulmonary embolism. *Am J Med,* 1981;70:17–22.

Genton E: Thrombolytic therapy of pulmonary thromboembolism. *Prog Cardiovasc Dis,* 1979;21:333–341.

Sharma DVRK, Sasahara AA: Diagnosis and treatment of pulmonary embolism. *Med Clin North Am,* 1979;63:239–250.

Hull RD, Hirsh J, Carder J, et al: Diagnostic value of ventilation-perfusion lung scanning in patients with suspected pulmonary embolism. *Chest,* 1985;88:819–828.

Asthma

Appel D, Rubenstein R, Schrager K, et al. Lactic acidosis in severe asthma. *Am J Med,* 1983;75:580–584.

Benatar SR. Fatal asthma. *N Engl J Med,* 1986;314:423–429.

Ben-Zvi Z, Lam C, Spohn WA, et al. An elevation of repeated injections of epinephrine for the initial treatment of acute asthma. *Am Rev Respir Dis,* 1983;127:101–105.

Bukowskyj M, Nakatsu K, Munt PW. Theophylline reassessed. *Ann Intern Med,* 1984;101:63–73.

Clark TJH, Hetzel MR. Diurnal variation of asthma. *Br J Dis Chest,* 1977;71:87–92.

Cohen CA, Zagelbaum G, Gross D, et al. Clinical manifestations of inspiratory muscle fatigue. *Am J Med,* 1982;73:308–316.

Edelson JD, Rebuck AS. The clinical assessment of severe asthma. *Arch Intern Med,* 1985;145:321–323.

Fanta CH, Rossing TH, McFadden ER. Emergency room treatment of asthma. Relationships among therapeutic combinations, severity of obstruction and time course of response. *Am J Med,* 1982;72:416–422.

Fiel SB, Swartz MA, Glarry K, Francis ME. Efficacy of short-term corticosteroid therapy in outpatient treatment of acute bronchial asthma. *Am J Med,* 1983;75:259–262.

Fischl MA, Pitchenik A, Gardner LB. An index predicting relapse and need for hospitalization in patients with acute bronchial asthma. *N Engl J Med,* 1981;305:783–789.

Haskell RJ, Wong BM, Hansen JE. A double-blind randomized clinical trial of methylprednisolone in status asthmaticus. *Arch Intern Med,* 1983;143:1324–1327.

Hopewell PC, Miller RT. Pathophysiology and management of severe asthma. *Clin Chest Med,* 1984;5:623–634.

Kaliner M. Mast cell mediators and asthma. *Chest,* 1985;87:2S–5S.

Karpel JP, Appel D, Breidbart D, Fusco MJ. A comparison of atropine sulfate and metaproterenol sulfate in the emergeny treatment of asthma. *Am Rev Respir Dis,* 1986;133:727–729.

Kelsen, SG, Kelsen DP, Fleezer RF, et al. Emergency room assessment and treatment of patients with acute asthma. *Am J Med,* 1978;64:622–628.

McFadden ER. Clinical appraisal of the therapy of asthma—An idea whose time has come [Editorial]. *Am Rev Respir Dis,* 1986;133:723–724.

McFadden ER, Kaiser R, DeGroot WJ. Acute bronchial asthma. *N Engl J Med,* 1973;288:221–224.

Millman M, Goodman AH, Goldstein IM, et al. Status asthmaticus: Use of acetylcysteine during bronchoscopy and lavage to remove mucous plugs. *Ann Allergy,* 1983;50:85–93.

Nowak RM, Pensler MJ, Sarkar DD, et al. Comparison of peak expiratory flow and FEV_1 admission criteria for acute bronchial asthma. *Ann Emerg Med,* 1982;11:64–69.

O'Rourke PP, Crone RK. Halothane in status asthmaticus. *Crit Care Med,* 1982;10:341–343.

Rose CC, Murphy JG, Schwartz JS. Performance of an index predicting the response of patients with acute bronchial asthma to intensive emergency department treatment. *N Engl J Med,* 1984;310:573–576.

Rossing TH, Fanta CH, Goldstein DH, et al. Emergency therapy of asthma: Comparison of the acute effects of parenteral and inhaled sympathomimetics and infused aminophylline. *Am Rev Respir Dis,* 1980;122:365–371.

Rossing TH, Fanta CH, Goldstein ER. Effect of outpatient treatment of asthma with beta agonists on the response to sympathomimetics in an emergency room. *Am J Med,* 1983;75:781–784.

Siegel D, Shepard D, Gelb A, Weinberg PF. Aminophylline increases the toxicity but not the efficacy of an inhaled beta-adrenergic agonist in the treatment of acute exacerbations of asthma. *Am Rev Respir Dis,* 1985;132:283–286.

Summer WR. Status asthmaticus. *Chest,* 1985;87:87S–94S.

Acute Decompensation of Chronic Respiratory Failure

Albert RK, Martin TR, Lewis SW. Controlled clinical trial of methylprednisolone in patients with chronic bronchitis and acute respiratory insufficiency. *Ann Intern Med,* 1980;92:753–758.

Bates DV. The fate of the chronic bronchitic: A report of the ten-year follow-up in the Canadian Department of Veterans Affairs coordinated study of chronic bronchitis. *Am Rev Respir Dis*, 1973;108:1043–1065.

Brackett NC Jr, Cohen JJ, Schwartz WB: Carbon dioxide titration curve of normal man: Effect of increasing degrees of acute hypercapnia on acid-base equilibrium. *N Engl J Med*, 1965;272:6–12.

Brackett NC Jr, Wingo CF, Muren O, et al. Acid-base response to chronic hypercapnia in man. *N Engl J Med,* 1969;280:124–130.

Campbell EJM: The J Burns Amberson Lecture: The management of acute respiratory failure in chronic bronchitis and emphysema. *Am Rev Respir Dis*, 1967;96:626–639.

Goldberg M, Green SB, Moss ML, et al. Computer-based instruction and diagnoses of acid-base disorders: A systematic approach. *JAMA*, 1973;223:269–275.

Graf H, Leach W, Arieff AL: Evidence for a detrimental effect of bicarbonate therapy in hypoxic lactic acidosis. *Science,* 1985;227:754–756.

Kassirer JP, Bleich HL: Rapid estimation of plasma carbon dioxide tension from pH and total carbon dioxide content. *N Engl J Med*, 1965;272:1067–1068.

Kettel LJ, Diener CF, Morse JO, et al. Treatment of acute respiratory acidosis in chronic obstructive lung disease. *JAMA,* 1971;217:1503–1508.

McNicol MW, Campbell EJM: Severity of respiratory failure: Arterial blood-gases in untreated patients. *Lancet,* 1965;1:336–338.

Roussos C, Macklem PT: The respiratory muscles. *N Engl J Med*, 1982;307:786–797.

CHAPTER **10**

Environmental Hazards

PETER L. GROSS, M.D.
NANCY WEBER-BORNSTEIN, M.D.
FRANK P. CASTRONOVO, Jr., Ph.D.
ANN S. BAKER, M.D.

Editor's note: Emergency problems involving humans and their environment are increasing, as the population grows and its activities become both far-ranging and bold. This chapter is not encyclopedic but illustrates basic principles of many of the problems. Some of the material in this topically wide-ranging treatise on environmental hazards is supplementary to other discussions: smoke inhalation in Chapter 31 (Thoracic Emergencies), carbon monoxide poisoning in Chapters 17 (Toxicologic Emergencies) and infections resulting from bites in Chapter 11 (Infectious Diseases in the Emergency Department), and frostbite in Chapter 38 (Thermal Injuries).

The emergency physician is often the key first responder in the diagnosis, treatment, and disposition of patients with medical emergencies related to environment hazards. This chapter focuses on selected environmental emergencies, including temperature disorders, drowning, carbon monoxide poisoning, smoke inhalation, barotrauma, radiation exposure, bites, and stings, and lightning injuries.

Although these emergencies are vastly different in terms of pathophysiology and treatment, their common denominator is the need for accurate diagnosis and often definitive initial therapy, beginning in the emergency department.

TEMPERATURE DISORDERS

Heat-related Illness

Three environmental, heat-related illnesses are seen in the emergency department. Heat cramps and heat exhaustion are relatively common conditions with little morbidity, but heat stroke is a catastrophic medical emergency with high mortality, accounting for approximately 4000 deaths annually in the United States. Whereas 80% of deaths occur in persons above the age of 50 years, there is still an appreciable mortality in young, otherwise healthy individuals. Survival depends on rapid diagnosis and initiation of definitive treatment, since morbidity and mortality from heat stroke correlate with the magnitude and duration of hyperpyrexia.

Heat stroke must be distinguished from two rare, but potentially catastrophic, nonenvironmental temperature disorders which occasionally may be seen in the emergency department: neuroleptic malignant syndrome and malignant hyperthermia. Neuroleptic malignant syndrome, discussed in Chapter 18 (Psychiatric Emergencies), is associated with the use of the phenothiazine, butyrophenone, or thiothixene neuroleptic agents and is characterized by hyperthermia, severe extrapyramidal reactions, muscle rigidity, altered sensorium, and potentially severe autonomic dysfunction. The pathogenesis of this condition is unknown, but it shares some of the same features as malignant hyperthermia, now determined to be an inherited disorder of skeletal muscle. Malignant hyperthermia is uncommonly seen in the emergency department but could present following ambulatory surgery where succinylcholine, inhalation anesthesia, or neuroleptic drugs may provoke a severe state of hyperpyrexia, muscle rigidity, hyperkalemia, and lactic acidosis leading to cardiorespiratory arrest if untreated. As in environmental heat-related illness, survival is improved with rapid treatment. Morbidity and mortality increase in direct relation to the magnitude of temperature elevation and the duration of the condition. In addition to supportive measures, dantrolene sodium, 2–3 mg/kg intravenously, has been effective in malignant hyperthermia and has also been used in neuroleptic malignant syndrome.

Physiology: Regulation of Heat Stress

Body temperature reflects the balance of physiologic heat production and the rate of heat loss modulated by the body thermostat in the hypothalamus and mediated through complex reflex changes involving the cardiovascular and central nervous systems. Figure 10.1 summarizes this interaction. The body can gain heat when the environment is warmer than body temperature or when physiologic responses that help dissipate heat are impaired. Increased heat production from metabolism can also occur, and combinations of these three variables can result in illness.

Increased body temperature may be dissipated by (*a*) evaporative heat loss secondary to sweating or (*b*) changes in cardiac output associated with peripheral vasodilatation that result in heat loss from the body surface by radiation, conduction, or convection. Only 5% of body heat loss occurs through the warming of urine, feces, or inspired air, whereas 30% is lost via the sweat mechanism and 65% by convection, conduction, or radiation.

As environmental temperatures approach body temperature, nonevaporative heat loss from the body surface is reduced. When high ambient humidity occurs with high environmental temperatures, evaporative heat loss becomes reduced as well. Other factors that contribute to diminished heat dissipation are listed in Table 10.1. Anticholinergic drugs can impair peripheral heat loss, propranolol hydrochloride can diminish normal cardiac responses, and

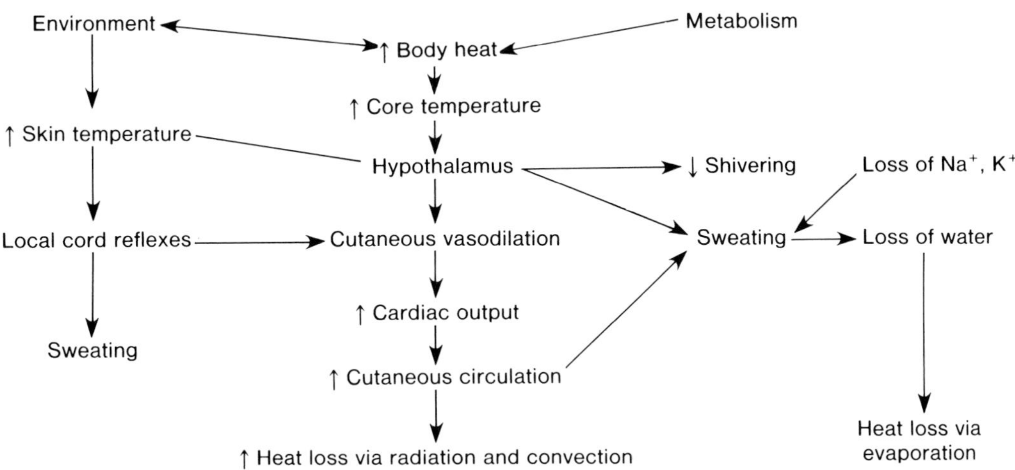

Figure 10.1. Physiologic response to heat stress. (Reproduced by permission from Stine RJ. Heat illness. *JACEP, 1979;8:154–160.)*

Table 10.1.
Factors in Heat-related Illness[a]

Increased heat production
Exercise, exertion
Infection (febrile state)
Agitation
Drugs
Amphetamines
LSD
Cocaine
Hyperthyroidism
Impaired heat dissipation
Lack of acclimatization
High ambient temperature
High ambient humidity
Obesity
Heavy clothing
Dehydration
Cardiovascular disease
Extremes of age
Drugs
Phenothiazines, anticholinergics, diuretics, propranolol hydrochloride
Sweat gland dysfunction

[a] Modified by permission from Stine RJ. Heat illness. *JACEP*, 1979; 8:154–160.

the hypothalamus can be affected by phenothiazine derivatives. Amphetamines, cocaine, hallucinogens, and other stimulants can cause increased heat production.

Acclimatization to heat stress occurs over time alter exposure on a regular basis. Myocardial efficiency improves, as does the sweat mechanism, which can elaborate higher volumes with better sodium preservation. Plasma volume can expand and be maintained in the face of heat stress, improving circulatory competence and diminishing heat dissipation.

Heat Stroke. In contrast to heat cramps and heat exhaustion, heat stroke, though uncommon, is a true medical emergency. Heat stroke is characterized by thermoregulatory failure after exposure to high environmental temperatures and humidity. The cardinal features are hyperpyrexia of 106°F (41.1°C) or higher, central nervous system disturbance (stupor, seizures, or coma), and absence of sweating (anhidrosis).

Anhidrosis is more common in "classical" heat stroke. In most series, sweating is absent in 90% of patients. Younger patients with "exertional" heat stroke associated with strenuous exercise can have preserved sweating. This has been reported in 50% of patients in some series. The features distinguishing classical from exertional heat stroke are summarized in Table 10.2. Overlap does occur.

Pathophysiology. Factors predisposing to heat stroke include both environmental conditions and difficulties in heat regulation, either impaired dissipation or increased production. The pathophysiology is incompletely understood. Four mechanisms have been suggested. It is likely that interaction of all four can contribute to this catastrophic condition in the proper environmental setting.

Since (*a*) cessation of sweating occurs in many patients, it has been suggested that sweat gland fatigue or failure causes a sudden lack of the capacity for evaporative heat loss with resultant hyperpyrexia. However, not all patients with heat stroke have anhidrosis, which has led others to postulate a (*b*) hypothalamic temperature-regulating dysfunction. Certain drugs, such as phenothiazines, have been reported to produce hyperpyrexia in this way. (*c*) Cellular effects at the extremes of hyperpyrexia can be a contributing factor, since enzyme systems and cellular permeability depend on the careful maintenance of cellular environmental temperature, pH, and solutes. At extremes of temperature, intracellular system failure can lead to cell, tissue, and organ dysfunction. Finally, (*d*) cardiovascular responses to hyperpyrexia can be inadequate, resulting in sudden heat stroke. Increase in heart rate and cardiac output occurs in response to heat stress, along with peripheral vasodilatation which hastens heat loss from the body surface area. If cardiac responses are limited by underlying disease and medications, heat stress is poorly tolerated. Physiologic studies have shown that extreme heat stress can contribute to markedly increased pulmonary vascular resistance with right-sided cardiac failure, diminished cardiac output, and sudden lack of peripheral heat loss through radiation, conduction, or convection. Although muscular exercise may be a factor in heat stroke, a muscle level defect, such as in malignant hyperpyrexia, has not been shown to be a factor.

Clinical Manifestations. The pathophysiologic effects of heat stroke often first become manifest with central nervous system alterations. Loss of consciousness occurs in 70% of patients and generalized seizures in 60%. Prodromes of headache, dizziness, faintness, and confusion can occur. Coma can last as long as 24 hours and then resolve without neurologic residual, but consciousness usually returns as the patient's temperature is brought to normal. The cerebellum is particularly sensitive to heat stress, and cerebellar ataxia can persist. Pathologic studies reveal diffuse edema of brain substance associated with petechial hemorrhage and Purkinje cell degeneration.

Hematologic effects occur in as many as 20% of heat stroke victims. In more severe cases, disseminated intravascular coagulation (DIC) can result in thermal injury to vascular endothelium and destruction of platelets. Hemolysis can occur. Reduction of temperature is the first priority in treating DIC.

Table 10.2.
Heat Stroke: Clinical Presentation

	Classical Heat Stroke	Exertional Heat Stroke
Age	Older	Younger
Activity	Sedentary life style	Strenuous exercise
Health	Underlying disease common, medications affecting temperature regulation	Good
Prodrome	2–36 hr	Brief or absent
Anhidrosis	Seen in 90%	Seen in 50–90%

Heparin has also been used to treat DIC (see Chapter 13).

Clowes and O'Donnell (see Suggested Readings) have described two hemodynamic states in heat stroke. Both show low total peripheral vascular resistance with peripheral vasodilation. More common is the hyperdynamic state with adequate blood pressure, tachycardia, a wide pulse pressure, and hot, dry, erythematous skin. These patients have an elevated cardiac index, and are often young, with exertional heat stroke. Severe volume depletion is less common. In such circumstances, the patient has a hypodynamic circulatory state with diminished cardiac output, high pulmonary arterial pressure and hot, dry, but ashen skin. Elderly patients can be hypovolemic from insensitive fluid losses or concurrent diuretic therapy, and present with manifestions of organ hypoperfusion.

Other organ effects in heat stroke include myocardial injury with possible infarction, skeletal muscle injury with rhabdomyolysis, and hepatocellular injury manifested by mild to moderate abnormality in liver function, usually not of clinical significance. Acute tubular necrosis can occur in 10–35% of heat stroke victims. In addition to thermal injury to renal parenchyma, other causes of acute renal dysfunction in these patients include hypotension with hypoperfusion and rhabdomyolysis with pigment-induced injury. Heat injury may induce polyuria secondary to tubular injury, even in the absence of acute renal failure.

Treatment. Since morbidity and mortality in heat stroke correlate with the degree and duration of hyperpyrexia, the first priority in therapy is to lower body temperature. For the emergency physician, the second priority is to assess specific organ injury and to institute appropriate therapy.

There should be little difficulty distinguishing heat stroke from other heat-related illnesses (Table 10.3) during a heat wave. However, in less severe extremes of atmospheric conditions, the physician must consider the differential diagnosis of the febrile patient with altered mental status, including consideration of meningoencephalitis, sepsis, and the noninfectious causes of catastrophic hyperpyrexia (malignant neuroleptic syndrome or malignant hyperthermia). The extreme of temperature elevation in adult heat stroke patients may be suggestive of the diagnosis but is by no means an absolute indication thereof. If circumstances seem to favor heat stroke, the first priority is temperature control, with deferral of diagnostic studies while the temperature is being lowered.

In the comatose patient, the airway is secured, a suitable intravenous cannula placed, and the temperature lowered, preferably in an ice bath with continuous monitoring of core temperature via a rectal probe thermometer. In the absence of an ice bath, the patient may be placed on a cooling blanket with ice packed around him or her. Profound shivering can occur, with subsequent temperature rebound from skeletal muscle activity. Chlorpromazine, 25–100 mg intravenously, usually controls shivering.

Control of the airway is important both for adequate oxygenation and for protection from aspiration, since severe vomiting occasionally occurs during the cooling process. The patient should be removed from the bath when body temperature reaches 101°F (38.3°C), since cooling to normal temperature often is followed by an overshoot to subnormal levels. This phenomenon is more common in the elderly.

Consciousness can return with restoration of temperature, but coma can persist. Persistent seizures should be controlled with intravenous phenytoin or alternative drugs, since uncontrolled seizure activity can contribute both to endogenous heat production with temperature elevation and to skeletal muscle injury with consequent rhabdomyolysis.

After body temperature is lowered, organ function should be assessed in terms of end-organ injury to the cardiovascular, hematologic, renal, and central nervous systems. Baseline renal function and coagulation parameters should be determined and the hemodynamic state stabilized. A pulmonary artery line is helpful in optimizing volume status and filling pressures, but requires transfer to an intensive care unit.

In most patients with exertional heat stroke, volume deficits are not severe and 1–2 liters of crystalloid solution over the first 2–4 hours with physiologic monitoring can be sufficient. Occasionally, volume deficits are greater, or cardiac disease with ventricular failure is limiting. Vasopressors are rarely necessary, but when they are required, pure or predominantly α-adrenergic agents should be avoided, since peripheral and splanchnic vasoconstriction can limit heat loss from the periphery, further compromising renal function. If volume expansion does not rapidly improve the hemodynamics and a sympathomimetic agent is to be added, dopamine in low to moderate doses can be tried.

An "intermediate syndrome" of heat stroke has been recognized, combining some of the features of heat exhaustion with elevated temperature but not catastrophic hyperpyrexia. Temperatures of 104–105°F (40–40.5°C) can occur and often are associated with strenuous exercise conditions, such as jogging or road racing in hot weather. These individuals can have less central nervous system dysfunction and a better prognosis after rapid cooling than a classic heat stroke patient but still require aggressive treatment of temperature and vigilance in the assessment of end-organ damage.

Prolonged temperatures in excess of 106°F (41.1°C), azotemia, hyperkalemia, and protracted coma are associated with poor prognosis. In the absence of these features, aggressive assessment and therapy in the emergency department should produce a satisfactory outcome.

Prevention. At times of environmental temperature and humidity extremes, preventative measures may help to limit heat-related illness. The elderly should make every effort to minimize exertional activities and maintain adequate hydration. Emergency physicians can play a useful role in the community with advice to those engaged in strenuous work or exercise programs in hot weather. Maintenance of adequate hydration before and during exercise, avoidance of the extremes of exposure whenever possible, and awareness of early symptoms of heat-related illness are among educational goals. The question of continued vigorous exercise for individuals who have survived heat stroke is more problematic. There is some evidence that thermoregulation and cardiac responses are abnormal in these individuals, although it is not clear whether such changes are causes or effects of heat stroke. In the absence of definitive data, heat stroke victims should use caution in exercise activities at times of environmental climate extremes.

Minor Heat-related Illness

Heat Cramps. Painful contractions in peripheral skeletal or abdominal muscles characterize heat cramps, which can occur in temperate ambient environment or with extremes of high temperature and humidity. The hallmark is strenuous exercise, usually without acclimatization or training.

Pathophysiology. Although serum electrolyte levels are usually normal, the pathophysiology of heat cramps appears to involve sweat-related electrolyte flux from tissues accompanied by enhanced muscle contractility, perhaps mediated by alkalosis and changes in calcium concentration. On clinical examination, patients have normal body temperatures with muscle cramps and a preserved sweat mechanism.

Treatment. Therapy involves reassurance, rest in a cool environment, and oral intake of fluids. Only rarely is parenteral fluid administration necessary. Gradual acclimatization, graded exercise, and maintenance of body hydration are usually sufficient to prevent this syndrome. Although advocated as a preventative measure, there is no proof that salt tablet pretreatment benefits this condition. Furthermore, preexercise hydration is best accomplished with water, rather than oral glucose-electrolyte solutions as there is evidence that added sugar delays gastric emptying and small bowel water absorption.

Heat Exhaustion. Heat exhaustion or heat prostration is the most frequent heat-related illness, occurring during environmental conditions of high ambient temperature and humidity in unacclimatized persons who often have some contributing element of impaired heat dissipation. This illness can be relatively sudden as in the "parade-ground faint," although commonly there is a prodromal period of 10–30 minutes. The patient feels weak, dizzy, sweaty, or nauseated, and can vomit, faint, or complain of headache. Muscle cramps can be associated, and the patient appears ashen, tachypneic, and profusely diaphoretic with clinical findings that resemble vagotonia except that the heart rate is usually elevated. Body temperature is normal, but when associated with extremes of ambient temperature or muscular exercise it can be elevated slightly to 101.5°F (38.6°C). Acute respiratory alkalosis is related to hyperventilation and is reflected in arterial blood gas studies. Most often, serum electrolyte levels are normal, although hyponatremia or hypernatremia can occur related to prolonged exposure and loss of varying proportions of salt and water. Hemoconcentration is seen occasionally.

Pathophysiology. The pathophysiology of heat exhaustion is incompletely understood. Beller and Boyd (see Suggested Readings) have suggested that the exaggerated ventilatory response derives from temperature-stimulated increases in respiratory rate and tidal volume and results in a hyperventilation-induced faint associated with a vasovagal syndrome. Others have suggested that changes in tissue levels of sodium and chloride ions and water play a role, though measurable serum electrolyte abnormalities are the exception.

Treatment. Treatment requires a cool environment and rehydration with reassurance by the emergency physician. Patients with mild heat exhaustion

Table 10.3.
Heat Syndromes

	Clinical Manifestations	Temperature	Sweat Mechanism	Central Nervous System Findings	Pathophysiology	Therapy
Heat cramps	Muscle cramps	Normal	Normal	Normal	Salt and fluid losses	Stop exercise Oral fluids
Heat exhaustion	Weakness Faintness	Normal to 101.5°F(38.6°C)	Diaphoresis	Normal or slight confusion	Salt and fluid losses Hyperventilation	Cool room Oral or intravenous fluids
Heat stroke	Stupor or sudden loss of consciousness	≥106°F (41.1°C)	Absent 50–90%	Coma Seizure Confusion	Unknown	Ice bath Maintain airway Support circulation

can be given oral fluids, whereas patients with more severe cases require parenteral rehydration with saline solution. Removal of the patient from the etiologic environmental conditions and rehydration in a cool environment cause symptoms to abate completely over 1–2 hours in most cases. In older patients, the emergency physician must be alert to specific organ stress that may develop secondary to heat prostration, such as myocardial ischemia.

Hypothermia

As in heat-related illness, the successful management of hypothermia begins in the emergency department with prompt recognition and rapid institution of appropriate therapy. Hypothermia, defined as a core temperature less than 95°F (35°C) can develop in a variety of circumstances. In otherwise healthy individuals, recreational activities with exposure to extreme cold, sometimes complicated by injury or immersion, are the most common precipitants of primary hypothermia. Secondary hypothermia occurs with medical illness, such as drug overdose combined with exposure, central nervous system dysfunction from stroke or spinal cord injury, and metabolic and endocrine disorders, including diabetic ketoacidosis, hypothyroidism, and hypopituitarism. In these circumstances, the exposure may not always be obviously cold stress but may involve the immobilized or injured patient unable to protect herself or himself from heat loss, due to underlying disease or to new injury or illness. Persons addicted to alcohol can be particularly prone to hypothermia caused by exposure and invariably associated with complications of alcohol abuse, including trauma, pancreatitis, seizures, or infection.

Secondary hypothermia can also occur in the emergency department where trauma or medical resuscitation involves the rapid administration of cold or room temperature volume expanders (blood, colloid, or crystalloid) in patients who are disrobed and prone to heat loss. While infants may be particularly affected, adult patients can rapidly become hypothermic as a consequence of shock and/or sepsis and their treatment.

The management of hypothermia is controversial. Therapeutic strategies depend first on an understanding of the physiologic consequences of hypothermia.

Pathophysiology

Decrease in core temperature results in a complex series of physiologic responses directed at conserving heat loss and increasing heat production. These responses are modulated by the temperature-regulating center in the hypothalamus. Reflex cardiovascular and central nervous system responses are necessary to maintain normothermia. In the presence of low environmental temperatures, excess heat loss and diminished heat production result in clinical hypothermia.

Heat loss occurs by conduction, convection, or radiation from the body surface. Conductive heat loss increases dramatically in water immersion, where heat loss may be 30 times more rapid than in air of comparable temperature.

Conservation of body temperature involves (*a*) peripheral vasoconstriction, which decreases heat loss, and (*b*) increased heat production in skeletal muscles. Increased heat production occurs most rapidly as a result of shivering which generates heat, central vasodilation, and the delivery of warmed blood to the core circulation. The endogenous catechol and neuroendocrine responses play a role in heat production, but at a slightly slower pace.

The physiologic and clinical consequences of hypothermia are summarized in Table 10.4. As body temperature is lowered to 95°F (35°C), heart rate, cardiac output, and respiration rate actually increase, and the metabolic rate can increase three to

Table 10.4.
Temperature Physiology

Temperature	Physiologic Response	Clinical Appearance
95°F (35°C)	↑ heart rate, ↑ respiratory rate, ↑ cardiac output, ↑ metabolic rate	Shivering, conscious
90°F (32.2°C)	↓ heart rate, ↓ respiratory rate, ↓ cardiac output, ↓ metabolic rate	Shivering ceases, confusion and stupor, muscle incoordination
86°F (30°C)	Metabolic rate—50% ↓, ↓ respiratory rate, ↓ blood pressure	Lethargy and coma, muscle rigidity, bradyarrhythmias, conduction disturbances
82°F (28°C)	Myocardial irritability, shock, ventilatory failure	Ventricular fibrillation
77° (25°C)	Respiratory arrest, cardiac arrest	Asystole, death

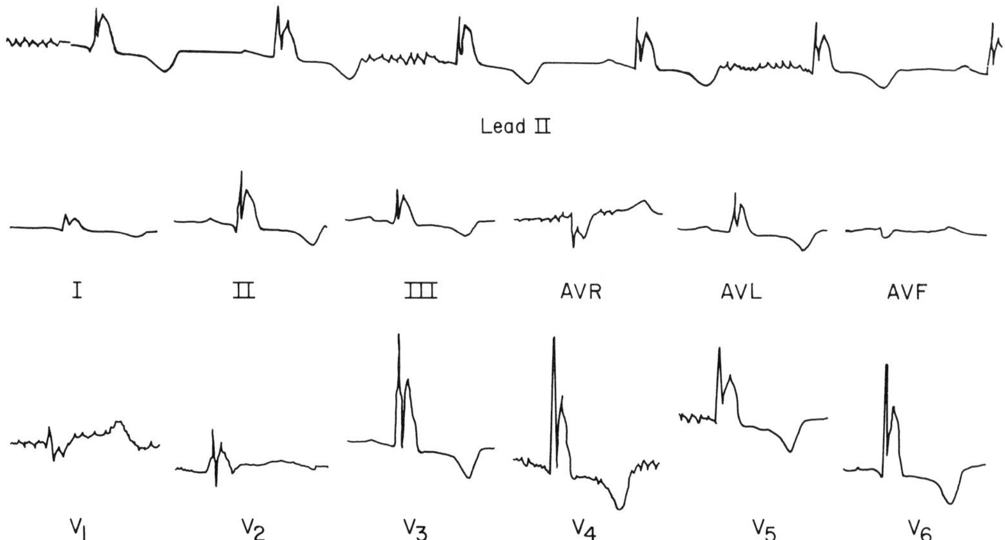

Figure 10.2. Electrocardiogram taken on admission. Rectal temperature was below 90°F (32.2°C). Rhythm is sinus bradycardia at 40 beats/min. PR, QRS, and QT intervals are prolonged and a prominent "J" deflection is seen in most leads. Intermittent oscillations of the baseline are identified in lead II. (Reproduced by permission from Trevino A, Razi B, Beller BM. The characteristic electrocardiogram of accidental hypothermia. *Arch Intern Med,* 1971;127:470–473.)

six times the basal rate in an effort to promote heat production in response to hypothermic stress. The patient is usually conscious and shivering. As temperature declines further, the metabolic rate decreases. At a body temperature of 90°F (32.2°C), heart rate, cardiac output, and respiration rate also are decreased and the shivering response can be lost at temperatures from 86 to 91°F (30 to 32.8°C). Confusion, stupor, or coma can develop at this stage. Hypothermia-induced altered judgment and associated fatigue, incoordination, weakness, and hallucinosis may lead to further exposure and severe consequences.

At temperatures approximating 86°F (30°C), muscular rigidity occurs and the basal metabolic rate can be 50% of normal. Respiration is depressed and hypoxemia results. Cardiac depression causes decreased cardiac output with associated bradyarrhythmias, conduction disturbances, and hypotension. Sinus bradycardia can give way to atrial fibrillation with a slow ventricular response and associated J or Osborne waves that are characteristic of the hypothermic effect on conduction (Fig. 10.2). As hypothermia progresses, absolute and relative refractory periods are prolonged and the rate of spontaneous cardiac depolarization slows. Myocardial irritability increases with hypothermia, and ventricular fibrillation becomes a major risk at about 82.4°F (28°C), particularly when the patient is moved or handled. The cold heart is sensitive to any such activity.

Hypothermia also causes bronchorrhea and depression of cough which become manifest at temperatures from 86 to 95°F (30 to 35°C). Aspiration pneumonitis can develop. At a temperature of 77°F (25°C) major respiratory depression occurs and asystole or ventricular fibrillation usually produce death.

Hypothermia can induce diuresis due to the effects of cold on renal tubules, and at extremes of hypothermia with hypotension and organ hypoperfusion, acute tubular necrosis can develop. Hemoconcentration occurs with intravascular sludging, and disseminated intravascular coagulation can be seen. As temperature lowers, cerebral blood flow diminishes and pupils dilate.

Either hyperglycemia or hypoglycemia may occur. Hypoglycemia can be a feature in the alcoholic, resulting from a malnourished nutritional state and the diminished hepatic gluconeogenesis of both hypothermia and alcoholism. Shivering utilizes glucose stores and contributes to hypoglycemia. Hyperglycemia develops because of the severe hypothermic effects on intermediary metabolism with blockage of insulin release and diminished peripheral glucose utilization. Blood glucose levels ranging from 300 to 400 mg/100 ml are not uncommon, but may not require insulin administration. These levels return to normal levels as rewarming reverses the altered physiology.

Arterial blood gas measurements must be corrected for temperature as neutrality is affected by

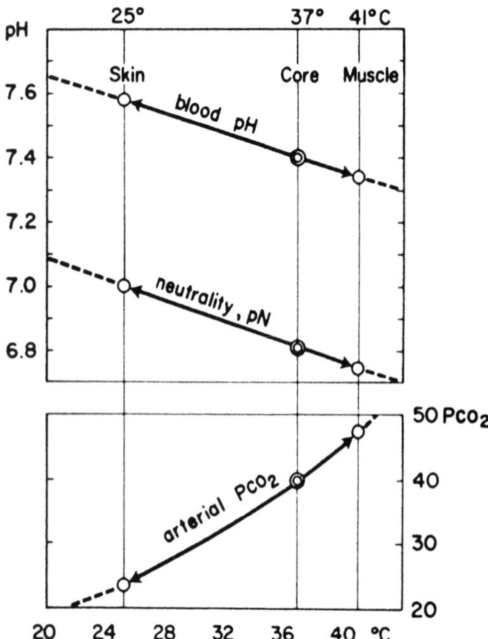

Figure 10.3. Changes in arterial pH and Pco_2 as 37°C blood arrives at the skin or exercising muscle at temperatures of 25 and 41°C, respectively. Neutrality of water, pN, changes in parallel with the changes in blood pH. Thus the relative alkalinity of the blood or the ratio between [OH⁻] and [H⁺] ion remains constant. (From Rahn, H. Body temperature and acid base regulation. In: Reeves RB, Howell BJ, Rahn H, eds. Protons, Proteins, Temperature. Department of Physiology, Buffalo: State University of New York at Buffalo, 1977).

hypothermia (Figure 10.3). Blood samples drawn from hypothermic patients but analyzed under standard conditions at 98.6°F (37°C) are subject to error. The Pao_2 and the $Paco_2$ will be falsely elevated, and the patient will appear more acidotic than is actually the case. The emergency physician must note the temperature of the patient when the arterial blood sample is drawn. With this information, the blood gas laboratory can correct the results for temperature using the Severinghaus nomogram.

In hypothermia, acidosis is caused by a combination of respiratory depression and resulting carbon dioxide retention and by lactate accumulation as circulatory failure ensues with hypotension and tissue hypoperfusion. Muscle activity with shivering adds to the accumulation of lactate, which is less efficiently metabolized by the liver in hypothermia. Metabolic and respiratory acidosis, in addition to hypoxemia, increase the risk of cardiac arrhythmias. Asystole occurs at temperatures of 68–77°F (20–25°C), sometimes preceding respiratory arrest.

Clinical Features

The emergency physician must be aware of the possibilities of occult primary hypothermia or physiologically significant secondary hypothermia, since environmental temperatures need not be dramatically low for hypothermia in the elderly or immobilized patient, in those with acute illness or injury superimposed on pituitary or thyroid dysfunction, or during medical or trauma resuscitation.

Hypothermia should be suspected in the stuporous patient with cold skin, slow pulse rate, low blood pressure, diminished deep tendon reflexes, and shivering, and also in the comatose patient with these features but muscular rigidity instead of shivering. Edema can also be a prominent feature with immersion or long-duration hypothermia. Whereas there is often a history of exposure or immersion to guide the emergency physician, the condition still can be unrecognized and the diagnosis delayed, since most clinical thermometers do not read below 94°F (34.4°C). Frostbite is occasionally the initial clue. Its treatment must be secondary to rewarming of the patient.

The emergency physician not only must be aware of the possibility of hypothermia but also must modify the usual criteria for attempting resuscitation. In the extreme situation, the patient can appear dead, with muscular rigidity, dilated pupils, barely discernible or absent pulse and respiration, and unobtainable blood pressure. However, recovery without significant sequelae has occurred despite prolonged hypothermic cardiopulmonary arrest. Patients with asystole or ventricular fibrillation lasting 2–3 hours have survived with continuous cardiopulmonary resuscitation (CPR) and rewarming efforts. If the patient has been rewarmed to more than 95°F (35°C) without restoration of cardiorespiratory function, resuscitative efforts should be halted.

Evaluation and Treatment

General Measures. Temperature should be monitored accurately, preferably with a rectal probe thermocouple providing continuous readings. In the stuporous or comatose patient, initial evaluation should include careful inspection for trauma that may have precipitated the exposure or followed a hypothermic state. All hypothermic patients should have cardiac monitoring, and patients should be handled very carefully because of the risk of ventricular arrhythmias or arrest. Arterial blood gas samples should be clearly marked with the patient's temperature, so that appropriate corrections can be made. Initial laboratory studies should include renal function tests, and determination of blood glucose, electrolytes, parameters for disseminated intravascular coagulation (prothrombin times, partial thromboplastin time, platelets, fibrinogen, and fibrinolysin), and liver function and amylase tests if there is evidence or history of chronic alcohol abuse.

Correction of acidosis in hypothermia requires the judicious use of sodium bicarbonate. Respiratory acidosis improves with restoration of ventilation, and to some extent, rewarming reverses metabolic acidosis as circulation is reestablished and normal metabolism returns. However, severe acidosis with cardiopulmonary arrest requires sodium bicarbonate in this particular situation of hypothermia. Extremes of acidosis and temperature make the heart resistant to many cardiac medications and maneuvers. Sympathomimetic amines have little effect below a pH of 7.15. If ventricular fibrillation is present, electrical defibrillation may not be effective. It is worthwhile to try defibrillation or cardioversion initially when the cardiac rhythm indicates such methods. If this is unsuccessful, further efforts should await rewarming of the patient to approximately 90–95°F (32.2–35°C).

Volume requirements vary. Patients with rapidly developing hypothermia after an immersion accident of short duration can have minimal volume needs. Blood pressure and organ perfusion often respond to rewarming alone. However, patients with hypothermia of longer duration or with underlying cardiac disease have high volume requirements. Third space volume loss often occurs, and invasive physiologic monitoring is required as the transition from emergency department to intensive care unit takes place. Placement of a central venous pressure or pulmonary artery line, however, may be associated with a risk of ventricular ectopy as the cold ventricle is stimulated by these lines. Under ideal circumstances, initial temperature resuscitation should be underway before these lines are placed.

Cardiopulmonary resuscitation is initiated in any hypothermic patient with asystole or ventricular fibrillation or tachycardia, but there is controversy over the initiation of CPR in severe hypothermia with an electrically organized but hemodynamically ineffectual cardiac rhythm. With slow atrial fibrillation or a nodal bradycardia, for example, the initiation of CPR at patient temperatures below 83°F (28.3°C) may convert the rhythm to ventricular fibrillation. In this circumstance, rewarming therapy precedes and may obviate the need for hemodynamic support by CPR. Airway management and ventilation, however, must be provided. At temperatures above 83°F (28.3°C) CPR may be initiated as needed with a lessened risk of ventricular dysrhythmias.

Rewarming Therapy. Specific rewarming therapy also continues to be controversial. In passive external rewarming, the patient is moved from the cold environment, protected from further heat loss by blankets, and allowed to warm slowly by normal body metabolism. Active external rewarming involves warming blankets or a heated bath, whereas active core rewarming attempts to warm the central circulation with hemodialysis, peritoneal dialysis, heated intravenous fluids, heated nebulized oxygen, and/or cardiopulmonary bypass.

Although all these methods have been used, no controlled randomized study has evaluated these techniques and their application. Passive external rewarming is slow, but for patients with mild hypothermia and a temperature higher than 95°F (35°C) without hemodynamic compromise, this may be sufficient. Those opposing active external rewarming argue that peripheral vasodilation may worsen hypotension and shock as the hypothermic heart and central circulation fail to meet the needs of the periphery. This type of rewarming has also been associated with "core temperature afterdrop," a phenomenon in which the core temperature decreases as the central circulation receives cold perpheral blood.

The emergency physician should evaluate each patient carefully in an effort to apply the most appropriate therapy available. In the emergency department, peritoneal dialysis is readily available to provide core rewarming. Dialysate tubing can be heated with a blood-warming coil, or dialysate in bottles heated to 113°F (45°C) can be used. Intravenous crystalloid, colloid, and blood products should also be warmed to 104°F (40°C) before administration. Oxygen heated to a temperature from 107.6 to 114.8°F (42 to 46°C) at the mouth can be applied via face mask or endotracheal tube. Gastric lavage with warmed saline solution has the early disadvantage of requiring a nasogastric tube, which may initiate ventricular ectopy. In extreme, resistant cases, open chest CPR, bathing the mediastinum in warmed physiologic saline, has been tried, but this invasive approach is not likely to be necessary when other core rewarming techniques are available nor is it advisable in the emergency department.

In severe hypothermia in which the temperature is less than 86°F (30°C) or in the presence of cardiopulmonary arrest, active core rewarming is the most rational approach. In peritoneal dialysis, for example, potassium-free 1.5% dialysate can be rapidly instilled and removed, providing a definite improvement in temperature in six to eight exchanges. The use of heated intravenous fluids and heated oxygen in the airway are adjunctive techniques while CPR is continued. Hemodialysis and cardiopulmonary bypass require preparation not available in the emergency department or even in some hospitals. Cardiopulmonary bypass, when available, however is the treatment of choice in the arrested patient.

When hemodynamics are stable and hypothermia

Table 10.5.
Treatment of Hypothermia

Condition	Temperature	Treatment
Mild hypothermia, stable cardiovascular status	T ≥ 95°F (35°C)	Passive rewarming, ± external rewarming
Moderate hypothermia, stable cardiovascular status, brief immersion injuries	T ≥ 90°F (32.2°C)	Active external rewarming, ± noninvasive core rewarming (i.v. heated O_2)
Severe hypothermia, unstable cardiovascular status, or cardiorespiratory arrest	T < 86–90°F (30–32.2°C)	Active core rewarming, CPR if arrested, defibrillation when T ≥ 95°F, CPR as needed when T > 83°F

is not severe [temperature from 90 to 95°F (32.2 to 35°C)], a combination of core rewarming (heated intravenous fluids and heated oxygen mask) and active external rewarming (warming blankets) is acceptable unless cardiac rhythm abnormalities develop, temperature decreases, or hypotension worsens. Table 10.5 summarizes these treatment methods.

Although there are no definitive guidelines regarding the duration of resuscitation in severe hypothermia, survival without major sequellae has occurred after asystole of 2 hours and ventricular fibrillation of 2–3 hours. Survival in these cases is related to the slowing of metabolic demands and to the protective effect of hypothermia on vital organ function. Within this time frame, the emergency physician should make every effort to restore approximately normal temperature before discontinuing resuscitation efforts.

When hemodynamics are stable and temperature is improved, complete assessment and treatment of other organ dysfunction can take place, with particular attention to frostbite injury, trauma, pneumonia, pancreatitis, and underlying diseases that may have precipitated or contributed to the hypothermic state.

DROWNING AND NEAR-DROWNING

At least 8000 drownings and many additional near-drownings occur annually in the United States. About 80% of these incidents are preventable, associated with faulty adult supervision or inadequate protective barriers (40% of deaths are in children under 4 years in bathtubs, pails, and backyard pools), alcohol and drug use, overestimation of swimming skills, and underestimation of environmental hazards.

Definitions

Drowning is defined as asphyxia and death resulting from submersion in fluid; near-drowning is survival for at least 24 hours after asphyxia due to submersion. Two other types of submersion injury are immersion hypothermia, which can occur with or without drowning, and the rare "immersion syndrome," in which ventricular fibrillation is precipitated by a sudden plunge into cold water. Some individuals, particularly young children, may be transiently protected from cerebral hypoxia by an active diving reflex, in which immersion in cold water produces bradycardia and intense vasoconstriction of all but coronary and cerebral blood vessels, temporarily preserving blood flow to the heart and brain despite the absence of respiration.

Pathophysiology

Two types of pathophysiology have been observed in drownings. In 10–20% of victims, "dry drowning" occurs, in which laryngospasm results in asphyxia and the glottis relaxes only after respiratory efforts have ceased; thus, no fluid is aspirated. In most cases, however, "wet drowning" occurs, in which variable amounts of fluid are aspirated. "Secondary drowning" refers broadly to the development of respiratory distress syndrome following survival after submersion; this may begin from 1 to 72 hours later.

The immediate result of submersion is asphyxia: Po_2 rapidly decreases, Pco_2 increases, and a combined metabolic and respiratory acidosis develops. Although much has been made of the difference between fresh and salt water drownings, only rarely is enough fluid (22 ml/kg) aspirated to cause clinically significant volume or electrolyte abnormalities. When fresh water is aspirated, the hypotonic fluid is quickly absorbed through the pulmonary capillary membrane, resulting in a washout of lung surfactant and subsequent alveolar collapse, intrapulmonary shunting, and hypoxemia. Since salt water is hypertonic to plasma, when it is aspirated, the osmotic gradient favors transudation of fluid into the alveoli, leading to pulmonary edema, intrapulmonary shunting, and hypoxemia. Hypertonic fluid also causes direct damage to the pulmonary capillary membrane with resultant leakage of plasma proteins into alveoli. Impurities and particulate matter, such as mud, sewage, detergents, chlorine, or vomitus, may be aspirated along with the water and add to the pulmonary insult. Despite the different mechanisms of pulmonary injury, the net result is ventilation-perfusion mismatch, intrapulmonary shunting, and hypoxemia.

In the rare case in which a large amount of fresh water is aspirated (more than 22 ml/kg), the metabolic abnormalities that can occur include decrease in serum sodium, chloride, calcium, and magnesium levels; volume overload; intravascular hemolysis leading to hyperkalemia, hemoglobinemia, and hemoglobinuria with potential hemoglobinuric renal failure; and disseminated intravascular coagulation. With salt water aspiration, hemoconcentration and hypovolemia can be seen, especially if a large volume of water has also been swallowed and absorbed through the gastrointestinal tract.

Aside from direct pulmonary damage from fluid aspiration and occasional metabolic abnormalities, the effects of drowning and near-drowning on the heart, kidneys, and brain are those of anoxia. The two most important prognostic factors for survival with good neurologic function are the duration of the anoxic episode (length of submersion plus time until effective CPR is begun) and the temperature of the water. In warm water submersion, several factors indicate a poor prognosis: submersion for more than 5 minutes, no CPR for 10 minutes, a pH less than 7.10 on arrival at the hospital, a continuing need for CPR in the emergency department, the presence of deep coma, and especially the presence of fixed dilated pupils. The profound protective effect of hypothermia on brain function is being increasingly appreciated, and the same prognostic factors cannot be applied to submersion in cold water. Many instances of full neurologic recovery after submersion in cold water for 20–40 minutes now have been reported, even when fixed dilate pupils were present on admission. Thus, vigorous attempts at resuscitation and rewarming are warranted in victims of cold water submersion, even when it is prolonged.

Treatment

Emergency treatment should begin with mouth-to-mouth resuscitation as soon as the rescuer reaches the victim, even before removal from the water. If a neck injury is suspected, the cervical spine should be immobilized. CPR and advanced life support, if available, should be instituted at the scene and continued en route. On arrival in the emergency department, vital signs should be checked, including an accurate temperature measurement and determination of pupil size. If the patient is in cardiopulmonary arrest, the usual advanced life support protocol (Table 10.6) should be instituted, with the addition of rewarming if hypothermia is present.

The indications for endotracheal intubation in a victim of near-drowning who has regained spontaneous respiration include coma with inability to protect the airway, the presence of copious secretions or gross aspiration of particulate matter, and an arterial P_{CO_2} over 45 mm Hg or an arterial P_{O_2} under 80–90 mm Hg on 40% oxygen by mask. Pulmonary drainage, though useful in dog studies, is not indicated. It interferes with CPR and has minimal benefit in humans where smaller amounts of fluid are aspirated. Intubated patients should be

Table 10.6.
Steps in Treatment of Near-drowning

Establish airway, breathing, and circulation (cardiopulmonary resuscitation, advanced life support)
Check for hypothermia; if present, begin rewarming
Perform appropriate laboratory tests
- Complete blood cell count
- Blood urea nitrogen, creatinine, calcium, magnesium, and electrolytes
- Arterial blood gases
- Prothrombin time
- Partial thromboplastin time
- Urinalysis
- Electrocardiogram
- Sputum culture

Place nasogastric tube
Obtain chest x-ray film
Perform adjunctive pulmonary therapy
- Ventilation with positive end-expiratory pressure
- Bronchodilation with aminophylline, inhaled or parenteral β-adrenergic agents
- Chest physical therapy and suction
- Bronchoscopy for gross aspiration of particulate matter

Correct fluid and electrolyte abnormalities
Place Foley catheter if indicated
Consider early transfer for intensive cerebral resuscitation
Admit and observe any patient with a significant episode of submersion and aspiration

maintained on a volume ventilator with positive end-expiratory pressure (the amount titrated for each patient). If the patient has spontaneous respiration, intermittent mandatory ventilation with continuous positive airway pressure may be tried, adjusting the Fio_2 to maintain an adequate arterial Po_2. In awake, cooperative patients with borderline blood gas levels, continuous positive airway pressure with a tight-fitting mask may be tried in an attempt to avoid intubation. A nasogastric tube should be placed, since a large amount of water and air could have been swallowed, further compromising ventilation. Blood samples should be obtained for a complete blood cell count, platelet count, and determination of electrolytes, blood urea nitrogen, creatinine, calcium, magnesium, prothrombin time, and partial thromboplastin time. The urine should be tested for hemoglobin. A chest x-ray film should be obtained, with the realization that in 25% of patients with significant pulmonary problems the initial chest x-ray film is normal. Thus, regardless of the chest x-ray findings, an arterial blood gas sample should be obtained. Most patients have radiographic evidence of perihilar or generalized pulmonary edema in the early hours, which later evolves to focal atelectasis or infiltrates.

Once the airway and adequate ventilation are assured, adjunctive therapy to improve gas exchange further should be instituted. This includes standard doses of aminophylline and inhaled or parenteral β-adrenergic agents to treat bronchospasm, chest physical therapy, and suction. When aspiration of particulate matter such as vomitus or mud is suspected, early bronchoscopy should be considered. Prophylactic administration of antibiotics or corticosteroids is not generally considered beneficial in the treatment of the pulmonary complications of near-drowning. Rather, initial and daily sputum cultures are recommended to guide antibiotic treatment should infectious complications develop.

An integral part of assessment and treatment is consideration of possible predisposing factors such as head trauma, cervical spine injury, alcohol or drug intoxication, seizure disorder, arrhythmia, suicide attempt, or child abuse. The prognosis for meaningful recovery after near-drowning has improved in recent years because of the increased availability of centers equipped to carry out intensive cerebral resuscitative measures such as intracranial pressure monitoring, controlled hypothermia, administration of barbiturates, mannitol, and corticosteroids, and careful fluid management to maximize intracranial perfusion pressure. The emergency physician should consider early transfer to such a unit if it seems indicated.

Since it often takes hours for the pulmonary complications of fluid aspiration to develop, all patients who have had a significant episode of submersion and aspiration should be observed at least 24 hours.

BAROTRAUMA AND DECOMPRESSION SICKNESS[1]

With the increasing popularity of scuba diving as a sport, diving-related emergencies will be more frequently encountered by the emergency physician. In sport scuba, the diver breathes air from a pressurized tank through a regulator that delivers air at the ambient pressure, which depends on the depth of the dive.

Physics Principles

To understand the causes and treatment of medical problems related to scuba diving, the emergency physician must be familiar with certain principles of physics concerning gases and pressure. The pressure at sea level is 760 mm Hg, defined as 1 atmosphere (atm). Each 33 feet of seawater (fsw) exerts 1 additional atm, so the pressure at a depth of 33 feet is 2 atm, and at 66 feet is 3 atm. Boyle's law states: "at a constant temperature, the volume of a given mass of gas is inversely proportional to its pressure," that is, $PV = K$, where K is a constant. Dalton's law states: "in a mixture of gases, the pressure exerted by each gas is the same as it would exert if it alone occupied the same volume, and the total pressure is the sum of the partial pressures of the component gases." As ambient pressure increases, the partial pressures of the component gases increase proportionately although their percentage in the gas mixture remains constant. For example, at sea level, the partial pressure of oxygen is 160 mm Hg (0.21×760 mm Hg). When air is breathed at 2 atm (33 fsw), the partial pressure of oxygen is 319 mm Hg (0.21×1520 mm Hg), and so on. Henry's law states: "at a given temperature, the amount of gas dissolved in a solvent is proportional to the pressure of the gas in equilibrium with the solvent." These laws form the basis of diving physiology and an understanding of diving emergencies.

Barotrauma

Barotrauma, the most common medical problem of divers, refers to injuries that result from changes in ambient pressure. Barotrauma, but not decompression sickness, may occur in shallow water. Numerous such injuries have occurred in swimming pools less than 12 feet deep. Because of their water content, body tissues are relatively incompressible,

[1]The original text of this section (Edition 2) was written by Eleanor T. Hobbs, M.D.

but air-filled spaces such as the middle ear, sinuses, respiratory tract, and to some extent the gastrointestinal tract are compressible and behave according to Boyle's law (PV = K).

Descent

During descent, as ambient pressure increases, unventilated air spaces such as the middle ear and sinuses are "squeezed" unless pressure in these spaces is equilibrated with ambient pressure. Divers are usually able to "equilibrate" by using various maneuvers to open the eustachian tubes. If pressure is not equilibrated, the diver experiences ear pain, followed by edema, hemorrhage into the middle ear, and ultimately, *rupture of the tympanic membrane,* a syndrome referred to as "middle ear squeeze." Otoscopic examination shows petechiae, blebs, and erythema of the tympanic membrane, and in more severe cases, gross hemorrhage or rupture. Treatment includes a systemic decongestant such as pseudoephedrine hydrochloride, 30–60 mg every 6 hours, nasal decongestant drops, and avoidance of further diving until symptoms have abated and the patient can easily equilibrate. Some physicians recommend prophylactic antibiotics to prevent bacterial otitis media. Patients with a ruptured tympanic membrane should receive antibiotics and be referred to an otolaryngologist for follow-up treatment.

A rarer injury that can occur during descent, usually as a result of a Valsalva's maneuver, is *rupture of the round window,* resulting in vertigo, tinnitus, and neurosensory hearing loss. When decompression sickness does not appear to be a likely cause of these symptoms, an otologic cause should be suspected. Treatment of round window rupture includes bed rest with the head elevated, avoidance of straining and noseblowing, and referral for evaluation by an otolaryngologist. Other forms of barotrauma of descent are *barosinusitis and barodontalgia,* usually associated with air pockets from carious teeth or recent dental work. Neither requires specific treatment.

Ascent

Barotrauma of ascent occurs when air spaces in the body expand as ambient pressure decreases. The most serious situation is pulmonary barotrauma. Overdistention of the lung may cause extravasation of air across alveolar membranes or frank lung rupture. Normally, a scuba diver prevents the development of such a gradient by continuously exhaling on ascent. If a diver holds his or her breath during ascent, or if there is air trapped in the lungs because of pulmonary disease, lung rupture may occur. There are four clinical presentations of lung rupture, which can occur singly or in combination and which are usually apparent immediately on surfacing from a dive. (*a*) Pneumothorax results from rupture of the visceral pleura. (*b*) Subcutaneous emphysema occurs as extravasated air tracks up the mediastinum into the neck. Mediastinal air may even dissect into the pericardium. Symptoms include hoarseness, dysphagia, dyspnea, syncope, and/or shock. Physical examination and radiologic evaluation confirm the presence of subcutaneous and mediastinal air. (*c*) Pulmonary tissue damage is manifested by cough, hemoptysis, and dyspnea as a result of widespread alveolar rupture. Finally, (*d*) air embolism occurs if air dissects into the pulmonary veins and is embolized into the systemic circulation, causing local vascular obstruction and infarction. Although any organ may be affected, the two most serious syndromes are cerebral air embolism, which presents as stroke, and coronary embolism with the typical symptoms of a myocardial infarction.

Treatment of suspected *air embolism* includes placing the victim on the left side with the head 30° lower than the feet, administration of 100% oxygen by mask *without* positive pressure, and rapid transport to a hyperbaric chamber for definitive treatment. Information about the location of the nearest hyperbaric chamber can be obtained by calling Brooks Air Force Base, San Antonio, TX (512-536-3281). If air transport is required, it is important that the patient be kept at an ambient pressure as close to 1 atm as possible by use of a low-flying or pressurized aircraft. Hyperbaric therapy has several effects. It reduces the size of emboli, allowing distal movement and speedier resolution. The use of 100% oxygen at 2.5 atm speeds the diffusion of inert nitrogen from the emboli, further enhancing resolution. Therapy in a hyperbaric chamber needs to be managed by someone familiar with the appropriate treatment schedules. Any patient with a pneumothorax should have a chest tube placed prior to hyperbaric therapy. Some authors recommend hyperbaric oxygen therapy for all divers with a head injury or near-drowning episode, electing to assume the incident was precipitated by an air embolus. Adjunctive measures for cerebral resuscitation, such as controlled hypothermia, corticosteroids, and mannitol, may be initiated in cases of severe cerebral air embolism.

Treatment of other forms of pulmonary barotrauma depends on the severity of symptoms. The patient should receive 100% oxygen by mask, since this will speed the diffusion of inert nitrogen from the abnormal gas pockets. Positive pressure should not be used since it may force additional gas into tissues. Pneumothorax requires thoracostomy tube drainage. Other general supportive measures are instituted as necessary.

Decompression Sickness

Pathophysiology

Decompression sickness, commonly known as "the bends," is caused by bubble formation within tissues and blood vessels, occurring under conditions of supersaturation. Gas that has been dissolved in tissue during a period of increased ambient pressure, according to Henry's law, will come out of solution and form bubbles when ambient pressure is decreased, that is, during ascent. Intravascular bubbles cause mechanical vascular obstruction with local ischemia. A variety of hematologic changes is initiated, most notably activation of the coagulation system and stimulation of platelet aggregation. The effect of extra vascular bubbles is not well-understood. Limb discomfort or actual pain is possible. Since the oxygen in air is constantly being utilized, it is inert nitrogen that causes the problem of supersaturation. The amount of nitrogen dissolved in body tissues during a dive depends on both time and pressure, in other words, the length and depth of the dive. The United States Navy Standard Air Decompression Tables, which should be familiar to all divers, establish guidelines for the depth and duration of a dive or series of dives, which, if observed, prevent decompression sickness in most divers. However, even with strict adherence to the guidelines, some divers will be afflicted.

Decompression sickness is divided into two clinical categories. Type I decompression sickness involves skin or joint symptoms, so-called skin-only or pain-only bends. Type II decompression sickness involves critical organ effects such as in the central nervous system and lungs.

Symptoms

Symptoms of decompression sickness may occur during ascent, particularly if ascent is at a rate of more than 60 feet/min, but they more commonly begin shortly after surfacing and evolve gradually over a period of several hours. Joint pain is a common symptom of decompression sickness. Shoulders, elbows, and any recently injured joint, such as a sprained ankle, are the most commonly affected in sport scuba. The pain usually is described as a steady ache or boring pain, the joint appears normal, range of motion is preserved, and x-ray films are unrevealing. Cutaneous symptoms include itching and burning. The skin characteristically appears mottled.

Central nervous system involvement can be in either the spinal cord or the brain. Spinal cord ischemia is thought to be caused by bubbles in the venous vertebral plexus, leading to stasis, obstruction to blood flow, and edema. The white matter of the cord, especially thoracic, upper lumbar, and lower cervical segments, most commonly is affected. The usual symptoms are transient back pain followed by lower extremity paresthesia, weakness, ataxia, and finally, urinary retention and paralysis. Brain involvement may present as a stroke or with subtle manifestations such as vertigo, difficult to differentiate from barotrauma. Pulmonary symptoms, which divers often refer to as "chokes," are thought to be caused by widespread bubble obstruction to pulmonary blood flow. These patients have dyspnea, chest pain, and other signs and symptoms of acutely increased pulmonary arterial pressure. Initially, it may be impossible to differentiate between chokes and pulmonary barotrauma.

Treatment

The initial treatment of type II decompression sickness is the same as that for suspected air embolism. This is fortunate, since early in the course of illness it may be difficult to distinguish the two. The patient should be positioned on the left side with the head 30° lower than the feet. 100% oxygen should be administered by mask, and arrangements made for transport to the nearest available hyperbaric chamber for recompression therapy. If air transport is necessary, it must be accomplished with as little decrease in ambient pressure as possible. Cardiopulmonary and circulatory support may be required. In addition, neurologic decompression sickness appears to improve with hydration (lactated Ringer's solution or normal saline, avoiding 5% dextrose in water (D_5W). It is routinely treated with corticosteroids. The importance of recompression therapy cannot be overemphasized, even when treatment has been delayed or a chamber is several hours away. Patients may show improvement even when neurologic deficits have been present for as long as 24 hours. When the diagnosis of decompression sickness is under consideration, it is always safer to initiate recompression therapy.

Although type I decompression sickness with joint pain only is less of an emergency, it should also be treated with recompression therapy. Skin-only bends can be treated without recompression, but the patient and physician must remain alert to the possible development of more serious symptoms in the ensuing hours.

SMOKE INHALATION

Pulmonary complications of smoke inhalation are usually associated with body burns, but may occur in isolation. It is estimated that more than half of the deaths due to fire are attributable to the effects of smoke inhalation.

Pathophysiology

Six mechanisms of respiratory compromise may be seen in victims of fire. (*a*) Early death due to asphyxia may occur as a result of breathing smoke—a gas with a variably reduced concentration of oxygen and increased concentrations of carbon dioxide and carbon monoxide. (*b*) Upper airway obstruction may develop within hours of exposure, as heat and noxious particulate matter and gases incite pharyngeal and laryngeal edema. (*c*) Circumferential thoracic burns can produce severe ventilatory restriction that must be relieved by escharotomies. (*d*) Carbon monoxide poisoning, and probably cyanide poisoning, frequently is associated with smoke inhalation and contributes to morbidity. (*e*) Inhalation injury, which in its narrower sense refers to the occurrence of either chemical tracheobronchitis or injury to small airways and alveoli as a result of exposure to smoke, may lead to progressive respiratory compromise. This serves as a substrate for (*f*) late pulmonary infection, often the cause of death in burn victims.

Pulmonary pathophysiology following smoke exposure can be classified as thermal or chemical. Heat and steam cause direct thermal injury that is usually confined to the supraglottic region, due to the cooling efficiency of the respiratory tract, producing pharyngeal and laryngeal edema, erythema, and blistering. More extensive thermal injury, involving the tracheobronchial tree, may be seen with steam which has 4,000 times the heat capacity of air. Chemical injury, often underestimated, occurs from the inhalation of particulate matter and noxious gases produced during combustion and pyrolysis. The deposition of carbonaceous material impregnated with organic acids and aldehydes causes direct mucosal damage. Exposure to toxic gases, such as chlorine, phosgene, nitrogen dioxide, sulfur dioxide, ammonia, and hydrogen cyanide, initiates a marked inflammatory response in the lung. Pulmonary capillary permeability increases, with leakage of protein-rich fluid into the alveoli and loss of lung surfactant, resulting in pulmonary edema, focal atelectasis, and intrapulmonary shunting.

Clinical Features

Certain historical factors suggest that a victim is at high risk for having sustained a significant inhalation injury. Patients exposed to smoke in a closed space, patients with impaired ability to protect themselves (infants, elderly, infirm, drug- or alcohol-intoxicated individuals, and those with head injuries or loss of consciousness), and patients with previous lung disease must be considered at high risk. Certain types of smoke and fumes are especially noxious, particularly those liberated by the burning or thermal degradation of polyvinyl chloride, which is present in plastics, telephone and electrical cables, and much upholstery.

The patient may complain of a sore throat or substernal burning (a prominent symptom in fires involving polyvinyl chloride). Hoarseness or stridor indicates upper airway edema and the potential for obstruction. Burns about the face and neck, a singed mustache, or singed nasal hairs frequently are associated with inhalation injury. Positive findings on physical examination include tachypnea and tachycardia; erythema, edema, and blistering of the oropharynx; and wheezing, rales, and cough producing carbonaceous sputum. It is important to remember that in some patients with normal findings on initial examination, real inhalation injuries may evolve.

Diagnosis

Certain laboratory and diagnostic tests are helpful in evaluating the presence, extent, and anatomic level of an inhalation injury. Early blood gas measurements with the patient breathing room air can be falsely reassuring—showing mild to moderate hypoxemia or even a normal $Pa{O_2}$, where $PA{O_2}$ is usually low, but may be normal or high. The calculation of an alveolar-arterial oxygen gradient on room air [$P^{(A-a)}O_2 = PA{O_2} - Pa{O_2}$, where $PA{O_2} = 150 - (1.25 \times P{CO_2})$ and $Pa{O_2}$ is that measured] reflects intrapulmonary shunting and increases the sensitivity of room-air arterial blood gas determination. A normal gradient is about 8 mm Hg; a gradient of higher than 28 mm Hg correlates well with inhalation injury documented by other means (see Petroff et al., Suggested Readings). The initial carboxyhemoglobin level is probably a better indicator of the severity of exposure than initial room-air arterial blood gas studies. Measurement of the alveolar-arterial gradient on an $Fi{O_2}$ of 1 increases the sensitivity of blood gas determinations even further. A $Pa{O_2}$ less than 250 mm Hg on 100% oxygen or a gradient that increases over time is highly predictive of significant pulmonary injury and early respiratory insufficiency (see Luce et al., Suggested Readings).

Initial chest x-ray findings are frequently normal, but within 24–48 hours, pulmonary edema and focal atelectasis or infiltrates may be seen. Three additional diagnostic techniques have been used to evaluate further the presence and extent of pulmonary injury. (*a*) Fiberoptic bronchoscopy, which can be performed transnasally at the bedside under local anesthesia, is helpful in assessing both upper and lower airway injury. Positive findings include mucosal erythema, edema, ulceration, hemorrhage, the presence of carbonaceous sputum, and bronchorrhea. For suspected mild injury, simple laryngoscopy may be helpful. (*b*) Xenon-133 ventilation lung scanning has been advocated to assess the presence of injury to small airways and alveoli. Positive results show a delay in clearance or an inequality of clearance of the isotope from the lungs. False-negative results may occur when the scan is obtained within 1–2 hours of exposure, since it often takes several hours for the pulmonary reaction to develop. False-positive results are seen in patients with preexistent obstructive lung disease (see Agee et al., Suggested Readings). (*c*) The most useful pulmonary function test in the assessment of pulmonary injury is the maximum expiratory flow volume curve. Normal spirometry essentially eliminates the possibility of real pulmonary injury. An expiratory flow rate at 50% of vital capacity, which is less than 50% of predicted, correlates highly with other evidence of pulmonary injury (see Petroff et al., Suggested Readings). Analysis of the curve can also be used to follow response to therapy. Unfortunately, spirometry is not always practical since it requires a cooperative patient without severe facial burns. Conventional spirometric measurements may be abnormal, but are less specific.

Treatment

Treatment begins with immediate attention to the upper airway. Experts differ on the timing of intubation in patients whose airway initially is patent but who have signs of upper airway injury and who are at risk for later obstruction. Some favor early prophylactic intubation; others, waiting until signs of early obstruction develop. Definite indications for intubation include upper airway obstruction, impaired consciousness with inability to protect the airway, elevated $Paco_2$, and hypoxia despite supplemental oxygen. Nasotracheal intubation is preferred. Tracheotomy should be avoided, especially in patients with body burns involving the upper body or neck. If a patient who is to be transferred for definitive care has evidence of upper airway injury, it is preferable to intubate the patient before transport (after consultation with the receiving facility). All patients, intubated or not, initially should receive as high a concentration of humidified oxygen as can be achieved to treat potential carbon monoxide poisoning. Ventilated patients should be maintained on positive end-expiratory pressure or continuous positive airway pressure to prevent terminal airway closure. Patients should be encouraged to cough and breathe deeply. Suctioning should be avoided unless absolutely necessary, since it adds to the potential for infection. Therapeutic bronchoscopy may be helpful in patients with copious bronchorrhea and carbonaceous sputum. Bronchodilators, such as aminophylline and β-adrenergic agents, are useful in treating associated bronchospasm. The current consensus is that neither prophylactic antibiotics nor prophylactic corticosteroids are indicated in the management of inhalation injuries. Corticosteroids may actually increase morbidity and mortality (see Moylan, Suggested Readings). Adjunctive measures include placement of a nasogastric tube, prophylactic use of cimetidine to protect against gastric ulceration, avoidance of fluid overload, and hyperbaric oxygen therapy for associated carbon monoxide poisoning.

Cyanide poisoning is being recognized as a frequent complication of inhaled smoke generated from such synthetic materials as nylon, asphalt, and polyurethane. Determination of cyanide levels is impractical, requiring a minimum of 2 hours. Cyanide poisoning may be suspected in patients with high carboxyhemoglobin levels and persistent metabolic acidosis despite treatment with 100% oxygen. The clinical significance of cyanide poisoning and the role of therapy in fire victims are currently unknown. Accordingly, considering the empiric nature and toxicity of treatment, specific therapy should be limited to (*a*) severely injured patients with (*b*) high carboxyhemoglobin levels and (*c*) a clinical presentation or history strongly suggestive of hydrogen cyanide gas exposure.

The decision regarding need for admission and length of observation can be difficult. Some guidelines are presented in Table 10.7, but within this framework, each case needs to be individualized.

CARBON MONOXIDE POISONING

Acute carbon monoxide poisoning accounts for about 3500 deaths per year in the United States and contributes to morbidity and mortality in an unknown number of victims of burns and smoke inhalation.

Pathophysiology

Because carbon monoxide is a colorless, odorless, nonirritating gas, it has been called a "silent killer." It is produced by the incomplete combustion of organic materials and is present in most fires, motor vehicle exhaust, and many factories. Methylene chloride, found in most paint strippers, is metabolized to carbon monoxide once it is absorbed through the skin. With an affinity for hemoglobin about 240 times that of oxygen, carbon monoxide rapidly binds to hemoglobin, forming carboxyhemoglobin. As carboxyhemoglobin levels rise, oxygen-carrying hemoglobin decreases proportionately, impairing oxygen transport. In addition, carboxyhemoglobin shifts the oxyhemoglobin dissociation curve to the left, so the oxygen bound to hemoglobin is less readily released to the tissues. At the cellular level, utilization of oxygen is impaired as dissolved carbon monoxide binds to the iron-containing molecules of the cytochrome system. Organs with the most active cellular metabolism, such as heart and brain, are the most susceptible to injury. Carboxy-

Table 10.7.
Protocol for Management of Victims of Smoke Inhalation

History: risk factors and symptoms
Physical examination: vital signs, body burns, special attention to nasal, oropharyngeal, and chest examinations
Categorization:

- Trivial exposure: Very low-risk history, no symptoms or signs of inhalation, normal vital signs; short emergency department observation and discharge
- Mild exposure: Some risk by history, minimal symptoms, normal physical examination, minimal tachycardia
  - Room-air, arterial blood gas, and carboxyhemoglobin levels
  - Humidified 100% oxygen by facemask
  - Electrocardiogram (especially if suspicious or elevated carboxyhemoglobin level)
  - Chest x-ray examination
  - Spirometry
  - Observe on oxygen for 4–6 hours from time of exposure; if no signs or symptoms develop and arterial blood gas and carboxyhemoglobin levels satisfactory, discharge with warning about possible late complications
  - If signs or symptoms develop, patient is moved up to next category
- Moderate exposure: Moderate-risk history; symptoms or signs such as singed nasal hairs, carbonaceous sputum, cough, tachypnea, tachycardia, wheezing
  - Arterial blood gas and carboxyhemoglobin levels, 100% humidified oxygen, electrocardiogram, chest x-ray examination
  - Admit and observe, follow arterial blood gas levels, perform physical examination, obtain chest x-ray film
  - Perform pulmonary toilet
  - Bronchodilators as needed
  - Consider further diagnostic workup to assess extent of injury: alveolar-arterial gradient, fiberoptic bronchoscopy, Xenon-133 scanning, maximum expiratory flow-volume curve analysis
- Severe exposure: High-risk history, multiple signs and symptoms of upper or lower airway injury
  - Assess need for intubation
  - Arterial blood gas and carboxyhemoglobin levels, 100% humidified oxygen, electrocardiogram, chest x-ray examination
  - Volume ventilator with positive end-expiratory pressure
  - Bronchodilators as needed
  - Nasogastric tube, cimetidine
  - Consider further diagnostic modalities as above

hemoglobin levels may not correlate with clinical status because dissolved carbon monoxide at the cytochrome level, responsible for the inhibition of cellular respiration, is unmeasured.

Clinical Features

The symptoms of carbon monoxide poisoning are those of hypoxia, which are nonspecific. At low levels of carboxyhemoglobin, the only symptom may be dyspnea on exertion or tightness across the head. With levels from 20 to 30%, patients complain increasingly of headache, nausea, fatigue, dyspnea, dizziness, and dimmed vision. As the carboxyhemoglobin level rises, these symptoms become more pronounced and the patient experiences vomiting, confusion, and syncope. Finally, loss of consciousness, seizures, and respiratory arrest develop (Table 10.8). Patients with coronary artery disease may have angina or arrhythmias, even at low carboxyhemoglobin levels.

It is important to remember that the carboxyhemoglobin level measured in the emergency department may be considerably lower than the peak carboxyhemoglobin level if sufficient time has elapsed since exposure or if oxygen has been administered at the scene or during transport. It is the peak level that carries prognostic significance. It should be estimated, if possible.

On physical examination, the patient usually is tachycardiac and may be tachypneic. The classic cherry-red hue of the lips and skin is not a reliable sign. More often, the patient appears pale. Because of the nonspecific and protean manifestations of carbon monoxide poisoning, the physician must maintain a high index of suspicion to avoid missing the diagnosis. Some unusual presentations include multiple family members with the simultaneous onset of what appears to be food poisoning or gastroenteritis, patients who appear intoxicated, and firefighters with angina. Carbon monoxide poisoning should always be assumed in victims of smoke inhalation and in patients with major body burns. Treatment should be started presumptively with a high concentration of oxygen while awaiting the results of blood gas and carboxyhemoglobin determinations. Blood gas studies usually show a normal Pao_2, a low $Paco_2$, and a lower pH than would be predicted by the $Paco_2$, that is, a combined respi-

Table 10.8.
Manifestations of Carbon Monoxide Poisoning

Carboxyhemoglobin Level	Symptoms[a]
≤ 10	Usually none; dyspnea on extreme exertion
11–20	Band-like or throbbing headache, dyspnea on moderate exertion
21–30	More severe headache, throbbing temples, dyspnea on mild exertion, nausea
31–40	All symptoms of previous level, plus visual dimming, dizziness, irritability, vomiting, tachycardia
41–50	All symptoms of previous levels plus tachypnea, dyspnea at rest, syncope
> 50	Coma, seizures, cardiorespiratory depression

[a] Patients with coronary artery disease may have angina at any level.

ratory alkalosis and metabolic acidosis. In most hospital laboratories, the oxyhemoglobin saturation reported with the blood gas analysis is calculated from the Pao_2, and is, thus, grossly incorrect in the presence of an elevated carboxyhemoglobin level. The electrocardiogram may show ischemic changes or ventricular arrhythmias, even when the patient has no cardiac symptoms.

Treatment

Oxygen is the mainstay of treatment. The two major decisions to be made are (*a*) which patients to intubate, and (*b*) when to employ hyperbaric oxygen therapy. The use of hyperbaric oxygen therapy has three major benefits. First, it greatly speeds the rate of carbon monoxide elimination, reducing the half-time for carboxyhemoglobin from 5 to 6 hours on room air to about 5 minutes on 100% oxygen at 3 atm (Table 10.9). Second, breathing 100% oxygen at 2.5–3 atm results in a dissolved oxygen content in plasma of 5.6–6.9 vol %, which is approximately the amount of oxygen extracted by the body under normal conditions (the normal arteriovenous oxygen content difference is 5–6 vol %). Finally, studies suggest a decrease in neurologic sequelae after hyperbaric oxygen therapy. Current indications for hyperbaric oxygen therapy include a carboxyhemoglobin level over 20%, cardiac ischemia or arrhythmias, persistent neurologic deficits, and a history of loss of consciousness. When a chamber is not readily available, awake cooperative patients with a carboxyhemoglobin level less than 40% can be treated with 100% oxygen by mask. Patients who are comatose, uncooperative, or hypoventilating, or who have a carboxyhemoglobin level over 40% require intubation and ventilation on 100% oxygen. Coma or a carboxyhemoglobin level over 40% indicates the need for transfer to a facility with a hyperbaric chamber, if available within a reasonable transfer time. Regardless of the method of oxygen administration, treatment should be continued until carboxyhemoglobin levels are less than 10%. Again, it is important to remember that carboxyhemoglobin levels may not correlate with the degree of carbon monoxide poisoning. Thus, strict reliance on carboxyhemoglobin levels to dictate therapy, without regard to clinical neurologic status, is inappropriate.

In addition to administration of oxygen, an attempt should be made to reduce oxygen demand by keeping the patient quietly at rest, with cardiac monitoring. In severe cases, further measures to reduce oxygen demand and to decrease cerebral edema have been advocated, including controlled hypothermia, corticosteroids, and fluid restriction.

Complications of carbon monoxide poisoning include late neuropsychiatric sequelae, and rarely, rhabdomyolysis with or without myoglobinuric renal failure as a result of either myonecrosis or generalized muscle hypoxia.

RADIATION ACCIDENTS

Basic Concepts

The primary purpose of this section is to provide the necessary information for treatment, at the emergency department level, of accident victims who may be contaminated with radioactive materials or who may have been exposed to high levels of radiation. Accidental radiation exposure may occur outside the hospital (as a result of a transportation or industrial accident, or use of atomic weapons, for example) or within the hospital in situations in

Table 10.9.
Half-life of Carboxyhemoglobin

Fio_2	PAo_2 mm Hg	Carboxyhemoglobin Half-time	Dissolved Oxygen (vol %)
0.21 (room air)	160	5–6 hr	0.3
1.0 at 1 atm (sea level)	760	80 min	2.09
1.0 at 3 atm (hyperbaric chamber)	2280	25 min	6.9

Table 10.10.
Ionizing Radiation Current Nomenclature

The recent adoption of special names and abbreviations for some units of the Systeme d'Unites International (SI) for use in the field of ionizing radiation follow:

Gy = Gray	=	SI unit for absorbed dose
SV = Sievert	=	SI unit for dose equivalent
Bq = Bequerel	=	SI unit for activity

To convert from one set of units to another, the following relationships are utilized

1 rad = 0.01 Gy = 10 mGy	=	1 cGy
1 rem = 0.01 Sv = 10 mSv	=	1 cSv
1 curie = 3.7 × 10^{10} Bq; 1 Bq	=	1 dps (disintegrations per second)

which radiation is utilized (as in the use of radiopharmaceuticals, radiotherapy, or diagnostic x-rays). The emergency department team should be well versed in the protocol for treating victims of a radiation accident. Realistic understanding of the biologic risks to themselves when treating these patients is also a necessity.

When radiation interacts with tissue, the atoms of the tissue become ionized. Ionization occurs when an orbital electron absorbs enough energy from radiation to escape all orbits around the atomic nucleus. The resultant "ion pair" consists of a free electron ("−" charge) and the ionized atom ("+" charge). Machines are one source of ionizing radiation (x-rays, γ-rays, and electrons); radionuclide decay is another (β-particles, x-rays, and γ-rays, for example). Nuclear reactors and cyclotrons generate more potent forms of ionizing radiation, such as neutrons and protons.

The number of ion pairs produced is a function of the intensity of the radiation interacting with the tissue. The greater the number of ion pairs produced, the greater the potential for biologic damage. The unit of biologic absorbed dose is the rad (Table 10.10) When corrections are made relative to the biologic effectiveness of the radiation in question (quality factor), the resultant unit is the rem: rem = (rad) × (quality factor). The quality factor for β-particles, x-rays, and γ-rays equals 1; for neutrons and protons, it is approximately 10. Therefore, a 10-rad dose of γ-rays equals 10 rem, and a 10-rad dose of neutrons equals 100 rem. A more common unit is the millirem (mrem) or millirad (mrad), which is 0.001 times the value of the rem and rad, respectively. To put these units into perspective, consider that the average whole-body dose from background radiation (natural and artificial) in the United States is approximately 200 mrem/year, a round-trip flight between Boston and London results in a whole-body dose of approximately 5 mrem, and a routine anteroposterior chest x-ray examination results in an entrance skin dose of approximately 20 mrem.

Persons who work with radiation are considered "occupationally exposed," and are permitted radiation exposure above that produced by background. The maximum permissible dose is the amount of ionizing radiation established by authorities below which there is no reasonable expectation of risk to human health. Table 10.11 lists maximum permissible doses for the general public and for occupationally exposed individuals as a function of organ type. The greater the radiosensitivity of an organ, the less its maximum permissible dose.

Radiation can be detected and measured with suitable equipment. The most common instrument for this purpose in the emergency department is a portable survey meter with an end-window Geiger-Müller (GM) probe to differentiate between particulate radiation (α and β-particles) and photons (x-rays and γ-rays). Particulate radiation is not usually detected when internally deposited, whereas photons traverse the tissue layers for subsequent detection. The meter should read directly in mrem units over a wide range, and it should be calibrated periodically to ensure its accuracy. It should be used

Table 10.11.
Maximum Permissible Doses of Ionizing Radiation per Year (in Adults)

Organ	Dose	
	Occupationally Exposed Persons	General Public
	mrem	
Whole body (including gonads, lens of eye, red bone marrow)	5,000	500
Forearms, hands, feet, and ankles	75,000	7,500
Skin of whole body	30,000	3,000

to monitor patients, personnel, and spaces within the emergency department.

The Radiation Accident

A radiation accident that qualifies for rapid medical treatment is defined as any unforeseen, unplanned, or unexpected event that causes acute whole- or partial-body radiation exposure with or without radioactive contamination. The radiation dose is usually large enough to result in injury, and when the individual is contaminated (internally or externally or both), rapid removal of the radioactive material is of primary importance.

Radiation accidents, therefore, can be divided into three basic categories: (*a*) single external radiation exposure; (*b*) contamination, either internal or external, with radioactive material; and (*c*) exposure to external radiation plus contamination with radioactive material.

External Exposure

External exposure to radiation produces clinical symptoms only if the dose is sufficient to produce such a response. Exposure to a high dose of radiation over a period up to 24 hours is termed acute exposure.

Acute whole-body radiation affects all systems and organs of the body. The pattern of biologic response is dictated by the intensity of the exposure and is termed acute radiation syndrome. Since all organs and biologic systems are not equally sensitive to ionizing radiation, the syndrome is presented clinically in order of increasing severity by the following categories: (*a*) subclinical (200 rem or less); (*b*) hematopoietic syndrome, mild (200–400 rem) or severe (400–600 rem); (*c*) gastrointestinal syndrome (600–1000 rem); and (*d*) central nervous system syndrome (1000 rem or more).

Biologic effects common to all four categories include nausea and vomiting, malaise, fatigue, increased temperature, and hematologic changes. Table 10.12 lists categories of acute radiation syndrome as a function of increasing whole-body radiation exposure.

The clinical management of acute radiation syndrome is a function of the type and extent of the clinical problems, for example, biologic and physiologic responses. Hospitalization is considered essential if the whole-body dose exceeds 100 rem. After a potentially lethal dose of radiation, the primary reason for hospitalization is to limit infection. Adequate fluid and electrolyte replacement is essential for the management of vomiting and diarrhea. If the possibility exists for rapid spread of infection (as evidenced by prolonged granulocytopenia), it may be necessary to administer antibiotics before identification of the organism and sensitivity studies. Hemorrhage will result from trauma, gastrointestinal denudation, or thrombocytopenia. Transfusions of whole blood or platelets or both may be indicated in the presence of severe anemia and thrombocytopenia.

Since 1945, the literature has reported several radiation accidents that have resulted in injury to individuals. The following are brief descriptions of two serious accidents, resulting from large acute external radiation exposures.

Pittsburgh, Pennsylvania, October 14, 1967: Three technicians employed by the Gulf Research Development Company were accidentally exposed to a high-energy electron beam while attempting to repair the cooling system of a Van de Graaff generator. Because of failure of the safety system, the machine was on without the knowledge of the operators. One hour after exposure, the three men suffered nausea, which they interpreted as a symptom of influenza. However, it soon became evident that they were victims of radiation sickness. One man had received an estimated dose of 6000 rad on his hands and 600 rad on the rest of the body. His life was saved with a marrow transplant from his identical twin. However, gangrene developed in his hands, and seven fingers had to be amputated. The other two men received whole-body doses of 300 and 100 rad, respectively. They suffered only mild radiation sickness and went back to work a few weeks after the accident.

On April 26, 1986, a reactor unit of 1000 megawatts (MW) in the Chernobyl Power Station (USSR) ignited following an explosion. During this episode substantial quantities of radioactive material (fusion products) were released in, near, and throughout Eastern and Western Europe. In fact, the deposition within the reactor building was so intense that bone marrow transplants were used as last resort when treating several exposed workers. United States travelers to the area have been reported to show ^{131}I elevations.

It must be emphasized that individuals exposed to *external* radiation are usually not "radioactive." Rarely, natural body atoms, such as sodium and phosphorus, may become radiactive if the human body absorbs a major dose of neutron radiation.

Contamination

Contamination is defined as the deposition of radioactive material (radionuclides) where the material is not desired and where its presence may be harmful. Radioactive contamination of the body may be either internal or external. The severity of the accident is a function of the type of radionuclide, its physical properties (half-life and decay emissions), and its chemical form. External contamina-

Table 10.12.
Acute Radiation Syndrome Classification

Category	Whole-body Dose, *rem*	Signs and Symptoms		Prognosis
		Early	Definitive	
Subclinical	≤ 200	Mild nausea and vomiting lasting 24 hr or less; lymphocytes > 1500/mm^3	Usually asymptomatic to minimal prodromal symptoms; depression of neutrophils and platelets by week 4–5 at higher dose range	Essentially 100% survival in healthy adults; evidence of some damage at higher dose range
Hematopoietic (mild form)	200–400	Intermittent nausea and vomiting in nearly all patients for 2–4+ days; lymphocytes > 1000/mm^3	Maximum hematopoietic depression at 3 weeks	Recovery in 5–6 weeks; complete recovery in 4–6 months
Hematopoietic (severe form)	400–600[a]	Severe hematopoietic complications; mild evidence of gastrointestinal damage on upper dose range	Severe neutrophil and platelet depression in 3–5 weeks; evidence of infection and hemorrhage may appear	Zero to 100% mortality in untreated cases; requires bone marrow transplants and other supportive measures; rarely fatal with adequate replacement therapy
Gastrointestinal	600–1000	Severe prodromal symptoms of nausea, vomiting, and diarrhea; difficult management of patient; lymphocytes < 500/mm^3	Some recovery, then return of severe diarrhea with blood and electrolyte loss; severe neutrophil and platelet depression by day 10 or earlier; hemorrhage and infection within 1–3 weeks	High mortality even among those given functional replacement therapy; progression to shock and death in 10–14 days; effectiveness of bone marrow therapy not yet evaluated
Central nervous system	≥ 1000	Severe, intractable nausea and vomiting; central nervous system symptoms; burning sensation at exposure and confusion; lymphocytes essentially lacking	Partial recovery, then progressive confusion and shock; central nervous system damage	100% mortality likely independent of therapy given; death in 14–36 hr; marrow therapy trial indicated

[a] The human whole-body LD_{50} at 60 days is approximately 400–500 rem.

tion can involve parts of the body, such as skin or hair, or can be primarily confined to clothing. Internal contamination results when radioactive material enters the body in one of the following ways: (*a*) inhalation—breathing radioactive dust, aerosol, and gas; (*b*) ingestion—drinking contaminated liquids, eating contaminated foods, and transferring radioactivity to the mouth by touch; and (*c*) absorption—absorbing radioactive material through the intact skin or through a wound.

The chemical form of the radionuclide determines the excretion pattern of the compound. For example, more than 70% of orally administered sodium iodide^{-131} is excreted in the urine within 48 hours, with a half-time of 21 hours (Fig. 10.4). Identification of the radionuclide and its chemical form will assist in predicting the biologic behavior of the radioactive material.

If the patient is *contaminated,* he or she is radioactive and represents a radiation source until decontaminated. Emergency department personnel, by increasing their distance from a source of radiation, lower their exposure for a given period. The physical principle that serves as a basis for dose reduction relative to distance is called the "inverse square law." The inverse square law relationship allows calculation of dose rates at any distance from a point source by application of the following equation:

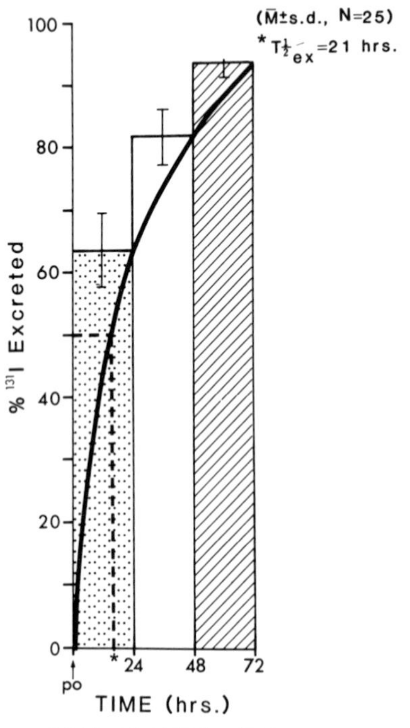

Figure 10.4. ^{131}I cumulative urinary excretion.

$$I_2 = I_1 \left(\frac{X_1^2}{X_2^2}\right)$$

where I_2 = dose rates at distance X_2, and I_1 = dose rates at distance X_1.

Example:

800 rem/hr is measured at 20 cm. Find the dose rate at 80 cm.

$$(800) \left(\frac{(20)^2}{(80)^2}\right) = (800) \left(\frac{400}{6400}\right) = 50 \textit{ rem/hr}$$

If the above equation is used for an extended source of radiation, such as a radioactive patient, it will give a good approximation of the dose rate.

The following is a brief description of an accident that resulted in internal contamination from the inhalation of radioactive material.

A worker inhaled airborne particles containing what must have been a relatively soluble compound of curium-244 (^{244}Cm) during removal of dry, solid, contaminated waste from a decontamination chamber. Filter papers used to smear the vestibules of his nose removed 0.016 μCi (microcurie) from the left nostril and 0.011μCi from the right. His nasal cavity was irrigated with isotonic saline solution, and external skin contamination was removed by swabbing. His lungs were chelated 2.5 hours after the incident with 4 ml of a 25% solution of trisodium diethylenetriaminepentaacetate (DTPA) with a nebulizer. Blood samples were taken for radioassay before and after treatment with DPTA. A catharic was given to hasten passage of the radioactive material through the gastrointestinal tract. About 4.5 hours after the incident, 0.014 μCi of ^{244}Cm was found by measuring the radioactive emissions from the worker's chest. Subsequent measurements showed that the amount of ^{244}Cm rapidly decreased to 0.005 μCi within 4 days.

Emergency Treatment

Types of radiation accident injuries which may be seen in the emergency department include: (*a*) simple trauma (no irradiation or contamination); (*b*) irradiation (without contamination); (*c*) internal contamination (with or without contaminated excreta); (*d*) contaminated wounds (possible hazard to attendants); and (*e*) external contamination (possible hazard to attendants).

Table 10.13 is a checklist of on-site emergency actions after radiation exposure. The sequence of these actions will vary with different accident conditions. Table 10.14 lists questions intended to provide useful medical information once the patient arrives in the emergency department.

The primary goals of the emergency department team are to remove from the victim any further sources of exposure (decontamination) and to pro-

Table 10.13.
On-site Radiation Accident Checklist

1. Provide emergency medical care immediately for serious injuries and preserve vital functions. Minor injuries can wait until after initial radiation survey has been completed.
2. Remove accident victim from contaminated radiation area. For assisting personnel, individual doses up to 100 rem may be permitted for lifesaving purposes, or up to 25 rem for less urgent purposes. Teams may be used in relays to remove injured persons from areas of very high radiation.
3. Survey victim for surface contamination levels.
4. Obtain smears of nasal mucus. Do this before the victim showers.
5. Remove contaminated clothes and replace with clean coveralls or wrap victim in blanket. Take victim to an area where skin can be decontaminated or a shower can be taken.
6. Decontaminate skin. Remove all transferable contamination if possible by cleansing contaminated skin areas and showering the accident victim.
7. Cover contaminated wounds with sterile dressings before and after decontamination.
8. Alert hospital and call for ambulance service as soon as it is determined that it is needed.
9. Identify radionuclide(s) involved, and if possible, ascertain the chemical form, solubility, and presumed particle size.
10. Send radiation dosimeters of involved personnel for processing.
11. Get complete history of accident, especially as it relates to the activities of the victim. Where was he/she? What was he/she doing? Exit path? Symptoms?
12. Evaluate possibility of penetrating radiation exposure.
13. Advise victim on collection of all excreta. Provide containers. Save other contaminated materials in appropriate leak-proof containers.
14. Be sure someone has assumed responsibility for management of the accident area. Is radiation safety assistance needed? Who will request it? From whom?
15. Report initial responses of assisting personnel and evaluation of situation to plant manager.
16. Obtain names of supervisory and health physics personnel who will remain on call in case additional information is needed.
17. Take victim to hospital if injuries require surgical care not available at plant or if further medical or dosimetric evaluation and treatment are required.
18. Take precautions to prevent spread of contamination during transport and movement of victim. Have transport vehicles, attendants, and equipment checked for residual radioactive contamination before release from hospital area.
19. If environmental contamination outside the scene of the accident has occurred, notify public health authorities.
20. Advise family or next of kin about extent of injuries and exposure. Plant management personnel and medical department personnel should agree on proper procedure.
21. Send bioassay specimens for analysis of radioactive content under the supervision of a safety officer. Specify who will receive results.

vide initial treatment for injuries. If contamination with radioactive material is present, decontamination procedures must be vigorously followed to avoid needless and serious spread of radioactive material throughout the hospital. After completion of initial emergency procedures, the team concentrates on additional patient management (Table 10.15).

The primary objective of the diagnostic workup is to determine whether biologically significant radiation exposure is present. If evidence is found, the next objective is to determine the immediate and anticipated biologic damage. As an aid in evaluation of the nature and seriousness of a radiation accident, Figure 10.5 illustrates the extent of injury in patient groups up to 6–9 days after radiation exposure. Clinical manifestations are correlated with patient groups in Table 10.16.

Decontamination

If the radiation accident occurred where there is an in-house physician or health physicist, this individual will often be able to provide specific information concerning the incident. Each patient should be identified with as much information as possible before decontamination is begun (Table 10.17). If a survey meter is immediately available, radiation monitoring should be accomplished. Decontamination room supplies are listed in Table 10.18.

Once the patient is ready for decontamination, procedures should be followed to minimize the radiation hazard to personnel and hospital facilities (Table 10.19). Removal of gross contamination is the recommended initial step in patient decontamination, and may be accomplished by removal of contaminated clothing, washing or removal of contaminated hair, and decontamination of wounds. Patients suspected of contamination should be washed as soon as possible. Useful detergent preparations, in order of increasing strength, are listed in Table 10.20. An intermediate stage in decontamination should include further local decontamination of any wounds and general support measures. Swabs of body orifices should be obtained to deter-

Table 10.14
Emergency Department Checklist[a]

1. When did the accident occur? What were the circumstances, and what were the most likely pathways for exposure? How much radioactive material is potentially involved?
2. What injuries occurred? What potential medical problems may be present besides radionuclide contamination?
3. Are toxic or corrosive chemicals involved in addition to radionuclides? Has any treatment been given for chemical exposure?
4. What radionuclides now contaminate the patient? Where? What are the radiation measurements at the surface?
5. What information is available about the chemistry of the compounds containing the radionuclides? Are they soluble or insoluble? Is there any information about probable particle size?
6. What radioactivity measurements have been made at the site of the accident, for example, air monitoring, smears, fixed radiation monitoring, nasal smear counts, and skin contamination levels?
7. What decontamination efforts, if any, have been attempted? With what success?
8. Have any therapeutic measures, such as administration of blocking agents or isotopic dilution agents, been attempted?
9. Was the victim also exposed to penetrating radiation? If so, what has been learned from processing personal dosimeters, such as film badges, thermoluminescent dosimetry badges, or pocket ionization chambers? If not yet known, when is the information expected?
10. Has clothing removed at the site of the accident been saved in case the contamination on it is needed for radiation energy spectrum analysis and particle-size studies?
11. What excreta have been collected? Where are the samples? What analysis are planned? When will they be performed?

[a] In industrial accidents, the best information is usually obtained from plant personnel, such as the health physicist or occupational physician familiar with the plant and with accident details.

Table 10.15
Guidelines for Patient Management after Completion of Initial Emergency Procedures

1. If there is radionuclide contamination, all exposed persons must be surveyed and decontaminated before additional patient management. If this step is neglected, personnel whose duty is to care for patients may become so contaminated themselves as to be rendered ineffective. Proper protective clothing must be available.
2. In performing decontamination procedures, personnel should wear coveralls or a scrub suit, shoe covers, gloves, cap, and respiratory mask as indicated by initial survey.
   Ambulatory patients
      Spread sheet of paper for patient to stand on. Have patient disrobe, putting clothing in suitable container (bag or wastebasket, for example) for later survey. Perform nose, mouth, and ear wipes. Have patient take shower, resurvey, and repeat procedure until patient is "clean."
   Nonambulatory patient
      Place patient on sheet and remove clothing. Save clothing as above for later survey. Wash patient, resurvey, and repeat procedure until patient is clean.
3. If there is evidence of massive exposure to external radiation, and if large numbers of persons are involved, perform triage. It may be necessary to limit any extensive medical care to moribund patients in order to use available facilities to care for patients whose lives may be saved. Dose estimates of more than 2000 rem for external radiation or more than 2000 rem/hr for radionuclide contamination indicate that little help can be offered. In such instances, contamination of treatment personnel may become a major problem.
4. Put patient in bed, obtain a detailed history, and perform a brief physical examination.
5. Obtain a routine blood cell count. If there has been neutron exposure, obtain an additional 20-ml sample of venous blood.
6. Hospitalize patients with severe nausea and vomiting.
7. No specific therapy is indicated for acute radiation injury within the first few days after exposure.
8. Patients with a dose estimate of less than 100 rads of external radiation do not require major emergency care.
9. Patients who have received external exposure only to α-, β-, γ-, and x-radiation are not radioactive.
10. Patients who have been exposed to neutron radiation are slightly radioactive, but are not hazardous to personnel caring for them.
11. Patients contaminated with radionuclides present a hazard to emergency personnel. The degree of hazard depends on the level and type of contamination.

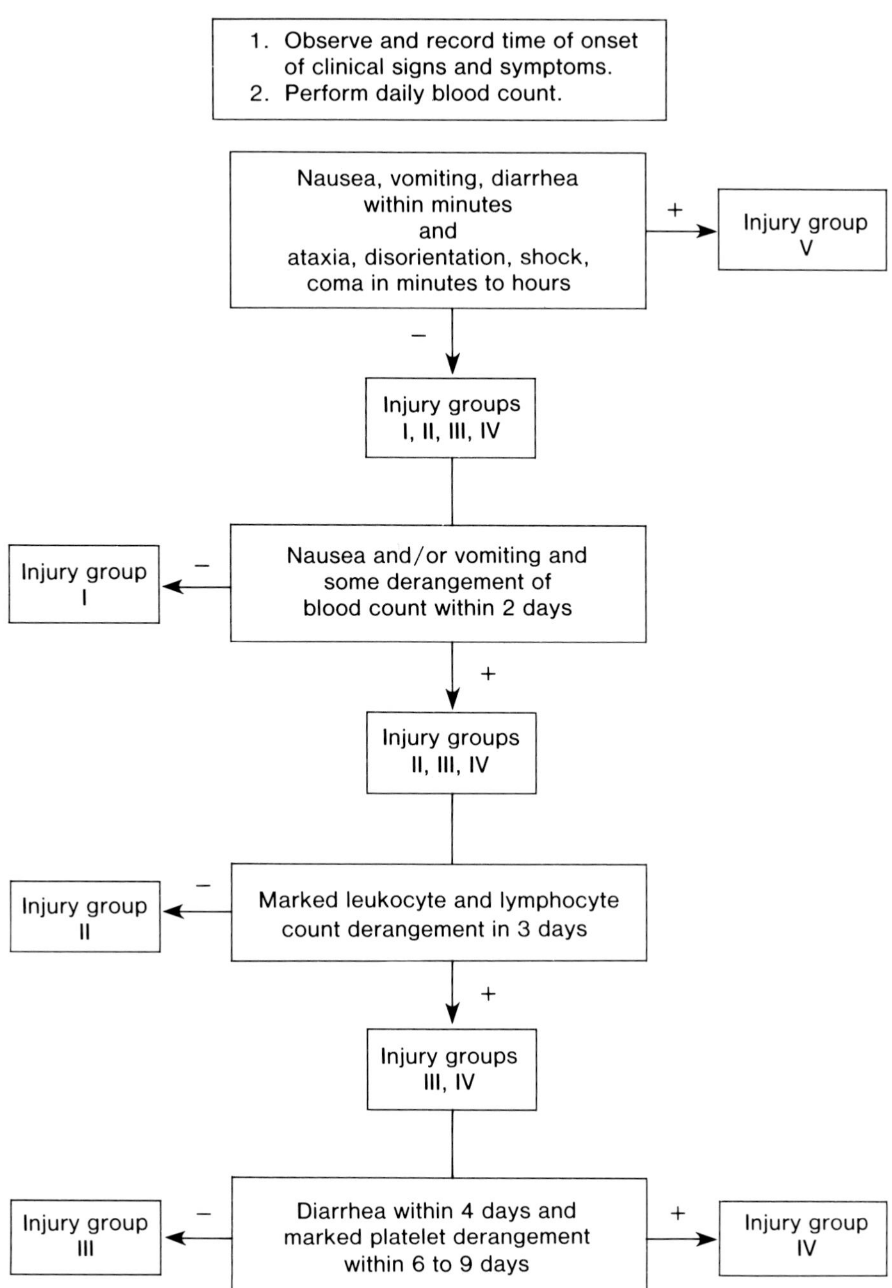

Figure 10.5. Preliminary evaluation of radiation injury with differentiation into patient groups. (Reproduced by permission from Thoma GE Jr., Wald N. The diagnosis and management of radiation injury. *J. Occup Med* 1959;1:421–447.)

mine whether internal contamination is present. More definitive surgical decontamination and other additional treatment might then be necessary.

A case study of a puncture wound contaminated with plutonium follows.

Intensive treatment of a plutonium-contaminated puncture wound in the right forefinger of a 26-year-old worker was effective in preventing major systemic deposits of plutonium in the first year following the injury. An estimated 1300 μCi of α activity

Table 10.16.
Correlation of Patient Groups with Clinical Manifestations of Radiation Injury

Patient Group	Clinical Manifestations
I	Mostly asymptomatic—occasional minimal prodromal symptoms
II	Mild form of acute radiation syndrome—transient prodromal nausea and vomiting, mild laboratory and clinical evidence of hematopoietic derangement
III	A serious course—severe hematopoietic complications, and some evidence of gastrointestinal damage in upper half of group
IV	Accelerated form of acute radiation syndrome—gastrointestinal complications dominate clinical presentation, severity of hematopoietic complications is related to time after exposure
V	Fulminating course with marked central nervous system impairment

(86% ^{239}Pu and ^{240}Pu, 11% ^{241}Am, 3% ^{238}Pu) was locally deposited in the finger by a puncture wound sustained within a glove box. Surgical excision within 7 hours of the injury removed approximately 25% of the activity. A second excision 9 days later removed an additional 50%. DTPA was first administered within 1½ hours of the injury. Daily injections of 1 gm Zn-DPTA were continued for 26 days, then reduced to five injections per week. At 5 months, treatment was reduced to three injections per week, and this frequency continued through 1 year post contaminated injury. Approximately 7% of the locally deposited α activity was excreted in urine during the first 15 days. After 9 months, urinary excretion of plutonium still exceeded 1 μCi/month. Direct in vivo measurements showed that ^{241}Am activity at the wound site appeared to reach a relatively stable level within 3 months following the injury. This case shows the effectiveness of intense chelation therapy over 1 year in preventing measurable systemic deposition. It also provides extensive data on DTPA-enhanced urinary excretion of ^{239}Pu and ^{241}Am, correlated to periodic wound, liver, axillary lymph node, and skull counts. Procedures and techniques used are valuable for management of future minor medical wounds having major radiological implications.

If radioactive contamination is internal, removal may be accelerated by a number of therapies. Radioactive material that has entered the gastrointestinal tract may be removed by administration of an emetic. To reduce tissue uptake, the emergency team may give large quantities of a stable isotope to cause "isotope dilution" or "metabolic blocking." An example of the latter is administration of stable po-

Table 10.17.
Patient Information That Should Be Readily Available to the Treatment Team

Name of patient, employer, employee number

Physical injuries and treatment

Skin surface contamination
- Location
- Dose rate and/or count rate measurements initially and after decontamination
- Decontamination methods and agents used

Internal contamination
- Radionuclide—chemical form, probable solubility, and possible particle character
- Suspected route of contamination
- Nasal smear counts
- Wound counts
- Whole-body counts
- Bioassay samples already collected
- Treatment

External exposure to penetrating radiation
- Precise location and position of patient relative to source of radiation at time of exposure
- Exact time and duration of exposure
- Was dosimeter being worn? Where? What type?
- Has dosimeter been collected? By whom? Where is it now?
- Symptoms—type and time of occurrence
- Other dosimetric studies underway
- Treatment

Name and telephone number of company health physicist or physician for additional information

tassium iodide to block the thyroidal uptake of radioactive iodine isotopes. An increase of fluids will promote rapid turnover and excretion of tritium (^{3}H) if the label is distributed throughout the body as tritiated water. Chelating agents form inactive complexes with certain metal ions that will accelerate the rate of renal excretion of certain radionuclides. They must be administered during the first 24–48 hours for optimum effect, and not all radioactive metals are sensitive to this therapy. A major disadvantage is the nephrotoxic effect of these agents. Bioassay procedures, including the collection of feces, urine, and sputum and the subsequent determination of radionuclide identity and content, as well as in vivo imaging or counting procedures, will assist the clinician in following the biologic release pattern of these radionuclides.

In summary, the medical treatment of a victim of radioactive accident can be a success only if the radiation treatment team is properly instructed. Appropriate use of hospital emergency space should be emphasized, along with methods of isolation, containment of contamination, adequate patient decon-

Table 10.18.
Decontamination Room Supplies

Coveralls or surgical scrub suits
Plastic aprons
Surgical caps
Plastic or rubber gloves
Sterile surgical gloves
Sterile suture sets with additional sterile scissors (2), forceps (4), scalpel (1), and hemostats (6)
Sterile irrigation sets
Sterile applicators and miscellaneous dressings.
Long patient gowns or coveralls, socks
Plastic shoe covers
Large towels
Ribbed or nonskid plastic sheets
Safety razor with extra blades and aerosol shaving soap
Bandage scissors (2)
Large plastic or cloth bags for collection for contaminated clothing
Respirators (prefit for team personnel)
Radiation tags
"Do Not Enter" signs for radiation area
Personal dosimeters (self-reading ionization chambers, 200-mR and 20-R levels) and dosimetry badges (thermoluminescent type)[a]
Masking tape, 2 inches wide
Labeled containers for collecting urine and fecal specimens
Blankets
Adhesive labels and tags for labeling tissue and contaminated material
Tissue specimen bottles (with formalin if freezing facilities are unavailable)
Felt-tipped pens (black for noncontaminated materials, red for contaminated materials).
Notebooks, paper, pencils
Portable radiation survey meters, both low-range (up to 25 mrem/hr) and high-range (up to 500 rem/hr)
Portable α scintillation detector
Large roll 36-inch-wide absorbent (blotter-type) paper or wrapping paper as used in stores (tear-off dispensers are available)
Specific decontamination supplies, with instructions on their use, in a separate labeled box
Detergents
Titanium dioxide (abrasive)
Potassium permanganate (and sodium acid sulfite to remove stain)
Household bleach (5% sodium hypochloride)
Fiberboard barrels or steel drums with tight-fitting tops for disposal of contaminated clothing and other contaminated items

[a] mR, milliroentgens; R, roentgens.

tamination procedures, the cleaning of wounds, and the care of patients who have internal contamination with radioactive material. In addition, emergency department personnel must be aware of the biologic risks when exposed to radiation and must understand basic radiation protection procedures, including the use of radiation detection instruments to monitor patients, personnel, and emergency department spaces.

BITES AND STINGS

More than 500,000 animal bites are reported yearly in the United States and dog bites constitute the largest group (93%). The human victim is usually a 7- to 9-year-old boy, often teasing or playing with the dog. The biting dog is usually 6- to 12-months-old, often female, and a working dog, such as a boxer, collie, German shepherd, Great Dane, or Saint Bernard, or a sporting dog, such as a pointer, setter, or retriever. Hounds are relatively safe.

The evaluation and treatment of all bites involves a careful history, including the type of animal, the site of the bite, and the geographic setting. Hand and puncture wounds become infected most often. Most bites should be cultured and a Gram's stain prepared. The wound should then be washed, irrigated well, and left open if possible. Selection of an antibiotic depends on the bite history and the Gram's stain results. Most patients with deep cat bites, deep cat scratches, and sutured wounds should be treated with penicillin, tetracycline or amoxicillin-clavulanate potassium (Augmentin) because of the increased incidence of infections with *Pasteurella multocida* and anerobic organisms. Dog bites in patients who have had splenectomy should be

Table 10.19.
Decontamination Guidelines for Protection of Hospital Personnel and Facilities

1. Personnel should wear surgical scrub suits of gowns, surgical caps, and rubber gloves. Gloves can be surgical, household, or industrial, depending on their use.
2. The team leader must be able to recognize the rare instance when masks, respirators, or airpacks may be needed because of high levels of α or β radionuclides.
3. Rubber or plastic shoe covers are desirable. Those persons performing the actual decontamination with water should wear plastic or rubber laboratory aprons. Temporary shoe covers for dry areas can be improvised from brown paper bags held on with adhesive or masking tape.
4. Unless a special filter system is available for use during decontamination, air conditioning and forced air heating systems should be turned off so that radioactive particles are not carried into ducts or other rooms.
5. Floors should be protected with a disposable covering both to reduce "tracking" by providing a cleaner surface and to aid cleanup. The covering should be changed when significant contamination is present. Brown paper rolls (36-inch-wide, 60-lb weight) are ideal where water is not used. Ribbed or nonskid plastic sheets are useful where spillage of liquids is a problem.
6. All contaminated clothing should be carefully placed in plastic or paper bags to reduce secondary contamination of area.
7. Splashing of solutions used in decontamination should be avoided.
8. Patients and potentially contaminated personnel should move to clean areas only after survey shows satisfactory decontamination.
9. All persons and property passing between contaminated and clean areas must be surveyed and regulated by monitoring teams.
10. Supplies should be passed through monitoring stations from clean areas to contaminated areas. Reverse flow must not occur unless supplies are monitored and found clean.
11. All persons on the decontamination team must be trained to radiologic monitoring and decontamination techniques. Persons not on the team should be excluded from the work area.
12. Fiberboard or steel drums with tight-fitting tops should be available for disposal of contaminated materials. Labels describing the contents should be affixed so that proper disposal can be carried out without reopening the drums. Lids should be taped to the drums with masking or other sealing tape.
13. All personnel in the decontamination area should have personal dosimeters (pocket ionization chambers, film badges, or thermoluminescent dosimeters). Personnel should be rotated after a dose of 5 rem (or less if possible)
14. Entry of individuals who are not part of the team, including family, visitors, and administrative personnel, should be restricted.

treated with penicillin for potential DF-2 infections. Tetanus immune status should be evaluated, and rabies immunization considered.

Table 10.20.
Detergent Preparations Used in Decontamination of Skin and Wounds

Aqueous preparations
- Soap and water
- Abrasive soap and water
- Commercial detergents (10% active ingredients): Tide, Dreft, Alconox, HemoSol
- Chelating agent (1% versene solution) with or without detergent

Waterless preparations
- Cornmeal and commercial powdered detergent in equal parts made into a watery paste and used without additional water (scrub with brush, remove with cotton or soft tissues)
- Waterless mechanics' hand cream, used without additional water (scrub with brush, remove with cotton or soft tissues)
- Homogenized cream of 8% carboxymethylcellulose, 3% commercial powdered detergent, 1% versene, and 88% distilled water, used without additional water (scrub with brush, remove with cotton or soft tissues)

Human and monkey bites deserve special mention, since 30% become infected with aerobic or anaerobic mouth organisms. Anaerobic infection can spread through the metacarpophalangeal space and cause severe damage. The same procedure should be followed as for other animal bites, that is, culture and Gram's stain, thorough washing, and wide incision. Wounds should be left open if possible, especially in the hand. Patients with human bites should be treated with penicillin, 500 mg four times a day, and dicloxacillin, 500 mg four times a day for 7–10 days. Clenched-fist injuries should be evaluated by a hand surgeon and admission considered for administration of intravenous penicillin and nafcillin.

Disease Caused by Pasteurella multocida

P. multocida is a common organism infecting bite wounds. Disease due to this organism is presently diagnosed more frequently. Thus, its presence in the nasopharynx in 50% of dogs and 75% of cats is of public health importance.

Most infections in humans fall into one of three clinical patterns.

1. The most common pattern is local infection with adenitis after a dog or cat bite or scratch. In patients with a cat bite, this can progress to tenosynovitis or osteomyelitis from inoculation of the organism into the periosteum by the long, sharp tooth of the animal. Canine teeth are more blunt and less likely to penetrate the periosteum.

2. In chronic pulmonary infection, *P. multocida* can occur as the primary pathogen or in association with other organisms. Bacteria may enter through the respiratory tract by inhalation of barn dust or infectious droplets sprayed by the sneeze of an animal. In such cases, the bacteria probably colonize the respiratory tract and lie dormant in patients with chronic lung disease. Acute infection occurs only after trauma to the bronchial tree. Bronchiectasis, emphysema, peritonsillar abscess, and sinusitis have all been described with this organism.

3. Systemic infection with bacteremia or meningitis may occur.

P. multocida is a small Gram-negative ovoid bacillus that grows well on blood agar but not on Gram-negative media, such as MacConkey agar. Because of its superficial resemblance to *Haemophilus influenzae* and *Neisseria* organisms, respiratory tract and central nervous system infections with *P. multocida* initially can be misdiagnosed. Failure of growth on routine Gram-negative media is an important clue.

Treatment of the patient with presumptive *P. multocida* infection (that is, any patient with a deep cat bite or scratch or a deep dog bite) includes careful washing and an attempt to leave the wound open. The antibiotic of choice is penicillin, 1.5 gm/day for 8–10 days orally, with careful follow-up of the wound. Ampicillin, tetracycline, and cephalosporins are alternative antibiotics. Oxacillin and erythromycin are less effective, but still beneficial, whereas clindamycin is least effective.

DF-2

Infections with DF-2 (dysgonic fermenter), a fastidious Gram-negative rod, are typically associated with dog contact or dog bites. There is often a necrotizing eschar at the bite site. Underlying disease or prior splenectomy are factors predisposing to severe infection with potentially fatal outcomes. Long, thin, slowly growing, oxidase-positive, catalase-positive Gram-negative rods that do not grow on MacConkey agar suggest DF-2. The drug of choice is penicillin.

Plague

Infection with *Yersinia pestis* usually results from a flea bite. Urban plague from *Y. pestis* occurs today as an important cycle only in devastated cities such as occurred in Vietnam. Sylvatic plague is the major source in the United States, and the major endemic area is the Southwest. The infected flea vector enters a community of susceptible rodents, such as ground squirrels, prarie dogs, marmots, wood rats, and rabbits, and transmits the bacteria. Mortality in these animals is high and transmission to humans has increased recently, as has been documented in New Mexico, California, Arizona, Colorado, and Utah.

Human plague occurs most often when an individual in a rural area is bitten by an infected flea. Infection also can occur in handling the carcasses of small mammals or by transfer of the vector from a domestic pet. In addition, direct skin contact with an infected mammal (as in skinning rabbits) may also result in infection.

Y. pestis is a Gram-negative bacillus that grows well in ordinary broth and agar. Bacteria are transmitted by the rat flea from the infected rodent. Immune rodents and humans maintain the organism in local vesicles. In less resistant hosts, spread occurs to lymph nodes and the blood stream.

The incubation period is 2–6 days. A local bubo and tender lymphadenitis then develop. Systemic onset is abrupt, with high fever. Bacteremia and shock occur in 3–5 days.

Diagnosis is made by Gram's stain and culture of the aspirate of a bubo and/or by blood culture. Other means include inoculation of the organism into mice or guinea pigs. Finally, acute and convalescent sera testing may be obtained.

All patients with plague should be isolated for the first 48 hours until secondary plague pneumonia is ruled out. Lymph nodes should not be incised and drained until the patient has been treated with antibiotics. Streptomycin is the preferred agent, 30 mg/kg/day intramuscularly in two divided doses, for 10 days. Alternative antibiotics include tetracycline and chloramphenicol.

Patients with plague pneumonia should be isolated, and all contacts should be quarantined and treated with oral tetracycline for 10 days.

Tick-borne Diseases

Ticks are small, oval, or round in shape, and along with mites and other insects, form the order of Acarina.

A tick uses its mouth parts to inflict the bite. In all cases of infected ticks, the tick feces, body juices, and blood are all infective. To remove a tick, the optimal way is the use of gentle traction with protected fingers, pulling the tick out completely. Ticks should not be crushed, either while attached to the patient, or after being removed. Substances such as acetone, gasoline, or aftershave lotion, if placed on the tick, will usually cause its retreat.

Ticks are vectors of diseases such as tularemia,

Rocky Mountain spotted fever, babesiosis, Lyme disease, and tick paralysis.

Tularemia

Francissella tularensis is a Gram-negative pleomorphic coccobacillus. Although the peak seasonal incidence varies with the geographic area, tick-borne tularemia is generally most common in summer, whereas in winter, contact with wild mammals (mainly rabbits during the hunting season) is the most frequent cause of disease.

Although infection with *F. tularensis* has been associated with at least 100 different species of mammal, wild rodents, especially cottontail rabbits, are the principal reservoir. Since transovarial passage occurs in ticks, they may serve as both reservoir and vector.

Three main types of human infection occur.

1. Cutaneous lesions (ulceroglandular). This form is most common, and occurs either after skinning or dressing rabbits or deer, or after a tick bite. Tularemia is an occupational hazard for hunters, butchers, sheepshearers, and felt hat manufacturers.

The typical lesion is macular and pruritic, and ulcerates within 2 days. Regional lymph nodes then enlarge, become tender, and drain, accompanied by fever from 104 to 106°F (40 to 41.1°C). The tick bite is not always easy to find. A case in point occurred in a 5-year-old boy from the Massachusetts coast with fever and occipital lymphadenopathy. After a long search, repeated, careful scalp examination revealed an engorged tick. High tularemia agglutination titers were later found.

2. Tularemic pneumonia. This form is less common, but may occur after inhalation of large amounts of infected particles, such as in a patient who skinned and eviscerated six rabbits. An outbreak of tularemic pneumonia occurred in August 1978 in a family vacationing in a cottage on Martha's Vineyard where mice were found inside and rabbits and ticks outside. The final premise was that dogs mangled the infected rabbits, then transmitted the bacteria via aerosolization of saliva in the cottage.

3. Typhoidal tularemia. This form occurs after ingestion of raw or improperly cooked meat. Symptoms include abdominal pain, diarrhea, fever, and bacteremia.

Tularemia is diagnosed mainly by a history of exposure to rabbits or ticks. Specific cysteine-dextrose blood agar is required for growth of the organism, but because laboratory propagation is potentially hazardous, culture is not routinely advised. When cultured, the organism may require 10 days for growth. Diagnosis may be confirmed by a fluorescent antibody test or by development of an elevated serum antibody titer of 1:640 or greater within a week.

Streptomycin, 30–40 mg/kg intramuscularly for 3 days, then 20 mg/kg/day, is the antibiotic of choice. Tetracycline may be used alternatively.

Rocky Mountain Spotted Fever

Another infection transmitted by ticks is Rocky Mountain spotted fever, a disease caused by *Rickettsia ricketsii.* There are two principal vectors in the United States. *Dermacentor andersoni,* the wood tick, is distributed in the Rocky Mountain states and is active in the spring and early summer. *Dermacentor variabilis,* the dog tick, is found mainly in the eastern half of the United States, especially in the southern portion, extending from Oklahoma to Tennessee, and northeast to Long Island and southern New England.

The clinical syndrome includes severe headache, then myalgia, followed by a maculopapular rash 2–3 days later. The rash starts typically on the wrists and ankles, extends to the palms and soles, and then becomes central. If allowed to progress without treatment, the rash may become petechial.

Complement fixation, indirect fluorescent antibody, indirect hemagglutination, latex agglutination, and microagglutination studies are now available. These tests are more specific and more sensitive than the Weil-Felix reaction.

Treatment for presumptive Rocky Mountain spotted fever is with chloramphenicol, 2–3 gm/day, or tetracycline, 2 gm/day for 10–14 days in adults.

Babesiosis

Babesiosis, a disease caused by the intracellular red blood cell parasite, *Babesia microti,* is also transmitted by ticks. Risk increases in patients with T-lymphocyte depression or after splenectomy, but cases have occurred in normal hosts. The clinical syndrome includes fever, myalgia, and hemolytic anemia. Diagnosis is made by observation of the intracellular red blood cell parasite on a Giemsa-stained smear. The tetrads may be confused with the findings in falciparum malaria, but Babesia-infected red blood cells do not have pigment granules. Antibody titers are helpful in making the diagnosis.

Treatment is symptomatic only. In splenectomized patients, exchange transfusions have been helpful. The combination clindamycin, 600 mg three times a day, and quinine, 650 mg, three times a day, has also been effective.

Lyme Disease

The infectious agent is a treponema-like spirochete that infests *Ixodes dammini* ticks, multiplies, and spreads through mice and squirrels to white-tailed deer, and inadvertently to humans via the tick feeding period.

Cases of Lyme disease cluster in summer in areas including the Connecticut shore, Long Island, Cape Cod, and the offshore islands. Cases have been reported from Arkansas, California, Georgia, Oregon, Texas, and Wisconsin. Person-to-person spread does not occur.

The common manifestation is erythema chronicum migrans (ECM). The rash consists of either single or multiple red annular-macular lesions of 2–5 cm in diameter. The lesions are warm and fade within about 3 weeks. There are no mucosal lesions but there may be constitutional symptoms, such as fever.

Arthritis is usually preceded on an average of 4 weeks by ECM. The arthritis is usually mild or uniarticular, occasionally migratory. The knee is most often involved, followed by other large joints. Arthritis may actually occur without ECM. The arthritis usually lasts about 1 week but may persist or develop into a chronic stage or recurring episodes with increasingly wider intervals.

The diagnosis is made by an indirect immunofluorescent test, testing for acute and convalescent sera from patients suspected of suffering from Lyme disease. A single dilution value of 1:256 is diagnostic; the enzyme-linked immunosorbent assay (ELISA) test is best. The IGM should be more than 1:200; it can be especially helpful since the illness is protracted and often perplexing, with or without the striking rash (ECM).

Antibiotics are helpful in shortening the duration of ECM and the associated symptoms and in avoiding the more serious problems of recurrent arthritis, meningoencephalitis, and myocarditis. Tetracycline is the most effective antibiotic, followed by penicillin. For treatment of established central nervous system (CNS) disease, penicillin is still the optimal therapy because of its access to the CNS, crossing the blood-brain barrier.

Toxin: Tick Paralysis

Tick paralysis may be caused by 43 different species of ticks, but most human cases in the United States arise from *Dermacenter* species. The paralysis is thought caused by a toxin secreted in the saliva of the tick that affects central as well as peripheral nerves. Typically, the tick is attached from 4 to 7 days before the onset of symptoms. The presentation is an ascending flaccid paralysis, acute ataxia, or a combination of the two. Diagnosis depends on a careful search of the scalp and body for the attached tick. Treatment consists of removing the tick, after which improvement is seen within a few hours.

Rat-bite Fever

Two bacteria that may cause disease after a rat bite are *Streptobacillus moniliformis* and *Spirillum minus. S. moniliformis* may be diagnosed by culture of the organism using special media supplemented with 20% rabbit or horse serum incubated in carbon dioxide.

Penicillin is the antibiotic of choice. Tetracycline, 500 mg orally four times per day, or streptomycin, 7.5 mg/kg intramuscularly twice a day, should be used in the penicillin-allergic patient. Table 10.21 illustrates the differences between the two forms of the disease.

Cat-scratch Disease

A bacterium may be the cause of cat-scratch disease. Its specific cause is not proved. Disease results from trauma, often from a cat scratch, less often from a dog or cat bite. The syndrome usually occurs in the early spring, transmitted by a young kitten. Cats act as vectors; they do not become ill themselves.

The incubation period is 3–10 days. The primary lesion is a tender papule. Lymphadenopathy then develops within 5 days to 2 months, usually unilaterally. The lymph node is tender, with erythema over the skin. About 20% of nodes drain sponta-

Table 10.21. Rat-bite Fever

	Streptobacillar Fever	Spirillar Fever
Organism	*Streptobacillus moniliformis*	*Spirillum minus*
Epidemiology	Bite, food	Bite
Incubation	>1 week	1–3 weeks
Bite site	Prompt healing	Healing followed by reactivation of the bite site
Rash	+	+
Arthralgia	+	−
Diagnosis	Culture, titer	Smear, dark field
Treatment	Penicillin × 10 days (1–2 gm/day)	Penicillin × 10 days (1–2 gm/day)

neously. Systemic symptoms include headache, fever, and malaise. Rarely, encephalitis or oculoglandular disease (Parinaud's syndrome) may develop.

The diagnosis of cat-scratch disease is made by a history of contact with cats or kittens, evidence of a primary lesion, and regional lymphadenopathy. A bacterium has been identified in Warthin-Starry stains of lymph node sections and skin lesions.

Treatment is supportive. Suppurative nodes should be aspirated for diagnostic and therapeutic purposes.

Rabies

The most notorious viral disease caused by an animal bite is rabies. The epidemiology has changed in the past few years, and now, nonimmune dogs account for only 16% of cases, whereas sylvatic animals, including skunks, foxes, bats, and raccoons account for more than 80% of cases in the United States. Skunks, raccoons, red and gray foxes, bats, and domestic dogs represent the greatest hazards; rodents, including squirrels and hamsters, are probably inconsequential.

Live virus is introduced into nerve tissue at the time of the bite. The virus persists 96 hours at the site and then spreads to the central nervous system. It replicates in gray matter and spreads along autonomic nerves to the salivary glands, adrenal glands, and heart. The incubation period varies with the site of the bite, from 10 days to as long as 1 year.

Clinical features include a prodromal period of 1–4 days, followed by a high fever, headache, and malaise. Paresthesias at the site of inoculation occur in 80% of patients. The rest of the sequence of events includes agitation, hyperesthesia, dysphagia, paralysis, and death.

The fluorescent antibody method for the viral antigen is the most rapid and sensitive means of diagnosis. Brain biopsy of the animal is also useful.

Preexposure prophylaxis is important for spelunkers, veterinarians, and virologists. Human diploid cell vaccine should be given, and the neutralizing antibody titer followed.

In postexposure prophylaxis, the following questions must be considered.

1. What is the status of animal rabies in the locale where the exposure took place?
2. Was the attack provoked or unprovoked?
3. Of what species was the animal?
4. What was the state of health of the animal?

Most animals transmit rabies virus in saliva only a few days before becoming ill themselves (dog and skunk, 5 days; fox, 3 days; cat, 1 day). Bats, however, may harbor the virus for many months.

The physician should regard the skunk, fox, raccoon, and bat as rabid, and should treat patients with bites from these animals with both human diploid cell vaccine and human rabies immune globulin. Healthy domestic dogs and cats should be observed.

Treatment of rabies includes the following.

1. The most important step is to scrub the wound vigorously with a brush and soap. Rinse well, then perform a second scrub with green soap or alcohol.

2. Active immunization is accomplished with human diploid cell vaccine (Merieux Institute, Inc.). Human diploid cell vaccine is more potent than duck embryo vaccine, and thus, fewer doses are needed. The dosage schedule is usually 1, 3, 7, 14, 30, and 90 days, and there are no known side effects. Following vaccination, antibody titers should be measured to assure protection. Further immunizations are indicated if titers remain low.

3. Finally, it is important to immunize the patient passively following a potentially rabid bite. Human rabies immune globulin should be given immediately, 50% around the site of the bite and 50% in the thigh or the arm. The dosage is 15–40 IU/kg. Passive immunization results in the early appearance of antibody, but also inhibits the development of the active antibody from the human diploid cell vaccine; this is the reason for prolonged dosage of the vaccines.

Although rabies has been regarded as uniformly fatal, several patients now have survived with prolonged cardiorespiratory support. An aggressive approach in the patient with known rabies infection certainly merits the effort.

Simian Herpes B Virus

Simian herpes B virus is found in old world monkeys, especially rhesus and cynomologus species. Infection occurs mainly by a bite and less commonly after inhalation of monkey saliva or contact with infected monkey cell cultures. A vesicular lesion develops at the wound site, with progressive lymphangitis and fever. Confusion, reduced tendon reflexes in lower extremities, and respiratory paralysis may follow.

Diagnosis depends on viral isolation or identification of intranuclear inclusion bodies in lymph nodes or brain biopsy from patient or animal, or a rise in neutralizing antibody titer to simian herpes B virus in the patient's blood. Treatment is supportive.

Orf (Contagious Ecthyma)

Orf is an endemic viral disease of sheep and goats. The disease in humans is contracted through direct cutaneous transmission. A nodular, vesicular, or pustular lesion develops at the site of contact. Regional lymphadenopathy follows. The lesions may progress to diffuse vesiculopapular rash.

Diagnosis is made by a complement fixation titer of more than 1:8 or isolation of virus on bovine kidney cell culture. Treatment is supportive.

Snake Bites

The two major poisonous snakes in the Americas are the pit viper and the coral snake. The coral snake belongs to the family *Elapidae*. The remainder of all poisonous snakes in this hemisphere belong to the family *Viperidae*. The subfamily of pit vipers includes the rattlesnake, water moccasin, and copperhead. There are about 7000 poisonous snake bites reported in the United States annually. The largest number occur in the Southwestern and Gulf states.

Two poisonous snakes are native to New England. The northern copperhead, also called the highland moccasin, is pink or reddish brown and is marked with large barrels of chestnut brown resembling dumbbells or hourglasses. The bite is painful but rarely fatal. The timber rattler is dark brown with chevrons of black and brown. The horny rattle on the tail buzzes when the snake is disturbed.

The degree of toxicity of a snake bite depends on the potency of the venom, the amount injected, the size and condition of the snake, and the size of the person bitten. There are instant clinical manifestations of the pit viper bite. Pain occurs at the site of the bite, as well as a wheal with local edema, numbness, and within moments, ecchymosis and painful lymphadenopathy. Nausea, vomiting, sweating, fever, drowsiness, and slurred speech may then develop. Bleeding of the gums and hematemesis are common hemorrhagic manifestations.

For proper treatment, it is extremely important to establish that the bite is from a poisonous snake. The patient should have distinct fang punctures and immediate local pain, followed by edema and dis-

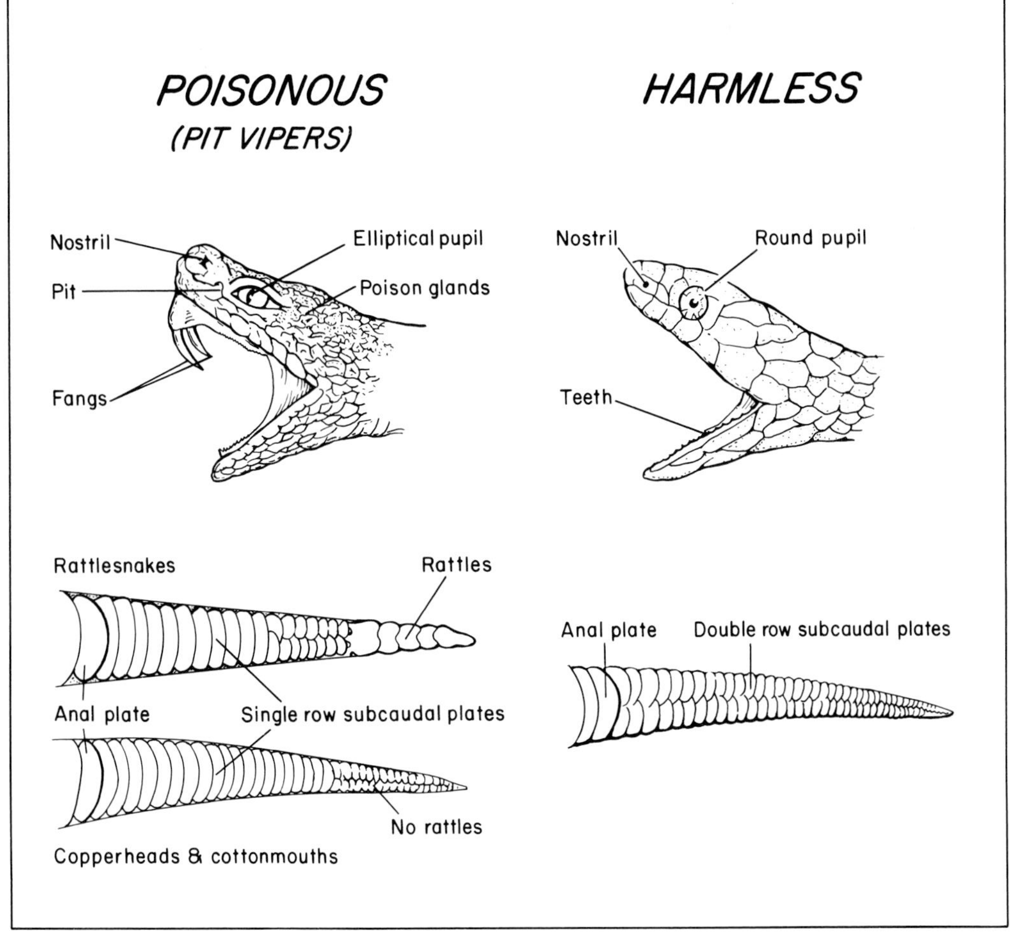

Figure 10.6. Ways to differentiate poisonous from harmless snakes. (Reproduced by permission from Wingert WA, Wainschel J. A quick handbook on snake bites. *Resident & Staff Physician,* May 1977:56. Reprinted with permission from *Resident & Staff Physician* © October 1988 by Romaine Pierson Publishers, Inc.)

Table 10.22.
Gradation of Envenomization

Grade	Signs	Antivenin
0	No local or systemic symptoms	None
Mild	Local swelling only	5 vials
Moderate	Progressive swelling, systemic symptoms, laboratory changes	10 vials
Severe	Marked local reaction, progressive edema, severe systemic symptoms, severe laboratory changes	15 vials

coloration within 30 minutes. It is helpful to inspect the snake, since those that are poisonous may be differentiated from those that are not by the presence of fangs and the elliptical shape of the pupils (Fig. 10.6). Most harmless snakes have round pupils.

The limb should be immobilized and a tourniquet applied proximal to the wound. The tourniquet should be released for 90 seconds every 15 minutes. The physician should make two long longitudinal incisions through the fang marks and apply suction intermittently for the first hour. An attempt should be made to neutralize the venom with immune serum. Emergency information and specific immune serum can be obtained from the Oklahoma City Poison Control Center (405-271-5454, 24 hours a day). A photograph of snakes common to a specific geographic area is important for all emergency departments. The severity of envenomization is graded for both adults and children as shown in Table 10.22.

Polyvalent pit viper antivenin can be used for the bites of all American snakes except the coral snake. If possible, it should be administered within 1 hour of the bite, and the patient should first undergo skin testing for hypersensitivity to horse serum. The dosage is usually 5 vials in 500 ml of normal saline solution intravenously over 30 minutes. Prophylactic antimicrobial therapy and tetanus prophylaxis are recommended for deep bites. Supportive treatment, including hospitalization and careful evaluation of the baseline hematocrit, platelet count, and prothrombin time, is important. Finally, surgical debridement is rarely necessary.

Spider Bites

Emergency physicians should be aware of two spiders in particular, the black widow and the brown recluse. The black widow spider, *Lactrodectus mactans,* may be found in basements and backyards all over the United States, especially in the South. The female is venomous and aggressive. The spider is jet black and globular, with a red mark shaped like an hourglass on the abdomen. The venom causes central and peripheral nervous system excitement, autonomic activity, muscle spasms, hypertension, and vasoconstriction.

Sharp pain occurs at the site of the bite, followed by cramping pain locally within about an hour, spreading to the extremities and the trunk. Severe abdominal pain may occur, causing a board-like abdomen that is rigid but not tender. This is an important differentiating point on examination. A fatal outcome is rare. Treatment is usually supportive only; antivenin may be needed in children or the elderly.

The brown recluse, *Loxosceles reclusus,* prefers dark, undisturbed places like old sofas and old fur coats. Commonly found in the Missouri valley, it is 0.5-inch long and 0.25-inch wide with a dark-brown, violin-shaped marking on the thorax. The brown recluse never attacks unless threatened. After the bite, there is immediate local pain. Extensive extravasation of blood may occur at the site in the next 24 hours. A generalized rash may appear over the body. The area of the bite may become deeply ulcerated, with ulceration extending down to the muscles. Treatment is supportive; there is no antiserum available. Several surgeons suggest early excision of the bite site to prevent the severe ulceration.

Scorpion Stings

There are about 650 species of scorpions, approximately 40 of which are found in the United States. Most of these are not venomous. The venomous scorpions belong to the family Buthidae. Particularly dangerous species include *Centruroides sculpturatus* and *Centruroides gertschi,* which are found in the southwestern United States.

The clinical symptoms of a scorpion sting are localized numbness at the site of the sting and, rarely, high blood pressure and respiratory impairment.

Therapy includes immersion of the limb in cold water and a tourniquet about the limb, as well as treatment of symptoms. Antivenin is available by calling Arizona State Antivenom Laboratory (602-965-3116).

Hymenoptera Stings

Twice as many persons die in the United States from Hymenoptera stings as from snake bites. Hymenoptera include bees, wasps, hornets, yellow jackets, and fire ants.

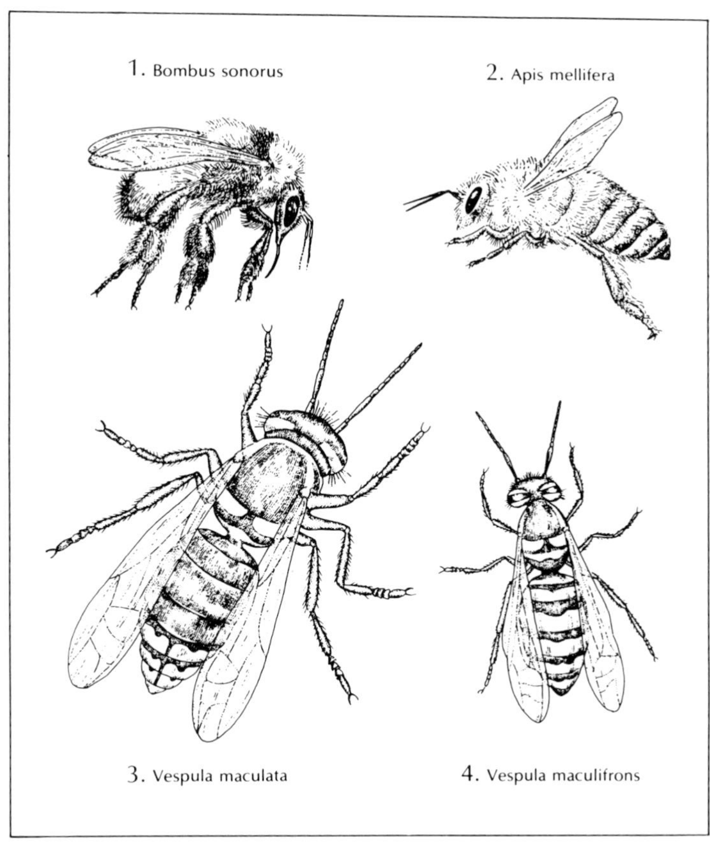

Figure 10.7. Four prominent members of the order Hymenoptera that cause many anaphylactic reactions are the *1,* bumblebee; *2,* honeybee; *3,* white-faced hornet; *4,* and yellow jacket. (Reprinted with permission from, Lichtenstein LM: Anaphylactic reactions to insect stings: A new approach. *Hosp Pract,* 1975;69.)

The emergency physician should be able to recognize four prominent members of the order Hymenoptera: (*1*) the bumblebee; (*2*) the honeybee, with a barbed stinger, fuzzy body, and brown, blunt abdomen; (*3*) the white-faced hornet; and (*4*) the yellow jacket, which has a black shiny thorax with long antennae (Fig. 10.7). Hymenoptera venoms contain histamines and other vasoactive substances. These are hemolytic and neurotoxic, in addition to being effective hypersensitizing agents.

The clinical syndrome after a sting includes sharp pain, a local wheal, erythema, and intense itching and edema. In the 1% of the population who are hypersensitive, a single sting may produce serious anaphylaxis with urticaria, nausea, abdominal pain, dypsnea, edema of the face and glottis, hypotension, and death.

Treatment requires removal of the venom sac (''stinger,'' if retained) and washing of the area, followed by local supportive care such as cool compresses. The allergic patient may need 0.3–0.5 ml of epinephrine (1:1000) injected subcutaneously.

The major factor in the consideration of insect stings is prevention. Desensitization with venom rather than with whole-body extract is now possible. The hypersensitive patient should have available an insect sting kit, such as that made by Hollister-Stier, containing medihaler epinephrine and chlorpheniramine maleate (Chlor-Trimeton).

Marine Diseases

Erysipeloid

Erysipeloid is an acute infection of traumatized skin, usually occurring in fishermen handling raw fish, but occurs also in butchers and those handling meat products and poultry. *Erysipelothrix rhusiopathiae* is a gram-positive bacillus found in the mouth of fish, swine, and poultry.

When it results from a bite, the initial symptom is burning pain at the site, followed by a warm, tender, raised, violaceous, or wine-colored area often associated with lymphangitis. As infection advances, the central lesion clears.

The antibiotic of choice is oral penicillin (1–2

gm/day) for 10 days, with immobilization and soaking of the limb for 2–3 days.

Seal Bites

Normally, seal bite is on the finger of a trainer or a seal hunter, thus the term "seal finger" or "Spaek finger." The etiologic agent is unclear; the result of a Canadian government study in an attempt to isolate the organism is not available at this writing.

The incubation period is 4–8 days, followed by throbbing pain, erythema, and swelling of the joint proximal to the bite. Untreated, Spaek finger produces cellulitis and progressive arthritis. The treatment before antibiotics was amputation of the affected finger to relieve the severe pain and deformity. Tetracycline, 500 mg orally four times a day for 10 days, is now the antibiotic of choice. It is also helpful to immobilize and elevate the finger, as well as to soak it several times a day.

Jellyfish Sting

Venom is discharged from nematocysts in the tentacles of the larger jellyfish. Stings are characterized by instant burning pain where the tentacles contact the skin, followed by the development of a red, elevated, linear lesion. In more severe cases, the victim experiences nausea, vomiting, abdominal and generalized muscular cramps, and difficulty in breathing. Stings of the sea wasps *Chironex fleckeri* and Chiropsalmus are extremely severe.

On-site resuscitation takes first priority. Weak solutions of acetic acid (or vinegar) then will inactivate the penetrating nematocysts.

LIGHTNING INJURIES

The emergency department physician should be concerned with the immediate life-threatening problems that the patient may suffer not only in the field but also in the emergency department. Vigorous efforts at resuscitation in the field are endorsed.

Injuries secondary to lightning are extremely uncommon with approximately 600 episodes reported each year in the United States resulting in 150 to 200 deaths. Survival from this environmental force is, therefore, possible. The electrical force is estimated to be between 10,000 and 200,000 amperes. The immediate life-threatening problems include respiratory paralysis, ventricular arrhythmias, asystole, and unconsciousness. Therapy at the scene necessitates standard assessment and initiation of basic and advanced life support which may include intubation and defibrillation. Sustained efforts at resuscitation are appropriate at the scene since successful outcomes have been reported.

Once in the emergency department, a complete secondary assessment is necessary. Injuries may result from the direct electric force as well as from a resultant fall or propulsive force. Fractures from the vigorous muscular contractions are possible. Extremities may suffer "compartment syndrome" with muscle necrosis and myoglobinuria.

Patients require hospitalization and consultation with general surgery and/or the burn service. Ideally, these patients are best managed in a designated burn facility. Routine support, monitoring, and burn wound care are essential and, when appropriately applied, can lead to successful outcome from these injuries. The reader is referred to Chapter 38 on burn management for a description of wound care.

The patients in the emergency department may present with combative behavior which will resolve over time. The electric force does not usually cause permanent myocardial damage and the arrhythmias are transient. The extremities should be very carefully examined and monitored for the development of compartment syndrome. Although unusual, the compartments may require fasciotomy. Routine monitoring of the urine for myoglobin is useful. A rare event is the very delayed development of cataracts as a result of these injuries.

SUGGESTED READINGS

Heat-related Illness

Beller GA, Boyd AE. Heat stroke. *Milit Med,* 1975;140:464–467.
Caroff SN. The neuroleptic malignant syndrome. *J Clin Psych,* 1980;41:79–83.
Clowes GHA, O'Donnell TF. Heat stroke. *N Engl J Med,* 1974;291:564–567.
Gottschalk PG, Thomas JE. Heat stroke. *Mayo Clin Proc,* 1966;41:470–482.
Gronert GA. Malignant hyperthermia. *Anesthesiology,* 1980;53:395–423.
Guze, BH, Baxter LR Jr. Neuroleptic malignant syndrome. *N Eng J Med,* 1985;313:163–166.
Knochel JP. Environmental heat illness—An eclectic review. *Arch Intern Med,* 1974;133:841–864.
Stine RJ. Heat illness. *JACEP,* 1979;8:154–160.
Wheeler M. Heat stroke in the elderly. *Med Clin North Am,* 1976;60:1289–1296.

Hypothermia

Danzl DF, Pozos RS, Auerbach PS, et al. Multicenter hypothermia survey. *Ann Emerg Med,* 1987;16:1042–1055.
Fitzgerald FT, Jessop C. Accidental hypothermia. *Adv Int Med,* 1982;27:127–150.
Haggers JP, Robson MC, Manavalen K, et al. Experimental and clinical observations on frostbite. *Ann Emerg Med,* 1987;16:1056–1062.
Kelman GR, Nunn JF. Nomograms for correction of blood PO_2, PCO_2, pH, and base excess for time and temperature. *J Appl Physiol,* 1966;21:1484–1490.
Paton BC. Accidental hypothermia. *Pharmacol Ther,* 1983; 22:331–377.
Reuler JB. Hypothermia: Pathophysiology, clinical settings and management. *Ann Intern Med,* 1978;89:519-527.
Reuler JB, Parker RA. Peritoneal dialysis in the management of hypothermia. *JAMA,* 1978;240:2289–2290.
Southwick FS, Dalglish PH. Recovery after prolonged asystolic cardiac arrest in profound hypothermia: A case report and review of the literature. *JAMA,* 1980; 243:1250–1253.

Stine RJ. Accidental hypothermia. *JACEP,* 1977;6:413–416.

Trevino A, Razi B, Beller BM. The characteristic electrocardiogram of accidental hypothermia. *Arch Intern Med,* 1971;127:470–473.

Weyman AE, Greenbaum DM, Grace WJ. Accidental hypothermia in an alcoholic population. *Am J Med,* 1974; 56:13–21.

Zell SC, Kurtz KJ. Severe exposure hypothermia, a resuscitation protocol. *Ann Emerg Med,* 1985;14:339–345.

Drowning and Near-Drowning

Calderwood HW. The ineffectiveness of steroid therapy for treatment of fresh water near-drowning. *Anesthesiology,* 1975;43:642–650.

Conn AW. Cerebral resuscitation in near-drowning. *Pediatr Clin North Am,* 1979;24:691–701.

Fandel I, Bancalari E. Near-drowning in children: Clinical aspects. *Pediatrics,* 1976;58:573–579.

Hoff BH. Multisystem failure: A review with special reference to drowning. *Crit Care Med,* 1979;7:310–320.

Knopp R. Near-drowning. *JACEP,* 1978;7:249–254.

Levin DL. Near-drowning. *Crit Care Med,* 1980;8:590–595.

Martin TG. Near-drowning and cold water immersion. *Ann Emerg Med,* 1984;13:263–273.

Modell JH. Biology of drowning. *Ann Rev Med,* 1978;29:1–8.

Orlowski JP. Prognostic factors in pediatric cases of drowning and near-drowning. *JACEP,* 1979;8:176–179.

Ports TA, Deueli TF. Intravascular coagulation in fresh water submersion. *Ann Intern Med,* 1977;87:60–61.

Young RSK. Zalnecaitis EL, Dooling EC. Neurological outcome in cold water drowning. *JAMA,* 1980;244:1233–1235.

Barotrauma and Decompression Sickness

Boettger ML. Scuba diving emergencies: Pulmonary overpressure accidents and decompression sickness. *Ann Emerg Med,* 1983;12:563–567.

Myers RA, Bray P. Delayed treatment of serious decompression sickness. *Ann Emerg Med,* 1985;14:254–257.

Myers RA, Schnitzer BM. Hyperbaric oxygen use: Update 1984. *Postgrad Med,* 1984;76:83–95.

Strauss RH, ed. Diving Medicine. New York: *Grune & Stratton,* 1976.

Strauss RH. Diving medicine. *Am Rev Respir Dis,* 1979; 119:1001–1023.

U.S. Navy Diving Manual, 1973.

Smoke Inhalation

Agee RN, Long JM III, Hunt JL, et. al. Use of xenon in early diagnosis of inhalation injury. *J Trauma,* 1976; 16:218–224.

Bartlett RH, Dressler DP, Horovitz JH, et. al. Consensus report on smoke inhalation. *J Trauma,* 1979;19:913–922.

Cahalane M, Demlong RH. Early respiratory abnormalities from smoke inhalation. *JAMA,* 1984;251:771–773.

Crapo RO. Smoke inhalation injuries. *JAMA,* 1981; 246:1694–1696.

Dyer RF, Esch VH. Polyvinyl chloride toxicity in fires. *JAMA,* 1976;35:393–397.

Hunt JL, Agee RN, Pruitt BA. Fiberoptic bronchoscopy in acute inhalation injury. *J Trauma,* 1975;15:641–649.

Luce EA, Chi Tsi SU, Hoopes JE. Alveolar-arterial oxygen gradient in the burn patient. *J Trauma,* 1976;16:212–217.

Moylan JA, Chan C-K. Inhalation injury, an increasing problem. *Ann Surg,* 1978;188:34–37.

Petroff PA, Hander EW, Clayton WH, et. al. Pulmonary function studies after smoke inhalation. *Am J Surg,* 1976; 132:346–351.

Pruitt BA, Erickson DR, Morris A. Progressive pulmonary insufficiency and other pulmonary complications of thermal injury. *J Trauma,* 1975;15:369–379.

Zawacki BE. Jung RC, Joyce J., et. al. Smoke, burns and the natural history of inhalation injury in fire victims. *Ann Surg,* 1977;185:100–110.

Carbon Monoxide Poisoning

Cohen MA, Guzzardi LJ. Inhalation of products of combustion. *Ann Emerg Med,* 1983;12:628–632.

Finley J. Van Beek A, Glover JL. Myonecrosis complicating carbon monoxide poisoning. *J Trauma,* 1977;17:536–540.

Goldbaum LR, Orellano T, Dergal E. Mechanism of the toxic action of carbon monoxide. *Ann Clin Lab Sci,* 1976; 6:372–376.

Kindwall E. Carbon monoxide poisoning. In: Dairs JC, Hunt TK, eds. *Hyperbaric Oxygen Therapy.* Bethesda, MD. Undersea Medical Society, Inc., 1977;177–190.

Radiation Accidents

Anonymous. Chernobyl meltdown. *Newsweek,* 12 May. 1986;20–30.

Beeson PN, McDermott W, eds. *Radiation Injury.* Textbook of Medicine, 14th ed. Vol. 1, Philadelphia: W. B. Saunders, 1976;66–72.

Bond VP, Fliedner TM, Cronkite EP. Evaluation and management of the heavily irradiated individual. *J Nuc Med,* 1960;1:221–238.

Carbaugh, E.W. A plutonium contaminated puncture wound cure study. *Health Phys,* 1986;50:541.

Casarett GW. *Radiation Histopathology,* Vols. I and II, Boca Raton, FL. CRC Press, 1980.

Castronovo FP Jr. Iodine-131 thyroid burdens of European travelers returning to Boston after the Chernobyl accident. *N Engl J Med,* 1986;315:1674–1680.

Catsch A, Kawin B. Pi *Radioactive Metal Mobilization in Medicine.* Charles C Thomas, 1964.

Cember H. *Introduction to Health Physics.* 2nd ed. New York: Pergamon Press, 1976.

Chernobyl Reactor Accident Report of a Consultation, May 6, 1986 (Provisional) Copenhagen: WHO, ICPCEH 129, 1986.

Dalrymple GV, Goulden ME, Kollmorgen GM, et al. *Medical Radiation Biology.* Philadelphia: WB Saunders, 1973.

Hounam RF. The removal of particles from the nasopharyngeal (NP) compartment of the respiratory tract by nose blowing and swabbing. *Health Phys,* 1975;28:743–750.

Húbner KF, Fry SA, eds. *The Medical Basis for Radiation Accident Preparedness.* New York: Elsevier/North-Holland, 1980.

International Atomic Energy Agency. *Handling of Radiation Accidents,* Proceedings of IAEA/WHO Symposium, Vienna, May 19–23, 1969, STI/PUB/229. Vienna: International Atomic Energy Agency, 1969.

International Atomic Energy Agency. *Manual on Radiation Haematology,* Technical Reports Series No. 123. Vienna: International Atomic Energy Agency, 1971.

International Atomic Energy Agency. *Manual on Early Medical Treatment of Possible Radiation Injury with an Appendix on Sodium Burns.* (IAEA Safety Series, No. 47) Vienna: International Atomic Energy Agency, 1978.

Joint Commission on Accreditation of Hospitals. *Accreditation Manual for Hospital*—1980 Edition, Chicago: JCAH, 1980.

Lincoln TA. Importance of initial management of persons internally contaminated with radionuclides. *Am Ind Hyg Assoc J,* 1976;37:16–21.

Love RA. Planning for radiation accidents. *Hospitals,* 1964;38:7–14.

National Council on Radiation Protection and Measurements. *Radiological Factors Affecting Decision Marking in a Nuclear Attack.* Report No. 42, Nov. 15, 1974. *Protection of the Thyroid Gland in the Event of Releases of Radioiodine.* Report No. 55, 1977. C/P NCRP Publications PO Box 3107, Washington, DC 20014.

National Council on Radiation Protection and Measurements. *Instrumentation and Monitoring Methods for Radiation Protection.* (NCRP Report No. 57), Washington, DC, 1978.

National Research Council, Committee on the Biological Effects of Ionizing Radiations. *The Effects on Popula-*

tions of Exposure to Low Levels of Ionizing Radiation: 1980. (BIER III) Washington, DC: National Academy Press, 1980.

NCRP Report 39, Basic Radiation Protection Criteria. Issued January 15, 1971.

Sanders, SM Jr. Excretion of Am^{241} and Cm^{244} following two cases of accidental inhalation. *Health Phys,* 1974;27: 359–365.

Saenger EL. Hospital planning to combat radioactive contamination. *JAMA,* 1963;112–113.

Saenger EL. Medical aspects of radiation accidents. United States Atomic Energy Commission, 1963.

United Nations. Report of the United Nations Scientific Committee on the Effects of Atomic Radiation (UNSCEAR), *Sources and Effects of Ionizing Radiation,* 1977 Report to the General Assembly, Publication Sales No. UN E. 77. IX. 1, New York, 1977.

U.S. Nuclear Regulatory Commission. Instruction Concerning Risks from Occupational Radiation Exposure, Regulatory Guide 8.29, July 1981.

U. S. Nuclear Regulatory Commission. Notices, Instructions and Reports to Workers: Inspections. Rules and Regulations, Title 10, Chapter 1, Code of Federal Regulations, Part 19.

U. S. Nuclear Regulatory Commission. Standards For Protection Against Radiation. Rules and Regulations, Title 10, Chapter 1, Code of Federal Regulations, Part 20.

Waldron RL, Danielson RA, Schultz HE, et al. Radiation decontamination unit for the community hospital. *AM J Roentgen,* 1981;136:977–981.

Weidner WA, Miller KL, Latshaw RF, et al. The impact of a nuclear crisis on a radiology department. *Radiology,* 1980;135:717–723.

World Health Organization. *Diagnosis and Treatment of Acute Radiation Injury,* Proceedings of a scientific meeting jointly sponsored by the IAEA and WHO, October 17–21, 1960. Geneva: World Health Organization, 1960.

Animal Bites

General

Baker AS. Infections on bites and trauma. In: Kass E, ed. *Current Therapy of Infectious Disease.* Ontario: BC Decker Co. 1984;187–196.

Berzon DR. Animal bites in a large city—A report on Baltimore, Maryland. *Am J Publ Health,* 1972;62:422–426.

Elliot DL, Toule SW, Goldberg L, et al. Pet associated illness. *N Engl J Med,* 1985;313:985–994.

Goldstein EJ. Bites. In: Mandell, et al., eds. *Principles of Practice of Infectious Diseases.* 2nd ed. New York: John Wiley & Sons, 1985.

Hubbert WT, McCullough WF, Schurrenberger PR. *Diseases Transmitted from Animal to Man.* Springfield, IL: Charles C Thomas, 1975.

Kahrs RF Holmes DN, Poppenseik GC. Diseases transmitted from pets to man: An evolving concern for veterinarians. *Cornell Vet,* 1978;68:422–459.

Rest JG; Goldstein EJ. Management of human & animal bite wounds. *Emerg Med Clin North Am,* 1985;(1)117–126.

Stelle JH. A bookshelf on veterinary public health. *Am J Publ Health,* 1973;63:291–311.

Dog Bites

Callahan M. Prophylactic antibodies in common dog bite wounds: A controlled study. *Ann Emerg Med,* 1980;9: 410–414.

Kalb R, Kaplan MH, Tenenbaum MJ. Cutaneous injection at dog bite wounds associated with fulminant DF2 septicemia. *Am J Med,* 1985;78:687–690.

Klein D. Friendly dog syndrome. *NY State J Med,* 1966;66: 2306–2309.

Human Bites

Goldstein EJC. Role of anerobic bacteria in bite-wound infections. *Rev Infect Dis,* 1984;6:S177–S183.

Mann RJ, Hoffeld TA, Farmer CB. Human bites of the hand: Twenty years of experience. *J Hand Surg,* 1977; 2:97–104.

Peeples E, Boswick JA, Scott, FA. Wounds of the hand contaminated by human or animal pasteurella saliva. *J Trauma,* 1980;20:383–389.

Pasteurella multocida

Hubbert WT, Rosen MN. *Pasteurella multocida* infection due to animal bite. *Am J Publ Health,* 1970;60:1103–1108.

Jarvis WR, Banko S, Snyder E, et al. *Pasteurella multocida* osteomyelitis following dog bites. *Am J Dis Child,* 1981; 135:625–627.

Lucas GL, Bartlett DH. *Pasteurella multocida* infection in the hand. *Plast Reconstr Surg,* 1981;67:49–53.

Tindall JP, Harrison CM. *Pasteurella multocida* infections following animal injuries, especially cat bites. *Arch Dermatol,* 1972;105:412–416.

Weber DJ, Wolfson JS, Swartz ML, et al. *Pasteurella multocida* infections: Report of 34 cases & review of the literature. *Medicine,* 1984;63:133–154.

DF-2

Case Records of the Massachusetts General Hospital. *N Engl J Med.* 1986;315:241–249.

Rubin SJ. DF-2: A fastidious fermentative gram-negative rod. *Eur J Clin Microbiol.* 1984;31:253–257.

Plague

Finegold KJ. Pathogenesis of plague. *Am J Med,* 1968;45: 549–554.

Kaufmann AF, Boyce JM, Martone WJ. Trends in human plague in the U.S. *J Infect Dis,* 1980;141:522–524.

Reed WP, Palmer DC, Williams RC Jr, et al. Bubonic plague in southwestern United States. *Medicine,* 1970;49: 464–486.

Werner SB, Weidmer CE, Nelson BC, et al. Primary plague pneumonia contracted from a domestic cat at South Lake Tahoe, California. *JAMA,* 1984;251:929–931.

Tularemia

Halperin SA, Gast T, Ferrieri P. Oculoglandular syndrome caused by *Francisella tularemsis. Clin Pediatr (Phila),* 1985;24:20–22.

Harrell RE Jr., Whitaker GR. Tularemia: Emergency department presentation of an infrequently recognized disease. *AmJ Emerg Med,* 1985;3:415–418.

Kloch CE, Olsen PF, Fukushima T. Tularemia epidemic associated with the deerfly. *JAMA,* 1973;266:149–152.

Markowitz LE, Hynes NA, De La Cruz P, et al. Tick-borne tularemia: An outbreak of lymphadenopathy in children. *JAMA,* 1985;254:2922–2926.

Teutsch SM, Martone WJ, Brink EW, et al. Pneumonic tularemia on Martha's Vineyard. *N Engl J Med,* 1979;301:826–828.

Young LS, Bicknell DS, Archer BG et al. Tularemia epidemic: Vermont 1968. 47 cases limited to contact with muskrats. *N Engl J Med,* 1969;280:1253–1260.

Rat-bite fever

Rat bite fever. *MMWR,* 1984;33:318–320.

Rogosa M. *Streptobacillus moniliformis* and *Spirillum minor.* In: Lennette EH, et al., eds. *Manual of Clinical Microbiology.* American Society for Microbiol, 1985.

Roughgarden JW. Antimicrobial therapy of rat-bite fever: A review. *Arch Intern Med,* 1975;116:39–54.

Cat-scratch Disease

Carithers HA, Carithers CM, Edwards RO Jr. Cat scratch disease. Its natural history. *JAMA,* 1969;207:312–316.

Gerber MA, Macalister TJ, Ballow M, et al. The aetiological agent of cat scratch disease. *Lancet,* 1985;1:1236–1239.

Life threatening cat-scratch disease in an immunocompromised host. *Arch Int Med,* 1986;394–396.

Margileth AM. Cat scratch disease: Bacteria in skin at the primary innoculation site. *JAMA,* 1984;252:928–931.

Margileth AM. Cat scratch disease: Non-bacterial regional lymphadenitis. The study of 145 patients and a review of the literature. *Pediatrics,* 1968;42:803–808.

Wear DJ, Margileth AM, Hadfield TL, et al. Cat scratch disease; Bacterial etiology. *Science,* 1983;221:1403–1405.

Rabies

Anderson LJ, Sikes RK, Langkos CW. Post exposure trial of human diploid cell strain. *J Infect Dis,* 1980;142:133–138.

Anderson, LJ, Nicholson KG, Tauxe RV, et al. Human rabies in the US, 1960–1979: Epidemiology, diagnosis & presentation. *Ann Int Med,* 1984;100:728–735.

Compendium of rabies. *MMWR,* 1985;33:51–52.

Corey L, Hattwick MA. Treatment of persons exposed to rabies. *JAMA,* 1975;232:272–275.

Houff SA, Burton RC, Wilson RW, et al. Human to human transmission of rabies virus by a corneal transplant. *N Engl J Med,* 1979;300:603–604.

Meyer HW. Rabies vaccine. *J Infect Dis,* 1980;2:287–289.

Rabies prevention. *MMWR,* 1984;33:393–402, 407–408.

Simian Herpes B Virus

Hull RN. The Simian herpes viruses. In: Kaplan AS, ed. *The Herpes Viruses.* New York: Academic Press, 1979:389–425.

Rocky Mountain Spotted Fever

Hechemy KE. Laboratory diagnosis of Rocky Mountain spotted fever. *N Engl J Med,* 1979;300:859–860.

Hazard GW, Ganz RN, Nevin RW, et al. Rocky Mountain spotted fever in the eastern United States. *N Engl J Med,* 1969;380:57–62.

Helmick GG, Bernard KW, D'Angelo LJ. Rocky Mountain spotted fever: Clinical, laboratory and epidemiologic features of 262 cases. *J Infect Dis,* 1984;150:480–488.

Rocky Mountain spotted fever. *MMWR,* 1985;34:195–197.

Babesiosis

Clindamycin and quinine treatment for *Babesia microti* infections. *MMWR,* 1983;32:65.

Gombert ME, Goldstein EJC, Benach JL, et al. Human babesiosis. *JAMA,* 1982;248:3004–3007.

Jacoby GA, Hunt JU, Kosinski KS. Treatment of transfusion-transmitted babesiosis by exchange transfusion. *N Engl J Med,* 1980;303:1098–1100

Ruebush TK, Spielman A. Human babesiosis in the U.S. *Ann Int Med,* 1978;88:263.

Lyme Disease

Burgdorfor W, Barbour AG, Hayes SF, et al. Lyme disease—A tick-borne spirochetosis? *Science,* 1982;216:1137–1319.

Magnarelli LA, Anderson JF, Barbour AG. The etiologic agent of Lyme disease in deer flies, horse flies, and mosquitoes. *J Infect Dis,* 1986;154:355–358.

Shrestha M, Grodzicki RL, Steere AC. Diagnosing early Lyme disease. *Am J Med,* 1985;78:235–240.

Steere AC, Malawista SE. Cases of Lyme disease in the US: Locations correlated with distribution of *Ixodes dammini. Ann Int Med,* 1979;91:730–733.

Steere AC, Grodzicki RL, Kornblatt AN, et al. The spirochetal etiology of Lyme disease. *N Engl J Med,* 1983;308:733–740.

Ticks

Needham GR. Evaluation of five popular methods for tick removal. *Pediatrics,* 1985;75:997–1002.

Ticks: Of public health importance and their control. Atlanta, GA, Centers for Disease Control, 1978; publication no. 79-8142.

Tick Paralysis

Gothe R. The mechanism of pathogenicity in the tick paralysis. *J Med Entomol,* 1979;16:357–362.

Tick paralysis. *MMWR,* 1981;30:217.

Snake Bites

Curry, SC, Kraner JC, Kunkel DB, et al. Noninvasive vascular studies in management of rattlesnake evenomation to extremities. *Ann Emerg Med,* 1985;14:1081–1084.

Goldstein EJC, Citron DM, Gonzalez H, et al. Bacteriology of rattlesnake venom and implications for therapy. *J Infect Dis,* 1979;140:818–821.

Grace TG, Omer GE. The management of upper extremity pit viper wounds. *J Hand Surg,* 1980;2:168–177

Minton SA. Present tests for detection of snake venom: Clinical applications. *Ann Emerg Med,* 1987;16:932–937.

Parrish HM, Badgley RF, Carr CA. Poisonous snake bites in New England. *N Engl J Med,* 1960;788–793.

Russell F. Jaws that bite. *Emerg Med,* 1978;10:25–40.

Russell F, Carlson RW, Wainschel J, et al. Snake venom poisoning in the U.S. *JAMA,* 1975;233:341–344.

Spider Bites

Burnett JW. Latrodectism: Black widow spider bites. *Cutis,* 1985;36:121.

Editorial. Spider bites. *Lancet,* 1969;2:509.

Gorham JR. The brown recluse spider, *loxosceles reclusa* and necrotic spider bite—a new public health problem in the U.S. *J. Environ Health,* 1968;31:138.

Hunt GP. Bites and stings of uncommon arthropods. 1. Spiders. *Postgrad Med,* 1981;70:91–102.

Rees R, Campbell D, Reiger E, et al. Diagnosis and treatment of brown recluse spider bites. *Ann Emerg Med,* 1987;16:945–955

Scorpion Stings

Horen WP. Insect and scorpion stings. *JAMA,* 1972; 221:894–898.

Kizer KW. Scorpaenidae envenomation. *JAMA,* 1985; 253:907–910.

Rimsza ME, Zimmerman DR, Bergson PS, et al. Scorpion envomization. *Pediatrics,* 1980;66:298–302.

Hymenoptera Stings

Emergency treatment of insect sting allergy. *JAMA,* 1978; 240:27–35.

Golden DE, Valentine MD, Sobotka AK, et al. Regimens of hymenoptera venom immunotherapy. *Ann Intern Med,* 1980;92:620–624.

Halstead BW. Poisonous and venomous marine animals of the world. Vols I & II, Washington: Government Printing Office, 1965, 1967.

Lichtenstein LM, Valentine MD, Sobotka AK, et al. A case for venom treatment in anaphylactic sensitivity to hymenoptera sting. *N Engl J Med,* 1974;290:1223–1227.

Schwartz HJ. Appropriate evaluation & therapy of stinging insect hypersensitivity. *Arch Int Med,* 1984;144:1560–1561.

Stawiski MA. Insect bites and stings. *Emerg Med Clin North,* 1985;3:785–808.

Erysipeloid

Erysipelothrix rhusiopathiae septicemia. *N Engl J Med,* 1978;298:957–962.

Grieco MH, Sheldon C. *Erysipelothrix rhusiopathiae. Ann NY Acad Sci,* 1970;174:523–532.

Klauder JV. Erysipeloid as an occupational disease. *JAMA,* 1938;11:1345–1348.

Nelson E. Five hundred cases of erysipeloid. *Rocky Mountain Med J,* 1955;52:40–42.

Price J, Bennett W. The erysipeloid of Rosenbach. *Br Med J,* 1951;2:1060–1062.

Seal Bite

Beck B, Smith TG. Seal finger: An unsolved medical problem in Canada. Technical report of the Fisheries Research Board of Canada. No. 625. Arctic Biological Station, Fisheries & Marine Service (Quebec: Ste Anne de Bellevue), 1976.

Hillenbrand FKM. Whale finger and seal finger. *Lancet, 1953;* 2:680–681.

Markham RB, Polk F. Seal finger. *J Infect Dis,* 1979;1:567–569.

Coelenterata

Drury JK, Noonan JD, Pollack JG, et al. Jelly fish sting with serious hand complications. *Injury,* 1980;12:66–68.

Burnett JW. Studies on the serologic response to jelly fish envenomation. *J Am Acad Dermatol,* 1983;9:229–231.

Burnett JW. Recurrent eruption following solitary envenomation by the cniderian stomolophous meleagris. *Toxicol,* 1985;23:1010–1014.

Hartwick R, Callanan U, Williamson J, et al. Disarming the box-jelly fish: Nemocyst inhibition in *Chironex fleckeri. Med J Aust,* 1980;1:15–20.

Howard RJ, Pessa ME, Brennaman BH, et al. Necrotizing soft-tissue injections caused by marine vibrios. *Surgery,* 1985;98:126–130.

Lightning Injuries

Apfelberg DB, Masters FW, Robinson DW. Pathophysiology and treatment of lightning injuries. *J Trauma,* 1974; 14:453–460.

Cooper MA. Electrical and lightning injuries. *Emerg Med Clin North Am,* 1984;2:489–501.

CHAPTER 11

Infectious Diseases in the Emergency Department

HARVEY B. SIMON, M.D.

Infectious diseases are among the most important problems for which patients seek medical care in the emergency department. The spectrum ranges from acute medical emergencies, such as bacterial meningitis and septic shock, to subtle diagnostic puzzles, such as fever of unknown origin. The etiologic agents span a diverse range of bacteria, viruses, fungi, and parasites, which may involve any organ system. Modern antimicrobial chemotherapy provides the means to eradicate many of these infections, but these drugs must be administered with care. The initial evaluation of the patient in the emergency department is often crucial. In the case of life-threatening sepsis, diagnosis and therapy must proceed without delay, and even in less dramatic situations, the emergency department workup may provide the only opportunity to collect diagnostic specimens before therapeutic intervention alters the microbial flora. Because of their frequency, seriousness, and treatability, this chapter will concentrate on the emergency management of acute bacterial infections.

GENERAL APPROACH TO THE PATIENT WITH SUSPECTED INFECTION

Evaluation of the patient with suspected infection is directed toward answering two basic questions: (*a*) What organ system is involved? Does the patient have a localized infection such as pneumonia or pyelonephritis or a generalized infection such as bacteremia? (*b*) What is the etiologic agent? Is the pneumonia, for example, caused by the pneumococcus or by a Gram-negative bacterium? The answers to these questions depend on a detailed history, a meticulous physical examination, and appropriate laboratory procedures, particularly Gram's stains and cultures.

History

Many items should be stressed when taking the history of a patient with suspected infectious disease:

1. Host factors. Is the patient normally healthy or does he or she have an underlying disease that may make the patient unusually susceptible to infection? For example, patients with malignant conditions (especially lymphoma, leukemia, and myeloma), acquired immunodeficiency syndrome (AIDS), diabetes, neutropenia, or sickle cell anemia and patients receiving corticosteroids or other immunosuppressive drugs may become infected with unusual, opportunistic pathogens or may be unable to respond normally, even to the common pathogens. For such patients, a vigorous approach to diagnosis and therapy is required. Patients with foreign material in place, such as a prosthetic heart valve, are also particularly vulnerable to infection.

2. Epidemiology. Has the patient traveled to areas where he or she may have been exposed to "exotic" infections such as typhoid fever or malaria? Has the patient been exposed to animals or birds that may transmit infection? Even common pets may be implicated, such as the cat (cat-scratch fever and *Pasteurella multocida* cellulitis from scratches or bites, toxoplasmosis from fecal contamination), parakeet (psittacosis), and turtle (salmonellosis). Bites of stray dogs, skunks, and bats are potentially serious because of the possibility of rabies. Has the patient been exposed to other persons with communicable diseases, such as influenza or tuberculosis? Have other persons in the community been ill recently? Does the patient's occupation provide clues to unusual infections, such as brucellosis or Q fever in slaughterhouse workers?

3. Antibiotics. Has the patient been receiving antibiotics that may alter susceptibility to infection by favoring growth of drug-resistant organisms? Does the patient have any drug allergies that may alter the physicians's choice of therapeutic agents? Are there underlying medical problems, such as renal failure, that may influence therapy?

4. Symptoms and clinical course. An important element in the history is to evaluate the course of the illness. Was the onset sudden or gradual? Is the illness rapidly progressing or smoldering? Symptoms such as headache, altered consciousness, cough, dyspnea, flank pain, and dysuria are especially helpful in localizing the infection. If the patient is unable to answer clearly, a friend or relative can often provide important information.

Physical Examination

A detailed physical examination is necessary. Vital signs must be measured carefully; hypotension, severe respiratory distress, or extreme hyperpyrexia may require immediate treatment. Although fever is an important clue to infection, the emergency physician must remember that many patients with infections are afebrile, and in other patients, fever may develop from noninfectious causes. Examination of the skin and mucous membranes may provide crucial information. For example, petechial eruptions may suggest meningococcemia or Rocky Mountain spotted fever, pustular lesions may indicate gonococcemia or staphylococcal endocarditis, an erythroderm with desquamation may suggest toxic shock syndrome, splinter hemorrhages and conjunctival petechiae may be clues to endocarditis, and macular or vesicular eruptions may reflect many viral infections. Similarly, the ocular fundi should be examined; Roth's spots suggest endocarditis, and choroidal tubercles may be the only physical finding in patients with miliary tuberculosis. Enlarged lymph nodes should be sought. Examination of the chest may disclose pneumonia or empyema, and cardiac examination may reveal evidence of endocarditis or pericarditis. Abdominal findings can disclose hepatomegaly or splenomegaly, or indicate an abscess or peritonitis, as can rectal and pelvic examinations. Evaluation of the musculoskeletal system can reveal septic arthritis or osteomyelitis, and neurologic evaluation can raise the possibility of meningitis or encephalitis.

Laboratory Evaluation

While a history should be taken and a physical examination performed in every patient with suspected infection, the clinical laboratory must be utilized more selectively. Once the infectious process can be localized to an organ system, that area should be studied intensively. In many patients, however, the history and physical examination fail to define the source of fever. In these patients and in patients with multiple problems or a systemic toxic reaction, certain laboratory studies are essential:

1. Compete blood cell count and differential. Polymorphonuclear leukocytosis with immature forms (a "shift to the left") suggests, but does not prove, bacterial infection. Toxic granulations, vacuoles, and Döhle inclusion bodies in polymorphonuclear leukocytes strongly indicate bacterial infection, and these should be sought in all blood smears.

2. Urinalysis. Pyuria and leukocyte casts suggest a urinary tract infection.

3. Posteroanterior and lateral chest x-ray films.

Such films may disclose pneumonitis even in the absence of abnormalities on physical examination.

4. Blood chemistries. Determination of the blood glucose level may reveal unsuspected diabetes and is important in evaluating the significance of the glucose concentrations in other body fluids. Liver function tests are often helpful in defining obscure fevers.

5. Examination of other body fluids. This is not always indicated, but may be lifesaving. If there is any possibility of meningitis, a lumbar puncture must be performed. Taps of pleural effusion, ascitic fluid, or joint effusion, may be extremely informative; whenever possible, these procedures should be performed in the emergency department before beginning antimicrobial therapy. Fluids should be examined directly by cell counts and differential studies, and the concentrations of glucose and protein should be determined. Gram's stains and cultures are mandatory.

6. Cultures and Gram's stains. These are critically important. The emergency department evaluation of a patient with fever of undefined origin should include cultures of blood (at least two cultures, each from a separate venipuncture), urine (a clean voided specimen), and sputum (together with a Gram's stain). If any other body fluids are obtained, they too should be examined by culture and a Gram's stain.

Bacteriologic Procedures in the Emergency Department

The cornerstone of management of an infectious disease is isolation and identification of the responsible pathogen. This requires the services of a professional bacteriology laboratory that can evaluate a specimen fully, which usually requires several days. However, because the physician is responsible not only for ordering the appropriate tests but also for interpreting the results, she or he must be familiar with bacteriologic principles. In addition, specimens should be collected and prepared for analysis before antimicrobial therapy is begun, and in many institutions, bacteriology technologists are not available during the evening and weekend hours when so many patients seek emergency care. The purpose of this section, therefore, is to discuss the bacteriologic procedures that the physician may have to perform. A few hours in the bacteriology laboratory will provide excellent practice.

Obtaining the Specimen

It is extremely important to obtain appropriate specimens before antibiotic therapy; in fact, antibiotic selection often depends on preliminary analysis of the specimen in the emergency department. Techniques for obtaining specimens of sputum, urine, and other body fluids are discussed in later sections.

Blood cultures are necessary for almost all patients with serious infections. Since the blood must not be contaminated with normal skin bacteria, meticulous preparation is required.

1. With tourniquet in place, select vein.
2. Prepare skin twice with iodine solution.
3. Prepare skin with alcohol.
4. Obtain 10 ml of blood. If venipuncture is difficult and requires excessive manipulation, the likelihood of contamination has increased, and an alternative site should be sought.
5. Place 5 ml of blood into each of two blood culture flasks. Ordinarily, one flask contains dextrose-phosphate broth, and the other, thioglycollate broth. The flasks should be prepared either by flaming (screw cap) or with alcohol swabs (rubber-stopped top). Incubate at 37°C.
6. Repeat blood culture, using a different site, preferably after waiting at least 30 minutes.

Examining the Specimen

The specimen can be examined in the emergency department within minutes. The macroscopic appearance may be very informative. Turbidity in cerebrospinal fluid, ascitic fluid, or urine often results from infection. A good sputum specimen from a patient with bacterial pneumonitis or bronchitis is usually thick, viscous, green, gray, or yellow. A foul odor from sputum or other body fluids is an important clue to the presence of anaerobic organisms that require specialized diagnostic techniques and chemotherapeutic agents.

Microscopic evaluation is critical. Ideally, all specimens of sputum, cerebrospinal fluid, and other body fluids should be examined using the Gram's stain technique; this is helpful but not mandatory for unspun specimens of urine, since urinalysis and quantitative cultures can frequently provide equivalent data.

Gram's Stain

1. Prepare smear by swabbing specimen on a clean glass slide. Air dry.
2. Heat fix by passing slide over Bunsen burner flame two or three times. Allow to cool.
3. Flood slide with gentian violet for 15 seconds. Rinse with water.
4. Flood slide with Gram's iodine for 15 seconds. Rinse with water.
5. Decolorize with 95% alcohol. This is the only step that requires experience. In the case of thin body fluids such as the cerebrospinal fluid, decolorization should render the specimen color-

Table 11.1.
Guide to Cultures

Specimen	Method of Procurement	Medium[a]	Other Studies
Blood	Sterile venipunture (10 ml blood)	Dextrose phosphate broth THIO	
Pharynx	Throat swab	BAP CAP if patient <6 years *(H. influenzae)* TM in 5% CO_2 or Transgrow if gonococcus suspected Loeffler if *C. diphtheriae* suspected	Methylene blue smear (if indicated) Rapid immunolgic tests for group A streptococcus
Middle ear	Myringotomy	BAP CAP	Gram's stain
Sinus	Surgical drainage or drainage from ostium	BAP CAP Anaerobic BAP	Gram's stain
Sputum	Expectoration Nasotracheal suction Transtracheal aspiration	BAP MacC or EMB CAP if patient <6 years or if *H. influenzae* suspected.	Gram's stain
		LJ if *M. tuberculosis* suspected[b] SAB if fungus suspected CYE if *Legionella* suspected	Acid-fast smear (if indicated) Fungal wet mount (if indicated)
Lung aspirate	Needle aspiration	As for sputum plus anaerobic BAP	Cytology Pathology
Pleural fluid	Thoracentesis	As for sputum plus anaerobic BAP	Cell count and differential Glucose, protein, lactate dehydrogenase Cytology Acid-fast smear (if indicated)
Peritoneal fluid	Paracentesis	BAP MacC or EMB THIO Anearobic BAP LJ if *M. tuberculosis* suspected[b]	Cell count and differential Glucose, protein, lactate dehydrogenase Cytology Acid-fast smear (if indicated)
Joint fluid	Arthrocentesis	BAP CAP in 5% CO_2 THIO LJ if *M. tuberculosis* suspected[b]	Gram's stain Cell count and differential Glucose, protein, crystals, mucin Acid-fast smear (if indicated)

Table 11.1—*continued*

Specimen	Method of Procurement	Medium[a]	Other Studies
Urine	Midstream clean voided specimen Bladder tap (especially in children) Urethral catheterization	BAP MacC or EMB	Urinalysis Gram's stain of unspun urine
Cerebrospinal fluid	Lumbar puncture	BAP CAS in 5% CO_2 THIO SAB if fungus suspected LJ if *M. tuberculosis* suspected[b]	Gram's stain Cell count and differential Glucose, protein Pressure (manometrics) India ink preparation (if indicated) Acid-fast smear (if indicated) Cytology (if indicated)
Wound Abscess	Swab or aspiration	BAP MacC or EMB CAS THIO Anaerobic BAP	Gram's stain
Urethra Cervix	Swab	TM in 5% CO_2 or Transgrow	Gram's stain
Skin	Aspiration	BAP MacC or EMB THIO	Gram's stain
Stool	Stool sample or rectal swab	SS Selenite BAP Campy	Direct examination for ova and parasites (if indicated) Gram's stain (if staphylococcal enterocolitis suspected) Methylene blue smear for leukocytes

[a] All specimens should be incubated at 37°C. THIO, thioglycollate broth; BAP, blood agar plate; CAP, chocolate agar plate; TM, Thayer-Martin agar; MacC, MacConkey agar; EMB, eosin-methylene blue agar; LJ, Löwenstein-Jensen slant; SAB, Sabouraud agar; CYE, charcoal yeast extract agar; CAS, chocolate agar slant; SS, Salmonella-Shigella agar; Campy, campylobacter (incubated at 42°C).
[b] Or other media for *M. tuberculosis* such as Middlebrook 7H10.

less; for this the alcohol should remain on the slide about 10 seconds. In the case of sputum or pus, the alcohol should be dropped onto the slide until the thinnest parts of the smear are colorless but the thickest parts retain a blue hue. After decolorization, rinse with water.

6. Flood slide with safranin for 15 seconds. Rinse with water.
7. Blot dry with filter paper and examine under oil immersion lens.

Interpretation of the Gram's stain requires practice. The polymorphonuclear leukocytes should be examined first; in a properly stained smear, they appear pink. Next, the numbers and types of inflammatory cells should be evaluated; abundant polymorphonuclear leukocytes often reflect bacterial inflammation. Finally, the bacterial flora should be examined. Are the organisms Gram-positive (blue) or Gram-negative (red)? Are they cocci (round), bacilli (rod-shaped), or do they have an intermediate shape (coccobacillary)? Is more than one type of organism present? It is important to remember that help in interpreting results is available; slides can be saved and reviewed with a bacteriologist or pathologist.

Although the Gram's stain is central to the evaluation of most bacterial infections, other procedures are required for the identification of certain organisms.

1. *Mycobacterium tuberculosis* and other mycobacteria—acid-fat stain.
2. *Cryptococcus meningitidis*—India ink preparation.
3. Fungi—fungal wet mount.
4. Nocardia and *Actinomyces israeli*—modified acid-fast stain.
5. *Corynebacterium diptheriae*—methylene blue preparation.
6. Intestinal parasites—stool examination.

Because they are used less frequently, these techniques are not discussed here, but can be reviewed in standard texts.

Culturing the Specimen

Since many pathogenic bacteria are fastidious, it is important to culture specimens promptly. Many types of media are available (Table 11.1). In general, solid media are useful in providing quantitative estimates of the organisms present and in allowing study of individual bacteria, while liquid media enable just a few organisms to grow readily. Some media are *enriched* to enhance growth of the more fastidious organisms, while other media are *selective,* that is, designed to inhibit growth of the normal flora, thus allowing the pathogens to grow.

When a specimen is inoculated on a solid medium, it should first be streaked across one quadrant of the culture plate with a sterile swab or loop (Fig. 11.1). Then, with a loop that has been flamed and allowed to cool, the specimen should be streaked across a second quadrant. This procedure should be performed twice more, flaming and cooling the loop each time. This will reduce the number of bacteria, enabling the technician later to select individual colonies for study.

When a liquid medium is used, the loop swab should be immersed in it and rotated several times. The mouth of the medium tube should be flamed before and after the specimen is introduced.

Anaerobic cultures require special mention. Numerous species of anaerobic bacteria reside in the upper part of the respiratory tract, in the gastrointestinal tract, and in the female genitourinary tract. It has become increasingly clear that these bacteria can be important pathogens. Infections that are particularly likely to be caused at least partly by anaerobes include abscesses, infections with foul-smelling pus, gas-forming infections, infections involving necrotic tissue, and other infections arising from respiratory, gastrointestinal, or genitourinary foci. Anaerobic bacteria will not grow in the presence of oxygen; hence, when they are suspected, specimens should be streaked on blood agar plates

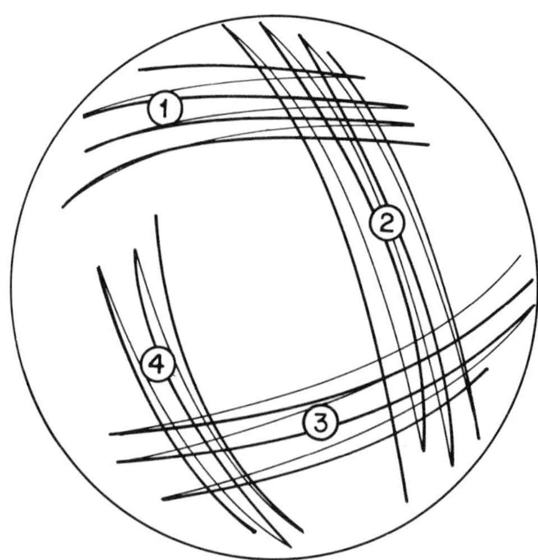

Figure 11.1. Technique of streaking specimen on agar plate.

and cultured in anaerobic jars. Many devices can be used to remove oxygen from such jars either chemically or nonchemically; in addition, numerous media are becoming available to preserve anaerobic conditions even while the specimen is en route to the laboratory.

Bacterial cultures must grow at least 24 hours before they can provide diagnostic information, and to obtain complete data usually takes 2–3 days. What data can the laboratory provide? Identification of the bacteria in the specimen is of utmost importance, as is antibiotic sensitivity testing of possible pathogens to ensure optimal antimicrobial therapy. However, interpretation of results is the responsibility not only of those in the laboratory but also of the physician. The presence of a microorganism does *not* automatically implicate it in the patient's disease. Four considerations may assist in interpreting results.

1. Contamination. Small numbers of organisms, unusual bacteria, or results inconsistent with clinical findings should raise the possibility of contamination.

2. Normal flora. Although the blood, cerebrospinal fluid, and urine are normally sterile, some areas of the body such as the skin, the gastrointestinal tract, the female genital tract, and the upper part of the respiratory tract teem with bacteria that are ordinarily harmless in those locations. The laboratory personnel must select possible pathogens from all these bacteria; the physician must differentiate pathogens from harmless saprophytes.

3. Tissue tropism. Certain bacteria are highly pathogenic in some areas of the body, but harmless in others. For example, the pneumococcus is a leading cause of otitis, sinusitis, and pneumonia, but

although it frequently inhabits the nasopharynx, it never causes pharyngitis. When the laboratory reports growth of pneumococci from a throat swab, the clinician's reaction should be different from his or her reaction to the same organism from a sputum culture.

4. Carrier state. Pathogens may be present without causing disease. For example, meningococci may be cultured from the throat, or salmonellae from the stool, of a healthy individual. Such findings may have greater significance for the epidemiologist than for the patient.

Thus far, only bacterial infections have been considered; the same laboratory principles apply to mycobacterial and fungal infections. Viruses, mycoplasmas, rickettsiae, and chlamydiae, however, are all important pathogens that require special culture techniques. The emergency physician can often suspect diseases caused by such organisms based on epidemiologic and clinical findings and can assist in the establishment of a definitive diagnosis by obtaining an "acute phase" serum sample and freezing it for later serologic study when a "convalescent phase" sample is also available.

SPECIFIC INFECTIOUS DISEASES

Before some of the infectious diseases seen in the emergency department are considered, some cautionary words are in order. First, patients are rarely seen with conditions as neatly defined as in this section; most patients pose problems of differential diagnosis. Second, spatial limitations make it necessary to emphasize problems that are common, serious, and treatable. Even so, generalizations are necessary, and the reader is invited to expand his or her understanding through the suggested readings. Third, neither diagnosis nor therapy stops in the emergency department. Both the patient who is sent home and the patient who is admitted to the hospital require follow-up study to reevaluate the validity of the emergency department diagnosis and the efficacy of initial therapy. This is particularly true of infectious diseases, since the cultures and sensitivity tests that are so crucial to therapy require at least 24–48 hours for interpretation.

Infections of the Respiratory Tract

Infections of the respiratory tract are among the most common infectious diseases seen in the emergency department. Although they range in location and severity from simple upper respiratory infection to overwhelming bacterial pneumonia, the approach to diagnosis and therapy remains similar.

Sinusitis and Otitis

Often, sinusitis and otitis are caused by the same viruses that cause the common cold. However, bacterial pathogens can produce more serious infections in the sinuses or ears; bacterial infection, in fact, often occurs after a milder viral process. The signs and symptoms of sinusitis and otitis, as well as the value of local therapy to ensure adequate drainage of these potentially closed spaces, are discussed in Chapter 42. Identification of the bacterial pathogens responsible for such infections is complicated by two problems. (*a*) As previously mentioned, the upper part of the respiratory tract teems with microorganisms that constitute its normal flora. (*b*) The involved anatomic parts are inaccessible for direct culture except during operation. Cultures of the nasopharynx do not accurately reflect the disease process. Hence, therapy often is educated guesswork based on knowledge of the usual pathogens. Fortunately, the range of possibilities is limited. In adults, most cases of bacterial sinusitis and otitis are caused by the Gram-positive cocci, including the pneumococcus, group A streptococci, and in occasional cases of sinusitis, *Staphylococcus aureus*. In children, the same organisms are frequently implicated, as well as *Haemophilus influenzae*. Recently, anaerobic bacteria have also been implicated in some cases of sinusitis. For acute sinusitis, ampicillin or amoxicillin are the preferred antibiotics; dicloxacillin may be useful in chronic sinusitis (Table 11.2). In the penicillin-allergic patient, cephalosporins, erythromycin, and clindamycin are acceptable alternatives; trimethoprim-sulfamethoxazole or erythromycin plus a sulfonamide may be especially useful in children. Table 11.3 lists appropriate dosages for mild infections. Most patients respond to oral administration of antibiotics without hospitalization.

Complications resulting from extension of infection to surrounding tissues include osteomyelitis, brain abscess, subdural empyema, and orbital cellutitis. These much more serious infections require immediate hospitalization, parenteral administration of large doses of antibiotics, and in the case of intracranial septic collections, surgical drainage.

Pharyngitis

In most patients, pharyngitis is mild; fever, sore throat, and occasionally dysphagia are the presenting symptoms. The major differential diagnosis is between viral infection and group A streptococcal pharyngitis. Even though high fever, cervical lymphadenopathy, pharyngeal exudate, and polymorphonuclear leukocytosis suggest streptococcal pharyngitis, throat culture is the definitive means of diagnosis. A rapid presumptive diagnosis of streptococcal pharyngitis can be made using kits which extract group A strepcococcal antigens from throat swabs, allowing immunologic identification. If "strep throat" seems likely, antibiotic therapy can

Table 11.2.
Characteristics of Some Common Bacterial Pathogens

Organism	Description	Medium[a]	Usual Location	Common Infections	Antibiotic of Choice[b]	Alternative Antibiotics[b]
Gram-positive cocci						
S. pneumoniae Pneumococcus	Lancet-shaped in pairs or short chains	BAP	Nasopharynx	Pneumonia, bronchitis, otitis, sinusitis, bacteremia, meningitis	Penicillin	Cephalosporins[c] Erythromycin Clindamycin Chloramphenicol (for meningitis)
S. aureus	Pairs, clusters, and clumps	BAP	Nasopharynx Skin Rectum	Skin infections, pneumonia, sinusitis, septic arthritis, bacteremia, endocarditis, osteomyelitis	Oxacillin[d]	Cephalosporins[c] Vancomycin Erythromycin Clindamycin
Group A streptococci	Pairs and chains	BAP	Nasopharynx	Pharyngitis, otitis, sinusitis, skin infection, osteomyelitis, septic arthritis, bacteremia, pneumonia	Penicillin	Cephalosporins[c] Vancomycin Erythromycin Clindamycin
S. viridans	Pairs and chains	BAP	Oral cavity	Endocarditis	Penicillin	Cephalosporins[c] Vancomycin (for endocarditis) Erythromycin Clindamycin
Enterococcus (group D streptococci)	Pairs and chains	BAP	Gastrointestinal tract Female genital tract	Urinary tract infection	Ampicillin	Variable
				Wound abscess, bacteremia, endocarditis,	Penicillin or ampicillin and gentamicin	Vancomycin alone or in combination with gentamicin (for

				peritonitis	(for serious sepsis)	serious sepsis)
Anaerobic streptococcus	Pair and chains	Anaerobic BAP	Oral cavity Gastrointestinal tract Female genital tract	Pulmonary, brain, and abdominal abscesses; empyema	Penicillin	Clindamycin Erythromycin Cephalosporins[c]
Gram-positive bacilli						
C. perfringens	Large rods	Anaerobic BAP	Gastrointestinal tract	Muscle, uterus, wound, bacteremia	Penicillin	Chloramphenicol Clindamycin Metronidazole
Gram-negative cocci						
N. gonorrhoeae	Bean-shaped diplococci	CAP or TM in 5%	Genitourinary tract	Urethritis, cervicitis, pharyngitis, septic arthritis, bacteremia	Penicillin, ampicillin, or tetracycline	Spectinomycin or ceftriaxone[c] Cefoxitin[c]
N. meningitidis	Bean-shaped diplococci	CAP or TM in 5% CO_2	Nasopharynx	Meningitis, bacteremia Carrier state	Penicillin Rifampin	Chloramphenicol A third generation cephalosporin[c] Minocycline
Gram-negative bacilli						
E. coli	Rods	BAP MacC	Gastrointestinal tract Female genital tract	Intraabdominal infection, urinary tract infection, bacteremia, neonatal meningitis, nosocomial pneumonia	Ampicillin	Cephalosporins[c] Chloramphenicol Gentamicin Tobramycin Tetracycline, sulfisoxazole, or trimethoprim-sulfamethoxazole (for urinary tract infection)
K. pneumoniae	Rods with thick capsules	BAP MacC	Gastrointestinal tract	Urinary tract infection,	Gentamicin or cephalosporins[c]	Tobramycin Kanamycin

Table 11.2—*continued*

Organism	Description	Medium[a]	Usual Location	Common Infections	Antibiotic of Choice[b]	Alternative Antibiotics[b]
			Female genital tract	pneumonia, intraabdominal infection, bacteremia		Amikacin Trimethoprim-sulfamethoxazole Chloramphenicol
P. mirabilis	Rods	BAP MacC	Gastrointestinal tract	Urinary tract infection, intraabdominal infection, bacteremia	Ampicillin	Cephalosporins[c] Gentamicin or tobramycin
Indole-positive Proteus species	Rods	BAP MacC	Gastrointestinal tract	Urinary tract infection, intraabdominal infection, bacteremia	Gentamicin or a second or third generation cephalosporin[c]	Tobramycin Amikacin Carbenicillin[e] or ticarcillin Chloramphenicol
P. aeruginosa	Rods	BAP MacC	Skin	Urinary tract infection, bacteremia, nosocomial infection	Gentamicin or tobramycin alone, or in combination with ticarcillin or piperacillin	Amikacin Carbenicillin, ticarcillin, or piperacillin Ceftazidime[c] Imipenim[c]
Bacteroides						
Oral strains	Thin filamentous rods	Anaerobic BAP	Oral cavity	Aspiration pneumonia, pulmonary and brain abscesses	Penicillin	Clindamycin Cefoxitin[c] Chloramphenicol Metronidazole
Gastrointestinal strains	Thin filamentous rods	Anaerobic BAP	Gastrointestinal tract Female genital tract	Intraabdominal infection, wound abcess, bacteremia	Clindamycin or chloramphenicol Cefoxitin[c] Metronidazole	Carbenicillin[e] Imipenim
H. influenzae	Small coccobacillary	CAP	Nasopharynx	Adults—bronchitis, epiglottitis Children—otitis,	Ampicillin[f] Chloramphenicol[f]	Cefuroxime and third generation cephalosporins[c]

				sinusitis, pneumonia, meningitis, bacteremia, pharyngitis, bronchitis, epiglottitis		Tetracycline Trimethoprim-sulfamethoxazole
L. pneumophila	Bacilli (not well seen with Gram's stain)	Charcoal-yeast extract agar	Lung	Pneumonia	Erythromycin	Rifampin Trimethoprim-sulfamethoxazole

[a] BAP, blood agar plate; CAP, chocolate agar plate; TM, Thayer-Martin agar; MacC, MacConkey agar.

[b] Antibiotic of choice depends on sensitivity testing. Antibiotics listed are mostly likely to be effective at present, but sensitivities should be confirmed.

[c] Cephalosporins and other β-lactam antibiotics such as imipenim *must be used with caution in penicillin-allergic patients*. The older cephalosporins are ineffective in meningitis but "third generation" drugs such as cefotaxime are effective in meningitis (due to susceptible pathogens).

[d] Nafcillin is an equally effective parenteral antistaphylococcal agent. Cloxacillin or dicloxacillin is preferred for oral administration in mild infections. If organisms are penicillin-sensitive, penicillin is drug of choice.

[e] Ticarcillin, mezlocillin, piperacillin, and azlocillin are similar to carbenicillin.

[f] Some strains of *H. influenzae* are ampicillin-resistant. In life-threatening *H. influenzae* infections, chloramphenicol should be administered until sensitivities are known. Parenteral third generation cephalosporins or cefuroxime are excellent alternatives. In mild *H. influenzae* infections in penicillin-allergic patients, tetracycline or trimethoprim-sulfamethoxazole are preferred.

Table 11.3.
Dosage Ranges for Selected Antibiotics[a]

Drug	Route	Adult Dosage	Pediatric Dosage	Comments and Typical Indications
Penicillins[b]				
Penicillin V	p.o.	250 mg every 4–6 hr	30–60 mg/kg/day divided into 4 doses	Bronchitis, otitis, pharyngitis
Penicillin G procaine	i.m.	600,000—1.2 millions units every 12 hrs	25,000–50,000 units/kg/day divided into 2 doses	Bronchitis, otitis, pharyngitis, pneumococcal pneumonia
Penicillin G	i.m.	600,000 units every 6 hr	25,000–50,000 units/kg/day divided into 4 doses	Bronchitis, otitis, pharyngitis, pneumococcal pneumonia
Aqueous crystalline	i.v.	1–4 million units every 4 hr	100,000–400,000 units/kg/day divided into 6 doses	Lower doses for streptococcal pneumonia, pulmonary abscess; highest doses for endocarditis, meningitis
Ampicillin	p.o.	250–500 mg every 4–6 hr	50–100 mg/kg/day divided into 4 doses	Otitis (pediatric), bronchitis, urinary tract infection
	i.v.	1–2 gm every 4–6 hr	100–400 mg/kg/day divided into 6 doses	Lower doses for pneumonia, pyelonephritis; highest doses for meningitis
Cloxacillin or dicloxacillin	p.o.	250–500 mg every 4–6 hr	50–100 mg/kg/day divided into 4 doses	Skin and soft tissue infections, sinusitis
Oxacillin or nafcillin	i.v.	1–2 gm every 4 hr	50–200 mg/kg/day divided into 6 doses	Highest doses for endocarditis, meningitis, osteomyelitis
Carbenicillin	p.o.	1–2 tablets (382 mg/tablet) every 6 hr	50–65 mg/kg/day divided into 4 doses	Urinary tract infection only
	i.v.	4–6 gm every 4 hr	100–600 mg/kg/day divided into 4 or 6 doses	Lower doses for urinary tract infection; higher doses for bacteremia, pneumonia; often used with an aminoglycoside; high sodium content
Ticarcillin, mezlocillin, piperacillin, or azlocillin	i.v.	2–3 gm every 4 hr	150–300 mg/kg/day divided into 4 or 6 doses	Similar to carbenicillin, except lower sodium content
Cephalosporins				
First generation				
Cephalexin	p.o.	250–500 mg every 6 hr	25–50 mg/kg/day divided into 4 doses	Urinary tract infection, pharyngitis, skin and soft tissue infections
Cephalothin Cephapirin	i.v.	0.75–2 gm every 4 hr	50–150 mg/kg/day divided into 4 doses	Lower doses for pyelonephritis; higher doses for pneumonia,

				bacteremia, endocarditis, osteomyelitis. Not effective for meningitis
Cefazolin	i.v., i.m.	0.5–1.5 gm every 6–8 hr	25–50 mg/kg/day divided into 3 or 4 doses	Similar to cephalothin except longer half-life, less painful i.m.
Second generation				
Cefaclor	p.o.	250–500 mg every 8 hr	40 mg/kg/day divided into 3 doses	Similar to cephalexin but more active against *H. Influenzae*
Cefoxitin	i.v.	0.75–2 gm every 6 hr	50–150 mg/kg/day divided into 4 or 6 doses	Most active against anaerobes; active against *N. gonorrhoeae*
Cefuroxime	i.v.	0.75–1.5 gm every 6 hr	100–200 mg/kg/day divided into 4 doses	Active against *H. Influenzae*; only second generation cephalosporin approved for meningitis
Third generation				
Cefotaxime	i.v.	0.75–2 gm every 4–6 hr	100–200 mg/kg/day divided into 4 doses	Typical spectrum of third generation cephalosporins, including *H. Influenzae, N. gonorrhoeae*, most enteric Gram-negative bacilli
Ceftazidime	i.v.	1–2 gm every 8–12 hr	100–200 mg/kg/day divided into 4 doses	Most active against *Pseudomonas*
Ceftriaxone	i.v.	1–2 gm every 12–24 hr	50–100 mg/kg given every 12 or 24 hr	Longest half-life; less active against *Pseudomonas* and *B. fragilis*
Imipenim	i.v.	0.5–1 gm every 6–8 hr	100–200 mg/kg/day divided into 4 doses	Extraordinarily broad spectrum, including most Gram-positive cocci, Gram-negative bacilli, and anaerobes
Erythromycin	p.o.	250–500 mg every 6 hr	20–50 mg/kg/day divided into 4 doses	Pharyngitis, otitis in penicillin-allergic patients Toxicity: hypersensitivity
	i.v.	0.25–1 gm every 6 hr	30–50 mg/kg/day divided into 4 doses	Pneumonia, cellulitis in penicillin-allergic patients Toxicity: hypersensitivity, phlebitis
Clindamycin	p.o.	150–300 mg every 6 hr	10–25 mg/kg/day divided into 4 doses	Infection with Gram-positive cocci in penicillin-allergic patients (except meningitis), anaerobic infection
	i.v., i.m.	300–600 mg every 6 hr	10–40 mg/kg/day divided into 4 doses	Toxicity: hypersensitivity, colitis

Table 11.3—*continued*

Drug	Route	Adult Dosage	Pediatric Dosage	Comments and Typical Indications
Vancomycin	i.v	250–500 mg every 6 hr	40 mg/kg/day divided into 4 doses	Life-threatening staphylococcal or enterococcal infection when penicillins and cephalosporins contraindicated
Tetracycline	p.o	250–500 mg every 6 hr	20–40 mg/kg/day divided into 4 doses	Nephrotoxic—dosage must be reduced if patient has renal failure
	i.v.	250–500 mg every 6 hr	10–20 mg/kg/day divided into 4 doses	Much overused, rarely drug of choice; may stain teeth in children
Chloramphenicol	i.v.	0.25–1 gm every 6 hr	50–100 mg/kg/day divided into 4 doses	Potential marrow toxicity, use in serious infection only; use cautiously in newborns Oral form available, but rarely indicated
Aminoglycosides				
Kanamycin, Amikacin	i.m. or i.v	7.5 mg/kg every 12 hr (maximal daily dose 1.5 gm)	Same as adult dosage	Toxicity: renal and VIII nerve
Gentamicin, Tobramycin	i.m. or i.v.	1.0–1.5 mg/kg every 8 hr	Same as adult dosage	Toxicity: renal and VIII nerve
Sulfisoxazole	p.o.	1 gm every 6 hr	150 mg/kg/day divided into 4 doses	Urinary tract infection Toxicity: hypersensitivity
Trimethoprim-sulfamethoxazole	p.o.	2 tablets every 12 hr	8 mg/kg/day (based on trimethoprim component) divided into 2 doses	Urinary tract infection Toxicity: hypersensitivity
	i.v.	3 mg/kg (based on trimethoprim component) every 8 hr	Same as adult dosage	Urinary tract infections and shigellosis (higher dose for *Pneumocystis carinii*)

[a] Dosage ranges are for average-size adults and for pediatric patients beyond neonatal period with normal renal and hepatic functions. Adult dosages are expressed per individual dose while pediatric dosages are expressed in amount per day. Pediatric doses are given in accordance with kilograms of body weight; in older children, care must be taken not to exceed normal adult doses. In all patients, dosage must be individualized; see manufacturer's literature for more details. In most cases, intravenous antibiotics should be diluted in at least 100 ml of fluid and administered over approximately 60 minutes. Avoid mixing more than one medication in each infusion bottle. Only major toxicities are listed; consult manufacturer's literature for details. In addition, all antibiotics predispose the patient to superinfection.

[b] Hypersensitivity is a major reaction; all cross-react—a patient allergic to one penicillin is allergic to all.

[c] Cephalosporins *must be used with caution in penicillin-allergic patients.* In general, the second and third generation cephalosporins have extended activity against Gram-negative organisms but less activity against Gram-positive bacteria in comparison to first generation drugs. First and second generation cephalosporins (except cefuroxime) are not effective in meningitis but third generation drugs are effective in meningitis caused by susceptible pathogens. The newer cephalosporins are more expensive and should be used only when the older agents are not effective.

be started in the emergency department. If the culture is positive, the patient should receive penicillin for 10 days to prevent rheumatic fever; if it is negative, antibiotics should be discontinued. In the penicillin-allergic patient, erythromycin is the drug of choice.

Both viral and streptococcal pharyngitis can sometimes become true medical emergencies. In patients with infectious mononucleosis, for example, the viral infection can cause sufficient edema to occlude the airway. These patients must be hospitalized and observed carefully, with tracheostomy immediately available. Fortunately, corticosteroids usually produce prompt improvement, obviating operation. Airway occlusion is also a threat if the streptococcus spreads from the pharynx to the soft tissues of the neck. Patients with this complication, called Ludwig's angina, are febrile and acutely ill, with a bullnecked appearance. Hospitalization and careful monitoring are mandatory; tracheostomy may be required but antibiotics alone can suffice. Penicillin is the traditional drug of choice, but since pathogens other than streptococcus have been reported, cefoxitin is an excellent choice for initial therapy. Streptococcal pharyngitis may lead to other serious local complications such as peritonsillar and retropharyngeal abscesses, but these infections have become rare since the introduction of penicillin.

Although many other bacteria can be cultured from the pharynx, only a few aside from the group A streptococci and *H. influenzae* in children cause pharyngitis. For example, pneumococci and *Staphylococcus aureus* do not cause pharyngitis although they may be present in large numbers. Two bacteria that can cause pharyngitis are *Neisseria gonorrhoeae* and *C. diphtheriae.* Gonococcal infection is suggested by a history of orogenital exposure, and should be confirmed by culture on Thayer-Martin or Transgrow media. Diphtheria, which is suggested in a nonimmunized patient by membranous pharyngitis sometimes accompanied by bull neck, should be confirmed with a methylene blue preparation and culture on Loeffler medium.

Epiglottitis

Another bacterial infection of the upper respiratory tract that is a true medical emergency is epiglottitis. This infection is much more common in children; when it occurs in adults, it is often fatal because of missed diagnosis. Presenting symptoms include fever, severe pharyngeal pain, dysphagia, and respiratory distress that can progress with alarming rapidity to asphyxia. The epiglottis is edematous, inflamed, and characteristically cherry red. Attempts to visualize the epiglottis directly can lead to severe spasm and airway obstruction. *Before a mirror, tongue blade, or culture swab is used, a lateral x-ray film of the neck should be taken.* If the epiglottis is edematous, instrumentation is contraindicated. If no edema is apparent and if respiratory distress is only mild, indirect laryngoscopic examination may be undertaken with caution. Tracheotomy or endotracheal intubation by an experienced person should be performed if any sign of respiratory decompensation occurs. Most epiglottitis is caused by *H. influenzae,* with Gram-positive cocci reported in a few cases. Ampicillin has traditionally been the drug of choice; however, ampicillin-resistant strains of *H. influenzae* are being recognized with increasing frequency, so chloramphenicol should also be administered until the sensitivity of the organisms is known. Cefuroxime and the third generation cephalosporins should also prove useful. Blood specimens should be cultured before therapy.

Bronchitis

Bronchitis is an infection of the lower part of the respiratory tract with typical presenting symptoms of cough, sputum production, and low-grade fever. Auscultation of the lungs may be normal or reveal diffuse rhonchi from large-airway secretions. The chest x-ray film is normal. Viruses frequently cause bronchitis; in such cases, the sputum is clear and antibiotics have no role in therapy. Bacterial infections of the tracheobronchial tree frequently are accompanied by production of purulent sputum and a higher fever. Examination of the sputum reveals the causative organism. In otherwise healthy adults, the pneumococcus is the leading bacterial cause of bronchitis; in patients with chronic pulmonary disease and in children, *H. influenzae* is also common. Examination of sputum and therapy are discussed later with the types of pneumonia. Most patients with bronchitis respond well to oral administration of antibiotics without hospitalization. In patients with chronic pulmonary disease, however, even mild infections can cause respiratory failure requiring intensive therapy. In addition, in children with bronchitis, bronchospasm may develop that is severe enough to require bronchodilators and hospitalization.

Bacterial Pneumonia

Bacterial pneumonia often follows a viral infection of the upper part of the respiratory tract. The cardinal features suggesting bacterial pneumonia are fever, cough, and sputum production. Shaking chills, dyspnea, and pleuritic chest pain are often present as well. Physical examination frequently reveals signs of pulmonary consolidation in addition to tachypnea and tachycardia. Hypoxemia may be present if infection is severe, and it may lead to delirium or stupor. The white blood cell count and differential typically reveal polymorphonuclear leukocytosis. The chest x-ray film usually demonstrates infiltration that may range from dense consolidation of one or more lobes to a patchy bronchopneumonic pattern; the film may also provide evidence of two of the local complications of pneumonia, pulmonary abscess and empyema. Systemic complications of pneumonia include bacteremia and blood-borne infections, such as septic arthritis and meningitis.

The differential diagnosis must take into consideration Legionnaire's disease and the types of nonbacterial pneumonia caused by viruses, mycoplasmas, and much less commonly, fungi. Tuberculosis occasionally may mimic acute bacterial pneumonia. Chronic pulmonary disease, including emphysema and bronchiectasis, may be misleading if previous chest x-ray films are unavailable. Noninfectious processes such as atelectasis, pulmonary infarction, pulmonary edema, and tumor also are confused sometimes with bacterial pneumonia.

In an emergency, the first concern is adequate oxygenation. Vital signs should be monitored, and arterial blood gas levels should be determined if there is respiratory distress, a depressed level of consciousness, or underlying pulmonary disease. Techniques for respiratory support are given in Chapter 9. General supportive measures such as suppression of fever, chest physical therapy, and administration of expectorants should be employed promptly when needed. Virtually all patients with bacterial pneumonia require hospitalization and parenteral antibiotic therapy; occasionally, otherwise healthy young adults with mild pneumococcal pneumonia may be treated at home if follow-up care is close by.

The key to diagnosis is examination of sputum. In patients with bacterial pneumonia, it is typically thick and green to brownish, and it may be tinged with blood. A good sputum specimen for microscopic examination and culture is crucial. If the patient cannot expectorate spontaneously, chest physical therapy, intermittent positive-pressure breathing with humidified air, or nasotracheal suction may be employed to obtain the specimen. If these fail, transtracheal aspiration may be performed. The Gram's stain usually reveals abundant polymorphonuclear leukocytes and often discloses the primary pathogen. The sputum should be cultured promptly, and blood cultures should also be obtained before administration of antibiotics (Table 11.1).

Pneumococcal Pneumonia. The pneumococcus is still the most common cause of bacterial pneumonia, accounting for from 30 to 60% of all cases. It affects all age groups, and is especially likely to be the agent infecting otherwise healthy ambulatory patients. Classic clinical features include abrupt onset of fever with a single rigor, cough with rusty sputum, and pleurisy. Radiologic evidence of lobar consolidation is typical, but infiltrates can be patchy, especially in patients with chronic pulmonary disease. Penicillin is the drug of choice (Tables 11.2 and 11.3). Tetracycline should *not* be administered because many pneumococci are now resistant to it. Therapy should be continued until the patient has been afebrile for 3–5 days; oral penicillin may be substituted in the last few days of treatment in uncomplicated cases. Bacteremia is a complication of pneumococcal pneumonia in about 30% of patients. Fortunately, conditions resulting from blood-borne sepsis (septic arthritis, peritonitis, meningitis, and the like) are much less common. Sterile pleural effusions occur often, empyema is less frequent, and pulmonary abscess is rare.

Streptococcal Pneumonia. Although pneumonia caused by group A streptococci is uncommon, it has occurred in epidemics. It usually begins abruptly with fever, cough, chest pain, and severe debility. The distinctive clinical and radiologic feature is rapid spread in the lung, resulting in early development of empyema. Penicillin is the drug of choice. Therapy should be continued until clinical manifestations of infection are resolved, which usually requires at least 2 weeks. Pulmonary abscess, bacteremia, and metastatic infection are uncommon complications, as is postinfectious acute glomerulonephritis.

Staphylococcal Pneumonia. *S. aureus* causes up to 10% of all cases of bacterial pneumonia. Except in infancy when it can be a primary infection, staphylococcal pneumonia most commonly follows a viral infection of the respiratory tract, particularly influenza. It may also occur as a nosocomial infection or as a result of bacteremic seeding of the lungs. These patients are usually extremely ill. *S. aureus* causes tissue necrosis, and the distinctive feature of staphylococcal pneumonia is the tendency to produce multiple small pulmonary abscesses. Healing usually leaves residual fibrosis. A semisynthetic penicillin such as oxacillin is the drug of choice; vancomycin is the drug of choice for methicillin-resistant strains of *S. aureus* (Tables 11.2 and 11.3). Therapy should be continued until both clinical and x-ray findings indicate healing; this usually requires at least 2–4 weeks. Empyema and pneumothorax are relatively common complications, and bacteremia with metastatic seeding of distant sites, including the endocardium, bones, joints, liver, and meninges, may also occur.

Haemophilus Pneumonia. *H. influenzae* commonly causes pneumonia in children less than 6 years old, often producing segmental or lobar consolidation or patchy bronchopneumonia; in older children, haemophilus pneumonia is rare. It is also uncommon in adults, except in the elderly or those with underlying chronic pulmonary disease; in these patients a bronchopneumonic pattern is typical. Ampicillin is the antibiotic of choice (Tables 11.2 and 11.3). Now that ampicillin-resistant strains of *H. influenzae* are appearing, however, sensitivity testing is important; chloramphenicol is the drug of choice for these strains, but cefuroxime and the third generation cephalosporins have also proven useful. For *H. influenzae* bronchitis, tetracyline and trimethoprim-sulfamethoxazole are useful alternatives to ampicillin for oral therapy. Therapy should be continued for 10–14 days. In children, bacteremia may develop, with metastatic infection (especially in the joints and meninges) or intrathoracic suppuration (pulmonary abscess or empyema). These complications are less common in adults, but hypoxia and respiratory failure may develop in elderly patients with chronic pulmonary disease.

Klebsiella Pneumonia. *Klebsiella pneumoniae* typically causes pulmonary infection in debilitated patients, especially alcoholics. Illness is usually acute, but chronic pneumonitis may occasionally occur. *K. pneumoniae* has a propensity to produce tissue necrosis, resulting in hemoptysis, dense lobar consolidation, and a high incidence of abscess. Gentamicin, tobramycin or a cephalosporin are the antibiotics of choice (Tables 11.2 and 11.3). Therapy should be continued until clinical and radiologic findings indicate resolution; this usually requires 2–4 weeks. Pulmonary abscess is part of the natural evolution of the disease, and empyema may also occur.

Other Gram-negative Bacillary Pneumonia. These serious infections, once rare, have increased over the past 15 years, accounting for up to 20% of cases of bacterial pneumonia in recent series. They occur typically as hospital-acquired infections in debilitated patients who frequently have received antibiotic therapy that has altered the respiratory flora. This type of pneumonia may result from aspiration of organisms from the upper part of the respiratory tract (often related to inhalation therapy) or from bacteremic seeding of the lungs. Bacteremic pneumonia is characterized by multiple small areas of infection in both lungs. Specific treatment depends on the etiologic agent. Gentamicin or tobramycin are the drugs of choice before the results of cultures and sensitivity testing are available; newer cephalosporins and imipenim have also been used. Most patients with pneumonia due to Gram-negative bacilli require at least 14–28 days of treatment. Complications include pulmonary abscess, empyema, and bacteremia with metastatic infection.

Aspiration Pneumonia. This type of pneumonia results from aspiration of bacteria from the mouth into the lower part of the respiratory tract. Infection is usually mixed, caused by the aerobic and anaerobic streptococci, Bacteroides, fusobacteria, and the like, that are normal flora in the mouth and upper airway but that are pathogenic in the parenchyma of the lung. Predisposing factors include alterations of consciousness resulting from drugs, anesthesia, alcohol, or trauma to the head, and diminution of the gag reflex. Patients usually are mildly to moderately ill, but can be severely ill, especially if pulmonary abscess or empyema occurs. In the usual aspiration pneumonia, the Gram's stain of sputum reveals abundant polymorphonuclear leukocytes and mixed bacterial flora including Gram-positive cocci in pairs and chains and pleomorphic Gram-negative bacilli. Penicillin is the drug of choice, and a 7-day course of therapy is usually sufficient. It must be stressed that both hospitalized and ambulatory patients receiving antibiotics may have altered respiratory tract flora, and aspiration of oral organisms in such individuals may result in staphylococcal or Gram-negative bacillary pneumonia. Hence, aspiration under these circumstances requires broader antimicrobial coverage. Complications of aspiration pneumonia include pulmonary abscess and empyema, which are fairly common if therapy is delayed.

Legionnaire's Disease. Although Legionnaire's disease is considered in the context of epidemics which occur during the warmer months, it is also an important cause of sporadic cases of pneumonia throughout the entire year in all parts of the country. Legionnaire's disease can also present as nosocomial pneumonia. In fact, as many as 5% of all pneumonias may be caused by *Legionella pneumophila.* All age groups can be affected, but attack rates appear higher in older patients and in those with underlying diseases such as chronic obstructive pulmonary disease, neoplasia, azotemia, and immunosuppression.

The typical patient with Legionnaire's disease becomes abruptly ill with high fever and rigors after a brief prodrome of myalgias, headache, and malaise. Cough is prominent but there is little, if any, sputum production; other pulmonary symptoms are tachypnea, dyspnea, and sometimes pleurisy. Diarrhea may be an important clue, and other extrapulmonary features may include encephalopathy and renal dysfunction.

The physical examination is usually nonspecific but may disclose confusion, rales, abdominal tenderness, and sometimes, relative bradycardia in addition to fever and "toxicity." Chest x-ray findings are variable, ranging from interstitial or patchy infiltrates to nodular consolidation; involvement may be confined to one lobe or may be diffuse. The white blood cell count is normal or mildly elevated. Other laboratory findings may include hypoxia, elevated liver enzymes, and abnormalities of the urinalysis and renal function tests.

In most cases, the emergency department diagnosis of Legionnaire's disease depends on these clinical features. Laboratory confirmation is difficult. The sputum examination fails to disclose a pathogen. Cultures can be helpful but require specialized media (charcoal-yeast extract) and techniques. An indirect fluorescent antibody stain can make a rapid diagnosis but this test is not widely available. Serologic tests can confirm the diagnosis but require acute and convalescent serum.

The differential diagnosis of Legionnaire's disease includes the other causes of pneumonia without sputum production (see "Nonbacterial Pneumonia"). If Legionnaire's disease is suspected in the emergency department, cultures and serologies should be obtained but treatment should not be delayed. Erythromycin is the drug of choice and is usually administered intravenously in doses of 500 mg to 1 gm every 6 hours. Rifampin is effective against most strains of *L. pneumophilia* in vitro, but clinical experience is limited.

Other Bacterial Pneumonia. Many other organisms, from *Bacillus anthracis* to the meningococcus, occasionally may cause bacterial pneumonia; patients require individualized therapy.

Other Intrathoracic Infections

Pulmonary Abscess. Patients with a pyogenic abscess of the lung are usually seen in the emergency department with fever, cough, and if the abscess communicates with the bronchial tree, copious production of sputum. Pleurisy, hemoptysis, and dyspnea also may occur. In this respect, these patients resemble patients with pneumonia. Diagnosis depends on the chest x-ray film, which reveals abscess formation, often with air-fluid levels. As with pneumonia, the etiologic diagnosis depends on the Gram's stain and culture of the sputum. The three basic causes of pulmonary abscess are as follows.

1. Aspiration of bacteria from the oropharynx into the lower part of the respiratory tract. This is the most common cause. Patients with the highest risk are those with depressed consciousness or an impaired gag reflex, such as alcoholics, patients who are heavily sedated or who are anesthetized, and patients with neurologic impairment. The α-hemolytic streptococci, together with the Gram-positive and Gram-negative oral anaerobes, are the causative organisms. The Gram's stain of sputum reveals abundant polymorphonuclear leukocytes and mixed flora. Penicillin is the drug of choice, and clindamycin is the preferred alternative in penicillin-allergic patients. Some authorities advocate oral therapy on an outpatient basis, but we recommend hospitalization and parenteral treatment with moderate dosages (Table 11.3). Patients should have chest physical therapy and should undergo postural drainage; many also require bronchoscopic examination to exclude the presence of an obstructing lesion.

2. Necrotizing bacterial pneumonia. Staphylococci, Klebsiella, and other Gram-negative bacilli are particularly likely to be the causative organisms of such abscesses, which are often small and multiple. Diagnosis and therapy are the same as for the underlying pneumonia, except that antibiotics dosage should usually be higher, with a longer duration of therapy.

3. Bronchial obstruction. Foreign bodies and neoplasms frequently obstruct the bronchi, and bronchoscopic examination is essential. If obstruction is complete, it may be impossible initially to obtain a specimen of sputum. Cefoxitin is an excellent antibiotic with which to begin therapy in this situation, but it is important to relieve the obstruction subsequently and to obtain specimens for a Gram's stain and culture.

Empyema. Patients with empyema typically are seen in the emergency department with fever and pleurisy. Dyspnea and respiratory insufficiency may occur, especially if the patient has underlying pulmonary disease. Although cough may be a prominent symptom, unless pneumonia is present such patients do not produce copious sputum.

Empyema may occur in several ways: it may be secondary to necrotizing pneumonia or a pulmonary abscess, in which case staphylococci, Gram-negative bacilli, or mixed oral organisms are the most common agents; it may be caused by diaphragmatic penetration of an intraabdominal septic process, such as a subphrenic abscess, in which case the intestinal flora are most common; or it may result from bacteremic seeding. The key to diagnosis and therapy is adequate drainage with thoracentesis performed in the emergency department. The fluid is typically thick and is foul-smelling if anaerobes are present. Polymorphonuclear leukocytes are numerous, the glucose level is depressed, and protein and lactate dehydrogenase levels are elevated. Specimens should be cultured both aerobically and anaerobically (Table 11.1), and a Gram's stain should be performed. If the source of infection is intestinal, antibiotic therapy should be directed at the gastrointestinal flora. Complete drainage is essential; if repeated thoracentesis is inadequate, drainage with a tube should be employed.

Nonbacterial Pneumonia. Patients with "atypical" or nonbacterial pneumonia are usually less acutely ill than those with bacterial pneumonia. This type of infection is most common in young adults, but can occur in any age group. Typically, patients are seen in the emergency department with fever and a cough that is nonproductive. Dyspnea, pleurisy, rigors, and frank pulmonary consolidation are uncommon; rales do occur. Chest x-ray examination can reveal infiltrates that are more extensive than suggested by physical findings; such infiltrates are often patchy and may be bilateral. The white blood cell count and differential are usually within normal limits.

The major causes of nonbacterial pneumonia are respiratory tract viruses and *Mycoplasma pneumoniae*. Epidemiologic findings are the key to diagnosis of the less common causes of nonbacterial pneumonia, such as Q fever in animal handlers and psittacosis in one exposed to an infected bird. In mycoplasmal pneumonia, an elevated cold agglutinin titer is a useful clue to diagnosis, but is absent in at least one-third of cases. Absolute diagnosis depends on either specific serologic tests available through most state laboratories or culture with special media and techniques. Mycoplasmal pneumonia should be treated with either erythromycin or tetracycline, and most patients can be treated at home with oral antibiotics. Tetracycline is the drug of choice for Q fever and psittacosis.

Tuberculosis. Patients with tuberculosis also may be seen in the emergency department with fever, cough, and pulmonary infiltrates. Primary tuberculosis, which is most common in children and young adults, may mimic atypical pneumonia clinically. Tuberculous pleuritis may occur. Postprimary or reactivation tuberculosis is a more frequent clinical problem and usually involves the upper lobes, with formation of cavities in advanced cases. Diagnosis depends on skin tests, acid-fast smears and cultures of sputum. The smears should be made and studied in the emergency department; however, cultures of these slow-growing organisms take 4–6 weeks. Patients with suspected pulmonary tuberculosis should be hospitalized for diagnosis and therapy. Respiratory precautions should be employed with well-ventilated single rooms and high-quality masks and if the diagnosis is confirmed, epidemiologic investigation must be undertaken.

Infections of the Central Nervous System

Bacterial Meningitis

A true medical emergency, bacterial meningitis is fatal in virtually all patients who do not receive prompt, expert therapy; however, most of those who do receive appropriate treatment recover. Most patients have systemic symptoms including fever and an acutely ill appearance. If the patient also has signs and symptoms of meningeal irritation including headache, stiff neck, and altered mentation, the diagnosis should be clear. Meningitis can be occult, however. Infants and very young children, for example, rarely have nuchal rigidity, and they may even be afebrile; elderly or debilitated patients may have only fever and altered consciousness. Because of the seriousness of this infection and the need for immediate therapy, any patient in whom bacterial meningitis is suspected should be vigorously evaluated.

Cardiovascular and pulmonary function must first be assessed. Many patients with meningitis have bacteremia, and septic shock may ensue (see this chapter and Chapter 3). A brief history should be obtained, usually from a friend or relative. The physician immediately should ascertain whether the patient has had any antecedent infection (particularly in the ears, sinuses, or lungs) and any drug allergies. Other details in the history will be important later, but because of the need for immediate action, the physician should next perform a physical examination. The skin should be examined for petechial or hemorrhagic lesions suggesting meningococcemia, and the ears and sinuses should be examined for a primary suppurative focus possibly extending to the meninges. Examination of the chest and even the abdomen may reveal a septic focus responsible for bacteremia and resultant meningitis. The neurologic examination is of utmost importance. Patients with bacterial meningitis usually display altered mentation ranging from confusion or delirium to stupor or coma. Seizures may occur. Signs of meningeal irritation may be demonstrated by the patient's resistance to passive flexion of the neck (Brudzinski's sign) or by pain on extension of the leg with the hip flexed (Kernig's sign). Localizing signs should be sought; these are absent in most patients with bacterial meningitis, and their presence should raise the possibility of a focal lesion such as a brain abscess.

If the abbreviated examination suggests meningitis, the physician should proceed with the crucial diagnostic procedure, the lumbar puncture (see Illustrated Technique 14). The pressure of the cerebrospinal fluid is typically elevated in these patients, but tentorial herniation is uncommon after lumbar puncture. Nevertheless, if the pressure exceeds 400 mm H_2O, mannitol should be given intravenously before the cerebrospinal fluid is collected (see Chapter 15).

The cerebrospinal fluid should be collected in at least four tubes. The fluid in the first tube should be used for a white blood cell count and differential, and if red blood cells are present, raising the possibility of a traumatic tap, the counts should be repeated with a sample from the fourth tube. The fluid in the second tube should be used for determination of glucose and protein levels, and a portion of the fluid in the third tube should be cultured using a blood agar plate, a chocolate agar slant, and thioglycollate broth (Table 11.1). The remaining fluid in the third tube should be used for a Gram's stain. Typical findings include an elevated white blood cell count usually between 500 and 20,000/mm^3. Most of these cells are polymorphonuclear leukocytes. In addition, the protein level is usually somewhat elevated, ranging from 70–150 mg/100 ml. An important finding is a glucose level depressed to less than 50 mg/100 ml or to less than 50% of a simultaneously determined blood glucose level (Table 11.4).

In the patient with meningitis, other laboratory studies should include a complete blood cell count, differential, and urinalysis, as well as determination of the levels of serum electrolytes, blood urea nitrogen, creatinine, and glucose. A platelet count, prothrombin time, and partial thromboplastin time are important if the patient has hypotension or hemorrhagic cutaneous lesions (see Chapter 13, for discussion of disseminated intravascular coagulation). Throat and blood cultures should be obtained, and sputum should be studied by a Gram's stain and culture if possible. X-ray films of the chest, skull, and sinuses should be taken to look for a primary septic focus. Cranial computed tomography (CT) scans are very useful to look for brain abscesses and parameningeal septic foci, but the lumbar puncture and antibiotic therapy should not be delayed to await a CT scan.

Definitive identification of the responsible bacterial pathogen requires 24–48 hours for culture results, but antibiotic therapy cannot wait. Ideally, the emergency department evaluation of a patient with meningitis should be completed quickly enough so that antibiotic administration can begin within 30–60 minutes. Fortunately, the Gram's stain of the cerebrospinal fluid and the clinical findings provide sufficient information for the physician to choose an antibiotic in the emergency department. Three major organisms account for most cases of bacterial meningitis.

1. Pneumococcus. These Gram-positive cocci, occurring in pairs or short chains, can cause meningitis in any age group, but particularly in adults. Meningitis results from direct extension of the pathogens from an infected ear or sinus or from bacteremic spread from a pulmonary focus. The antibiotic of choice is penicillin, administered intravenously in high doses. In the penicillin-allergic patient, chloramphenicol should be administered, 4 gm/day in four doses for adults. Remember that all first and most second generation cephalosporins are ineffective therapy for meningitis, and even the third generation cephalosporins are not recommended for pneumococcal meningitis.

2. Meningococcus. On the Gram's stain, these organisms appear as bean-shaped, Gram-negative diplococci. Meningococcal meningitis can occur at any age, but is particularly common in children and young adults. This potentially fulminating infection spreads from the pharynx to the meninges via the bloodstream; even if meningitis does not develop, meningococcemia can be fatal within hours. Petechial lesions on the skin may indicate disseminated intravascular coagulation. In hypotensive patients, corticosteroids may be helpful because of the possibility of associated adrenal hemorrhage. Cardiac function should be monitored in all patients; meningococcemia can cause myocarditis, resulting in arrhythmias and congestive heart failure, as well as purulent pericarditis with tamponade. Meticulous circulatory and respiratory support is vital. Penicillin is the drug of choice. In the penicillin-allergic patient, chloramphenicol should be administered (Table 11.3).

Meningococcal meningitis is the only form of bacterial meningitis that is contagious, and in these patients, mask and gown precautions should be taken for the first 24 hours of therapy. Prophylactic treatment of contacts is difficult. Penicillin is ineffective when administered to persons in the carrier state, and many meningococci are now resistant to the sulfonamide compounds. The only effective antibiotics in this situation are minocycline and rifampin, but because of fewer side effects rifampin is generally preferred, 600 mg twice a day for a total of four doses in adults, 10 mg/kg twice a day for a total of four doses in children from 1–12 years, and 5 mg/kg twice a day for a total of four doses in children less than 1 year. Because of cost, side effects, and emerging drug resistance, therapy should be reserved for close contacts.

3. *H. influenzae*. These small, Gram-negative, coccobacillary organisms vary in size and shape. Bacterial meningitis caused by *H. influenzae* is common in children between 6 months and 6 years of age, but is uncommon in other age groups. The infection may originate in either the upper or lower part of the respiratory tract. Until recently, ampicillin was the drug of choice. In the last few years, however, ampicillin-resistant strains of *H. influenzae* have been isolated with increasing frequency. Because there is no room for error in the management of bacterial meningitis, it is best to begin treatment with chloramphenicol in the same doses as for meningococcal meningitis; cefuroxime and the third generation cephalosporins are also very useful. If the causative organism is then proved sensitive to ampicillin, this drug can be administered instead, 12 gm/day intravenously in six doses for adults and 400 mg/kg/day in six doses for children.

Table 11.4.
Typical Cerebrospinal Fluid Findings in Infectious Meningitis

Type	Pressure	White Blood Cells/mm^3	Differential	Glucose	Protein	Other
Bacterial	Normal-elevated	500–20,000	Mostly polymorphs	Low, usually <50 mg/100 ml	Elevated	Gram's stain positive in 80%
Partly treated	Normal-elevated	Usually <1000	Variable	Normal	Elevated	
Viral	Usually normal	Usually <1000	Polymorphs early, mostly mononuclear cells later	Normal	Normal-elevated	Viral cultures may be positive; blood serologies required for specific diagnosis
Tuberculous	Elevated	Usually <500	Mostly mononuclear cells	Low	Elevated	Acid-fast smears, culture on tuberculosis medium
Fungal	Elevated	Usually <500	Mostly mononuclear cells	Low	Elevated	India ink preparation, crytococcal serologies on blood and cerebrospinal fluid

While the three organisms discussed account for most cases of bacterial meningitis, in special circumstances other bacteria may be implicated.

1. In the newborn, bacterial meningitis may be caused by a wide range of pathogens, including group B streptococci, *Escherichia coli* and other enteric Gram-negative bacilli, and *Listeria*. It may be manifested by nothing more specific than failure to feed, often with hypothermia. Meningitis must be suspected in all newborns with sepsis, and a lumbar puncture must be performed. Neonates with streptococcal or Listerial meningitis should be treated with ampicillin and gentamicin. If Gram-negative bacilli are present, or if the pathogen is not identified, ampicillin and cefotaxime or ceftriaxone should be used.

2. Staphylococcal meningitis is uncommon. Except in newborns, Gram-negative bacillary meningitis is also rare. These both occur almost exclusively in the immunosuppressed, debilitated patient or as a complication of a neurosurgical procedure or penetrating head trauma. Until results of sensitivity testing are available, patients whose cerebrospinal fluid reveals Gram-negative bacilli should be treated with a third generation cephalosporin in maximal doses (see Table 11.3). Patients with staphylococcal meningitis should receive a semisynthetic penicillinase-resistant penicillin such as oxacillin.

3. Other bacteria can also cause meningitis under special circumstances; examples include *Listeria monocytogenes* in immunosuppressed patients and *S. epidermidis* in patients with cerebrospinal fluid (CSF) shunts. Therapy for these specialized circumstances must be individualized.

In some patients with bacterial meningitis, the initial Gram's stain of the cerebrospinal fluid does not reveal the causative organism. As stated previously, most cases of bacterial meningitis beyond the neonatal period are caused by *H. influenzae,* pneumococci, or meningococci. In adults in whom the pathogen is unidentified, ampicillin is usually sufficient, but in children, initial therapy with both ampicillin and chloramphenicol is preferred because of the existence of ampicillin-resistant strains of *H. influenzae.* If the patient is allergic to penicillin, therapy with chloramphenicol is recommended; as noted previously, third generation cephalosporins are also extremely useful, but they must be administered with caution in penicillin-allergic patients. If cultures of the cerebrospinal fluid become positive, therapy should then be directed toward the organism isolated.

Partly treated bacterial meningitis is a difficult problem for the emergency physician. Often, these patients have received oral antibiotics before being seen in the emergency department. As a result, Gram's stains and cultures of the cerebrospinal fluid may be negative, and the cerebrospinal fluid may even show a predominance of lymphocytes and a nearly normal glucose level. If blood and cerebrospinal fluid cultures remain negative, these patients should be treated in the manner discussed above for bacterial meningitis of uncertain cause.

Viral Meningitis

The course of viral meningitis is usually much milder than that of bacterial meningitis. Patients are commonly seen with fever and headache with or without photophobia and vomiting. Nuchal rigidity may be severe, but these patients are mentally alert and free of focal neurologic signs. Identical clinical findings can be produced by many viruses, including enteroviruses, some of the herpesviruses, and mumps virus. The specific diagnosis is usually difficult, but examination of the cerebrospinal fluid should suggest that a viral agent is responsible (Table 11.4). Typical findings include normal pressure, a normal glucose level, and a normal to slightly elevated protein level. The white blood cell count is usually less than 1000/mm^3; early in the course of viral meningitis, polymorphonuclear leukocytes may predominate, but within 24 hours, almost all cells should be lymphocytes. Gram's stains and bacterial cultures are negative. In general, patients with viral meningitis should be hospitalized for observation. There is no antibiotic treatment yet available.

If polymorphonuclear leukocytes predominate in the cerebrospinal fluid from the initial lumbar puncture and if the patient appears ill, it is best to start administration of antibiotics before culture results are available. However, if polymorphonuclear leukocytes predominate in the cerebrospinal fluid but other findings are typical of viral meningitis, antibiotics may be withheld, with the patient closely observed and a lumbar puncture repeated in 12–24 hours.

Tuberculous and Fungal Meningitis

These are much less common than bacterial and viral meningitis. Patients typically are seen with a history of several days or weeks of fever, headache, confusion, and personality changes. Physical examination may reveal nuchal rigidity and cranial nerve palsies. Examination of the cerebrospinal fluid suggests the diagnosis. Typical findings include elevated pressure, an elevated protein level, a decreased glucose level, and fewer than 500 white blood cells/mm^3 with a predominance of lymphocytes. In the most common fungal meningitis, cryptococcal meningitis, the Gram's stain may reveal yeast forms; however, the India ink preparation is more specific. Cryptococcal polysaccharide may also be detected in the cerebrospinal fluid by immunologic tests. Specimens should be inoculated on Sabouraud agar if fungal meningitis is suspected and on Löwenstein-Jensen slants if tuberculosis is a possibility. Acid-fast smears should always be made when tuberculous meningitis is suspected, and chest x-ray films and skin tests can provide additional useful data. Amphotericin B is the drug of choice for most types of fungal meningitis; 5-fluorocytosine is a new agent that is proving useful in combination with amphotericin B. Combination therapy with isoniazid, rifampin, and ethambutol is recommended for tuberculosis of the central nervous system.

The differential diagnosis of nonbacterial (aseptic) meningitis includes many conditions. Carcinomatous meningitis, sarcoidosis, Lyme disease, syphilis, and leptospirosis can all cause lymphocytic meningitis with a low glucose level in the cerebrospinal fluid; viral encephalitis, syphilis, vasculitis, brain abscess, subdural empyema, and osteomyelitis of the cranial bones can cause lymphocytic meningitis with a normal glucose level. Diagnosis and therapy of these conditions take place in the emergency department rarely.

Gastrointestinal and Intraabdominal Infections

The normal gastrointestinal tract has abundant bacterial flora; colonization is most dense in the colon, where fecal material contains approximately 1×10^{11} bacteria/gm. Infectious diseases involving the abdomen may be divided into very different categories: (*a*) serious acute infectious processes, such as peritonitis, cholecystitis, and intraabdominal abscess, that result from entry of intestinal bacteria into normally sterile areas and that usually require surgical treatment; and (*b*) gastroenteritis caused by ingestion of toxins or pathogenic organisms that are not part of the normal flora. The diarrhea and vomiting that result from such ingestion may require rehydration in the emergency department and occasionally hospitalization.

Surgical Abdominal Infections

Included in this category are many processes in which the integrity of the gastrointestinal tract is disrupted by an anatomic defect such as a perforated viscus or impaired drainage of the biliary tract that leads to bacterial overgrowth and infection. The clinical features of these illnesses, including appendicitis, diverticulitis, cholecystitis, peritonitis, and intraabdominal abscess, are considered elsewhere in this text (Chapter 33). Prompt surgical therapy is required to correct the underlying anatomic defect in almost all of these situations; however, antibiotics also have an important role in treatment.

The proper choice of antibiotics in intraabdominal infections depends on knowledge of the fecal bacteria. In all cases, blood cultures should be obtained in the emergency department, and cultures and Gram's stains at operation. Even before a specific pathogen is isolated, antibiotics can be chosen directed at the "usual suspects." The most well-known constituents of the intestinal flora are the enteric Gram-negative bacilli. *E. coli* is the most important of these aerobic organisms; others include Klebsiella, Proteus, and Enterobacter. Antibiotic sensitivities vary, but most strains of *E. coli* are sensitive to ampicillin, chloramphenicol, gentamicin and cefoxitin. A second group even more common in feces are the anaerobic Gram-negative organisms, particularly *Bacteroides fragilis.* Because these slender bacilli are often involved in intraabdominal infections, abscesses must specifically be cultured for anaerobes. The Bacteroides species present in the intestine are *not* sensitive to ampicillin or aminoglycosides, and a high percentage are now resistant to tetracycline. The antibiotics effective against most strains of *B. fragilis* are clindamycin, chloramphenicol, cefoxitin, metronidazole, and imipenim. A third group of organisms present in the intestine are the Gram-positive bacteria. Anaerobes are also found in this category, including the clostridia and streptococci. Most organisms in this group are sensitive to ampicillin, penicillin, and clindamycin and cefoxitin. Finally, an aerobic streptococcus, the enterococcus, represents a special problem. Enterococci can be adequately treated with ampicillin alone in uncomplicated urinary tract infections, but in serious tissue infections or bacteremia, a combination of a penicillin (such as ampicillin) and an aminoglycoside (such as gentamicin) is required.

With this information, guidelines can be established for the initial choice of antibiotics in intraabdominal infections. In the mildly to moderately ill patient with a localized condition, such as appendicitis, cholecystitis, or diverticulitis, ampicillin alone can suffice, 1–1.5 gram intravenously every 4 hours for adults. In the more seriously ill patient with generalized peritonitis and possible bacteremia, a combination of antibiotics should be administered. Several combinations have proved effective, and at present, no one method is favored. Traditional combinations include: (*a*) clindamycin (600 mg intravenously every 6–8 hours) with gentamicin (1.5 mg/kg intravenously every 8 hours in patients with normal renal function), and (*b*) ampicillin (1–1.5 gm intravenously every 4 hours) with chloramphenical (500 mg intravenously every 6 hours), or (*c*) ampicillin with metronidazole (500 mg intravenously every 6 hours). All dosages are for adults. Another approach would be to administer cefoxitin alone in a dose at 1–2 gm intravenously every 4–6 hours. None of these approaches, however, is effective against the enterococcus, so in the extremely ill patient, it may be necessary to start therapy with three antibiotics simultaneously—ampicillin and gentamicin plus clindamycin, chloramphenicol or metronidazole. Because of problems concerning toxic reactions, hypersensitivity, superinfection, and cost, simultaneous administration of three drugs should be restricted to special circumstances, such as critical abdominal sepsis in the immunosuppressed patient.

Primary Peritonitis. Most cases of bacterial peritonitis result from perforation of an abdominal viscus, involve multiple enteric organisms and require surgery as well as antibiotics for successful therapy. In contrast, primary bacterial peritonitis (spontaneous bacterial peritonitis) results from hematogenous seeding at the peritoneum. Patients with preexisting ascites are at greatest risk; primary peritonitis is seen most often in cirrhotics but can occur in patients with nephrotic syndrome or systemic lupus erythematosus (SLE). In primary peritonitis, a single bacterial species is recovered from the infected ascites; *E. coli* or other enteric organisms are present most often, but pneumococci and other respiratory pathogens may be responsible.

Two-thirds of patients with spontaneous peritonitis present with fever, abdominal pain and tenderness, but in the remainder infection is occult. Laboratory findings include leukocytosis in the peripheral blood and ascitic fluid. A single bacterial species is present on Gram's stain and culture. The distinction between primary and secondary peritonitis can be difficult but is important because patients with primary peritonitis should be managed with antibiotics without surgery.

Percutaneous Abscess Drainage. Until the mid-1970s, surgical drainage of intraabdominal abscesses was mandatory. However, the treatment of these abscesses has changed dramatically within just a few years of the introduction of percutaneous abscess drainage under ultrasound or CT guidance. Many studies have demonstrated that percutaneous abscess drainage is safe and effective for a broad range of intraabdominal collections; success rates range from 47 to 92%, with most studies reporting greater than 80% success. For example, in one study of 250 percutaneous drainage procedures 84% were complete successes and 6% were partial successes in which the patient improved but surgery was eventually necessary because of recurrences or complications. Failures were most common in patients with poorly defined phlegmons, multiloculated abscesses, thick hematomas or organized infections, or abscesses with associated fistulous tracts. Minor complications occurred in 8%, and major complications (hemorrhage, sepsis, and bowel perforation) in 2.8%.

Prospective trials comparing surgical and percutaneous abscess drainage have not been performed, and in view of the widespread acceptance of the percutaneous technique, future studies of this sort are unlikely. Retrospective studies comparing the two approaches have not demonstrated clear differences between them in success rate, duration of drainage, or mortality, Radiographic features alone cannot predict which abscesses will respond to percutaneous drainage; even abscesses with low output fistula production may respond to percutaneous drainage. Hence it seems reasonable to institute percutaneous drainage in all patients who have a safe access route, providing that skilled personnel are available and that the patient does not otherwise need surgery. Surgical drainage may then be used in patients with recurrences, failures, or complications.

Gastroenteritis

Diarrhea and vomiting cause many patients to seek emergency care, and gastroenteritis is an important part of the differential diagnosis in these patients (see Chapter 12). Many can be treated adequately at home, but children and elderly or debilitated persons may require hospitalization and intravenous rehydration. Measurement of vital signs, an abdominal examination, a hemogram, and determination of serum electrolyte levels serve to indicate whether a patient should be hospitalized. An epidemiologic history is important, and examination and culture of stool specimens may establish the etiologic diagnosis. Several important categories of gastroenteritis are caused by infectious agents.

Intoxication ("Food Poisoning"). Food products may be contaminated with bacteria that produce toxins. Since ingestion of the toxin rather than actual bacterial infection is responsible for the illness, these patients are afebrile, have normal white blood cell counts, do not have blood or leukocytes in the stool specimen, and do not require antibiotic therapy. Most cases of food poisoning are due to either *Clostridium perfringens,* with a 12- to 24-hour incubation period and diarrhea predominating, or *S. aureus,* with a 4- to 16-hour incubation period and vomiting predominating. *Clostridium botulinum* may cause mild diarrhea, but this uncommon intoxication usually is seen as a neurologic emergency in which the patient has ocular and respiratory symptoms. Stool cultures are not helpful in the diagnosis of food poisoning; an epidemiologic history must be taken, food samples must be cultured, and assays for toxins must be performed.

Toxicogenic Bacterial Gastroenteritis. In some infections of the gastrointestinal tract, disease results from local production of bacterial toxins. Cholera is the best known example, but certain strains of *E. coli* and *Vibrio parahemolyticus* can also cause diarrhea by toxin production. Such patients are afebrile and have no blood or white blood cells in the stool specimen. Cholera is not endemic in the United States, but should be considered in patients who have been in endemic areas if symptoms include copious diarrhea, dehydration, and electrolyte imbalance.

Invasive Bacterial Gastroenteritis. Some bacterial pathogens cause diarrhea by invading the intestinal mucosa. In this manner, *S. aureus* sometimes causes enterocolitis in patients receiving broad-spectrum antibiotics. These patients are febrile, and stool specimens often reveal blood and polymorphonuclear leukocytes. Stool cultures yield abundant staphylococci. These patients require intravenous rehydration plus parenteral administration of antistaphylococcal antibiotics such as oxacillin or cephalothin.

Patients receiving antibiotics may also develop antibiotic-induced enterocolitis, which is caused by *Clostridium difficile.* The stool may contain blood and leukocytes but no enteric pathogens can be cultured. The diagnosis can be made by assaying the stool for *C. difficile* toxin. Oral vancomycin or metronidazole is the treatment of choice.

Certain strains of *E. coli* can also cause diarrhea by invading the mucosa. In these patients, clinical features resemble those of Salmonella gastroenteritis; diagnosis requires special techniques. Patients with nontyphoidal Salmonella gastroenteritis are seen with fever and diarrhea 1–3 days after ingesting contaminated food. Diarrhea may be bloody, and the stool specimen contain leukocytes. Such patients may require intravenous rehydration and antidiarrheal treatment, but antibiotics prolong the carrier state and should be reserved only for very sick persons; ampicillin is generally used in these circumstances, *Campylobacter jejuni* causes gastroenteritis, which is clinically very similar to salmonellosis, and is among the most common causes of bacterial enteritis. The diagnosis requires culturing the stool on special media at 42°C (see Table 11.1). Many patients recover spontaneously; but erythromycin is recommended for severe or protracted cases. *Shigellosis* has similar clinical features, although bloody diarrhea may be more severe. Most of these patients recover without antibiotics, but if the patient is seriously ill, trimethoprim-sulfamethoxazole is an acceptable initial choice. The symptoms of *typhoid fever* are usually systemic rather than gastrointestinal; hospitalization and antibiotic therapy are mandatory. Parenteral therapy with chloramphenicol or ampicillin is recommended, but in special circumstances, oral trimethoprim-sulfamethoxazole may suffice.

Parasitic Gastroenteritis. *Giardiasis* and *amebiasis* are examples of such conditions. Diagnosis depends on epidemiologic findings and microscopic examination of a fresh stool specimen for ova and parasites. For further discussion, please see the section on protozoal gastroenteritis in medical gastrointestinal emergencies (Chapter 12).

Genitourinary Infections

Urinary Tract Infections

Infections of the urinary tract are much more common in females, except in infancy when anatomic anomalies increase the incidence in males, and in the elderly when prostatism and bladder outlet obstruction predispose to infections in men. In all age groups, instrumentation of the urinary tract is a major cause of infection.

Although urinary tract infections (UTI) may be asymptomatic, patients are likely to seek medical attention in the emergency department because of local or constitutional symptoms or both. Suprapubic pain, dysuria, frequency of urination, and urgency usually reflect infection of the lower part of the urinary tract (cystitis); flank pain, fever, chills, nausea, and vomiting suggest infection of the upper part (pyelonephritis). In patients with cystitis, physical findings are absent or confined to suprapubic tenderness. Patients with prostatitis may have prostatic tenderness and sponginess on rectal examination, and patients with acute pyelonephritis may have high fever, prostration, and flank tenderness. Hypotension can occur and suggests bacteremia. Although absolute differentiation of cystitis and pyelonephritis can be difficult based on clinical findings, the distinction is important because of differences in management.

In all patients, the key to diagnosis is the urine specimen. Urinalysis may reveal white blood cells or red blood cells or both. White blood cell casts suggest pyelonephritis. Hematuria may occur even with cystitis and prostatitis. If the pH of the urine is alkaline, infection with a urea-splitting organism such as Proteus is likely. Normal results of urinalysis in a patient with signs and symptoms of pyelonephritis may indicate infection above a completely obstructed ureter.

Although urinalysis may strongly suggest a urinary tract infection, urine must be cultured to confirm the diagnosis and to identify the responsible pathogen. Because the perineum and distal part of the urethra are colonized by numerous bacteria, a clean voided "midstream" specimen is essential. In infants and children, percutaneous suprapubic aspiration of urine from the bladder may be the best way to obtain an uncontaminated specimen. In adults, urethral catheterization is occasionally necessary, but because this procedure carries a significant risk of introducing pathogens, it should be avoided when possible. Urine should be cultured on both blood agar and on MacConkey or eosin-methylene blue agar. If specimens cannot be inoculated promptly, the urine should be refrigerated. In addition to urinalysis and culture, a Gram's stain of *unsedimented* fresh urine can be extremely valuable in making a rapid diagnosis. The presence of organisms on such a stain suggests significant bacteriuria, with more than 100,000 organisms/ml.

Urinary cultures reveal Gram-negative bacilli in most patients with infection of the urinary tract. *E. coli* is the most common pathogen, especially in women with uncomplicated infections. Other enteric Gram-negative bacilli can also cause uncomplicated UTIs. Among the Gram-positive organisms, the enterococcus (a group D streptococcus) is most likely to be the etiologic agent. *S. aureus* is an uncommon pathogen in the urinary tract, and its presence may indicate either bacteremic seeding of the kidney with or without abscesses or a prostatic abscess. Although other pathogens can also cause urinary tract infection, unusual organisms should raise the possibility of contaminated specimens, and cultures should be repeated. Negative cultures in patients with pyuria or other urinary tract symptoms are sometimes encountered in prostatitis, urethritis, vaginitis, cervicitis, or urinary tract tuberculosis. Rarely, infection with fastidious bacteria such as *H. influenzae* or Brucella species can result in "sterile" pyuria. Adenovirus infection can cause hemorrhagic cystitis.

Although urinary cultures and sensitivity testing determine the optimal choice of antibiotics, administration of antibacterial agents should be started as soon as the specimen is cultured, and the choice should be reevaluated when results become available. Patients with cystitis respond well to oral antibacterial therapy. First infections in ambulatory patients are almost always caused by *E. coli* with broad antibiotic sensitivities. Patients with uncomplicated cystitis respond well to either conventional 10–14 day treatment regimens or to single-dose therapy with amoxicillin, trimethoprim-sulfamethoxazole, or sulfisoxazole (Table 11.3).

In patients who have recurrent infections, who have recently been receiving antibiotics, or who have been hospitalized and catheterized, infection may be due to sulfa-resistant organisms. Single-dose treatment is not appropriate. Antibiotic sensitivity testing is mandatory for these patients, before results are available, ampicillin, cephalexin, tetracycline, and trimethoprim-sulfamethoxazole are all acceptable agents. Some physicians prefer nitrofurantoin; we have found this drug useful for chronic and recurrent infections. Intravenous pyelograms should be obtained in patients with recurrent cystitis. High fluid intake should be encouraged in all patients, and all should be instructed to return for follow-up urinalysis and culture after completing therapy.

Although patients with acute pyelonephritis respond to a similar range of antibiotics, most should initially be treated in the hospital with parenteral antibacterial agents. These patients may be severely ill, with high fever and leukocytosis. Since Gram-negative bacteremia may occur, blood cultures should be obtained before antibiotic therapy. Septic shock may develop, and vital signs must be closely monitored. In the severely ill patient and when Proteus, Pseudomonas, or Enterobacter is suspected, gentamicin or tobramycin is generally the drug of choice for initial therapy. Results of sensitivity testing may then allow a change to a potentially less toxic drug. In less critically ill patients, intravenous ampicillin or a parenteral cephalosporin may be administered initially. Other useful drugs include chloramphenicol, amikacin, and trimethoprim-sulfamethoxazole. Maintenance of adequate hydration is important and often requires administration of intravenous fluids in the first few days of treatment. Renal function must be evaluated, and intravenous pyelograms are indicated in most patients. Because pyelonephritis tends to recur, follow-up urinalysis and culture are important.

In addition to requiring medical therapy, some patients with urinary tract infections require emergency surgical evaluation. This occurs most often when urinary flow is obstructed by a calculus, stricture, or tumor, or by prostatic hypertrophy, as discussed in Chapter 35.

Sexually Transmitted Infections

Infections of the genital organs are common. Many are minor conditions that can be managed with topical agents on an outpatient basis, such as vaginitis due to *Candida albicans*. Others, such as prostatitis and epididymitis, usually are caused by the same organisms that cause urinary tract infections and may be managed with the same oral antibiotics. Because of good tissue penetration, trimethoprim-sulfamethoxazole is particularly valuable for prostatitis. In young, sexually active males, epididymitis is often caused by chlamydia or by *N. gonorrhoeae*; therapy with amoxicillin, 3.0 gm, and probenacid, 1.0 gm orally, followed by tetracycline, 500 mg four times daily for 10 days is ideal. A single dose of ceftriaxone, 250 mg intramuscularly, may be substituted for amoxicillin and probenecid. In older men, a broad range of Gram-negative bacilli can cause epididymitis. In some cases, epididymitis can progress to extreme local swelling with intense inflammation and pain as well as fever and leukocytosis; these patients require hospitalization, parenteral antibiotics, immobilization, analgesics, and sometimes operation.

Syphilis. Caused by *Treponema pallidum,* syphilis is an increasingly common venereal disease. Asymptomatic patients may be seen because of recent sexual exposure to a person with known or suspected syphilis; serologic testing should be performed, and these patients should also be examined to exclude gonorrhea. If exposure is certain, patients can be treated on epidemiologic grounds. In primary syphilis, patients are seen with a highly infectious, painless, ulcerated chancre, usually on the genitalia. In secondary syphilis, patients have systemic illness that includes fever, malaise, lymphadenopathy, and cutaneous lesions characteristically involving the palms and soles. Secondary syphilis is also infectious. All patients with syphilis should be reported to local public health authorities, and contacts should be identified and treated. The treatment for incubating primary and secondary syphilis is the same, consisting of benzathine penicillin G, 2.4 million units total by intramuscular injection at a single session. Penicillin-allergic patients should receive tetracycline or erythromycin, 500 mg four times a day for 15 days. Follow-up evaluation with repeated serologic testing is necessary to ensure adequacy of treatment. The optimal treatment for syphilis of more than one year's duration is less well-established; three successive weekly injections of 2.4 million units benzathine penicillin should be given. Patients with neurosyphilis should be hospitalized and treated with high dose intravenous penicillin.

Gonorrhea. This is the most common venereal disease seen in the emergency department; caused by *N. gonorrhoeae,* it may display a broad spectrum of clinical features. Both men and women may be asymptomatic; diagnosis of the carrier state depends on urethral and cervical cultures and epidemiologic history. Urethritis in men and cervicitis in women often are indicated by pain, discharge, and dysuria. In men, a Gram's stain of the urethral discharge is highly diagnostic, revealing Gram-negative intracellular diplococci; in women, the Gram's stain is less reliable. Specimens from all patients should be inoculated promptly on Thayer-Martin or Transgrow media; cultures from the urethra in men and from the cervix and anus in women are best. A serologic test for syphilis should also be performed.

The therapy of gonorrhea must take into account the increasing prevalence of gonococcal strains which are resistant to penicillin and, less often, other antibiotics. Another important factor is the increasing prevalence of chlamydial infections, which can be difficult to diagnose. Uncomplicated gonococcal urethral, cervical, and pharyngeal infections may be treated with several regimens: (*a*) Ampicillin, 3.5 gm orally, or amoxicillin, 3.0 gm orally, or aqueous procaine penicillin, 4.8 million units intramuscularly, plus probenecid, 1.0 gm orally, or (*b*) ceftriaxone, 250 mg intramuscularly. Each of these regimens should then be followed by (*c*) tetracycline, 500 mg orally four times daily for 7 days, or doxycycline, 100 mg orally twice daily for 7 days. In pregnancy and in other situations in which tetracyclines are contraindicated, erythromycin is substituted, 500 mg orally four times daily for 7 days. Rectal gonorrhea in women will respond to any of these regimens, but in homosexual men only the intramuscular regimens listed above or spectinomycin, 2.0 gm intramuscularly, should be used. Patients who are allergic to penicillins, cephalosporins, or probenecid should be treated with tetracycline or doxycycline as outlined above, or with spectinomycin, 2.0 gm intramuscularly, followed by erythromycin, 500 mg orally four times daily for 7 days. All patients should have follow-up cultures of infected sites 4 to 7 days after treatment; treatment failures should be retreated with ceftriaxone, 250 mg intramuscularly, or spectinomycin, 2.0 gm intramuscularly. Sexual partners of all patients should be cultured and treated as outlined above. All patients and their partners should have serologic tests for syphilis.

Disseminated Gonococcal Infections. Gonococcal bacteremia may present with fever, leukocytosis, pustular or petechial rash, and arthritis. Patients with the gonococcal arthritis-dermatitis syndrome may be treated with one of several regimens: penicillin, 2.5 million units intravenously four times daily for at least 3 days, followed by amoxicillin or ampicillin, 500 mg four times daily to complete 7 days of therapy, or ceftriaxone, 1.0 gm intravenously once daily for 7 days, or cefoxitin 1.0 gm intravenously four times daily for at least 7 days. In reliable patients who are not severely ill, outpatient treatment is acceptable using amoxicillin, 3.0 gm orally, or ampicillin, 3.5 gm orally, plus probeneced, 1.0 gm orally, followed by ampicillin or amoxicillin, 500 mg orally four times daily for at least 7 days. In patients who are allergic to penicillins and cephalosporins, tetracycline, 500 mg orally four times daily for 7 days, or doxycycline, 100 mg orally twice daily for 7 days, may be used.

Chlamydial Infections. *Chlamydia trachomatis* has become the most prevalent sexually transmitted pathogen in the United States today. Clinical features range from asymptomatic infection to nongonococcal urethritis (NGU) and epididymitis in men and mucopurulent cervicitis and pelvic inflammatory disease (PID) in women. Serious complications include infertility due to tubal scarring and neonatal conjunctivitis and pneumonia. Patients and their sexual contacts should be treated with tetracycline, 100 mg orally four times daily for 7 days, or doxycycline, 500 mg two times daily for 7 days. Pregnant women and tetracycline-allergic patients should receive erythromycin, 500 mg orally four times daily for 7 days.

Pelvic Inflammatory Disease. PID may be caused by a broad range of pathogens including the gonococcus, *C. trachomatis, Bacteroides fragilis* and other anaerobes, *E. coli* and other enteric Gram-negative bacilli, and Gram-positive cocci. In most cases, it is not possible to identify one causative organism, so therapy should be directed against a broad range of pathogens with careful clinical follow-up to monitor results. Women with moderate to severe PID should be hospitalized and treated with parenteral antibiotics. Doxycycline, 100 mg intravenously twice daily and cefoxitin, 2.0 gm intravenously four times daily, is an excellent regimen. Women with clearcut but mild salpingitis who are reliable about adherence to therapy may be treated as outpatients with ceftriaxone, 250 mg intravenously, followed by doxycyline, 100 mg twice daily for 14 days.

Genital Herpes Simplex. Although no therapeutic regimen will eradicate herpes simplex virus or prevent recurrent infections, therapy can ameliorate symptoms and shorten the duration of viral shedding. Acyclovir, 200 mg by mouth five times daily for 7 to 10 days, may be administered to patients with primary or recurrent genital herpes. The occasional patient who is ill enough to require hospitalization may be treated with acyclovir, 5 mg/kg intravenously every 8 hours for 5 to 7 days.

Acquired Immunodeficiency Syndrome (AIDS). AIDS is surely the most dramatic new disease of this century, and it threatens to become one of the most devastating epidemics of human history. Because of the intense study of AIDS, textbooks cannot keep pace with new information, and current journals should be consulted.

The emergency department has only a limited role in the management of patients with AIDS. Three priorities can be identified: *a*) recognizing patients at risk for infection with human T cell lymphotropic virus type III (HTLV-III), the organism which causes AIDS; *b*) instituting appropriate precautions to prevent transmission of HTLV-III to emergency department personnel; *c*) initiating the studies necessary to diagnose the numerous potential infectious and neoplastic processes which can afflict patients with the syndrome.

Individuals with increased risk for infection with HTLV-III include homosexual and bisexual men, intravenous drug abusers, patients transfused with infected blood or blood products, children born to infected mothers, and heterosexual contacts of patients infected with HTLV-III. Before invasive procedures are performed on any patient in the emergency department, a brief history should be obtained to learn if risk factors are present; if so, appropriate precautions should be instituted.

Although HTLV-III can be detected in many body fluids of infected individuals, transmission of the virus appears to require sexual or parenteral exposure to infected blood or semen (or transplacental transmission to children of infected mothers). Hence, health care workers can be protected with precautions similar to those used to prevent hepatitis B transmission. If exposure to blood or other body fluids is anticipated, gloves should be worn; gowns, masks, and eye coverings should be worn if extensive exposure is possible (endoscopies, dental procedures, etc). If gloves are torn, they should be replaced as quickly as possible. Gloves should be discarded and replaced between patient contacts. Extreme care should be used in handling needles, scalpel blades, and other sharp items. Disposable needles, blades, and instruments must be placed in puncture-resistant containers for disposal.

Whereas these precautions are extremely important to prevent exposure to infected body fluids, casual contact with HTLV-III-infected individuals does not appear to increase risk for infection; hence, special precautions in examination rooms, registration desk, and waiting rooms are not necessary.

Because patients with AIDS are at risk for a wide range of unusual infections and neoplasms, even mild symptoms may require an unusually comprehensive approach in the emergency department. For example, a cough, without sputum production, which might seem quite innocent in a healthy individual, could be the presenting feature of pneumocystis pneumonia in a patient with AIDS. Problems of special concern in AIDS patients include pulmonary infiltrates, central nervous system symptoms, cutaneous infiltrates, gastrointestinal symptoms, and fever. The list of potential causes of these complaints is long and growing; processes and pathogens of concern include *Pneumocystis carinii, Toxoplasma gondii, Mycobacterium tuberculosis* or *avium-intracellulare, Candida albicans, Cryptococcus neoformans* and other fungi, cytomegalovirus, herpes simplex and other viruses, Salmonella, *Legionella pneumophila* and other bacteria, Kaposi's sarcoma, lymphoma, and other neoplasia. Even if the underlying HTLV-III infection cannot be treated, many of these complicating processes will respond to treatment. Clearly, patients with AIDS, like other immunosuppressed patients, require a vigorous approach to the diagnosis of these problems. Whereas management of these processes is not within the scope of the emergency department, early triage for diagnostic studies and hospitalization are extremely important.

A précis of the cutaneous manifestations of human immunodeficiency virus infection is given in Chapter 19.

Infections of Bones and Joints

Bacterial infections of bones and joints are among the most important infections seen in the emergency department. Although these infections are rarely life-threatening, a vigorous approach to diagnosis and treatment is required to preserve joint function and to avoid chronic osteomyelitis.

Acute pyogenic infections of the skeletal system usually produce constitutional symptoms, including fever, chills, and anorexia. Pain, swelling, and inflammation, together with impaired function of the infected bone or joint, often pinpoint the site of infection. In such patients the diagnosis is not difficult, although the differential diagnosis must include crystalline arthritis (gout and pseudogout), rheumatic disease and other hypersensitivity states, as well as trauma, viral infection (especially rubella and mumps), and tuberculosis. Occasionally the diagnosis may be occult; this is especially true in children and when the axial skeleton is involved.

Laboratory evaluation reveals leukocytosis and an elevated erythrocyte sedimentation rate in most patients. Workup should also include blood cultures, studies directed at the noninfectious diseases just mentioned, and a search for other sites of infection that may have led to bacteremic seeding.

Acute Osteomyelitis

Hematogenous seeding or direct extension from a contiguous focus may result in acute osteomyelitis. *S. aureus* is the most common cause of this disease, but other organisms may be involved, such as Salmonella in patients with sickle cell anemia, Pseudomonas in drug users, Gram-negative bacilli in persons with vertebral osteomyelitis, and even rare organisms such as *P. multocida* after a cat bite. Because of this range of organisms, direct examination of the infected tissue is necessary unless other studies such as blood cultures or Salmonella agglutination titers are diagnostic; this involves either needle biopsy or open surgical biopsy. Histologic examination is important to exclude other processes such as tumor and tuberculosis. Roentgenograms do not show bony changes for several weeks, although soft-tissue swelling may be apparent. Bone scans may indicate osteomyelitis earlier, and the serum alkaline phosphatase level may be elevated. Again, the Gram's stain and cultures are diagnostic. Pus or bone specimens or both should be inoculated on blood agar and chocolate agar, in thioglycollate broth, and also on a blood agar plate to be incubated anaerobically. If *M. tuberculosis* or fungi are suspected, special media must be used. The choice of antibiotics follows the principles discussed in relation to septic arthritis to follow. High-dose parenteral therapy is required, usually for 4–6 weeks. Such vigorous and prolonged treatment is necessary to avoid chronic osteomyelitis, which responds poorly to antibiotics and which may require multiple surgical procedures.

Septic Arthritis

The cause of septic arthritis may be bacteremic seeding, direct spread of infection from contiguous bone or muscle, a penetrating injury, or postoperative infection. This disease can occur in all age groups, and may involve any joint, although infections of the knees, hips, elbows, and shoulders are most common. X-ray examination usually reveals only soft-tissue swelling. Pyogenic arthritis is most often monoarticular, but multiple joints may be involved, especially in patients with gonococcal arthritis.

The gonococcus is the most common cause of septic arthritis in sexually active persons. The meningococcus can also cause septic arthritis, but does so much less commonly. In all age groups, Gram-positive cocci are important causes of this disease; *S. aureus* is more common than the pneumococcus or streptococcus. *H. influenzae* may cause septic arthritis in children. Enteric Gram-negative bacilli may be responsible in debilitated patients and in drug addicts, as well as after trauma and in infections of the vertebral disc spaces.

The key to diagnosis is examination of the joint fluid. Arthrocentesis should be performed as soon as possible (see Illustrated Techniques 24 and 25). In the patient with typical septic arthritis, the joint fluid is viscous and purulent with a high number of white blood cells (usually 20,000–200,000/mm^3), most of which are polymorphonuclear leukocytes. The glucose level is depressed (less than 50 mg/100 ml, or less than 50% of the blood glucose level), and the mucin clot is poor. A Gram's stain of the joint fluid is essential, and fluid should promptly be inoculated on blood agar and chocolate agar and in thioglycollate broth (Table 11.1).

The choice of antibiotics depends on the organism isolated. If analysis of the joint fluid and the clinical findings suggest septic arthritis, antibiotic therapy should not be delayed until culture results are available. If the gonococcus or meningococcus is suspected, penicillin is the drug of choice. For Gram-positive cocci, oxacillin or nafcillin should be administered initially, with a change to penicillin if pneumococci or sensitive streptococci are cultured. In the presence of *H. influenzae,* ampicillin, a newer cephalosporin, or chloramphenicol should be administered, depending on the results of sensitivity testing. These results also determine the choice of drug for Gram-negative bacilli, but gentamicin or tobramycin is acceptable until these data are available. Antibiotics should be administered parenterally in high doses. Intraarticular administration is unnecessary and can be harmful.

Pyogenic arthritis is a closed-space infection, and drainage is required to avert permanent damage. In peripheral joints, immobilization and repeated arthrocentesis are usually sufficient, but if an effusion cannot be completely tapped, operation is necessary for drainage. Because of its delicate blood supply, early surgical drainage of the hip joint is advisable.

Lyme Disease

First described in Connecticut in 1975, Lyme disease is a systemic infection caused by the spirochete *Borrelia burgdorferi.* The infection is transmitted by the bite of Ixodes ticks and is commonest between May and November. Most cases have been reported from the east coast (Massachusetts to Maryland) but the disease has also been recognized in the midwest and west, as well as in Europe. The clinical manifestations include a destinctive skin rash, erythema chronicum migrans (ECM), which begins with a small red papule and expands to a large circular lesson with a diameter that can exceed 12 inches before clearing in about 3 weeks. Neurologic features range from a septic meningitis to peripheral neuropathies. Arthritis can appear within weeks of infection but may be delayed for as long as 2 years; recurrent bouts of acute arthritis of large joints is typical, but chronic joint inflammation can occur, especially in the knees. Cardiac manifestations include myocarditis, pericarditis, and conduction abnormalities. Constitutional symptoms, including fever, myalgias, and arthralgias, are common.

If a patient presents with full-blown Lyme disease from an endemic region, the diagnosis should not be difficult. But patients may also present to the emergency department with aseptic meningitis, acute arthritis, or myopericarditis alone or in combination; if there is no history of a tick bite or the characteristic rash, the diagnosis may be difficult. Serologies should be used to diagnose Lyme disease; penicillin or tetracycline should be administered.

Infections of Skin and Soft Tissue, Including Wounds

The skin is unique among the organ systems in that many of its pathologic conditions are visible on

Table 11.5.
Rash and Fever in the Acutely Ill Patient: Diagnosis According to Type of Lesion[a]

Macules or Papules	Vesicles, Bullae, or Pustules	Purpuric Macules, Papules, or Vesicles
Drug hypersensitivities	Drug hypersensitivities	Drug hypersensitivities
Scarlet fever	Dermatitis from plants	Bacteremia[b]
Erythema infectiosum (fifth disease)	Rickettsial pox	Meningococcemia (acute or chronic)
Measles (rubeola)	Varicella (chicken pox)[c]	Gonococcemia
German measles (rubella)	Generalized herpes zoster[c]	Staphylococcemia
Enterovirus infections (ECHO and Coxsackie)	Disseminated herpes simplex[c]	Pseudomonas bacteremia
Adenovirus infections	Eczema herpeticum[c]	Subacute bacterial endocarditis
Typhoid fever	Disseminated vaccinia[c]	Enterovirus infections (ECHO and Coxsackie)
Secondary syphilis	Eczema vaccinatum[c]	Rickettsial diseases
Typhus, murine (endemic)	Variola[c]	Rocky Mountain spotted fever
Rocky Mountain spotted fever (early lesions)	Enterovirus infections (ECHO and Coxsackie), including hand-foot-mouth disease	Typhus, louse-borne (epidemic)
Pityriasis rosea	Toxic epidermal necrolysis	Allergic cutaneous vasculitis
Erythema multiforme	Erythema multiforme bullosum	
Erythema marginatum		
Systemic lupus erythematosus		
Dermatomyositis		
"Serum sickness" (manifested only as wheals)		

[a] Reproduced by permission, from Fitzpatrick TB, Eisen AZ, Wolff K, et al, eds. Dermatology in General Medicine. 3rd ed, 1987, New York: McGraw-Hill Book Company.
[b] Often present as infarcts.
[c] Characteristic lesion is an umbilicated papule or vesicle on an erythematous base.

direct inspection. Since rash is a symptom that many patients find alarming, cutaneous lesions often cause patients to go to the emergency department for care.

Table 11.5 lists the possible causes of rash and fever in the acutely ill patient. Many of these diseases are viral infections or drug-induced hypersensitivity states (see Chapter 19).

Cutaneous Infections

Cutaneous infections may result from direct inoculation of bacteria or from hematogenous seeding. The cutaneous stigmata of meningococcemia and gonococcemia were mentioned earlier; it is important to remember that in either of these infections, fever and petechial, purpuric, or pustular lesions may be the presenting symptoms. Blood cultures are essential, as is a full workup that includes careful examination for primary sites of infection. In addition, fluid should be aspirated from pustular lesions, since a Gram's stain may disclose Gram-negative diplococci and culture may reveal Neisseria.

Similar cutaneous lesions may result from other types of bacteremia. Staphylococcal sepsis may cause pustules, and endocarditis due to any organism can lead to hemorrhagic, pustular, or infarcted lesions resembling those in some patients with vasculitis. Sepsis due to Pseudomonas may lead to ecthyma gangrenosum, with large necrotic lesions. Any bacteremia, but especially those due to Gram-negative bacilli, can cause purpuric lesions that often indicate disseminated intravascular coagulation.

Certain bacterial infections which are localized to areas of the body remote from the skin can produce fever and a systemic illness with prominent rash by the mechanism of toxin production. Well known examples include scarlet fever (usually resulting from group A streptococcal pharyngitis) and the scalded skin syndrome (*S. aureus* of phage group II).

Another disorder which belongs in this category is the *toxic shock syndrome* (TSS). TSS occurs primarily in menstruating women using tampons but has occurred occasionally in nonmenstruating women and men with localized staphylococcal infections. Clinical features include high fever, hypotension, and a diffuse scarlatiniform eruption with hyperemia of mucous membranes, involvement of palms and soles, and late desquamation. Diarrhea, myalgias, headaches, encephalopathy, abnormal liver function tests, azotemia, and pulmonary infiltrates often are present and reflect the characteristic involvement of multiple organ systems. Blood cultures almost always are negative since the disease is caused by a circulating toxin rather than bacteremic spread of infection. However, staphylococci often can be isolated from the vagina of menstruating females or from localized infections in others. Therapy should include antistaphylococcal antibiotics and vigorous cardiovascular support.

Among the other illnesses that can cause fever and petechial lesions of the skin, *Rocky Mountain spotted fever* deserves special mention. Despite its name, this disease is found nationwide, with most cases coming from the Atlantic seaboard, especially Virginia and North Carolina. Rocky Mountain spotted fever is caused by a rickettsia transmitted to human beings by the bite of infected ticks, usually between the months of April and August. Patients are seen with fever, chills, severe headache, photophobia, myalgia, and rash that often involves the palms and soles. Mental changes are common, and approximately 50% of patients have splenomegaly. Characteristic laboratory findings include thrombocytopenia and normal white blood cell counts, although polymorphonuclear leukocytes and band forms can predominate. Meningococcemia and atypical measles are the most common misdiagnoses in these patients. Because rickettsiae cannot be cultured under ordinary conditions, serologic tests are needed to confirm the diagnosis. However, mortality is high and therapy must be immediate; if the diagnosis seems probable according to clinical and epidemiologic findings, tetracycline or chloramphenicol should be administered, 2 gm/day for adults.

Direct inoculation of organisms into the skin may produce several other disease syndromes. The most common organisms involved are *S. aureus* and group A streptococci. Either of these may cause impetigo, with crusting, superficial lesions. Deep, localized abscesses such as furuncles, carbuncles, and paronychial lesions are caused by staphylococci. Patients with these infections are usually free of systemic findings and respond well to hot soaks and oral antistaphylococcal antibiotics, although surgical drainage may hasten recovery. These same organisms can also cause much more serious infections of the skin, including erysipelas, cellulitis, and lymphangitis. Such patients require hospitalization, parenteral administration of antibiotics, and a full workup including blood cultures. Antistreptolysin O titers may sometimes be helpful in diagnosing streptococcal infections. Aspiration of infected skin for a Gram's stain and culture should be attempted, although these studies are often negative; if no material can be obtained by direct aspiration, a small amount of sterile saline *without* antibacterial preservatives can be injected and then aspirated. The bacteria causing these infections are so characteristic that administration of antistaphylococcal antibiotics may be started before culture results are available; patients should receive high-dose parenteral therapy until the infection is considerably resolved.

Although streptococci and staphylococci are responsible for most primary cutaneous infections, many other bacteria can cause cellulitis. In children, cellulitis due to *H. influenzae* has a characteristic blue to purple appearance. In immunosuppressed patients, Gram-negative bacilli can occasionally cause devastating cutaneous infections. Perirectal and perineal infections may be caused by these and other intestinal flora. *C. diphtheriae* is a rare cause of skin infection in nonimmunized patients. Finally, animal contact may be responsible for many uncommon infections, including cellulitis from *P. multocida* (cats), lesions due to Erysipelothrix (fish), anthrax (cattle and sheep), and tularemia (many wild species). An epidemiologic history provides the essential clue in these cases.

Wound Infections

Thus far, the focus has been on normal skin, but when the integrity of the skin is altered by trauma, burns, or operation, virtually any organism can cause infection; often, multiple species produce synergistic infection. Accurate etiologic diagnosis requires a Gram's stain and aerobic and anaerobic cultures of any exudate, blood cultures, and x-ray examination for gas and foreign bodies. Early surgical drainage and débridement of infected wounds and abscesses are important. A few organisms cause relatively characteristic infections in these circumstances. For example, group A streptococci typically cause early infection (sometimes within 12–24 hours of injury) associated with high fever and a watery, nonpurulent exudate. Therefore, low doses of penicillin or other antistreptococcal antibiotics are recommended during the first few days after a contaminated wound or burn is sustained. *Pseudomonas aeruginosa* is one of the most common pathogens of burned skin. The resultant infection produces a characteristic musty, sweet odor, and illumination of the infected area with Wood's light reveals green fluorescence due to bacterial pigment. Cultures are necessary to confirm the diagnosis, and gentamicin or tobramycin, alone or with antipseudomonal penicillins are the drugs of choice. Anaerobic infections may produce foul-smelling pus. A variety of organisms, including group A streptococci, anaerobic streptococci, and Gram-negative bacilli, either singly or in combination, can cause many serious necrotizing infections of the skin, subcutaneous tissue, and muscle, including cutaneous gangrene, necrotizing fasciitis, and necrotizing myositis. Patients with these conditions have pronounced systemic toxic reactions and rapidly advancing infections. In addition to administration of high doses of parenteral antibiotics (usually a penicillinase-resistant penicillin and an aminoglycoside until culture results are available), these patients require immediate aggressive surgical débridement of all devitalized tissues.

Clostridial species can cause many types of wound infection. Wound botulism caused by *C. botulinum* is rare. *Tetanus,* which can result from contamination with either the vegetative cells or spores of *C. tetani,* may occur even in patients with minor lesions, but is more common after contamination of deep wounds that have devitalized tissues. The key to management of this disease is prevention. The wound must first be cleaned and debrided. The need for active immunization with tetanus toxoid or passive immunization with tetanus immune globulin (human) is determined by the patient's immunization history and the nature of the wound (Table 11.6). *C. perfringens, C. welchii,* and other species may be present in wounds as surface contaminants without causing significant disease. However, these same organisms can cause localized infection or spreading anaerobic cellulitis. Such patients are febrile, but do not have systemic toxic reactions.

Table 11.6.
Summary Guide to Tetanus Prophylaxis in Routine Wound Management—United States[a]

History of Adsorbed Tetanus Toxoid (Doses)	Clean, Minor Wounds		All Other Wounds[b]	
	Td[c]	TIG	Td[c]	TIG
< three or unknown	Yes	No	Yes	Yes
≧ three[d]	No[e]	No	No[f]	No

[a] Modified with permission from *Morbidity and Mortality,* 1981;30:420.
[b] Such as, but not limited to, wounds contaminated with dirt, feces, soil, saliva, etc.; puncture wounds; avulsions; and wounds resulting from missiles, crushing, burns and frostbite.
[c] Td, tetanus and diphtheria toxoids, adult type; TIG, tetanus immune globulin (human) 250–500 units intramuscularly. For children under 7 years old, DTP (diphtheria, tetanus, pertussis toxoids, child type) (DT, if pertussis vaccine is contraindicated) is preferred to tetanus toxoid alone. For persons 7 years old and older, Td is preferred to tetanus toxoid alone.
[d] If only three doses of *fluid* toxoid have been received, a fourth dose of toxoid, preferably adsorbed toxoid, should be given.
[e] Yes, if more than 10 years since last dose.
[f] Yes, if more than 5 years since last dose. (More frequent boosters are not needed and can accentuate side effects.)

Gas is produced in the involved areas, but pain is minimal and the skin is not discolored. High doses of penicillin with local drainage produce excellent results. Much more serious is *clostridial myonecrosis* or *gas gangrene,* in which patients are febrile, delirious, and often hypotensive. The infected tissues are edematous, with discoloration of skin and often bleb formation. Gas is produced deep in the tissue planes, and infection advances rapidly. Pain is intense. Large Gram-positive bacilli are evident in Gram's stains of the exudate, but spore formation is rare and polymorphonuclear leukocytes are characteristically scant. Specimens must be cultured anaerobically when clostridial infection is suspected. Therapy requires high doses of penicillin. 20–30 million units/day for adults, and immediate, aggressive surgical débridement with complete excision of all infected tissues. Hyperbaric oxygen therapy should be considered if available.

Not all gas-forming infections are caused by Clostridia. Many aerobic and anaerobic bacteria, especially the Gram-negative bacilli, can produce gas in tissues. Patients with diabetes are particularly susceptible to gas-forming infections. The choice of antibiotics is dictated by the results of Gram's stains and cultures, but broad coverage by oxacillin and chloramphenicol or clindamycin and gentamicin is usually advisable until results are available. Surgical drainage and débridement are important.

A final problem concerning wound management is the possibility of rabies in the patient with an animal bite. Human rabies is rare in the United States today, with only one or two cases reported each year, and rabies in domestic animals has also become uncommon. However, rabies among wild animals appears to be increasing. Because this disease is almost invariably lethal, the main concern is prevention. Any wound should immediately be washed thoroughly with copious amounts of soap and water. If bacterial infection is present or seems likely, antibiotics should be administered; penicillin is the recommended antibiotic for many animal and human bites. The need for prophylactic immunization against rabies depends on the species of animal involved (see Chapter 10).

Fortunately, human rabies immune globulin is now available and should be administered when antiserum is required. Similarly, the new human diploid cell rabies vaccine (HDCV) is a major advance in active immunization against rabies.

Cardiac Infections

Bacterial Endocarditis

Patients with bacterial endocarditis constitute only a small minority of individuals receiving medical care in the emergency department; however, the emergency physician must be fully knowledgeable in the management of these life-threatening infections. Endocarditis is classically divided into two types. First is *subacute bacterial endocarditis,* which usually occurs in patients with congenital or acquired (rheumatic or calcific) valvular heart disease. The most common causative organism is *Streptococcus viridans.* These streptococci, whose virulence is ordinarily low, are part of the normal oral flora; however, they commonly cause transient bacteremia, especially after dental manipulations, and they then may establish foci of infection on the previously damaged valve. Many other organisms can also cause subacute bacterial endocarditis. Symptoms include fever, anorexia, and weight loss, often of weeks' or even months' duration; congestive heart failure may also develop or may worsen as a result of infection. Neurologic manifestations may be striking, and subacute bacterial endocarditis should be considered in any patient with a cerebrovascular accident and fever. Physical examination usually reveals a murmur, but this may seem insignificant or may even be absent. Classic features include petechiae, Roth's spots, splinter hemorrhages in the nails, painful lesions of the fingertips (Osler's nodes), and splenomegaly. These findings require weeks to evolve, however, and are often absent when the patient is first examined. The same is true of abnormalities revealed by laboratory testing. Anemia is common, and the white blood cell count may be elevated or normal. Urinary sediments are often abnormal, and subacute bacterial endocarditis should be considered in patients with fever and renal failure of uncertain cause, especially in the elderly. The erythrocyte sedimentation rate is elevated, and the rheumatoid factor, reflecting chronic inflammation, is positive in about half the patients.

The second type of endocarditis is *acute bacterial endocarditis.* The pace of this condition is greatly accelerated because the disease classically results from more virulent organisms that produce destructive lesions, even on previously normal valves. Many organisms have been implicated in acute bacterial endocarditis. *S. aureus* is the most common; endocarditis due to this pathogen may follow bacteremia from even a minor infection such as a furuncle, or it may arise from an inapparent primary site. This is an extremely serious infection, and most patients with high-grade bacteremia due to *S. aureus* should be treated for it even if murmurs and other traditional indications of endocarditis are absent. Enterococci also cause acute bacterial endocarditis, often after a primary gastrointestinal or genitourinary disorder. Pneumococci are now uncommon causative agents. Among drug addicts a broad variety of organisms, including Gram-negative bacilli, have been implicated. Although the clinical and laboratory features of acute bacterial endocarditis may include all the findings of the subacute type, in typical cases the peripheral manifestations are less pronounced and fever and acute systemic illness are more prominent. Congestive heart failure can fulminate if valve damage is severe.

The role of the emergency physician is to suspect the diagnosis of endocarditis and to order the crucial diagnostic procedure, the blood culture. In patients with indolent illness consistent with subacute bacterial endocarditis, six specimens for culture can be drawn in a 24- to 48-hour period before instituting antibiotic therapy. However, in acute disease the patient's condition may rapidly deteriorate, and therapy should not be so delayed. If acute bacterial endocarditis appears likely, four to six specimens for culture can be obtained with separate vein punctures in the course of 2–3 hours, and administration of antibiotics can be started. Most patients with endocarditis have high-grade bacteremia, and blood cultures are often all positive. In all patients, high doses of antibiotics should be administered parenterally for 4–6 weeks, with patients carefully observed for complications, including congestive heart failure, emboli, and mycotic aneurysms. Antibiotic therapy should be guided by sensitivity testing, and whenever possible, serum bactericidal levels should be determined. Until these data are available, penicillin, 20 million units/day, is the ideal first choice for adults with subacute bacterial endocarditis. Oxacillin, 12 gm/day, with gentamicin, 1.0–1.5 mg/kg every 8 hours if renal function is normal, is acceptable for initial treatment of patients with suspected acute bacterial endocarditis.

Pericarditis

Another cardiac condition that may require emergency treatment is pericarditis (see Chapter 6). Many of the causes of pericarditis are noninfectious, including myocardial infarction, tumor, trauma, uremia, myxedema, and vasculitis. Among the infectious causes, viruses are most common. Patients with viral pericarditis usually have pericardial pain and may be febrile, but they usually do not have leukocytosis or severe systemic reactions. Pericardial tamponade is uncommon. Diagnosis is usually based on clinical criteria, but can sometimes be confirmed by serologic testing or, if specialized facilities are available, viral isolation. Therapy depends on symptoms, with antiinflammatory agents such as indomethacin being particularly useful. Prognosis is generally excellent, although pain may recur in some patients, and rarely, early tamponade or late constrictive pericarditis may develop. Tuberculous pericarditis, which is much less common, may be indicated by fever and hemodynamic compromise. Pain is often less severe and the course is usually subacute, with the possibility of late calcific pericarditis. The tuberculin skin test is positive in most patients, but pulmonary tuberculosis may or may not be coexistent. Pericardiocentesis (see Illustrated Technique 10) or biopsy or both provide the definitive diagnosis. A final form of pericarditis, which is also rare but which constitutes a true emergency, is purulent pericarditis. This can develop after a thoracic operation, from direct extension of bacterial pneumonia or deep plane neck infections, or by bacteremic seeding. Patients are usually febrile and acutely ill; the condition rapidly progresses to tamponade and death if untreated.

Pericardiocentesis is necessary for diagnosis in most cases. The fluid contains a high number of white blood cells with a predominance of polymorphonuclear leukocytes, a low glucose level, and a high protein level. A Gram's stain and aerobic and anaerobic cultures are mandatory (Table 11.1). Studies for tuberculosis and fungal processes should be performed if there is any doubt as to diagnosis. Surgical drainage of the pericardium is required in almost all patients. Although *S. aureus* and pneumococci were previously the most common causes of purulent pericarditis, many organisms have been implicated recently; antibiotic therapy must therefore be individualized, based on the Gram's stain, presence or absence of another septic focus, and clinical features.

Bacteremia and Septic Shock

Many of the acute infections that have been discussed may be accompanied by *bacteremia,* the clinical expression of which may be obvious or occult. Often, patients have a serious underlying disease such as diabetes, cirrhosis, or leukemia, or they may have had recent medical or surgical therapy involving Foley catheters or intravenous lines. The signs and symptoms of a primary infectious process, such as pyelonephritis, cholecystitis, or pneumonia, can predominate. High fever is common, and shaking chills are suggestive of bacteremia. Neither finding is invariable, however; patients with uremia and those receiving corticosteroids may even be afebrile. As mentioned earlier, patients with bacteremia may have purpuric, pustular, or necrotic cutaneous lesions. Even in the absence of pulmonary infection, tachypnea may be striking and often may lead to respiratory alkalosis. Confusion and disorientation may be pronounced, especially in the elderly; although these signs should always raise the possibility of infection of the central nervous system, the metabolic and circulatory effects of bacteremia alone can produce toxic encephalopathy. Tachycardia is characteristic, and in patients with underlying heart disease, angina or congestive heart failure may develop.

A dread complication of bacteremia, *septic shock* constitutes a true medical emergency. All the clinical considerations just discussed apply to the bacteremic patient in whom septic shock develops. In the earliest stages, clinical findings may be those of "warm shock"; the patient is alert, with warm, dry skin. However, without treatment the classic syndrome of "cold shock" ensues; the skin becomes clammy and cold, with mottled cyanosis, and the patient becomes obtunded. Hypotension is a cardinal feature of septic shock, although some patients may have normal blood pressure early in the process. Even more common is the patient who has hypotension without true septic shock; however, management of hypotension in the presence of fever and possible bacteremia should always be approached vigorously.

True septic shock involves inadequate tissue perfusion, the clinical manifestations of which vary. Inadequate renal perfusion results in oliguria and a low concentration of sodium in the urine, poor perfusion of the coronary arteries can lead to myocardial ischemia or arrhythmias or both, and compromised cerebral perfusion may cause confusion or coma. Impaired peripheral blood flow results in vasoconstricted cutaneous vessels and diminished pulses.

The laboratory manifestations of septic shock are variable. Polymorphonuclear leukocytosis with band forms often occurs. Thrombocytopenia may develop with or without coagulation disorders, suggesting disseminated intravascular coagulation. Hypoxia may be present, and blood gas levels may indicate respiratory alkalosis or metabolic acidosis or both. The level of lactate in the blood is often elevated in acidotic patients. Azotemia develops if renal perfusion remains poor.

The patient with septic shock requires immediate attention. Vital functions should be supported (see Chapters 2 and 3), first securing an adequate airway. Arterial blood gas levels should be determined and oxygen should be administered if indicated. A Swan-Ganz catheter is indispensable, and an intra-arterial line to monitor blood gases and pressure is helpful. A Foley catheter should be inserted to monitor urinary output. A rapid history and physical examination are essential, as is laboratory evaluation to determine a primary site of infection. The importance of complete cultures, especially of the blood and urine, cannot be overemphasized. It is also important to screen for noninfectious causes of shock, including myocardial failure, pulmonary emboli, pericardial tamponade, hemorrhage, and other causes of volume depletion such as pancreatitis.

Therapy for septic shock is multifaceted. Volume replacement is of primary importance. Because left ventricular function may be depressed as a result of sepsis, careful hemodynamic monitoring is required during volume expansion. Crystalloids, such as normal saline and Ringer's lactated solutions, can be administered on a trial basis, but colloids such as albumin and whole blood are usually more effective. Volume expanders should be administered rapidly until the pulmonary artery wedge pressure reaches 12–16 mm Hg. Some patients with chronic pulmonary disease may require even higher filling pressures, but further volume expansion must be approached with caution. Acidosis and other metabolic abnormalities should be corrected. If shock persists after fluid and electrolyte therapy, vasoactive drugs must be administered. There is no consensus as to which agents are best, and therapy must be individualized. Dopamine is the mainstay of therapy. Occasionally, epinephrine or norepinephrine is necessary when other drugs fail to provide satisfactory perfusion. Detailed information about these drugs is presented in Chapter 3. Even more controversy surrounds the use of corticosteroids in patients with septic shock. Some physicians advocate large doses of glucocorticoids, but these have not been shown to enhance survival. Experimental approaches to therapy include the use of human antiserum to endotoxin, nalaxone, prostaglandin inhibitors, and vasodilators. None of these has yet been found effective in human septic shock.

In patients with septic shock, although survival often depends on metabolic, respiratory, and circulatory support, vigorous antimicrobial therapy is also necessary. The initial choice of antibiotics should be based on the primary site of infection. The choice of antibiotics for specific infectious processes has been detailed earlier in this chapter. But what of the patient whose condition appears septic and in whom no focus can be identified in the emergency department? Although cultures and other tests may provide an etiologic diagnosis within a few days, antibiotic therapy must be administered much sooner. Even though most cases of septic shock are caused by Gram-negative organisms, Gram-positive bacteria can cause clinically identical syndromes, so initial antibiotic coverage must be broad. High doses of nafcillin and gentamicin or tobramycin are recommended in these circumstances. In the penicillin-allergic patient, a cephalosporin or vancomycin can be substituted for nafcillin (Table 11.3). If anaerobes seem likely, as in abdominal or pelvic sepsis, a third drug such as clindamycin, metronidazole or chloramphenicol should be added, or cefoxitin can be substituted for nafcillin. If pseudomonas seems likely, as in the neutropenic cancer patient, an anti-pseudomonal penicillin should be added. Single drug therapy with imipenim or third-generation cephalosporins may prove useful, and is under study. Because muscle perfusion is inadequate for reliable drug absorption in patients with septic shock, drugs should be administered intravenously. If gentamicin or tobramycin is administered, the dosage must be adjusted to the patient's renal function. The first dose should be 1.5 mg/kg, but the time between doses should be prolonged according to the severity of renal failure; in many patients it may be better to substitute another drug.

Hyperpyrexia

Thus far, fever has been discussed only as a sign of an underlying disease process. While infectious diseases are the most common causes of fever, it can also be caused by many other processes. In fact, extremely high body temperatures are often due to noninfectious causes such as heat stroke, thyroid storm, malignant hyperthermia of anesthesia (see Chapter 10), and disorders of the hypothalamus.

In otherwise healthy patients, temperatures of 103°F (39.4°C) or 104°F (40°C) may be well-tolerated and may not require treatment. However, fever often causes deleterious effects that do indicate a need for antipyretic therapy. Uncomfortable symptoms such as anorexia, myalgia, confusion, lethargy, and chills respond to lowering of the body temperature. In young children, febrile convulsions can result from temperatures higher than 104°F (40°C) even without underlying neurologic problems; therefore, antipyretic therapy should be employed routinely in this age group. Hyperpyrexia has profound metabolic consequences, including elevation in oxygen consumption and accelerated tissue catabolism. As a result, the cardiovascular system is faced with increased demands, and fever can precipitate myocardial ischemia or congestive heart failure or both in patients with heart disease. Extreme hyperpyrexia with a temperature of 105°F (40.6°C) or higher may directly cause tissue damage, including changes in the vascular endothelium. In patients with extreme hyperpyrexia, disseminated intravascular coagulation, acidosis, and cardiovascular collapse can develop.

In the emergency department, the patient's respiratory, metabolic, and circulatory status must first be stabilized. Since extremely high fever can cause shock, these patients should be treated like patients with septic shock. A workup to diagnose the underlying disorder should be undertaken without delay, and specific therapy should be directed by the findings. Any complications, such as seizures, congestive heart failure, or disseminated intravascular coagulation, should be treated, as well as the fever itself. Antipyretic therapy may include both chemical agents and physical cooling. Among the drugs available, both aspirin and acetaminophen act directly on the hypothalamus to lower its thermal set point. Doses up to 1.2 gm can be given to adults orally or rectally and repeated every 4 hours. Caution must be exercised, since elderly patients and those with certain conditions, such as Hodgkin's disease and typhoid fever, may react adversely to antipyretic agents. Phenothiazine compounds are sometimes useful, but their effectiveness has not been completely elucidated and their use in extreme pyrexia is still experimental. The technique of physical cooling depends on the seriousness of condition. If the fever is being well-tolerated, a hypothermic mattress or sponging with alcohol or ice water may suffice. Since these are uncomfortable procedures, they should be reserved for patients in whom rapid reduction of temperature is mandatory. Under even more serious circumstances such as heat stroke, more extreme cooling may be required, in which case immersion in an ice water bath is recommended. Other measures such as iced gastric lavage, ice water enemas, and iced peritoneal dialysis are both less effective and more cumbersome. Once body temperature has been reduced to a safe level, physical cooling should be discontinued to avoid hypothermia.

GUIDELINES FOR ANTIBIOTIC THERAPY IN THE EMERGENCY DEPARTMENT

The number of antimicrobial agents available to the physician is great, and new drugs are rapidly being marketed. This section is not intended to provide a comprehensive review of antibiotics but rather to present some guidelines likely to be useful in the emergency department.

1. Antibiotics treat bacterial infection, not fever. It is important to evaluate the condition of each patient following the general approach on pp 209–211 to arrive at a tentative diagnosis before starting administration of antibiotics.
2. In general, antibiotics do not *prevent* infection. "Prophylactic antibiotics" are beneficial only in few special circumstances.
3. Antibiotics have disadvantages, including possible toxic effects, potential sensitization of the patient, and selection of resistant organisms that can superinfect the patient. Capricious use of antibiotics can result in resistant organisms

throughout the hospital and community. In addition, many antibiotics are expensive.

4. New antibiotics should be compared critically with established agents. Many "new" drugs are minor modifications of standard drugs and are often more expensive. Toxic reactions may become apparent long after introduction of the new agent.
5. Appropriate cultures and Gram's stains should be obtained *before* starting antibiotic therapy.
6. The patient must be treated specifically. Although the acutely ill patient may initially require broad antibiotic therapy, the goal should always be to select as specific a program of treatment as possible. Results of cultures and sensitivity testing and any other data that may become available should always be used to reevaluate therapy.
   a. Administer as few drugs as possible. Direct therapy at the specific pathogen or pathogens isolated from the patient.
   b. Administer drugs that will penetrate the infected tissues.
   c. Administer the least toxic drugs available. If the patient also has renal or hepatic disease, this should be considered in choosing the drug and its dosage.
   d. Administer bactericidal rather than bacteriostatic drugs when possible.
   e. Choose the route of administration, dosage, and duration of therapy appropriate for the specific infection being treated.
   f. Monitor the patient's condition for effectiveness of treatment, toxic reactions, hypersensitivity, and superinfection.
   g. Administer the least expensive drugs available when possible.
   h. Beware of drug incompatibilities.

Table 11.3 summarizes some properties of selected antibiotics. This material is not exhaustive; alternative drugs of similar efficacy may be available, and new drugs are being introduced frequently. The current literature should be consulted for details.

Suggested Readings

American Academy of Pediatrics. Report of the Committee on Infectious Disease, 20th ed. Evanston, IL: American Academy of Pediatrics, 1986.

Gardner P, Provine HT. Manual of Acute Bacterial Infections: Early Diagnosis and Treatment. Boston: Little, Brown & Co., 1984.

Mandell GL, Douglas RG, Bennet JE, eds. Principles and Practice of Infectious Diseases, ed. 2, New York: John Wiley & Sons, 1985.

Medical Letter on Drugs and Therapeutics, Choice of antimicrobial drugs. 1986;28:33–40.

Petersdorf RA, Adams RD, Brownwald E, et al., eds. Harrison's Principles of Internal Medicine. ed 10, Part 4, Disorders Caused by Biologic and Environmental Agents. New York: McGraw-Hill, 1983;839–1255.

Rubenstein E, Federman DD, eds. Scientific American Medicine. Section 7, Infectious Diseases. New York: Scientific American, 1986.

Wyngaarden JB, Smith LH, eds. Textbook of Medicine. ed. 16, Part 14, Infectious Diseases. Philadelphia: WB Saunders, 1982;1391–1778.

CHAPTER 12

Medical Gastrointestinal Disorders

JAMES M. RICHTER, M.D.

Editor's note: This medical chapter on gastrointestinal disease includes the broad and diverse subjects of diarrhea, hemorrhage, vomiting, peptic disease, swallowed foreign bodies, and hepatic and proctologic disorders. The separation of gastrointestinal diseases into medical and surgical components is arbitrary. Additional coverage is provided, therefore, in Chapter 33 (Abdominal Emergencies), and in Chapter 11 (Infectious Diseases).

The emergency physician has to cope with an increasing variety of medical disorders related to the digestive tract. This chapter reviews some common gastrointestinal problems seen in the emergency department requiring diagnostic and therapeutic intervention.

DIARRHEA

One of the most common problems seen in the emergency department is diarrhea. Because therapy for diarrhea varies with the clinical findings, it is important to gather historical, physical, and laboratory information.

The history should include information about the foods eaten during the previous 72 hours, recent travel, contacts with other persons with diarrhea, current medical problems (for example, diabetes mellitus), and medications. In addition, the patient should be questioned about the onset of the diarrhea (acute or gradual), the amount and duration, the character of stool (including presence of blood or pus), and any concomitant fever, nausea, vomiting, or abdominal pain.

Physical examination initially is directed toward assessing the state of hydration and clinical toxicity of the patient. The seriously ill patient requires careful observation and fluid replacement regardless of the cause of the diarrhea. A complete examination is optimal, but special attention should be directed toward the abdomen and rectum. The stool specimen should be examined for gross and occult blood; in addition, a methylene blue stain for polymorphonuclear leukocytes is helpful in the diagnosis of inflammatory and infectious diarrheas (Table 12.1 and 12.2).

The following sections discuss common causes of

Table 12.1.
Causes of Acute Infectious Diarrhea

Virus
Rotavirus
Adenovirus
Parvovirus
Enterovirus
Bacterial toxins
Staphylococcal toxin
Clostridial toxin
Bacteria
Salmonella
Shigella
Escherichia coli
Campylobacter fetus
Yersinia enterocolitica
Vibrio cholerae
Protozoa
Amoeba
Giardia lamblia
Cryptosporidium

diarrhea with regard to their clinical features and treatment.

Viral Gastroenteritis

The most common causes of acute sporadic diarrhea are viruses such as the rotavirus, parvovirus, enterovirus, and adenovirus. Typically the patient has fever, headache, and malaise, and may have nausea, vomiting, or upper respiratory tract symptoms. The stools are watery with no blood or pus.

Table 12.2.
Fecal Leukocytes in Acute Diarrhea

Present	Absent
Salmonella	Viruses
Shigella	Staphylococcal toxin
Escherchia coli, invasive	*Clostridial* toxin
Campylobacter fetus	*E. coli,* toxinogenic
Amebiasis[a]	Cholera
Pseudomembranous colitis	Giardiasis
Ulcerative colitis	Amebiasis
Crohn's disease	Cryptosporidiosis
	Most drug-associated diarrhea

[a] When invasive.

Diarrhea usually resolves in 5–7 days. Because these illnesses are self-limited and since viral isolation techniques are expensive, a specific etiologic diagnosis is not indicated. Recently an enzyme-linked immunosorbent assay (ELISA) for rotavirus in stool has become available and may be helpful when confirmation of a viral diarrhea is needed. Therapy is principally directed at symptoms, with fluid replacement being of primary importance, especially in children. Aspirin or acetaminophen is taken for fever and myalgias. Bismuth subsalicylate (Pepto-Bismol), 30 ml every 4 hours, or diphenoxylate hydrochloride with atropine sulfate (Lomotil), 2.5–5.0 mg every 6 hours, may be taken for control of symptoms.

Table 12.3.
Etiology of Food-borne Disease Outbreaks by Food, Season, and Geographic Predilection[a]

Etiology	Foods	Season	Geographic Predilection
Bacterial			
Salmonella	Beef, poultry, eggs, dairy products	Summer	None
S. aureus	Ham, poultry, egg salads, pastries	Summer	None
C. jejuni	Raw milk, poultry, beef, frosting, clams	Spring, summer	None
C. botulinum	Vegetables, fruits, fish, honey (infants)	Summer, fall	West, Northeast
C. perfringens	Beef, poultry, gravy, Mexican food	Fall, winter, spring	None
Shigella	Egg salads	Summer	None
V. parahaemolyticus	Crabs	Spring, summer, fall	Coastal states
B. cereus	Fried rice, meats, vegetables	Year round	None
Y. enterocolitica	Milk, tofu	Unknown	Unknown
V. cholerae 01	Shellfish	Variable	Tropical, Gulf Coast
V. cholerae non-01	Shellfish	Unknown	Tropical, Gulf Coast
Viral			
Norwalk agent	Shellfish, salads	Year round	Unknown

[a] From Hughes JM. Food poisoning. In Mandell GL, Douglas RG Jr., and Bennet JE, eds. Principles and Practice of Infectious Diseases. New York: John Wiley & Sons, © 1985, p. 914.

Bacterial Gastroenteritis

Bacteria may cause acute diarrhea by producing a toxin in contaminated food, invading the gastrointestinal mucosa, or producing a toxin after ingestion. Foods contaminated by staphylococcal toxin, often custard-filled pastries or processed meats, produce nausea, vomiting, abdominal cramps, and diarrhea within a few hours of ingestion. Symptoms usually last less than 12 hours. Similarly, foods contaminated by *Clostridium perfringens* toxin, which have often been warmed on steam tables, induce diarrhea and abdominal cramps, beginning 8–24 hours after ingestion and lasting about 24 hours. Both conditions are distinguished by common-source outbreaks and the lack of fever.

In the United States, acute diarrheal illness often is caused by ingestion of Shigella, Salmonella, *Escherichia coli,* or *Campylobacter fetus* (Table 12.3). These diseases are most common among children, but may occur at any age. Typically, shigellosis begins 24–72 hours after ingestion of the bacteria, with fever, toxicity, bloody diarrhea, nausea, vomiting, and cramps. Frequently, the disease is more subtle and may be difficult to distinguish clinically from other diarrheal illnesses. It usually resolves in less than 7 days. Symptoms of salmonellosis develop 12–36 hours after ingestion of the bacteria, with watery diarrhea, cramps, nausea, vomiting, and fever. Salmonellosis is often nonspecific, and there is often no visible blood in the stool. It usually improves in less than 5 days, but may persist for up to 2 weeks. *E. coli* carries a wide spectrum of diarrheal illness resulting from mucosal invasion or toxin production. Toxinogenic strains cause a profuse watery diarrheal syndrome with cramps and low-grade fever. This is commonly experienced as traveler's diarrhea. Invasive strains, which are unusual in the United States, produce a disease characterized by fever, severe cramps, and bloody diarrhea. Recently, *C. fetus* has been recognized as a major cause of acute diarrhea in the United States. The clinical illness is similar to shigellosis, often with prominent rectal bleeding. The illness resolves spontaneously over 7–14 days, but may recur for 6–8 weeks.

Sigmoidoscopic examination of patients with invasive bacterial diseases reveals diffuse erythema, edema, and friability of the mucosa, but no discrete ulceration and is indistinguishable from ulcerative colitis. *Campylobacter* may be detected by finding wing-shaped Gram-negative bacteria on a smear of rectal pus or stool.

Most acute diarrheal illnesses should be managed by hydration, waiting for spontaneous resolution. Hydration often can be maintained by oral administration of fluids, even in patients with profuse diarrhea. Solutions containing electrolytes and sugars are best, but milk products should be avoided since acquired lactase deficiency is common, particularly in children. Patients in whom dehydration or electrolyte abnormalities develop should be admitted for parenteral therapy.

Antibiotics should *not be used routinely* for acute bacterial diarrhea. They have little effect on the course of the disease, and they may prolong an asymptomatic bacterial carrier state. Ampicillin is the first choice for the treatment of salmonellosis, but patients who are very ill or allergic to penicillin may require chloramphenicol. Elderly, debilitated patients and those who may not tolerate bacteremia, such as patients with sickle cell anemia or prosthetic heart valves, may benefit from the ability of antibiotic therapy to limit distant complications. Trimethoprim-sulfamethoxazole, ampicillin, or a single dose of tetracycline may be given for shigellosis. Erythromycin is presently recommended for campylobacterosis. Its role in the treatment of this disease is not clearly defined, but it probably should be given to toxic patients or individuals who are at risk for transmitting the disease. Traveler's diarrhea may be prevented by taking doxycycline, 100 mg daily prophylactically. See Chapter 11 for further discussion of antibiotic choices in bacterial diarrheas.

Absorbent preparations commonly are used to treat the symptoms of uncomplicated acute diarrhea. Solutions of kaolin and pectin have no proved benefit, but seem to be harmless; they should not be relied on, however, in the treatment of severe diarrhea. Bismuth subsalicylate has been effective therapy for the symptoms of traveler's diarrhea and may be helpful in other forms of simple diarrhea. Diphenoxylate hydrochloride and loperamide hydrochloride effectively decrease most diarrhea by directly inhibiting the motility of the gastrointestinal smooth muscle. They should be used cautiously, if at all, in conditions in which toxic megacolon is possible. Use also should be restricted in bacterial diarrheas because they may prolong the course of shigellosis. The usual dose of diphenoxylate is 2.5–5.0 mg every 4 hours up to 20 mg/day. Loperamide is given in a dose of 2 or 4 mg every 4 hours up to 16 mg daily. Dosage often can be decreased for maintenance after initial control of the diarrhea. Opiates are potent antidiarrheal agents, but carry a higher risk of abuse. They are particularly useful when their coincident analgesic activity is needed. Tincture of opium, 0.5–1.0 ml, paregoric, 4 ml, or codeine, 30–60 mg, is given orally every 4 hours.

Protozoal Gastroenteritis

Amebiasis

Amebiasis can cause an intermittent, chronic diarrheal syndrome or a severe fulminating condition presenting similarly to that of acute ulcerative colitis. A history of travel is important because acute disease occurs primarily in persons who have been in tropical areas. Recently, amebiasis has become common among sexually active male homosexuals in the United States without a history of travel. Findings on physical examination are usually nonspecific, and in many patients, sigmoidoscopic examination may be negative because the cecum is the primary site of infection. In some patients, however, shallow ulcers may be seen, with normal mucosa between them. Other patients may have diffuse ulceration similar to that seen in ulcerative colitis or bacillary dysentery. Microscopic examination of fresh stool specimens by an experienced parasitologist is the primary diagnostic test. Examination of at least three specimens usually is necessary to exclude the diagnosis of amebiasis. Examination of a wet saline stool preparation or of a scraping from the base of a rectal ulcer is most likely to show typical trophozoites with ingested red blood cells. Recently, serologic tests for amebiasis have proved helpful, especially in patients with coincident hepatic disease. A plain x-ray film of the abdomen should be obtained in seriously ill patients to exclude the possibility of toxic megacolon or intestinal perforation. Once the diagnosis of amebic disease is established, the patient should be treated with metronidazole (Flagyl), 250 mg three times a day for 10 days. Alternative therapy is diiodohydroxyquin (Diodoquin), 650 mg three times a day for 21 days, tetracycline, 250 mg every 6 hours for 10 days, and chloroquine, 500 mg twice a day for 2 days followed by 250 mg twice a day for 19 days. Severe intestinal infection may be treated with dehydroemetine, 1.0–1.5 mg/kg to a total of 1 gm, tetracycline, 1 gm/day in four divided doses, and diiodohydroxyquin, 650 mg four times a day for 21 days, followed by chloroquine, 500 mg twice a day for 2 days and then 250 mg twice a day for 19 days.

Giardiasis

Giardia lamblia is a frequent cause of acute or chronic diarrhea in the United States. A history of travel in areas with uncertain water supplies or in endemic areas should alert the physician to the possibility of giardiasis. Giardiasis is often asymptomatic, and diarrhea may be intermittent. Stools are loose, greasy, or watery. Mucus often is present, but blood is rare. Mild steatorrhea and malabsorption occasionally may develop. Although some stool specimens contain cysts or trophozoites, diagnosis often depends on microscopic examination of biopsy specimens from the small intestine or duodenal aspirates. Metronidazole, 250 mg three times a day for 7 days, or quinacrine hydrochloride (Atabrine), 100 mg three times a day for 7 days, is effective therapy.

Cryptosporidiosis

Cryptosporidiosis is now recognized as a common diarrheal illness especially in children and homosexual males. It is manifested by frequent watery, nonbloody stools which usually resolve spontaneously in several days to a few weeks. The diagnosis is confirmed by an acid-fast stain of a stool smear. Currently there is no effective treatment.

Drug-associated Diarrhea

Because drugs are frequently associated with acute diarrhea (Table 12.4), a careful medication history should be obtained by the emergency physician. Ingestion of large amounts of caffeinated beverages or alcohol may cause diarrhea. Patients frequently experience diarrhea in the course of taking medications such as magnesium-containing antacids or quinidine. Some patients who take laxatives are seen with diarrhea because of misunderstanding or the psychological need to be ill and to receive attention.

Antibiotics are an important cause of acute diarrhea. Almost all antibiotics have been associated with diarrhea, but most cases are associated with clindamycin or ampicillin. The diarrhea may vary from a mild disease with a few soft stools to a toxic reaction and acute pseudomembranous colitis. In most cases, examination of the stool specimen reveals a cytotoxin produced by *Clostridium difficile*. The diagnosis is based on clinical findings, the presence of pseudomembranes on sigmoidoscopic examination, and *C. difficile* cytotoxin in the stool specimen. Withdrawal of the antibiotic is the mainstay of therapy, but vancomycin, 125–500 mg orally every 6 hours, bacitracin, 200,000 units four times daily, or metronidazole, 250 mg four times daily, are quite valuable for most patients.

Cholestyramine (Questran), 2–4 gm orally every 6 hours, is often helpful in milder cases.

Inflammatory Bowel Disease

Diarrhea is a cardinal symptom in several chronic inflammatory diseases of the intestine including ulcerative colitis or Crohn's disease.

Table 12.4.
Drugs Associated with Acute Diarrhea

Magnesium-containing antacids
Caffeine
Antibiotics, especially clindamycin and ampicillin
Quinidine
Alcohol
Colchicine
Guanethidine
Laxatives

Ulcerative Colitis and Toxic Megacolon

Patients with ulcerative colitis have mild to severe bloody diarrhea, crampy abdominal pain, and tenesmus. A history of diarrhea, rectal bleeding, or pain for months or years is often present. Symptoms persisting more than 2 weeks help exclude bacterial or viral causes of diarrhea. Extracolonic manifestations may include fever, uveitis, dermatitis, and arthritis. Sigmoidoscopic examination is important because the rectum is inflamed in virtually all patients with ulcerative colitis. A fiery red, friable mucosa that bleeds easily with the touch of a cotton swab or has frank ulceration is characteristic of ulcerative colitis. Methylene blue stain of the mucosal exudate demonstrates polymorphonuclear leukocytes, and culture of the stool specimen or exudate is negative for enteropathogenic bacteria. Stool specimens should be examined to exclude amebiasis. Leukocytosis and anemia are present in more severe cases. Serum electrolyte levels should be measured and corrected if needed. In patients with clinical toxicity, a plain x-ray film of the abdomen should be examined for toxic dilatation of the colon to more than 5.5 cm. Seriously ill patients should be hospitalized for replacement of fluids, electrolytes, and blood if necessary. High doses of corticosteroids (prednisone or prednisolone, 50–60 mg/day) should be administered orally or parenterally. Patients with toxic megacolon are difficult to treat, but available data favor advocating colectomy soon after correction of fluid and electrolyte imbalances. Barium enemas, anticholinergic drugs, and opiates should not be administered to seriously ill patients because of the possibility of precipitating toxic megacolon. Less severely ill patients can be treated with lower doses of corticosteriods or sulfasalazine, depending on their clinical status. Except in severely ill patients, corticosteroid therapy should be withheld until infectious diseases can be excluded and the diagnosis firmly established.

Crohn's Disease

Patients with Crohn's disease often have mild to severe diarrhea with or without blood, and with abdominal pain that may be indistinguishable from ulcerative colitis. Intestinal obstruction and acute ileitis are other common emergency presentations of Crohn's disease. Frequent clinical features include perirectal fistulas and tenderness in the lower right periumbilical area. A mass of thickened, tender small intestine sometimes may be palpated. Sigmoidoscopic examination is helpful if the rectum is involved, but this is much less frequent than in ulcerative colitis. Inflammation secondary to Crohn's disease characteristically shows focal ulcerations and a cobblestone appearance in the mucosa with areas of normal appearing mucosa. A complete blood cell count may show leukocytosis, and the hematocrit may be decreased secondary to blood loss.

Therapy includes parenteral fluid and electrolyte replacement in the acute phase and administration of corticosteroids in doses similar to those given for acute ulcerative colitis. Sulfasalazine is helpful in milder cases with principally colonic inflammation. Patients with intestinal obstruction are treated with nasogastric suction, intravenous fluid and electrolyte replacement, and parenteral administration of prednisone or prednisolone, 40–60 mg/day initially. If these measures fall, surgical resection of the involved area is indicated.

Neoplastic Disease

Patients with colonic carcinoma or adenomatous polyps may seek treatment in the emergency department for diarrhea due to partial obstruction of the intestinal lumen. These patients often have a history of rectal bleeding, anorexia, weight loss, constipation, or pain. Physical examination may reveal an abdominal mass or tenderness with an enlarged, hard liver and a friction rub. On rectal examination, the physician palpates the tumor or a rectal shelf. A fecal occult blood test is usually positive. When cancer or polyps are suspected, sigmoidoscopic examination, followed by a barium enema or colonoscopy, usually demonstrates the lesion.

Malabsorptive Disease

A common reason for diarrhea and intestinal gas in many patients is lactose intolerance. It may be difficult to obtain an exact historical correlation between milk or milk-product ingestion and diarrhea. If the physician suspects this problem, a lactose tolerance test can be performed or the patient can be advised to omit lactose-containing foods.

Patients with steatorrhea usually complain of chronic diarrhea and weight loss. The stools are often large, foul-smelling, pasty, and floating. The patient should be questioned about problems in childhood that may suggest celiac disease. A history of living in the Caribbean or India suggests tropical sprue. A history of alcohol abuse or chronic pancreatitis points toward pancreatic insufficiency. In patients in whom malabsorption is suspected, a thorough physical examination is necessary, as well as complete blood cell counts, serum chemistries, and examination of stool for fat. After fat malabsorption is documented, studies are directed toward distinguishing small bowel disease from pancreatic insufficiency. The usual initial test is the D-xylose test, which is abnormal in small bowel disease. Direct measurements of pancreatic function are difficult, but an indirect measure of protease secretion (Chymex Test) may be helpful. A therapeutic trial of pancreatic enzymes usually is sufficient. Small bowel biopsy and radiographs are indicated when results of the D-xylose test are abnormal. Pancreatic calcifications on a plain x-ray film suggest chronic pancreatitis, but more extensive study with ultrasonography and pancreatography may be needed to exclude pancreatic cancer.

Celiac disease is treated with gluten restriction, and tropical sprue responds to administration of vitamin B_{12}, folic acid, and broad-spectrum antibiotics. Treatment of pancreatic insufficiency includes a low-fat, high-caloric diet and pancreatic enzyme replacement.

Functional Bowel Disease

Fecal impaction should be suspected when diarrhea occurs in a patient who is chronically constipated. In such a case, diarrhea is resolved soon after disimpaction. A high-fiber diet or bulk laxative help prevent recurrence.

Many patients have crampy abdominal pain with a history of alternating diarrhea and constipation, and no change in weight or bleeding; this is characteristic of the irritable bowel syndrome. After appropriate clinical, laboratory, and x-ray examinations, these patients should be treated with reassurance and a high-fiber diet. They should take bran or a bulk laxative such as psyllium hydrophilic mucilloid (Metamucil), the dosage of which must be adjusted relative to bowel movements. Anticholinergic medications alone or in combination with sedatives may help patients with cramps.

Certain patients who have chronic diarrhea and irritable bowel syndrome may have decreased absorption of bile salts in the ileum, and this may cause a detergent effect in the colon, resulting in diarrhea. This most often occurs after cholecystectomy. Cholestyramine, 4–16 gm/day, is helpful.

Diarrhea may be the presenting complaint of an underlying psychiatric condition. Medical history, mental status, and physical examination may suggest a need for referral to a psychiatrist as well as to an internist or gastroenterologist.

GASTROINTESTINAL HEMORRHAGE

Upper Gastrointestinal Hemorrhage

Patients with upper gastrointestinal hemorrhage usually present with hematemesis, melena, hematochezia, or shock. Prompt evaluation of blood loss is the key to initial management of acute hemorrhage. Emergency management begins with placement of large intravenous catheters, rapid infusion of fluids, cross-matching of blood, and monitoring of vital signs. Every patient with gastrointestinal bleeding should be treated for impending hypovolemic shock. Once sufficient data have accumulated to justify a less urgent approach, emergency measures can be modified.

History

After volume resuscitation is initiated, the specific source of the bleeding may be evaluated. A history of dyspepsia or previous peptic ulcer disease often is obtained in patients bleeding from ulcers. Patients with hematemesis usually have lesions above the ligament of Treitz. Recent violent vomiting followed by hematemesis suggests a gastroesophageal mucosal tear (Mallory-Weiss phenomenon). A history of alcohol abuse predisposes the patient to esophageal varices, gastritis, or gastroduodenal ulceration. Therapy with aspirin, nonsteroidal anti-inflammatory agents, or high-dose corticosteroids may cause erosions or ulcerations of the stomach or duodenum. Previous gastric surgery raises the possibility of an anastomotic ulceration or recurrent carcinoma.

Examination

Physical examination may reveal orthostatic hypotension, a decrease in systolic blood pressure more than 10 mm Hg, and a pulse rate increase more than 20 beats/min, indicating significant blood volume loss. The presence of jaundice, hepatosplenomegaly, ascites, or spider angiomas indicates chronic hepatic disease and suggests the possibility of variceal bleeding. Enlarged lymph nodes, liver, or spleen may suggest a malignant disease. Black tarry stool in the rectum is characteristic, but a normal stool, negative for occult blood, may be found early in acute upper hemorrhage. Hematochezia is seen in rapid upper gastrointestinal bleeding and in many episodes of lower intestinal bleeding, especially from the right colon. If there is no history of hematemesis, a nasogastric tube must be passed to determine whether the blood is coming from the upper gastrointestinal tract and to ascertain whether bleeding is active. A nasogastric aspirate is considered negative when nonbloody bilious material is obtained or if only nonbloody fluid is found after 2 hours of gastric suction.

Laboratory

A complete blood cell count, platelet count, prothrombin time, and partial thromboplastin time should be obtained, as well as cross-matching for as many as 8 units of blood.

Endoscopy

When a specific diagnosis is needed to guide surgical or medical management, esophagogastroduodenoscopy should be performed. This is best done after fluid resuscitation and the patient is hemodynamically stable. Although routine endoscopic examination has not been shown to prolong short-term survival, gastrointestinal hemorrhage is a sign of a serious pathologic process, and a specific diagnosis allows more intelligent management. This is especially true in the patient with hepatic disease. If endoscopy fails to provide a diagnosis, angiographic examination may be helpful. Bleeding usually must be greater than 0.5 ml/min to be localized angiographically. Barium contrast studies are not helpful in the emergent situation because, although they may demonstrate a lesion, they provide no evidence that the lesion is the bleeding source.

Major Causes

Mallory-Weiss Tear. Although initial therapy for all patients with upper gastrointestinal bleeding is fluid replacement and supportive care, subsequent therapy is aimed at the cause of the bleeding. Gastroesophageal mucosal bleeding secondary to a Mallory-Weiss tear is treated conservatively with adequate fluid and blood replacement, because 80% of these patients stop bleeding spontaneously.

Peptic Ulcer. The most common cause of copious upper gastrointestinal bleeding is peptic ulcer disease. An ulcer may erode into a large artery, causing massive blood loss. Many patients with bleeding from a peptic ulcer have no previous history of ulcers. If there is a large amount of bleeding into the proximal portion of the duodenum, blood usually refluxes into the stomach and is vomited or recovered on aspiration of gastric contents. Occasionally, however, the blood passes distally and is manifested by melena with black or maroon stools. Signs of hypovolemia provide the best evidence of continuing blood loss. Lavage of the stomach is useful in clearing blood clots and in judging the rate of blood loss, but recovery of only small amounts of blood from the stomach does not exclude extensive ongoing loss into the distal portion of the gastrointestinal tract. If bleeding is ongoing, endoscopic or angiographic examination will either establish the diagnosis or provide sufficient information for the physician to infer the presence of a bleeding ulcer.

Endoscopic thermal coagulation of bleeding peptic ulcers and gastroesophageal mucosal tears using the Nd:YAG laser, Keater probe, or electrocoagulator can stop bleeding and decrease the need for subsequent surgery. Patients with active bleeding from visible vessels probably will benefit by coagulation but most good diagnostic endoscopists are still inexperienced with these techniques. Very large and rapidly bleeding arteries are difficult to treat endoscopically and may be best treated surgically.

When bleeding appears to be due to peptic ulcer disease, medical therapy usually is begun, although it probably has little effect on the bleeding itself. Cimetidine, an inhibitor of acid secretion, is given, 300 mg orally or intravenously every 6 hr. Alternatively, antacid can be given hourly by nasogastric tube, the amount depending on the pH of the gastric fluid. The gastric contents are aspirated before every hourly instillation and the pH is checked and sufficient antacid is instilled to keep the pH above 4.

Varices. Hemorrhage from esophageal varices often is severe and requires prompt and effective therapy. Many patients have a history of previous upper gastrointestinal bleeding, chronic liver disease, alcohol abuse, hepatitis, or jaundice. Esophageal varices should be suspected in all patients with portal hypertension and bleeding. All patients with hepatic disease and hemorrhage should have special attention directed to the blood clotting function and correction with vitamin K, fresh frozen plasma, and platelets as necessary. If hemorrhage is substantial or continuing, early endoscopic examination usually is wise in order to document the presence of varices and to exclude a bleeding coexistent peptic ulcer or gastritis.

Endoscopic injection sclerosis of varices has emerged as the primary treatment of bleeding esophageal varices. Optimally, the patient is examined and treated as soon as she or he is stable. If there is rapid bleeding, circulatory compromise, or altered mental status, an endotracheal tube is usually needed to protect the airway from aspiration.

If an endoscopist skilled with injection sclerosis of varices is not readily available or if sclerosis fails to control the bleeding, vasopressin is then infused intravenously through a peripheral line at the rate of 0.1–0.4 unit/min. If this does not control the bleeding quickly, a Sengstaken-Blakemore tube (with Boyce modification of the esophageal component) should be passed for tamponade of the bleeding varices. The tubing should be well-lubricated and passed via the nose into the stomach. The gastric balloon is inflated with 200–300 ml of air and pulled back into the gastroesophageal junction under 1–2 lb of traction. After the position of the tube is checked by x-ray study, the esophageal balloon is inflated to 40 mm Hg. When bleeding stops, the balloon is deflated to the minimum pressure necessary for control of any further bleeding. The use of intermittent suction helps monitor the rate of bleeding. If bleeding is controlled for 24 hours, the esophageal balloon is decompressed, but suction is maintained. If no bleeding occurs for 24 additional hours, the gastric balloon is decompressed. An alternative method of balloon tamponade is use of the Linton balloon tube. This is a single gastric balloon tube, the effectiveness of which is based on compression of the collateral veins supplying the esophageal varices by distention of the balloon in the gastric fundus coupled with traction on the tube; 200–300 ml of air is placed in the balloon and 1–2 lb of traction are applied to the tube. Variceal hemorrhage and the use of balloon tubes pose a substantial threat of aspiration. Most patients require endotracheal intubation to protect the airway. Caution must be exercised in the use of any tube that involves balloon distention of the lower part of the esophagus. A balloon that is overdistended in the distal esophagus or a gastric balloon that is drawn back into the esophagus may result in esophageal necrosis or rupture. When medical therapy does not stop the bleeding, either the portal circulation should be decompressed via a surgical portosystemic shunt or varices should be obliterated by endoscopic sclerosis or operative ligation depending on the status of the patient and the experience of the attending personnel.

Aortic Fistula. Aortoenteric fistulas are almost always a complication of an implanted graft after aortic resection. The diagnosis should be considered in any patient with gastrointestinal bleeding and previous operation on the aorta or iliac artery. Initially, bleeding from such fistulas is not always profuse. Surgical repair of the fistula is the only treatment.

Lower Gastrointestinal Hemorrhage

History

Intestinal bleeding below the ligament of Treitz usually presents by the passage of bright red blood or maroon stools. Similar to acute upper gastrointestinal hemorrhage, the initial assessment must quickly focus on the hemodynamic status of the patient and the rate of the bleeding. Initial therapy and further evaluation then may proceed simultaneously. An accurate history is important to determine the onset, duration, and character of the bleeding, as well as associated symptoms, such as abdominal pain or diarrhea.

Examination

Physician examination may reveal telangiectasias (hereditary hemorrhagic telangiectasia), osteomas or lipomas (Gardner's syndrome), rectal polyps, or carcinoma. Laboratory tests include a complete blood cell count, prothrombin time, partial thromboplastin time, platelet count, and blood typing and cross-matching. A nasogastric tube should be passed and gastric contents aspirated for an hour or until blood or bile is recovered in order to rule in or out hemorrhage from the upper gastrointestinal tract. Sigmoidoscopic examination then should be performed to ascertain the presence of carcinoma, polyps, inflammatory disease, or hemorrhoids in the rectum and sigmoid colon. In patients with bloody diarrhea, infectious causes should be investigated. If the bleeding site is not determined by sigmoidoscopy, further evaluation is indicated. Most patients can have their colons prepared and examined by colonoscopy semiemergently. Patients who are bleeding more rapidly or who are hemodynamically unstable should have angiography to look for a bleeding site.

Colonoscopy

Colonoscopy is being used increasingly in patients with lower gastrointestinal bleeding in whom the rate of bleeding is not fast enough for it to be seen during angiography. This technique also has been helpful in patients who bleed from inflammatory bowel disease, because the site can be observed and a biopsy specimen taken. In patients with angiodysplasia, the physician may be able to cauterize the bleeding point in the arteriovenous malformation at colonoscopic examination.

Angiography

If the site of intestinal bleeding is found by angiography, vasopressin can be infused to attempt control of blood loss. If these measures do not stop the bleeding, the involved area should be surgically excised. The barium enema in patients with lower gastrointestinal bleeding is the least effective method of determining the cause or site of hemorrhage, and if it is used initially, it can preclude angiography or colonoscopy for an extended period while the patient has cleansing enemas.

Major Causes

Meckel's Diverticulum. The small intestine may be the source of massive bleeding from an ulcerated Meckel's diverticulum, or from Crohn's disease, benign or malignant tumors, and diverticula. Angiographic examination is the most accurate method and is often the only means other than laparotomy by which the site of small intestinal bleeding can be established. In young patients the possiblity of Meckel's diverticulum should be a major consideration. This lesion should be demonstrated by angiographic examination in the actively bleeding phase. At other times, it may be detected by technetium scanning.

Colonic Diverticula. Massive colonic bleeding may originate from diverticula. Many diverticula arise at sites where major blood vessels penetrate the muscle wall, and bleeding is usually the result of erosion into one of these vessels. The typical history of bleeding diverticula is the passage of huge, bloody stools without preceding symptoms, followed by faintness.

Angiodysplasia. Angiodysplasia of the colon is an important cause of bleeding. Patients are typically elderly and may have valvular heart disease. There is often a history of previous bleeding with an inconclusive evaluation. Presently, the diagnosis depends on angiography or colonoscopy that demonstrate the arteriovenous malformations even in the absence of active bleeding. Lesions are usually present in the right colon, but may be found in the remainder of the colon or small intestine. Multiple lesions are often found. Treatment is endoscopic thermal coagulation, if reachable by colonoscopy, or by surgical resection of the involved bowel.

Inflammatory Disease. Inflammatory bowel disease may present as acute lower gastrointestinal bleeding. The patient has a history of diarrhea, abdominal pain, or previous colitis. Diagnosis usually is established by sigmoidoscopy.

Hemorrhoids. Hemorrhoidal bleeding occasionally may be profuse enough to be frightening. In this instance, sigmoidoscopic examination is of primary importance. Portal hypertension or some form of bleeding disorder should be suspected in the patient whose bleeding is voluminous enough to constitute an acute, serious hemorrhage.

Tumors of the colon, including polyps, may bleed, but seldom enough to produce hypovolemia.

VOMITING

Vomiting is a common complaint in the emergency department. It usually accompanies other symptoms which are more discriminating and point to an underlying cause. Thus, fever and diarrhea point to gastroenteritis; dyspepsia suggests gastric outlet obstruction; and pain and jaundice suggest pancreatic or biliary tract disease. Infectious and alcoholic gastroenteritis are by far the most common causes of vomiting. The initial goal in assessing these patients is to determine the state of hydration. If their intravascular volume is seriously compromised, they should be admitted for intravenous rehydration. Most patients, however, enter prior to serious dehydration and can be managed with oral rehydration. Cola beverages at room temperature with a minimum of effervescence are best tolerated. Clear fruit juices and water may also be taken. Patients should be instructed not to take solid food until their nausea and vomiting is clearly improved. Compazine or Tigan suppositories are useful in the early stages when it is uncertain whether the patient will be able to take any medication by mouth. Later, Compazine, Tigan, or metoclopramide may be taken by mouth to decrease the nausea and associated vomiting. Vomiting from an infectious gastroenteritis rarely lasts longer than 2–3 days. If it persists, it bears more extensive evaluation for other coincident or complicating conditions.

Patients with unremitting vomiting, particularly in whom an underlying process such as cholecystitis, pancreatitis, or a gastric or intestinal obstruction exists, should have a nasogastric tube placed for continuous suction. Further therapy is discussed elsewhere in this chapter and in Chapter 33 under the specific disease process causing the vomiting.

ACID PEPTIC DISEASE

Patients with acid peptic disease often present to the emergency department complaining of dyspepsia. This is a burning, nauseous, epigastric distress which is either improved or exacerbated by eating. Acid peptic disease may also present as abdominal pain, vomiting, and hemorrhage. The most common causes of acid peptic disease and symptoms are duodenal and gastric ulcer, gastritis, and gastroesophageal reflux with esophagitis. These conditions have multiple contributing causes but the principal insult is the action of acid on an insufficiently protected mucosal surface. Mild and moderately severe disease is common and can be treated medically on an ambulatory basis. Most patients who do not have vomiting, dehydration, bleeding, or weight loss can be treated empirically with abstinence from alcohol, tobacco, coffee, and nonsteroidal anti-inflammatory drugs. They are treated with acid neutralization using a potent antacid 1 and 3 hours after meals and at bedtime, or with an H_2 blocker such as cimetidine or ranitidine.

Patients greater that 65 years of age or those with early satiety, weight loss, vomiting, or bleeding are at particular risk for complications of acid peptic disease or from gastric carcinoma. These patients require a more extensive evaluation of the anatomy of their upper digestive tract using both upper gastrointestinal radiography and endoscopy.

Patients who have symptoms of gastroesophageal reflux with discomfort located in the lower chest should be treated with antireflux postural measures. These include eating small frequent meals sitting upright or maintaining an upright position for 2 hours after each meal. They also include abstinence from bedtime snacks and raising the shoulders with pillows or the head of the bed with 6-inch blocks.

Because all acid peptic conditions tend to be chronic or recurrent and because the manifestations of the disease may not be apparent at first, adequate medical follow-up must be arranged. For the emergency physician, this means consultation with an internist.

SWALLOWED FOREIGN BODIES

In adults the history of foreign body ingestion or impaction of food in the esophagus is not difficult.

Foreign matter lodged in the esophagus produces a sense of fullness and anxiety. Most patients attempt to wash the object down by drinking liquids. If the obstruction is complete or near-complete the patient may then choke, cough, or aspirate.

The detection of foreign body ingestion by a child is more difficult because it occurs most commonly between the ages of 6 months and 3 years, when the children are largely unable to give a description of their difficulty. The most common symptoms are gagging, choking, the inability to swallow, or distress in the neck or chest. Sometimes the child may simply refuse to eat or even swallow.

Physical examination should focus on examination of the hypopharynx and larynx with direct laryngoscopy. The neck is evaluated for subcutaneous air which suggests perforation. Radiographs of the neck and chest may demonstrate radiopaque foreign bodies or air outside the esophagus, suggesting a perforation even more strongly. If the diagnosis remains uncertain, an esophagogram should be performed with gastrografin.

A vast majority of ingested foreign bodies will traverse the entire digestive tract without difficulty. Once the foreign body has passed the pylorus, treatment can be expectant. Any foreign body that becomes lodged in the esophagus or does not pass the pylorus should be removed by esophagogastroscopy, or by surgery if necessary.

In individuals with narrowings of the esophagus, such as stricture, web, ring, or tumors, food, particularly bread and meat, may lodge. Food that is lodged in the esophagus that does not pass spontaneously in 4 to 6 hours should be removed by fiberoptic esophagoscopy, where available. The enzyme papain in 2½% solution has been used to digest protein food. A reported 3% incidence of perforation using proteolytic enzymes is substantially higher than the morbidity of endoscopic retrieval. The coincident esophageal disease requires further evaluation.

HEPATIC DISEASE

Patients with hepatic disease are seen in the emergency department with jaundice, upper abdominal pain, abdominal swelling, encephalopathy, or malaise. The first two symptoms also may be due to primary obstructive biliary disease, which is discussed in more detail in Chapter 33.

History

The nature of the course of the illness should be determined. The onset of fever, anorexia, malaise, dark urine, abdominal discomfort, and perhaps jaundice over a few days is characteristic of viral hepatitis. A long history of intermittent abdominal pain or indigestion can suggest cholelithiasis, which coupled with jaundice points to choledocholithiasis. Sudden onset of high fever, jaundice, and clinical toxicity, especially with the history of gallstones, is characteristic of cholangitis. Previous hepatobiliary disease may suggest a recurrence or exacerbation of a more chronic disease.

Careful questioning regarding alcohol consumption is always important. Drug use, especially of antituberculous chemotherapeutic agents, methyldopa, phenothiazines, and estrogens (including oral contraceptives) may provide important insights (Table 12.5). An occupational history should be taken, particularly regarding work in institutions where hepatitis is endemic or where potential hepatotoxins, such as carbon tetrachloride or vinyl chloride, are used. Needle exposure to drugs, receipt of blood products, or persons with known hepatitis can point to viral hepatitis. A recent operation on the biliary tract can suggest a surgical complication. A history of a malignancy suggest metastatic disease.

Examination

Physical examination is important to assess the patient's general health and to determine the presence of fever and manifestations of chronic hepatic disease, such as spider angiomas. For jaundice to be clinically apparent, the serum bilirubin level must be more than 2.0–2.5 mg/100 m. An offensive, sweet smell of the breath (fetor hepaticus) also may indicate chronic hepatic disease. Lymphadenopathy suggests mononucleosis, viral hepatitis, or malignant disease. Arthritis and dermatitis may indicate acute or chronic viral hepatitis. The abdomen should be examined for signs of ascites, such as distention, fluid wave, or shifting dullness. Shifting dullness can be determined by percussing the abdomen with the patient supine and then with the patient on his or her side. Next, the breadth of the liver should be measured by percussing it over the right side of the chest onto the right side of the abdomen; normal breadth is 8–10 cm. The liver should be palpated to determine whether it is tender, and the firmness, smoothness, or nodularity of its edge should be noted. The presence of a palpable gallbladder and splenomegaly should be determined. A positive fecal occult blood test can indicate a gastrointestinal tumor metastatic to the liver or obstructing the bile ducts. Neurologic examination always should be performed to determine neuropathy, ophthalmoplegia, the level of consciousness, and the presence of asterixis.

Laboratory

Patients with jaundice should have a complete blood cell count, including reticulocytes. Blood urea nitrogen and serum electrolyte levels are helpful in determining the severity of hepatic dysfunction and

Table 12.5.
Drugs Reported to Cause Hepatic Injury[a]

Drug	Incidence	Mechanism	Pattern of Injury	Comment
Anesthetic agents				
Choloroform	High, dose-related	Direct toxicity	Hepatocellular	
Halothane	Low	Hypersensitivity	Hepatocellular	May cause massive hepatic necrosis
Antibiotics				
Erythromycin estolate	Low	Hypersensitivity	Cholestatic	
Tetracycline, oral	Low	Indirect toxicity	Hepatocellular	
Tetracycline, intravenous	High, dose-related (>2 gm/24hr)	Indirect toxicity	Hepatocellular	Particularly in pregnancy, characterized by small fat droplets in hepatocytes
Sulfonamides	Low	Hypersensitivity	Mixed	
Penicillin	Very low	Hypersensitivity	Hepatocellular	
Anti-inflamatory agents				
Acetaminophen	High, dose-related	Direct toxicity	Hepatocellular	Only seen with overdose, when fulminant hepatic failure may occur
Salicylates	High	Direct toxicity (?)	Mixed	Clinical disease rare, transaminase elevations with levels >25 mg/100ml
Antimetabolites and immunosuppressive agents				
Azathioprine	Low	Indirect toxicity	Mixed	Irreversible hepatic failure reported
Chlorambucil	Low	Indirect toxicity	Cholestatic	
6-Mercaptopurine	10–35%	Indirect toxicity	Mixed	
Methotrexate	High, dose-related	Indirect toxicity	Mixed	Progression to cirrhosis suggested but not proved
Antituberculous agents				
Isoniazid	Low	Metabolic idiosyncrasy (related to acetylation rate)	Hepatocellular or mixed	
Rifampin	Low		Hepatocellular	
Paraaminosalicylic acid	1%	Hypersensitivity	Mixed	
Ethionamide	3–5%	Metabolic idiosyncrasy	Hepatocellular	
Hormones				
Methyltestosterone	Jaundice: low	Metabolic idiosyncrasy	Bland cholestasis	No evidence for hepatic inflammation, but jaundice may be severe

	High, dose-related interference with hepatic excretory function	Indirect toxicity	Peliosis	
Synthetic estrogens (e.g., mestranol)	Jaundice: very low	Metabolic idiosyncrasy	Bland cholestasis	
	High, dose-related interference with hepatic excretory function	Indirect toxicity		
Synthetic progestational agents ("19-Nor" compounds)	Jaundice: low	Metabolic idiosyncrasy	Cholestatic	May be potentiated by estrogens
	High, dose-related interference with hepatic excretory function	Indirect toxicity		
Psychotropic drugs				
Phenothiazines	Low (exception: 1–3% with chlorpromazine)	Hypersensitivity	Cholestatic	
Miscellaneous				
α-Methyldopa	Low	Hypersensitivity	Mixed	
Phenytoin	Low	Hypersensitivity	Mixed	
Oxyphenisatin	Low	Metabolic idiosyncrasy	Mixed	Reversible chronic active hepatitis reported
Propylthiouracil	Low	Hypersensitivity	Hepatocellular	
Methimazole	Low	Hypersensitivity	Cholestatic	
Thiazide diuretics	Very low	Hypersensitivity	Cholestatic	

[a] Modified by permission from Zimmerman HJ. Drug-induced hepatic injury. In Samler M, Parker C, eds. Hypersensitivity to Drugs. Vol. 1. Elmsford, NY. Pergamon Press, 1974.

of fluid and electrolyte disturbances that often occur. The prothrombin time and platelet count are frequently abnormal and reflect the severity of hepatic injury and the bleeding potential. Liver function tests should be performed, depending on the historical and physical findings and the questions that the clinician needs answered. The adolescent with a few days of malaise and dark urine may require only a serum glutamic oxaloacetic transaminase (SGOT) determination to confirm the diagnosis of acute hepatitis and a prothrombin time to assess the severity of the hepatic damage. The older adult with abdominal pain and jaundice needs fractionated bilirubin and alkaline phosphatase determinations, as well as an SGOT measurement. If the alkaline phosphatase and direct bilirubin levels are elevated, suggesting biliary tract disease, an ultrasound study may be indicated as well. Patients with chronic hepatic disease require assessment of hepatic synthetic function such as albumin and prothrombin time.

Hepatitis

Viral Hepatitis

Several viruses may produce acute hepatitis. Hepatitis virus A is a frequent cause of acute hepatitis, especially in children and young adults. Formerly known as infectious hepatitis or short incubation hepatitis, viral hepatitis type A is passed by fecal-oral transmission. The illness is usually not severe and has an excellent prognosis. There is no known carrier state, and illness never progresses to chronic hepatitis. Hepatitis virus B causes serum hepatitis or long incubation hepatitis in persons of all ages. The virus often is passed by parenteral contact with blood products, but nonparenteral transmission has frequently been reported, particularly between sexual contacts. Hepatitis B surface antigen is often detectable early in the disease, and usually disappears as hepatitis B surface antibody is produced. In about 5% of patients, the antigen persists. Hepatitis B surface antibody provides immunity to subsequent infection. Usually the precise virologic diagnosis is not needed initially, except for prognosis and prophylactic treatment of contacts.

Patients who chronically carry hepatitis B virus may also contract ∂-hepatitis virus. This is a defective virus which requires hepatitis B virus to replicate. It is transmitted primarily by contaminated needles among intravenous drug abusers. It is often a very severe form of hepatitis.

As serologic techniques for identifying cases of hepatitis due to virus A and virus B have improved, it is now clear that there is a third principal hepatitis virus. Sufficient studies have been performed to demonstrate that it is not another widely recognized virus. Therefore, until it is identified and characterized, it has been designated "non-A, non-B." This agent (or these agents) is responsible for 90% of viral hepatitis occurring after blood transfusion and probably 20% of sporadic hepatitis in the community. The disease tends to be indolent, with a significant number of anicteric cases and a substantial frequency of subsequent chronic hepatitis, especially in posttransfusion cases. Infectious mononucleosis (Epstein-Barr virus) can also produce hepatitis. In this type of infection, pharyngitis and adenopathy are evident.

The diagnosis of acute viral hepatitis is based on the clinical features and a serum SGOT level that is characteristically very high. The alkaline phosphatase level usually is elevated moderately, but is less strikingly abnormal than the SGOT level. The bilirubin level is often high and is composed of both direct and indirect reacting fractions.

Most patients with viral hepatitis can be cared for at home. Pregnant or elderly patients may do better in the hospital with bed rest. Patients with abnormal clotting ability or encephalopathy should be admitted for observation and treatment for possible complications. Patients who cannot maintain hydration by themselves also should be hospitalized for parenteral fluid administration. The principal therapy for all patients is supportive and includes rest, fluids, good nutrition, and abstinence from alcohol.

The complications of acute viral hepatitis usually arise from infection with hepatitis virus B. A prothrombin time greater than 2 seconds more than control and a bilirubin level greater than 20 mg/dl are the most reliable predictors of poor prognosis. In the early period, acute or subacute hepatic necrosis can develop, which is indicated by symptomatically severe hepatitis complicated by signs of hepatic failure such as ascites, encephalopathy, or coagulopathy. Recent data suggest that corticosteroids are not beneficial and that they actually may be detrimental. Supportive care is probably the only treatment available.

Patients with viral hepatitis should maintain good personal hygiene to limit transmission of the virus. When blood is drawn from patients with viral hepatitis type B, needles and syringes should be disposed of carefully and the tubes of blood should be labeled as potentially infectious. Household contacts of patients with viral hepatitis type A should be treated with immune serum globulin, which is approximately 90% effective in inhibiting the clinical manifestations of acute hepatitis (Table 12.6). The recommended dose is 0.5 ml for patients weighing less than 50 lb, 1 ml for patients weighing from 50 to 100 lb, and 2 ml for patients weighing more than 100 lb; this will protect contacts for 4–8 weeks. Larger doses protect longer and are appro-

Table 12.6.
Recommendations for Acute Viral Hepatitis Immunoprophylaxis

Exposure	Type	Immune Serum Globulin, Dosage
Household or intimate contacts	Hepatitis A	0.02 ml/kg intramuscularly up to 2 ml
	Hepatitis B	0.07 ml/kg intramuscularly up to 5 ml; repeat in 1 month for sexual contacts
	Unknown or non-A, non-B	0.07 ml/kg intramuscularly up to 5 ml
Percutaneous (needle-stick)	Hepatitis B (exposed person, hepatitis B surface antigen and antibody negative)	Hyperimmune globulin 5 ml intramuscularly; repeat in 1 month
	Unknown or non-A, non-B	0.07 ml/kg intramuscularly up to 5 ml
	No evidence of hepatitis B or clinical hepatitis	No prophylaxis

priate for persons traveling to or residing in endemic areas. Close contacts, especially sexual partners of patients with viral hepatitis type B, should receive immune serum globulin, 0.07 ml/kg, if their test results are negative for hepatitis B surface antigen and antibody. Persons exposed to viral hepatitis B via needle should be given hyperimmune serum globulin when available. A hepatitis B vaccine is now available for preexposure prophylaxis and is probably also helpful for postexposure prophylaxis.

Alcoholic Hepatitis

Some persons who drink substantial quantities of alcohol over prolonged periods develop liver disease. The liver may acquire fatty change, hepatitis cirrhosis, or frequently, combinations of these. In the emergency department, alcoholic hepatitis or complications of cirrhosis are frequently encountered problems. Patients with alcoholic hepatitis are seen with jaundice, dull pain in the right upper abdominal quadrant, vomiting, and fever. The SGOT level invariably is elevated, but is not as high as often is observed in viral hepatitis. In addition, the alkaline phosphatase level is significantly elevated and is often three to five times the upper limit of the normal range. Because of the coincidence of chronic liver disease, evidence of hepatic insufficiency, such as a prolonged prothrombin time and hypoalbuminemia, frequently is present. Therapy includes abstinence from alcohol, supportive care, and specific therapy for complications, such as encephalopathy, bleeding, and ascites. Hospitalization is usually required.

Toxin-induced Hepatitis

Patient may be seen in the emergency department with hepatitis induced by toxins such as acetaminophen or carbon tetrachloride. Many drugs also cause hepatitis either because of hypersensitivity or because of toxic metabolism of the drug. Table 12.5 lists certain medications and their hepatotoxic effects. The principal treatment is withdrawal of the offending agent and supportive care. Corticosteroids occasionally are given for hypersensitivity reactions, but the efficacy of this therapy is unclear.

Acetaminophen is emerging as an important cause of toxic liver injury, because of its increasing use. It is safe in normal doses, but in massive overdose—more than 25 gm but sometimes as little as 10 gm in adults—serious toxic injury of the liver regularly occurs (Fig 12.1). This can be substantially prevented if treatment with *N*-acetylcysteine is begun in 12 to 24 hours. The presently recommended regimen is 140 mg/kg orally followed by 70 mg/kg every 4 hours for 3 days. Current information is available at the Rocky Mountain Poison Center (1-800-525-6115).

Cirrhosis

In the United States, cirrhosis is caused primarily by alcohol or chronic hepatitis. The major related problems in the emergency department are its associated complications—bleeding, encephalopathy, and ascites. Bleeding already has been discussed; encephalopathy and ascites are considered in the following sections.

Hepatic Encephalopathy

Hepatic encephalopathy is a complex metabolic disturbance in neurologic function characterized by alterations of consciousness, neurologic signs, and asterixis. It occurs in patients with severe acute or chronic hepatocellular disease, often with extensive portosystemic shunts. Disturbances in mentation with forgetfulness and elation are the earliest signs. This state is followed by confusion, drowsiness, and asterixis. The stages of hepatic encephalopathy are listed in Table 12.7. The emergency physician must be careful to exclude other causes of altered consciousness such as meningitis in a febrile patient or

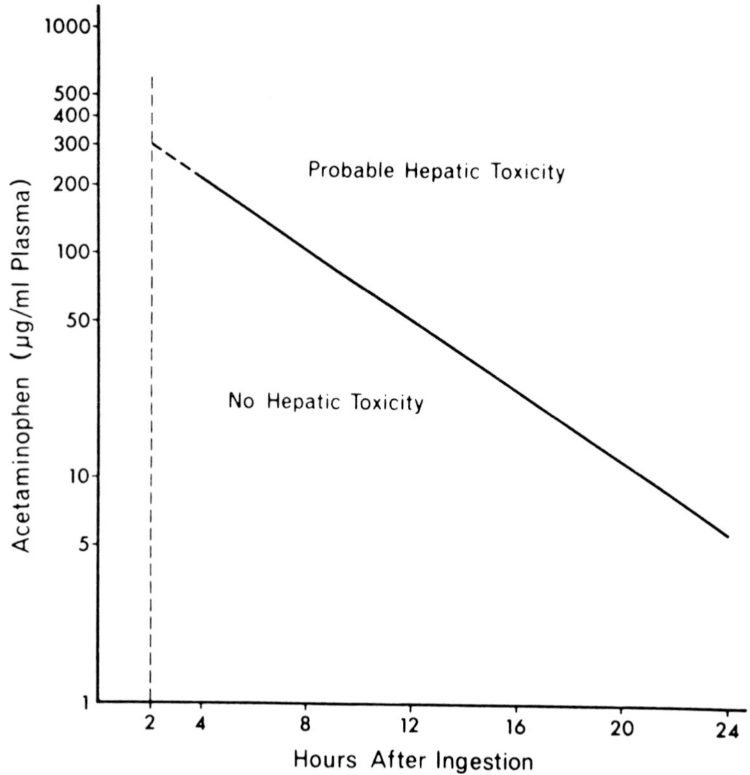

Figure 12.1. Semilogarithmic plot of plasma acetaminophen levels versus time. (Adapted from Rumack OH, Matthew H. Acetaminophen poisoning and toxicity. *Pediatrics,* 1975;55:871–876.)

intracranial hemorrhage in a trauma victim (see also Chapter 16).

After hepatic encephalopathy is recognized, the nature of the underlying hepatic disease and the precipitants of the encephalopathy need to be defined. Hepatic failure may occur acutely in patients with fulminant hepatitis due to viruses or hepatotoxins such as alcohol or acetaminophen. In children, one must consider Reye's syndrome, in which upper respiratory tract illness typically precedes coma and hypoglycemia. In patients with chronic hepatic disease with portosystemic shunting, hepatic coma may develop as a result of intestinal bleeding, increased protein ingestion, hypokalemia secondary to diarrhea or diuretics, hypovolemia, viral or bacterial infection, drug ingestion (for example, narcotics or sedatives), or abdominal disease (for example, acute pancreatitis or a perforated viscus).

Family or friends should be questioned about previous medical history, exposure to toxins, diet, intravenous and other drug usage, exposure to others with hepatitis, and use of alcohol. Physical examination is helpful in determining signs of chronic hepatic disease, such as spider angiomas, jaundice, hepatosplenomegaly, and ascites. Evidence of trauma is critical because of the possibility of intracranial hemorrhage. Fever indicates the possibility of infection, such as peritonitis or pneumonia. The physician should assess the degree of dehydration, including a central venous pressure measurement. A stool specimen should be studied for occult blood, and a nasogastric aspirate obtained to determine the presence of active or previous bleeding (coffee-ground material) or recently ingested drugs.

Patients with encephalopathy may be seen in the emergency department in markedly varying conditions ranging from mild confusion to coma (Table 12.7). In the patient with impending coma, the physician may elicit asterixis, difficult in the stuporous or comatose patient, who cannot maintain a sustained posture. The blood ammonia level frequently is elevated in patients with hepatic encephalopathy and is useful when the cause of the encephalopathy is not clearly hepatic. The electroencephalogram is abnormal in patients with either impending coma, stupor, or actual coma, but this tool is not usually available to the emergency physician.

X-ray films of the chest and abdomen should be taken to exclude the possibility of pneumonia or a perforated viscus. Lumbar puncture should reveal

Table 12.7.
Stages of Hepatic Encephalopathy[a]

Stage	Mental State	Tremor (Asterixis)	Electroencephalogram[b]
Prodrome	Euphoria, mild confusion, slow mentation	Often present, but slight	Changes usually absent
Impending coma	Confusion, drowsiness	Present	Changes usually present
Stupor	Marked confusion; sleepy but arousable	Present if patient can cooperate	Changes almost always present
Coma	Unconsciousness; may respond to pain	Absent (no muscle tone)	Changes often present

[a] Adapted by permission from Schiff L. Diseases of the Liver. ed. 3. Philadelphia: JB Lippincott Co., 1969:378.
[b] The electroencephalogram abnormalities are characterized by paroxysms of bilaterally synchronous high-voltage slow waves in the Δ range (1.5–3/sec), alternating with normal α waves.

normal cerebrospinal fluid in patients with hepatic coma.

All patients with hepatic coma should be admitted to an area of the hospital where they will receive constant attention from nurses and physicians. Therapy consists of withdrawal of the offending drug, reduction of dietary protein, and correction of electrolyte and fluid imbalance. Hypokalemia can require administration of large amounts of potassium chloride, 100–300 mEq orally or intravenously during the first 2–3 days. The patient with hyponatremia, peripheral edema, and ascites may require fluid restriction to less than 1500 ml/day and dietary sodium restriction to less than 500 mEq/day. Bacterial infections should be treated with the appropriate antibiotics. Gastrointestinal bleeding should be managed as discussed previously. In addition, cathartics and enemas should be administered on the first day of hospitalization to decrease the intestinal absorption of nitrogenous substances. Lactulose, 30 ml every 4 hours, is given until diarrhea begins and then is decreased to a dose that produces two soft bowel movements daily. Alternatively, neomycin, 500–1000 mg, with sorbitol may be given every 6 hours.

Ascites

Patients with acute alcoholic hepatitis, fulminant viral hepatitis, or chronic hepatic disease may be seen in the emergency department with ascites or peripheral edema or both. These patients are typically hypoalbuminemic and have an increased portal venous pressure. They behave as if they are dehydrated with an active secondary aldosterone mechanism, resulting in peritoneal and interstitial fluid retention. In addition to a full clinical and serum chemical evaluation, it is important to perform an examination of peritoneal fluid to exclude the diagnosis of bacterial, mycobacterial, or carcinomatous peritonitis.

Ascitic fluid in patients with cirrhosis should have less than 100 polymorphonuclear leukocytes or 300 total white blood cells. The presence of more cells suggests bacterial peritonitis; antibiotics are indicated.

The treatment of ascites secondary to cirrhosis includes restriction of sodium, usually to 500 mg/day, and often restriction of fluid to 1200–1500 ml/day to prevent hyponatremia. Diuretic therapy is begun with spironolactone and is increased until sodium diuresis begins and urinary potassium loss decreases below 20 mEq/liter. Later, thiazides or loop diuretics may be given to raise the urine output to 400 ml daily. Loop diuretics must be used carefully because they can cause hypokalemia and depletion of extracellular fluid with resultant encephalopathy. Therapeutic paracentesis should be reserved for patients with significant respiratory embarrassment due to pressure under the diaphragm. When used, it should be limited to the removal of 1 liter because a rapid shift of fluid from the plasma into the peritoneal cavity can lead to circulatory compromise.

PROCTOLOGIC CONDITIONS

A variety of anorectal problems commonly are seen in the emergency department. A thorough history and an appropriate physical examination are required to determine the nature and cause of symptoms. Inspection of the perianal area and anoproctoscopic examination are necessary diagnostic procedures. Familiarity with these techniques is essential.

Hemorrhoids

Patients with hemorrhoids are seen with bleeding, perianal pain, or pruritus ani. Most pain and bleeding arise when the vascular anal cushions prolapse through the anal canal and are congested by the internal sphincter on forceful defecation. Such prolapsed hemorrhoids should be reduced manually, as promptly as possible. Stool softeners and bulk laxatives are the mainstay of long-term treatment. A painful thrombosed external hemorrhoid can be treated by injecting 1% lidocaine hydrochloride (Xylocaine) with epinephrine into the hemorrhoid and incising it, evacuating the clot, coagulating the bleeding areas, and using Gelfoam or Oxycel to control hemorrhage (see Illustrated Technique 26). Bleeding internal hemorrhoids are treated with stool softeners, bulk laxatives, hot tub baths, lubricants and medicated or hydrocortisone suppositories. The bleeding from hemorrhoids is virtually never hemodynamically compromising except in the presence of portal venous hypertension or vascular coagulopathy. The emergency physician must resist the temptation to attribute all anorectal bleeding to hemorrhoids unless the bleeding from the hemorrhoid can be visualized. Patients with rectal carcinoma or polyps too often are diagnosed initially as having hemorrhoidal bleeding.

Fissure-in-Ano

Patients with acute anal fissures usually are seen in the emergency department because of rectal pain (especially with defecation) or mild bleeding or both. In men, acute fissures tend to occur in the posterior midline; in women, anterior fissures tend to be more common. Fissures secondary to Crohn's disease are typically multiple, and less likely to be acute. Acute fissures are diagnosed visually with the patient in the prone or lithotomy position, the buttocks gently drawn apart. Proctoscopic examination is helpful, but may not be possible because of the pain. Acute fissures are treated with bulk laxatives, stool softeners, topical anesthetics, and sitz baths. Gentle anal dilatation under topical anesthesia is helpful, if tolerated, in relieving the painful spasm.

Chronic fissures extend to the internal sphincter and are associated with an edematous skin tag (''sentinel pile''). This type of fissure may be related to Crohn's disease, and these patients need to be examined thoroughly because of this possibility. Other possibilities include carcinoma and infectious ulcers. Patients with chronic fissures should be referred to the surgeon for further evaluation.

Anorectal Fistula

Anorectal fistulas are inflammatory tracts which originate in an abscess in the longitudinal muscle layer and have an internal opening in the mucosa of the anal canal or rectum and an external opening in the perianal skin. Diagnosis often is made by a history of recurrent rectal discharge and perianal abscesses. The examiner should note the position of the fistulas in relation to the anal opening to determine the expected position of the internal opening. Next, by palpating the skin between the fistula and the anal canal, the physician may feel an indurated area that indicates the direction of the fistula. When digital examination of the anal canal is performed, then the extension of the fistula may be felt. If Crohn's disease is suspected as a result of examination, a thorough evaluation is indicated for this possibility. Definitive therapy is surgical.

Pruritus Ani

Perianal itching has several causes. It is necessary to take a broad history and to examine the patient with particular attention to dermatologic lesions in other parts of the body. Many patients may have pruritus ani because of improper cleansing after defecation, or because of hemorrhoids, fissures, fistulas, or rectal prolapse.

Candidiasis

Candida albicans can cause perianal irritation and pruritus, especially in patients with poorly controlled diabetes mellitus, receiving broad-spectrum antibiotics or corticosteroid therapy. Diagnosis is confirmed by microscopic examination of a scraping of the lesion.

Anogenital Warts

Infectious anogenital warts of viral origin that cause perianal itching are frequent in homosexuals. Patients with this condition should undergo anoscopic examination because the warts can extend upward to the dentate line. Treatment consists of weekly applications of 25% podophyllin in benzoin until the warts have disappeared.

Herpes Simplex

Herpes simplex also occurs in the perianal area and is manifested by erythematous macules and vesicles. This infection can be treated by keeping the lesions clean and dry. The use of acyclovir is discussed in Chapter 11.

Parasites

Pinworms can cause pruritus ani and are diagnosed by placing a piece of transparent tape against the anus in the early morning for several hours and then examining it with a microscope. Scabies and infestation with crab lice are other problems that causes pruritus. Both conditions can be treated with gamma benzene hexachloride (Kwell) lotion or shampoo.

Psoriasis

Psoriasis may be seen in the perianal area without the scales seen in other parts of the body, but examination of the remainder of the skin suggests the diagnosis. Topical corticosteroids and coal tar preparations are standard treatment for this condition.

Lichen planus occurs in the perianal area and almost always is manifested in other areas of the skin as well. It must be differentiated from secondary syphilis.

Venereal Disease

Many bacterial infections can occur in the anorectal area. Common among these is the primary chancre of syphilis in the anal canal of homosexuals. This may appear to be only a superficial erosion in the anorectal area. On further examination, these patients are noted to have enlarged inguinal nodes. Specific diagnosis is made by demonstrating *Treponema pallidum* by means of darkfield microscopy of serum from the area of the chancre. Results of serologic testing may not be positive until several weeks after the occurrence of the primary chancre. Secondary syphilis is manifested by anal macules and condyloma latum in the perianal area, macules on the hands and soles of the feet, and generalized lymphadenopathy. The diagnosis of secondary syphilis is made by means of positive serologic testing.

Therapy is directed at treating not only the patient but also the patient's contacts for the previous 3 months in the case of primary syphilis and for the previous year in the case of secondary syphilis. Antibiotic therapy consists of benzathine penicillin G, 2.4 million units intramuscularly at a single session, or erythromycin, 500 mg orally four times a day for 15 days (see also Chapter 11). The patient definitely requires follow-up care.

Gonorrheal infection of the rectal mucosa also is seen in emergency department patients. This disease causes pain on defecation, tenesmus, and rectal discharge. On examination, the sphincter is lax, and proctoscopy reveals mild inflammation, friability of the rectal mucosa, and mucus. Specific diagnosis is made by a Gram's stain of the pus showing intracellular Gram-negative diplococci, or by culture of *Neisseria gonorrhoeae* on Thayer-Martin agar.

The treatment of gonorrheal proctitis is procaine penicillin G, 4.8 million units intramuscularly, with probenecid, 1 gm orally. Patients allergic to penicillin can be treated with 2 gm of spectinomycin. These patients and their sexual contacts should receive follow-up care, including repeated cultures (see also Chapter 11).

A common problem in homosexual men is nonspecific proctitis, which may have a clinical presentation similar to that of gonococcal proctitis. These patients should be evaluated thoroughly for parasitic and less common venereal diseases. If no cause is found, tetracycline, 1 gm/day for 10 days may be tried. The sexual partner also should be evaluated for venereal disease.

SUGGESTED READINGS

Black M. Acetaminophen hepatotoxicity. *Gastroenterology,* 1980;78:382–392.

Blaster MJ, Berkowitz ID, LaForce FM, et al. Campylobacter enteritis: Clinical and epidemiological features. *Ann Intern Med,* 1979;91:179–185.

Boley SJ, DiBiase A, Brandt LJ, et al. Lower intestinal bleeding in the elderly. *Am J Surg,* 1979;137:57–64.

Cello JP, Grendell JH, Crass RA, et al. Endoscopic sclerotherapy versus portocaval shunt in patients with severe cirrhosis and variceal hemorrhage. *N Engl Med,* 1984;311:1589–1594.

Eastwood GL. Does early endoscopy benefit the patient with active upper gastrointestinal bleeding? *Gastroenterology,* 1977;72:737–739.

Jokipii L, Jokipi AMM. Timing of symptoms and oocyst excretion in human cryptosporidiosis. *N Engl J Med,* 1986;315:1643–1647.

Seeff LB, Hoofnagle JH. Immunoprophylaxis of viral hepatitis, *Gastroenterology,* 1979;77:161–182.

Sleisenger RH, Fordtran JS, eds. Gastrointestinal Disease: Pathophysiology, Diagnosis, and Management. 3rd ed. Philadelphia: WB Saunders, 1983.

Wolfson JS, Richter JM, Waldron MA, et al. Cryprosporidiosis in immunocompetent patients. *N Engl J Med* 1985;312:1278–1282.

Wright R, Alberti KGMM, eds. Liver and Biliary Disease. London: WB Saunders, 1979.

CHAPTER 13

Hematologic Emergencies

LEONARD ELLMAN, M.D.

This chapter focuses on hematologic conditions that require immediate diagnostic or therapeutic intervention and that are likely to be seen in the emergency department. An effort is made to present the basic laboratory tests necessary for effective diagnosis.

HEMOLYTIC ANEMIA

Signs of Hemolysis

Hemolysis refers to premature destruction of red blood cells. The hallmark of hemolysis is a decreasing hematocrit without signs of blood loss. If erythroid production in the bone marrow increases sufficiently to compensate for the hemolysis, the hematocrit remains stable, but the reticulocyte count will be persistently elevated and suggest the presence of hemolysis. An elevated reticulocyte count immediately suggests hemolysis. However, the absence of reticulocytosis does not exclude hemolytic anemia since the bone marrow may be suppressed for a variety of reasons and may be unable to respond appropriately to the decreasing red blood cell count. Most cases of hemolysis are due to *extravascular* destruction of red blood cells by phagocytic cells in the liver and spleen, in which case hemoglobin is largely converted to bilirubin. Less commonly, hemolysis is *intravascular* and is characterized by the unique finding of free hemoglobin in the plasma and urine; if hemoglobinemia and hemoglobinuria persist, hemosiderinuria may develop. This is detected by performing the Prussian blue stain test on the urinary sediment. Signs com-

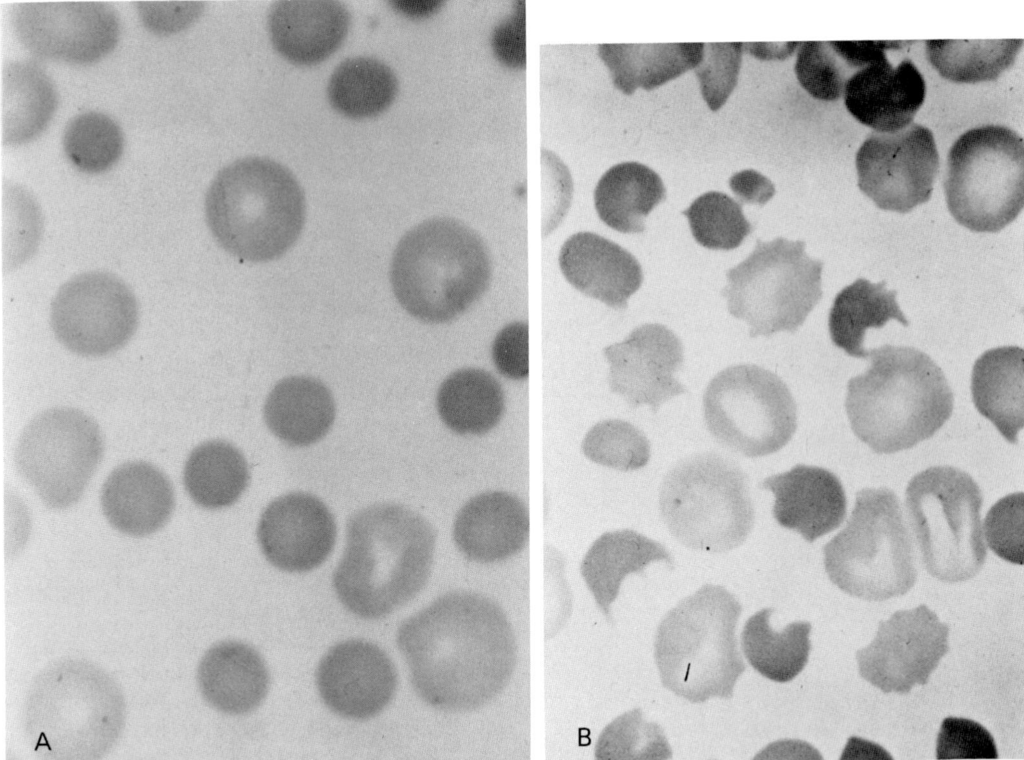

Figure 13.1. Hemolytic anemia. A, Spherocytes, which are generally smaller than normal red blood cells, perfectly round, and lacking in central pallor. They are the hallmark of immune hemolytic anemia and hereditary spherocytosis. B, Fragmented red blood cells, which result from shearing trauma to red cell membrane and which indicate microangiopathic hemolytic anemia.

mon to both intravascular and extravascular hemolysis include depressed or absent serum haptoglobin, indirect hyperbilirubinemia, the presence of serum methemalbumin, and elevated concentrations of serum lactate dehydrogenase (particularly in intravascular hemolysis) and urinary urobilinogen. The routine blood smear may also strongly suggest hemolytic anemia if spherocytes or fragmented red blood cells are present (Fig. 13.1). Intracellular organisms that cause hemolysis may also be seen (Fig. 13.2). On physical examination, jaundice, scleral icterus, and splenomegaly suggest a hemolytic process.

If hemolytic anemia develops suddenly (for example, after a transfusion reaction), presenting features may include back and abdominal pain, vomiting, headache, chills and fever, and occasionally shock. In the presence of hemoglobinuria, oliguria and renal failure may develop. More commonly, acquired hemolytic anemia develops insidiously and is characterized by pallor, jaundice, and the usual signs and symptoms of anemia, such as fatigue, dyspnea, and palpitation.

Conditions That May Mimic Hemolysis

Certain conditions can occasionally be confused with hemolytic anemia. Occult hemorrhage with a brisk bone marrow response may be difficult to distinguish from hemolysis, particularly if the hemorrhage has occurred internally so that hyperbilirubinemia results from the reabsorption of hemoglobin breakdown products. Brisk recovery from iron, folate, or vitamin B_{12} deficiency may also mimic hemolysis because of the combination of anemia and a high reticulocyte count. Myoglobinuria resulting from severe muscle injury may suggest hemolysis because the red urine may be mistaken for a sign of hemoglobinuria. Myoglobin, however, is a protein of small molecular weight, and it is rapidly cleared from the plasma. In contrast, when hemoglobinuria is present, the plasma usually remains pink for several hours since the larger size of the hemoglobin molecule leads to a slower clearance by the kidney. Definitive identification of the urinary pigment can be made by means of electrophoresis or spectrophotometry.

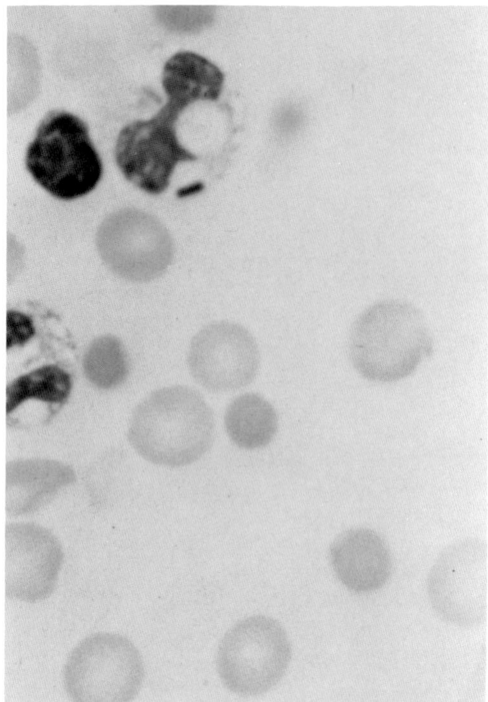

Figure 13.2. Hemolysis may result from *Clostridium perfringens* septicemia. Ingested bacteria may be present in polymorphonuclear leukocytes. Also note presence of spherocytes.

Classification of Hemolytic Anemia

Discussion of all the causes of hemolytic anemia is beyond the scope of this chapter. Distinctions can be made, however, that will assist the physician in making a differential diagnosis. *Intravascular hemolysis* versus *extravascular hemolysis* is one such distinction. Hemoglobinemia, hemoglobinuria, and hemosiderinuria in patients with intravascular hemolysis immediately call attention to the disorders listed in Table 13.1, many of which require immediate therapy. Hemolytic anemia may also be classified as *inherited* or *acquired.* The inherited disorders are frequently characterized by a family history of the disease, and are usually due to a fundamental defect in synthesis of the red blood cell membrane, an enzyme, or globin. Patients with congenital hemolytic anemia frequently have a history of recurrent anemia and icterus, often first noted in childhood. Congenital hemolytic anemia may be first suspected because of gallstones at a young age.

Major categories of inherited hemolytic disorders include:

1. Defects in the red blood cell membrane, as in hereditary spherocytosis, elliptocytosis, and stomatocytosis. These disorders are readily diagnosed by examination of the blood smear.
2. Defects in the Embden-Meyerhof pathway of glycolysis, as in pyruvate kinase deficiency. These disorders are rare, and special enzyme tests are required to confirm the diagnosis.
3. Defects in the hexose monophosphate shunt pathway, the most common of which is glucose-6-phosphate dehydrogenase deficiency.
4. Defects in globin structure, as in unstable hemoglobin disease. These disorders are also rare and require specialized tests.

Inherited Hemolytic Anemia

Glucose-6-Phosphate Dehydrogenase Deficiency. Among the inherited disorders, the most likely to be encountered in an emergency setting is a deficiency of glucose-6-phosphate dehydrogenase (G-6-PD), a key enzyme in monophosphate shunt. Normal function of this pathway is required for the red blood cell to withstand oxidative stress that otherwise leads to denaturation of hemoglobin and intravascular hemolysis.

Disorders due to G-6-PD deficiency are common in the black population and to a much lesser extent in persons from the Mediterranean basin, the Middle East, and Thailand. Since the gene for G-6-PD activity is carried on the X chromosome, inheritance is sex-linked. In the United States, 10–12% of black males and 1–2% of black females have G-6-PD deficiency.

The mechanism of hemolysis in the common variety of G-6-PD deficiency occurring in blacks is due to premature loss of G-6-PD activity as the red

Table 13.1.
Conditions in Which Hemolytic Anemia is Predominantly Intravascular

Immunohemolytic anemia
Acute or delayed transfusion reaction
Paroxysmal cold hemoglobinuria
Some cases of Coombs'-positive, warm autoimmune hemolytic anemia
Some cases of cold agglutinin disease
Disorders associated with red blood cell fragmentation: e.g., malfunctioning prosthetic heart valve
Infection
Falciparum malaria
Clostridial sepsis
Complications due to chemical agents
Acute drug reaction in patient with glucose-6-phosphate dehydrogenase deficiency
Arsine poisoning
Snake and spider venoms
Intravenous infusion of distilled water
Thermal injury
Physical injury: e.g., march hemoglobinuria
Paroxysmal nocturnal hemoglobinuria

blood cell ages. As the bone marrow responds with the production of reticulocytes, G-6-PD activity increases because of the younger population of red blood cells. As a result, episodes of G-6-PD hemolysis in the black population are usually mild and self-limited. No specific therapy is required except omission of drugs that induce hemolysis; blood transfusion is rarely required. In contrast, in many of the forms of G-6-PD deficiency in the white population, there is severe lack of G-6-PD activity; these forms are characterized by chronic hemolytic anemia with severe exacerbations after exposure to oxidative stress.

In the absence of oxidative stress, the peripheral blood of blacks with G-6-PD deficiency appears normal. During a hemolytic crisis, cells containing Heinz bodies (globules of denatured hemoglobin) may be transiently present when blood smears are made with supravital stains such as brilliant cresyl blue. Heinz bodies may be noted while performing a reticulocyte count since the stain used is a supravital stain. Many screening tests for G-6-PD deficiency are widely available; results may be falsely negative during the acute phase of hemolysis as a result of the elevated reticulocyte count.

Table 13.2 lists the principal agents causing G-6-PD hemolysis. If these agents are taken in sufficient amounts by normal persons, a similar hemolysis may develop. It is important to note that stressful physical situations in general, such as bacterial infections and diabetic ketoacidosis, can induce hemolysis in G-6-PD-deficient individuals in the absence of the ingestion of oxidative medications.

Table 13.2.
Drugs Associated with Hemolysis in Persons with Glucose-6-Phosphate Dehydrogenase Deficiency

- Antimalarial agents
  - Primaquine phosphate
  - Pamaquine
  - Chloroquine
  - Quinacrine hydrochloride (Atabrine)
- Sulfonamide compounds
  - Sulfanilamide
  - Sulfisoxazole (Gantrisin)
  - Salicylazosulfapyridine (Azulfidine)
  - Sulfacetamide (Sulamyd)
  - Sulfamethoxypyridazine
  - Sulfamethoxazole (Gantanol)
- Antibiotics
  - Nitrofurantoin (Furadantin)
  - Chloramphenicol[a]
  - Paraaminosalicylic acid
  - Nalidixic Acid (NegGram)
- Analgesics
  - Aspirin
  - Phenacetin
- Miscellaneous
  - Quinine[a]
  - Quinidine[a]
  - Procainamide hydrochloride (Pronestyl)
  - Probenecid
  - Vitamin K (water-soluble analogues)

[a] Not hemolytic in blacks.

Table 13.3.
Immune Hemolytic Anemia

- Acute or delayed transfusion reaction due to incompatible blood
- Autoimmune hemolytic anemia due to warm-reactive antibodies
  - Idiopathic
  - Secondary
    - Lymphoproliferative disease
    - Other malignant disease
    - Systemic lupus erythematosus and other autoimmune disorders
- Drug-induced (penicillin, quinidine, quinine, chlorpropamide, α-methyldopa (Aldomet), L-dopa)
- Autoimmune hemolytic anemia due to cold-reactive antibodies
  - Cold agglutinin disease
    - Idiopathic
    - Secondary
      - Lymphoproliferative disease
      - Mycoplasmal infection
      - Infectious mononucleosis
  - Paroxysmal cold hemoglobinuria

Acquired Hemolytic Anemia

Although acquired hemolytic anemia may have an insidious onset, it is not associated with the features that suggest a congenital hemolytic anemia, such as episodes of anemia and jaundice in childhood, a family history of anemia, and gallstones. The acquired hemolytic anemias that have clinical importance may be classified into two main groups: immune disorders in which antibodies and complement play a major role in red blood cell destruction, and secondary conditions in which red blood cell destruction results from physical trauma to the cell from chemicals and toxins, infectious agents, or microangiopathic processes. Tables 13.3 and 13.4 list the types of acquired hemolytic anemia and their causes.

Autoimmune Hemolytic Anemia. The hallmark of autoimmune hemolytic anemia (AIHA) is a positive *direct Coombs' test* which reveals the presence of antibody and complement on the red blood cell surface. If such antibody is also present in the serum, it can be detected by means of the *indirect Coombs' test.*

In terms of clinical presentation and laboratory findings, it is convenient to divide AIHA into warm AIHA, in which the antibody combines with the red blood cell optimally at 37°C, and cold AIHA, in which the antibody combines optimally at 0–4°C and shows progressively decreased affinity for the

Table 13.4.
Additional Types of Acquired Hemolytic Anemia

Microangiopathic hemolytic anemia
Prosthetic valves and cardiac abnormalities
Hemolytic-uremic syndrome
Disseminated intravascular coagulation
Thrombotic thrombocytopenic purpura
Hemangioma
Disseminated carcinoma
Malignant hypertension
Infectious disease
Clostridial sepsis
Bartonellosis
Malaria
Toxoplasmosis
Leishmaniasis
Anemia due to chemicals, drugs, or venoms
Chemicals and toxins
Naphthalene
Nitrofurantoin (Furadantin)
Sulfonamides
Sulfones
Phenacetin
Phenylhydrazine
Paraaminosalicylic acid
Phenol derivatives
Arsine
Water
Copper
Anemia due to physical agents
Thermal injury
March hemoglobinuria
Miscellaneous
Hypophosphatemia
Paroxysmal nocturnal hemoglobinuria
Spur-cell anemia in severe hepatic disease

red blood cell antigens at higher temperatures. In addition to a positive direct Coombs' test, cold AIHA is characterized by a higher titer of cold agglutinins (more than 1:200). In this test the highest dilution of the patient's serum is determined that will cause agglutination of type O red blood cells in the cold. In contrast with warm AIHA, in which the antibody is of the IgG class, cold agglutinin disease is due to an IgM antibody.

AIHA can be acute and fulminating, but more commonly it is chronic and insidious. In patients with cold agglutinin disease, acute exacerbations with hemoglobinemia and hemoglobinuria may occur after exposure to the cold. In such patients, Raynaud's phenomenon or passing dark urine after cold exposure may be the first recognized abnormality. Slight to moderate splenomegaly is the most common physical finding in both warm and cold types. Examination of the blood smear is of considerable value. In warm AIHA, the characteristic findings are large numbers of spherocytes and often many polychromatophilic cells representing reticulocytes. In cold AIHA, spherocytosis is less common, and the blood smear more frequently shows large clumps of red blood cells. Both warm and cold AIHA may be secondary to underlying disorders (Table 13.3), and the precipitating factor should be sought in any patient with this diagnosis.

In the management of AIHA, transfusions should be avoided if possible, since the transfused cells will be hemolyzed just as rapidly as the patient's red blood cells. In fact, cross-matching may be very difficult since the autoantibody, which is frequently present in the patient's serum, may react with virtually all units of blood in the blood bank. In this case the unit of blood showing the weakest reaction pattern in vitro can be administered, with careful monitoring and cessation of the transfusion if signs of increased hemolysis develop.

Three-fourths of patients with warm AIHA respond initially to prednisone, 1 mg/kg/day. Unfortunately, most patients relapse as the corticosteroid is tapered, and splenectomy often becomes necessary. Most patients with cold AIHA related to infection require no treatment aside from warmth and rest, since the illness is transient. Management of chronic cold agglutinin disease is not very satisfactory, however, since corticosteroids and splenectomy are usually of little value. Keeping the patient warm and transfusing packed red blood cells when necessary is often the principal form of therapy. Red blood cells should be washed in saline before transfusion to remove complement, which may exacerbate the hemolysis in cold AIHA. In all chronic hemolytic states the folic acid requirement increases, and folic acid should be administered prophylactically.

SICKLE CELL ANEMIA

Pathophysiologic Principles

Sickle cell anemia (homozygous sickle cell disease) is the most common genetic disease seen in clinical practice. As a result of many years of research, much is now known about the cause of this condition. Normal adult human hemoglobin (hemoglobin A) consists of two α and two β chains. In sickle cell anemia, a single amino acid substitution of glutamic acid for valine occurs on the β chains, resulting in substantial alterations in the physicochemical properties of the hemoglobin molecule (hemoglobin S). In addition to a change in the electrophoretic mobility of the hemoglobin, erythrocytes from patients with homozygous sickle cell disease assume the sickle shape when they are deprived of oxygen. Sickling is also fostered by a decrease in pH. When enough cells have assumed the sickle shape, blood viscosity increases considerably and reduced blood flow results. Local impairment of circulation leads to further hypoxia and acidosis, and this engenders further sickling. A cycle occurs in which more and more cells become sickled, causing local blockage of the circulation and ischemic infarction. This sequence can occur in virtually any organ of the body, leading clinically to the painful "sickle crisis."

Sickle Cell Trait

Sickle cell anemia is inherited as a recessive gene according to Mendelian law. In the heterozygous state, sickle cell trait, only one β locus is affected and the red blood cell contains approximately equal amounts of hemoglobin A and hemoglobin S. The structure of the red blood cell is normal, and no anemia is present. Sickle cell trait is found in 8–11% of the black population in the United States and to a much smaller extent in persons of Greek, Italian, and Middle Eastern ancestry. Since the red blood cells in a person with sickle cell trait contain both hemoglobin A and hemoglobin S, they require much greater deoxygenation before sickling develops. As a result, sickle crises occur only during extreme conditions of deoxygenation such as flying in an unpressurized aircraft.

There are few established complications of sickle cell trait. The structure of Henle's loop facilitates sickling in this area, leading to dysfunction of the loop and hyposthenuria. Painless hematuria, more commonly from the left kidney, is the most frequent complication of medical significance. Hematuria may occasionally be prolonged and recurrent and may respond to treatment with diuretics or intravenous alkali. Priapism, occlusion of the central retinal artery, and splenic infarction are rarely reported. The longevity of persons with sickle cell trait appears to be normal.

Homozygous Sickle Cell Disease

In homozygous sickle cell disease, both β loci are affected, and the patient has only hemoglobin S, except for residual amounts of fetal hemoglobin (hemoglobin F). The clinical problems of sickle cell anemia can be divided into three major categories.

1. *Repeated episodes of vascular occlusion* with pain, fever, and end-organ damage (sickle crisis). The pain, which is usually described as gnawing, gradually increases in the course of several hours; it commonly involves the extremities, the joints, the abdomen, and the chest, although it may affect virtually any organ. There are generally no specific clinical or laboratory findings that identify the episode as sickle crisis. Diagnosis may be aided by the prior experience of the patient, since many have a consistent pattern of pain. At times, however, it may be extremely difficult to differentiate sickle crisis from other conditions such as pulmonary embolism, appendicitis, or cholecystitis.

2. *Chronic hemolytic anemia* due to the short survival time of the rigid sickle cells. The hematocrit value is usually from 20 to 30%.

3. *Frequent, severe infections,* including Salmonella osteomyelitis, pneumococcal pneumonia, pneumococcal meningitis, and mycoplasma pneumonia. Many factors appear to contribute to the high incidence of severe infection; the factors include functional asplenia, lack of bacterial opsonins, impairment of activity of the complement pathway, and defective phagocytic activity. Local factors such as stasis and tissue necrosis may also be important in bacterial growth. Persons with sickle cell anemia respond to infection poorly, and prompt antibiotic therapy should be started for presumed infection, especially if the pneumococcus is suspected.

Special mention should be made of *pulmonary complications.* In persons with sickle cell anemia, occlusive phenomena may develop in the pulmonary arteries. In addition, marrow and fat emboli from infarcted bone marrow, as well as emboli from peripheral veins, occur with considerable frequency. Pulmonary infection is also extremely common. Hence, elucidation of the cause of chest pain and lung infiltrates may be extremely difficult. The value of lung scanning and pulmonary angiographic examination in this setting has not yet been clearly established. Transtracheal aspiration and bronchial brushing may be helpful in recognizing bacterial infection, and possible sepsis should be treated vigorously.

Neurological manifestations of sickle cell disease are primarily related to vascular occlusion. Hemiplegia and confusion are the most common manifestations. One should also be alert to the possibility of narcotic overdosage and withdrawal syndromes in the sickle cell patient with lethargy or confusion.

Acutely tender and inflamed *joints* are usually the result of synovial or periarticular thrombosis. However, septic arthritis, aseptic necrosis, osteomyelitis, and gout are possibilities. Diagnostic arthrocentesis (see Illustrated Techniques 24 and 25) should be considered in patients who are febrile or who have a monoarticular arthritis.

Priapism is an uncommon complication requiring immediate urological consultation. Analgesia and ice compresses are helpful as initial treatment.

Laboratory Tests

Sickle cells (Fig. 13.3) are not seen on a routine blood smear of the peripheral blood from a patient with sickle cell trait. Thus, the presence of sickle cells indicates sickle cell anemia or a major variant such as sickle cell-hemoglobin C disease.

The sickling phenomenon can be induced by several maneuvers that depend on the deoxygenation of hemoglobin. Sodium metabisulfite is the classic

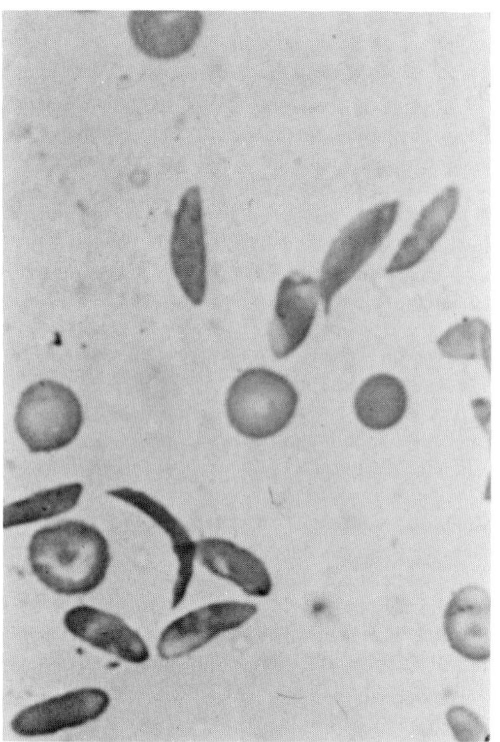

Figure 13.3. Sickle cell anemia. Peripheral blood smear with sickle cells characterized by pointed configuration at both ends of cell.

agent used to induce sickling in sickle cell anemia or sickle cell trait. This screening test has largely been replaced by commercially prepared tests, such as the Sickledex test that allow rapid detection of hemoglobin S on the basis of its decreased solubility in high phosphate buffer solutions. Electrophoresis of hemoglobin on various media such as paper or cellulose acetate remains the definitive method for identification of hemoglobin S. It also readily allows differentiation between sickle cell trait and homozygous sickle cell anemia.

Therapy

Since painful episodes are often precipitated by infection, fever, and perhaps excessive cold, measures that prevent or remedy these conditions are important. Vigorous hydration and analgesics have remained the mainstay of therapy for the painful crisis. Patients with sickle cell anemia are likely to become dehydrated because of chronic hyposthenuria. Dehydration is a particular danger because it increases the concentration of hemoglobin S in the red blood cells, and therefore increases the tendency for sickling. Since acidosis enhances sickling, some physicians recommend administration of sodium bicarbonate and sodium lactate for alkalization. However, use of these agents remains controversial.

Transfusion with several units of normal blood or exchange transfusion to dilute the percentage of sickled cells is probably beneficial in patients with life-threatening complications such as impending cerebral infarction. Transfusion therapy before a surgical procedure is useful in decreasing sickle crises during and after operation and may also be useful in patients with almost constantly recurring crises. Limited exchange transfusion may also decrease the duration of painful crises. Transfusion therapy, however, has the associated complications of hepatic and iron overload and may lead to development of minor blood group incompatibilities that make future transfusions more difficult.

Administration of oxygen to patients with painful crises offers little benefit and, if continued, may lead to suppression of red blood cell production and exacerbation of anemia. Oxygen, however, should be given liberally to patients with cardiopulmonary disease or pneumonia. Hyperbaric oxygen therapy has been utilized with uncertain results in intracerebral sickling.

Many agents have been employed in attempts to abort painful crises, usually without significant benefit. Enthusiasm for urea, one of the newer agents, has largely disappeared. Potassium cyanate prevents sickling in vitro as a result of ''carbamylation'' of the terminal nitrogen atom on the hemoglobin molecule. Carbamylation inhibits the sickling process, and also increases the oxygen affinity of hemoglobin S, which indirectly decreases the tendency for sickling. Unfortunately, clinical trial with potassium cyanate has failed to show a decrease in the incidence of painful crises and has been associated with the development of cataracts and peripheral neuropathy.

Related Syndromes

Other types of hemoglobin present in the red blood cell along with hemoglobin S can influence the extent of sickling. For example, hemoglobin S-thalassemia tends to be milder than sickle cell anemia because the presence of hemoglobin F, hemoglobin A, and hemoglobin A_2 tends to solubilize the hemoglobin S. Similarly, sickle cell-hemoglobin C disease is usually milder than sickle cell anemia because hemoglobin C has a lesser tendency for sickling than hemoglobin S. Homozygous hemoglobin C disease is also milder than sickle cell anemia, but vascular occlusive crises do occur. Hemoglobin C trait is asymptomatic.

MEGALOBLASTIC ANEMIA

Diagnosis

Clinical Features

Anemia due to vitamin B_{12} or folic acid deficiency is a common cause of severe anemia encountered in the emergency department. Because megaloblastic anemia develops gradually, there is sufficient time for hemodynamic compensation to occur, and patients may look well despite profound anemia. Moderate *neutropenia* and *thrombocytopenia* are also frequently present, although complications due to infection and bleeding are uncommon. In addition to the general features of anemia such as weakness and shortness of breath, patients with megaloblastic anemia often have glossitis and mild jaundice. Patients with vitamin B_{12} deficiency often suffer from peripheral neuropathy or degeneration of the posterior and pyramidal tracts of the spinal cord (combined systems disease), resulting in paresthesia, loss of vibration and position sense, muscular weakness, difficulty in walking, and occasionally, psychotic behavior. Folic acid deficiency may cause mental slowness and, rarely, mild dementia, but does not cause significant organic nervous system disease.

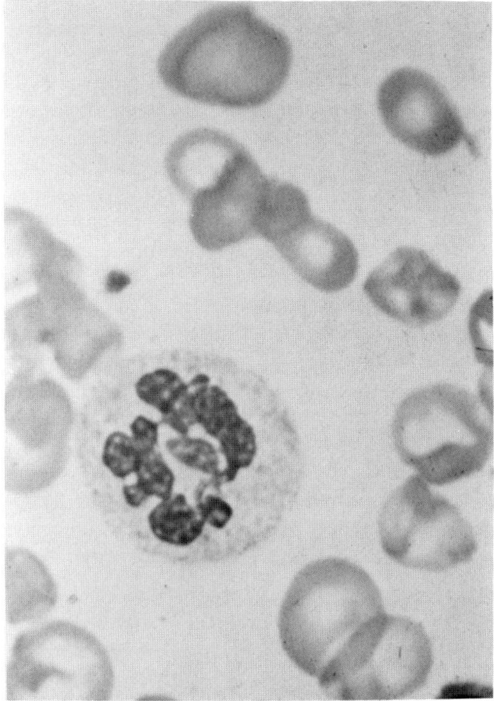

Figure 13.4. Megaloblastic anemia. Blood smear is noteworthy because of hypersegmented polymorphonuclear leukocytes and macrocytes.

Laboratory Tests

The diagnosis of megaloblastic anemia is usually easy to make from the blood smear and from the bone marrow aspirate (sternal or iliac crest). The peripheral smear is characterized by *giant macrocytes* and *hypersegmentation of the neutrophils,* that is, neutrophils with six or seven nuclear lobes or more than 5% with five nuclear lobes (Fig. 13.4). As a result of the macrocytes, the mean corpuscular volume is elevated, often with values as high as 120–130. The bone marrow is also characteristic, with a hypercellular appearance and dissociation between nuclear and cytoplasmic development of the erythroblasts, the nucleus maintaining a primitive appearance with fine, lacy chromatin despite normal maturation of the cytoplasm. The myeloid series is characterized by large, abnormally shaped bands and metamyelocytes. The reticulocyte count is very low, particularly when the degree of anemia is considered. The serum lactate dehydrogenase concentration is frequently substantially elevated, and the indirect bilirubin level is mildly elevated.

Table 13.5.
Causes of Megaloblastic Anemia

- Vitamin B_{12} deficiency
  - Pernicious anemia
  - Gastrectomy
  - Intestinal absorptive defects
    - Ileal resection
    - Regional enteritis
    - Celiac disease
    - Malabsorption syndrome
  - Competitive parasites
    - Fish tapeworm
  - Diverticula and blind loop syndrome
  - Vegetarian diet very deficient in vitamin B_{12}
- Folic acid deficiency
  - Poor diet
    - Alcoholism
    - Food faddism
    - Gastrectomy
    - Other
  - Impaired absorption
    - Intrinsic intestinal disease
    - Malabsorption syndrome
  - Increased requirement
    - Pregnancy
    - Tumor
    - Hemolytic anemia
  - Drugs
    - Folate antagonists
      - Methotrexate
      - Trimethoprim
      - Pyrimethamine
    - Phenytoin
    - Oral contraceptives
    - Triamterene
    - Barbiturates
    - Tetracycline

It is often possible to determine whether vitamin B_{12} or folic acid deficiency is present from the patient's history (Table 13.5). However, confirmation depends on measurement of the serum levels of the two vitamins, and it is essential to obtain results of these tests before starting therapy. The presence of achlorhydria and the absence of gastric intrinsic factor as demonstrated in the Schilling's test help confirm the diagnosis of pernicious anemia.

Therapy

It is usually possible to establish which of the two deficiencies is the cause of megaloblastic anemia and to treat the patient with the appropriate vitamin. Vitamin B_{12}, 100–1000 μg/day intramuscularly for 7–10 days, or folic acid, 2–5 mg/day orally, is adequate initial therapy. If the cause of megaloblastic anemia is unclear, treatment can be started with both vitamins until the results of serum folate and B_{12} determinations are available. Transfusion is usually unnecessary because of the rapid response to the hematinics. If symptoms such as angina or congestive heart failure are due to severe anemia, packed red blood cells should be administered slowly.

Potassium supplements are also recommended in patients with normal renal function along with vitamin replacement because of the danger of hypokalemia that may develop during the initial hematologic response. Sudden death during this period may result from arrhythmias induced by hypokalemia.

ERYTHROCYTOSIS AND POLYCYTHEMIA

Classification

The upper limit of the hematocrit value in healthy men is 54%, and in healthy women it is 49%. *Relative erythrocytosis* refers to the situation in which the hematocrit is elevated because of a decrease in plasma volume. Relative erythrocytosis usually has a brief course and is due to such causes as excessive diuresis, severe diarrhea or vomiting, and profuse sweating. Therapy consists of fluid replacement and correction of the underlying cause of volume depletion.

A few persons, who are usually young men, have a chronic form of pseudoerythrocytosis that has been referred to as *Gaisböck's syndrome* or *stress erythrocytosis*. Although the hematocrit level may be as high as 60%, the red blood cell mass is not increased. Complaints include headache, dizziness, and paresthesia, but symptoms are usually not alleviated by phlebotomy. It is doubtful that stress erythrocytosis is a true clinical entity, and no specific therapy is indicated.

Table 13.6.
Causes of Secondary Erythrocytosis

Causes
Appropriate erythropoietin production due to decreased oxygen transport
High altitude
Inadequate functioning hemoglobin
Hemoglobin Chesapeake
Congenital methemoglobinemia
Pulmonary disease with oxygen saturation < 90%
Cyanotic congenital cardiac disease with right-to-left shunt
Cigarette smoking with elevated carbon monoxide level in blood
Inappropriate erythropoietin production unrelated to oxygen transport
Malignant lesion in kidney, liver, adrenal gland, lung
Benign disease
Uterine myoma
Renal cyst
Hydronephrosis
Cerebellar hemangioma
Pheochromocytoma
Cushing's syndrome
Exogenous agents
Cobalt
Testosterone

True increases in the red blood cell mass occur in *secondary erythrocytosis* and *polycythemia vera*. Secondary erythrocytosis refers to an absolute increase in the red blood cell mass unassociated with a myeloproliferative disorder. The white blood cell count and the platelet count are normal. Causes of secondary erythrocytosis can be divided into two major categories (Table 13.6). The first category includes conditions associated with appropriate increases in the erythropoietin concentration resulting from tissue hypoxia. Severe pulmonary disease, in which oxygen saturation is less than 90%, and cyanotic congenital heart disease are the most common examples. The second category includes lesions resulting in inappropriate erythropoietin elaboration, such as tumors, cysts, and various renal conditions.

The absolute erythrocytosis of polycythemia vera is part of a panmyelopathy characterized by leukocytosis, thrombocytosis, basophilia, splenomegaly, hepatomegaly, and pruritus, especially after bathing.

Therapy

The relation between blood viscosity and hematocrit is characterized by a steep curve; small increases in the hematocrit level above 60% lead to substantial increases in the blood viscosity. The symptoms and signs of polycythemia vera can be attributed primarily to the expanded blood volume and to the slowing of the blood flow that results from the increased viscosity. The main form of emergency therapy for polycythemia vera is phlebotomy. Morbidity and mortality are considerably decreased by lowering the hematocrit to the normal range, and this fact is particularly important for patients with polycythemia vera who are to undergo a surgical procedure. In these patients, phlebotomy should be performed on an emergency basis, if necessary, before operation. Blood obtained by phlebotomy may be stored and then used for replacement during operation if it is needed. Long-term treatment of polycythemia vera may involve use of radioactive phosphorus or alkylating agents to suppress the bone marrow in addition to phlebotomy.

The decision to perform phlebotomy for secondary erythrocytosis resulting from appropriate elaboration of erythropoietin, as in chronic pulmonary disease or cyanotic congenital heart disease, is less clear-cut. Erythrocytosis in these situations is usually regarded as a compensatory response to tissue hypoxia. Nonetheless, phlebotomy should be performed if the increased blood volume and viscosity appear to be related to symptoms such as congestive heart failure or impending vascular thrombosis. Return of the red blood cell mass to normal improves pulmonary vascular resistance in patients with cor pulmonale and erythrocytosis. If phlebotomy is performed, time must be allowed for equilibration of vascular volume.

HYPERVISCOSITY SYNDROME

Blood viscosity increases substantially in both polycythemia and sickle cell anemia. However, the term ''hyperviscosity syndrome'' is usually applied only to situations in which serum viscosity increases as a result of greatly increased concentrations of abnormal plasma proteins. The hyperviscosity syndrome is a prominent feature of Waldenström's macroglobulinemia and is less commonly seen in patients with multiple myeloma and Sjögren's syndrome. The hyperviscosity syndrome has certain characteristic features, including bleeding from mucous membranes; visual disturbance and retinopathy consisting of venous engorgement, hemorrhages, and occasionally papilledema; neurologic disorders such as headaches, seizures, and coma; congestive heart failure; and severe lethargy. *It is unusual for a patient to become symptomatic until the serum becomes four times as viscous as water* (normal viscosity of serum is less than 1.5 that of water). In an emergency, the viscosity of water and serum can be estimated with a white blood cell pipette and a stopwatch by measuring the time it takes the meniscus to fall from above the bulb to below the bulb of the pipette.

A patient with symptomatic hyperviscosity syndrome should undergo *plasmapheresis*. Two to four units of plasma daily can be removed, allowing time for equilibration of the plasma volume; if necessary, saline solution or colloid can be infused to maintain vascular volume. Plasmapheresis is greatly facilitated on the centrifugal type of cell separator (Celltrifuge, American Instrument Company). This device was developed to allow selective isolation and removal of granulocytes or platelets, but it also allows efficient plasma exchange. Plasmapheresis tends to be less effective for hyperviscosity due to multiple myeloma or Sjögren's syndrome, since the abnormal protein is less restricted to the intravascular compartment. Long-term therapy for the hyperviscosity syndrome involves chemotherapy, usually with an alkylating agent.

GRANULOCYTOPENIA

Leukopenia refers to depression of the total white blood cell count to fewer than 3500 cells/mm^3; *neutropenia* and *granulocytopenia* refer to a total neutrophil (or granulocyte) count of fewer than 1500 cells/mm^3. Susceptibility to infection becomes a serious problem when the neutrophil count decreases to fewer than 1000 cells/mm^3 and is extremely hazardous when the count is fewer than 500 cells/mm^3. *Agranulocytosis* describes almost complete disappearance of granulocytes from the blood.

Neutropenia

The major causes of neutropenia are listed in Table 13.7. Biopsy of the bone marrow is often valu-

Table 13.7.
Causes of Neutropenia

- Infection
  - Typhoid fever
  - Rickettsial infection
  - Malaria
  - Kala azar
  - Viral infection
  - Overwhelming infection
    - Miliary tuberculosis
    - Septicemia, especially in debilitated patients
- Aplastic anemia
- Myelophthisis
  - Myelofibrosis
  - Leukemia
  - Carcinoma or granuloma involving bone marrow
- Hypersplenism
- Megaloblastic anemia
- Felty's syndrome
- Systemic lupus erythematosus
- Drugs
- Miscellaneous
  - Cyclic neutropenia
  - Hypothyroidism
  - Anaphylactoid shock

Table 13.8.
Drugs and Physical Agents Causing Neutropenia and Agranulocytosis

Agents that produce marrow hypoplasia in all persons if given in sufficient doses
Ionizing radiation
Benzene
Chemotherapeutic agents
Nitrogen mustard
Chlorambucil
Cyclophosphamide
Phenylalanine mustard
Methotrexate
6-Mercaptopurine
5-Fluorouracil
Cytosine arabinoside
Daunorubicin (daunomycin)
Adriamycin
Drugs that occasionally cause neutropenia as result of individual sensitivity
Analgesics
Aminopyrine
Phenylbutazone
Indomethacin
Sulfonamide compounds
Thiazide diuretics
Oral hypoglycemic agents
Phenothiazines
Antithyroid drugs
Propylthiouracil
Methimazole
Antimicrobial agents
Chloramphenicol
Isoniazid
Cephalothin
Semisynthetic penicillins
Antihistamines
Pronestyl sustained release (Procan)

able in the evaluation of leukopenia, particularly in determining whether a primary disorder of the marrow is present. Neutropenia may be due to severe sepsis and is associated with a high mortality in this setting. A careful drug history is a necessity since drugs are the principal cause of acute neutropenia in clinical practice. Table 13.8 lists the most important drugs causing neutropenia.

Agranulocytosis

The form of neutropenia with the most striking presentation is acute drug-induced agranulocytosis. This is usually due to myeloid suppression in the bone marrow after many days to weeks of drug therapy. Less commonly, acute agranulocytosis develops almost immediately after use of a drug as a result of an immune form of peripheral granulocyte destruction mediated by an antibody.

The onset of agranulocytosis is indicated by high fever, shaking chills, sore throat, and oral ulceration. The appearance of the bone marrow is variable; there may be a substantial decrease in myeloid elements or there may be adequate numbers of promyelocytes and myelocytes but markedly decreased numbers of more mature forms (so-called maturation arrest). Occasionally, the bone marrow appears entirely normal. Other diseases that may be confused with acute agranulocytosis include aleukemic leukemia, aplastic anemia, and overwhelming bacterial infection with secondary severe granulocytopenia due to bone marrow suppression.

Initial therapy for agranulocytosis is omission of the offending agent or drug. Table 13.8 lists the more common drugs causing agranulocytosis, but since virtually any drug can induce this condition, it is usually necessary to omit all the drugs that the patient is taking. Intensive broad-spectrum antibiotic coverage with bactericidal agents such as oxacillin and gentamicin should be instituted after bacteriologic cultures have been obtained. Lack of granulocytes may make the site of infection difficult to detect. For example, minimal infiltrates on a chest film and anal ulcers may be significant and should be monitored. High-grade septicemia is common in this group of patients and is the usual cause of death. The general care of the patient is important, and careful attention should be given to oral and anal hygiene to prevent the occurrence of serious ulceration. Corticosteroids have not been proved effective in the treatment of agranulocytosis, and their use should be discouraged. With prompt omission of the offending agent, good supportive care, and antibiotic therapy, the condition of most patients can be kept stable until the granulocyte count becomes normal. For the patient whose infection is advancing and becomes life-threatening, consideration should be given to the daily administration of granulocyte transfusions harvested on a cell separator from a healthy ABO compatible donor.

LEUKOSTASIS CRISIS IN ACUTE MYELOID LEUKEMIAS

Patients with acute myeloid leukemia and acute monocytic leukemia who present with blast cell counts greater than 100,000/mm^3 are at high risk of developing intravascular leukostasis. This leukostasis occurs in the small arteries of the lung or brain, but also may occur in other organs. The leukemic aggregates are associated with hemorrhage and infarction in the white matter of the brain and, to a lesser extent, in the lung. The leukostasis syndrome must be considered a medical emergency and physicians should be aware of the need for prompt treatment. A single, daily, oral dose of hydroxyurea, 50–100 mg/kg with a maximum dose of 6 gm/day, is effective in rapidly reducing the blast count and can be instituted in the interval before consultation or referral. Conventional chemotherapy for acute leukemia can be initiated simultaneously, but its peak effect does not occur for several days. If central nervous system symptoms have already become evident, emergency cranial irradiation is indicated; leukopheresis of the patient on a cell separator machine should also be considered since it is highly effective at rapidly reducing the white count on a temporary basis.

The risks of cerebral and pulmonary leukostasis are much less in patients with acute lymphoblastic (lymphocytic) leukemia, probably because myeloblasts and monoblasts are larger than lymphoblasts and the mass of circulating leukocytes is much greater. The leukostasis syndrome does not appear to occur despite the height of the white count when the cells are mature, as in chronic lymphocytic or chronic myelogenous leukemia.

COMPLICATIONS OF CHEMOTHERAPY

The armamentarium of chemotherapeutic agents is rapidly expanding and the potential toxicity of these agents is very large. The majority of chemotherapeutic agents are cytotoxic and affect all rapidly dividing cells. Hence, bone marrow depression with thrombocytopenia and granulocytopenia is very common and is the most frequently encountered serious complication of chemotherapy. Patients may require intensive supportive care including platelet and granulocyte transfusions for periods of intense or prolonged bone marrow depression associated with bleeding or infection.

Mucositis involving the mouth, alimentary tract, and vagina manifested as oral and vaginal sores, and nausea and diarrhea are also frequently encountered. Treatment is supportive. Certain chemotherapeutic agents have unique toxicities unrelated to mucositis and bone marrow depression and these problems are summarized in Table 13.9.

BLEEDING DISORDERS

The rapid arrest of hemorrhage after injury is an extremely important defense mechanism. Although it is customary to consider platelets and the coagulation factors separately, the distinction is largely one of convenience since there is an integral relation between platelets and the coagulation cascade.

Platelets are essential for sealing tiny leaks that continuously develop in the walls of small blood vessels. In addition, they are the first defense in the presence of tissue injury. When tissue injury occurs and endothelial tissue is exposed, platelets adhere at the injured site. After adhesion, other platelets aggregate, adding to the adherent platelets. Aggregation is mediated both by adenosine diphosphate released by adherent platelets and possibly by collagen from the exposed vascular wall. Thus, platelets are essential for the formation of a primary hemostatic plug. Platelet aggregation may also induce constriction of the injured vessel wall through release of serotonin, a powerful vasoconstricting agent. Vasoconstriction assists hemostasis by reducing blood flow in the injured vessel.

While the primary hemostatic plug is forming, the exposed vascular endothelium and thromboplastins released by the injured tissue activate the coagulation cascade, which leads to deposition of fibrin in and around the platelet plug. The fibrin strengthens the plug and helps anchor it to the wall of the blood vessel. The clot then begins to contract, and a permanent hemostatic plug is formed.

The coagulation cascade (Fig. 13.5) involves the sequential interaction of the coagulation factors, each factor being activated by the one preceding it. The end point of the process is generation of large amounts of fibrin clot. The coagulation cascade has traditionally been divided into two overlapping pathways, the intrinsic and the extrinsic. All of the factors required for the intrinsic system are present in the circulating blood, and the system is assayed by the partial thromboplastin time (PTT). Injury to the vessel wall exposes collagen, which initiates the intrinsic system by activating Factor XII (Hageman factor). Lipid from platelets and calcium are required at several points in the pathway.

The extrinsic coagulation system, which is monitored by the prothrombin time (PT) and by the thrombin time (TT), depends on release of tissue thromboplastin from damaged cells or vascular endothelium. The tissue thromboplastin together with Factor VII activates Factor X. The remainder of the sequence is identical to that of the intrinsic system, with generation of fibrin clot. Although called the extrinsic system, this pathway is also intravascular and contributes to fibrin formation along with the intrinsic system.

Evaluation of the Bleeding Patient

History

The clinical evaluation of a bleeding patient must include a careful history. It is important to determine whether the patient has a newly acquired bleeding disorder or a life-long disorder associated with bleeding at the time of circumcision, dental extraction, or menstruation, or after trauma. A family history of bleeding may also be informative in determining the presence of a congenital coagulation disorder. Hemophilia and Christmas disease occur almost exclusively in males since these are inherited, sex-linked conditions. In contrast, von Willebrand's disease is inherited as a dominant disorder and occurs equally in males and females. A history of drug use should be obtained to determine

Table 13.9.
Nonhematologic Complications of Commonly Used Chemotherapeutic Agents

Agents	Complications
Vincristine (Oncovin)	Peripheral neuropathy Constipation, ileus Syndrome of inappropriate antidiuretic hormone secretion
Doxorubicin (Adriamycin)	Cardiac arrhythmia
Daunorubicin (Cerubidine)	Congestive heart failure
Bleomycin (Blenoxane)	Pulmonary infiltrates Pulmonary fibrosis Erythroderma Fever Hypotension
Busulfan (Myleran)	Pulmonary fibrosis
Cyclophosphamide (Cytoxan)	Sterile hemorrhagic cystitis Syndrome of inappropriate secretion of antidiuretic hormone Pulmonary fibrosis
Mithramycin (Mutamycin)	Renal toxicity
Nitrosoureas (BCNU, CCNU, methyl CCNU)	Renal toxicity Hepatic toxicity Pulmonary fibrosis
Methotrexate	Hepatic toxicity
Streptozitocin	Renal toxicity
cis-Platinum	Renal toxicity Hemolytic anemia Ototoxicity
Procarbazine (Matulane)	Dermatitis Myalgias Arthralgias
Dimethyl-triozeno-imidazole-carboxamide (DTIC)	Influenza-like syndrome

whether the patient is receiving anticoagulants or drugs that impair platelet function. It is also important to seek information by means of the history and physical examination relating to possible underlying disease such as leukemia, uremia, and hepatic disease, since they affect the hemostatic process in well-defined ways.

Further information may be obtained from the type of bleeding (Table 13.10). Most petechiae are due to thrombocytopenia. Widespread ecchymoses with hematuria and melena are common in patients with acquired coagulation defects such as defects resulting from sodium warfarin (Coumadin) or heparin excess and disseminated intravascular coagulation. In contrast, hemarthrosis and soft-tissue bleeding are characteristic of congenital coagulation defects such as hemophilia.

Laboratory Tests

The platelet count, bleeding time, PT, and PTT are an excellent set of screening tests for the bleeding patient. If results are normal, it is extremely unlikely that bleeding can be attributed to a coagulation defect.

Platelet Count. In most hospitals, platelet determinations are performed by direct count with a phase-contrast microscope or on an electronic counter. The normal count is 150,000–350,000 platelets/mm^3. Bleeding due to thrombocytopenia is unusual if the value is more than 70,000–90,000 platelets/mm^3. If a platelet count is not immediately available, a good estimate can be obtained from the blood smear; the oil immersion field normally contains 10–30 platelets, and significant thrombocytopenia can easily be detected.

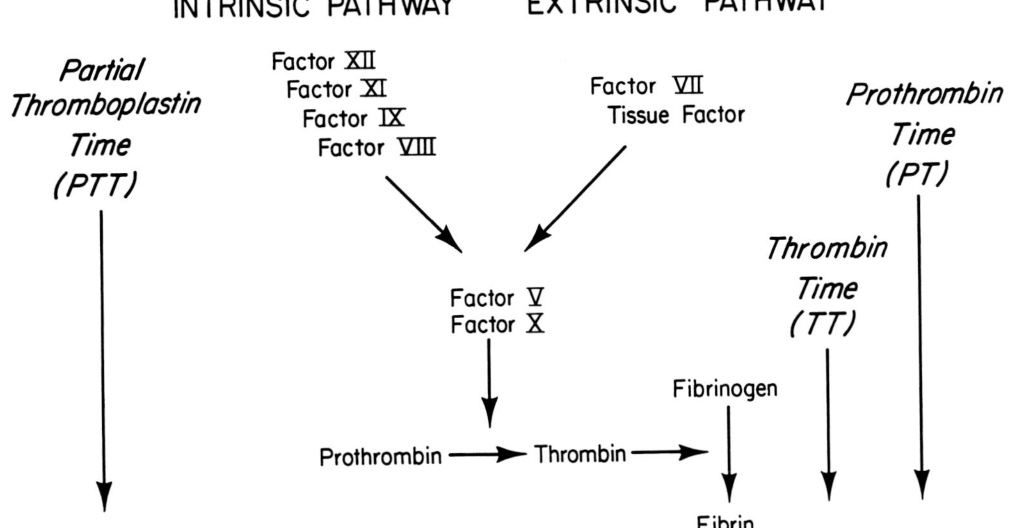

Figure 13.5. Coagulation cascade, which involves sequential interaction of coagulation factors with generation of fibrin. Both the intrinsic pathway, monitored by partial thromboplastin time, and the extrinsic pathway, monitored by prothrombin time, operative in vivo.

Bleeding Time. It is necessary to have not only adequate numbers of platelets but also platelets that function normally. Platelet function can be determined by measuring the bleeding time with Ivy's method: 40 mm Hg of pressure is maintained on the arm with a blood pressure cuff, and an incision 1 cm long and 1 mm deep is made on the volar surface of the forearm. The edge of the incision is gently blotted with filter paper at 30-second intervals. Bleeding for longer than 9–10 minutes suggests a disorder of platelet number or function. The bleeding time can be made more reproducible and accurate through use of a commercially available spring-activated bleeding time device (Fig. 13.6). The bleeding time is not influenced by anticoagulation with sodium warfarin or by coagulation factor deficiencies with the exception of von Willebrand's disease.

Table 13.10.
Signs of a Bleeding Diathesis

Diffuse petechiae or ecchymoses
Spontaneous bleeding from mucous membranes of the mouth, rectum, vagina, nose, and conjunctivae.
Spontaneous development of a hemarthrosis or hematomas
Multisystem bleeding: e.g., melena and hematuria
Profuse or prolonged bleeding after minor injury
Delayed bleeding several hours after surgery or trauma

Prothrombin Time. Tissue thromboplastin (whole brain extract) is added to plasma, and the time required for clotting is measured; the normal range is 11–13 seconds. The PT tests the integrity of the extrinsic system and is routinely used to monitor oral anticoagulant therapy with coumarin derivatives.

Partial Thromboplastin Time. This test monitors the intrinsic system and is performed in a similar manner to the PT except that an "incomplete" thromboplastin such as cephalin is substituted for whole brain extract. A surface-active agent such as kaolin is added to ensure complete activation of the contact factors (XII and XI). The normal PTT ranges from 25 to 40 seconds, depending on the technique employed. The PTT becomes prolonged when a factor in the intrinsic or common portion of the pathway is less than 25%.

Specific Factor Assay. A sample of the patient's plasma is mixed with plasma from a congenitally deficient individual with zero factor activity. The clotting time of the mixture allows determination of the amount of the coagulation factor in the patient's plasma. Pooled plasma from a large number of healthy persons is used to define 100% activity. However, there is considerable variation of factor levels in healthy individuals, and the normal range for each factor is approximately 50–150%.

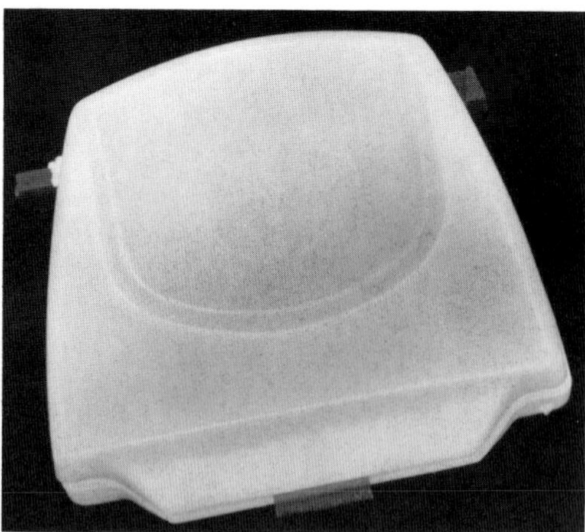

Figure 13.6. Bleeding-time kits that make the test more accurate and reproducible are now commercially available (Simplate, General Diagnostics Co.).

Normal Plasma Mix. This test determines whether abnormal results of a coagulation test are due to deficiency of a coagulation factor or are due to a circulating anticoagulant such as heparin or an antibody to a coagulation factor. A 1:1 mixture of the patient's plasma and normal plasma is made, and a PT, PTT, or specific factor assay is then performed. The 50% concentration of normal plasma in the mixture is adequate to correct for any factor deficiencies in the patient's plasma. Alternatively, if a circulating anticoagulant is present, the coagulation test will remain prolonged despite the addition of normal plasma.

Thrombin Time. A standardized amount of commercial thrombin is added to the patient's plasma. This test examines only the terminal portion of the coagulation cascade. The clotting time is usually about 20 seconds, depending on the technique. Prolonged thrombin times occur in severe hypofibrinogenemia, in the presence of heparin, and in the presence of large amounts of fibrin degradation products, such as occurs with the use of streptokinase or tissue plasminogen activator. The rare disorders in which fibrinogen fails to function normally (dysfibrinogenemia) are also characterized by a prolonged thrombin time. The thrombin time is not influenced by coumarin anticoagulants.

Fibrin Degradation Products. Increased amounts of fibrin degradation products (also called fibrin split products) occur in conditions in which there is excessive activation of the fibrinolytic system with digestion of fibrin. Increased concentrations of these substances are the hallmark of disseminated intravascular coagulation and primary fibrinolysis. Several methods are available for determination of the fibrin degradation products, including rapid, accurate slide agglutination techniques.

Fibrinogen Level. Fibrinogen can be determined quantitatively by several techniques that measure the fibrin clot directly, or it can be estimated less accurately by tests such as the thrombin time.

Fibrin Stabilizing Factor (Factor XIII). Factor XIII deficiency, a rare disorder associated with delayed bleeding, is detected by determining the stability of the clot in either a 1% solution of monochloroacetic acid or a 5 M solution of urea for 2 hours. Premature dissolution of the clot indicates Factor XIII deficiency.

Vascular Purpura

If results of coagulation tests are normal, the bleeding patient may have a vascular defect. These are usually associated with underlying systemic illnesses (Table 13.11). Careful examination of the skin is necessary to note the pathognomonic findings of telangiectases in Osler-Weber-Rendu disease, palpable petechiae in Henoch-Schönlein purpura, and corkscrew hairs in scurvy, as examples of the more common types of vascular purpura.

Thrombocytopenia

The risk of bleeding increases in patients with fewer than 70,000–80,000 platelets/mm^3, and spontaneous hemorrhage is common with fewer than 30,000 platelets/mm^3. In patients with fewer than 10,000 platelets/mm^3, life-threatening hemorrhage is frequent.

Classification

In evaluating thrombocytopenia, the physician must distinguish between impaired production of

Table 13.11.
Classification of Vascular Purpura According to Defect

- Vascular defects
  - Henoch-Schönlein purpura
  - Infection
    - Bacterial endocarditis
    - Rocky Mountain spotted fever
  - Nonthrombocytopenic drug purpura
  - Hereditary hemorrhagic telangiectasia (Osler-Weber-Rendu disease)
- Extravascular defects
  - "Senile" purpura
  - Ehlers-Danlos syndrome
  - Marfan's syndrome
  - Cushing's syndrome
  - Scurvy
- Unclassified
  - Dysglobulinemic purpura
  - Purpura simplex
  - "Autoerythrocyte sensitization"

Table 13.12.
Causes of Thrombocytopenia

Decreased platelet production
Bone marrow replacement
Neoplastic disease
Leukemia
Megaloblastic anemia
Marrow injury from drugs, radiation, or chemicals
Aplastic anemia
Advanced uremia
Acute alcohol ingestion
Severe sepsis
Drug toxicity
Abnormal distribution
Splenomegaly
Dilution
Transfusion with large amounts of thrombocytopenic blood and colloid
Increased platelet destruction
Purpura after viral infection
Drug-induced purpura
Idiopathic thrombocytopenic purpura
Secondary immunologic purpura: e.g., lymphoma
Purpura after transfusion
Nonimmune platelet consumption
Disseminated intravascular coagulation
Thrombotic thrombocytopenic purpura

platelets by the bone marrow and accelerated peripheral sequestration or destruction of platelets. A classification of the causes of thrombocytopenia according to this distinction is provided in Table 13.12.

Bone marrow examination is important in the evaluation of thrombocytopenia. When thrombocytopenia is due to *decreased marrow production* of platelets, the bone marrow usually shows hypoplasia, infiltration with malignant cells or granuloma, fibrosis, or megaloblastic changes. In cases of excessive peripheral destruction of platelets, the bone marrow usually appears normal and contains normal or increased numbers of megakaryocytes. The megakaryocytes characteristically appear young—nonbudding and with few nuclear segments. In such cases the blood smear usually shows the platelets to be large, often as large as red blood cells, reflecting the increased production rate of young platelets, which are larger than platelets that have circulated for a few days.

The response to transfusion with 8–10 units of platelets may be helpful in distinguishing the two mechanisms of thrombocytopenia. In patients with thrombocytopenia due to excessive peripheral destruction of platelets, little or no increase in the platelet count is evident 2–3 hours after transfusion. In patients with impaired marrow production of platelets, however, an increase of approximately 10,000 platelets/mm^3 for each transfused unit may be expected in the absence of brisk bleeding, high fever, or prior sensitization to platelet antigens by multiple transfusions or pregnancy.

Increased peripheral destruction of platelets can be divided into two categories: *immune* and *nonimmune.* The most frequent cause of nonimmune peripheral thrombocytopenia is hypersplenism. The spleen normally acts as a reservoir for approximately one-third of the peripheral platelet pool, but with splenomegaly this proportion may increase to 75 or 80%. Abrupt thrombocytopenia due to traumatic injury to platelets occurs after extracorporeal circulation in cardiac operations. Thrombocytopenia is also frequently encountered as a result of severe bleeding followed by massive blood transfusion with products that are relatively platelet poor. This cause of thrombocytopenia can be corrected by platelet transfusion. Thrombocytopenia is also characteristic of disseminated intravascular coagulation and of thrombotic thrombocytopenic purpura, a rare illness in which the patient has microangiopathic hemolytic anemia, fever, renal failure, and neurologic symptoms.

If thrombocytopenia appears to be immune, a careful search should be made for an underlying cause such as a drug, systemic lupus erythematosus, or a lymphoproliferative disease. Thrombocytopenia after a viral illness is common in children and is usually self-limited. If no underlying cause is apparent, the illness is considered idiopathic.

Among the causes of immune thrombocytopenia, it is important to consider that drug-induced thrombocytopenia can occur even after years of symptom-free use of a drug. Although certain drugs such as quinine, quinidine, and sulfonamide derivatives are the most common offending agents, any drug may be implicated. In a patient with thrombocytopenia without a clear-cut cause, all current medications should be omitted. If the thrombocytopenia is drug-induced, it should disappear within 2 weeks after withdrawal of the drug. However, the patient may maintain a life-long susceptibility to recurrence of thrombocytopenia with use of the same drug.

Post-transfusion purpura is extremely rare and occurs almost exclusively in women. Thrombocytopenia develops about 1 week after blood transfusion. This entity may easily be confused with idiopathic thrombocytopenic purpura, and the diagnosis depends on the temporal relation to transfusion and demonstration of a unique antibody to platelet antigen. Exchange transfusion has been proposed as a means of treating the thrombocytopenia.

Prolonged heparin administration has been associated with thrombocytopenia through both immunologic and nonimmunologic mechanisms. Patients receiving heparin should have periodic platelet counts determined, and the heparin may need to be discontinued in the presence of a falling count.

Table 13.13.
Drugs That Inhibit Platelet Function and Potentially Prolong Bleeding Time

Aspirin and other non-steroidal anti-inflammatory agents[a]	Dextran
Naprosyn	Anticoagulants
Motrin	Heparin (high concentrations inhibit collagen-induced aggregation)
Phenylbutazone	Androgens
Sulfinpyrazone	Phenformin hydrochloride (DBI)
Phenothiazines[a]	Clofibrate (Atromid-S)
Chlorpromazine	Sympathetic blocking agents
Promethazine hydrochloride	Phentolamine
Tricyclic antidepressants[a]	Dihydroergotamine
Imipramine hydrochloride (Tofranil)	Dibenzylchlorethamine (Dibenamine)
Amitriptyline hydrochloride (Elavil)	Phenoxybenzamine hydrochloride (Dibenzyline)
Desipramine hydrochloride (Norpramin)	Propranolol
Nortriptyline hydrochloride (Aventyl)	Colchicine
Antihistamines[a]	Vinca alkaloids
Diphenhydramine hydrochloride (Benadryl)	Vinblastine sulfate (Velban)
Chlordiazepoxide hydrochloride (Librium)	Vincristine
Diazepam (Valium)	Glyceryl guaiacolate
Flurazepam hydrochloride (Dalmane)	Monoamine oxidase inhibitors
Dipyridamole (Persantine)	Nialamide
Methylxanthines	Diuretics
Caffeine	Ethacrynic acid
Theobromine	Nitrofurantoin (Furadantin)
Aminophylline (high doses)	Carbenicillin
Local anesthetics	
Cocaine	
Procaine	
Lidocaine (Xylocaine)	
Dibucaine (Nupercaine)	

[a] Major offenders that commonly prolong the bleeding time test.

Therapy

General Measures. Avoidance of trauma, especially to the head, is important. All intramuscular injections and any medications, such as salicylates, that interfere with platelet function should be avoided. Straining at bowel movements should be prevented by liberal use of stool softeners and laxatives. Platelet transfusions may be of great value in patients with thrombocytopenia due to decreased marrow production of platelets; platelet transfusions are unlikely to be of more than transient value when the cause is hypersplenism, disseminated intravascular coagulation, or immune peripheral destruction. However, in the patient with significant bleeding, large numbers of platelet transfusions may be of some benefit despite the short survival time of the transfused platelets. If chronic thrombocytopenia is likely, as in aplastic anemia, persons matched for HL-A antigen are the most suitable platelet donors, and platelet transfusion may be feasible for a long period without development of sensitization to the transfused platelets.

Corticosteroids. High-dose corticosteroid therapy—usually prednisone, 1 mg/kg—is generally effective in raising the platelet count (within 7–10 days) in patients with *immune thrombocytopenic purpura*. Unfortunately, many patients relapse as the dosage is tapered, and splenectomy then becomes necessary.

Splenectomy. If life-threatening bleeding develops before corticosteroids have become effective, emergency *splenectomy* is indicated. Approximately three-fourths of patients respond well to splenectomy, and the platelet count improves substantially within 24 hours of operation in most of these patients. Once the splenic pedicle has been clamped, transfused platelets can be expected to have a relatively normal survival time and can be administered to support the patient during operation. Platelet transfusion may also be of benefit before splenectomy for the patient with severe bleeding despite the very short survival of the infused platelets in immune thrombocytopenia.

Platelet Dysfunction

Despite adequate numbers of platelets, a bleeding diathesis may develop if the platelets fail to function properly. In recent years, several congenital platelet disorders have been delineated that usually cause mild to moderate bleeding syndromes characterized by easy bruising, menorrhagia, and excessive bleeding after operation. Many drugs impair platelet aggregation (Table 13.13), and with some, such as aspirin, the defect is present for the life of the platelet. Significant bleeding due to the antiplatelet

Table 13.14.
Congenital Disorders of Blood Coagulation Factors

Factor	Inheritance	Sex Distribution	Frequency	Comments
XII (Hageman)	Recessive	Male Female	$1/10^6$	No bleeding disorder
XI	Recessive	Male Female	$1/10^6$	Often mild and not discovered until adulthood
IX Christmas disease Hemophilia B	Sex-linked	Male	$10/10^6$	Frequently severe
VIII				
Hemophilia A	Sex-linked	Male	$60–80/10^6$	Frequently severe
von Willebrand's disease	Dominant	Male Female	$60–80/10^6$	Also has a platelet defect manifested by prolonged bleeding time, decreasing platelet adhesiveness, and abnormal aggregation to ristocetin
X	Recessive	Male Female	$1/10^6$	Usually mild Acquired variety with amyloidosis
V	Recessive	Male Female	$1/10^6$	Usually mild to moderately severe
VII	Recessive	Male Female	$1/10^6$	Usually mild to moderately severe
II (prothrombin)	Recessive	Male Female	Rare	Moderately severe
I (fibrinogen)	Recessive	Male Female	Rare	Usually severe

effect of drugs is unusual, but cannot be ignored if the bleeding time is prolonged and results of other coagulation tests are normal. In this situation, more sophisticated tests of platelet function such as use of platelet aggregometry may confirm the defect. Transfusion with 8–10 units of normal platelets corrects the prolonged bleeding time. Advanced uremia and dysproteinemia also cause acquired platelet dysfunction. Uremic patients require dialysis to correct the platelet functional defect.

Thrombocytosis

Considerable increase in the platelet count is associated with both thrombosis and hemorrhage. The risk of complications becomes great when the count exceeds 2–3 million platelets/mm^3. Thrombocytosis may be due to a primary myeloproliferative disease, or it may result from several other disorders, including hemorrhage, iron deficiency, a malignant process, arthritis, and infection. Complications due to thrombocytosis are more commonly associated with the myeloproliferative disorders. Treatment is not well-established. If the increased platelet count is directly associated with a hemorrhagic or thrombotic complication, it may rapidly be decreased by thrombocytopheresis. After thrombocytopheresis, nitrogen mustard, 10 mg/m^2, should be administered intravenously. If the need for reducing the platelet count is less urgent, nitrogen mustard or an oral alkylating agent such as busulfan (Myleran), 6–8 mg/day, may be administered without thrombocytopheresis. Heparin, aspirin, and dipyridamole have been used as prophylactic agents against thrombosis, but may aggravate hemorrhage. Splenectomy may severely accentuate thrombocytosis and should be performed only after careful consideration in a patient with significant thrombocytosis.

Congenital Coagulation Factor Deficiencies

Table 13.14 lists the features of the congenital coagulation factor disorders. With the exception of hemophilia and Christmas disease, which are sex-linked, and von Willebrand's disease, which is inherited as a dominant trait, the congenital coagulation deficiency states are inherited as autosomal recessive traits and are extremely uncommon. Since the coagulation factors are required for generation of the fibrin that supports the primary platelet plug, deficiencies in any of the coagulation factors may be expected to lead to development of a fragile clot. Delayed bleeding after trauma is characteristic of coagulation factor deficiencies. The severity of the disorder depends on the amount of the coagulation factor present. The normal range for each coagulation factor is approximately 50–150%. Levels of

0–2% are associated with severe disease and are characterized by spontaneous bleeding into joints and soft-tissue spaces and severe hemorrhage after trauma. Persons with levels from 3 to 5% have moderate disease with less frequent episodes of spontaneous bleeding, and persons with levels more than 5% often have mild disease that may not be detected until operation.

Therapy

Local measures such as *immobilization* and application of *cold compresses* to a joint with hemarthrosis are important. Persons with congenital coagulation factor deficiencies should avoid drugs that impair platelet function, since they may exacerbate the tendency to bleed. The major form of therapy, however, is replacement of adequate amounts of the deficient factor.

Concentrates of plasma coagulation factors are available for the major congenital coagulation deficiencies, allowing replacement therapy without the risk of volume overload. The intensity of replacement therapy depends on the severity of the deficiency and the site of bleeding. For example, spontaneous bleeding into a joint in a hemophiliac patient can usually be managed on an outpatient basis with a single large infusion of Factor VIII concentrate, which corrects the factor deficiency for several hours. Bleeding into vital organs or into soft-tissue spaces that threatens to cause nerve compression or other serious damage, trauma to the head, and major surgical procedures require vigorous replacement therapy to maintain the factor level at more than 30% (the level at which the PTT is normalized) for 7–10 days.

Calculation of Replacement Therapy. Replacement therapy is calculated in terms of the "unit," which represents the amount of coagulation factor in 1 ml of normal plasma. The number of units administered depends on the patient's size, the half-life of the infused factor in the circulation, and the distribution between intravascular and extravascular compartments. Pertinent data on replacement therapy for major bleeding episodes are given in Table 13.15. In each case it is imperative to test the adequacy of replacement therapy by ascertaining that the specific factor assay increases to the appropriate level or that the screening test—such as PTT in hemophilia A, von Willebrand's disease, Christmas disease, and Factor XI deficiency—remains corrected at all times.

Hemophilia. Two forms of Factor VIII concentrate are available. When frozen plasma is thawed at 4°C, the fibrinogen precipitates as a sludge containing much of Factor VIII. When this cryoprecipitate is removed, the Factor VIII of a unit of plasma can be concentrated into a volume of 10–15 ml. The major disadvantage of the cryoprecipitate is that the amount of Factor VIII may vary greatly, leading to difficulty in accurate replacement therapy. In addition, cryoprecipitate must be preserved at −40°C. The second source of Factor VIII for replacement therapy, glycine precipitate, is assayed by the manufacturer, and the number of units of Factor VIII is printed on the container. This preparation is usually more expensive.

Different clinical situations require different levels of circulating Factor VIII.

1. Minor episodes such as spontaneous hemarthrosis usually respond to a single large infusion, which maintains the level of Factor VIII above 30% for 12 hours and above 5% for 36–48 hours.
2. Moderate bleeding or bleeding after minor trauma requires Factor VIII replacement until it is clear that bleeding has stopped.
3. Major surgical procedures and significant trauma require full, therapeutic doses for 7–10 days.

A new approach to the treatment of bleeding in patients with *mild* hemophilia and von Willebrand's disease is the use of the vasopressin analogue, desmopressin (DDAVP, Stimate), which stimulates release of factor VIII material as well as the fibrinolytic system. Desmopressin is administered as an intravenous infusion at a dose of 0.3 μg/kg diluted in 50 ml normal saline infused slowly over 15–30 minutes. Nausea, headache, abdominal cramps, facial flushing, and transient hypertension are relatively uncommon complications. ϵ-Aminocaproic acid (Amicar) is often used in conjunction with desmopressin in order to inhibit the fibrinolytic system.

Inhibitors of Factor VIII. In a small percentage of patients with severe hemophilia and occasionally in patients with mild disease, specific antibodies against Factor VIII develop, leading to resistance to Factor VIII infusions. This is detected either by failure of the PTT or Factor VIII assay to return to normal after replacement therapy or by development of a progressively larger requirement for Factor VIII. Specific assays to quantitate the level of inhibitor are available.

Development of an inhibitor severely complicates management. The traditional approach has been to try to overwhelm the inhibitor by administering enough Factor VIII to saturate all inhibitor molecules. This massive amount of Factor VIII is usually administered along with immunosuppressive agents such as cyclophosphamide and corticosteroids to prevent a further anamnestic increase in the amount of inhibitor. The higher the titer of the inhibitor, the less likely it is that this form of therapy will be successful. A new approach involves the administration of commercially prepared prothrombin concentrate (Factors II, VII, IX, and X) (autoplex) which contains activated coagulation factors able to

Table 13.15.
Replacement Therapy

Deficiency	Replacement	Initial Dosage/ kg Body Weight	Maintenance Dosage/ kg/day	Metabolic Half-life
				hr
Factor II (prothrombin)	Plasma	20 units twice a day	15–20 units	50–80
	Prothrombin concentrate	40 units	15–20 units	
Factor V	Fresh-frozen plasma	15–25 units	15–20 units	24
Factor VII	Plasma	5–10 units	5 units four times a day	5
	Prothrombin concentrate	5–10 units	5 units four times a day	
Factor VIII				
Hemophilia A	Cryoprecipitate	1 bag/2–4 kg	1 bag/4–8 kg twice a day	12
	Glycine precipitate	40 units	20 units twice a day	
	Desmopressin (DDAVD)[a]	0.3 μgm/kg in 50 ml saline over 15–30 minutes	0.3 μgm/kg in 50 ml saline over 15–30 minutes	
von Willebrand's disease	Plasma	10 units	10 units	24
	Cryoprecipitate	1 bag/10 kg	1 bag10 kg	
	Desmopressin (DDAVP)	0.3 μgm/kg in 50 ml saline over 15–30 minutes	0.3 μgm/kg in 50 ml saline over 15–30 minutes	
Factor IX				
Christmas disease	Plasma	30–60 units	5–10 units twice a day	20–30
	Prothrombin concentrate	30–60 units	5–10 units twice a day	
Factor X	Plasma	10–15 units	10 units	20–60
	Prothrombin concentrate	10–15 units	10 units	
Factor XI	Plasma	10–20 units	5 units	40–80
	Prothrombin concentrate	20 units	10 units	

[a] For mild cases.

''bypass'' the inhibitor. Several promising reports have appeared regarding this approach in patients with high titers of inhibitor, but complications such as thrombosis, disseminated intravascular coagulation, and a high incidence of hepatitis have also been reported. The risk of thrombosis or disseminated intravascular coagulation appears particularly high in patients with hepatic disease, and prothrombin concentrate should be used in this condition only when the patient has life-threatening bleeding. Since prothrombin concentrate contains prothrombin, thrombin can appear spontaneously during transit or storage. It is therefore important to perform the preinfusion stability check as outlined in the package insert. To decrease the risk of thrombotic complications further, 5 units of heparin should be added for each milliliter of reconstituted material. This amount of heparin does not prolong the clotting time after infusion. The patient's condition should be monitored during infusion to detect intravascular clotting, and infusion should be stopped promptly if any signs of this occur.

von Willebrand's Disease. A mild to moderately severe bleeding disorder, von Willebrand's disease is characterized by deficiency of Factor VIII and a prolonged bleeding time. The severity of the condition often fluctuates. Platelet aggregation is normal with the standard aggregating reagents such as adenosine diphosphate and epinephrine, but is decreased with ristocetin; platelet adhesiveness is also decreased. In contrast with hemophilia A, von Willebrand's disease is inherited as an autosomal dominant trait, and is thus found in both females and males. Recent investigations have demonstrated that Factor VIII antigenic material is present in normal amounts in hemophilia A, but is functionally

Table 13.16.
Conditions Associated with Disseminated Intravascular Coagulation

Sepsis, especially Gram-negative bacteremia
Malignant disease, especially prostatic carcinoma and acute promyelocytic leukemia
Obstetric complication
Brain injury
Burns
Hemolytic transfusion reaction
Fat embolism
Severe hepatic disease
Extensive operation involving prolonged hypotension
Purpura fulminans
Microangiopathic hemolytic anemia
Thrombotic thrombocytopenic purpura

inactive. In contrast, in von Willebrand's disease the amount of Factor VIII antigenic material is decreased in proportion with the decline in Factor VIII functional activity. Patients with von Willebrand's disease appear to lack an early intermediary compound in Factor VIII synthesis that can be supplied to them in cryoprecipitate or plasma, including plasma from a patient with hemophilia A. As a result, these patients have an increase in Factor VIII after transfusion that is larger than would be predicted from the amount of Factor VIII infused. Plasma and cryoprecipitate lead to correction of both the Factor VIII deficiency and the bleeding time, but glycine precipitate does not lead to correction of the latter. Because of this, plasma or cryoprecipitate is recommended (Table 13.15).

As previously mentioned in the section on hemophilia, desmopressin commonly corrects the hemostatic defect in von Willebrand's disease without the need to resort to cryoprecipitate. In a rare form of von Willebrand's disease, Type IIB, there may be platelet aggregation resulting in thrombocytopenia following desmopressin infusion. If a patient is known to have type IIB von Willebrand's disease, desmopressin should be avoided and cryoprecipitate is the agent of choice to correct the factor VIII level and prolonged bleeding time.

Christmas Disease (Hemophilia B). Deficiency of Factor IX shows striking similarities to hemophilia A in terms of clinical manifestations and replacement therapy. Factor IX equilibrates with the extravascular compartment to a greater extent than Factor VIII, necessitating a larger initial infusion. This is counterbalanced by the longer metabolic half-life of Factor IX. Factor IX deficiency can be corrected by plasma infusion (often requiring simultaneous diuretic administration) or prothrombin concentrate (Table 13.15). Because of the potential complications associated with prothrombin concentrate, this material should be reserved for major bleeding episodes.

Factor XI Deficiency. This deficiency can usually be corrected with infusion of plasma (Table 13.15). Potential volume overload can be managed with diuretics. Prothrombin concentrate is frequently contaminated with Factor XI and may be useful for the patient with large plasma requirements. Before administration, the prothrombin concentrate should be assayed to determine its Factor XI content.

Disseminated Intravascular Coagulation

This is a paradoxical disorder involving both abnormal clotting and bleeding. Disseminated intravascular coagulation results from aberrant activation of the coagulation cascade, leading to depletion of coagulation factors and platelets. The fibrinolytic system is activated secondarily, and as a consequence, hemostasis is compromised further because of lysis of fibrin, fibrinogen, and Factors V and VIII, as well as elaboration of fibrin degradation products that impair fibrin polymerization and platelet aggregation. Table 13.16 lists the major clinical situations in which disseminated intravascular coagulation is encountered, and Table 13.17 lists criteria for diagnosis.

Disseminated intravascular coagulation may range

Table 13.17.
Criteria for Diagnosis of Disseminated Intravascular Coagulation and Primary Fibrinolysis

Finding	Disseminated Intravascular Coagulation	Primary Fibrinolysis
Thrombocytopenia	+	−
Prolonged prothrombin time	+	+
Prolonged partial thromboplastin time	+	+
Prolonged thrombin time	+	+
Hypofibrinogenemia	+	+
Elevation of level of fibrin degradation products	+	+ +
Depression of Factors V and VIII	Usually substantial	Usually moderate
Microangiopathic blood smear	±	−

in severity from an asymptomatic state to fulminant hemorrhage. Treatment emphasizing cure or palliation of the underlying disorder may be sufficient. Replacement therapy with platelets, fresh-frozen plasma, and a source of fibrinogen such as cryoprecipitate may improve hemostasis, although it may exacerbate thrombotic complications. Use of heparin remains controversial. Although heparin may frequently improve coagulation, its effect on survival appears to be negligible since patients tend to die from the underlying disorder. Heparin should probably be reserved for patients who have significant hemorrhage as a result of well-documented disseminated intravascular coagulation. In this instance, continuous intravenous infusion of heparin, 10,000–24,000 units/day, is indicated with monitoring of coagulation and adjustment of dosage. Signs of improvement include increase in fibrinogen and platelet levels, decrease in fibrin degradation products, and improvement in hemostasis. Fresh-frozen plasma should be administered along with the heparin to replace depleted coagulation factors. If bleeding appears to increase as a result of heparin, protamine sulfate should promptly be administered (see below).

Primary Fibrinolysis

This is a rare disorder that may be difficult to distinguish from disseminated intravascular coagulation. However, patients with primary fibrinolysis do not have thrombocytopenia or fragmented red blood cells on blood smears, and they have somewhat higher levels of Factors V and VIII. Primary fibrinolysis is much less common than disseminated intravascular coagulation and should only be considered in the setting of prostatic carcinoma or operation, severe hepatic disease, or a thoracic operation. In patients with well-established primary fibrinolysis, anti-fibrinolytic therapy may be started with ε-aminocaproic acid (EACA, Amicar), 4 gm initially followed by 1 gm/hr either intravenously or orally. EACA therapy has on rare occasion been associated with thrombotic complications, especially in patients with disseminated intravascular coagulation who have not received prior heparin therapy.

Circulating Anticoagulants

In addition to their occurrence in congenital coagulation disorders, circulating anticoagulants against Factors V, VIII, IX, and XI may occur spontaneously or associated with a collagen vascular disease. They are detected by finding that prolonged coagulation times and factor assays fail to be corrected when the plasma is mixed with an equal volume of normal plasma. Rarely, severe hemorrhage will require the type of measure discussed under "Inhibitors of Factor VIII."

Bleeding Associated with Massive Transfusion

Massive transfusion is characterized by transfusion of one-half or more of the patient's blood volume at one time or the entire blood volume within a 24-hour period. Bleeding in this situation is usually related to consumption of the coagulation factors and platelets and their dilution by transfused products. *Refrigerated blood is deficient in factors V and VIII.* Dilution of other coagulation factors can also occur if only packed red blood cells and crystalloid are utilized in large volume. The PT and PTT are both commonly prolonged in this situation. Hence, good prophylaxis is to infuse 1 unit of fresh-frozen plasma (FFP) for every 5–6 units of packed red blood cells. Dilutional thrombocytopenia is less common, but if present should be rapidly corrected by transfusion of 10 platelet packs.

ANTICOAGULATION

The decision to use anticoagulants involves consideration of the risks of hemorrhage versus the risks of thrombosis and embolism. In general, anticoagulants should not be administered to patients with active bleeding from the gastrointestinal, genitourinary, or pulmonary tracts; severe hypertension; a hemorrhagic diathesis; cerebrovascular hemorrhage; or pericarditis complicating acute myocardial infarction. Hemorrhage in a patient receiving anticoagulants should raise the suspicion that an occult pathologic process may have been uncovered as a result of anticoagulation, especially if the results of coagulation tests used to monitor the anticoagulation are in the therapeutic range.

Heparin

Heparin is the drug of choice for anticoagulation in the acute situation. A naturally occurring mucopolysaccharide derived principally from beef lung and hog intestine, heparin interferes with coagulation at several points in the coagulation cascade; among its effects are inhibition of the action of thrombin and inhibition of activated Factors XI, IX, and X. Sodium heparin is available in solutions containing 1,000, 5,000, 10,000, 20,000, and 40,000 USP units/ml. In most solutions, 1 mg of heparin contains approximately 150 units. Dosage should be prescribed in units rather than in milligrams.

Administration

Intravenous injection is the preferred route of administration. The initial dose is usually a bolus of 5,000–10,000 units, followed by either a continuous infusion of 500–2,000 units/hr by a pump or repeated injections of 5,000–10,000 units every 4–6 hours. Although the intermittent method is more convenient, recent studies have suggested that continuous infusion is associated with fewer hemorrhagic complications. Anticoagulation with heparin should be monitored by means of coagulation tests. The most commonly employed are the PTT, with a therapeutic range from 1.5 to 2.5 times the control value, and the Lee-White method for determination of clotting time, with a therapeutic range from 2 to 3 times the control value. If heparin is administered by continuous infusion, the coagulation test may be performed at any time; if administration is intermittent, blood should be drawn just before the next dose of heparin.

Toxicity

Hemorrhage is the major side effect, occurring in approximately 3–7% of patients in large series. Allergic reactions such as urticaria, conjunctivitis, bronchospasm, and hypotension are uncommon. Thrombocytopenia has recently been reported as a frequent complication of prolonged heparin infusion, and the platelet count should be monitored. Osteoporosis may occur after prolonged used.

Antidote

Heparin is rapidly metabolized in the liver and kidney. A heparin antagonist is necessary, therefore, only when anticoagulation must be reversed within 4 hours after a dose. Protamine sulfate is the agent of choice, completely reversing the effect of heparin within minutes. It is administered slowly in the course of 3–5 minutes in a solution of 2 mg/ml. Immediately after a dose of heparin is administered, the number of milligrams of protamine sulfate necessary to neutralize the heparin is equal to the heparin dose in milligrams, which is calculated by dividing the number of USP units in the heparin dose by 150. Protamine sulfate neutralizes more heparin units derived from hog intestine than from beef lung. Hence, knowledge of the source of the heparin is helpful for accurate neutralization. One hour after the dose of heparin has been administered, the amount of protamine sulfate should be decreased by half. The maximal amount safely administered is 100 mg. As a result of its highly basic charge, large amounts of protamine sulfate interfere with coagulation and may lead to a hemorrhagic diathesis.

Coumarin Derivatives

The coumarin derivatives, such as sodium warfarin (Coumadin) and bishydroxycoumarin (Dicumarol), antagonize vitamin K, resulting in depression of hepatic synthesis of prothrombin (Factor II) and Factors VII, IX, and X. After coumarin therapy is started, the individual factor activities decrease at varying rates; Factor VII is the first to decrease in activity because of the short half-life. As a result of the longer half-life of Factors X and II, it may take from 40 to 90 hours for amounts to decrease to therapeutic levels. Although coumarin therapy is monitored by the PT, it also leads to prolongation of the PTT.

Administration

Dosage is regulated by the PT. The therapeutic range of the PT should be established by each laboratory, but is usually 1.5–2.5 times the control value, which corresponds to 10–25% of control activity. Initiation of anticoagulation can be efficiently undertaken by administering 10 mg of sodium warfarin daily for 3 days, with further adjustment of anticoagulation by means of daily PT determination and sodium warfarin doses until a stable maintenance dose is established.

Toxicity

The major toxic reaction is hemorrhage. The principal drugs that interact with coumarin compounds are listed in Table 13.18. Coumadin crosses the placental barrier, and its use during pregnancy must be monitored carefully to prevent neonatal hemorrhage. Coumarin compounds are also teratogenic during the first trimester of pregnancy. Necrosis of subcutaneous fatty tissue (coumarin necrosis) is a rare complication occurring on the 3rd to 10th day of therapy. Coumarin skin necrosis may be particularly common in the rare group of individuals who have a congenital deficiency of protein C, a vitamin K-dependent inhibitor of the coagulation cascade. It is not related to excessive anticoagulation, and its mechanism is unclear. Other

Table 13.18.
Drugs That Interact with Coumarin Compounds

Potentiation of action
Indomethacin
Cimetidine
Sulfinpyrazone
Clofibrate
Quinidine, quinine
Salicylates
Sulfisoxazole
Tolbutamide, chlorpropamide
Phenytoin
Chloramphenicol
Cholestyramine
Dextrothyroxine
Retardation of action
Barbiturates
Ethanol
Oral contraceptives
Griseofulvin
Glutethimide
Rifampin

unusual reactions include rash, nausea, diarrhea, fever, jaundice, leukopenia or thrombocytopenia, and vasculitis.

Antidote

The effect of a coumarin derivative can be neutralized by administration of vitamin K. For moderate or severe bleeding, 10–25 mg may be given slowly intravenously. The PT may begin to be corrected within 1 hour, and is often within normal limits by 8 hours. A somewhat slower response occurs after intramuscular injection. For mild bleeding, 5–10 mg can be administered orally with correction expected within 12–24 hours.

Immediate correction of a prolonged PT due to a coumarin derivative can be achieved by infusion of 2–6 units of plasma along with vitamin K administration; this is often indicated for major hemorrhagic complications. Plasma infusion alone is also useful for partial correction of an excessively prolonged PT without interrupting anticoagulation with administration of vitamin K.

Elective Operation

The anticoagulant should be discontinued. After the PT decreases to less than 1.5 times the control value, operation can be performed. Therapy can be resumed after the procedure has been completed.

THROMBOLYTIC THERAPY FOR ACUTE PULMONARY EMBOLISM AND DEEP VENOUS THROMBOPHLEBITIS

A National Institutes of Health Consensus Conference in 1980 recommended thrombolytic therapy rather than heparin anticoagulation as the primary treatment for certain patients with deep venous thrombophlebitis and pulmonary embolism. Although heparin is effective in reducing the formation of venous clot and decreasing the likelihood of recurrent embolism, it does not dissolve the thrombus. In contrast, thrombolytic agents are able to lyse clot and potentially are able to alleviate the hemodynamic and vascular complications of thrombosis. Streptokinase (SK) and urokinase (UK) are two commercially available agents that induce thrombolytic activity by activating plasminogen with generation of the proteolytic enzyme plasmin. Both agents are expensive; since UK is several times more expensive than SK, it is recommended that the use of UK be restricted to individuals who have become sensitized to SK as a result of streptococcal infections or prior use of SK.

A major prospective, controlled study has investigated the use of SK in pulmonary embolism. Although a 24-hour infusion of SK was shown to result in more rapid lysis of embolic clot than heparin, ventilation perfusion scans were no different after 7 days and the mortality was no different between the heparin and SK-treated groups. Hence, the use of SK in pulmonary embolism probably should be limited to those patients with massive pulmonary embolism showing hemodynamic instability who would normally be candidates for pulmonary embolectomy.

In patients with deep vein thrombophlebitis, SK reduces the risk of pulmonary embolism to the same degree as heparin, but also helps to preserve venous valves and prevent the postphlebitic syndrome, particularly in the more serious cases involving the femoral or iliac veins. SK, therefore, can be recommended in any patient with deep thrombophlebitis involving the femoral or iliac veins which is less than 7 days old.

To limit the bleeding complications of SK, the drug should be administered only in an area where close monitoring and supervision are available. All invasive procedures should be avoided except carefully performed venipuncture. No anticoagulants or drugs which impair platelet function should be given concurrently with SK. Major contraindications to the use of SK include surgery less than 10 days ago, signs of recent trauma, ongoing menses, recent gastrointestinal bleeding, and intraarterial diagnostic procedure within the past 10 days (excluding uncomplicated arterial blood gas studies), cerebrovascular accident within the past 2 months, and severe hypertension. Some of these contraindications may be outweighed in patients with massive pulmonary emboli and hemodynamic instability.

A fixed dosage schedule of SK has been found to result in sufficient activation of plasminogen in 95% of patients. The initial loading dose of 250,000 units in normal saline is administered over 30 minutes followed by a constant infusion of 100,000 units/hr via an infusion pump. It is recommended that 4 hours after initiation of SK, and every 12 hours thereafter, a thrombin time and hematocrit be checked. A thrombin time test two to six times normal indicates an appropriate fibrinolytic state. If the thrombin time remains normal, or if it is greater than six times normal, one should seek consultation for dosage adjustment. The SK is continued for 24 hours for pulmonary embolism and 72 hours for phlebitis. Thrombolytic therapy should not be considered a substitute for anticoagulant therapy, and following completion of SK, anticoagulation is mandatory. Heparin, without a loading dose, is begun once the thrombin time is less than twice control, which is usually 2–4 hours after stopping the SK. This is followed by conventional coumadin therapy.

Mild allergic reactions occur in up to 15% of patients treated with SK, usually in the form of urticaria, pruritus, flushing, nausea, and headache.

Mild fever occurs in up to one-third of patients given SK. The most feared complication is bleeding which most often occurs at the sites of skin incisions and blood vessel punctures. Serious bleeding may be controlled by stopping the SK infusion, and the administration of fresh frozen plasma and/or the antifibrinolytic agent, EACA (Amicar), 4 gm over 1 hour followed by 1 gm/hr by continuous infusion.

A multicenter pilot study of recombinant tissue type plasminogen activator for the treatment of acute emboli is underway (1987).

SUGGESTED READINGS

Allgood JW, Chaplin H Jr. Idiopathic acquired autoimmune hemolytic anemia: A review of forty-seven cases treated from 1955 through 1965. *Am J Med,* 1967;43:254–273.

Bell WR, Meek AG. Guidelines for the use of thrombolytic agents. *N Engl J Med,* 1979;301:1266–1270.

Beutler E: Glucose-6-phosphate dehydrogenase deficiency. *Br J Haematol,* 1970;18:117–121.

Blatt PM, Lundblad RL, Kingdon HS, et al: Thrombogenic materials in prothrombin complex concentrates. *Ann Intern Med,* 1974;81:766–770.

Brody, JI, Goldsmith MH, Park SK, et al: Symptomatic crises of sickle cell anemia treated by limited exchange transfusion. *Ann Intern Med,* 1970;72:327–330.

Colman RW, Robboy SJ, Minna JD: Disseminated intravascular coagulation (DIC): An approach. *Am J Med,* 1972;52:679–689.

Corrigan JJ Jr, Jordan CM: Heparin therapy in septicemia with disseminated intravascular coagulation: Effect on mortality and on correction of hemostatic defects. *N Engl J. Med,* 1970;283:778–782.

Fairbanks VF, Fernandez MN: The identification of metabolic errors associated with anemia. *JAMA,* 1969;208:316–320.

Fillmore SJ, McDevitt E: Effects of coumarin compounds on the fetus. *Ann Intern Med,* 1970;73:731–735.

Fuente B, Kasper C, Rickles FR et al: Response of patients with mild and moderate hemophilia A and von Willebrand's disease to treatment with desmopressin. *Ann Intern Med,* 1985;103:6–14.

Grund FM, Armitage JO, Burns CP: Hydroxyurea in the prevention of the effects of leukostasis in acute leukemia. *Arch Intern Med,* 1977;137:1246–1247.

Harris JW, Kellermeyer RW: The Red Cell; Production, Metabolism, Destruction: Normal and Abnormal, revised ed. Cambridge: Harvard University Press, 1970.

Jacobson LB, Longstreth GF, Edgington TS: Clinical and immunologic features of transient cold agglutinin hemolytic anemia. *Am J Med,* 1973;54:514–521.

Kabins SA, Lerner C: Fulminant pneumococcemia and sickle cell anemia. *JAMA,* 1970;211:467–471.

Koch-Weser J. Coumarin necrosis, Editorial. *Ann Intern Med,* 1968;68:1365–1367.

Koch-Weser J, Sellers EM: Drug interactions with coumarin anticoagulants. *N Engl J Med,* 1971;285:487–498, 547–558.

Livio M, Mannucci PM, Vigano G et al: Conjugated estrogens for the management of bleeding associated with renal failure. *N Engl J Med,* 1986;315:731–735.

Ratnoff OD: Prothrombin complex preparations: A cautionary note [Editorial]. *Ann Intern Med,* 1974;81:852–853.

Salzman EW, Weinstein MJ, Weintraub RM et al: Treatment with desmopressin acetate to reduce blood loss after cardiac surgery. *N Engl J Med,* 1986;1402–1406.

Sherman LA: Therapeutic problems of disseminated intravascular coagulation. *Arch Intern Med,* 1973;132:446–453.

Solomon A, Fahey JL: Plasmapheresis therapy in macroglobulinemia. *Ann Intern Med,* 1963;58:789–800.

Sullivan LW. Differential diagnosis and management of the patient with megaloblastic anemia. *Am J Med,* 1970;48:609–617.

Wasserman LR: The management of polycythaemia vera. *Br J Haematol,* 1971;21:371–376.

Wessler S: Anticoagulant therapy—1974. *JAMA,* 1974;228:757–761.

Yankee RA, Grumet FC, Rogentine GN: Platelet transfusion therapy: The selection of compatible platelet donors for refractory patients by lymphocyte HL-A typing. *N Engl J Med,* 1969;281:1208–1212.

CHAPTER **14**

Metabolic and Endocrine Emergencies

GILBERT H. DANIELS, M.D.

The metabolic problems encountered in an emergency department encompass a broad spectrum of biophysiologic abnormalities. Any presentation of the subject is based on an arbitrary classification of the disease processes and endocrine organs involved. This discussion is divided into five components: (*a*) metabolic emergencies involving carbohydrate metabolism and ketoacidosis, (*b*) adrenal emergencies, (*c*) thyroid emergencies, (*d*) emergencies of hypercalcemia and hypocalcemia, and (*e*) a consideration of hyponatremia and hyperkalemia.

METABOLIC EMERGENCIES

Diabetic Ketoacidosis

Diabetic ketoacidosis was almost always fatal 50 years ago, but today, knowledge of the relevant pathophysiologic processes, combined with the availability of insulin, permits remarkably successful therapy. In most medical centers, the overall mortality due to diabetic ketoacidosis is less than 10%, and in uncomplicated series, mortality should be less than 2%.

Pathophysiologic Principles

The central role of insulin in normal intermediary metabolism is depicted in Figure 14.1, which schematically shows the three major target and storage tissues to be considered—the liver, muscle, and adipose tissue. Insulin serves as the "storage" (anabolic) hormone for glucose, amino acids, and free fatty acids, which are stored as glycogen, protein, and triglycerides, respectively.

A steady supply of *glucose* is mandatory for normal function of the central nervous system. The so-called counterregulatory hormones (for example, epinephrine, glucagon, growth hormone, and cortisol) maintain or elevate the blood glucose level to help ensure the supply. Insulin is the only major hormone that lowers the blood glucose level. This is accomplished in part by promoting storage of glucose as glycogen in the liver and inhibiting the de novo formation (gluconeogenesis) and release of glucose by this organ. Insulin also facilitates glucose transport into muscle and subsequent glycogen synthesis and stimulates passage of glucose into fat cells, where it is converted to glycerol phosphate and free fatty acids and then stored as triglycerides.

Transport of *amino acids* into muscle, their subsequent conversion into protein, and inhibition of degradation of these proteins also result from the action of insulin.

Free fatty acids, the major energy source of the body, are stored as triglycerides in the fat cells. Insulin facilitates transfer of these triglycerides from the plasma into the fat cells and prevents their breakdown (lipolysis) to free fatty acids and glycerol by inhibiting the enzyme responsible for such degradation. This enzyme is called the "hormone-sensitive lipase" because it is stimulated by many of the counterregulatory hormones.

Given these considerations, it is easy to perceive the ultimate consequence of insulin deficiency to be diabetic ketoacidosis. Diabetic ketoacidosis results from an absolute lack of insulin or from a relative lack associated with "stress" and increased concentrations of the counterregulatory hormones. The inhibition of lipolysis and glycogenolysis by insulin occurs at much lower insulin concentrations than stimulation of glucose transport and storage. Gluconeogenesis seems to have intermediate sensitivity to insulin. Although the effects of insulin deficiency on carbohydrate and lipid metabolism are complex and intertwined, for the purposes of discussion, they may be dissociated and considered separately (Fig. 14.2); clinically, these effects may be dissociated as well.

Carbohydrate Metabolism. Insulin deficiency, in conjunction with stress-related increases in the counterregulatory hormones, leads to marked hyperglycemia. Initially, increased glucose production is most important. This is due to increased conversion of hepatic glycogen to glucose (glycogenolysis), as well as to increased gluconeogenesis. Insulin deficiency stimulates hepatic glucose production by (*a*) increasing the activity of appropriate hepatic enzymes, (*b*) increasing hepatic extraction of appropriate substrates for glucose production (e.g. alanine from muscle), and (*c*) facilitating lipolysis in adipose tissue (yielding glycerol). In addition, insulin deficiency prevents the utilization of the increased glucose, by decreasing peripheral uptake, particularly in muscle cells.

Lipid Metabolism. With severe insulin deficiency, insulin restraint on lipolysis is lost and triglycerides in the fat cells are hydrolyzed to glycerol and free fatty acids. The free fatty acids are transported to the liver, where they are oxidized to acetyl coenzyme A and preferentially utilized for ketone body production. Acetoacetic acid and β-hydroxybutyric acid are the "ketone bodies" pro-

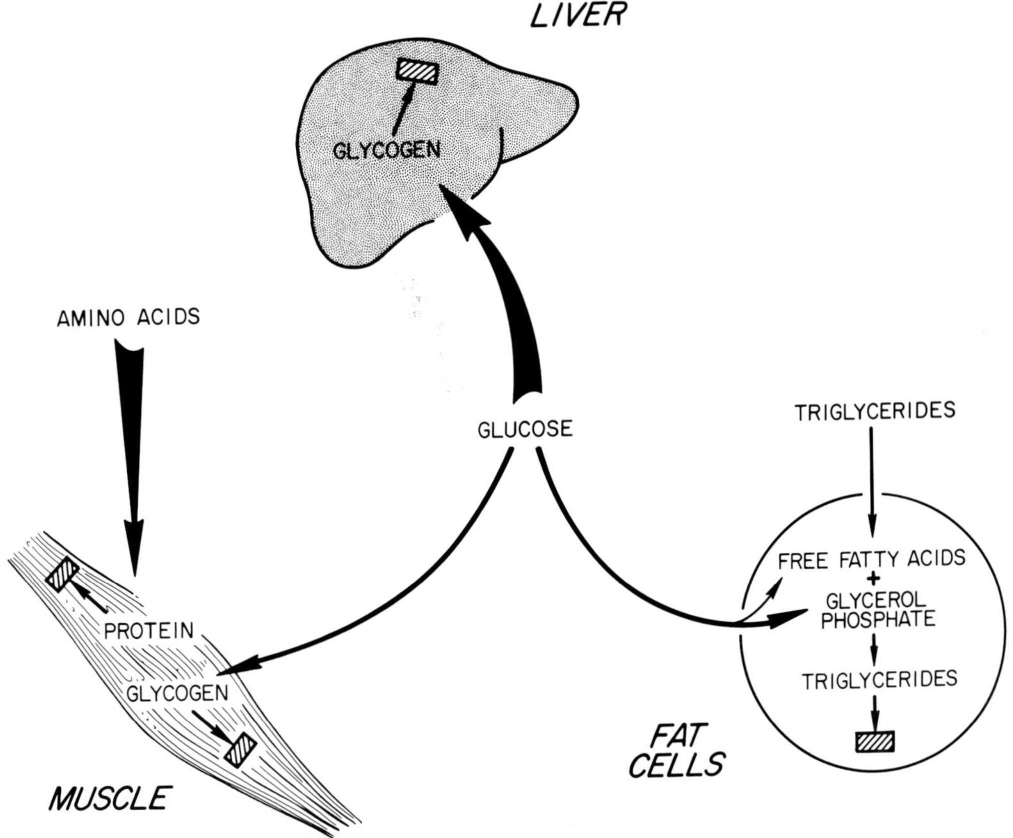

Figure 14.1. Effects of insulin

duced by the liver, acetone being generated from acetoacetic acid by nonenzymatic decarboxylation. The preferential shunting of free fatty acids to ketone body production is facilitated by glucagon excess. Released from the liver, the ketone bodies apparently overwhelm their usual disposal mechanism, namely, oxidation by muscle. It is likely that insulin is necessary for the normal peripheral utilization of ketone bodies.

Clinical Correlations. As the blood glucose level increases, so does the serum osmolality. Water moves out of the cells, and cellular dehydration can occur. As the capacity of the kidney for glucose reabsorption is exceeded, glycosuria develops. Osmotic diuresis results in the loss of water and electrolytes, more water being lost than sodium or potassium. Acetoacetic acid and β-hydroxybutyric acid are strong acids whose increased production results in metabolic acidosis. Excreted in the urine as sodium and potassium salts, these ketone bodies further exacerbate the electrolyte losses. The intravascular volume contraction leads to secondary hyperaldosteronism which exacerbates the potassium loss.

Diagnosis

Clinical Features. Diabetic ketoacidosis may develop during the course of known diabetes or may be the initial indication of disease. A history of the "three Ps" may be obtained from the patient or the patient's relatives or friends. An episode of *p*olyuria and *p*olydipsia of several days' duration consequent to loss of a large amount of glucose in the urine, as well as *p*olyphagia, can precede ketoacidosis. Unexplained recent weight loss is common in younger patients, reflecting both muscle and adipose tissue breakdown. A history of visual disturbances can be a clue to new onset diabetes or worsening control. Muscle cramps can occur, perhaps related to fluid and electrolyte losses.

Anorexia follows the development of ketosis; nausea and vomiting can occur, thereby exacerbating the dehydration. If the patient is ketotic and unable to maintain oral intake, he or she should be

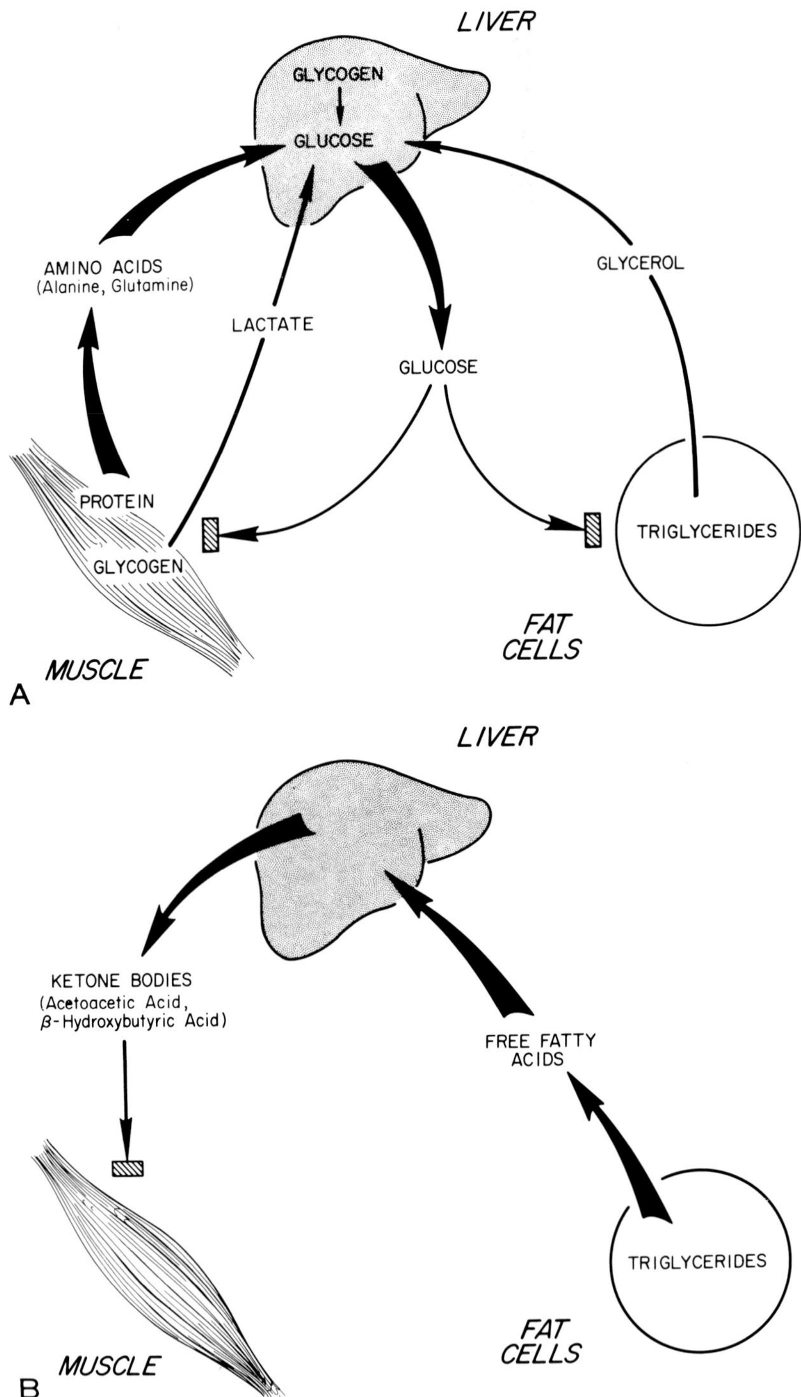

Figure 14.2. Effects of insulin deficiency on carbohydrate metabolism (A) and lipid metabolism (B).

hospitalized for intravenous fluid replacement even if frank acidosis has not yet developed. Although abdominal pain may occur related to ketoacidosis and abdominal tenderness is common, especially in children, in adults such symptoms should suggest an underlying precipitating event, such as pancreatitis or cholecystitis.

Whenever an acute abdominal emergency is suspected in a patient with diabetic ketoacidosis, the ketoacidosis should be vigorously treated for 3–4 hours. If the abdominal signs disappear, the metabolic derangement is the important clinical situation. If the abdominal findings persist, the patient will be better able to tolerate surgery after treating the ketoacidosis.

The patient's appearance is often dominated by signs of dehydration. The combination of dehydration and good urinary output should always suggest diabetic ketoacidosis. Dehydration may be mild, manifested by decrease in skin turgor or orbital resistance or absence of axillary sweat; moderate, with postural tachycardia or hypotension; or severe, resulting in frank shock. Despite hypotension, the skin often remains warm, flushed, and dry because of metabolic acidosis.

If the patient is febrile, infection must be assumed. However, hypothermia may be present in diabetic ketoacidosis even in the presence of serious infection. Deep, labored respiration (Kussmaul's respiration) is a consequence of metabolic acidosis that is usually evident when the pH of the arterial blood is between 7.0 and 7.24. With more profound degrees of acidosis, respirations may become shallow. The patient's breath may have a fruity ketone (acetone) odor, and the patient may be alert, lethargic, or, less commonly, comatose. Hypertonic dehydration leading to brain cell dehydration and ketosis itself are probably both contributory. It is important to remember that in all cases of coma, hypoglycemia should be considered and prophylactically treated.

Clinical Studies. A rigorous definition of diabetic ketoacidosis would include a blood glucose concentration over 250 mg/dl, serum ketones strongly positive in an undiluted serum specimen with an arterial pH less than 7.25, or a serum bicarbonate concentration less than 10 mEq/l. However, the attending physician can diagnose diabetic ketoacidosis within minutes with the aid of glucose oxidase strips (e.g., Dextrostix or Chemstrips) and nitroprusside reagent for serum ketones (e.g., Acetest tablets or acetone test). Therapy, thus, can commence before definitive laboratory confirmation has been made.

Several caveats are worth noting. Glucose oxidase strips are sensitive to heat, light, and moisture and should be kept fresh in a tightly closed container. Fluoride-containing tubes should not be used to collect blood for this test. The accuracy of the strips is enhanced with the aid of a reflectometer. The Acetest tablets should be crushed prior to use. Undiluted serum may interfere with the reagent and a dilution of serum should be used before concluding that serum ketones are negative. The nitroprusside reagents react to acetoacetate and less so to acetone (a nonacidic neutral compound). However, the dominant ketone body in the circulation is β-hydroxybutyrate and is not measured by this reagent. Reagent strips for ketones (e.g., Ketostix) should not be employed.

Although the initial blood glucose level may be less than 250 mg/dl and rarely less than 100 mg/dl in diabetic ketoacidosis, this situation almost always occurs in patients with known diabetes who have continued on a regimen of insulin. It has recently been recognized in patients on the ambulatory insulin pump as well. Thus, a blood glucose level less than 250 mg/dl does not exclude the possibility of diabetic ketoacidosis, but indicates that intravenous administration of glucose should be started immediately to permit administration of additional insulin without the hazard of hypoglycemia.

A strongly positive test for serum ketones can occur in alcoholic ketoacidosis as well. However, the blood glucose is usually less than 250 mg/dl in such patients. In alcoholic ketoacidosis, intravenous glucose is usually sufficient without concomitant insulin. However, whenever the distinction between alcoholic ketoacidosis and diabetic ketoacidosis is in doubt, with only slight elevation of the blood glucose, it is safer to administer both glucose and insulin.

The magnitude of serum ketone elevation is one important indication of the severity of the ketoacidosis. For determination of the serum ketone level, five crushed Acetest tablets should be placed separately on a sheet of filter paper. Serum from a centrifuged, clotted blood sample is then diluted serially with 2, 4, 8 and 16 parts of water or saline solution, and one or two drops of each dilution and of the undiluted serum are placed on the respective tablets. After 3 minutes, the color is determined. Deep purple represents a strong reaction, and the highest dilution at which a strong reaction is noted is the value recorded—a serum ketone test strongly positive at 1:8 dilution, for example. β-Hydroxybutyrate is not detected by this test.

Other immediate studies should include: measurement of blood glucose, sodium, potassium, chloride, bicarbonate, blood urea nitrogen, amylase, and arterial blood gas levels; a complete blood cell count; urinalysis; and an electrocardiogram. Appropriate specimens for culture, including blood, should be taken.

Therapy

The hallmarks of comprehensive therapy include an admission to an intensive care setting, individualization of treatment, and monitoring of the clinical and chemical progress of the patient so that appropriate adjustments can be made. A flow sheet

Table 14.1.
Diabetic Ketoacidosis: Treatment

Therapy	Dosage	Comments
Volume replacement	Moderate: 1 liter of normal saline intravenously over 30–60 min; 500–1000 ml/hr subsequently until central venous pressure increases or dehydration disappears Severe: Add plasma, albumin (Albumisol) to above	Usual fluid deficit: 5–7 liters Usual sodium deficit: 300–500 mEq Monitor central venous pressure if indicated Subsequent fluids should be hypotonic (0.45% saline)
Insulin (alternatives)[a]		
Constant intravenous infusion	50 units in 500 ml of normal saline, 100 ml/hr (10 units/hr); may give 10 units intravenous bolus	Discard first 10 ml If blood glucose does not respond in 1–2 hr, double the insulin dosage
Intramuscular insulin	15–20 units initially; 10 units/hr subsequently	Do not use in hypotensive patients If blood glucose does not respond in 1–2 hr, double the insulin dosage
Hourly intravenous insulin	10 units intravenous bolus each hour	If no response in 1–2 hr, double the insulin dosage or change to constant infusion
Bicarbonate	88–125 mEq intravenously over 1 hour; repeat as necessary	Indications: shock, pH < 7.1, serum bicarbonate < 5 mEq/liter
Potassium	Potassium chloride, 20–40 mEq/liter	Administer when serum potassium enters normal range if urinary output satisfactory Usual potassium deficit: 200–500 mEq
Glucose	5 or 10% dextrose intravenously in water or saline, depending on blood glucose level and volume status 50 ml of 50% dextrose for hypoglycemia	Indication: when blood glucose concentration decreases to 250 mg/dl, particularly with persistent ketosis.

[a] Use only regular insulin (e.g. crystalline zinc insulin (CZI)).

recording the patient's status, laboratory data, and therapy is indispensable.

Initial Adjunctive Therapy. At the outset of therapy, several simple measures should be considered. If the Po_2 is less than 80 mm Hg, administration of oxygen may increase tissue oxygenation, thereby improving mental status. In obtunded patients, an endotracheal tube may be needed. Gastric atony is a regular finding that often results in aspiration; a nasogastric tube should be passed and the stomach emptied. If the patient is alert, the nasogastric tube can then be removed, but in the obtunded patient, it should be left for further suctioning. The gastric contents can be black and viscous, and guaiac tests can be positive. A Foley catheter should not be placed initially; however, if the patient does not urinate after 2–4 hours, a catheter should be placed. In the obtunded, severely hypotensive patient, a Foley catheter may be necessary. Elderly patients and children with longstanding diabetes can require a central venous pressure line during fluid administration to avoid circulatory overload. Rarely, a pulmonary artery catheter will be necessary in patients with severe cardiac or pulmonary disease.

Specific Therapy. In the specific therapy for diabetic ketoacidosis (Table 14.1), administration of insulin alone is insufficient, even though insulin deficiency precipitated the metabolic and clinical abnormalities. In sequence, the patient must receive volume replacement, insulin, possibly bicarbonate, potassium, and glucose. In practice, both insulin and volume replacement must be started simultaneously as soon as the diagnosis is established.

Volume Replacement. The volume deficits are surprisingly large, averaging 10% of body weight or 6–8 liters of water, and from 300–500 mEq or more of sodium. Initial therapy is determined by the severity of the dehydration. For patients with frank shock or a minimal urine flow, plasma expanders are necessary. With moderate dehydration, normal saline is sufficient, the first liter given over 30 minutes. The subsequent choice of fluids remains controversial. However, preservation of intravascular volume seems to be of paramount importance. A second liter of normal saline can be given over 1 hour. Subsequent infusions should be either normal saline or half-normal saline (0.45%) at a rate of 500–1000 ml/hr, until the central venous pressure reaches 5–7 cm of water or the clinical signs of dehydration begin to disappear. When the patient is nearly adequately rehydrated, half-normal saline at 250 ml/hr can be administered. If the initial sodium concentration is greater than 150 mEq/liter or rises to 155 mEq/liter during therapy, half-normal saline should be substituted at that time. Extremes of hypo- and hypernatremia are to be avoided. In fully alert patients who are no longer nauseated, oral fluids can supplement intravenous infusion.

Insulin. Insulin therapy is critical in reversing the spiraling sequence of metabolic decompensation. However, much of the initial fall in blood glucose concentration is due to dilution of intravenous fluids. Only insulin will inhibit lipolysis and help correct ketosis. Insulin too is necessary to inhibit the ongoing gluconeogenesis. There is no "correct" amount of insulin and the optimal route of administration is still controversial. Only rapidly acting insulin [e.g., crystalline zinc insulin (CZI), Actrapid, or others] should be used. Although fears of "insulin resistance" in diabetic ketoacidosis led to the use of heroic doses of insulin in the past, it appears that "low" or "modest" dose intravenous insulin by infusion provides a simple, reliable means of controlling diabetic ketoacidosis. Although doses as low as 4 units/hour can control the situation there is no merit to picking the lowest possible dose and no harm in using somewhat higher doses.

An intravenous bolus of 10 units can be given, followed by an infusion of 0.15 units/kg/hr or 10 units/hr. Although a variable quantity of insulin adheres to glass and plastic tubing, if a sufficiently concentrated solution is employed (e.g., 50 units in 500 ml), this is not a practical problem. Additional safety can be achieved by running the initial 10 ml out through the tube to "saturate" insulin binding sites. A pediatric infusion set is quite effective in delivering the insulin. If an infusion pump is available, 100 units of insulin can be added to 100 ml normal saline. Although albumin has been recommended to prevent insulin binding, a small amount of the patient's blood drawn into the infusion apparatus will suffice. Insulin can then be infused at a similar rate as above.

This regimen provides for a controlled fall in the blood glucose. Independent of dilution effects, the blood sugar can be expected to fall at the rate of 75–100 mg/dl/hr. The use of intravenous insulin by constant infusion provides great flexibility in the management of uncontrolled diabetes, whether it be diabetic ketoacidosis or early decompensation in a hospitalized or ambulatory diabetic.

It is obvious that, if the intravenous line stops or becomes disconnected, the patient will receive no insulin. If the blood glucose does not begin to fall in 1 hour, the concentration or the rate of the infusion should be doubled, and so on each hour. The intravenous infusion systems are superior to traditional methods of intravenous plus subcutaneous insulin in that hypoglycemia and hypokalemia appear to be minimized.

The half-life of insulin is short (4–6 minutes), hence the effect of an intravenous bolus of insulin is only 20–30 minutes. Despite this theoretical reservation, hourly intravenous insulin boluses (e.g., 10 units/hr) appear to be as effective as insulin infusions. Another alternative is hourly intramuscular (deltoid) injections. After an initial dose of 15–20 units, approximately 10 units/hr can be administered. Intramuscular insulin should not be employed in patients with severe hypotension.

The more traditional methods of insulin administration (e.g., intravenous plus subcutaneous insulin) are also effective; however, the variable rate of delivery of insulin from the subcutaneous sites makes these regimens somewhat less desirable.

Although these schedules simplify the initial decision regarding insulin administration, they do not alter the need for intensive monitoring of the patient's condition, and subsequent decisions regarding insulin administration must be determined by assessing the patient's response. If no change in blood glucose level is noted in the course of 1–2 hours, the dosage must be increased.

Bicarbonate. Acidosis in diabetic patients results from ketone body production (ketoacidosis) and, to a lesser degree, from poor tissue perfusion (lactic acidosis). In most cases, the acidosis is easily corrected with insulin and volume replacement alone. However, if peripheral vascular collapse is present, bicarbonate should be administered, 88–125 mEq intravenously in the course of 15–30 minutes. Also, if the pH of the arterial blood is less than 7.1 or if the serum bicarbonate concentration is less than 5mEq/liter, bicarbonate should be administered at the rate of 44–88 mEq/hr until those values are exceeded. The bicarbonate should be added only to hypotonic fluids [e.g., 0.5 N (0.45%) saline] to prevent severe hypernatremia. Profound acidosis antagonizes the action of catecholamines, such as norepinephrine, that are required for normal peripheral vasoconstriction and maintenance of blood pressure, and in patients with profound shock, bicarbonate may be lifesaving.

Most patients do not require bicarbonate therapy. Furthermore, excessive administration of bicarbonate may result in metabolic alkalosis and arrhythmias. In addition, hypokalemia may develop precipitously after bicarbonate therapy, increasing early potassium requirements substantially. Theoretical dangers of bicarbonate therapy include development of paradoxical cerebrospinal fluid acidosis and unfavorable shifts in the oxygen-hemoglobin dissociation curve.

Potassium. Striking potassium deficits are almost invariably present in patients with diabetic ketoacidosis. Deficits average about 5 mEq/kg of body weight (350 mEq in a person weighing 70 kg), but may range up to 10 mEq/kg. Although large quantities of potassium are lost in the urine, the serum potassium concentration is usually normal or elevated. This paradox is a consequence of the acidosis, which causes a shift of potassium ions from cells to plasma, as well as a consequence of insulin deficiency *per se,* which prevents the entry of potassium into cells. Although peaked T waves on the electrocardiogram indicate an elevated serum potassium concentration, they may also occur with acidosis alone. Less than 5% of patients have initial hypokalemia; those who do should receive vigorous potassium replacement therapy immediately.

Once therapy with insulin and fluid replacement has been started, the serum potassium concentration may plummet. This is partly due to dilution by fluids that do not contain potassium and partly due to entry of potassium into the cells. As acidosis is corrected and insulin administered, potassium enters cells. As stated previously, bicarbonate therapy may accelerate the development of hypokalemia.

As soon as the serum potassium concentration enters the normal range (3.5–5.0 mEq/liter)—provided that good urinary output has been established—potassium chloride, 20–40 mEq/hr should be administered. Oral potassium salts may be given as well. The serum potassium level should be monitored at least every 2 hours to avoid a fatal arrhythmia, especially if the patient is receiving digitalis.

Glucose. If insulin therapy is adequate, a decrease in the blood glucose level should be noted within a few hours. When the blood glucose concentration decreases to between 250-300 mg/dl (usually between 4–8 hours), glucose should be given. If the acidosis and ketosis have disappeared, insulin therapy can be diminished but must not be stopped. If ketosis persists, intravenous glucose should be administered to allow insulin to be given to speed the clearance of ketone bodies and yet avoid hypoglycemia. When glucose is required, it should be given at a rate of 250 ml/hr of 5% dextrose solutions or 125 ml/hr of 10% dextrose solutions (12.5 gm/hr of glucose), depending upon the volume status of the patient at the time.

Although the serum ketones are an important indicator of the severity of the diabetic ketoacidosis, they are somewhat less useful in following the course of the disease. The disappearance of ketones in the blood and urine is, of course, a favorable clinical sign. However, the ketones may be slow to clear due to the shift in the equilibrium between acetoacetate and β-hydroxybutyrate. As the acidosis is corrected, the ratio of acetoacetate to β-hydroxybutyrate rises as the concentration of β-hydroxybutyrate falls. Only the acetoacetate is measured by the nitroprusside reagent and its concentration may not change while the total ketone bodies decline. This improved state should be reflected by a decline in the anion gap, which does measure the hidden anion (β-hydroxybutyrate).

Phosphate. Severe phosphate deficits may occur in diabetic ketoacidosis. Although serum phosphate concentrations are often normal or elevated, intracellular organophosphates are depleted, including 2,3-diphosphoglycerate (2,3-DPG), the red cell organophosphate which facilitates oxygen unloading from hemoglobin. During the course of therapy for diabetic ketoacidosis, serum phosphate concentrations often fall dramatically. There has been a recent trend to supplement phosphate with intravenous therapy in nonoliguric patients (e.g., 5 mmol/hr of intravenous phosphate as the potassium salt). Although theoretically attractive, such therapy does not appear to be necessary and has not been shown to influence morbidity or mortality. Furthermore, symptomatic hypocalcemia may occur if the phosphate infusion rate is too vigorous.

Subsequent Management. The nasogastric tube, Foley catheter, and central venous pressure line should be removed as soon as possible, if it has been necessary to use them. The nasogastric tube may be removed when the patient becomes alert, and the central venous pressure line need not be left in place once normal volume status has been reestablished.

Increased cerebrospinal fluid pressure occurs commonly during the course of therapy of diabetic ketoacidosis. Fortunately, coma or death due to documented cerebral edema is rare. If the mental state begins to deteriorate after a period of improvement, the fundi should be examined for papilledema. Although their efficacy has not yet been demonstrated, therapy for cerebral edema with mannitol and high-dose glucocorticoids should be considered in the appropriate clinical setting. Hyponatremia may predispose to this dreaded complication and should be avoided.

Arterial blood gases should be monitored. As in all cases of metabolic acidosis, a rising P_{CO_2} and a falling pH constitute a poor prognostic sign; they suggest that the patient is tiring and mandate assisted ventilation.

Table 14.2.
Diabetic Ketoacidosis: Common Errors in Management

Failure to individualize therapy
Insulin infusions becoming disconnected
Failure to increase rate of insulin infusion if patient not responding
Insufficient salt and volume replacement
Failure to begin potassium therapy when (K^+) enters normal range
Excessive bicarbonate
Failure to administer glucose when blood glucose levels enter 250–300 mg/dl range
Premature cessation of insulin therapy
Inadequate surveillance for delayed hypoglycemia
Failure to begin intermediate-acting insulins (NPH or lente) when ketosis has cleared
Inadequate search for precipitating cause
Failure to follow laboratory abnormalities in serial fashion and to maintain flow sheet of progress

A vigilant watch for hypoglycemia must continue, although this is less likely if insulin has not been administered subcutaneously. It is worth reemphasizing the need for continuous glucose infusion once the blood glucose enters the range of 250–300 mg/dl. Once acidosis has been corrected, insulin should be administered subcutaneously at 4-hour intervals, based on the blood glucose, until the serum ketone test is no longer strongly positive and urinary ketones are no longer present in large amounts. Administration of intermediate acting insulin (e.g., NPH or lente insulin) should be started the following morning. Common errors in the management of diabetic ketoacidosis are summarized in Table 14.2.

Vascular thrombosis is a common concomitant of diabetic ketoacidosis, either as a precipitating event or a consequence of the dehydration. Low-dose subcutaneous heparin therapy may be considered in appropriate situations. Renal failure can develop during the course of therapy and dialysis may need to be instituted in certain cases.

Precipitating Factors

Once therapy has been started, the cause of the decompensation must be sought (see Table 14.3). Newly diagnosed diabetes, insulin omission, and infection are the most common offenders. The temperature may not be elevated despite infection, and the white blood count may be elevated in the absence of infection. Prophylactic antibiotics should not be used, but a careful search for infection, particularly of the urinary and respiratory tracts, should be initiated. The serum amylase is commonly elevated in diabetic ketoacidosis, although pancreatitis is rare. Salivary rather than pancreatic amylase may account for the confusing amylase elevation. Virtually any major stress can lead to diabetic ketoacidosis in a predisposed individual. It is equally important to remember that other conditions can cause coma, for example, subdural hematoma, presence of drugs including ethanol, and meningitis. These must be considered even if frank ketoacidosis is evident. Although no precipitating cause is found in 10-20% of patients with diabetic ketoacidosis, a vigilant search must be made in every case.

Diabetic ketoacidosis is easier to prevent than to treat. Patients must be instructed not to omit insulin therapy when they become ill; rather, insulin dosage often needs to be increased. Oral intake must be sustained and perhaps augmented if additional insulin is administered. If the patient is nauseated, fruit juices, soft drinks, and bouillon can provide palatable sources of fluid, glucose, and sodium. Home monitoring of blood glucose and urine ketones is of great importance.

Hyperglycemic Hyperosmolar Nonketotic Coma

Severe hyperglycemia without ketosis is being recognized with increasing frequency, although unfortunately, often in its late stages. In contrast, with diabetic ketoacidosis, hyperglycemic hyperosmolar nonketotic coma (HHNC) has a mortality that still approaches 50%. It is unproven, but seems likely, that the long delay in recognition, advanced age of the patients, and severity of underlying medical conditions are all important in this unacceptably high mortality. This syndrome often occurs in "mild" diabetics or in those with previously unrecognized diabetes, leads to initially subtle and then progressive deterioration in mental status, and is most commonly misdiagnosed as "stroke" in the emergency department.

Pathophysiologic Principles

Although relative insulin deficiency is present, only the carbohydrate side of the insulin deficiency schema is apparently affected (Fig. 14.2*A*). The explanation for the absence of ketosis remains elusive. It is possible, but unlikely, that sufficient insulin is present to prevent lipolysis, but insufficient

Table 14.3.
Diabetic Ketoacidosis: Precipitating Factors

Newly diagnosed diabetes
Insulin omission
Infection
Myocardial infarction (may be silent) or cerebrovascular accident
Intraabdominal emergencies including pancreatitis
Trauma
Pregnancy
Surgery

to prevent gluconeogenesis and stimulate glucose uptake. Additional effects of increased osmolality on intermediary metabolism are being explored.

As the blood glucose begins to rise, glycosuria develops. If renal perfusion is adequate, the kidney serves as a "drain" for the excess glucose, but if urinary output begins to decrease or if renal failure is present, the blood glucose increases substantially. The increased thirst often results in drinking of fruit juices or other high sugar beverages, further raising the blood glucose. Although intrinsic renal disease may account for a reduced urinary output, such a decrease more commonly represents decreasing glomerular filtration as a consequence of these fluid losses. Progressive lethargy, dehydration, and obtundation result and oral intake diminishes. The consequence is a striking elevation of the blood glucose and often the serum osmolality, resulting in profound cellular dehydration. The impaired mental state is best correlated with the magnitude of the serum osmolality elevation.

Diagnosis

The diagnosis can be unsuspected until an elevated blood glucose level is revealed by a "routine" laboratory test. Kussmaul's respiration and an acetone odor to the breath are absent. Patients tend to be middle-aged or older and can have a history of Type II ("maturity-onset") diabetes. Signs of dehydration can provide the only clinical clue. Coma is common, and focal neurologic abnormalities, including seizures, may dominate the clinical findings. The common misdiagnosis is stroke.

To meet accepted criteria for hyperosmolar nonketotic coma, the blood glucose concentration must be more than 600 mg/dl, the serum osmolality more than 350 mEq/l, and the serum ketone reaction less than strong in undiluted serum. Lesser degrees of hyperglycemia and hyperosmolality may of course be present and should be treated with similar care. At the other end of the scale, a severe hyperosmolar state may be part of diabetic ketoacidosis. Since the advent of intravenous insulin infusions, the arbitrary distinction between these syndromes is of somewhat less importance.

The osmolality may be measured precisely in the clinical laboratory, but a quick estimation is often helpful in establishing a diagnosis:

$$\text{serum osmolality} = 2\,[\text{Na}^+] + \frac{\text{BUN}}{2.8} + \frac{\text{blood glucose}}{18}$$

The osmolality and the serum sodium concentration $[\text{Na}^+]$ are both expressed as mEq/liter, and the blood urea nitrogen (BUN) and blood glucose concentrations are expressed as mg/dl.

Therapy

Although mild to moderate degrees of acidosis may be present in patients with hyperosmolar nonketotic coma, profound acidosis is usually absent. With this exception, the therapeutic considerations are similar to those pertaining to diabetic ketoacidosis.

Volume Replacement. Volume deficits often exceed those of diabetic ketoacidosis, perhaps reflecting a longer prodromal period before clinical recognition. Deficits in excess of 10 liters are not unusual. Half of the volume lost should be replaced within the first 8–12 hours if possible. If profound dehydration with hypotension is present, the initial solutions should include plasma expanders. Although 0.9% (normal) saline is a hypertonic fluid (308 mosm/liter), it is relatively hypotonic for these patients and is the initial therapy of choice to maintain adequate intravascular volume. Guidelines are similar to those for initial fluid management in diabetic ketoacidosis. In this older age group, close attention to volume status is of even greater importance, to prevent extremes of intravascular volume depletion and circulatory overload.

Insulin. The initial fall in blood glucose concentration in these patients reflects dilution by intravenous fluids and increased urinary losses secondary to improved renal perfusion. Insulin should be administered as in diabetic ketoacidosis, with constant intravenous infusions providing a controlled method of decreasing the blood glucose. When the blood glucose reaches 300 mg/dl, however, constant infusions of insulin can be discontinued. Regular insulin (CZI) can be given subcutaneously at 4-hour intervals based on the blood glucose, until the next morning when intermediate acting insulins (e.g., NPH or lente) should be started.

Bicarbonate. The mild to moderate degrees of acidosis that have been noted are not adequately explained by decreased tissue perfusion (lactic acidosis) or renal insufficiency (uremic acidosis). Unless shock is present, bicarbonate therapy is rarely indicated.

Potassium. Severe potassium deficits are the rule. The initial serum potassium concentration is often closer to normal than those in diabetic ketoacidosis, reflecting the lack of severe acidosis. Potassium chloride, 20–40 mEq/hr, should be added to intravenous infusions once a good urinary output has been established.

Glucose. Intravenous administration of glucose should be started when the blood glucose concentration has decreased to between 250 and 300 mg/dl.

Phosphate. Profound phosphate depletion is

much less common than in diabetic ketoacidosis, with normal red blood cell 2,3-DPG levels usually being present. Although controversy continues about the utility of phosphate in patients with diabetic ketoacidosis, there is even less indication for this therapy in patients with hyperglycemic hyperosmolar coma.

Precipitating Factors

Some of the initiating events are similar to those that can precipitate diabetic ketoacidosis. Infection is important, and a rather high prevalence of Gram-negative bacterial infection has been noted, especially pneumonia and urinary tract infections. Drugs play a more important role here, including thiazide diuretics or furosemide, phenytoin, glucocorticoids and occasionally propranolol and diazoxide. In addition, peritoneal dialysis patients, burn patients, and demented or obtunded individuals, particularly those receiving intravenous glucose (e.g., hyperalimentation), are all prevalent in series of patients with this diagnosis. The increased intake of solutions containing carbohydrates early in the course of dehydration may be important in ambulatory patients. Myocardial infarction, cerebrovascular disease, and renal failure are particularly prevalent in these patients. Of the surviving patients, many require no diabetic therapy after the episode of hyperglycemic hyperosmolar coma has resolved.

Alcoholic Ketoacidosis

Alcoholic ketoacidosis is not a manifestation of diabetes but may be confused with diabetic ketoacidosis. In this situation, persons with chronic alcoholism, who have been drinking continually, become nauseated and increasingly anorexic. Food intake ceases, and alcohol intake usually ceases as well. Nausea increases and vomiting develops, often with abdominal pain. Other presenting features include hyperpnea and possibly pancreatitis.

These patients are generally dehydrated with rapid Kussmaul's respirations. The breath is free of ethanol odor. The abdomen is usually tender, especially in the epigastrium. Hepatomegaly is common. The mental status is generally normal or slightly impaired, but severe obtundation or coma may occur.

It appears that the lipid or ketone body pathway (Fig. 14.2*B*) is activated without necessarily activating the carbohydrate pathway. Acidosis is often severe. Although this is a ketoacidosis, the serum ketone concentration may be only mildly increased as assessed by testing with Acetest tablets; for example, there may be less than a 4+ reaction for undiluted serum. This is due to a predominance of β-hydroxybutyrate (not measured by Acetest tablets) over acetoacetate, as well as concomitant lactic acidosis. The blood glucose concentration ranges from hypoglycemic to moderately hyperglycemic levels.

The pathophysiologic mechanisms are unclear. During starvation, insulin deficiency is present and this permits lipolysis and ketogenesis to occur. However, ketoacidosis is not a concomitant of the "normal" starved state, and the role of ethanol, volume depletion, and stress on the release of free fatty acids, inhibition of insulin release, and hepatic ketogenesis remains unresolved. In most patients, the glucose tolerance test is normal after recovery.

The nondiabetic patient with such a typical history should receive intravenous or intramuscular thiamine (25 mg), intravenous fluid and electrolytes, large quantities of intravenous glucose, and bicarbonate if the arterial blood pH is less than 7.1. If the blood glucose level is greater than 250 mg/dl, it appears judicious to administer insulin (CZI, 10 units/hr by intravenous infusion) along with intravenous glucose (12.5 gm/hr).

Lactic Acidosis

Lactic acidosis is a syndrome, not a disease. Severe metabolic acidosis due to accumulation of lactate may occur in many diseases.

Pathophysiologic Principles

Lactic acid is the end product of anaerobic glycolysis. All lactic acid is derived from pyruvic acid, a reaction catalyzed by lactate dehydrogenase (LDH):

$$\text{NADH} + \text{pyruvate} + \text{H}^+ \overset{\text{LDH}}{\leftrightarrows} \text{NAD}^+ + \text{lactate}$$

where NADH = nicotinamide adenine dinucleotide. Under aerobic conditions, glucose in muscle and other tissues is partly oxidized to pyruvate. Under anaerobic conditions, the pyruvate is preferentially converted to lactate and released into the bloodstream. The liver has a great capacity for lactate metabolism, lactate being converted back to pyruvate. Several alternative pathways are available for pyruvate, including further oxidation to carbon dioxide and water with the storage of energy in the form of ATP, free fatty acid synthesis, and resynthesis into glucose (followed by release from the liver, completing the Cori cycle).

Under normal circumstances, skeletal muscle, the gut, red blood cells, and skin are the major contributors to the blood lactate pool. The liver and kidney are instrumental in lactate removal. In pathologic states, cellular oxidation of glucose may be impaired by poor tissue perfusion, poor tissue oxygenation, or metabolic poisons. Under these circumstances, virtually any tissue may produce a large amount of lactic acid. Impaired lactate removal is usually present in pathologic states, as the removal capacity for lactate is quite high under normal circumstances.

Lactic acidosis is now commonly separated into *type A,* in which circulatory collapse or hypoxia are primary, and *type B,* where the lactic acidosis has other causes. The clinical situation may be confusing, in that profound lactic acidosis can secondarily result in vascular collapse.

Diagnosis

The recognition of lactic acidosis depends on the recognition of metabolic acidosis. Vascular collapse or unexplained air hunger require assessment of acid-base status by means of arterial blood gas determination. The presence of vasodilation and "warm shock" should suggest the presence of severe acidemia or overwhelming sepsis. Arterial blood with a pH less than 7.4, with a decreased P_{CO_2} or serum bicarbonate level, establishes the diagnosis of metabolic acidosis. Even if the pH is close to normal (e.g., 7.35–7.39), a decreased P_{CO_2} or serum bicarbonate concentration is still a valuable indication of ongoing metabolic acidemia (with respiratory compensation).

When a strong acid (such as lactic acid, represented by HA) is added to a solution of bicarbonate (such as plasma), carbon dioxide is produced:

$$HA + NaHCO_3 \rightleftharpoons Na^+ A^- + H_2CO_3 \rightarrow H_2O + CO_2 \uparrow$$

Neutralization of the acid results in the formation of anions (A^-); these are the anions that contribute to the anion gap. In the presence of metabolic acidosis, the anion gap should be determined. The anion gap is equal to the serum sodium concentration minus the sum of the serum bicarbonate and serum chloride concentrations, normal being less than 12 mEq/liter. (If the serum potassium concentration is also considered, normal is less than 15 mEq/liter.) If the anion gap is more than 12 mEq/liter, one of the causes listed in Table 14.4 must be considered. It is usually fairly easy to exclude uremia, ketoacidosis, and drug ingestion, leaving lactic acidosis as the diagnosis.

Lactate can be measured directly as well, and in most clinical laboratories, the result can be known within several hours. A lactate concentration greater than 5 mEq/liter in a sick patient with metabolic acidosis indicates that lactic acidosis is at least contributory. Determination of the pyruvate level is more time-consuming, adds little information, and is unnecessary for diagnosis. The white blood cell count is often elevated in acute metabolic acidosis. The uric acid level is often markedly elevated, due to inhibition of renal excretion of urate by the elevation of blood lactate.

Table 14.4.
Metabolic Acidosis with Anion Gap

Type	Anion in Excess
Lactic acidosis	Lactate
Ketoacidosis (diabetic or alcoholic)	β-Hydroxybutyrate Acetoacetate
Uremic acidosis	Phosphate Sulfate
Drug-induced acidosis	
Ethylene glycol	Glycolate, oxalate
Methyl alcohol	Formate, ? lactate
Paraldehyde	Uncertain
Salicylates	? Lactate

Precipitating Factors

Increased lactate production is a regular finding in the shock state and frequently occurs with regional underperfusion as well. Frank lactic acidosis is less common. With type A lactic acidosis, 70% of patients are in shock at the time of presentation and 90% of these will die. If the shock or underperfusion can be corrected, the lactic acidosis will disappear as well. Profound hypoxia, whether local or systemic, stimulates increased lactate production and depresses lactate clearance by the liver.

Type B lactic acidosis is much less common and can be further subdivided. In type B1, a number of common disorders are found, including diabetes mellitus, renal failure, infections, liver disease, and leukemia. Type B2 includes drug-induced lactic acidosis and is less prevalent now that phenformin is no longer prescribed. Ethyl alcohol (ethanol) inhibits the hepatic disposal of lactic acid presumably by increasing the levels of NADH in the liver. Lactic acidosis may be precipitated or exacerbated by ethanol. Infusion of sorbitol or fructose, total parenteral nutrition in patients with malignancies, poisoning with cyanide, carbon monoxide, isoniazid, salicylate, or lye and streptozotocin administration have all been associated with lactic acidosis. Type B3 includes a disparate group of hereditary enzyme defects.

Cardiovascular collapse often supervenes in type B lactic acidosis. When the blood pressure falls to less than 100 mm Hg, recovery is uncommon.

Therapy

Therapy must be directed at the underlying disorder. In type A lactic acidosis, tissue perfusion should be improved with volume replacement or cardiotonic agents when indicated. Hypoxia should be corrected, with assisted ventilation if necessary. Bicarbonate should be administered intravenously to maintain the arterial pH above 7.2. Some investigators point out that bicarbonate may worsen intracellular acidosis and hence cause clinical deterioration. However, viable alternative therapies are not yet available.

The quantities of bicarbonate necessary will be quite variable (see below). Arterial blood gas determinations must be serially repeated to monitor the effects of therapy.

In type B lactic acidosis the offending drugs should be omitted and any treatable underlying disease identified and treated as well. With vascular collapse, volume replacement will be necessary. Bicarbonate is required, often in heroic amounts, with thousands of milliequivalents administered in some cases. If the acidemia is severe and ongoing, 5% (600 mmol) $NaHCO_3$ may be required.

Loop diuretics such as furosemide or ethacrynic acid are often necessary to prevent volume overload. If sodium overload occurs in the face of such therapy, peritoneal dialysis may be necessary to remove excess sodium. The use of vasodilator therapy to allow adequate bicarbonate therapy has been successful and has the theoretic advantage of opening unidentified areas of regional underperfusion. Nitroprusside has been used but other vasodilators may be tried. Methylene blue (1–5 mg/kg intravenously) can decrease hepatic levels of NADH and may help correct the lactate accumulation but is rarely lifesaving. The experimental drug dichloracetate holds promise as a stimulator of pyruvate dehydrogenase, providing an alternative route for pyruvate other than to lactate production. It is effective in correcting lactic overproduction in experimental situations and its role in clinical lactic acidosis is being explored. Thiamine administration (several hundred milligrams intravenously) seems reasonable, particularly in alcoholic patients. The role of insulin with glucose therapy is being explored as well.

Hypoglycemia

The challenge of hypoglycemia lies in its recognition rather than its management. The type of hypoglycemia requiring treatment in the emergency department is usually that which occurs after a variable period of fasting. Reactive hypoglycemia occurring within 4–5 hours after a meal is a benign condition and rarely requires immediate therapy; it may occasionally accompany fasting hypoglycemia. By far, the most common cause of hypoglycemia is insulin administration.

The immediate treatment is administration of glucose. Once treatment has been started, the amount of glucose and the duration of therapy can safely be determined. The physician must then also seek the underlying cause. Although the manifestations of hypoglycemia may vary considerably, one specific rule must be followed: any obtunded or comatose patient seen in the emergency department should be treated immediately with 50 ml of a 50% glucose solution after blood has been drawn for determination of the glucose content.

Pathophysiologic Principles

During the normal fasting state (4 or more hours after the last meal), the blood glucose level begins to decrease and insulin release is inhibited. The liver provides glucose to maintain the amount in the blood, preventing hypoglycemia. Glycogen breakdown, and synthesis and release of glucose are both contributory. The substrates for glucose synthesis (lactate, the amino acids alanine and glutamine, and glycerol) are derived from muscle and fat breakdown. Cortisol, glucagon, growth hormone, and epinephrine—the counterregulatory hormones—may provide substrates for glucose production. This process is similar to that occurring in insulin deficiency described in Figure 14.2*A*, and the net result is provision of an adequate glucose supply for the brain. Most instances of hypoglycemia are caused, in part, by inability of the liver to provide the necessary glucose. Rarely, increased peripheral utilization alone is at fault.

Insulin. Inappropriate elevation of insulin can cause substrate flow to the liver to halt and increase peripheral utilization of glucose, as well as terminate glucose production by the liver. The net result is severe hypoglycemia. This situation is most commonly due to insulin injections, oral hypoglycemic therapy with sulfonylurea compounds, and insulinomas. Drug interactions (for example, between sulfonamides and sulfonylureas) and hepatic or renal insufficiency may precipitate hypoglycemia in patients receiving long-term oral hypoglycemic therapy. Liver glycogen is adequate or increased in insulin-induced hypoglycemia, and alternative substrates such as free fatty acids or ketones are diminished by the action of insulin on fat cells.

Inhibition of Glucose Synthesis. Alcohol is the most common drug known to inhibit glucose synthesis; inhibition occurs because the increased NADH generated by ethanol oxidation depletes hepatic pyruvate by converting it to lactate. As long as the alcoholic continues to eat, hypoglycemia will not develop. However, when hepatic glycogen reserves are depleted, after a variable period of starvation, alcohol-induced inhibition of glucose synthesis can result in profound hypoglycemia. It is easy to confuse the clinical findings with those of alcoholic stupor, and this lethal error has often been made. Severe starvation may result in decreased gluconeogenic substrates and hence hypoglycemia.

Salicylates in massive quantities can produce hypoglycemia, perhaps by inhibition of glucose synthesis. The glycogen storage diseases of infancy are rare causes of hypoglycemia. In these conditions, hereditary defects are present in the enzymes necessary for glucose production by the liver.

Intrinsic Hepatic Disease. Hypoglycemia is rare in patients with cirrhosis unless terminal hepatic failure develops. However, acute yellow atrophy, toxic hepatic damage, and Reye's syndrome can produce severe hypoglycemia.

Lack of Counterregulatory Hormones. Cortisol deficiency alone, as in Addison's disease, or in association with growth hormone deficiency, as in hypopituitarism, may result in fasting hypoglycemia, especially in children. Patients with longstanding diabetes often develop deficiencies of glucagon and epinephrine, making them particularly prone to insulin-induced hypoglycemia.

Other. Fasting hypoglycemia may develop during pregnancy since the fetus has an obligatory glucose requirement. In infants with ketotic hypoglycemia, the liver is apparently insufficiently provided with substrates. Rarely, hypoglycemia is a consequence of nonpancreatic neoplasms, but the mechanism remains elusive. Prolonged exertion such as marathon running may result in hypoglycemia. Hypoglycemia may be a manifestation of sepsis or severe renal failure. Drugs such as propranolol and disopyramide (Norpace) have rarely been implicated.

Clinical Features

For convenience, the symptoms of hypoglycemia may be considered as "catechol-like" and "neuroglucopenic." A rapid fall in the blood glucose level results in release of the catecholamines epinephrine and norepinephrine, which tend to increase the amount of blood glucose. The symptoms and signs of catecholamine excess include anxiety, palpitations, tremor, diaphoresis, weakness, hunger, cool moist skin, pallor, and tachycardia. Increased systolic and decreased diastolic blood pressure may be present. Catechol-mediated symptoms occur when the blood glucose level falls rapidly, being absent with gradual decrease in the blood glucose level or with sustained or chronic hypoglycemia. Autonomic neuropathy in the diabetic patient or β-adrenergic blockade with propranolol will prevent signs and symptoms of catechol excess. Propranolol should be avoided or used with great caution in insulin-requiring diabetics; other drugs such as metoprolol may be safer. Alcohol-induced hypoglycemia often lacks signs of catechol excess, for unclear reasons.

When the central nervous system is deprived of its principal source of energy, glucose, a variety of neuroglucopenic signs and symptoms may develop. Mental changes are common, and range from lethargy, mild confusion, or difficulty in concentrating to personality changes or profound coma. Grand mal seizures may occur, and unilateral signs identical with those of a cerebrovascular accident may be present. These are all reversible if therapy is not delayed too long. However, it is important to recognize that, whereas response to glucose infusion is diagnostic, lack of response to a single bolus does not exclude the diagnosis of hypoglycemia.

Additional signs and symptoms may also be helpful. Nocturnal hypoglycemia may be characterized by nightmares, night sweats, early morning headaches, or occasionally, angina during sleep. Hypoglycemia causes hypothermia probably due to increased peripheral vasodilatation and sweating, which may be appreciated by studying the patient's temperature chart for inappropriate dips or failure of the temperature to rise from early morning to late evening. Chronic hypoglycemia, as in patients with insulinoma, may lead to increased caloric intake and weight gain, and may occasionally be associated with chronic sensory-motor neuropathy. Trismus may occur in patients with alcoholic hypoglycemia.

Specific Diagnosis and Therapy

If hypoglycemia is suspected or in acute neurologic conditions (such as seizures, cerebrovascular accidents, or coma), blood should be drawn for a glucose determination by the laboratory and for testing by glucose oxidase strips; 50 ml of a 50% glucose solution should be administered intravenously. If it is certain that insulin-induced hypoglycemia is present, an alternative therapy is glucagon, 1 mg by intramuscular injection, a rapidly acting therapy which can spare veins in diabetics with recurrent hypoglycemia. In suspected alcoholics, 25–50 mg of thiamine should also be administered to prevent an acute episode of Wernicke-Korsakoff syndrome. Even in the absence of obvious response to intravenous glucose, the blood glucose concentration should be estimated quickly with glucose oxidase reagent strips. A laboratory determination revealing a blood glucose level less than 40 mg/dl or a plasma glucose level less than 45 mg/dl is diagnostic.

Coma which is apparently due to hypoglycemia but does not reverse after glucose administration can be quite difficult to manage. Continued intravenous glucose to maintain the blood glucose level around 150–180 mg/dl is advisable, often requiring 10% dextrose solutions with concomitant insulin. Therapy for cerebral edema should be instituted with dexamethasone and/or mannitol. A search for other causes of coma, including drugs, trauma, and continued seizure activity should be performed. A computed tomogram of the brain should be performed.

When the blood is drawn, a specimen should be set aside in a heparinized tube for possible insulin assay. The combination of fasting hypoglycemia and inappropriately elevated insulin levels indicates insulin-induced hypoglycemia, which may be due to insulin therapy, oral hypoglycemic agents, or insulinoma. Much time can be saved and expense avoided if this simple expedient is followed. Surreptitious insulin injections (factitious hypoglycemia) in a nondiabetic patient can be detected if anti-insulin antibodies are present in serum. Proinsulin, the larger precursor molecule for insulin, circulates in the plasma of patients with insulinomas but is absent in patients with factitious hypoglycemia. A blood specimen should also be set aside for cortisol assay if the cause of hypoglycemia is not obvious. In hypoglycemia, cortisol secretion and therefore the plasma cortisol level normally increase; if this does not occur in the presence of hypoglycemic symptoms, adrenal insufficiency or hypopituitarism is likely, especially in children. The possibility of willful insulin overadministration in a suicide attempt should be kept in mind.

If insulin therapy is the cause of the hypoglycemia, intramuscular glucagon (1 mg) or intravenous glucose (25 gm) will suffice for the acute management. Dietary instructions and a careful review of the insulin regimen should be undertaken as well. If an oral hypoglycemic drug is responsible, the patient must be hospitalized. The hypoglycemia may last for days or weeks, particularly if chlorpropamide is the etiologic agent, and it may recur several times after initial seemingly successful therapy. This may, in part, be related to increased insulin release by the sensitized pancreatic β cell in response to bolus glucose therapy. In these patients, continuous intravenous infusion of glucose, adequate oral food intake, and frequent monitoring of the blood glucose level are mandatory. Since a liter of 5% dextrose in water contains only 50 gm of glucose, a 10 or 20% solution should be administered with intravenous boluses of 50% dextrose as necessary. If hyperglycemia (blood glucose level more than 100 mg/dl) cannot be established in 4–6 hours with this therapy, hydrocortisone hemisuccinate (100 mg) should be added to each liter of solution. In particularly refractory situations, diazoxide, a drug which inhibits insulin release from the pancreas, should be administered.

Alcohol-induced hypoglycemia is particularly treacherous because the diagnosis is often missed.

The alcoholic who is stuporous from hypoglycemia may be thought to be drunk, and grand mal seizures may be interpreted as withdrawal seizures ("rum fits"). Alcoholics should not be permitted to "sleep it off" unsupervised. Glucose and thiamine should be administered intravenously, and patients should be observed for increasing obtundation. After correction of alcoholic hypoglycemia, hospitalization is not required. The brain utilizes 5–6 gm/hr of glucose. In this situation, in contrast to the insulin-induced hypoglycemia, increased peripheral utilization is not playing a role and 10 gm/hr of glucose should suffice for maintenance therapy until the patient is eating. It is important to realize that alcoholic ketoacidosis rarely can coexist with alcoholic hypoglycemia.

Profound hepatic failure is usually obvious and must be managed with adequate caloric intake, at least 100 gm of carbohydrates each day, either orally or parenterally, to spare muscle protein. With persistent hypoglycemia, larger quantities of glucose may be required.

Hypoglycemia is preventable in many patients. Otherwise healthy persons with diabetes should not decrease oral intake or increase exercise without decreasing the dosage of insulin. Diabetics with intermittent symptoms at home should be taught to test their blood by finger-stick analysis to exclude hypoglycemia. Chlorpropamide should not be administered to any patient with renal failure, and tolbutamide should not be given to patients with abnormal hepatic function. Drugs known to potentiate the action of the sulfonylurea compounds must be avoided.

ADRENAL INSUFFICIENCY AND HYPOPITUITARISM

Adrenal Physiology

The adrenal cortex produces three major classes of hormones: glucocorticoids or "sugar" hormones, mineralocorticoids or "salt" hormones, and androgens or "sex" hormones. Deficiency of either glucocorticoids or mineralocorticoids may be life-threatening. Adrenal androgen deficiency is of less consequence and is not considered in this chapter.

Cortisol is the major glucocorticoid in human beings. Adrenocorticotropic hormone (ACTH), a pituitary hormone, controls the synthesis and release of cortisol from the adrenal gland. Normally, decrease in cortisol production leads to increased release of ACTH, and cortisol administration leads to decreased release of ACTH. ACTH deficiency, as in hypopituitarism, leads to cortisol deficiency.

As the principal glucocorticoid, cortisol has many functions. It is required to sustain a normal blood glucose level and is also necessary for maintenance of blood pressure, permitting normal sympathetic control of arterial tone. In addition, it contributes to normal appetite, sense of well-being, energy, mental acuity, and the ability of the kidneys to excrete extra water. In the absence of cortisol, the percentage of eosinophils and lymphocytes in the peripheral circulation increases.

Most importantly, cortisol enables the body to respond adequately during stress. The unstressed adrenal glands secrete 15–20 mg of cortisol daily, but they are capable of at least 10 times that output.

In the presence of major stress, such as an operation, sepsis, or trauma, 200–300 mg of cortisol must be produced to sustain life. With lesser degrees of stress, smaller amounts of cortisol are required. It is this ability to respond to stress that makes the adrenal cortex so critical. Lesions of the adrenal cortex may be difficult to diagnose since destruction of 90% of the tissue may result in few or no everyday symptoms, although profound debility will occur in times of stress.

Aldosterone is the most potent of the mineralocorticoids. Volume depletion is the major stimulus for aldosterone production, mediated by angiotensin II. Decrease in either intravascular volume or renal perfusion causes renin production by the kidney and subsequent generation of angiotensin II in the blood. Since ACTH does not contribute substantially to aldosterone control, aldosterone production tends to be unaffected by pituitary disease.

The role of the mineralocorticoids aldosterone and desoxycorticosterone is more limited than that of cortisol, but is equally important, since these hormones defend against loss of intravascular volume by promoting sodium reabsorption in the distal renal tubules. Sodium is conserved, and in its place, potassium and hydrogen ions are excreted. It is logical, therefore, that hyperkalemia is another important stimulus for release of aldosterone, and aldosterone is important in defending against hyperkalemia.

Addison's Disease

Destruction of the adrenal cortex (Addison's disease) may occur relatively slowly, as in patients with tuberculosis or autoimmune disease, or it may occur more rapidly, for example, as a result of bilateral adrenalectomy or adrenal hemorrhage. With destruction of this tissue, both mineralocorticoid and glucocorticoid functions are lost.

Diagnosis

Clinical Features. The history may include weight loss with poor appetite, fatigue, lethargy, arthralgias, postural dizziness, and impaired ability to concentrate. Delayed recovery from either a minor illness, such as influenza or gastroenteritis, or a major stress, such as an operation, is important historically. Salt craving develops as a consequence of salt loss via the kidneys. Severe symptoms may develop in the summer months, as additional salt is lost through the skin, or during hospitalization, when access to salty snacks or oral intake may be limited. The patient may have gastrointestinal symptoms, such as nausea, vomiting, and severe abdominal pain; the mechanism of such symptoms is uncertain. Acute symptoms may develop in a patient with known Addison's disease when concurrent illness develops, and the patient neglects to increase his or her dose of glucocorticoids.

Hyperpigmentation is the most valuable clue to Addison's disease, although with rapid adrenal destruction there may not be sufficient time for hyperpigmentation to develop before the patient becomes critically ill. As cortisol deficiency develops, ACTH is secreted, causing the skin to darken. Pigmentation may be generalized, with the appearance of a suntan that is often sustained, and brownish, almost dirt-like pigmentation may also appear over the extensor surfaces, such as knuckles, elbows, and knees. Pigmentation of the lips and buccal mucosa is characteristic. Scars formed since the onset of Addison's disease become hyperpigmented, but older scars do not. Vitiligo, a patchy depigmentation of the skin, may also be present, suggesting the autoimmune nature of adrenal destruction.

High fever may be present with severe illness, even in the absence of infection. Hypotension is common, ranging from mild postural hypotension to frank shock, and is due to loss of arterial tone (cortisol deficiency) and diminished intravascular volume (mineralocorticoid deficiency). The combination of low blood pressure with fever and abdominal pain may mimic a surgical emergency.

Hyponatremia occurs frequently and results from renal salt loss and impaired renal excretion of water. Hyperkalemia is a consequence of the decreased exchange of sodium, potassium, and hydrogen ions. Metabolic acidosis may result for similar reasons. Hypoglycemia is more likely to develop in infants with Addison's disease than in adults. Lymphocytosis and eosinophilia may be present. Suprarenal calcifications on plain x-ray films of the abdomen may be a valuable indication of tuberculous Addison's disease.

The manifestations of Addison's disease are summarized in Table 14.5, and the pathogenesis of Addisonian crisis is given in Table 14.6. In the absence of a classic presentation, the diagnosis should be considered in every patient with unexplained hypotension, hyperpigmentation, "failure to thrive" after a major or minor stress (especially a surgical procedure), unexplained weight loss, tuberculosis, hyponatremia, hyperkalemia, hypoglycemia, or eosinophilia.

Clinical Studies. Since Addison's disease requires lifelong therapy, establishment of a definitive diagnosis is mandatory after the crisis has passed. A plasma cortisol level within normal limits (approximately 10–15 μg/dl) during major stress is inappropriately low, and a value below normal at such a time is almost diagnostic of Addison's disease. In unstressed patients, a normal plasma cortisol level or 24-hour excretion of 17 hydroxysteroids is com-

Table 14.5.
Addison's Disease: Manifestations

Site	History	Physical Examination	Laboratory Finding
General	Anorexia Lethargy Weight loss Salt craving[a] Delated recovery from illness or operation Impaired ability to concentrate	Fever	Hyponatremia Hyperkalemia[a] Acidosis[a] Hypoglycemia Lymphocytosis Eosinophilia
Cardiovascular	Postural dizziness	Postural hypotension or shock Volume depletion[a]	
Skin	Prolonged suntan[a]	Hyperpigmentation[a] Vitiligo[a]	
Gastrointestinal	Nausea Vomiting Abdominal pain		
Genitourinary		Absent axillary and pubic hair in women	
Musculoskeletal	Myalgias, arthralgias	Muscle weakness	

[a] Absent in ACTH deficiency (hypopituitarism or ACTH suppression).

patible with decreased adrenal reserve and does *not* exclude the diagnosis of adrenal insufficiency.

Initial therapy (see below) should not be discontinued during diagnostic testing, but dexamethasone, 2–4 mg/day in four divided doses, should be administered rather than cortisol; 1 mg of dexamethasone is equivalent to 20–30 mg of cortisol. Such small amounts of this potent glucocorticoid do not interfere with plasma or urinary corticosteroid measurements.

An attempt to stimulate the adrenal gland with ACTH is the diagnostic test of choice. ACTH should be administered according to a standard protocol such as synthetic ACTH (1–24), 25 units intravenously in 500 ml of 5% dextrose in saline solution in the course of 8 hours on 3 consecutive days. In persons without adrenal insufficiency, the plasma cortisol level will increase to more than 30 μg/dl and the 17-hydroxysteroids will at least double to a value of 15 mg/day by the end of the 3rd day's infusion.

In ambulatory patients in whom Addison's disease appears unlikely, a rapid test can be performed to exclude it conclusively. Synthetic ACTH, 25 units, is administered by intravenous bolus or intramuscular injection and the plasma cortisol level is measured before and 1 hour after injection. Only synthetic ACTH should be given. An increase to more than 17 μg/dl excludes the diagnosis of Addison's disease. If these results are not achieved, however, more prolonged ACTH stimulation should be carried out.

Once the diagnosis is established, patient education is extremely important. In addition to wearing a Medic Alert bracelet or necklace, the patient should have an identification card providing the diagnosis and current therapy.

Therapy

Although the definitive diagnosis of Addison's disease depends on measurement of corticosteroid levels in plasma or urine, therapy must be started immediately in sick patients with the suspected diagnosis. Blood should be drawn for a cortisol determination, and cortisol then should be administered intravenously. Dextrose and saline solutions are required as well.

Glucocorticoids. Intravenous administration of cortisol in the form of hydrocortisone sodium succinate may be lifesaving (Table 14.7). The dose should approximate the normal adrenal output during maximal stress, namely, 300 mg/day. Since the half-life of cortisol is at most a few hours, injections should be repeated, 75 mg intravenously or intramuscularly every 6 hours after an initial 100-mg intravenous bolus of cortisone hemisuccinate. A similar regimen of cortisol administration is required in patients with known Addison's disease who are about to undergo a major surgical procedure or who have another major illness. In the presence of persistent hypotension a continuous intravenous infusion of cortisone hemisuccinate should be employed.

The emergency situation often subsides within a few days; as this happens, the dosage of cortisol should be tapered by 50% each day until maintenance therapy is reached.

Table 14.6.
Addisonian Crisis: Pathogenesis

Condition	Cause
Hypotension	↓Cortisol ↓Mineralocorticoid
Hyperpyrexia	↓Cortisol (?)
Hyperpigmentation	↑ACTH
Hyponatremia	↓Cortisol ↓Mineralocorticoid
Hyperkalemia	↓Mineralocorticoid
Hypoglycemia	↓Cortisol

Volume Replacement. Cortisol alone is insufficient in the presence of volume depletion. More than 20% of the extracellular fluid volume may be lost. Deficits of 3 liters or more are common in hypotensive patients. The choice of fluid is 5% dextrose in saline to restore sodium and to prevent hypoglycemia. The rate of administration depends on the age and clinical status of the patient; central venous pressure monitoring is desirable in elderly patients and in those with known cardiac disease. Hospitalized patients with Addison's disease should receive saline solution intravenously if oral intake is limited for any reason.

The response to saline administration may be dramatic. In fact, in hypotensive patients, Addison's disease is often unrecognized because of the favorable response to saline administration. The cycle of alleviation of hypotension with saline solution followed by recurrence when administration is discontinued may occur several times before adrenal insufficiency is recognized.

Mineralocorticoids. Administration of mineralocorticoids may help prevent further loss of sodium. In large dosages, 200–300 mg/day, cortisol does have significant mineralocorticoid effects, particularly when saline solution is administered concomitantly. However, mineralocorticoids should be administered: (*a*) if the blood pressure remains low despite saline; (*b*) if hyperkalemia persists; and (*c*) if a synthetic glucocorticoid such as prednisolone is used instead of cortisol (1 mg of prednisolone is the equivalent of 4 mg cortisol). Mineralocorticoid is often required as the dosage of cortisone is diminished. Desoxycorticosterone acetate, 5 mg intramuscularly twice a day, or fludrocortisone acetate (Florinef), 0.05–0.2 mg/day orally, is recommended.

Long-term therapy is considered in Table 14.7. Patients with adrenal insufficiency must be instructed to increase corticosteroid dosage during illness or stress, however minor. Any patient who has a decreased oral intake or a severe fluid loss such as might result from vomiting or diarrhea should be hospitalized. Patients should be instructed in injection technique and provided with injectable drugs so that corticosteroids can be administered intramuscularly before arriving at the hospital. In such a situation, 100 mg of hydrocortisone sodium succinate is recommended.

ACTH Suppression and Hypopituitarism

ACTH deficiency results in cortisol deficiency, mineralocorticoid function being spared. The most common cause of ACTH lack is pituitary suppression after long-term corticosteroid (glucocorticoid) therapy. After weeks to months of therapy with su-

Table 14.7.
Addison's Disease: Therapy

Type	Dosage	Comments
Emergency[a]		
Volume and glucose replacement	5% dextrose in normal saline to replenish volume	
Glucocorticoid	Hydrocortisone hemisuccinate, 100 mg intravenously, and hydrocortisone hemisuccinate, 75 mg intramuscularly or intravenously every 6 hr	
Mineralocorticoid	Desoxycorticosterone acetate (DOCA), 5 mg intramuscularly two times a day, or fludrocortisone acetate (Florinef), 0.05–0.2 mg/day orally	For persistent hypotension or hyperkalemia
Long-term		
Glucocorticoid	Hydrocortisone or cortisone acetate, 20–35 mg/day orally (2/3 dose at 8 AM, 1/3 dose at 3 PM) or prednisone, 5–10 mg/day orally (2/3 dose at 8 AM, 1/3 dose at 3 PM)	For minor stress, double dosage; for major stress, see above (Emergency)
Mineralocorticoid	Fludrocortisone acetate, 0.05–0.02 mg/day orally	

[a] Only glucocorticoid therapy is required in patients with hypopituitarism or ACTH suppression.

praphysiologic doses of corticosteroids, the ability of the pituitary gland to release ACTH during stress is lessened for as long as 6–9 months, and adrenal cortisol response is similarly impaired. The therapeutic implementations are clear.

1. All patients being treated with pharmacologic doses of corticosteroids (for example, more than 25 mg of cortisone or 5 mg of prednisone daily) need additional therapy during stress. If the stress is major, such as an operation or sepsis, 300 mg of cortisol or an equivalent corticosteroid are required—hydrocortisone sodium succinate, 75 mg intramuscularly every 6 hours, or methylprednisolone sodium succinate, 20 mg intramuscularly or intravenously every 6 hours. Patients with known adrenal insufficiency or hypopituitarism require similar therapy.
2. Any patient who has received pharmacologic doses of corticosteroids for more than 4 weeks during the past year may need similar therapy during stress and should be prophylactically treated with corticosteroids during any surgical procedure.

If the pituitary-adrenal axis has been shown to be normally responsive, stress doses of glucocorticoids are not necessary.

Diagnosis

In adults, pituitary surgery and pituitary tumors are the most common causes of panhypopituitarism. Single or multiple hormone deficiencies may develop slowly or rapidly. Although growth hormone production ceases first, the consequences of this deficiency are usually recognized in adults. Gonadotropin (follicle-stimulating hormone and luteinizing hormone) deficiency usually occurs next, resulting in amenorrhea or oligomenorrhea in women and loss of libido in men. Thyroid-stimulating hormone and ACTH deficiencies usually develop last, and the consequences may be life-threatening. The presence of multiple hormone deficiencies should always suggest the possibility of hypopituitarism. Visual field abnormalities, especially bitemporal hemianopsia, may be a valuable clue to a pituitary tumor. Patients with pituitary tumors causing acromegaly, Cushing's disease, or galactorrhea may have pituitary insufficiency as well. Pituitary apoplexy (sudden hemorrhage into a pituitary tumor), which is rare, may be manifested by severe headache, visual field defects, depression of consciousness, meningismus, and occasionally other cranial nerve palsies. Sudden loss of adrenal cortical function may occur, whereas other pituitary deficits, even when present, are slow to develop clinically.

Sheehan's syndrome, postpartum pituitary insufficiency, is easily recognized by the failure of menses to resume, inability to breast-feed, and generalized debility from thyroid and adrenal insufficiency that may follow postpartum hemorrhage. Pituitary insufficiency during pregnancy is particularly likely to develop in diabetic patients.

The life-threatening consequences of hypopituitarism are those of cortisol and thyroid hormone deficiency. Cortisol deficiency from hypopituitarism or ACTH suppression may be extraordinarily difficult to diagnose if it occurs alone. Many of the most valuable clinical indications leading to the recognition of Addison's disease are lacking, including hyperpigmentation and hyperkalemia. Although hypotension is present, volume depletion is not, unless the patient has had recurrent vomiting or diarrhea. Hypopigmentation may be present. Hyponatremia is often noted and may be profound. The explanation for these findings is the lack of ACTH with preservation of aldosterone function. A history of weight loss, poor response to stress, gastrointestinal symptoms, and "collapse" all may be recorded. The presence of concomitant hormone deficiencies (for example, thyroid or gonadal) may be a valuable finding. Patients in whom corticosteroids have recently been discontinued may experience arthralgia.

The presence of clinical Cushing's syndrome in a severely ill patient should suggest the possibility of exogenous glucocorticoid therapy with possible cortisol deficiency syndrome due to glucocorticoid withdrawal.

The definitive diagnosis of hypopituitarism or ACTH suppression requires pituitary stimulation by means of an insulin tolerance test or a metyrapone test or, by inference, short or prolonged ACTH stimulation tests, details of which can be found in standard endocrinology texts.

Therapy

The immediate therapy is intravenous glucocorticoid replacement as in Table 14.7, or with Solumedrol (60–80 mg/day in divided doses), since mineralocorticoid activity is unnecessary. Patients usually do not require volume replacement, and indeed, water restriction may be necessary because of hyponatremia. If concomitant adrenal and thyroid deficiencies are present, corticosteroid replacement must be started first. Thyroid hormone replacement can precipitate adrenal crisis in such a situation unless glucocorticoids are administered at the same time.

THYROID EMERGENCIES

Thyroid Storm or Decompensated Thyrotoxicosis

The drama and crisis of thyroid storm are implicit in its name. This exaggerated state of hyperthyroidism is, fortunately, now rare. Modern advances in the diagnosis and therapy of conventional hyperthyroidism, as well as intensive care for the decompensated thyrotoxic patient, have had a significant impact.

Early recognition and prompt therapy of hyperthyroidism are of utmost importance. When hyperthyroidism is complicated by concomitant illness, symptoms are likely to be exacerbated and early hospitalization is recommended. Long-standing untreated hyperthyroidism is likely to result in failure of specific organ systems. Although the decompensated thyrotoxic patient is critically ill, an excellent response to an orderly sequence of therapeutic maneuvers may be expected.

Pathophysiologic Principles

The thyroid gland produces both thyroxine and triiodothyronine. In addition, thyroxine released from the gland is converted to triiodothyronine. Approximately 99.98% of thyroxine, as well as 99.8% of triiodothyronine, is bound to protein. It is the free, nonprotein-bound hormone that is metabolically active. The manifestations of severe hyperthyroidism are related to overproduction of thyroxine and triiodothyronine and apparent overactivity of the sympathetic nervous system. The distinction between severe hyperthyroidism and thyroid storm is qualitative: the blood levels of thyroid hormones do not differ in these conditions. The failure of various thyroid hormone target organs may be due to either untreated thyrotoxicosis itself or concomitant illness and indicates the need for intensive medical care.

Diagnosis

Clinical Features. The diagnosis of hyperthyroidism may be obvious in the younger patient with classic signs and symptoms (Table 14.8). However, in the elderly, only minor indications may be present, many of which are cardiovascular. Exacerbation of underlying heart disease, atrial fibrillation refractory to digitalis, insidious onset of congestive heart failure, unexplained sinus tachycardia, atrial tachyarrhythmias, or progressive angina pectoris may be the only sign in conjunction with a slightly enlarged thyroid gland. Elderly patients may seem apathetic, with weakness, weight loss, and debility often mimicking neoplastic disease. When an additional illness or insult is present, the manifestations may become more severe (Table 14.9).

Although fever may be present in uncomplicated

Table 14.8.
Hyperthyroidism: Manifestations

	History	Physical Examination
General	Weight loss with good appetite Heat intolerance	
Skin		Warm, moist, smooth Onycholysis Pretibial myxedema (Graves' disease)
Eyes	Burning Tearing Diplopia	Lid lag, stare Exophthalmos, soft-tissue swelling, extraocular muscle paresis, corneal involvement (Graves' disease)
Neck	Enlargement	Goiter Diffuse Nodular
Respiratory	Dyspnea	
Cardiovascular	Palpitations Angina pectoris	Sinus tachycardia Atrial fibrillation Increased systolic blood pressure Decreased diastolic blood pressure Scratchy systolic ejection murmur Congestive heart failure, right-sided more severe than left-sided
Gastrointestinal	Diarrhea	
Genitourinary	Nocturia Hypomenorrhea	Gynecomastia
Neuromuscular	Tremor Weakness	Peripheral and bulbar myopathy Brisk deep tendon reflexes
Psychiatric	Emotional instability Hyperkinesia Insomnia Anxiety	

Table 14.9.
Decompensated Thyrotoxicosis: Manifestations

High fever
Cardiac decompensation
  Failure
  Arrhythmias
Gastrointestinal decompensation
  Diarrhea
  Vomiting
Neurologic deterioration
  Agitation
    Restlessness
    Delirium
  Apathy
    Myopathy
    Torpor
    Stupor
    Coma

hyperthyroidism, an elevated temperature should be considered as a sign of a potentially serious process. Even minor infections may produce a dramatic febrile response, and a careful search for sepsis is mandatory. The pulse rate is usually elevated disproportionately in relation to the temperature.

The cardiac, gastrointestinal, and sympathetic nervous systems are most likely to become decompensated. Overwhelming congestive heart failure—particularly right-sided—may develop, as well as the other cardiac symptoms mentioned. Vomiting may occur, and diarrhea may be debilitating. Although the blood flow to most organs increases in patients with hyperthyroidism, flow to the liver remains relatively constant despite increased metabolic demands, and hepatic decompensation may result. Central nervous system activation may be indicated by restlessness, severe agitation, or delirium. On the other hand, myopathy both of the peripheral and bulbar musculature may be so profound that patients become lethargic, stuporous, or comatose; this is often complicated by repeated aspiration.

Iodine excess may precipitate hyperthyroidism in patients with nodular goiters. This situation may be particularly treacherous in patients with coronary disease undergoing angiographic procedures or patients with arrhythmias treated with iodine containing drugs such as amiodarone.

Clinical Studies. Laboratory tests can confirm the diagnosis of hyperthyroidism, but are usually not a good index of its severity. In patients with hyperthyroidism, the total serum thyroxine level is usually elevated. To separate hyperthyroidism from other conditions that falsely elevate the total serum thyroxine level (namely, an elevated level of binding protein, which is commonly due to estrogens), either the triiodothyronine resin (T_3 resin) or the free thyroxine level is determined, both of which are usually elevated in hyperthyroidism. With an elevated level of binding protein, the patient is not hyperthyroid, the T_3 resin is decreased, and the free thyroxine is normal. Patients occasionally have so-called T_3 toxicosis, in which the concentrations of total and free thyroxine in the blood are normal, but the total triiodothyronine level is elevated. These tests take one to several days to complete. However, in an emergency, therapy must be started before laboratory confirmation.

Therapy

The prognosis for the patient with severe decompensated thyrotoxicosis has improved substantially as specific therapeutic measures have become available (Table 14.10).

General Measures. The hyperpyrexic patient may require acetaminophen or cooling blankets while the search for infection proceeds. Attention to hydration is of utmost importance. Copious amounts of hypotonic fluid may be lost through the skin, and occasionally, large amounts of sodium and potassium may be lost if the patient has diarrhea. Glucose and soluble B vitamins should also be administered.

Blockade of Thyroid Hormone Synthesis. Both propylthiouracil (PTU) and methimazole (Tapazole) block the synthesis of thyroid hormone. Methimazole is 10 times as potent and has a longer half-life, but propylthiouracil prevents some of the peripheral conversion of thyroxine to triiodothyronine. When large doses are used at frequent intervals, as in thyroid storm, propylthiouracil is the drug of choice. These agents are not commercially available for parenteral administration, although hospital pharmacies may be able to formulate such a preparation in an emergency. Patients with decompensated thyrotoxicosis should receive propylthiouracil, 200–250 mg, or methimazole, 20–25 mg, every 4 hours either orally or by nasogastric tube if necessary. In contrast, patients with uncomplicated hyperthyroidism receive propylthiouracil, 100 mg, or methimazole, 10 mg, every 6 or 8 hours.

Although complete blockade of thyroid hormone synthesis can be achieved within hours, clinical response may not be apparent for weeks or months because the large stores of thyroid hormone within the thyroid gland must be dissipated before euthyroidism is achieved, and neither propylthiouracil nor methimazole blocks release of these hormones.

Blockade of Thyroid Hormone Release. Although iodide is the substrate for thyroid hormone synthesis, in pharmacologic doses it blocks the release of hormone from the thyroid gland, especially from the diffuse toxic goiter. To prevent the administered iodide from being directed into new hormone stores, synthesis must be ade-

Table 14.10.
Decompensated Thyrotoxicosis: Therapy

Measure	Agent
General	
Reduction of fever	Acetaminophen, cooling blanket, sponge bath
Hydration	Intravenous fluids as necessary
Administration of vitamins	Soluble B vitamins
Administration of glucose	5% dextrose solution
Blockade of thyroid hormone synthesis	Propylthiouracil, 200–500 mg every 4 hr orally or by nasogastric tube or Methimazole, 20–25 mg every 4 hr orally or by nasogastric tube
Blockade of thyroid hormone release	Iodides Sodium iodide, 1–2 gm/day intravenously or Supersaturated solution of potassium iodide, 5 drops orally every 4 hr
Blockade of peripheral effects	Sympatholytics Propranolol, 1–5 mg intravenously or 20–200 mg orally every 4 hr or Reserpine, 0.25–2.5 mg intramuscularly every 4–6 hr or Guanethidine, 1–2 mg/kg/day orally
Inhibition of thyroxine to triiodothyronine conversion	Propylthiouracil (see above) Propranolol (see above) Glucocorticoids (e.g., Dexamethasone, 2 mg intravenously or intramuscularly every 6 hr)
Therapy for cardiac disease	Ipodate, 1 gm/day
Atrial fibrillation	Digoxin (increased requirements) Propranolol or other β-adrenergic blockers as required
Congestive heart failure	Digoxin plus diuretics Sympatholytics subsequently, if necessary

quately blocked. For this reason, iodides should be given approximately 1 hour after therapy with propylthiouracil or methimazole. Sodium iodide, 1–2 gm/day intravenously, or a supersaturated solution of potassium iodide, 5 drops orally every 4 hours, is effective. In general, the use of iodides is reserved for emergency situations.

Lithium shares with iodide the ability to block release of thyroid hormone. Although still considered an experimental agent for thyrotoxicosis, it has the potential advantage over iodides of not serving as a hormone substrate.

The half-life of thyroxine in plasma is approximately 7 days; that of triiodothyronine is 1 day. Although these periods are somewhat shortened in hyperthyroidism, it is obvious that the effects of blockade of hormone release are relatively slow to appear.

Blockade of Peripheral Effects. There is no known specific antagonist to the actions of thyroid hormone. Many of the manifestations of thyroid hormone excess mimic those of an overactive sympathetic nervous system, for example, tachycardia, tremor, diaphoresis, and weight loss. Although there is no direct evidence for sympathetic overactivity, several sympatholytic agents have been introduced into the therapeutic regimen for severe thyrotoxicosis. Used in conjunction with the previously mentioned modes of therapy and less commonly by themselves, these agents have proved remarkably successful.

The most effective agent appears to be propranolol, a β-adrenergic antagonist. Propranolol has the additional advantage, not shared by other β-adrenergic blockers, of partially inhibiting conversion of thyroxine (T_4) to triiodothyronine (T_3). Intravenous doses of 1–5 mg or oral doses of 20–40 mg every 4 hours may dramatically improve the patient's condition within minutes to hours. In some situations, 200 or more mg by mouth every 4–6 hours may be necessary. The lower doses should be tried first. In the presence of congestive heart failure, propranolol should be administered very cautiously, and it is possible that newer β-adrenergic antagonists will be safer. Propranolol is contraindicated in patients with asthma, and may not be of benefit in the hyperthyroid patient without tachycardia.

Reserpine, 2.0–2.5 intramuscularly every 4–6 hours, is an alternative. However, a lower dose, such as 0.25-1.0 mg, may be effective and should be tried first. Reserpine should not be administered when sedation is considered undesirable.

Guanethidine, 70–100 mg/day orally, is also effective. Although hypotension may develop, significantly low blood pressure has not been common.

Inhibition of T_4 to T_3 Conversion. Under ordinary circumstances, 85% or more of circulating T_3 is derived from peripheral conversion of T_4. T_3 is a more active hormone with T_4 possibly serving as a prohormone or precursor hormone for T_3. In hyperthyroidism, relatively more T_3 is produced from the thyroid gland. However, peripheral tissue T_3 production contributes a significant amount to the circulating T_3 concentration. Glucocorticoids have been part of the regimen for thyroid storm for years. Thyroid hormone accelerates the degradation of cortisol. However, frank adrenal insufficiency has not been recognized in thyroid storm in the absence of established Addison's disease. Recently, glucocorticoids such as dexamethasone have been shown to partially impair T_4 to T_3 conversion, providing a reasonable excuse to continue this firmly entrenched modality of therapy. Propranolol but not other β-adrenergic agents contributes to this impaired conversion as well. Glucocorticoids are additive to propylthiouracil in terms of peripheral T_4 to T_3 conversion. Iodinated contrast materials (e.g. ipodate) inhibit T_4 to T_3 conversion as well.

Therapy of Congestive Heart Failure. In addition to exacerbating underlying heart disease, thyrotoxicosis can precipitate congestive heart failure in a previously normal heart. The striking increase in cardiac output often results in predominantly right-sided failure, and treatment may be difficult. The initial therapy should be administration of digitalis and diuretics. Sympatholytic agents may be administered later if response to therapy is inadequate. Since propranolol has myocardial depressant effects that are independent of its β-adrenergic blocking effects and that may exacerbate congestive heart failure, guanethidine and reserpine may be safer in this situation. Administration of these agents should follow conventional therapy. Newer, pure β blockers will surely receive additional trials in this situation.

Digitalis must be administered to patients with atrial fibrillation. Since the space of distribution for digoxin is increased in patients with hyperthyroidism, larger doses than usual may be required. The ventricular response may slow to between 100 and 120 beats/min, but further increases in dosage are more likely to result in digitalis toxicity than in ventricular slowing. β-Adrenergic blocking agents such as propranolol may be helpful in reducing the rate further.

Removal of Thyroid Hormone. Large quantities of thyroid hormone can be removed by peritoneal dialysis or plasmapheresis. This is usually not necessary and has not been shown to improve the prognosis in decompensated thyrotoxicosis.

Precipitating Factors

Untreated hyperthyroidism may range from mild to severe, and exacerbations are usually related to an identifiable precipitating factor. In patients with hyperthyroidism, the following may be particularly dangerous: operation, infection, trauma, delivery, diabetic ketoacidosis, and certain drugs such as parasympatholytic and sympathomimetic agents. Symptoms of hyperthyroidism may worsen for a few days after therapy with iodine 131, and radioactive therapy is best deferred in acutely ill patients.

Before the development of effective antithyroid drugs, thyroid storm usually occurred as a result of thyroidectomy in untreated or iodide-treated thyrotoxic patients. Even now, extrathyroidal operation on patients with unrecognized hyperthyroidism can precipitate a crisis, particularly if atropine is used as a preanesthetic agent. Sepsis represents the major decompensating event today, and thyrotoxic patients with infections require special care. As stated previously, hospitalization should be considered for any patient with thyrotoxicosis and a concurrent illness.

Preparation for Operation

Currently, every thyrotoxic patient who undergoes operation—whether thyroidectomy or other surgical procedure—must receive specific preoperative preparation. Patients should be treated with propylthiouracil or methimazole until a euthyroid state is achieved. In addition, a supersaturated solution of potassium iodide, 3 drops orally twice a day, should be administered to reduce the vascularity of the thyroid gland during the 10 days before thyroid operation. Recently, patients have successfully been treated with β blockade alone before thyroidectomy. Sufficient drug must be given to decrease the pulse (after exercise if possible) to the 80–90 beats/min range. This may require 1000 mg or more of propanolol per day. The drug must be given up to and including the morning of surgery and continued for several postoperative days, even if a thyroidectomy has been performed. If tachycardia appears in the patient in the recovery room, intravenous propranolol should be administered. Failure to adhere to these rigid guidelines may allow thyroid storm to develop.

Emergency operation for an unrelated condition is occasionally necessary in thyrotoxic patients. Survival in such a situation may depend on the use of sympatholytic agents, especially the β-adrenergic blocking agents. Atropine and scopolamine should be avoided as preanesthetic drugs. Haloperidol has recently been implicated as a precipitant of thyroid storm. In addition, prophylactic administration of propylthiouracil or methimazole, as well as iodides, is recommended.

Myxedema Crisis

Severe, complicated hypothyroidism (myxedema crisis) usually develops as a result of the body's inability to handle additional insults, either endogenous or exogenous. It may occur with or without coma and is a highly lethal disorder, with reported

Table 14.11.
Hypothyroidism: Manifestations

	History	Physical Examination	Laboratory Findings
General	Intolerance to cold Weight gain with decreased appetite Obesity (rare) Radioactive iodine therapy	Hypothermia	Decreased thyroxine, free thyroxine, T_3 resin Increased thyroid-stimulating hormone (primary hypothyroidism) Elevated cholesterol, triglycerides, sedimentation rate, creatinine phosphokinase, cerebrospinal fluid protein
Cardiovascular		Sinus bradycardia Increased diastolic blood pressure Cardiomegaly Distant heart sounds	
Skin		Dry, cool, coarse, thickened Carotenodermia Patchy alopecia Periorbital edema	
Mouth		Enlarged tongue	
Neck	Thyroidectomy	Goiter Scar	
Gastrointestinal	Constipation	Ileus	
Genitourinary	Menorrhagia (primary hypothyroidism) Amenorrhea (secondary hypothyroidism)		
Neurologic	Muscle cramps Paresthesias Unsteadiness	Ataxic gait Delay in relaxation of deep tendon reflexes Obtundation	
Psychiatric	Lethargy Depression Mental slowing	Apathy Psychosis Myxedema "wit"	

mortalities between 50 and 75%. Death from severe hypothyroidism is particularly tragic in light of the ease with which uncomplicated hypothyroidism can be treated. The fact that myxedema crisis develops after admission to the hospital in about 50% of cases emphasizes the need for early recognition and treatment of hypothyroidism. Although myxedema may be easy to recognize, mild hypothyroidism is often an extremely subtle process. Symptoms may be nonspecific or absent, and clinical indications may be easily overlooked.

Pathophysiologic Principles

As soon as hypothyroidism is suspected, the question of primary versus secondary disease must be raised. Primary hypothyroidism refers to failure of the thyroid gland itself. It is most commonly caused by Hashimoto's thyroiditis (autoimmune thyroiditis), radioactive iodine therapy, and thyroid operation, and it accounts for 95% of all cases of hypothyroidism. As the thyroid gland begins to fail, the pituitary gland attempts to compensate with increased production of thyroid-stimulating hormone (TSH). The earliest sign of a failing thyroid gland, therefore, is an increase in the serum TSH level. Secondary hypothyroidism results from disease of the pituitary gland or hypothalamus, with resultant failure of TSH release.

Goiter usually indicates primary disease; loss of axillary and pubic hair, diminished libido, or amenorrhea may indicate a pituitary origin. An elevated radioimmunoassay TSH level confirms the diagnosis of primary hypothyroidism. If the TSH level is not elevated in a hypothyroid patient, secondary hypothyroidism is present.

The distinction between primary and secondary disease is important in the selection of therapy. Thyroid hormone accelerates the metabolism of cortisol in the liver, and normally, this results in release of ACTH from the pituitary gland and compensatory cortisol secretion. When the pituitary gland fails, many trophic hormones in addition to TSH are not produced, ACTH being particularly notable. If ACTH release is deficient, the addition of thyroid hormone may precipitate adrenal failure by inactivating the small amounts of cortisol that are being produced. In this setting (hypopituitarism), cortisol must be administered before thyroid hormone.

Diagnosis

Clinical Features. The cardinal features of hypothyroidism are listed in Table 14.11. Apathy may dominate the clinical findings, and as a result, the patient may deny all symptoms. On the other hand, depression may be striking and may be accompanied by many somatic complaints.

The pulse rate may be normal, and the diastolic blood pressure is often elevated. Hypothermia is frequently not diagnosed because of failure to shake the mercury in the thermometer to below 96°F (35.6°C). Exophthalmos may be the only residual manifestation of previously treated hyperthyroidism (Graves' disease). Cutaneous manifestations such as dryness, swelling, and carotenodermia are common, and periorbital edema is a regular finding. A thyroidectomy scar may be a valuable clue to early hypothyroidism; however, radioactive iodine therapy leaves no clues. Delay in the relaxation phase of the deep tendon reflexes (especially of the ankle and biceps) is helpful, but may occur in hypothermia from any cause. Proptosis (exopthalmos) may be a clue to previously treated Graves' disease. The absence of any of these findings does not exclude the diagnosis of hypothyroidism.

Clinical Studies. In general, in patients with severe hypothyroidism, values for the conventional thyroid function, such as serum thyroxine and serum free thyroxine, are all low. These tests, however, may fail to confirm the diagnosis of hypothyroidism even when clinical evidence is present. For example, the normal range of the serum thyroxine is 4–11 μg/dl. However, each individual maintains a serum thyroxine level within a narrower range, for example, 8–9 μg/dl. If the thyroid gland fails, this level will decrease, but will stay within the "normal" range. In addition, pregnant women and those using oral contraceptives normally have an elevated serum thyroxine level because of an elevated level of binding proteins, and such patients may have thyroid failure with a thyroxine level in the range of 8–9 μg/dl. Thus, since the serum TSH level increases concomitantly with decrease in serum thyroxine, the only way to diagnose early hypothyroidism may be to measure the serum TSH in every patient with suspected hypothyroidism. The clinical recognition of such patients is important if one is to diagnose hypothyroidism early. However, such mild hypothyroidism is unlikely to precipitate myxedema crisis.

Many patients with a low serum thyroxine measurement do not have hypothyroidism. Such patients may have a deficiency of thyroxine-binding globulin, in which case the T_3 resin will be elevated. In hypothyroid patients, low normal or frankly low T_3-resin values are the rule.

Impaired T_4 to T_3 conversion is common in starved and "sick" individuals, the so called "sick euthyroid syndrome". This may be a homeostatic attempt by the body to decrease catabolism under these circumstances. With the fall in serum T_3 concentration, an inactive metabolite of T_4, called reverse T_3, rises in the circulation.

Low serum thyroxine concentrations are increas-

Table 14.12.
Myxedema Crisis: Manifestations, Prevention, and Therapy

Manifestation	Prevention	Therapy
HYPOventilation	Monitor blood gases Avoid sedatives	Institute assisted ventilation Perform tracheotomy early if necessary
HYPOmetabolism of drugs	Avoid sedative, narcotics, iodides, lithium, preanesthetic medications Delay elective operation Alert anesthesiologist if emergency operation required If digitalis required, use in decreased dosage	
HYPOthermia	Avoid cold exposure Suspect infection with normal temperature	
HYPOresponsiveness	Suspect infection even with normal temperature and physical examination Monitor frequently: chest x-ray, white blood cell count, urinalysis	Administer antibiotics as infections are identified
HYPOnatremia	Avoid excess fluids	Restrict fluid
HYPOadrenalism		Administer hydrocortisone sodium hemisuccinate, 75 mg intramuscularly or intravenously every 6 hr after 100 mg intravenously (sick primary hypothyroidism and all secondary hypothyroidism)
HYPOglycemia	Monitor blood glucose	Administer dextrose solution intravenously
HYPOtension	Administer steroids to sick hypothyroid patients Avoid sedatives Search for infection	Avoid pressor agents Administer cortisol Administer colloid Treat infection as indicated
HYPOtonia	Suspect ileus with "surgical abdomen" Administer mild laxatives as prophylaxis Search for silent urinary tract infection	
HYPOthyroidism	Place patient in intensive care unit	Administer L-thyroxine, 100–200 μg intravenously, then 100 μg/day either orally or intravenously. Consider L-triiodothyronine 12.5–25 μg/day.

ingly being recognized in critically ill patients in intensive care units: the "low T_4, sick-euthyroid syndrome." Although these patients have an extremely high mortality rate, they are not hypothyroid and do not seem to be helped by thyroid hormone administration.

The decreased T_4 concentration is due to the tissue release of a substance (? fatty acid) which inhibits the binding of T_4 to its binding proteins. Although the T_3 resin is often slightly elevated in this situation, the free T_4 index and occasionally the direct free T_4 concentrations may be slightly low. A serum TSH greater than 20 microunits/ml is diagnositc of primary hypothyroidism and is not found in the "sick euthyroid" states. Elevated serum reverse T_3 concentrations are found in the sick euthyroid states but not in hypothyroidism.

Radioactive iodine uptake studies are of almost no value in the diagnosis of hypothyroidism and are not recommended.

Therapy

The factors precipitating myxedema crisis, the manifestations, and therapy (Table 14.12) are closely related and are discussed together in this section. Therapy must begin before laboratory confirmation of the diagnosis. Myxedema crisis or coma is a problem of general medical care, and the components can be treated even if the diagnosis of hypothyroidism is not initially considered.

Hypoventilation. Carbon dioxide retention and narcosis commonly cause coma in the patient with myxedema. Arterial blood gas levels must be monitored in the hospitalized hypothyroid patient. Respiratory failure in this setting has several causes. Hypothyroid patients have a decreased respiratory response to conventional stimuli such as hypoxia and carbon dioxide elevation. An enlarged tongue may fall back into the oropharynx, causing obstruction of the upper part of the respiratory tract. Sedative drugs administered either routinely or because of bizarre behavior can easily depress respiration in these patients. Patients with borderline hypothyroidism may become profoundly hypothyroid when exposed to iodides. This is particularly devastating when the iodides are prescribed for underlying pulmonary disease (for example, expectorants with iodides or a supersaturated solution of potassium iodide) since the subsequent hypothyroidism exacerbates the preexistent respiratory problem.

Myxedema develops and reverses slowly. Several weeks may be required to reverse the clinical state. Patients with severe ventilatory failure require intubation. If oversedation is not a causative factor, tracheotomy may be necessary until the underlying hypothyroidism responds to therapy.

Hypometabolism of Drugs. Many drugs are metabolized or excreted more slowly in the hypothyroid patient. Routine administration of sedatives, narcotic analgesics, or preanesthetic drugs, as well as anesthesia itself, can precipitate coma in the borderline or frankly hypothyroid individual. Sedatives and narcotics are contraindicated in patients with suspected hypothyroidism, and elective operation should be avoided until the patient is almost euthyroid. If emergency operation is required, preanesthetic medications can be omitted, and the anesthesiologist should be notified of the diagnosis. It is surprising how well surgery is tolerated in patients with moderate and even severe hypothyroidism, particularly when the diagnosis is recognized preoperatively and adequate precautions are taken.

Certain drugs can precipitate hypothyroidism in susceptible persons or cause myxedema in patients with borderline hypothyroidism. The most notable agents are the iodides, which inhibit thyroid hormone synthesis and release, and lithium, which also inhibits thyroid hormone release.

The heart size is often enlarged in patients with hypothyroidism. In myxedematous patients this may be due to a benign pericardial effusion requiring no specific therapy (tamponade is extraordinarily rare). Congestive heart failure is unusual in hypothyroidism, but digitalis might mistakenly be administered because of cardiac enlargement. Digoxin metabolism is impaired because of a decreased space of distribution; if conventional doses are administered, higher blood levels of digoxin will result, and digitalis toxicity will develop. If digitalis is required in the hypothyroid patient, it should be used sparingly and with great caution.

Hypothermia. Myxedema should be considered in any hypothermic patient. Hypothermia is important for several reasons. The lower the temperature, the worse the prognosis. Fewer than 15% of patients survive temperatures less than 90°F (32.2°C) in the setting of myxedema crisis. Cold weather and exposure may precipitate coma. Also, infection may be undetected because of the absence of fever. A "normal" temperature in a profoundly hypothyroid patient should always prompt a careful search for infection.

Hyporesponsiveness to Infection. The placid demeanor, apparently stable temperature, and lack of complaints of the hypothyroid patient may be misleading. Pneumonia will be missed on the basis of physical examination alone, since shallow respirations make examination difficult and cough is often absent. Patients will not complain of dysuria.

Frequent chest x-ray films, white blood cell counts, and urinalyses are necessary if infections are to be recognized early and if fatal sepsis is to be avoided. Prophylactic administration of antibiotics is not indicated, however.

Hyponatremia. The glomerular filtration rate is diminished in patients with hypothyroidism, probably because of decrease in intravascular volume. This results in impaired ability to excrete water. Hyponatremia results if hypotonic fluids are administered in excess. Inappropriate secretion of antidiuretic hormone is an alternative explanation for the hyponatremia.

The therapy and prevention of hyponatremia involve avoidance of an excess of free water. In severe cases, fluids must be restricted to less than 800-1000 ml/day. Although the intravascular space is contracted in hypothyroidism, there is an excess of whole body sodium that is located in the myxedema fluid. Therefore, sodium should be avoided as well. If volume replacement is necessary, colloid is the therapy of choice.

Hypoadrenalism. Patients with secondary hypothyroidism due to failure of the pituitary gland commonly have adrenal insufficiency as well. It is less recognized, however, that patients with severe primary hypothyroidism have relative adrenal insufficiency. Although their basal production of cortisol is adequate, hypothyroid patients may have an inadequate cortisol response to stress. Cortisol therapy is recommended, therefore, not only in all patients with secondary hypothyroidism but also in acutely ill patients with primary hypothyroidism. The doses are similar to those for ACTH deficiency. If emergency operation is necessary, corticosteroids should be administered.

Hypotension. Drug sensitivity, relative or absolute adrenal insufficiency, or occasionally sepsis may induce hypotension in the myxedematous patient. The intravascular volume tends to be decreased, making colloid the initial therapy of choice. The myxedematous patient is thought to be refractory to catecholamines unless thyroid hormone is administered first. In addition, arrhythmias may develop if pressor agents and thyroid hormone are administered simultaneously. Given these two considerations, pressor agents are probably best avoided.

Hypotonia. Intestinal hypotonia may lead to ileus and may mimic obstruction; prophylactic administration of a mild laxative is recommended. Distension of the intestine may result in seeding of the blood by Gram-negative organisms and, occasionally, gastrointestinal bleeding. In patients with atony of the bladder, stasis and infection may develop. To treat these complications properly, the underlying cause must be recognized.

Hypoglycemia. Hypoglycemia is a rare complication of hypothyroidism. It is much more common in patients with secondary hypothyroidism, but may complicate primary hypothyroidism with devastating consequences. The therapy is intravenous glucose. Seizures are common in the presence of hypoglycemia.

Hypothyroidism. It is not an error to consider hypothyroidism last. Most patients with coma or hypothyroid crisis respond favorably if attention is paid to all the complications previously mentioned.

In patients with uncomplicated hypothyroidism, small doses of L-thyroxine orally are recommended, with increments at 2- to 4-week intervals. The severity of the hypothyroidism, the duration of symptoms, the extent of cardiac disease, and the increasing age of the patient all dictate a lower initial dose. Recommended doses of L-thyroxine are 25–50 μg/day for older or sicker patients and 100–150 μg/day for younger patients or those with milder disease. Full replacement therapy with L-thyroxine varies with the individual, but commonly ranges from 50 to 200 μg/day.

Higher doses of L-thyroxine have been recommended for myxedema crisis—up to 500 μg as initial intravenous therapy. This approximates the whole body deficit of thyroxine in patients with hypothyroidism. We, however, are not convinced that the dose of thyroid hormone is the critical variable and recommend an intermediate dose, 100–200 μg intravenously followed by 100 μg/day intravenously or orally.

Others have advocated administration of triiodothyronine. This agent is not commercially available for parenteral administration, although it can be prepared in hospital pharmacies. Although the rapid termination of action that occurs after stopping this drug is thought to be an advantage, the rapid onset of action may be a considerable disadvantage, leading to cardiac arrhythmias and death.

Careful studies on thyroxine to triiodothyronine conversion have not been reported in myxedema crisis. In the face of sepsis or shock, impaired conversion might play a clinically important role. Although there are no data to suggest that it is helpful or necessary, triiodothyronine therapy (12.5–25 μg/day) should be strongly considered.

Some patients who show considerable improvement after a few days of therapy die within a few weeks. The reason for this is unclear. We recommend intensive care monitoring for at least 2 weeks in all such critically ill patients with hypothyroidism. Although the patient may not appear to be critically ill, the presence of severe hypothyroidism with the above complications warrants such precautions.

Surgery in Hypothyroid Patients

We prefer to avoid elective surgery in patients with moderate or profound hypothyroidism. However, the risks of surgery in mild to moderate hypothyroidism have been overstated; the risks of surgery with profound hypothyroidism are unknown. When emergency surgery is required, it should not be delayed. We do not advocate emergency thyroid hormone repletion in hypothyroid patients with angina requiring bypass surgery.

Surgical mortality is not increased in patients with moderate *clinical* hypothyroidism (serum T_4 as low as 1 μg/dl without myxedema). With hypothyroidism increased surgical morbidity includes mild intraoperative hypotension in noncardiac surgical patients and mild increased congestive heart failure in cardiac surgical patients. Postoperative morbidity includes increased constipation and confusion with decreased ability to manifest a fever.

CALCIUM EMERGENCIES

Physiologic Principles

Calcium in the blood circulates in bound, complexed, and ionized forms. Although all three are measured when the serum calcium level is determined, only the ionized calcium exerts important biologic effects. In some laboratories, the ionized calcium can be measured directly; this may be helpful in certain situations.

Approximately 45% of circulating calcium is bound to serum proteins. Roughly 0.8 mg is bound to each gram of albumin and 0.2 mg to each gram of globulin. For simplicity, the following rule can be adopted: an increase or decrease of 1 gm/dl in the serum albumin concentration causes a corresponding increase or decrease of approximately 1 mg/dl in the serum calcium concentration.

The serum calcium level, together with the serum albumin level, becomes elevated with dehydration or with prolonged tourniquet application before blood letting, but the ionized calcium concentration remains normal. Similarly, hypoalbuminemic states result in decrease in the total serum calcium concentration. With a normal serum albumin level of approximately 4.5 gm/dl, the normal serum calcium concentration is 8.5–10.5 mg/dl. However, an albumin concentration of 2 gm/dl corresponds to a total calcium concentration of 6.5–8.4 mg/dl, the ionized calcium remaining within normal limits. To correct for this, a second rule must be invoked: the serum albumin concentration must be measured whenever the serum calcium concentration is determined.

The concentration of ionized calcium is maintained within narrow limits in the blood, predominantly through the action of parathyroid hormone. Increase in the serum calcium concentration suppresses parathyroid hormone production; decrease stimulates production. Parathyroid hormone mobilizes calcium from bone with the aid of vitamin D. Bone resorption releases phosphate in addition to calcium, and since parathyroid hormone facilitates urinary excretion of phosphate, a low serum phosphate value may indicate excess parathyroid hormone. In addition, parathyroid hormone increases absorption of calcium from the urine and, indirectly, from the diet.

Calcium is absorbed from the duodenum and upper part of the small intestine predominantly under the influence of vitamin D. Absorbed from the diet or synthesized in the skin, vitamin D must be hydroxylated by the liver (25-hydroxylation) and subsequently by the kidneys (1-hydroxylation) to become fully active. Decreased serum phosphate and parathyroid hormone appear to contribute to 1-hydroxylase activation. The fully active compound, 1,25-dihydroxycholecalciferol, both increases bone resorption and is necessary for the action of parathyroid hormone on bone resorption.

Calcitonin, a peptide hormone synthesized by the thyroid gland, retards bone resorption. In pharmacologic doses, calcitonin can lower the serum calcium level. However, its role in normal physiology remains unclear.

Table 14.13.
Hypercalcemia: Causes[a]

- Common
  - Spurious
    - Laboratory error
    - Tourniquet
    - Dehydration (e.g., with Addison's disease)
  - Malignant condition (especially breast and lung carcinoma, multiple myeloma)
    - With bony metastases
    - Without bony metastases (?ectopic hormone production)
  - Primary hyperparathyroidism
- Uncommon
  - Granulomatous disease (sarcoidosis, berylliosis, tuberculosis, histoplasmosis, blastomycosis)
  - Vitamin A or D intoxication
  - Thyrotoxicosis
  - Milk-alkali syndrome
  - Immobilization with increased bone turnover
  - Renal transplantation

[a] Any of these may be exacerbated by thiazide diuretic therapy.

Hypercalcemia

Recognition of severe hypercalcemia without laboratory testing is extremely difficult if not impossible. Therefore, the serum calcium level of every patient with a disordered state of consciousness must be determined. The physician should also remember that a normal serum calcium level in the presence of hypoalbuminemia may, in fact, represent early or important hypercalcemia. Awareness of the possibility of hypercalcemia often leads to early and successful therapy.

Hypercalcemia can often be prevented if appropriate precautions are observed. Patients with hyperparathyroidism, cancer, or accelerated bone resorption as in Paget's disease may be susceptible to lethal hypercalcemia if they are immobilized, dehydrated, or treated with thiazide diuretics, since immobilization increases resorption of calcium from bone, and dehydration and thiazide diuretics prevent excretion of calcium in the urine. Growing children are particularly susceptible to immobilization hypercalcemia; this problem is more common now that quadriplegics have improved survival. Hypercalcemia is particularly likely to develop after therapy for certain neoplasms, for example, breast carcinoma treated with estrogens or androgens. A surprising number of patients who enter the hospital with a normal serum calcium level become hypercalcemic as a result of immobilization or fasting, and all patients at risk should be kept well hydrated and should be encouraged to walk. Thiazide diuretics should not be administered to such patients.

Diagnosis

To provide optimal therapy, the physician must estimate the probable cause of the hypercalcemia (Table 14.13). In our experience, more than 90% of hypercalcemic patients have either a malignant tumor or primary hyperparathyroidism.

Clinical Features. Prodromal symptoms may develop with slight to moderate elevation of the serum calcium level. These symptoms depend on the level of calcium itself and not on the cause. Gastrointestinal symptoms include constipation, anorexia, nausea, and vomiting. Nausea and vomiting may cause dehydration, reducing renal calcium excretion and exacerbating hypercalcemia. As a result, a cycle may develop, terminating in coma or death. Polyuria and polydipsia are apparently related to the impaired renal concentrating ability induced by hypercalcemia, and increased urinary losses may begin a similar dehydration cycle. Central nervous system changes range from subtle depression, impaired memory, or difficulty in concentrating to lethargy, stupor, or coma. A history of any of these symptoms in a comatose patient should raise the suspicion of hypercalcemia.

Physical examination is rarely informative. Hypertension may develop with acute hypercalcemia. Tachycardia and, less commonly, bradycardia or irregular rhythms may occur, but are also nonspecific. Chronic hypercalcemia may cause band keratopathy, that is, calcific deposits at the limbus of the eye. These deposits occur at the junction of the cornea and the sclera, in the parenthesis distribution of ("3 o'clock and 9 o'clock") and can occasionally be demonstrated by shining a penlight obliquely at these areas. The absence of deep tendon reflexes may be another clinical sign. A parathyroid adenoma is rarely palpable. A careful search for malignant neoplasms is imperative, with particular attention to breast nodules or mastectomy scars.

Clinical Studies. The electrocardiogram may provide the first clinical indication of hypercalcemia. A shortened Q-T interval suggests this condition, particularly when a prior normal electrocardiogram is available for comparison. It is important to remember that hypercalcemia sensitizes the myocardium to digitalis, and digitalis toxicity may develop in this setting.

In general, any feature indicating chronic hypercalcemia favors primary hyperparathyroidism as the diagnosis; examples include prior laboratory confirmation of hypercalcemia, renal calculi, and nephrocalcinosis. It is extremely unusual for a malignant tumor to cause sustained hypercalcemia of several years' duration. A deceased glomerular filtration rate is regularly observed with severe hypercalcemia itself; therefore, an elevated blood urea nitrogen level does not necessarily imply chronicity of hypercalcemia or irreversible renal failure. A low fasting serum phosphate value favors but does not establish the diagnosis of hyperparathyroidism. Oral or intravenous glucose also lowers the serum phosphate level, and values determined while the patient is receiving glucose or after meals should be ignored. Parathyroid hormone causes loss of bicarbonate through the kidneys, and an elevated serum chloride level with a decreased serum bicarbonate concentration suggests parathyroid hormone excess. Although ability to measure parathyroid hormone has aided differential diagnosis considerably, this test takes too long to be of benefit in a hypercalcemic emergency.

Rouleaux on a peripheral blood smear suggest multiple myeloma, which should be confirmed with protein electrophoresis or immunoelectrophoresis or both. Diffuse hyperglobulinemia is characteristic of sarcoidosis.

When the clinical condition permits, the following radiologic studies should be obtained: chest films (pulmonary malignant process, hilar adenopathy, or interstitial pattern of sarcoidosis); kidney-ureter-bladder films (renal stones or nephrocalcinosis); bone survey or scan (metastatic disease or Paget's disease); hand and clavicular films (subperiosteal resorption pathognomonic of hyperparathyroidism); intravenous pyelogram (hypernephroma); and mammograms (cancer). Normal radiologic results exclude neither hyperparathyroidism nor a malignant lesion.

Therapy

Hypercalcemia may result from excess calcium absorption, excess bone resorption, or decreased calcium excretion (Table 14.14). A combination of these factors is often at fault. Therapy should not be more toxic than the disease. The therapy of hy-

Table 14.14.
Hypercalcemia: Physiologic Mechanisms

Increased calcium absorption
Vitamin D intoxication
Sarcoidosis
Milk-alkali syndrome
Increased bone resorption
Hyperparathyroidism
Malignant disease
Hyperthyroidism
Immobilization, especially with Paget's disease or in children
Vitamin D intoxication
Sarcoidosis
Decreased calcium excretion
Hyperparathyroidism
Above conditions in combination with dehydration or administration of thiazide diuretics

percalcemia due to a malignant process is usually based on hope for other therapeutic inverventions in the future. Patients who were clearly dying before development of hypercalcemia should probably not be treated, but whenever the prognosis is in doubt, hypercalcemic patients should receive treatment (Tables 14.15 and 14.16).

Prevention of Calcium Absorption. To eliminate excess calcium from the diet, consumption of dairy products and calcium-containing antacids such as Tums should be discontinued. Except in patients with the milk-alkali syndrome, this unfortunately has little immediate effect on the serum calcium level. Vitamin D and newer analogues should be discontinued.

The effects of vitamin D on calcium absorption may last for months. In patients with vitamin D intoxication or hypersensitivity (for example, sarcoidosis), rapid reversal of hypercalcemia may be accomplished with administration of glucocorticoids, such as prednisone, 40–60 mg/day in divided doses. Drugs such as phenytoin or phenobarbital may accelerate the metabolism of vitamin D to less active products.

Increase in Urinary Calcium Excretion. Calcium appears in the urine in conjunction with sodium. Dehydration rids the urine of sodium and prevents calcium excretion. Rehydration with oral fluids and salty foods may be adequate for prevention or treatment of mild hypercalcemia. Potassium should be replaced, and thiazide diuretics should not be prescribed.

With markedly symptomatic or severe hypercalcemia, large amounts of intravenous fluid containing sodium are often required. "Forced diuresis" with saline solution and potent diuretics, such as furosemide or ethacrynic acid, is effective, but is potentially dangerous and should never be performed outside of an intensive care setting. The central venous pressure should be monitored to prevent fluid overload. In severe cases, a minimum of 200 ml/hr of normal saline solution with intravenous furosemide in sufficient quantity (40–100 mg every 2 hours) is necessary to sustain the diuresis. Fluid administration must match urinary volume. In addition, urine should be analyzed for potassium and magnesium, and the amounts lost should be replaced, potassium replacement being mandatory.

Isotonic sodium sulfate solution has been suggested as an alternative to normal saline because it contains more sodium per liter and because sulfate complexes calcium in the urine. However, these advantages are outweighed by the disadvantages of sodium overload and hypernatremia. Ethylenediaminetetraacetic acid (EDTA) complexes calcium, facilitating its urinary excretion, but nephrotoxicity limits its use.

If other measures fail, peritoneal dialysis or hemodialysis with calcium-free solutions should be considered.

Decrease in Bone Resorption or Increase in Bone Formation. Corticosteroids have an important but limited role in the treatment of hypercalcemia. Prednisone in vitamin D intoxication and sarcoidosis has already been discussed. Similar doses of corticosteroids are sometimes effective in hypercalcemia due to a malignant process, especially multiple myeloma, lymphoma, leukemia, or breast cancer; they have no effect on hypercalcemia due to hyperparathyroidism, however. Although they are part of the emergency therapy for hypercalcemia, corticosteroids should never be the only therapy in that setting, because of variable efficacy and delayed clinical response.

Mithramycin, an antineoplastic agent, is one of the most effective agents in the correction of hypercalcemia. The recommended dosage, 25 μg/kg intravenously, is much lower than the tumoricidal dose of this drug. Although we prefer to reserve this therapy for hypercalcemia due to a malignant condition, mithramycin may be the therapy of choice for emergency treatment of hypercalcemia refractory to rehydration. The effects of a single injection appear in the course of hours and last for 2–5 or more days. Therapy should not be repeated in less than 48 hours, and repeated therapy is reserved almost exclusively for patients with carcinoma. Toxic effects include thrombocytopenia, as well as renal and hepatic damage.

Salmon calcitonin is a safe, but only modestly effective means of lowering the serum calcium; a simple therapeutic regimen is 100 Medical Research Council (MRC) units intramuscularly every 8 hours. This will usually lower the serum calcium level acutely but rarely to within the normal range. The therapeutic effect often wears off after 48 hours. Recently, it has been suggested that prednisone (30–60 mg/day in three divided doses) may be synergistic with calcitonin and appears to prevent the loss of effectiveness of calcitonin or "escape" phenomenon. Calcitonin's safety makes it the initial drug of choice in patients with cardiac, renal, or hepatic disease.

Phosphate can be quite effective in the management of hypercalcemia. The mechanism of action is not completely known, but increased deposition of calcium in bone is one of the effects. Unfortunately, calcium tends to be deposited in other tissues as well. If the patient has hyperphosphatemia, this mode of therapy should be avoided.

With moderate, symptomatic hypercalcemia, 1–4 gm/day orally of elemental phosphate is preferred. Antacids bind phosphate and should not be given concurrently. Diarrhea may develop and limit

Table 14.15.
Hypercalcemia: Drug Therapy

Agent	Dosage and Route	Indications	Contraindications	Comments	Toxic Reactions
Corticosteroids Prednisone or Hydrocortisone	15 mg four times a day orally or intravenously 75 mg four times a day orally or intravenously	Sarcoidosis, vitamin D intoxication, malignant disease, in emergency	None in acute situation	Never sole form of emergency therapy PPD prior to chronic use if possible[a]	Hyperadrenocorticism
Mithramycin	25 μ/kg intravenously as bolus or over 4 hr	Emergency only, ideally in hypercalcemia of malignancy	Thrombocytopenia, bleeding disorders	Wait 48–72 hr before repeating dose	Thrombocytopenia, renal and hepatic damage
Normal saline with Furosemide	200 ml/hr intravenously (minimum) 40–100 mg intravenously every 2 hr as needed	Emergency only	Cardiac disease, congestive heart failure, renal failure	Requires intensive care unit, replacement of urinary volume and electrolytes	Congestive heart failure, hypokalemia, hypomagnesemia
Salmon calcitonin	2–8 MRC units/kg intramuscularly, subcutaneously or intravenously every 8 hr	Emergency only	None	Limited efficacy May be potentiated by glucocorticoids	Nausea, vomiting
Phosphorus Oral	1–4 gm/day elemental phosphate orally	Symptomatic moderate hypercalcemia		Avoid antacids Administer between meals	Diarrhea
Intravenous	50 mmol elemental phosphate intravenously over 6–8 hr	Emergency only	Renal failure, hyperphosphatemia		Metastatic calcifications, renal failure, hypocalcemia

[a] PPD, purified protein; MRC, Medical Research Council.

Table 14.16.
Hypercalcemia: Therapeutic Protocol

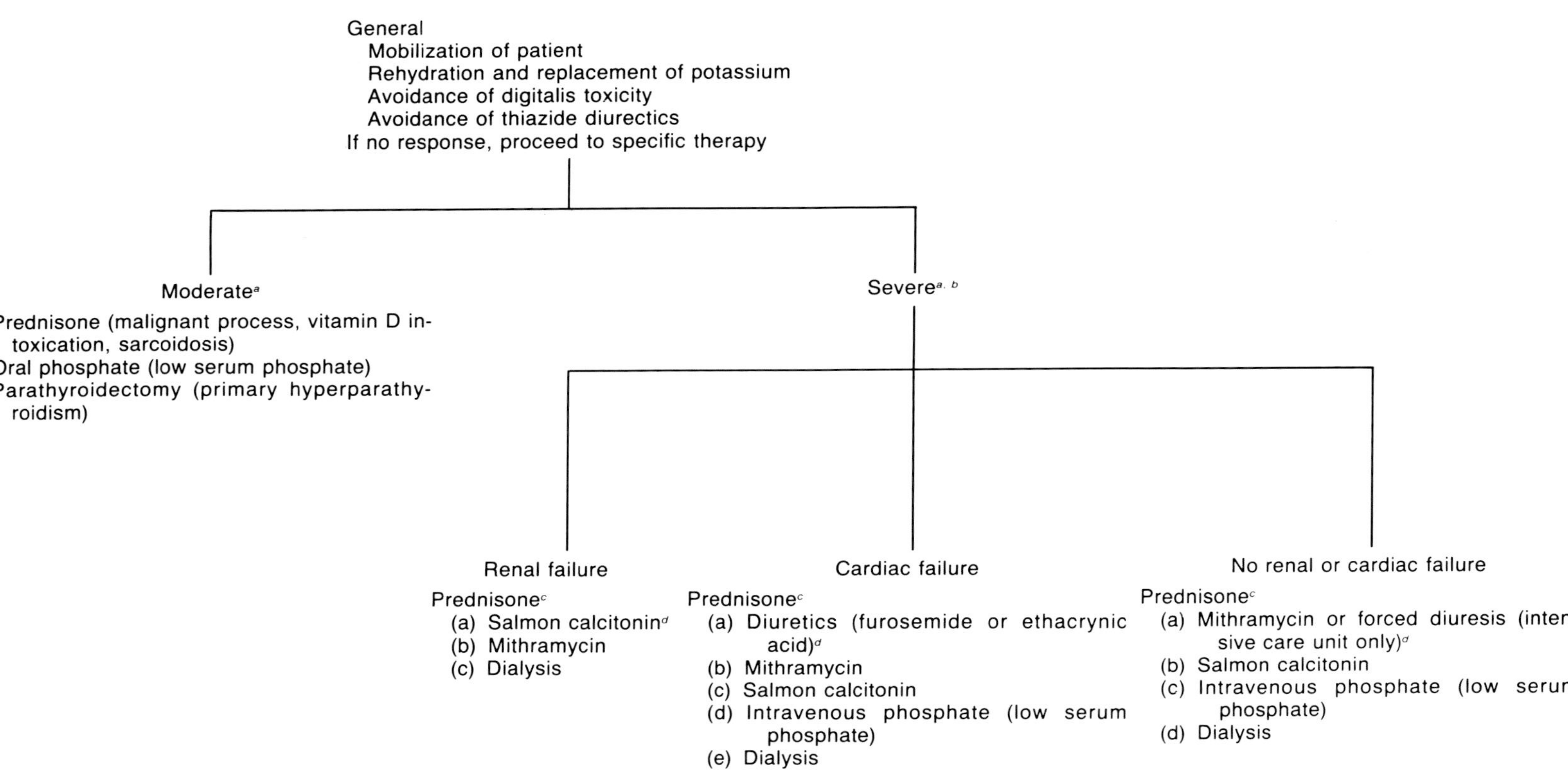

General
- Mobilization of patient
- Rehydration and replacement of potassium
- Avoidance of digitalis toxicity
- Avoidance of thiazide diurectics
- If no response, proceed to specific therapy

Moderate[a]
- Prednisone (malignant process, vitamin D intoxication, sarcoidosis)
- Oral phosphate (low serum phosphate)
- Parathyroidectomy (primary hyperparathyroidism)

Severe[a, b]

- Renal failure
  - Prednisone[c]
  - (a) Salmon calcitonin[d]
  - (b) Mithramycin
  - (c) Dialysis
- Cardiac failure
  - Prednisone[c]
  - (a) Diuretics (furosemide or ethacrynic acid)[d]
  - (b) Mithramycin
  - (c) Salmon calcitonin
  - (d) Intravenous phosphate (low serum phosphate)
  - (e) Dialysis
- No renal or cardiac failure
  - Prednisone[c]
  - (a) Mithramycin or forced diuresis (intensive care unit only)[d]
  - (b) Salmon calcitonin
  - (c) Intravenous phosphate (low serum phosphate)
  - (d) Dialysis

[a] Moderate: serum calcium < 15 mg/100 ml, alert but symptomatic patient. Severe: serum calcium > 15 mg/100 ml or comatose patient.
[b] Emergency parathyroidectomy may be lifesaving in patients with primary hyperparathyroidism.
[c] Prednisone should never be the sole therapeutic agent in hypercalcemic emergencies, but should always be administered in conjunction with one or more of the measures listed below.
[d] If no response, proceed to (b), etc.

the dosage. Intravenous phosphate has been employed in comatose patients, the magnitude of calcium decrease being directly proportional to the amount of phosphate infused. The dangers of intravenous phosphate are significant, and this therapy should be considered only in extreme emergencies. It is recommended that no more than 50 mmol of phosphate be infused in the course of 6–8 hours. When larger amounts are administered, therapy is more effective, but renal failure and soft-tissue calcification become more frequent. The serum calcium level may continue to decrease for several hours after an infusion of intravenous phosphate is completed, and this must be kept in mind if additional phosphate is being considered.

In rare cases of "ectopic hormone hypercalcemia," prostaglandins appear to mediate the hypercalcemia, in the absence of bony metastases. Prostaglandin inhibitors such as indomethacin are occasionally effective in decreasing the serum calcium in such patients and are worth a 24- to 48-hour trial. Although the humoral hypercalcemia of malignancy is not due to parathyroid hormone production, inhibitors of parathyroid hormone action may prove effective in treating such hypercalcemia.

The diphosphonates are pyrophosphate analogues which inhibit bone resorption. The currently licensed diphosphonates are effective in treating Paget's disease, but ineffective in hypercalcemia. The newer analogues (particularly dichloromethylene diphosphate) are still experimental but appear to be very effective when administered intravenously in treating the hypercalcemia of malignancy. As oral agents, they hold great promise for the outpatient chronic treatment of hypercalcemia of malignancy when antitumor therapy has failed or is being tried.

The definitive therapy for parathyroid hormone-induced hypercalcemia is parathyroidectomy. Emergency operation is indicated if progressive renal failure appears or if the calcium level is refractory to the above modes of therapy. If possible, the patient's condition, including the calcium level, should be stabilized before surgery is performed. Additional medical adjuncts prior to the surgical therapy of hyperparathyroidism include estrogen administration (appears to inhibit action of parathyroid hormone), cimetidine therapy (appears to inhibit release of parathyroid hormone), and dichloromethylene diphosphonate (inhibits bone resorption).

Therapeutic Protocol. In the alert patient whose serum calcium level is less than 15 mg/dl (mild or moderate hypercalcemia), hydration and mobilization may be adequate therapy (Table 14.16). If there is no response and the patient is symptomatic, phosphorus should be administered orally, particularly if the serum phosphate value is low. Corticosteroids are an alternative in patients with a malignant process or a condition considered responsive to corticosteroids.

In the comatose patient or the patient whose serum calcium level is more than 15 mg/dl (severe hypercalcemia), intravenous hydration and corticosteroids are required initially. If no decrease in the serum calcium level is noted during the next several hours, the decision regarding further therapy may be difficult. For a malignant condition, mithramycin is clearly the therapy of choice. It may also be useful as one-time therapy in hypercalcemia of unknown cause. If an intensive care unit is available, forced diuresis is an acceptable alternative in young patients without heart disease. In the presence of renal failure, only calcitonin, mithramycin, or dialysis is effective. In patients with refractory hypercalcemia, intravenous phosphate can be administered. It should not be administered to patients with renal failure and is most effective when the serum phosphate level is diminished. Emergency parathyroidectomy is occasionally lifesaving if the diagnosis is firm and if the situation continues to deteriorate.

Hypocalcemia

Although the causes of hypocalcemia are many, the therapy, in general, is simple: administer calcium. In contrast with hypercalcemia, severe hypocalcemia is relatively easy to recognize because of signs of neuromuscular irritability; however, neuromuscular irritability alone does not necessarily imply hypocalcemia.

Diagnosis

Clinical Features. Numbness and tingling of the fingers and toes with perioral paresthesia are among the earliest symptoms of hypocalcemia, and are often accompanied by signs of tetany, such as carpal and pedal spasms. These findings, however, are nonspecific, the most common causes of such neuromuscular irritability being hyperventilation with metabolic alkalosis and, less often, hypomagnesemia. In patients with these signs and symptoms, the serum calcium should be measured immediately. Severe hypocalcemia may result in laryngeal spasm with stridor or in grand mal seizures and should be treated as a genuine medical emergency. Decreased ionized calcium due to rapid infusion of citrated blood may result in severe myocardial depression which responds to intravenous calcium. Total serum calcium may not be increased in this situation.

Chronic hypocalcemia is associated with many nonspecific symptoms. Changes in mental status include general malaise, torpor, anxiety, neurosis, depression, delusions, and even psychosis. Spasms may occur in both smooth and voluntary muscles, and patients may complain of vague muscle cramps, diplopia, difficulty in swallowing, abdominal cramps, or bronchospasm.

Physical examination may be very informative. In the absence of obvious signs of neuromuscular irritability such as twitching, latent tetany can be unmasked with the Chvostek or Trousseau maneuver. The Chvostek test is performed by tapping the facial nerve anterior to the ear. Unilateral contraction of a facial muscle, such as twitching of the lip, is a positive sign; ipsilateral contraction of the eyelid is a more specific response. The Trousseau test renders nerves temporarily ischemic, bringing out latent tetany. An arm blood pressure cuff is inflated to a pressure above systolic and maintained at that level for 3 minutes. Carpal spasm with wrist flexion and finger adduction (main d'accoucheur) is a positive response. Chovstek and Trousseau tests can be negative in hypocalcemic patients, and positive tests need not indicate hypocalcemia. These tests may provide important information, however, when hypocalcemia is suspected.

An operative scar on the neck should suggest the possibility of hypocalcemia, whether it is the result of surgical treatment for thyroid disease, parathyroid disease, or an unrelated neoplasm. The deep tendon reflexes may be hyperactive in patients with mild to moderate hypocalcemia, but often disappear when hypocalcemia is profound.

Cutaneous changes indicating chronic hypocalcemia include dry scaly skin, eczema, brittle nails, thin or patchy scalp and eyebrow hair, absent axillary and pubic hair, and candidiasis. Dental hypoplasia suggests hypocalcemia dating from infancy. Cataracts regularly develop with sustained hypocalcemia. Pseudohypoparathyroidism, a rare syndrome of resistance to parathyroid hormone, is characterized by short stature, mental retardation, and short metacarpal bones. Although these findings may help establish the onset and duration of hypocalcemia, they are rarely useful in an emergency situation.

Clinical Studies. Lengthening of the Q-T interval on the electrocardiogram after correction for heart rate is a significant indication of hypocalcemia. In contrast with the Q-T lengthening seen with hypokalemia, no U waves are present. The serum albumin, creatinine, phosphate, magnesium, and blood urea nitrogen must be measured to determine the cause of the hypocalcemia.

Therapy

Emergency therapy for symptomatic hypocalcemia is intravenous administration of calcium. Vitamin D should *not* be administered in the emergency situation; with its long duration of action, it tends to complicate subsequent management by obscuring the cause of the hypocalcemia. In tetanic patients 200 mg of elemental calcium (20 ml of calcium gluconate or 22 ml of calcium glucoheptonate) should be administered over 5 minutes. In cases of severe hypocalcemia, this should be followed by 800–1000 mg of elemental calcium in 1000 ml of 5% dextrose solution to be infused over 12–24 hours. Calcium glucoheptonate and calcium gluconate contain 9 and 10%, respectively, calcium by weight; that is, 100 ml of a 10% solution contains 9–10 gm of compound, but only 900–1000 mg of elemental calcium. Patients without parathyroid glands can be treated with 400 mg elemental calcium every 24 hours by constant intravenous infusion. However, in patients with bones avid for calcium, so called "hungry bones", up to 2000 mg or more per 24 hours will be required intravenously. It is important that serum calcium values be determined serially and the clinical response be monitored to ensure the desired therapeutic effect and to avoid overshoot. A serum calcium level of 7–8 mg/dl usually eliminates symptoms.

When hungry bones are not present, 400 mg of intravenous (elemental) calcium/24 hr will usually suffice even in a parathyroidectomized patient. After parathyroid surgery with hungry bones, after parathyroid trauma or removal post-thyroidectomy, or after parathyroidectomy in renal failure patients, vitamin D or its derivatives will usually be required. Vitamin D, 50,000 units/day will suffice, but the newer derivative, 1,25-dihydroxyvitamin D has the advantage of more rapid onset. Initial dosages of 1,25-dihydroxyvitamin D range from 0.5 to 2.0 μg/day. As soon as possible, calcium supplements should be changed from parenteral to oral. For chronic therapy, 1,25-dihydroxyvitamin D is still quite expensive and a switch to vitamin D is reasonable.

Thiazide diuretics are occasionally helpful in the chronic therapy of hypoparathyroidism. These agents facilitate calcium reabsorption by the kidneys.

A few warnings are necessary. Calcium chloride is sclerosing to veins and should not be administered intravenously. Bicarbonate should never be added to a solution containing calcium, since calcium carbonate will precipitate. If the serum phosphate level is elevated when calcium therapy is begun, it must be lowered to avoid deposition of calcium in tissues. Oral antacids are recommended for this purpose. When calcium is being administered, the myocardium becomes sensitized to digitalis, and digitalis intoxication may develop. If neuromuscular irritability persists during calcium administration or if hypocalcemia develops rapidly after cessation of calcium therapy, magnesium de-

Table 14.17.
Hypocalcemia: Etiology

Spurious
- Laboratory error
- Hypoalbuminemia

Decreased calcium absorption (increased parathyroid hormone production)
- Vitamin D deficiency
  - Dietary lack
  - Malabsorption (sprue, chronic pancreatitis)
- Vitamin D resistance
  - Renal failure
  - Phenytoin or phenobarbital administration
  - Hereditary condition

Decreased bone release of calcium (decreased effect of parathyroid hormone)
- Severe vitamin D deficiency or resistance
- Parathyroid hormone absence
  - Idiopathic
  - Postoperative (parathyroidectomy)
    - Permanent
    - Transient (edema, ischemia, parathyroid gland suppression)
  - Magnesium deficiency
- Parathyroid hormone resistance
  - Pseudohypoparathyroidism
  - Magnesium deficiency

Increased bone deposition
- Hungry bones
- Blastic tumors

Acute pancreatitis

Decreased ionized calcium (citrated blood)

ficiency may be at fault, requiring administration of magnesium sulfate, 40–60 mEq intravenously in the course of 4–6 hours if renal function is normal.

After the acute situation has been treated, the cause of the hypocalcemia must be determined.

Precipitating Factors

The differential diagnosis of hypocalcemia is listed in Table 14.17. The most common cause of a low serum calcium level is hypoalbuminemia. The ionized calcium value is normal in this situation, the patient is asymptomatic, and no therapy is indicated.

Hypocalcemia is a regular feature of renal failure, but emergency therapy is rarely required. The neuromuscular irritability of uremia is usually not due to the hypocalcemia. In patients with renal failure, lack of hypocalcemic symptoms is probably related to acidosis; hydrogen ions displace calcium bound to albumin, increasing the ionized form. Conversely, rapid administration of alkali in such a setting can substantially decrease the ionized calcium, precipitating seizures or severe neuromuscular irritability.

Malabsorption of Vitamin D in conditions such as sprue or chronic pancreatitis is a common cause of hypocalcemia. Phenytoin (diphenylhydantoin) and phenobarbital have recently been shown to divert Vitamin D metabolism, preventing formation of active metabolites and causing functional Vitamin D deficiency. Inhibition of Vitamin D effect on bone is another possible mechanism of phenytoin-induced hypocalcemia and osteomalacia. In patients lacking Vitamin D, additional parathyroid hormone is secreted in response to hypocalcemia, and the serum phosphate level decreases because of the phosphaturic effect of parathyroid hormone.

In contrast, all forms of hypoparathyroidism are accompanied by hyperphosphatemia, the phosphaturic effect of parathyroid hormone being absent. Idiopathic parathyroid hormone deficiency is rare, and may be accompanied by mucocutaneous candidiasis and Addison's disease. Iatrogenic hypoparathyroidism is far more common and most often occurs after parathyroid or thyroid operation. Parathyroid hormone resistance (pseudohypoparathyroidism) has already been mentioned.

Hypocalcemia after operation on the neck (especially parathyroid or thyroid operation) raises several important considerations. Permanent hypoparathyroidism may result from removal or destruction of the parathyroid glands. In patients who have undergone removal of a parathyroid adenoma, transient hypoparathyroidism may develop a few days after operation because of prior suppression of the parathyroid glands by the neoplasm, or it may develop days, weeks, or months later, resulting from ischemia of the residual parathyroid glands. Hyperphosphatemia is the indicator that one of these two situations exists. In patients with hyperparathyroidism or thyrotoxicosis, the serum calcium and phosphate levels may both decrease after operation, requiring temporary calcium therapy. This is due to hungry bones, that is, diversion of large amounts of calcium and phosphate into bone formation. The magnesium deficiency associated with hyperparathyroidism may result in hypocalcemia after operation, and postoperative hyperparathyroidism in rare cases is complicated by severe pancreatitis with attendant hypocalcemia. As in other instances of pancreatitis, the cause of hypocalcemia is unclear.

Severe hypomagnesemia may result from alcoholism, malabsorption, or diuretics and has been shown to inhibit the release of parathyroid hormone or its action or both, resulting in hypocalcemia. Calcium administration transiently elevates the serum calcium level in this situation; however, hypocalcemia recurs rapidly unless magnesium is administered. Furthermore, neuromuscular irritability may not subside unless magnesium is administered as well as calcium.

SODIUM AND POTASSIUM EMERGENCIES

Hyponatremia

Renal Physiology

Hyponatremia is a consequence of impaired ability of the kidneys to exrete adequate amounts of dilute urine. In this setting, administration or ingestion of hypotonic fluids dilutes the serum sodium concentration and hyponatremia develops. To understand this fully, the manner in which kidneys excrete dilute urine must be considered.

The tonicity or osmolality of the blood is normally maintained within narrow limits, 280–295 mosm/liter (technically mosm/kg); electrolytes constitute most of the osmotically active particles. The serum osmolality equals approximately twice the serum sodium concentration if the blood urea nitrogen and blood glucose concentrations are normal, these components also being osmotically active.

Antidiuretic hormone (ADH) stimulates conservation of water by the kidneys. It is secreted from the posterior part of the pituitary gland and is very sensitive to changes in the osmolality of the blood. Increased osmolality stimulates ADH release, resulting in concentration of the urine and correction of the increased tonicity of the blood by reabsorbed water. Severe volume depletion or nausea are nonosmotic stimuli for ADH release by which intravascular volume is replaced.

Conversely, decreased serum osmolality inhibits release of ADH. If a healthy person drinks too much water, the excess is rapidly excreted by the kidneys in the form of dilute urine. This is because renal cells in the distal tubes and collecting ducts become relatively impermeable to water in the absence of ADH. In the absence of this hormone, when sodium is reabsorbed from the tubular fluids, water is left behind and dilute urine is excreted. The integrity of the barrier to water reabsorption requires the presence of cortisol as well as the absence of ADH; therefore, impaired ability to excrete dilute urine can result from the *presence of ADH* or the *absence of cortisol.*

Excretion of sufficient amounts of dilute urine also requires an adequate glomerular filtration rate, by which the filtrate is delivered to the diluting segments. In conditions in which renal perfusion is decreased, such as hypotension, increased sodium and water reabsorption occurs in the proximal renal tubules in an attempt to preserve or to expand the intravascular volume. As a result, flow to the distal segments is inadequate, and the ability to excrete normal quantities of dilute urine is impaired. Furthermore, the urine that *is* excreted may be less dilute than expected, and may even be hypertonic. There are two possible explanations for this. One is the imperfect barrier to water presented by the distal sites. If the urinary flow is sufficiently low, enough water will be reabsorbed that concentrated urine will result. Although the urine may be free of sodium, it will contain urea, the major solute in hypertonic urine. The other explanation is release of ADH by volume contraction; resultant water retention serves as a partial defense against hypotension. In such a situation, the attempt to preserve volume may override the usual osmotic stimulus to ADH release.

Thus, four requirements must be fulfilled for the excretion of sufficient amounts of dilute urine; the glomerular filtration rate must be adequate, ADH release must be inhibited, cortisol must be present, and the renal cells must remain impermeable to water.

Diagnosis and Therapy

The symptoms of hyponatremia are variable and to some extent nonspecific. Hyponatremia that develops rapidly is more likely to produce symptoms than that occurring more slowly. Acute severe hyponatremia may cause brain swelling with attendant delirium, convulsions, or coma. Occasionally, focal neurological symptoms may develop. When hyponatremia develops more slowly, the brain can compensate with loss of intracellular solute (sodium, potassium, and chloride) which protects against swelling. Additional symptoms include weakness, lethargy, anorexia, nausea, vomiting, headache, dizziness, muscle twitching, and restlessness. Most patients will demonstrate symptoms when the serum sodium is less than 115 mEq/liter.

Decisions regarding therapy depend on clinical assessment of the state of sodium balance (Table 14.18). Excess and deficiency of whole body sodium can only be determined in this way, laboratory studies being of little help. The report of a low serum sodium value often results in routine administration of isotonic or hypertonic saline; this approach to therapy is irresponsible and may have dire consequences. The serum sodium concentration bears *no* relation to the amount of sodium in the body (Fig. 14.3). A low serum sodium level may be a consequence of water excess alone, in which case the sodium balance is normal and the only therapy required is water restriction. Hyponatremia may also occur with an excess of both water and sodium, the water excess predominating. Therapy in this instance consists primarily of water and sodium deprivation, but diuretics are often administered as well. Last, decrease in the serum sodium level may result from deficits of both salt and water

Table 14.18.
Hyponatremia: Differential Diagnosis and Therapy

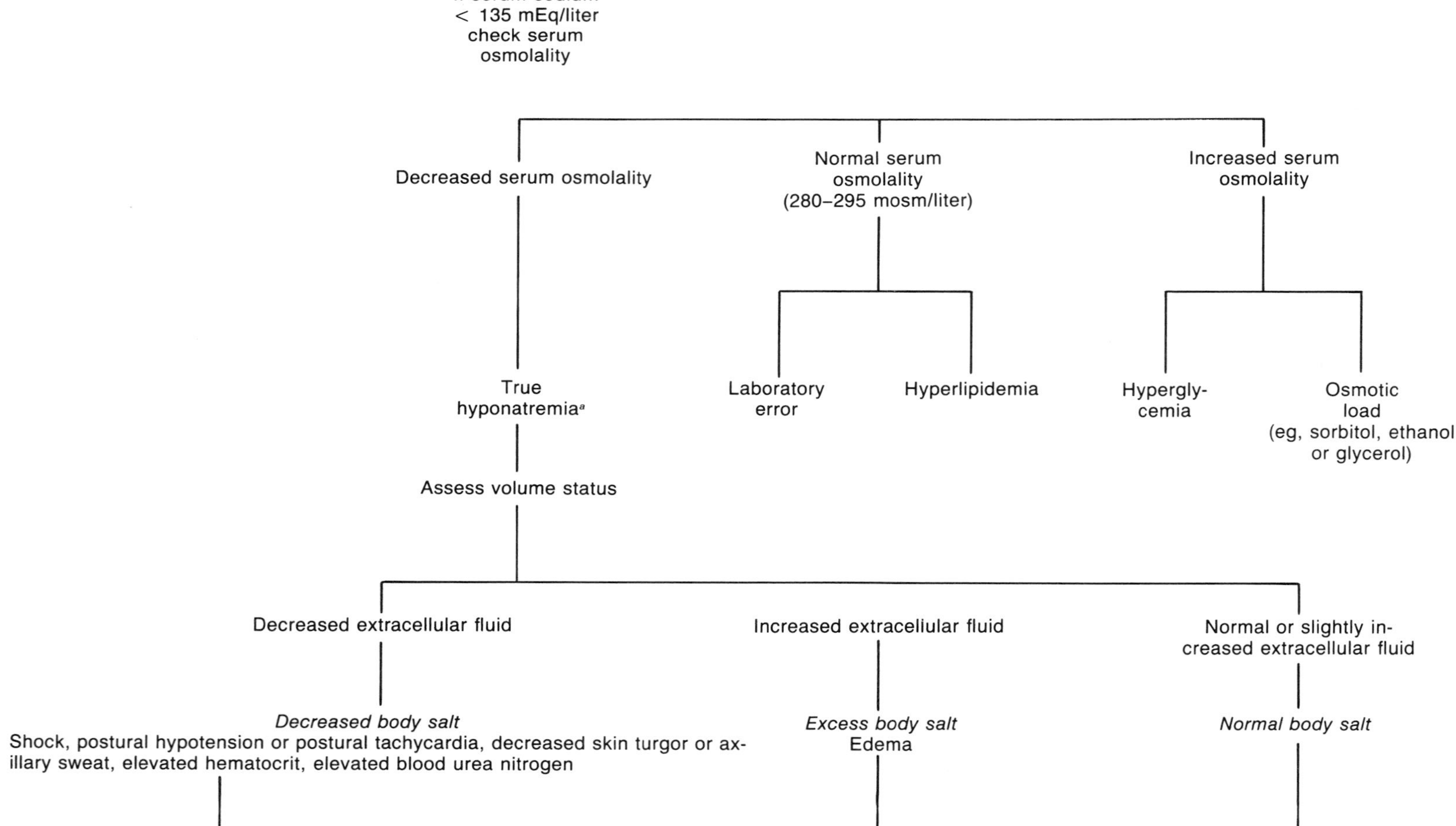

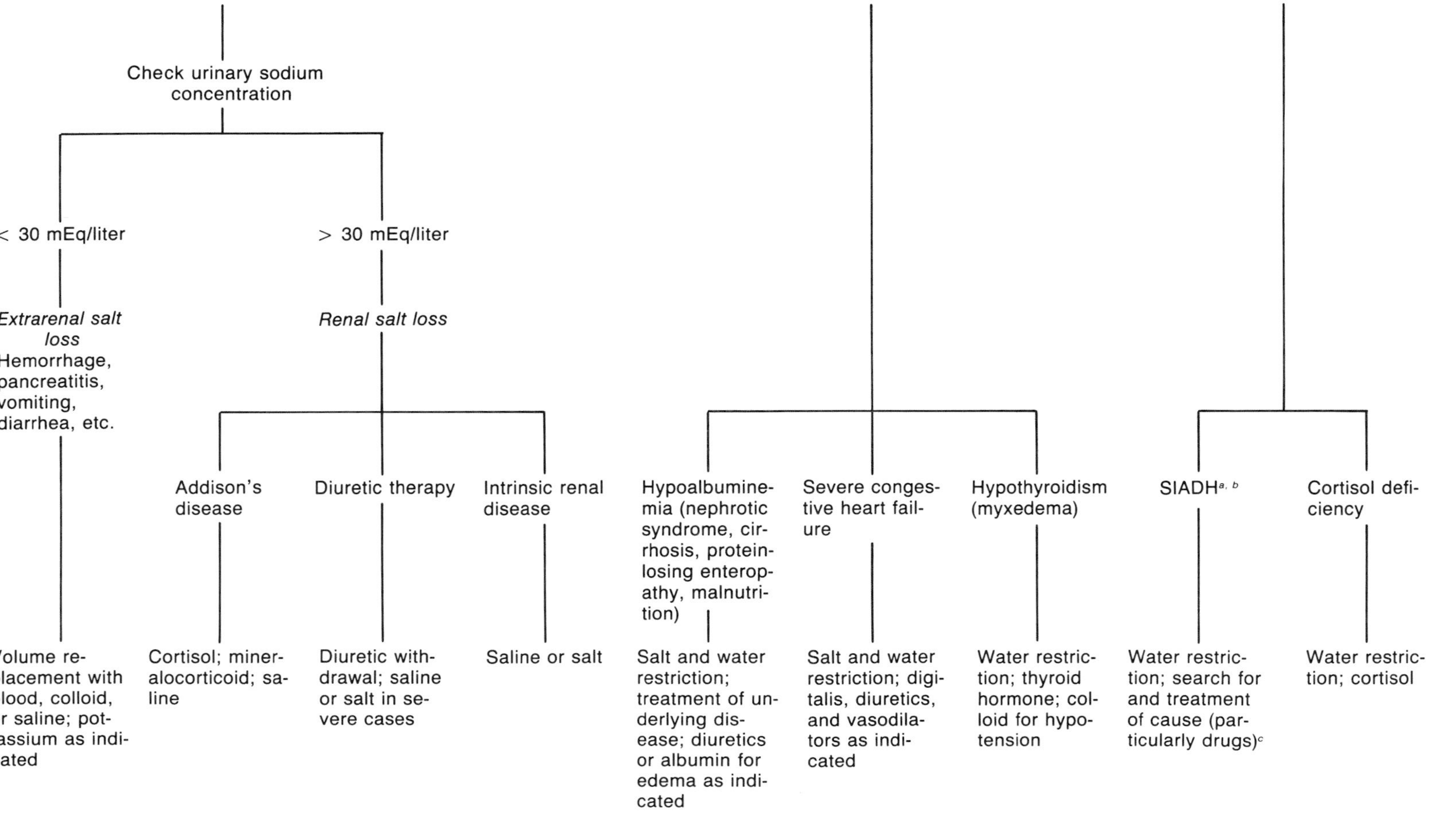

[a] In an emergency, administer 3% saline solution, intravenously to raise serum sodium by 2 mEq/liter/hr until serum sodium reaches 128. In the presence of volume overload, diuretics should be administered as well

[b] SIADH syndrome of inappropriate antidiuretic hormone secretion; normal renal, adrenal, and thyroid function; blood urea nitrogen usually < 10 mg/dl, urinary sodium usually > 30 mEq/liter, urinary osmolality elevated inappropriately.

[c] Occasionally, demeclocycline or lithium are useful for chronic therapy.

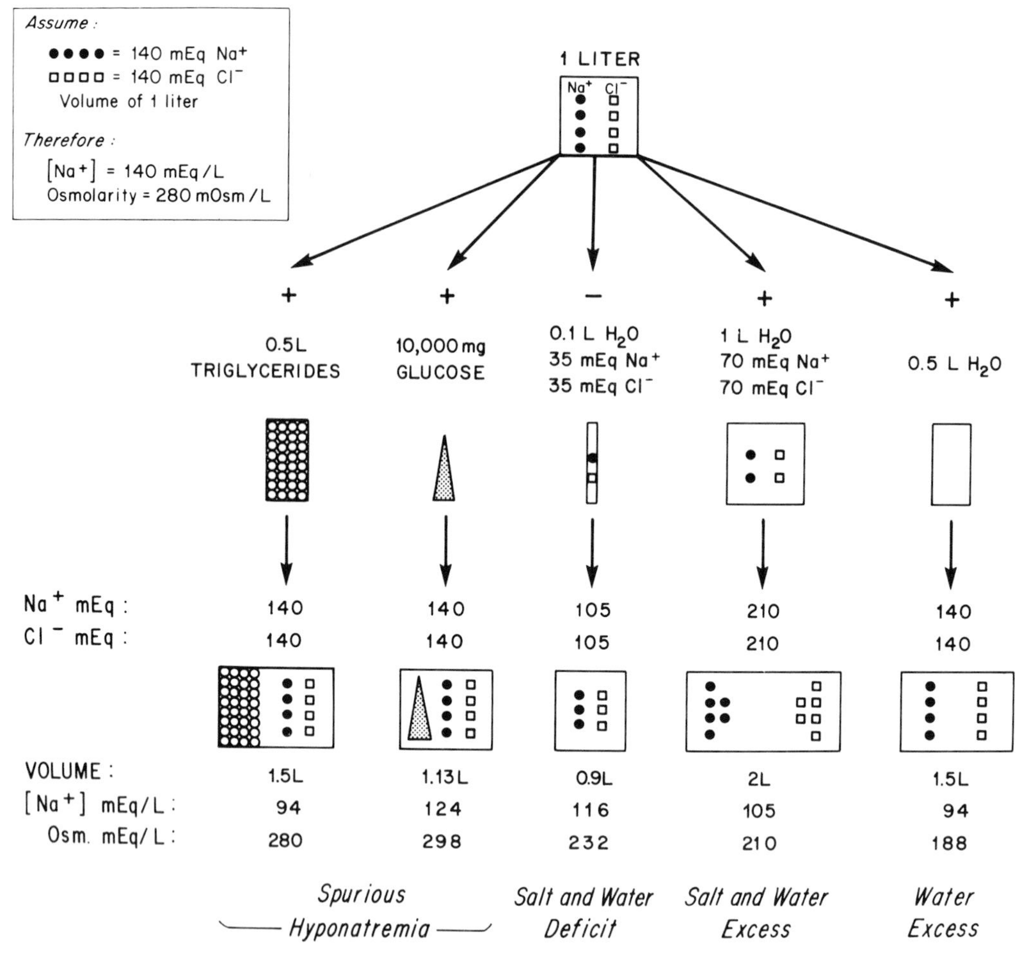

Figure 14.3. Mechanisms of hyponatremia.

followed by hypotonic fluid ingestion or therapy. Saline or salt administration is then necessary.

Spurious Hyponatremia. When hyponatremia is reported, the serum sodium should immediately be measured again along with the serum osmolality. If the serum osmolality is not diminished, the hyponatremia is probably spurious (Table 14.18). Common causes of spurious hyponatremia include laboratory error and improper sampling—blood may have been drawn downstream from a rapidly flowing intravenous line, for example.

Severe hyperlipidemia may result in artifactual hyponatremia. The additional triglycerides separate the blood into a lipid compartment and an aqueous compartment. The sodium concentration and osmolality of the aqueous phase are normal. Since the serum sodium concentration depends on the volume of the sample, the aqueous sodium content is diluted by the lipid compartment. The serum osmolality, however, is not influenced by the additional lipid, and is normal (Fig. 14.3). As a guide, an increase in the triglyceride concentration of 6000 mg/dl will result in a 5% decrease in the serum sodium concentration. The creamy appearance of the plasma will establish the diagnosis, and a search for the cause of the elevated triglyceride concentration can then be instituted.

When glucose is added to the intravascular compartment, it remains osmotically active and draws water to it. This movement of water out of the cells results in a decrease in the serum sodium concentration. An increase in the blood glucose level of 100 mg/dl will result in a serum sodium decrease of 1.6 mEq/liter. For example, a blood glucose level of 1000 mg/dl (900 mg/dl above baseline) will decrease the serum sodium concentration from 144 to 130 mEq/liter independent of any sodium or water losses from the body. (Since 100 mg/dl of glucose represents 5 mosm/liter, if enough water were attracted by the increase to maintain a constant blood osmolality, the electrolyte concentration would be expected to decrease by 5 mosm/liter, half of which would be sodium. However, such a shift of water out of the cells would make the intracellular compartment hyperosmolar, and the osmolality must be constant throughout the body. Therefore, in actuality, a slight increase in the blood osmolality results from administration of glucose, and the sodium concentration decreases less than the theoretical 3 mosm/liter.) Therapy in this situation must be directed toward the hyperglycemia rather than the hyponatremia.

Unmeasured osmotically active particles such as sorbitol or glycerol may cause similar changes.

Hyponatremia with Sodium Deficiency. Sodium is primarily an extracellular cation, and sodium deficits result in a decrease in both intravascular and interstitial fluid volumes. Acute, severe depletion of intravascular volume, as in blood loss or pancreatitis, is easily recognized by a low central venous pressure in the presence of shock. Less severe volume loss may result only in postural hypotension or tachycardia.

Recognition of mild, chronic sodium depletion may be difficult. Such a deficit may be suggested by a history of vomiting, diarrhea or diuretic intake; weight loss or persistently negative fluid balance in a hospitalized hyponatremic patient; and lack of axillary sweat. Decreased skin turgor in a well-nourished patient should also suggest sodium deficiency; the skin of the forehead should be pinched and then released, a slow relaxation rate indicating decreased turgor. The blood urea nitrogen value is commonly elevated, as is the hematocrit value if acute blood loss has not occurred.

Sodium loss may be extrarenal or renal. With extrarenal salt loss—as in sweating, vomiting, diarrhea, or pancreatitis—the glomerular filtration rate decreases, the blood urea nitrogen level may increase, and the urine is relatively free of sodium (less than 30 mEq/liter) because of salt conservation by the kidneys. Ability to dilute the urine is impaired, and hyponatremia will result *if* hypotonic fluids are ingested by the patient or administered by the physician.

Therapy for extrarenal salt loss is replacement of the underlying deficits. Severe loss of volume may require blood or plasma expanders. Lesser amounts of volume can be replaced with normal saline solution. Mild chronic sodium deficits can be managed with sodium-containing foods and fluids, salt tablets, or judicious administrations of saline. Concomitant potassium deficits should be corrected as well. Hypotonic fluids should be excluded until volume is replaced, at which time the kidneys will be able to excrete dilute urine again. If the serum sodium level is less than 110mEq/liter or if seizures are noted, 500–1000 ml of a 3% solution of hypertonic saline should be administered in addition to brisk volume expansion.

Hyponatremia in the presence of renal sodium loss can occur as a result of intrinsic renal disease, diuretic administration, or Addison's disease. Despite hyponatremia and clinical evidence of sodium deficiency, the urinary sodium concentration will be more than 30 mEq/liter. Diuretics and renal disease with salt-wasting results in excretion of isotonic urine. Even mild diuretics such as hydrochlorthiazide can lead to profound, often lethal, hyponatremia, particularly in older patients. If excess hypotonic fluids are provided, hyponatremia will result. In patients with Addison's disease, impaired ability to excrete dilute urine is a consequence of cortisol lack, resulting in "leaky" distal tubules as well as volume depletion itself. Saline administration may correct the volume depletion but not the hyponatremia, and renal salt-wasting in this setting may strongly indicate Addison's disease. Therapy with cortisol may be lifesaving for such patients.

Hyponatremia with Sodium Excess. Hyponatremia with total body sodium excess is characterized by edema. Severe hypoalbuminemia, as in patients with cirrhosis, nephrotic syndrome, protein-losing enteropathy, or severe malnutrition, leads to extravasation of fluid out of the intravascular compartment. Despite peripheral edema, the intravascular volume and glomerular filtration rate are diminished, resulting in impaired ability to excrete excess water. The hyponatremia is corrected with fluid restriction, and salt should be limited as well. Diuretic therapy or albumin administration is not necessary for the hyponatremia, but may be required for the edema.

In patients with severe congestive heart failure, the kidneys may be underperfused despite an increased intravascular volume, and hyponatremia may result. Therapy for heart failure includes digitalis, diuretics, vasodilators, and salt restriction; rigorous water restriction is required to treat the hyponatremia. Although not all patients with congestive heart failure have an impaired ability to excrete dilute urine, careful monitoring of the serum sodium levels is imperative if hyponatremia is to be prevented.

Hypothyroidism is another special example of this syndrome. The intravascular volume is often diminished, although the excess sodium is present in the myxedema fluid. Impaired ability to excrete dilute urine is probably related to the diminished glomerular filtration rate, although inappropriate secretion of ADH has been postulated as well. Therapy requires fluid restriction and thyroid hormone administration. If hypotension is present, colloid may help replace volume and correct hyponatremia.

Hyponatremia with Normal Amounts of Body Sodium. This situation represents a state of water intoxication. There is no evidence for volume depletion, edema is absent, and renal function is normal. Such patients have a normal sodium balance, the urinary sodium excretion being equal to the sodium intake. This condition often results from inappropriate secretion of ADH; it may be mimicked by administration of certain drugs and by isolated cortisol deficiency. In the presence of adequate sodium intake, lack of urinary sodium (less than 30 mEq/liter) probably implies sodium depletion, and in this circumstance the diagnosis of water intoxication alone is suspect.

Inappropriate Secretion of ADH. The criteria for this syndrome include: (*a*) decreased serum sodium and serum osmolality; (*b*) normal renal function (glomerular filtration rate), with a blood urea nitrogen value usually less than 10 mg/dl; (*c*) normal adrenal and thyroid function; and (*d*) urinary osmolality inappropriately elevated in relation to the serum osmolality.

The last criterion requires amplification. A healthy person should be able to dilute urine to an osmolality of 50–75 mosm/liter if large amounts of water are ingested. Blood hypotonicity should inhibit ADH release and result in similarly dilute urine. When the serum osmolality is decreased, a urinary osmolality more than 150 mosm/liter is inappropriate and indicates inability to dilute the urine maximally. Note that all forms of hyponatremia will be associated with inappropriately elevated urine osmolality, not just the syndrome of inappropriate antidiuretic hormone secretion (SIADH). Criteria *a*–*c* establish the diagnosis of SIADH.

Etiology. Inappropriate secretion of ADH has many causes. ADH release from the normal hypothalamus appears to be tonically inhibited. Central nervous system (CNS) lesions, including those resulting from trauma, which interrupt the inhibitory flow to the hypothalamus can cause ADH release. Pulmonary lesions, including tuberculosis, abscess, and rarely pneumonia may initiate this syndrome. Ectopic production of ADH by malignant neoplasms—especially oat cell carcinoma of the lung—is being recognized with increasing frequency. Many drugs produce the syndrome by releasing ADH and these include: chlorpropamide, clofibrate, nicotine, vincristine, cyclophosphamide, and narcotics (probably through their effect of producing nausea). Vasopressin (ADH) infusion for gastrointestinal bleeding or overly vigorous therapy for diabetes insipidus with pitressin tannate in oil (ADH) or desmopressin (DDAVP, an ADH analogue) provide exogenous sources for the hormone. Diuretic therapy, particularly in the elderly can mimic SIADH. *Remember*, although ADH production may be constant, the hyponatremic state will occur only with excess water ingestion or intravenous administration.

Therapy. When hyponatremia is associated with volume contraction, normal saline should be administered. With SIADH, when hyponatremia is mild or asymptomatic, the therapy is simple: restrict water while searching for a correctable cause, particularly drug intake. Total fluid intake may have to be decreased to 500–800 ml/day and this may be difficult. Continuous intravenous fluid administration is a notorious means of perpetuating hyponatremia. Even if normal saline is administered, hypertonic urine will be excreted and hyponatremia may worsen.

Demeclocycline (but not other tetracyclines) and lithium both cause a partial defect in water conservation by the kidney, which can be utilized to advantage in the SIADH situation. Demeclocycline is probably safer and can be administered in doses of 0.6–1.2 gm/day in divided dosages. This may be useful in chronic hyponatremia due to SIADH. In the future, synthetic inhibitors of ADH action should supplant all other therapies in the SIADH.

The therapy for profound hyponatremia is more important, but also more controversial. Hyponatremia may be lethal, but certain investigators have suggested that the therapy of hyponatremia may in itself be harmful. The syndrome of central pontine myelinolysis has been reported to occur with "rapid" correction of hyponatremia. This syndrome is generally found in malnourished alcoholics and is characterized by myelin destruction in the pons with attendant flaccid quadriplegia, facial weakness, inability to speak or swallow, and impaired response to painful stimuli. Although the issue is unresolved, at this time it appears that the hyponatremia is more likely to be dangerous than is the therapy.

If the hyponatremia is life-threatening (serum sodium less than 110 mEq/liter or hyponatremia with coma or seizures), then hypertonic saline (3%, 514 mmol/liter) should be administered. The infusion should be controlled at a rate which causes a mean rise in serum sodium of 2 mEq/liter/hr until a serum sodium of 125–130 mEq/liter is achieved. Frequent serum sodium determinations will be necessary. Free water restriction should be instituted at the same time.

With SIADH, where circulatory overload is feared or develops, a loop diuretic such as furosemide should be administerd before or with the hypertonic saline. Although furosemide will not allow for excretion of a dilute urine (the urine will be approximately isotonic—300 mosm/liter), the excretion of isotonic urine with hypertonic fluid replacement will result in a rising serum sodium. Osmotic diuretics such as mannitol or glycerol have the theoretical advantage of allowing water excretion out of proportion to solute.

Cortisol Insufficiency. Cortisol deficiency alone due to hypopituitarism or pituitary suppression is a rare but important cause of water intoxication. In contrast with Addison's disease, lack of pigmentation and volume depletion may delay the diagnosis. The low serum sodium level responds to water restriction; however, cortisol must be administered to achieve a satisfactory clinical response.

Hyperkalemia

Physiologic Principles

Of the body potassium, 98% is intracellular; the low potassium concentration in the extracellular fluid is maintained within fairly narrow limits, 3.5–5.0 mEq/liter. Acidosis favors a shift of potassium from intracellular to extracellular sites, and alkalosis favors the reverse. Insulin deficiency is associated with decreased potassium tolerance (i.e., impaired ability to dispose of potassium loads), as in α-adrenergic stimulation or β-adrenergic blockade.

Most urinary potassium results from the sodium/potassium-hydrogen ion exchange that occurs in the distal renal tubules and collecting ducts. This exchange requires the presence of aldosterone, the major mineralocorticoid. Hence, urinary potassium excretion is a consequence of tubular secretion, little being derived directly from glomerular filtration.

The requirements for normal potassium excretion include: *a*) adequate glomerular filtration to deliver sodium to the distal tubules; (*b*) aldosterone or other mineralocorticoid hormones; and (*c*) renal tubules that respond to mineralocorticoid hormones.

Precipitating Factors

If spurious causes are excluded, hyperkalemia can be considered to result from either excessive potassium input or impaired potassium excretion (Table 14.19). A combination of these two possibilities often exists.

Spurious Hyperkalemia. Miminal test tube hemolysis may strikingly elevate the serum potassium concentration; this is a consequence of the extremely high intracellular potassium levels. Potassium release from platelets in vitro may lead to pseudohyperkalemia in patients with severe thrombocytosis. Heparin prevents such platelet lysis, and a normal plasma potassium level (heparinized tube) simultaneous with an elevated serum potassium level confirms the diagnosis of pseudohyperkalemia.

Excessive Potassium Input. Moderate to substantial increase in the serum potassium concentration may result from exogenous or endogenous sources. Exogenous sources include oral and intravenous potassium salts, salt substitutes, low-sodium milk (potassium concentration of 60 mEq/liter) and penicillin G (potassium concentration of 1.7 mEq/million units). Although low-dose penicillin therapy represents little hazard, high-dose therapy, 20–40 million units/day, may lead to severe hyperkalemia unless the sodium salt is utilized. Banked blood is another important potassium source, the potassium leaking from the red blood cells with time. All these agents should be used with extreme caution in patients with an impaired ability to excrete potassium.

Endogenous sources of potassium are equally important. Acidosis may lead to profound hyperkalemia, as in diabetic ketoacidosis. Insulin deficiency in itself may prevent the translocation of potassium into cells. Tissue destruction, such as a crush injury or gangrene, may release massive amounts of potassium from damaged cells. Brisk intravascular hemolysis, as in clostridial sepsis, may result in death from hyperkalemia. The rare syndrome of hyperkalemic periodic paralysis is due to a potassium shift out of the cells, but the mechanism is unknown.

Table 14.19.
Hyperkalemia: Mechanisms and Diagnostic Possibilities

- Spurious
  - Laboratory error
  - Hemolysis in vitro
  - Platelet lysis associated with thrombocytosis (pseudohyperkalemia)
- Excessive potassium input
  - Exogenous
    - Potassium salts
    - Salt substitutes and low-salt milk
    - Penicillin G therapy
    - Transfusions with long-stored blood
  - Endogenous
    - Severe tissue injury (trauma, gangrene)
    - Acidosis
    - Insulin deficiency
    - Intravascular hemolysis (clostridial sepsis)
    - Hyperkalemic periodic paralysis
- Decreased potassium excretion
  - Decreased glomerular filtration rate
    - Acute renal failure
    - Chronic renal failure
    - Sodium restriction
    - Volume depletion producing poor renal perfusion
  - Decreased sodium and potassium exchange
    - Addison's disease
    - Isolated aldosterone deficiency (renin deficiency, biosynthetic defect, heparin therapy)
    - Drugs (spironolactone, triamterene or amiloride, digitalis intoxication)

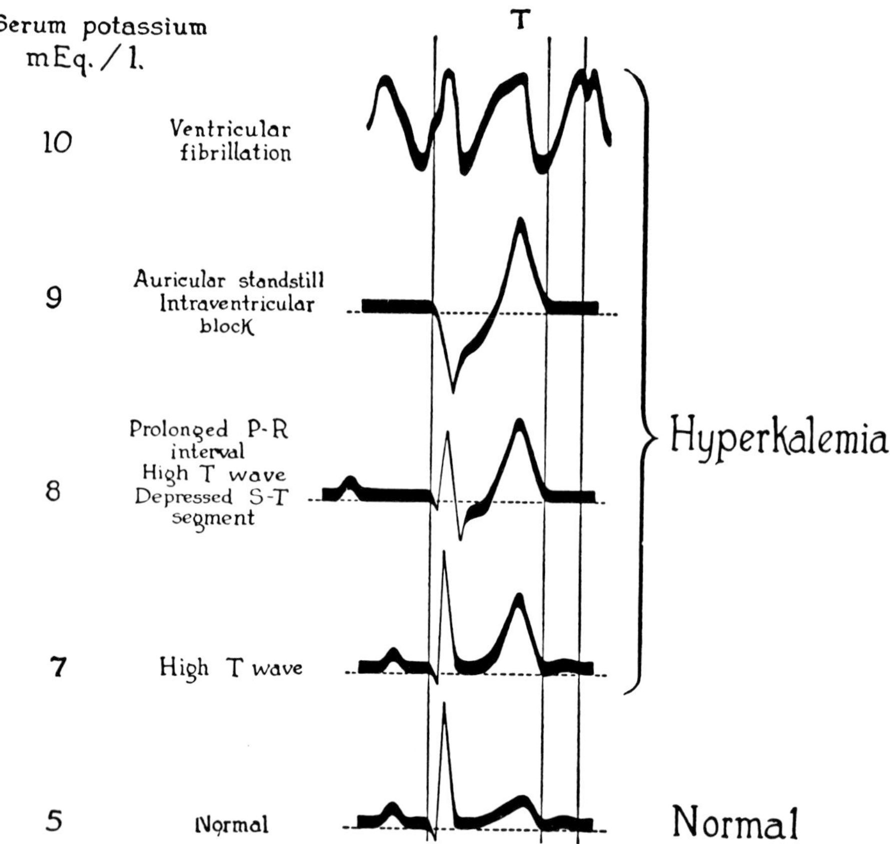

Figure 14.4. Electrocardiographic manifestations of hyperkalemia. (Modified with permission, from Burch GE, Winsor T. A Primer of Electrocardiography, 4th ed. Philadelphia: Lea & Febiger, 1960)

Impaired Excretion of Potassium. The simplest example of this is anuric renal failure, in which potassium excretion ceases and hyperkalemia develops. Acidosis soon follows and exacerbates the hyperkalemia. The physician should not only be aware of the possibility of hyperkalemia in patients with anuric renal failure but should also realize that with even minor decreases in the glomerular filtration rate, as in severe sodium restriction or minor volume depletion, sodium does not reach the distal tubules and potassium excretion is impaired.

When aldosterone is absent or its effect is blocked, potassium excretion diminishes. Aldosterone deficiency may occur with cortisol deficiency as part of Addison's disease, or it may be isolated, as in renin deficiency, biosynthetic defects, or heparin therapy.

Isolated aldosterone deficiency, due to decreased renin release or synthesis, has been recognized with increased frequency (so-called hyporeninemic hypoaldosteronism). It is particularly common in the elderly, especially those with renal insufficiency and/or diabetes mellitus. It may be exacerbated or unmasked by β-adrenergic blocking agents and by nonsteroidal anti-inflammatory agents (such as indomethacin) which inhibit prostaglandin biosynthesis. The clinical presentation is usually that of isolated hyperkalemia without significant volume contraction, the latter being poorly explained. Despite hyperkalemia, a potent aldosterone stimulant, serum or urine aldosterone concentrations are low. Aldosterone antagonism due to drug therapy with spironolactone is far more common, however. Both triamterene and amiloride are mild diuretics which appear to inhibit sodium-potassium exchange, independent of aldosterone. In general, potassium should *not* be administered with any of these drugs, unless hypokalemia is present.

The urinary sodium concentration may help establish the cause of hyperkalemia. A urinary sodium concentration less than 30 mEq/liter implies decreased sodium delivery to distal sites, and sodium replacement is likely to help lower the serum potassium level by providing substrate for the sodium-potassium exchange. If the urinary sodium concentration is high, excessive administration of

Table 14.20.
Hyperkalemia: Therapeutic Protocol

	Findings	Therapy	Agent and Dosage	Comments
General		Stop potassium administration Correct acidosis Stop drugs impairing potassium excretion Increase urinary sodium excretion by increasing sodium intake or by administering diuretics Remove necrotic tissue	Fludrocortisone acetate (0.1–0.2 mg/day orally) for isolated aldosterone deficiency	Check for spurious hyperkalemia
Specific				
Mild	Serum potassium < 6.5 mEq/liter	Follow above steps		Consider diagnosis of Addison's disease if urinary sodium > 30 mEq/liter
Moderate	Serum potassium 6.5–8.0 mEq/liter or peaked T waves on electrocardiogram	Follow above steps Administer ion-exchange resins	Sodium polystyrene sulfonate, 20 gm, plus sorbitol, 20 ml, four times a day orally, or sodium polystyrene sulfonate, 50 gm in 50 ml of 70% sorbitol solution, plus 100–150 ml water as retention enema	With circulatory overload or severe renal insufficiency, consider using calcium resin Retain enema at least half hour, repeat in 4 hours after a cleansing enema if necessary
Severe	Serum potassium > 8.0 mEq/liter or widened QRS complex, heart block, or ventricular arrhythmia on electrocardiogram	Follow above steps Administer specified agents Employ peritoneal dialysis or hemodialysis if drug therapy is ineffective Administer ion-exchange resins as above when crisis passes	Sodium bicarbonate, 88 mEq/liter over 5 min intravenously and/or 50% glucose, 50–100 ml, plus insulin (CZI), 8–15 units as intravenous bolus[a] If above therapy ineffective, administer calcium gluconate, 1–2 gm over 5 min intravenously	Repeat in 15–20 min as needed Peak effect after 30 min Contraindicated in patients receiving digitalis, requires electrocardiographic monitoring

[a] In the absence of circulatory overload, an alternative to sodium bicarbonate and glucose in combination is 5% dextrose in 1 liter of normal saline, plus sodium bicarbonate, 88 mEq/liter intravenously over 30 min.

potassium or aldosterone deficiency or antagonism is likely.

Diagnosis and Therapy

The important manifestations of hyperkalemia are cardiac. Sudden death may occur without any previous clinical signs, although the electrocardiogram often contains important information regarding early potassium toxicity.

As the serum potassium level begins to increase, peaked T waves appear on the electrocardiogram (Fig. 14.4). In contrast with other causes of symetrically peaked T waves, hyperkalemia is associated with a normal or decreased Q-T interval. With more profound hyperkalemia (serum potassium usually more than 8 mEq/liter), the P-R interval lengthens, P waves may disappear, and complete heart block may develop. The QRS complex widens and may progress to sine waves. Ventricular arrhythmias are common. When exposed to hyperkalemia, the heart is more sensitive to vagal influences, and such stimulation may lead to cardiac arrest. Hyponatremia, hypocalcemia, and acidosis all may exaggerate the cardiac effects of hyperkalemia.

If the serum potassium concentration is elevated, an electrocardiogram should be obtained immediately. Abnormalities compatible with the diagnosis of hyperkalemia dictate immediate therapy while the laboratory data are verified. A urinary sodium determination is helpful in planning therapy in this situation. If no electrocardiographic abnormalities are noted, the potassium in both serum and plasma (heparinized tube) should be measured again. Tubes should be carried to the laboratory immediately to minimize hemolysis.

In the hyperkalemic patient, administration of potassium and drugs that impair potassium excretion must be discontinued; large areas of necrotic tissue should be removed. However, these measures do not suffice in the emergency management of hyperkalemia (Table 14.20). If the serum potassium level is more than 8 mEq/liter or if electrocardiographic changes *other than peaked T waves* are present, such as widening of the QRS complex or indications of heart block or a ventricular arrhythmia, administration of either sodium bicarbonate, insulin plus glucose, or intravenous calcium should be considered.

Sodium bicarbonate drives potassium into the cells even in the absence of acidosis and may be lifesaving. Glucose with insulin is effective therapy because insulin transports potassium into cells, and the glucose prevents hypoglycemia. The peak effect of glucose plus insulin occurs after 30 minutes, however, and this may be too slow if the electrocardiogram shows signs of worsening hyperkalemia. Calcium directly antagonizes the effect of potassium on the heart, although it does not influence the serum potassium concentration. Calcium therapy is potentially hazardous, requires careful electrocardiographic monitoring, and should be avoided if the patient is receiving digitalis. Hypertonic saline solution antagonizes the effect of potassium on the heart to a lesser degree, and an alternative form of therapy is a "cocktail" containing dextrose, normal saline, and bicarbonate. If heart block is present and is not immediately reversed with medical therapy, a transvenous pacemaker should be inserted.

The effect of these agents are short-lived. Although with moderate hyperkalemia (serum potassium value from 5.6 to 8.0 mEq/liter and peaked T waves the only electrocardiographic indication) these slower forms of therapy may suffice, therapy directed toward a more sustained decrease in the serum potassium level should be instituted as well. Sodium intake should be increased if renal and cardiac functions are adequate. If the urinary sodium concentration is low, oral or parenteral salt administration will help return the potassium to normal levels. Ion-exchange resins such as sodium polystyrene sulfonate (Kayexalate) are effective, removing approximately 1 mEq of potassium for each gram of resin; the route of administration may be oral or rectal. Sorbitol is often administered in conjunction with resins to prevent constipation and to decrease absorption of the sodium leaving the resin. In patients with circulatory overload, the calcium form of the resin may be safer than the sodium form. If these measures do not suffice, hemodialysis or peritoneal dialysis against potassium-free solutions should be started.

It is important to avoid hypokalemia as a result of too vigorous therapy, particularly in patients receiving digitalis. The diagnosis of Addison's disease should be considered. Desoxycorticosterone acetate, 5 mg twice a day intramuscularly, or fludrocortisone acetate, 0.1–0.2 mg/day orally, in addition to cortisol is effective therapy. The latter is quite effective in hyporeninemic hypoaldosteronism as well.

SUGGESTED READINGS

Diabetic Ketoacidosis and Hyperosmolar Nonketotic Coma

Alexander E: Metabolic acidosis. Recognition and etiologic diagnosis. *Hosp Pract,* 1986;21(1):100E–100R.

Arieff AL, Carroll HJ: Nonketotic hyperosmolar coma with hyperglycemia. *Medicine,* 1972;51:73–94.

Barrett EJ, De Fronzo RA: Diabetic ketoacidosis: Diagnosis and treatment. *Hosp Pract,* 1984;19(4):89–104.

Fisher JN, Kitabchi AE: A randomized study of phosphate therapy in the treatment of diabetic ketoacidosis. *J Clin Endocrinol Metab,* 1983;57:177–180.

Fisher JN, Shahshahani MN, Kitabchi AE: Diabetic ketoacidosis: Low-dose insulin therapy by various routes. *N Engl J Med,* 1977;297:238–241.
Foster G: From glycogen to ketones—and back. *Diabetes,* 1984;33:1188–1199.
Foster DW, McGarry JD. The metabolic derangements and treatment of diabetic ketoacidosis. *New Engl J Med,* 1983;309:159–169.
Hare JW, Rossini AA: Diabetic comas: The overlap concept. *Hosp Pract,* 1979;14:95–108.
Johnston DG, Alberti KGMM: Diabetic emergencies: Practical aspects of the management of diabetic ketoacidosis and diabetes during surgery. *Clin Endocrinol Metab,* 1980;9:437–460.
Schade DS, Eaton RP: Diabetic ketoacidosis—pathogenesis, prevention and therapy. *Clin Endocrinol Metab,* 1983;12:321–338.

Alcoholic Ketoacidosis and Lactic Acidosis

Cohen RD, Iles RA: Lactic acidosis: Diagnosis and therapy. *Clin Endocrinol Metab,* 1980;9:513–527.
Kreisberg RA, Wood BC: Drug and chemical-induced metabolic acidosis. *Clin Endocrinol Metab,* 1983;12:391–411.
Narins RG, Rudnick MR, Basti CP: Lactic acidosis and the elevated anion gap (I) and (II). *Hosp Pract,* May, 1980;15:125–135, June, 1980;15:91-98.
Olivia PB: Lactic acidosis. *Am J Med,* 1980;48:209–225.
Palmer JP: Alcoholic ketoacidosis: Clinical and laboratory presentation, pathophysiology and treatment. *Clin Endocrinol Metab,* 1983;12:381–389.
Park R, Arieff AI: Lactic acidosis: Current concepts. *Clin Endocrinol Metab,* 1983;12:339–358.
Stacpoole PW, Harman EM, Curry SH, et al: Treatment of lactic acidosis with dichloroacetate. *N Engl J Med,* 1983;309:390–396.
Warner A, Vaziri ND: Treatment of lactic acidosis. *S Med J,* 1981;74:841–847.

Hypoglycemia

Fajans SS, Floyd JC. Jr: Fasting hypoglycemia in adults. *N Engl J Med,* 1976;294:766–772.
Gale E: Hypoglycemia. *Clin Endocrinol Metabol,* 1980; 9:461.
Malouf R, Brust JCM: Hypoglycemia: Causes, neurological manifestations and outcome. *Ann Neurol,* 1985;17:421–430.
Miller SI, Wallace RJ Jr, Musher DM, et al: Hypoglycemia as a manifestation of sepsis. *Am J Med,* 1980;68:649–654.
Seltzer HS: Drug-induced hypoglycemia: A review based on 473 cases. Diabetes 1972;21:955–966.

Adrenal Insufficiency

Bayliss RIS: Adrenal cortex. *Clin Endocrinol Metabol,* 1980;9:477–486.
Burke CW. Adrenocortical insufficiency. *Clin Encodrinol Metab,* 1985;14:947–976.
Dixon RB, Christy NP: On the various forms of corticosteroid withdrawal syndrome. *Am J Med,* 1980;68:224–230.
Mason AS, Meade TW, Lee JA, et al: Epidemiological and clinical picture of Addison's disease. *Lancet,* 1968; 2:744–747.
Melby JC: Drug spotlight program: Systemic corticosteroid therapy: Pharmacology and endocrinologic considerations. *Ann Intern Med,* 1974;81:505–512.

Thyroid Storm or Decompensated Thyrotoxicosis

Das G, Kreiger M: Treatment of thyrotoxic storm with intravenous administration of propranolol. *Ann Intern Med,* 1969;70:985–988.
Menendez CE, Rivlin RS: Thyrotoxic crisis and myxedema coma. *Med Clin North Am,* 1973;57:1463–1470.

Myxedema Crisis

Blum M: Myxedema coma. *Am J Med Sci,* 1972;264:432–443.
Hausmann W: Myxoedema crisis. *Hormones,* 1970;1:110–128.
Ladenson PW, Levin AA, Ridgway EC, et al. Complications of surgery in hypothyroid patients. *Am J Med,* 1984;77:261–268.
Senior RM, Birge SJ, Wessler S, et al: The recognition and management of myxedema coma. *JAMA,* 1971;217:61–65.

Calcium Emergencies

Elias EG, Evans JT: Hypercalcemic crisis in neoplastic diseases: Management with mithramycin. Surgery 1972; 71:631–635.
Evans RA. Hypercalcemia. What does it signify? 1986; 31:64–74.
Heath DP: The emergency management of disorders of calcium and magnesium. *Clin Endocrinol Metab,* 1980; 9:487–502.
Muggia FM, Heinemann HO: Hypercalcemia associated with neoplastic disease. *Ann Intern Med,* 1981;94:312–316.
Schneider AB, Sherwood LM: Calcium homeostasis and the pathogenesis and management of hypercalcemic disorders. *Metabolism,* 1974;23:975–1007.
Suki WN, Yium JJ, Von Minden M, et al: Acute treatment of hypercalcemia with furosemide. *N Engl J Med,* 1970;283:836–840.

Hyponatremia

Anderson RJ, Chung H-M, Kluge R, et al. Hyponatremia: A prospective analysis of its epidemiology and pathogenetic role of vasopressin. *Ann Intern Med,* 1985;102:164.
Arieff AJ. Central nervous system manifestations of disordered sodium metabolism. *Clin Endocrinol Metab,* 1984;13:269–294.
Arieff AJ. Hyponatremia, convulsions, respiratory arrest and permanent brain damage after elective surgery in healthy women. *N Engl J Med,* 1986;314:1529–1535.
Ashraf N, Locksley R, Arieff AI: Thiazide-induced hyponatremia associated with death or neurologic damage in outpatients. *Am J Med,* 1981;70:1163–1168.
Ayus JC, Olivero JJ, Frommer JP: Rapid correction of severe hyponatremia with intravenous hypertonic saline solution. *Am J Med,* 9182;72:43–48.
Baylis PH: Hyponatremia and hypernatremia. *Clin Endocrinol Metabol,* 1980;9:625–637.
Narins RG: Therapy of hyponatremia: Does haste make waste? *N Engl J Med,* 1986;314:1573–1574.
Schrier RW: Treatment of hyponatremia. *N Engl J Med,* 1985;312:1121–1123.
Weinberg MS, Donohoe JF: Hyponatremia in the syndrome of inappropriate secretion of antidiuretic hormone: Rapid correction with osmotic agents. *Med J,* 1985;78:348–351.

Hyperkalemia

DeFronzo RA: Hyperkalemia and hyporeninemic hypoaldosteronism. *Kidney Int,* 1980;17:118–134.
Sterns RH, Cox M, Feig PU, et al. Internal potassium balance and the control of the plasma potassium concentration. *Medicine,* 1981;60:339–354.

CHAPTER **15**

Neurologic Emergencies

Amy A. Pruitt, M.D.

INTRODUCTION

The emergency physician is presented with a vast range of potentially neurologic conditions, many of which can be confused with psychologic, metabolic, or other nonneurologic problems. Competence in neurologic emergency medicine requires recognition that many benign and critical, acute and progressive symptoms can be considered emergencies by the patient. The patient may present with the first onset of a serious symptom such as a seizure or a headache or may seek attention when a long-standing headache worsens, when a recurrent convulsion occurs, or when a preexisting condition like dementia is exacerbated by fever or metabolic derangement. Progressive pain or weakness that began many weeks before may reach a stage that causes the patient to seek emergency help. It is the task of the emergency department physician to recognize conditions that require immediate attention, differentiating them from problems that can be dealt with in a more leisurely fashion.

This chapter is designed to help direct emergency department evaluations along the lines of a neurologist's thinking in the differential diagnosis of nontraumatic neurologic emergency problems. Spinal cord compression, head trauma, altered consciousness, toxicologic, pediatric neurologic, and psychiatric emergencies are covered elsewhere in this volume.

Specifically, the often very brief or unavailable history and the screening physical examination should lead the physician to decide (*a*) *WHERE is the lesion?* Thus, is the problem in the nervous system or outside the nervous system? If in the nervous system, is the problem in the peripheral or the central nervous system? If peripheral, is the problem at the nerve root, nerve, neuromuscular junction, or muscle level? If central, is it the brain or in the spinal cord? If in the spinal cord, is the problem intramedullary or extramedullary? If in the brain, is the lesion in the brainstem, cerebellum, or cerebral hemispheres? If the lesion is in the hemispheres, is it superficial or deep, right or left, anterior or posterior?; and (*b*) *WHAT is the lesion?* (tumor, hemorrhage, stroke, etc.).

HISTORY

The history is designed to help the physician answer the question "WHAT is it?" that is causing the patient's problem. If possible, it is best to have a family member or witness in the examining room to assist the patient, to corroborate the patient's story, and to give an idea about the patient's premorbid level of function. It should be remembered that the patient's report of symptoms may be inaccurate either because of mental status impairment or because the very nature of the lesion may be difficult to describe. A patient with a Bell's palsy, for example, may report numbness of the affected side of the face, a binocular visual disturbance involving the left visual field may be called "left eye trouble," or the autonomic discharges accompanying a partial complex seizure may be termed "stomach upset," "anxiety," or "queasiness."

The *pace* of onset is of critical importance in giving a clue to the etiology. *Abrupt onset* over minutes to seconds characterizes seizure, hemorrhagic stroke, embolic stroke, and subarachnoid hemorrhage. Onset over minutes to hours could be indicative of a lacune or of large vessel thrombotic stroke. *Progressive deterioration* over days to weeks should lead to suspicion of a degenerative process, of an expanding intracranial process such as neoplasm or subdural hematoma, or of a toxic exposure. *Episodic neurologic dysfunction* leads to such diagnostic possibilities as transient ischemic attacks, seizures, or neuromuscular junction disorders like the myasthenic syndromes.

A history of trauma should always be sought. Likelihood of suicide attempt should be ascertained, and prior drug use or other major metabolic problems such as diabetes should be investigated to refine further diagnostic considerations.

PHYSICAL EXAMINATION

A basic neurologic screening examination in the patient with a general neurologic complaint should evaluate six areas: (*a*) mental status (see Chapter 16), (*b*) cranial nerves, (*c*) motor function, (*d*) coordination, (*e*) sensation, and (*f*) reflexes. However, an organizational plan is required lest the physician end up with bits and pieces of seemingly unrelated physical examination data. The following plan is offered to help direct the screening examination.

Organizing Principles of Physical Examination

Eight principles will organize the examination for maximum efficiency.

1. *Are there mental status abnormalities present?* If so, are they diffuse (delirium, disorientation), or are they focal (receptive aphasia, isolated memory loss)? If the cognitive functions are disturbed, the problem is likely to be cerebral in origin (rather than in brainstem or peripheral nervous system).
2. *Are cranial nerve signs present?* If so, the problem must lie at least at brainstem or cerebral level and, with rare exceptions, cannot be confined to spinal cord or peripheral nervous system.
3. *Are there unilateral or bilateral signs?* If a hemiparesis is present, the problem could originate in brainstem or in one hemisphere. If a paraparesis is present, the problem could arise in lumbar or thoracic spinal cord or in the parasagittal area of the cerebrum. Quadriparesis implies dis-

ease at the level of the cervical cord or a location rostral to this region.

4. *Is the problem upper or lower motor neuron?* Upper motor neuron lesions are associated with spasticity, hyperreflexia, and, in the lower limbs, Babinski signs. The lesion may be in the cerebrum, brainstem, cervical, thoracic, or upper lumbar spinal cord. Lower motor neuron lesions are characterized by flaccidity, fasciculations, and hypoactive or absent deep tendon reflexes. The lesion may be in nerve root or peripheral nerve.
5. *If the problem is in the peripheral nervous system, is there evidence of nerve or of muscle disease?* Weakness, usually most pronounced in the distal extremities, in conjunction with depressed deep tendon reflexes and abnormal sensation, suggests nerve disease. Primary muscle pathology results in preserved reflexes and normal sensation often with characteristic patterns of predominantly proximal muscle weakness.
6. *Are there motor signs only, sensory signs only, or a mixture of both?* Pure motor involvement is expected in Bell's palsy and internal capsule lacunar strokes. Pure sensory dysfunction is anticipated in a thalamic lacunar stroke. Both motor and sensory symptoms are found with a middle cerebral artery stroke.
7. *Are there local signs only or is there evidence of widespread neurologic abnormality?* The patient may notice only tremor in one limb, but the physician may discover cogwheel rigidity, masked facies, and abnormal gait suggestive of a widespread extrapyramidal problem. Conversely, diagnosis of a Bell's palsy demands that no other cranial nerve or corticospinal signs be present to implicate a central rather than a peripheral origin for the facial weakness.
8. *Does the examination suggest a nonanatomic picture?* For example, the complaint of complete blindness in the presence of normal gait, orientation, fundi, and pupillary reflexes is hard to localize to any specific area, and cortical blindness can usually be differentiated from hysterical visual loss. Similarly, "body-splitting" vibration sense loss or whole head numbness is not compatible with a specific locus of neurologic disease and should raise suspicion of psychiatric overlay to the complaint.

As the physician goes through the screening examination of patients with a general neurologic

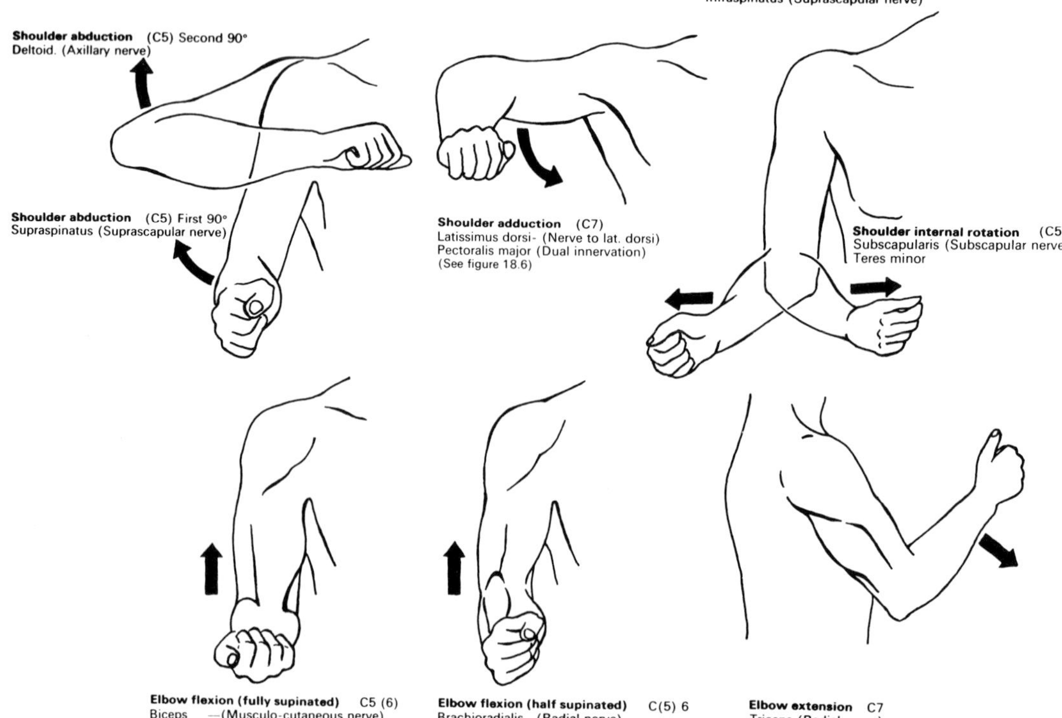

Figure 15.1. Shoulder and arm movements.

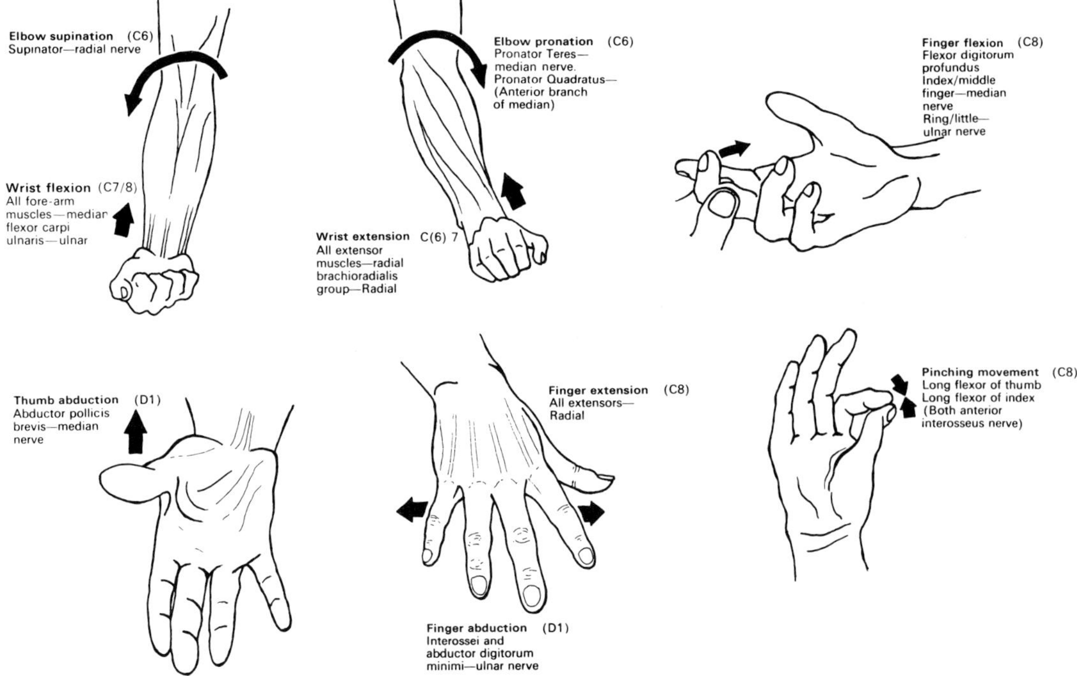

Figure 15.2. Forearm and hand movements.

complaint, detailed below, he or she should keep in mind the organizing principles and try to relate them to the history obtained. Frequent, deliberate examination of patients for neurologic dysfunction gives the examiner a feeling for the expected range of normal strength in patients of different builds and ages and produces confidence in the grading of reflexes, strength, and coordination.

Neurologic Screening Examination

Mental Status

A detailed mental status examination is outlined in Chapter 16. Elaborate testing for hemispheric functions and memory is not necessary in a patient who is conversing normally, responding appropriately to questions, and is oriented. Observations of speech, reasoning, and memory for details of history is sufficient.

Cranial Nerves

Cranial nerve I (olfactory nerve) is not usually assessed in the emergency department. Cranial nerve II (optic nerve) should be tested in every patient. Assessment of visual acuity in each eye can be performed with a hand-held or wall eye chart. Fundi should be examined for papilledema or embolic material. Visual fields can be assessed grossly by having the patient look at the examiner's nose from the distance of an arm's length. The examiner flicks both index fingers individually and then simultaneously in the superior and inferior quadrants of vision, both medially and temporally for each eye.

Cranial nerves III, IV, and VI (oculomotor, trochlear, and abducens nerves, respectively) are tested together by observing the extraocular movements. The patient is asked to look up, down, left, and right and then is asked to follow the examiner's finger all the way to the right and in this plane of gaze to look fully up and down. The same method is repeated in full left lateral gaze. This allows the examiner to isolate extraocular muscles. If the patient is complaining of double vision, but no ocular movement abnormality can be detected, a red glass over the right eye may help reveal the problem (see ''Visual Problems'' later in this chapter). Pupillary size and reactivity are assessed and recorded. Nystagmus is noted.

Cranial nerve V (trigeminal nerve) is assessed by testing the corneal reflex with a wisp of sterile cotton, noting both direct and consensual responses. Each of the three divisions of the trigeminal nerve on both sides is tested quickly for equality of sensation to light touch and pinprick (see Fig. 15.5).

Facial muscle movement (cranial nerve VII) is assessed by having the patient show his or her teeth and squeeze his or her eyes tightly against resistance. Upper motor neuron lesions are characterized by unilateral weakness predominantly or exclusively of the lower half of the face, while lower motor neuron (peripheral nerve) lesions involve the entire side of the face.

Cranial nerve VIII (auditory and vestibular nerve) is tested if the patient complains of vertigo or hearing difficulty or if there is evidence of cranial nerve V or VII dysfunction. Examination of the tympanic membranes, is always indicated. Tests for cranial nerves IX-XII are not usually part of a screening examination. However, palatal function is assessed in a patient with recent stroke because dysphagia is often present. If the patient has other signs localizing the problem to brainstem level, careful examination of palatal movement and sensation is performed. If the patient complains of dizziness, hoarseness, dysphagia, or altered voice, full-scale lower cranial nerve function testing is in order.

Motor Function

Evaluation of general strength, tone, and movement is the objective of the screening examination. The patient is watched as he or she walks in, maneuvers onto the table, and changes clothes. Abnormal movements, such as tics, tremors, asterixis, and myoclonus, are noted. Evidence of atrophy or asymmetry of muscle bulk is easily observed. Assessment of lower extremity tone is performed by having the patient lie on his or her back. The knee is quickly lifted from the stretcher and the heel dragged along the surface. Increased tone is indicated if the leg comes up as a single unit or bends with difficulty. Individual muscle strength testing is done in the patient with any complaint of weakness. The examiner should have a plan in mind: Is the pattern of weakness unilateral (hemiparesis), bilateral in the lower extremities (paraparesis), confined to a specific peripheral nerve, consistent with a known pattern of muscle disease? A sensitive indicator of pyramidal weakness is the pronator drift. The patient is asked to extend both arms in front of the body, palms up, eyes closed. If there is any downward movement of the hand with pronation of the arm, there may be contralateral hemispheric trouble. Another screen of gross muscle power in the lower extremities is to have the patient walk on heels and toes and to ask if he or she perceives any unilateral difficulty with this maneuver.

Specific muscle testing takes another few minutes. Figs. 15.1–15.4 demonstrate the important muscles to be surveyed. The examiner tests muscles about the shoulder, wrist, hand, hip, knee, and foot. The patient's upper extremities are assessed while he is seated; lower extremities, in the supine position. A useful emergency department book is *Aids to the Diagnosis of Peripheral Nerve Injuries.*

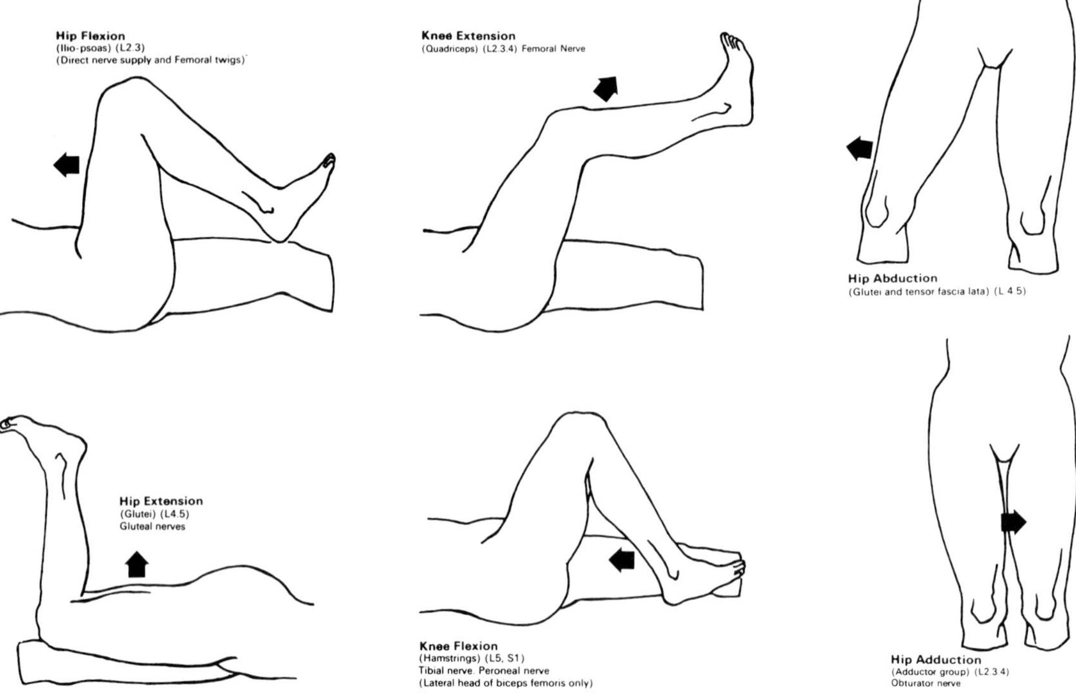

Figure 15.3. Hip and knee movements.

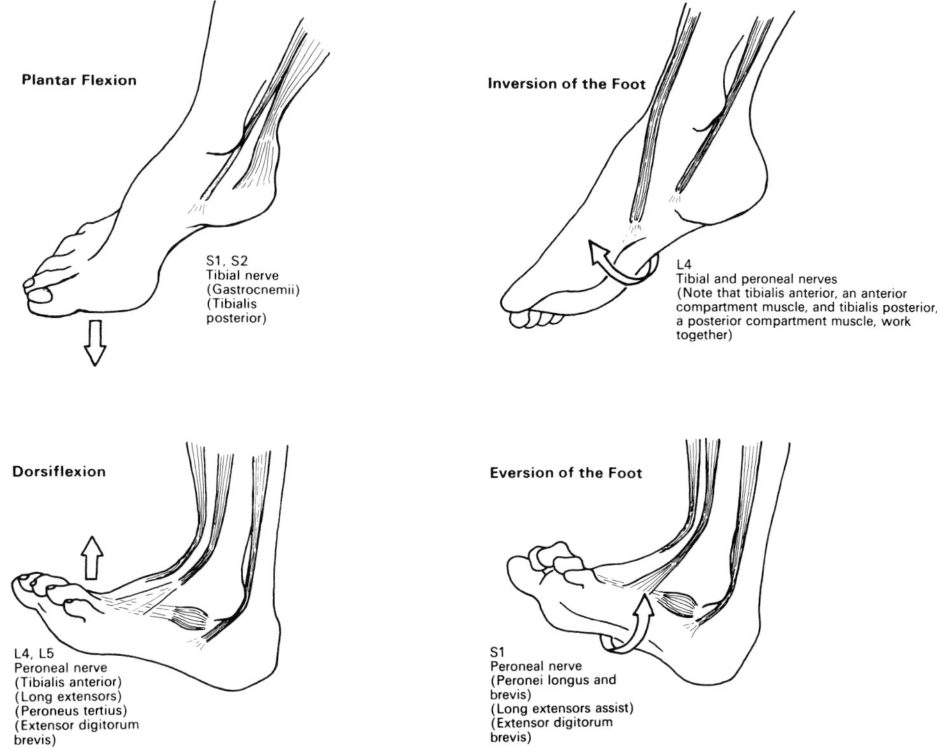

Figure 15.4. Movements of the foot.

Coordination

Coordination testing presumes that the patient's gross motor power is sufficient to perform the tasks required. Screening tests include observation of gait for ataxia. Finger-to-nose testing and heel-knee-shin testing are good indicators of cerebellar hemispheric dysfunction. The abnormal response is an increase in oscillation of the limb as the target is approached. Having the patient tap his or her foot quickly while standing with the heel on the floor or with the middle finger against the tip of the thumb gives good indications of fine motor control. Abnormal test performance indicates either cerebellar dysfunction or corticospinal tract abnormality and is commonly seen well after major motor recovery has occurred following stroke or other upper motor neuron lesion. Romberg testing is an appropriate screen in patients with a complaint of instability of walking or dizziness. The patient stands with feet together. If balance is maintained in this position, the patient is then asked to close his or her eyes. Patients with primarily cerebellar problems will have difficulty maintaining balance even with eyes open. A positive Romberg, i.e., inability to maintain balance with eyes closed but adequate balance with eyes open, is seen with posterior column dysfunction or with peripheral vestibular dysfunction. The patient falls consistently to one side. Other signs of cerebellar dysfunction include dysarthria, scanning speech, and pronounced ocular dysmetria with overshoot of eyes on attempted fixation.

Sensory Examination

The sensory examination is least helpful either in screening or in detailed testing because it is the most subjective. It is not a major part of the screening examination and is used in more detailed testing only after the history and physical examination at that point indicate a specific localization. The patient is asked to outline the area of perceived sensory abnormality; words of description are particularly heeded. Spinothalamic lesions may be described as burning, searing, or numbness. Posterior column dysfunction may be expressed as tightness, constriction, or swelling of the affected part. The examiner should have a plan as simple sensory modalities are tested (pin and temperature sensation, joint position, vibration, and light touch). Patterns are sought (see Figs. 15.5 and 15.6 for dermatomes and peripheral nerves). Is there stocking-glove sensory loss in several modalities suggesting a peripheral nerve problem? Is the sensory loss con-

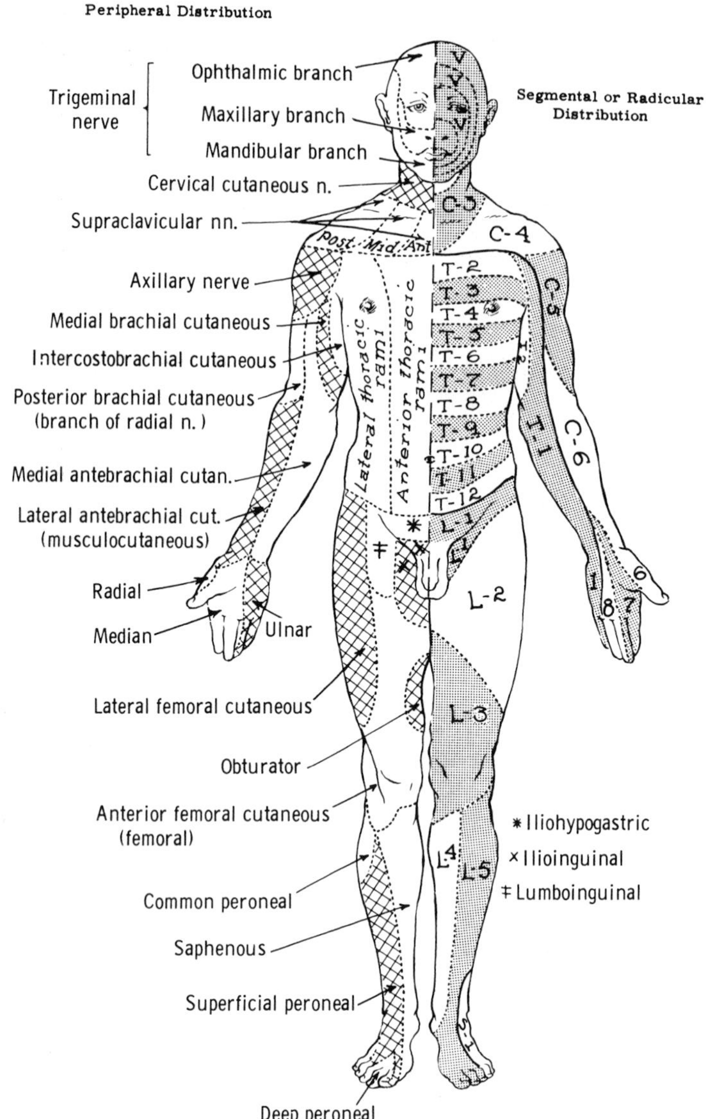

Figure 15.5. Sensory innervation. (From Chusid JG. *Correlative Neuroanatomy and Functional Neurology.* 19th ed. Los Angeles: copyright Lange Medical Publications, 1979.)

fined to one dermatome or to a single peripheral nerve distribution? Key areas to remember in the sensory examination are: C2-3, back of head; C6, thumb; T4 nipple level; T10, waist level; L1, groin level; L5, web space between great and first toes; and S1, lateral foot. Cortical sensory modalities including stereognosis, graphesthesia, double simultaneous stimulation, and two-point discrimination are tested if primary sensation is preserved and only if confirmation or cortical dysfunction is essential to diagnostic accuracy (i.e., the distinction between a lacunar and a cortical stroke).

Reflex Testing

Deep tendon reflex testing is a part of the emergency department screening examination, providing a useful baseline for future reference should the patient's condition change. The muscle stretch reflexes represent specific levels of reflex arc function. Those routinely tested include biceps (C5), brachioradialis (C6), triceps (C7), patellar (L4), and ankle (S1). The grading scale comprises: 0 = no response, 1 = hypoactive, 2 = normal, 3 = brisk but not pathologic, and 4 = abnormally brisk with or without

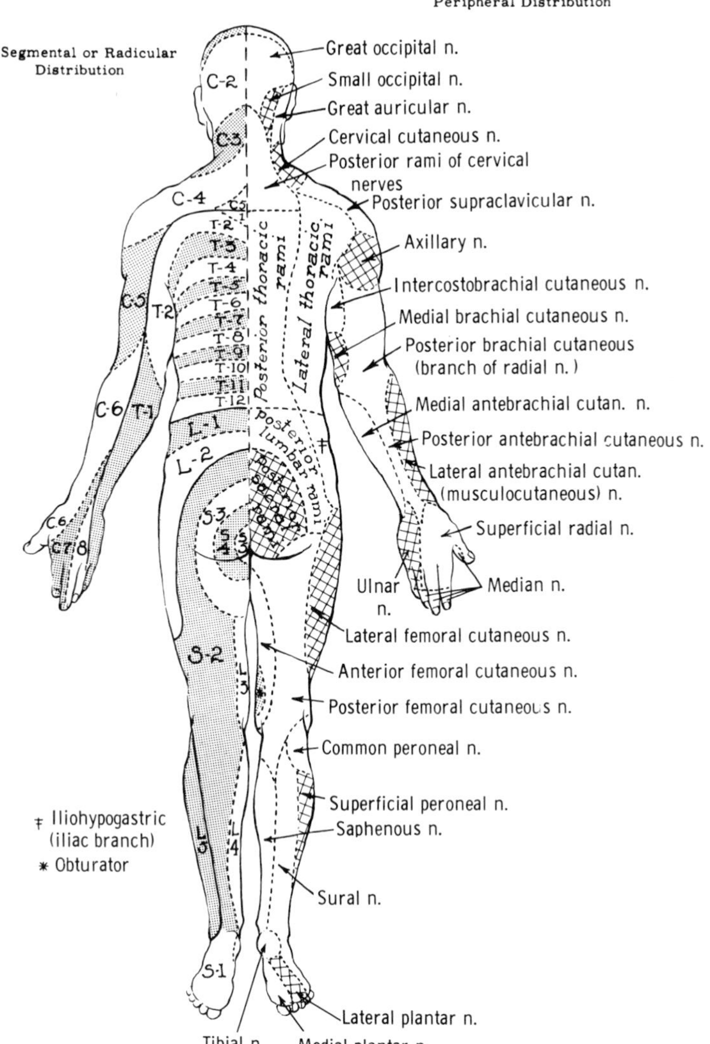

Figure 15.6. Sensory innervation. (From Chusid JG, *Correlative Neuroanatomy and Functional Neurology.* 19th ed. Los Angeles: copyright Lange Medical Publications, 1979.)

clonus. Asymmetry is the important finding. One patient can have very brisk reflexes, while another can have diffusely hypoactive reflexes, both normal. A difference in reflexes between the arms and legs, with legs brisker, suggests a lesion of the spinal cord. Depression of reflexes in only one limb is consistent with a peripheral nerve or root lesion. Pathologic reflexes, such as the Babinski, snout, root, and grasp, all indicate failure of inhibition from higher cortical and spinal centers to the lower reflex arcs. Babinski signs are elicited by stroking the lateral aspect of the foot gently, moving forward toward the great toe across the ball of the foot. The abnormal response is extension of the great toe, with or without fanning of the other toes. It must be differentiated from a withdrawal response.

Table 15.1 summarizes a neurologic screening examination. Subsequently sections of this chapter ("Symptom-Oriented Management") present the more detailed accessory tests employed for specific types of neurologic complaints.

DIAGNOSTIC TESTS

The history and physical examination identify patients who require emergency diagnostic procedures. Increasingly, sophisticated neurologic diagnostic equipment is accessible to the emergency

Table 15.1.
Neurologic Screening Examination

Function	Test
Mental status	Normal orientation, speech, affect (see Chapter 16)
Cranial nerves	II—visual acuity, fundi, fields
	III, IV, VI—extraocular movements, pupillary response, nystagmus
	V—corneal reflexes, facial sensation
	VII—facial muscle strength
	Tympanic membrane examination
Motor function	Pronator drift, tone, heel and toe walking
	Muscle survey—shoulder, arm, hand, hip, knee, foot
	Abnormal movements (tics, tremors, chorea)
Coordination	Gait, finger-to-nose testing
Sensation	Pinprick on areas indicated by patient
Reflexes	Deep tendon reflexes: biceps, brachioradialis, triceps, patellar, ankle
	Babinski response

physician. However, the history and physical examination dictate the appropriate circumstances under which these tests are utilized.

Computed Tomography

Computed tomography (CT) scans are often available to emergency physicians. The CT scan without contrast infusion detects blood, cerebral edema, hydrocephalus, atrophy of brain, calcification, and shift of midline structures. It clearly outlines the supratentorial structures, and newer CT scanners provide an outline of the base of the brain and the posterior fossa. CT scans with infusion of iodinated contrast medium give further information about cerebral structures. Cerebral vessels can be seen, and some aneurysms and arteriovenous malformations can be visualized. Neoplasms may take up contrast because of defects in the blood-brain barrier. Other conditions that result in uptake of contrast (''enhancement'') include recent cerebral infarction (10 days to several weeks), abscess, meningitis, and postsurgical changes (5 days to several weeks). *An emergency CT scan is always done without contrast first.*

Indications for CT scans include sudden acute neurologic deterioration with altered consciousness or mentation, or evidence of raised intracranial pressure, progressive deficits consistent with an expanding intracerebral process, new onset seizure disorder in an adult, papilledema, and constellations of cranial nerve deficits referrable to a specific area of the brainstem or posterior fossa. Further diagnostic information is obtained in any of these situations by a second scan with contrast infusion. Dye has been known to precipitate seizures in patients with epilepsy or intracranial lesions. The patient with seizures is given a parenteral anticonvulsant before CT scanning if medical circumstances allow. The clinician's judgment is required in the emergency utilization of CT scans in a number of other circumstances. A severe headache may be a muscle contraction headache, a migraine, or a subarachnoid hemorrhage. Detailed history and physical examination obviate the need for many CT scans. For example, physicians routinely order a CT scan in the diagnosis of stroke. Several studies have shown that agreement among observers on stroke type (hemorrhage, ischemic, lacunar, embolic) based on history and physical examination alone is quite good. However, CT scanning does produce refinement of diagnosis, and the occasional hemorrhage or hemorrhagic infarction clinically unsuspected can be diagnosed by CT scanning. (see ''Stroke'' for further discussion of the differential diagnosis of stroke by CT scan).

Magnetic Resonance Imaging

The magnetic resonance imaging (MRI) scan, formerly termed nuclear magnetic resonance (NMR), is a newcomer to the neurologic diagnostic armamentarium. At this point it is not used in the emergency department setting. It can be anticipated that this technique will follow the same course as CT scanning and that soon a majority of hospitals will have access to it. The MRI is based on ferromagnetic characteristics of the molecules of the brain and its surrounding structures. The apparatus is a large magnet. Patients with indwelling implants (excluding dental fillings) such as metallic joint prostheses, pacemakers, and cerebral aneurysm clips cannot have this study. For others, the technique may be very useful. The MRI images tumors, particularly those of the posterior fossa, brainstem, and skull base better than CT. Stroke abnormalities appear earlier on MRI than on CT. MRI studies are changing our understanding of the transient ischemic attack and infarction process. Hemorrhages, aneurysms, and arteriovenous malformations are imaged well. No contrast enhancement is required. The MRI is particularly useful for the spinal cord. *Developing indications* for MRI include early diagnosis of stroke when surgical intervention or anticoagulation are being considered. A patient with history of malignant tumor presenting with a spinal cord syndrome, can be evaluated by MRI and spared a myelogram at a time when the presence of cerebral metastases makes subarachnoid puncture un-

Table 15.2.
Cerebrospinal Fluid Formulas

Disease	WBC[a]	RBC[a]	Protein *mg %*	Sugar *mg %*	Comment
Bacterial meningitis	100–3,000[b]	0	100–1000	Reduced	+ smear, culture
Aseptic (viral) meningitis	10–500[c]	0	40–300	Normal or slightly reduced	Formula may be consistent with chemical, fungal, or infective endocarditis associated disease
Tuberculous meningitis	20–200[c]	0	100–1000	Reduced	+ smear, culture
Carcinomatous meningitis	5–300[d]	0	50–2000	Reduced	+ cytology, but several samples often necessary
Guillain-Barré syndrome	0–4	0	50–1000	Normal	Protein may be normal early in disease
Herpes simplex encephalitis	100–500	0–5000	100–500	Normal	CSF culture negative, brain biopsy positive

[a] WBC, White blood cell count; RBC, red blood cell count.
[b] Polymorphonuclear leukocyte predominance.
[c] Lymphocyte predominance.
[d] Lymphocytes, polymorphonuclear leukocytes, and nonhematic cells.

desirable. Patients with acutely evolving cervical myelopathies due to tumor or cervical spondylosis have been diagnosed and treated on the basis of MRI alone.

Lumbar Puncture

The technique of lumbar puncture is described in Illustrated Technique 14. Lumbar puncture permits determination of cerebrospinal fluid (CSF) pressure, protein content, cells, and sugar. The spinal tap is potentially useful in diagnosing or excluding conditions that either involve the meninges or cause secondary changes in the cerebrospinal fluid through disruption of the blood-brain barrier. Four major classes of diseases, meningeal infection, subarachnoid hemorrhage, central nervous system malignancy, and demyelinating disease (includng the Guillain-Barré syndrome) have distinctive and differentiating CSF formulas. Although the CSF may show changes in other conditions, the changes are neither sufficiently consistent nor specific to be definitive. The lumbar puncture is critical to the diagnosis of suspected bacterial meningitis (see Table 15.2). It is suggestive in fungal and mycobacterial infection, but its immediate effectiveness is diminished by lower sensitivity and long culture time. The role of lumbar puncture is changing in the diagnosis of subarachnoid hemorrhage. The test is usually deferred until after a CT scan. In many cases the CT is of sufficient quality to obviate the lumbar puncture. Therefore, the use of this invasive procedure involves an assessment of the risks versus benefits. The strongest indications are signs pointing to bacterial meningitis: fever, headache, meningismus. The strongest contraindications are signs suggesting a high risk for serious complications: papilledema, posterior fossa signs, and known disorders of hemostasis (anticoagulation, a platelet count less than 40,000).

If the CSF pressure is greater than 400 mm Hg and there is reason to suspect that the patient has an expanding intracranial process that could produce a pressure cone, the patient should be given mannitol intravenously, 1–2 gm/kg. Only the CSF in the manometer should be removed for examination. Emergency department examination of CSF includes: pressure recording, cell count, Gram's stain and culture, sugar and protein determinations, and an India ink preparation if cryptococcus infection is a consideration. Cytology, testing for syphilis, and γ-globulin cannot be determined in time for useful emergency department diagnosis. Red blood cells may not be found in cases of hemorrhage if blood is deep in the cerebral parenchyma and has not reached the ventricular or hemispheric surface *or* if the lumbar puncture is done more than 4 days after the hemorrhage. The normal CSF total protein is approximately 0.5% that of the serum protein. Increased CSF protein produced by lysing red blood cells adds about 1 mg % for every 500 red blood cells counted in the CSF.

Cervical Spine and Skull Radiographs

Plain radiographs of the neck and skull provide useful information in traumatic neurologic emergencies, but are occasionally indicated in nontraumatic disease as well. Anteroposterior, lateral, and oblique views of the cervical spine to outline the neural foramina may be used to investigate radicular pain with neck discomfort. Arthritic change is seen in virtually all persons over the age of 50, but more specific diagnositic changes, such as the presence of cervical spondylosis, foraminal encroachment by bone spurs at a level consistent with symptoms, or evidence of lytic or blastic metastatic disease, can be discovered. Skull radiographs should be obtained if there is any history or physical evidence of trauma. Often CT scans are not available, the skull film may give clues to the presence of an expanding intracranial process (displacement of a calcified pineal gland, erosion of the sella turcica, or abnormal calcification with the cranium). Metastatic bone lesions, particularly common in multiple myeloma and prostatic carcinoma, are seen on plain radiographs of the skull.

Electroencephalography

Electroencephalography (EEG) is seldom used in the emergency department. However, a portable machine with a trained recording technician can be used after only 10 minutes of setup time. The EEG does have several emergency department indications. EEG distinguishes patients with true seizures from those with hysterical attacks simulating epileptic activity. It also differentiates ongoing seizure activity from a postictal state. Recording of brain waves aids in the differential diagnosis of patients with acute psychosis. Tracings of patients with acute schizophrenia or manic illness are always nearly normal. Acute psychosis, presenting as a metabolic derangement, such as hypoglycemia, is suggested by the presence of generalized EEG slowing. Encephalitis, particularly caused by herpes simplex virus, is often manifested by psychotic behavior even before other symptoms are present. In these cases, the EEG characteristically shows generalized sharp slowing over one temporal lobe. Behavioral disorders also occur in children with subacute sclerosing panencephalitis and adults with Creutzfeldt-Jakob disease. In both these situations, characteristic paroxysmal EEG activity is present. The differential diagnosis of comatose patients may also be aided by the EEG. Patients with severe, bilateral lower brainstem disease may appear to be comatose, but are actually wide awake and paralyzed (''locked-in'' syndrome); the EEG is normal. The presence of therapeutic or toxic amounts of several medications can be suggested by anterior fast (β) wave activity on the EEG. Most notable among these drugs are barbiturates and benzodiazepine compounds, diazepam hydrochloride (Valium), chlordiazepoxide hydrochloride (Librium), and flurazepam (Dalmane).

The EEG is one element in the diagnosis of ''cerebral death'' or irreversible cerebral cortical damage. Such a diagnosis is suspected when the patient meets rigid clinical criteria. In this instance such criteria must be met for at least 6 to 12 hours before a confirmatory EEG is undertaken, and, thus, is not a situation to be confronted in the emergency department.

Angiography

Angiography, either retrograde femoral arteriography or digital subtraction intravenous angiography, occasionally is indicated on an emergency basis when a patient with atherosclerotic cartoid artery disease presents with recent transient ischemic attacks or with an evolving stroke. Appropriate surgical backup consultation, of course, is mandatory. These techniques and their indications and complications are further discussed in the section of this chapter devoted to cerebrovascular disease.

SYMPTOM-ORIENTED MANAGEMENT

This section directs the physician to a more detailed history and physical examination based on the patient's initial complaint (or the observer's history) and the screening physical examination. Common symptoms, such as seizures and headaches, are covered first. Other neurologic conditions are grouped according to the pace of onset and the generalized or focal nature of the symptoms. Clearly, there is overlap in these categories. For example, weakness due to a tumor of the spinal epidural space can develop very quickly in a period of hours, but also may be preceded by several weeks of back pain. In this chapter, ''acute'' conditions are those coming on over a period of minutes to 48 hours, e.g., subarachnoid hemorrhage. ''Progressive'' deficits leading to emergency attention are problems of more than 48 hours symptom duration or problems of a relapsing, recurring nature such as myasthenia gravis.

Seizures

A seizure is a symptom of disordered neuronal function and therefore implies neurologic disease originating in the cerebrum. Epilepsy is a condition of recurring seizures, and status epilepticus is a seizure activity that is prolonged (greater than 20 minutes) or repetitive. Epilepsy may be primary or secondary. Primary or idiopathic epilepsy is defined as recurring convulsions of any type without definable cause and secondary epilepsy, convulsions occurring as a symptom of any disease.

Since 1% of the adult population in the United States suffers from recurring seizures and since seizures can be the first manifestation of a wide variety of conditions, the emergency physician must be comfortable with both the acute management of a patient actively experiencing seizures and with the follow-up and appropriate workup and triage of patients whose seizures have been controlled.

Table 15.3.
Treatment of Status Epilepticus

Drug	Initial Dose		Rate	Repeat Doses[a]		24 Hr Maximum Dose	
	Adult	Child		Adult	Child	Adult	Child
	mg		*mg/min*	*mg*		*mg*	
Diazepam	5–10	5	1–5	5–10	5	100	100
Phenytoin	500	5–8/kg	30–50	250–500	1.5/kg	18/kg	12/kg
Phenobarbital	150–400	5–8/kg	30–60	30	3/kg	1000	12/kg
Lorazepam	2–4	2	2	4[b]	2[b]	Not established	

[a] mg every 20–30 minutes.
[b] mg every 15–20 minutes.

Status Epilepticus

Status epilepticus is a state of recurring or continuous seizures. Though epileptic status may occur as a manifestation of any type of seizure (see Table 15.4), it is tonic-clonic status which is the most life-threatening medical emergency. Even when adequate ventilation and blood pressure are maintained, status epilepticus for more than 1 hour can mean permanent cerebral damage because of the enormous metabolic demands on the brain. Thus, an organized, deliberate approach to seizure control is essential. Table 15.3 outlines a protocol for the management of status epilepticus. After adequate airway and blood pressure are assured, thiamine, 50 mg intravenously, is given, followed by 50 gm of glucose, into a rapidly running normal saline intravenous line. Normal saline is chosen for the intravenous fluid because phenytoin, the usual first choice of medication, is soluble only in this fluid. Initial seizure control may be achieved with diazepam, but since the serum half-life of this drug is short, a longer-acting anticonvulsant is started immediately. Unless the patient is known to be allergic to the medication, phenytoin is the drug of choice. Phenytoin must be infused slowly since excessive infusion rates may cause hypotension. A full loading dose in a patient previously not treated with phenytoin is 18 mg/kg and a therapeutic level is maintained for 24 hours after such a dose. At the recommended rates, this takes approximately 25 minutes to deliver. If the patient is still having seizures, some sodium bicarbonate is given at this point. Most often the patient has been intubated by this time. Phenobarbital is the next drug administered for continuing seizures; its disadvantage is alteration of the level of consciousness for subsequent examination. Up to 1 gm of phenobarbital can be given to an adult at the rates indicated in Table 15.3. A less potent, but useful adjunctive medication for seizures is paraldehyde. It is particularly recommended for seizures due to alcohol withdrawal. If care is taken to use glass syringes for this organic solvent, 7 ml can be administered deeply into each buttock. Rectal paraldehyde dissolved in oil is frequently used to control seizures in children.

Other drugs for the control of resistant status epilepticus are lorazepam and valproic acid. The latter is sometimes given rectally, but is really too cumbersome for therapeutic adjunctive use. In some centers, lorazepam is recommended as the drug of choice for initial status epilepticus control. Two to four mg of this medication are given as an intravenous injection with repeat doses in 15–20 minutes. Respiratory depression from lorazepam is less common than with diazepam. It is reasonable to intersperse some lorazepam with phenytoin or phenobarbital.

By the time the physician has administered two or three anticonvulsant drugs, preliminary screening metabolic studies are likely to be ready. Hyponatremia and hypocalcemia are metabolic derangements particularly likely to cause intractable seizures. A few patients in whom no correctable metabolic disorder is found fail to respond to full doses of medication as outlined. At this point, general anesthesia must be induced because of the threat of brain damage from continued generalized convulsions. Cessation of seizures can then be guaranteed with confirmatory EEG monitoring. It may be hours before it is possible to decrease the amount of anesthetic without seizure recurrence. Paralytic agents, such as curare, stop the somatic expression of the seizure by neuromuscular blockade, but they do not solve the major difficulty of excessive cerebral activity. They are therefore not recommended. After the seizures are controlled, the possible medical consequences of prolonged seizure activity, including acidosis, hyperkalemia, hyperthermia, hypoglycemia, and rhabdomyolysis leading to renal failure, must be anticipated.

Once the seizures are stopped, the physician considers the underlying etiology for the episode of status epilepticus. In 50% of patients with status epilepticus no prior seizure disorder is known. Noncompliance with medication accounted for 53% of those with prior seizure histories, and intercurrent infection or alcohol ingestion was the probable precipitating factor in the majority of the others (see Aminoff and Simon, Suggested Readings). After thorough investigation no cause could be found in 15% of patients. Drugs, tumors, trauma, and cerebrovascular disease all contributed to the onset of status epilepticus in some patients. An appropriate workup for status epilepticus includes a CT scan and then a lumbar puncture. Many patients have fever following their convulsions, most will have leukocytosis in the peripheral blood, and many, when studied with lumbar puncture, will have a CSF pleocytosis with a predominance of polymorphonuclear leukocytes. The presence of fever and CSF pleocytosis does not usually indicate infection, but coverage with broad-spectrum antibiotics is necessary until culture results are returned. In a patient with a prior seizure history a repeat CT scan is not necessary unless there is a history of trauma. If fever is present, a lumbar puncture and metabolic studies are indicated.

Seizure Control

More often the physician treating seizures is confronted with a patient who had a seizure (or allegedly had a seizure) but is no longer having them. In this situation the physician has more leisure to consider possible etiologies and to weigh treatment plans.

Differential Diagnosis. The examiner must consider the possibility that what he or she observed or was observed by others was not a seizure. Episodes of *syncope* can look very much like seizures, and there are no absolute criteria by which to distinguish the two entities. However, the presence of a remembered aura of any sensory type, urinary incontinence, head turning, or staring, and postevent confusion all suggest a convulsion. Episodic focal dysfunction with a sensory or motor ''march'' is seen with transient ischemic events and migraine as well as with seizures. True vertigo is unlikely to be a seizure manifestation. One should also be aware that the variety of frontal and temporal lobe seizures with partial complex symptomatology is large and that the autonomic manifestations of partial complex seizures can stimulate anxiety attacks, cardiac events (even with accompanying EEG changes), or gastrointestinal disorders. Sleep paralysis and narcolepsy or cataplexy can be misconstrued as seizure phenomena, but a careful history minimizes this possibility. Pseudoseizures have many appearances, but it must be remembered that some patients with hysterical seizures can also have organic seizures.

Workup. The *history* of seizure should include description of (*a*) aura (any sensory modality such as olfaction or vision, déjà vu, palpitations); (*b*) focal motor or sensory onset; (*c*) duration and lateralization of tonic-clonic convulsions; (*d*) witnessed head trauma; (*e*) prior, or family history of seizures; and (*f*) drug use. The immediate *postical examination* may give a clue to the focal onset of a secondarily generalized seizure. A unilateral Babinski reflex may be the only clue suggesting the origin of the convulsion. The physician should also look for evidence of extracranial pathologic processes, such as hyperthermia or decreased temperature, anoxic damage, drug use, or metabolic disorders.

Though imperfect, the phenotype of the seizure, as witnessed or remembered, gives all important diagnostic information determining the workup, the expected diagnostic yield, prognosis, and therapy. Table 15.4 outlines a classification of seizures, EEG findings, etiology, prognosis, and drugs of choice. A first seizure requires different diagnostic considerations and workup from a recurrent seizure in a previously controlled seizure patient. A focal seizure raises different considerations from a generalized one. A rough idea of seizure etiology by age is given in Table 15.5. At no time in life is a general convulsion consistent primarily with a brain tumor, but a new onset of seizures in an adult is usually symptomatic of an underlying problem other than idiopathic epilepsy.

The *CT scan* is recommended for any patient with a first seizure. However, several studies have questioned this routine policy. In one series of 148 patients, a structural lesion was found in 37% of patients, including 15% of those with nonfocal findings on physical examination. Another study found abnormal CT scans in 47% of patients with none of these patients between the ages of 16 and 30. Of patients with a normal physical examination and a normal EEG, only 12% had a structural CT abnormality and, again, none was in the young adult age group. In patients over age 60 the diagnostic yield of CT scanning increased, revealing stroke or hemorrhage in some patients. A reasonable standard of care dictates a CT scan without and then with contrast (after ''loading'' with anticonvulsants) in any patient over age 30. For those between 16 and 30 years of age in whom the examination and EEG are normal, CT may show an abnormality (e.g., atrophy) but it is unlikely to provide information essential to patient care. Irrespective of seizure type, if the physical examination is abnormal, a CT is not only useful but mandatory. A repeat CT scan in an adult over age 30 should be arranged 4 to 6 months after the original scan, even if the EEG and physical examination are normal, since some of the patients may be harboring a slowly growing malignancy.

The *electroencephalogram* (EEG) remains an im-

Table 15.4.
Types of Seizures

Type	EEG	Etiology	Prognosis	Drugs of Choice
I. *Primary generalized*				
Tonic-clonic (grand mal)	Normal 20% Nonspecific 40% Localizing 40%	Cause found in 15–20%	Age-related overall, 25% seizure-free 5 yr off medication	Phenytoin Carbamazepine Valproate
Tonic or clonic				Same
Absence (petit mal)	Abnormal, 80% 3/sec spike and wave	?autosomal dominant with age-related penetrance	Absences stop by age 20 in 50%, but many continue to have grand mal	Ethosuximide Valproate Clonazepam
Atypical absence	2–4 Hz during attack; polyspikes interictally[b]		May have generalized seizures as well or myoclonic seizure	Valproate/ ethosuximide Clonazepam Trimethadione
Myoclonic	Frontal or frontotemporal high voltage bursts	Uremia/hepatic/ CJ disease[a]	Disease-related	Valproate Clonazepam ?carbamazepine
II. *Partial or focal*				
Simple (motor, sensory, visual)	Focally abnormal in 66%	Increasing in CT era, 40% roughly divided trauma, tumor, vascular	Related to etiology, overall more difficult to control than generalized	Phenytoin Carbamazepine Clonazepam
Complex partial (psychomotor/TLE ± loss of consciousness[c]	Awake abnormal 50% Asleep abnormal 80%	Cause defined in ~ 50%: trauma, neoplasm, grand mal evolution	Psychoses: 30% without family history of seizure, 17% with family history	Phentytoin or carbamazepine and phenobarbital or primidone
Secondary generalized, partial seizures		*Beware* the history: the initial focal event may have been missed!		Carbamazepine or phenytoin Valproate/ phenobarbital

[a] CJ disease, Creutzfeldt-Jakob disease.
[b] Hz, unit of frequency = one cycle per second.
[c] TLE, temporal lobe epilepsy.

portant diagnostic tool in epilepsy. The timing of this test depends on the situation. An EEG should be done as soon as possible, if not actually during a spell when the diagnosis is still in question. It should be done expeditiously (i.e., 1 week) during the evaluation of a clear-cut seizure for prognostic, therapeutic (absence versus partial complex), and legal implications. A normal EEG may help the physician decide about the likelihood of seizure recurrence. The EEG should be done at least 2 to 3 weeks after the seizure in situations in which drugs are implicated. If the EEG is abnormal at this point, anticonvulsants may be continued, but if it is now normal, no further drug therapy is indicated if abstention from the abused substance can be assured.

A *lumbar puncture* is of limited value for the emergency evaluation of seizures (except for status epilepticus). In a series of 100 consecutive patients in the emergency department of the Massachusetts General Hospital with a first seizure, no patient was diagnosed by the findings on the lumbar puncture (Kaminski M, Beal M, unpublished data). Fever or prolonged convulsions do mandate CSF examination.

A *metabolic screen* is appropriate in all patients with a seizure. Many patients with a structural cause for the seizure have a concurrent metabolic problem and many with solely a metabolic problem, particularly hypoglycemia, have focal convulsions.

Therapy. A major question in emergency departments involves the decision to hospitalize a patient who has had a seizure but is now stable. Since

Table 15.5.
Etiology of Seizures by Age

Infancy (0–2)	Birth injury, malformation, infection, metabolic (sugar, calcium, pyridoxine deficiency)
Childhood (2–12)	Idiopathic, infection, trauma, febrile
Adolescence (12–18)	Idiopathic, trauma, drug, arteriovenous malformation
Early adult (18–35)	Idiopathic, trauma, drug, neoplasm
Middle age (35–60)	Neoplasm, trauma, metabolic, drug, vascular
Late life (> 60)	Vascular, neoplasm, trauma

one cannot know what the likelihood of seizure recurrence will be and since it is sometimes impractical to obtain a CT scan in the emergency department, hospitalization for all the initial workup, a 24-hour requirement, is ideal. If the patient is to be sent home, he or she should be given some anticonvulsant therapy parenterally and should be observed for several hours following the convulsion, or until metabolic studies have returned, before discharge.

Since the patient is not experiencing seizures, the physician can decide how fast to start medication and may even decide that treatment is not mandatory. Statistics about the likelihood of recurrent seizures in adults with a first convulsion have been provided by Hauser (see Suggested Readings). Only 27% of patients with a first seizure had recurrent convulsions when followed for 3 years either on or off medication. However, if the EEG shows generalized spike and slow wave activity, if a sibling has a seizure disorder, or if there is a history of prior neurological derangement, the incidence of recurrent seizures rises to 34%. In the absence of all risk factors, seizure recurrence is only 17%. However, since the likelihood of recurrent convulsion cannot be predicted from the data available in the emergency department, it is standard practice to give a patient anticonvulsants for the moment and to assure neurologic follow-up or provide admission for workup. The exception to this rule is a patient known to be having seizures from alcohol withdrawal. No medication is generally required in this situation.

An oral loading dose of medication may suffice for a patient who is not actively experiencing seizures. An appropriate oral schedule for phenytoin gives the patient 1000–1200 mg of the drug in the first 12 hours of treatment. Thus, 300 mg could be given every 4 hours for four doses. The patient then begins a daily adult dose of 300 mg/day. Another applicable schedule, particularly if the patient is being discharged, involves one-half of the first gram of phenytoin by vein at 100 mg every 5 minutes and then completion of the loading with oral phenytoin.

For the patient with a known seizure disorder, it is important to obtain a history about medication compliance or the addition of another mediation that might alter anticonvulsant levels. Drugs known to increase phenytoin levels include coumadin, isoniazid, disulfiram, chloramphenicol, chlorpromazine, and alcohol ingested acutely. Drugs which decrease phenytoin concentrations include valproic acid, folic acid, antihistamines, and carbamazepine. Phenytoin levels usually fall in the second trimester of pregnancy. Phenytoin also may cause inhibition of its own biotransformation so that a previously therapeutic dose becomes excessive. Blood should be

Table 15.6.
Anticonvulsant Drug Doses and Metabolism

Drug	Initial Level Check after Loading	Therapeutic Level	Adjustment Dose[a]	$T_{1/2}$	Time to Steady State
	days	*µg/ml*	*mg*	*hr*	*days*
Phenytoin (Dilantin)	8–10	5–20	100 qod	10–36	5–9
Phenobarbital (Luminal)	14–21	15–50	30 qd	46–136	14–21
Primidone (Mysoline)	7–10[b]	5–11 primidone 10–30 phenobarbital	125 qd	6–18	4–7
Carbamazepine (Tegretol)	5	4–12	100–200 qd	14–27	3–4
Valproic acid (Depakene)	5	50–100	250 qd	6–15	2–4

[a] Additional amount of drug to be given on a daily or every other day basis to boost a subtherapeutic level into the correct range.
[b] If patient has just started primidone, primidone level will be in steady state level before phenobarbital level.

Table 15.7.
Commonly Abused Drugs Associated with Seizures[a]

Drug	Overdose Seizure	Withdrawal Seizure	Dose Required to Provoke Seizure
			per day
Alcohol	−	+	Depends on prior drinking or underlying epilepsy
Meperidine (Demerol)	+	+	1 gm[b] 2–3 gm[c]
Propoxyphene (Darvon)	+	+	Variable
Pentazocine (Talwin)	−	+	Variable; may precipitate withdrawal from other opiates with as little as 100 mg
Barbiturates	−	+	600 mg/day (short acting)
Meprobamate (Miltown)	−	+	1.2 g/day
Chlordiazepoxide (Librium), diazepam (Valium)	−	+	Unknown; may have 7–8-day latency
Phenothiazines, haloperidol (Haldol)	+	−	Variable
Cocaine	+	−	May be idiosyncratic, usually with intravenous abuse

[a] −, does not occur; +, occurs
[b] Overdose seizure.
[c] Withdrawal seizure.

drawn in all cases for anticonvulsant levels and sent for stat determination. Remember that alcohol and infection are the next offenders in the exacerbation of a previously well-controlled seizure disorder. If the anticonvulsant level is not therapeutic, the physician may give the patient about double the usual daily dose of medication orally or parenterally. If the levels are adequate and no exacerbating metabolic or infectious feature can be found, the physician should consider adding a second medication. In general, it is preferable to increase one anticonvulsant into the high therapeutic range rather than adding a new medication. Thus, if the phenytoin level is at a midtherapeutic level of 13 μgm%, it is preferable to increase the phenytoin level to 18–20 μgm% than to start immediately on a new medicine. If a new medication is added, it should be remembered that anticonvulsants do not follow strict first-order kinetics, that they influence each other's levels, and that the time to steady state is five plasma half-lives. These considerations are summarized for the commonly used adult anticonvulsants in Table 15.6. The correct adjustment doses per day and the time at which the physician must arrange for the patient to return for a repeat level check are also given. Follow-up is extremely important, because anticonvulsant changes may affect the proper doses of many other medications, prominent among them coumadin.

Drug-related Seizures. Drugs are common causes of seizures. Table 15.7 summarizes the commonly abused drugs associated with convulsions either in overdose or withdrawal. Substances less likely to be associated with abuse but capable of causing seizures in therapeutic doses include penicillin, aqueous iodinated contrast agents, anticholinergics (physostigmine), lidocaine, sympathomimetics (amphetamines, ephedrine, terbutaline), isoniazid, methotrexate, methylxanthines, baclofen, lithium, salicylates, nalidixic acid, and metronidazole. However, among the common precipitants of seizures are the tricyclic antidepressants and hypoglycemic agents. Drug-induced seizures accounted for 1.7% of seizures during a 10-year period in the study by Messing (see Suggested Readings). Forty-five percent of these patients had single seizures, 40% suffered multiple convulsions, and 15% had status epilepticus. Generalized seizures were most common. Antidotes and agents that increase drug elimination may be added to anticonvulsants in the treatment of drug-induced seizures. Pyridoxine reduces the severity of isoniazid-induced convulsions. Physostigmine reverses the neurologic manifestations of tricyclic antidepressant toxicity, but can also cause asystole, hypotension, and convulsions. Bicarbonate is useful in promoting urinary excretion of tricyclic antidepressants and phenobarbital, while acidification of urine increases phencyclidine elimination. Mortality correlates with the combined cardiovascular toxicity of the offending drugs, anticonvulsants, and antidotes rather than with the number or duration of seizures. Treatment of blood pressure fluctuations and cardiac arrhythmias is of prime importance in assuring a favorable outcome.

Headache and Facial Pains

Headache and pains in the face are among the more commonly evaluated emergency department complaints. It is the objective of the emergency physician to sort out ominous headaches from the more common ones that require only symptomatic treatment and reassurance.

History

The headache history should include age at onset, location and radiation of type of pain (throbbing, stabbing, steady, aching, tight), severity, and duration. The time of buildup of pain to maximal intensity, first warning, aura, course of pain, and associated symptoms (nausea, scotomas, strange odors, stiff neck, confusion, parasthesias, faintness, vertigo) are additional important features. Prior headaches and their frequency, precipitating factors (menses, pregnancy, sound, odor, foods, position), ameliorating factors (rest, compression of temples, darkness), and similarity of the current headache to previous ones give the physician an idea about the chronicity of the complaint. Family history (headache, seizures, psychiatric problems) and social history contribute to a judgment about the urgency of the current headache. At this point in the history, the physician should have a good idea of the type of headache being presented and probably will be able to classify the problem. A standard classification of headaches is given in Table 15.8.

The *warning signs* for serious intracranial pathology include (*a*) headaches of new onset in a patient not previously prone to such problems; (*b*) sudden, explosive onset (possible subarachnoid or intracerebral hemorrhage), focal accompanying signs (tumor, stroke), scalp sensitivity in an elderly person (temporal arteritis), and fever with or without nuchal rigidity (meningitis, encephalitis). These types of headaches will require emergency evaluation with a CT scan and possibly with a lumbar puncture. However, as summarized in Table 15.9, there is considerable symptom overlap and both "benign" and "ominous" causes of headache can present with many of the same symptoms.

Vascular Headaches

Migraine Headache. Migrane headache is the classic example of a headache defined by prior history, family history, and temporal and qualitative characteristics of the pain and its accompanying phenomena. A prodrome may begin minutes to days before the actual onset of the pain and can be quite specific with scintillating scotomata or sensory phenomena on one side of the body or can be nonspecific with emotional alterations, malaise, nausea, hunger, or thirst. It is theorized that vasospasm and ischemia of branches of the intracranial arteries cause the aura and that vasodilatation is responsible for the subsequent throbbing, initially often lateralized headache. Throbbing may be improved by

Table 15.8.
Classification of Headache

I. Vascular
  A. Migrainous
    1. Common
    2. Classic
    3. Complicated
      a. Hemiplegic
      b. Basilar
      c. Ophthalmoplegic
      d. Retinal
    4. Cluster
  B. Nonmigrainous
    1. Hypertension
    2. "Hangover"
    3. Hypoglycemia
    4. Fever
    5. Hypoxia
    6. Postconvulsive
    7. Posttraumatic
    8. Vasodilating drugs
    9. Exertional
    10. Benign orgasmic cephalgia
II. Muscle contraction (tension)
III. Combined vascular and muscle contraction
IV. Traction
  A. Space-occupying lesions
    1. Tumor
    2. Hematoma
    3. Abscess
  B. Pseudotumor cerebri
  C. Postconcussive
  D. Post lumbar puncture
  E. Post shunt
V. Inflamatory
  A. Meningitis
  B. Arteritis
  C. Subarachnoid hemorrhage
VI. Cranial neuralgias
  A. Trigeminal
  B. Glossopharyngeal
VII. Diseases of other cranial structures
  A. Eyes
  B. Teeth
  C. Ears
  D. Sinuses
  E. Temporomandibular joint
  F. Cervical spine

Table 15.9.
Common Symptoms, Signs, and Causes of Headache

Symptoms and Signs	Benign Causes	Serious Causes
Onset after age 55	Temporal arteritis Depression	Tumor Cerebrovascular disease
Sudden, severe pain	Migraine	Subarachnoid hemorrhage Meningitis/encephalitis
Morning headache	Hypertension Migraine	Tumor
Nocturnal headache	Cluster	Tumor
Paroxysmal cough or exertional headache	Exertional headache	Posterior fossa tumor Hydrocephalus
Paroxysmal positional headache	Sinusitis	Obstructive hydrocephalus
Photophobia	Migraine	Meningitis/encephalitis Subarachnoid hemorrage
Nausea and/or vomiting	Migraine	Tumor Raised intracranial pressure
Nuchal rigidity	Muscle contraction Migraine	Meningitis Subarachnoid hemorrhage
Oculomotor nerve palsy	Ophthalmoplegic migraine Diabetes	Aneurysm Tumor
Scalp sensitivity	Muscle contraction Migraine	Temporal arteritis
Horner's syndrome	Cluster headache Paroxysmal hemicrania	Carotid artery dissection Tolosa-Hunt syndrome Cerebral metastases due to lung cancer[a]

[a] *The Horner's syndrome in this instance would be due to apical lung involvement by tumor.*

direct digital compression of the painful area or by pressure on the ipsilateral common carotid artery. In older patients the pain component of the migraine may be less severe, leaving only the prodrome that must be distinguished from transient ischemic events or from seizure activity. The most frequently used prophylactic medications, β blockers, tricyclic antidepressants, and methysergide, are not appropriate for treatment of the acute attack. Ergotamine compounds, administered rectally, intramuscularly, sublingually, and orally, can abort the painful part of the episode if they are given during the aura, but once the pain is developed they are not useful. It is reasonable to consider parenteral opiate analgesics coupled with antiemetics, such as phenergan, to break the acute attack. Some 80% of patients with migraine have the so-called common variant and do not experience any clearcut focal aura prior to the development of the headache. This type of headache may be difficult to distinguish from a muscle contraction headache, though the emergency treatment of the two will be the same.

Cluster Headache. Cluster headache is another recurring headache with a pathognomonic time and quality profile. The patient is more likely to be male and the peak age of onset is in the mid-30s. The attacks tend to occur at the same time of the year and go on for several weeks, typically occurring at night. Each attack lasts between 30 and 90 minutes and is invariably on the same side of the face during a particular cluster. The patient describes intense retroorbital or frontal pain accompanied by lacrimation or rhinorrhea sometimes with an associated transient Horner's syndrome. Treatment of the acute episode is similar to the treatment for a migraine headache with pain control by opiates and, for those attacks occurring exclusively or predominantly at night, oral ergotamine at bedtime. β blockers and calcium channel blockers have been less successful for prophylactic use with this type of vascular headache than with migraine headache, and methysergide maleate must frequently be used. The usual daily adult dose of this medicine is 2 mg three times a day. It should not be given for more than 3 months at a time lest the patient incur the risk of retroperitoneal fibrosis.

Muscle Contraction Headache

Muscle contraction headache, also called *tension headache,* results from sustained contraction of the deep neck muscles and muscles of mastication. Such muscle spasm often reflects no serious intracranial pathology, but may be a response to a primary organic pain of cerebral (tumor, trauma) or cervical origin (tumor, spondylosis). The pain is constant and the muscle spasm is often palpable. The head pain may be described as constrictive. When no primary cause can be discovered, the symptom itself can be treated with analgesics and muscle relaxants, sometimes with the addition of psychotropic drugs, or longer range planning for biofeedback or psychologic counselling to address contributing psychosocial causes.

Headache Due to Intracranial Space-occupying Lesions

This headache results from direct pressure, traction, or displacement of pain-sensitive structures on the surface of the brain, the blood vessels at the base of the brain, the falx, the tentorium, and/or the venous sinuses. Headache from supratentorial structures is usually referred to the side of the head on which the lesion lies. The headache is usually steady, possibly worse at night and worse with movement of the head. A tumor below the tentorium is more likely to cause pain in the occiput or in the neck and often is aggravated when the patient lies down.

Toxic-Metabolic Headaches

The majority of toxic-metabolic headaches, or headaches due to infection, metabolic derangement, or medications, resemble vascular headaches with pulsatile throbbing made worse by lying down. Foods containing monosodium glutamate, tyramine, or nitrates may be the culprits. Alcohol consumption on the previous day may contribute. Withdrawal from a vasoconstrictor, such as caffeine, can cause rebound vascular headache. Hypoxia and hypercapnia are both potent cerebral vasodilating stimuli; the latter may play a role in exertional or postcoital headaches. The headaches accompanying fever and infection may be caused by released compounds similar to those implicated in the inflammatory process accompanying migraine. Analgesics are not very effective, and a thorough search for the underlying etiology is in order. Fever accompanying headache or significant nuchal rigidity in the absence of any other signs or symptoms are indications for a lumbar puncture (with a preceding CT scan if there is reason to suspect an intracranial mass lesion).

Headache is often a prominent feature of encephalitis or meningitis. Therefore, these two conditions will be covered in this section.

Encephalitis. Encephalitis is most frequently viral. Fever and meningeal irritation are commonly present. Alteration in mental status, usually with delirium and without focal cognitive deficit, distinguishes encephalopathic conditions from those with just meningeal alteration. The most common nonepidemic etiologic agent for encephalitis is herpes simplex virus. The medial temporal lobe is a common site of infection. The olfactory apparatus is another preferred site of the necrotizing process that occurs with this virus. The patient may exhibit disordered behavior with acute psychosis. Cerebral edema can be severe and the CT scan may show these changes quite early in one temporal lobe. The EEG is always abnormal, with diffuse, sharp slowing over the affected hemisphere. The CSF may show both red and white blood cells. The antiviral agent adenine arabinoside (Vidarabine) is effective in the treatment of herpes simplex encephalitis (15 mg/kg/day intravenously for 10 days). Since this is the one commonly occurring form of encephalitis for which there is specific treatment, early use of CT scanning and consideration of brain biopsy along with vigorous treatment of cerebral edema (see "Cerebral Tumors" for use of mannitol and corticosteroids) is appropriate in any patient presenting with symptoms suggesting encephalitis. Emergency neurosurgical and infectious disease consultations should be sought. Intravenous phenytoin is recommended to prevent seizures. Fluid restriction should be strictly maintained to help combat cerebral edema.

Encephalitis may accompany almost all common viral diseases. Some agents, such as the virus that causes infectious mononucleosis, typically produce mild illness, while others, such as that responsible for eastern equine encephalitis, cause devastating disease. Most often, the precise etiologic agent is not recovered, but samples of CSF, blood, throat washings, and stool should be collected in the emergency department for viral studies.

Meningitis. Bacterial meningitis is discussed in Chapter 11. A CSF pleocytosis with moderate elevations of CSF pressure may be found in many viral meningitides. In the spring and summer, many cases of meningitis occur due to the enteroviruses. Typically, the patient has a severe headache without focal neurologic findings. The lumbar puncture is done because of the new onset headache and the worsening of headache when the patient is recumbant. The CSF shows five to several hundred white blood cells, predominantly lymphyocytes. If the process is a viral meningitis, other than herpes simplex, there is no specific therapy except pain medication for the headache. However, other etiologies for meningitis must be excluded. These include infective endocarditis, Lyme disease, cryptococcal meningitis, mycobacterial meningitis, and chemical meningitis. Thus, if the epidemiologic setting suggests some process more ominous than a viral meningitis or if the peripheral white blood cell count is elevated, it is appropriate to admit the patient for observation and to prescribe antibiotics for the 24-hour period required for culture results to be reported.

Post Lumbar Puncture Headache

Headache following a lumbar puncture begins within hours of the spinal tap or may be delayed by several days. Once developed, it can persist for several weeks. It is usually intense and throbbing, referred to the occiput and down the neck and back, and made much worse with standing. Since it is a low pressure headache caused by CSF leakage from the previous puncture site, it should be much better, if not entirely relieved, when the patient lies down. Augmented fluid intake, bed rest, and analgesics usually solve the problem, though the headache may recur after the patient has been upright for several hours even weeks after the lumbar puncture.

Cranial Arteritis

Cranial arteritis is an inflammatory process of the cerebral arteries usually occurring in patients over the age of 60 and sometimes accompanied by the diffuse myalgias and arthralgias characteristic of polymyalgia rheumatica. The involved blood vessels can be palpable and tender, and the whole scalp can be sensitive to touch. Pain is described as burning. An erythrocyte sedimentation rate is the diagnostic test and should be obtained in all middle-aged and elderly patients with new onset headache regardless of the precise description of symptoms. Immediate treatment with corticosteroids (before confirmatory temporal artery biopsy) can eliminate the risk of blindness due to central retinal artery occlusion. If the erythrocyte sedimentation rate is greater than 50 mm/hr and there is no better explanation for the headache, it is wise to begin prednisone, 40 mg/day, and to make arrangements for urgent follow-up of the patient with plans for a temporal artery biopsy.

Ocular Headache

Inflammation of the cornea, conjunctiva, or eyelids, or raised intraocular pressure produces intense pain in the distribution of the first branch of the trigeminal nerve. Pain in this area should always be considered a possible manifestation of ocular disease (see Chapter 43). Pain on movement of the eye with decreased visual acuity in that eye suggests optic neuritis.

Trigeminal Neuralgia

Neuralgic pain is characteristically sudden, excruciating, electrical, and in the distribution of one or more divisions of the fifth cranial nerve. The pain lasts for only a few seconds, recurs frequently, or lasts up to several minutes. It is triggered by chewing, washing the face, brushing the teeth, or exposure to cold or hot substances. The irritable lesion may be in the nerve itself or in the gasserian gangloin or spinal nucleus. The typical age of onset is in the fifth decade, twice as common in females as in males. In the 20- to 30-year-old patient, the physician must consider multiple sclerosis. If the pain is typical of neuralgia and the examination discloses no motor or sensory localizing findings, it is reasonable to forego CT scanning and to treat symptomatically, usually with carbamazepine or phenytoin. However, dental and sinus problems should be excluded before the diagnosis of idiopathic trigeminal neuralgia is entertained. The more successful drug is carbamazepine, but its use requires a baseline assurance of normal complete blood cell count (CBC), platelets, and liver function tests followed by weekly CBC and platelet count for at least 6 weeks. The initial carbamazepine dose is 200 mg twice per day, though lower doses may be employed. Arrangements for follow-up of hematologic parameters and dose-response assessment should be made before the patient leaves the emergency department. If there is any atypical feature of the pain, if the patient has a sensory loss in the distribution of the trigeminal nerve, or if the pain is in the first division of the trigeminal nerve, further workup is indicated. A CT scan with particular attention to the posterior fossa is in order and, in patients with first division trigeminal pain, consideration should be given to the possibility of developing herpes zoster of the cornea.

Glossopharyngeal Neuralgia

Neuralgic pain in the distribution of the ninth cranial nerve produces discomfort in the jaw, neck, base of the throat, and ear. The pain has the same features as trigeminal neuralgia. This neuralgia is particularly prone to produce a reflex vagus-mediated bradycardia. The patient can thus present with a syncopal spell. Carbamazepine is an effective medication for this neuralgia as well as for the more common tic douloureux of the trigeminal nerve, but referral to an otolaryngologist is also mandatory to exclude pathology in the throat or neck.

Dizziness

History

Dizziness is a vague term that means many different things to different patients. It can be used to describe a condition arising from otologic, neurol-

Table 15.10.
Clinical Spectrum of Dizziness

- "I am dizzy"
  - Sensation of motion (vertigo) → Disturbances of vestibular function
    - Peripheral
      - Vestibular neuronitis
      - Labyrinthitis
      - Benign positional vertigo
      - Ménière's disease
      - Posttraumatic vertigo
    - Central
      - Brainstem ischemia/infarct
      - Posterior fossa tumors
      - Multiple sclerosis, etc.
  - Sensation of impending faint (syncope) → Cardiovascular disorders
    - Orthostatic hypotension (various causes)
    - Cardiac arrhythmias
    - Hypersensitive carotid sinus
    - "Vasovagal attacks," etc.
  - Dysequilibrium → Neurologic disorders
    - "Multiple sensory deficits"
    - Cerebellopontine angle or posterior fossa tumors
    - Cerebellar degeneration, etc.
  - Ill-defined lightheadedness other than vertigo, syncope, or dysequilibrium → Psychiatric disorders
    - Hyperventilation syndrome
    - Anxiety neurosis
    - Hysterical neurosis
    - Affective disorders, etc.

Table 15.11.
Nylen-Bárány Maneuver for Positional Nystagmus

	Peripheral (Vestibular) Disorder	Brainstem-Posterior Fossa Disorder
Latent period before onset of positional nystagmus	2–20 seconds	None
Duration of nystagmus	< 1 minute	> 1 minute
Fatigability	Nystagmus disappears with repetition of the maneuver	Nonfatiguing
Direction of nystagmus in one head position	One direction	May change direction in a given head position
Intensity of vertigo	Severe	Slight or none
Head position	A single vertical position	More than one position
Clinical examples	"Benign positional vertigo" Vestibular neuronitis	Acoustic neuroma Vertebrobasilar insufficiency Multiple sclerosis

ogic, metabolic, or psychiatric abnormalities. The physician's first task is to have the patient define what is meant by dizziness. Table 15.10 uses the patient's description to guide the examiner toward possible etiologies. In general, if the patient is experiencing true spinning dizziness, the physician is likely to be able to make a more specific anatomic diagnosis than if the patient reports vague unsteadiness. The examiner should take a detailed drug history looking, in particular, for drugs commonly associated with unsteadiness: anticonvulsants, sedatives, alcohol, quinine, quinidine, salicylates, and aminoglycoside antibiotics.

Examination

The examination of the patient with dizziness concentrates on definition of the locus for the patient's problem, and, if possible, on stimulation of the sensation. Orthostatic blood pressure and pulse are recorded, Valsalva's maneuver is tried, carotid sinus pressure is performed (after auscultation for carotid bruits) with recording of pulse changes, and hyperventilation is attempted for 3 minutes. If the patient complains of a presyncopal sensation, thorough cardiac evaluation is indicated. If there are complaints of positional dizziness, in addition to the maneuvers outlined below, the physician thinks of and looks for possible peripheral neuropathy, extrapyramidal disease, or cerebellar signs.

The presence or absence of spontaneous and positional nystagmus are recorded, tilting the patient's head straight back over the edge of an examining table for 30 seconds and repeating the maneuver (Bárány's test) with the right ear and then the left ear down. Table 15.11 indicates some of the features of this maneuver that differentiate "central" from "peripheral" causes of vertigo. Tests for speech discrimination and Weber and Rinne's tests are performed to screen for hearing disorders. The tympanic membranes are visualized to exclude infection.

Serious Causes of Dizziness

The majority of patients with dizziness have either benign, presumably viral, self-limited disorders of the labyrinth or are found eventually to have drug-related or "multiple sensory" abnormalities to explain the symptoms. However, sources of misdiagnosis in the emergency evaluation of dizziness arise from those conditions that have profound spinning vertigo as a major component and are therefore called vestibular neuronitis or labyrinthitis when, in fact, there are subtle neurologic abnormalities that have been overlooked. The most serious misdiagnosis is calling a brainstem or cerebellar infarction an episode of labyrinthitis. A posterior inferior cerebellar artery infarction can produce profound vertigo with only minimal ipsilateral ataxia or incoordination. On a day following an infarction there can be serious intracranial swelling leading to cerebellar tonsillar herniation. In an adult with profound vertigo and subtle incoordination on examination, CT is mandatory and a period of observation in hospital is wise. The CT should exclude a cerebellar hemorrhage immediately, but the signs of an ischemic cerebellar infarction may not be visible on the immediate CT. *The subtle signs of cerebellar hemorrhage or infarction include slight ataxia of the limb on the side to which the patient feels he or she is falling, a VIIth nerve (facial nerve) palsy, a diminished corneal reflex on that side, and asymmetric nystagmus.* Satisfactory outcome from surgical decompression is correlated with early intervention so CT scanning is advisable on the least suspicion.

Treatment

For the majority of patients with true vertigo on a peripheral basis, the etiology can remain unknown and, thus, the diagnosis of vestibular neuronitis is made. This is a disturbing, but benign, condition which, untreated, can correct itself or can respond to a number of medications. Useful drugs for the symptomatic treatment of vertigo include: meclizine (Bonine, Antivert), 25 mg three times per day; phenergan, 25 mg four times per day; scopolamine, 0.6 mg dermal patch; dimenhydrinate (dramamine), 50 mg four times per day; or benadryl, 50 mg up to four times per day by mouth or intramuscularly at the same intervals. The patient can be reassured that the symptoms are always worse at the beginning of the illness and should be counselled to avoid alcohol and to abstain from airplane travel until the symptoms have subsided.

Visual Symptoms

Field Defects

While the patient may be quite accurate about reporting sudden loss of vision in one eye (see Chapter 43 for vascular and ophthalmic causes of monocular visual loss as well as for papilledema and papillitis), binocular visual field problems may be less accurately characterized. The problem may have been present for some time before attracting the patient's attention. The patient may perceive a left homonymous hemianopsia, for example, as "loss of vision in the left eye" or be entirely unaware of the visual problem in such a situation because of associated parietal lobe dysfunction and because central vision is preserved. Bedside confrontation visual field testing as described earlier in this chapter reveals only the basic visual field defects, but the physician should get an adequate idea of the general locus of this problem as summarized in Figure 15.7.

General rules of defect localization in visual field problems are: (*a*) Monocular visual defects, whether whole field or partial (quadrant, altitudinal, or central scotoma), imply disease at the retina, retinal artery, or optic nerve; (*b*) bilateral whole visual field loss places the defect either in both optic nerves, retinal arteries or retinae (an unlikely simultaneous occurrence except in trauma or burn injuries), or in the occipital cortex; (*c*) bitemporal field cuts place the problem at the optic chiasm; (*d*) superior homonymous quadrant vision loss localizes the lesion to the opposite temporal lobe; and (*e*) a hemianopsia is of less specific localizing value than other defects. Hemianopsias can be due to lesions in the optic tract, optic radiations, or occipital cortex. The common stroke syndromes giving rise to hemianopsias involve the inferior division of the middle cerebral artery. In this situation associated parietal lobe sensory deficits are likely to be present. When the posterior cerebral artery is the locus of the pathology, the field defect may be the only neurologic deficit.

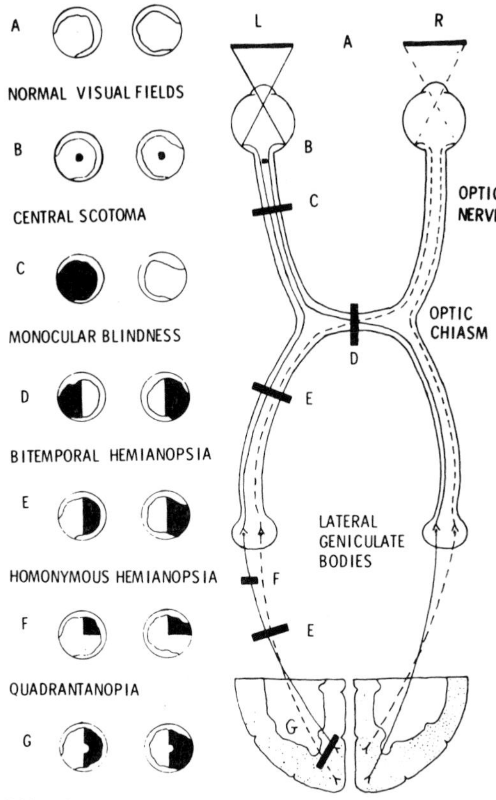

Figure 15.7. Field defects resulting from lesions at different sites in the optic pathways. (Reprinted by permission of the publisher from Pryse-Phillips W, Murray TJ. Field defects resulting from lesions at different sites in the optic pathways. *Essential Neurology,* 3rd ed. Copyright 1986 by Elsevier Science Publishing Co., Inc., New York.)

Diplopia

Diplopia refers to the subjective perception of two images when only one object is present. It occurs because the image falling on the retina of the abnormal eye lands away from the macula. Thus, the image is interpreted by the patient as lying in a position peripheral to the point of fixation. The patient may be unable to characterize the visual problem as diplopia and may simply call the problem "blurred vision," or may be experiencing some other symptom such as profound vertigo with associated nystagmus that so disorients him or her to express the symptom in visual terms.

There are several useful rules governing the relationship of the images; (*a*) displacement of the false image may be horizontal, vertical, or oblique, and the first question should be aimed at defining this relationship; (*b*) the separation of the images is greatest in the direction in which the weak muscle has its purest action; and (*c*) the false image (the image from the abnormal eye) is maximally displaced in the direction in which the weak muscle normally should move the eye.

Approach to the Diagnosis of Diplopia. The physician should remember that double vision may result from nerve, neuromuscular junction or muscle dysfunction, or from mechanical limitation of eye movement. Therefore, it should be assumed that the problem is within the central or peripheral nervous system. Several general rules are helpful in determining the muscle pair involved. (*a*) If the eye cannot move outwards, there is a lateral rectus muscle (VIth nerve) or an associated neuromuscular junction problem. If the maximal displacement of the images is on lateral gaze to the right, but no limitation of extraocular movement can be discerned by the examiner, then the pair to be considered is the left medial rectus and the right lateral rectus muscles. The next step is to determine which of the two images is displaced more laterally. This is made easier for the patient when a red glass is placed over the right eye. (*b*) If the eye, when deviated inwards, will not move down, there is a trochlear (IVth) nerve or muscle problem. The patient may develop a corrective head tilt to the opposite side from the defective eye. (*c*) All other defects in eye movements are due to oculomotor (IIIrd) nerve or associated muscle disease.

Table 15.12.
Causes of Oculomotor Palsies

Brainstem	Vascular disease (stroke)[a] Encephalitis Multiple sclerosis[a] Wernicke's encephalopathy
Base of skull	Basal meningitis Clinoid fracture, meningioma Nasopharyngeal carcinoma[a] Raised intracranial pressure, uncal or central herniation syndrome[a] Posterior communicating aneurysm[a] Concussion[a]
Cavernous sinus	Internal carotid artery aneurysm Carotid-cavernous fistula Extrasellar extension of pituitary tumor Meningioma Granulomatous inflammation (Tolosa-Hunt syndrome)
Orbit	Fracture of orbital wall Periostitis of superior orbital fissure Paget's disease Orbital mass lesions, edema (pseudotumor)
Neuromuscular disease	Hyperthyroidism Myasthenia gravis
Site uncertain	Cranial arteritis Ophthalmoplegic migraine Diabetic ischemic neuropathy Collagen vascular Diphtheria Botulism Guillain-Barré

[a] More common lesions.

IIIrd Nerve Lesions. Tumor, trauma, and vascular problems represent the three large categories of disease affecting the oculomotor nerve. Table 15.12 summarizes the causes and localizations of IIIrd nerve and associated muscle problems. The most common cause of a IIIrd nerve lesion is diabetes mellitus or atherosclerotic microvascular disease. It is important to distinguish a diabetic IIIrd nerve palsy from one due to an expanding aneurysm, usually of the posterior communicating artery. A diabetic IIIrd nerve palsy frequently begins with pain, but by the time the defect is maximally developed the pain is usually gone. The pupil is usually, but not always, spared in the diabetic IIIrd nerve palsy. When the time sequence of the pain and the defect is typical, the pupil is spared. When the patient is known to have diabetes, an arteriogram can usually be obviated, but otherwise any painful IIIrd nerve palsy must be considered due to aneurysm until proven otherwise by arteriography.

IVth Nerve Palsies. Nerve or muscle conditions involving the superior oblique muscle produce an oblique diplopia, partially or completely corrected by having the patient tilt the head to the opposite side. Such a palsy is common after traumatic head injury and neurosurgical procedures. It also may be due to the vascular or diabetic problems discussed in IIIrd nerve lesions. More ominous etiologies include cavernous sinus and superior orbital fissure tumors or inflammation, and posterior fossa tumors.

Abduction Deficits. Failure of one or both eyes to abduct can result from VIth nerve palsies, muscle or neuromuscular junction problems such as dysthyroidism and myasthenia gravis, orbital inflammation (pseudotumor), or orbital trauma with medial rectus entrapment. As is the case with all extraocular movement problems, decompensation of a congenital phoria or tropia can occur if the patient has received sedative-hypnotic drugs or if some other metabolic derangement interferes with visual focusing.

Table 15.13.
Causes of Abducens Palsies

Nonlocalizing
- Increased intracranial pressure
- Head trauma
- Lumbar puncture or spinal anesthesia
- "Vascular-hypertensive" ischemic neuropathy
- Diabetes
- Parainfectious (postviral, middle ear infections in children)
- Basal meningitis

Localizing
- Pontine syndromes (infarction, demyelination, tumor)
- Cerebellopontine angle lesions (acoustic neuroma, meningioma)
- Clivus lesions (nasopharyngeal carcinoma, clivus chordoma)
- Middle fossa disorders (tumor, inflammation of petrous bone)
- Cavernous sinus or superior orbital fissure (tumor, inflammation, aneurysm)
- Carotid-cavernous or dural arteriovenous fistula

When the abduction problem is due to an abducens (VIth) nerve palsy, a wide range of localizing and nonlocalizing abnormalities can be at fault. These are summarized in Table 15.13. The common cause of a VIth nerve palsy is the diabetic or vascular problem. Though the nerve may be severely affected, recovery to normal or nearly normal is the rule within 6–8 weeks. More serious causes of localizing VIth nerve palsies include pontine stroke or demyelination syndromes in which there are almost always associated neurologic signs and symptoms, cerebellopontine angle lesions, and clivus lesions, almost always due to tumor. The VIth nerve can be affected unilaterally or bilaterally by a number of processes not immediately anatomically related to it. Thus, increased intracranial pressure from tumor or pseudotumor may present with horizontal double vision due to VIth nerve dysfunction. Occasionally, the nerve is injured after head trauma and in some cases of meningitis the VIth nerve can be affected.

Workup of Diplopia. Remembering that metabolic and muscle problems can be present as well as nerve lesions, the physician should proceed with treatment for all immediately threatening possibilities while narrowing the differential diagnostic field and planning necessary studies. Thus, a Tensilon (edrophonium) test is indicated in all instances of pupil-sparing extraocular movement abnormalities, particularly when the defects are fluctuating or do not fit neatly into the territory of one extraocular nerve or muscle. The technique of Tensilon administration is fully discussed in this chapter in the section on myasthenia gravis. The double vision and/or ptosis can clear rapidly, coincident with the development of epigastric cramping and rhinorrhea or lacrimation. Severe coronary artery disease may be a relative contraindication to this procedure. Thiamine, 50 mg intravenously, is given, since Wernicke's encephalopathy may present with a combination of both abduction weakness and other eye movement deficits. This dose of thiamine is sufficient to correct both the extraocular movement abnormality and to prevent incipient Korsakoff's psychosis. A blood glucose level and erythrocyte sedimentation rate should be obtained in all patients with an isolated extraocular movement problem since cranial arteritis can also present with such a symptom. Skull series, once recommended with serial laminagraphy of the superior orbital fissure, cavernous sinus, and clivus have been replaced by CT scans. If the etiology of an isolated cranial nerve palsy is not apparent, an emergency CT scan should be performed. This should be done, as always, first without contrast and then with dye infusion. This can reveal an intracranial aneurysm. The painful IIIrd nerve palsy is then referred for arteriography. If the diagnosis remains unclear, ancillary studies, such as a full glucose tolerance test and studies of thyroid function are scheduled.

Painful Ophthalmoplegia Syndromes. Less common than isolated cranial neuropathies, the painful ophthalmoplegia syndromes involving multiple cranial nerve lesions present a different diagnostic spectrum. Etiologic processes in the orbit include contiguous sinusitis, mucormycosis or other fungal infections, inflammatory pseudotumor, and metastatic tumor. Superior orbital fissure or anterior cavernous sinus diseases include nonspecific granulomatous inflammation (Tolosa-Hunt), metastatic or nasopharyngeal tumor, herpes zoster, cavernous sinus thrombosis, and carotid-cavernous fistula. Parasellar region problems include pituitary adenoma, intracavernous aneurysm, tumors (including meningioma and chordoma), and petrositis (Gradenigo's syndrome). Diabetic ophthalmoplegias and cranial arteritis also produce simultaneous dysfunction of multiple cranial nerves. A contrast-enhanced CT scan is always indicated, followed by a lumbar puncture, in the presence of the constellation of these findings.

Ptosis. Ptosis or drooping of the upper eye lid can be partial or complete, unilateral or bilateral. There is a wide variation in the normal appearance of eyelids; asymmetry, if not different from the patient's usual appearance, is accepted as normal. The upper eyelid is kept elevated by the levator palpebrae superioris muscle (IIIrd nerve) and Mueller's muscle. Interference with sympathetic innervation results in partial ptosis. Table 15.14 outlines the causes of unilateral and bilateral ptosis. Horner's

Table 15.14.
Causes of Ptosis

I. Unilateral ptosis
    Voluntary suppression of diplopia
    Local abnormality of lid
    Horner's syndrome
    Gunn's phenomenon (jaw-winking)[a]
    IIIrd nerve lesion
    Ophthalmoplegic migraine
    Myasthenia gravis
II. Bilateral ptosis
    Normal variation
    Myopathies (ocular forms and myotonic dystrophy)
    Myasthenia gravis
    Tabes dorsalis
    Bilateral IIIrd nerve or sympathetic lesions
III. Causes of Horner's syndrome
    1st neuron
        Hypothalamic lesions
        IIIrd ventricle tumor
        Pituitary tumor
        Basal meningitis
        Brainstem or cervical cord disease (infarction, syrinx, tumor, multiple sclerosis)
    2nd neuron
        Cervical rib
        Pancoast tumor
        Aortic aneurysm
        Supraclavicular or cervical adenopathy
        Klumpke's paralysis
        Thyroid mass lesions
    3rd neuron
        Internal carotid artery occlusion, arteritis, dissection, or aneurysm
        Cavernous sinus lesion
        Paratrigeminal syndrome
        Orbital tumor or infection

[a] Actually due to a VIIth nerve lesion with faulty reinnervation.

syndrome, partial ptosis with miosis of the pupil and variable decrease in sweating on the ipsilateral face, is also covered in Table 15.14. In general, complete ptosis is more likely due to a IIIrd nerve lesion than to Horner's syndrome. Thus, complete ptosis is usually accompanied by pupillary and/or extraocular movement abnormalities.

ACUTE FOCAL NEUROLOGIC DEFICITS

Stroke

Definitions

Stroke is the sudden or rapid onset of a neurologic deficit lasting more than 24 hours due to one of several types of vascular diseases. A *transient ischemic attack* (TIA) is defined as the sudden onset of a neurologic deficit due to vascular disease, resolving within 24 hours. However, the advent of CT and MRI scanning has revealed a considerable overlap between the two entities. Thus, 16–19% of patients who have no residual neurologic deficit may have a radiographically visible defect. The term *cerebral infarction with transient signs* (CITS) defines this group. It is the tempo of the disorder that stamps the process as vascular. The deficit evolves over seconds to minutes in the case of hemorrhage and embolism, or over minutes to hours to 1 or 2 days in the case of a thrombotic stroke. Sudden focal neurologic deficit resulting from vascular disease must be differentiated from other sudden permanent or transient focal neurologic disturbances, such as those occurring with migraine, seizure, mass lesions, subdural hematoma, arteritides, venous occlusion, and local or peripheral diseases (e.g., Bell's palsy), radiculopathies due to herniated intervertebral discs or peripheral nerve disease, and peripheral vestibular disorders.

Types of Vascular Diseases

There are five general types of vascular conditions involving cerebral arterial pathology. Each has a characteristic clinical setting with associated risk factors, pattern of onset, findings on clinical examination and in the laboratory profile, and emergency treatment. The goal of the emergency physician is to define the deficit as a stroke, to characterize the type of stroke whether completed or evolving, to recognize the territory and pathophysiology involved, and to triage those patients who can be helped immediately by medical or surgical intervention while controlling blood pressure and other medical parameters in all stroke victims.

Large Artery Thrombosis. The most common type of vascular pathology in several large series of stroke patients, large artery thrombosis occurs in the clinical setting of hypertension, advanced age, heart disease, diabetes, and risk factors associated with atherosclerosis elsewhere. Specific risk factors for thrombotic stroke include polycythemia, the use of oral contraceptive agents, alcohol abuse, the postpartum period, sickle cell disease, ulcerative colitis, hypotension, collagen vascular diseases (e.g., arteritis), and trauma to extracranial vessels (e.g., arterial dissection).

The *onset* of stroke may be gradual or stuttering. TIAs occur in more than three-quarters of patients who proceed to have a completed infarction. A bruit may be heard over the affected carotid artery. Clinical syndromes reflect the distribution of arteries in the anterior circulation (see Fig. 15.8). Internal carotid syndromes include varying combinations of hemiparesis, hemisensory deficit, hemianopsia, aphasia (if on the dominant side), and cortical sensory dysfunction (inattention to double simultaneous stimulation, absent graphesthesia). Middle cerebral artery syndromes, similar to internal carotid artery disease, usually affect the face and arm more than the leg. With basilar artery thrombosis a constellation of quadriparesis, dizziness, internuclear ophthalmoplegia, bilateral blindness, dysphagia, and coma can be found in any combination. A particularly common posterior circulation stroke is the so-called lateral medullary syndrome due either to vertebral artery or posterior inferior cerebellar artery thrombosis. The patient experiences profound vertigo, hoarseness, dysphagia, and facial numbness and is found to have nystagmus as well as facial numbness, Horner's syndrome, and palatal paresis on one side with contralateral truncal and limb numbness. Laboratory evaluation initially shows no deficit on the CT scan, but an area of low density evolves between 12 and 24 hours after onset of the stroke. The EEG shows ipsilateral slow waves and an arteriogram shows occlusion, ulcer, or stenosis of the appropriate blood vessel.

Treatment of a maximal fixed deficit involves fluid restriction, mannitol for acutely evolving cerebral edema which peaks at 2–5 days from the stroke, gentle blood pressure reduction, and a decision about anticoagulation. For a maximal fixed deficit there is no role for urgent arteriography, and for very large edmatous strokes anticoagulation may be dangerous (see below under "Cerebral Embolism"). For less than maximal deficits, if the patient begins to improve, more urgent intervention with arteriography for carotid deficits can be considered. Some physicians advocate anticoagulation immediately for victims of the lateral medullary syndrome, since some of these patients progress to involve more of the vertebrobasilar territory. Acute anticoagulation with heparin followed by 6 months of anticoagulation with coumadin has been suggested, but there have been no controlled trials.

Lacunes. Another type of thrombotic arterial pathology involves the occlusion of small penetrating endarteries producing small deep infarctions in characteristic territories. This occurs almost always in the setting of hypertension. The onset is abrupt or fluctuating, often mimicking large vessel thrombosis. The syndromes are almost diagnostic of the process: pure motor hemiparesis (internal capsule), pure unilateral sensory loss (thalamus), ataxic hemiparesis (pons), and the multiple lacunar state with bilateral corticospinal signs, pseudobulbar affect, gait ataxia, and dementia. However, in recent years it has become clear that there are many other lacunar syndromes, many of which can involve both sensory and motor signs and, thus, can resemble large artery thrombosis. Except for the multiple lacunar state, lacunar disease should not involve any alteration in visual or cortical function. This fact helps to distinguish lacunes from large artery thromboses or cerebral embolism.

The CT scan can be normal even several days after the event, but the most recent generation of the CT scanning machines can show the small infarctions deep in subcortical territory. MRI has proved to be even more sensitive than CT in detecting multiple small lacunes. The EEG and CSF are normal. Angiography reveals no major stenoses. Treatment consists of reduction in blood pressure and the performance of tests to exclude large vessel thrombosis as a cause for the syndrome. Thus, in some instances it may be necessary to proceed to arteriography because what is eventually diagnosed as a lacunar syndrome looks like carotid artery thrombosis in evolution. There is no established role for anticoagulation in lacunar stroke.

Cerebral Embolism. Cerebral embolism occurs in several clinical settings, including atrial fibrillation due to valvular or ischemic heart disease, recent myocardial infarction, cardiomyopathy, calcific aortic stenosis, mitral valve prolapse, prosthetic valves, infective endocarditis, myxoma, congenital heart disease, ventricular aneurysm, tumor emboli or marantic endocarditis, or trauma (e.g., air or fat embolus). Embolism to the cerebral arteries from other atherosclerotic arteries or from the heart is the presumed pathogenesis when no clearcut embolic source can be identified. The onset

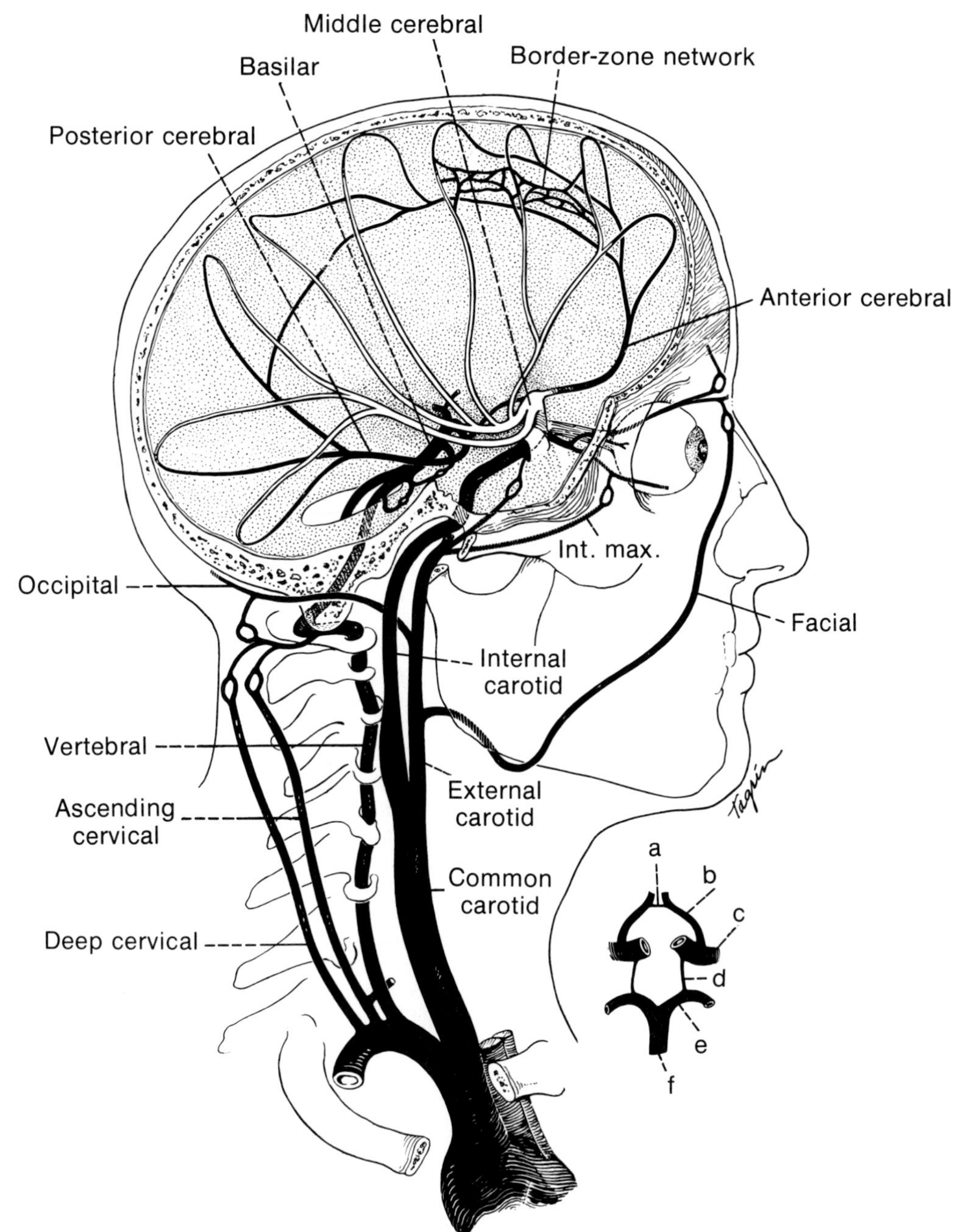

Figure 15.8. Arterial supply to the brain. Internal carotid artery gives rise to anterior cerebral and middle cerebral arteries, which supply most of the cerebral hemispheres. Internal carotid artery and all its branches are sometimes referred to as the "anterior circulation" of the brain. The "posterior circulation" consists of the intracranial branches of the two vertebral arteries, the midline basilar artery and its branches, and the posterior cerebral arteries arising from the "top" of the basilar. Anastomotic communications between major surface arterial territories occur via a border-zone network of vessels. In addition, the major cerebral arteries usually efficiently communicate, close to their origins, into a seven-sided polygon termed the circle of Willis (*inset, a,* anterior communicating artery; *b*, anterior cerebral artery; *c*, internal carotid artery; *d*, posterior communicating artery; *e*, posterior cerebral artery; *f*, basilar artery). (Courtesy of C. Miller Fisher, M.D., Massachusetts General Hospital.)

Table 15.15.
Common Syndromes of Cerebral Embolism

Location	Symptoms
Superior division, middle cerebral artery	Face and arm weakness Expressive dysphasia if on the dominant side
Inferior division, middle cerebral artery	Hemisensory deficit Hemianopsia Neglect of the opposite side to sensory testing Receptive aphasia if on the dominant side.
Posterior cerebral artery	Hemianopsia Memory loss and dysnomia if on the dominant side Movement disorder and sensory loss if proximal part of the posterior cerebral artery with involvement of thalamic penetrating branches
Anterior cerebral artery	Leg weakness

of cerebral embolic stroke is sudden without antecedent TIA (see Table 15.15 for common syndromes).

Infarction is visible on CT scan at 12 to 24 hours after the onset of the stroke. Hemorrhage into the infarction may be seen on subsequent scans. Arteriography reveals a branch artery occlusion if the procedure is performed early in the course of the disease, although this is not usually indicated in the emergency setting.

Treatment of cerebral embolic stroke first involves determination of the source of embolism. Blood cultures should be obtained, cardiac examination performed, and carotids auscultated. A more extensive search for arrhythmias with Holter monitoring or assessment of structural cardiac disease with echocardiography is beyond the scope of the emergency department investigation. *Anticoagulation* may be considered for patients in atrial fibrillation in whom the risk of recurrent stroke outweighs the risk of hemorrhage into the infarction. There are no absolutely convincing data on the risks versus benefits of acute anticoagulation for completed embolic stroke, but the following statistics can help to influence individual decisions. The recurrence rate of stroke for patients in atrial fibrillation with a valvular problem is 33% with up to 15% of second strokes occurring within 1 week after the first event. Hemorrhagic lesions large enough to appear on CT scan occur in only 2% of embolic strokes, but hemorrhage may be delayed for 24 to 48 hours following onset of the stroke. Retrospective studies suggest that the risk of converting a bland infarction to a hemorrhagic one is small. The group at higher risk for this complication consists of those patients with large, edematous infarctions and uncontrolled hypertension. Thus it is sound practice to heparinize those patients with a negative CT scan at 24 hours from the onset of the stroke in the setting of atrial fibrillation or valvular heart disease and a stable deficit. Indications for heparinization during the 1st day after the stroke, for subsequent coumadin, and for long-term anticoagulation in other groups of patients with embolic stroke remain less clear. It is generally established that all patients with mitral valve disease in atrial fibrillation should take coumadin, while it is also agreed that heparinization in the presence of infective endocarditis is unwise. The role of antiplatelet agents in the prevention of recurrent embolic stroke has never been studied.

Intracerebral Hemorrhage. Major cerebral hemorrhage can occur with uncontrolled hypertension, anticoagulation, congophilic angiopathy, coagulation abnormalities, or brain tumor. The onset is generally sudden with gradual worsening over minutes to hours, usually with nausea, vomiting, headache, and an altered level of consciousness. Prior to the availability of antihypertensive regimens, the typical syndromes reflecting the site of hemorrhage were: (*a*) putamen: hemiparesis; (*b*) thalamus: hemiparesis, hemisensory deficit, stupor; (*c*) pons: quadriparesis, loss of consciousness; and (*d*) cerebellum: headache, nausea, limb ataxia, and inability to walk. Small lobar hemorrhages may mimic embolic or lacunar infarctions. The CT scan reveals a high density area of blood in the affected territory. The CSF may be hemorrhagic if the hemorrhage has occurred near the ventricular or convexity surface. *Treatment* includes mannitol to reduce cerebral edema acutely and corticosteroids to continue the edema reduction effect for several days. Blood pressure should be controlled, and coagulation defects corrected. Emergency surgery may be considered for cerebellar hemorrhages when the patient is not yet stuporous, for some nondominant lobar and putamenal hemorrhages, and for more massive hemorrhages with acute obstructive hydrocephalus (ventriculostomy or shunting procedure). A substantial literature about the prognosis of cerebral hemorrhages based on the size and location of the initial lesion as defined on CT scan has developed. Emergency decision-making could be aided by familiarity with some of these data (see Suggested Readings).

Subarachnoid Hemorrhage. Sudden headache with or without immediate altered consciousness or neurologic deficit raises the specter of hemorrhage into the subarachnoid space from either an intracranial aneurysm or from an arteriovenous malformation. This occurs in a younger age group than other vascular syndromes. There may be a family history of aneurysm or of sudden death. Cocaine snorting is a recent epidemiologic feature in some young victims of subarachnoid hemorrhage. The onset is abrupt without TIA. Headache, nausea, and vomiting are nearly always present. Syncope may occur. The patient may then become more alert or may remain stuporous. A partial IIIrd nerve palsy involving the pupil raises suspicion of a posterior communicating aneurysm. Gait disorder and abulia or memory disturbance may indicate an aneurysm of the anterior communicating artery. Middle cerebral artery or internal carotid artery aneurysms may produce hemiplegia. The CT scan shows blood in the subarachnoid space. There can also be a parenchymal hematoma. The CSF is usually bloody and the pressure is elevated. The presence of blood in the basilar cisterns on CT scan has been correlated with increased risk for vasospasm with a worsening neurologic deficit several days following the hemorrhage.

Effective *treatment* of subarachnoid hemorrhage requires blood pressure control, mannitol, corticosteroids, sedation, and possibly the intravenous use of ϵ-aminocaproic acid (Amicar) to reduce the incidence of rebleeding. Until recently, arteriography was delayed for 1 or 2 weeks until the peak risk of vasospasm had passed, but recent surgical practice has tended toward early arteriography and clipping of the aneurysm in patients who are neurologically intact after the initial hemorrhage.

Comparison of Vascular Syndromes

The previous discussion shows that there are several types of arterial pathology responsible for strokes. However, clinical features alone do not always distinguish these types. Table 15.16 outlines some of the major characteristics of the five different types of cerebral arterial vascular diseases. Some generalizations can be emphasized. (*a*) Patients with lacunes and with large vessel thrombotic stroke have the same risk factors of age, hypertension, and coronary artery disease, the same incidence of prior stroke, and the same lack of atrial fibrillation and valvular heart disease. (*b*) The type of onset of stroke is not absolutely predictive of stroke mechanism, as stuttering onset occurred in one-third of all lacunes and a fluctuating deficit was equally common in lacunes and large vessel thromboses. (*c*) Atrial fibrillation is found in up to 15% of all patients with cerebral ischemic events. (*d*) Coma is almost never present with lacunes, emboli, or thrombotic stroke. (*e*) A surgically remediable lesion accounts for about 15% of all strokes.

Figure 15.9 outlines an overview of the approach to management of the stroke patient. The physician first should be sure that the problem is a stroke. Believing that vascular disease is one problem, the physician should ascertain whether the stroke is a TIA, or completed stroke, or a CITS. If it is a TIA, is it in the carotid or vertebrobasilar artery territory? If it is a stroke, in what area of the brain is it and is it still evolving? The physician should triage those stroke victims who can be helped immediately, sorting out those with hemorrhages, particularly in the cerebellum, and consulting neurosurgical colleagues promptly for these. The physician should

Table 15.16.
Comparison of Vascular Syndromes[a]

	Incidence of Findings in Type of Stroke (numbers of patients)				
	Thrombosis 34%	Lacune 19%	Embolism 31%	Hematoma 10%	Aneurysm/ Arteriovenous Malformation 6%
History of hypertension	55	75	40	72	19
Atrial fibrillation	8	5	34	6	2
Vomiting	10	5	4	51	47
Coma	4	0	0	24	24
Headache	21	5	20	52	95
Grossly bloody CSF	0	2	1	70	94
TIA	50	23	11	8	7
Stuttering onset	34	32	11	3	3
Smooth onset	13	20	5	63	14
Fluctuations	13	10	5	0	3

[a] From Mohr, JP et al. The Harvard Cooperative Stroke Registry: A prospective study. *Neurology*, 1978;28:754–762.

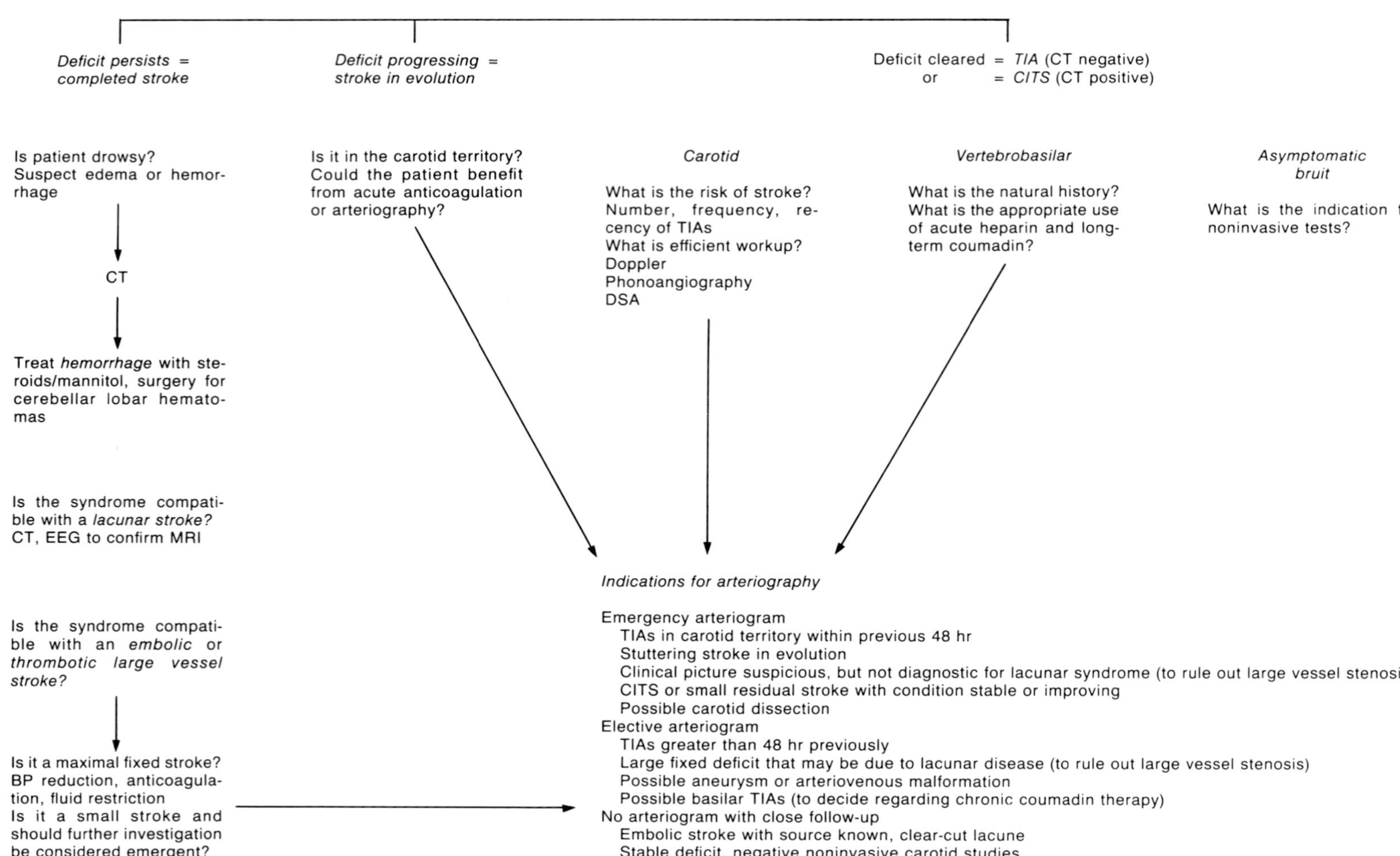

Figure 15.9. Overview of approach to stroke. *DSA,* digital subtraction angiography.

look for deficits that might be minimized by the findings of emergency arteriography. If he or she feels the stroke is clinically consistent with a lacune, confirmatory tests may be necessary. These include CT scanning, EEG, and even arteriography in some instances of ambiguous clinical findings.

Transient Ischemic Attacks

Transient ischemic attacks (TIAs) require separate consideration. TIAs related to impairment of the carotid circulation are characterized by sudden transient monocular blindness or transient hemispheric signs. Transient monocular blindness is defined as temporary visual loss in one eye, typically described as a "curtain descending" over the affected eye. Transient hemispheric attacks involve temporary face or arm numbness, weakness of face or arm, or dysphasia. Vertebrobasilar TIAs may present as sudden bilateral visual loss, bilateral weakness, numbness, dizziness, diplopia, dysarthria, transient global amnesia, drop attacks, loss of consciousness, or any combination of the above. It is rare for a vertebrobasilar TIA to consist solely of true vertigo, a symptom that in isolation bespeaks peripheral vestibular (labyrinthine) disease. The pathogenesis of the TIA is thought to be transient flow reduction through a stenotic area, plaque ulceration with embolism, or less commonly, a "steal" phenomenon. Unusual causes of TIAs (and some strokes) include fibromuscular dysplasia, chiropractic neck manipulation, Paget's disease, dissection of arteries following trauma, and radiation therapy to the neck.

The natural history of carotid TIAs involves a 5–8%/year incidence of stroke. Spontaneous cessation of attacks may occur, possibly coincident with ipsilateral carotid artery occlusion in as many as one-third of patients. The greatest risk for stroke may be in the first few months after onset of TIAs. Twenty-one percent occur in the first month and 50% of all strokes in the first year after onset of TIA. Age, hypertension, and cardiac disease all increase mortality with the leading cause of death myocardial infarction. In most studies, about 50% of patients with symptoms of carotid TIA had significant carotid stenosis. Positive arteriograms are more likely to be found in patients with transient monocular blindness (amaurosis fugax) than in those with hemispheric spells. The occurrence of both hemispheric attacks and amaurosis fugax correlates with an 80% likelihood of significant carotid stenosis. However, the incidence of major hemispheric stroke over a 7-year period in patients with "eye TIAs" was only 14%. Lightheadedness accompanying the spells or spells brought on by exertion tend to correlate strongly with bilateral severe carotid stenosis.

Thus, except for relatively uncommon features such as exertional precipitation of a spell or coincidence of amaurosis fugax with a hemispheric symptom, clinical features predicting progress to stroke with carotid TIA are imperfect. Such predictors are even more imprecise with vertebrobasilar TIAs. There are no adequately prospective controlled studies of anticoagulation versus surgery for carotid TIAs. The incidence of complications of emergency arteriography and surgery varies with radiographers and surgeons, but is probably no lower than a combined 3% in the best institutions. Faced with these statistics, the emergency physician evaluating a patient with carotid TIAs must decide on the urgency of confirming a stenotic carotid artery. Clinical examination for a bruit is imperfect; and the flow may be critically reduced without an audible bruit. Similarly, only about 50% of bruits represent significant carotid artery stenosis. Doppler examination of the carotids is available on an emergency basis in some hospitals, but does not differentiate total from nearly total carotid occlusion and will not always pick up an ulcerated plaque. Digital subtraction angiography (DSA) with intravenous contrast injection may provide adequate visualization of the carotid bifurcation, but does not offer an accurate estimate of intracranial collateral flow, and can have a higher incidence of complications than arteriography. These complications include dye reactions, precipitation of angina, and intimal dissection of the subclavain vein. Arteriography is the definitive procedure for the patient who has a carotid transient ischemic event and who is a candidate for a carotid endarterectomy, in a center in which the combined radiographic and surgical morbidity is less than 3%. The urgency of this procedure depends on several features which are summarized in Figure 15.9. Aspirin or coumadin may be offered to those patients who are not surgical candidates, but no definitive studies have compared these two medications. Patients with acutely fluctuating vertebrobasilar TIAs should be hospitalized for heparin therapy, placing the patient in the head-down position to maximize blood flow. Subsequent arteriography can be considered to define the pathologic anatomy and to help decide about chronic anticoagulation.

Asymptomatic Bruits

In the course of an emergency department evaluation, the physician may hear a bruit in an artery that is not the current source of the patient's symptoms. He or she then must decide how to advise the patient. The following section is designed to provide information relevant to that decision.

As many as 4% of patients over age 40 years will have an audible bruit in the neck without symptoms. Studies have tried to assess the risk of stroke and to offer management suggestions for these patients. Most investigators concur that the risk of stroke in the region of brain supplied by a vessel with a bruit is actually quite low. The most recent information comes from a study by Chambers (see Suggested Readings). Among 500 asymptomatic patients with cervical bruits followed prospectively by clinical and Doppler examination, 36 had stroke or TIA (7.2%), 51 had cardiac ischemic events (10%) and 45 died (9%). Neurologic outcome correlated best with the degree of carotid artery stenosis. At 1 year, patients with severe carotid artery stenosis, i.e., greater than 75% narrowing of carotid lumen, had an 18% incidence of cerebral ischemic events (TIA and/or stroke) and a 5% incidence of completed stroke. The incidence of stroke without a preceding TIA was only 3%. The severity of carotid artery stenosis, the presence of ischemic heart disease, and male sex were the best predictors of cerebral ischemic events. Most of the symptomatic patients (78%) presented with TIA. Invasive evaluation and carotid endarterectomy could therefore be deferred until the occurrence of such attacks. Most studies have concluded that there is no subgoup of patients identifiable for whom the risks associated with prophylactic carotid endarterectomy are justified. *Patients with newly discovered neck bruits should undergo noninvasive carotid evaluation to determine the site, extent, and severity of extracranial arterial disease.* If severe carotid artery stenosis is found, the patient should be educated about possible symptoms and asked to report any transient cerebral ischemic symptoms in order to facilitate early carotid angiography. In view of the very low risk of unheralded stroke, carotid endarterectomy is not justified in any group of asymptomatic patients.

Unusual Etiologies of Stroke

Venous Thrombosis. Cerebral venous thrombosis is much less commonly encountered as a cause of stroke than is arterial disease. It may follow parturition, or a consequence of infection of the middle ear or mastoids, or a concomitant of pseudotumor cerebri. It may accompany purulent meningitis or malignant infiltration of the central nervous system and tends to occur in all situations involving the superior sagittal sinus. The infarction is almost always hemorrhagic and occurs on the cortical surface. Seizures are common. Diagnosis of cerebral venous disease requires close observation of the venous phase of cerebral arteriography.

Low Cerebral Perfusion. A special type of ischemic damage can occur during systemic hypotension. Sustained low blood pressure during massive blood loss, surgical procedures, or cardiovascular arrest causes strokes limited to "watershed" or "border-zone" territories. The most common syndrome involves the watershed between middle cerebral artery and anterior and posterior cerebral artery branches. Weakness of the upper extremities is the most common feature of anterior hemispheric border-zone infarctions. Blindness or partial visual loss occurs with the posterior hemispheric syndrome. Prevention of further hypotension and administration of oxygen are the only indicated therapies.

Nonvascular Causes of Acute Focal Cerebral Disease. Acute focal cerebral disease encompasses a few nonvascular conditions. Perhaps the most common is an acute attack of *multiple sclerosis.* A history of this illness or of other characteristic transient episodes is often obtained, simplifying the emergency diagnostic workup. Acute optic neuritis, sudden weakness of one limb, sudden diplopia, ataxia, and dizziness are among the neurologic presentations of this illness, and cognitive functions can be impaired. Emergency therapy is not crucial, but diagnostic studies are required to exclude other conditions. For example, a myelogram is necessary to exclude a compressive spinal cord lesion. Exacerbation of multiple sclerosis can be precipitated by local or systemic infection. Urinary tract infection is particularly likely to occur in multiple sclerosis patients with myelopathy. Elevation of body temperature worsens the neurologic condition of many patients with multiple sclerosis.

Many *metabolic abnormalities* may cause asymmetric or focal cerebral symptoms. Hypoglycemia and hyponatremia are the common etiologic agents. In patients with previous focal cerebral disease such as stroke with complete recovery, symptoms of the earlier focal cerebral lesion may reappear in the presence of a metabolic derangement, such as uremia or hepatic failure.

Acute Myelopathies

When the examination points to the spinal cord as the source of the neurologic problem, the physician is confronted with a spectrum of diagnostic possibilities. Many disease processes, whether intrinsic to the spinal cord or pressing on the spinal cord externally, produce clinical symptoms of partial or complete cord transection. Table 15.17 summarizes the disease process. While the examination can point to the sensory level of the problem and the hyperreflexia and Babinski signs may confirm the upper motor neuron nature of the lesion, reflexes can initially be entirely absent (spinal shock). There are no reliable bedside rules to determine whether an acute or subacute segmental cord syndrome is due to a lesion that is intrinsic or extrinsic to the spinal cord. Depending on the period of time

Table 15.17.
Myelopathy

Paraplegia or Quadriplegia of Acute Onset (hours to days)
- Traumatic (fracture-dislocation, ischemia, contusion, hematoma)
- Prolapsed intervertebral disc
- Spinal collapse (carcinoma, infection of vertebral body)
- Acute myelitis (postinfectious, viral or postvaccination)
- Cord ischemia
- Poliomyelitis[a]
- Guillain-Barré syndrome[a]
- Tick paralysis[a]

Paraplegia or Quadriplegia of Slow Onset
- Cervical spondylosis
- Multiple sclerosis
- Spinal tumor
- Subacute combined degeneration of the spinal cord (B_{12} deficiency)
- Motor neuron disease[a]
- Foramen magnum lesions (Paget's disease, tumor)
- Spinocerebellar degenerations
- Parasagittal meningioma
- Bilateral lacunar strokes

[a] Lower motor neuron process or combined upper and lower motor neuron disease.

over which the lesion evolved, weakness below the level of the problem can be spastic or flaccid, and the distribution can be asymmetric. Extramedullary compression can occur as a result of *trauma* with vertebral fracture, acute *midline disc herniation, abscess* (often associated with vertebral osteomyelitis), and *tumor,* usually metastatic tumor. *Hematoma* can occur as a result of neck injury or as a complication of anticoagulation therapy. *Cervical spondylosis* from progressive arthritic disease occasionally can present with a relatively short course of progressive weakness and tingling in both hands and variable neck pain. Intrinsic (primary) cord tumors tend to present more slowly over a period of months, but sudden neurologic deterioration can occur due to bleeding into the tumor. Rarely, the *anterior spinal artery* can be the site of thromboembolic disease. The ventral part of the spinal cord can become ischemic at any level, most commonly near the 6th thoracic vertebra, resulting in features of cord transection with paralysis and sensory loss below the level with relative sparing of joint position and vibration which are supplied by the posterior spinal arteries. Transfemoral angiography now allows visualization of the anterior spinal arteries, but the diagnosis is based on clinical findings. Acute spinal cord ischemia can be seen following trauma, with expanding thoracic aortic aneurysm or following surgery, in the descending thoracic aorta.

Many illnesses have *transverse myelitis* as a part of the symptom complex. *Multiple sclerosis* and *postinfectious myelitis* are among the more common. Some lymphocytes are typically observed in the CSF, and the protein may be slightly elevated. Seldom can the diagnosis of the extrinsic spinal cord compression be excluded with such confidence in these cases that myelographic examination is obviated. MRI scanning is used to exclude cord compression with a high degree of efficiency, but this technique is not available widely. Vertebral body metastases and meningeal carcinomatosis can also be diagnosed with MRI. Acute, severe necrotizing myelopathy can occur in heroin addicts. However, since addicts have a greater risk for infection, the diagnosis of vertebral osteomyelitis with eipdural abscess must be excluded by myelography or MRI. Progressive ascending myelitis has been the presenting feature of the acquired immunodeficiency syndrome (AIDS) due to cytomegalovirus and to herpes simplex virus type 2.

The *treatment* of all acute spinal cord syndromes is similar. Catheterization of the bladder must be considered since urinary retention is quite common. Corticosteroids, usually dexamethasone, 20 mg intravenously, or its equivalent in methylprednisolone, is administered prior to lumbar puncture for myelography in all cases of suspected spinal cord compression. Corticosteroids should be continued, at the dose of dexamethasone 4 mg four times per day, in all patients with documented compression. The use of steroids in patients with transverse myelitis due to multiple sclerosis or to infectious etiologies is less well-established.

Acute Peripheral Neurologic Lesions

While most peripheral neuropathies are slowly developing processes, there is a sizable number of relatively rapidly evolving conditions which affect peripheral nerves diffusely or weakening muscles throughout the body, progressing over hours or days, even worsening acutely. Such patients are likely to appear first in an emergency department. It is the task of the emergency physician to define the distribution of the polyneuropathy or mononeuropathy and to separate these conditions from central nervous system diseases.

Mononeuropathies

A mononeuropathy is dysfunction in the distribution of one peripheral, cranial, or spinal nerve. Lesions involving cranial nerves III, IV, and VI have been discussed in the section of this chapter concerning visual problems.

Facial Nerve. Sudden onset of facial weakness involving both upper and lower facial musculature may be due to pathology at any level in the course of the nerve from the facial nucleus to the neuromuscular junction. The most common lesion

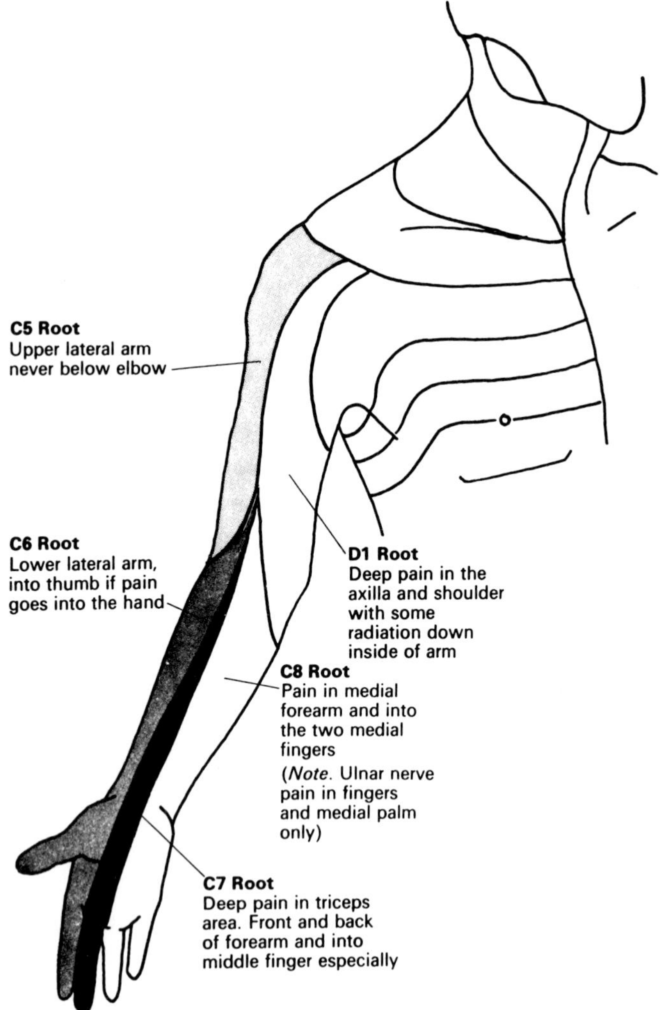

Figure 15.10. *Left,* Distribution of root pain and paresthesia. *Right,* Distribution of peripheral nerve pain and paresthesia. (From Patten, J. *Neurological Differential Diagnosis.* New York: Springer-Verlag, 1977.)

occurs during an upper respiratory infection and evolves over several hours, often with pain in the ipsilateral ear. When acute otitis, parotitis, and central facial weakness have been excluded, idiopathic or Bell's palsy is the likely problem. For idiopathic facial palsy, a short course of prednisone beginning at 60 mg/day and tapering every 3 days by 10 mg, has been shown to hasten recovery and to improve cosmetic outcome, if the steroid is started within 24 hours of the onset of the problem. The presence of bilateral facial lesions raises the possibility of sarcoidosis or Lyme disease and a history of arthralgias, headache, and tick bite should be sought. Prognosis for recovery of facial palsy of the idiopathic variety is very good with 90% of patients achieving a cosmetically acceptable result. If lid closure is greatly affected by the facial palsy, artificial tears should be supplied and the patient should be instructed to tape the eye shut at night and to report pain or foreign body sensation immediately. Tarsorrhaphy to close the lid may be considered, if complete weakness of lid closure is present, to prevent corneal damage.

Cervical Radiculopathy. Osteophytic spurs may develop that encroach on nerve roots of the cervical spinal cord. The C5, C6, and C7 roots are most frequently involved with characteristic patterns of pain and variable sensory and motor findings (see Fig. 15.10). Radiologic assessment usually includes cervical spine films, but abnormalities seen on these films may not correlate with symptoms. If only radicular signs and symptoms are present, the patient may benefit from cervical traction, with analgesics, muscle relaxants, and abstinence from

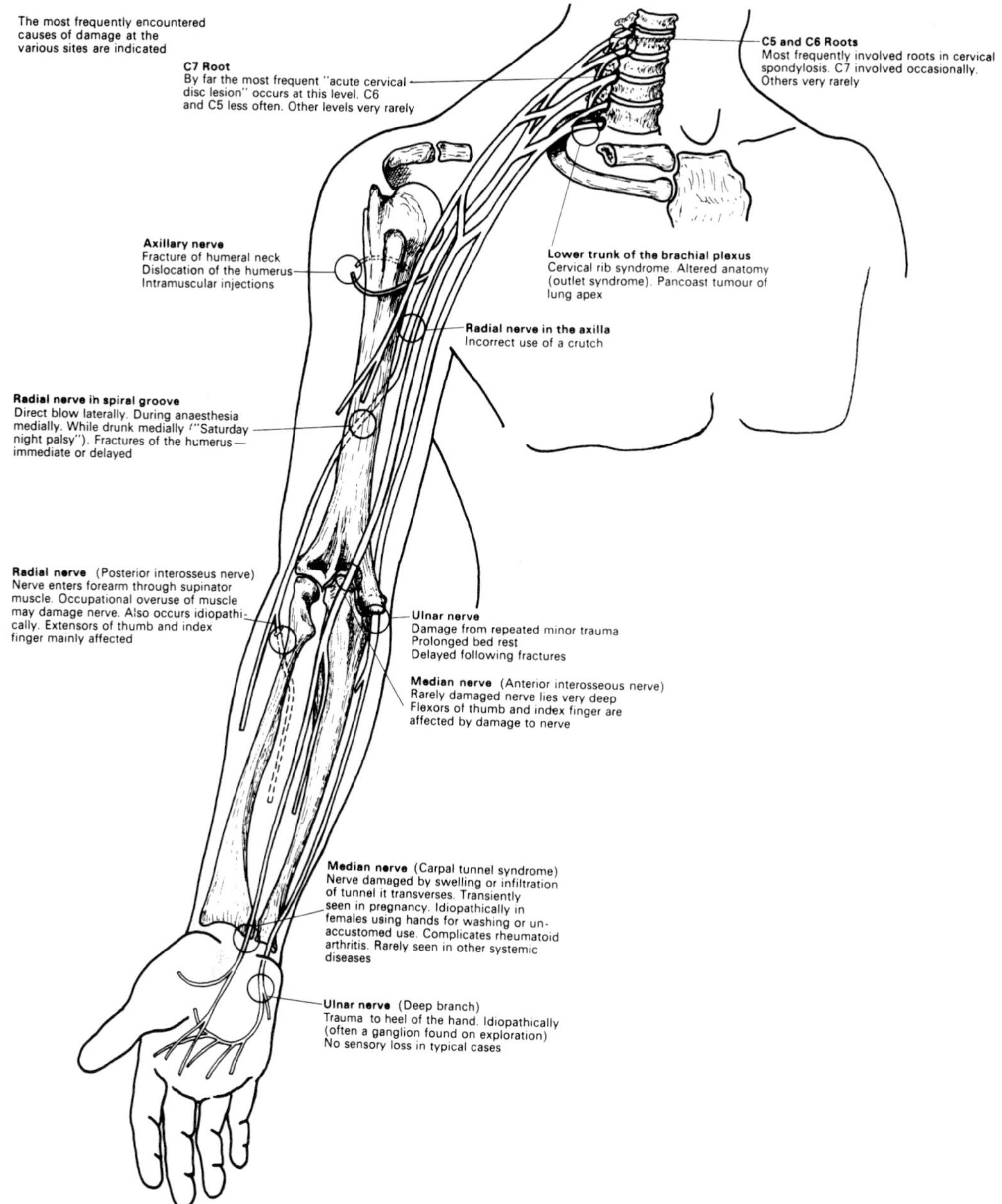

Figure 15.11. Peripheral nerve distribution to the upper limb. (From Patten, J. *Neurological Differential Diagnosis*. New York: Springer-Verlag, 1977.)

physical activity. Cervical nerve radiculopathies must be differentiated from other upper extremity nerve involvement at the brachial plexus or peripheral nerve level. Electromyography is helpful in distinguishing the level of the problem in some instances.

Carpal Tunnel Syndrome. The median nerve is entrapped at the carpal tunnel because of pressure from ligamentous thickening (see Fig. 15.11). In most cases there is no underlying disease, though the syndrome is associated with rheumatoid arthritis, pregnancy, acromegaly, hypothyroidism, fractures of the carpal bones, amyloidosis, myeloma, and occupational trauma (jack hammers, percussion instruments). A combination of pain, paresthesias, and numbness in the median nerve

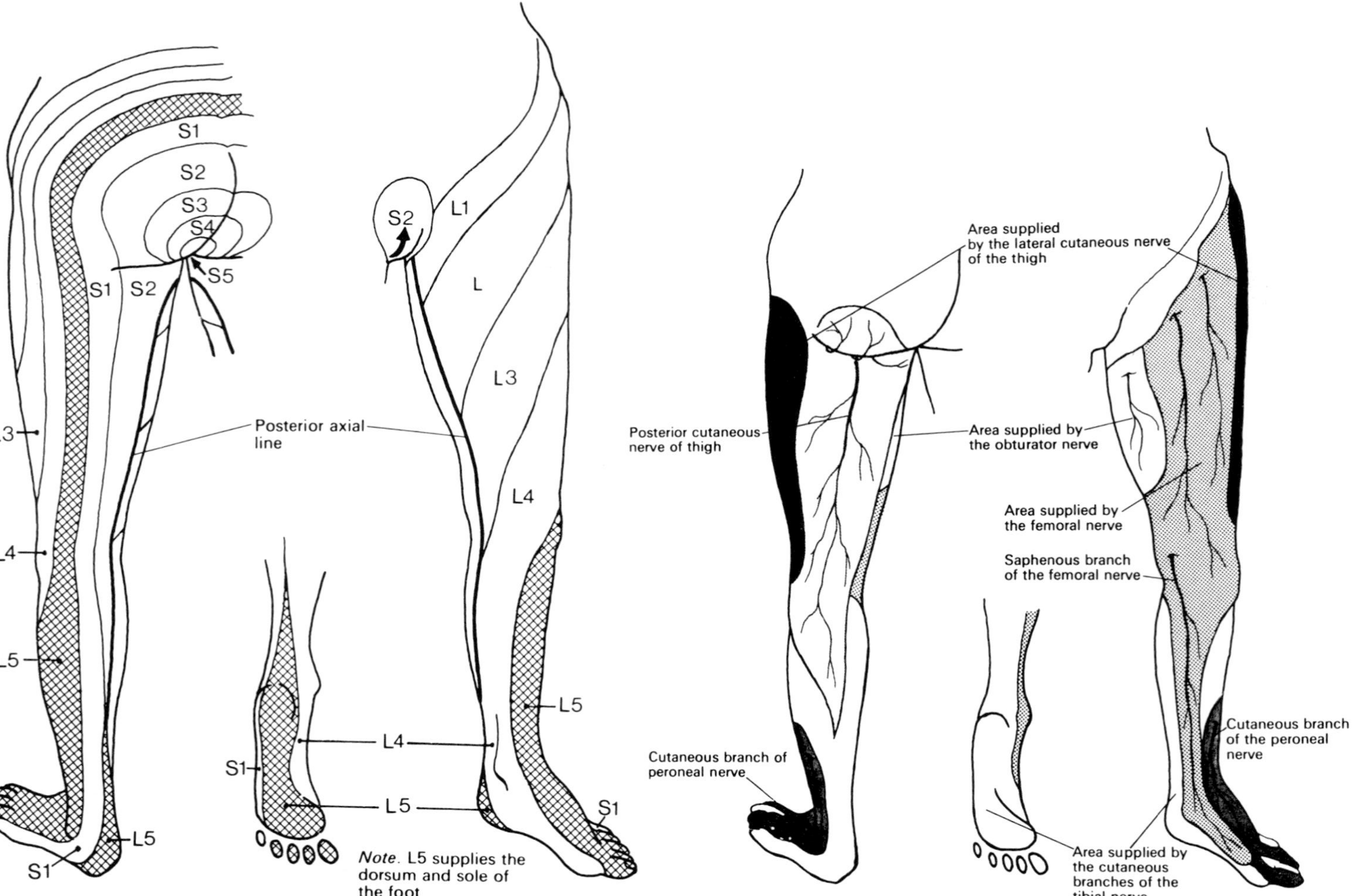

Figure 15.12. *Left,* Lumbosacral dermatomes. *Right,* Lower limb peripheral nerve distribution. (From Patten, J. *Neurological Differential Diagnosis*. New York: Springer-Verlag, 1977.)

distribution, often worse at night and accompanied by some swelling of the hand, is reported and may have been present for several weeks by the time the patient seeks emergency attention. Later, weakness of thumb abduction and opposition occurs and then atrophy can be seen. Aching pain can be felt as far up as the arm and shoulder and should not distract the examiner's attention from the wrist. Tapping on the wrist over the course of the nerve can reproduce the pain (Tinel's sign).

The differential diagnosis includes radiculopathy from C6 or C7 cervical root compression, but comparison of the distribution of pain and paresthesias (see Fig. 15.10) should help distinguish this. Wrist splints and anti-inflammatory medications are useful emergency adjuncts, but following electromyographic confirmation of the level of the problem, surgical relief is easily accomplished and effective. An electromyogram (EMG) is necessary because the median nerve can be entrapped at more proximal levels, though the carpal tunnel region is by far the most common site.

Ulnar Nerve Injury. The ulnar nerve is most frequently injured at the elbow. Causes include fracture deformities, arthritis, faulty positioning of the arm during surgery, or repetitive occupational or recreational trauma (holding a telephone, playing tennis). The development of paresthesias and weakness may postdate an injury by many months. Sensation is usually spared in the forearm, but there is sensory loss in the fifth and ulnar half of the fourth finger. Wasting of the intrinsic muscles of the hand occurs later. Nerve conduction studies can accurately localize the site of compression. The condition must be differentiated from thoracic outlet syndrome or from C8-T1 cervical root lesions. Treatment is avoidance of the positions that irritate the nerve, but in cases of severe pain or weakness, surgical repositioning of the ulnar nerve at the elbow may be necessary for relief.

Radial Nerve Injury. Radial nerve damage most often occurs in the axilla or upper arm. It can be seen with improperly used crutches, with prolonged pressure during sleep (the Saturday night palsy), or as a result of direct injury including fracture of the mid-humoral shaft. Wrist drop is the prominent feature. A short "cock-up" wrist splint will make the hand more comfortable and functional until spontaneous recovery, predictable within 6–8 weeks, occurs. Nerve disruption requires surgical correction.

Lateral Femoral Cutaneous Nerve Compression. Also known as meralgia paresthetica, lateral femoral cutaneous nerve compression involves a purely sensory nerve formed by branches arising from the second and third roots of the lumbar plexus. The nerve supplies the anterolateral and lateral aspects of the thigh almost to the knee (see Fig. 15.12). Compression causes an extremely unpleasant, burning pain with cutaneous hypersensitivity. Standing or walking exacerbates the pain. The syndrome often occurs in obese people or when tight corsets are worn. It is common in diabetics and may begin during pregnancy. Differential diagnosis includes a lesion in the second or third lumbar roots or arthritic or traumatic hip disease. Weakness and reflex changes do not occur in meralgia paresthetica. The neuropathy tends to regress spontaneously over a long period of time. Recovery can be hastened with weight loss. Emergency workup should include lumbosacral spine and hip radiographs. If the pain persists, trials of tricyclic antidepressants have been advocated with modest success.

Femoral Neuropathy. The femoral nerve derives from the second, third, and fourth lumbar roots. Its posterior division is the major innervation to the quadriceps femoris muscle and terminates as the saphenous nerve which supplies sensation to the medial aspect of the leg as far as the medial malleolus (Fig. 15.13). Onset of femoral neuropathy is frequently sudden, painful, and followed quickly by wasting and weakness in the quadriceps, loss of patellar reflex, and sensory impairment over the medial thigh and leg. The most common cause is probably infarction of the small blood vessels supplying the nerve, and the syndrome is most commonly seen in diabetics. Entrapment of the femoral nerve can occur in the inguinal region and in the retroperitoneum due to compression by tumor or hematoma. While some improvement occurs, the patient is often left quite weak. The speed of onset of weakness and the degree of weakening of the quadriceps differentiates this syndrome from a pure L4 radiculopathy. If there is also hip flexion weakness, the site of the lesion is usually in the lumbar plexus. EMG studies may be indicated, and tumor must be excluded, usually with a CT scan of the retroperitoneum, but these are not studies that would be indicated on an emergency basis. Lumbosacral spine radiographs are appropriate in the emergency department to exclude major vertebral body abnormalities.

Sciatic Nerve Syndromes. The sciatic nerve arises from the lumbosacral plexus (L4 to S3). It terminates in the common peroneal and tibial nerves (Fig. 15.13). The tibial nerve supplies the gastrocnemius, soleus, and popliteus muscles, while its extension into the calf, the posterior tibial nerve, supplies the calf muscles involved in plantar flexion. The common peroneal nerve divides into superficial and deep peroneal nerves. The latter supplies the muscles that dorsiflex the foot and toes, while the superficial peroneal nerve innervates the muscles of foot eversion.

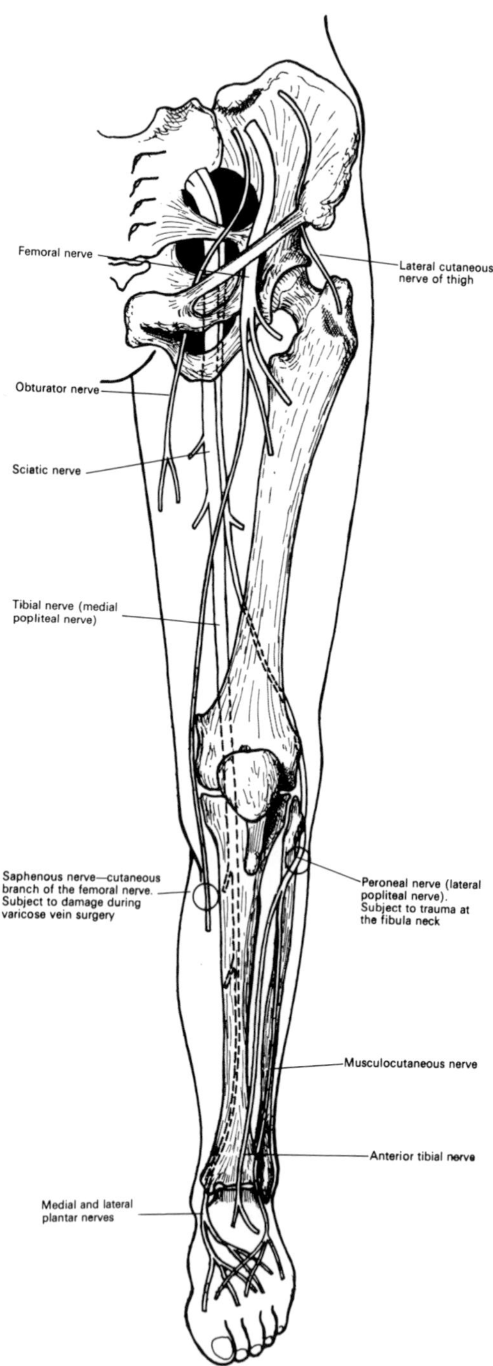

Figure 15.13. Peripheral nerve distribution to the lower limb. (From Patten, J. *Neurological Differential Diagnosis,* New York: Springer-Verlag, 1977.)

Sciatic nerve compression can result from tumors within the pelvis or from prolonged pressure from lying or sitting on the buttocks, particularly in states of stupor, coma, or anesthesia. Gluteal abscesses or misplaced buttock injections have also caused sciatic nerve injury. Weakness of the gluteal muscles implies compression within the pelvis, while lesions just beyond the sciatic notch cause weakness in the hamstrings and in all the muscles of the lower leg.

Common peroneal compression usually occurs at the level of the fibular head (Fig. 15.13) and is seen in cachectic patients following prolonged bedrest, in alcoholics, in diabetics, and in patients placed in tight casts. Injury leads to faulty dorsiflexion and eversion of the foot, producing a foot drop. Complete or partial recovery can be expected when the paralysis results from transient pressure. Treatment consists of a foot-drop brace and avoidance of positions that put pressure on the fibular head.

Lumbar Disc Syndromes. Compressive neuropathies of the peripheral nerves to the lower limbs must be distinguished from the very common lumbar disc syndromes. In the lumbar region the discs between the L4 and L5 and the L5 and S1 vertebral bodies are most frequently affected, leading to dysfunction of the L5 and S1 nerve roots, respectively. Pain can be sudden and clearly subsequent to an inciting traumatic event or can evolve more gradually with or without back pain. The pain is worsened by bending forward, sneezing, or straining and by sitting. The herniated disc can compress one or more nerve roots. L4-L5 disc herniation, affecting the L5 root, produces pain over the sciatic notch, lateral thigh and leg, numbness of the webspace between the great and adjacent toes and in the lateral leg, and weakness of dorsiflexion of the great toe and foot without reflex changes (see Fig. 15.12). L5-S1 disc herniation catches the S1 root, producing pain down the back of the leg to the heel, numbness of the lateral heel, foot, and toe, weakness of plantar flexion, and loss of the ankle reflex. Straight leg raising may worsen the pain in the characteristic radiating pattern or can even produce pain on the opposite side of the back or in the opposite leg (crossed positive straight leg raising, sometimes indicative of a "free fragment" of disc). Unless there is pronounced weakness, uncontrollable pain, or bladder and bowel dysfunction, the usual treatment is a trial of bed rest with anti-inflammatory and analgesic drugs. If sphincter dysfunction or pronounced weakness is present, early myelography is indicated to define the pathology and to exclude more unusual causes of radiculopathy, such as tumor.

Herpes Zoster. Pain along the distribution of any sensory nerve root, including the trigeminal nerve, can be due to herpes zoster. The pain can cause diagnostic confusion prior to the emergence of the rash, but should be suspected particularly when the anatomic site of involvement is unusual for other disc or entrapment syndromes or if the patient is immunocompromised. Typical sites include the first (ophthalmic) division of the trigeminal nerve and thoracic nerve roots. The pain is confined strictly in a dermatomal distribution and stops at the midline. The rash usually erupts within a few days of the pain, but can be delayed as long as 2 weeks. Some physicians advocate a trial of oral acyclovir to lessen the likelihood of postherpetic neuralgia.

Acute Toxic Polyneuropathies

Most peripheral polyneuropathies evolve slowly over weeks to months. A few, however, can present acutely and a limited number of life-threatening illnesses will present early with severe peripheral neurologic findings. Because both pain and autonomic involvement can be features of these illnesses, syncope or pain can bring the patient to the emergency department. The *history* should include exposures to toxins such as arsenic, lead, triorthocresylphosphate (TOCP), solvents, glue, vincristine, cisplatinum, amiodorone, isoniazid, nitrofurantoin, hydralazine, gold, quinine, quinidine, and phenytoin. Recent immunizations, systemic disease, and family history are all necessary parts of questioning in the history. The polyneuropathy can involve a stocking-glove distribution of sensorimotor dysfunction. The legs are usually more severely affected than the arms. Reflexes can be absent, normal, or diminished. Cranial nerve findings can be present. The distribution can be predominantly sensory (amyloidosis, carcinoma, vitamin E deficiency, herpes zoster, myelomatosis, diabetes, early uremia), predominantly motor (late uremia, diphtheria, TOCP poisoning, porphyria, lead poisoning, Guillain-Barré syndrome), or may have a prominent autonomic component with diarrhea, orthostatic signs, gastric dysfunction, and impotence (diabetes, vincristine toxicity, Guillain-Barré syndrome). Cranial nerve involvement may be prominent (diabetes, diphtheria, botulism, tetanus, and tick, spider, and ciguatera poisoning).

Rapid paralysis may occur for many reasons in these varied conditions. The common critical element in therapy is respiratory maintenance. In emergency care, adequate ventilatory support has priority over measures dealing with the specific disease. This section presents the neurologic diseases associated with rapid onset of diffuse weakness. The sites of abnormality differ among the disease processes: motor neuron (amyotrophic lateral sclerosis, poliomyelitis), peripheral nerve (Guillain-Barré syndrome, diphtheria), or neuromuscular junction (botulism, tick and shellfish poisoning). Because the rapidity of onset and multiple sites of clinical findings cause diagnostic confusion, these diseases are all grouped together.

Acute Intermittent Porphyria. The only common type of porphyria that affects the nervous system is acute intermittent porphyria. Total paralysis may develop during an acute attack. Many substances, the most common being barbiturates, can precipitate an attack. Barbiturates may inadvertently be administered during an attack of severe abdominal pain, which is typical of the illness. Diagnosis can be established rapidly by testing the urine for porphobilinogen (Watson-Schwartz test) and this test should be carried out in all patients with sudden, unexplained paralysis. Respiratory support may be necessary and barbiturates, sulfonamide derivatives, griseofulvin, and estrogens must be eliminated.

Acute Idiopathic Polyneuritis (Guillain-Barré Syndrome). Paralysis from acute idiopathic polyneuritis (Guillain-Barré syndrome) is the most common form of acute paralytic neurologic disease to confront the emergency physician. It occurs in all seasons and at all ages, sometimes associated with infectious mononucleosis or infectious hepatitis, diseases which should be considered in all patients with the syndrome. The history can reveal recent inoculation or upper respiratory infection. Weakness and tingling paresthesias begin distally in the lower extremities and ascend over a period of days; paralysis can eventually be total and muscles innervated by the cranial nerves can be involved with bifacial paresis, extraocular muscle abnormalities, and weakness of phonation, chewing, swallowing, and breathing. On examination, the motor findings are always more prominent than are the sensory findings, but posterior column dysfunction with loss of joint position and vibration sense can be present. An important diagnostic finding is the early depression or absence of all deep tendon reflexes. Thus, while the early symptoms of nonspecific weakness and paresthesias can lead the physician to consider a diagnosis of a viral syndrome or a psychiatric problem with hyperventilation, the absence of reflexes in a young patient should raise the possibility of early Guillain-Barré syndrome. Although emergency studies of nerve conduction are usually unnecessary, the slowing of motor nerve conduction velocity is usually profound and can rapidly provide diagnostic evidence since few other illnesses, and certainly no common illnesses, produce such extreme slowing. The CSF contains increased amounts of protein without cells (''albuminocytologic dissociation''), but early in the course of the illness the CSF protein level may be normal. The presence of large numbers of white blood cells (lymphocytes) leads the physician to consider other illnesses associated with rapid onset of weakness (see paralytic infections below). Autonomic dysfunction is common in the Guillain-Barré syndrome and wide alterations in blood pressure occur spontaneously, even in only moderately weak patients. Cardiac arrhythmias have been documented. Progress of the disease is unpredictable: the disease can progress rapidly to respiratory embarrassment without the steady ascending pattern that is more typical of the syndrome or can begin with the cranial musculature (Miller Fisher variant). Vital capacity should be measured frequently and admission is advisable even if the patient has only mild distal weakness. Prognosis is good for nearly complete recovery, though the patient with severe acute idiopathic polyneuritis can remain paralyzed for months and require tracheotomy for respiratory support. Steroids are useful in the relapsing remitting variety of polyneuritis. Plasmapheresis can help in limiting the severity of the disease if it is performed early during the presentation.

Paralytic Infectious Diseases. The Guillain-Barré syndrome should be distinguished from several much less common illnesses due either to bacterial toxins or to invasion of the central nervous system (CNS) by neurotropic viruses. In the diseases caused by toxins (tetanus, botulism, diphtheria, spider bite, and shellfish poisoning), full neurologic recovery is the rule if the patient can be brought safely through the acute phase of the illness. The CSF is normal in the toxin-produced illnesses. However, in the diseases caused by viral invasion of the CNS (rabies and poliomyelitis), the CSF contains cells and often has an elevated protein level. When the acute illness is past, permanent neurologic sequelae are common in the viral diseases.

Poliomyelitis. Poliomyelitis is now rarely seen in the United States. However, approximately 15 cases per year of this once epidemic disease are still reported. Half or more develop as a complication of oral poliovirus vaccine, and a few instances of the disease have occurred in persons in close contact with recent recipients of this vaccine. A minor upper respiratory tract illness or gastrointestinal upset with fever may precede the neurologic illness. In most patients with CNS involvement, the clinical presentation is simply one of aseptic meningitis, with stiff neck, fever, and inflammatory cells in the CSF. No single feature distinguishes this syndrome from other viral meningitides. In a small number of patients, the disease takes the form of encephalomyelitis with rapid progression of paresis or paralysis of bulbar and limb musculature, usually asymmetric. In the earliest stages, coarse twitches and fasciculations of muscles occur, superseded shortly by paralysis. Although paresthesias are common, no sensory loss can be documented. It is important to exercise the patient's muscles as little as possible. Serum should be set aside and pharyngeal washings and stool specimens cultured as soon as possible to attempt to isolate the virus.

Rabies. Rabies is a viral encephalitis that appears months after the virus enters the body at the site of the rabid animal bite. In recent years a greater threat to human beings has been posed by bats, squirrels, raccoons and skunks. Most domestic dogs have now been vaccinated. From 1 month to 1 year following the animal bite, the patient experiences paresthesias and pain at the site of the bite with a prodromal syndrome of fever and malaise. Within a few days of premonitory symptoms, the encephalitic syndrome ensues. There is alternating agitation and depression and severe muscle spasms, especially reflex spasms of the larynx that make drinking painful (hydrophobia). Other cranial nerves are affected, resulting in disorders of the ocular and facial movement. Some persons do recover if respiratory assistance, sedation, and treatment of other medical complications are vigorously carried out.

Tetanus. Tetanus is strictly a "paralytic" disease, although the patient with clinical manifestations of this illness can suffer such spasms of somatic musculature as to preclude normal muscular function. Death can result from respiratory failure. The wound can be inapparent, and since only about one-third of patients with tetanus have cultures positive for *Clostridium tetani,* the diagnosis is made primarily on the basis of the clinical presentation. After an incubation period of a few days to more than 2 weeks, neurologic signs and symptoms develop. Spasms of cranial and cervical muscles are prominent, generally with clenching of the teeth (trismus) and painful spasms of limbs and trunk, leading to opisthotonic posturing triggered by afferent stimuli, such as touch, bright light, and noise. Involvement of the autonomic nervous system produces profuse sweating. There are potentially dangerous swings in blood pressure and temperature. In the United States, noteworthy portals of entry for the bacteria are the venous puncture sites of drug addicts, the pelvis in cases of septic abortion, and wounds inflicted by lawnmowers. Women more than 60 years of age are a group at greatest risk because of inadequate prior immunization.

Human tetanus immune globulin is recommended therapy (see Chapter 11). This globulin does not counteract toxin already bound to nervous tissue. The painful spasms are best treated with small amounts of intravenous diazepam (2–5 mg). If complications including secondary infection and hypoxia can be avoided, total recovery is the rule.

A syndrome of generalized muscular rigidity with severe trismus and sweating can occur as an idiosyncratic reaction to phenothiazine medications, and a history of the use of this class of drug must be questioned in every case of a suspected tetanus. Parenteral administration of diphenhydramine hydrochloride (Benadryl), 25–50 mg intravenously, or benzatropine (Cogentin) 1–2 mg intravenously, can quickly reverse this idiosyncratic drug reaction.

Botulism. Botulism, a rare but often fatal condition caused by the potent neurotoxin produced by *Clostridium botulinum,* exists in two forms. The more common type is due to the ingestion of preformed toxin associated with poor food processing techniques. This form is most common in Colorado because boiling food in the high level of the Rocky Mountains does not provide a high enough temperature to destroy the spores of the organism. Killing spores requires temperatures of 120°C for 30 minutes. Six toxigenic types of *C. botulinum* are recognized (A–F) but disease is almost always caused by types A, B, and E. The uncommon type of botulism is due to wound or gastrointestinal infection by the organism.

Adult botulin intoxication follows the ingestion of food by 12 to 48 hours. The adult patient develops blurred vision, diplopia, dysphonia, dysphagia, dyspnea, and then experiences generalized weakness with nausea, vomiting, and abdominal cramps. The blurred vision is due to failure of pupillary accommodation. Despite severe motor involvement, sensory abnormalities are absent and the sensorium is clear. Botulism paralysis differs from that of the Guillain-Barré syndrome in that reflexes are usually preserved until the patient is quite weak and that botulism paralysis tends to descend through the body. Botulism differs from diphtheria in the absence of oropharyngitis in an acute febrile illness.

The clinical diagnosis is confirmed by serum collection before antitoxin (trivalent ABE) is administered. This latter can be obtained most rapidly by telephoning the Center for Disease Control in Atlanta, GA (404-329-3311 during the day or 404-329-3644 at night and on weekends). Since most laboratories require at least 24 hours to report results of tests for toxin, treatment must start on clinical indications alone. A diagnosis of wound botulism should be considered if no food item can be implicated epidemiologically. The incubation period for wound botulism ranges from 4 to 14 days.

A patient suspected of botulism should be hospitalized. The toxin is flushed from the gastrointestinal tract by inducing vomiting, gastric lavage, and cathartics (avoiding magnesium salts, however, since they could augment the toxin-produced prevention of presynaptic acetylcholine release at the neuromuscular junction. The earlier the antitoxin is administered, the better the prognosis. The serum should be checked for toxin the day after antitoxin therapy. If toxin persists, repeat the treatment with antitoxin with the type-specific antitoxin indicated. Attention to respiratory care, infection control, bowel and bladder care, and nutrition make full recovery theoretically possible. However, some patients complain of dry mouth and fatigue even after several years.

Botulism in infants presents as an acute, transient hypotonia. These cases are caused by colonization of the gastrointestinal tract by *C.botulinum* organisms and local production of toxin. Finding the toxin or the organism in the feces confirms the clinical diagnosis in infants. (Adult colon normally contains clostridium.) Affected children usually present within the first 4 months of life with hypotonia, weakness of cranial and somatic muscles, hyporeflexia, and respiratory failure, with or without ophthalmoplegia and autonomic dysfunction. The infants recover spontaneously. A common source of the organism is honey which should be avoided in children under 1 year of age.

Diphtheria. Because of decreasing levels of immunity in the United States, almost 250 cases of *diphtheria* occur each year. Membranous pharyngitis or laryngitis is the key to diagnosis, but the toxin can produce several different syndromes. Cranial motor neuropathy with prominent dysphagia and dysphonia may develop several weeks after the pharyngitis, and a peripheral neuritis clinically identical to the Guillain-Barré syndrome can appear up to 3 months after the acute episode. All the neuropathic consequences of diphtheria are totally reversible.

Tick Paralysis. Tick paralysis produced by scrub tick bites causes a profound neuromuscular paralysis. The toxin acts locally on the nerves reducing nerve action potentials. It has a botulin-like effect at the neuromuscular junction. The clinical picture is very much like the Guillain-Barré syndrome. The typical patient develops paresthesias in the hands and feet, along with ascending weakness, over a period of 24-48 hours. There may be bulbar and respiratory paralysis. Reflexes are absent. Tick paralysis also can present as a subacute ataxia. The diagnosis should be considered in the differential diagnosis of Guillain-Barré syndrome, particularly in children and especially in young girls with long hair. Recovery after removal of the tick occurs rapidly and most patients are well within 2 days.

Spider Bites. Bites by black widow spiders (in the United States) and funnel web spiders (Australia) produce venom-induced neurologic syndromes. Within 10 minutes of a bite on a limb, the patient experiences generalized piloerection and widespread fasciculations. Excessive sweating, salivation, lacrimation, tachycardia, trismus, and laryngeal spasm occur. The latter is combatted with large doses of diazepam and atropine to permit intubation. Consciousness returns slowly after the twitching subsides. The victim can then develop progressive hypotension which should be treated with intravenous fluids. There are no specific antidotes.

Scorpion Stings. Scorpions are arachnids and their stings inflict a toxin on the nervous system that is similar to that of spider toxins, releasing central and peripheral neurotransmitters with consequent excessive nervous system discharge followed by transmission block. Most bites occur in the warm months from April through July. There can be local pain and swelling associated with fever, muscle spasms, salivation, diarrhea, restlessness, and convulsions. Electrocardiograms can show changes of myocardial infarction and congestive heart failure. Pulmonary edema can develop. Diazepam and atropine can be given supportively. A specific antivenom is available but may produce a hypersensitivity reaction. Meperidine (Demerol), morphine, and paraldehyde may augment the lethal effects of scorpion venom and should be avoided.

Fish and Shellfish Poisoning. Fish and shellfish poisoning is incurred after the ingestion of fish containing toxin derived from dinoflagellates. *Ciguatera fish poisoning* occurs a few minutes to 30 hours after eating any of a number of popular game fish, such as red snapper and grouper. Acute symptoms include abdominal cramps, nausea, diarrhea, numbness, paresthesias of the lips, tongue, and throat, a metallic taste, myalgias, blurred vision, photophobia, sharp pains in the extremities, and the odd sensation of looseness of the teeth. Autonomic instability and respiratory paralysis occur. Mortality may be as high as 12%. *Ciguatoxin* resists heat destruction and inhibits cholinesterase. Treatment is supportive with induction of vomiting and administration of a cathartic to remove the toxin. *Tetrodotoxin,* a heat-stable toxin present in puffer fish, newts, goby, frogs, and octopus blocks action potentials by interfering with the increase in sodium permeability associated with excitation. Human paralytic disease may result in a nearly "locked-in" syndrome. Tetrodotoxin has been invoked as the responsible agent in some remarkable Haitian cases of "zombiism" with full recovery from what appeared to be a state of coma. Treatment is supportive.

Paralytic shellfish poisoning occurs within 30 minutes of eating either raw or cooked shellfish. Acute symptoms include burning, tingling, and prickling of the lips, gums, tongue, and face, succeeded by paralysis. In severe cases dysphonia and dyspnea develop. Reflexes and consciousness are preserved. *Saxitoxin* causes the illness and withstands heat and commercial canning, acting much like tetrodotoxin. Purgation and ventilatory support are critical. Preventive measures prohibiting shellfish consumption during "red tides" and strict control of shellfish processing reduce outbreaks.

Periodic Paralysis. No group of patients is more often misdiagnosed as having a psychiatric disorder than are those rare individuals with periodic paralysis. There are three forms, hyperkalemic, hypokalemic, and normokalemic. Hypokalemia in patients without a history of periodic paralysis can also produce profound weakness. Serum potassium determination should be part of the evaluation of any patient with generalized weakness of uncertain cause (see section of this chapter on metabolic disturbances). The onset of periodic paralysis disorders is usually between ages of 7 and 21. A family history of the disease is often obtained. Rapid onset of limb weakness and respiratory distress can follow certain precipitating events. In patients with hypokalemic paralysis, episodes of diarrhea or vomiting can lower the serum potassium to a critical level. Some of these patients have coexistent and possibly causative hyperthyroidism. Attacks of hypokalemic periodic paralysis tend to last many hours, longer than those of patients with hyperkalemic paralysis. Some patients with hyperkalemic periodic paralysis have associated myotonia: sharp percussion of an affected muscle produces a slight depression and contraction that may be slow to relax. Treatment of the paralyses consists of correcting the serum potassium level. Acetazolamide can be useful in patients with hyperkalemic paralysis, while those with the hypokalemic variety should be treated with potassium replacement and possibly with β-blocking drugs. They should avoid strenuous exercise and meals heavy in carbohydrate.

PROGRESSIVE NEUROLOGIC DEFICITS

Progressive Focal Neurologic Deficits

While vascular processes fluctuate and progress over a period of hours to a day, these processes evolve more gradually, in a stuttering or smooth fashion, over a period of days to weeks. Retrospective history discloses that the patient was symptomatic well before the acute worsening that led him or her to seek emergency attention. The major categories of intracranial process producing a focal neurologic deficit are tumor, subdural hematoma, and abscess.

Cerebral Tumors

Symptoms of intracranial masses reflect tumor expansion within a fixed bony vault impinging on space normally occupied by brain, blood vessels, and CSF. Although normal brain tissue accommodates the presence of slowly growing tumors, both benign and malignant masses more than 3 cm in diameter increase intracranial pressure. The pressure rise can impair venous return from the optic nerve causing papilledema. Fluid extravasates through fenestrations in the blood vessels of a growing tumor producing a plasma filtrate or "vasogenic cerebral edema" that in some cases trebles the tumor volume.

Symptoms leading to the diagnosis of intracranial tumor occur both in patients with and without a previously diagnosed systemic cancer. Patients with intracranial tumor usually present with one or more of the following groups of symptoms: (*a*) headache with or without evidence of increased intracranial pressure; (*b*) progressive generalized decline in cognitive abilities or impairment of specific neurologic functions affecting speech, gait, or memory; (*c*) adult onset seizures or increased frequency or severity of previously documented seizure activity; and (*d*) regional symptoms reflecting the particular anatomic site of the tumor, such as those caused by acoustic neuroma in the cerebellopontine angle, meningioma in the olfactory groove, or nuchal rigidity with focal cranial nerve deficit from a tumor in the vicinity of the foramen magnum. A tumor may present with a very short history of symptoms if there is (*a*) obstructive hydrocephalus from a strategically positioned, usually posterior fossa tumor; (*b*) hemorrhage into a previously unsuspected tumor; and (*c*) seizure activity in a patient not previously known to have a tumor.

The syndrome of chronic subdural hematoma and of cerebral abscess is essentially the same, with epidemiologic features of trauma or infection pointing to etiologies other than neoplasm. A patient may be seen in the emergency department at any stage in the evolution of an expanding intracranial mass. In most patients with supratentorial expanding processes, head pain radiates to the side of the mass, whereas patients with posterior fossa masses describe retroorbital, retroauricular, or occipital pain. Tumors of the frontal and temporal lobes can attain considerable size before symptoms develop.

The initial diagnostic test in patients suspected of an expanding intracranial process is a CT scan without contrast, followed by a contrast-enhanced CT scan. The addition of contrast helps differentiate tumor from stroke, can reveal a chronic isodense subdural collection with an enhancing membrane, and can provide evidence of multiple cranial tumors though symptoms are referrable to only one of these masses. The unenhanced CT scan provides information about the presence of calcium and blood and, by identifying tumors whose density is greater than that of surrounding brain, can give a clue to the histologic identity of the tumor.

Treatment of Intracranial Masses. The acutely decompensating patient should be given intravenous mannitol, 1–2 gms/kg, and intubated, if necessary, with respirator-assisted hyperventilation. (See Chapter 16 for a discussion of the herniation syndromes). Corticosteroids, such as dexamethasone, 20 mg, or methylprednisolone, 100 mg, are given intravenously as a bolus followed by maintenance dexamethasone or methylprednisolone at doses determined by the tumor size and location. Less acutely ill patients can be started on corticosteroids at maintenance dose levels judged appropriate from the CT scan. Their symptoms improve rapidly in 1 to 2 days. They should be counselled to take the steroids with an antacid. Anticonvulsants are prescribed prophylactically by some physicians and should be given parenterally in loading doses (see section of this chapter about seizures) for patients with a known intracranial mass who have already experienced a seizure. Coagulopathy should be corrected if a hematoma is demonstrated. Catheterization is wise in the drowsy patient to be treated with vigorous mannitol diuresis.

Pseudotumor Cerebri

Symptoms of increased intracranial pressure can occur in the absence of demonstrable parenchymal tumor. A lumbar puncture can reveal leptomeningeal tumor. If the CSF is under increased pressure and the CT scan is normal or shows "slit-like" ventricles, the diagnosis of pseudotumor or "benign" intracranial hypertension may be considered. There is little that distinguishes the presentation of pseudotumor from that of true tumor with headache, papilledema, visual obscurations, diplopia, and nausea. Pseudotumor cerebri usually afflicts young, often obese women. The marked increase in intracranial pressure can reflect impaired venous drainage within the brain or can accompany the hormonal alterations of pregnancy, oral contraceptive use, or obesity. Endocrinologic illness including both hypothyroidism and hyperthyroidism, adrenal insufficiency and exogenous steroid use has been implicated in the condition, as well as drugs such as vitamin A, tetracycline, nalidixic acid, nitrofurantoin, and sulfonamide preparations. The diagnosis is one of exclusion of intracranial mass lesion, meningeal tumor, or infection, in the presence of raised CSF pressure. The CSF is otherwise unremarkable, although the protein can be unusually low. Treatment is directed at prevention of visual deficits. If the pressure is over 300 mg Hg or if visual field defects are present (usually a central scotoma), the patient should be admitted for serial lumbar punctures with removal of sufficient CSF (usually about 40 ml at a time) to decrease CSF pressure below 200 mm Hg. Patients refractory to repetitive lumbar puncture can benefit from acetazolamide or furosemide. Lumboperitoneal shunting and surgical decompression are reserved for patients with progressive visual impairment who have failed medical therapy. The outlook for most patients with pseudotumor cerebri is excellent, but as many as 10% will have permanent visual deficits.

Progressive Generalized Weakness

The most vexing of emergency department complaints may be those voiced by the patient who, without more specific elaboration, simply complains of generalized weakness. The possible causes range from the psychological (depression, anxiety, conversion reactions) to upper or lower motor neuron lesions, or even to severe proprioceptive disorders impeding the patient's perception of his or her movement. Many patterns of weakness and sensory loss appear in conversion syndromes and in malingering, but common organic syndromes can be quite similar. For example, paresthesias and weakness in the feet can indicate hyperventilation, but can also be early indications of a demyelinating neuropathy or of an acute idiopathic polyneuritis (Guillain-Barré syndrome). It is therefore essential to define the nature of the patient's weakness and to characterize particular patterns of affected movements: the duration, fluctuation, and progression of the symptoms and the presence or absence of associated pain or stiffness.

This section presents those types of weakness confined to muscle and to neuromuscular junction.

Motor Neuron Disease

Motor neuron disease, or amyotrophic lateral sclerosis, is a chronic neurologic condition. However, the patient with such a problem can present in the emergency department, without prior diagnosis, when fasciculations are suddenly noticed or when weakness has developed to the point that the patient stumbles or is unable to perform some other routine task. A previously diagnosed patient can present with rapid lessening of strength or with a fall or an episode of aspiration as the result of bulbar involvement. The etiology of motor neuron disease is unknown, and the disease frequently results in death within 1–2 years from the onset of symptoms. The upper motor neurons of the corticobulbar and corticospinal tracts can be involved with spastic weakness, hyperreflexia, and Babinski signs. Lower motor neuron involvement is marked by flaccid weakness, atrophy, and visible fasciculations. Often the patient has both upper and lower motor neuron signs. The differential diagnoses includes cervical myelopathy and subacute combined degeneration.

Myopathies

Like most polyneuropathies, myopathies progress slowly. The relatively rapidly progressive, acquired myopathies are few in number and confront the emergency department physician with a limited range of possibilities. Neuropathies tend to give distal symptoms first. Myopathies tend to affect the large proximal muscle groups at the same time or before they affect distal musculature. A second important differentiating feature is that myopathies rarely include sensory symptoms. There can be aching or cramps in the involved muscles, but paresthesias and decreased sensation are not noted. In myopathies, despite rather pronounced weakness, the patient has preserved deep tendon reflexes.

A screening history for endocrinologic symptoms (those of hyperthyroidism, hyperparathyroidism, hypothyroidism, Cushing's syndrome), drug use (steroids, alcohol, colchicine, chloroquine, clofibrate, vincristine, cathartics, diuretics), recent anesthesia, and family history of muscle disease should be obtained. Pain in joints should raise suspicion of polymyalgia rheumatica. The presence of severe cramping should raise suspicion of a viral (ECHO, Coxsackie), or metabolic disorder, or trichinosis.

Polymyositis Syndrome. This myopathy evolves rapidly within a few weeks but can develop over several days. Many patients have muscle tenderness and some have dysphagia. Accompanying symptoms, such as fever, Raynaud's phenomenon, and arthralgia, all further the diagnosis of polymyositis. Many infections, including trichinosis and toxoplasmosis, have been implicated. All the collagen vascular diseases have been associated with this condition. In approximately 10% of adults, predominantly males over the age of 50, polymyositis occurs as a paraneoplastic manifestation of an underlying carcinoma. Steroids may produce such a syndrome, though painless myopathy is more common. The diagnosis depends on the determination of elevated creatinine phosphokinase (CPK) and aldolase levels and is confirmed by a characteristic electromyogram and muscle biopsy. There is no specific emergency treatment for this condition, but appropriate diagnostic studies including CBC, erythrocyte sedimentation rate (ESR), serum magnesium, potassium, and calcium levels, and renal and thyroid function tests should be requested.

Polymyalgia Rheumatica. Polymyalgia rheumatica is a more painful condition than is polymyositis with prominent arthralgias or myalgias and less severe weakness. Temporal arteritis or cranial neuropathy can be present. The syndrome is difficult to distinguish from painful viral myopathies. ESR elevation is essential and overnight improvement with corticosteroids strengthens diagnostic suspicion. Recovery is gradual over many weeks or months.

Alcoholic Myopathy. Alcoholics are prone to a type of unique myopathic syndrome. During prolonged periods of heavy alcohol intake, a patient can experience severe muscle tenderness and swelling, muscle cramps, and rapid onset of weakness. The symptoms can be diffuse or focal. There is diffuse necrosis of skeletal muscle or acute rhabdomyolysis leading to life-threatening hyperkalemia, hypocalcemia, and hypophosphatemia with myoglobinuria resulting in renal failure. With acute muscle pain and weakness, determination of serum electrolyte levels and of muscle enzymes and urinalysis for myoglobin are necessary. No other specific intervention is indicated.

Neuromuscular Manifestations of Electrolyte and Metabolic Disorders. A metabolic screening of the blood is always indicated in patients with acute muscle weakness. The primary electrolytic disorders associated with profound weakness are hypokalemia, hypophosphatemia, hypercalcemia, and uremia, although hyponatremia and magnesium variations in either direction from normal also have been implicated (see myasthenic syndromes below). Fasciculations, cramps, myalgias, tetany, and myotonia have been reported with various metabolic derangements. Table 15.18 summarizes the clinical manifestations of skeletal muscle dysfunction in specific electrolytic disturbances. Early uremia is also characterized by cramps, fasciculations, muscle twitching, asterixis, and myoclonus or chorea.

Myasthenia Gravis

Myasthenia gravis is a condition marked by periodic weakness, or apparent paralysis, of voluntary musculature with preservation of deep tendon reflexes and pupillary responses. The disease is associated with the presence of antiacetylcholine receptor antibodies that block postsynaptic acetylcholine receptor sites. Myasthenia gravis affects extraocular muscles, bulbar muscles, and limb muscles either singly, in a group, or in any combination. Females are affected two to three times as commonly as males, with a peak female incidence in the third decade of life and a peak male incidence in the sixth and seventh decades. Ten to fifteen percent of myasthenic patients have a thymoma.

Diagnosis. The hallmark of the condition is fluctuation. Episodic weakness is brought on by fatigue or exertion, is improved with rest, and usually is worse later in the day. Bulbar musculature may be affected resulting in dysphagia and dysphonia. Weakness of facial muscles may lead to difficulty with lid closure and drooping of the jaw.

The diagnosis is suspected from the characteristic history and is confirmed by temporary improvement of the weakness after administration of an acetylcholinesterase inhibitor. An intravenous line is started and the patient is asked to exercise the suspected muscle group, i.e., to look up until ptosis develops or to grip until the hand fatigues. Then 1–2 mg of edrophonium (Tensilon) is injected over a period of 1 minute. Objective improvement accompanied by lacrimation, rhinorrhea, or abdominal cramping should start 20–30 seconds after the injection. If there is no change, an additional 8 mg is given over 2 minutes. Most patients require the entire 10-mg dose. Atropine should be available (0.5 mg) for immediate administration if bradycardia, hypotension, profound salivation, or fasciculations appear. An intramuscular injection of 1.5 mg of neostigmine with 0.5 mg of atropine to reverse the muscarinic symptoms has equivalent but longer lasting effects noticeable after a few minutes and persisting 3–4 hours.

If the diagnosis is suggested by the Tensilon test, the patient should have further studies including a chest radiograph, planar tomography or CT for thymoma, antiacetylcholine receptor antibody titers, thyroid function tests, ESR, antinuclear antibody test (ANA), and EMG with repetitive stimulation technique or with single fiber study.

The common precipitant of decompensation in a known myasthenic patient is respiratory tract infection. Patients may feel weaker before there are any manifestations of pulmonary infection. Generally, if a known myasthenic patient feels weaker, he or she should be hospitalized and infection should be suspected.

Treatment. Treatment of myasthenia gravis is with cholinergic drugs. Medication is usually started at a moderate dose of Mestinon (pyridostigmine bromide), 60 mg three times per day increasing gradually to 180 mg at 3-hour intervals. This is coupled with a 180-mg time-release capsule of Mestinon for overnight use. The maximum effect is seen in approximately 1 hour and lasts 2–6 hours. Neostigmine can be given in 30-mg doses three times per day with meals, but may range up to 60 mg every 3 hours.

Adjunctive medications, such as ephedrine, guanidine, and potassium chloride have been used to supplement the cholinergic medicines. Corticosteroids given initially under hospital conditions can be very useful in patients who are poorly controlled with maximum anticholinesterase drugs. Plasmapheresis (plasma exchange therapy) plays an increasing role in the management of myasthenic crisis. Many patients can be temporarily strengthened for surgical procedures or carried through a severe infection with this technique. For others, chronic periodic plasmapheresis every 3–4 weeks minimizes anticholinesterase and corticosteroid drug requirement. An established diagnosis of thymoma is an indication for thymectomy. Many experts believe that thymectomy is indicated in debilitating myasthenia that is poorly responsive to medical therapy.

Table 15.18.
Neuromuscular Manifestations of Electrolyte Abnormalities[a]

	Hypo-kalemia	Hyper-kalemia	Hypo-phospha-temia	Hypo-magne-semia	Hyper-magne-semia	Hypo-calcemia	Hyper-calcemia	Hypo-natremia	Hyper-natremia
Weakness	+ +	+	+ +	+	+	+	+ +	+	+
Paralysis	+	+	−	−	+	−	−	−	−
Myalgias	+	−	+	+	−	+	−	−	+
Fasciculations	+	+	+	+	−	+	−	+	−
Cramps	+	−	−	+	−	+	−	+	+
Restless legs	+	−	−	−	−	−	−	−	−
Tetany	−	−	−	+[b]		+	−	−	−
Myotonia	−	+[e]	−	−		−	−	−	−
Areflexia	+	+	+	−		−	−	−	−
Hyperreflexia	−	+	−	+		+	+	+	+
Choreoathetosis	−	−	−	+		−	−	−	−
Rhabdomyolysis	+	−	+	+[d]		−	−	+[e]	+

[a] From Knochel, JP. Neuromuscular manifestions of electrolyte disorders. *Am J Med,* 1982;72:521–533
[b] Indefinite, may be due to associated hypocalcemia.
[c] Myotonia may occur in familial hyperkalemic periodic paralysis.
[d] Experimental animals (dog, rat) only.
[e] Biochemical evidence only (CPK increase, creatinuria).

Cholinergic Crisis. Cholinergic crisis is due to depolarizing block from cholinergic drugs. The patient can gradually have increased the medication in response to an infection, and, while getting weaker, may have taken an inordinate dose of his or her cholinergic drugs. Weakness of the respiratory and bulbar muscles ensues with hypersecretion and bronchospasm. If the weakness in a myasthenic patient is attended by bronchospasm, bradycardia, hypotension, miosis, hypersalivation, and fasciculations, cholinergic excess can be suspected. Tensilon will not help the situation, but a rapid response can be seen with 1 mg of intravenous atropine. Cholinergic drugs are withheld for several days.

Differential Diagnosis. Toxins affecting the neuromuscular junction, such as botulism, have been discussed earlier in this chapter. A few other conditions simulate myasthenia gravis. The Eaton-Lambert syndrome is characterized by fluctuating weakness, recovery with rest, but also improvement after mild continuation of exercise. The cranial muscles are spared, though pharyngeal muscle weakness can be prominent. This condition is associated with occult carcinoma, usually small cell carcinoma of the lung. Therapy consists of guanidine hydrochloride. The condition does not usually improve with anticholinesterase medication. Steroids and azathioprine can be useful, however. Distinction between this syndrome and myasthenia gravis is made by EMG examination, since increment in motor unit action potential occurs on repetitive stimulation of a motor nerve in patients with Eaton-Lambert syndrome. Deep tendon reflexes are frequently depressed in this syndrome, whereas they are normal in myasthenia gravis.

Alterations in Magnesium Concentration. Alterations in magnesium concentration can profoundly affect neuromuscular transmission. *Hypermagnesemia* can cause symptoms ranging from diffuse weakness and areflexia to paralysis and coma. Magnesium salts used as cathartics or as antacids may raise the magnesium level. Usually, decreased renal excretion of magnesium is required, in addition to ingestion of magnesium salts, to achieve sufficient elevation of magnesium level to produce neuromuscular problems. Thus, patients with renal failure receiving antacids or cathartics are most often affected, although magnesium therapy for eclampsia has produced hypermagnesemia in both mother and child. Magnesium blocks neuromuscular transmission by interfering with calcium-dependent presynaptic release of acetylcholine and by decreasing postsynaptic sensitivity to acetylcholine. The paralytic effect can be reversed by administering calcium, by reducing serum magnesium levels, or by increasing acetylcholine effectiveness with acetylcholinesterase inhibitors. For magnesium elevation with mild neuromuscular symptoms, discontinuation of the offending magnesium source should suffice. Emergency therapy includes administration of calcium salts and glucose (100 gm) with 20 units of insulin in 1 liter of water to increase intracellular magnesium flux.

Magnesium deficiency occurs with diuretic use, hyperaldosteronism, sprue, diabetic acidosis, and in regional ileitis and colitis where magnesium is lost in gastrointestinal fluids. Excessive vomiting, administration of parenteral fluids and mechanical suctioning can cause magnesium depletion. Alcoholic patients characteristically develop hypomagnesemia because of poor dietary intake and gastrointestinal loss from malabsorption and vomiting. Delirium tremens and withdrawal convulsions, however, may develop despite magnesium replacement therapy.

The clinical picture of magnesium deficiency ranges from diffuse hyperreflexia, fasciculations, cramping, and myocolonic jerks to altered personality, confusion, and seizures. Chvostek's and Trousseau's signs may be present. Very low magnesium levels with profound neurologic symptoms should be treated with 2 gm (16.2 mEq) of magnesium sulfate intravenously over 2 hours (administered as a 0.4% solution in 5% glucose). Oral magnesium replacement can begin with 3 gm daily, given as a 4% solution in orange juice.

Neurologic Complications of Drug Therapy

Many medications used in the treatment of medical illnesses can have adverse effects on the central and peripheral nervous system. Drugs causing seizures, peripheral neuropathy, pseudotumor cerebri, myopathies, and delirium are covered elsewhere in this chapter and in Chapter 16. Although there is no room for extensive discussion of drug interactions, this section summarizes other drugs that provoke neurologic symptoms or exacerbate preexisting neurologic disorders.

Vestibular and Ototoxicity

Many antibiotics, including virtually all the aminoglycoside drugs, can cause cochlear or vestibular dysfunction. Table 15.19 summarizes the relative cochlear and vestibular toxicity of these drugs. Improvement can be expected when the drug is discontinued, but some permanent damage can remain. Other drugs known to cause hearing loss are aspirin and cisplatinum.

Table 15.19.
Drugs Affecting VIIIth Nerve Function[a]

Drug	Cochlear Toxicity	Vestibular Toxicity
Kanamycin	+ + +	+
Amikacin	+ + + +	
Neomycin	+ + +	+
Streptomycin	+	+ + +
Gentamicin	+	+ + +
Tobramycin	+	+ + +
Vancomycin	+ + + +	
Ethacrynic acid	+ + +	+
Furosemide	+ + + +	
Quinine	+ + + +	
Minocycline		+ + + +
Aspirin	+ + +	
Cisplatinum	+ + + +	

[a] + + + +, maximum toxicity; +, minimum toxicity.

Movement Disorders

Movement disorders can be brought on by a number of medications. *Tremor* is caused by lithium, aminophylline, terbutaline, valproic acid, moxalactam, methylphenidate, phenytoin (both cerebellar action tremor and asterixis/myoclonus), and carbamazepine. *Chorea* can be seen with methadone, oral contraceptives, phenytoin, and L-dopa. *Dystonias* can be produced by phenothiazines, butyrophenones, L-dopa, and α-methyldopa. *Orofacial dyskinesias* are also associated with antihistamines, phenytoin, methylphenidate, and tricyclic antidepressants. Both choreiform movements and tardive dyskinesia with exacerbation of Parkinson's disease have been reported from use of metoclopramide.

Several patients have developed chronic severe Parkinson's disease after repeatedly injecting themselves with 1-methyl-4-phenyl-1,2,3,6-tetrahydropyridine (MPTP) intravenously. The compound is a biproduct of the synthesis of a meperidine analogue. Levodopa and bromocriptine can control the symptoms, but many patients experienced dyskinesias or on-off fluctuations. The neurotoxic effects of MPTP seemed limited to the substantia nigra.

Myasthenic Syndromes

Myasthenic syndromes in previously nonmyasthenic patients have been induced by neomycin, streptomycin, kanamycin, polymyxin, bacitracin, dihydrostreptomycin, colistin, tobramycin, and amikacin. Penicillin, bacitracin, chloramphenicol, and tetracycline also have weak neuromuscular blocking effects, but the clinical problems induced by these agents are not as severe as those produced by the first group. Synergism with hypokalemia, hypocalcemia, and neuromuscular blocking agents, such as succinylcholine and decamethonium, is usually required for the complete effect. The route of administration of drug seems to matter very little in the production of myasthenia. Lithium, mysoline, and penicillamine can cause neuromuscular transmission defects resembling myasthenia.

Myasthenic patients are susceptible to all of the above drugs, and choice of antibiotic medication is a difficult one for some of these patients. In patients known to have myasthenia gravis, quinine, quinidine, phenytoin, procainamide, propranolol and other β blockers, thiotepa, nitrogen mustard, corticosteroids, and thyroid hormone have all been reported to worsen the condition.

SUGGESTED READINGS

Aminoff MR, Simon RP. Status epilepticus: Causes, clinical features and consequences in 98 patients. *Am J Med,* 1980;69:637–666.

Ausman JI. Vertebrobasilar insufficiency: A review. *Arch Neurol,* 1985;42:803–808.

Cerebral Embolism Task Force. Cardiogenic brain embolism. *Arch Neurol,* 1986;43:71–84.

Chambers BP, Norris JW. Outcome in patients with asymptomatic neck bruits. *N Engl J Med,*1986;315:860–865.

Hauser, WD. Seizure recurrence after a first unprovoked seizure. *N Engl J Med,* 1982;307:522–528.

Kistler JP, Ropper AH. Therapy of ischemic cerebrovascular disease. *N Engl J Med,* 1984;311:27–34, 100–105.

Marton, KI, Gean AAD. The spinal tap: A new look at an old test. *Ann Intern Med,* 1986;104:840–848.

Medical Research Council of the United Kingdom. *Aids to the Diagnosis of Peripheral Nerve Injuries.* 3rd ed. Palo Alto, CA: Pendragon House, 1976.

Messing RO, Classor RG, Simon RP. Drug-induced seizures: a 10-year experience. *Neurology,* 1984;34:1582–1586.

Patten J, *Neurologic Differential Diagnosis.* New York: Springer-Verlag, 1978.

Ramirez-Lassepas, M. Value of computed tomographic scan in the evaluation of adult patients after their first seizure. *Ann Neurol,* 1984;15:536–543.

CHAPTER **16**

Approach to the Patient with Altered Consciousness

AMY A. PRUITT, M.D.

Editor's note: This chapter supplements the preceding chapter on neurologic emergencies by presenting a systematic approach to the patient with any alteration in state of consciousness. It thus concentrates on one very troublesome aspect of neurology and psychiatry for the emergency physician: the approach to the delirious or comatose patient.

Patients with acutely altered mental status present the physician with an array of medical, neurologic, and psychiatric diseases that challenge his or her emergency diagnostic and therapeutic skills. More than 10% of patients admitted for medical and surgical problems have a component of confusion superimposed on their illness, and conversely, 18% of patients seen in psychiatric outpatient settings have a medical illness that explains a significant part of their psychiatric problem. The accurate triage of such patients can mean the difference between successful reversal of the impairment and permanent neurologic damage. This chapter presents a general emergency department approach to confused, agitated, stuporous, and comatose patients and offers a multidisciplinary differential diagnosis of delirium and coma.

DELIRIUM

Presentation

The confused patient is brought to the hospital because he or she is behaving inappropriately. Delirium is defined as a clouding of consciousness with reduced awareness of the environment. Prominent alterations in arousal and attention are the hallmarks: the patient may alternate between hyperalert agitation and somnolence. Frequently worse at night, perceptual disturbances with hallucinations or misinterpretations are common. The patient may have increased or decreased psychomotor activity. These fluctuating features develop over minutes to a few days.

Certain patients are more susceptible to delirium, such as elderly patients, alcohol and other drug abusers, and patients with structural brain damage. Situations in which delirium is likely to develop include sleep deprivation, psychologic stress, sensory deprivations, drug changes, and seemingly trivial alterations in metabolic balance. The recognition of delirium should alert the examiner to begin a thorough medical evaluation, *since delirium is most often due to a primary problem outside the central nervous system.*

Differential Diagnosis

The differential diagnosis of delirium includes an extensive list of medical illnesses, a small group of psychiatric conditions, and a limited number of structural neurologic defects (Table 16.1).

"Medical" Delirium

Medical delirium has the largest number of causes. The apparent neurologic nature of the presentation should not fool the physician into neglecting basic cardiopulmonary and metabolic examination. Hypothermia or hyperthermia may be sufficient to greatly disorient an elderly patient and may indicate sepsis. Similarly, hypoperfusion states with diminished cerebral blood flow due to a new myocardial infarction or cardiac arrhythmia may masquerade primarily as agitation rather than somnolence. Hypertensive encephalopathy with raised intracranial pressure may do the same.

A comprehensive list of metabolic abnormalities producing delirium would include every metabolic

Table 16.1.
Causes of Delirium

Medical delirium
- Altered temperature
- Hypoxia, hypercapnia
- Hypoperfusion—new myocardial infarct, slower heart rate
- Hypertensive encephalopathy
- Hypoglycemia
- Electrolyte imbalance
  - Hypernatremia, hyperosmolar states
  - Hyponatremia
  - Hypercalcemia
- Endocrine imbalance
  - Hyperthyroidism
  - Hypothyroidism
  - Addisonian crisis
  - Cushing's syndrome
- Organ failure
  - Liver
  - Kidney
- Deficiency states
  - Thiamine—Wernicke's encephalopathy
- Drugs
  - Anticholinergics
  - Barbiturates, opiates, sedative-hypnotics
  - Alcohol
  - Amphetamines, cocaine
  - Carbidopa-Levodopa (Sinemet)
  - Zomax
  - Cimetidine
  - Lithium
  - Withdrawal syndromes

Psychiatric delirium
- Acute manic states
- Acute schizophreniform psychoses
- Hysteria
- Homosexual panic
- Ganser's syndrome

Neurologic delirium
- Postictal states
- Psychomotor status epilepticus
- Postconcussive states
- Posthypoperfusion states
- Subarachnoid hemorrhage with acute hydrocephalus
- Infection
  - Encephalitis (herpes simplex)
  - Meningitis (viral, bacterial, tuberculous)
- Vascular syndromes
  - Nondominant parietal lobe infarct
  - Mesial occipital or temporal cortex infarct
  - Aphasia
    - Wernicke's encephalopathy
    - Transcortical motor and sensory
  - Transient global amnesia
- Mass lesions
  - Tumor
  - Abscess
  - Subdural hematoma

imbalance known, but the most common offending conditions are hypoglycemia, hyperglycemia, electrolyte imbalances, and organ failure with ammoniemia or hyperuricemia. In all these cases, rapid development of the metabolic abnormality results in a more florid presentation of central nervous system dysfunction, sometimes including seizures.

Although other vitamin deficiencies such as niacin and B_{12} deficiencies may produce delirious states, the most common deficiency that causes delirium is diminished thiamine reserve in alcoholic and malnourished patients. This critical syndrome is characterized by acute or subacute onset of confusion, nystagmus, oculomotor palsies (usually bilateral abducens palsies), and variable ataxia. Even if the syndrome is not seen on initial examination, it may be precipitated by a glucose load. Thus, in the emergency setting, any patient suspected to have thiamine deficiency should be given parenteral thiamine, 100 mg, before being given glucose. A smaller dose of thiamine may be sufficient to relieve the ocular symptoms, but the above dose with continued supplementation is advisable to prevent development of the irreversible memory deficit known as Korsakoff's syndrome.

The drugs causing delirium are listed in Table 16.1. Major offenders include drugs with central and peripheral anticholinergic properties, such as scopolamine, tricyclic antidepressants, antihistamines, phenothiazines, butyrophenones, and antidiarrheal compounds such as Donnagel and Lomotil. Peripheral signs of these drugs are mydriasis, tachycardia, urinary retention, fever, ileus, and dry mouth; central signs include hallucinations, ataxia, dysarthria, and myoclonus. Acute confusion and peripheral side effects may be reduced by administration of physostigmine, which should not be given in the presence of coronary artery disease, hyperthyroidism, bronchial asthma, or peptic ulcer. Administration of physostigmine results in lacrimation, salivation, and rhinorrhea. The acute dystonias seen with phenothiazines and butyrophenones such as haloperidol (Haldol) may be rapidly reversed by intravenous administration of benztropine mesylate (Cogentin) or diphenhydramine hydrochloride (Benadryl).

Barbiturates, opiates, and sedative-hypnotic agents are less likely to cause a delirious state, but paradoxical reactions may occur. An excited, hyperalert state, often with headache, tachypnea, and dysesthesias, may be seen with cocaine ingestion, and a similar state is produced by amphetamines. Withdrawal syndromes from any of the above medications may produce confusion, mydriasis, tachycardia, or seizures. The examiner should carefully take an ingestion history, looking particularly for medications with a long half-life (''tranquilizers'' such as diazepam (Valium) and chlordiazepoxide hydrochloride). Of particular importance is alcohol withdrawal, alcohol being the most commonly abused drug in most emergency department presentations. Peaking at 12–24 hours after the last ingestion, withdrawal is marked by restlessness, tremors, and confusion with auditory and visual hallucinations. Actual seizures may occur in this same time interval and the patient may have a quiet, oriented period between the "rum fits" and full-blown delirium tremens.

A final reminder: the physician can never be too thorough in taking a medication history. Particularly in the organically impaired brain, very small changes in medication or very low doses of sedative-hypnotic agents may be sufficient to alter mental status.

"Psychiatric" Delirium

Psychiatric delirium is a component of a smaller but equally difficult group of diagnoses. The hallmarks of psychiatric disease in this setting include inconsistencies in the mental status examination, with some high-level responses or consistently abnormal responses indicating that the patient has some understanding of the question. There may be highly variable performance, and the patient may have auditory rather than visual hallucinations. Ganser's syndrome is a denial of specific events, usually with the intent of avoiding prosecution. Several psychiatric medications, including lithium and tricyclic antidepressants, can be associated with tremors, agitation, and in some cases, seizures.

"Neurologic" Delirium

The group of neurologic disorders causing delirium is relatively small. Immediately after a seizure, patients may be confused, amnesic, and extremely agitated. Progressive improvement should occur over several hours. Psychomotor status epilepticus has been confused with psychiatric disease; its hallmarks are a trance-like appearance, rhythmic move-

Table 16.2.
Emergency Mini Mental Status Examination

Procedure	Abnormalities and Significance
Describe the patient's condition Include level of consciousness, coherence of speech, and types of movement (purposeful, asterixis, tremor) ?Hallucinations	Establishes baseline
Ask about orientation	Disorientation to person implies psychiatric disease
Test attention[a] Digit span—recite numbers in monotone and have patient repeat immediately; recite random letters, asking patient to raise a hand every time you say certain letters	Normal = 7 digits forward, 5 backward
Test short-term memory Ask patient to memorize three to five objects and ask him 5–10 minutes later to repeat them	Selective disturbance of new memory Postictal, postconcussive states, transient global amnesia, temporal infarction, herpes simplex encephalitis
Test long-term memory Ask about remote historical or biographic events	Tests general level of intelligence/education and may indicate acute deterioration
Test object-naming ability Ask patient to identify several objects in room, including body parts	Specific nominal aphasia seen with left temporooccipital defects Word salad in Wernicke's aphasia to be distinguished from schizophrenic speech Echolalia to be distinguished from transcortical aphasia Look for associated visual field defects.
Test ability to draw simple objects: square, star, cube, house	Tests right hemisphere function

[a] If patient is unable to perform these tests, it is unlikely he or she will be able to perform subsequent tests.

ments of the tongue or lips, and repetitive, often complex stereotypical movements. Intravenous administration of diazepam may abruptly reverse the abnormality and clarify the situation. The classic temporal lobe features of disagreeable odor or lip smacking may be seen in patients without a history of seizures who have acute herpes simplex encephalitis.

Focal signs may be absent in many neurologic disorders. Posttraumatic confusion and confusion after an episode of hypoxic or ischemic injury should be suspected with the appropriate history. Steady improvement is expected, and deterioration should raise suspicion of epidural, subdural, or intracerebral hematoma. The sudden onset of hydrocephalus from a subarachnoid hemorrhage or third ventricular tumor may also be unaccompanied by headache or focal signs.

Neurologic syndromes with focal deficits indicating the underlying cause are predominantly vascular, although patients are occasionally seen who have a frontal or temporal lobe mass with an acutely altered mental state independent of seizure activity. Specific vascular syndromes are listed in Table 16.1. Right middle cerebral artery disease with nondominant parietal lobe infarction may result in agitation and concomitant left-sided weakness with inattention to the deficit. However, denial of illness occurs frequently in delirious patients. Similarly, although many delirious patients have word-finding difficulty, mesial occipital and temporal cortex infarction, particularly on the dominant side, may result in inability to form new memories and in localizing symptoms of nominal aphasia and homonymous hemianopsia. Fluent aphasias may produce difficult diagnostic dilemmas, since schizophrenic speech must be distinguished from the "word salad" of Wernicke's aphasia or the echolalia of transcortical aphasia. A careful screen for primarily verbal problems (Table 16.2) should separate patients with a focal lesion from those without a focal deficit who may have some word-finding difficulty as part of the delirious state. Transient global amnesia is a syndrome of complete inability to form new memories that may last up to several hours. This may be a symptom of basilar artery insufficiency, or it may occur after head trauma or seizures.

A final word of caution concerning the differential diagnosis of delirium: *there frequently may be more than one reason for the delirious state.* Thus, a patient with Wernicke's encephalopathy may also be withdrawing from alcohol and may have ceased to eat and drink because of an infection or a subdural hematoma. A patient with seizures may fail to waken rapidly because of anoxic damage suffered during the seizure, and a patient with a markedly altered mental state with apparently trivial medication change or metabolic alteration may harbor an underlying dementia or other structural neurologic problem.

Evaluation

History

The confused patient frequently has little insight into the problem, and often a relevant history must be obtained from bystanders. Points of immediate significance include: (*a*) mode of onset, whether abrupt or insidious; (*b*) history of trauma; (*c*) history of cerebrovascular or cardiovascular disease (*d*) history of underlying metabolic disease such as diabetes or renal failure; (*e*) history of seizures; (*f*) use of anticoagulants or presence of coagulopathy; (*g*) likelihood of intoxication or a suicide attempt (psychiatric history); and (*h*) knowledge of any complaint in the days or weeks preceding the illness such as headache, loss of balance, depression, visual disturbance, or memory loss.

Examination

The delirious state can be assessed quickly with a "mini" mental status examination. Excellent expanded versions are available, but Table 16.2 allows quantitation of the degree of the disturbance and aids in the triage of the medical, psychiatric, and neurologic causes of delirium, providing a hemispheric localization for the last.

The mental status examination can be performed only in patients whose level of attention permits it. A wide variety of focal neurologic findings should not be expected in metabolic delirium, and aphasia, apraxia, or memory disturbance should raise suspicion of a focal deficit. Isolated inability to form new memories in patients who do not appear agitated or confused may indicate Korsakoff's syndrome. Inconsistent performance should raise the suspicion of psychiatric delirium.

The general physical and neurologic examination of the delirious or comatose patient is directed toward distinguishing between medical and neurologic diseases. Unlike in the comatose patient, some tests such as visual field testing can also be included.

Treatment

Emergency therapeutic maneuvers depend on assessment of the underlying cause for the altered mental state. General principles dictate a calm approach to the confused patient. A family member or other familiar person should be present with the patient in a well-lighted environment. Minimal restraint should be used, if possible, and the examination should be conducted at a pace that does not frustrate the patient. Sedation should be avoided until the underlying problem is evident. Electrolyte determinations and other metabolic studies should be performed early, and thiamine may be administered without harmful effects. If initial examination suggests a focal deficit or if the patient has a history of trauma, computed tomography (CT) without contrast enhancement should be performed to look for hematoma or edema. Although sedation is undesirable, it may be necessary to obtain a high-quality scan. Lumbar puncture is required in all but a few settings. If there is a clear metabolic problem such as hypoglycemia and if the patient appears to be improving rapidly with correction of the abnormality, or if a patient with a known seizure disorder was witnessed to have a seizure and is improving rapidly, lumbar puncture may be omitted. Even if alcohol ingestion has been established, lumbar puncture should be considered, to rule out infection. Repetitive seizures or psychomotor status epilepticus can be stopped with intravenous diazepam, 5 mg every 5–10 minutes with respiratory support on hand. Long-acting anticonvulsant agents should be started simultaneously (see Chapter 15). Acute psychiatric management is discussed in Chapter 18; antipsychotic agents with sedative properties such as chlorpromazine (Thorazine) may be useful in many agitated patients as soon as the type of disease underlying the altered mental state has been determined.

COMA

At the other end of the spectrum from the hyperalert, delirious patient is the person who over a period of minutes to days has become sleepy but rousable (stuporous) or unrousable (comatose). Perhaps even more than in the case of the delirious patient, rapid action is essential. The physician requires a systematic approach to focus actions quickly and effectively.

Neuroanatomy

Whereas the list of diseases leading to coma is lengthy (Table 16.3), the neuroanatomic variations in altered consciousness are few. For any pathologic process to cause coma, it must produce bilateral dysfunction of the cerebral hemispheres either structurally or metabolically *or* it must damage the reticular activating system in the upper brainstem and diencephalon, again either structurally or metabolically. Thus, supratentorial lesions, infratenorial lesions, and metabolic processes may all lead to coma.

Table 16.4 summarizes the anatomic areas whose dysfunction leads to coma and indicates the appropriate terminology. Finally, psychiatric unresponsiveness should be considered a fourth cause of "coma."

Table 16.3.
Causes of Coma

- Outside the central nervous system
  - Metabolic causes
    - Hypoxia
      - Cardiopulmonary disease
      - Carbon monoxide poisoning
    - Ischemia
      - Decreased cerebral blood flow due to myocardial infarction, congestive heart failure, pulmonary disease, hyperviscosity
    - Hypoglycemia
    - Hepatic failure
    - Renal failure
    - Hypothyroidism
    - Adrenal insufficiency
    - Acid-base or electrolyte imbalance
      - Hyponatremia, hypernatremia
      - Acidosis, alkalosis
      - Hypercalcemia
      - Hypophosphatemia
      - Hypermagnesemia, hypomagnesemia
    - Hypothermia, hyperthermia
  - Exogenous poisons
    - Barbiturates, opiates, alcohol, tranquilizers, bromides
    - Psychotropic agents
      - Tricyclic antidepressants
      - Lithium
      - LSD
    - Heavy metals
    - Organic phosphates
  - Infection
    - Meningitis
    - Encephalitis
- Within the central nervous system
  - Supratentorial lesions
    - Hemorrhage, traumatic and nontraumatic
      - Subdural, epidural
      - Intracerebral (lobar)
      - Basal ganglia (putamen, thalamus)
      - Intraventricular
      - Subarachnoid
    - Infarction
      - Middle cerebral occlusion with edema or hemorrhage or both
    - Tumor
    - Abscess
  - Infratentorial lesions
    - Hemorrhage
      - Cerebellar
      - Pontine
      - Posterior fossa (subdural, epidural)
    - Infarction
      - Basilar thrombosis
      - Cerebellar infarction with edema
    - Posterior fossa tumor
    - Posterior fossa abscess
    - Demyelinating disease
    - Basilar migraine

Table 16.4.
Relationship of Neuroanatomy to Coma

Damaged Site	Resulting State
Cortex	
Bilateral cerebral hemispheres	Coma (metabolic, structural)
Frontal lobes	Abulia, akinetic mutism
Unilateral hemispheric lesion plus edema or hemorrhage	Early local signs leading to coma
Brainstem/diencephalon	
Hypothalamus	Hypersomnia
Brainstem reticular formation	Coma
Basis pontis	Locked-in or "de-efferented" state: patient awake but unable to respond

Differential Diagnosis

Initial diagnosis depends on the integration of available history and physical data to place the cause of coma into one of the general categories just discussed. This will lead to effective initial emergency treatment. Using laboratory and radiologic data, the emergency physician can then make a more specific diagnosis.

Supratentorial lesions are usually accompanied by early signs and symptoms of focal cerebral dysfunction. Motor signs may be asymmetric, or the observer's history may suggest focal dysfunction at an early stage. Thus, the patient with an expanding right subdural hematoma will have early left hemiparesis followed by altered consciousness as both hemispheres are affected. As pointed out in Table 16.4, unilateral hemispheric disease alone is insufficient to cause coma. A patient with a large left middle cerebral infarct may be densely aphasic and hemiplegic, but is not comatose. Later deterioration in level of consciousness may be due to hemorrhage into the infarcted area or to edema caused by ischemic cell death.

Infratentorial lesions lead to more rapid onset of coma. The patient may briefly experience headache, vertigo, nausea, vomiting, diplopia, or other brainstem symptoms before losing consciousness. Localizing brainstem signs such as cranial nerve palsies and oculovestibular abormalities may accompany coma. Unusual respiratory patterns such as hyperventilation or extremely irregular breathing are characteristic.

Metabolic causes of coma are heralded by more gradual progression from confusion or delirium through stupor to coma. Pupillary reactions may be preserved (unless a drug effect is present), and abnormal (symmetric) motor findings, such as asterixis, myoclonus, and tremor, may be seen. There may be increased ventilation (due to hypoxia or acidosis) or hypoventilation.

Psychogenic unresponsiveness is characterized by preserved pupillary reactions, active lid closure, nystagmus with caloric stimulation, normal motor tone, normal deep tendon reflexes, and either normal ventilation or hyperventilation.

Examination

The goal of physical examination is to determine which type of coma is present. The *general examination* seeks to establish a metabolic or infectious origin of the coma, and the *neurologic examination* attempts to characterize the type of intracranial abnormality leading to the comatose state.

Table 16.5 summarizes the sequence of the physical examination in the comatose patient. The patient is observed for signs of shock, metabolic derangement, or sepsis. The neurologic examination then attempts to sort out neurosurgical emergencies and to separate brainstem disease from bilateral cerebral hemispheric disease. The patient is quickly observed for level of responsiveness and rousability. Assessment of eyes and pupils then localizes the lesion within the brainstem. A problem in diagnosis is failure of the pupils to react, caused by mydriatic agents such as atropine, glutethimide, or other anticholinergics. Pinpoint, barely reactive pupils are seen both in pontine dysfunction and in opiate overdose.

Spontaneous eye movements and resting position offer many clues to localization. Skew deviation of the eyes can arise from an intraaxial brainstem lesion or from a compressive lesion in the posterior fossa. More specific clues to the level of brainstem dysfunction in the unresponsive patient are obtained by irrigating the external canals with ice water. In the comatose patient, intact brainstem function is indicated by conjugate deviation of the eyes toward the irrigated ear. Dysconjugate responses to caloric stimulation should suggest an infratentorial cause of coma. When eye movements and pupillary movements are disproportionately preserved compared with level of function, metabolic coma is likely. Observation of nystagmus with a cold water irrigation indicates either light stupor or an awake patient (who will be very nauseated).

Spontaneous movement indicates the patient's level of responsiveness, as well as laterality. Reflex movements to noxious stimuli may fall into recognizable patterns: extension of all limbs is consistent with decerebration, and flexion of arms with extension of legs indicates decortication. Asymmetries of tone should be recorded, and adventitial movements such as tremor or myoclonus suggest a metabolic origin. Deep tendon reflexes give further evidence of laterality.

The abbreviated neurologic examination outlined in Table 16.5 should provide the examiner with an idea of which part of the brain has malfunctioned. The physical examination should also give the physician a sense of the pace of the disease. The examiner should be aware of progressive signs warning of incipient herniation. The syndrome of *uncal herniation* results from intracranial lesions in the temporal lobe or lateral part of the cranium. Unilateral dilatation of the pupil from oculomotor nerve compression occurs early in the patient's course. Impaired consciousness is not necessarily present at

Table 16.5.
Physical Examination of the Comatose Patient

General examination: Is there an extracranial cause for the coma?

Observations	*Abnormalities and significance*
Vital signs	Hypotension: shock, sepsis Hyperthermia: tricyclics, lithium, monoamine oxidase inhibitors, sepsis Hypothermia: phenothiazines, exposure, alcohol, myxedema
Head	Evidence of trauma, odor of alcohol, old burr holes
Eyes	Papilledema
Skin	Shock, needle tracks, hepatic disease, bleeding disorders, suicide attempts, endocarditis
Cardiopulmonary evaluation	Shock, arrhythmia, pneumothorax, pneumonia
Abdomen	Acute abdominal event precipitating shock

Neurologic examination: Is this a neurosurgical emergency? Is coma due to brainstem disease or to bilateral cerebral hemispheric disease?

	General description
Responsiveness	Occasional appropriate verbal response Garbled speech No speech
Arousal	Opens eyes to voice Opens eyes to gentle stimulation Opens eyes to noxious stimulation No response Brainstem assessment

Observations	*Abnormalities and significance*
Pupillary reaction	
Equal and reactive	Likely metabolic cause for coma
Large, often fixed	Midbrain dysfunction or mydriatics
Pinpoint	Pontine dysfunction
Fixed, dilated	Medullary dysfunction or mydriatics
Spontaneous eye position and movements	Skew deviation: posterior fossa
Oculovestibular testing with warm and cool or ice water (check eardrums)	Dysconjugate response: infratentorial lesion
Corneas	Unilateral loss: infratentorial lesion
Respiratory pattern	Hyperventilation: acidosis, hypoxia, pontine disease, psychogenic origin Cheyne-Stokes: supratentorial or metabolic
Motor assessment	
Check tone, spontaneous movements—myoclonus, seizures, opisthotonos, swallowing, chewing	Lateralization: supratentorial origin, suggest metabolic low-level function
Blinking	Pons intact
Yawning, sneezing	Light coma
Deep tendon reflexes	Lateralization: supratentorial origin

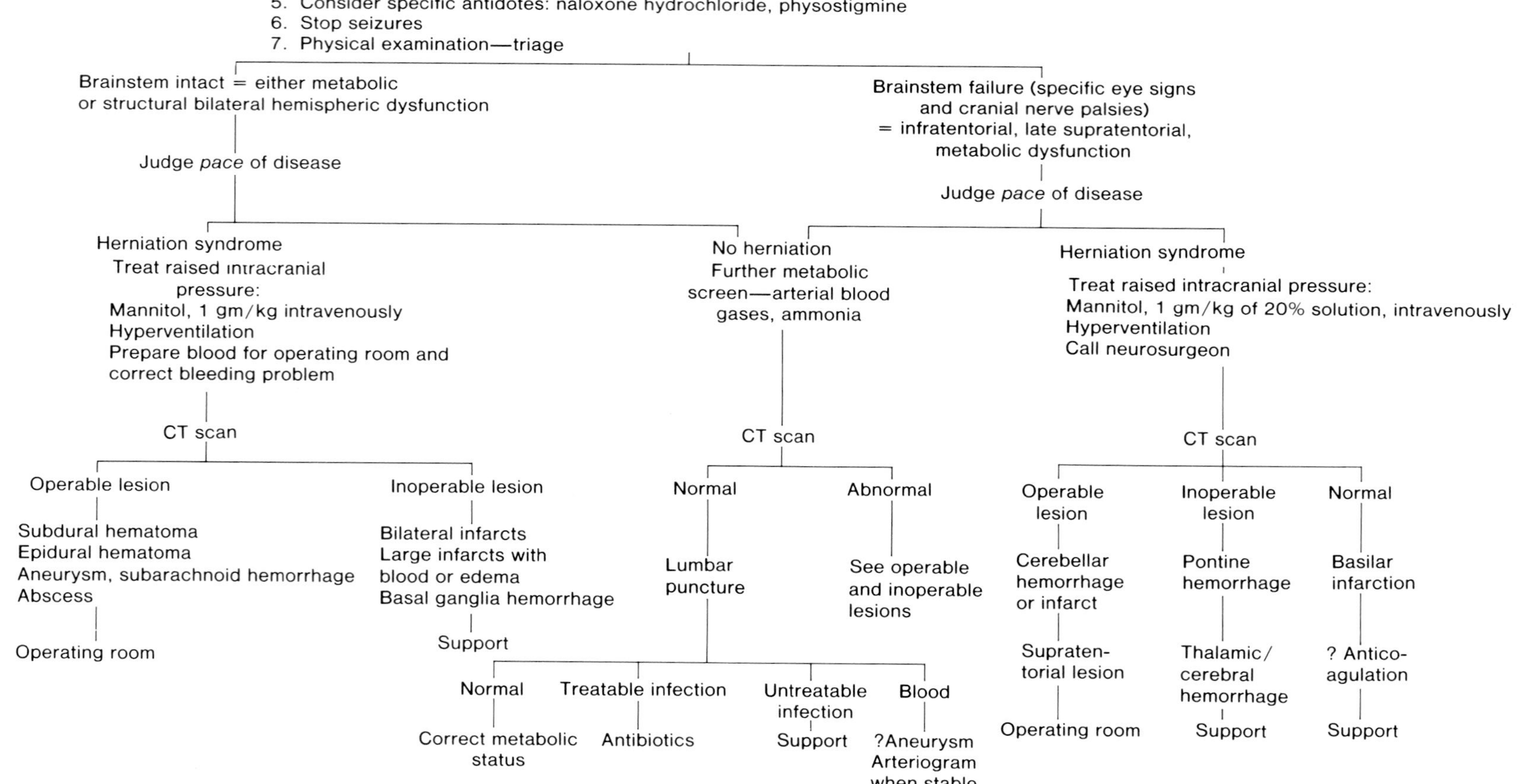

Figure 16.1. Schema (algorithm) of steps in triage/treatment of the comatose patient.

this stage, but motor signs will then appear, frequently with ipsilateral hemiparesis due to compression of the cerebral peduncle against the tentorium. Signs of brainstem compression then develop rapidly.

The *central herniation* syndrome results from more medial supratentorial lesions. Unlike in uncal herniation, drowsiness occurs early as a result of direct pressure on the diencephalon from above. Respiration may be the Cheyne-Stokes pattern. Eye movements are full, pupils small and reactive, and motor signs possibly bilateral. With progression, level of consciousness decreases, respiration rate increases, pupils become midsized and unreactive, and decerebration may be observed, which then gives way to flaccidity with ataxic respirations in the medullary stage. *The early stage of the central herniation syndrome may be mistaken for metabolic coma with drowsiness, periodic respirations, and preserved eye movements.*

Treatment

The physician may have to perform several steps of the evaluation at once. While obtaining a history from family or friends, he or she must begin general supportive measures and carry out the examination that will lead to definitive therapy. Figure 16.1 summarizes the steps in initial emergency support and triage based on the physical examination.

Brainstem failure with incipient herniation is the most critical situation. The patient should be given mannitol, 1 gm/kg of 20% solution intravenously, followed by intubation and hyperventilation to decrease cerebral blood flow. Dexamethasone, 20 mg intravenously, may be given in addition, although its effects will not begin for several hours. A neurosurgeon may need to place a burr hole on the side of the dilating pupil in patients with uncal herniation before CT scanning. A CT scan without contrast enhancement should be obtained immediately. Potentially operable lesions include cerebellar hemorrhage and infarction. The former is usually seen in the setting of systemic hypertension or anticoagulation. Hallmarks are sudden occipital headache, nausea, vomiting, dizziness, and difficulty walking. Similar although usually less acute findings occur with ischemic infarction, which later can compress the contents of the posterior fossa and compromise brainstem function. Since it is virtually impossible to distinguish intraaxial brainstem lesions, such as stroke, from compressive lesions, such as cerebellar hemorrhage, or from late compressive effects of supratentorial lesions, the patient should be treated for a compressive lesion because these processes are potentially reversible. If the patient has a fluctuating ischemic deficit in the basilar territory, immediate anticoagulant therapy with heparin should be considered and blood pressure should be kept at adequate levels to assure perfusion.

If the brainstem is intact (eye movements, pupils, and oculovestibular movements preserved), the examiner should judge the pace of deterioration. A potential hazard at this point in the evaluation is that, in the early stages of central herniation, the patient may appear to be in metabolic coma. If there is no clear reason to suspect metabolic coma, the examiner should proceed as if treating raised intracranial pressure. If there is reason to suspect a coagulation disturbance, the patient should be given vitamin K, 10 mg intramuscularly, and fresh-frozen plasma and typed blood should be made available for use in the operating room. A CT scan should then be obtained. Operable lesions such as subdural hematoma or epidural hematoma should be treated immediately. Acute obstructive hydrocephalus can be relieved and abscesses drained. Inoperable lesions resulting in supratentorial coma include bilateral cerebral infarcts, large unilateral infarcts with edema or blood, and basal ganglia hemorrhages (see Chapter 37).

If herniation is not imminent, the examiner has more time to obtain further metabolic screening information. If data are unrevealing, a CT scan should be obtained. CT scanning will frequently reveal blood in subarachnoid hemorrhage and may give information about the location of an arteriovenous malformation or aneurysm. If findings are normal, a lumbar puncture should be performed to rule out treatable infection. Lumbar puncture should be a primary diagnostic procedure in coma only when infection is suspected. If CT scanning is unavailable in the emergency department, arteriography or ultrasound studies should be performed if raised intracranial pressure is suspected.

At this point in the evaluation, all structural causes of coma should be excluded and any infection discovered, with laboratory studies in process that will reveal the metabolic abnormality in need of correction. In many cases, it is impossible to be sure of the diagnosis after examination alone. Late stages of any supratentorial or infratentorial lesion result in brainstem failure. Similarly, early stages of central herniation may mimic metabolic coma. In no patient in whom a structural lesion is suspected should a CT scan be omitted because of absence of focal signs, nor should any of the initial resuscitative and general support measures listed at the top of Figure 16.1 be omitted, no matter how focal the findings.

Some statistics may be useful for the emergency physician to remember as he or she begins examination and treatment of the comatose patient: of 500 consecutive patients with coma treated at New York Hospital, 326 had a metabolic cause, 101 had supratentorial lesions, 65 had infratentorial lesions, and 8 had psychogenic unresponsiveness. Attention to examination and careful supportive therapy at each step should allow appropriate triage of each patient and should maximize the possibility of successful recovery from this life-threatening situation.

SUGGESTED READINGS

McEvoy JP. Organic brain syndromes in DSM-III (letter). *Am J Psychiatr,* 1981;138:124–125.

Strub RL, Black FW. The Mental Status Examination in Neurology. Philadelphia: F.A. Davis Co., 1977.

CHAPTER 17

Toxicologic Emergencies

PETER L. GROSS, M.D.

Acute poisoning is a common medical emergency requiring rapid assessment and well-organized treatment. A successful outcome depends on (*a*) appropriate application of basic management principles and (*b*) recognition and treatment of specific complicating clinical problems. This chapter reviews the basic management principles and discusses the complicating clinical syndromes. Space does not allow a complete review of all poisons, drugs, and toxins, but selected agents are highlighted in an attempt to review both common and controversial management problems.

With more than 1 million poisonings each year, resulting in approximately 5000 deaths, emergency departments are frequently required to provide information as well as medical consultation concerning intentional and accidental overdose, poisoning, and toxic exposure. In some geographic areas, poison control centers also provide valuable assistance in answer to public and professional needs.

The emergency physician must have extensive knowledge of clinical toxicology and be prepared to assess and treat poisonings in all age groups. Approximately 70% of reported cases of poisoning in the United States involve children under the age of 5 years, the most common situation being accidental ingestion. Although unintentional poisoning also occurs in adults (as the result of factors such as confusion in medication dose and treatment schedules or the accidental ingestion or inhalation of toxins), deliberate toxic exposure is more likely in this age group.

Suicide is now the third leading cause of death among adolescents, with self-injury secondary to poisoning, the most common method. Although adolescents and adults represent less than 30% of patients with overdoses and poisonings presenting to emergency departments, they are the groups most likely to have both serious intent and major morbidity as a consequence of their action.

Suicide attempts or drug abuse problems require concurrent medical and psychiatric treatment and evaluation. The patient with intentional poisoning can be difficult to evaluate because of depression or behavioral abnormalities. The underlying psychiatric state or the effect of the poison or toxin often makes history unreliable and compliance with treatment difficult. In addition, some patients are repeatedly seen with ingestions or complaints of drug abuse, perhaps diminishing the physician's suspicion of a true suicidal intent and making objective evaluation more difficult. Each patient must be approached calmly and dispassionately with a rational plan of assessment and treatment.

BASIC MANAGEMENT PRINCIPLES

Treatment of the poisoned patient may be divided into four parts: (*a*) general support, (*b*) removal of the drug by decreasing absorption or increasing elimination, (*c*) specific treatment of complicating medical conditions, such as shock, seizure, cardiac arrhythmias, and respiratory failure, and (*d*) psychiatric assessment of suicidal intent. The emergency physician must be skilled in all of these phases of patient evaluation and treatment including the assessment of suicidal intent because immediate psychiatric consultation may not always be available. Further discussion of this aspect of treatment is found in Chapter 18 (Psychiatric Emergencies).

General Support

The first priority for the emergency physician is general supportive care and resuscitative measures. Rapid attention must be given to the airway and adequacy of ventilation, as well as to blood pressure, cardiac rhythm, and level of consciousness. Once basic resuscitative or supportive measures have been instituted, attention can be given to specific management of the poisoning. Consideration of the pharmacokinetics and specific characteristics of the drug or toxic substance is secondary to the initial general support of the patient in almost all circumstances.

Estimation of Severity

The emergency physician must make an initial determination of the severity of a drug ingestion or poisoning and must then continually reassess the patient's condition for signs of improvement or deterioration. Three factors contribute to the initial determination: (*a*) the patient's general status and level of consciousness on arrival, (*b*) the alleged drug and dose involved, and (*c*) any specific complicating clinical situations already present or possible with the particular agent.

Status. Adequacy of cardiorespiratory function and level of consciousness should be noted and recorded. The published literature on emergency department poisonings indicates that up to 50% of all patients with overdoses will have some alteration in mental status, and a continuum from wakeness to coma may be seen. Table 17.1 provides a more detailed grading for depth of coma, but actual staging is less important than the recorded statement concerning reflexes, response to pain, and level of consciousness. Changes with time are extremely important indicators of improvement or deterioration.

Table 17.1.
Evaluation of Level of Consciousness

Grade	Description
0	Fully conscious
1	Drowsy, but responds to verbal commands
2	Unconscious, but responds to minimal painful stimuli[a]
3	Unconscious, responds only to maximal painful stimuli
4	Unconscious, no response, loss of all reflexes

[a] Sternal rubbing with a knuckle is an adequate painful stimulus and is less dangerous than other methods.

Drug Identification. The history from the patient may be unreliable, but it should be obtained and compared with available information from family, friends, or ambulance personnel in the attempt to determine the drug, dose, and time of ingestion or exposure. In the circumstance of illicit drug use, persons accompanying the patient tend to leave as soon as the patient is under a physician's care. The physician should obtain any information in a nonjudgmental manner, with attention to any home remedies already tried that might complicate the patient's clinical course.

The use of a toxic screen analysis of blood, urine, or gastric contents may help in the identification of the poisoning agent but such laboratory support may not be readily available in all geographical areas with a sufficiently rapid response to provide information during the time in which the patient is in the emergency department. The medical literature indicates frequent nonconcordance between the patient history and actual drug levels, and there are also reports of variability in the reliability of commercial toxic screens. Furthermore, there are some ingested agents for which a quantitative toxic screen level will actually indicate a specific change in therapy, a specific intervention, such as diuresis, dialysis, alkalization, acidification, or the use of a specific antidote.

When toxicologic laboratory support is available in a reasonable time period, the emergency physicians can often improve the yield and shorten the time to obtain a toxic screen by indicating to the laboratory possible specific drugs suspected. However, in general, the emergency physician will often be required to make a clinical assessment and initiate intervention without the benefit of such data. When toxic screen information is available promptly, the result must be interpreted cautiously and in light of the patient's clinical status. Given the potential for errors in such results, treatment of the patient is the first priority.

A rough guideline for toxicity in adults with sedative, hypnotic, antipsychotic, or antidepressant overdose is ingestion of 10–20 times the usual daily therapeutic dose. However, the adolescent and adult patient with intentional ingestion or overdose is most likely to have polydrug poisoning, and the clinical picture of the combination may obscure the clinical appearance resulting from pure ingestion of individual agents. Alcohol is the most common secondary agent in poisoning and overdose, in addition to multiple pharmaceuticals, but the increasing use of fixed combination drugs (e.g., propoxyphene, codeine, or oxycodone plus acetaminophen and aspirin) represents another special area of dual toxicity for which the emergency physician must initiate proper intervention. Standard toxicology texts and information resources, such as poison control center telephone numbers, should be readily available to the emergency physician to help with the patient's assessment, determination of the extent of toxicity, and estimation of severity.

Admission Criteria. Deep stupor, coma, or the presence of one or more of the conditions listed in Table 17.2 increases the gravity of the situation and may require admission of the patient for medical intensive care. Local institutional resources may vary, and some patients with mild ingestion or toxic exposure may be observed in the emergency department and released after appropriate psychiatric assessment. Many patients who are still stuporous after several hours require brief hospital admission, and patients in whom the particular agent may cause ongoing or delayed complications require admission as well.

Emergency physicians can expect to admit up to 50% of overdose patients presenting to their department. The literature indicates that approximately one in five drug overdose patients in an emergency department may require admission for intensive medical care, and another 30% will require at least short-term psychiatric hospitalization. The criteria for psychiatric admission after medical evaluation are discussed in Chapter 18 (Psychiatric Emergencies).

Table 17.2.
Clinical Situations Complicating Drug Ingestion

Hypotension or hypertension
Hypothermia or hyperthermia
Respiratory failure
Pulmonary edema
Aspiration pneumonia
Cardiac arrhythmia
Agitation, hyperactivity, or seizure
Anticholinergic syndromes
Oliguria or renal failure
Clinical relapse

Initial Therapeutic Measures

When no history is available, drug overdose should always be considered in comatose patients with or without localizing neurologic findings, but rapid assessment to exclude other causes of this state is necessary. Possible diagnostic considerations include hypoglycemia, hyperglycemia, postictal state, head injury, hypothermia, intracranial bleeding, hepatic or uremic coma, meningoencephalitis, myxedema, and electrolyte imbalance. Some of these conditions may exist as complications of drug overdose when trauma, exposure, infection or underlying disease is present.

The physician must immediately attend to airway, ventilation, and circulatory support of the presumed overdose patient while simultaneously considering the use of available antidotes.

Dextrose/Thiamine. In all patients with coma of unclear cause, 50–100 ml of 50% dextrose in water should be rapidly administered after blood is drawn for glucose determination, since it may be lifesaving should the diagnosis prove to be hypoglycemia. In debilitated or malnourished patients in whom Wernicke-Korsakoff syndrome may be a possibility, dextrose administration should be preceded by thiamine, 50–100 mg intravenously.

Narcotic Antagonists. Naloxone hydrochloride (Narcan) is a narcotic antagonist without agonist properties that will effectively reverse narcotic-induced respiratory depression, unless irreversible end-organ injury has occurred. Hypotension and central nervous system depression will be reversed less predictably but may well respond to naloxone. It should certainly be tried in the presence of such clinical signs, even in the absence of respiratory depression. Signs of narcotic abuse, such as pinpoint pupils or needle tracks, may be present, but the emergency physician should note that certain narcotics may produce pupillary dilatation (meperidine hydrochloride) and that certain nonnarcotic analgesics may produce naloxone-reversible respiratory depression (e.g., propoxyphene and pentazocine).

The initial dose of naloxone hydrochloride should be 1–2 ampules (0.4 mg/ampule), but some narcotic and narcotic-like poisonings may require up to 5 ampules (2 mg) for an initial response. Naloxone is best given intravenously, but intramuscular injection may be used if there is adequate tissue perfusion. The half-life of the narcotic may be considerably longer than the effect of Narcan, and vigilant assessment of the patient for the timing of repeat doses is necessary. Although naloxone by intravenous infusion can be used for long-acting narcotics, the emergency physician is best advised to use intermittent doses until the clinical course and requirement for antagonist therapy is established.

Table 17.3.
Selected Antidotes in Poisoning and Overdose

Poison	Antidote	See Page
Acetaminophen	Acetylcysteine	406
Atropine		
Anticholinergic poisonings	Physostigmine	401
Carbon monoxide	Oxygen	Chapter 10
Carbamates	Atopine	420
Cyanide	Amyl nitrite	
	Sodium nitrite	
	Sodium thiosulfate	419
Ethylene glycol	Ethanol	414
Fluorides	Calcium gluconate	419
Iron	Deferoxamine mesylate	418
Methanol	Ethanol	413
Narcotics	Naloxone	403
Nitrites, nitrates	Methylene blue	420
Organophosphates	Atropine	
	Pralidoxime	420

Other Antidotes. If there is specific knowledge or clinical evidence of the identity of the ingested substance, consideration should be given to the use of specific antidotes after basic resuscitation measures have been applied to provide airway and circulatory support and after the administration of thiamine, dextrose, and naloxone. However, the vast majority of patients with overdoses will not require such "antidote" treatment, and rarely, with the exception of cyanide poisoning, will such therapies be required in the initial minutes of management. A full assessment of the patient's clinical status must be undertaken by the emergency physician, and the use of other antidotal treatment must be utilized carefully with clear understanding of the risks and benefits of such treatments and their potential impact. Table 17.3 is a partial listing of some of these therapies.

Initial Laboratory Studies

Measurements of blood glucose, calcium, and electrolyte levels are often necessary in evaluation of the obtunded patient in whom the cause is unclear. Arterial blood gas analysis is extremely useful both for assessment of ventilatory adequacy and for determination of acid-base disturbance that might lead to the suspicion of certain drugs with metabolic toxicity, such as methanol, ethylene glycol, and salicylates.

Creatine phosphokinase levels become elevated with rhabdomyolysis and should be determined along with renal function when uncontrolled seizures occur or when ingested drugs have the potential to cause muscle injury, which may lead to renal failure. Pink or red urine may be an early clue to this possibility.

Drug Removal

Decreased Absorption

Induced emesis or gastric lavage may remove significant amounts of orally ingested drug if utilized properly. Data on the benefit of these techniques are limited to a small number of drugs, but the following guidelines are relevant to many common drug ingestions.

Depressed mental status contraindicates use of induced emesis or lavage because of the risk of aspiration. If the patient is stuporous or comatose, he or she should be intubated first with a cuffed endotracheal tube. Gastric lavage may then be performed safely. With most drugs, the efficacy of induced emesis or gastric lavage decreases with time, as gastric emptying and absorption take place. After approximately 4 hours, only an insignificant amount of drug may be returned unless the agent has enough anticholinergic potential to slow gastric emptying and absorption.

Gastric lavage and induced emesis should never be utilized as punitive measures to discourage future ingestion. The inappropriate application of invasive procedures may lead to disastrous consequences. Patients who have ingested a minor amount often do well with supportive care only, with no attempt to remove drug from the gastrointestinal tract. A more serious ingestion, however, warrants consideration of induced emesis or lavage. Contraindications to these techniques include ingestions of strong alkali, corrosive agents such as lye or ammonia, and strong acids. Emptying the stomach after petroleum distillate ingestion remains controversial.

Emesis. Ipecac is the first choice for inducing

emesis in a serious overdose, if the patient is alert and relatively cooperative, and if fewer than 4 hours have elapsed since ingestion. It is a safe drug with little toxicity. The dose of syrup of ipecac is 15 ml orally in a 1- to 5-year-old, 30 ml in older children, and 30–60 ml in adults. This must be followed by 6–8 ounces of water in children and four or five 8-ounce glasses of water in adults. Emesis will follow in approximately 20 minutes.

Apomorphine may be used alternatively. It is given parenterally in a dose of 0.1 mg/kg in adults and also requires that the stomach be filled with water. Emesis occurs in 3–5 minutes. Although its onset of action is faster than that of syrup of ipecac, it can produce hypotension and respiratory depression, and it requires time to prepare in fresh solution. In general, ipecac is preferred. Respiratory depression and hypotension secondary to apomorphine administration are reversible with naloxone hydrochloride.

Gastric Lavage. This technique may be utilized if there is no response to ipecac. This may occur with anticholinergic poisonings that are antiemetic. The patient must be alert and cooperative. If mental status is depressed even slightly, endotracheal intubation is necessary.

Data from animal experiments suggest that spontaneous emesis is more effective in removing drugs, but serious ingestions may require lavage. Efficacy in humans demands proper technique. An Ewald or similar large-bore tube (at least 28 French or larger) must be used to remove pill fragments. The patient should be in the left lateral decubitus position. With the stomach dependent and the pylorus uppermost, adequate mixing of lavage fluid and stomach contents occurs without excessive loss of fluid into the duodenum. The tube is passed through the mouth, preferably after topical anesthesia in the pharynx to diminish the likelihood of gagging and vomiting. Physiologic saline solution is preferred since water can induce a hypotonic intravascular state in children. In adults, a total of 5–10 liters of fluid is used, although many European centers advocate more than 20 liters. Lavage fluid should be brought to a temperature of approximately 37°C to avoid hypothermia.

Activated Charcoal. This agent is a very useful adjunct in the management of drug overdose, and recent literature suggests that it may be as effective as emesis or lavage and possibly safer. Activated charcoal will absorb almost all inorganic and organic chemicals with the exception of cyanide, and it may be used after the stomach has been emptied by either emesis or lavage. It should never be given simultaneously with ipecac since it may absorb ipecac and prevent its action. Charcoal, 20–50 gm, is mixed in a slurry with 100–200 ml of water. The slurry can be given orally to a cooperative patient, or it can be instilled via the orogastric tube used for lavage or with a smaller nasogastric tube if lavage has not preceded its use. It should be followed with a saline cathartic to decrease transit time of drug already in the intestine or bound to charcoal. Magnesium sulfate, 15 gm in adults and 250 mg/kg in children, is effective, as is sorbitol, 50–100 ml of a 70% solution.

The use of repetitive doses of activated charcoal in the intestinal tract (30 gm given every 2–6 hours) has now been shown to increase the clearance of some drugs and poisons. Repetitive charcoal doses may produce this result because certain agents may be subject to enterohepatic circulation, active secretion, or simple passive diffusion into the gastrointestinal tract. Continued charcoal therapy appears most applicable to drugs that are relatively nonprotein bound and are water-soluble with small volumes of distribution. Data showing enhanced clearance now exist for phenobarbital, theophylline, carbamazepine, and digitoxin where the half-life may be reduced by approximately 50%. Less significant reductions in half-life have also been reported with nadolol and digoxin. However, only limited data exist on the important question of improvement in the clinical course of the overdosed patient when continued charcoal is used, and it has yet to be shown that shortening the half-life of the drug shortens the duration of coma, of respiratory support, or of time in intensive care units.

Increased Elimination

Forced Diuresis. Some drugs may be removed by increasing urinary excretion. Forced diuresis refers to vigorous administration of intravenous fluids to rates of 200–400 ml/hour in adults, or 5 ml/kg. This technique along with addition of potent loop diuretics is of benefit only with water-soluble, weakly protein-bound drugs that are excreted by the kidneys such as phenobarbital, meprobamate, amphetamines, and lithium salts. Forced diuresis is contraindicated in patients with congestive heart failure, shock, or renal failure. The procedure may be started in the emergency department, but requires careful monitoring in an inpatient unit to assure electrolyte balance and prevention of volume overload.

Alkalization and Acidification. Alkalization with sodium bicarbonate to produce a urinary pH of 8 further enhances removal of a drug whose pK is such that it remains ionized in the renal tubule at this pH. This is a useful adjunct to the treatment of overdoses with long-acting barbiturates, salicylates, and isoniazid. Excretion of certain other toxins is enhanced with systemic acidification. Phencyclidine hydrochloride and amphetamine excretion can be increased by acidifying the urine to a pH of less than 5 with ascorbic acid, 8 gm/day, or ammonium chloride, 2.75 mEq/kg every 6 hours orally or intravenously.

Dialysis and Hemoperfusion. Although dialysis is not performed in the emergency department, it is important for the emergency physician to recognize its place in the treatment of the poisoned patient. In general, peritoneal dialysis or hemodialysis is rarely necessary in most poisonings since supportive management usually suffices. Standard peritoneal dialysis or hemodialysis is only useful for removal of weakly protein-bound drugs and water-soluble substances. Phenobarbital, salicylates, lithium, and meprobamate, for example, can be removed by dialysis, but the technique has no advantage over forced diuresis and may result in increased morbidity. Standard dialysis is of no benefit with lipid-soluble drugs such as glutethimide or highly protein-bound drugs such as short-acting barbiturates, phenothiazine derivatives, tricyclic antidepressants, and benzodiazepines. Charcoal hemoperfusion (dialysis across a column of activated charcoal) is a specialized technique that may be of use with lipid-soluble or protein-bound drugs, but it requires systemic anticoagulant therapy and is associated with coagulation-factor consumption. It should be reserved for life-threatening overdoses with associated renal failure.

In the presence of renal failure, dialysis may be necessary both to support the patient and to remove a water-soluble, weakly protein-bound toxin. Dialysis is also indicated in methyl alcohol and ethylene glycol poisonings and may be required in heavy-metal intoxications after administration of chelating agents. Table 17.4 summarizes the indications for dialysis and the potential applications.

Table 17.4.
Dialysis Indications and Potential Applications

- Indications
  - Poisoning with water-soluble, poorly protein-bound drugs
  - Extreme toxicity with hypotension or renal compromise
  - Potentially lethal dose determined by history or blood levels
- Dialyzable drugs with markedly increased clearance
  - Acetaminophen
  - Amphetamines
  - Bromides
  - Ethanol
  - Ethchlorvynol
  - Ethylene glycol
  - Lithium
  - Meprobamate
  - Methanol
  - Phenobarbital
  - Salicylates

Complicating Medical Conditions

Many clinical situations can complicate the management of serious drug ingestions, and knowledge of the pathophysiology of these conditions can help the emergency physician administer proper therapy.

Blood Pressure

Hypotension is commonly seen in overdoses of sedatives, hypnotics, antipsychotics, and antidepressants; it is principally caused by dilatation of venous capacitance vessels. Unreplaced volume losses in the comatose patient can also contribute to hypotension. Phenothiazines produce venous pooling, but in high doses they can also cause decreased peripheral vascular resistance due to α-adrenergic blockade. In this setting, sympathomimetic amines with β-adrenergic actions, such as isoproterenol hydrochloride, epinephrine, and dopamine, may worsen the shock state by causing vasodilatation. Volume replacement is often all that is necessary in drug overdose-induced hypotension. If a pressor amine is required for a patient with phenothiazine ingestion, predominantly α-adrenergic agents such as phenylephrine hydrochloride or levarterenol bitartrate should be used.

Drug overdoses can also cause hypertension. This may be a direct effect, as occurs with tricyclic antidepressants or monoamine oxidase inhibitors, or it may be a consequence of hypoxic brain injury. Drug-induced hypertension is often of short duration and requires treatment only if there is evidence of end-organ damage to the brain or heart. For drug-induced hypertension, rapidly acting agents such as nitroprusside should be used so that the effect may be quickly reversed.

Respiratory Failure

In the setting of poisoning or overdose, respiratory failure may have several causes, which may be independent or related. Most often, drug ingestion causes central nervous system depression with hypoventilation and carbon dioxide retention. Naloxone hydrochloride administration and assisted ventilation comprise the primary treatment.

Pulmonary edema may be responsible for respiratory failure in patients with drug overdose, most commonly when there has been parenteral narcotic abuse with heroin but also in instances of high-dose salicylate toxicity. The pathophysiology involves an alveolar-capillary leak syndrome, and in parenteral narcotic abuse, it may be a reaction to the adulterants of the drug mixture. The cause is unclear in salicylate poisoning, but in both circumstances, left ventricular function may be adequate and treatment consists of intubation and positive-pressure ventilation. High-dose corticosteroids have been advocated, but are not of proven benefit. Aspiration pneumonia can contribute to respiratory failure as a primary event or as an additional factor in ventilatory depression or pulmonary edema.

Temperature Variations

Hypothermia may complicate treatment of the poisoned patient and is most commonly due to exposure of a comatose patient to ambient temperature below body temperature. Iatrogenic hypothermia may result from vigorous lavage with fluids at room temperature, and some drugs, such as phenothiazine derivatives, may have a direct effect on the hypothalamic temperature-regulating center. Hypothermia may contribute to the comatose state and to cardiorespiratory depression and may be initially overlooked unless accurate rectal probe temperatures are obtained. Rapid core rewarming with cardiopulmonary bypass or peritoneal dialysis is preferred in the presence of cardiorespiratory arrest, but for mild hypothermia (T > 90°C), heated nebulized oxygen, warmed intravenous fluids, and passive rewarming techniques may be sufficient. Vigorous external rewarming should be avoided since it may cause peripheral vasodilatation, vascular compromise, and further temperature drop.

Elevated temperature may be a direct effect of some drugs, such as salicylates, tricyclic antidepressants, and other anticholinergic agents. Temperature elevation with salicylates is related to the associated hypermetabolic state; with tricyclic antidepressants and other anticholinergic drugs, peripheral heat loss is reduced and central nervous system thermoregulation may be affected.

Uncontrolled seizures or unrecognized infection may also contribute to hyperthermia. Fever always demands careful consideration of occult infection as a primary or secondary problem. Significant hyperpyrexia should be reduced with external cooling to minimize insensitive fluid losses and to reduce the impact of heat stress on already compromised organ systems.

Table 17.5.
Sources of Anticholinergic Poisoning

Drugs and chemicals
Atropine
Belladonna
Benactyzine hydrochloride
Chlorpheniramine maleate
Cyclopentolate hydrochloride
Dicyclomine hydrochloride
Diphenhydramine hydrochoride
Homatropine
Hyoscine (scopolamine)
Hyoscyamus
Isopropamide iodide
Mepenzolate bromide
Methantheline bromide
Methapyrilene
Phenothiazine derivatives
Pipenzolate methylbromide
Propantheline bromide
Pyrilamine maleate
Stramonium
Tricyclic antidepressants
Amitriptyline hydrochloride
Desipramine hydrochloride
Doxepin hydrochloride
Imipramine hydrochloride
Nortriptyline hydrochloride
Protriptyline hydrochloride
Plants
Amanita muscaria
Belladonna (deadly nightshade)
Bittersweet
Black henbane
Jerusalem cherry
Jimson weed
Lantana
Potato tuber
Wild tomato

Anticholinergic Syndromes

Atropine, antihistamines, phenothiazine derivatives, and tricyclic antidepressants may cause a spectrum of complications that are commonly referred to as anticholinergic syndromes. In addition, certain plants such as jimson weed, belladonna (deadly nightshade), bittersweet, and the *Amanita muscaria* mushroom may have anticholinergic properties (Table 17.5). Commonly available proprietary sleep aids contain various antihistamines, usually pyrilamine maleate (Table 17.6). Scopolamine, previously present in proprietary sleep aids, has been removed by order of the Food and Drug Administration, but the antihistamine alone is capable of producing anticholinergic effects.

Peripheral and central nervous system effects as well as cardiac arrhythmias are seen in patients with anticholinergic poisoning. Classical features include dry skin, flushing, mild fever, urinary retention, confusion, tachycardia, and mild hypertension. Hypotension may also occur in patients with a large overdose. Blurred vision with secondary mydriasis is common. Central nervous system effects include agitation, seizures, and confusion leading to stupor and coma in high doses. These drugs cause atrial and ventricular arrhythmias, as well as conduction disturbances, because of their quinidine-like effect on the heart. Cardiac and central nervous system features may be increased by coexistent fever, hypoxemia, or electrolyte imbalance.

Physostigmine, a cholinesterase inhibitor, has been used to reverse temporarily peripheral, central, and cardiac effects of anticholinergic poisoning. Quarternary cholinesterase inhibitors, such as neostigmine and edrophonium chloride, are not ef-

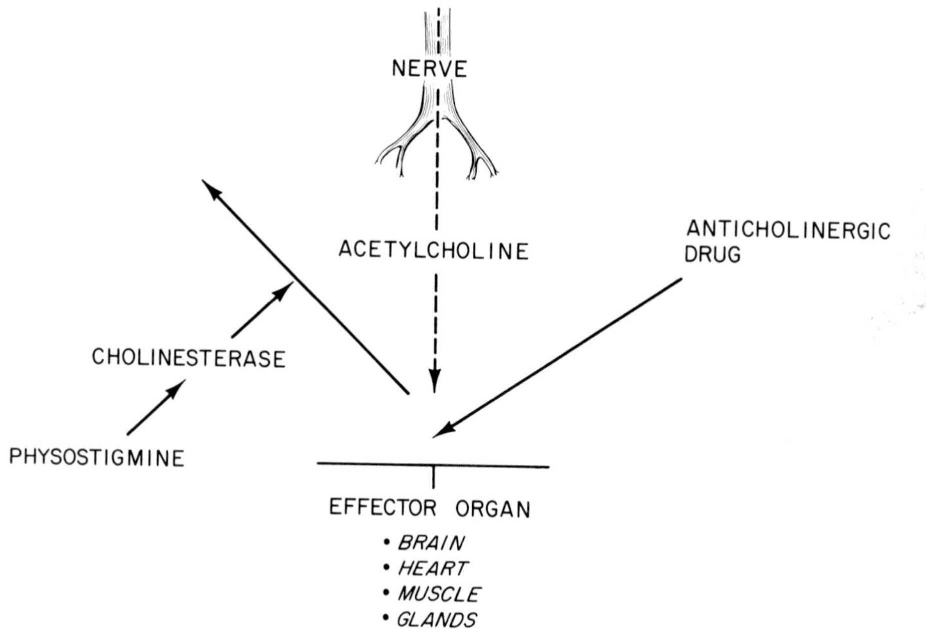

Figure 17.1. Pathophysiology of anticholinergic syndrome.

fective in the reversal of central nervous system effects since they do not cross the blood-brain barrier. Anticholinergic drugs block parasympathetic nerve endings and motor endplates and prevent the action of acetylcholine on muscle, glands, heart, and brain. Physostigmine reverses this effect by diminishing the cholinesterase-mediated metabolism, resulting in increases in acetylcholine (Fig. 17.1).

After initial popularity as an antidote for anticholinergic poisoning, it is clear that physostigmine must be given with caution since cholinergic excess can result and too rapid infusion can cause seizures. Physostigmine may cause bronchospasm, as well as nausea, vomiting, and abdominal pain, and it is contraindicated in patients with asthma. It should only be given after initial stabilization of the airway and ventilation. Alternative strategies for patients with anticholinergic poisoning should be tried before physostigmine is used. These therapeutic options involve use of lidocaine hydrochloride, propranolol hydrochloride, or phenytoin for serious cardiac arrhythmias and conduction disturbances, which may also benefit from sodium bicarbonate administration. Seizures may be treated with phenytoin, and severe hypertension with end-organ compromise will respond to rapidly acting agents such as nitroprusside, but appropriate monitoring should be available.

In patients with peripheral or central manifestations of excessive anticholinergic response who do not respond to alternative therapy, physostigmine may be tried for the following conditions: malignant cardiac arrhythmias uncontrollable with standard drugs, hypertension with end-organ compromise, and uncontrolled seizures. Patients in coma may respond to physostigmine given as a diagnostic test, but coma alone is not an indication for ongoing treatment, nor is a response totally diagnostic of anticholinergic poisoning. In adults, 2 mg intravenously can be given slowly over approximately 3–5 minutes. The half-life of the drug is 1–2 hours, and repeated doses may be necessary since the duration of action may be less than that of the anticholinergic compound.

Seizures

Agitation, hyperactivity, and seizures may complicate drug overdose. Dystonic movements and extrapyramidal reactions may be seen with phenothiazine overdose and should be distinguished from seizures. Careful observation of the patient after assuring adequacy of the airway often provides the clue, since posturing is frequently characteristic. Dystonic reactions may be reversed by diphenhydramine hydrochloride (Benadryl), 25–50 mg intravenously, or benztropine mesylate (Cogentin), 1–2 mg intravenously. Restraints should be applied to any patient in danger of injuring him- or herself, but sedation should be used with great care, lest it be additive to the central nervous system depressant effects of the drug overdose.

Overdoses of propoxyphene, tricyclic antidepressants, and phenothiazine derivatives may cause seizures directly, but central nervous system hypoxemia, coexistent trauma, electrolyte disturbances, and underlying seizure disorders may also be contributory. Uncontrolled seizures can lead to rhabdomyolysis and pigment-induced renal failure; hyperthermia may also result. Intravenous phenytoin is the treatment of choice for seizures in patients with drug overdose. Diazepam and barbiturates should be avoided because they may contribute to central nervous system depression.

Renal Failure

Commonly abused drugs are usually not nephrotoxic, and when oliguria and acute renal failure occur, the condition is often a consequence of renal hypoperfusion and shock. Rhabdomyolysis may occur with phencyclidine hydrochloride and drugs associated with prolonged seizures, and it may contribute to renal failure. With anticholinergic drugs, urinary retention may occur. The bladder should be palpated; if it is distended, use of a Foley catheter will establish the diagnosis.

Clinical Relapse

Clinical relapse is a feature of many drug ingestions. A patient who awakens after several hours of care may still require observation. Anticholinergic drugs may have slowed gastrointestinal uptake because of drug-induced ileus or delayed gastric emptying, and the patient's condition may deteriorate after initial improvement. In a multiple drug overdose, the effect of one agent may wane before the effect of a second agent becomes maximal. In addition, drugs such as glutethimide and phencyclidine hydrochloride are highly lipid-soluble and have enterohepatic circulation resulting in a waxing and waning course.

Psychiatric Considerations

Treatment of the poisoned patient does not end with control of clinical complications. Psychiatric evaluation is essential to establish the intent or suicidal risk and to determine the social supports available to the patient. Many overdoses that are medically not serious are actually high risk because of the psychiatric implications.

After a patient's medical condition becomes satisfactory, a psychiatrist or trained psychiatric nurse or social worker should assist in the determination of suicidal intent. The patient must have a clear mental status for the psychiatrist or psychiatric worker to make a complete assessment. If an emergency department does not provide space for supportive care in a holding unit, the patient will often have to be admitted until a complete psychiatric evaluation, unencumbered by a drug-depressed mental state, is possible. The environment in the emergency department and hospital must offer protection from further self-induced injury as well. Restraints may be necessary, and such equipment as knife blades, needles, and drugs should not be in the immediate vicinity of the patient.

Each patient must be viewed as being at a high risk until all of the data are available to judge completely the potential for serious injury. It is far better to admit the patient for supportive short-term care than to run the risk of a repeated attempt with a fatal outcome.

Many patients do not have to be hospitalized if supportive help is available on an outpatient basis and if family supports are strong. The elderly, alcoholic, drug-dependent, or psychiatrically high-risk patient with a violent method or with an attempt involving little likelihood of rescue will usually require hospitalization, as will psychotic and severely depressed patients.

Whereas poisonings in children are most often accidental, such an event may be a manifestation of social disorder in the home, parental neglect, or frank child abuse by a parent or sibling. The emergency physician and psychiatric staff must be alert to this phenomenon and must involve appropriate community resources if further injury is to be prevented.

SPECIFIC POISONINGS

In this section, the treatment of selected poisonings is discussed. The selections represent an effort to address both common and controversial problems facing the emergency physician. A list of clinical papers relating to these and to less common poisonings is supplied at the end of this chapter. Toxicity resulting from lithium, amphetamines, hallucinogens, barbiturates, and narcotics is also discussed in Chapter 18 (Psychiatric Emergencies).

Narcotics

Poisoning with narcotics is a common problem in the United States. When it is associated with parenteral drug abuse, there is often coexistent medical illness. When the patient's condition is stabilized, the physician must be alert to common infectious complications. Hepatitis is often seen, as well as local and systemic bacterial infections such as skin abscess, cellulitis, septicemia, endocarditis, septic thromboembolism, osteomyelitis, acquired immunodeficiency syndrome, and, occasionally, tetanus. These patients require precautions in the handling of blood and secretions.

Overdose with opiates results in central nervous system and respiratory depression with hypotension. Gastric hypomotility may occur with ileus; nausea and vomiting may result from central nervous system stimulation. Noncardiogenic pulmo-

Table 17.6.
Sleep Aid and Sedative Product Table[a]

Product (Manufacturer)	Antihistamine	Other Ingredients
Alva Taranquil-Span (Alval Amco)	Chlorpheniramine	Potassium bromide, potassium salicylate, L-tryptophan, niacin, niacinamide, thiamine
Alva Tranquil (Alval Amco)	Chlorpheniramine	Potassium bromide, potassium salicylate, L-tryptophan, niacin, niacinamide, thiamine
Compoz Tablets (Jeffrey Martin)	Pyrilamine maleate, 25 mg	
Nervine Capsule-shaped Tablets (Miles)	Pyrilamine maleate, 25 mg	
Nytol Capsules and Tablets (Block)	Pyrilamine maleate 25-mg tablet 50-mg capsule	
Quiet Tabs (Commerce)	Pyrilamine maleate, 25 mg	
Quiet World Tablets (Whitehall)	Pyrilamine maleate, 25 mg	Aspirin, 227.5 mg; acetaminophen, 162.5 mg
Relax-U-Caps (Columbia Medical)	Pyrilamine maleate, 25 mg	
Sedacaps (Vitarine)	Pyrilamine maleate, 25 mg	
Sleep-Eze Tablets (Whitehall)	Pyrilamine maleate, 25 mg	
Sominex (J. B. Williams)	Pyrilamine maleate, 25 mg	
Somnicaps (American Pharmaceutical)	Pyrilamine maleate, 25 mg	
Tranquil Capsules (North American)	Pyrilamine maleate, 25 mg	
Unisom (Leeming)	Doxylamine succinate, 25 mg	

[a] From *Handbook of Non-prescription Drugs*, ed 7. Washington, DC: American Pharmaceutical Association, 1982.

nary edema may occur, perhaps related to adulterants in the injected mixture, such as quinine, lactose, and fruit sugars; however, pulmonary edema has also been reported with ingestion of propoxyphene and methadone. The pupils are commonly pinpoint, except in the case of meperidine hydrochloride where the pupils are normal to slightly dilated. Support of the airway and administration of the narcotic antagonist naloxone hydrochloride to reverse respiratory depression are first measures. Repeated doses of naloxone are often required, since the half-life of the drug is often longer than that of the antagonist. Continuous naloxone infusion may have a role in the intensive care unit setting once the response to treatment and dose needs have been established, but in general, it will not have application in the emergency department setting. A mixture of 2–4 mg of naloxone in 500 ml of normal saline produces a concentration of 0.4–0.8 mg in 100 ml and is titrated at approximately 0.4 mg/30 min to reverse cardiorespiratory depression with long-acting narcotics.

Determination of the route of overdose administration is very important. Emesis or lavage has no efficacy if the drug has been parenterally injected, but should be utilized in oral ingestions if the patient is alert. In comatose patients with oral ingestions, the stomach should be emptied after the airway has been intubated. Concurrent aspirin or acetaminophen toxicity can complicate the patient's course when a narcotic has been ingested in fixed combinations with these agents. Blood levels are necessary to determine coexistent toxicity and to guide therapy. The emergency physician must also be alert to "street resuscitation methods," usually seen with intravenous heroin abuse, as those may complicate the clinical course with aspiration (oral milk), hypothermia (ice packing), or cellulitis (injection of milk or saline).

Corticosteroids have been advocated for pulmonary edema resulting from opiate overdose, but there are no good scientific data to support this. These patients require intubation, positive-pressure ventilation, and intensive care.

Barbiturates

Barbiturates are sedative drugs that are frequently abused in the United States and elsewhere. They are responsible for nearly 20% of the hospitalizations resulting from acute poisoning in the United States. Barbiturates are usually classified according to the duration of clinical action, which is determined by the rate of absorption, lipid solubility, serum binding, and mode of metabolism. Absorption from the intestine is limited by the rate of dissolution and dispersal in the gastrointestinal contents. Barbiturates are absorbed more rapidly if taken with ethanol or on an empty stomach.

Short-acting barbiturates, such as amobarbital, sodium pentobarbital, and secobarbital, have a duration of therapeutic action of 4–6 hours. They are primarily metabolized to inactive products by the liver. Toxic effects usually occur at blood levels of 3 mg/dl and higher; in most cases, this requires ingestion of 5 mg/kg of drug in children and 4 mg/kg in adults.

The long-acting barbiturates, such as phenobarbital, are subject to liver hydroxylation up to 75%, but 25% or more of the drug is excreted unchanged by the kidneys with a therapeutic life of 12–24 hours. Serum levels above 8 mg/dl are toxic if the barbiturate is taken "acutely," but tolerance occurs and many patients on long-term therapy are asymptomatic with high blood levels. Ingestion of 8–10 mg/kg acutely produces a toxic level.

Respiratory depression is the major toxic effect assessed clinically and with arterial blood gas analysis. Aspiration pneumonia is common, and necrotizing pneumonia is a frequent cause of death in these patients. Pulmonary edema is seen occasionally and is usually due to fluid overload and coexistent myocardial impairment. Hypothermia may occur as a result of depression of temperature regulation in the brainstem. Cutaneous bullae are seen frequently and are helpful in diagnosis, although they are not specific for barbiturate intoxication. They occur over pressure areas within a few hours after drug ingestion.

Treatment is primarily supportive, with attention to airway management. Positive-pressure ventilation is necessary if ventilatory failure is present; the patient should be observed for pneumothorax throughout the hospital course since many pulmonary infections are necrotizing and cause blebs that can rupture into the pleural space.

Shock should be treated by correction of hypoxemia and acidosis and by plasma expansion. Forced diuresis with systemic alkalization to produce a urinary pH of 8 enhances excretion of long-acting barbiturates. Urinary output should be advanced to 3–6 ml/kg/hr with careful attention to electrolyte and volume status. This may require infusion rates of 200–400 ml/hr, best accomplished in an intensive care unit setting and adjusted accordingly for patients with underlying cardiac, renal, or pulmonary disease. Diuresis can be initiated with furosemide, 20–40 mg, or with mannitol, 12.5–25 gm, each given intravenously.

Hemodialysis can be used but should be reserved for extreme toxic reactions and for the patient with renal failure. With short-acting barbiturates, forced diuresis or hemodialysis offers no benefit since these drugs are relatively more protein-bound and liver-metabolized. Charcoal resin hemoperfusion can be considered for patients with severe intoxication from short-acting barbiturates.

Salicylates

Salicylate poisoning remains the most commonly reported poisoning in the United States, occurring frequently in children less than 6 years old. Intentional poisoning in adults is common, but accidental overdose occurs in the adult population as well. In such a situation, the patient is seen in the emergency department with altered mental status, and the major indicator as to cause is an unexplained metabolic acidosis.

A dose of 150 mg/kg is usually associated with toxicity (35 tablets or 10 gm in adults), although toxicity can very, with fatalities in adults reported after ingestion of 10–30 gm but survival reported with a single dose in excess of 100 gm. The prevalence of salicylates in poisonings relates in part to the large number of salicylate products on the market. Among these is the highly toxic methyl salicylate found in wintergreen oil and linaments. One teaspoon of this preparation provides 6 gm of salicylate and is a source of considerable toxicity in children, who may be attracted to the bottle by its color or smell. The multiplicity of pharmaceuticals containing aspirin in fixed combination demand attention to coexistent toxicity to more than one drug. The clinical picture may be obscured by combination effects of oxycodone (Percodan), propoxyphene (Darvon compound), barbiturate (Fiorinal), or over-the-counter preparations of antihistamines.

With either purposeful or accidental mild salicylate intoxication, salicylism occurs, characterized in the clinical setting by tinnitus, diminished hearing, and vertigo. With more moderate doses, nausea and vomiting occur along with hyperventilation and confusion. More severe toxicity is associated with tachycardia, hyperpyrexia, and mental torpor, with seizures, coma, cardiorespiratory compromise, and pulmonary edema at the extreme.

Salicylic acid salts are rapidly absorbed from the gastrointestinal tract, but absorption of commercial products varies in relation to tablet dissolution and gastric motility. Although the drug is usually well-absorbed in the stomach and small intestine and bound in part (50–80%) to albumin, tablets occasionally combine to form a large bolus that may continue to be absorbed for several days. Free salicylate is conjugated in the liver and eventually excreted by the kidneys.

Saturation of hepatic metabolic pathways occurs rapidly in overdoses, but may also occur slowly with increased therapeutic doses or decreased intervals of administration. The half-life of the drug is therefore variable, increasing from 4 hours with a low dose to as much as 30 hours in patients with salicylate toxicity. Accidental self-poisoning in the adult is produced by this changing half-life that allows a progressive increase in the level of salicylate in the blood.

Salicylates stimulate the central respiratory drive center, causing hyperventilation, hypocapnia, and initially, respiratory alkalosis in adults. Renal loss of bicarbonate occurs in compensation. Children are more commonly acidemic on presentation, with buffering capacity overwhelmed. In mild cases, adults may have a relatively normal pH along with renal compensation. In extreme situations, however, respiratory center depression occurs, with carbon dioxide retention and respiratory acidosis adding to the metabolic acidosis caused by the lactate and keto acids produced by the effect of salicylate on the Krebs cycle.

Salicylate excess also interferes with carbohydrate metabolism. Depletion of tissue stores of glucose may result in hypoglycemia, but hyperglycemia may also occur because of the variability of metabolism, level of tissue stores, and rate of consumption. Hypoglycemia may be worsened by nausea, vomiting, and diminished oral intake.

Hyperpyrexia can occur and is occasionally severe. Increased heat production by inefficient oxidative phosphorylation may not be eliminated rapidly enough to maintain homeostasis since the sweating mechanism may be impaired in a dehydrated, vomiting patient.

Microscopic gastrointestinal bleeding is common with therapeutic doses of salicylates, and increased bleeding has been assumed for larger toxic doses. The incidence of massive bleeding is low despite the multiple effects that salicylates produce on the hematologic system, including interference with prothrombin production and platelet function and an increase in capillary permeability. Acute renal failure occurs rarely and is usually a result of dehydration and hypotension.

Laboratory studies are helpful in the evaluation and treatment of salicylate poisoning. A ferric chloride test may give a quick qualitative screen to indicate the presence of salicylate (5–10 drops of 10% ferric chloride in 10 ml of urine produce a purple color), but exact serum salicylate levels are essential. Pending salicylate levels, electrolytes, determination of the anion gap, and arterial blood gas levels should be used to determine the acid-base status of the patient. Substantial hypoglycemia and hypokalemia occasionally develop and should be treated. Hypokalemia may be due to intracellular shifts owing to early alkalosis or to renal and gastrointestinal losses. If the patient is acidotic, the degree of hypokalemia may be underestimated.

Table 17.7.
Clinical Features of Salicylate Intoxication

Level of Toxicity	Manifestations
Mild (<30 mg/dl)	Salicylism with tinnitus, deafness, nausea
Moderate (30–70 mg/dl)	Salicylism, vomiting, confusion, fever, acid-base and electrolyte disturbances
Severe (>70 mg/dl)	Pulmonary edema, cardiorespiratory failure, coma

Plasma salicylate levels of more than 30 mg/dl can cause a toxic reaction, with moderate toxicity usually seen at levels of 30–70 mg/dl and severe toxicity at levels in excess of 70–100 mg/dl (Table 17.7). Because of the variability of absorption and tissue saturation, one blood level determination may not reflect the peak, and reliance should be placed more on serial determinations and on other clinical and laboratory findings. A rising blood level may also suggest that tablets have agglomerated in the stomach. Even after 4–6 hours, gastric lavage or emesis may be of benefit. Forced diuresis should be employed with attention to cardiac status to avoid volume overload, particularly in patients with severe poisoning in whom pulmonary edema may develop as the result of an alveolocapillary leak syndrome and in whom it may be worsened by volume excess. Sodium bicarbonate, 2–3 mg/kg intravenously, to normalize or slightly alkalize serum pH and increase urinary pH to 8, enhances urinary excretion in the acidemic patient. Hemodialysis is indicated in cases of severe toxicity with cardiac impairment and pulmonary edema or when there is major compromise to renal function.

Acetaminophen

Increased use of acetaminophen as an antipyretic and analgesic has led to its appearance as a common overdose agent, either alone or in fixed combination with other analgesics such as propoxyphene, oxycodone, glutethimide, and co-

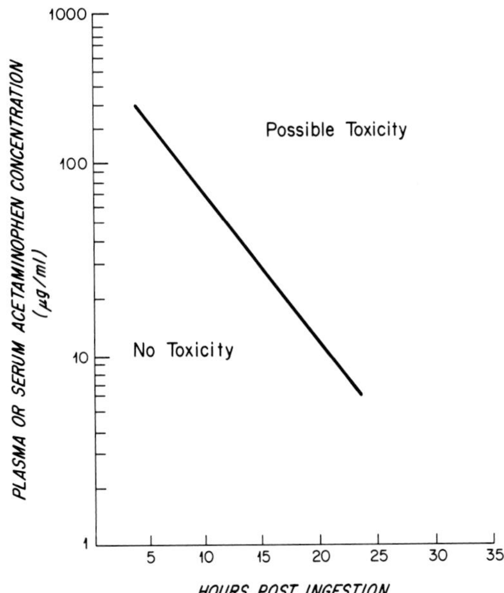

Figure 17.2. Blood level of acetaminophen over time.

deine. In adults, 10–15 gm can produce serious toxicity and may be fatal. The blood level is the key to determination of potential toxicity; ideally, the blood level should be determined and then repeated after several hours to confirm the need for therapy (Fig. 17.2).

The liver is the major organ affected by acetaminophen toxicity, and the clinical features of the poisoning may be divided into three phases. In the early phase, up to 24 hours after ingestion, the patient may have mild anorexia, nausea, vomiting, and diaphoresis, but occasionally there may be little evidence of toxicity unless other drugs have been simultaneously ingested. This underscores the importance of the history, since the patient may be seen in the emergency department with depression or suicidal ideation without the usual signs of drug overdose. Early recognition of this poisoning is important to the therapeutic outcome.

In the second phase of acetaminophen toxicity, from 24–48 hours, the patient may feel initially improved, but abnormal liver function will be detectable and pain in the right upper abdominal quadrant may develop as hepatic toxicity proceeds. In the third phase, from 2–5 days, the sequelae of hepatic necrosis occur, with jaundice, coagulopathy, and encephalopathy.

Acetaminophen is rapidly absorbed from the gastrointestinal tract, with peak levels occurring in 30–60 minutes at therapeutic doses. The drug is metabolized in the liver by the cytochrome P-450 mixed function oxidase system to an active intermediate metabolite that is normally detoxified by conjugation with glutathione. In overdose situations, glutathione is depleted, allowing increased intermediate metabolites that are toxic to liver cells. These intermediate metabolites bind to hepatic microsomes and cause cell death.

Table 17.8.
Treatment of Acetaminophen Poisoning

Empty stomach with induced emesis or lavage as appropriate.
Avoid activated charcoal or remove it by lavage.
If < 24 hours since ingestion, administer acetylcysteine in a 20% solution diluted 1:3 in cola, grapefruit juice, orange juice, or water:
140 mg/kg orally in loading dose
70 mg/kg orally every 4 hours for 68 hours (17 doses)
Start treatment pending confirmation by blood level determination. If > 24 hours since ingestion, provide supportive measures.

Treatment of acetaminophen poisoning requires administration of a sulfhydryl-containing substitute for glutathione. If it is given early after ingestion, hepatic injury may be substantially reduced. Methionine and cysteamine have been shown to be effective, but acetylcysteine is currently the drug of choice. These agents provide sulfhydryl groups that bind the toxic intermediate metabolites. The stomach should be emptied, but charcoal should be avoided since it will absorb acetylcysteine. If charcoal has already been administered or if it is utilized purposely in the circumstance of a mixed ingestion, it is preferable either to delay the administration of acetylcysteine by 1–2 hours or to lavage charcoal from the stomach so that acetylcysteine can then be given. Blood samples should be drawn for determination of acetaminophen level, but if the history suggests the potential for toxicity and less than 24 hours have passed since ingestion, therapy should be started and either continued or stopped when blood-level results are available. Table 17.8 summarizes the dosage schedule for acetylcysteine, which may be given orally or by nasogastric tube. If more than 24 hours have passed since ingestion, supportive measures should be used without acetylcysteine. Nausea and vomiting may occur as side effects, but in general, the drug is adequately tolerated.

Benzodiazepines

The benzodiazepine group of drugs (diazepam, chlordiazepoxide hydrochloride, oxazepam, and others) are among the most commonly prescribed pharmaceuticals in the United States. Used primarily as antianxiety agents or as muscle relaxants, they are also frequently prescribed indiscriminately and patients are commonly seen in emergency departments with minor and major overdoses. In fact, overdose with benzodiazepine and alcohol represents one of the most frequent combination ingestions seen in the emergency department.

These drugs have a wide therapeutic range and are relatively safe. Mild to moderate overdoses are associated with initial excitement followed by drowsiness, dysarthria, and confusion; more severe overdoses result in coma with respiratory depression. Overdoses of 1–2 gm require supportive measures, but fatalities have not been reported resulting solely from these drugs.

However, when these drugs are seen in overdoses involving multiple pharmaceuticals or street drugs plus alcohol, major morbidity may occur, and death, which is often due to ventilatory depression, can ensue. Toxicologic assays may determine the presence of these agents, but should not be solely relied on in clinical decision making both because of the difficulty in assaying for the agents and because of the inherent unreliability of commercial assays themselves.

Reports of response to physostigmine have been published, but sufficient data are not available to warrant this treatment, with its risks of cholinergic excess. Supportive measures usually suffice.

Glutethimide

Glutethimide (Doriden) causes serious poisoning because a very small amount of the drug yields significant toxicity, particularly in combination with alcohol or other sedative hypnotic agents. As few as 10–20 500-mg tablets may cause death in adults.

The drug is highly lipid-soluble, with relatively rapid intestinal uptake and concentration in brain and adipose tissue. Although blood levels are easily determined, they do not always correlate with the clinical findings or with the severity of the poisoning.

Gluetethimide overdose is similar to barbiturate intoxication in that stupor, coma, respiratory depression, and hypotension are key features. Glutethimide may be associated with a fluctuating mental status that is probably related to changing levels of the drug in the blood and brain. Hyperthermia is associated with coma and may develop slowly over 24 hours. The skin may be dry and flushed as in anticholinergic poisonings, and the pupils are often widely dilated.

The stomach should be emptied with emesis or lavage. Authors have advocated lavage with castor oil emulsion, which can theoretically absorb the drug in the stomach, but there are no good data to indicate significant drug removal with this technique. Standard lavage followed by administration of activated charcoal is preferable, because the efficacy of castor oil lavage is unproven, and aspiration of this mixture increases morbidity. The airway must be scrupulously protected to prevent aspiration of lavage material if the patient is stuporous or comatose.

Since the drug is lipid-soluble, forced diuresis is of no benefit, and vigorous volume expansion may overwhelm a hypokinetic cardiovascular system and result in pulmonary edema. Lipid hemodialysis has been attempted, but charcoal hemoperfusion is probably the preferred treatment in severe cases complicated by hypotension and shock.

Glutethimide-Codeine Combinations (''Pacs'')

Fixed combinations of glutethimide and codeine are now being sold illicitly as an oral putative heroin substitute. Clusters of use in Los Angeles, Newark, and Chicago have led to a more widespread availability of this street drug combination. Pharmaceutically pure sources may provide more bioavailability of this combination narcotic-hypnotic than heroin, and in some areas fatal cases are being reported with alarming frequency, second only to heroin. Users are younger and less experienced than heroin users, although they have often tried intravenous drugs as well. ''Advantages'' of this combination include cost and availability. The onset of the high or rush is slower than with heroin, occurring over 20–40 minutes, and is often enhanced by alcohol. The user apparently experiences dream-like euphoria followed by somnolence. Initial duration may be up to 12 hours, but tolerance may reduce its effect to 3 hours.

Because codeine is often acquired for this preparation in fixed combination with acetaminophen or aspirin, overdose may well have coexistent toxicity with these drugs. Known on the street as ''loads'' or ''hits,'' the combination is also referred to as Pacs because of the sale of the pills in packages of ''3s and 8s'' (three glutethimide 500-mg tablets and eight acetaminophen-codeine 30-mg tablets). While the average user may consume three Pacs in a day, tolerance may lead to use of up to eight Pacs in a 24-hour period, with the unintended toxicity of approximately 10–20 gm of acetaminophen or aspirin depending on the pill combination. With heavy use or overdose, the emergency physician may expect to see narcotic-hypnotic-induced stupor or coma with coexistent acetaminophen-induced liver injury or salicylism. Hypotension leading to acute tubular necrosis and renal failure has been reported, and seizures may occur. Treatment is directed at reversal of hypotension with volume replacement and sympathomimetic amines, if necessary, and support of the airway by intubation and ventilatory assistance in the circumstance of respiratory depression.

Seizures can be controlled with phenytoin and salicylate. Tylenol levels must be determined. In the circumstance of associated acetaminophen toxicity, hepatic injury may be well-established if the ingestion took place more than 24 hours before, and supportive measures should be used because acetylcysteine will be of no benefit. If oliguria does not respond to volume and leads to acute tubular injury and renal failure, dialysis is required. In this event the prognosis is poor.

Amphetamines

The amphetamines are noncatecholamine sympathomimetic drugs that stimulate both the α- and β-adrenergic nerve endings, producing central nervous system and cardiorespiratory stimulation. In therapeutic doses, these drugs may temporarily diminish fatigue and improve the patient's sense of well-being, but in overdoses of 15–25 mg/kg, a toxic delirium may give way to seizures, hyperpyrexia, and cardiovascular compromise.

Chronic amphetamine abuse may lead to amphetamine psychosis manifested by paranoia, delusions, and hallucinosis, but with preservation of orientation and memory. Chronic abuse may also be associated with nausea, vomiting, diarrhea, and weight loss. In chronic intravenous use, necrotizing angiitis and intracerebral hemorrhage have been described.

The drug is rapidly absorbed over 1–2 hours. Metabolism of 30–40% of the parent drug takes place in the liver, followed by excretion of metabolites along with free drug via the kidneys. With a pK of 9.9, amphetamines have a pH-dependent urinary excretion pattern that is enhanced by acidification and delayed by alkalization.

If the drug has been taken orally, the stomach should be emptied and charcoal administered. Patients who are extremely agitated or anxious can be calmed with haloperidol, 2–5 mg, or chlorpromazine, 1 mg/kg every 4–6 hours. Severe hypertension with end-organ compromise should be treated with either phentolamine or phenoxybenzamine hydrochloride, nitroprusside, or diazoxide. Severe hyperthermia can mimic heat stroke and can be associated with coagulopathy and acute renal failure. Temperature elevations will respond to vigorous external cooling, with chlorpromazine administration to prevent shivering and further temperature elevation.

Since some of the drug is excreted unchanged in the urine, forced diuresis with systemic acidification will enhance removal. Either ammonium chloride, 2.75 mEq/kg every 6 hours intravenously or by nasogastric tube, or ascorbic acid, 8 gm/day, can be given in both acute and chronic poisonings. Dialysis greatly enhances clearance but is rarely needed if adequate supportive measures are instituted.

Phenylpropanolamine

Like amphetamines, phenylpropanolamine is a noncatecholamine sympathomimetic used in nasal decongestant and over-the-counter diet preparations. Its abuse, however, stems largely from its marketing as an amphetamine substitute, body stimulant, and putative aphrodesiac in numerous pornographic magazines and mail order catalogues. Available in large lots for a low price, those capsules and tablets are then resold on the street as "street speed," "uppers," or stimulants and in fact may have shape, color, and numerical imprint codes identical to prescription amphetamines.

Phenylpropanolamine and its combinations with caffeine are rapidly absorbed from the gastrointestinal tract with a variable half-life of 3–6 hours depending on the preparation, some existing in time-release capsules. The drug is only minimally metabolized in the liver, and up to 90% may be excreted unchanged in the urine. Therapeutic and toxic blood levels are not well-established, but qualitative confirmation of the presence of the drug is possible with gas chromatographic toxic screen techniques. The enzyme multiplied immunoassay technique (EMIT) toxic screen technology may mistakenly identify phenylpropanolamine as amphetamine.

The clinical features of phenylpropanolamine abuse or overdose include hypertension, headache, dizziness, and blurred vision with confusion or apparent psychosis. Unlike anticholinergic delirium, these patients are usually sweating, not dry. Supraventricular and ventricular cardiac arrhythmias and seizures have been seen, and scattered cases of intracranial hemorrhage have been reported. Mortality is generally low in overdoses with this agent.

The treatment of phenylpropanolamine excess is supportive. Patients who are still alert may be able to identify the preparations by their street names (street speed, "magnums," "pink hearts"), or poison control centers can assist the emergency physician in identifying the pills or capsules if they are available. As always, toxic screen information must be interpreted with caution but can be useful in identifying other agents ingested simultaneously.

Hypertension with central nervous system, cardiac, or renal end-organ toxicity can be treated with phentolamine, an α-adrenergic blocker, or with nitroprusside, the latter offering rapid control. Seizures can be controlled with phenytoin, phenobarbital, or a benzodiazepine. Toxicity is usually of brief duration, and more aggressive measures, such as forced diuresis with acidification, while theoretically of benefit, are generally not needed.

Tricyclic Antidepressants

Drugs of this group (amitriptyline hydrochloride, imipramine hydrochloride, nortriptyline hydrochloride, protriptyline hydrochloride, desipramine hydrochloride, doxepin hydrochloride, and others) are common causes of hospitalization for drug overdose in the adult population.

The large number of tricyclic or polycyclic antidepressants should not be a source of confusion in management since their clinical presentation is similar. Poisoning with tricyclic antidepressants usually occurs as a suicide attempt by a depressed individual and is not generally part of street drug abuse.

Doses of 1.5–3.0 gm of tricyclic drugs result in serious poisonings with potentially fatal outcomes. The clinical features are those of initial central nervous system excitation followed by depression with seizures and anticholinergic syndromes, hypertension followed by hypotension, and cardiac effects including atrial and ventricular arrhythmias and conduction disturbances. There may be mild temperature elevation, urinary retention, and a progressively deteriorating course despite good initial management.

Blood levels of more than 1000 mg/ml correlate with true toxicity. Biggs et al. (see Suggested Readings) has shown that this level, which is associated with risk of serious cardiac arrhythmias, seizures, coma, and need for ventilatory support, correlates with 0.10 second or greater prolongation of the QRS interval on the electrocardiogram. In a prospective study of tricyclic overdoses, Boehnert and Lovejoy (see Suggested Readings) have further shown that seizures occurred in 34% of patients with QRS prolongation of 0.10 second or longer but not in individuals with QRS intervals of less than 0.10 second. Ventricular arrhythmias in that series occurred in 14% of patients with QRS prolongation, all of whom had QRS durations of 0.16 second or longer. Since serum levels have been shown to be an unreliable predictor of seizures or arrhythmias and such measurements are usually not rapidly available, the emergency physician should serially assess cardiac conduction as an essential indicator of major toxicity.

Treatment of tricyclic ingestions involves standard initial supportive measures. These drugs are antiemetic, but administration of ipecac early after ingestion may still be of benefit. In more serious ingestions with central nervous system and respiratory depression, the airway should be intubated, the stomach lavaged, and activated charcoal instilled, followed by administration of a saline cathartic. The anticholinergic properties of the drugs result in ileus with delayed gastric emptying and possibly delayed intestinal uptake; as a result, efforts to remove drug from the gastrointestinal tract may be beneficial even after 3–4 hours.

Cardiac arrhythmias are most often supraventricular, but serious ventricular arrhythmias (ectopy, tachycardia, and fibrillation) occur because of the quinidine-like effect of these drugs. These arrhythmias are more likely in the setting of hypoxemia, acidosis, and underlying ischemic cardiac disease. The concern for the possible risk of late cardiac arrhythmias with tricyclic antidepressant poisoning has led to many hospital admissions for cardiac monitoring. However, new studies show that the risk of late arrhythmias is probably low and occurs when the patient has arrhythmias, abnormal conduction, coma, or need for ventilatory support in the initial phase of management in the emergency department. Patients who have ingested tricyclic antidepressants but who remain alert in 6–8 hours of observation with normal electrocardiograms or only sinus tachycardia are not likely to need admission for cardiac monitoring, although psychiatric admission may be required depending on suicide intent and available social support.

Suggested guidelines regarding this issue include the following.

1. Patients with ventricular arrhythmias or conduction disturbances on admission to the emergency department or developing within several hours of observation should be admitted and monitored until arrhythmias cease.
2. Patient with anticholinergic findings and sinus tachycardia of more than 110 beats/min may require monitoring until the clinical course is defined more clearly, particularly if there is central nervous system depression or ventilatory impairment.
3. Patients with no anticholinergic findings or cardiac arrhythmias more troublesome than sinus tachycardia, who are sufficiently alert mentally for psychiatric treatment, have a low risk for late significant arrhythmias.

Physostigmine can be administered to reverse the central and peripheral anticholinergic effects of tricyclic antidepressants, but most tricyclic poisonings can be treated conservatively without it. Rapid bolus administration may precipitate seizures in patients with tricyclic poisoning, and severe bradyarrhythmias or asystole may occur. In general, physostigmine should be utilized for diagnosis in patients with unexplained coma and associated anticholinergic findings, since better alternatives exist for treatment of cardiac arrhythmias, seizures, and hypertension. Hypotension resulting from anticholinergic and tricyclic agents is generally poorly responsive to physostigmine, unless it is strictly due to reversible tachyarrhythmia.

Serious ventricular arrhythmias in patients with tricyclic antidepressant poisoning should be treated with intravenous lidocaine hydrochloride, 50–75 mg intravenously, followed by a 1–4 mg/min infusion.

Bretylium tosylate, 5–10 mg/kg intravenously, may be used for refractory ventricular tachycardia or fibrillation, and small doses of propranolol hydrochloride, 1 mg/min up to 5 mg total, may be of benefit in the absence of cardiac failure and volume overload. Systemic alkalization with 1–2 ampules of sodium bicarbonate or by means of transient hyperventilation of the intubated patient has been reported to be successful adjunctive therapy for ventricular arrhythmias caused by tricyclic antidepressants, even in the absence of acidosis. The mechanism of this effect is not completely understood. Quinidine and procainamide are contraindicated.

Phenytoin can reverse tricyclic-induced atrioventricular block and conduction disturbances and can also diminish ventricular ectopy. However, its use in patients with tricyclic-related QRS interval prolongation and a stable hemodynamic pattern has not yet been fully evaluated.

Hypotension usually responds to intravenous volume expansion with crystalloid or colloid. In general, sympathomimetic agents should be avoided, but when necessary, levarterenol bitartrate is a good choice since it provides some α-adrenergic peripheral vasoconstriction without significant cardiac effects.

Seizures should be treated with intravenous phenytoin, a 50- to 100-mg bolus slowly over 5 minutes, repeated to a total dose of 800–1000 mg as necessary. Barbiturates and diazepam should be avoided because of their additive effect to central nervous system or respiratory depression. Physostigmine, 1–2 mg given slowly intravenously, may help to abort seizures in tricyclic antidepressant overdose that have not responded to phenytoin or diazepam, but it should be used only as a last resort since a more rapid bolus may precipitate or prolong seizures.

These drugs are highly protein-bound and poorly water-soluble, so forced diuresis and standard hemodialysis are of no benefit. In severely poisoned patients with refractory hypotension, charcoal hemoperfusion should be considered.

Phenothiazines

Phenothiazine derivatives are commonly given for their antipsychotic effects and for the treatment of nausea and vomiting. These drugs may be divided into three classes: aliphatic, piperidine, and piperazine compounds. The pharmacologic effects of each group are slightly different, but in general, piperidine compounds (for example, thioridazine hydrochloride) and aliphatic compounds (for example, chlorpromazine) produce sedation and hypotension rather than central nervous system excitation in overdoses, whereas piperazine compounds (for example, perphenazine) tend to have an excitatory phase with agitation and extrapyramidal effects before central nervous system depression occurs.

In major overdoses of 2–4 gm, the clinical features include confusion, delirium, seizures, and coma with anticholinergic stimulation. Extrapyramidal reactions, including posturing, oculogyric crisis, and muscle spasm in the face and neck, may be confused with seizure activity. Hyperthermia may occur on an anticholinergic basis or secondary to hypothalamic effects, but hypothermia has also been reported with exposure.

Neuroleptic malignant syndrome with hyperthermia, muscular rigidity, and coma may mimic phenothiazine overdosage and should be considered in the differential diagnosis. In general, the temperature will be higher with neuroleptic malignant syndrome (often 105°F or greater), the muscles of the extremities more rigid, and the toxic screen will be in the therapeutic range or below (see Chapter 18).

Cardiac effects are in part anticholinergic, with a quinidine-like toxicity producing conduction disturbances and atrial and ventricular arrhythmias. Hypotension is due to both phenothiazine-induced α-adrenergic blockade and splanchnic vasodilatation with relative hypovolemia. Respiratory depression occurs when the doses are sufficient to cause coma.

Although as little as 2 gm of a phenothiazine derivative can cause death in adults, patients on chronic maintenance therapy may survive much higher single overdoses. In children, ingestion of 350 mg of chlorpromazine has been reported to cause death.

Although these agents are antiemetic, ipecac may be of benefit soon after ingestion and before the development of sedation. If a major overdose is suspected and the patient is stuporous or comatose, the airway should be secured, lavage performed, and activated charcoal instilled. Extrapyramidal reactions often respond rapidly to diphenhydramine hydrochloride, 25–50 mg intravenously, or benztropine mesylate, 1–2 mg, which may be repeated if necessary. Seizures should be treated with phenytoin.

The emergency physician should treat phenothiazine-induced hypotension with volume expansion. Sympathomimetic agents are rarely needed. However, if a pressor agent is required, agents with β-adrenergic activity, such as low doses of dopamine or isoproterenol hydrochloride, should be avoided. These agents may worsen hypotension because of peripheral β-adrenergic vasodilatation in the setting of phenothiazine-induced α-adrenergic blockade.

Patients with ventricular ectopy and conduction disturbances require cardiac monitoring. Supraventricular tachycardia is common but rarely requires treatment. Quinidine and procainamide hydrochloride should be avoided in the treatment of ventricular ectopy since they may add to the cardiotoxic effects. Lidocaine hydrochloride, phenytoin, bretylium tosylate, or propranolol hydrochloride may be given, with sodium bicarbonate as an adjunctive agent as in tricyclic antidepressant poisonings. Physostigmine may be of benefit in patients with these arrhythmias but only after other standard agents have been tried.

Phenothiazine derivatives may be ingested in fixed combination with tricyclic antidepressants (Triavil) or as part of a multiple drug ingestion. Qualitative analysis for the presence of phenothiazines is not difficult for most toxicology laboratories, but quantitative analysis is unreliable since blood levels may not correlate with the patient's clinical course. Because these drugs are protein-bound, treatment with forced diuresis is of no benefit.

Cocaine

Increasing numbers of patients are being treated in emergency departments for toxic effects from cocaine, one of the most common recreational drugs of abuse. Although it has been advocated as a relatively safe drug when used intranasally, deaths have occurred by this route as well as by smoking, oral ingestion, and intravenous injection. Increased availability of cocaine has reduced its cost as has the dramatic increase in the free-based form of cocaine called "crack" or "rock," which is sold for a small unit price in the form of chips or "rocks" that can be smoked.

Cocaine is an alkaloid extract of the leaves of *Erythroxylon coca.* A topical anesthetic, it blocks peripheral nerve conduction. Cocaine also has prominent central nervous system stimulation properties, and its illicit use depends on this phenomenon.

The drug is usually sold as a powder of the cocaine hydrochloride salt, adulterated with mannitol, sugars, or such other drugs as lidocaine hydrochloride, phencyclidine, or amphetamine. It is most often taken by intranasal insufflation, which is followed in 5–20 minutes by pharmacologic effects. Intravenous and pulmonary absorption is also rapid; oral administration results in absorption in the small intestine at a pK of 8.5. but gastric hydrolysis may diminish the effect.

Free-based cocaine in the form of crack is almost pure cocaine in its alkaloidal form, produced by mixing a solution of cocaine hydrochloride with ammonia or sodium bicarbonate. The rock crystal produces a popping or cracking sound when heated, and the name derives from this sound. Crack can be smoked directly in a pipe or mixed with tobacco and smoked with a rapid onset of an intense stimulation more like intravenous cocaine with onset of action within minutes. The brief duration of effect may lead to frequent repeat doses or "runs" with a major addiction potential.

Central nervous system stimulation begins rapidly, with a sense of euphoria and excitement associated with pupillary dilation and increased heart rate, blood pressure, and respiration rate. Occasionally, dysphoria occurs acutely, with confusion, apprehension, and hallucinosis. Chronic use can be associated with hallucinosis and a syndrome of schizophrenia with paranoia. In addition, the nasal septum may become perforated as a result of vasoconstriction and tissue loss.

Pharmacologic effects depend on dosage and route of administration, but major life-threatening complications of cocaine in all its forms are being recognized and reported with increasing frequency. In excessive doses, hyperthermia, seizures, coma, respiratory arrest, angina pectoris, coronary spasm or occlusion, and ventricular arrhythmias may occur. However, convulsions or cardiac arrhythmias may also follow small doses. Free-based forms appear to have increased risks of seizures and cardiac arrest. Intracranial hemorrhage has occurred, possibly related to the hypertensive response. Underlying cerebrovascular and cardiovascular disease increase the risk of morbidity and mortality.

Cocaine-filled condoms ingested by drug dealers in smuggling activities have ruptured in the gastrointestinal tract, leading to sudden massive absorption and rapid cardiac arrest. Because of the risk of rupture with handling, operation rather than endoscopic examination is recommended for intact ingested condoms, if there is any sign of toxicity. Catharsis may be tried in the stable patient, but there is risk of rupture with any of these approaches.

Treatment of cocaine ingestion involves protection of the airway, observation, and appropriate treatment of the cardiac rhythm with cardioversion or antiarrhythmic drugs. Residual drug on the nasal mucosa should be removed. Persistent seizures should be treated with phenytoin, body temperature should be lowered with external cooling, and severe hypertension with end-organ compromise should be treated with rapid-acting antihypertensive agents, Paranoia and agitation may respond to haloperidol, in cautious doses.

Small doses of intravenous propranolol hydrochloride may antagonize the cardiopressor effects of cocaine, and some have advocated its use in patients with casual cocaine intoxication with hypertension, tachycardia, and behavioral changes. In animal experiments, pretreatment with chlorpromazine has been shown to block some of the cardiotoxic effects. Data to support clinical administration of these drugs are not yet available, and the emergency physician should proceed cautiously, with provision of supportive measures as the first priority.

Phencyclidine

Phencyclidine hydrochloride is an analgesic anesthetic agent similar to ketamine hydrochloride. Because of severe dysphoric reactions during its development, phencyclidine was discontinued for application in humans, although it is still used in veterinary medicine as Sernylan. The major current source in drug abuse and overdose is illicit manufacture. Phencyclidine is sold on the street in pill or powder form (usually misrepresented as tetrahydrocannabinol, mescaline, or LSD) or in marihuana mixtures (''supergrass''). Street vernacular referring to phencyclidine includes such terms as angel dust, crystal, goon, surfer, peace weed, and cyclones.

The clinical features of this intoxication depend on dose and route of administration, with smoking and inhalation in general causing a milder course than oral ingestion or the less common intravenous use. At low doses, agitation, excitement, and incoordination may be present, but a predominant feature is a blank stare with occasional catatonic mutism. The patient may appear inebriated. The pupils are usually in midposition and reactive with prominent nystagmus. Disorganized thoughts and a sense of altered body image may be present along with paranoid ideation.

At moderate to high doses, seizures, stupor, or coma with respiratory depression may occur. The eyes may remain open with reactive pupils, and nystagmus and vomiting may occur with risk of aspiration. Myoclonus and muscular rigidity can mimic seizure activity, and the anesthetic effect of the drug can cause diminished sensation. Considerable agitation may result, and the patient can be easily provoked into assaultive behavior, which can include homicide. Clinical findings can be marked by a relapsing course, and rhabdomyolysis can produce pigment-induced renal failure.

A dose of 5–10 mg of phencyclidine can produce moderate symptoms, with severe manifestations occurring after ingestions in excess of 10 mg. The drug produces sensory dissociation and blockade and is highly lipid-soluble with a pK of 8.6. Phencyclidine is metabolized in the liver, with urinary excretion of metabolites in low doses and excretion of free drug in high doses. The half-life varies with the dose, as hepatic metabolism becomes limiting. Enterohepatic circulation may prolong the half-life as well. As a weak base, the drug is readily ionized in an acidic environment and trapped within cells.

Low-dose intoxication should be treated in a quiet environment. Haloperidol may be used for sedation in cases of extreme agitation. The patient must be monitored carefully for central nervous system and respiratory depression at higher doses of phencyclidine. Intubation may be required and seizures should be controlled with phenytoin. If the drug has been taken orally, the stomach should be emptied.

Done and associates (see Aronow and Done, 1978, Suggested Readings) have advocated continuous gastric suction and systemic acidification. Urinary concentration can be increased by acidification to 200 times the concentration in the blood to produce a urinary pH less than 5. Either ascorbic acid, 8 gm/day orally, or ammonium chloride, 2.75 mEq/kg by nasogastric tube or intravenously every 6 hours, can be given, and forced diuresis with the addition of a loop diuretic will maximize urinary excretion of the drug.

Methanol

Methyl alcohol or wood alcohol intoxication produces serious poisoning associated with severe metabolic acidosis. The degree of acidosis is disproportionate to the amount of acid produced by the toxin and is due to interference with normal intermediary metabolism with consequent overproduction of metabolic acids (lactate and keto acids). The usual sources of methanol in poisonings are solvents, paint thinner, and Sterno. Methanol may be accidentally consumed as an ethanol substitute or taken in a purposeful suicide attempt.

Methanol is less inebriating than ethanol. It is oxidized to formaldehyde by alcohol dehydrogenase and then to formic acid. The toxicity of methanol is due to formaldehyde and formic acid, and becomes manifest slowly, usually appearing 12–24 hours after ingestion. Headache, nausea, vomiting, and dizziness are followed by central nervous system and respiratory depression. Visual impairment results from the toxic effects of formaldehyde and formic acid on the optic nerve and retina. The pupils may be dilated and optic disc hyperemia develops. Ingestions of 10–15 ml may result in significant visual impairment, and death has occurred after a 20-ml ingestion. The toxicity may vary, however, and survival has occurred after ingestions in excess of 100 ml.

Blood levels of 20–50 mg/dl suggest major toxicity, and treatment includes lavage or induced emesis in the first few hours after ingestion. Sodium bicarbonate must be administered intravenously to reverse acidosis.

Ethanol and methanol are both metabolized by alcohol dehydrogenase, but the metabolic rate of methanol is only 15% that of ethanol. Because of its affinity for alcohol dehydrogenase, ethanol competitively inhibits the metabolism of methanol and should be used in therapy when blood levels of methanol exceed 20 mg/dl. For intravenous treatment, a loading dose of absolute ethanol, 1 ml/kg, is given in 5% dextrose solution over 15 minutes, followed by 7–10 ml/hr to maintain a blood level of ethanol at 100 mg/dl. Oral ethanol may also be used with the same blood level goal. When methanol levels exceed 50 mg/dl or when acidosis is severe and resistant to bicarbonate therapy, hemodialysis is indicated in addition to ethanol therapy. On dialysis, intravenous administration of ethanol may have to be increased up to 50% to maintain the blood level of ethanol at 100 mg/dl.

Ethylene Glycol

Ethylene glycol, like methanol, produces severe anion gap acidosis due to the contribution of its metabolic products (aldehydes, glycolic acid, and oxalic acid) and its effect on intermediary metabolism, which causes the elaboration of lactic acid and keto acids. As in methanol ingestion, mild inebriation may occur without the odor of alcohol, but unlike methanol poisoning, ethylene glycol toxicity becomes manifest rapidly over several hours. Death in adults can occur with ingestions of approximately 75–100 gm of ethylene glycol.

Headache, nausea, vomiting, ataxia, and stupor can be followed by convulsions and coma in the first 6 hours. Cardiac failure, pulmonary edema, and respiratory failure often ensue by 24 hours, with oliguria leading to acute renal failure. Oxalate crystals can be present in the urine sediment and be a clue to diagnosis. Diffuse oxalate crystal deposition occurs in other organs as well. Hypothermia and hypocalcemia may develop.

The treatment of ethylene glycol poisoning requires rapid diagnosis. In the absence of corroborative history, the diagnosis should be suspected in comatose patients with severe anion gap metabolic acidosis. Toxicologic analysis will confirm the diagnosis and exclude salicylate, methanol, and paraldehyde ingestions. The clinical data and history will often help exclude causes of anion gap acidosis unrelated to poisoning, such as diabetic ketoacidosis, lactic acidosis, and chronic renal failure.

The stomach should be emptied after the airway is protected, and vigorous sodium bicarbonate therapy can be required to control acidosis. The metabolic breakdown of ethylene glycol, like that of methanol, depends on alcohol dehydrogenase and can be blocked by the concurrent administration of ethanol. A blood level of 100 mg/dl of ethanol should be maintained with intravenous therapy; loading and maintenance doses are the same as for methanol. Intravenous administration of pyridoxine, 100 mg, and thiamine, 100 mg, has been advocated to direct metabolism of glycol to nontoxic metabolites, although this effect is not proven. Like methanol, ethylene glycol can be removed with dialysis, which should be undertaken promptly. Ethanol infusion rates must be increased on dialysis to maintain a blood level of 100 mg/dl.

In contrast to ethylene glycol and methanol, isopropyl alcohol (rubbing alcohol) does not produce metabolic acidosis. It is metabolized to acetone, and is inebriating like ethanol. Coma, gastritis, and aspiration pneumonitis may occur, but death is uncommon. Treatment is supportive.

Petroleum Distillates

Petroleum distillate ingestion frequently occurs in children. Approximately 100 deaths occur yearly from this poisoning, 90% of which are in children less than 5 years old, but almost 20,000 hospitalizations related to petroleum distillate exposure or ingestion occur annually, so emergency physicians will commonly deal with this toxic exposure.

The most commonly ingested products are kerosene, charcoal lighter fluids, mineral seal oil preparations, turpentine, and gasoline. As little as 0.5 ounce of ingested petroleum distillate has occasionally caused death. Death is produced by central nervous system depression, cardiotoxic reactions, and complications of aspiration. The viscosity and surface tension of the fluid determine the aspiration hazard. Distillates with lower viscosity and surface tension tend to "creep" along the mucous membranes. This is much more likely in patients who are lethargic or convulsing.

The clinical findings are related to the respiratory central nervous, and gastrointestinal systems. Respiratory findings may be as mild as the frequent upper respiratory tract infections in this age group, or they may be severe, with cyanosis, pulmonary edema, and hemorrhage. Breath holding usually signals an attempt to protect the airway from further aspiration of distillate and indicates severe ingestion. Central nervous system depression and seizures are infrequently seen unless more than 30 ml have been ingested. Local irritation of the mucous membranes in the mouth and pharynx occurs. Vomiting is frequent and is usually accompanied by the characteristic odor of the hydrocarbon product. Diarrhea may also occur and occasionally may be bloody. Furniture polish containing mineral seal oil products produces particularly severe gastrointestinal symptoms.

Blood levels of hydrocarbons are extremely difficult to determine, but x-ray evaluation is helpful. An x-ray film of the chest should be obtained in all suspected cases, since there is often evidence of pneumonitis in the absence of clinical signs and symptoms. A double gastric fluid shadow on an upright abdominal x-ray film can be seen after giving the patient 4–8 ounces of water. This can detect as little as 5 ml of petroleum distillate in the stomach, thereby identifying cases of potential toxicity.

Treatment of petroleum distillate ingestions has been controversial, with gastric lavage, emesis, and cathartics being both favored and opposed. The controversy has been heightened by the product labels on petroleum distillate packages. A typical label states: *"In case of accidental ingestion, do not induce vomiting. Call your physician immediately."* Cautious gastric lavage has been advocated, but few physicians can perform this procedure in a struggling, frightened child.

If the patient is coughing, wheezing, or dyspneic with pulmonary findings on presentation, aspiration is likely to have already occurred, and further gastric emptying is not necessary. If more than 1 ml/kg has been ingested, the current trend favors gastric emptying with emesis induced by ipecac in the alert patient. There is a risk of aspiration with this method, but it is less than the risk of aspiration after depression of consciousness. If the patient is comatose, gastric lavage should be performed after the airway is protected by a cuffed endotracheal tube. Sympathomimetic drugs should be avoided in these patients since life-threatening arrhythmias may develop in a sensitized myocardium. Charcoal is of no benefit, but a saline cathartic may help to reduce gastrointestinal absorption. There is no proven benefit to prophylactic antibiotics and no data to support use of high-dose corticosteroids.

Data on decision making for hospitalization suggest that all patients with respiratory symptoms and chest x-ray evidence of pneumonitis should be admitted, whereas children who are asymptomatic with normal physical findings and x-ray films and who remain asymptomatic for 6–8 hours of observation may be safely discharged. Patients with x-ray evidence of minor aspiration but without symptoms may not require hospitalization, but the emergency physician should base this decision on the patient's availability for follow-up care and on the family's reliability.

The toxicity of aromatic hydrocarbons (xylene, toluene) and halogenated hydrocarbons (carbon tetrachloride, trichloroethane) is distinct from that of petroleum distillates. The aromatic hydrocarbons affect the gastrointestinal tract, the central nervous system, and the bone marrow (marrow suppression). Chronic use may also be associated with renal tubular injury. The halogenated hydrocarbons cause severe hepatic and renal injury. Aromatic and halogenated hydrocarbons should be removed from the gastrointestinal tract as a definite priority. Table 17.9 summarizes the decision-making process for toxin removal in petroleum distillate ingestion.

Mushrooms

Although there are more than 3000 species of mushrooms, only about 50 are known to cause toxic reactions, and more than 90% of lethal mushroom poisonings are attributed to the genus *Amanita.* Mushroom poisoning may vary from mild gastrointestinal symptoms to severe hepatic, renal, and neurologic toxicity. Table 17.10 summarizes seven groups of toxic mushrooms according to their toxin.

The emergency physician can best judge the severity of these poisonings by combining clinical assessment with identification of the mushroom. Knowledge of local toxic species is of benefit, and often, poison control centers maintain a list of experts who are able to identify mushrooms from description or direct examination. Local mycologic societies are usually willing to provide such consultation, and the emergency department should maintain a call list. Identification involves gross examination of the mushroom cap, stem, and bulb, and occasionally, microscopic examination of the spores.

Amanita phalloides (death cup), *Amanita verna,* and *Amanita virosa* (destroying angel) are among the most poisonous mushrooms. They produce toxins, phalloidin and α-amanitin, that interfere with RNA synthesis and cellular metabolism in the liver, kidneys, brain, and striated muscle. The clinical manifestations are divided into three phases. The first phase begins 10–20 hours after ingestion and is characterized by nausea, vomiting, abdominal pain, and profuse watery diarrhea. During the second phase, from 24 to 48 hours, the patient's condition improves as electrolytes and volume are replenished, but hepatic and renal damage occurs as evidenced both by liver function tests showing progressive hepatocellular dysfunction and by renal impairment. Within 3–4 days, marked liver failure ensues, with coagulopathy, acidosis, oliguric renal failure, and acute tubular necrosis. Cardiac arrhythmias and conduction disturbances may occur.

The use of emesis, gastric lavage, or charcoal is rarely of benefit in *Amanita* poisonings since ingestion has often occurred 8–10 hours before the onset of symptoms. Supportive measures, volume and electrolyte replacement, and attention to the end-organ effects of coagulopathy, hepatic failure, and renal failure are necessary. Renal failure may require dialysis, but the toxins themselves are poorly dialyzable. Thioctic acid has been used in Europe and in the United States for *Amanita* poisoning. The mechanism of action is not completely understood, nor is there complete agreement as to its efficacy. Early administration seems to correlate with the best results. The mortality rate among patients with *Amanita* poisoning ranges from 50 to 80%.

Table 17.9.
Hydrocarbons

Petroleum Distillates				
High viscosity	Low viscosity	Halogenated	Aromatics	"Dangerous Additives"
Low toxicity	*Moderate toxicity*	*High toxicity*	*High toxicity*	*High toxicity*
Tar Paraffin Motor oil Diesel fuel Transmission oil Petroleum liquid jelly	Gasoline Kerosene Mineral seal oil (Furniture polish) Varnish Naphtha	Carbon tetrachloride Trichloroethylene Trichloroethane Halothane	Benzene Toluene Xylene Styrene	Pesticides Organophosphates Camphor Nitrobenzene Methyl chloride
		Gastric Emptying		
No	Possible with doses >1–2 ml/kg	Yes	Yes	Yes

Table 17.10.
Classification of Mushroom Groups[a]

	Group						
	Cyclopeptide	Ibotenic	Muscarine	Psilocybin	Disulfiram-like	Gastrointestinal Irritant	Gyromitrin
Mushroom genus and species	*Amanita phalloides, verna, virosa* *Galerina autumnaus, marginata, venenata*	*Amanita muscaria, pantherine*	*Inocybe* many species *Clitocybe dealbata, virulosa*	*Psilocybe cubensis, eaerulescens, silvatic* *Panaeolus subbalteus*	*Coprinus atramentarius*	Many varied genera	*Gyromitra* many species
Toxin	α-Amanitin phalloidin	Ibotenic acid, muscimol, pantherin	Muscarine	Psilocybin, psilocin, baeocystin	Monomethyl hydrazine	Unidentified	Gyromitrin
Onset of symptoms	10–20 hr	15–30 min	15–30 min	30–60 min	5–10 min	30–90 min	6–8 hr
Predominant signs and symptoms	Initial gastrointestinal toxicity, transient clinical improvement, terminal hepato- and nephrotoxicity	Anticholinergic and CNS disturbances	Cholinergic	CNS disturbances[b]	Antabuse-like reaction, gastrointestinal toxicity	Gastrointestinal toxicity	Gastrointestinal toxicity
Treatment	Thioctic acid, supportive	Supportive, atropine contraindicated	Suppportive, atropine	Supportive	Supportive, avoid alcohol	Supportive	Supportive
Prognosis	Poor; fatalities have been reported from one mushroom cap	Good; recovery is rapid and complete; deaths are rare	Good; death infrequently results from cardiac arrest and respiratory failure	Good; recovery is rapid and complete	Good; recovery is rapid and complete	Good; recovery is rapid and complete	Fair to poor; mortality may range from 2–4%

[a] Reproduced, with permission, from McCormick DJ, Avbel AJ, Gibbons RB: Nonlethal mushroom poisoning. *Ann Intern Med,* 1979;90:332–335.
[b] CNS, central nervous system.

Nonlethal mushroom poisonings tend to have an earlier onset of symptoms and can be characterized by either gastrointestinal symptoms of nausea, vomiting, pain, and diarrhea or by neurologic dysfunction related to either cholinergic or anticholinergic manifestations. Hallucinosis, delirium, and coma may occur with bronchorrhea, lacrimation, and bronchospasm in cholinergic excess; tachycardia, fever, and seizures characterize the anticholinergic toxins.

Anticholinergic poisonings respond to supportive measures, and improvement has been reported after physostigmine administration in comatose and delirious patients. The toxin muscarine in the genus *Clitocybe* produces cholinergic excess that responds to supportive measures and atropine, 0.6–1.0 mg intravenously. The genus *Coprinus* produces an acute Antabuse-type reaction with alcohol, resulting in moderately severe gastrointestinal symptoms but usually relatively rapid recovery over 24 hours.

Poisons with Specific Antidotes

Several poisons require antidotes promptly to decrease morbidity and mortality. The emergency physician will frequently utilize the previously described antidotal applications of naloxone for narcotics and acetylcysteine for acetaminophen. While anticholinergic poisonings are common, the use of physostigmine as an antidote remains limited. Carbon monoxide poisoning, with or without body burns, encountered in the emergency department and its treatment with oxygen are described in Chapter 10.

However, several less frequently encountered poisonings require specific antidotal therapies, which are discussed in this section. These include iron, fluorides, cyanide, nitrites and nitrates, and organophosphate and carbamate insecticide compounds.

Iron

Fatal iron poisoning is uncommon, but iron ingestion may be seen frequently because of the multiple preparations of iron salts or multivitamins containing iron that are found in the home. Purposeful ingestion in adults is occasionally seen, but the emergency physician will more commonly encounter smaller ingestions in children who may be attracted to the brightly colored or sugar-coated tablets.

Iron salts cause a corrosive-like injury to the intestinal tract that is followed by hemorrhage, volume loss, and shock. Metabolic acidosis results from hypotension, from the formation of ferric hydroxides with the release of hydrogen ion, and from interruption of intermediary metabolism. As the binding capacity of ferritin is exceeded, free iron is found in the serum and subsequently deposited in the intestine, liver, and spleen. Hemorrhage into various organs may occur because of effects on both prothrombin clotting mechanisms as well as platelets and fibrinogen. Lethargy and stupor may develop in significant overdoses due to the direct effects of iron on the central nervous system and to cerebral hypoperfusion.

Toxicity is related to the amount of elemental iron ingested. Ferrous sulfate tablets (300 mg) contain 20% elemental iron (60 mg), whereas ferrous gluconate tablets (350 mg) contain 12% elemental iron (36 mg). Potential toxicity can occur with as little as 200 mg of elemental iron in children or in any patient with ingestion of 30–60 mg/kg. Fatality may occur in high-dose ingestions approaching 300 mg/kg. As indicators of toxicity, the serum iron level and total iron-binding capacity should be determined. A serum iron level exceeding total iron-binding capacity by 350 mEq/dl or greater is an indication for chelation therapy, particularly if clinical symptoms of bleeding, shock, or central nervous system depression are present. When iron levels are not readily available, a provocative chelation test may be utilized to establish the presence of free circulating iron. After the administration of 25–50 mg/kg of deferoxamine intramuscularly (maximum 1 gm), the urine turns pink or "rosé" if the iron level exceeds the total iron-binding capacity. This test may not be reliable in hypotensive, oliguric patients. They are treated empirically, while awaiting level determination, if the clinical symptoms are severe. Abdominal x-rays revealing radiopaque tablets in the intestinal tract support the clinical diagnosis.

There are several phases in the clinical course of iron poisoning. Within the first 2 hours, there may be nausea, vomiting, and abdominal pain leading to bloody diarrhea. With high doses patients may be lethargic. A transient phase of improvement may occur over 6–24 hours, but fever, shock, and severe metabolic acidosis may develop in the same time frame in severe ingestions. Later phases include liver necrosis with coagulopathy and encephalopathy, renal failure (2–4 days), and the more delayed intestinal obstruction (2–4 weeks) in surviving patients.

Therapy of iron ingestion should begin with efforts to remove drug from the intestinal tract with emesis in awake persons and lavage with airway protection in obtunded patients. Lavage with a 5% solution of sodium bicarbonate is recommended to encourage formation of the less toxic ferrous carbonate salt. Activated charcoal is not beneficial. Serial plain x-rays of the abdomen indicate whether radiopaque tablets are still present in the stomach. Catharsis can be utilized early if there is no sign of intestinal bleeding. Chelation therapy is indicated with serious ingestions, with associated clinical symptoms, with iron levels greater than 350 μg/dl, or with ingestions of 300 mg/kg or greater. Levels of 350–500 μg/dl may require brief chelation therapy. Levels of 500–1000 μg/dl may require more vigorous treatment, while levels in excess of 1000 μg/dl require chelation treatment and possibly hemodialysis or exchange transfusion. Deferoxamine is infused intravenously in doses of 15 mg/kg/hr or, if the patient is not hypotensive, intramuscularly at 20 mg/kg every 4 hours. The initial intramuscular dose should not exceed 1 gm, and the total dose should not exceed 6 gm in 24 hours. Too rapid infusion may produce hypotension. The iron-deferoxamine complex is excreted in the urine, and when the urine color turns from pink to normal, the chelation process is complete. A repeat iron level less than the total iron-binding capacity confirms this endpoint. Dialysis may be required with renal failure, but chelation therapy will still be necessary.

Fluorides

Hydrofluoric acid is a corrosive inorganic acid used in the glass-etching and semiconductor industries. Fluoride salts are used in insecticides. Hydrogen fluoride and fluorine gas also cause toxicity in their corrosive action on tissues and cellular effects on enzymatic pathways. The toxicity of these agents depends on the preparation and route of exposure.

Direct contact with hydrofluoric acid can produce a devitalizing corrosive burn with severe pain. High concentration hydrofluoric acid dissociates in the tissues and binds calcium, producing calcium fluoride, with the potential for systemic hypocalcemia and cardiac arrhythmia. Inhalation of fluorine or hydrogen fluoride produces a noxious pulmonary irritant injury with delayed chemical pulmonary edema over 24–48 hours depending on the concentration of the gas and the duration of exposure. Associated upper airway and facial burns complicate the course. Oral ingestion of fluoride salts (e.g., sodium fluoride) produces nausea, vomiting, and abdominal pain because the corrosive action of the fluoride injures gastrointestinal tissues. Seizures can occur and carpopedal spasm heralds systemic hypocalcemia. Severe exposure results in shock and respiratory arrest.

Hydrofluoric acid skin exposures should be vigorously irrigated with water and then covered with a dressing soaked in calcium gluconate. If there is evidence of burn or local pain, 10% calcium gluconate should be infiltrated locally via a 25-gauge needle into the wound after local or regional anesthesia, and the patient should be admitted for close observation of such systemic complications as hypocalcemia or delayed pulmonary injury (see Chapter 38 for a discussion of burn management). With oral fluoride salt ingestion, milk, lime water, or calcium gluconate can be given orally in an effort to inactivate the fluoride ion. Charcoal can be given and followed by 10 gm of calcium gluconate and an osmotic cathartic. Serial serum calcium determinations are necessary with treatment of hypocalcemia by intravenous calcium gluconate or chloride. The usual clinical signs of hypocalcemia (carpopedal spasm, Chvostek's sign) can be absent. Patients should have continuous cardiac monitoring.

Cyanide

Cyanide is one of the most rapidly acting of all poisons. It inhibits cytochrome B, one of the enzymes in cellular oxygen transport, by binding with the ferric (Fe^{3+}) component of cytochrome oxidase. Cyanides are present in rodent poisons and in the seeds of many fruits, including the peach, apple, plum, cherry, and apricot, and they are used industrially in electroplating and mining. They are absorbed through the skin and mucous membranes, and toxic amounts can be absorbed quickly via inhalation.

Symptoms appear soon after exposure; although most deaths are rapid, patients may survive for several hours and can be saved with prompt and proper treatment. An odor of bitter almonds is classic, but is not always present. Signs are due to the rapid development of tissue hypoxia.

Treatment is based on the principle of providing competitive ferric sites with which the cyanide can bind, thus freeing some of the ferric components of cytochrome oxidase. This is done by converting hemoglobin containing ferrous (Fe^{2+}) iron to methemoglobin with ferric sites, producing methemoglobinemia. Care must be taken to prevent a lethal level of methemoglobin. Methemoglobinemia can be produced by inhalation of amyl nitrite or intravenous infusion of sodium nitrite:

$$\underset{(Fe^{2+})}{\text{hemoglobin}} + \text{nitrite} \rightarrow \underset{(Fe^{3+})}{\text{methemoglobin}}$$

Some of the cyanide then binds to the methemoglobin:

$$\text{methemoglobin} + \text{cytochrome oxidase-cyanide} \rightarrow \text{methemoglobin-cyanide} + \text{cytochrome oxidase}$$

If thiosulfate is made available, thiocyanate is formed, which is nontoxic and can be excreted:

$$\text{methemoglobin-cyanide} + \text{thiosulfate} \rightarrow \text{methemoglobin} + \text{thiocyanate} + \text{sulfite}$$

The methemoglobin is reduced to hemoglobin by erythrocytic enzyme systems.

A prepackaged kit containing the necessary drugs is available (Eli Lilly & Co.). The amyl nitrite should be replaced yearly. Amyl nitrite pearls should be broken and held under the nose while the sodium nitrite is being drawn into a syringe, and should be removed after the sodium nitrite is given. Oxygen should be administered during treatment. Sodium nitrite is infused intravenously, 10 ml of a 3% solution in a 2-minute period. Ideally, such treatment will produce a methemoglobin level of approximately 30% in adults. The adult dose produces fatal methemoglobinemia in children. The pediatric dose is 10 mg/kg or 0.33 ml/kg of the 3% solution. Immediately after administration of sodium nitrite, 50 ml of a 25% solution of sodium thiosulfate are given intravenously in the course of 1–2 minutes.

If the poisoning was the result of ingestion, gastric lavage should be performed with a 1:5000 solution of potassium permanganate. After lavage, 300 ml of the 25% solution of sodium thiosulfate should be instilled in the stomach. Symptoms can recur and be treated in a manner similar to the initial treatment with half the dose.

Contaminated skin and clothing can be cleansed with soap and water. Since cyanide can be absorbed through the skin, personnel must avoid becoming contaminated.

Nitrites and Nitrates

Nitrite and nitrate poisoning is unusual. Poisoning can result from nitrite-containing drugs used as coronary vasodilators. Nitrite is also used in meat processing for preservation and for prevention of discoloration. Nitrates are found in fertilizers and feedstock and are converted to nitrites by intestinal bacteria. Beets, spinach, and carrots grown in soil containing large amounts of nitrite or nitrate have high concentrations of the toxin. Accidental poisoning also occurs in children whose milk formula has been contaminated with *Bacillus subtilis*.

The toxic state is produced by development of methemoglobinemia. Clinical findings include considerable cyanosis unresponsive to the administration of oxygen. Diagnosis can be confirmed by drying a drop of blood on filter paper and observing a brown color. A 1% solution of methylene blue can be infused intravenously, 0.2 ml/kg in the course of 5 minutes. Exchange transfusion may be required in severe cases. Surface decontamination is important because the chemicals can be absorbed through the skin.

Organophosphorus Compounds and Carbamates

Organophosphorus compounds are used as insecticides, and the incidence of poisoning with them has increased since they have replaced banned DDT. These compounds are extremely toxic; one drop of undiluted parathion can be fatal. Most poisoning is due to occupational exposure in crop dusters, farmers, and florists, with absorption through the mucous membranes, skin, and lungs.

Organophosphates block the action of cholinesterase, so the action of acetylcholine released from nerve endings is unopposed. Cholinesterase activity in red blood cells can be measured, and is usually less than 30% of normal. Poisoning is manifested by the SLUD syndrome: *s*alivation, *l*acrimation, *ur*ination, and *d*efecation. Pupils are usually small, but this sign can be unreliable. Other effects are fasciculations, muscular weakness, paralysis, ataxia, and coma. Death may be due to depression of central respiratory or circulatory centers, bronchoconstriction, excessive bronchial secretion, or paralysis of the respiratory muscles.

Treatment should not wait for confirmation from the laboratory. The initial treatment in a cyanotic patient is oxygen, after which intravenous or intramuscular atropine sulfate can be given, 2 mg initially (0.05 mg/kg in children). If atropine is given to a cyanotic patient, ventricular fibrillation may occur due to myocardial sensitivity to atropine in the setting of hypoxemia and acidosis. Lack of a clinical response to small amounts of atropine is further evidence for poisoning of this type. The amount of atropine administered depends on the given patient, and salivation can be used as a clinical factor. When salivation decreases substantially, enough atropine has been given. Large amounts are often necessary, and a total dose of more than 500 mg has been reported often. Usually, a total of 25–50 mg is necessary in a 24-hour period. Artificial ventilation with a respirator is usually indicated since the atropine often does not reverse the muscular paralysis. Frequent suction of the lower part of the respiratory tract is necessary to keep the patient from drowning in secretions.

After the diagnosis is confirmed and the symptoms are controlled with atropine sulfate, reactivation of cholinesterase can be accomplished by the use of oximes, which cleave the bond between the organophosphate and the cholinesterase. Pralidoxime chloride (Protopam), 1 gm intravenously in adults, can be given in a 2-minute period. This dose can be repeated after 1 hour if the exposure was severe. The dosage in children is 25–50 mg/kg. Pralidoxime chloride is effective if given within several hours of exposure.

Mild cases of poisoning can usually be treated with oral administration of pralidoxime chloride, and symptoms usually abate within 1 hour. The dose may be repeated as necessary. All patients, however mild the toxic state, should be closely supervised in the hospital for 24 hours. Seizures can be controlled with small doses of short-acting barbiturates since the anticholinesterase sensitizes the medullary depressant center. Morphine, aminophylline, succinylcholine, and phenothiazines are contraindicated.

Decontamination of skin and clothing is important. An alkaline solution should be used since this accelerates hydrolysis of the phosphate. Leather cannot be decontaminated and must be discarded properly.

Carbamates are used as insecticides, and poisoning produces signs and symptoms similar to those seen with organophosphorus compounds. The carbamates also combine with cholinesterase, but binding is reversible and the complex usually rapidly dissociates spontaneously. Treatment is similar to that for organophosphorus poisoning, with use of atropine sulfate as needed. However, oximes are not indicated and may be harmful.

SUGGESTED READINGS

Arena JM. Poisoning—treatment and prevention *JAMA,* 1975;232:1271–1275; 233:358–363.

Arieff A. Coma following non-narcotic overdose: Management of 208 adult patients. *Am J Med Sci,* 1973;266:405–426.

Greenblatt DJ, Shader RI. Acute poisoning with psychotropic drugs. In Shader RI, et al. (eds): *Psychotropic Drug Side Effects: Clinical and Theoretical Perspectives,* Baltimore; Williams & Wilkins, 1970:214–234.

Haddad LM, Winchester JF (eds). *Clinical Management of Poisoning and Drug Overdoses.* WB Saunders: Philadelphia, 1983.

Nicholson DP. The immediate management of overdose. *Med Clin North Am,* 1983;67:1279–1293.

Park GD, Spector R. Goldberg MJ, et al. Expanded role of clinical therapy in the poisoned and overdosed patient. *Arch Intern Med, 1986;146:969–973.*

Smith RP, Gosselin RE. Current concepts about the treatment of selected poisonings: Nitrite, cyanide, barium and quinidine. *Annu Rev Pharmacol Toxicol,* 1976;16:189–199.

Stern TA, Mulley AG, Thibault GE. Life threatening drug overdose: Precipitants and prognosis. *JAMA,* 1984;251:1983–1985.

Winchester JF, Gelfand MC, Knepshield JH, et al. Dialysis and hemoperfusion of poisons and drugs—update. *Trans Am Soc Artif Intern Organs,* 1977;23:762–842.

Specific Poisonings

Acetaminophen

Acetylcysteine for acetaminophen overdosage. *Med Lett,* 1979;21:98–100.

Ameer B, Greenblatt DJ. Acetaminophen. *Ann Intern Med,* 1977;87:202–209.

Rumack BH, Peterson RG, Koch GG, et al. Acetaminophen overdose: 662 cases with evaluation of oral acetylcysteine treatment. *Arch Intern Med,* 1981;141:380–385.

Amphetamines

Angrist BM. Managing amphetamine toxicity. *Psychiatr Ann,* 1978;8:443–446.

Aspirin

Anderson RJ, Potts DE, Gabow PA, et al. Unrecognized adult salicylate intoxication. *Ann Intern Med,* 1976;85:745–748.

Done AK. Aspirin overdose: Incidence, diagnosis and management. *Pediatrics,* 1978;63(suppl):890–897.

Hill JB. Salicylate intoxication. *N Engl J Med,* 1973;288:1110–1113.

Barbiturates

Greenblatt DJ, Allen MD, Harmatz JS, et al. Overdosage with pentobarbital and secobarbital: Assessment of factors related to outcome. *J Clin Pharmacol,* 1979;19:758–768.

Carbon Monoxide

Turino GM. Effect of carbon monoxide on the respiratory system. *Circulation,* 1978;63:253A-259A.

Winter PM, Miller JN. Carbon monoxide poisoning. *JAMA,* 1976;236:1502–1504.

Caustics

Campbell GS, Burnett HF, Ransom JM, et al. Treatment of caustic burns of the esophagus. *Arch Surg,* 1977;112:495–500.

Chodak GW, Passano E. Acid ingestions. *JAMA,* 1978;239:225–226.

Rumack BH, Burrington JD. Caustic ingestions: A rational look at solvents. *Clin Toxicol,* 1977;11:27–34.

Cocaine

Cohen S. Cocaine. *JAMA,* 1975;231:74–75.

Crack. *Med Lett,* 1986;28:69–70.

Haddad LM. Cocaine in perspective: 1978. J Am Coll Emerg Phys, 1978;8:374–376.

Kossowsky WA, Lyon AF. Cocaine and acute myocardial infarction: A probable connection. *Chest,* 1984;86:729–731.

Pasternack PF, Colvin SB, Bauman FG. Cocaine-induced angina pectoris and acute myocardial infarction in patients younger than 40 years. *Am J Cardiol,* 1985;55:847–850.

Wetli CV, Wright RK. Death caused by recreational cocaine use. *JAMA,* 1979;241:2519–2522.

Cyanide

Chen KK, Rose CL. Treatment of acute cyanide poisoning. *JAMA,* 1956;162:1154–1155.

Ethchlorvynol

Teehan BP, Jaher JF, Carey JH, et al. Acute ethchlorvynol (Placidyl) intoxication. *Ann Intern Med,* 1970;72:875–882.

Ethylene Glycol

Levinsky NG. Severe metabolic acidosis in a young man—case records of MGH. *N Engl J Med,* 1979;301:650–657.

Parry MF, Wallach P. Ethylene glycol poisoning. *Am J Med,* 1974;57:143–150.

Peterson CD, Collins AJ, Himes JM, et al. Ethylene glycol poisoning: Pharmacokinetics during therapy with ethanol and hemodialysis. *N. Engl J Med,* 1981;304:21–24.

Fluorides

Mayer TG, Gross PL. Fatal systemic fluorosis due to hydrofluoric acid burns. *Ann Emerg Med,* 1985;14:149–153.

Tintinalli JE. Hydrofluoric acid burns, Emergency Care Conference. *J Am Coll Emerg Phys,* 1977;7:24–26.

Glutethimide

Chazan JA, Garella S. Glutethimide intoxication: A prospective study of 70 patients treated conservatively without hemodialysis. *Arch Intern Med,* 1971;128:215–219.

Greenblatt DJ, Allen MD, Harmatz JS, et al. Correlates of outcome following acute glutethimide overdosage. *J Foren Sci,* 1979;24:76–86.

Wright N, Roscoe P. Acute glutethimide poisoning: Conservative management of 31 patients. *JAMA,* 1970;214:1704–1706.

Glutethimide-Codeine (Pacs)

Fever E, French J. Descriptive epidemiology of mortality in New Jersey due to combinations of codeine and glutethimide. *Am J Epidemiol,* 1984;119:202–207.

Khajawall AM, Sramek JJ, Simpson GM. Loads alert. *West J Med,* 1982;137:166–168.

Heavy Metals

Chisholm JJ. Poisoning due to heavy metals. *Pediatr Clin North Am,* 1970;17:591–597.

Iron

Haddad LM. Iron poisoning. *J Am Coll Emerg Phys,* 1976;5:691–693.

LaCouture PG, Lovejoy FH, Haddad LM, et al. (eds). *Clinical Management of Poisoning and Drug Overdose.* Philadelphia: WB Saunders, 1983:644–648.

Methanol

Bennett IL Jr, Cary FH, Mitchell GL Jr, et al. Acute methyl alcohol poisoning: A review based on experiences in an outbreak of 323 cases. *Medicine,* 1953;32:431–463.

Keyvan-Larijarni H, Tannenberg AM. Methanol intoxication: Comparison of peritoneal dialysis and hemodialsis treatment. *Arch Intern Med,* 1974;134:293–296.

McCoy HG, Cipolle RJ, Ehlere SM, et al. Severe methanol poisonings. Application of a pharmacokinetic model for methanol therapy and hemodialysis. *Am J Med,* 1979;67:804–807.

Mushrooms

Lampe KF, McCann MA. Differential diagnosis of poisoning by North American mushrooms with particular emphasis on Amanita phalloides-like intoxication. *Ann Emerg Med,* 1987;16:956–962.

McCormick DJ, Avbel AJ, Gibbons RB. Non-lethal mushroom poisoning. *Ann Intern Med,* 1979;90:332–335.

Paaso B, Harrison DC. A new look at an old problem: Mushroom poisoning. Clinical presentations and new therapeutic approaches. *Am J Med,* 1975;58:505–509.

Narcotics

Frand UI, Shim CS, Williams MH. Heroin induced pulmonary edema. *Ann Intern Med,* 1972;77:29–35.

Moore RA, Rumack BH, Conner CS, et al. Naloxone underdosage after narcotic poisoning. *Am J Dis Child,* 1980;134:156–158.

Martin WR. Naloxone. *Ann Intern Med,* 1976;85:765–768.

Thornton WE, Thornton BP. Narcotic poisoning: A review of the literature. *Am J Psychiatry,* 1974;131:867–869.

Pesticides

Haddad LM. Organophosphate poisoning. In Haddad LM, Winchester JF (eds): *Clinical Management of Poisoning and Overdose.* Philadelphia: WB Saunders, 1983;704–710.

Milby TH. Prevention and management of organophosphate poisonings. *JAMA,* 1971;216:2131–2133.

Zavon M. Poisoning from pesticides: Diagnosis and treatment. *Pediatrics,* 1974;54:332–336.

Petroleum Distillates

Anas N, Namasonthi V, Ginsburg CM. Criteria for hospitalizing children who have ingested products containing hydrocarbons. *JAMA,* 1981;246:840–843.

Beamon RF, Siegel CJ, Landers G, et al. Hydrocarbon ingestion in children: A six-year retrospective study. *J Am Coll Emerg Phys,* 1976;5:771–775.

Brown J, Burke B, Dajani AS. Experimental kerosene pneumonia. *J Pediatr,* 1974;84:396–441.

Shirkey H. Treatment of petroleum distillate ingestion. *Mod Treat,* 1971;8:580–592.

Phencyclidine

Aronow R, Done AK. Phencyclidine overdose: An emerging concept of management. 1978; *J Am Coll Emerg Phys,* 1978;7:56–59.

Cohen FC, Rigg G, Simmons JL. Phencyclidine-associated rhabdomyolysis. *Ann Intern Med,* 1978;88:210–212.

McCarron MM, Schulze BW, Thompson GA, et al. Acute phencyclidine intoxication: Clinical patterns, complications and treatment. *Ann Emerg Med,* 1979;90:428–430.

Pearlson GD. Psychiatric and medical syndromes associated with phencyclidine (PCP) abuse. *John Hopkins Med J,* 1981;1:25–33.

Phenothiazines

Barry D, Muyskens, FL, Becker CE. Phenothiazine poisoning. *Calif Med,* 1973;118:1–12.

Benowitz NC, Rosenberg J, Becker DE, et al. Phenothiazine poisoning, *Med Clin North Am,* 1979;63:276–296.

Tricyclic Antidepressants and Anticholinergic Poisonings

Biggs JT, Spiker DG, Petit JM, et al. Tricyclic antidepressant overdose: Incidence of symptoms. *JAMA,* 1977;238:135–138.

Boehnert MT, Lovejoy FH Jr. Value of QRS duration versus the serum drug level in predicting seizures and ventricular arrhythmias after an acute overdose of tricyclic antidepressants. *N Engl J Med,* 1985;313:474–479.

Callahan M, Kasser D. Epidemiology of fatal tricyclic antidepressant ingestion: Implications for management. *Ann Emerg Med,* 1985;14:29–37.

Goldberg RJ, Capone RJ, Hunt JD. Cardiac complications following tricyclic antidepressant overdose: Issues for monitoring policy. *JAMA,* 1985;254:1772–1774.

Granacher RP, Baldessarini RJ. Physostigmine. *Arch Gen Psychiatry,* 1975;32:375–380.

Holten BA, Heath A. Clinical aspects of tricyclic antidepressant poisoning. *Acta Med Scand,* 1983;213:275–278.

Rumack BH. Physostigmine: Rational use. *J Am Coll Emerg Phys,* 1976;5:541–542.

Rumack BH. Anticholinergic poisoning: Treatment with physostigmine. *Pediatrics,* 1973;52:449–451.

Stern TA, O'Gara PT, Mulley AG, et al. Complications after overdose with tricyclic antidepressants. *Crit Care Med,* 1985;13:672–674.

CHAPTER **18**

Psychiatric Emergencies

WILLIAM H. ANDERSON, M.D.
THEODORE A. STERN, M.D.

Psychiatric emergencies refer to medical and psychologic disturbances manifested chiefly by acute alteration of behavior, thought, or feeling. Some of the conditions are life-threatening and, therefore, require immediate diagnosis and vigorous management. Others are less severe conditions that nevertheless are defined subjectively as emergencies by the patient or family, and so are likely to be seen by the emergency physician. The task of the emergency physician is to identify those conditions with risk of mortality or serious morbidity, to institute treatment, and to arrange adequate continued inpatient or outpatient care. In addition, the time and situation permitting, the physician may have the opportunity to intervene effectively in those less severe conditions that are defined as emergencies by patients or their social environment. Among the first questions to address is "What acute disturbance has there been in this patient's medical, psychologic, or social condition that causes him or her to appear for emergency care today?" The problem of specific diagnosis usually presents little difficulty provided that general principles of patient management are observed. All too often the patient with an acute behavioral disturbance is evaluated inadequately because of staff assumption that the disturbance is willful or deliberate. Careful attention to standard examination procedures is essential. A complete history should be taken from the patient or persons accompanying the patient, the mental status should be evaluated, and an appropriate physical examination and relevant laboratory studies should be performed. The physician in charge must make every effort to resist the temptation to make a rapid and perhaps unsatisfactory disposition in an effort to rid the emergency department of a disruptive patient. Numerous acute physiologic conditions can simulate the behavioral manifestations of schizophrenia, manic-depressive disease, or other "functional" psychiatric illnesses.

MAJOR LIFE-THREATENING CONDITIONS

This section considers emergency situations that have the potential for fatality or serious morbidity. These include acute psychosis and suicidal and homicidal states.

Acute Psychosis

This condition constitutes a medical emergency. Victims of these disorders are in constant danger of acting on distorted perceptions or delusional ideas with the result that serious injury or death may occur inadvertently. In addition to this cardinal indication for early intervention, three other considerations demand that diagnosis and treatment proceed without delay. First, acute psychosis is generally a mental state of intense discomfort. Second, family and social relationships may be strained severely in the course of the episode. Third, psychotic symptoms may be the most visible indicators of subtle but serious acute medical conditions.

Acute psychosis refers to a spectrum of aberrant mental states characterized by rapid development of major disturbances of perception, cognition, affect, and reality testing. Schizophrenia, manic-depressive illness, and psychotic depression usually are classified as functional psychoses and are separated conceptually from organic psychoses that represent those disturbances of mental state that can be attributed to disorders of brain tissue function. The most critical problem for the emergency physician who evaluates the psychotic patient is differentiating between these two general classifications. Guidelines are summarized in Table 18.1.

Initial Examination

Exclusion of Organic Brain Disease. The first step is to take all of the necessary measures to obtain a thorough history and to perform an adequate physical examination. Two problems must be overcome to accomplish this—the patient's agitation and discomfort, and on occasion, the resistance of the emergency department staff. The patient's cooperation usually can be obtained by an attitude of gentle firmness on the part of the physician, who

Table 18.1.
Differential Diagnosis of Acute Psychosis

Clinical Information	Organic	Functional
History		
Age	Most often >40 years	Most often <40 years
Onset	Can be sudden	Usually over weeks
Physical examination		
Vital signs		
Temperature	Often elevated	Usually normal
Pulse, blood pressure	Often elevated	Usually normal
Head	Injury may be present	Injury absent
Autonomic signs (pathologic)	Present	Can be present
Tympanic membranes	Bloody (with skull fracture)	Normal
Ocular fundi	Can be papilledematous	Normal
Mental status		
Orientation	Impaired	Preserved
Recent memory	Impaired	Preserved
Hallucinations	Often visual, tactile, or olfactory	Usually auditory
Intellectual function	Impaired	Preserved
Insight	Often present	Usually absent
Neurologic examination		
Nystagmus	Can be present	Absent
Pathologic reflexes	Can be present	Absent
Tremor	Can be present	Absent
Asterixis	Can be present	Absent
Response to caloric test	Can be impaired (coma)	Normal
Laboratory findings		
Complete blood cell count and sedimentation rate	Can be abnormal	Normal
Urinalysis	Can be abnormal	Normal
Chest and skull x-ray films	Can be abnormal	Normal
Blood chemistries	Can be abnormal	Normal
Electroencephalogram	Often abnormal	Normal

should explain procedures in a matter-of-fact, unambiguous manner without excessive discussion, exhortation, or argument. Occasionally, a patient may be so agitated that chemotherapy may be required before full examination. In such case, the best choice of medication is a high-potency antipsychotic drug such as haloperidol (Haldol), 5–10 mg intramuscularly. Drugs of this class have relatively little sedative or hypotensive effect and, therefore, are less likely to complicate the clinical presentation than are barbiturates or other sedatives.

At times, the patient may resist an adequate medical evaluation, leaving the physician with the dilemma that to perform an examination despite the patient's protest may constitute an assault, whereas to avoid examination may be negligence. In general, a patient who comes to the emergency department with an acute psychosis should be presumed to have a potentially life-threatening condition. Good practice, therefore, requires that an evaluation be performed that, at the very least, can exclude a major medical illness. While every effort must be made to be courteous, diplomatic, and gentle, the "assault" of performing an examination usually is more defensible than the negligence of refusing to assess an incapacitated patient.

The other problem that may make full evaluation difficult is the occasional negative attitude of the emergency department staff. There is a tendency to regard the acute psychotic patient as having a "psychiatric" problem, by which some persons imply that the patient has no business in a medical emergency department. Professional judgment may be impaired by anger or fear. The physician in charge may feel subtle pressure to make a quick disposition rather than a thorough evaluation. Under such circumstances, the physician may find that the ancillary help to which he is accustomed may not be forthcoming. Initial identifying data may not be collected by desk clerks, vital signs may not be evaluated, or the patient may not be assigned to an appropriate examining area. Such difficulties are

Table 18.2.
Metabolic and Structural Disorders That May Have Psychotic Features

- Space-occupying lesions in brain
  - Primary tumor
  - Metastatic carcinoma (lung, breast)
  - Subdural hematoma
  - Brain abscess (bacterial or fungal infection, gumma, cysticercosis)
- Cerebral hypoxia
  - Pulmonary insufficiency
  - Severe anemia
  - Diminished cardiac output
  - Toxicosis (e.g., carbon monoxide)
- Metabolic and endocrine disorders
  - Electrolyte imbalance
  - Hypocalcemia
  - Thyroid disease (thyrotoxicosis and myxedema)
  - Pituitary insufficiency
  - Adrenal disease (Addison's disease and Cushing's syndrome)
  - Hypoglycemia
  - Diabetes mellitus (ketoacidosis)
  - Uremia
  - Hepatic failure
  - Porphyria
- Use of exogenous substances
  - Alcohol (intoxication and withdrawal)
  - Barbiturates and other sedatives (intoxication and withdrawal)
  - Amphetamines
  - LSD, PCP, and other similar compounds
  - Anticholinergic agents
  - Heavy metals
  - Digitalis
  - Corticosteroids
  - L-Dopa
  - Reserpine
  - Cocaine
  - Bromide compounds
  - Marihuana
  - Carbon disulfide
  - Isoniazid
  - Cycloserine
  - Disulfiram
  - Cimetidine
  - Antiarrhythmics
  - Cancer chemotherapy
- Nutritional deficiencies
  - Thiamine (Wernicke-Korsakoff syndrome)
  - Niacin (pellagra)
  - Vitamin B_{12}
  - Folate
- Vascular abnormalities
  - Intracranial hemorrhage
  - Lacunae due to hypertension
  - Collagen disorders
  - Aneurysm
  - Hypertensive encephalopathy
- Infections
  - Meningitis (bacterial, fungal, tuberculous)
  - Encephalitis (viral, e.g., herpetic)
  - Syphilis
  - Subacute bacterial endocarditis
  - Typhoid fever
  - Malaria
- Miscellaneous conditions
  - Normal-pressure hydrocephalus
  - Temporal lobe epilepsy
  - Huntington's chorea
  - Alzheimer's disease
  - Remote effects of carcinoma
  - Wilson's disease
  - Pancreatitis

understandable, and the specialist in emergency medicine ought to anticipate them. If the emergency physician is not prepared to do all of the necessary procedures him- or herself, continuing staff education may be required.

History. Every potential source of relevant present and past medical information must be explored. Most frequently, this information can be obtained from the patient, family, or friends. Hospital records, when available, are usually helpful. Special inquiry should be directed to the possibility of head injuries, epilepsy, diabetes mellitus, endocrine disorders, ingestion of drugs or other foreign substances, cardiopulmonary disease, electrolyte imbalance, and hepatic and renal dysfunction (Table 18.2). Use of a mnemonic, ''rule out the WHHHIMP,'' helps one to recall the acute life-threatening causes of delirium or psychosis (Table 18.3).

Even if the patient is mute or has a florid thought disorder, he or she may be able to provide some history. Such patients may be asked to show identification. Examination of the patient's wallet may provide medical information, phone numbers of relatives, or names of physicians. A severely depressed patient may be unable to give oral answers, but may be able to write ''yes'' and ''no'' or short sentences.

The patient's age is an important consideration. Acute functional psychosis is typically a disorder with onset after puberty and before age 40. The most common exception to this is major depressive disorder, which may be suspected by the presence of profound depression, often with agitation, with onset after age 40. Excluding this entity, psychotic features appearing for the first time in the older age group should be presumed initially to have an organic cause.

Mode of onset is also a helpful feature in the history. Acute psychosis that has developed in the course of minutes or hours suggests either a vascular, metabolic, toxic, infectious, or epileptic cause. Thus, intracranial hemorrhage, hypoglycemia, meningitis, temporal lobe epilepsy, or intoxications (for example, from amphetamines, cocaine, phencyclidine, lysergic acid diethylamide (LSD), or anticholinergic agents) should be suspected. Psychosis in a young person in whom florid symptoms develop over several weeks suggests the likelihood of a schizophrenic or manic-depressive condition. Insidious onset with barely perceptible personality change over months suggests a dementing illness. Since some of these are remediable, the cause always should be sought, although this is not usually the task of the emergency physician.

Table 18.3.
Life-threatening Causes of Delirium

*W*ernicke's encephalopathy
*H*ypoxia or hypoperfusion of the central nervous system
*H*ypoglycemia
*H*ypertensive encephalopathy
*I*ntracerebral hemorrhage
*M*eningitis/encephalitis
*P*oisoning

Physical Examination. A complete physical examination should be performed, although rectal and pelvic examinations are best deferred in the absence of specific indications. Although vital signs frequently are neglected because of real or assumed lack of patient cooperation, they are of utmost importance and should always be recorded. The temperature is most critical. Mild elevations may exist (99–100°F; 37.2–37.8°C) in functional states such as acute catatonia, but fever usually implies an acute organic process and deserves full investigation. In such a case, meningitis and encephalitis, subacute bacterial endocarditis, collagen diseases, thyrotoxicosis, delirium tremens, neuroleptic malignant syndrome, and anticholinergic poisoning should receive special consideration.

The scalp should be examined carefully for evidence of laceration, contusion, or penetrating injury. Such injuries may not be noted in the history because of traumatic amnesia. Ecchymoses around the orbits or behind the ears may be suggestive evidence of bleeding behind the tympanic membranes and should be sought. The optic fundi should be examined for signs of papilledema.

Signs of autonomic dysfunction may suggest a specific cause. The combination of fixed, dilated pupils, tachycardia, dry mucous membranes, urinary retention, and abdominal distention with absent bowel sounds is highly suggestive of anticholinergic poisoning or delirium of the anticholinergic type. Profuse cold sweat, tachycardia, and peculiar brightness of the eyes suggest hypoglycemia and are consistent with manifestations of adrenergic excess. Acute amphetamine overdose may cause dilated pupils and tachycardia.

Mental Status. Performing a careful systematic evaluation of the patient's mental status is often the most helpful procedure in making the differential diagnosis between organic and functional psychosis. Orientation, the ability of the patient to recognize time and place, should be tested first. Disturbance of spatial and temporal orientation usually indicates acute organic disease. The patient with functional psychosis typically retains knowledge of the day of the week and of the place even in the presence of profound thought disorder. Severe temporal disorientation, such as incorrect identification of the year, suggests a more insidious organic disorder of brain function.

Recent memory should be evaluated next. The physician should ask the patient about recent actions and experiences, verifying the answers by consulting independent sources. Another method is to instruct the patient to name three objects and to request him or her to name them again after 5 minutes. Patients with functional psychosis usually have intact recent memory, but delirious and demented patients usually do not. A useful means of testing and quantifying several areas of cognitive function is by administering the Mini-mental State Examination (MMSE), an easy to use, brief objective test that involves testing of attention, memory, orientation, and calculation ability (Table 18.4).

Preservation of intellectual function is typical of schizophrenia and manic-depressive illness. Measurements must be judged against standards of premorbid function, that often must be inferred from a patient's educational history.

Hallucinations frequently accompany an acute psychotic process. The patient in the acute phase of schizophrenia typically experiences auditory hallucinations. Visual, tactile, and olfactory phenomena are uncommon in acute functional psychosis, but often are present in acute organic brain syndromes, especially those secondary to a toxic or metabolic disturbance, infection, or complex partial seizures.

A patient's insight is determined by evaluating the degree to which he or she appreciates the extent of the illness. Patients with organic brain disease, even though they may be delusional, have hallucinations, or both, often recognize that illness is present, but patients with schizophrenia or manic-depressive illness frequently do not. However, this criterion is perhaps the least reliable in the evaluation of mental status.

Neurological Examination. A full neurologic examination should always be attempted. Certain aspects of this type of examination are more likely to yield positive findings in patients with an acute psychosis. Pathologic reflexes require little time to check and are highly suggestive of organic brain dysfunction when present. The plantar flexion, grasping, snout, sucking, and palmomental reflexes, as well as the glabellar response, should be investigated.

Myoclonus suggests diffuse brain dysfunction, and nystagmus suggests intoxication with sedative-hypnotics or Wernicke's encephalopathy. Tremor and asterixis indicate organic brain disease. In comatose or unresponsive patients in whom hysteria or catatonia cannot be excluded readily, the response to caloric stimulation of the external auditory canals may be helpful. Patients who generally are unresponsive because of hysteria or catatonia show a normal response. Irrigation with ice water normally causes nystagmus with the quick component away from the irrigated ear. In unconscious patients with intact brainstem function, conjugate tonic deviation toward the irrigated ear suggests a metabolic cause.

Before proceeding further, the physician should consider the possibility that the abnormal mental status may be early evidence of Wernicke-Korsakoff syndrome. This condition deserves special attention since its reversal requires early aggressive diagnosis and treatment in the emergency department. Early in the course of the disease, patients may be confused without prominent evidence of alcohol intoxication or other signs such as nystagmus, ophthalmoplegia, or ataxia. This syndrome may occur in alcoholic patients and in those otherwise deprived of thiamine. When it is suspected, an initial dose of 100 mg of thiamine should be given intravenously.

Laboratory Evaluation. In some patients, diagnosis continues to be difficult despite the aforementioned methods of evaluation, and it usually is best to hospitalize such patients for further evaluation. Laboratory studies that may be helpful include an electroencephalogram (including a sleep study when temporal lobe epilepsy is suggested) and a computed tomographic (CT) scan or magnetic resonance imaging (MRI) of the head. On admission, other tests should routinely be performed and include a complete blood cell count, sedimentation rate, urinalysis, chest film, electrocardiogram, serologic studies, and measurement of serum electrolytes, calcium, blood urea nitrogen, and blood glucose. Thyroid studies, vitamin B_{12} and folate levels, liver function tests, and screening for toxic exogenous substances complete the work-up.

Patients with signs and symptoms of organic brain disease should be admitted to establish an etiologic diagnosis. In other patients, the diagnosis of functional psychosis may be made, although the possibility of an organic cause must not be forgotten.

Suicidal and Homicidal Potential. The next problem that the emergency physician must evaluate is the risk of suicidal or homicidal activity. Any acute psychotic process increases the possibility of such behavior. Patients with severe depressive symptoms in addition to psychosis should be presumed to have high suicidal potential. It is of cardinal importance to inquire directly about such ideas or intentions. Psychotic patients with persecutory delusions may have increased potential for homicide, since they may respond to the imagined threat with a preemptive defense. Patients with high risk should be hospitalized in a setting that provides security appropriate to their condition. Those in whom the risk of suicide or of harming others is less may

Table 18.4.
Mini-mental State Examination[a]

Maximum Score	Score	Mini-mental State
		Orientation
5	( )	What is the (year) (season) (date) (day) (month)?
5	( )	Where are we: (state) (county) (town) (hospital) (floor).
		Registration
3	( )	Name three objects: 1 second to say each. Then ask the patient all three after you have said them. Give 1 point for each correct answer. Then repeat them until he or she learns all three. Count trials and record. Trials: ______
		Attention and Calculation
5	( )	Serial 7s. 1 point for each correct. Stop after 5 answers. Alternatively spell "world" backwards.
		Recall
3	( )	Ask for the three objects repeated above. Give 1 point for each correct.
		Language
9	( )	Name a pencil, and watch (2 points). Repeat the following: "No ifs, ands or buts" (1 point). Follow a three-stage command: "Take a paper in your right hand, fold it in half, and put it on the floor" (3 points). Read and obey the following: "Close your eyes" (1 point). Write a sentence (1 point). Copy design (1 point).
______		Total Score
		Assess level of consciousness along a continuum ______ Alert Drowsy Stupor Coma

at times be treated on an outpatient basis; this requires an adequate system of social support during the acute phase of treatment.

Evaluation of Social Supports. Not every acutely psychotic patient requires hospitalization. Many can be treated effectively as outpatients with appropriate chemotherapy. For this to be a feasible option, however, a social support system of concerned and capable family members and/or friends is essential. Those patients who live alone or whose relatives and friends are of dubious helpfulness should be hospitalized. Family members often wish to deny the nature and severity of an acute psychotic illness and, therefore, are vulnerable to the patient's rationalizations that treatment is unnecessary. If, however, family or friends can provide ongoing supervision and protection and ensure the patient's adherence to medication and appointment schedules, then outpatient management may be considered.

Initial Treatment

In patients with acute schizophrenic or manic psychosis, the cornerstone of initial treatment is the timely aggressive use of antipsychotic chemotherapy. With this type of regimen, the acute symptoms may subside substantially within 4–6 hours. Time and situation permitting, it is worth such a trial in the hope that hospitalization may be avoided or that the illness may be brought toward remission more quickly.

Despite modern advances, hospitalization in a psychiatric department carries with it certain disadvantages: social opprobrium is always present, undue pessimism concerning prognosis sometimes results, and finally, the cost of inpatient treatment is high. To avoid these disadvantages, the physician must first establish that (*a*) the cause is not organic, (*b*) suicidal and homicidal danger is minimal, and

Table 18.4—*continued*

Instructions for Administration of Mini-mental State Examination

Orientation

1. Ask for the date. Then ask specifically for parts omitted, e.g., "Can you also tell me what season it is?" One point for each correct.
2. Ask in turn "Can you tell me the name of this hospital?" (town, county, etc.). One point for each correct.

Registration

Ask the patient if you may test his or her memory. Then say the names of three unrelated objects, clearly and slowly, about 1 second for each. After you have said all three, ask the patient to repeat them. This first repetition determines the score (0–3) but keep saying them until the patient can repeat all three, up to six trials. If he or she does not eventually learn all three, recall cannot be meaningfully tested.

Attention and Calculation

Ask the patient to begin with 100 and count backwards by 7. Stop after 5 subtractions (93, 86, 79, 72, 65). Score the total number of correct answers.

If the patient cannot or will not perform this task, ask for the spelling of the word "world" backwards. The score is the number of letters in correct order, e.g., dlrow = 5, dlorw = 3.

Recall

Ask the patient to recall the three words you previously asked him or her to remember. Score 0–3.

Language

Naming: Show the patient a wrist watch and ask what it is. Repeat for pencil. Score 0–2.

Repetition: Ask the patient to repeat the sentence after you. Allow only one trial. Score 0 or 1.

Three-stage command: Give the patient a piece of plain blank paper and repeat the command. Score 1 point for each part correctly executed.

Reading: On a blank piece of paper print the sentence "Close your eyes," in letters large enough for the patient to see clearly. Ask him or her to read it and do what it says. Score 1 point only if the patient actually closes the eyes.

Writing: Give the patient a blank piece of paper and ask him or her to write a sentence for you. Do not dictate a sentence, it is to be written spontaneously. It must contain a subject and a verb and be sensible. Correct grammar and punctuation are not necessary.

Copying: On a clean piece of paper, draw intersecting pentagons, each side about 1 inch, and ask the patient to copy it exactly as it is. All 10 angles must be present and 2 must intersect to score 1 point. Tremor and rotation are ignored.

Estimate the patient's level of sensorium along a continuum, from alert on the left to coma on the right.

[a] Folstein MF, Folstein SE, McHugh PR. "Mini-Mental State." A practical method for grading the cognitive state of patients for the clinician. *J Psychiatr Res,* 1975; 12:189–198.

(*c*) social supports for outpatient treatment are satisfactory. If these criteria are fulfilled, the physician may attempt to induce symptomatic remission with chemotherapy.

As a general rule, the high potency antipsychotic medications such as haloperidol, trifluoperazine hydrochloride (Stelazine), and fluphenazine hydrochloride (Prolixin) are the drugs of choice in this situation. They are potent in their antipsychotic effect without the major side effects of sedation or hypotension that characterize the lower-potency antipsychotic agents such as chlorpromazine (Thorazine) and thioridazine hydrochloride (Mellaril). Sedation is not an essential feature in the treatment of acute psychosis. In fact, sedation may be counterproductive since patients may feel more discomfort in an obtunded state. While every antipsychotic drug has some sedative effect, it is minimal with the high potency preparations. Hypotension occasionally limits the dosage of antipsychotic medication. Use of the high potency preparations also minimizes this side effect when compared with the lower potency drugs of equal therapeutic effect.

A frequent side effect of the chemotherapy of psychosis is development of acute extrapyramidal reactions of the dystonic type. These usually occur within the first hours or days of antipsychotic drug use and are uncommon after the first 2–4 weeks. They consist of involuntary contraction of the muscles of the face, neck, and throat. Swallowing may be difficult, and occasionally the airway is impaired. The incidence of this complication is markedly reduced by prophylactic treatment with benztropine mesylate (Cogentin), 1 mg orally twice a day beginning with the first dose of antipsychotic drug. Should the reaction occur despite this therapy, it may be treated with intravenous diphenhydramine hydrochloride (Benadryl), 50 mg.

Having chosen an appropriate antipsychotic drug, the physician should consider the dosage schedule and route of administration. The intramuscular route usually is preferred because of rapid onset of action and a high initial level in the blood. If this is not feasible, oral liquid medication may be satisfactory. Tablets are not always swallowed and may be hidden easily, with resulting uncertainty about the dose received. The intravenous use of haloperidol has become more widely accepted in recent years despite the lack of Federal Drug Administration approval for this route of administration. It has been used safely and effectively to treat agitation, even in critically ill patients (e.g., those in cardiogenic shock) in intravenous bolus doses of up to 150 mg and doses as high as 975 mg in 24 hours.

An appropriate initial dose of haloperidol is 5 or 10 mg, depending on age, weight, and severity of illness. This dose may be repeated every 60 minutes until satisfactory improvement occurs or the patient sleeps. Improvement usually occurs at doses between 15 and 40 mg, although higher doses occasionally are required. Under circumstances in which doses greater than 40 mg appear to be required, the accuracy of the working diagnosis should be reassessed. Trifluoperazine hydrochloride is about half as potent as haloperidol, and fluphenazine is about 1½ times as potent. Doses may be adjusted accordingly. Careful observation during this period is necessary to note signs of excessive sedation, extrapyramidal reactions, or hypotension.

The goal of initial treatment is to reduce psychotic symptoms sufficiently to make outpatient management feasible or to ensure patient and staff safety upon patient transfer to an inpatient psychiatric unit. Many patients respond favorably to the regimen described. Those in whom the psychosis is not abated must receive inpatient treatment.

Outpatient Follow-up Care

If the psychotic process has been brought into remission and if the other appropriate criteria are fulfilled (Fig. 18.1), outpatient follow-up care should be arranged. Outpatient treatment must include a combination of monitoring of chemotherapeutic requirements, and psychotherapy directed at restoration of premorbid function and reparation of the social and family turmoil that was brought about by the psychotic illness. A psychiatrist is usually best able to satisfy these requirements, and appropriate referral should be made. Pending transfer of the patient to the care of another physician, the emergency physician may find it necessary to continue chemotherapy for several days. Usually the total initial dose that was effective in bringing about remission should be continued on a daily basis by the oral route. The most frequent cause of relapse is the premature reduction of medication. If sedation and extrapyramidal reactions are not excessive, this dose may be continued for days or weeks until reliable follow-up care is arranged. Occasionally, a larger dose is required. Recurrence of psychotic thinking or insomnia suggests the need for additional medication. A reduction of dosage or a change in class of neuroleptic agent is indicated when excessive sedation or extrapyramidal reactions occur.

If the patient has manic-depressive illness, maintenance chemotherapy might include lithium carbonate. This treatment is usually outside the scope of the emergency physician, and should properly be monitored by the psychiatrist to whom the patient is referred.

Suicide

Self-destruction is a common event frequently preceded by incomplete or "unsuccessful" attempts. Although it is listed as the tenth leading cause of death, the actual incidence is virtually impossible to determine since many apparent accidents may be suicides.

Since these considerations are well known and generally appreciated, it is curious that the patient who has attempted suicide receives remarkably little sympathy from medical personnel. Emergency department staff often become angry when a patient with a self-inflicted injury arrives. The feeling that the patient should have "finished the job" and other such attitudes must be recognized since they may lead to improper care. It is not difficult to appreciate the origin of such notions in the harassed emergency department physician who may be busy with many medical emergencies and injuries and who may, therefore, view the attempted suicide patient as unnecessary extra work. Those whose lives are dedicated to the cure and amelioration of illness may find it difficult to have empathic feeling for those whose actions so openly reject life as worthy of preservation. Although the emergency department physician cannot always prevent the emergence of these feelings, he or she should make every effort to avoid letting these feelings compromise the patient's care.

Such subjective attitudes notwithstanding, evaluation and treatment would be relatively simple if all suicide attempts were equally serious. However, the task is complicated by the fact that, like all other human illness, the degree of severity falls within a spectrum. At one end, there is the psychotic de-

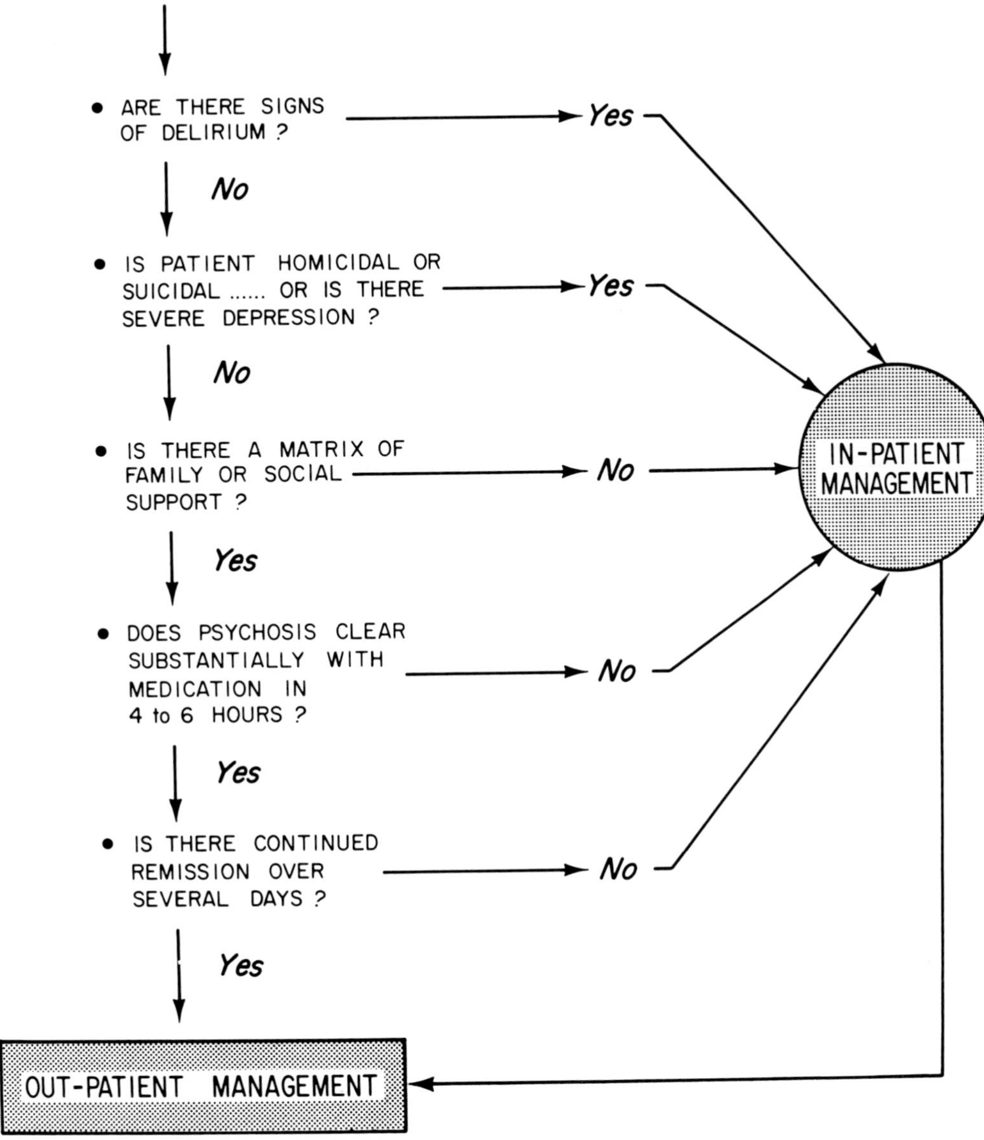

Figure 18.1. Flow sheet for determination of appropriate inpatient/outpatient management.

pressive who has swallowed a lethal dose of barbiturates before jumping in front of a subway train. He or she should obviously be hospitalized and intensively treated. At the other end, there is the adolescent who fails a minor examination and takes 6 aspirin before calling an ambulance. This individual may not require hospitalization. Seldom is the situation so clear-cut, however. Even attempts that appear minor may be an early warning of a serious psychopathologic disturbance. In the emergency department, it is best to assume that suicidal thoughts or actions are evidence of a serious morbid process. Ideally, every suicide attempt should be investigated by a psychiatric consultant called to the emergency department. Since this is not always feasible, some guidelines are necessary to gauge the degree of imminent danger so that appropriate treatment plans can be made (Table 18.5). An assessment of the risk of an attempt (e.g., its potential lethality) and the potential for rescue is essential and helps determine the level of intervention that is required. The following criteria should be considered before disposition of the patient.

Assessment of Suicidal Risk

Suicidal Intention. The simplest, most important means of evaluation is to ask the patient his or her intention; however, this is frequently neglected. By assessing the content and quality of the patient's answer, the physician obtains the single most valuable piece of information. Patients who state that they intend to take their lives should be believed, at least in the emergency department evaluation. Physicians are often reluctant to question patients directly on this point, with the erroneous assumption that it may plant an idea in the patient's mind. Clinical experience shows that virtually every depressed person has entertained suicidal thoughts at some time and that the patient may be reassured by receiving implicit permission to discuss these thoughts or intentions. Questions such as "Have you been thinking of harming yourself or taking your life?" tactfully stated can do no harm and may provide information not available by any other means. Those who state their intention to attempt or to repeat suicidal behavior must have immediate psychiatric consultation.

Psychosis. As noted, the psychotic patient, especially when symptoms are acute, is in serious danger of either intentional or inadvertent self-harm because of disordered perception and thought process. When suicidal ideation or a recent attempt on one's life is superimposed on an ongoing psychotic episode, the risk of self-destruction is great. A protective environment is mandatory at least until the major overt manifestations of the psychosis are controlled. Psychoses with manic features are especially dangerous because of their intensity of affect, lability of mood, and poor ability to control actions. Even marked elevations of mood contain the seeds of profound irritability and depression. Patients with schizophrenia may have imperative or command auditory hallucinations ("Jump out the window!") or such intense persecutory delusions that death may seem a preferable alternative.

Major Depression. Depression is a common illness that frequently results in suicide. It is manifest not only by the subjective feelings of sadness or loss but by a syndrome replete with neurovegetative symptoms. Whenever suicidal ideation is present, a diagnosis of depression should be considered. This is especially important because depression is successfully treated in the vast majority of cases. Its symptoms can be recalled by use of a mnemonic SIGECAPS, i.e. "SIG" the Latin for the information on the prescription label, "E" for energy, and "CAPS" for capsules. Each letter stands for a separate symptom of depression (see Table 18.6). A diagnosis of depression is confirmed when four or more symptoms are present for a duration of 2 weeks or longer, in the presence of depressed mood. Sleep is frequently impaired with a pattern of early morning awakening, although difficulty falling asleep may also occur. Interests (e.g., libido) are decreased, guilt or preoccupation of thought may be present, energy is decreased, concentration ability is decreased, a disturbance in appetite may occur (either increased or decreased), and psychomotor agitation or retardation may be present. When depression is substantial and accompanied by these symptoms, the risk of suicide is greatly increased. In a given patient, the risk can be

Table 18.5.
Factors Associated with an Increased Rate of Suicide[a]

Affirmation of suicidal intention
Psychosis (especially acute schizophrenia or manic-depressive illness)
Major depression (i.e., with a full complement of neurovegetative symptoms)
History of impaired impulse control
Contemplation or use of a violent method (e.g., jumping in front of a subway train or from a height, or shooting or hanging oneself)
Alcohol or drug dependence
Social isolation (divorce, separation, friendlessness)
Previous suicide attempts
Family history of suicide or affective illness
Recent major loss of self-esteem (e.g., loss of love or employment)
Subjective perception of helplessness and hopelessness
Presence of suicide note
Concurrent medical disease (serious, chronic, incurable)
Age (greater with advancing age, although on the increase in adolescents)
Sex (men more than women)

[a] Factors are listed in descending order of seriousness.

Table 18.6.
Neurovegetative Symptoms of Depression

*S*leep disturbance (usually with early morning awakening)
*I*nterests and libido decreased
*G*uilt or preoccupation of thought
*E*nergy decreased
*C*oncentration ability decreased
*A*ppetite disturbance (usually decreased, but it may be increased)
*P*sychomotor agitation or retardation
*S*uicidal thoughts or thoughts of death

greatest either as a depression is deepening or as it is getting better.

History of Impaired Impulse Control. Suicide or its attempt is often an impulsive act. Unlike similar acts, it is irreversible—a notion which, curiously, may elude the patient. Those whose risk is greatest are those whose life-style is marked by the tendency to avoid realization of the implications of their actions. Examples are reckless drivers, heavy drinkers, those with a poor employment history, and those with considerable family turmoil. Deficiencies of personality development that characterize the patient with poor impulse control not only make a specific suicidal act more probable but also suggest that other risk factors are likely to be increased. A majority of overdose admissions to the Massachusetts General Hospital medical intensive care unit manifest such an impairment in impulse control, rather than manifesting symptoms of major depression.

Contemplation of Use of a Violent Method. Investigators in the area of the psychodynamics of suicide have repeatedly emphasized the importance of anger as a concomitant of self-destruction. Anger may provide the energy for the attempt to succeed. An index of the magnitude of the anger is the degree of violence it requires for its expression. Self-mutilation, shooting, or hanging oneself, or the use of painful corrosive poisons not only increases the likelihood of a successful suicide attempt but also suggests a high degree of anger.

Alcohol or Drug Dependence. For several reasons, victims of alcohol or drug addiction have an increased risk for completed suicide. Impulse control is diminished during acute intoxications, social supports may be transitory or nonexistent, and there is a diminished capacity for adaptive restoration because of impaired sensorium.

Social Isolation. Those who can share distress are more fortunate than those who must bear it alone. The well-adjusted person with difficulties can nevertheless sustain him- or herself by drawing on the psychic and material resources of friends and relatives. Those without families or friends have no such reserves on which to draw. While others may be rescued from the intention or consequences of a suicidal act, the isolated person enjoys no such likelihood.

Previous Suicide Attempts. Some physicians may believe that a history of previous suicide attempts suggests that future risk is less serious, presumably on the misconception that the first could not have been serious since the patient did not succeed. To the contrary notwithstanding, there is about a 10% chance of successful suicide within 10 years after a significant attempt. In addition, it is noteworthy that a majority of cases of life-threatening drug overdose at Massachusetts General Hospital have been previously treated for a drug overdose.

Family History of Suicide or Affect Disorder. As a family history of suicide has taught the individual, perhaps at an early age, that this method of ultimate escape is not without precedent and perhaps does not hold special personal, social, or religious opprobrium. Furthermore, suicide in first-degree relatives suggests the likelihood of an affective illness which has strong genetic components.

Recent Major Loss of Self-esteem. Some persons depend on one or more extrinsic evidences of self-worth for their ego identity. These may include financial status, social position, or family harmony. Sudden and irrevocable loss of one of these supports may provide sufficient impetus for a major suicide attempt. Such an act may also be manipulative in the sense that it may be an attempt to restore the lost support. It is nevertheless perilous for the physician to assume that an attempt is manipulative and that it is therefore not serious.

Presence of a Suicide Note. Investigators have repeatedly noted an association between the use of a suicide note and the success of the attempt. One suggestion is that the note represents an emotional testament to express the patient's intent after his death.

Concurrent Medical Disease. Maintenance of a well-integrated life with continued rewards requires acceptable physical health. When pain, weakness, and incapacity become constant companions, adaptive resources become depleted.

Age. In general, older patients are more vulnerable to completed suicide than are younger patients. However, suicide is the second leading cause of death in adolescents, exceeded only by accidents, and the prevalence of suicide in adolescents and young adults is rising dramatically.

Sex. Although women are more likely to attempt suicide, men are more likely to carry the attempt to completion.

Treatment

An expressed suicide intention or overt attempt should ideally be managed by a psychiatrist in the emergency department situation. Since this is not always possible, the emergency physician must make the best choices available, given the resources of time and personnel. Those patients who by virtue of one or more of the previously discussed criteria are judged to be at high risk should be hospitalized and observed pending psychiatric consultation. Psychotic patients may be evaluated and aggressively treated on a medical floor. The physician may elect to transfer the patient to a psychiatric service of a general hospital (ideally) or may elect to send the patient to a psychiatric hospital. The physician is urged to become familiar with the available resources for management and with the guidelines for involuntary admission in one's community.

The Homicidal and the Assaultive Patient

These patients can present the most disruptive and most difficult situations that the emergency physician must face. The usual routines of emergency department personnel can become paralyzed in the presence of either threatened or overt violence.

General Considerations and Initial Management

Regardless of the cause of the episode, the most reasonable initial assumption is that overwhelming anger is the phenomenologic substrate. The physician must try to understand the anger before accurate diagnostic evaluation can proceed. Statements such as "Stop acting like a child" and "Control yourself" are not helpful. Instead, the physician should try to assume that the anger may be partly justified, at least in principle if not in mode of expression or intensity. If possible, a relevant history should first be obtained from relatives or police officers. The patient should then be interviewed in surroundings of reasonable privacy and security. An initial statement such as "You appear very angry. Could you explain your feelings to me?" is often helpful. This allows the patient the opportunity to substitute verbal aggression for physical violence and suggests the possibility that the physician may become an ally. After reasonable opportunity for expression of feelings, the patient is usually much more amenable to further history-taking and examination. Medication may then be offered with the suggestion that it will help the patient to be calm.

On rare occasions, violence may become overt in the emergency department before peaceful methods of solution can be utilized. Since the safety of other patients and staff cannot be compromised, physical methods of control must be employed. Should this become necessary, the best strategy is use of overwhelming force. Several persons must work together to apply needed restraint. Ideally, these are security personnel with special training. Avoidance of unnecessary injury is sometimes facilitated by use of a mattress to immobilize the patient while restraint is applied.

Adjunctive chemotherapy is often indicated in the emergency department. For patients in whom the diagnosis is unclear, the best choice is usually a parenteral high-potency antipsychotic drug, such as haloperidol or thiothixene. The parenteral route is preferred because of its rapid rate of absorption. If the physician's judgment is to use oral medication, liquid preparations are preferable to tablets. One important exception to the use of antipsychotic agents is psychosis produced by large doses of drugs with anticholinergic side effects. Antipsychotic drugs make this condition worse. Fortunately, such a diagnosis is usually easy to make with history and physical findings. Barbiturates and other sedative-hypnotics are inappropriate and may worsen assaultive behavior, unless it can be determined that the underlying cause of agitation and assaultiveness is a withdrawal phenomenon, e.g. barbiturate withdrawal or delirium tremens.

Oral medication should be administered in liquid form to ensure that it is swallowed by the patient. It has the advantage that the patient begins to participate in his care but has the disadvantage of somewhat slower absorption than the parenteral route. Choices of drug and dosage must be individualized to the person and the situation. Chlorpromazine may be given in doses of 50 mg intramuscularly or 100 mg orally, repeated every half-hour if necessary. Haloperidol may be given in doses of 5–10 mg intramuscularly or orally every 30–60 minutes.

Specific Causes of Violent Behavior

Each of the following may represent the underlying cause of violent episodes.

Catatonic Excitement. A patient with a history of psychosis (more commonly from affective illness than from schizophrenia) who has an unmanageable violent episode is likely to be experiencing the excited form of catatonia. The patient is usually oblivious to surroundings and, if untreated, may die of exhaustion or injury. Treatment involves the aggressive use of chemotherapy as discussed. On some occasions, electroconvulsive therapy may be necessary.

Delirious Mania. The patient has a history of manic-depressive illness. Treatment of the acute episode is the same as that for catatonic excitement.

Paranoid Delusions. The actively delusional patient is in constant danger of acting as if the delusions were true; the patient can plan and carry out an aggressive defense against his or her imagined persecutors. In the emergency department, the patient can appear brooding and quiet, but can be able to act out homicidal plans. The danger is increased if symptoms are relatively acute and if delusions relate to a specific person or group. Imperative or command auditory hallucinations ("Kill your patients!") are likewise an ominous sign. Such patients require antipsychotic chemotherapy and a protective hospital environment until symptoms subside.

Sedative-Hypnotic Intoxication and Withdrawal. Sedatives can be responsible for acutely diminished impulse control. Such disability may occur as a result of either intoxication or acute withdrawal from an addicting substance. Alcohol is the most common offending agent, but barbiturates and other sedatives must be considered as well. Some persons are susceptible to "pathologic" intoxication that occurs with small amounts of alcohol.

Intoxicated states can usually be recognized by slurred speech, incoordination, ataxia, and nystagmus. Treatment requires a quiet, protective environment with special nursing if possible to avoid such secondary emergencies as aspiration of vomitus. Physical restraint should be kept to a minimum and must not be used if the patient cannot be watched constantly. If chemical restraint cannot be avoided, the best choice is a high-potency antipsychotic agent such as haloperidol, which has relatively little hypotensive effect and sedative potentiation. An initial dose is often 5 mg intramuscularly.

Withdrawal states can be recognized by tremor, autonomic hyperactivity, diaphoresis, disorientation, visual hallucinosis, seizures, hyperreflexia, and mydriasis. Treatment requires controlled administration of a cross-tolerant sedative-hypnotic. Diazepam (Valium) is a good choice. The initial dose may be 5 mg intravenously, administered slowly. Careful observation is required to avoid and monitor oversedation, hypotension, or respiratory depression. Oral diazepam may be used after initial control is obtained.

Phencyclidine Intoxication. This is a common cause of extreme or episodic violence. It may be suspected by a history of drug ingestion or inhalation. Physical findings include blank stare, labile mental status, nystagmus, ataxia, hypertension, and anesthesia (see Chapter 17).

Temporal Lobe Epilepsy. While frequently suspected as an underlying cause of violence, seizure activity rarely provides an adequate explanation. When it is suspected on historical grounds or because of the presence of aura, an electroencephalogram recorded during sleep may be confirmatory, but often is not. Anticonvulsant medication may be useful.

Antisocial Personality. Violent behavior occasionally may arise without any evidence of illness. This usually occurs in patients with a long history of criminal offenses or antisocial behavior. If no other evidence of medical or psychiatric illness is found, appropriate limit-setting should be employed, including consultation with law enforcement authorities.

Hospitalization

Hospitalization may be voluntary or involuntary. The latter is implemented only as a last resort when the physician has compelling evidence that the patient is in imminent danger of causing himself or another person serious harm because of the disordered mental state. The physician must become familiar with the law concerning involuntary hospitalization within his or her jurisdiction.

Psychosis in and of itself is insufficient to justify involuntary hospitalization. If the possibility of serious harm is not imminent, the patient may refuse treatment as for any medical condition. However, patients who are not formally homicidal or suicidal may require involuntary hospitalization if their judgment is so impaired that their safety is seriously compromised. For example, a manic patient can believe it is possible to walk 100 miles in subzero weather with inadequate clothing.

In most cases, voluntary hospitalization is accepted when the physician states the recommendation with conviction and firmness. Any ambiguity or uncertainty is likely to be magnified by the patient, who probably has a pathologic degree of ambivalence. It is essential to involve the family as much as possible in the decision to hospitalize. This is not always easy, since family perceptions and concerns often vary considerably from those of the hospital staff. Some family members become excessively worried about minor symptoms, such as an acute extrapyramidal reaction, while others deny the significance of the most florid psychosis. All too often, family members resist acceptance of a psychiatric diagnosis with the outdated belief that such a diagnosis implies culpability for improper childrearing or suggests the possibility of genetic taint.

Having accepted in principle the physician's recommendation for hospitalization, the patient or family may enter a phase of bargaining. The argument often consists of such statements as "I will stay in the hospital, but not tonight," "I must put my affairs in order first," or "I want to be on a medical floor but not a psychiatric service." Such behavior can be symptomatic of the original illness or be an attempt to deny the seriousness of the situation. Occasionally, it is a test of the physician's judgment and firmness. Once the decision to hospitalize is made, however, there must be no ambiguity in the decision to implement it. The patient must not be allowed to leave the hospital with the promise to return later.

Finally, those who resist all recommendations and who cannot be hospitalized involuntarily should be asked to indicate their intention by signing out "against advice." Since many patients are unwilling to do even this, a careful note should be made and witnessed in the hospital record.

LESS SEVERE DISORDERS

Acute Anxiety Attacks and Hyperventilation

Anxiety is a symptom of many psychiatric conditions and some organic diseases. In addition, it may occur episodically in entirely healthy persons. Psychiatric conditions with manifest anxiety include incipient and acute schizophrenia, agitated depression, and transient situational disturbances. As always, the first concern of the emergency physician is to consider the possibility of an acute medical condition with psychiatric symptoms. The organic differential diagnosis includes effects of exogenous substances, metabolic disturbances, and cardiorespiratory conditions. Among exogenous substances, caffeine, amphetamines, cocaine, and corticosteroids and withdrawal from alcohol or sedative-hypnotics must be considered. Metabolic conditions of importance are hypoglycemia, electrolyte disturbances, hyperthyroidism, and pheochromocytoma. Cardiovascular and respiratory disturbances may include arrhythmia, mitral valve prolapse, asthma, congestive heart failure, and pulmonary embolism.

In the majority of cases of acute anxiety in the emergency department none of these conditions is apparent. Typically, the patient appears very frightened and agitated, with a history of shortness of breath of acute onset. The sensation may be described as the inability to take a deep-enough breath. Chest pain or pressure can be present, and muscular symptoms suggestive of hypocalcemia, such as carpopedal spasm, can occasionally occur. The subjective sensation is one of impending doom. Sensory changes consist of paresthesias of the distal extremities and of the circumoral region. Most commonly, the acute anxiety or panic attack is seen in young adults. It is unusual for a first attack to occur over the age of 35 years. When this constellation of findings appears without indication of other illness, the diagnosis of an acute anxiety attack is made.

Immediate treatment is directed at removal of physical symptoms. Since these are brought about by a shift in the acid-base balance secondary to hyperventilation, restoring the balance brings quick relief. Among the most popular and inexpensive methods is use of a paper bag, which the patient holds over his mouth to rebreathe expired air and consequently to increase alveolar carbon dioxide. Rapid relief of symptoms is usual.

The next task is to demonstrate to the patient that his or her symptoms have resulted from simple hyperventilation. This is not always easy, and patients may cling for some time to the idea that they have had a "heart attack." One of the dramatic and effective educational methods is to have the patient deliberately hyperventilate for several minutes or until symptoms are reproduced. This usually requires considerable encouragement by the physician, but is well worth the effort on those occasions when the patient is initially refractory to acceptance of a "nonmedical" explanation.

By this time, the patient may be ready to accept the suggestion that "nerves" may have something to do with the symptoms. If approached diplomatically, most patients can relate some information concerning emotional turmoil that might have contributed to the emergent symptoms. However, a substantial number of patients manifest spontaneous panic attacks. The physician may now be tempted to prescribe one of the commonly used high-potency antianxiety agents such as alprazolam (Xanax) or clonazepam (Klonopin). Generally, such prescription is premature at best. Often the attack is an isolated episode, and a few minutes of discussion will elucidate the psychodynamic or environmental cause. The physician does the patient much more service by sympathetic listening followed by firm reassurance than by mechanically prescribing a pill. Chemotherapy is seldom required. However, if a diagnosis of panic disorder is made, i.e. if three or more episodes occur within a span of 3 weeks, then more rigorous treatment with antipanic agents, behavioral therapy, or psychotherapy is required.

Antianxiety agents do, however, occasionally have value in other situations. Benzodiazepines are effective in the treatment of occasional anticipatory anxiety. Patients with phobias for air travel or public speaking, for example, may achieve satisfactory relief in a much more economical way than might be the case with psychotherapeutic treatment.

Chronic anxiety is a different problem. If anxiety is severe and prolonged, psychiatric referral is appropriate for definitive diagnosis and management. Chronic use of sedative-hypnotics and antianxiety agents is seldom effective, since tolerance grows and habituation is a possibility. Despite advertising claims, phenothiazines and other neuroleptics have little demonstrable effect on relieving chronic anxiety. The unfortunate terms "major" and "minor" tranquilizers have increased confusion about this issue. It is good to remember that there are no "tranquilizers"—there are antipsychotic, antidepressant, and antianxiety agents. Each has its indications and its limits of usefulness.

Insomnia

Difficulty with sleep is a frequent complaint late at night in the emergency department, occasionally to the ironic amusement of a sleepy physician, who is tempted to prescribe a single dose of a sedative and hope that the matter will end there. A better strategy is to investigate the problem and review the differential diagnosis of insomnia. Difficulty in sleeping (i.e. a difficulty of initiating and maintaining sleep, a disturbance of excessive somnolence, a manifestation of a circadian rhythm problem, or disrupted sleep secondary to a parasomnia) can be a presenting symptom of virtually any psychiatric condition and numerous medical problems. Among the major psychiatric conditions frequently implicated are acute schizophrenia, affective illness, chronic abuse of amphetamines or cocaine, and incipient delirium tremens. Each of these usually presents no diagnostic difficulty after a brief history and examination.

Having excluded major disturbances, the emergency physician is faced with treating a patient who gives a history of recent onset of inability to sleep with an absence of other symptoms. Occasionally a history of recent situational difficulty may be elicited—perhaps tension relating to an examination, a change in occupation, or family disharmony. Sometimes the cause of insomnia may be as simple as excessive use of caffeine or a restless new baby in the house. On careful history-taking and examination, most cause of insomnia may be elucidated without serious difficulty. There are, nevertheless, certain cases that remain refractory to investigation. The possibility must be considered that the patient may be a drug abuser hoping for a prescription for sedatives or even seeking sedatives for the purpose of suicide.

The general approach to treatment is to attempt specific therapy for the underlying condition if possible. Schizophrenic patients should receive antipsychotic medications on either an inpatient or outpatient basis. Manic patients can similarly benefit from such medications. Those with endogenous depression most often benefit from tricyclic antidepressants. In general, however, it is not reasonable to begin treatment for these conditions in the emergency department.

Insomnia as a result of environmental events may respond to brief psychotherapy or to a short course of small amounts of sedatives at bedtime. Advice and reassurance, as well as courtesy and empathy, may have much more desirable long-term benefits than a casually written prescription for sedatives. After exclusion of specific clinical entities as causes of insomnia, the physician must decide what treatment, if any, is appropriate for so-called primary insomnia. Specific guidelines are as follows.

1. Sedatives are not prescribed if the cause of insomnia is inapparent. A transient situation occasionally can suggest the desirability of short-term bedtime sedation.
2. Prescription of barbiturates should be avoided. They have a high abuse potential and relatively low index of safety. They can agitate elderly patients.
3. Prescription of sedatives for longer than a few days is avoided. They lose effectiveness, and in addition, the potential for abuse is present.
4. Flurazepam hydrochloride (Dalmane), a long-lasting agent, and related benzodiazepine compounds are among the safest and most effective short-term sedative-hypnotic agents. However, one must be aware of drug accumulation, especially in the elderly.
5. Although numerous hypnotic preparations have been marketed with considerable advertising fanfare, none shows special advantage over preparations mentioned previously; those with intermediate half-lives are more likely to lead to withdrawal syndromes and to habituation.
6. Sedatives are not prescribed for patients with a history of alcohol abuse. Not only can alcohol and sedatives act synergistically with dangerous results (i.e., leading to central nervous system and respiratory depression), but also alcoholism that is currently in remission can be reactivated by the prescription of cross-tolerant drugs.
7. When in doubt, medication should not be prescribed. For the physician to do otherwise is much more likely to complicate the situation than to help it.

Pain and Hypochondriasis

Occasionally, a patient will appear in the emergency department with a complaint of severe pain for which no cause is immediately obvious or which seems disproportionate to the visible lesion or injury. If the patient is hostile or demanding or exhibits marked dramatic or histrionic behavior, the physician may be persuaded that the pain is psychogenic—often a euphemism for saying that the patient is lying. Such patients represent extremely challenging diagnostic problems.

It must be remembered that pain is always "in the head" and that, while personality factors may color its mode of expression or intensity, no reliable information as to its cause necessarily need be implied. To assume otherwise sets the stage for the possibility of serious error.

The physician may be under the impression that the situation can be clarified by administration of a "pain-killing" placebo. *This practice should be abandoned* since it provides no useful information, and on discovery, which is frequent, it almost invariably leads to irreparable rupture of any rapport with the patient. This is not to say that placebo trials have no place. Approximately one-third of patients respond to placebos, experiencing increased pain relief from inactive injections, regardless of the cause of pain. The properly executed trial requires informed consent, a well-controlled schedule of various analgesics as well as placebo, and an inpatient setting with the goal of determining the most effective schedule of medication for chronic pain. Such trials are inappropriate and impractical in the acute situation in the emergency department.

Finally, it is wise to avoid the essentially pejorative labeling of a patient as hysterical or hypochondriacal. This not only interferes with clarity of diagnostic thinking but also may compromise future care if unsupported assumptions are made in the medical record. In a survey of 74 patients so labeled, Slater and Glithero found that three-fourths were seriously ill or had died in a 5- to 10-year follow-up period. Good medical practice demands suspension of such judgments before thorough diagnostic evaluation.

Family Turmoil

That couples and families come to the emergency department for aid in solving domestic crises gives testimony to the frequent absence of other sources of counsel. On some occasions, one of the members first presents a nonspecific medical complaint, while on other occasions the physician is simply asked for emergency family therapy.

Most often, one member of the family is defined as the patient at the outset. The best strategy is usually to interview this person alone at first. Depending on the circumstances, the physician may then wish to interview other parties separately or together. This process is not always excessively time-consuming, although it can be. The most important task is to identify the possibility of such serious conditions as incipient psychosis, assault, and child abuse. Having excluded such possibilities, the physician may make appropriate referral to available family counseling. The main pitfall is coming to a premature conclusion and giving advice based on inadequate information. The emergency physician must not expect to be an accomplished single-visit family counselor and should avoid accepting such a role if it is thrust on him or her. The obligations of the emergency physician are to intercept nascent emergencies and to make impartial referrals when indicated.

Grief Reactions

Psychologic reaction to major personal loss is a commonly encountered difficulty in emergency practice. The reaction may be acute, as is the case when a relative is brought to the hospital dead on arrival. Alternatively, symptoms may be delayed, causing a later visit to the emergency department with symptoms either directly felt or displaced (e.g., insomnia or gastrointestinal disturbance).

Often it is the unhappy task of the emergency physician to speak to relatives immediately after the death of a loved one. Occasionally, the physician may be under a mistaken impression that the relatives are already aware of the death. It is the physician's duty to inform them. This is best done in a gentle manner in a private setting. It is best to avoid unnecessary and unsolicited details, but all relevant questions should be answered. The well-integrated family may require little further assistance. Families without interpersonal resources may need the help of other professionals, such as a clergyman or lawyer. The physician should attempt to recognize this need and to arrange the appropriate referral. Occasionally, a sedative is helpful especially if a severe reaction is noted.

Persons with protracted, delayed, or displaced grief reactions also may seek emergency assistance. The immediate task is to identify such grief as a probable cause for nonspecific symptoms such as insomnia, anorexia, anxiety, or depression. If the reaction appears unusually intense or if the patient does not show the expected gradual recovery over the course of several weeks, referral for short-term psychotherapy may be helpful.

SPECIAL PROBLEMS

Extrapyramidal Reactions

Reactions of the extrapyramidal system to phenothiazine compounds and related drugs are frequently encountered. Drugs most commonly implicated are the high-potency phenothiazines, such as trifluoperazine, prochlorperazine (Compazine), fluphenazine, and perphenazine (Trilafon), and haloperidol, a butyrophenone. The most common reaction seen in the emergency department is dystonia that usually involves the facial muscles, the tongue, and the sternocleidomastoid muscles. Torticollis or an oculogyric crisis can occur. Also seen are akathisia, a syndrome of motor restlessness visible chiefly in the legs, and classic parkinsonian tremor.

Diagnosis is not difficult when a history of drug intake is known. Dystonia has been mistaken for a conversion reaction, possibly because the muscle spasm may respond transiently to suggestion or to treatment with a placebo. Occasionally, tetanus may be suspected. The manifestations may provoke intense anxiety. Oculogyric crisis is especially troublesome in this regard.

Fortunately, the most severe symptoms of dystonia may be reversed readily by intramuscular injection of diphenhydramine hydrochloride (Benadryl), 50 mg, which brings about remission within 15 minutes. Intravenous administration is preferred if symptoms are very distressing or if there is any suggestion of respiratory difficulty. In such cases, the same dose should be given over 3–5 minutes. Complete remission of symptoms usually occurs within a few minutes.

The physician must then address the question of whether to maintain or to discontinue administration of the neuroleptic compound. It is helpful to contact the prescribing physician for guidance. If the drug has been given for a benign and self-limiting condition, such as nausea or vomiting, it may be best to discontinue the offending agent. If, however, the medication has been prescribed for the treatment of psychosis, it is usually better to continue the neuroleptic, perhaps at a reduced dosage, allowing the prescribing physician to make further changes. The treatment of psychosis often requires use of neuroleptics in doses that may be expected to cause extrapyramidal reactions. These usually can be controlled satisfactorily with appropriate medication for drug-induced parkinsonism, such as benztropine mesylate (Cogentin), 1 or 2 mg twice a day.

After emergency treatment of the dystonia, remembering that neuroleptic compounds have a longer duration of action than diphenhydramine hydrochloride, the physician should prescribe benztropine mesylate or a similar agent for several days to avoid recurrence, even if the offending drug is to be discontinued.

Lithium Toxicity

Widespread use of lithium carbonate for the treatment and prophylaxis of manic-depressive illness raises the possibility that the emergency physician may see a patient with acute or subacute lithium toxicity. The therapeutic serum range is 0.6–1.2 mEq/liter. Levels more than 1.5 mEq/liter may be in the toxic range, although some patients may become toxic even at "therapeutic" levels. Clinical expression of excess serum lithium concentration begins with tremor and proceeds to nausea, vomiting, slurred speech, ataxia, seizures, coma, and death.

Lithium concentration in excess of the therapeutic range may occur as a result of several situations. Acute suicidal overdose is the most serious and may result in very high serum concentrations. Chronic mild overdose due to the patient's misunderstanding of directions or the theory that "if a little is good, a lot is better" is also possible. Lithium-treated patients inadvertently placed on a thiazide diuretic or on low-salt diet may have a toxic reaction. Finally, diminished renal function that is primary, or that is secondary to decreased cardiac output, can promote a toxic state due to failure of excretion. In mild and moderate states of toxicity, treatment is directed at removal of the cause and administration of saline solution. In severe intoxications, lithium excretion may be enhanced by urea-induced diuresis, alkalization of urine, and administration of aminophylline.

Chronic Brain Syndromes

Patients with chronic brain syndromes are frequently brought to the emergency department by frustrated, desperate, or angry relatives with the demand that the hospital "do something." The precipitating event may be acute, such as an episode of assaultive behavior, or it may be a chronic accumulation of family frustrations. Frequently, the situation presents itself during night or weekend hours when the resources of the emergency department are less than optimal.

This situation requires the services of a skilled and compassionate physician. On the one hand, giving in to inappropriate family demands must be avoided, while on the other, due consideration must be given the family's problems within the context of providing optimal patient care.

The first consideration is to determine, if possible, whether the precipitating event could have been brought about by a sudden deterioration of function from an ongoing medical illness that might have a remedy. If this is the case, delicate negotiation with the family often can proceed to a conclusion that is satisfactory to all. Cardiopulmonary or renal failure and other metabolic derangements are common causes to be investigated.

In many cases, identification of a specific medical precipitant is not possible. The task then is to determine what balance of medical, psychologic, and social remedies best serves the patient within the context of the current situation. Paranoid ideation may be diminished or eliminated by relatively small amounts of antipsychotic medication. Often the best choice is a high-potency drug such as trifluoperazine or haloperidol, which may have little direct sedative or hypotensive effect. Night wandering or irritable agitation similarly may be diminished to an acceptable level.

Throughout the evaluation it must be remembered that nothing tends to upset patients with chronic brain disease more than calling attention to their disabilities or asking them to perform mental status tasks that are beyond their ability. Extreme diplomacy is required during and after the examination.

Optimal care of the patient may require a change in social environment. A family that is unable or unwilling to provide satisfactory care may make placement in a nursing home the most reasonable alternative. Decisions of this nature that have major long-term consequences are best deferred for a few days until the situation can be clarified by further investigation of the social as well as medical status. If no immediate medical remedy can be found, a brief admission might be the most satisfactory alternative.

Neuroleptic Malignant Syndrome

This rare, potentially lethal disorder, occurs as an idiosyncratic reaction to the administration of neuroleptic agents. Although the more potent neuroleptics account for the majority of cases, even therapeutic doses of low potency neuroleptics may give rise to the syndrome.

The hallmark of the disorder is a catatonic-like state, replete with muscular rigidity, fever, autonomic instability (hypertension, hypotension, or lability of blood pressure), tachycardia, diaphoresis, and tremor. Fatalities have been reported in approximately 20% of patients, usually secondary to complications of dehydration, aspiration, hypotension, or respiratory failure. Central nervous system damage can also result from hyperthermia. Myonecrosis, from peripheral muscular rigidity, can increase hyperthermia and lead to myoglobinuria and renal failure.

It must be distinguished from other illnesses rapidly so that appropriate treatment may be initiated. Other disorders that have similar manifestations include neuroleptic-induced catatonia, malignant hyperthermia, encephalitis, and anticholinergic delirium. Among these conditions the presence or absence of several features may help clarify the diagnosis. In neuroleptic-induced catatonia, high fever is usually absent. Those having malignant hyperthermia often have a family history of the disorder or a prior adverse reaction to anesthetic agents. A lumbar puncture, performed when encephalitis is suspected, shows the presence of white blood cells in the cerebrospinal fluid (CSF). Anticholinergic delirium more commonly presents with prominent anticholinergic symptoms (confusion, dry mouth, fever, ileus, midriasis, flushing). A diagnostic trial of physostigmine salicylate, given intravenously in doses of 1–2 mg over 1–2 minutes, may help determine the extent to which anticholinergic symptoms contribute to the clinical picture.

Treatment involves the immediate discontinuation of neuroleptics. However, it must be remembered that neuroleptics can have effects that last for several weeks, especially when depot preparations are administered. Supportive care needs to be initiated promptly. High fevers can be treated with ice packs and hypotension should be treated with intravenous fluids. Other complications of the catatonic state should be prevented (e.g., aspiration, pulmonary embolism, decubitus ulcers). During the treatment of the hyperthermic phase, electrocardiographic monitoring is recommended.

Although no specific treatments have been proven successful in all cases, anecdotal reports provide evidence of the efficacy of dantrolene (a muscle relaxant that has been effective in the treatment of malignant hyperthermia), in doses of 0.8–1.0 mg/kg every 6 hours orally or intravenously, and bromocriptine mesylate (a dopamine agonist), given initially as 2.5 mg twice daily and increased gradually to 5 mg three times a day. With either of these agents treatment should continue for a duration of 2 weeks.

Factitious Illness

The voluntary presentation of physical or psychologic symptoms that is not understandable in the light of an individual's circumstances (e.g., malingering) is termed factitious illness. Although the dramatic exhibition of pain is often the first step toward hospital admission for individuals with factitious disorders (e.g., Munchausen syndrome), signs and symptoms pertaining to any organ system may be simulated or created. Most cases resemble organic emergencies. They include (*a*) the acute abdominal type (laparotomaphilia migrans); (*b*) the hemorrhagic type (hemorrhagica histrionica or, depending on the alleged site of bleeding, "hemoptysis merchants" or "hematemesis merchants"); (*c*) the neurologic type (neurologica diabolica) frequently presenting with a report of loss of consciousness or seizures; (*d*) dermatitis autogenica; and (*e*) hyperpyrexia figmentatica. Endocrinologic presentations consistent with hyperinsulinemia, hypoglycemia, and hyperthyroidism have been noted. The complaint of chest pain can also serve as a reason for admission. However, psychiatric presentations occur with reports of hallucinations, depression, and suicidal ideation.

Typically, these individuals have an extensive knowledge of medical jargon and capitalize on any real organic disturbance to make their case more interesting. They frequently demand immediate attention and express irritation when it is not forthcoming. Complaints of misdiagnosis and mistreatment are often made before their hoax is discovered. At that point it is difficult for the physician to recognize and empathize with the psychological suffering of the patient. As a result, few of these individuals receive psychiatric evaluations and fewer still enter ongoing treatment.

Few physicians have avoided being fooled by such patients, in part because physicians tend to believe what their patients tell them. While it is almost impossible to be certain of the diagnosis at first, there are several useful diagnostic aids: (*a*) a multiplicity of scars; (*b*) an evasiveness in manner; (*c*) an acute but not entirely convincing history; (*d*) numerous forms of identification; and (*e*) a history of having worked in the medical field.

Many of these individuals have a history of childhood deprivation, chronic illness, or institutionalization and have a wide range of psychiatric diagnoses. Their willingness to undergo unnecessary medical and surgical interventions has been thought to reflect masochistic tendencies and a pathologic way of loving. It is also important to realize that their behavior may be driven by unconscious and environmental factors. Physicians who fail to view this disorder as an illness end up contributing to it. Successful treatment is rare. However, attention to the physician's own countertransference reaction to the patient (often involving first protectiveness and then rage) may reduce unproductive struggles, unnecessary surgery, and premature discharge and increase the chance for a successful referral.

Drug Abuse

For the past 15 years, drug abuse, especially among the young, has come increasingly to the attention of physicians. The original cause is obscure, and patterns of incidence are constantly changing. Results of treatment are dubious. For the emergency physician there are two problems: (*a*) diagnosis and treatment of the acute effects of drug overdose and the possible medical complications and (*b*) referral of patients for ongoing treatment when this is appropriate.

Medical Complications

In addition to the specific pharmacologic hazards of each of the various drugs of abuse, there are general complications that can occur secondary to septic parenteral injection. Hepatitis is the most widely recognized, but tetanus, septic pulmonary embolism, pulmonary granulomatosis, and malaria are also possibilities. Subacute bacterial endocarditis and septicemia can occur. Organisms most frequently seen are coagulase-positive *Staphylococcus aureus,* enterococcus, *Staphylococcus albus,* and Candida species, and occasionally, *Escherichia coli,* Klebsiella, and Pseudomonas. Recently, the risk of infection with the acquired immunodeficiency syndrome (AIDS) virus has been added to the list of complications secondary to sharing needles with infected intravenous drug abusers.

Heroin and Other Opiates

Overdose is the most serious acute complication to opiate abuse. Within the subculture of the abuser, a variety of myths concerning treatment has developed. As a result the arrival of patients at the emergency department can be delayed by attempts to resuscitate with home remedies, such as bathing in ice and intravenous injection of saline solutions. Diagnosis is made by history from friends, sclerosis of veins, respiratory depression, and pinpoint pupils, except in the case of meperidine hydrochloride (Demerol) overdose, in which pupils may be normal or dilated. Treatment requires a narcotic antagonist, preferably naloxone hydrochloride (Narcan), 0.4 mg initially. This may be repeated two or three times as necessary in the first few minutes after arrival. Naloxone hydrochloride does not have respiratory depressant properties and, therefore, is safer than other narcotic antagonists. Supportive cardiorespiratory care is required.

Pulmonary edema secondary to opiate overdose is variable in its time of presentation. Because delayed onset is a possibility, patients with severe opiate intoxication should be observed carefully for 24 hours even if they respond quickly to narcotic antagonists.

During the withdrawal phase of opiate abuse, the patient may be seen in the emergency department with profound subjective distress but without major evidence of physiologic compromise. The typical pattern of most opiate abusers is such that florid symptoms of withdrawal seldom occur. The presenting symptoms are usually agitation, nausea, and muscle cramps with concurrent signs of mydriasis, diaphoresis, and goose flesh. The patient may insist on receiving narcotics. If the emergency physician is to admit the patient for other reasons or specifically for detoxification, it is appropriate to administer methadone hydrochloride, 5–10 mg intramuscularly, to diminish unnecessary suffering. Since this is a long-acting preparation and since habituation to large doses is unusual, these injections are seldom required more than two or three times in 24 hours. Symptoms of narcotic withdrawal may be greatly diminished by administration of clonidine, 0.1 mg three times a day for a period of 1–2 weeks, usually without risk of hypotension. In some centers, outpatient withdrawal schedules using oral methadone hydrochloride have had some success when combined with a highly structured program of group therapy. Without such a program, outpatient withdrawal is hazardous and should not be attempted. Only certified detoxification programs should engage in the outpatient maintenance or detoxification of narcotic addiction.

Amphetamines

Psychiatric emergencies after amphetamine abuse are of two types. First, as the result of a single acute overdose, a toxic delirium may be seen, with disorientation, visual and auditory hallucinosis, change in vital signs, tremor, and autonomic hyperactivity. The patient may have mydriasis, elevated blood pressure and pulse, and diaphoresis. Activity usually is frenetic. When these signs are prominent with a history of acute amphetamine abuse, the diagnosis is clear. Treatment requires supportive care and administration of antipsychotic medication. Unlike the treatment of functional psychosis, small doses are effective. Haloperidol, 2–5 mg, or trifluoperazine, 5 mg administered intramuscularly, usually brings about rapid resolution.

Second, when amphetamines are taken in moderate doses for several weeks, another toxic syndrome may develop. Termed amphetamine psychosis, it is a chronic paranoid condition suggestive of schizophrenia with insidious onset and without the usual signs of organic psychosis. Orientation and recent memory are preserved. Auditory hallucinations, delusions, and ideas of reference are prominent. Physical signs are absent. Indeed, it is usually impossible to separate this condition from paranoid schizophrenia except by a history of chronic amphetamine use or by urinary screening for amphetamines. This syndrome usually disappears a few weeks after discontinuing the drug. Hospitalization is generally advised during this time period.

Cocaine

Over the past few years, cocaine has become one of the most popular illicit drugs used in this country. Initially, its high cost limited its availability, but with the advent of cheaper forms (e.g., alkaloid cocaine or "crack") it has become accessible even to those in grade school.

Cocaine is most commonly ingested by snorting, free-basing (smoking), or injecting intravenously. However, its danger is greatest via the latter two routes of administration. Its stimulant effect (i.e., feelings of confidence, alertness, high energy, and euphoria) lasts between 20 minutes and 1 hour. The predominant physical effects involve dilatation of the pupils, increases in heart rate and blood pressure, constriction of peripheral blood vessels, and loss of appetite. Serious adverse physical reactions can occur and include cardiac arrhythmias, myocardial infarction, stroke, seizures, and death. Repeated usage or high doses can result in a maniform state with hyperactivity, rapid pressured speech, impaired judgment, and paranoia. Excessive anxiety and/or panic may also result.

In addition, the desire for repeated use is quite high, and craving for the drug often leads to social dysfunction. Tolerance develops rapidly and a higher dose is needed to produce its stimulant effects.

Chronic cocaine abuse may lead to headaches, loss of appetite, malnutrition, irritability, and exhaustion. A paranoid psychosis may develop, usually in the presence of a clear consciousness. It is also likely that chronic (and especially intermittent) use of cocaine will result in a seizure disorder, a consequence of cocaine's potent ability to kindle limbic system structures.

Although there is no physically dangerous abstinence syndrome, depressive symptoms may last for several days after discontinuing prolonged or intensive use. In the acute phase, high potency neuroleptics (e.g., haloperidol) are effective in the treatment of paranoia, while longer term treatments have included self-help groups (e.g., Cocaine Anonymous), psychotherapy, and pharmacotherapy. Lithium carbonate and a tricyclic antidepressant [desipramine hydrochloride (Norpramin)] have been noted to reduce the craving for cocaine in some, and depressive symptoms in others. For a more extensive discussion of cocaine and its effects see Chapter 17.

LSD and Similar Hallucinogens

Abuse of hallucinogens appears to be declining. Patients with dysphoric phenomena associated with their use may be seen in the emergency department after friends have made unsuccessful attempts to "talk down" the patient. Typically, patients are manifestly anxious with signs of sympathetic hyperactivity. Visual hallucinosis is the chief finding. Some delusional activity also may be present. Insight is usually preserved at least partly, so the patient is able to give a history of drug ingestion. Treatment requires supportive care and reassurance from a sympathetic person in a quiet, private, moderately lighted room. Diazepam, 5–15 mg orally, is the medication currently favored by experienced clinicians. Phenothiazine compounds have been reported to exacerbate the psychotic reaction.

Phencyclidine

This pernicious analog of ketamine has sedative, anesthetic, hallucinatory, and seizure-generating effects. It is produced cheaply in small illicit laboratories. It cannot be detected reliably by the usual toxic screening procedures. Clinical findings include extreme lability of mental status, from catatonia to violence; a blank stare, nystagmus, and sympathetic overactivity. The patient must be protected by all available means, including rest in a moderately lighted room, with close supervision and possibly the use of restraints. Medical management is discussed in Chapter 17.

Marihuana

Adverse reaction to marihuana is uncommon despite widespread use of the drug. Like all intoxicants, it can produce variations in mental status, not always with a pleasurable result. Panic attacks and paranoid reactions have been seen. Usual signs and symptoms of intoxication include euphoria, changes in perception of time and space, hunger, dry mucous membranes, tachycardia, and conjunctival injection. Use of potent preparations such as hashish can cause more profound effects, including hallucinosis. Treatment is supportive, with rest and reassurance, and recovery can be expected in a few hours. The occasional paranoid reaction, if persistent beyond that time, should be investigated further in an inpatient setting.

Barbiturates and Other Sedative-Hypnotics

Acute overdose with rapid progression to coma is a medical emergency, whereas chronic abuse can provoke more of a psychiatric emergency. All of the sedative-hypnotics, including alcohol, tend to bring about cortical release phenomena with consequent diminution of impulse control and deterioration of social behavior. Barbiturates and other drugs may cause episodic violent outbursts.

In addition, withdrawal from barbiturates and other sedative-hypnotics may be particularly dangerous. The patient can become tremulous, hyperreflexic, and hallucinatory and in severe cases can have clinical features similar to those seen with delirium tremens. Such patients require hospitalization, carefully controlled reintoxication, and slow, controlled withdrawal. The schedule of withdrawal depends on the particular sedative involved, but can be calculated by performing a barbiturate tolerance test. Frequent examination is necessary. It is wise to depend on physical signs for dosage decisions rather than on subjectively reported symptoms, since sedative abusers are not noted for truthfulness. Outpatient withdrawal attempts virtually always fail.

Anticholinergic Drugs

A wide variety of prescription drugs as well as over-the-counter medications contain anticholinergic substances that may be implicated in psychiatric emergencies. Overdoses can be accidental or deliberate, either with suicidal or recreational intention. Atropine, scopolamine (hyoscine), and stramonium are the active ingredients and can be found in antisecretory preparations and sleep medications. Symptoms of overdose are dry skin and mucous membranes, mydriasis, tachycardia, gastrointestinal atony, tactile and visual hallucinations, and delusional activity. Physostigmine is a specific antidote, but should be used with caution as discussed in Chapter 17. Because it has a shorter duration of action than some anticholinergic compounds, multiple injections may be necessary. Quaternary compounds such as neostigmine are ineffective in reversal of central nervous system effects since they do not cross the blood-brain barrier.

Follow-up Care

Having resolved medical psychiatric emergencies of drug abuse, the physician must address the question of further care. Unfortunately, the current state of treatment can point to few concrete results. The best strategy for the emergency department physician is to become familiar with regional facilities that specialize in drug problems.

SUGGESTED READINGS

American Psychiatric Association. Diagnostic and Statistical Manual of Mental Disorders, 34d ed. Washington, DC: American Psychiatric Association, 1980.

Anderson WH. The physical examination in office practice. *Am J Psychiatry,* 1980;137:1188–1192.

Anderson WH, Kuehnle JC. Diagnosis and early management of acute psychosis. *N Engl J Med,* 1981;305:1128–1130.

Anderson WH, Kuehnle JC, Catanzano DM. Rapid treatment of acute psychosis. *Am J Psychiatry,* 1976;133:1076–1078.

Detre TP, Jarecki HC. Modern Psychiatric Treatment. Philadelphia: JB Lippincott, 1971.

Folstein MF, Folstein SE, McHugh PR. "Mini-mental state," a practical method for grading the cognitive state of patients for the clinician. *J Psychiatr Res,* 1975;12:189–198.

Hackett TP, Cassem EH, eds. Handbook of General Hospital Psychiatry. St Louis: CV Mosby, 1978.

Hyman SE, ed. Manual of Psychiatric Emergencies. Boston: Little, Brown & Co, 1984.

Louria DB, Hensle T, Rose J. The major medical complications of heroin addiction. *Ann Intern Med,* 1967;67:1–22.

Murray GB. Complex partial seizures. In: Manschreck TC, ed. Psychiatric Medicine Update. New York: Elsevier, 1981:103–118.

Plum F, Posner JB. The Diagnosis of Stupor and Coma. 2nd ed. Philadelphia: FA Davis, 1972.

Rosenbaum JF. Current concepts in psychiatry: The treatment of anxiety. *N Engl J Med,* 1982;306:401–404.

Shader RI, ed. Manual of Psychiatric Therapeutics. Boston: Little, Brown & Co, 1975.

Slater ET, Glithero E. Follow-up of patients diagnosed as suffering from "hysteria". *J Psychsom Res,* 1965;9:9–13.

Soreff SM, ed. Emergency Psychiatry. Philadelphia: WB Saunders, 1983.

Stephenson JN, Moberg DP, Daniels BJ, et al. Treating the intoxicated adolescent: A need for comprehensive services. *JAMA,* 1984;252:1884–1888.

Stern TA. Munchausen's syndrome revisited. *Psychosomatics,* 1980;21:329–336.

Stern TA, Anderson WH. Benztropine prophylaxis of dystonic reactions. *Psychopharmacology,* 1979;61:261–262.

Stern TA, Murray GB. Complex partial seizures presenting as a psychiatric illness. *J Nerv Ment Dis,* 1984;172:625–627.

Stern TA, Mulley AG, Thibault GE. Life-threatening drug overdose: Precipitants and prognosis. *JAMA,* 1984;251:1983–1985.

Tesar GE, Stern TA. Evaluation and treatment of agitation in the intensive care unit. *J Intensive Care Med,* 1986;1:137–148.

Tesar GE, Murray GB, Cassem NH. Use of high-dose intravenous haloperidol in agitated cardiac patients. *J Clin Psychopharmacol,* 1985;5:344–347.

CHAPTER **19**

Acute Rash and Fever: Differential Diagnosis

RICHARD A. JOHNSON, M.D.
THOMAS B. FITZPATRICK, M.D., PH.D.

Approximately 10% of patients who seek emergency medical care do so with a dermatologic complaint. Many of these acute disorders, such as contact dermatitis or sunburn, are managed more appropriately in an ambulatory care center other than the emergency department. Some dermatologic disorders, however, because of their life-threatening nature or because they are part of the syndrome of a life-threatening disorder, require prompt diagnosis and therapy. Cutaneous findings range from the subtle but diagnostic erythematous macules and pustules that occur with gonococcemia to toxic epidermal necrolysis in which the entire epidermis is necrotic.

Patients may complain of acute onset of both rash and fever. Many times the cutaneous findings may be diagnostic in the emergency department before confirmatory laboratory data are available. As in the problem of the acute abdomen, the results of the laboratory tests, such as microbiologic cultures, serologic titers, and skin biopsy, may be available only after days to weeks. On the basis of a differential diagnosis, appropriate therapy, whether antibiotics or corticosteroids, can be started. One approach that has been effective in this differential diagnostic challenge has been to consider diseases according to the basic lesions: (*a*) *macules and papules;* (*b*) *bullae and/or pustules;* and (*c*) *purpuric lesions—macules, papules, and/or vesicles.* It must also be understood that the morphology of lesions is by no means static. Erythema multiforme begins with formation of macules and papules which may quickly progress to bullae; the early lesions of Rocky Mountain spotted fever are erythematous macules which evolve to purpuric papules. The physician must scrutinize the types of primary lesion, their configuration, and their distribution when the patient is first examined. The temporal evolution of the eruption may be the key in establishing the definitive diagnosis.

DISEASES MANIFESTED BY MACULES AND/OR PAPULES (TABLE 19.1)

Drug Hypersensitivity

Eruptions due to drugs are common problems that may be accompanied by fever. Although about 30 different patterns of drug eruption occur, only a few types are of sudden enough onset that the patient seeks emergency evaluation.

A period of sensitization is required with most drugs. Eruptions frequently appear 1 to 2 weeks after initiation of drug therapy. If the patient has been exposed to the drug previously, however, the eruption may begin within minutes to hours of reinstatement of the agent. In addition, eruptions may occur several weeks after drug administration has ceased.

Predictably, certain diseases are associated with much higher risk of sensitization to a specific drug than the general population. Patients who have an atopic disorder such as hay fever, asthma, or eczema or who have systemic lupus erythematosus appear to become sensitized to drugs, especially the penicillins, much more frequently. Acquired immunodeficiency syndrome (AIDS) patients given the sulfonamide combination, trimethoprim-sulfamethoxazole, for *Pneumocystis carinii* pneumonitis frequently experience an adverse drug eruption. Infectious mononucleosis patients who receive ampicillin or amoxicillin develop an exanthematous drug eruption in up to 100% of cases in some series. From a series of 446 patients with adverse drug reactions, clinical types and frequencies are reported in Table 19.2.

The differential diagnosis of a febrile patient with an exanthematous eruption can often be narrowed to either a drug eruption or a viral exanthem. Both viral and drug eruptions may appear abruptly. Both types often appear symmetrically and centripetally, suggesting a systemic cause rather than a topical or local cause. Drug eruptions are often a deeper "drug" red, compared with viral exanthems. Concomitant conditions, such as coryza, an enanthem, pharyngitis, or gastroenteritis, are helpful in distinguishing between the two eruptions. However, often the patient with these symptoms has taken an antibiotic, making the distinction between a viral or drug etiology difficult-to-impossible. When detected in a differential white blood count, peripheral eosinophilia with drug eruptions is helpful evidence.

The specific drug-induced eruptions, erythema multiforme, serum sickness, toxic epidermal necrolysis, and allergic cutaneous vasculitis are discussed separately.

At times patients are taking multiple drugs. Certain drugs such as ampicillin often cause a drug eruption; however, digoxin rarely (see Tables 19.3 and 19.4).

In most situations a suspected drug can be withdrawn, and if indicated, administration of an alternative agent can be started. Drug eruptions frequently begin to fade within a few days of discontinuance. Therapy for drug eruptions is for the most part based on symptoms. Topical corticosteroids are beneficial for eczematous drug eruptions. An evolving extensive eruption may resolve more quickly with oral prednisone, 60–120 mg in divided doses initially.

Viral Exanthems

Many viral infections cause systemic illness accompanied by eruptions on both the skin (exanthem) and the mucosa (enanthem). The morphology of an exanthem may be indistinguishable in viral exanthems and drug eruptions, which are thus referred to as measles-like or morbilliform. Temporal evolution of the exanthem is often helpful in the identification of a specific viral syndrome in comparison with a single observation.

Rubella (German Measles)

Because of widespread childhood immunization the incidence of rubella is now considerably reduced. Still at risk are those children who have not been immunized and young adults who have not had the illness or undergone immunization. Rubella alone is an inconsequential infection, except for the developing fetus, who following maternal transmission and intrauterine infection, is subject to all the malformations of the congenital rubella syndrome. A rubella-like illness in women frequently follows administration of the attenuated live rubella virus.

After an 18-day incubation period, a mild prodromal illness occurs. Adolescents and adults may complain of anorexia, malaise, conjunctivitis, headache, low-grade fever, and mild upper respiratory tract symptoms. These symptoms are absent or mild in young children. Lymphadenopathy is frequently present at this time. Postauricular, suboccipital, and posterior cervical lymph nodes are enlarged and tender. Mild generalized lymphadenopathy, as well as splenomegaly, may occur. Enlargement of lymph nodes usually persists for 1 week, but may last for months.

Table 19.1.
Differential Diagnosis for the Patient with Acute Onset of Rash and Fever: Diseases Manifested by Macules and Papules

		Physical Examination			
Disease	Clinical History	General	Dermatologic	Diagnostic Signs	Laboratory Data Available within 8 Hours
Drug hypersensitivity	More likely in atopy and in systemic lupus erythematosus Recent administration of new drug	Variable clinical presentation	Exanthematous eruption Fixed eruption Urticaria/angioedema Eczematous eruption Erythema multiforme Generalized erythroderma Toxic epidermal necrolysis SLE-like reactions	Variable laboratory findings	White blood cell count for eosinophilia
Rubella	Older children, young adults May follow rubella immunization in women Prodrome to rash may be absent or consist of mild headache, malaise, sore throat Arthralgia, especially women	Suboccipital, postauricular, and posterior cervical lymph nodes enlarged Periarticular tenderness or arthritis with effusion	Red macules or petechiae on soft palate (Forchheimer's sign) Exanthem appears as pink macules that coalesce on face; rash spreads during 24 hr to involve trunk and extremities as face clears; by 4th day, trunk and extremities clear	Eruption spreads rapidly from face to trunk and legs; clears within 3 days (compare with measles)	
Measles	Malaise, photophobia, dry hacking cough, upper respiratory tract catarrh	Conjunctivitis Fever to 40°C	Exanthem appears on forehead and behind ears on 4th day of illness; evolves inferiorly and centrifugally during next 72 hr to involve face, trunk, and extremities Initial pink discrete macules evolve into dull red confluent papules Exanthem fades during 6th–10th day of illness (compare with rubella) with residual brown staining and fine desquamation	Koplik's spot on buccal mucosa *before* rash; cluster of bluish white spots with bright red ring Eruption persists 6–10 days	

Nonspecific viral syndromes	Malaise Nausea and vomiting Diarrhea Sore threat Headache	Fever Variable clinical presentations	Exanthematous or vesicular rash Possible enanthem (discrete inflamed ulcers on palate or buccal mucosa)		
Erythema infectiosum	Relatively asymptomatic	Fever to 38°C Unremarkable	Early slapped-cheek butterfly erythema of face Later, pink macules and papules become confluent to form reticulate pattern on trunk and extremities Rash may recur over several weeks	Slapped-cheek appearance in otherwise well child	
Exanthem subitum	Child 6 months to 4 years old who is febrile but asymptomatic for 3–5 days	Fever to 38–40°C Unremarkable	As defervescence occurs, exanthem appears Discrete pink macules and papules mainly on trunk but also on proximal extremities Exanthem disappears in 24 hr	Exanthem following defervescence	
Primary human immunodeficiency virus type I infection	Incubation period 6 weeks to 5 years, male homosexual, parenteral drug user, hemophiliac Mononucleosis-like or flu-like syndrome lasting 2–3 weeks Malaise, severe headache, myalgia, arthralgia, sore throat, diarrhea, abdominal cramps	Stiff neck Generalized lymphadenopathy	Macular erythematous truncal eruption lasting up to 1 week Urticaria		Seroconversion of HTLV-III antibody, thrombocytopenia, lymphopenia, CSF lymphocytic pleocytosis
Infectious mononucleosis	Malaise, fatigue, sore throat Drug eruption if given ampicillin/ amoxicillin	Fever to 39°C Lymphadenopathy, possibly tender Splenomegaly (50%) Pharyngitis, exudative tonsillitis	Urticarial, morbilliform, or erythema multiforme-like rash Bilateral supraorbital edema Petechiae at border of hard and soft palate	Early in course, resembles rubella	Differential shows many atypical lymphocytes (>10% of WBC) Heterophil test
Cytomegalovirus infection	Nonspecific viral illness	Fever, lymphadenopathy,	Exanthematous eruption (6%)		Atypical lymphocytes Negative heterophil test

Table 19.1—*continued*

Disease	Clinical History	Physical Examination: General	Physical Examination: Dermatologic	Diagnostic Signs	Laboratory Data Available within 8 Hours
	Mononucleosis syndrome Multiple blood transfunsions, bone marrow transplant Reactivation of latent CMV in immunocompromised patient Drug eruption if given ampicillin/amoxicillin	splenomegaly, pneumonia, hepatitis, lymphocytosis No tonsillar pharyngitis			
Hepatitis B	Male homosexual, recent blood transfusions, parenteral drug abuser, laboratory or medical personnel Malaise, fatigue, arthralgia, headache	Fever, subsequent jaundice, arthritis	Urticaria-like lesions for 2–7 days, i.e., serum sickness, before jaundice Gianotti-Crosti syndrome in children Polyarteritis nodosa (PAN) Palpable purpura		Positive hepatitis B surface antigen (HBsAg), eosinophilia with PAN
Gianotti-Crosti syndrome	Early childhood	Fever, malaise, generalized lymphadenopathy, hepatomegaly	Coppery-red, flat-topped firm papules (1–5 mm), symmetric on face, buttocks, limbs (excluding palms and soles)	Distinctive rash in child	Positive HBsAg (commonly except in North America)
Scarlet fever	Sore throat in patient in 1st decade of life Possible wound infection	Fever Follicular or membranous tonsillitis Painful regional lymph node enlargement	Punctate erythema on upper trunk, generalized within hours to days Face flushed, with perioral pallor Petechial lesions possible at body folds, especially antecubital fossae (Pastia's lines)	Strawberry tongue, initially white with enlarged filiform papillae, then bright red	Immunofluorescence test of throat for group A β-hemolytic streptococcus

			Perifollicular hyperkeratosis resulting in sandpapery feel to skin Desquamation of palms and soles		
Erythema multiforme (EM)	Recent herpes simplex or mycoplasma infection Prior history of erythema multiforme with recurrent herpes Drug exposure	Fever to 40°C	Target lesions characteristically on distal extremities, palms, soles Wide spectrum of lesion morphology Wide spectrum of severity—EM major, EM minor Lesions may become bullous Bullous and erosive lesions of conjunctival, oropharyngeal, nasal, and anogenital mucosa possible	Target lesions on extremities	Skin biopsy
Erythema marginatum	Fever, possible migratory arthritis, cardiac involvement, chorea Usually a child	Fever to 40°C New murmurs, cardiomegaly, pericardial rub	Usually, flat or slightly raised erythema on trunk Macules enlarge by 1 cm/day with central clearing, resulting in polycyclic or geographic pattern	Rapidly evolving circinate rash	
Toxic shock syndrome	Menstruation (90%), previous episode Nasal packs Influenza B infection	Fever over 38.9°C Hypotension with systolic blood pressure 90 mm Hg Abnormalities of gastrointestinal, hepatic, muscular, renal, cardiovascular, neurologic systems (three or more)	Conjunctival hyperemia, red strawberry tongue Palms and soles, erythema and swelling Desquamation after first week of illness	Characteristic syndrome in a menstruating female	*S. aureus* producing toxic shock syndrome toxin
Secondary syphilis	Sexually active individual Possible history of chancre occurring within 21 days after sexual exposure Sore throat, malaise,	Residual chancre, at times Inguinal lymphadenopathy associated with genital chancre Lymphadenopathy (suboccipital, postauricular,	Pink-tan macules to papules to scaling papules on trunk and extremities, especially palms and soles Moth-eaten alopecia of scalp Condylomata lata in anogenital area, mucous patches in mouth, split papules of lips Annular lesions	Positive serology Pink-tan macules to papules on palms and/or soles highly characteristic Herxheimer reaction	Darkfield microscopy of lesion is diagnostic (except in mouth) Rapid plasma reagent (RPR) card test

Table 19.1—*continued*

Disease	Clinical History	Physical Examination: General	Physical Examination: Dermatologic	Diagnostic Signs	Laboratory Data Available within 8 Hours
	headache, fever, myalgias occurring 6–12 weeks after chancre	posterior cervical, epitrochlear)			
Lyme disease	Tick bite, incubation period 3–32 days Living in or visiting endemic area; June through early fall Malaise, headache, stiff neck, arthralgias, myalgias	Fever to 40°C, lymphadenopathy (regional or generalized) Late manifestations: joints, nervous system, heart	Erythema chronicum migrans at site of tick bite Multiple annular secondary lesions Malar rash	Erythema chronicum migrans	
Systemic lupus erythematosus	Fatigue, rash, photosensitivity, Raynaud's phenomenon SLE-inducing drug (hydralazine, procainamide, penicillin, anticonvulsants, sulfonamides, birth control pills) Psychosis or convusions	Fever, low grade or to 40°C Pleural or pericardial rub, arthritis	Butterfly rash, maculopapular eruption on trunk Scaling, erythematous, atrophic plaques (discoid lesions) on scalp, face, ears, shoulders Alopecia; ulcers, oral or nasopharyngeal	Discoid lesion, butterfly rash	Skin biopsy Antinuclear antibody positive, anemia, leukopenia, thrombocytopenia
Rocky Mountain spotted fever	History of tick bite Endemic area Incubation period of 7 days Malaise, severe fever, chills, severe headache,	Fever to 40°C Muscle tenderness Stiff neck Splenomegaly	Erythematous macules begin on wrists and ankles in sick patient; in 6–18 hr, rash spreads centrifugally to involve palms and soles, and centripetally to extremities and trunk	Site of origin of rash (wrists and ankles are unique sites of origin among exanthems)	Skin biopsy shows *R. rickettsii* within vascular endothelial cells

	myalgia, toxic reaction for 3–4 days		During next few days, lesions may become papular and purpuric		
Typhus (epidemic) fever	History of travel to Central or South America, endemic area Headache, malaise	Fever	Pink macular eruption appearing in axillae, then trunk, and spreading centrifugally to extremities May become petechial and confluent Purpura fulminans with disseminated intravascular coagulation		Weil-Felix reactions, specific serologic tests
Murine (endemic) typhus	Excoriated rat flea bite Endemic area	Fever to 39°C Splenomegaly in 25% of patients	Rash appears on 5th day of illness Centripetal erythematous macular and papular discrete eruption Duration—evanescent to several days	Centripetal eruption in patient in endemic area	
Salmonella infection	Fever, chills, headache, and constipation of 1 week's duration followed by diarrhea and abdominal pain	Fever 39–40°C Abdominal tenderness	Crops of 10–20 pink macules (rose spots) and papules 1–3 mm in diameter on lower chest, abdomen, midback	Rose spots (2nd week)	
Sweet's syndrome	Prior respiratory infection Underlying myeloproliferative disorder	Spiking fever, arthralgia, conjunctivitis	Abrupt onset of tender red plaques or nodules on face and extremities Enlarge with very edematous borders and central clearing	Rapid resolution with systemic corticosteroids but not antibiotics	Skin biopsy shows dense dermal neutrophilic infiltrate Mature neutrophilic leukocytosis
Kawasaki disease	Child Diarrhea, arthralgia, arthritis, meatitis, tympanitis, photophobia, meningeal irritation	Fever for 5 or more days Cervical lymphadenopathy Pericarditis, myocarditis, hepatitis, urethritis, coronary artery aneurysms	Bilateral conjunctival injection Fissured lips, injected pharynx, strawberry tongue Erythema of palms or soles, edema of hands or feet, generalized or periungual desquamation	Diagnostic criteria	
Serum sickness	Drug or serum exposure	Fever to 39–40°C Migratory polyarthritis	Commonly, urticaria-like eruption		Skin biopsy

Table 19.1—*continued*

Disease	Clinical History	Physical Examination: General	Physical Examination: Dermatologic	Diagnostic Signs	Laboratory Data Available within 8 Hours
	Malaise, headache, myalgia, anorexia Serum sickness-like syndrome as prodrome of hepatitis B infection	Generalized lymphadenopathy Uncommon, splenomegaly			
Trichinosis	History of ingestion of undercooked pork or bear meat Diarrhea, myalgia	Fever Abdominal tenderness, muscle weakness	Periorbital edema, subungual splinter hemorrhages Transient exanthematous eruption	Biopsy of splinter hemorrhage in nail bed reveals *T. spiralis*	Differential of WBC shows eosinophilia

Table 19.2.
Adverse Drug Reactions in a Series of 446 Patients

Clinical Types[a]	Frequency
	%
Exanthematous eruptions	42.4
Fixed eruption	20.6
Urticaria/angioedema	12.8
Eczematous eruption	10.5
Erythema multiforme	4.0
Generalized erythroderma	2.2
Toxic epidermal necrolysis	1.8
Photosensitivity reactions	1.1
Drug fever	1.1
Purpuric eruption	1.0
SLE-like reaction	0.5
Erythema nodosum	0.2

[a] SLE, systemic lupus erythematosus.

An enanthem of petechiae on the soft palate (Forchheimer's sign) may be seen during the prodromal illness. This finding is not pathognomonic for rubella, since petechiae may be seen in this location in infectious mononucleosis, which also is accompanied by prominent lymphadenopathy.

The exanthem begins as pink macules and papules at the hairline, which spread during the first 24 hours to involve the face, trunk, and extremities. By the second day, the facial exanthem may fade, whereas the discrete lesions on the trunk become confluent, creating a scarlatiniform eruption. The exanthem usually remains discrete on the extremities. Unlike measles, by the end of the 3rd day the eruption has faded with a residual yellow-tan color or fine scaling.

The diagnosis can be confirmed by isolation of the rubella virus from the throat and demonstration of a rise in rubella antibody titer. Serologic studies indicate that the exanthem may not appear in 10–40% of known cases of rubella.

Rubeola (Morbilli, Measles)

Rubeola is a highly contagious viral infection of childhood. Because of infant immunization, the incidence has strikingly declined from a preimmunization annual figure of 500,000 cases (1963) in the United States to 2,813 cases (1985). Large outbreaks presently do occur in inadequately or unimmunized groups such as preschool-aged children and junior or senior high school and university students.

Within 10–15 days after exposure to measles, symptoms of an upper respiratory tract infection with coryza and a hacking, bark-like cough occur, accompanied by photophobia, malaise, and fever. If the patient is examined on or after the 2nd day of febrile illness, Koplik's spots may be observed on the buccal mucosa opposite the premolar teeth.

Table 19.3.
Agents Causing Drug Eruptions in a Series of 430 Patients

Agent	Frequency
	%
Antimicrobial agents	53
Antipyretic/anti-inflammatory analgesics	14
Central nervous system depressant drugs	12
Gold	6
β-Adrenoreceptor blocking agents	5.5
Other	9.5

This pathognomonic enanthem is characterized by a cluster of tiny bluish-white papules with an erythematous areola. By the 4th day the characteristic exanthem appears as erythematous macules and papules on the forehead and behind the ears. By the 3rd to 5th day of rash, the eruption spreads centrifugally and inferiorly to involve the face, trunk, and extremities. The initial discrete lesions may become confluent. The exanthem fades gradually with residual yellow-tan stain due to mild extravasation and faint desquamation.

Measles can be complicated by encephalitis (1 in 800 cases), thrombocytopenia, and secondary bacterial infections. A late complication is subacute sclerosing panencephalitis.

A clinical diagnosis of measles is made with findings of generalized rash lasting 3 or more days, and at least one of the following: cough, coryza and/or conjunctivitis. Laboratory confirmation is by isolation of measles virus from blood, urine, or pharyngeal secretions or by a 4-fold or greater rise in measles antibody.

Nonspecific Viral Syndromes

Coxsackie viruses of both groups A and B, ECHO virus, reoviruses, respiratory syncytial virus, and adenoviruses are associated with exanthems. In most cases the symptoms and physical findings suggest a

Table 19.4.
Antibiotics Causing Skin Reactions in a Series of 74 Patients

Antibiotic	Frequency
	%
Ampicillin	42
Penicillin	27
Tetracyline	15
Amoxicillin	4.0
Choramphenicol	2.7
Dicloxacillin	1.4
Doxycycline	1.4
Dimethylchlortetracycline	1.4
Erythromycin	1.4
Streptomycin	1.4

viral infection, which can only be confirmed by viral cultures or immunofluorescence techniques. Most of the exanthems are characterized by pink macules or papules, or both, on the trunk and extremities; vesicles and petechiae are rare. Enanthems are also seen. The cutaneous findings may be accompanied by fever, malaise, gastroenteritis, pharyngitis, or aseptic meningitis.

The diagnosis of a viral syndrome is made on clinical grounds, usually by excluding treatable bacterial agents.

Erythema Infectiosum (Fifth Disease)

Erythema infectiosum is an acute mild illness with a characteristic exanthem. A viral cause is probable. Human parvovirus has been detected by DNA hybridization and immune electron microscopy in patient serum. Human parvovirus infection can be asymptomatic or cause a variety of clinical manifestations, including nonexanthematous illness. The disease usually occurs in epidemics and in that setting is easier to identify. Sporadic cases may be difficult to diagnose with certainty.

Erythema infectiosum occurs most frequently in girls from 5 years of age to puberty, but is also seen in boys and in adults. Prodromal symptoms are absent to mild. Malaise, headache, nausea and vomiting, coryza, sore throat, and musculoskeletal pain do occur. Adults tend to have more severe constitutional symptoms. The temperature is rarely higher than 38°C.

The exanthem begins with an erythematous plaque in a butterfly distribution on the face, creating a "slapped-cheek" appearance. The skin is hot and the eruption must be distinguished from erysipelas, scarlet fever, and lupus erythematosus. The plaque fades within a few days, leaving a dusky violet hue. As the facial eruption fades, an exanthem appears on the buttocks and extremities. Macular or urticarial lesions develop, which become confluent to form a characteristic annular, gyrate, or reticulate pattern. This latter eruption fades in 3 to 5 days, but may recur.

Usually a definitive diagnosis can be made by following the course of the illness over a week. Treatment of symptoms at times may be required.

Exanthem Subitum (Roseola Infantum)

Exanthem subitum, as the name suggests, is characterized by the sudden appearance of a rash. Although thought to be viral, the agent has not been isolated. The disease is usually seen in children from 6 months to 4 years of age. Either the degree of contagiousness is low or the subclinical attack rate is high, since epidemics do not occur and the incidence of secondary cases within families is low. A temperature from 38–40°C develops suddenly while the infant is otherwise asymptomatic. The fever is relatively constant for 3–5 days, after which defervescence occurs abruptly.

The exanthem develops coincidentally with defervescence; it appears mainly on the trunk and to a lesser extent on the proximal extremities, neck, and face. Discrete pink macules and papules are seen. The exanthem is short-lived, usually lasting only 24 hours.

No confirmatory laboratory tests are available. Unless the patient has been examined during the febrile phase and subsequently with the exanthem, the diagnosis cannot be confirmed on clinical grounds.

Human Immunodeficiency Virus Type I (HIV-I) Infection

Primary infection by the human immunodeficiency virus type I (HIV-I) is often asymptomatic but may be an acute flu-like or mononucleosis-like illness. Individuals at risk for HIV-I infection, identical to those at risk for hepatitis B virus infections, are as follows: (*a*) homosexual men or others with frequent and multiple sexual contacts; (*b*) percutaneous drug abusers who share needles; (*c*) patients receiving blood transfusions, blood products, or requiring hemodialysis; and (*d*) laboratory or medical personnel exposed to blood or blood products. The clinical incubation period from known HIV-I exposure to onset of febrile illness ranges from 3 to 6 weeks, but may be much longer.

A flu-like illness of fever, chills, arthralgia, and myalgia can occur following the incubation period in at-risk individuals and persist for 2–3 weeks. A maculopapular truncal eruption may accompany the acute illness and persist for up to 1 week. Urticaria may occur in the 3rd week of illness. Severe headache, stiff neck, sore throat, nausea, diarrhea, and abdominal cramps occur in some patients. Generalized lymphadenopathy can follow the initial symptoms. Localized lymphadenitis has occurred following an infecting needle stick.

Laboratory abnormalities associated with primary HIV-I infection include mild leukocytosis and lymphopenia, relative monocytosis, mild thrombocytopenia, and elevated erythrocyte sedimentation rate. Patients with a HIV-I meningitis characterized by headache and stiff neck may have cerebrospinal fluid (CSF) lymphocytic pleocytosis. Definitive diagnosis is made by isolating HIV-I from blood and/or CSF, during the acute illness. Seroconversion following presumed exposure occurs somewhat later, as early as 6–8 weeks.

The Center for Communicable Diseases has proposed the following classification system for the broad spectrum of clinical manifestations and laboratory findings which may eventuate from life-long HIV-I infection.

Group I. Acute HIV-I Infection. Acute HIV-I infection is defined as a mononucleosis-like syndrome, with or without aseptic meningitis, associated with seroconversion for HIV-I antibody. Antibody seroconversion is required as evidence of initial infection; current viral isolation procedures are not adequately sensitive to be relied on for demonstrating the onset of infection.

Group II. Asymptomatic HIV-I Infection. Asymptomatic HIV-I infection is defined as the absence of signs or symptoms of HIV-I infection. To be classified in Group II, patients must have had no previous signs or symptoms that would have led to classification in Groups III or IV. Patients whose clinical findings cause them to be classified in Groups III or IV should not be reclassified in Group II if those clinical findings resolve.

Patients in this group may be subclassified on the basis of a laboratory evaluation. Laboratory studies commonly indicated for patients with HIV-I infection include, but are not limited to, a complete blood cell count (including differential white blood cell count) and a platelet count. Immunologic tests, especially T-lymphocyte helper and suppressor cell counts, are also an important part of the overall evaluation. Patients whose test results are within normal limits, as well as those for whom a laboratory evaluation has not yet been completed, should be differentiated from patients whose test results are consistent with defects associated with HIV-I infection [e.g. lymphopenia, thrombocytopenia, decreased number of helper (T_4) T-lymphocytes].

Group III. Persistent Generalized Lymphadenopathy (PGL). PGL is defined as palpable lymphadenopathy (lymph node enlargement of 1 cm or greater) persisting for more than 3 months at two or more extrainguinal sites in the absence of a concurrent illness or condition other than HIV-I infection to explain the findings. Patients in this group may also be subclassified on the basis of a laboratory evaluation, as is done for asymptomatic patients in Group II. Patients with PGL whose clinical findings caused them to be classified in Group IV should not be reclassified in Group III if those other clinical findings resolve.

Group IV. Other HIV-I Disease. The clinical manifestations of patients in this group can be designated by assignment to one or more subgroups (A–E) listed below. Within Group IV, subgroup classification is independent of the presence or absence of lymphadenopathy. Each subgroup may include patients who are minimally symptomatic, as well as patients who are severely ill. Increased specificity for manifestations of HIV-I infection, if needed for clinical or research purposes or for disability determinations, may be achieved by creating additional divisions within each subgroup.

Subgroup A. Constitutional Disease. Constitutional disease is defined as one or more of the following: fever persisting more than 1 month, involuntary weight loss of greater than 10% of baseline, or diarrhea persisting more than 1 month; and the absence of a concurrent illness or condition other than HIV-I infection to explain the findings.

Subgroup B. Neurologic Disease. Neurologic disease is defined as one or more of the following; dementia, myelopathy, or peripheral neuropathy; and the absence of a concurrent illness or condition other than HIV-I infection to explain the findings.

Subgroup C. Secondary Infectious Diseases. Secondary infectious disease is defined as the diagnosis of an infectious disease associated with HIV-I infection and/or at least moderately indicative of a defect in cell-mediated immunity. Patients in this subgroup are divided further into two categories.

Category C-1. Category C-1 includes patients with symptomatic or invasive disease due to one of 12 specified secondary infectious diseases listed in the surveillance definition of AIDS: *P. carinii* pneumonia, chronic cryptosporidiosis, toxoplasmosis, extraintestinal strongyloidiasis, isosporiasis, candidiasis (esophageal, bronchial, or pulmonary), cryptococcosis, histoplasmosis, mycobacterial infection with *Mycobacterium avium* complex or *Mycobacterium kansasii,* cytomegalovirus infection, chronic mucocutaneous or disseminated herpes simplex virus infection, and progressive multifocal leukoencephalopathy.

Category C-2. Category C-2 includes patients with symptomatic or invasive disease due to one of six other specified secondary diseases: oral hairy leukoplakia, multidermatomal herpes zoster, recurrent *Salmonella* bacteremia, nocardiosis, tuberculosis, or oral candidiasis (thrush).

Subgroup D. Secondary Cancers. Secondary cancers are defined as the diagnosis of one or more kinds of cancer known to be associated with HIV-I infection as listed in the surveillance definition of AIDS and at least moderately indicative of a defect in cell-mediated immunity: Kaposi's sarcoma, non-Hodgkin's lymphoma (small, noncleaved lymphoma or immunoblastic sarcoma), or primary lymphoma of the brain.

Subgroup E. Other Conditions in HIV-I Infection. Other conditions are defined as the presence of other clinical findings or diseases, not classifiable above, that can be attributed to HIV-I infection and/or can be indicative of a defect in cell-mediated immunity. Included are patients with chronic lymphoid interstitial pneumonitis. Also included are those patients whose signs or symptoms could be attributed either to HIV-I infection or to another course or management of which may be complicated or altered by HIV-I infection. Examples include: patients with constitutional symptoms not meeting the criteria for subgroup IV-A; patients with infectious diseases not listed in subgroup IV-C; and patients with neoplasms not listed in subgroup IV-D (see Appendix).

Infectious Mononucleosis (Epstein-Barr Virus)

Infectious mononucleosis is an acute infectious process caused by the Epstein-Barr virus (EBV) and is characterized by fever, sore throat, lymphadenopathy. Young adults, 15 to 25 years of age, have the highest rate of infection. The majority of cases are subclinical. In children the incubation period is 10 to 14 days; however, it can range up to 50 days in adult.

The prodrome consists of fever, malaise, fatigue, and headache. Up to 10% of symptomatic patient may have a faint, transient, erythematous, morbilliform eruption on the trunk and proximal extremities. Bilateral edema of the upper eyelids also occurs early in the course. Less commonly urticarial, scarlatiniform, or hemorrhagic eruptions occur. A high percentage of patients with infectious mononucleosis given ampicillin or amoxicillin develop an extensive morbilliform eruption.

Most symptomatic patients experience a sore throat during the first week of illness, which is associated with a gray-white exudative tonsillitis in half of cases. Constitutional symptoms vary and include fever, fatigue, malaise, and headache. In a third of patients with infectious mononucleosis, a characteristic enanthem occurs and consists of 5–20 circumscribed petechial hemorrhages at the border of the soft and hard palates. Tender lymphadenopathy of the anterior and posterior cervical nodes occurs most frequently, but generalized lymphadenopathy may occur. Fifty percent of patients develop splenomegaly during the 2nd and 3rd weeks.

During the prodromal stage of infectious mononucleosis differentiation from rubella or cytomegalovirus (CMV) infection may be impossible. The presence of a large number of atypical lymphocytes and demonstration of rising or elevated titers of heterophil or EBV antibodies confirms the diagnosis of infectious mononucleosis. Cytomegalovirus mononucleosis can be differentiated by isolation of CMV from the urine and an antibody rise. The differential diagnosis of bilateral periorbital edema in the patient with rash and fever includes infectious mononucleosis, Lyme disease (also with conjunctival suffusion), toxic shock syndrome, trichinosis, and leptospirosis.

Cytomegalovirus Infections

Cytomegalovirus infections are extremely common and usually subclinical. An infection occurring in utero or in an immunocompromised host can, however, be devastating.

Rash and fever are seen in several clinical syndromes caused by the cytomegalovirus. Although primary infection in an adult is most commonly asyptomatic, cytomegalovirus can cause a mononucleosis syndrome virtually identical with Epstein-Barr mononucleosis. Sore throat is a common complaint in CMV mononucleosis but signs of pharyngeal exudation, especially exudative tonsillitis, are not seen. Mucosal petechiae are also absent. However, a transient morbilliform eruption can be seen on the trunk in about 5% of CMV mononucleosis patients. Tender cervical lymphadenopathy is not characteristic of CMV mononucleosis; however, splenomegaly, liver involvement, and atypical lymphocytes do occur. Seroconversion or a 4- to 8-fold rise in CMV antibody titer is required for diagnosis of active infection.

Post-pump perfusion syndrome is a primary CMV infection resembling CMV mononucleosis, transmission occurring through multiple blood transfusions. A morbiliform eruption, similar to that in CMV mononucleosis, occurs in the prodrome. Immunosuppressed renal allograft transplantation patients are at additional risk, both from blood transfusion as well as organ transplant, from a donor strain of CMV.

Chronic CMV infections in immunocompromised patients (i.e. acquired immunodeficiency syndrome) are not associated with rash.

Hepatitis B

Infection with hepatitis B virus (HBV) is associated with four distinct dermatologic syndromes: a serum sickness-like prodrome, polyarteritis nodosa, essential mixed cryoglobulinemia, and papular acrodermatitis of childhood (Gianotti-Crosti syndrome). Each of these four syndromes is related to the presence of circulating immune complexes of HBV antigen and anti-HBV antibody. HBV surface antigen (HBsAg) can be detected from 1 to 12 weeks following time of infection, and evidence of hepatitis appears from 1 to 7 weeks following appearance of HBsAg.

The population at risk for HBV infection, nearly identical for human T cell lymphotrophic virus type III (HTLV-III) infection, is as follows: (*a*) homosexual men or others with frequent and multiple sexual contacts, (*b*) percutaneous drug abusers who share needles, (*c*) patients receiving blood transfusions or requiring hemodialysis, (*d*) laboratory or medical personnel exposed to blood or blood products. The clinical incubation period from exposure time to the appearance of clinical jaundice is variable from 30 to 130 days. However, the serologic incubation period from exposure to appearance of HBsAg in the serum can be as short as 6 days.

HBV prodromal symptoms include anorexia, nausea and vomiting, malaise, headache, fatigue, a distaste for cigarettes, myalgia, and coryza. During the preicteric period, a serum sickness-like prodrome occurs in 20 to 30% of infected patients, manifesting as fever, urticarial-like rash, angioedema, arthropathy, and proteinuria or hematuria. Unlike classical urticaria which is evanescent, lasting less than 24 hours, an urticaria-like lesion of the serum sickness-like prodrome may persist for several days (so called "urticaria perstans"). The urticarial lesions, which correlate with the serologic existence of antigen-antibody complexes, resolve in 2 to 7 days, but may be the sole clinical manifestation of HBV infection. The onset of HBV hepatitis is usually insidious with jaundice noted 1–6 weeks after the prodrome.

The arthropathy is commonly acute symmetric arthralgia of the small joints of the hands, ankles, knees, and shoulders. Frank arthritis and synovitis may occur. Less commonly monarticular involvement of large joints may occur. Joint symptoms usually resolve within 3 weeks.

Polyarteritis nodosa is associated with HBsAg positivity in 40–50% of cases and can occur in one of each 500 HBV infections. This systemic vasculitis is characterized by dermatologic manifestations in 10–15% of cases: fever, polyarthralgia, and neurologic and renal involvement. This chronic progressive vasculitis eventually can cause mononeuritis multiplex and other neuropathies, hypertension, eosinophilia, hematuria, and azotemia. Depending on the size of the artery involved in polyarteritis nodosa, livido, nodules, and ulceration occur, as well as urticaria and angioedema. With distal artery vasculitis, acral necrosis can be seen. Vasculitis lesions in the leg panniculus can result in linear subcutaneous nodules, 1–2 cm in diameter, and can evolve into painful ulcerations.

Essential mixed IgG and IgM cryoglobulinemia occurs with prolonged HBsAg antigenemia, but correlates with easily recognizable cold sensitivity in only one-third of patients. "Palpable" purpura (95%) is seen on the lower extremities; less commonly, erythrocyanosis and Raynaud's phenomenon. Systemic involvement of a necrotizing vasculitis results in arthropathy (45%) and nephropathy (48%).

Uncommonly, hepatitis A virus (HAV) infection is associated with a similar transient serum sickness-like prodrome.

Gianotti-Crosti Syndrome (Papular Acrodermatitis of Childhood)

Gianotti-Crosti syndrome or papular acrodermatitis of childhood is characterized by a nonrelapsing papular eruption on the face and extremities, lymphadenopathy, anicteric HBV hepatitis, and HBsAg subtype ayw-antigenemia. The classic syndrome is rarely reported outside of Italy and Japan. However, Gianotti-Crosti syndrome is also associated with respiratory syncytial virus, Epstein-Barr virus, poliovirus of vaccine origin, and probably other viral infections.

Gianotti-Crosti syndrome occurs in children 2–6 years of age, and rarely after 10 years, and usually as isolated, nonepidemic cases. Patients may experience low-grade fever and malaise, but constitutional symptoms do not commonly occur. Axillary and inguinal lymphadenopathy can occur.

The characteristic eruption occurs on the face and extensor surfaces of the extremities, including the palms and soles. The trunk, antecubital, or popliteal fossae are rarely involved. Nonpruritic, dusky to coppery red, flat-topped, firm papules 2–3 mm in diameter appear at these sites over 2–3 days and may enlarge to 5 mm. Even though many papules form on the face and extremities, they do not tend to coalesce. The eruption does persist for 15–20 days, and the lesions remain monomorphic throughout the course. At times the papules may become more infiltrated, or even purpuric, and exhibit the Koebner phenomenon. The oral mucosa is not involved. In cases of HBV-associated Gianotti-Crosti syndrome, hepatitis is anicteric and occurs concurrently with the eruption or within 7–14 days.

Diagnosis is made on clinical grounds, and confirmed by demonstration of HBsAg antigenemia. Skin biopsy shows capillary endothelial swelling and a mononuclear perivascular infiltrate.

Scarlet Fever

Scarlet fever is an acute infection of the tonsils or skin, the syndrome of which is caused by an erythrogenic exotoxin-producing strain of group A streptococcus, occurring most commonly in the first decade of life. Staphylococcal scarlet fever is a rare but well-recognized disease which may range over the full spectrum of severity to the toxic shock syndrome. Erythrogenic toxin production depends on the presence of a temperate bacteriophage. Patients with prior exposure to the erythrogenic toxin have antitoxin immunity and neutralize the toxin. The scarlet fever syndrome therefore does not develop in these patients. Since several erythrogenic strains of β-hemolytic streptococcus cause infection, it is theoretically possible to have a second episode of scarlet fever. Strains of *Staphylococcus aureus* can synthesize an erythrogenic exotoxin producing a scarlatiniform exanthem. Pharyngeal infection is manifested by acute follicular or membranous tonsillitis with anterior cervical lymphadenitis. Less frequently the β-hemolytic streptococcus infects a surgical or other wound.

Vasodilatation induced by erythrogenic toxin becomes clinically apparent within 2–3 days after the onset of infection. Finely punctate erythma is first noted on the upper part of the trunk. The face becomes diffusely flushed, contrasted with a perioral pallor. The eruption becomes confluent (scarlatiniform) on the chest as it spreads to the extremities. Erythema is most intense at pressure points and in the body folds. Linear petechiae (Pastia's sign) may be noted in the antecubital and axillary folds. The clinical intensity of the exanthem varies from mild erythema confined to the trunk to a more extensive purpuric eruption. Within 4–5 days the exanthem fades and is followed by brawny desquamation on the body and extremities and by sheet-like exfoliation on the palms and soles. In subclinical or mild infections the exanthem may pass unnoticed. In this case the patient may seek medical advice only when exfoliation on the palms and soles is noted.

Erythrogenic toxin also produces a characteristic enanthem. Early in the illness the lingular mucosa becomes hyperkeratotic. Scattered red swollen papillae give the tongue the appearance of a white strawberry. By the 4th or 5th day the hyperkeratotic membrane has been sloughed, and the lingular mucosa appears bright red, resembling a red strawberry. Punctate erythema and petechiae may occur in the palate.

The diagnosis can be confirmed by a rapid test for streptococcal antigen, throat or wound culture, or rise in the antistreptolysin O titer. With adequate antibiotic therapy the suppurative complications resolve and the nonsuppurative complications are greatly reduced.

Erythema Multiforme

Erythema multiforme (EM) is a clinical syndrome, which is triggered as an adverse drug reaction or by infection with herpes simplex virus or mycoplasma and is manifested by a diverse list of cutaneous and mucosal findings. The pathogenesis is not clearly understood but is most likely a delayed type of hypersensitivity. Depending on the clinical severity of the syndrome, the terms *erythema multiforme minor* or *erythema multiforme major* are used. Erythema multiforme major replaces the older, less well-defined Stevens-Johnson syndrome. The target or iris lesions may occur in only a quarter of patients, with 75% of cases showing erythematous macules, papules, plaques, or vesiculobullous lesions. The multiple forms of the lesions in EM initially referred to the morphologic evolution over the time courses of the eruption.

The EM syndrome occurs in three well-described clinical settings: (*a*) associated with herpes simplex infection and, as with the herpetic infection, the EM may be recurrent; (*b*) associated with mycoplasma infection; and (*c*) occurring as an adverse drug eruption.

Herpes simplex-associated EM accounts for up to 75% of cases, depending on the population studied. Herpes simplex virus (HSV) antigen has been identified in both biopsied skin lesions and in circulating immune complexes in these patients. Cases are associated with both type 1 and type 2 herpes infection and probably account for most cases of recurrent EM minor in young adults. Precipitating factors of EM including upper respiratory infections, tuberculosis, other infections, sunlight, x-ray, and menses all can reactivate herpes simplex virus and thus initiate EM.

Mycoplasma pneumonitis, occurring usually in children and young adults, can be followed by EM. The onset of EM correlates with the appearance of antibodies to mycoplasma. However, the organism has been cultured from bullous skin lesions. Characteristically, multiple mucosal erosive lesions and large bullous skin lesions occur sometimes associated with marked prostration. Recurrences of mycoplasma-associated EM have not been documented.

EM as an adverse drug reaction occurs with sulfonamides, especially the trimethoprim-sulfamethoxazole combination, diphenylhydantoin, penicillin derivatives, and phenylbutazone. In previously nonsensitized patients EM occurs after 7–14 days of drug administration, but once sensitized, the reaction can appear within hours of readministration. Drug-induced EM may be severe, accompanied by fever, prostration, and large bullous lesions on skin and mucosa.

A prodrome of malaise, fever, headache, sore throat, rhinorrhea, and cough may precede the cutaneous lesions by a week or more. However, it may be impossible to distinguish the prodrome from symptoms associated with the precipitating factor.

The spectrum of morphologic patterns occurring in erythema multiforme is wide and makes simple description difficult. Initial erythematous macules evolve quickly to papules and plaques. Marked edema and bulla formation may result in iris or target lesions, with multiple zones of concentric color changes. However, these pathognomonic findings occur only in one-quarter of patients with erythema multiforme. Classically, iris or target lesions occur symmetrically, especially on the dorsum of the hand and extensor surface of the extremities. Palm and sole involvement is frequent. Truncal involvement is often minimal except in erythema multiforme major.

Mucosal involvement of the conjunctivae, nose, oropharynx, and genitalia occurs in more severe cases of erythema multiforme. Initial erythema and edema quickly evolve with resultant erosions. Although usually concurrent with cutaneous involvement, mucosal lesions can precede or follow those on the skin. Extensive oropharyngeal involvement can have a bad prognosis because of the increased risk of pulmonary aspiration and infection.

The duration of erythema multiforme varies according to the extent of cutaneous and mucosal involvement. EM minor usually resolves within 2 weeks and EM major, within 6 weeks.

Diagnosis of EM is made by clinical and pathologic criteria, which are subjective in that no specific diagnostic markers for EM are known at this time.

Recurrent herpes simplex-associated EM can be prevented by oral administration of acyclovir, either as daily prophylaxis for frequent outbreaks or episodic use with the first sign of skin lesions. When drug-induced EM occurs, the causative drug should be identified and discontinued. Patients with EM major usually require supportive care in a hospital. Corticosteroids are administered in an attempt to halt evolving EM but their efficacy is not clearly determined.

Erythema Marginatum (Erythema Circinatum)

Erythema marginatum is part of the syndrome occurring in children with acute rheumatic fever, including fever, carditis, chorea, and possibly, migratory arthritis. Fortunately, the incidence of rheumatic fever and erythema marginatum has declined markedly in the past few decades. Erythema marginatum is noted in approximately 10% of patients with rheumatic fever. Macular or slightly raised erythema appears on the trunk and proximal extremities. While the borders of the erythema advance rapidly, the central area resolves. The evolving lesions result in annular, polycyclic, or geographic configurations. The rash may appear intermittently for months, but its presence does not correlate with the activity of the carditis.

Subcutaneous nodules on the extensor surfaces can also be seen in patients with acute rheumatic fever, especially in children with severe carditis. Epistaxis and abdominal pain, mimicking acute appendicitis, occur uncommonly in rheumatic fever.

The diagnosis of erythema marginatum is made by the clinical characteristics of the lesions and by the findings on skin biopsy. Erythema marginatum is one of the major manifestations in the modified Jones criteria for the diagnosis of rheumatic fever, but can occur in isolation. The differential diagnosis for erythema marginatum occurring in a 6–12-year-old child should include erythema chronicum migrans of Lyme disease and other figurate erythemas, urticaria, and erythema multiforme.

Toxic Shock Syndrome

Toxic shock syndrome (TSS) is defined on a clinical case definition and should be suspected in a febrile, hypotensive patient with conjunctival hyperemia and swollen hands in the presence of a rash. Colonization of a local site by exotoxin-producing *S. aureus* with subsequent toxin release, absorption, and hematogenous dissemination causes the toxic shock syndrome. Delay in diagnosis and therapy can lead to severe organ dysfunction and death.

Seventy percent of cases of toxic shock syndrome occur around menstruation and are related to tampon use. *S. aureus* multiplies in this intravaginal foreign body and elaborates the toxic-shock-syndrome toxin, which is absorbed and causes the clinical changes. Many women have a history of milder symptoms of TSS associated with prior menstrual periods and tampon use. The remaining cases of toxic shock syndrome have been associated with use of a contraceptive sponge, with nasal packing, and with influenza B infection.

Patients with toxic shock syndrome present with fever, hypotension, and often during the course of the illness, skin and mucosal changes. The clinical case definition of the toxic shock syndrome is as follows: (*a*) body temperature over 102°F (38.9°C); (*b*) rash that is characteristically an erythroderma with swelling of the palms and soles; (*c*) desquamation, usually after the 1st week of illness; (*d*) hypotension with a systolic blood pressure of 90 mm Hg or less, an orthostatic decrease of 15 mm Hg or more, or orthostatic dizziness or syncope; (*e*) the presence of clinical or laboratory abnormalities involving at least three organ systems, including gastrointestinal, hepatic, muscular, renal, cardiovascular, and neurologic systems and the mucous membranes (conjunctival hyperemia, strawberry tongue); and (*f*) absence of evidence of other causes of illness including bacteremia.

Prodromal constitutional symptoms, a "flu-like" syndrome of fever, headache, arthralgia, myalgia, nausea, vomiting, and malaise occur frequently. The patient is often a young, otherwise healthy woman, currently menstruating and using a tampon, or there can be a history of current nasal packing or contraceptive sponge usage. Similar symptoms may have been associated with previous menstrual periods.

Presenting to the emergency department, the patient appears acutely ill with fever and marked hypotension. The truncal rash is present early in the course and can be scarlatiniform or morbilliform. Much more characteristic are findings on the face, hands, and feet, and on the mucosa of the conjunctiva, oropharynx, and genital area. Marked edema and induration may occur on the face, hands, or feet with erythema. The bulbar conjunctiva is often markedly injected. The oropharynx shows similar erythema, which may be associated with tenderness. A red "strawberry" tongue may be seen. Similarly the vaginal and labial mucosa may be red and tender. Desquamation of the hands and feet, as well as of the trunk, is frequently seen in the healing stage of toxic shock syndrome and is confirmatory in the clinical diagnosis. In some cases of toxic shock syndrome the rash is not apparent initially and only the desquamation may be noted near the end of the illness.

The diagnosis of toxic shock syndrome is made on clinical criteria. Gram's stain of local exudate shows many leukocytes and Gram-positive cocci in clusters. The culture eventually yields *S. aureus*. Skin biopsy may be diagnostic showing a superficial perivascular and interstitial mixed-cell infiltrate that contains neutrophils and occasional eosinophils, spongiotic foci that contain neutrophils as well, and scattered necrotic keratinocytes arranged in clusters within the epidermis. The following is the differential diagnosis of the young patient with fever, rash, and hypotension: (*a*) toxic shock syndrome, (*b*) Kawasaki's disease, (*c*) drug eruption, (*d*) staphylococcal scalded-skin syndrome, (*e*) streptococcal scarlet fever, (*f*) staphylococcal scarlet fever, (*g*) erythema multiforme, (*h*) toxic epidermal necrolysis, (*i*) systemic lupus erythematosus, and (*j*) viral exanthems.

Treatment of the toxic shock syndrome consists of treatment of the hypotension, the life-threatening result of the staphylococcal toxemia. Removal of any foreign body, such as a tampon, sponge, or nasal pack, and irrigation of the site with povidone-iodine solution helps prevent additional toxin absorption. An adequate course of antistaphylococcal antibiotic is the primary therapy which prevents recurrence of the toxic shock syndrome.

Secondary Syphilis

Asymptomatic dissemination of *Treponema pallidum* via the blood and lymphatics occurs from the inoculation site within the first few days after exposure. A chancre usually appears at the inoculation site within 21 days (range 7–90 days) and heals spontaneously in 3–4 weeks.

Symptoms and lesions of secondary syphilis may develop 6–12 weeks after appearance of the chancre. Constitutional symptoms are present in fewer than half of patients with secondary syphilis. Early symptoms are sore throat (53%), malaise (42%), headache (24%), fever (14%), and musculoskeletal pain (9%). These symptoms alone are nonspecific. The incidence of syphilis, which doubled during the decades of the 1960s and 1970s and peaked in the early 1980s, is now declining presumably associated with decreasing sexual promiscuity in response to the AIDS epidemic. A serologic test for syphilis (STS) should be considered for all patients with headache, sore throat, and lymph node enlargement.

Lymphatic involvement occurs in 70% of patients; in addition to the inguinal nodes, which can remain enlarged following a penile chancre, the suboccipital, postauricular, posterior cervical, and epitrochlear lymph nodes are frequently enlarged, but not tender. Generalized lymphadenopathy occurs less frequently. In the evaluation of a patient with generalized lymphadenopathy, qualitative and quantitative STS should be performed with initial noninvasive studies. It is preferable to make the diagnosis at this stage of the evaluation than after a lymph node biopsy. Rarely, the nodes may be tender. A tender mass in the inguinal region may be diagnosed as an incarcerated inguinal hernia, and emergency operation performed. Histologic study of the removed mass can show luetic lymphadenitis, which would then be confirmed by a STS and a fluorescent treponemal antibody-absorption (FTA-ABS) test.

The earliest cutaneous lesions of secondary syphilis are symmetrical, discrete, pink-tan macules, which appear first on the chest and abdomen. The eruption is easily overlooked and is difficult to detect in blacks. The initial eruption may fade, reappear, or evolve into a papular eruption. The papules become rather firm and change from reddish brown to brown in older lesions. The surface initially is shiny, but later forms a thin scale. At this time secondary syphilis may resemble pityriasis rosea. In time the lesions may become hyperkeratotic. In the papular stage the lesions may be round, oval, or annular. On the palms and soles, early lesions become infiltrated and papular, covered with scale. Typical papules are seen on the penile shaft and glans.

Large, soft, moist papules (condylomata lata) occur on mucosal or macerated surfaces in the perianal and vulvar regions. These lesions have a high density of viable organisms. Darkfield examination can be performed within a few minutes to confirm the diagnosis. Hypertrophic papules occur on the oral mucosa as mucous patches and at the corners of the mouth as split papules. Perifollicular inflammation in the scalp results in patchy, "moth-eaten" alopecia.

Laboratory confirmation of syphilis can be made by indentification of *T. pallidum* from a cutaneous lesion with a darkfield microscope. Qualitative and quantitative STS are virtually always positive in secondary syphilis. Early in this stage the quantitative titer can be low, and therefore not separable from a biologic false-positive (BFP) test. The specific FTA-ABS test should be performed. The quantitative serologic test should be repeated at intervals for at least a year; in adequately treated cases of secondary syphilis the test usually becomes negative in 6–18 months.

Secondary syphilis can be treated with benzathine penicillin G, a total of 2.4 million units intramuscularly at a single session, or procaine penicillin G, 600,000 units/day for 8 days. Patients should be informed of Herxheimer's reaction, occurring 12–24 hours after penicillin therapy. This reaction is characterized by a temperature up to 104°F (40°C) and a flu-like syndrome. In the penicillin-allergic patient, tetracycline or erythromycin, 500 mg orally four times a day for 15 days, should be prescribed.

Lyme Disease

Lyme disease is a spirochetal infectious disease transmitted to humans by the bite of an infected tick. The clinical syndrome begins with a pathognomonic rash, erythema chronicum migrans (ECM), and includes later involvement of the joints, nervous system, and/or heart.

During the past decade, Lyme disease (LD) has become the most common tick-borne disease in the United States, occurring in three geographic areas: the northeast coast (Massachusetts, Rhode Island, Connecticut, New York, New Jersey, Pennsylvania, Delaware, Maryland), the midwest (Minnesota, Wisconsin), and the west (California, Oregon, Nevada, Utah). An estimated 1500–3000 cases occur per year (1986). The vector on the northeast coast and the midwest is the pinhead-sized deer tick *Ixodes dammini* and, in the northwest, *Ixodes pacificus*. The infecting spirochete, *Borrelia burgdorferi,* is transmitted to humans following biting and feeding of the tick. The Ixodes ticks cling to vegetation, are most numerous in brushy, wooded, or grassy habitats, and are not found on open sandy beaches. The ticks are dormant during the winter months and begin and continue feeding from late May through early fall, with the onset of 80% of cases of LD in June and July.

In endemic areas 20–60% of Ixodes ticks carry *B. burgdorferi* in comparison to *Dermacentor variabilis*, the tick vector for Rocky Mountain spotted fever, carrying 1% of *Rickettsia rickettsii.* Ixodes tick bites are not pruritic or painful; only one-third of LD patients are aware of a preceding tick bite. Removal of the pinhead-sized tick within 18 hours of attachment may preclude transmission. It is not known whether the increase in numbers and widening geographic distribution of cases reflect increased recognition or increased reporting.

About 7 days following the tick bite (range 7–32 days), LD begins with the skin lesion, *erythema chronicum migrans,* at the site of the bite. ECM can occur at any site, but the trunk and proximal extremities are the most common. An initial erythematous macule or papule enlarges within days to form an expanding annular lesion, with a distinct red border and partially clearing middle. The median maximum diameter is 15 mm with a range of 3–68 mm. Half of primary lesions of ECM are symptomatic with complaints of burning sensation, itching, or pain. Alternately, the center becomes intensely red and indurated, vesicular, or necrotic, or remains an even red, or blue before clearing. At times, concentric rings form. When occurring on the scalp, only a linear streak may be evident on the face or neck.

Within several days after the onset of the primary ECM, about 50% of patients with LD develop multiple annular secondary lesions, ranging in number from several to more than 100. Secondary lesions resemble ECM but are smaller, less migratory, and lacking central induration. They are seen at any site except the palms and soles; they can become confluent. In addition, 13% of patients have a malar rash, 11% conjunctivitis, and 1% diffuse urticaria.

Untreated ECM and secondary lesions fade in a median time of 28 days (range 1 day to 14 months). Both ECM and secondary lesions can fade and recur during this time. However, following adequate treatment, early lesions resolve within several days and late manifestations are prevented.

Lyme disease is a systemic infection, constitutional symptoms occurring simultaneously with ECM and secondary lesions. The following early symptoms have been noted: malaise, fatigue and lethargy (80%), headache (64%),fever and chills (59%), stiff neck (48%), arthralgia (48%), myalgia (43%), backache (26%), anorexia (23%), sore throat (17%), nausea (17%), dysesthesia (11%), vomiting (10%), abdominal pain (8%), and photophobia (6%). Typically, fever in adults is low-grade and intermittent; however, in children it may be high and persistent.

Early clinical findings of LD are as follows: erythema chronicum migrans (virtually 100%), multiple secondary lesions (48%), regional lymphadenopathy (41%), generalized lymphadenopathy

(20%), pain on neck flexion (17%), malar rash (13%), erythematous throat (12%), conjunctivitis (11%), right upper quadrant tenderness (8%), frank arthritis (8%), splenomegaly (6%), hepatomegaly (5%), muscle tenderness (4%), periorbital edema (3%), and abdominal tenderness (2%). Rarely, LD occurs without ECM or secondary lesions and presents only with the late manifestations.

Late manifestations of LD involving the joints, nervous system, and heart occur weeks to months following the tick bite and are mediated by the immune system. Arthritis occurs in 60% of untreated cases, 4–6 weeks after the tick bite (range 1 week to 22 months) and is sudden in onset, involving one or a few joints. Knees, shoulders, and elbows are commonly affected. Neurologic involvement occurs in 10–20% of untreated LD cases, 1–6 weeks following the tick bite, and are manifested by excruciating headache, neck pain, meningitis, cranial neuropathies, and sensory and motor radiculopathies. Neurologic abnormalities occur without erythema chronicum migrans, making the diagnosis less apparent. Cardiac abnormalities occur in 6–10% of untreated cases, usually within 4 weeks, and are manifested by fluctuating degrees of atrioventricular block, myopericarditis, and left ventricular dysfunction. These cardiac manifestations are usually transient and not associated with long-term sequellae.

Diagnosis is made on the characteristic clinical findings in a person living in or having visited an endemic area and can be confirmed by skin biopsy and indirect immunofluorescence assay (IFA). Direct visualization of *B. burgdorferi* in ECM is difficult due to the paucity of organisms; however, the histopathology is characteristic. Early in LD when only ECM has occurred, as few as 50% of patients have positive IFA titers, and adequate treatment may block seroconversion. Virtually all cases with late manifestation are IFA-positive with a titer of 1:256 or greater.

Early infection with *B. burgdorferi* is cured with adequate antibiotic treatment and the later immune-mediated manifestations prevented. In adults tetracycline (250 mg four times daily for 10 days) is usually curative. In children 50 mg/kg/day is given in divided doses for 10 days. In penicillin-allergic children or tetracycline-intolerant adults, erythromycin can be substituted.

Leptospirosis (Weil's Disease)

Leptospirosis, which is caused by a spirochete, is usually biphasic. In the initial phase headache is the major manifestation and is associated with severe myalgia. The rash of leptospirosis is usually maculopapular, petechial, or purpuric, although it is occasionally macular. Patients with leptospirosis typically have conjunctival suffusion, which usually appears on the 3rd or 4th day. The CSF abnormalities usually do not occur until the second phase of leptospirosis, an immune phase that correlates with the appearance of circulating IgM antibodies. Usually, the CSF contains neutrophils or mononuclear cells, frequently as many as hundreds to thousands. Most patients with leptospirosis have an elevated CSF protein. The specific diagnosis of leptospirosis is made by isolation of the spirochete from the blood during the first phase of the illness or the urine during the second phase. Serologic methods are helpful diagnostically during the second phase of the illness.

Rocky Mountain Spotted Fever

Rocky Mountain spotted fever, the most severe of the spotted fevers, (RMSF) is caused by *R. rickettsii.* Transmission to humans is by the wood tick, *Dermacentor andersoni* in the western United States and by the dog tick, *Dermacentor variabilis,* in the eastern United States. Ninety-five percent of patients report onset of illness between April 1 and September 30, with 66% becoming ill in May, June, and July, when humans and the wood tick have the greatest mutual exposure. The patient lives in or has recently visited an endemic area and may have knowledge of a recent tick bite. Despite its name, most cases of RMSF occur in the southeastern quadrant of the United States with endemic areas centered in Virginia-the Carolinas-Georgia and Kansas-Oklahoma-Texas and in Massachusetts on Cape Cod and the islands.

After an incubation period of 7 days (range 3–12 days), the onset of RMSF begins abruptly with high fever, severe headache, chills, malaise, myalgia, and arthralgia. During this time rickettsemia occurs with seeding of the endothelial cells of capillaries, arterioles, and venules. The diffuse vasculitis results in occlusion of vessels of various sizes with tissue infarction. Signs and symptoms referable to the pulmonary system (cough or rales), the gastrointestinal system (nausea, vomiting, or abdominal pain), or the central nervous system (stupor, meningismus, or ataxia) do occur with RMSF as the clinical course becomes more fulminant.

The characteristic rash, which is the most helpful diagnostic sign, appears on the 4th day of the illness (range 2–6 days). The earliest lesions are macular, nonfixed, pink, and irregular, 2–6 mm in diameter, and are *characteristically first noted on the wrists, forearms, and ankles, and somewhat later the palms and soles.* Within 6–18 hours the rash spreads centripetally to the arms, thighs, trunk, and face. In 1–3 days the macular lesions evolve into deep red papules. In 2–4 days the lesions may become hemorrhagic and no longer blanch. With extensive cutaneous vascular involvement, areas of necrotic skin may occur, particularly over the fingers, toes, earlobes, nose, scrotum, or vulva. The temporal evolution of the rash is extremely helpful in the diagnosis. However, in 16% of cases of RMSF a rash was never detected, and in 10% of cases the characteristic rash appeared after the 5th day of illness.

Patients with RMSF may present in the emergency department with findings of an acute abdomen, either at the onset or in the fulminant phase of the illness. The signs and symptoms probably relate to the effects of inflammatory reaction, edema, and ischemia on the gastrointestinal tract nerves. Especially in the elderly and in the black patient (in whom the rash may not be noticed), the diagnosis of RMSF can be easily missed. Acute cholecystitis or appendicitis may be diagnosed, and the patient subjected to unnecessary laparotomy.

Skin biopsy may be helpful since rickettsiae can at times be demonstrated within the endothelial cells of the dermal vasculature, or specific *R. rickettsii* antigen can be detectable. Specific complement fixation studies on acute and convalescent sera, or indirect flourescent antibody assays for IgM or IgG, confirm the diagnosis.

Treatment with tetracycline or chloramphenicol, 2 gm/day for adults, should be started early, especially if the patient has a history of tick bite in an endemic area, prodromal symptoms, and an exanthem on the wrists and ankles. Overall mortality is 4%, but higher in blacks (16%) than whites (3%), and higher in patients 40 years of age or older (9%) than in younger individuals (2%).

Epidemic Typhus

Epidemiic typhus is caused by *Rickettsia prowazekii* and is transmitted to humans by the body louse. The disease is not currently endemic in the United States but does occur in Central and South America. The initial constitutional symptoms of chills, fever, headache, and malaise are followed by a pink macular rash appearing in the axillae and then trunk, spreading centrifugally to the extremities. The macules may become petechial and confluent. The face, palms, or soles are rarely involved. In severe cases disseminated intravascular coagulation may occur, resulting in acral gangrene. The definitive diagnosis for epidemic typhus is made serologically by the Weil-Felix reaction. Treatment is with tetracycline or chloramphenicol. Untreated or inadequately treated patients may experience recurrence of a mild form of epidemic typhus, the recrudescent disease referred to as Brill's disease.

Murine (Endemic) Typhus

Murine typhus is a mild systemic disease caused by *Rickettsia mooseri*. This rickettsia is transferred from infected rats and mice to humans by the bite of the rat flea. In the United States, reservoirs of infection occur along the southeast coast and along the Gulf of Mexico. In a 1-year period, 44 cases of murine typhus were reported to the Centers for Disease Control (CDC) in Atlanta, Georgia, compared to 844 cases of Rocky Mountain spotted fever, a more serious and more frequently detected rickettsial disease.

After an incubation period of 8–16 days, the patient experiences a fever to 102.2°F (39°C), with chills, malaise, headache, nausea, and vomiting. The rash appears about the 5th day of illness and is characterized by a centripetal, truncal, macular, or papular eruption. Involvement of the distal extremities is unusual. The rash may be evanescent or may last several days. Symptoms resolve in 9–14 days. The diagnosis is confirmed by detection of rising titers of specific complement-fixing antibodies.

The mortality from murine typhus is low. Administration of tetracyline or chloramphenicol, 2 gm/day, is followed by defervescence in 24–48 hours, together with abatement of the rash and symptoms.

Systemic Lupus Erythematosus

Systemic lupus erythematosus (SLE) is an intermittent, recurrent, systemic inflammatory disease in which 10% of patients have fever or rash or both at any one period. Patients may present acutely with arthritis, pleuritis, pleural effusion, pericarditis, myocarditis, thrombocytopenia, seizures, or psychosis. Cutaneous involvement can be of clinical diagnostic value before laboratory confirmation is available.

Discoid lesions, scaling red plaques, occur on the face, ears, scalp, and upper trunk, and after months and years of activity, show atrophic changes with telangiectasia, depressed scars, and follicular plugging. The majority of patients with discoid lesions have a localized cutaneous variant of lupus erythematosus referred to as *chronic discoid lupus erythematosus* and do not, even after decades of local activity, progress to systemic lupus erythematosus. Fever occurring in a patient with long-standing chronic discoid lupus erythematosus is most likely associated with a different disease process.

In SLE 85% of patients have cutaneous or mucosal involvement at some period in the course of the disease. As seen in Table 19.5, six of the 14 American Rheumatism Association (ARA) preliminary criteria for the classification of SLE involve the skin and mucosa. Periungual erythema and telangiectasia are not specifically diagnostic of SLE, but suggest a connective tissue disorder, that is, SLE, dermatomyositis, rheumatoid arthritis, or rarely progressive systemic sclerosis (sclerodema). Urticaria is a nonspecific finding.

Table 19.5.
Incidence of Cutaneous Manifestations of SLE

Manifestations of the ARA Preliminary Criteria for the Classification of SLE[a]	Percentage of 365 SLE Patients Meeting the Criteria with Each Manifestation	
	At the Time of Diagnosis	At Diagnosis or during Subsequent Course of Disease
1. Facial erythema (butterfly rash). Diffuse erythema, flat or raised, over the malar eminence(s) and/or bridge of the nose; may be unilateral.	52	55
2. Discoid LE. Erythematous raised patches with adherent keratotic scaling and follicular plugging; atrophic scarring can occur in older lesions; can be present anywhere on the body.	18	19
3. Raynaud's phenomenon. Requires a two-phase color reaction, by patient's history or physician's observation.	16	20
4. Alopecia. Rapid loss of large amount of scalp hair, by patient's history or physician's observation	58	71
5. Photosensitivity. Unusual skin reaction from exposure to sunlight, by patient's history or physician's observation.	37	41
6. Oral or nasopharyngeal ulceration.	25	36

[a] ARA, American Rheumatology Association, SLE, systemic lupus erythematosus.

The diagnosis of lupus erythematosus involving the skin is confirmed by histopathology and direct immunofluorescence studies of skin biopsies.

Salmonella Infections (Enteric Fever)

Salmonella typhi and other less virulent Salmonella species cause gastroenteritis followed by systemic illness. Following travel to an endemic area or epidemic exposure, symptoms begin days to several weeks after ingestion of contaminated food or water. Fever, headache, musculoskeletal aches, bronchitis, and constipation occur during the first week of illness. The temperature ranges from 102.2 to 104°F (or 39 to 40°C).

During the course of infection, the "rose spots" of typhoid fever (described by Osler) develop in 75% of patients and are accompanied by abdominal pain and diarrhea. In the second week of illness, successive crops of 10–20 pink papules 2–5 mm in diameter appear on the abdomen, lower part of the chest, and middle of the back. These lesions do not evolve further and fade in 3–4 days. New crops appear in the next 2–3 weeks. The lesions follow bacteremia, and salmonellae can be cultured and demonstrated on a Grams's stain of a scraping from a lesion.

Today, most patients are treated early in the illness with the result that the classic lesions do not appear. Administration of chloramphenicol or ampicillin is begun, based on the presumptive diagnosis, and the diagnosis is confirmed by blood, stool, or urine cultures. A 4-fold or greater increase in agglutinin titer, especially against the O antigen, in the absence of recent typhoid immunization, is confirmatory.

Sweet's Syndrome (Acute Febrile Neutrophilic Dermatosis)

Sweet's syndrome, or acute febrile neutrophilic dermatosis, is a rare hypersensitivity reaction characterized by spiking fever, painful red plaques, rapid resolution in response to systemic corticosteroids, leukocytosis, and a neutrophilic dermal infiltrate. This hypersensitivity reaction is associated with both bacterial and viral antigens as well as tumor antigen, following respiratory infections or underlying myeloproliferative disorders.

An initial viral-like syndrome or prodrome of high fever, malaise, episcleritis, and arthralgia occurs initially. Painful, bright red plaques typically occur on the face and extremities and enlarge with very edematous borders and central clearing. Lesions vary in size from 0.5 to 4 cm and can coalesce, forming large geographic plaques. Mucosal lesions are not seen. Untreated, the plaques may persist from 1 to 6 months and can recur.

Diagnosis of Sweet's syndrome is confirmed by skin biopsy which shows a pathognomonic dermal infiltrate composed of mature neutrophilic polymorphonuclear leukocytes, which may invade the epidermis and subcutaneous fat. Often a neutrophilic leukocytosis to 24,000 mm^3 is seen with mature polymorphonuclear leukocytes.

Treatment with prednisone, 60 mg/day, arrests the progression of the painful red plaques, and resolution occurs quickly. However, unless this rare hypersensitivity reaction is considered and diagnosis confirmed by skin biopsy, patients with Sweet's syndrome are inappropriately treated with antibiotics.

Kawasaki Disease (Acute Febrile Mucocutaneous Lymph Node Syndrome)

Kawasaki disease, or acute febrile mucocutaneous lymph node syndrome, is an acute disease of young children, characterized by cutaneous and mucosal inflammation, cervical lymphadenitis, and complicated by coronary artery aneurysms (20%). The disease was first described in Japan in 1961, and in the United States in 1971. It is idiopathic. Person-to-person transmission has not been shown. However, seasonal peaks in incidence occur in winter and spring. During the latter half of 1984, 10 outbreaks of Kawasaki disease occurred in the United States in 10 states and the District of Columbia with 262 suspected cases. The age ranged from 7 weeks to 12 years (mean 2.6 years), with a male predominance (59%).

The initial illness begins with fever, frequently accompanied by mucocutaneous findings and cervical lymph node enlargement. The diagnostic criteria for Kawasaki disease of the Center for Disease Control are as follows. Fever lasting 5 or more days without more reasonable explanation associated with at least four of the following five criteria:

1. Bilateral conjunctival injection;
2. At least one of the following mucous membrane changes:
   a. injected or fissured lips;
   b. injected pharynx;
   c. strawberry tongue;
3. At least one of the following extremity changes:
   a. erythema of palms or soles;
   b. edema of the hands or feet;
   c. generalized or periungual desquamation;
4. Rash:
   a. diffuse scarlatiniform erythroderma, in some cases diffuse centrally but with sharply demarcated borders on the extremities;
   b. deeply erythematous maculopapular rash, morbilliform;
   c. with iris lesions as in erythema multiforme;
5. Cervical lymphadenopathy (at least one lymph node 1.5 cm or greater in diameter).

Constitutional symptoms of diarrhea, arthralgia, arthritis, meatitis, tympanitis, photophobia, signs of meningeal irritation, and pneumonia can occur during the acute illness.

Uneventful recovery occurs in the majority of cases of Kawasaki disease. However, in 20% of children cardiovascular complications develop. Two to eight weeks following the onset of the disease, coronary artery aneurysms may be detected and are associated with myocarditis, myocardial infarction, pericarditis, angina, peripheral vascular occlusion, small bowel obstruction, and stroke. Case fatality ratios are low (1–2%).

The efficacy of any single therapeutic regimen has not been established.

Serum Sickness

Serum sickness is a systemic immunologic reaction associated with the formation of antibody-antigen complexes. The initial cases occurred following the administration of horse serum (antidiphtheria, antitetanus) at 8–12 days. Currently, serum sickness is seen as an adverse drug reaction with the protein antigen, horse antithymocyte globulin, antilymphocyte globulin (ALG), snake antivenin, and infrequently with many nonpolypeptide drugs. The following may cause serum sickness: penicillins, various sera, streptomycin, sulfonamides, thiouracil, apresoline, barbiturates, hydantoins, iodides, phenylbutazone, quinidine, quinine, and salicylates. The antibody source for immune-complex formation may be viral as in the serum sickness-like syndrome occurring in 10–20% of preicteric hepatitis B infections.

Serum sickness is accompanied by fever and a pruritic urticaria-like eruption, which can fade and recur over several week in 75% of patients. Patients receiving horse antithymocyte globulin can experience a morbilliform truncal eruption and erythema of the hands, feet, fingers, and toes, which become purpuric. Constitutional symptoms of headache, myalgia, malaise, and anorexia occur frequently. Characteristically, generalized lymphadenopathy and migratory polyarthritis, involving the distal large joints, are seen. Scarlatiniform eruptions occur less frequently, and cutaneous vasculitis rarely. Splenomegaly has been reported in severe cases of serum sickness.

Trichinosis

Ingestion of *Trichinella spiralis* encysted pork or bear meat may be followed by symptomatic trichinosis. A wide spectrum of symptoms may occur with fever, periorbital edema, abdominal pain and tenderness, cramping, diarrhea, myalgia, neurologic symptoms, and in up to 20% of symptomatic patients, a maculopapular rash. Subungual splinter hemorrhages are also seen. The diagnostic criteria for trichinosis are: an individual with a history of ingesting implicated pork or bear meat and signs and symptoms compatible with trichinosis and either *(a)* an elevated eosinophil count, or *(b)*serologic proof.

DISEASES MANIFESTED BY VESICLES, BULLAE, AND/OR PUSTULES (Table 19.6)

Varicella (Chickenpox)

Herpesvirus varicellae is the cause of two distinct clinical infections: *(a)* varicella or chickenpox, a primary systemic infection, and *(b)* herpes zoster or "shingles," which is usually an endogenous infection limited to cranial or peripheral sensory nerves and their corresponding dermatomes. Varicella is highly contagious, and most cases occur during childhood, when the constitutional symptoms and exanthem tend to be mild to moderate. In adults, however, systemic and cutaneous involvement may be more severe.

After an incubation period of 14–15 days a prodromal illness of low-grade fever and mild constitutional symptoms occurs. Patients are infectious from 1–2 days before the exanthem to 4–5 days after (or until the last crop of vesicles has crusted). In 1–2 days the exanthem appears on the trunk with initial erythematous macules, or rarely, urticarial papules evolving into small vesicles in 24 hours; sometimes large bullous lesions occur. The contents of the vesicles become turbid, and the vesicles become pustular with central umbilication. The lesions may rupture with crust formation. During the following 3–4 days, successive crops of vesiculopustules appear and further involve the trunk, the proximal extremities, and the face. Characteristically, lesions in all stages of evolution are present. With extensive involvement, lesions appear on the distal extremities, palms, and soles. Vesicles and erosions occur frequently on the oral mucosa. The ultimate number of vesiculopustules varies from few to profuse.

Crusted lesions usually heal in 1–3 weeks without scarring. Pruritus is common. Scratching the lesions increases the depth of cutaneous involvement and facilitates secondary impetiginization. If this occurs, scarring may result, especially on the face. Second episodes of varicella are rare and probably represent cutaneous dissemination of herpes zoster or suboptimal host-immune response during the primary infection.

Adults and immunocompromised patients, especially those with defects in cell-mediated immunity, frequently have more severe disease. Both are more likely to develop other manifestations of varicella infection, such as purpura, visceral disease, and neurologic signs. They are at risk for progressive varicella and can die of overwhelming viral infection. Asymptomatic pneumonitis occurs in half of the patients. Severe symptomatic varicella pneumonitis can develop. Varicella hepatitis frequently occurs in fatal cases.

The diagnosis of varicella can be confirmed in the emergency department by demonstration of multinucleated giant epidermal cells within the vesicular fluid. This procedure, the Tzanck test, is performed by unroofing an intact vesiculopustule, gently scraping the base with a curved scalpel blade, and smearing the contents on a slide. After air drying, the smear is stained with Wright's or Giemsa stain and examined for multinucleated giant cells. Disseminated infection with herpes simplex virus is the only other cause of a generalized vesiculopustular eruption with multinucleated giant cells. Chest x-ray study is indicated in adults.

Treatment of uncomplicated varicella should be directed at alleviating pruritus and preventing secondary infection of erosions. An antihistamine may be given to sedate the patient and minimize excoriation. Impetiginization by a β-hemolytic streptococcus or *S. aureus* should be suspected in crusted lesions that increase in size or persist and confirmed by Gram's stain and bacterial culture. Patients with secondary bacterial infection may be treated with chlorhexidine gluconate topically and erythromycin orally.

Herpes Zoster

Zoster or shingles is considered to be a reactivation of a latent *Herpesvirus varicellae* infection residing in the posterior root or cranial nerve ganglion after an episode of varicella. Most patients are in their 6th to 9th decades, which probably reflects a waning immunologic surveillance against the virus. Most patients are otherwise healthy adults without precipitating factors. However, herpes zoster may be triggered by surgery or trauma, irradiation and other immunosuppressive agents, malignancies, and certain infections. If the immune mechanism declines below a certain critical level and is unable to confine or eliminate the virus, the activated virus within the sensory ganglion can cause neuronal necrosis, inflammation, and neuralgia. The virus replicates within the peripheral sensory nerve, and once the cutaneous nerve endings are reached, the characteristic dermatomal pattern of grouped vesicles on an erythematous base appears.

Associated with neuronal viral replication and neuronal inflammation is local pain, which may be dull, sharp, burning, or shooting. At this time, with no skin eruption, misdiagnosis can be made. The patient is afebrile. Crops of vesiculopustules on an erythematous base appear posteriorly, along the posterior branch of the intercostal nerve. A specific diagnosis can usually be made at this point with the history of pain and the demonstration of multinucleated giant epidermal cells in the vesicular fluid (Tzanck test.) During the next few days, crops of grouped vesicles continue to appear on the dermatome. The frequency of dermatomal involvement is as follows: thoracic (53–56%), trigeminal (10–15%), cervical (12–20%), lumbar (8–9%), and lumbosacral (2–4%). The extent of cutaneous involvement varies from scattered vesicles to confluent necrosis.

Mild hematogenous dissemination with a few vesicles outside the involved dermatome can occur in approximately 15% of patients.

Generalized Herpes Zoster

Generalized herpes zoster involving skin and viscera can develop in the immunocompromised patient with lymphoma, leukemia, acquired immunodeficiency syndrome, or immunosuppressive therapy. The prognosis for patients with generalized herpes zoster depends on control of the underlying disease. Generalized herpes zoster can usually be diagnosed by noting a zosteriform eruption, a generalized vesiculopustular eruption, and multinucleated giant cells within the pustules. Rarely, there may be sensorineural involvement without a zosteriform eruption (zoster sine zoster) in patients with generalized herpes zoster. Visceral involvement is most pronounced in the liver, lung, and brain. In such cases, generalized infection with *H. varicellae* can be distinguished from infection with herpes simplex virus by immunofluorescence technique or by viral tissue cultures of vesicular fluid, sputum, biopsy tissue, or blood.

Herpes Simplex Virus Infections

Herpes simplex virus (HSV) causes the following clinical syndromes that are characterized by both rash and fever: (*a*) primary herpetic gingivostomatitis, (*b*) primary genital HSV infections, (*c*) eczema herpeticum, and (*d*) generalized herpes simplex infection. Only 10–15% of persons have symptomatic primary herpesvirus infection. The incidence of past infection, indicated by the presence of antibodies, varies according to conditions of overcrowding, hygiene, and sexual promiscuity. In more affluent social groups, 25% have evidence of past infection, compared with 95% in poorer socioeconomic groups.

The most frequent symptomatic manifestations of primary HSV-1 infection are gingivostomatitis and pharyngitis, occurring most often in children and young adults. There may be a history of recent exposure to someone with a cold sore. The patient experiences sudden fever, malaise, myalgias, inability to eat, and cervical lymphadenopathy. On examination, vesiculopustules can be seen at any site on the oropharyngeal mucosa, lips, and skin about the mouth. The submandibular lymph nodes are usually enlarged and tender. In addition, primary infection with HSV-1 or HSV-2 causes exudative or ulcerative pharyngitis in the posterior pharynx or tonsillar pillars. Constitutional symptoms usually resolve within a week and oral erosions within 2 weeks. Subsequent to this, herpesvirus may remain latent for a lifetime. Reactivated oral-labial HSV infection occurs on the cutaneous surface of the lip, and very rarely on the oropharyngeal mucosa.

The diagnosis is confirmed by demonstration of multinucleated giant cells with a Tzanck test, immunofluorescence test, or by herpesvirus culture. Oral acyclovir, 200 mg every 4 hours (five doses/day) given for 10 days early in the infection, can alter the natural course of the primary infection and cause marked symptomatic improvement within 24–48 hours. Symptomatic treatment of oral erosions and gingivitis includes aspirin, hydrogen peroxide irrigations of the mouth, and application of topical anesthetics, such as viscous lidocaine (Xylocaine) or dyclonine hydrochloride (Dyclone).

In patients with atopic dermatitis or thermal burns, large areas of skin may become infected with herpesvirus. Patients with minimal or even inactive atopic dermatitis are subject to endogenous or exogenous infection of extensive areas of skin (eczema herpeticum). Since patients with eczema may scratch and rupture herpetic vesicles, both intact vesicles and sharply demarcated erosions can be seen. The patient can have fever and lymph node enlargement. Acyclovir should be given either orally or intravenously. Since the lesions are frequently impetiginized with *S. aureus*, crusted lesions should be cultured and the patient begun on erythromycin or dicloxacillin. Symptomatic treatment includes baths or moist compresses to help debride crusted areas. Topical corticosteroid ointment can be applied to the eczematous areas after the herpetic lesions resolve.

Some patients experience recurrent erythema multiforme with each episode of recurrent herpes labialis. Patients can be febrile and have two types of vesiculobullous disease simultaneously. Erythema multiforme following herpes labialis or genitalis can usually be aborted if the patient begins oral acyclovir upon appearance of symptoms of an early cold sore.

Generalized herpes simplex infection may follow a primary or recurrent herpetic infection or eczema herpeticum. A temperature to 104°F (40°C), headache, and severe malaise may be accompanied by lymphadenopathy, hepatosplenomegaly, and signs of meningeal irritation or mental deterioration. Involvement of the bone marrow may result in leukopenia and thrombocytopenia. Concomitant with a primary

Table 19.6.
Differential Diagnosis for the Patient with Acute Onset of Rash and Fever: Diseases Manifested by Vesicles, Bullae, and Pustules

Disease	Clinical History	Physical Examination: General	Physical Examination: Dermatologic	Diagnostic Signs	Laboratory Data Available within 8 Hours
Varicella	Exposure: chickenpox or shingles In children, mild constitutional symptoms In adolescents and adults, more severe constitutional symptoms	Fever 39°C	Exanthem appears 1–2 days after onset of illness Vesiculopustules appear centripetally in crops over next 3–5 days Palms, soles, and oropharynx can be involved Crusted lesions heal in 1–3 weeks	Characteristic exanthem	Tzanck test shows multinucleated giant epidermal cells in vesicular fluid
Zoster, disseminated and generalized	Immunocompromised: AIDS, chemotherapy, lymphoma, leukemia, carcinoma	Fever	Dissemination outside dermatome occurs in 15% of patients with zoster Generalized to liver, lung, brain Grouped vesicles on erythematous base in dermatomal distribution Generalized vesicles	Characteristic eruption	Tzanck test shows multinucleated giant epidermal cells
Herpes simplex virus infection	Active or history of atopic dermatitis Exposure to cold sore	Fever to 39°C Regional lymphadenitis	Gingivostomatitis with vesicles and erosions Vesicles or well-demarcated erosions in eczematous skin with varying involvement	Vesicles in eczematous skin	Tzanck test shows multinucleated giant epidermal cells, immunofluorescence test
Hand-foot-and-mouth disease	Exposure during epidemic summer months	Low-grade fever	Tender vesicles on hands and feet, oropharynx, buttocks	Tender oval vesicles with peripheral red ring on palms or soles	Negative Tzanck test
Staphylococcal scalded-skin syndrome	Infants <2 years old May have preceding purulent	Mild fever and constitutional symptoms	In infant, erythema and tenderness initially of face and flexural skin, which shears off with minimal trauma; large bullae formed;	Nikolsky's sign (skin can be rubbed off in sheets)	Gram's stain of bulla fluid shows no organisms

	conjunctivitis, otitis media, or occult nasopharyngeal infection		red moist erosions Generalized desquamation with recovery No mucosal involvement		
Toxic epidermal necrolysis	Age: middle-aged to elderly	Prodromal fever and constitutional symptoms Following epidermolysis, may become obtunded	In 24–48 hr, tender macular erythema evolving rapidly to extensive painful exfoliation Oral, nasal, conjunctival mucosa sloughs and becomes eroded	Nikolsky's sign	Skin biopsy diagnostic; Gram's stain negative for organisms
Rickettsial pox	Inoculation papule (eschar) present 3–7 days before onset of fever	Fever to 40°C Tender lymphadenitis in nodes draining inoculation papule	Generalized vesiculopapular lesions		Negative Tzanck test

or recurrent herpetic lesion, a generalized Tzanck-positive vesicular eruption is seen. The specific diagnosis is made by culture of *Herpesvirus hominis* from skin, blood, or tissue, or by immunofluorescence test.

Enteroviral Infections

Hand-foot-and-mouth disease is a mild condition caused by the Coxsackie A 16 enterovirus that produces characteristic mucocutaneous findings. As with other enteroviral infections, hand-foot-and-mouth disease occurs in epidemic outbreaks in late summer.

Systemic symptoms are mild to minimal and include low-grade fever, vague malaise, and tenderness of the lesions. In a few patients these symptoms may be more intense and may be accompanied by myalgia, arthralgia, or diarrhea.

Within 24 hours after the prodromal symptoms, a vesicular eruption appears on the hands and feet and in the oropharynx. On the palmar and plantar surfaces the vesicles are characteristically elongated or linear. The individual vesicles are tender and are surrounded by a red areola. There may be fewer than a dozen lesions confined to the hands and feet or there may be hundreds of lesions involving the extremities and buttocks. When an extensive exanthem occurs, varicella may be considered, but is ruled out by the centrifugal density of the lesions and a negative Tzanck test. The mucosal lesions may appear at any site in the oropharynx, and unlike herpetic gingivostomatitis, they are not associated with submandibular lymphadenopathy. Oral vesicular lesions are fragile and quickly evolve into erosions. Although the three sites frequently demonstrate vesicles, some patients do not simultaneously have lesions on the hands and feet and in the mouth. Treatment is based on symptoms.

The *Boston exanthem* is a fairly characteristic clinical syndrome associated with ECHO 16 virus. Epidemics occur during the summer. The disease is more frequent in young children; adults, however, are more symptomatic. Children become mildly febrile with a temperature to 102.2°F (39°C) for 1–2 days. Youngsters may complain only of a mild sore throat associated with chills, headache, muscle aches and pains, prostration, and cramping abdominal pain. Associated with defervescence, a pink- to salmon-colored macular and papular eruption appears on the face and upper part of the chest. In some patients the exanthem becomes generalized, involving the palms and soles but clearing in 1–5 days. Treatment is based on symptoms.

Staphylococcal Scalded-skin Syndrome

Staphylococcal scalded-skin syndrome (SSSS) is characterized by bulla formation and exfoliation, occurring mainly in newborns and infants under 2 years of age. Severity ranges from a localized form, bullous impetigo, to a generalized form with extensive epidermolysis and desquamation. Clinical forms of staphylococcal scalded-skin syndrome have been classified as follows: (*a*) bullous impetigo (*b*) bullous impetigo with generalization, (*c*) scarlatiniform syndrome, and (*d*) generalized scalded-skin syndrome.

Only staphlyococci of phage group II (mostly type 71) produce the exfoliative toxin and are responsible for the staphylococcal scalded-skin syndrome. Local production and diffusion of the exfoliative toxin (epidermolysin) results in bullous lesions with *S. aureus* detected on Gram's stain and culture. The scarlatiniform syndrome results from local production of the exfoliative toxin followed by hematogenous transport to all the skin, analogous to streptococcal scarlet fever. Fever does occur with widespread bullous impetigo and in the staphylococcal scarlatiniform syndrome. In contrast to streptococcal scarlet fever, oral mucosal involvement with a strawberry tongue is rarely seen in staphylococcal scarlatiniform syndrome.

In newborns and infants, staphylococcus may colonize the nose, conjunctivae, or umbilical stump without causing clinically apparent infection, but produces an exotoxin that is transported hematogenously to the skin. At times purulent conjunctivitis, otitis media, or occult nasopharyngeal infection is the site of toxin production. The exfoliative toxin causes necrosis of the upper half of the viable epidermis. The few cases of SSSS reported in adults were associated with immunologic or renal insufficiency.

Clinically, initial tender erythema occurs around the mouth and on the neck, axillae, and groin. In 24–48 hours, the tender erythema becomes much more widespread, and, if untreated, the epidermis appears wrinkled and either shears off with gentle pressure (Nikolsky's sign) or forms large bullae. The unroofed epidermis has a red, moist base. The epidermal injury is caused by the hematogenous exotoxin, and therefore Gram's stain and culture fail to show staphylococcus. Following adequate antibiotic treatment, the superficial denuded areas heal in 5–7 days with generalized desquamation in large sheets of skin. In contrast to drug-induced toxic epidermal necrolysis the oral mucosa is rarely involved.

Staphylococcal scalded-skin syndrome is diagnosed by the clinical findings and responds quickly to antibiotics. In the newborn, hospitalization and treatment with intravenous oxacillin, 200 mg/kg/day in divided doses every 4 hours, is preferable. Hospitalization is also indicated for infants when there is extensive sloughing of skin or if parental compliance to treatment is questioned. With reliable home care and mild involvement, dicloxacillin, 30 to 50 mg/kg/day, can be given orally. Baths or compresses to exfoliating or crusted areas, followed by application of a topical agent such as bacitracin or silvadene, will optimize the rate of epidermal regrowth. Prognosis is excellent.

Toxic Epidermal Necrolysis

Toxic epidermal necrolysis (TEN) is a cutaneous reaction pattern characterized by skin tenderness and generalized erythema, followed by extensive exfoliation. TEN is most often drug-induced. However, it is also associated with various infections, neoplastic diseases, and graft-host reaction. It may also be idiopathic. TEN is rare, occurring in middle-aged or elderly patients, more common in women than men.

Drugs frequently implicated in TEN are as follows (*a*) antibiotics, (*b*) barbiturates, (*c*) hydantoins, (*d*) pyrazolon derivatives (phenylbutazone), (*e*) sulfonamides, and (*f*) sulfones. Although TEN can occur after days or even years of use of these drugs, a newly added drug is more suspect. If the patient survives the first episode of TEN, reexposure to the causative drug can be followed by recurrence within hours to days, more severe than the initial episode.

Prodromal symptoms of mild or moderate skin tenderness, fever, malaise, headache, conjunctival burning or itching, myalgias, arthralgias, nausea and vomiting, and/or diarrhea occur in the majority of patients. The brevity and severity of the prodrome is distinctive.

Following 24–48 hours, a morbilliform eruption or discrete macular erythema appears initially on the face and extremities and subsequently becomes generalized. The entire thickness of the epidermis becomes necrotic and shears off in large sheets (Nikolsky's sign), but frank bulla formation does not occur. The epidermal sloughing may be generalized, resembling a second degree thermal burn. The patient may be alert and in severe pain following epidermal necrosis and denuding, but often becomes obtunded. The mucosa of the oropharynx, nose, and conjunctivae may also contain sloughs.

Skin biopsy confirms the clinical diagnosis of TEN. Early skin lesions show vacuolization and necrosis of both individual basal epidermal cells and cells scattered throughout the epidermis. There is little or no inflammatory infiltrate in the dermis.

Optimal care is provided by hospitalization and treatment in a burn unit. Epidermal necrosis usually stops within a few days. Once the diagnosis is established by biopsy and the implicated drug stopped, parenteral corticosteroids have little if any effect on the natural course of TEN. Intravenous fluid replacement is not of the magnitude required in a burned patient since blood vessels sustain little damage and there is little leakage of interstitial fluid. Because mucosal involvement occurs, bacterial conjunctivitis may be prevented with topical erythromycin ointment. Frequent suctioning helps prevent aspiration pneumonitis when the oropharynx is denuded and the patient obtunded. The mortality in older patients with drug-induced TEN approaches 50%.

Rickettsial Pox

A mild, self-limited urban disease, rickettsial pox is caused by *Rickettsia akari.* The rickettsia is transmitted from the host, the mouse, to humans through the bite of the mouse mite. One to two weeks after the bite, a firm papule develops at the site of inoculation. The papule enlarges to 10–15 mm in diameter and quickly undergoes central vesiculation. After crusting with eschar formation, healing with residual scar formation takes place in 3 weeks. Tender regional lymphadenitis is associated with the inoculation papule.

Three to seven days after the appearance of the inoculation papule, which may be aymptomatic but detectable in 95% of patients, systemic symptoms of temperature of 104°F (40°C), chills, sweats, malaise, and myalgias develop. A papular eruption usually accompanies the constitutional symptoms; it may be generalized, involving the palms, soles, and oropharynx. Within 24 hours, vesicles appear atop the papules. The exanthem and symptoms usually resolve in 7–10 days.

Rickettsial pox is often misdiagnosed as varicella; however, varicella can be ruled out by the absence of multinucleated giant cells in a Tzanck test. The diagnosis can be confirmed by serologic titers for specific complement-fixing antibodies.

Rickettsial pox resolves spontaneously. Tetracycline, 2 gm/day, will arrest the natural course of the disease within 24 hours of administration.

DISEASES MANIFESTED BY PURPURIC MACULES, PAPULES, AND/OR VESICLES (Table 19.7)

Septicemia

The presence of microorganisms or microbial products in the blood results in many possible cutaneous pathologic reactions. Some reactions are nonspecific, whereas other lesions are pathognomonic of the infecting bacterium, i.e. *Neisseria meningitidis* and *Neisseria gonorrhoeae.*

Meningococcus

N. meningitidis may colonize the oropharynx and spread hematogenously causing meningitis and cutaneous lesions. Carriers of meningococci usually are over 21-years-old. However, attack rates of

Table 19.7.
Differential Diagnosis for the Patient with Acute Onset of Rash and Fever: Diseases Manifested by Purpuric Macules, Papules, and/or Vesicles

		Physical Examination			
Disease	Clinical History	General	Dermatologic	Diagnostic Signs	Laboratory Data Available within 8 Hours
Acute meningococcemia	Exposure Headache Confusion	Fever to 104°F (40°C), hypotension Meningismus	Petechiae axillary folds, belt line, back Scattered macules to papules to hemorrhagic vesicles; small infarcts Numerous large infarcts (purpura fulminans)	Petechiae and small infarcts with signs of meningeal irritation	Gram's stain or pustular aspirate or CSF reveals Gram-negative cocci
Gonococcemia	Sexual exposure Commonly a menstruating woman Periarticular joint pains	Fever to 102.2°F (39°C) Tenosynovitis Septic arthritis Possible cervicitis or pelvic inflammatory disease	5–20 tender acral macules evolving to hemorrhagic pustules	Few scattered pustules associated with tenosynovitis or arthritis	Gram's stain of pustular aspirate may reveal Gram-negative cocci Immunofluorescence test of pustular aspirate for *Neisseria gonorrhoeae*
Necrotizing angiitis or vasculitis	Drug exposure Prior streptococcal pharyngitis Arthralgia Abdominal pain	Fever to 102.2°F (39°C) Possible arthritis Abdominal tenderness Peripheral neuritis	Palpable purpura, most pronounced in dependent areas May become bullous	Palpable purpura	Skin biopsy Frank or occult blood in stool or urine

meningococcemia and meningitis are highest in children. The disease occurs either epidemically in groups or sporadically.

Meningococcemia lacks a prodrome, the onset of fever, rash, and hypotension being abrupt. Bacteremia originating in the oropharynx may result in widespread vasculitis. During the first 3 days of illness 30–60% of patients demonstrate petechial or other purpuric skin lesions. There is no characteristic distribution of the petechiae. The lesions are more frequent in mechanically traumatized skin, such as the axillary folds, the belt line, and the back. Petechiae may be seen on oral and conjunctival mucosa.

Purpura fulminans, ranging from hemorrhagic, purpuric lesions with a geographic border to hemorrhagic lesions evolving into bullae, are associated with endotoxin-initiated disseminated intravascular coagulation. These cutaneous infarctions occur more commonly over pressure points and acral areas, but may be seen anywhere.

The diagnosis of meningococcemia is made clinically. Gram's stain of scraping of early skin lesions may show meningococcus in 30–50% of cases. The diagnosis is confirmed by cultures of the blood and/or cerebrospinal fluid.

Gonococcus

N. gonorrhoeae may disseminate hematogenously from the penile urethra, endometrium, oropharynx, or anorectum causing acute or subacute arthritis-dermatitis syndrome. Dissemination occurs in 1% of males and 3% of females with gonorrhea. However, most patients with urogenital, pharyngeal, or anorectal gonococcal colonization are asymptomatic.

Gonococcemia is characterized by fever, rash, and polyarthropathy. Three to twenty tender erythematous acral macules evolve into hemorrhagic pustules during the following 24–48 hours. The cutaneous lesions are associated with tenosynovitis of the wrist or ankle, arthralgia, or frank septic arthritis. Currently, gonococcal arthritis is the most common type of septic arthritis in the 16–50-year-old group. In menstruating women, bacteremia originates from the infected, sloughing, denuded endometrium, and in subacute cases, symptoms may recur monthly. Gonococcal meningitis or endocarditis may complicate gonococcemia.

The diagnosis is made on clinical criteria. However, immunofluorescent staining of exudate from the hemorrhagic skin lesions shows gonococci in two-thirds of cases. Gram's stain of mucus from the male urethra or from the cervix may show gonococci. The diagnosis is confirmed by culturing *N. gonorrhoeae* from the blood, and/or metastatic skin lesions.

Staphylococcus aureus

S. aureus bacteremia can produce metastatic cutaneous infections ranging from pustules to subcutaneous abscesses to purulent hemorrhagic lesions. Gram-positive clustered cocci may be seen in a smear of the pustular aspirate and its presence confirmed by culture. An adequate number of blood cultures must be obtained, and if they are positive, the patient is presumed to have *S. aureus* endocarditis, even in the absence of a new murmur.

Streptococcus viridans

Subacute bacterial endocarditis caused by *S. viridans* produces several types of vascular lesions, which are immunologically modulated rather than septic emboli. Petechiae occur in crops on the skin or on the mucosa of the conjunctivae or palate. These lesions do not blanch with pressure, but fade in several days. The diagnostic significance of subungual splinter hemorrhages is highly overrated. Such lesions can be detected in 10% of patients admitted to a medical service, and by far the most common cause is nail trauma. Such hemorrhage in the proximal or midnail area is more noteworthy. *Osler's nodes* are tender pink papules 6–8 mm in diameter occurring on the digital pads and lasting 12–24 hours. *Janeway lesions* are small pink or slightly hemorrhagic macules on the palms or soles. Because of the widespread use of antibiotics, these cutaneous findings are observed far less frequently.

Pseudomonas aeruginosa

P. aeruginosa septicemia occurs in immunocompromised hosts, who often have received cancer chemotherapy and corticosteroids within the 2 weeks prior to bacteremia. The respiratory and genitourinary tracts are the most common sites of origin of the sepsis. Intravenous heroin users are also at risk for pseudomonas bacteremia and endocarditis.

The characteristic lesion of pseudomonas sepsis is *ecthyma gangrenosum,* which begins as an erythematous macule and quickly evolves into a large bulla or pustule. Eventually, the epidermis sloughs and the dermal base becomes indurated resulting in a gunmetal gray, indurated, relatively painless ulcer with surrounding erythema. The lesion frequently occurs in the axilla or anogenital area. Ecthyma gangrenosum occurs in patients who are very ill with high fever, chill, and septic shock.

In addition to ecthyma gangrenosum the following dermatologic manifestations of pseudomonas septicemia have been reported: (*a*) hemorrhagic bullae, (*b*) cellulitis, (*c*) plaques, (*d*) small papules on the trunk resembling rose spots of typhoid fever, (*e*) grouped petechiae, and (*f*) erythematous or violaceous subcutaneous nodules.

The initial diagnosis of pseudomonas septicemia is made on clinical suspicion and confirmed by cultures of blood or biopsied skin tissue. Early diagnosis and treatment is imperative for survival.

Candida albicans

C. albicans sepsis is seen much more frequently due to the increasing incidence of AIDS, organ transplantation with immunosuppressive therapy, and cancer chemotherapy. Colonization of the oropharynx and, indeed, the entire gastrointestinal tract, the respiratory tract, and the genitourinary tract occurs commonly in the immunocompromised patient. Superficial mucosal invasion of the oropharynx and esophagus results in thrush (candidiasis). Deeper invasion results in candidemia and systemic candidal infection.

Erythematous papules and nodules, single or multiple, localized or generalized, are seen in up to 13% of patients with disseminated candidiasis. They are often accompanied by fever and muscle tenderness. Disseminated intravascular coagulation with the pathognomonic infarctive skin lesion, purpura fulminans, and an ulcerative ecthyma gangrenosum-like lesion have also been reported in disseminated candida sepsis.

Biopsy of skin lesions in candidal septicemia shows pseudohyphae in the deep dermis and subcutaneous fat, indicating that the invasive route is hematogenous and not by superficial invasion. Biopsy of other organs has significant morbidity. Blood cultures may be positive for *C. albicans* only after several weeks.

Cutaneous Necrotizing Venulitis

Necrotizing vasculitis can involve only the venules in the dermal plexus (cutaneous necrotizing venulitis), or it can involve any organ. The characteristic cutaneous finding is palpable purpura. These lesions appear first where the venous pressure is greatest, that is, on the lower legs. They do not blanch with pressure. With sufficient vascular involvement, purpuric vesicles and even infarcts occur with formation of ulcers.

The pathogenesis of necrotizing venulitis results from immunologic or undefined inflammatory mechanisms. Associated etiologic factors are: (*a*) coexistent disorders (rheumatoid arthritis, Sjögren's syndrome, systemic lupus erythematosus, hypergammaglobulinemic purpura, lymphoproliferative disorders, cryoglobulinemia, ulcerative colitis, cystic fibrosis; (*b*) recent precipitating event (drug-induced reactions, certain bacterial and viral infections), and (*c*) Henoch-Schönlein syndrome (chronic urticaria/angioedema and variants, genetic C2 deficiency, erythema elevatum diutinum, nodular vasculitis, livedoid vasculitis, idiopathic causes).

In patients with the rash of cutaneous necrotizing venulitis, the extent of systemic involvement must be determined by the history, physical examination, and laboratory studies. In patients with Henoch-Schönlein purpura, periarticular vasculitis is common with arthralgia or frank arthritis. Gastrointestinal involvement is manifested by colicky pain or, if there is intestinal obstruction, by intussusception or intramural hemorrhage. The stool specimen may be bloody or tarry, or may give just a positive test for occult blood. Renal involvement with glomerulitis is supported by urinalysis showing erythrocytes.

Systemic corticosteroid therapy is not indicated for cutaneous involvement alone, but can be indicated with involvement of other organs.

Appendix
Précis of the Cutaneous Manifestations of Human Immunodeficiency Virus (HIV) Infection[a]

Part I. Infectious Diseases

Organism	History	Physical Examination	Laboratory Examination
Viral			
HIV—primary infection	Risk group (promiscuous homosexual, i.v. drug abuser, child born to HIV-infected mother, history of blood transfusion in 1978–1985) Incubation period of primary infection 1–6 weeks Chills, headache, arthralgia, myalgia, abdominal cramps, diarrhea Incidence of symptomatic primary HIV infection, uncommon	Fever, stiff neck Truncal maculopapular exanthem Urticaria	Seroconversion of HIV on ELISA or Western blot Culture of HIV from blood and/or CSF Later, lymphopenia, T4: T8 ratio reversed, increased sedimentation rate, polyclonal gammopathy
Herpes simplex (HSV)	Prior genital or labial herpes Painful perioral or perianal lesions for weeks or months Ulcers heal with oral acyclovir Dysphagia Incidence, very common	Initial group vesicles on erythematous base May evolve into many confluent painful perioral or perianal ulcers Enlarged regional lymph nodes Dissemination results in widespread vesicles	Tzanck prep positive for multinucleated giant cells HSV culture positive Biopsy shows multinucleated giant keratinocytes Barium swallow shows HSV esophagitis
Cytomegalovirus (CMV)	Painful perianal lesions for weeks or months Diarrhea from coexistent CMV colitis or proctitis Incidence, common	Painful, deep, confluent ulcers with raised borders Less commonly, petechiae, purpura, vesiculobullous eruption, morbilliform eruption	CMV culture or urine and/or ulcer positive Skin biopsy shows CMV-infected fibroblast or endothelial cell
Herpes zoster	Childhood history of varicella Prior history of zoster in same dermatome Severe dermatomal or multidermatomal pain; progressive encephalitis Incidence, common	Zosteriform eruption may be confluent in dermatome or multidermatome May have disseminated cutaneous vesicles	Tzanck prep positive for multinucleated giant cells
Epstein-Barr virus (EBV)	Asymptomatic tongue lesion in homosexual Incidence, very common No response to anticandida treatment	Oral hairy leukoplakia (HL)—corrugated white plaques on lateral tongue Oral squamous cell carcinoma (?)	Biopsy HL shows flat wart Biopsy shows squamous cell carcinoma

Appendix—*continued*

Organism	History	Physical Examination	Laboratory Examination
Human papillomavirus (HPV)	Genital or perianal condylomata for months or years; extensive Asymptomatic tongue lesion (HL) Asymptomatic anal lesion Incidence, very common	Voluminous condylomata, especially perianal Intraoral warts Oral HL Anal mass lesion	Biopsy shows condyloma Biopsy shows flat wart Biopsy shows invasive squamous cell carcinoma
Molluscum contagiosum	Asymptomatic papules Incidence, very common	Many clustered, shiny, umbilicated papules on face, neck, and especially beard area Giant molluscum	Curetting shows molluscum bodies Biopsy shows molluscum contagiosum
Vaccinia virus	Recent history of vaccination in a soldier Constitutional symptoms Incidence, rare	Primary vaccination site Disseminated varioliform pustules	Biopsy of pustule shows Guarnieri bodies Viral culture of pustule grows vaccinia
Arthropod			
Sarcoptes scabiei	Asymptomatic to severe generalized pruritus Incidence, uncommon	Generalized papulosquamous or eczematous eruption especially in skin folds; burrows Norwegian or "exaggerated" scabies	Oil prep and biopsy show sarcoptic mites
Fungus			
Candida albicans	Oropharyngeal, may be asymptomatic or associated with sore tongue or throat, loss of taste, dysphagia Vulvovaginal soreness, vaginal discharge Incidence, nearly 100%	White curdlike colonies on the oropharyngeal mucosa; angular cheilitis; thick plaques on back of throat; deep erosions on tongue White curdlike colonies on vulvar and vaginal mucosa	KOH positive for spores and hyphae
Pityrosporum orbiculare	Often intensely pruritic eruption (folliculitis) Asymptomatic discoloration of trunk (tinea versicolor) Incidence, common	Folliculitis on chest, upper arms, lateral neck, face, scalp, axillae, thighs Extensive confluent scaling, hyper- and/or hypopigmented areas on trunk	KOH or biopsy shows large numbers of yeast KOH positive for hyphae and spores
Pityrosporum ovale	Asymptomatic mild to severe rash in seborrheic areas; clears with topical or oral ketoconazole but poor response to topical corticosteroids (seborrheic dermatitis) Incidence, very common	Mild to severe papulosquamous eruption in typical seborrheic areas (scalp, face, midchest, back, groin)	Biopsy of lesion resembles histopathology of seborrheic dermatitis but with scattered necrotic keratinocytes
Dermatophytes	Asymptomatic to pruritic rash on face, hands, feet	Keratoderma blennorrhagicum-like lesions on hands and/	KOH positive for septated hyphae

Appendix—*continued*

Organism	History	Physical Examination	Laboratory Examination
	Incidence, common	or feet; red, scaling patch on face	
Cryptococcus neoformans	Headache Altered mental status Incidence, uncommon	Numerous molluscum-like or herpetiform lesions follow hematogenous dissemination Single or multiple reddish-purple papules, nodules, or plaques resembling cellulitis Discrete papular lesions with central keratotic areas on sides of palms and soles	Biopsy of lesion shows *C. neoformans* Culture of biopsied skin grows *C. neoformans*
Coccidioides immitis	Residence in or travel to California or American Southwest Incidence, uncommon (regional)	Scanty, scattered papular pustules on arms, legs, trunk	Biopsy of lesion shows *C. immitis* Culture of biopsied skin grows *C. immitis* Fungal culture of lesion grows *C. immitis*
Histoplasma capsulatum	Asymptomatic lesions Incidence, rare	Scattered acneiform papules Few indurated pinkish-red crusted plaques	Biopsy of lesion shows intrahistiocytic *H. capsulatum* Culture of biopsied skin grows *H. capsulatum*
Bacterial			
Staphylococcus aureus	Early in course (impetigo) Tenderness at catheter site Abscess at site of intravenous, intradermal, or subcutaneous injection Large tender area of skin Botryomycosis Incidence, rare	Crusted lesions on neck or beard area Inflamed, tender catheter insertion site Local abscess over vein, old needle tracts, thrombosed veins Red, hot, tender area of cellulitis Prurigo nodularis-like lesions on trunk, upper arms	Bacterial culture grows *S. aureus* Biopsy of lesion shows granules in dermis with Gram-positive cocci
Haemophilus influenzae	Swelling of arms Incidence, rare	Both arms may be red, hot, tender (cellulitis)	Blood culture grows *H. influenzae*
Enteric Gram-negative rods	Tenderness at catheter site	Inflamed, tender catheter insertion site	Bacterial culture grows *Pseudomonas aeruginosa* or *Enterobacter aerogenes*
Mycobacterium avium/ intracellulare	Kaposi's sarcoma (KS) Incidence, rare	Ill-defined macular, discolored lesions on forearms resembling KS	Biopsy of lesion shows innumerable acid-fast organisms within histiocytes
Protozoan			
Acanthamoeba castellanii		Nonspecific papular lesion	Biopsy of lesion shows amebic trophozoites

Appendix—*continued*

Part II. Neoplastic, Hyperproliferative, Hypersensitive, Vascular, and Miscellaneous Disorders

Type of Disorder	History	Physical Examination	Laboratory Examination
Neoplastic			
Kaposi's sarcoma (KS)	Asymptomatic but cosmetically unacceptable lesions appearing over weeks to months Predominantly in homosexual men (up to 80%); much less common in other risk groups	Initially, dermal nodules with faint yellow-green halos Later, violaceous to brown epidermal-dermal nodules to tumors expecially on upper trunk, neck, scalp, face, penis Mucosal violaceous nodules visible on conjunctivae, hard palate, gingiva Edema (periorbital, genital) secondary to lymph node obstruction	Biopsy shows KS
Basal cell epithelioma (BCE), metastatic	Asymptomatic skin nodule usually on the face; recurring BCE Incidence, uncommon	Pearly to ulcerating tumor Possible enlarged regional lymph node	Biopsy of lesion shows BCE Regional lymph node biopsy shows metastatic BCE
Oral squamous carcinoma	Asymptomatic to tender oral mass Incidence, 2%	Tumor, either ulcerated or hyperkeratotic on the tongue or floor of the mouth	Biopsy shows squamous cell carcinoma
Squamous carcinoma of anal canal	Melena, diarrhea, pruritus Incidence, uncommon	Focal, indurated mass to large exophytic lesion, 2–10 cm above the anal verge Bowen's papulosis on penis	Biopsy shows squamous cell carcinoma
Benign Epidermal Hyperproliferative			
Psoriasis	Prior personal or family history of psoriasis may be lacking Explosive, extensive flares Therapeutically, difficult to control with usual topicals or phototherapy Treatment with methotrexate may precipitate rapid deterioration Incidence, uncommon	Atypical distribution, with prominent involvement of axillae, groin, scalp, soles, palms Guttate or pustular pattern that rapidly becomes confluent or erythrodermic	Biopsy shows psoriasis
Reiter syndrome	May precede or follow diagnosis of AIDS Skin lesions recalcitrant to topical treatment Incidence, uncommon	Urethritis or cervicitis Conjunctivitis or uveitis Balanitis circinata, painless oral ulcerations, keratoderma blennorrhagicum involving palms or soles	Biopsy shows keratoderma blennorrhagicum

Appendix—*continued*

Type of Disorder	History	Physical Examination	Laboratory Examination
		Asymmetric oligoarthritis (large joints of legs, sacroiliac joint)	
Xeroderma, ichthyosis	Possible pruritus, malnourishment Incidence, common	Generalized xeroderma	Biopsy shows hyperkeratosis or ichthyosis
Adverse Drug Reaction			
Trimethoprim/ sulfamethoxazole	*Pneumocystis carinii* pneumonia Incidence, up to 60%	Generalized exfoliative eruption 8–12 days after treatment begun; generalized urticaria	Biopsy shows drug reaction
Sulfadiazine/ pyrimethamine	Toxoplasma chorioretinitis, encephalitis, brain abscess	Generalized macular and papular eruption	Biopsy shows drug reaction
Pyrimethamine/ sulfadoxine	Toxoplasma chorioretinitis, encephalitis, brain abscess	Erythema multiforme	Biopsy shows erythema multiforme
Pentamidine	*P. carinii* pneumonia Incidence, up to 20%	Urticaria and erythema Sterile abscess at site of injection	Biopsy shows drug reaction
Rifampin	*Mycobacterium tuberculosis* infection Pruritus, weakness, myalgia, diarrhea, abdominal pain, vomiting Onset within 30 days of administration Incidence, 52%	Fever Exanthematous eruption	Biopsy shows drug eruption
Methotrexate	Psoriasis, Reiter syndrome Fulminant development of KS Rapid downhill course with infection	Extensive KS	Biopsy shows KS
Prednisone	Vasculitis, Burkitt's lymphoma KS resolves spontaneously when prednisone discontinued	Sudden appearance of KS	Biopsy shows KS
Nonmalignant Vascular			
Immune thrombocytopenic purpura	Asymptomatic nonblanching lesions Incidence, uncommon	Petechiae	Thrombocytopenia
Immune-complex vasculitis	Asymptomatic nonblanching lesions Incidence, uncommon	Palpable purpura	Biopsy shows necrotizing vasculitis
Hyperalgesic pseudothrombo-phlebitis syndrome	KS, painful calf Resolves in 1 month Incidence, rare	Painful, swollen calf, Homan's sign positive Overlying skin red and exquisitely tender	Venography shows *no* evidence of venous occlusion

Appendix—*continued*

Type of Disorder	History	Physical Examination	Laboratory Examination
		Palpable tender, indurated cord overlying superficial veins	
Miscellaneous			
Papular eruption	Chronic pruritic eruption, which may wax and wane	Noncoalescing 2- to 5-mm skin-colored papules of the head, neck, and upper trunk	Biopsy shows perivascular mononuclear cell infiltrate
Folliculitis	Asymptomatic to pruritic eruption	Follicular papules or pustules presenting as widespread acneiform eruption, axillary folliculitis, and eosinophilic pustular folliculitis	Bacterial culture shows *S. aureus* in 50% of cases Biopsy may show a mixed perifollicular infiltrate, eosinophilic infiltrate, a severe necrotizing folliculitis with vasculitis, or Pityrosporum
Pruritus	Intractable generalized itching	No skin findings to explain pruritus Excoriations	No metabolic cause for pruritus detected
Yellow nail syndrome	Associated with *P. carinii pneumonia* Yellowing usually of less than 1 year's duration	Yellow discoloration of distal finger- or toenails	

[a] From Johnson RA.

SUGGESTED READINGS

Arndt, KA. *Manual of Dermatologic Therapeutics,* 3rd ed. Boston: Little, Brown & Co., 1983.

Asbrink E. Erythema chronicum migrans Afzelius and acrodermatitis chronica atrophicans: Early and late manifestations of *Ixodes ricinus* borne Borrelia spirochetes. Acta Derm Venereol (Suppl) (Stockh) 1985;118:1–63.

Benson M, Walker, DH. Rocky Mountain spotted fever in the differential diagnosis of the acute abdomen. *Contemp Surg,* 1984;24:79–83.

Berger BW. Erythema chronicum migrans of Lyme disease. *Arch Dermatol*, 1984;120:1017–1021.

Bielory L, Yancey KB, Young NS, et al. Cutaneous manifestations of serum sickness in patients receiving antithymocyte globulin. *J Am Acad Dermatol*, 1985;13:411–417.

Caughman W, Stern R, Haynes H. Neutrophilic dermatosis of myeloproliferative disorders: Atypical forms of pyoderma gangrenosum and Sweet's syndrome associated with myeloproliferative disorders. *J Am Acad Dermatol*, 1983;9:751–758.

Center for Disease Control. Rubella and congenital rubella syndrome—United States, 1984–1985. *MMWR*, 1986;35:129–135.

Center for Disease Control. Multiple outbreaks of Kawasaki's syndrome—United States. *MMWR*, 1985;34:33–35.

Center for Disease Control. Classification system for human T-lymphotropic virus type III/lymphadenopathy-associated virus infections. *MMWR*, 1986;35:334–349.

Center for Disease Control. Rocky Mountain spotted fever—United States, 1985. *MMWR*, 1986;35:247–249.

Center for Disease Control. Toxic shock syndrome associated with influenza—Minnesota. *MMWR*, 1986;35:143–144.

Chesney PJ, Davis JP, Purdy WK, et al. Clinical manifestations of toxic shock syndrome. *JAMA*, 1981;246:741–748.

Cohen AS, Reynolds WE, Franklin EC, et al. Preliminary criteria for the classification of systemic lupus erythematosus. *Bull Rheum Dis*, 1971;21:643–648.

Cooper PH, Innes DJ Jr, Greer KE. Acute febrile neutrophilic dermatosis (Sweet's syndrome) and myeloproliferative disorders. *Cancer*, 1983;51:1518–1526.

Davis AE Jr, Bradford AD. Abdominal pain resembling acute appendicitis in Rocky Mountain spotted fever. *JAMA*, 1982;247:2811–2812.

Ekenstam E, Callen JP. Cutaneous leukocytoclastic vasculitis: Clinical and laboratory features in 82 patients seen in private practice. *Arch Dermatol*, 1984;120:484–489.

Elias PM, Fritsch PM, Epstein EH Jr. Staphylococcal scalded skin syndrome: Clinical features, pathogenesis, and recent microbiological and biochemical developments. *Arch Dermatol*, 1977;113:207–219.

Fitzpatrick TB, Elsen AZ, Wolff K, et al, eds. *Dermatology in General Medicine*. 3rd ed. New York:McGraw-Hill, 1986.

Flick MR, Cluff LE. Pseudomonas bacteremia: Review of 108 cases. *Am J Med*, 1976;60:501–508.

Greene SL, Su WPD, Muller SA. Ecthyma gangrenosum: Report of clinical, histopathologic, and bacteriologic aspects of eight cases. *J Am Acad Dermatol*, 1984;11-781–787.

Greene JA, Spruance SL, Wenerstrom G, et al. Post-herpetic erythema multiforme prevented with prophylactic oral acyclovir. *Ann Intern Med*, 1985;102:622–623.

Helmick CG, Bernard KW, D'Angelo LJ. Rocky Mountain spotted fever: Clinical, laboratory and epidemiological features of 262 cases. *J Infect Dis*, 1984;150:480–488.

Hermans PE. The clinical manifestations of infective endocarditis. *Mayo Clin Proc*, 1982;57:15–21.

Hoeprich PD, et. *Infectious Diseases: A Modern Treatise of Infectious Processes* 3rd ed. Philadelphia:Harper & Row, 1983.

Huff JC, Weston WL, Tonnesen MG. Erythema multiforme: A clinical review of characteristics, diagnostic criteria, and causes. *J Am Acad Dermatol*, 1983;8:763–775.

Jawitz JC, Hines HC, Moshell AN. Treatment of eczema herpeticum with systemic acyclovir. *Arch Dermatol*, 1985;121:274–275.

Kaplowitz LG, Fischer JJ, Sparling PF. Rocky Mountain spotted fever: A clinical dilemma. *Curr Clin Top Infect Dis*, 1981;2:89–108.

Kauppinen K. Cutaneous reactions to drugs with special reference to severe bullous mucocutaneous eruptions and sulphonamides. *Acta Derm Venereol (Suppl) (Stockh)*, 1972;52:68.

Kauppinen K. Stubb S. Drug eruptions: Causative agents and clinical types. *Acta Derm Venereol (Stockh)*, 1984;64:320–324.

Lawley TJ, Bielory L, Gascon P, et al. A prospective clinical and immunologic analysis of patients with serum sickness. *N Engl J Med*, 1984;311:1407–1413.

Lemak MA, Duvic M, Bean SF. Oral acyclovir for the prevention of herpes-associated erythema multiforme. *J Am Acad Dermatol*, 1986;15:50–53.

Levin DL, Esterly NB, Herman JJ, et al. The Sweet syndrome in children. *J Pediatr*, 1981;99:73–78.

Liesegang TJ. The varicella-zoster virus: Systemic and ocular features. *J Am Acad Dermatol*, 1984;11:165–191.

Longley S, Caldwell JR, Panush RS. Paraneoplastic vasculitis: Unique syndrome of cutaneous angiitis and arthritis associated with myeloproliferative disorders. *Am J Med*, 1986;80:1027–1030.

McElgun PSJ. Dermatologic manifestations of hepatitis B virus infection. *J Am Acad Dermatol*, 1983;8:539–547.

Michels TC. Mucocutaneous lymph node syndrome in adults: Differentiation from toxic shock syndrome. *Am J Med*, 1986;80:724–728.

Ororato IM, Morens DM, Martone WJ, et al. Epidemiology of cytomegaloviral infections: Recommendations for prevention and control. *Rev Infect Dis*, 1985;7:479–487.

Orton PW, Huff JC, Tonnesen MG, et al. Detection of a herpes viral antigen in skin lesions in erythema multiforme. *Ann Intern Med*, 1984;101:48–50.

Reik L Jr, Burgdorfer W, Donaldson JO. Neurologic abnormalities in Lyme disease without erythema chronicum migrans. *Am J Med*, 1986;81:73–78.

Reingold AL, Hargrett NT, Dan BB, et al. Nonmenstrual toxic shock syndrome: A review of 130 cases. *Ann Intern Med*, 1982;96:871–874.

Reyes MP, Palutke WA, Wyline RF, et al. Pseudomonas endocarditis in the Detroit Medical Center, 1969–1972. *Medicine*, 1973;52:173–194.

Schad GA, Leiby DA, Duffy CH, et al. Swine trichinosis in New England slaughterhouses. *Am J Vet Res*, 1985;46:2008–2010.

Schmid GP. The global distribution of Lyme disease. *Rev Infect Dis*, 1985;7:41–50.

Shands KN, Schmid GP, Dan BB, et al. Toxic-shock syndrome in menstruating women: Association with tampon use and *Staphylococcus aureus* and clinical features in 52 cases. *N Engl J Med*, 1980;303:1436–1442.

Silverman RA, Rhodes AR, Dennehy PH. Disseminated intravascular coagulation and purpura fulminans in a patient with candida sepsis: Biopsy of purpura fulminans as an aid to diagnosis of systemic candida infection. *Am J Med*, 1986;80:679–684.

Soter NA, Baden HP. *Pathophysiology of Dermatologic Diseases.* New York: McGraw-Hill, 1984.

Spear KL, Winkelmann RK. Gianotti-Crosti syndrome: A review of ten cases not associated with hepatitis B. *Arch Dermatol*, 1984;120:891–896.

Steere AC, Bartenhagen NH, Craft JE, et al. The early clinical manifestations of Lyme disease. *Ann Intern Med*, 1983;99:76–82.

Steere AC, Grodzick RL, Kornblatt AN, et al. The spirochetal etiology of Lyme disease. *N Engl J Med*, 1983;308:733–740.

Steere AC, Hutchinson GJ, Rahn DW, et al. Treatment of the early manifestations of Lyme disease. *Ann Intern Med*, 1983;99:22–26.

Straus SF, Rooney JF, Sever JL, et al. Herpes simplex virus infection biology, treatment, and prevention. *Ann Intern Med*, 1985;103:404–419.

Walker DH, Lesesne HR, Varma VA, et al. Rocky Mountain spotted fever mimicking acute cholecystitis. *Arch Intern Med*, 1985;145:2194–2196.

Westerman RL: Rocky Mountain spotless fever: A dilemma for the clinician. *Arch Intern Med*, 1982;142:1106–1107.

Westly ED, Wechsler HL. Toxic epidermal necrolysis: Granulocytic leukopenia as a prognostic indicator. *Arch Dermatol*, 1984;120:721–726.

Williams CL, Curran AS, Lee AC, et al. Lyme disease: Epidemiologic characteristics of an outbreak in Westchester County, NY. *Am J Public Health*, 1986;76:62–65.

Yanagihara R, Todds JK. Acute febrile mucocutaneous lymph node syndrome. *Am J Dis Child*, 1980;134:603–614.

SECTION 3

Pediatrics

PATRICIA J. O'MALLEY, M.D.
Associate Editor

CHAPTER 20

Approach to the Emergency Pediatric Patient

PATRICIA J. O'MALLEY, M.D.

Emergency department staff experienced in caring for adults may find the pediatric patient difficult to predict, to interpret, and to manage. This chapter reviews some of the fundamentals of caring for children in an acute care situation, the normals and abnormals on examination, indices of illness, and suggestions for examination procedures with a brief discussion of some particular pediatric differential diagnoses. It concludes with a formulary of commonly used pediatric drugs (see Appendix).

CARING FOR CHILDREN IN THE EMERGENCY DEPARTMENT

The Child

Caring for children, above all, requires calm, gentleness, and patience. Children demand that we consider and deal directly with emotions that adult patients feel but frequently repress: anger, fear, pain, and loss of control. A child adapts to new situations by using members of his or her family, toys, and other belongings, and by active engagement of fantasy and imagination. Care should be taken to respect the modesty, privacy, and individuality of the child. Like adults, children are often fearful of situations they do not understand. They need to be told about their illness, its evaluation, and treatment in terms that they can understand, avoiding jargon or technical terms which may have no meaning. For example, "I'm going to take your blood pressure" may sound threatening to a 3- or 4-year-old child whereas, "This wraps around your arm and gives it a squeeze" prepares the child for what may happen.

Fear and anger are normal reactions to new situations and painful procedures. The understanding emergency physician is not threatened by these reactions: rather, he or she can guide the child by giving fair warning and by setting limits. For a venipuncture, for example, one may say, "This may hurt for a minute, and it is all right to cry if you get scared, but it is very important that you hold still." Deceiving a child about painful procedures ultimately results in loss of trust far more certainly than the procedure itself.

The Parent

Parents are key to successful care of the pediatric patient. They know their child better than the emergency department staff and they are the ones who must continue therapy after the acute intervention in the emergency department. Eliciting their observations and concerns, making them feel comfortable, and advising them of what is to be expected in the emergency department supports the emotional resources they need in order to help their child. During the examination and during any procedures, the medical staff enlists the cooperation of the parents by explaining what is needed. Most parents understand that procedures such as lumbar puncture, bladder tap, or intravenous line placement may be technically easier to perform without their presence. However, they may feel that it is more important to be present to reassure the child; in fact, the calm and reassuring parent is very helpful during a procedure. On the other hand, if a parent has conflicting feelings about whether to stay or to go during a procedure, the emergency department staff should help resolve the dilemma in a supportive fashion.

THE PEDIATRIC EXAMINATION

General Evaluation

Performing an examination of the pediatric patient under 3 years of age can challenge a physician's skill and patience. It is important with all children to establish social contact before medical contact, in a nonconfronting fashion and in a way that allows the child to read his parents' reaction to the situation and be reassured by their acceptance of the physician. Establishing eye contact and making some gentle physical contact such as offering an improvised toy, a stethoscope or an examination glove blown up as a balloon, while talking to the parents to obtain history, not only allows the physician to form an alliance with the child but also yields important clinical information. The infant or toddler who smiles, plays, or alerts normally to the interaction is statistically less likely to be seriously ill than the inconsolable or apathetic infant. This preexamination period, in fact, has been defined as a period of "optimal observation," resulting in a scale of observations items (Fig. 20.1) that are predictive of the presence of serious bacterial disease in the febrile child (see McCarthy, et al., Suggested Readings).

In the child 3½ years or older, the physical examination can usually proceed in much the same top-to-toe orderly and expeditious fashion as in the adult, particularly if care if taken to explain and reassure along the way. This is not the case in the toddler, where order is determined by the potential discomfort of the examination and by willingness to cooperate. Much of the examination can be performed with the child in the parent's arms. Listening to the heart and lungs, feeling the abdomen, checking extremities for injury or infection, and ob-

Predictive Model: Six Observation Items and Their Scales

Observation Item	1 Normal	3 Moderate Impairment	5 Severe Impairment
Quality of cry	Strong with normal tone OR Content and not crying	Whimpering OR Sobbing	Weak OR Moaning OR High pitched
Reaction to parent stimulation	Cries briefly then stops OR Content and not crying	Cries off and on	Continual cry OR Hardly responds
State variation	If awake → stays awake OR If asleep and stimulated → wakes up quickly	Eyes close briefly → awake OR Awakes with prolonged stimulation	Falls to sleep OR Will not rouse
Color	Pink	Pale extremities OR Acrocyanosis	Pale OR Cyanotic OR Mottled OR Ashen
Hydration	Skin normal, eyes normal AND Mucous membranes moist	Skin, eyes-normal AND Mouth slightly dry	Skin doughy OR Tented AND Dry mucous membranes AND/OR Sunken eyes
Response (talk, smile) to social overtures	Smiles OR Alerts (≤2 mo)	Brief smile OR Alerts briefly (≤2 mo)	No smile Face anxious, dull, expressionless OR No alerting (≤2 mo)

Figure 20.1. McCarthy scale of observations.

Table 20.1.
Classification of Hypertension by Age Group[a]

Age Group	Significant Hypertension (mm Hg)[b]	Severe Hypertension (mm Hg)
Newborn		
7 days	Systolic BP ≥96	Systolic BP ≥106
8–30 days	Systolic BP ≥104	Systolic BP ≥110
Infant (<2 yr)	Systolic BP ≥112 Diastolic BP ≥74	Systolic BP ≥118 Diastolic BP ≥82
Children (3–5 yr)	Systolic BP ≥116 Diastolic BP ≥76	Systolic BP ≥124 Diastolic BP ≥84
Children (6–9 yr)	Systolic BP ≥122 Diastolic BP ≥78	Systolic BP ≥130 Diastolic BP ≥86
Children (10–12 yr)	Systolic BP ≥126 Diastolic BP ≥82	Systolic BP ≥134 Diastolic BP ≥90
Adolescents (13–15 yr)	Systolic BP ≥136 Diastolic BP ≥86	Systolic BP ≥144 Diastolic BP ≥92
Adolescents (16–18 yr)	Systolic BP ≥142 Diastolic BP ≥92	Systolic BP ≥150 Diastolic BP ≥98

[a] From Task Force on Blood Pressure Control in Children. Blood pressure control—1986. *Pediatrics,* 1987; 79:1–25.
[b] BP, blood pressure.

taining accurate vital signs cannot be done when the child is screaming; however, examining the ears and mouth and observing neurologic function can. Advising the parents beforehand about which parts of the examination may cause discomfort will enlist their cooperation. In checking for meningism or for bone and joint pathology, it is important to elicit and observe spontaneous flexion of the neck or use of the limb; forced movement may be misleading by producing voluntary resistance or even overcoming involuntary resistance in the small infant.

Special Evaluation

Fruitful parts of the pediatric examination which are frequently overlooked include: *a*) observing the child walk; *b*) examining the skin completely for rash or bruising; *c*) genital, rectal, and perianal examination; and *d*) careful joint examination for possible infection in the febrile child. Every effort should be made to include these simple items in the examination.

It is unrealistic to expect a child under 6 years of age to comply voluntarily with requests to hold still for painful procedures or examinations. If a child is unable or unwilling to cooperate for an uncomfortable part of the examination, such as looking in the ears or mouth, careful holding minimizes discomfort and the chance of injury to the child. Swaddling the child in a sheet may be helpful for venipuncture or intravenous placement. For ear and mouth examination, restraining by pinning the arms securely above the head as the child lies supine frequently allows for a safe examination. When wax precludes visualizing the tympanic membrane and checking its mobility, there are several methods for removal. Flushing the ear with water or a mixture of water and dilute peroxide using a Water Pik or an improvised set with a syringe and tubing from a "butterfly" needle may take 5 or 10 minutes but is relatively atraumatic. Calgi swabs or ear currettes are effective, but frequently cause bleeding from the external canal which may obliterate the examination and dismay the parents. When using an instrument or swab introduced into the ear, the physician must be sure that the child is lying down, carefully restrained, and only the force of gravity is used to introduce the swab or instrument.

Tables 20.1 and 20.2 and Fig. 20.2 list the range of expected values for vital signs by age and some

Table 20.2.
Normals for Age

Age	Heart Rate	Respiratory Rate
Newborn	90–160	30–50
6 months	80–150	20–30
2 years	80–130	20–30
6 years	75–115	18–25
10 years	70–110	12–20

Table 20.3.
Interpretation of Abnormal Vital Signs

Heart rate	Increased in fever, shock, anxiety, primary cardiac disease
Blood pressure	Increased in renal disease, drugs, ingestions, increased intracranial pressure
	Decreased in shock, dehydration, prearrest situation
Respiratory rate	Increased in respiratory compromise, acidosis, Reye's syndrome, anxiety, aspirin overdose, fever
	Decreased in seizures, drug overdose, sepsis, prearrest situation, (apnea, gasping)
Weight	Increased in fluid overload states, renal and cardiac disease
	Decreased in chronic failure to thrive, dehydration
Capillary refill	Increased in fever, high cardiac output states
	Decreased in shock, hypothermia

causes of abnormal values. One cause of abnormal values is difficulty in obtaining them; it is worthwhile to obtain repeated signs over a period of time and when the child is distracted or sleeping. Body weight and observation of capillary refill are *vital signs* in the pediatric patient and should be obtained on all pediatric patients admitted to the emergency department. In addition to abnormal vital signs (Table 20.3) and the features on "optimal observation" examination, three other warning signs are useful in signaling real disease in the pediatric patient: *a*) the child who, although awake, prefers to lie down; *b*) the child with grunting respirations; and *c*) the child with mottled skin and poor capillary refill.

Sedation of the pediatric patient presents some specific problems, but is occasionally necessary such as in trying to accomplish repair of lacerations or to obtain optimal cooperation for radiographic or computed tomography (CT) that requires the child to hold still for a long time. The characteristics of a sedative drug that are most desirable, i.e. rapid onset, short duration, reversibility, and absence of respiratory depression, are unfortunately not available in a single medication. Table 20.4 displays some of the options for sedating the pediatric patient.

THE PRESENTING COMPLAINT: A PEDIATRIC DIFFERENTIAL DIAGNOSIS

This section deals with a limited number of acute presentations with particular pediatric etiologies.

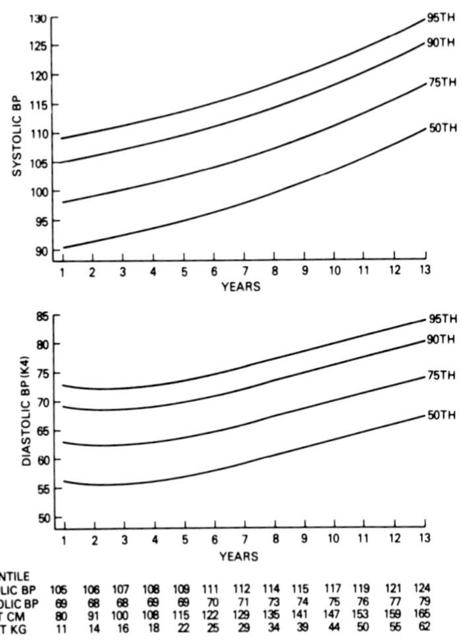

90TH PERCENTILE	1	2	3	4	5	6	7	8	9	10	11	12	13
SYSTOLIC BP	105	106	107	108	109	111	112	114	115	117	119	121	124
DIASTOLIC BP	69	68	68	69	69	70	71	73	74	75	76	77	79
HEIGHT CM	80	91	100	108	115	122	129	135	141	147	153	159	165
WEIGHT KG	11	14	16	18	22	25	29	34	39	44	50	56	62

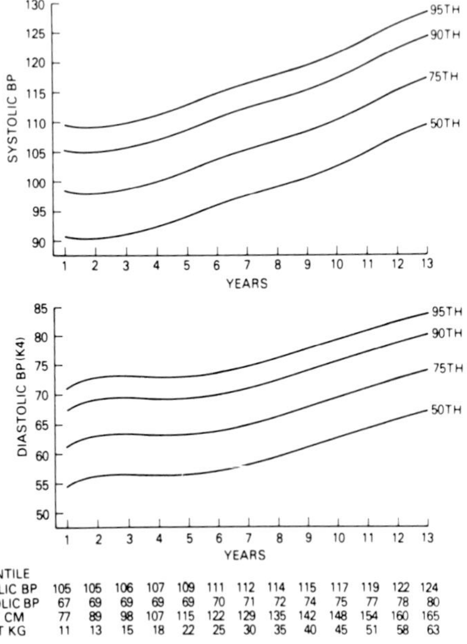

90TH PERCENTILE	1	2	3	4	5	6	7	8	9	10	11	12	13
SYSTOLIC BP	105	105	106	107	109	111	112	114	115	117	119	122	124
DIASTOLIC BP	67	69	69	69	69	70	71	72	74	75	77	78	80
HEIGHT CM	77	89	98	107	115	122	129	135	142	148	154	160	165
WEIGHT KG	11	13	15	18	22	25	30	35	40	45	51	58	63

Figure 20.2. Task force blood pressure norms. *Left panel,* Age-specific percentiles of blood pressure *(BP)* measurements in boys, 1 to 13 years of age; Korotkoff phase IV (*K4*) used for diastolic BP. *Right panel,* Age-specific percentiles of BP measurements in girls, 1 to 13 years of age; K4 used for diastolic BP. From Task Force on Blood Pressure Control in Children. Blood pressure control—*Pediatrics,* 1987; 79:1–25.

Table 20.4.
Options for Sedation in Children

Chloral hydrate
  30–50 mg/kg/dose
    Oral or rectal
    Irregular onset ½–1 hr
    Safe, minimal side effects
    No analgesia
    No reversal
DPT or "Pedi Cocktail" or "Lytic Cocktail"
  *D*emerol, 25 mg/ml
  *P*henergan, 6.25 mg/ml
  *T*horazine, 6.25 mg/ml
  1 ml/15 kg dose, maximum 2 ml
    i.m. shot, analgesic and sedative
    Irregular onset ½–1 hr
    Poly pharmacy
    No reversal
i.v. Morphine/Demerol
  Morphine, 0.1–0.2 mg/kg/dose
  Demerol, 1.5 mg/kg/dose
    Rapid onset, requires i.v.
    Sedative and analgesic
    Reversible
i.v. Valium
  0.05–0.2 mg/kg/dose
    Rapid onset
    No analgesia
    May take large total dose
Brevital (methohexital)
  i.v. 1–2 mg/kg/dose
    May cause apnea
    Rapid onset, within 1 minute, duration 5–10 minutes
  Rectal 10–15 mg/kg dose
    Onset in 5–10 minutes, duration ½ hr
    Requires physician's presence by either route

Subsequent chapters in this section deal with other specific pediatric problems in more detail. There are several excellent books written on the subject of pediatric differential diagnosis; the reader is referred to them for a more complete discussion.

The Child Who Won't Walk

The child who won't walk has likely suffered some traumatic injury, trivial or significant, but may also be unable to walk from weakness or refuse to walk because of ataxia. The physician should therefore consider the following possibilities:

1. Pain from "toddler's fracture," splinter, toxic synovitis, septic hip, polyarthritis;
2. Weakness from Guillain-Barré syndrome, transverse myelitis, spinal cord lesion;
3. Ataxia from acute cerebellar ataxia, tumor, drugs.

The history should therefore focus on possible trauma, prodromal illness or fever, ingestions, tempo of the presentation, and the child's level of illness. The examination should focus on vital signs, neurologic examination with particular attention to strength, cerebellar function, sensation, and relexes; and orthopedic evaluation of the lower extremities, especially the range of motion of the hip, pain, resistance on logrolling the leg, the tibia for point tenderness, the soles of the feet for foreign body, and the joints for pathology. The examiner should try to get the child to bear weight and walk, crawl, or pull to stand. Laboratory tests are guided by the findings on history and physical assessment, but should include a complete blood cell count, erythrocyte sedimentation rate, and if indicated, radiographs of the hip.

The Child with Abdominal Pain

Apart from the usual intraabdominal pathology causing acute abdominal pain (appendicitis, gastroenteritis, intussusception, pyelonephritis), the physician should consider the possibility of streptococcal pharyngitis, pneumonia, Henoch-Schönlein purpura (HSP), child abuse, and diabetic ketoacidosis in the differential diagnosis.

In addition to vital signs and a careful abdominal examination, including observing the child walk and jump to elicit peritoneal signs, one must include a detailed throat examination, a check for cervical adenopathy, and chest examination noting respiratory rate, the most sensitive sign of pneumonia. The lower extremities are examined for the typical rash of HSP (a palpable petechial or purpuric rash in dependent areas, such as buttocks and lower extremities), and for joint edema and pain typical of HSP.

Laboratory evaluation should include a urinalysis for sugar, ketones (frequently present in the fasting child), red blood cells (which may occur with streptococcal pharyngitis, appendicitis, pyelonephritis, or HSP), and leukocytes. A chest x-ray should be obtained if there is any reason to suspect an occult pneumonia, such as fever with vomiting and tachypnea.

The Very Sick Infant under 2 Months of Age

Although fortunately uncommon, the problem of the very sick infant involves a very wide range of possible acquired and congenital problems and is one of the most frightening problems encountered in the emergency department. The most common cause of severe illness in the infant under 2 months of age is bacterial infection, usually bacteremic sepsis associated with meningitis, pyelonephritis, or bacterial enteritis, although viral infections occasionally cause severe illness in this age group. Infants are brought with either fever or hypothermia when septic; therefore, an abnormal temperature in either direction is cause for concern. Several other etiologies must be considered, however, even in the face of fever, which may simply be due to a trivial intercurrent infection tipping the balance in the presence of other underlying pathology. The same pattern of a gray, grunting, hypothermic infant presumed septic may, in fact, represent an infant with (*a*) underlying heart disease, such as ventricular septal defect, critical coarctation of the aorta, or paroxysmal atrial tachycardia; (*b*) unsuspected metabolic disease, such as renal tubular acidosis, organic or amino acidopathies, such as maple syrup urine disease, or adrenal insufficiency due to congenital adrenal hyperplasia; or (*c*) a perforated abdominal viscus, as in Hirschsprung's disease, malrotation of the gut, volvulus, or child abuse.

Immediate attention to the airway with oxygenation and early consideration of intubation, intravenous access, antibiotics, possible volume support, if there is no reason to suspect congestive heart failure, and thermal support are key. Vital signs and examination should be performed as quickly as possible and should focus on possible causes of infection as well as careful cardiac, abdominal, and neurologic evaluation. Blood pressure in upper and lower extremities should be documented.

Laboratory evaluation should take into account that, regardless of etiology, the infant may be acidotic, hypoglycemic, hypocalcemic, and at risk for disseminated intravascular coagulation. A full septic workup including bladder tap, blood culture, lumbar puncture, and chest x-ray is desirable, but may not be tolerated before initiating antibiotics and stabilizing the patient. Serum electrolytes, blood glucose, arterial blood gases, electrocardiogram, evaluation for disseminated intravascular coagulopathy (DIC), and serum for blood typing should be obtained.

Treatment is aimed at any identified underlying etiology, which is discussed in more detail in subsequent chapters, but must include airway support, antibiotics, metabolic correction, and volume resuscitation when necessary.

The Child with Altered Mental Status

The likelihood of any cause for altered mental status in the child varies with age. In the toddler or infant, infection (central nervous system or systemic), dehydration, shock, and trauma are more common; in the older child drug ingestion, trauma, seizure, metabolic disorders, including diabetic ketoacidosis or Reye's syndrome, and brain tumor become more likely. Mental confusion, with normal blood pressure but other signs of shock, poor capillary refill, tachycardia, tachypnea, acidosis, and decreased urine output, and subtle abdominal findings, is an infrequent but potentially overlooked presentation of perforated appendix in this pediatric age group. Cerebral vascular accidents are uncommon but occur at any age; however, the entire range of differential diagnoses must be considered in each child who presents with altered mental status.

As with an adult patient with this problem, the vital signs, airway, breathing, circulation, and vascular access need to be assessed and stabilized rapidly. Although their application may be more limited in the pediatric population, the standard therapy of dextrose, 0.5 gm/kg, and naloxone, 0.01 mg/kg, should be considered. The neurologic examination should include assessment of the fontanel turgor and the presence/absence of meningism, a fundoscopic examination, assessment of the level of coma using the Glascow Coma Scale where applicable, and brainstem function (extraocular eye movements, gag and corneal reflexes, and assessment of any focal defect on motor examination).

Laboratory studies should include a toxicology screen, Dextrostix test and serum glucose, electrolytes, blood gases, and serum ammonium or liver function tests. If there is concern for intracranial trauma, mass, or pressure, a CT scan will be far more productive than a skull film. Beyond initial stabilization, treatment should be aimed at managing increased intracranial pressure if the history or examination point to trauma or Reye's syndrome. In the febrile child with focal neurologic findings and suspicion of intracranial infection, waiting for CT scan results should not delay the appropriate antibiotic therapy, with or without spinal fluid results.

Appendix
A Pediatric Formulary: Dosage Schedule[a]

Resuscitation

Oxygen	100% O_2
Atropine	0.02 mg/kg i.m./i.v./ETT: maximum 1.0 mg
Bicarbonate	1–2 mEq/kg i.v.: repeat prn
Epinephrine	0.1 ml/kg (1:10,000) i.v./ETT/intracardiac
Calcium chloride	10 mg/kg elemental Ca^{++} i.v. slow push; 0.3 ml/kg $CaCl_2$ or 1.0 ml/kg calcium gluconate. Start with 1/3 dose
Glucose	1 gm/kg = 4 ml/kg $D_{25}W$ i.v. push
Lidocaine	1 mg/kg i.v. bolus, then 20–40 µgm/kg/min i.v. drip
Fluid bolus	10–20 ml/kg NS/LR/colloid i.v. push
Defibrillation	V Fib./V Tach. = 2 watt-sec/kg

Cardiovascular

Pressors	Dopamine	2–5 µgm/kg/min (renal effect); 5–20 µgm/kg/min (cardiac effect)
	Dobutamine	5–20 µgm/kg/min
	Isoproterenol (Isuprel)	0.1 µgm/kg/min starting dose; titrate increase, keep HR<200 BPM
	Epinephrine	0.1 µgm/kg/min i.v.; titrate increase
	Norepinephrine (Levophed)	0.1 µgm/kg/min i.v.; titrate increase
	Phenylephrine (Neo-Synephrine)	0.1 µgm/kg/min i.v.; titrate increase
Vasodilators	Tolazoline (Pristoline)	2 mg/kg i.v. push test dose, then 1–2 mg/kg/hr i.v. drip
	Nitroprusside (Nipride)	1 µgm/kg/min i.v.; titrate increase, monitor BP and cyanide levels
	Prostaglandin	0.1–0.2 µgm/kg/min i.v.
	Nitroglycerine	1 µgm/kg/min i.v.; titrate increase

Drug Drip Infusions

0.1 µgm/kg/min = 1 mg/100 ml @ 2/3 BW (kg) ml/hr
1.0 µgm/kg/min = 6 mg/100 ml @ BW (kg) ml/hr
5.0 µgm/kg/min = 30 mg/100 ml @ BW (kg) ml/hr
20 µgm/kg/min = 120 mg/100 ml @ BW (kg) ml/hr

Digoxin — TDD = premature 20 µgm/kg i.v.; full-term newborn 30–50 µgm/kg i.v.; <2 yr, 40–60 µgm/kg i.v. or 60–80 µgm/kg p.o.; >2 yr, 20–40 µgm/kg i.v. or 40–60 µgm/kg p.o. Give 1/2 TDD stat, then 1/4 dose q6–8hr × 2. Maintenance = 1/4 TDD ÷ q12hr

Antibiotics	**1st week of life**	**1–4 weeks**	**4+ weeks**
Ampicillin	100–200 mg/kg/d ÷ q12hr	200 mg/kg/d ÷ q8hr	200–300 mg/kg/d ÷ q4–6hr
Cefotaxime	100 mg/kg/d ÷ q12hr	150 mg/kg/d ÷ q6–8hr	200 mg/kg/d ÷ q6hr
Cefuroxime			200 mg/kg/d ÷ q6–8hr
Chloramphenicol[b]	....................not for neonate	....	75 mg/kg/d ÷ q6hr
Gentamicin[b,c]	5 mg/kg/d ÷ q12hr	5–7.5 mg/kg/d ÷ q8hr	6mg/kg/ ÷ q8hr
Nafcillin	50 mg/kg/d ÷ q12hr	100 mg/kg/d ÷ q6–8hr	200 mg/kg/d ÷ q4–6hr
Penicillin G	100,000 U/kg/d ÷ q12hr	200,000 U/kg/d ÷ q6–8hr	200,000–300,000 U/kg/d ÷ q4–6hr
Ticarcillin	150 mg/kg/d ÷ q12hr	200–300 mg/kg/d ÷ q6–8hr	300–400 mg/kg/d ÷ q4–6hr
Tobramycin[b]	4 mg/kg/d ÷ q12hr	6 mg/kg/d ÷ q8hr	6 mg/kg/d ÷ q8hr
Vancomycin[b]	20–30 mg/kg/d ÷ q12hr	30–45 mg/kg/d ÷ q8hr	30–45 mg/kg/d ÷ q8hr

Anticonvulsants

Phenobarbital	10 mg/kg i.v. load × 2; maintenance 5 mg/kg/d ÷ bid; therapeutic level 20–40 µgm/ml
Phenytoin (Dilantin)	10 mg/kg i.v. slow load × 2; maintenance 5 mg/kg/d ÷ bid; therapeutic level 15–30 µgm/ml

Appendix—*continued*

Diazepam (Valium)	0.1–0.3 mg/kg i.v. **slow**; contraindicated in hyperbilirubinemia
Paraldehyde	300 mg (0.3 ml)/kg PR; 150 mg (0.15 ml)/kg i.v.; maximum dose 8 ml
Pyridoxine	50 mg i.v. (for neonate)
Antihypertensives	
Hydralazine	0.1–0.2 mg/kg/dose i.m./i.v. q4–6hr
Diazoxide (Hyperstat)	5 mg/kg/dose rapid i.v. push
Nitroprusside (Nipride)	1 μgm/kg/min; titrate increase to effect. Monitor BP and cyanide levels
Propranolol	0.05–0.1 mg/kg/dose i.v.; maximum single dose = 10 mg
Muscle Relaxants	
Curare	0.5 mg/kg/dose i.v., repeat prn with ½ dose
Pancuronium (Pavulon)	0.1 mg/kg/dose i.v., repeat prn with ½ dose
Metacurine (Metubine)	0.25 mg/kg/dose i.v., repeat prn with ½ dose
Succinylcholine (Anectine)	$<$1 yr, 2 mg/kg dose i.v.; $>$1 yr, 1 mg/kg/dose i.v.; 5 mg/kg/dose i.m.
Reversal	
Atropine	0.02 mg/kg i.v.
Prostigmine	0.06 mg/kg i.v. (*always* precede with atropine)
Analgesics/Narcotics	
Aspirin/acetaminophen	10 mg/kg/dose
Meperidine (Demerol)	1 mg/kg/dose i.m./i.v. q2–4hr
Morphine	0.1 mg/kg/dose i.m./i.v./s.c. q2–4hr
Fentanyl	5–10 μgm/kg/dose i.v. q2–3hr; 5–40 μgm/kg/hr i.v. drip
Reversal	
Naloxone (Narcan)	0.01 mg/kg/dose, repeat prn
Sedatives/Anesthetics	
Benadryl	0.25–0.5 mg/kg/dose i.v. q4–6hr or 5 mg/kg/d ÷ q6hr p.o.
Chloral hydrate	10–30 mg/kg/dose p.o./p.r. q4–8hr; maximum 100 mg/kg/d
Phenobarbital	10 mg/kg i.v. load × 2; maintenance 5 mg/kg/d ÷ b.i.d.; level 20–40 μgm/ml
Pentobarbital (Nembutal)	2 mg/kg dose i.v. "Barb Coma" - load 5–10 mg/kg i.v.; maintenance 1–2 mg/kg/hr i.v. drip
Methohexital (Brevital)	1.0 mg/kg of 1% solution i.v.; 20 mg/kg 10% solution p.r.
Pentothal (thiopental)	3–5 mg/kg of 2.5% solution i.v.
Asthma/Anaphylaxis	
Epinephrine	0.01 ml/kg (1:1000) s.c.; maximum 0.5 ml
Sus-Phrine	0.005 ml/kg s.c.; maximum 0.15 ml
Aminophylline	5–7 mg/kg i.v. bolus over 20 min; repeat q6hr or follow by infusion 0.9–1.4 mg/kg/hr; therapeutic level 10–20 μgm/ml
Isoproterenol (Isuprel)	0.1 μgm/kg/min i.v. increase to effect, keep HR $<$ 200 BPM
Bronkosol/Isoproterenol	0.25–0.5 ml in 2.5 ml saline by nebulizer
Metaproterenol (Alupent)	0.2–0.3 ml in 2.5 ml saline by nebulizer
Diuretics	
Furosemide (Lasix)	1–2 mg/kg/dose p.o./i.m./i.v.
Aldactone	2–3.5 mg/kg/d p.o. ÷ q6–12hr
Diuril	20–30 mg/kg/d p.o. ÷ q12hr
Mannitol	0.25–1.0 gm/kg/dose; repeat q2–4hr

Steroids	**Standard Doses**	**Shock Doses**
Prednisone	2 mg/kg/d	
Dexamethasone (Decadron)	0.3–1.0 mg/kg/dose q8hr	10 × standard dose
Hydrocortisone (Solu-Cortef)	10 mg/kg/d ÷ q4–6hr	10 × standard dose
Methylprednisolone (Solu-Medrol)	1 mg/kg/dose q6hr	10 × standard dose

Appendix—*continued*

Intoxications	
Ipecac	<1 year, 10 ml; 1–12 years, 15 ml; >12 years, 30 ml; repeat × 1 after 20 minutes
Activated charcoal	1 gm/kg
Magnesium citrate	4 ml/kg/day

[a] This Appendix is a formulary of commonly used emergency pediatric drugs. Drugs for cardiac resuscitation are specifically reviewed in Chapter 21. ETT, endotracheal tube; PRN, as necessary; $D_{25}W$, 25% dextrose in water; NS, normal saline solution; LR, lactated Ringer's solution; BPM, beats per minute; HR, heart rate; BP, blood pressure; BW, body weight; TDD, total daily dose; U, units; p.r., per rectum.

[b] Monitoring blood levels required.

[c] <34 weeks, 2.5 mg/kg/dose q18hr. <30 weeks, 2.5 mg/kg/dose q24hr.

SUGGESTED READINGS

Green M. *Pediatric Diagnosis.* 4th ed. Philadelphia: WB Saunders, 1986.

Illingsworth RS. Common Symptoms of Disease in Children. London: Blackwell Scientific Publications, 1979.

McCarthy PL, Sharpe MR, Spiesel SZ et al. Observation scales to identify serious illness in febrile children. *Pediatrics,* 1982;70:802–809.

CHAPTER 21

Pediatric Cardiopulmonary Resuscitation

PATRICIA J. O'MALLEY, M.D.
I. DAVID TODRES, M.D.

This chapter reviews pediatric resuscitation as needed in the emergency department. Newborn resuscitation, in the delivery room or the emergency department, is reviewed in Chapter 22. Although the principles of pediatric resuscitation parallel those of adult resuscitation, important differences in etiology, pathophysiology, and in age-related technical difficulties, make the infrequent pediatric resuscitation a most challenging problem. The similarities and differences between adult and pediatric resuscitation are reviewed and strategies for dealing with practical difficulties presented.

DIFFERENCES BETWEEN ADULT AND PEDIATRIC RESUSCITATION

Etiology

The most striking difference between adult and pediatric resuscitation is in the *etiology* of cardiopulmonary arrest. In the 1st month of life congenital anomalies, infection, and metabolic diseases are the problems most likely to bring an infant critically ill or in cardiopulmonary arrest to the emergency department. Sudden Infant Death Syndrome (SIDS) is the commonest cause of death in the 1st year of life. Along with trauma, infection, and respiratory obstruction, SIDS is a problem most likely to be encountered in the emergency department. Trauma, inflicted or accidental, is an important cause of cardiopulmonary arrest throughout the pediatric and young adult years. Unlike the adult, the pediatric patient has a primary cardiac dysfunction as cause of cardiopulmonary arrest less than 10% percent of the time. The commonest pathophysiologic pathway for the pediatric arrest, in over 60% of the cases, is a primary respiratory insufficiency leading to hypoxemia, hypercarbia, and bradyarrhythmia or asystole. Hypovolemia (from dehydration, hemorrhage, or septic shock), leading to acidosis, respiratory insufficiency, hypotension and then to bradyarrhythmias or asystole, is a primary factor in another 30% of cases. Even where a cardiac dysrhythmia is the apparent initial cause, underlying metabolic derangements such as acidosis, hyper- or hypokalemia, or hypocalcemia will frequently be found rather than a primary cardiac pathology.

Differences

There are important lessons to learn from these differences in etiology and pathophysiology. First of all, pediatric arrest can frequently be *anticipated* in the patient with progressive respiratory insufficiency, inadequate perfusion, or severe acidosis. When anticipated, arrest can often be *prevented* by early respiratory and intravascular volume support and metabolic correction. Arrhythmia management directed at cardiac causes is frequently of secondary importance. Finally, understanding these differences may improve the relatively poor outcome of most pediatric arrests. Recent studies have documented from 70 to 90% mortality for out of hospital pediatric cardiopulmonary arrest.

A second important differences between adult and pediatric arrest is that *age- and weight-related differences* among pediatric patients necessitate understanding per kilogram dosage schedules and size choices of airway equipment, intravenous site and equipment, ventilation, and fluid support. Although nonpediatricians find this aspect of pediatric care intimidating, there are simple strategies to minimize these difficulties, some of which are discussed in this chapter.

A third important difference is the relative *infrequency* with which pediatric arrests occur. In the Massachusetts General Hospital Emergency Department there are two to three adult arrest patients per day and perhaps one pediatric arrest per month. This paucity of cardiopulmonary arrest means that principles not frequently put into practice are at risk of being forgotten. Because of this, it is strongly urged that every emergency department caring for children use regular "mock code" practice sessions that not only allow staff to rehearse and to retain training, but also may uncover deficiencies in the resuscitation system correctable prior to actual need.

PRINCIPLES OF PEDIATRIC RESUSCITATION

Reviewing pediatric resuscitation along the ABC (airway, breathing, cardiac compressions) principles of adult resuscitation highlights the differences and similarities.

Airway

Airway management is vital in the pediatric patient and since many pediatric "arrests" are respiratory arrests only, without actual loss of cardiac function, securing the airway to provide oxygenation and ventilation may be all that is required to save a life. Although endotracheal intubation is the most secure way of providing airway control, the pediatric patient can often be easily managed for a long period of time with bag and mask ventilation alone, particularly if care is taken to vent the stomach of air. Bag and mask ventilation with 100% oxygen and *a clear airway* for 1–2 minutes should precede any intubation attempt.

In airway management of any compromised pediatric patient, *arrested or not,* the first step is to provide the optimal airway position. The pediatric airway is smaller in caliber than in the adult, more anterior in position, with softer cartilage and with a tongue relatively large for the size of the oropharynx. Because of these differences, the "sniffing position," with slight flexion of the neck and extension of the head, is the optimal position for maintaining the airway (see Fig. 21.1). This position is helpful for the obtunded but spontaneously breathing patient, for bag and mask or mouth-to-mouth ventilation, and for intubation. After airway positioning, it is mandatory to lift the tongue clear of the posterior pharyngeal wall by pulling the mandible up with the chin lift maneuver or pushing the mandible forward at the angles (see Fig. 21.2).

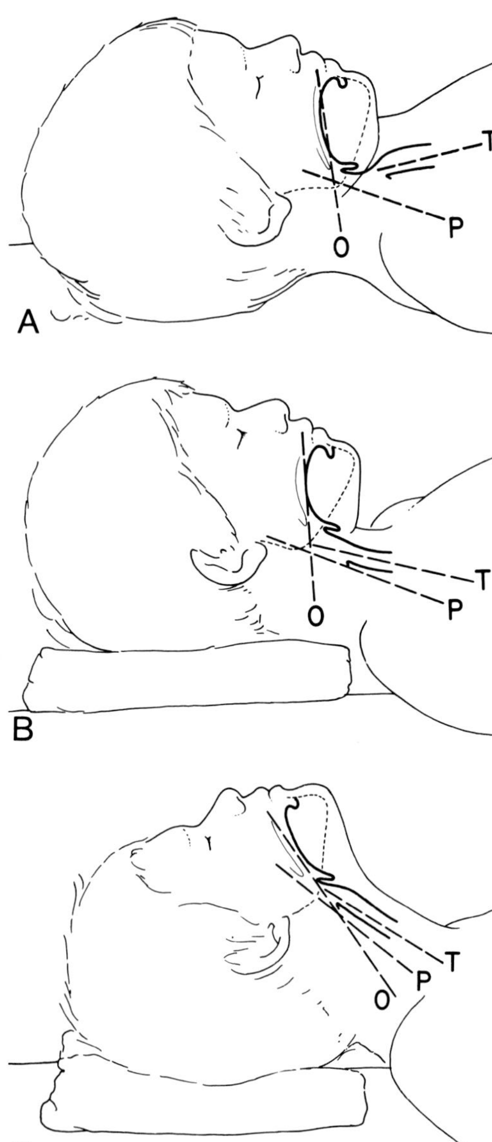

Figure 21.1. Position for tracheal intubation. Oral (*O*), pharyngeal (*P*), and tracheal (*T*) axes (*A*) are aligned through flexion of the neck (*B*) and extension of the head (*C*).

The ideal pediatric face mask has a clear, soft, inflatable rim which frequently gives the best fit. This mask should be applied first over the nose and then the face lifted into the mask by supporting the jaw with the last two or three fingers of the left hand, applying the mask to the face with a squeezing or pincer grip between the thumb and index finger. *Lifting* the face into the mask insures that the sniffing position and mandible thrust are maintained as the mask is applied. At times an oropharyngeal airway is necessary in addition to the chin-lift maneuvers (see Fig. 21.3). If prolonged bag and mask management is anticipated, such as after unsuccessful intubation attempts, then passage of a decompressing gastric tube and firm pressure over the

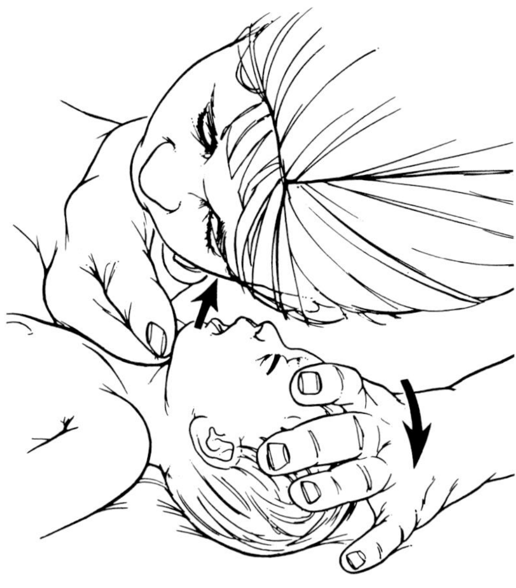

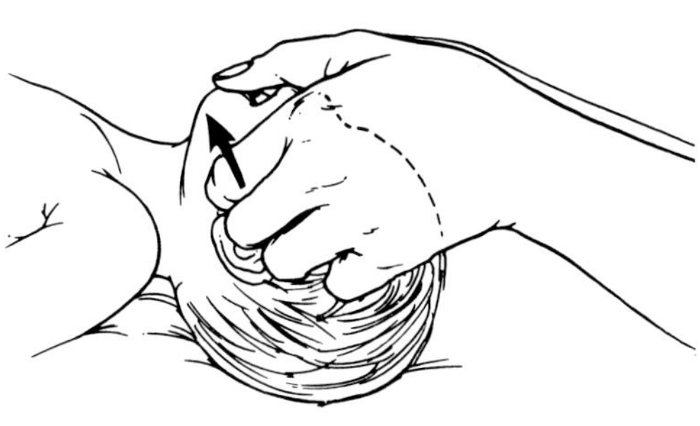

Figure 21.2. Determination of whether the child is breathing. (From Standards and guidelines for cardiopulmonary resuscitation (CPR) and emergency cardiac care (ECC). *JAMA* 1986;255:2905–2989

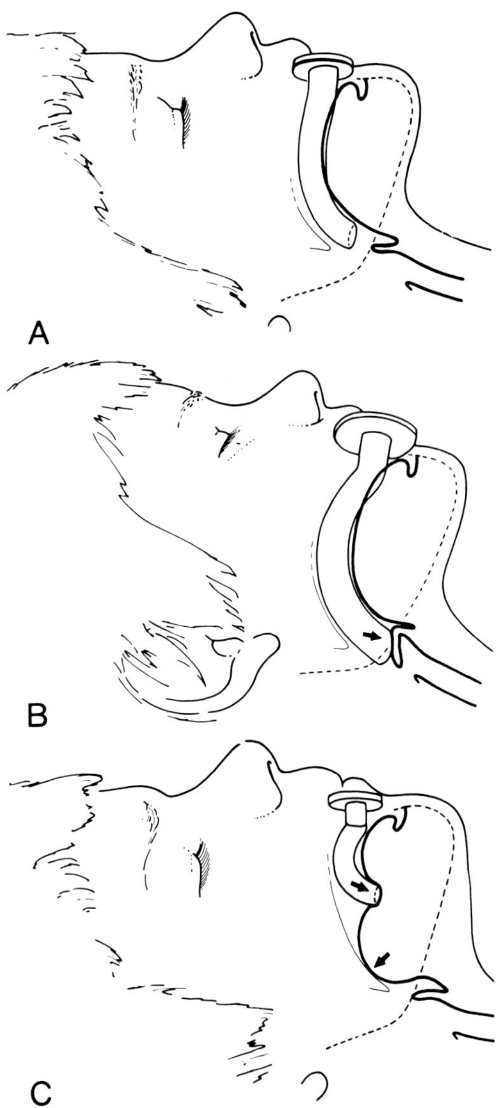

Figure 21.3. Oropharyngeal tube placement. (*A*) Proper length and placement, over tongue and above epiglottis. (*B*) Overly long tube abuts epiglottis. (*C*) Short tube abuts tongue and aggravates airway obstruction by base of tongue.

cricothyroid cartilage (Sellick's maneuver) minimize gastric and abdominal distention. This, in turn, means better diaphragmatic excursion with ventilation and a decreased risk of aspiration of stomach contents. Tracheal intubation provides the optimal route for suctioning secretions and blood, and avoiding gastric distention. The appropriate equipment for intubation should be assembled beforehand; the mnemonic SOAP may be helpful in

Table 21.1.
SOAP Mnemonic for Assembling Intubation Equipment

Suction—(tonsil tip, flexible oral, endotracheal, and gastric suction catheters)
Oxygen source
Airway equipment—(bag and mask, oral airway, endotracheal tubes and laryngoscope with blade of correct size, stylet, tape, benzoin, and stethoscope)
Pharmacopeia–(atropine, other resuscitation medicines, succinycholine, rapidly acting sedative if paralysis is necessary)

Table 21.3.
Strategies for Determining Proper Endotracheal Tube Size for Age[a]

Age	Internal Diameter
	mm
Premature	2.5
Term	3.0–3.5
<1 year	3.5–4.0
1–2 years	4.0–4.5
>2 years	(age in years + 16)/4

[a] "Rule of thumb and little finger" endotracheal tube (ETT) size falls between size of the child's thumb and little finger.

remembering the necessary equipment (Table 21.1). Suggested laryngoscope blade sizes for age and strategies for determining the proper endotracheal tube size for age are listed in Table 21.2 and 21.3, respectively.

There is controversy concerning the safest and most effective emergency maneuvers for the child with airway obstruction from a foreign body. Although there is no concensus, the recent American Heart Association Standards and Guidelines for Cardiopulmonary Resuscitation (CPR) recommends back blows and chest thrusts for infants less than 1 year of age and the Heimlich maneuver beyond 1 year of age. In the emergency department when a pediatric patient is suspected by history of having a foreign body or when adequate bag and mask ventilation is not possible, the first attempt at resuscitation should involve direct laryngoscopy, visualization, and removal of the foreign body with Magill forceps before proceeding to the sequence of back blows and chest thrusts. *a*) With the patient positioned prone and head down, along the rescuer's arm or knee, four blows are delivered to the interscapular area. *b*) If the airway is still obstructed, the patient is repositioned supine along the rescuer's arm or on the floor, or stretcher as for external cardiac compression, and four chest thrusts done in the same manner as a cardiac compression are delivered. *c*) Using the jaw thrust, the mouth is inspected and a foreign body removed if seen. *d*) If obstruction persists, mouth-to-mouth, mouth-to-nose, or bag and mask ventilation is attempted. This sequence may be repeated by the first responder in the field. However, in the emergency department, in the child who cannot be intubated, cannot be managed by bag and mask ventilation or mouth-to-mouth ventilation, and is not spontaneously breathing, needle cricothyrotomy is the recommended technique for obtaining emergency transcervical airway in the pediatric patient. This technique is described in Illustrated Technique 4. The emergency physician should practice locating the necessary landmarks for needle cricothyrotomy on healthy children because they are often difficult to appreciate in the prepubertal child.

The technique of laryngoscopy and intubation in the pediatric patient is similar to that performed in the adult, although the equipment will necessarily be different. Three maneuvers may be particularly helpful to the intubating physician and can be performed by an assistant (Table 21.4). (*a*) Insure that the sniffing position with slight flexion of the neck and extension of the head is maintained to permit optimal visualization of the larynx. (*b*) Offer cricothyroid pressure in an attempt to lower the anterior airway into the field of vision. (*c*) Apply traction on the right corner of the mouth to enlarge the field of vision as the laryngoscope is used to visualize the larynx. The endotracheal tube is inserted into the right side of the mouth and guided through the cords under direct visualization. The tip of the tube is passed only 1–2 centimeters beyond the cords in infants and 3–4 centimeters in children.

The best sign that the endotracheal tube is in good position is improvement in the patient's condition. Adequate and symmetric chest movements should

Table 21.2.
Laryngoscope Blade Sizes for Age

Miller 0	Premature/term infant
Miller 1	Term to 4 years
Miller 2	4 to 8 years
Macintosh 3	8 years to adolescent

Table 21.4.
Assistance in Intubation

Maintain sniffing position
Offer cricothyroid pressure
Apply traction to the right corner of oral cavity
Grip tube and soft palate to stabilize tube after intubation

Table 21.5.
Cardiac Compression and Ventilation Rates

Age	Compressions	Respirations	Ratio
Newborn	120/min	40	3:1
Infant	100/min, 1, 2, 3, 4, etc.	20	5:1
Child	80/min, 1 & 2 & 3 & 4 &, etc.	16	5:1
Adult	60/min, one thousand 1, one thousand 2, one thousand 3, etc.	12	5:1

be confirmed as breath sounds may be difficult to interpret, especially in young infants and small children. This is carried out by auscultating laterally and toward the axilla on each side. The commonest complications of endotracheal intubation in the pediatric patient are hypoxia during the procedure, aspiration, esophageal intubation, and bronchial intubation. Continuous monitoring of the airway is essential to avoid later accidental and undetected extubation. Therefore, the person responsible for airway management should not only secure the endotracheal tube once in good position with adequate benzoin and tape, but should also maintain a simultaneous grip on the tube and soft palate of the child at all times during the resuscitation effort.

Breathing

Recent studies of the effect of simultaneous ventilation and cardiac compression and abdominal binding during cardiopulmonary resuscitation in adults cannot be extrapolated to pediatric patients. The current recommendations in the pediatric patient are to maintain a ''programmed'' breath, allowing a pause between cardiac compressions to give sufficient time for adequate ventilation. The recommended ratio of cardiac compressions to breaths for pediatric patients is 5:1 except in newborns, (Table 21.5); however,the pediatric patient may benefit from early hyperventilation. Subsequent respiratory rates should be guided by blood gas determinations. Increased ventilating pressures may be necessary for an endotracheal tube that is too small for an obstruction to the airway, for the drowning victim, or for severe alveolar collapse. An in-line manometer is recommended in the management of all intubated pediatric patients to avoid overexpansion and the risk of pneumothorax. However, bilateral symmetrical chest excursion is the primary aim and the manometer is used as an indicator of poor airway compliance or high airway resistance to help titrate the inspiratory pressures necessary for adequate ventilation. As stressed in the airway section, continuous monitoring of airway management in terms of patient improvement, symmetrical chest movements, and symmetrical breath sounds is necessary throughout the pediatric resuscitation.

Circulation

Cardiac compressions to maintain circulation are initiated in the pediatric patient when there is no palpable pulse or when the heart rate is steadily dropping below a rate of *50*. The pulse is best palpated at the brachial or axillary arteries, and the precordial impulse should not be used; it is not reliable in determining effective circulation. Chest compression technique varies with the size of the patient but all methods require that the patient be on a hard surface, except for the technique in small infants of encircling the chest (see Fig. 21.4). The operator compresses the chest approximately one-quarter of the anterior-posterior diameter of the chest at a point one finger breadth below the nipple line, using both encircling thumbs or two fingers—one or two hands depending on the size of the patient. The rate of compressions and ventilations per minute according to age is listed in Table 21.5.

Access to the circulation for drug and volume support can be difficult in the pediatric patient. Fortunately, two of the three drugs most commonly used, epinephrine and atropine, may be given via the endotracheal tube. The third, sodium bicarbonate, *cannot* be given this way, but the inability to administer bicarbonate via the endotracheal tube can be compensated by hyperventilating the patient.

Valuable time can be wasted in an arrest in attempting to place a large secure catheter intravenously. A ''butterfly i.v.'' needle may be an appropriate means of gaining initial intravenous access. Although not a stable line, the butterfly i.v. can be quickly placed in a surface vein on the back of the hand or foot and give rapid access for initial drug and volume support. This then facilitates obtaining more secure access elsewhere.

The optimal sites for a large bore intravenous catheter, placed either percutaneously or via cutdown, are the femoral vein, the basilic vein, and the internal jugular vein. The subclavian vein may also be used; however, this site has the highest complication rate, even in experienced hands. The tech-

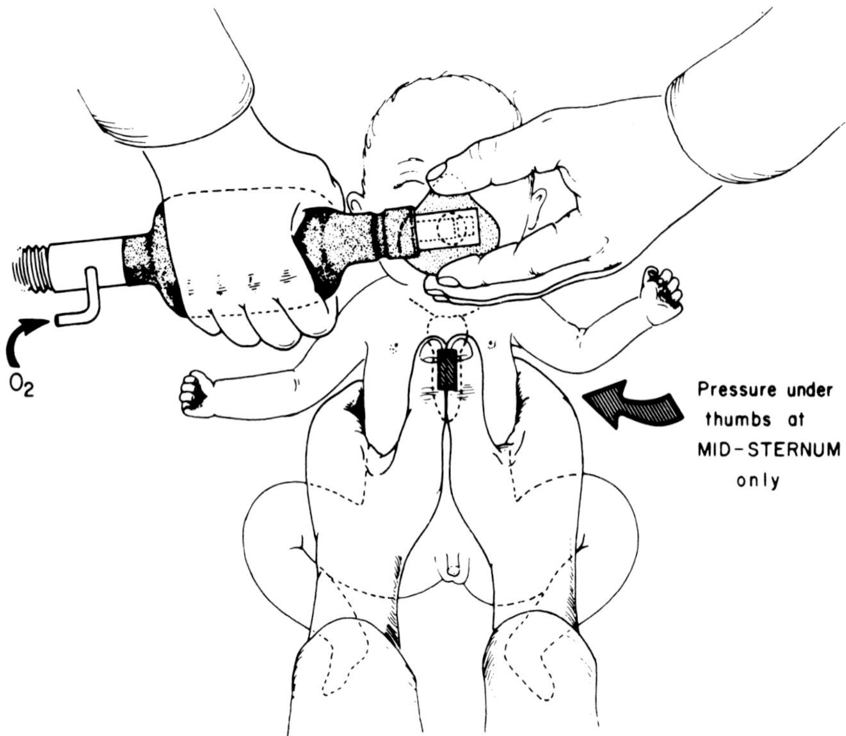

Figure 21.4. Chest encircling method for cardiac compression of the neonate. Note: Pressure under thumbs at a point one finger's breath below nipple line. (Modified after Todres ID, Rogers MC. Methods of external cardiac massage in the newborn infant. *J Pediatr* 1975;86:781–782.)

nique for intravenous placement in these sites is described in Illustrated Techniques 5, 6, and 7. The external jugular vein, although frequently easily visualized, is an unstable and capricious vein for peripheral intravenous placement. It may be used to gain access to the central circulation. The Seldinger technique of intravenous catheter placement using a catheter over a guide wire, passed through an initial small introducer needle, is ideal for small pediatric veins and is preferable to the catheter-through-a-needle technique. Ideally, vascular access can be obtained within 5 minutes; Figure 21.5 displays a protocol for vascular access that may aid in achieving this goal.

In the event that vascular access is not possible through percutaneous or cutdown techniques, when fluid and pressor support is vital, interosseus bone marrow infusion of fluid and vaspressor infusions is possible. This simple technique (see Fig. 21.6) was common in the 1920–1940 era and has recently enjoyed new publicity in the pediatric literature. More widespread use undoubtedly will result in increased awareness of potential complications, including infection, embolic phenomena, and bony defects; at this time, therefore, it cannot be recommended as a first line vascular access technique but rather a simple technique to be employed if standard vascular access is not successful within a short period of time.

Drugs/Defibrillation

The weight-adjusted dosages and indications of drugs and defibrillation are listed in Table 21.6. A frustrating aspect of pediatric resuscitation for nonpediatricians is the difficulty of remembering and accurately calculating the appropriate drug dosages. Every emergency care facility with pediatric patients should develop a strategy for dealing with this problem. A per kilogram dosage chart should be clearly posted in the resuscitation room. If pediatric arrests are common, it may be worthwhile to set up a resuscitation cart with different drawers for representative ages or weights, containing the proper-sized airway equipment, blood pressure cuff, intravenous catheters, and drug dosages. A less expensive alternative is a booklet or index card of advanced cardiac life support (ACLS) worksheets, such as pictured in Table 21.6 with calculations for

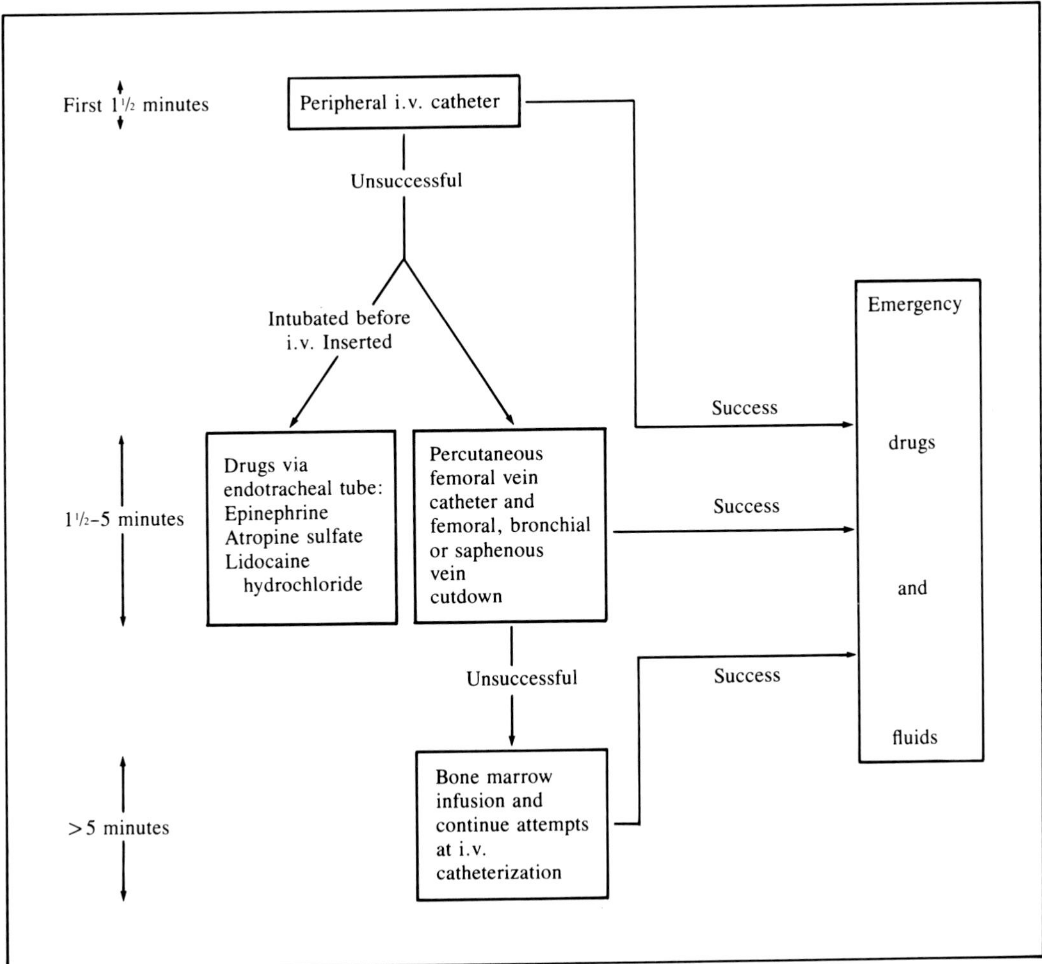

Figure 21.5. Protocol for emergency intravenous (i.v.) access during pediatric resuscitations. (Modified from Kanter RK, Zimmerman JJ, Strauss RH, et al. Pediatric emergency intravenous access. *Am J Dis Child,* 1986;140:132–134.)

representative weights or ages. In the event of a pediatric arrest, weight is estimated (Table 21.7) and the precalculated sheet appropriate to that weight is utilized by the staff person drawing up medications. The Massachusetts General Hospital pediatric worksheet includes endotracheal tube size, bolus drug dosages, continuous infusion recipes and rates, defibrillation dosages, fluid bolus amounts, and an estimate of total circulating blood volumes.

The recognition and management of dysrhythmia in the arrested pediatric patient is usually simple compared with the adult cardiac arrest patient. The algorithm pictured in Figure 21.7 should be reviewed. Oxygenation, acid-base balance, intravascular volume status, and vasopressor support are much more likely to be important to the outcome than is defibrillation, lidocaine, pacemakers, or specific antiarrhythmic treatment. Producing adequate cardiac output and tissue perfusion, whether the pulse is slow or fast, is more important than the precise arrhythmia diagnosed at the time of the arrest. In any pediatric arrest, if resuscitative efforts are not successful in obtaining a recognizable electrocardiographic complex or a cardiac output, review of oxygenation, ventilation, acid-base balance, and volume status must be undertaken, and the possibility of obstruction to cardiac output, such as pneumothorax or pericardial effusion, considered. Electromechanical dissociation, in the absence of any of these factors, is rare in the pediatric patient with arrest.

Environmental Factors

A concern particularly pertinent to the pediatric patient, rarely considered in the adult with arrest, is relative hypothermia due to environmental loss of

Table 21.6.
Pediatric Cardiopulmonary Resuscitation Sheet[a]

Weight ____ Endotracheal tube size ____ Laryngoscope blade size ____	Endotracheal suction catheter size ____ Estimated blood volume (80 ml/kg) ____
Atropine (0.4 mg/ml)	0.02 mg/kg = ____ mg = ____ ml (maximum 0.5 mg, single dose)
Bicarbonate (1 mEq/ml, child) (0.5 mEq/ml, infant)	1 mEq/kg = ____ mEq = ____ ml (child) 0.5 mEq/kg = ____ mEq = ____ ml (infant)
Calcium chloride (27 mg elemental Ca^{++}/ml)	0.15 ml/kg = ____ ml
Dextrose (25% = 0.25 gm/ml)	0.5 gm/kg = ____ gm = ____ ml (child) 0.25 gm/kg = ____ gm = ____ ml (infant)
Epinephrine (1:10,000)	0.1 ml/kg = ____ ml (maximum 5 ml, single dose)
Lidocaine (100 mg/5 ml)	1 mg/kg = ____ mg = ____ ml
Isotonic fluid bolus (Lactated Ringer's or normal saline)	10–20 ml/kg/bolus = ____ ml
Maintenance fluid infusion	4 ml/kg/hr for 0–10 kg plus = ____ ml/hr 2 ml/kg/hr for 10–20 kg plus = ____ ml/hr 1 ml/kg/hr for over 20 kg = ____ ml/hr
Dopamine infusion (40 or 80 mg/ml vials)	Standard mixture 6 × body weight = ____ mg in D_5W to 100 ml 5 μg/kg/min = 5 ml/hr 10 μg/kg/min = 10 ml/hr 20 μg/kg/min = 20 ml/hr[b]
Epinephrine infusion	Standard mixture 0.6 × body weight = ____ mg in D_5W to 100 ml 0.1 μg/kg/min = 1 ml/hr 0.5 μg/kg/min = 5 ml/hr
Isoproterenol infusion	Standard mixture 0.6 × body weight = ____ mg in D_5W to 100 ml 0.1 μg/kg/min = 1 ml/hr 0.5 μg/kg/min = 5 ml/hr
Lidocaine infusion	Standard mixture 6 × body weight = ____ mg in D_5W to 100 ml 20 μg/kg/min = 20 ml/hr[b] 50 μg/kg/min = 50 ml/hr[b]
Defibrillation	2–4 joules/kg = ____ joules
Physician's signature ____________ Nurse's signature ____________ Date ____________	

[a] This standard sheet can be precalculated as part of a booklet of representative weights from 0 to 50 kg. Care must be taken, when adapting this sheet to any particular setting, that the drug solutions and concentrations (which may not be standard) are correct for the particular preparation available at that site. D_5W, 5% dextrose in water.

[b] In infants and small children a sustained infusion at this rate may represent an excessive fluid load if continued over several hours; the solution should therefore be reconstituted in a more concentrated form if it is to be used for longer than 20–30 minutes.

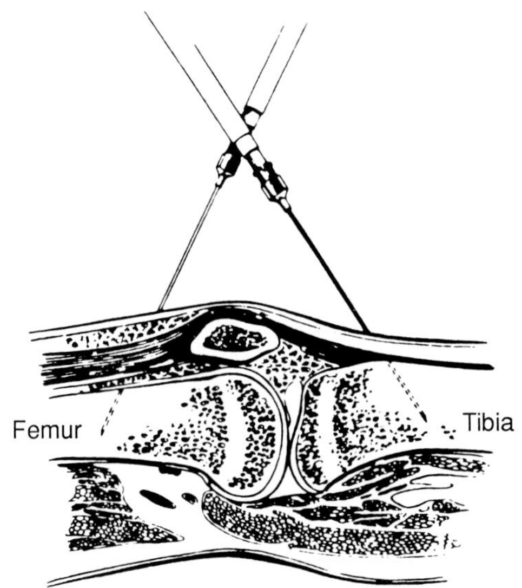

Figure 21.6. Needle placement for intraosseous infusion. (From Rossetti V, Thompson BM, Miller J, et al. Intraosseous infusion: an alternative route of pediatric intravenous access. *Ann Emerg Med,* 1985;14:885–888.)

body heat. Because of a large surface area to mass ratio, the pediatric patient may rapidly become hypothermic when deprived of an adequate circulation, unclothed in a cool emergency department. Therefore, emergency department staff must pay attention to the maintenance of careful environmental control of the core temperature of the pediatric patient.

Fluid

Because hypovolemia and/or circulatory collapse is an important precipitating factor in pediatric arrest, volume and circulatory support are critical. Nevertheless, it is a common mistake either to overhydrate or underhydrate the pediatric patient. A volume push is rarely detrimental to an arrested pediatric patient, even if volume loss was not the precipitating factor; therefore, a bolus of 20 ml/kg of lactated Ringer's solution or normal saline is indicated for any arrested pediatric patient if hypovolemia cannot be excluded by history. Isotonic crystalloid solutions diffuse out of the vascular space into the interstitium, leaving only one-third of the salt solution in the vascular space. For this reason, if greater than 30 to 40 ml/kg is required for fluid resuscitation, it is advisable to begin administration of colloid in the same bolus amounts of 10 to 20 ml/kg. The total circulating blood volume in the pediatric patient is approximately 80 ml/kg; these figures can be used to guide the total amount of fluid administration. For example, the trauma victim may have lost nearly half his circulating blood volume; if an isotonic solution is used, he or she may require two or three times the 40 ml/kg blood loss that was sustained. The most rapid way of restoring the circulating blood volume by bolus administration is to draw the fluid into a 50–60-ml syringe and push it rapidly through the intravenous line. This causes no harm, so long as the solution is isotonic crystalloid or colloid. Five percent dextrose in water solution should never be used in a pediatric resuscitative effort because it is not an effective expander of intravascular space. In addition, particularly in infants, small amounts of dextrose/water solution may cause significant hyponatremia and disruption of cellular membranes.

Gastric Dilatation

Because the pediatric patient uses diaphragmatic muscles primarily to breathe, gastric dilatation can have significant consequences for ventilatory support. Whether from bag and mask ventilation or from the poorly understood gastric reflex reaction to stress, gastric dilatation should be anticipated and treated early in the pediatric arrest victim by placement of a naso- or orogastric tube (sizes 10–14 Fr) to vent the stomach. This optimizes attempts at ventilatory support and minimizes the risk of aspiration of stomach contents during the procedure.

Other Considerations

When a pediatric patient dies in the emergency department, autopsy is an important final step in the care of the patient. Unsuspected trauma, congenital anomalies, or infection may influence subsequent counseling and management of the family. Because a pediatric death is rarely anticipated, support for the family regardless of the cause of death is also an important part of care of the pediatric patient. If a child dies in the emergency department, the staff should take responsibility for long-term follow-up for the family by arranging for counseling if needed or desired and for review of autopsy results when they later become available.

Table 21.7.
Relationship of Age and Weight

Age	Weight
yr	*kg*
1	10
3	15
5	19
7	23

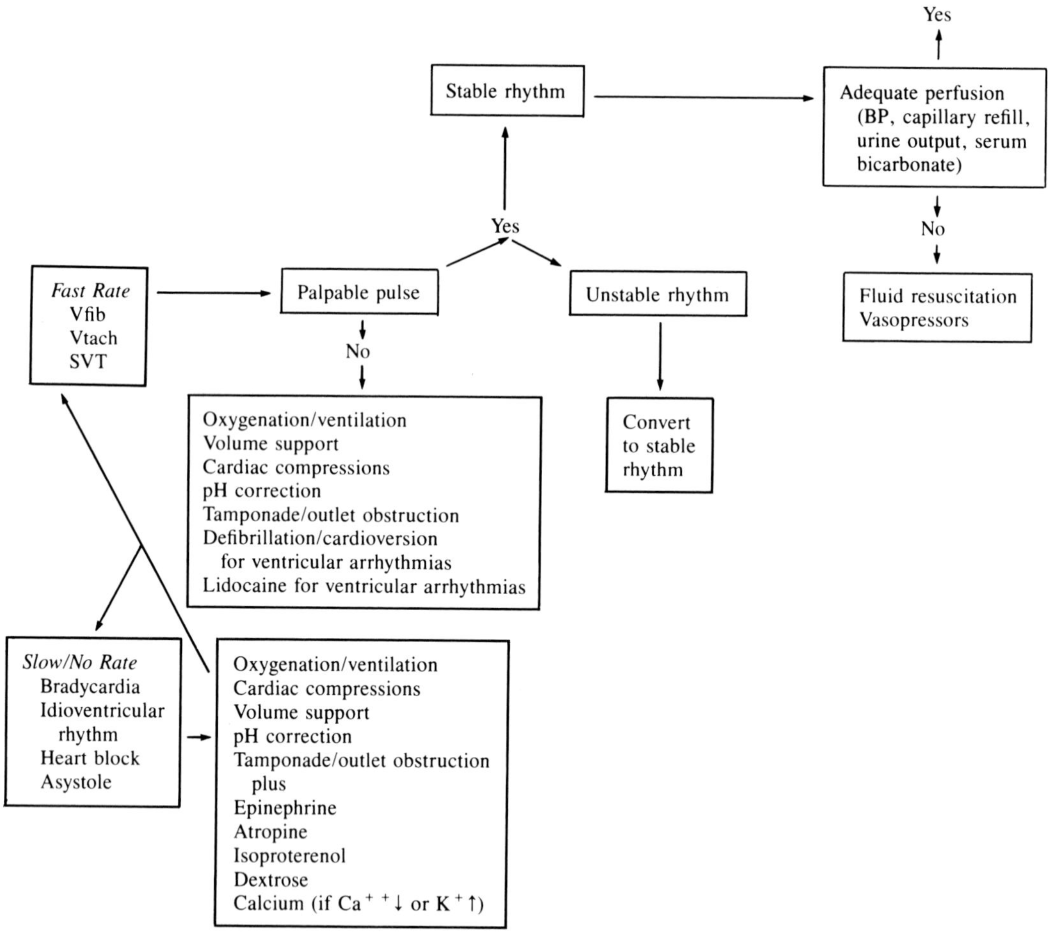

Figure 21.7. Algorithm for arrhythmia management in a pediatric cardiopulmonary resuscitation. *BP,* blood pressure; *Vfib,* ventricular fibrillation; *Vtach,* ventricular tachycardia; *SVT,* supraventricular tachycardia. (Read from *left* to *right.*)

SUGGESTED READINGS

Babbs CF: New versus old theories of blood flow during CPR. *Crit Care Med* 1980;8:191–196.

Berg RA: Emergency infusion of catecholamines into bone marrow. *Am J Dis Child,* 1984;138:810–811.

Cavallaro DL, Melker RJ: Comparison of two techniques for detecting cardiac activity in infants. *Crit Care Med* 1983;11:189–190.

Chernow B, Holbrook P, D'Angona DS Jr, et al: Epinephrine absorption after intratracheal administration. *Cum Res Anesth Analg* 1984;63:829–832.

Eisenberg M, Bergner L, Hallstrom A: Epidemiology of cardiac arrest and resuscitation in children. *Ann Emerg Med* 1983;12:672–674.

Graf H, Leach W, Arieff AI: Evidence for a detrimental effect of bicarbonate therapy in hypoxic lactic acidosis. *Science* 1985;227:754–756.

Harris CS, Baker SP, Smith GA, et al: Childhood asphyxiation by food: A national analysis and overview. *JAMA* 1984;251:2231–2235.

Hedges JR, Barsan WB, Doan LA, et al: Central versus peripheral intravenous routes in cardiopulmonary resuscitation. *Am J Emerg Med* 1984;2:385–390.

Kanter RK, Zimmerman JJ, Strauss RH, et al. Pediatric emergency intravenous access. *Am J Dis Child,* 1986;140:132–134.

Lewis JK, Minter MG, Eshelman SF, et al: Outcome of pediatric resuscitation. *Ann Emerg Med* 1983;12:297–299.

Ludwig S, Kettrick RG, Parker M. Pediatric cardiopulmonary resuscitation: a review of 130 cases. *Clin Pediatr,* 1984;23:71–75.

Melker RJ. Asynchronous and other alternative methods of ventilation during CPR. *Ann Emerg Med,* 1984;13:758–761.

Orlowski JP: Optimal position for external cardiac massage in infants and children. *Crit Care Med* 1984;12:224.

O'Rourke, PP: Outcome of children who are apneic and pulseless in the emergency room. *Crit Care Med* 1986;14:466–468.

Rossetti V, Thompson BM, Aprahamian C, et al: Difficulty and delay in intravascular access in pediatric arrests. *Ann Emerg Med* 1984;13:406.

Rudikoff MT, Maughan WL, Effron M, et al: Mechanism of

blood flow during cardiopulmonary resuscitation. *Circulation* 1980;61:345–352.

Spivey WH, Lathers CM, Malone DR, et al: Comparison of intraosseous, central, and peripheral routes of sodium bicarbonate administration during CPR in pigs. *Ann Emerg Med* 1985;14:1135–1140.

Steuven HA, Thompson B, Aprahamian C, et al. The effectiveness of calcium chloride in refractory electromechanical dissociation. *Ann Emerg Med,* 1985;14:626–629.

Todres ID, Rogers MC: Methods of external cardiac massage in the newborn infant. *J Pediatr* 1975;86:781–782.

Torphy DE, Minter MG, Thompson BM: Cardiorespiratory arrest and resuscitation of children. *Am J Dis Child,* 1984;138:1099–1102.

Ward JT Jr: Endotracheal drug therapy. *Am J Emerg Med* 1983;1:71–82.

Zaritsky A, Chernow B: Use of catecholamines in pediatrics. *J Pediatr* 1984;105-341–350.

CHAPTER **22**

Neonatal Emergencies

ELIZABETH A. CATLIN, M.D.

The emergency department intermittently doubles as a delivery room (DR) and therefore equipment and personnel must be rapidly mobilized for such an event. This chapter reviews management of the normal term delivery, neonatal resuscitation in specific emergency situations, emergency department care of fetal demise, and preparation for neonatal transport.

NORMAL TERM DELIVERY

For an imminent delivery the equipment detailed in Table 22.1 should be assembled.

Cord Clamping and Resuscitation

Once the infant's body is delivered it should be held approximately at the level of the introitus or slightly below and the cord clamped 1 minute after initiation of respirations. Be sure to leave at least 6 cm of cord when clamping and cutting for vascular access in the event of particular need. Each newborn's blood volume varies with the volume of blood transferred from the placenta at birth. Immediate clamping of the cord results in a decrease in blood volume to 70–80 ml/kg (instead of 85–90 ml/kg obtained with clamping 1 minute after initiation of breathing). Following clamping and cutting of the umbilical cord, the newborn infant should be systematically *assessed* and *resuscitated* (Tables 22.2 and 22.3).

Airway Management

Bag and mask ventilation is the starting point in resuscitation of the apneic or ineffectively ventilating newborn. The face mask must cover the nose and mouth without a leak. An anesthesia bag (half-liter, Mapleson) with an in-line manometer provides precise control of inflating pressures and positive end-expiratory pressure (PEEP). If the self-inflating bags are used, the pop-off valve should be set at 40 cm H_2O. While specific treatment must be individualized for each baby, inflating pressures of 25 cm H_2O in preterm babies and 30 cm H_2O in term babies are reasonable initial values at rates of 30–40 breaths per minute (BPM) in premature infants and 20–30 BPM in term babies. It cannot be overemphasized that, particularly following delivery, the infant's airway *must be cleared/suctioned* prior to initiating artificial ventilation.

If endotracheal intubation is indicated, the infant should be positioned with his or her chin up and nose in the so-called sniffing position. Care should be taken not to overextend the newborn's neck. A proper-sized endotracheal tube should be inserted (see Table 21.3) under direct laryngoscopy and both sides of the chest auscultated for the presence of equal breath sounds. Ventilatory rates and pressures outlined in the previous section on bag-mask ventilation are also appropriate for the intubated newborn, bearing in mind that adequate air excursion, chest wall movement, and "pinking up" of the infant are desirable end points.

Routine Postnatal Care

Healthy newborns should be kept warm, dry, and near mother if possible. Vitamin K_1 oxide is given at birth (1 mg intramuscularly or 0.5 mg if body weight is <1.5 kg) to prevent hemorrhagic disease of the newborn. Eye care is provided with instillation of 2 drops of 1% silver nitrate into each conjuctival sac.

Table 22.1.
Delivery Room Neonatal Resuscitation Equipment

1. Prewarmed blankets and dry towels
2. Radiant warmer or stretcher with flannel sheet covering
3. Bag and mask attached to O_2 supply[a]
4. Bulb syringe, DeLee suction catheter, stethescope, cord clamp
5. Laryngoscope and no. 0 and no. 1 Miller (straight) blades
6. Endotracheal tubes (sizes 2.0, 2.5, 3.0, 3.5 mm)
7. Drugs: epinephrine (1:10,000); 10% dextrose; atropine, 0.1 mg/ml; naloxone; sodium bicarbonate, 1 mEq/ml; 10% calcium gluconate
8. Syringes; needles (butterflies), tape, umbilical catheters (sizes 3.5, 5)

[a] Appropriate newborn sizes of bag and mask.

SPECIFIC DELIVERY ROOM EMERGENCIES

Shock

Shock in the neonate is a clinical syndrome encountered when the metabolic demands of the baby outstrip his or her circulatory supply. Its etiologies are multiple but they break down primarily into intrapartum hemorrhage and/or fetal asphyxia. These infants are pale, tachycardic, and apneic or tachypneic with poor capillary filling (>3 seconds) and thready pulse.

Treatment

1. Stabilizing the cardiorespiratory system; first clearing the airway, providing supplemental oxygen via face mask, bag and mask, or intubation, and proceeding with full resuscitation, if needed, as outlined in Table 22.3. The infant must be kept warm and dry.
2. Volume expansion via an umbilical venous catheter starting with 10 ml kg intravenously of:
   a. whole blood;
   b. fresh-frozen plasma;
   c. 5% albumin;
   d. lactated Ringer's; or
   e. 5% dextrose in 0.5 N saline.

   This dose of 10 ml/kg may be repeated if perfusion remains inadequate.
3. If the above measures are ineffective, check liver edge and consider the possibility of pump (i.e. the heart) failure secondary to asphyxia. Dopamine may be useful at 5–20 μgm/kg/min intravenously.

Meconium

Meconium may be released in utero by postmature fetuses and fetuses experiencing acute or chronic hypoxia. In an effort to reduce the volume of meconium aspirated, (*a*) the infant's oropharynx and nose should be suctioned while the head is still on the mother's perineum, and (*b*) prior to initiation of breathing, the larynx should be visualized, intubated, and suctioned of obvious meconium. Depending upon the severity of the aspiration, the infant may require continued oxygen and airway support, as well as antibiotics.

Prematurity

Infants born prior to 37 weeks gestation are classified as preterm/premature; their delivery room management may be complicated, requiring attention to a number of issues simultaneously. Decisions regarding any infant's viability, (*a*) should not hinge on size/body weight, as a proportion of extremely premature infants now survive the neonatal period; and (*b*) are best deferred until well after the delivery, since experienced/expert input is essential. In other words, resuscitate any newborn with

Table 22.2.
Apgar Scoring[a]

	Score[b]		
	2	1	0
Heart rate	>100 BPM[c]	<100 BPM	Absent
Respiratory effort	Vigorous or crying	Irregular or <30/min	Absent
Muscle tone	Active motion	Some flexion of extremities	Limp
Reflex irritability (response to nasal suctioning)	Grimacing, coughing, sneezing	Inconsistent grimace/ avoidance	Absent response
Color	Pink	Blue extremities and central pinkness	Blue or pale

[a] Apgar, V. A proposal for a new method of evaluation of the newborn infant. *Curr Res Anesth Analg* 1953;32:260.
[b] The actual score is a total of the points assigned for each characteristic and thus may vary from 0 to 10.
[c] BPM, beats per minute.

or without signs of life (the cardiac impulse may have ceased just moments earlier) unless it is apparent (e.g. macerated skin) that the child expired antenatally.

Treatment

1. Resuscitate premature newborns using the newborn resuscitation format in Table 22.3, remembering that respiratory distress and apnea are common in these babies.
2. Maintain thermal neutrality [i.e. maintenance of a normal core temperature with minimal metabolic work. (see Table 22.4 for specifics)] via:
   a. gentle drying (avoid rough materials because the skin of premature infants is very fragile) and placing a hat on infant;
   b. positioning under radiant warmer and/or using dry, warm-water-filled gloves against baby;
   c. frequent monitoring of body temperature to avoid hypo- and hyperthermia; and
   d. transferring into prewarmed isolette as soon as baby has been stabilized.
3. If transport to a nursery is delayed, start fluid therapy (10% dextrose in water at 80 ml/kg/day) via peripheral intravenous or umbilical catheter.
4. Because premature infants are more likely to be infected at birth, obtain cultures of blood and gastric aspirate (obtain blood cultures via peripheral venipuncture or scalp vein puncture and obtain gastric aspirate by passing a no. 5 or 8 French feeding tube orally or nasally and aspirating stomach contents) and administer broad-spectrum antibiotics (ampicillin, 100 mg/kg/day

Table 22.3.
Algorithm for Newborn Resuscitation[a]

1. Place infant supine on flat, dry surface
   ↓
2. Suction mouth and nares with bulb syringe
   ↓
3. Assess respiratory effort/heart rate/pulses while towel-drying the baby. (Use Apgar system if familiar, see Table 22.2)

4\. (*a*) (Apgar 7–10) Regular breathing, heart rate > 100/min, reasonable color
↓
Observe, keep warm

(*b*) (Apgar 4–6) Apnea or poor respiratory effort with HR > 100[a]
↓
(Give naloxone 0.01 mg/kg i.m./i.v. if indicated)
↓
Stimulate gently by drying with towel, provide blow-by O_2 and several breaths via bag-mask
- Regular breathing commences, go to 4 (*a*)
- Apnea/poor respiratory effort persists, go to 4 (*c*)

(*c*) (Apgar ≤ 3) Apnea or poor respiratory effort with HR < 100/min
↓
Begin bag-mask ventilation with 100% O_2 at 40 breaths/minute. Intubate if HR < 100 after 1–2 min
↓
If baby's HR < 70, cardiac compressions at 120/min should be performed, check for equal breath sounds with bagging and femoral pulses with cardiac massage
↓
Drug/fluid therapy (*seldom required with adequate CPR*) should be started if bradycardia persists:
- Sodium bicarbonate, i.v./ET 1–2 mEq/kg diluted 1:1 with 10% dextrose in H_2O[b]
- Epinephrine, i.v./ET 0.01 mg/kg
- Calcium gluconate, i.v. 1 ml/kg
- Colloid, i.v. 10 ml/kg
- Atropine, i.v./ET 0.02 mg/kg

Note:
- Towel-drying reduces evaporative heat loss and makes the infant easier to handle
- The best place for palpating the pulse and determining heart rate is at the base or 2 cm from the base of the umbilical cord

[a]HR, heart rate.
[b]ET, endotracheal.

every 12 hours intravenously, gentamicin, 2.5 mg/kg/dose every 12–18 hours intravenously or intramuscularly, if indicated (e.g. premature rupture of membranes, maternal infection, suspicion of neonatal sepsis, premature babies with respiratory distress).

Pulmonary Air Leaks

Pulmonary air leaks may occur spontaneously in an otherwise well newborn but more commonly develop in infants with hyaline membrane disease, meconium aspiration, and particularly those requiring bag-mask ventilation. These infants present with signs of respiratory distress (expiratory grunting, nasal flaring, cyanosis with tachypnea, retractions). The chest x-ray is diagnostic, but decreased breath sounds on the affected side and positive transillumination (using a high intensity fiberoptic procedure lamp briefly held against each hemithorax and watching for "lighting up" of extrapleural air) are very suggestive.

Treatment

Evacuation of symptomatic pneumothorax (pneumomediastinum is rarely treated) can be initiated using a 21-gauge butterfly needle (attached to a 3-way stopcock and a 50-ml syringe) inserted shallowly in the anterior axillary line of the 4th intercostal space. A chest tube (no. 10) may then be placed while continually drawing back on the syringe. Supplemental oxygen should be administered to the baby as needed.

Surgical Emergencies

(See also Chapter 30.) Infants noted in the delivery room to have ventral wall defects (gastroschesis, omphalocele, ectopic bladder), neural tube defects (encephalocele, meningomyelocele), or diaphragmatic hernia require attention to specific resuscitative issues: *A*irway, *B*reathing, *C*irculation, + *D*rugs, and thermal neutrality (Table 22.4).

Multiple Congenital Anomalies

A major congenital defect occurs in as many as 4 of 100 liveborn infants. Nevertheless, these infants should be resuscitated in standard fashion, with the exception of specific major surgical emergencies, following the newborn resuscitation format (Table 22.3). A variety of problems may arise during these resuscitations. Infants with cleft palates may be difficult to intubate. Babies with renal agenesis/oligohydramnios/compression deformities (Potter's sequence), babies with cyanotic heart disease, and certain dwarves tend to remain cyanotic despite maximal intervention.

A calm and supportive attitude is crucial for parents in these circumstances. The physician should refrain from making definitive diagnoses in the delivery room. For example, there may be marked, though transient, distortion of an infant's craniofacial features during a long labor, resulting in an alarming appearance to parents and less experienced care providers.

Cyanosis

Peripheral cyanosis is common in the immediate newborn period in neonates and need not be treated. Central cyanosis, however, should be addressed immediately. Common *causes* of central cyanosis in the newborn include respiratory failure, polycythemia, hypothermia, and congenital heart disease. Fetal blood oxygen tensions range from 20 to 30 mm Hg, and therefore, at the moment of transition to extrauterine life the baby is normally cyanotic.

Treatment

1. If the baby is crying lustily, has good bilateral air excursion on auscultation, and has a regular heart rate, administer "blow-by" O_2 and observe initially, then obtain an hematocrit, arterial blood gas, and serum glucose.
2. Respiratory failure (primary or secondary apnea, airway obstruction, severe respiratory distress) is treated by clearing the airway, then using bag and mask ventilation with 100% O_2, followed by intubation if effective breathing with pinking up has not occurred after several minutes. Always auscultate the chest and consider the possibility of pneumothorax.
3. Body temperature must be monitored in newborns to avoid hypothermia and associated duskiness. Upon rewarming, a cold-stressed newborn is at risk for hypoglycemia; if hypoglycemic, it may remain dusky. A Dextrostix or serum glucose should be checked, if indicated, and an appropriate infusion of 10% dextrose in water begun.
4. Polycythemia in newborns is present when the venous hematocrit is greater than 65%. These infants may appear cyanotic without being hypoxic. Obtain a venous hematocrit, a serum glucose, and arterial blood gases. Polycythemic babies are often hypoglycemic and may require supplemental O_2. Thus, they should receive a glucose infusion and oxygen prior to partial exchange transfusion.
5. Congenital heart disease (CHD) occurs in 7–8 of 1000 babies. Distinguishing cyanosis of CHD from pulmonary disease may be very difficult. A chest x-ray, arterial blood gas on 100% oxygen, careful physical examination, and ECG are reasonable starting points when respiratory disease or failure seems *unlikely*. Remember that intravenous infusion of prostaglandin E_1 (0.1 μgm/kg/min) may be useful in certain ductal-

Table 22.4.
Neutral Thermal Environmental Temperatures[a]

Age and Weight	Starting Temperature	Range of Temperature
	°C	°C
0–6 hr		
Under 1200 gm	35.0	34.0–35.4
1200–1500 gm	34.1	33.9–34.4
1501–2500 gm	33.4	32.8–33.8
Over 2500 (and >36 weeks)	32.9	32.0–33.8
6–12 hr		
Under 1200 gm	35.0	34.0–35.4
1200–1500 gm	34.0	33.5–34.4
1501–2500 gm	33.1	32.2–33.8
Over 2500 (and >36 weeks)	32.8	31.4–33.8
12–24 hr		
Under 1200 gm	34.0	34.0–35.4
1200–1500 gm	33.8	33.3–34.3
1501–2500 gm	32.8	31.8–33.8
Over 2500 (and >36 weeks)	32.4	31.0–33.7
24–36 hr		
Under 1200 gm	34.0	34.0–35.0
1200–1500 gm	33.6	33.1–34.2
1501–2500 gm	32.6	31.6–33.6
Over 2500 (and >36 weeks)	32.1	30.7–33.5
36–48 hr		
Under 1200 gm	34.0	34.0–35.0
1200–1500 gm	33.5	33.0–34.1
1501–2500 gm	32.5	31.4–33.5
Over 2500 (and >36 weeks)	31.9	30.5–33.3
48–72 hr		
Under 1200 gm	34.0	34.0–35.0
1200–1500 gm	33.5	33.0–34.0
1501–2500 gm	32.3	31.2–33.4
Over 2500 (and >36 weeks)	31.7	30.1–33.2
72–96 hr		
Under 1200 gm	34.0	34.0–35.0
1200–1500 gm	33.5	33.0–34.0
1501–2500 gm	32.2	31.1–33.2
Over 2500 (and >36 weeks)	31.3	29.8–32.8
4–12 days		
Under 1500 gm	33.5	33.0–34.0
1501–2500 gm	32.1	31.0–33.2
Over 2500 (and >36 weeks)		
4–5 days	31.0	29.5–32.6
5–6 days	30.9	29.4–32.3
6–8 days	30.6	29.0–32.2
8–10 days	30.3	29.0–31.8
10–12 days	30.1	29.0–31.4
12–14 days		
Under 1500 gm	33.5	32.6–34.0
1501–2500 gm	32.1	31.0–33.2
Over 2500 (and >36 weeks)	29.8	29.0–30.8
2–3 weeks		
Under 1500 gm	33.1	32.6–34.0
1501–2500 gm	32.1	31.0–33.2
3–4 weeks		
Under 1500 gm	32.6	31.6–33.6
1501–2500 gm	31.4	30.0–32.7
4–5 weeks		
Under 1500 gm	32.0	31.2–33.0
1501–2500 gm	30.9	29.5–32.2
5–6 weeks		
Under 1500 gm	31.4	30.6–32.3
1501–2500 gm	30.4	29.0–31.8

[a] From Klaus M. Fanaroff A. Care of the High Risk Neonate. Philadelphia: WB Saunders, 1979:102–103.

Table 22.5.
Check List for Neonatal Transport

1. Written permission for transport from parents, copies of maternal/baby's records (include x-rays), and sample of maternal blood for type/cross-matching
2. Qualified transport personnel, usually one nurse and one physician
3. Stable newborn (check vital signs, temperature, dextrostix/serum glucose, CBC with differential, blood gases if indicated) with a functioning intravenous line of 10% dextrose and a secured ETT (if intubated)[a]
4. Telephone communication with receiving physician prior to departure
5. Obtain cultures and administer first dose of antibiotics prior to transport, if infection is suspected
6. Show the parent(s) their baby briefly prior to departure
7. Transport isolette should be adequately warm and fully equipped with oxygen tank, anesthesia or/Ambu-bag, cardiac monitor

[a] CBC, complete blood count; ETT, endotracheal tube.

dependent lesions, such as pulmonary atresia. Transport to a tertiary facility should be accomplished quickly for the newborn with cyanotic heart disease.

Neonatal Transport

Neonatal transport to a tertiary facility is required for newborns with respiratory distress, prematurity, multiple anomalies, cardiac disease, or other complex problem. The goal in transporting the sick newborn is to provide a controlled, safe, and efficient transition from referring to receiving hospital. Table 22.5 is a checklist.

Fetal Demise

Stillbirths comprise 50% or more of perinatal deaths. A stillbirth is defined as the complete expulsion or extraction from the mother of a fetus greater than 20 weeks gestation or 500 gm birth weight that shows no signs of life at or after birth. Following intrauterine fetal death, the majority of women deliver spontaneously within 2 weeks. Unless it is apparent that the fetus in question has been long dead (e.g. obvious maceration), then the newborn without pulses or respirations should be resuscitated as if cardiorespiratory arrest occurred just prior to delivery. A birth certificate must be completed for every stillbirth and forwarded to the local registrar. The possibility for postmortem examination of the stillborn should be offered to the parent(s). Emergency department personnel should assist the parent(s) with contacting a funeral home and recommend appropriate follow-up with the obstetrician, family doctor, or pediatrician. Delivering a stillborn is a wrenching, sorrowful experience for parents; support and kindness are required.

SUGGESTED READINGS

Bose CL, ed. Current Concepts in Transport. Columbus, OH: Ross Laboratories, 1982.

Cloherty JP, Stark AR, eds. Manual of Neonatal Care. 2nd ed. Boston: Little, Brown & Co., 1985.

Dazé AM, Scanlon JW. Code Pink: A Practical System for Neonatal/Perinatal Resuscitation. Baltimore: University Park Press, 1981.

CHAPTER 23

Acute Upper Airway Obstruction in the Child

I. DAVID TODRES, M.D.
ROLAND D. EAVEY, M.D.

The child with acute airway obstruction presents a treacherous situation. On the one hand, the condition may be benign and self-limited and require no therapeutic intervention. On the other hand, the child may slip quickly into severe respiratory distress and death by asphyxiation. The child is often unable to verbalize a history or describe the symptoms well, placing the clinician in a challenging situation.

ANATOMY AND PHYSIOLOGY

Anatomic Differences from the Adult

The pediatric anatomy and physiology of respiration make the child more susceptible to potential compromise of function. Anatomically, the child is initially a nasal breather. The choanae at the junction of the posterior nose and the nasopharynx are tiny portals through which the child must exert an effort to breathe. Even in a resting state, an infant works much harder to breathe than does an adult. The child additionally has a disproportionately large tongue fitting into a relatively small oral cavity, with a proportionately retruded mandible. The larynx also sits much higher in a child. The adult larynx at rest may sit, for example, at approximately the 5th cervical vertebral body. In an infant, it may sit at the 3rd cervical vertebral body and with swallowing elevates even higher. This means that, because the food and air passages share a common conduit, an infant must, by quick and accurate reflex, deflect air through the larynx, and liquid and solid materials posteriorly into the esophagus, with less room for error than an adult. Furthermore, the laryngeal anatomy is not aligned along a straight vertical axis parallel to the vertebral bodies. Instead it is somewhat bowed. The bow string parallels the vertebral bodies but the actual air conduit follows a tract more akin to the actual bow. The anterior attachment of the vocal cords is somewhat slanted from the horizontal so that, should an endotracheal intubation be attempted, the tube may potentially hang up in that region. The subglottic region, immediately beneath the vocal cords, is much smaller in a child than in an adult. Therefore, the tube may pass through the cords but hang up in the region immediately beneath the cords. In an adult, the subglottic region is more spacious. Additionally, any compromise of the subglottic region may have a profound impact on the cross-sectional diameter of the airway. A similar degree of swelling in an older patient has practically no effect on respiration.

Pathophysiology

An appreciation of the physiological behavior of the compromised upper airway provides a rational approach to therapy. With normal breathing, the inspiratory phase is associated with negative intrathoracic pressure. This negative pressure is transmitted to the upper airway. Thus, in the extrathoracic upper airway there is a pressure differential between the negative intratracheal pressure and the outer atmospheric pressure. This results in a slight narrowing of the upper airway on inspiration. With expiration, the reverse occurs, causing a narrowing

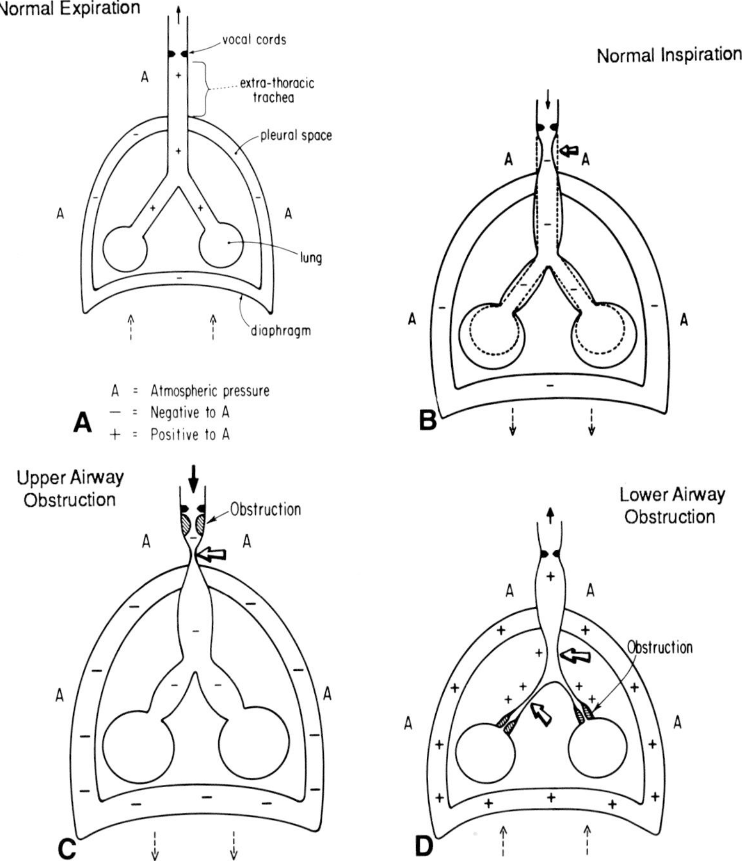

Figure 23.1. Diagrammatic representation of child's airway, lungs, and chest cage. Shown are changes in pressures within the airways and the chest with normal expiration (*A*), normal inspiration (*B*), upper airway obstruction (*C*), and lower airway obstruction (*D*). Note the effects of dynamic collapse—the airway causing increasing obstruction.

of the lower airway and a slight expansion of the upper airway.

With obstruction of the upper airway, as in croup, foreign body, or epiglottitis, greater negative pressure is exerted during inspiration resulting in an even greater differential between the upper airway and surrounding atmospheric pressure. This leads to greater collapse of the upper airway and increasing distress on inspiration. For this reason the stridorous child who becomes agitated with crying may experience increasing airway compromise, in some cases resulting in total airway obstruction. Thus, efforts must be made to relieve anxiety and crying and, in this way, minimize dynamic collapse of the airway. From this aspect too we can appreciate the value of positive pressure breathing in the child with severe airway obstruction, to counteract dynamic collapse of the airway and thereby facilitate gas exchange (Fig. 23.1).

HISTORY

The Three Basic Questions

In the evaluation of a child with respiratory obstruction, there are certain questions that must be addressed. One should think of the three functions of the larynx as a framework from which to ask questions. These questions may be embellished by the usual demographic information. The *three basic functions* of the larynx are: (*a*) to help with breathing, (*b*) to phonate, and (*c*) to prevent aspiration. Therefore, all questions should spring from those three considerations (Table 23.1). For example, questions of respiration include stridor, apnea, cyanosis, and respiratory rate. Phonatory questions revolve around voice changes, aphonia, and hoarseness. Laryngeal competence is questioning regarding cough and aspiration with feeding.

Table 23.1.
History of Laryngeal Function for the Pediatric Patient[a]

Breathing	Feeding		Voice
Normal breathing Abnormal breathing Is the noisy breath stridor (vs. snoring, wheezing, etc.)? Is stridor Inspiratory, Expiratory, To-and-fro? Not breathing Central Obstructive Cyanosis Degree of respiratory distress	Normal feeding Abnormal feeding Choking Coughing Vomiting Refuses to feed Foreign body Caustic ingestion	(with swallowing or later)	Normal voice/cry Abnormal voice (hoarse, weak, muffled) Absent voice

[a] Also, prior respiratory problems including history of intubation, prematurity, and need for an apnea monitor.

Demography

Important demographic information include questions: how long has the airway been abnormal; with what is it associated, i.e. crying; has this been more severe; is it becoming worse, better, or stable; was a foreign body ingested, by any chance; was it abrupt or gradual onset?

PHYSICAL EXAMINATION

Only a few moments are actually necessary to evaluate the child during the physical examination. This involves looking at the child and listening to the child. Looking informs the examiner of the severity of the problem and helps to determine whether or not immediate therapeutic intervention is necessary. Listening to the patient informs the examiner of the approximate location of the obstruction.

Table 23.2.
Physical Examination—Looking

General appearance—degree of agitation/distress (normal, mild, moderate, severe)
Retractions (mild, moderate, severe)
Nasal flaring
Suprasternal
Intercostal
Subcostal
Respiratory rate
Cyanosis—nail beds, circumoral region, skin
Position
Mouth open or closed
Drooling
Oral intake—accepts or refuses
Neck appearance—normal, swelling, trauma
Gross neurological abnormalities or dysmorphic features

Looking

The child should be visually evaluated by *looking* for the following characteristics (Table 23.2): respiratory rate, cyanosis, open mouth, drooling, leaning forward, nasal flaring, and retractions in the suprasternal, intercostal, or subcostal areas. If the child is judged to be in respiratory distress, this can generally be classified as mild, moderate, or severe. In the severe situation the airway may require treatment before the exact analysis of the problem has been completed.

Listening

Listening to the patient helps inform the examiner of the location of the difficulty (Table 23.3). The airway, if compromised, has a characteristic sound—stridor. Inspiratory stridor suggests an upper respiratory tract problem: epiglottitis, vocal cord paralysis, and subglottic edema, such as with croup, produce inspiratory stridor. Expiratory stridor comes from lower tract problems and includes such problems as a foreign body lodged in a bronchus, or a vascular ring. In severe situations, a to-and-fro stridor may be audible. However, even in these there is usually a predominant direction which can help guide the clinician to localization of the problem.

Direct examination of the throat should be undertaken only by skilled personnel who can deal immediately with further compromise of the airway. If epiglottitis is likely, direct examination is best avoided; attempts at trying to view the pharynx with a tongue depressor may precipitate acute obstruction.

Signs and Symptoms

Symptoms and signs relating to airway obstruction and the resulting systemic effects are:

Table 23.3.
Physical Examination—Listening

Symptom	Site of Obstruction
1. Stridor	
Inspiratory	Extrathoracic trachea (high)
Expiratory	Intrathoracic trachea (low)
To-and-fro	Predominantly inspiratory = extrathoracic Predominantly expiratory = intrathoracic
2. Voice quality	Normal—no pathology in vicinity of glottis (exception bilateral abductor paralysis) Abnormal (hoarse, weak, muffled)—pathology in vicinity of glottis
3. Cough quality	Croupy (high pitched)—subglottic narrowing Croupy (low pitched)—tracheal narrowing

1. Stridor—the cardinal sign of airway obstruction. With exhaustion and poor respiratory efforts the intensity of the stridor diminishes although the child's condition has deteriorated.
2. Tachypnea—increased respiratory rates are common. Rates above 60/minute in the young child are indicative of severe airway obstruction.
3. Retractions—suprasternal, substernal, and intercostal.
4. Tachycardia—heart rates above 160/minute are indicative of severe and potentially life-threatening obstruction.
5. Cyanosis—a manifestation of severe hypoxemia.
6. Agitation—may be due to hypoxemia.
7. Drooling of secretions—occurs typically in the child with epiglottitis because of an inability to swallow.
8. Dysphagia—occurs with epiglottitis and obturating esophageal foreign bodies.

LABORATORY EVALUATIONS

Inspection and listening have been completed; the degree of distress and approximate location of the problem have been determined. The exact type of problem may not be clear, however. This presents the option of x-ray assistance or endoscopy. For the child with mild distress, one has the luxury of further studies. For the child with severe distress, the patient may need artificial airway maintenance with bag and mask, intubation, or some form of transcervical airway, such as cricothyroid needle puncture (see Illustrated Technique 4).

X-Rays or Not

Roentgenograms of the upper airway should not be performed in the child in severe respiratory distress. Clinical judgment must determine therapeutic management. Roentgenograms of the upper airway must be evaluated carefully in diagnosing epiglottitis because of the possibility of false positive interpretation. Roentgenograms can be of value in demonstrating a retropharyngeal mass or radiopaque foreign body. As discussed in Chapter 47, the lateral neck film is most useful for diagnosing epiglottitis; the anteroposterior neck film, for demonstrating the typical "pencil" or "steeple" sign of croup. Airway fluoroscopic examination may be necessary to confirm the presence of a retropharyngeal mass.

Should x-ray studies be contemplated, it is important that the child always be accompanied by a physician with instant access to equipment for airway maintenance. The airway may be further obstructed suddenly; the x-ray department is often not the safest place for the patient in that situation. The emergency medical staff must avoid agitating the child into crying which exaggerates airway collapse. Therefore, venipunctures and arterial blood gas sampling are usually avoided in cases of acute airway obstruction until a more secure diagnosis and management plan has been established. Careful consideration must always be given to the risks versus benefits in each particular situation.

DIFFERENTIAL DIAGNOSIS

A useful approach to the problem of stridor is to think of the airway as an open tube and to consider the ways in which its patency may be affected (Table 23.4).

1. Mechanical obstruction from within, e.g. foreign body, vomitus, blood, mucus;
2. Obstruction associated with pathology of the airway leading to encroachment on the lumen:
    - congenital, e.g. hemangioma
    - inflammatory, e.g. croup, epiglottitis
    - traumatic, e.g. chemical burn smoke inhalation;
3. Obstruction due to compression of the airway from without, e.g. vascular ring, tumor, retropharyngeal mass.

Table 23.4.
A List of the More Common Causes of Upper Airway Obstruction

Congenital anomaly
Laryngomalacia
Vocal cord paralysis
Subglottic stenosis
Trauma
Caustic ingestion
Foreign body
Infection
Supraglottitis
Laryngotracheobronchitis (croup)
Tumor
Hemangioma
Cystic hygroma
Allergy (angioneurotic edema)

Epiglottitis

Epiglottitis is a life-threatening infection in children usually between the ages of one and 8 years. It can occur in older children and adults. Pathologically, there is an acute inflammation of the epiglottis and the aryepiglottic folds. Therefore, it is more appropriately termed supraglottitis. The organism responsible is usually *Haemophilus influenzae,* type B. The condition needs differentiation from laryngotracheobronchitis (croup) (Table 23.5).

The condition is acute in onset, rapidly progressive, and potentially life-threatening. Thus, urgent diagnosis and treatment are necessary. The child is acutely ill with high fever and has difficulty swallowing; as a result, drooling develops, a very important sign in the clinical diagnosis of this condition. The child prefers to sit up with the head pushed forward to maintain the best possible airway. Rapid progression of the inflammation may cause total obstruction within hours.

Acute epiglottitis is a medical emergency and personnel in the emergency department must adopt an organized multidisciplinary approach to treat it. Laryngeal obstruction may be precipitated by crying, leading to respiratory arrest. Situations which can provoke distress in the child, throat examination and arterial blood gas sampling, should be deferred until control of the airway has been established, specifically placement of an endotracheal tube or tracheotomy. Restraining the child for a satisfactory roentgenogram in a remote x-ray facility is hazardous. Poor interpretation of the films leads to errors in diagnosis. The emphasis should therefore be placed on clinical evaluation and the therapeutic approach based on the clinical picture.

An artificial airway should be established in all cases of childhood epiglottitis with an endotracheal tube. Tracheotomy is preferred in some centers. The endotracheal tube is placed under controlled conditions in the operating room using general anesthesia with the surgical team in attendance, should there be need for bronchoscopy or tracheotomy. In some centers the endotracheal tube placement is performed in the pediatric intensive care unit. Once the artificial airway is placed, cultures are taken from the epiglottis and blood. The blood culture is positive in 90 to 95% of cases for *Haemophilus influenzae,* type B. Antibiotic therapy is initiated with ampicillin and chloramphenicol. Once bacterial sensitivity is known, the appropriate antibiotic is continued for 10 days. These patients are always admitted to the hospital, preferably to an intensive care unit.

Complications of epiglottitis are potentially serious and should be suspected if toxicity and fever do not readily resolve or if new symptoms appear. There is a 25% incidence of concomitant pneumonia. Meningitis is rarely associated with acute epiglottitis but may be overlooked when the child is heavily sedated to prevent accidental extubation. Other related infections include pericarditis, pleural effusions/empyema, and periarticular abscess.

The use of corticosteroids in this disease remains controversial. Rifamycin (rifampin) should be administered to intimate contacts and siblings under 8

Table 23.5.
Clinical Features in the Differential Diagnosis of Epiglottitis and Laryngotracheobronchitis

	Epiglottitis	Laryngotracheobronchitis
Age	2–12 yr, occasionally adult	3 months to 5 yr
Onset	Sudden	Slow
Preceding symptoms	Uncommon	Upper respiratory infection
Toxicity	Marked	Mild-moderate
Temperature	High	Moderate
Stridor	Mild-moderate	Marked
Position	Sitting up, "tripod"	Variable
Drooling	Common	Rare
Course	Rapid	Slow

years of age. The patient should also receive rifamycin to eliminate a carrier state.

Laryngotracheobronchitis

Laryngotracheobronchitis is a common cause of upper airway obstruction in children from 3 months to 6 years of age. The condition is usually benign but may, on occasion, become life-threatening. The cause is usually viral, predominantly a parainfluenza virus. The staphylococcus is responsible for more recent cases of severe tracheitis presenting with the symptoms of croup.

The onset of the disease is insidious with an upper respiratory tract infection for 3–4 days followed by the inspiratory stridor associated with airway obstruction. The child usually has a mild fever and a "croupy" cough. Other differential conditions with the typical barking cough include subglottic stenosis, hemangioma or cyst of the airway, or foreign body lodged below the cords. Intercostal retractions are an indication of airway obstruction and increase with worsening of the disease. If the child is cyanotic in room air, treatment becomes urgent. Close monitoring of vital signs, heart rate, respirations, skin color, stridor, retractions, and mental status, is essential. The approach to therapy depends upon the degree of airway obstruction and its effect on the cardiopulmonary and cerebral status of the child.

In the early stages of the illness an enriched oxygen environment is necessary. This is often provided in a well-humidified atmosphere. Oxygen therapy is essential because laryngotracheobronchitis has been shown to be associated with hypoxemia due to ventilation/perfusion mismatch. Recent studies question the value of humidification. Further appraisal of this traditional mode of therapy is required.

Other therapeutic measures, such as corticosteroids and helium/oxygen mixtures, have not been proved effective with sound scientific support. Recurrent croup occurs more often in families with a positive history of allergy. When respiratory obstruction becomes more severe, as manifested by increasing heart rate, respiratory rate, and intercostal retraction, inhalation of racemic epinephrine (0.5 ml in 3 ml saline) may be beneficial, although the duration of the illness may not be shortened. Repeated inhalations are usually necessary 1–3 hours apart with continued close monitoring of the cardiorespiratory status. Rebound swelling may follow a treatment and, therefore, children requiring racemic epinephrine in the emergency department should not be discharged. They must be closely observed in the hospital.

Should the child deteriorate with increasing obstruction, an artificial airway may be essential. Further obstruction usually results from increasing edema with formation of thick inspissated secretions which the exhausted child is unable to raise up. An endotracheal tube or tracheotomy is placed under controlled conditions in the operating room. Roentgenographic evaluation may be helpful in the differential diagnosis but it should be stressed again that establishment of the airway in the severely distressed child takes precedence over radiographic studies.

Foreign Body Aspiration

Foreign body aspiration must always be considered in all cases of acute respiratory distress. The foreign body may cause asphyxia resulting in death or severe morbidity. Infants under 2 years of age are particularly susceptible to food asphyxial death. Candy, hot dogs, raisins, and peanuts are common offending food items. Foreign body aspiration may be multiple. Movement of the foreign body from its original position is common.

Early diagnosis, in some two-thirds of cases, is associated with a history of violent coughing and gagging with severe airway obstruction and cyanosis. Wheezing may be noted. The classic triad of wheezing, coughing, and decreased breath sounds over the affected side are more commonly seen in the late diagnosed cases and only in bronchial lodging of the foreign body. However, in the majority of cases this classic presentation is incomplete. Roentgenograms may be helpful but the majority of foreign bodies are not radiopaque. Atelectasis or obstructive emphysema may be seen on the affected side. In late-diagnosed cases, pneumonitis recurring in a localized area not responding to standard therapy should suggest the diagnosis. Impaction of a foreign body in the esophagus may occasionally compress the trachea with resulting airway obstruction.

Emergency management of the child with a foreign body lodged in the extrathoracic airway consists of applying abdominal thrusts in the Heimlich maneuver. In infants under 1 year of age back thrusts are recommended, followed by chest thrusts if needed. In the child who is relatively stable, not in an acute life-threatening situation, removal of the foreign body is carried out under general anesthesia in the operating room. If symptoms persist, follow-up is necessary to check for residual foreign body.

SUGGESTED READINGS

Baker AS, Eavey RD. Adult supraglottitis (epiglottitis). *N Engl J Med,* 1986;314:1185–1186.

Bas JW, Fajardo JE, Brien JH, et al. Sudden death due to acute epiglottitis. *Pediatr Infect Dis,* 1985;4:447–449.

Blazer S, Naveh Y, Friedman A. Foreign body in the airway: A review of 200 cases. *Am J Dis Child* 1980;134:68–71.

Cohen SR, Herbert WE, Lewis GB, et al. Foreign bodies in the airway: Five year retrospective study with special reference to management. *Ann Otol Rhinol Laryngol* 1980;89:437–441.

Cotton E, Yasuda K. Foreign body aspiration. *Pediatr Clin North Am,* 1984;31:937–941.

Dajani AS, Asmar BI, Thirumoarta MC. Systemic Hemophilus influenzae disease—An overview. *J Pediatr,* 1979;94:353–364.

Friedman EM. Supraglottitis and concurrent Hemophilus meningitis. *Ann Otol Rhinol Laryngol,* 1985;94:470–472.

Hawkins DB. Corticosteroids in the management of laryngotracheobronchitis. *Otolaryngol Head Neck Surg,* 1980;88:207–2l0.

Henry R. Moist air in the treatment of laryngotracheitis. *Arch Dis Child,* 1983;58:572.

Kimmons HC, Peterson BC. Management of acute epiglottitis in pediatric patients. *Crit Care Med,* 1986;14:278–279.

Kresch MJ. Pericarditis complicating Hemophilus epiglottitis. *Pediatr Infect Dis,* 1985;4:559–561.

MayoSmith MF, Hirsch PJ, Wodzinsky SF, et al. Acute epiglottitis in adults, An eight-year experience in the state of Rhode Island. *N Engl J Med,* 1986;314:1133–1139.

Skrinkas GJ, Hyland RH, Hutcheon MA. Using helium oxygen mixtures in the management of acute upper airway obstruction. *Care Med Assoc J.* 1983;128:555–558.

Standards and guidelines for cardiopulmonary resuscitation and emergency cardiac care—Airway obstruction management. *JAMA,* 1986;255: 2905–2989.

Stankiewiez JA, Bowes AK. Croup and epiglottitis, a radiologic study. *Laryngoscope,* 1985;95:1159–1160.

Vernon DD, Sarnaik AP. Acute epiglottitis in children: A conservative approach to diagnosis and management. *Crit Care Med,* 1986;14:23–25.

Wesbley CR, Cotton EK, Brooks JG. Nebulised racemic epinephrine by IPPB for treatment of croup. *Am J Dis Child,* 1978;132:484–487.

Whisnant JK, Rogentine GN, Gralnick MA, et al. Host factors and antibody response in Hemophilus influenzae, type B meningitis and epiglottitis. *J Infect Dis,* 1976;133:446–455.

Wiseman NE. The diagnosis of foreign body aspiration in childhood. *J Pediatr Surg,* 1984;19:531–535.

CHAPTER **24**

Emergency Department Management of Apnea of Infancy and Sudden Infant Death Syndrome

DOROTHY H. KELLY, M.D.
DANIEL C. SHANNON, M.D.

The emergency physician is frequently the first physician to evaluate the infant who has had a frightening episode of apnea or to deal with the infant found lifeless in the crib, the apparent victim of sudden infant death syndrome (SIDS). This chapter discusses the clinical presentation, the present understanding of pathophysiology, evaluation, and management of both apnea of infancy and SIDS.

APNEA OF INFANCY (AOI)

Clinical Presentation

The usual presentation of apnea of infancy (AOI) is an episode of apnea accompanied by a change in color and tone. Often the caretaker has intervened in some way to terminate the episode and to help the infant to begin to breathe again. With the typical sleep onset episode, the caretaker usually fortuitously finds the infant. With the typical awake onset episode, the caretaker generally witnesses the entire event, which frequently follows choking or regurgitation and is commonly associated with stiffening, redness, and a frightened look. Often the mouth is opened in these episodes as if trying to breathe. If uninterrupted, some awake episodes can proceed to cyanosis, central apnea, limpness,and unconsciousness. Occasionally, infants present with a history of shallow or irregular breathing during sleep, accompanied by a significant color change or with a history of numerous episodes of sleep apnea without a change of tone or color. With any of the above presentations, the infant may appear completely normal by the time of arrival in the emergency department.

Pathophysiology

Numerous studies of infants with AOI have reported abnormal control of ventilation in some of these infants. The abnormalities include a decreased ventilatory response to hypercapnea, mild hypoventilation in quiet sleep, absent arousal response to hypoxia and hypercarbia, prolonged sleep apnea, occasionally obstructive sleep apnea, excessive short apnea, and excessive periodic breathing. Some AOI infants with one or more of these abnormalities have subsequently died. The cause(s) of these abnormalities remain(s) unknown. On autopsy, increased muscularity of the pulmonary vasculature was documented in five infants with AOI, and gliosis in the brainstem in one. Both findings are associated with chronic hypoxia, either as cause or effect of the physiologic abnormalities in these infants.

Evaluation

We are able to determine the cause of the event in approximately 35% of those infants referred to

Name ____________________

HISTORY OF EVENT (leading to evaluation): Please circle features and complete as needed.

Date: ____________; Age: ________; # hours after feed: ____________

Last Immunization (specify date / type): ____________; Medications; ____________

Recent illness: ____________________

OBSERVER	**LOCATION**	**INFANT POSITION**	**STATE**	**COLOR**	**COLOR CHANGE**
Parent	Holding infant	Prone	Asleep	Cyanotic	Entire body
MD	Same room	Supine	Awake	Grey	Extremities
RN	Audible distance	Upright	Drowsy	Pale	Face
Other ______	In car	Infant seat	Feeding	Red	Perioral
	Other ______	Other ______	Other ______	Purple	Lips
				Normal	Other ______

BREATHING	**TONE**	**EYES**	**NOISE**	**FLUID**	**HEART RATE**
No effort	Limp	Closed	Cough	Milk	Bradycardia @ ____bpm
Shallow	Stiff	Dazed	Choke	Vomitus	Tachycardia @ ____bpm
Struggling	Tonic/clonic	Scared	Stridor	Mucus	Normal
Rapid	Normal	Rolled	Gasp	Blood	Unknown
Normal	Other ______	Staring	Cry	None	
Other ______		Normal	None	Other ______	
		Other ______	Other ______		

STIMULATION	**DURATION OF EVENT:**	**ABNORMALITIES FOLLOWING EVENT**
None	________ sec / min	Abnormal breathing x ________ min / hrs
Gentle		Color change x ________ min / hrs
Vigorous		Behavior ____________
MTM: # breaths ______		None
CPR: # cycles ______		

EMT/ER Observations:

Figure 24.1. Features of the history of an infant with apnea of infancy. *MTM,* mouth-to-mouth; CPR, cardiopulmonary resuscitation.

the Pediatric Pulmonary Laboratory at the Massachusetts General Hospital. The following diseases known to cause apnea should be considered in the differential diagnosis of AOI: *congenital*—anatomic airway abnormalities, vascular anomalies causing airway obstruction, congenital heart disease (patent ductus arteriosus or congestive heart failure in the young infant), and cardiac arrhythmias; *infectious*—sepsis, meningitis, pneumonia, and respiratory syncytial virus (RSV) bronchiolitis; *toxic*—botulism, sedative drug usage, and/or overdose; *metabolic*—hypothermia, hypoglycemia, and some inborn errors of metabolism; *neoplastic*—tumors resulting in obstruction of the airway or seizure disorders with apnea; and *other*—gastroesophageal reflux, primary seizure disorder, idiopathic hypoxemia, anemia in the preterm infant, and abnormalities in the control of ventilation.

A careful evaluation including this differential diagnosis should be undertaken as soon as possible in these infants since physical, neurologic, and biochemical abnormalities may be transient. Initially, a meticulous history taken from every person who observed the infant during or immediately following the episode should be obtained. A detailed history is necessary to help determine the cause of the episode, as well as the severity, judged by the amount and duration of the intervention needed to terminate the event. A thorough past history and family history should also be obtained and a careful physical examination performed to identify signs of partial airway obstruction, congenital anomalies, intercurrent illness, or metabolic or neurologic abnormalities. Figure 24.1 displays in detail the features of history which are important to obtain.

Most episodes occurring awake with a component of coughing, choking, and/or upper airway obstruction are caused by gastroesophageal reflux.

Episodes occurring quietly during sleep are more likely to be related to an abnormal control of ventilation. Seizure disorders, the cause in a small number of these infants, can occur either during sleep or while awake. The remaining disorders can result in an apneic event while awake or asleep and are usually associated with an abnormality detectable on physical examination.

Appropriate laboratory tests should be performed to identify a cause of the event and to determine if there is any acidosis, hypoxemia, hypercapnea, or neurologic abnormality present. If the latter was found even transiently, it indicates that the episode was severe. The laboratory evaluation includes a complete blood cell count with a differential white cell count; serum sodium, potassium, chloride, bicarbonate, glucose, and urea nitrogen measurement; urinalysis, arterial blood gas measurement; chest radiograph; electrocardiogram; electroencephalogram; and a barium esophagogram under fluoroscopic or videotaping guidance. Other studies such as blood and urine cultures, lumbar puncture, bronchoscopy, computed axial tomography (CAT) scan, and viral cultures should be obtained when specifically indicated.

If by a careful history, physical examination, and laboratory examination no cause can be identified, tests to determine if the infant has an abnormality in control of ventilation include polysomnography, pneumogram, studies of ventilatory and arousal responses to hypercapnea and hypoxia. These are beyond the scope of the emergency department and necessitate referral to a center specializing in evaluation and management of infants with AOI. The emergency physician has full responsibility for arranging a prompt referral, with hospital admission if necessary.

Thus, the emergency physician's approach to an infant with an episode considered "frightening and/or life-threatening" by the caretaker is to stabilize the infant, obtain a careful history and physical and neurologic examination, and initiate the appropriate laboratory studies. All infants who have had an apparent life-threatening episode should be hospitalized for a further evaluation. During hospitalization, continuous cardiorespiratory monitoring should be performed for both hospital evaluation and management of these infants.

Management

For infants in whom a cause of the apneic episode has been identified, specific treatment is indicated. For infants whose episodes are significant and remain unexplained, the decision to treat with methylxanthines and/or home monitoring is based on the gestational and chronologic age of the infant as well as the characteristics of the initial episode. This decision is made only after the results of the evaluation are available. In general, infants with idiopathic AOI, who are <44 weeks postconceptional age and have documented abnormalities in control of ventilation, are treated with a methylxanthine; such as theophylline, 2–4 mg/kg/day in three divided doses. If such treatment resulted in a resolution of clinical and laboratory abnormalities, they are discharged on methylxanthines and without a monitor. The referring physician is instructed to maintain carefully the methylxanthine trough level that was documented to resolve the abnormalities. This treatment is continued until approximately 52 weeks postconceptional age at which time the infant is retested to determine if the abnormalities have resolved.

For all other infants with idiopathic AOI, a home cardiorespiratory monitor is prescribed and the caretakers are carefully taught the use of the equipment and infant cardiopulmonary resuscitation. Anticonvulsants, esophageal antireflux measures, and/or methylxanthines are also prescribed as indicated. Monitoring is continued until the infant is free from all serious apneic episodes for 3 months and all minor episodes for 2 months and until any physiologic abnormalities found on initial or subsequent evaluations have resolved.

Infants with AOI with High Mortality Rates

We have analyzed our experience with 13,400 referrals. Twenty-two infants who were monitored at home have died. The majority (82%) of those infants who died have presented with an unexplained episode of sleep onset apnea which did not respond to gentle stimulation but did resolve after the caretakers instituted vigorous stimulation or mouth-to-mouth resuscitation. Seventy-two percent of the deaths, however, occurred when there was a delay in the caretaker response to a subsequent episode of apnea during home monitoring. Thus, infants with severe sleep onset apnea seem to be at higher risk than all other infants with AOI and we, therefore, recommend immediate consultation with an apnea center for these infants coming to the emergency department.

Indications for Admission/Referral

All infants who have had an episode of apnea accompanied by a cyanotic or pale color change should be admitted for evaluation and for continued cardiorespiratory monitoring by medical personnel trained in infant monitoring and cardiopulmonary resuscitation. Infants requiring tests to determine abnormalities of ventilation, other than a pneumogram, are best referred to centers specialized in the evaluation of AOI. Finally, referral and possible transfer is recommended for those infants who are in the high mortality rate groups. The tertiary neonatal and infant referral center must be identified by all emergency departments.

Outcome

For many infants experiencing an apneic episode, the etiology can be discovered with careful searching. For those with idiopathic AOI, treatment with methylxanthines and/or home monitoring with appropriate teaching and support has been successful. Approximately 21% of the infants who were monitored at home had a subsequent successful resuscitation for apnea. Ninety-two percent of infants are well by 12 months of age. However,a few infants with severe AOI have died during home monitoring and 72% of these deaths occurred when intervention was not timely or was incorrectly performed.

SUDDEN INFANT DEATH SYNDROME (SIDS)

Introduction

Unexpected and unexplained infant deaths are known to have occurred since biblical times. With improved control of infectious causes of death in this age group, SIDS has become the leading cause of death in infants aged 1 month to 1 year, accounting for approximately 7000 deaths per year in the United States. By definition, SIDS is a sudden death, unexpected, and unexplained after careful autopsy. Abnormalities in control of ventilation described in the section on apnea provide a possible explanation for the etiology, although many other mechanisms have been proposed.

Clinical Presentation

The victim of apparent SIDS is usually found lifeless in the crib, unresponsive to parental or emergency personnel attempts at resuscitation, dead on arrival, or unresuscitatable in the emergency department. The infant may also die within several days of an apparently successful resuscitation resulting in irreversible brain damage. The history is strikingly similar from case to case; 90% are infants 1–6 months of age; the infant is thought to be asleep; and, death occurs without noise sufficient to wake a parent who may be sleeping in the same room. Most appear to have been in good health prior to death, although approximately 50% have a history of preceding trivial upper respiratory tract infection. SIDS is more common in the winter months, in male infants, in infants of mothers who smoke, in premature infants, and in families of lower socioeconomic status.

Pathologic findings have been nonspecific for a consistent etiology and some of the proposed pathophysiologic considerations are similar to those proposed in apnea of infancy; although it is not clear that AOI represents one end of a spectrum, we have reported sudden death in several infants with idiopathic apnea of infancy. However, there are likely to be several mechanisms contributing to SIDS.

Management

The emergency physician responsibility for the victim of SIDS and family extends beyond the attempt to resuscitate. The history preceding the event must be reviewed in detail and with compassion. Postmortem x-rays should be obtained to rule out the possibility of occult child abuse. Parents should be given a provisional diagnosis of SIDS and told that it is a definite, although poorly understood, clinical entity for which there is at present no known prevention. They should be told that this diagnosis can be confirmed only by autopsy to exclude occult injury, infection, or metabolic disorder and that referral of the case to the medical examiner is required by law in most jurisdictions.

The emergency physician is responsible for establishing liaison between the family and appropriate support systems (such as family clergy, family physician, professional counseling, and/or specific counseling on SIDS) and for arranging for future discussion of autopsy results with the family and the infant's physician, if there is one.

SUGGESTED READINGS

American Academy of Pediatrics: Task force on prolonged infantile apnea. Prolonged infantile apnea: 1985. *Pediatrics,* 1985;76:129–131. (This is the official statement of the American Academy of Pediatrics on the evaluation and management of infants with apnea.

Haight BF, Kelly D, and McCabe KC. Manual for home monitoring. Distributed by Massachusetts Sinai Hospital and National SIDS Foundation, 1982, Bethesda, MD. (A manual for the home training program for the infant's caretakers which is necessary before an infant can be discharged with a monitor.)

Kelly DH, Shannon DC. Treatment of apnea and excessive periodic breathing in the full-term infant. *Pediatrics* 1981,68:183–186. (This study demonstrates that pneumogram abnormalities in full-term infants normalize with theophylline.)

Kelly DH, Shannon DC. Sudden infant death syndrome and near sudden infant death syndrome: A review of the literature, 1964 to 1982. *Pediatr Clin North Am* 1982;29:1241–1261. (This article reviews the epidemiology of SIDS, recent research of the cause of SIDS and research of the pathophysiology and management of infants with apnea of infancy.)

Kelly DH, Shannon DC, O'Connell K. Care of infants with near-miss sudden infant death syndrome. *Pediatrics* 1978;61:511–514. (This article describes an approach to the evaluation and management of infants with apnea and the outcome of home monitoring, including four case studies.)

Oren J, Kelly DH, Shannon DC. Follow-up of infants who were resuscitated for sleep apnea: Identification of a high risk group. *Pediatrics* 1986;77:495–499. (This study identifies the characteristics of the infants with AOI who have a very high mortality rate (13–57%) and suggests methods of managing the infants to decrease this mortality.)

Steinschneider A. Prolonged apnea and the sudden infant death syndrome: Clinical and laboratory observations. *Pediatrics* 1972;50:646–654. (This is a report of the first two cases of sudden and unexplained death during sleep in two siblings who had apnea.)

Valdes-Dapena MA. Sudden infant death syndrome: A review of the medical literature 1974–1979. *Pediatrics, 1980;66:597–614.* (This is a state of the art review of the epidemiology and the current theories and research of the causes of SIDS.

CHAPTER **25**

The Wheezing Child

RAN D. ANBAR, M.D.
DENISE J. STRIEDER, M.D.

DEFINITIONS

Infants and children are often brought to an emergency department because of wheezing, which must be distinguished from other respiratory noises. Wheezing is a high-pitched, continuous, musical sound, heard most often during *expiration* alone, but occasionally during both expiration and inspiration. In contrast, stridor is a harsh, low-pitched vibration dominant during *inspiration*. Stridor reflects airway obstruction above the thoracic inlet, while wheezing indicates intrathoracic airway obstruction. Management of children presenting with inspiratory stridor is discussed in Chapter 23. Infants with upper or lower respiratory tract congestion may make a gurgling or rasping inspiratory sound while sucking, which parents may incorrectly refer to as wheezing.

Wheezing originates in large intrathoracic airways and is thought to be caused by vibration of both the air column and the airway walls. Vibrations are amplified during expiration, as the airway lumen narrows. Vibrations are further magnified by active expiration (dynamic compression), associated with widespread airway obstruction. Severe airway obstruction at times presents without wheezing, because air flow is insufficient to cause vibrations of the airway walls.

The term airway obstruction refers not only to complete obstruction but also to narrowing of the lumen. Possible causes are mucus accumulation, inflammation in the airway walls, bronchial smooth muscle contraction, peribronchial edema, congenital anomalies, foreign body, or any combination of these. Infants have more severe respiratory distress secondary to airway obstruction than older children. Since resistance to air flow through an airway is inversely related to the 4th power of its radius, an equal amount of narrowing causes a much greater degree of airway obstruction in infants whose airways are small.

DIFFERENTIAL DIAGNOSIS OF WHEEZING

The differential diagnosis of wheezing in children should be considered in relation to age. Bronchiolitis is a cause of wheezing, usually in infancy, resulting in marked distress because of the small airway size. Wheezing in infancy can also be the presenting symptom of congenital structural anomalies, extrinsic compression of the airways, congestive heart failure, or aspiration secondary to gastroesophageal reflux. Foreign body aspiration occurs most often in toddlers. Table 25.1 summarizes the differential diagnosis of the wheezing child, with reference to age.

History and physical examination suggest the proper diagnosis in most cases of wheezing (Table 25.2). A history of acute onset suggests foreign body aspiration or anaphylaxis. Rapid onset of wheezing suggests asthma. Recurrent wheezing may be associated with aspiration, asthma, bronchopulmonary dysplasia, or cystic fibrosis, and in these diseases cough is often associated with wheezing. In contrast, structural anomalies of the airways, which usually do not cause an increase in mucus production, frequently cause wheezing without a cough.

On physical examination, unilateral wheezing indicates foreign body aspiration, or localized airway narrowing below the trachea, such as in lobar emphysema or lymphadenopathy due to primary tuberculosis. Hyperinflation and associated flattening of the diaphragms displace the liver lower into the abdomen.

All children who present with their first episode of wheezing should have a chest x-ray to help identify congenital anomalies, interstitial edema, or cardiomegaly. If foreign body aspiration is suspected, fluoroscopy is indicated to establish unequal aeration.

MANAGEMENT OF THE WHEEZING CHILD

Some general rules apply to all patients presenting with wheezing. Obvious cyanosis is an indication for supplemental oxygen. Respiratory failure necessitates endotracheal intubation and transfer to an intensive care unit. Signs of respiratory failure include decreased or absent inspiratory breath sounds, severe inspiratory intercostal retractions and use of accessory muscles, depressed level of conciousness, decreased response to pain, and cyanosis persisting despite 40% inhaled O_2. Worsening obstruction or respiratory muscle fatigue is heralded by a rapid rise of Pco_2, i.e. more than 5 mm Hg/hr. Respiratory failure can also be defined as a Po_2 $<$ 50 mm Hg on 100% inhaled O_2, or Pco_2 $>$ 60 mm Hg. However, many infants with bronchiolitis will tolerate a Pco_2 of 60 mm Hg in the acute phase of the disease without further decompensation. Improvement of respiratory distress in the wheezing

Table 25.1.
Differential Diagnosis of Children Presenting with Wheezing

Age	Common and Acute	Uncommon and Recurrent	Uncommon	Rare[a]
<6 months	Bronchiolitis	Aspiration pneumonia[b] Bronchopulmonary dysplasia Congestive heart failure Cystic fibrosis		Asthma Foreign body aspiration
6 months to 2 years	Bronchiolitis Foreign body aspiration	Aspiration pneumonia[b] Asthma Bronchopulmonary dysplasia Cystic fibrosis		Congestive heart failure
2–5 years	Asthma Foreign body aspiration		Bronchopulmonary dysplasia Cystic fibrosis Viral pneumonia	Aspiration pneumonia[b] Bronchiolitis Congestive heart failure Mycoplasma pneumonia
5–18 years	Asthma		Cystic fibrosis Mycoplasma pneumonia Viral pneumonia	Aspiration pneumonia[b] Bronchiolitis Bronchopulmonary dysplasia Congestive heart failure Foreign body aspiration

[a] Rare for all ages; anaphylaxis, broncheal/tracheal stenosis, chondromalacia, endobronchial lesion, extrinsic airway compression (enlarged lymph nodes, mediastinal masses, vascular ring or sling), interstitial edema secondary to an extracardiac shunt, lobar emphysema, and toxic inhalation.
[b] Aspiration pneumonia may be secondary to gastroesophageal reflux, transient or permanent uncoordinated swallowing or, rarely, tracheoesophageal fistula.

Table 25.2.
Valuable Points in the History of the Wheezing Child

Was the onset of wheezing acute?
Has patient wheezed before? If so, is this the usual wheezing?
Is the wheezing associated with a cough?
Did the wheezing follow choking on food or a toy?
Was there evidence of vomiting or gagging prior to wheezing?
Was patient exposed to an allergen or toxic fume prior to wheezing?
Has the patient been drinking adequate oral fluids?
Does patient have any other significant medical conditions?
Do wheezing or other illnesses run in the family?

Important Features on Physical Examination of the Wheezing Child

1. Tachypnea, retractions, cyanosis, alertness, fatigue, vital signs, including pulsus paradoxus
2. Hyperinflation and wheezing, diffuse vs. focal
3. Conjunctivitis, rhinitis, dermatitis, failure to thrive, digital clubbing
4. Heart murmur, hepatomegaly, hemangiomas

child can be detected by an improvement in color and mental status, a decrease in tachypnea and intercostal retractions and, when appropriate, an improvement in peak expiratory flow rates.

Proper management of the wheezing child depends on an accurate diagnosis. Response to therapy can be misleading. For example, bronchodilators such as theophylline, given to a wheezing infant prone to gastroesophageal reflux, can worsen the symptoms, while bronchodilators given to a patient with an inhaled foreign body can improve symptoms and delay diagnosis.

Aspiration Pneumonia

Aspiration pneumonia is caused by inhalation of a foreign substance (usually food or gastric contents), with subsequent changes secondary to inflammation or obstruction. Aspirations may be due to gastroesophageal reflux, incoordinated swallowing secondary to neurological disorders, or a fistula between the tracheobronchial tree and the gastrointestinal tract. Gastroesophageal reflux may also cause wheezing in the absence of tracheal aspiration, by direct stimulation of esophageal vagal receptors, leading to reflex bronchospasm.

Recurring aspiration is not necessarily accompanied by frequent vomiting or choking but it should be suspected in any young child with recurring pulmonary symptoms, in whom asthma is unlikely and cystic fibrosis has been ruled out. A barium swallow, esophageal pH probe testing, or a milk technetium scan study are tests to help verify the diagnosis of reflux. A successful antireflux therapeutic trial supports the diagnosis.

The most common cause of recurring aspiration in infants is gastroesophageal reflux. Treatment includes frequent feedings thickened with 1–2 teaspoons of cereal per ounce (formula), positioning the child after meals either upright or prone with head and chest elevated. If these measures fail, metoclopramide is the drug of choice in a concentration of 1 mg/ml, 0.5 mg/kg/day divided in equal doses, 15 minutes before meals. Metoclopramide enhances gastric motility and raises the lower esophageal sphincter tone. Serious side effects are uncommon, but do include acute dystonic reactions, which may lead to an emergency department visit. Treatment therefore consists of diphenhydramine (Benadryl), 1 mg/kg, which takes effect within 3–5 minutes intravenously, or within 30 minutes if given intramuscularly.

Surgical correction of gastroesophageal reflux by gastric fundoplication is not an emergency department consideration.

Asthma

Asthma is a reversible obstructive airway disease, characterized by increased mucus production, peribronchial edema, and bronchial smooth muscle contraction. Precipitating factors include upper respiratory tract infections, environmental allergens, exercise, and exposure to cold or certain drugs. Children with asthma often present a history of atopic dermatitis and/or bronchiolitis, and a family history of asthma or hay fever. The disease affects approximately 5% of children in the United States. The patient presents with recurring episodes of dyspnea characterized by prolonged expiration, suprasternal and intercostal retractions, tachypnea and wheezing, recurring cough, or a feeling of constriction in the chest. Severe attacks may cause cyanosis and acute respiratory failure. Further elaboration considering triggering events and pathophysiology of asthma is found in Chapter 9.

Table 25.2 lists the baseline information to be gathered for all wheezing children. The following questions are important to be answered in the emergency department: What medication(s) is the child taking? Has there been good compliance and tolerance for this medication(s)? Have corticosteroids been required within the past 12 months? Has the patient been hospitalized for asthma? If so, was intensive care required?

A flow sheet is useful in gauging the effectiveness of treatment for the asthmatic patient and in planning succeeding management steps. All therapeutic maneuvers are noted on the flow sheet and findings on physical examination are recorded at 15-minute intervals: pulse rate, respiratory rate, pulsus paradoxus (systolic pressure variance of 20–50 mm Hg or more between inspiration and expiration), extent of retractions, inspiratory:expiratory (I:E) ratio, quality of air movement, and degree of wheezing. It must be remembered that wheezing may be absent when air movement is very poor. In such a circumstance improvement can actually be heralded by the onset of wheezing.

Unless too ill, children over 5 years of age cooperate for effort-dependent measurements of their peak expiratory flow rate (PEFR), measured with a pediatric Wright peak flow meter. This measurement provides an objective assessment of the clinical status of the asthmatic child. It is recorded on the asthma flow sheet. Fig. 25.1 shows expected PEFR values based on the patient's height. A chest x-ray is not necessary in assessing an uncomplicated recurrent asthma attack. The film would show hyperinflated lungs, flattened diaphragms, increased peribronchial markings, a small cardiac shadow, and occasionally migratory atelectasis. If a concurrent infection is suspected, a complete blood cell count should be obtained prior to administration of β agonists. The white blood cell count can actually be elevated in asthma because of stress, unrelated to infection.

Dehydration

Dehydration is common in asthmatic children because of increased insensible water loss, decreased fluid intake, and increased incidence of vomiting. Deficits should be corrected and maintenance fluids provided intravenously. Overhydration should be avoided; it does not improve mucus clearance and can lead to interstitial pulmonary edema.

Atelectasis

The most common complication of asthma is atelectasis. It occurs in 10% of children hospitalized with asthma, predominantly in the middle and upper lobes of the right lung. Atelectasis should be differentiated from pneumonia. Percussion respiratory therapy and postural drainage are helpful in the management of atelectasis. Antibiotics are not indicated.

Pneumomediastinum/Pneumothorax

Pneumomediastinum, occurring in 5% of children hospitalized with asthma, usually resolves, with improvement in clinical symptoms over a period of 7–10 days. On the other hand, pneumothorax is rare, except in patients requiring assisted ventilation. A small pneumothorax may be managed conservatively with careful observation. A large or tension pneumothorax with respiratory distress necessitates placement of a chest tube.

Metabolic Acidosis

Metabolic acidosis in young children with asthma is usually due to ketoacidosis. It is corrected with dextrose and fluid administration and, when possible, resumption of oral caloric intake.

Medications

Sympathomimetics, theophylline, and steroids are the major drugs utilized in the emergency management of children presenting with asthmatic wheezing.

Sympathomimetics (Table 25.3). Sympathomimetic agents cause bronchodilation by stimulating the β_2 receptors on bronchial smooth muscle and secretory cells. Sympathomimetics are avail-

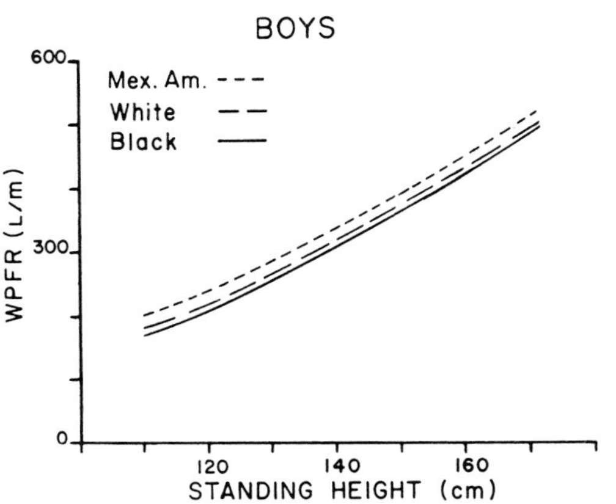

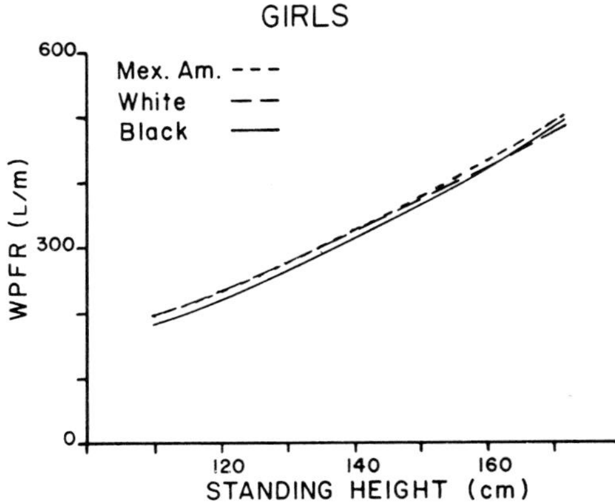

Figure 25.1. Prediction curves of Wright peak flow rate (WPFR) for each race and sex versus standing height. (From Hsu KHK, Jenkins DE, Bartholomew PH, et al. Ventilatory functions of normal children and young adults—Mexican-American, white, and black. *J Pediatr,* 1979;95:192–196).

Table 25.3.
Selected Sympathomimetic Drugs for Asthmatic Patients, Listed in Ascending Order of β_2 Specificity

	Subcutaneous	Aerosolized	Metered Dose Inhaler	Oral Preparation
Epinephrine	1/1000 solution 0.01 ml/kg/dose Maximum dose 0.3 ml q 20 minutes × 3	Available in racemic form: only ½ of the dose is active	AsthmaHaler Bronkaid Primatene (All over the counter)	Not available
Isoetharine (Bronkosol)	Not available	1% solution 0.25 ml for <20 kg 0.5 ml for ≥20 kg in 2.5 ml saline	Bronkometer 1 or 2 puffs q 4 hr	Not available
Metaproterenol (Alupent, Metaprel)	Not available	5% solution 0.15 ml for <20 kg 0.3 ml for ≥20 kg in 2.5 ml saline	2 puffs q 3–4 hr	5 mg tid for <10 kg 10 mg tid for 10–25 kg 20 mg tid for >25 kg
Terbutaline (Brethine, Bricanyl)	1/1000 solution 0.005 ml/kg/dose Maximum dose 0.25 ml q 30 minutes × 2	0.1% solution 0.25 ml for <20 kg 0.5 ml for ≥20 kg in 2.5 ml saline	Brethaire Brethancer 2 puffs q 4–6 hr	Not recommended for children under 12 years 2.5 mg tid for 30–50 kg 5 mg tid for >50 kg
Albuterol (Ventolin, Proventil, Salbutamol)	Not available	0.5% solution 0.25 ml for <20 kg 0.5 ml for ≥20 kg in 2.5 ml saline	2 puffs q 4–6 hr	1 mg tid for <10 kg 2 mg tid for 10–25 kg 4 mg tid for >25 kg

able in aerosolized, parenteral, and oral forms. Aerosolized forms have been shown to be as effective as parenteral and oral forms, even in patients with poor air movement. In providing a similar clinical response, inhaled β_2 agonists have a lower incidence of side effects than the same drugs administered orally or parenterally. Therefore, in most cases, treatment of an asthmatic attack should begin with inhalation of aerosolized β_2 agonists.

Young children seem to be less threatened by a Styrofoam cup mounted onto a nebulizer than by a face mask. They usually allow the cup close to their nose and mouth and inhale sufficient medication to produce a clinical response.

Dosages for selected sympathomimetics are listed in Table 25.3. In general, predominantly β_2 specific agents should be used to maximize bronchodilation with minimal side effects.

Inhalation treatments can be repeated three times in the 1st hour and subsequently on a 3–4 hour basis—even more frequently, if necessary, so long as close attention is paid to vital signs and other parameters included on the asthma flow sheet. In most cases, if two treatments do not improve the status of the patient, a nonsympathomimetic medication is added.

Indications for parenteral administration of β agonists are few: (*a*) patients in respiratory failure; (*b*) older children who insist, despite patient education, that subcutaneous treatment is more effective for them than an inhalation; and (*c*) patients who do not cooperate in the administration of an inhaled treatment.

β_2 agonists, delivered by a metered dose inhaler, are also the first-line drug for continued management of the acute asthmatic episode after discharge from the emergency department. Children who are unable to use inhalers may be given an oral β agonist.

Theophylline (Table 25.4). The bronchodilating effect of theophylline is no longer thought secondary to its inhibition of phosphodiesterase, because concentrations 10-fold higher than attained clinically would be required to effect this mechanism. It is more likely that theophylline causes bronchodilation by its effects on intracellular calcium ion concentration and its antagonism of adenosine.

The therapeutic range of serum theophylline concentration is 10–20 μg/ml. Achievement of a therapeutic level should be considered a guideline rather than an imperative. Side effects, especially nausea

Table 25.4.
Aminophylline and Theophylline Starting Dosages

Pediatric Intravenous Aminophylline Starting Dosages

Loading dose: 7 mg/kg in 25 ml saline over 20 minutes (3.5 mg/kg if child has received oral theophylline less than 6 hours before presentation)
Maintenance rate: 1/1000 or 1 mg/ml solution; e.g., 250 mg aminophylline/250 ml saline

Age	Dosage
	mg/kg/hr
Less than 1 year	0.0125 × age in weeks + 0.33
1–3 years	1.1
3–6 years	1.0
6–9 years	0.9
9–12 years	0.8
12–18 years	0.7

Pediatric Oral Theophylline Starting Dosages[a]

Age	Dosage q 6 hr	Dosage q 8 hr	Dosage q 12 hr
		mg/kg/dose	
0–1 years	0.3 × age in weeks + 8[b]		
1–5 years	6	8	12
5–10 years	5	6.5	10
10–15 years[c]	4.5	6	9
15–18 years[c]	3	4	6

[a] Dosages above these require serum theophylline level checks.
[b] Total daily dose.
[c] Total daily dose not to exceed 800 mg regardless of body weight.

and vomiting, can be manifest below the therapeutic range. Seizures usually occur only with serum levels exceeding 20 μg/ml. However, theophylline lowers the seizure threshold at any concentration in susceptible individuals. Therapeutic effect in children has been noted at serum concentrations of less than 10 mg/ml but some children need serum levels in excess of 20 mg/ml to achieve optimal physiologic effect without side effects.

Children arriving at the emergency department have often been taking a theophylline preparation for chronic management of asthma. If the theophylline dose was appropriate (Table 25.4), if the preparation used was short-acting, and if the last dose was taken more than 6 hours before the visit, the serum level can be assumed low because of the relatively short half-life of theophylline. These children can be given regular emergency department loading doses (Table 25.4). For children who received higher than recommended doses prior to arrival or have taken a recent dose, the loading dose is halved. If a serum theophylline level is quickly obtainable, a precise loading dose can be calculated using the rule: *1 mg/kg of theophylline raises the serum concentration by approximately 2 μg/ml.* For children who have been taking a sustained-release theophylline, the serum level may peak 3–4 hours after the last dose, and absorption from the gut may continue for 10–12 hours. Safe administration of additional theophylline to these children requires frequent monitoring of serum level.

Treatment begins with a loading dose of 7 mg/kg given orally as a short-acting preparation or intravenously over 20 minutes as aminophylline (85% theophylline). (If the intravenous loading dose is delivered over a longer period of time, the peak serum level will be lower than expected.) The choice between oral and intravenous routes depends on the severity of the asthmatic attack and the clinical response to β_2 agonists. If the child remains in respiratory distress, a second theophylline bolus may be indicated but should be given only after a serum theophylline level has been checked. If this level is below 10 μg/ml, another intravenous aminophylline bolus can be given to raise the serum level into the 15–20 μg/ml range. During intravenous administration of an aminophylline bolus, children should be monitored for the uncommon development of tachyarrhythmias and hypotension.

An aminophylline bolus is best followed by a constant drip at a rate which varies with age and weight (Table 25.4). Serum theophylline levels should be monitored because individual patients have differing clearance rates. If a constant infusion pump is not available, the patient may be given quadruple the hourly dose as a 30-minute bolus every 4 hours.

Children who show a good clinical response to theophylline in the emergency department may be discharged with a prescription for an 8–10-day course of oral theophylline. There are many oral preparations of theophylline. A particular brand is chosen on the basis of tolerance and bioavailability. Theophylline is available as (*a*) a liquid, short-acting preparation, often disliked by children; (*b*) capsules, containing sustained-release beads which can be mixed with food but have an erratic absorption pattern; and (*c*) tablets, which are available as short-acting or sustained-release. The short-acting tablet may be crushed and mixed in jam for younger children (the sustained-release tablet will lose its long-acting character if crushed). Short-acting forms are given every 6 hours; and long-acting, every 8–12 hours. The long-acting theophylline capsule is prescribed for children unable to swallow a sustained-release tablet or because of poor compliance with the more frequent administration required for short-acting preparations. The same total daily dose of theophylline is given whether the short or long-acting preparation is prescribed (Table 25.4).

Theophylline dosage should be reduced in the presence of congestive heart failure or liver disease because clearance is decreased in these circumstances. Theophylline metabolism is also affected by several drugs in common pediatric use: erythromycin and cimetidine decrease theophylline clearance; phenobarbital, phenytoin, and carbamazepine (Tegretol) increase clearance.

Corticosteroids (Table 25.5). Corticosteroids are valuable in the treatment of asthma because of their anti-inflammatory properties and their inhibition of prostaglandin and other vasoactive substance release. Corticosteroids make the bronchial smooth muscle more responsive to β agonists within an hour of parenteral administration. Inhaled steroids should generally not be used in the management of acute asthma.

Corticosteroids are used in the asthmatic child if: (*a*) symptoms persist after sympathomimetic and theophylline administration; (*b*) the child has a history of relapse if steroids are not used; or (*c*) the child has required steroids, including inhaled preparations, for asthma control within the past 6 months. Oral corticosteroids may be given in a short course (3–7 days) without a dose tapering for an acute asthma attack. If an intravenous line has already been placed for an aminophylline bolus in a child to be discharged, the first dose of a corticosteroid should be given as an intravenous push to allow for rapid action. Table 25.5 lists the dosages for commonly used corticosteroids.

Cromolyn. Cromolyn is the drug of choice for long-term control of chronic asthma. It does not help resolve an acute attack. Cromolyn treatment should be recommended or initiated in the emergency department if a patient develops an acute attack despite adequate maintenance doses of sympathomimetics and theophylline at home. Cromolyn can be administered by metered dose inhaler (MDI) or by nebulizer. By MDI the dosage is 3 puffs, three times per day, regardless of patient weight. By nebulizer cromolyn is also administered three times per day, 20 mg/dose, regardless of weight. After 2 months without recurrence of asthma, its administration may be reduced to twice daily.

Table 25.5.
Selected Corticosteroids Used in Treatment of Acute Pediatric Asthma

Intravenously		
Methylprednisolone[a]	1 mg/kg/dose	q 6 hr
Hydrocortisone[b]	2.5 mg/kg/dose	q 6 hr
Orally		
Prednisone	1 mg/kg/dose (maximum = 60-mg dose)	q A.M.

[a] Less mineralocorticoid effect than hydrocortisone.
[b] Less than half the price of methylprednisolone.

Anticholinergic agents, antihistamines, expectorants, mucolytic agents, and *cough suppressants* are not indicated in management of asthma.

Discharge Plans. A child is ready to be discharged from the emergency department when most symptoms have abated and when he or she can drink fluids and tolerate oral medications. The parent, or an older patient, should compare the current status to previous experience and take part in the decision to discharge.

Most children with an acute asthmatic attack improve enough in response to emergency department treatment to allow discharge. However, the therapeutic effects of sympathomimetic agents and/or theophylline given in the emergency department last only for 2–6 hours. Maintenence therapy must be prescribed, to prevent a symptomatic relapse. In addition, even though a child's symptoms may have dramatically improved, the underlying lung pathology persists. Therefore, continued medication is needed to control symptoms and allow complete recovery from the attack.

If a child is not currently taking medication for asthma, he or she should be started on a sympathomimetic agent. Children older than 8 years can be instructed in use of a MDI (Table 25.3). Younger children can be given an oral form of albuterol (Table 25.3), which is the most specific oral β_2 agent. If a child was taking medication prior to presentation, the dose should be optimized or another drug added to the treatment regimen (Table 25.6). With the exception of cromolyn, which is prescribed for long-term prevention, medications are usually prescribed in the emergency department for a 5–10-day course. The patient must be seen within that time by the primary care provider. The primary provider must educate the patient and family regarding the early signs of an asthma attack, such as retractions or tachypnea, and encourage them to seek early help. The follow-up plan should be clearly explained to the parents and arranged by contact with the primary care provider.

Status Asthmaticus

Patients who fail to improve or continue to deteriorate despite emergency department treatment with an adrenergic agent and theophylline are considered to be in status asthmaticus. They require hospitalization. All patients in status asthmaticus are hypoxic while breathing room air, secondary to perfusion of poorly ventilated or atelectatic regions

Table 25.6.
Algorithm for Treating an Acute Pediatric Asthma Attack

Treat with a sympathomimetic agent (Table 25.3); if improved, *end ED treatment.*
If not improved, add theophylline (Table 25.4); if improved, *end ED treatment.*
If not improved, begin aminophylline maintenance drip (Table 25.4) and corticosteroids (Table 25.5)

Upon sending home:
If patient presented with no medications: send home on a *sympathomimetic.*
If patient presented taking a sympathomimetic *or* theophylline: send home on a *sympathomimetic and theophylline.*
If patient presented taking a sympathomimetic *and* theophylline: send home on a *sympathomimetic and theophylline* and a short course of *corticosteroids;* recommend or initiate *cromolyn.*
If patient presented taking a sympathomimetic *and* theophylline *and* corticosteroids: send home on optimal dose of *all medications* and a *higher* short-term dose of *steroids;* recommend or initiate *cromolyn;* recommend or initiate *consultation* (pediatric allergy or pulmonology).

in their lungs. Arterial blood gases are obtained in the emergency department as a baseline. Humidified oxygen is administered even before results of the blood gases are known. The Po_2 should be maintained above 70 mm Hg; it is seldom necessary to use more than 30% O_2. Mist tents are *not* indicated because water droplets irritate the airways of many asthmatics.

While the patient is awaiting admission, treatment is continued with inhaled sympathomimetics (Table 25.3), aminophylline drip or regular boluses (Table 25.4), and intravenous corticosteroids (Table 25.5). Antibiotics are indicated only if there is evidence of infection: fever above 101°F, leukocytosis prior to β agonist administration, purulent sputum with a dominant bacterial form on Gram's stain, or radiographic evidence of pneumonia. Sedation is contraindicated because of the danger of respiratory depression.

Respiratory Failure

Children with asthma who present to the emergency department in extreme distress or even respiratory arrest, in need of immediate ventilatory support, must be managed differently from other patients needing resuscitation. Mouth-to-mouth breathing is usually ineffective because of inability to generate sufficient pressures; even if adequate ventilation is achieved initially, the resuscitator quickly tires because of the necessary high inflation pressure. Self-inflating ventilation bags are generally inadequate because they usually have a safety ("pop-off") valve opening at pressures below those required for ventilating an asthmatic patient. Because of their lung disease, these patients should be resuscitated with an anesthesia or Mapleson bag that does not have a safety valve. One hundred percent oxygen should be used. Adequate time for expiration can be judged by allowing chest movement almost to cease prior to initiation of insufflation. Effectiveness of the resuscitation is gauged by assessment of chest movement, auscultation for breath sounds, and resolution of clinical cyanosis. As soon as cyanosis resolves and an intravenous line has been secured, a comatose patient should have an endotracheal tube placed.

An asthmatic patient in combined respiratory and metabolic acidosis should *not* be given bicarbonate. If ventilation is ineffective, conversion of bicarbonate to carbon dioxide worsens the respiratory acidosis. On the other hand, if ventilation and oxygenation are effective, respiratory and lactic acidosis resolves as the resuscitation progresses. The remaining ketoacidosis does not require immediate correction in these circumstances.

Bronchiolitis

In infants, viral lower respiratory tract infections are clinically manifested as bronchiolitis. The illness usually occurs during winter and early spring and is associated with a respiratory syncytial virus (RSV) infection. The typical infant is between 2 and 6 months of age, and has had a low-grade fever (less than 102°F), coryza, and cough for a few days. In an occasional patient the symptoms develop over as little time as several hours. With spread of the infection to the distal airways, the destruction of epithelial cells, inflammatory cell infiltration of the airway walls, and peribronchial edema all result in severe obstruction. The infant is most vulnerable during the first 72 hours of illness, after which rapid improvement can be expected.

On physical examination, the bronchiolitic patient is tachypneic with a respiratory rate > 40 and demonstrates retraction and wheezing. Hyperinflation of the lungs and an increased anterior-posterior diameter are usually noted on physical examination and chest x-ray. In addition, the child may exhibit signs of dehydration secondary to inadequate fluid intake. Arterial blood gases reveal hypoxemia, which correlates with the respiratory rate. The white blood cell count is usually normal.

Small areas of atelectasis are usually seen on the chest x-ray of bronchiolitic infants. Pneumothorax and pneumomediastinum are rare, except in patients treated with assisted ventilation. Prolonged

Table 25.7.
Criteria Which Must Be Fulfilled Prior to Discharging a Child with Bronchiolitis from the Emergency Department

The child must:
Be well-hydrated
Drink fluids well
Void normally
Not be cyanotic while breathing room air
Appear comfortable in parent's arms
Have a respiratory rate less than 60 per minute
Not have a history of apnea during the illness
Not have a past history of prematurity or bronchopulmonary dysplasia
The parents must:
Be comfortable in following the child's respiratory and hydration status at home

(> 20 seconds) and frequent apneic spells occur early in the course of the illness, possibly as the presenting complaint, such as a cyanotic spell, in an infant with an otherwise unremarkable upper respiratory tract infection. This complication is probably related to an RSV-specific impairment of central control of respiration, since apnea is seldom seen with bronchiolitis caused by other viral agents. Infants with underlying medical disorders, such as prematurity, bronchopulmonary dysplasia, or congestive heart failure, have increased morbidity and mortality rates.

Bronchiolitis is usually a mild disease, diagnosed by the primary physician and managed at home. Serious illness is recognized from respiratory distress, requirement for oxygen, and inability to take adequate oral fluids. Such patients must be admitted to the hospital. Table 25.7 lists the criteria which should be fulfilled prior to sending an infant with bronchiolitis home from the emergency department. Parents must be instructed to monitor fluid intake and respiratory rate and to return to the emergency department if these deteriorate. Discharged patients should be seen within 24 hours for reevaluation.

The hospital management of bronchiolitis is mostly supportive. Humidified oxygen (Fio_2 of 40%) is provided by mask, hood, or tent. Nasal prongs tend to cause reflex bronchospasm and should not be used. Maintenance intravenous hydration is needed for infants who cannot drink because of their respiratory distress. Overhydration is not helpful.

Bronchiolitic infants under 2 months of age with rectal temperatures over 102°F and infants who appear clinically toxic should be treated with broad-spectrum antibiotics, because they may have acquired a bacterial superinfection. Before antibiotic administration, tracheal secretions and blood are obtained for bacterial culture.

If a trial of a sympathomimetic drug improves the symptoms of a child with bronchiolitis, maintenance sympathomimetics (Table 25.3) or theophylline (Table 25.4) can then be given. In infants older than 6 months, bronchiolitis may be difficult to distinguish from an episode of asthma on the basis of history and physical findings. The clinical response to bronchodilators does not rule out bronchiolitis.

A new antiviral agent, ribavirin, improves symptoms of bronchiolitis in patients with RSV infection. The drug is administered by a small particle aerosol generator for 12–20 hours/day for 3–7 days. Candidates for such treatment are infants in severe respiratory distress and infants who are at high risk of severe illness because of a history of premature birth, congenital heart disease, or an underlying pulmonary disorder, such as bronchopulmonary dysplasia. Infants considered for treatment with ribavirin should have nasotracheal aspirates analyzed by immunoflorescent staining for confirmation of RSV. Infants requiring intubation for respiratory failure can be given ribavirin, only when special precautions are taken to limit precipitation of drug in the respirator. On rare occasion, pulmonary function worsens after administration of the drug.

Corticosteroids are *not* helpful in the management of bronchiolitis. Sedatives are contraindicated because of suppression of the respiratory drive.

Patients with bronchiolitis should be isolated from other infants by contact precautions because they shed RSV in sputum for several weeks after contracting the illness.

Bronchopulmonary Dysplasia

Bronchopulmonary dysplasia (BPD) is a chronic obstructive lung disease, resulting from prolonged mechanical ventilation of a premature infant. The parents are usually aware of the diagnosis.

Many infants with BPD are chronically tachypneic, have intercostal retractions, and wheeze. The wheezing may be exacerbated by viral infections or by interstitial pulmonary edema. If a viral infection is causing respiratory distress in an infant or toddler with BPD, that child should be admitted for close observation and treatment because of the high risk of respiratory decompensation. A chest film should be obtained to detect interstitial pulmonary edema, the presence of which indicates the need for fluid restriction and diuretics. If the child is responsive to bronchodilator therapy, this form of treatment should be pursued (Tables 25.3–25.5).

Congestive Heart Failure

Pulmonary congestion secondary to heart failure can present as tachypnea, cough, cyanosis, and wheezing. In infants, the most common cause of congestive heart failure (CHF) is a congenital heart lesion associated with a large left-to-right shunt.

Other causes of CHF include myocarditis, endocarditis, or rheumatic heart disease, arrhythmias, doxorubicin (Adriamycin) therapy, large extracardiac left-to-right shunts (hemangioma or pulmonary sequestration), and iatrogenic fluid overload.

Cystic Fibrosis

Cystic fibrosis (CF) is an autosomal recessive disorder affecting primarily Caucasians. In this disease, abnormal function of exocrine glands results in the secretion of abnormally thick mucus. Bronchial mucus is poorly cleared, with resulting airway obstruction which causes dyspnea, hyperinflation, a prolonged inspiratory:expiratory ratio, and in some children expiratory wheezing. Mucus stasis predisposes to chronic bacterial infections, which ultimately lead to destruction of bronchial walls and bronchiectasis, and pulmonary scarring.

Patients with undiagnosed CF who come to the emergency department with wheezing usually have a history of chronic cough. They may also have a history of recurrent bronchopulmonary infections, failure to thrive, and/or chronic production of large greasy stools, which parents often describe as diarrhea. On physical examination, clubbing, nasal polyps, barrel chest appearance, or a prominent abdomen raise suspicion of CF. Chest x-ray in the young child shows hyperinflation and peribronchial cuffing, occasionally with segmental atelectasis or pneumonitis. Sputum cultures are likely to yield *Staphylococcus aureus, Haemophilus influenzae,* or *Pseudomonas aeruginosa.* Any child suspected of having CF should be referred to a CF center for a diagnostic sweat chloride test and evaluation.

Patients with previously diagnosed CF can come to the emergency department with wheezing because of intercurrent respiratory viral infection or because of associated asthma. These patients are often responsive to bronchodilators (Tables 25.3–25.5). Hydration is essential to improve mobilization of the thick secretions. Chest physiotherapy is a valuable adjunct to clearing the secretions.

Acute pulmonary complications of CF include exacerbations of chronic bronchial infection, atelectasis, hemoptysis, lung abscess, pneumonia, and pneumothorax. Patients on long-term oral antibiotic treatment for control of their airway disease are likely to harbor *Pseudomonas* species as the dominant organisms in their sputum. When antibiotic treatment is needed, antipseudomonal drugs are usually given intravenously. These include the semisynthetic penicillins, third generation cephalosporins, and aminoglycosides. Recently, ciprofloxacin has become available as an effective oral agent in the treatment of acute exacerbations due to *Pseudomonas.* This drug should not be administered without consultation with a CF specialist.

Foreign Body Aspiration

Toddlers are candidates for foreign body aspiration, but infants have been known to inhale objects placed in their grasps or in their mouths. Older children also accidentally inhale small objects, such as paper clips, peanuts or seeds. A history of choking in a child, who presents with sudden onset of wheezing, suggests a foreign body aspiration.

Noting asymmetry of the chest and evidence of localized air trapping on physical examination, review of inspiratory and expiratory chest films, or chest fluoroscopy are the principal methods of diagnosing foreign body aspiration. The foreign body is infrequently radiopaque and visible on chest film. Bronchoscopy is diagnostic and in most instances the foreign body can be removed through the open, rigid bronchoscope. Bronchial mucoid impaction in asthmatics may cause localized air trapping, decreased breath sounds, and wheezing, mimicking foreign body aspiration.

So long as the child is effectively moving air, *no attempt* should be made by the emergency department staff to remove the foreign body. Attempts by inexperienced persons to remove a foreign body from a bronchus may result in complete obstruction of the trachea or larynx or distal impaction of the foreign body. If obstruction of trachea or larynx is complete, the Heimlich maneuver should be performed on children older than 1 year of age. Back thumps and chest thrusts should be used in children less than 1 year of age, instead of the Heimlich maneuver, which may result in injury to abdominal organs in infants. (See Chapter 24 for management of the pediatric upper airway obstruction.)

On rare occasions children arrive several weeks after foreign body aspiration, with wheezing, pneumonia, or chest pain. A choking spell may not have been observed or it may not be recalled. Foreign body aspiration should be suspected in children of all ages with pulmonary disease of acute onset that fails to resolve spontaneously or to clear completely with therapy.

Toxic Inhalation

Many chemicals, if inhaled in sufficiently high concentrations, cause acute interstitial pulmonary edema and inflammation, which present as a sudden onset of cough, wheezing, cyanosis, and chest pain. Chemicals associated with illness in children include hydrocarbons (in kerosene and some furniture polishes), shellac, gum arabic, polyvinylpyrrolidone (in some hair sprays), ammonia, and chlorine (in bathroom cleaning fluids and swimming pool maintenance fluids). Other toxic inhalants are found at the work place, where a child occasionally might encounter them.

The local poison control center should be consulted when a particular offending agent has been identified. Treatment is generally supportive: oxygen, chest physiotherapy, fluids, and antibiotics for bacterial superinfections.

Rare Causes of Wheezing

Anaphylaxis

Anaphylaxis occurs within minutes of exposure to an allergen to which the child is sensitized. The degree of reaction may vary from pruritus, urticaria, nausea, and abdominal pain to laryngeal edema and stridor, small airways obstruction with wheezing, shock, and even death within as few as 10 minutes of the onset of symptoms. Following injection of an antigen, such as with drug administration, or a bee sting, symptoms can start within 30 seconds; following ingestion or inhalation, symptoms begin within several minutes.

Anaphylaxis is caused by a type I, IgE-mediated reaction. The allergen combines with IgE on the surface of mast cells, causing release of histamine and other mediators of immediate hypersensitivity. These cause increased capillary permeability, resulting in tissue edema. The increased capillary leak causes loss of intravascular fluids, which may lead to circulatory collapse. Histamine release causes bronchospasm.

Causes of anaphylaxis include certain antibiotics (penicillins, cephalosporins, tetracycline, streptomycin), other drugs (aspirin, dextran), biologic agents (insect venoms, allergen extracts, human gamma globulin, blood transfusion, hormones), diagnostic agents (iodinated contrast media), and foods (eggs, milk, citrus fruit, shellfish, peanuts, and chocolate). Inhaling the products of cooking foods, such as broiling fish or roasting nuts, has been reported to cause anaphylaxis.

Treatment of an anaphylactic reaction must begin immediately upon recognition of the process:

1. Discontinue administration of any possible agents of anaphylaxis.
2. Administer epinephrine 1:1000 (aqueous solution, 1 mg/ml), 0.01 ml/kg/dose subcutaneously (maximum dose 0.4 ml). If laryngeal edema impairs respirations at this time, give the first dose of epinephrine, diluted with 10 ml normal saline by intravenous push.
3. Inject 0.01 ml/kg aqueous epinephrine 1:1000 into the antigen introduction site to slow absorption of the antigen. Repeat every 20 minutes three times.

For more severe anaphylactic reactions:

4. Begin intravenous line.
5. Provide oxygen by mask.
6. Inject 1 mg/kg (up to 50 mg) diphenhydramine (Benadryl) intravenously slowly, to inhibit further histamine release. This may be followed by 1 mg/kg/doses (up to 50 mg) diphenhydramine every 6 hours by mouth, or intravenously, or by intramuscular injection.

For very severe anaphylactic reactions:

7. If there is evidence of hypotension, provide an isotonic solution in a 20 ml/kg "wide-open" intravenous bolus, preferably with 5% albumin.
8. Persistent hypotension can be treated with vasoconstrictors such as norepinephrine (0.1–0.5 μg/kg/min) or dopamine (10–30 μg/kg/min).
   - 1.0 mg of norepinephrine mixed in 100 ml normal saline yields a solution which, when run at body weight (number of ml = body weight in kg) per *hour* is equivalent to 0.17 μg/kg/min.
   - 60.0 mg of dopamine mixed in 100 ml normal saline yields a solution which, when run at body weight (number of ml = body weight in kg) per *hour* is equivalent to 10.0 μg/kg/min.
9. Give 10 mg/kg hydrocortisone intravenously, followed by 5 mg/kg every 6 hours.
10. Bronchospasm should be treated initially with β_2 inhalants (Table 25.3). If bronchospasm persists, 4 mg/kg aminophylline may be given intravenously over 30 minutes, followed by a constant drip as outlined in Table 25.4. However, aminophylline should be not administered concurrently with β_1 agonists such as intravenous epinephrine, because of an increased likelihood of cardiac arrhythmias. *Caution:* aminophylline is a potent vasodilator during rapid administration.

Bronchial or Tracheal Stenosis

Bronchial or tracheal stenosis can cause chronic wheezing in the infant. Usually congenital in origin, bronchial stenosis can occur as a complication of thoracic surgery or of endobronchial tuberculosis. Tracheal stenosis, on the other hand, occurs either as a congenital lesion or as a complication of prolonged endotracheal intubation. Definitive diagnosis is accomplished at bronchoscopy.

Chondromalacia

Chondromalacia is associated with hypercompliant airways and wheezing. The chest x-ray is normal. Flexible bronchoscopy, allowing for spontaneous breathing during the examination, identifies the characteristic expiratory collapse of the lower trachea and main bronchi. As children become older, the airways usually stiffen and symptoms disappear.

Endobronchial Lesion

An endobronchial lesion, such as a bronchial cyst, hemangioma or web, or tumor can obstruct airflow during expiration, leading to *lobar emphysema*. The obstruction may be associated with wheezing. Clinical and radiologic findings are indistinguishable from a foreign body, but the history usually suggests persistent or slowly progressive symptoms.

Extrinsic Compression of the Airways

Extrinsic compression of the airways can be caused by a vascular anomaly, enlarged hilar nodes, mediastinal masses, or any other process that impinges on the airway. An enlarged thymus very rarely causes compression. A chest x-ray, tuberculin skin test, barium swallow, computed chest tomography, and/or bronchoscopy should identify the cause for the airway compression.

Left-to-Right Extracardiac Shunt

A left-to-right extracardiac shunt (systemic arteriovenous fistula, hemangioma) can cause interstitial pulmonary edema and respiratory symptoms including tachypnea and wheezing, as an early manifestation of congestive heart failure.

Pneumonia

Pneumonia is uncommonly associated with wheezing. Only viral and *Mycoplasma* pneumonias may be accompanied by wheezing, because of widespread airway involvement associated with the pneumonic process. Primary tuberculosis and, very rarely, bacterial pneumonia may cause hilar lymphadenopathy large enough to compress the trachea or lobar bronchi, causing focal wheezing. Wheezing associated with pneumonia may represent infection in a child suffering from an acute asthma attack. The evaluation and management of childhood pneumonias are discussed in Chapter 26.

SUGGESTED READINGS

Becker AB, Nelson NA, Simons FER. Inhaled salbutamol (albuterol) vs. injected epinephrine in the treatment of acute asthma in children. *J Pediatr,* 1983;102:465–469.

Blazer S, Naveh Y, Friedman A. Foreign body in the airway. *Am J Dis Child,* 1980;134:68–71.

Eigen H. Pulmonary function testing: A practical guide to its use in pediatric practice. *Pediatr Rev* 1986;7:235–245.

Ellis EF. Asthma in childhood. *J Allergy Clin Immunol* 1983;72:526–538.

Fireman, P. The wheezing infant. *Pediatr Rev* 1986;7:247–254.

Hall CB, McBride JT, Walsh EE, et al. Aerosolized ribavirin treatment of infants with respiratory syncytial viral infection. *N Engl J Med* 1983;308:1443–1447.

Hendeles L, Massanari M, Weinberger M. Update on the pharmacodynamics and pharmacokinetics of theophylline. *Chest* 1985;88(suppl 2):103S–111S.

Hsu KHK, Jenkins DE, Bartholomew PH, et al. Ventilatory functions of normal children and young adults—Mexican-American, white, and black. II. Wright peak flowmeter. *J Pediatr* 1979;95:192–196.

Nelson, HS. Adrenergic therapy of bronchial asthma. *J Allergy Clin Immunol* 1986;77:771–785.

Nickerson BG. Bronchopulmonary dysplasia: Chronic pulmonary disease following neonatal respiratory failure. *Chest,* 1985;87:528–535.

Siegel SC. Overview of corticosteroid therapy. *J Allergy Clin Immunol* 1985;76:312–320.

Standards and Guidelines for Cardiopulmonary Resuscitation (CPR) and Emergency Cardiac Care (ECC). Part IV: Pediatric basic life support. *JAMA* 1986;255:2954–2960.

Stempel DA, Mellon M. Management of acute severe asthma. *Pediatr Clin North Am* 1984;31:879–890.

Stern RC. Cystic fibrosis: Recent developments in diagnosis and treatment. *Pediatr Rev* 1986;7:276–286.

Wright PF. Bronchiolitis. *Pediatr Rev* 1986;7:219–222.

CHAPTER **26**

Evaluation of the Febrile Child

PATRICIA J. O'MALLEY, M.D.

Fever is one of the most common complaints bringing a child to medical attention, accounting for 20–30% of pediatric emergency department visits. Although trivial infections may present with high fever, the height of the fever is roughly proportional to the risk of serious bacterial infection. Fever may be the only clue to illness in the young infant who localizes signs and symptoms poorly. The emergency physician must therefore differentiate the febrile child with a trivial or self-limited infection from the child with possible sepsis, bacteremia, or other serious bacterial infection.

The workup of fever in the pediatric patient is based on age, signs and symptoms, and familiarity of the patient and family to the physician. This chapter discusses the evaluation of fever as a presenting symptom in children of different ages, the management of fever without apparent focus, occult bacteremia, and several specific common pediatric febrile syndromes.

THE INFANT LESS THAN 3 MONTHS OF AGE

Pathophysiology

For any infant less than 3 months of age with a rectal temperature greater than 100.5°F (38°C), a prudent and conservative approach dictates a full workup for septic possibilities, hospitalization, and expectant antibiotic therapy. Fever is an uncommon problem in this age group, accounting for less than 1% of all visits to the Boston City Hospital Pediatric Walk-in Clinic (see Klein et al., Suggested Readings). Nevertheless, the category defined by age less than 3 months and fever greater than 100.5°F (38°C) yielded a 14% incidence of serious bacterial infection in the Boston City study, and comparable figures in other studies. Although height of fever, age less than 1 month, male sex, prematurity, and birth complications have all been statistically associated with higher risk of infection, intensive study of this age group has failed to find reliable indices to identify the infant at risk for serious infection. The highest incidence of serious infection in this age group occurs in infants less than 1 month of age with temperatures greater than 101°F (38.3°C). Infections in this age group are most commonly acquired household infections, but late onset disease from infection in utero, at delivery, in the nursery, or secondary to anatomic or physiologic abnormalities may also present in the period from birth to 3 months. Common bacterial agents in this group include Group B *Streptococcus* found in blood, spinal fluid, or bone and joint infections; *Escherichia coli* in blood and urine; *Staphylococcus* in skin and blood infections; organisms causing bacterial enteritis, especially *Salmonella,* in blood and stool; and *Chlamydia* conjunctivitis and pneumonia.

The *evaluation* of an infant in this age group includes the history of pregnancy, delivery, nursery experience and household contacts, and assessment of the nonspecific signs of illness at this age (lethargy, irritability, poor feeding, vomiting, diarrhea, decreased urinary output, and any signs of respiratory distress, such as cough, tachypnea, grunting, or apnea). Specific signs of focal infections should also be sought, considering congenital infections (jaundice, hepatosplenomegaly, rash, pneumonia, and unusual head size), bone and joint infections, and meningitis. Appropriate laboratory evaluation includes spinal fluid for culture, Gram's stain, cell count, and protein and glucose analysis; blood for culture and complete blood count; urine for culture obtained by suprapubic aspiration or catheterization; and stool for culture if positive for red and white blood cells. Chest x-ray is indicated if the infant is tachypneic, even if there are no significant auscultatory findings.

Treatment

Treatment should be carried out in a hospital. It is indicated for any ill infant, any infant with a defined focus of infection, or even for well-appearing infants in this age group, whether or not there is a defined focus. Experience and study indicate that it is not possible to identify the infant at low risk with sufficient accuracy. Discharge from the emergency department should not be considered without consultation with and defined follow-up by a pediatrician. The choice of drugs for treatment depends on the gestational maturity of the infant. Infants under 4 weeks of age should receive penicillin and an aminoglycoside (see formulary in Chapter 20 for dosage schedule); premature infants or infants with perinatal complications should receive the same choice of drugs until 2 months of age. After this time, Gram-negative bacilli are less likely to cause infection other than urinary or intestinal tract disease; *Haemophilus influenzae* becomes a greater threat for blood and soft tissue infections. After the 2nd month of life, therefore, the aminoglycoside is usually replaced by chloramphenicol. Although a third generation cephalosporin may be a reasonable alternative before or after the 1st month, a penicillin is still required in the treatment of the infant under 1 month because of the concern for infection caused by Listeria.

THE INFANT FROM 3 TO 24 MONTHS

In this age group, more reliable data are available to predict the presence of serious bacterial infection than in the younger infant. However, several serious bacterial infections peak in incidence in this age group, including occult pneumococcal bacteremia, *Haemophilus influenzae* type B soft tissue and blood infections, and bacterial meningitis. These infections may often be occult, as demonstrated by a study of 330 febrile children in this age group with temperature greater than 104°F (40°C), in which 95% of the occult pneumococcal bacteremia cases, 52% of the pneumonias, and 100% of the urinary tract infections were not suspected by history or examination. Otitis and viral syndrome were the most frequent erroneous diagnoses. In this age group, the observation scale devised by McCarthy (see Chapter 20) is helpful in predicting the likelihood of serious bacterial infection. Using this scale in three prospective studies of 881 children, all 10 cases of bacterial meningitis were identified on examination. However, previous studies have documented that 11 of 152 children with bacterial meningitis did not have meningismus, a Brudzinski's sign, bulging fontanel, nor altered mental status. Therefore, the evaluation and treatment of febrile children in this age group still present many hazards for the emergency physician.

In children who score low on the McCarthy scale and are therefore acting quite well, who have no focus for infection on examination other than coryza, the syndrome of occult pneumococcal bacteremia (OPB) is likely to be present in 10–20% of children who meet the following criteria: white blood cell count greater than 15,000, temperature greater than 102°F (38.9°C), and sedimentation rate greater than 30. The natural history of OPB is that approximately one third of children seen on repeat visit within 48–72 hours will be well and afebrile without treatment, and the remaining two thirds will be persistently febrile, the majority with a definable focus. Those infants at risk for OPB by laboratory criteria, and who appear well may be treated as outpatients with one dose of ampicillin 50 mg/kg intravenously, followed by oral amoxicillin, provided that a blood culture and sterile urine sample have been obtained and that careful follow-up has been arranged. Although this regimen has been shown to be effective in reducing the suppurative complications of pneumococcal bacteremia (otitis, facial cellulitis, pneumonia, meningitis), it is still controversial therapy. Many physicians recommend that such a child simply be seen again if he or she is still febrile in 24 hours. Whether or not a prophylactic antibiotic is prescribed, the emergency physician should advise fever therapy, good fluid intake, and repeat examination in 24 hours, unless afebrile.

In this age group, it is sometimes difficult to decide when it is necessary to examine the spinal fluid for the possibility of meningitis. Any child with meningismus, unexplained lethargy and fever, or with a high score on the McCarthy scale, should undergo lumbar puncture. Fever greater than 105.8°F (41°C) bears a greater risk of bacterial meningitis (10% of 100 consecutive children with temperatures greater than 41°C had meningitis). Again, children under the age of 18 months do not consistently have meningismus; therefore, particularly in this age group, lumbar puncture should be considered in any ill-appearing child. A full septic workup including spinal tap, blood culture, urine by bladder tap or catheterization, as well as hospitalization and presumptive treatment, should be performed on any child scoring high on the McCarthy scale, regardless of whether or not a focus has been identified.

Figure 26.1 displays an algorithm for the evaluation and treatment of children in this age range who present with fever.

THE CHILD OVER 2 YEARS OF AGE

In the child over 2 years old, the repertoire of behaviors and the reliability of history and physical examination increase so that management of the febrile child in this age range proceeds as for an adult, provided that a careful search for common pediatric febrile syndromes has been undertaken. Table 26.1 lists some of the common recognizable

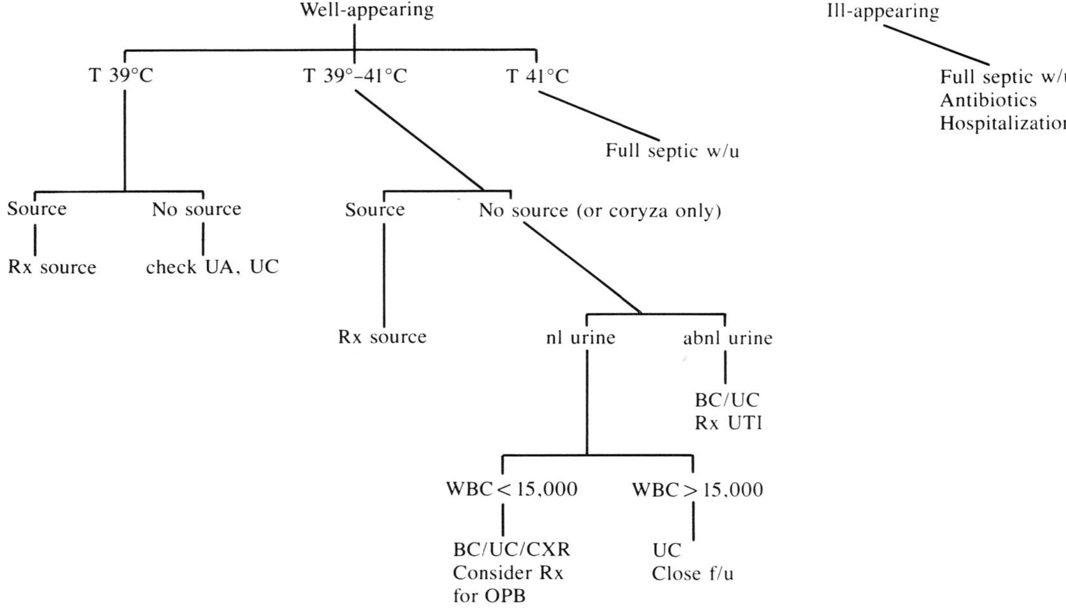

Figure 26.1. Evaluation of the febrile child, age 3 months to 24 months. w/u, workup; T, temperature; UA, urinalysis; UC, urine culture; Rx, prescription; nl, normal; abnl, abnormal; BC, blood culture; CXR, chest x-ray; WBC, white blood count; UTI, urinary tract infection; OPB, occult pneumonia bacteremia; f/u, follow-up.

pediatric febrile syndromes. Several specific infections are discussed in more detail.

Otitis Media

Although it is one of the common infections in infants and children, otitis media is a diagnosis that is frequently overused in the emergency department. In the verbal child who complains of ear pain, fullness, or hearing loss and who complies with the requirements of examination, the diagnosis is straightforward. However, in the child under 2 or 3, the diagnosis can be very difficult. The symptoms of fever, rhinorrhea, and irritability, although commonly associated with otitis media, are also least specific. Examination of the tympanic membrane and its mobility are key, but this may be difficult because of wax or discharge in the canal, because of lack of patient cooperation, or because of parental intolerance. The most reliable finding on examination is loss of mobility of the drum, bulging of the pars tensa and flaccida, and loss or distortion of the light reflex and bony landmarks. Erythema of the drum is not a reliable sign by itself. Bilateral otitis media is not common and suggests either chronic disease or overzealous diagnosis.

The most common organisms over the age of 1 month include pneumococcus and nontypable *Haemophilus influenzae;* in the child over 6 years, Group A *Streptococcus* also becomes common. Up to 25% of ear aspirates are sterile, suggesting virus or *Mycoplasma* as the etiologic agents.

There are many effective antibiotic regimens for the treatment of acute suppurative otitis media, including amoxicillin 50 mg/kg/day three times a day, trimethoprim-sulfamethoxazole, sulfisoxazole and erythromycin (Pediazole) and cefaclor. Two to 3 days of treatment may be necessary before there is resolution of symptoms, and fluid behind the drum may persist for weeks. The ear should be reexamined in 2 weeks to confirm that the infection has cleared and that the fluid has resolved. Antihistamines and decongestants are of no value in acute otitis media. Aspirin or acetaminophen for control of pain and fever are helpful.

Oral Infections

Two distinctive viral infections of the oropharynx are worth searching for in the febrile infant and toddler: Coxsackie herpangina and herpetic gingivostomatitis. Both may cause fever, toxic appearance, cervical adenopathy, and distinctive oral lesions; neither requires specific therapy, other than attention to fluid status, fever control, and topical analgesia with viscous xylocaine or a mixture of liquid Benadryl and Kaopectate. Coxsackie lesions are typically clustered in the posterior pharynx, appearing as shallow yellow or white ulcers sur-

Table 26.1.
Common Febrile Syndromes in Infants and Children

Meningitis
Osteomyelitis
Septic Arthritis
Otitis Media
Facial Cellulitis
Orbital and Periorbital Cellulitis
Streptococcal Pharyngitis
Viral Gingivostomatitis (Herpes and Coxsackie)
Cervical Adenitis
Croup
Epiglottitis
Retropharyngeal Abscess
Bronchiolitis
Pneumonia
Cystitis
Pyelonephritis
Common Viral Exanthemata
Varicella
Measles
Rubella
Fifth Disease
Roseola
Kawasaki's Syndrome

rounded by a rim of erythema. Herpetic lesions are vesicular and often involve the tongue, lips and gums, as well as the pharynx. Streptococcal pharyngitis is very uncommon in children under 2, and there is little reason to obtain a throat culture in this age group.

Bacterial Meningitis

Bacterial meningitis has its peak incidence between 6–12 months of age, with 90% of cases occurring before the age of 5 years. The predominant organisms beyond the neonatal period are *Haemophilus influenzae* type B, *Neisseria meningitidis,* and *Streptococcus pneumoniae.* Although *Haemophilus* is overall the most common, infants with sickle cell disease have greater than 300 times the risk of pneumococcal meningitis than do white infants.

Vomiting, lethargy, irritability, seizures and focal neurologic findings in the presence of fever suggest meningitis. Photophobia, headache, and meningismus may be reported in older children, and a bulging fontanel may be present in the infant under 10 months. In the child suspected of having meningitis, a complete septic workup should be performed, and antibiotics should be administered as promptly as possible following the confirmation of a pleocytosis of the cerebrospinal fluid. The choice of antibiotics is dictated by age, as just described for infants under 1 month; ampicillin (200–400 mg/kg/day) and chloramphenicol (50–100 mg/kg/day) are used for older infants and children. Children with meningitis are frequently dehydrated, and fluid deficits should be corrected; however, maintenance fluids should be restricted to two thirds maintenance requirement to prevent the complication of secretion of inappropriate antidiuretic hormone (SIADH) and increased intracranial pressure. The only exception to this guideline is the child who also demonstrates signs of septicemia and shock, with tachypnea, tachycardia, decreased urinary output, prolonged capillary refill, acidosis, hypotension, and a disseminated intravascular coagulopathy (DIC). Septic shock commonly complicates meningitis caused by Neisseria and infrequently in meningitis caused by *Haemophilus* or pneumococcus, except in the child with sickle cell anemia. If septic shock is present, aggressive fluid resuscitation is administered in 10–20 ml/kg boluses, preferably as colloid. Fresh frozen plasma or platelets will be necessary to treat concomitant DIC. In addition, early consideration should be given to endotracheal intubation and dopamine infusion (10–25 μg/kg/min) for blood pressure support. Bicarbonate therapy may temporarily correct metabolic acidosis but will not be sufficient treatment unless the underlying shock can be reversed. Progressive depression of the serum bicarbonate and a diminished absolute neutrophil count are ominous prognostic signs in septic shock.

SUGGESTED READINGS

Anbar RD, Richardson deCorral V, O'Malley PJ. Difficulties in universal application of criteria identifying infants at low risk for serious bacterial infection. *J Pediatr,* 1986;109:483–485.

Bratton L, Teele DW, Klein JO. Outcome of unsuspected pneumococcal bacteremia in children not initially admitted to the hospital. *J Pediatr,* 1977;90:703–706.

Carroll W, Farrell MK, Singer JI, et al. Treatment of occult bacteremia: A prospective randomized clinical trial. *Pediatrics,* 1983;72:609–612.

Klein JO, Schlesinger PC, Karasic RB. Management of the febrile infant three months of age or younger. *Pediatr Infect Dis,* 1984;3:75–79.

McCarthy PL. Controversies in pediatrics: what tests are indicated for the child under 2 with fever. *Pediatrics Rev,* 1979;1:51–56.

McCarthy PL and Dolan TP. Hyperpyrexia in children: Eight-year emergency room experience. *Am Dis Child,* 1976;130:849–851.

Samson JH. Febrile seizures and purulent meningitis. *JAMA,* 1969;210:1918–1919.

CHAPTER **27**

Fluid, Electrolyte, Metabolic, and Renal Emergencies in the Pediatric Patient

JOHN T. HERRIN, M.B.B.S.
DANIEL G. HELLER, M.D.
DAVID A. LINK, M.D.

Editor's note: Considerable space is taken in this chapter for inpatient management of particular pathologic states. This is done to provide the reader with a spectrum of therapy into which the emergency department management logically and more understandably fits.

FLUID, ELECTROLYTE, AND METABOLIC EMERGENCIES

The treatment of children with life-threatening metabolic emergencies presents opportunities for therapeutic misadventures in the emergency department. Emergency physicians must calculate the degree of metabolic disturbance accurately, interpret the laboratory results correctly, and initiate therapy with appropriate volume and composition of fluids. Errors in managing fluid disturbances or correcting electrolyte derangements pose additional stress to the delicate physiologic homeostasis of the child. Mistakes often produce immediate, serious, and life-threatening complications which further aggravate a precarious condition. The child with a grave metabolic imbalance faces dangers ranging from seizures, renal impairment, and permanent central nervous system deficits, to cardiac arrhythmias and shock. Vital systems and cellular integrity are threatened with temporary or permanent damage, or even death.

Classification

Clinical findings in these situations (Table 27.1) are often similar, despite chemical differences. Symptoms include failure to feed or to gain weight, persistent vomiting, weakness, somnolence, altered consciousness, or seizures. These symptoms mandate immediate attention to both emergency diagnosis and treatment. In the absence of trauma, the differential diagnosis lies among overwhelming sepsis, circulatory failure, and a metabolic crisis. The initial therapeutic approach follows this scheme of *priorities:*

1. Establish and maintain an adequate airway and respiration;
2. Restore circulatory volume;
3. Establish and sustain urine output;
4. Draw appropriate blood samples for diagnosis of the underlying condition;
5. Correct fluid, electrolyte, and acid-base disturbances as guided by test results.

Table 27.1.
Classification of Pediatric Metabolic Emergencies

Fluid imbalances
- Dehydration
- Water intoxication
- Hyperosmolar state

Electrolyte abnormalities
- Hypernatremia
- Hyponatremia
- Hyperkalemia
- Hypokalemia
- Hypercalcemia
- Hypocalcemia

Acid-base disturbances
- Acidosis
- Alkalosis

Disorders of carbohydrate metabolism
- Hyperglycemia
- Hypoglycemia
- Diabetic ketoacidosis
- Galactosemia

Inherited aminoacidopathy

Urea cycle abnormality

Reye's syndrome

Iatrogenic emergency
- Parenteral nutrition without adequate laboratory control
- Hypernatremia due to overadministration of sodium bicarbonate in neonatal emergency or in salicylate intoxication emergency
- Fluid overload—especially with renal failure

To initiate prompt management, insert a large bore intravenous line, preferably via central vein, to obtain blood for appropriate laboratory studies and to start volume replacement. Screening tests include electrolyte profile, glucose, ketones, blood urea nitrogen, creatinine, pH, Pco_2, bicarbonate, and calcium. Complete blood count, differential white blood cell count, and blood culture are mandatory; other cultures are obtained as indicated.

The initial step in *resuscitation* is to administer 20 ml/kg of lactated Ringer's solution or normal saline with 5% albumin intravenously over 20–30 minutes. In the majority of cases, the child will respond to such fluid administration with signs of circulatory improvement and an improved urinary output (Table 27.2). If there is no improvement, repeat the fluid load and consider using a central venous line for volume monitoring and vasopressor therapy if needed. If this yields no improvement, consider a broader spectrum of diagnostic problems beyond simple dehydration. After the first hour, as circulation returns, adjust the rate of fluid administration to 10 ml/kg/hr; then make further decisions based on the electrolyte profile.

After initial resuscitation, diagnostic workup may continue with qualitative testing of the serum ketone level with Acetest tablets and the blood glucose level with Dextrostix reagent strips. Urine should be analyzed for glucose, electrolytes, and sediment. The patient should be hospitalized for further workup and therapy.

Table 27.2.
Adequacy of Therapy

Urine output 40 ml/m²/hr (1.5 ml/kg/hr)
Urine Na^+ 40 mEq/liter
Normal circulation
Restoration of weight

Management schemes for specific abnormalities—dehydration, hypernatremia, diabetic ketoacidosis, hyponatremia, hyperkalemia, hypokalemia, and metabolic abnormalities of Reye's syndrome—follow.

Specific Abnormalities

Dehydration

Acute gastroenteritis in children may reach life-threatening dimensions due to severe dehydration, chemical imbalance, acid-base disturbance, and acute renal failure. Although dehydration in childhood usually results from loss of enteric fluids by vomiting and/or diarrhea, this occurs most often in a mild form. Emergency physicians examining children with dehydration must characterize the child's disturbance with respect to both quantitative and qualitative aspects. They must rapidly make the distinction between mild and more severe cases because treatment will be guided by this assessment. Because a child's fluid reserve is limited (Table 27.3), and a small volume deficit makes a large physiological difference, therapy requires a calculated approach. The most appropriate route, oral or intravenous, and type of replacement fluid solution depends on the particular fluid and electrolyte status.

Infants have a large insensible water loss and large daily water turnover; hence, reduced intake or increased losses result in major body fluxes that do not occur in adults (Table 27.3).

Pathophysiology. Except in cases of critical dehydration, where fluid resuscitation is paramount, the physician's assessment aims to gauge the *extent*

Table 27.3.
Body Water

	Child	Adult
Water anatomy		
Total body water	70–80%	60%
Extracellular fluid	35–45%	15%
Intravascular fluid	5%	5%
Intracellular fluid	30%	40%
Turnover Rate		
Extracellular fluid	½ per 24 hr	⅐ per 24 hr

Table 27.4.
Signs and Symptoms of Gauging Severity of Dehydration

	Mild	Moderate	Severe
% Weight loss			
Infant	5%	10%	15%
Child	3–4%	6–8%	10–12%
Behavior	Normal	Irritable	Hyperirritable to lethargic
Thirst	Slight	Moderate	Intense
Mucous membranes	May be normal	Dry	Parched
Tears	Present	Variable	Absent
Anterior fontanel	Flat	Variable	Sunken
Skin	Normal	Variable	Tenting (doughy with hypertonic)
Circulation	Normal	Variable	Incipient shock
Urinary specific gravity (SG)	Slight increase SG 1.020	Increased SG 1.025–1.030	Greatly increased SG greater than 1.035
Urine flow	Decreased	Oliguria	Oliguria

of dehydration (mild, moderate, severe—see Table 27.4) and to determine the *type of dehydration* (hypotonic, isotonic, hypertonic—see Table 27.5) to plan proper treatment.

For qualitative assessment, it is useful to separate dehydration states based on the amount of sodium and potassium lost in relation to the amount of water lost. This diagnostic distinction determines the proper tempo of fluid replacement and also alerts the physician to children with hypertonic states, which require more careful, phased management because they carry a worse prognosis.

In *hypotonic* dehydration, serum sodium less than 125 mEq/liter net loss of salt from: (*a*) intestine (infantile diarrhea or intestinal obstruction); (*b*) urine (salt-losing renal disease, adrenal failure or diabetic ketoacidosis); or (*c*) rarely, sweat (cystic fibrosis) is followed by extracellular fluid (ECF) contraction. Hypotonic dehydration also occurs when fluid losses are replaced with high volumes of low-solute fluids (e.g., fruit juice, cola soft drinks). Progressive losses lead to ECF depletion and circulatory inadequacy. The falling ECF tonicity creates an osmotic gradient with respect to the intracellular fluid (ICF) compartment, which favors a water shift from the circulation into the cell. This further depletes ECF; subsequent poor renal perfusion follows and leads to oliguria (with loss of the kidney's ability to regulate the ionic composition of body fluids). In addition, these children may develop a metabolic acidosis secondary to poor tissue perfusion, renal retention of organic acids plus chloride, sulfate and phosphate anions, and high bicarbonate losses in the stool.

In contrast, predominant or net pure loss of water gives rise to intracellular dehydration and a *hypertonic state* (serum sodium greater than 155 mEq/liter). This problem usually results when high solute fluids, such as boiled skim milk or chicken broth, are given to replace losses or when large free-water losses are secondary to a renal concentrating defect.

However, even some children receiving low solute fluid replacement may become hypertonic. The reason for this apparent paradox is unclear. Increasing ECF tonicity resulting from a hypertonic state produces movement of water out of the cell to the vascular space preserving circulation despite advancing dehydration. Unfortunately, the brain withstands such intracellular dehydration poorly; these children present with a clinical picture of neuromuscular dysfunction, rather than with the circulatory failure seen with hypotonic dehydration. The mortality in hypertonic dehydration is substantial, with reports as high as 30–40%; hence, great effort is required for the management and monitoring of children so afflicted.

Isotonic (serum sodium 130–150 mEq/liter) dehydration is the most common form of pediatric dehydration. It follows replacement of enteric losses

Table 27.5.
Types of Dehydration

Hypotonic
- Serum Na^+ less than 125 mEq/liter
- ECF depletion with relative sparing of intracellular contents: hence, early vascular compromise with early signs of dehydration.[a]

Isotonic
- Serum Na^+ 130–150 mEq/liter
- Balanced loss of water and ions

Hypertonic
- Serum Na^+ greater than 155 mEq/liter
- Intracellular fluid depletion; allows more severe chronic dehydration before signs are obvious.

[a] ECF, extracellular fluid.

Table 27.6.
Clinical Laboratory Assessment of Dehydration[a]

History—stool/vomiting pattern and description: voiding pattern; intake; infectious disease contacts; weight loss.
Examination—weight, mucous membranes, skin turgor, fontanel, tachycardia, hypotension, level of activity, and behavior.
Laboratory Profile
Blood
- CBC, differential—sepsis, DIC, hemolytic-uremic syndrome
- Na^+—identifies type of dehydration
- K^+—serum level not predictable
- Cl^-—for calculation of anion gap (e.g., ketoacidosis)
- pH/CO_2—acid-base derangement is common
- BUN/creatinine—baseline for monitoring; warns of unsuspected renal impairment—ATN, obstruction, infection, hemolytic-uremic syndrome
- Osm—direct measurement of tonicity of body water
- Glucose—may be low with enteric losses; often elevated in hypernatremic dehydration; diabetic ketoacidosis
- Ca^+—sometimes depressed in hypernatremic dehydration
- Blood culture—any patient in shock

Urine
- Volume flow/minute
- SG—if less than 1.025, consider underlying concentrating defect
- pH—renal tubular acidosis
- Glucose—diabetes
- Ketones—diabetes or poor intake
- Culture—pyelonephritis masquerading as enteritis
- Amino acids and ferric chloride—inborn error of metabolism presenting as enteritis

Stool
- Cultures may be indicated for *Shigella, Salmonella, E.coli, Yersinia, Campylobacter, Rotavirus,* parasites *(Giardia, Amoeba).*

[a] CBC, complete blood count; DIC, disseminated intravascular coagulopathy; BUN, blood urea nitrogen; ATN, acute tubular necrosis; SG, specific gravity; Osm, osmolarity.

with an intermediate solute load, such as breast milk, Lytren or Pedialyte. Fewer symptoms occur in isotonic dehydration per a given weight loss than are seen for hypotonic dehydration. Nonetheless, moderate or severe isotonic dehydration can cause morbidity.

Clinical Assessment. The first priority in clinical assessment (Table 27.6) is to identify the child in shock and to restore the circulation. In less severe cases, it is best to characterize quantitative and qualitative measures of dehydration, as outlined in Table 27.4.

In reviewing the history, parents should be asked about the frequency and amount of diarrhea, maintenance of urinary flow, intake, including type of formula, solids, supplements, and details of preparation (''home-made,'' or proprietary preparation). In infants, marked fluid losses and/or poor fluid intake lead to a decrease in ECF and oliguria. Continuation of urinary output with isotonic or dilute urine in the presence of severe diarrhea suggests a polyuric state associated with renal or hormonal abnormality (diabetes insipidus).

Clinical assessment or review of weight record assists in determination of the degree of dehydration. Infants more often have a record of frequent weights available.

In hypertonic dehydration, the degree of dehydration is notoriously difficult to estimate clinically except by noting changes in eyeball tension and by reviewing the weight record. The skin may have decreased turgor with a peculiar ''doughy'' consistency. Most infants who have hypernatremia associated with diarrhea have some concurrent salt depletion, but the water loss has exceeded the salt loss. On the other hand, if the infant's weight has remained stable, indicating that water loss has not occurred, or if salt replacement has been excessive, salt intoxication may be present. Thus, weight review is extremely important because treatment of salt intoxication requires removal of salt rather than replacement of water.

In general, one attempts to depict clearly the child's chemical status while differentiating other underlying conditions that present clinically as acute gastroenteritis, but require specific therapy (Table 27.7).

Treatment. After assessing the extent and na-

Table 27.7.
Conditions That Mimic Acute Gastroenteritis

Disease	Associated Features
Diabetic ketoacidosis	Urinary ketones + glucose
Acute pyelonephritis	Bacteriuria/pyuria
High bowel obstruction	Pyloric stenosis
Hemolytic–uremic syndrome	Pallor, bloody diarrhea, hemolysis, thrombocytopenia
Chronic renal disease, especially with concentrating defect or salt wastage	Specific gravity inappropriately low in the presence of dehydration
Adrenogenital syndrome	Neonate: examine genitalia, elevated K^+, depressed Na^+

Table 27.8.
Acute Fluid Management and Resuscitation

1. Weigh the patient.
2. If shock is present or urine output is questionable, give 20–30 ml/kg lactated Ringer's or 5% albumin i.v. over 15 minutes, and assess circulatory return. Repeat if blood pressure does not improve.
3. Then give 10 ml/kg/hr of D5 lactated Ringer's until shock is alleviated and actual fluid and electrolyte picture can be accurately determined and appropriate replacement therapy planned.[a]
4. Use multiple electrolyte solution for repair; rule of thumb:

Moderate dehydration	2500–3500 ml/m²/24 hr	(twice maintenance)
Severe dehydration	3500–4500 ml/m²/24 hr	(three times maintenance)

5. If the patient is stable and dehydration is *hyponatremic* or *isotonic,* give ½ total calculated fluid in the first 8 hours. The remaining half should be administered over the next 16 hours.
6. *If hypertonic dehydration is present,* after restoring circulation, correct the deficit slowly and evenly over 48 hours.
7. Body temperature will affect fluid losses, and total maintenance needs require modification; with fever, add 10% of maintenance amount per °C elevation.
8. Ongoing fluid losses will increase fluid requirements.

[a] D5, 5% dextrose.

ture of the dehydration and identifying the underlying conditions, rational fluid therapy may be planned (Table 27.8). The first considerations are (*a*) should the child be admitted to the hospital? (Indications are outlined in Table 27.9); and (*b*) will oral fluid therapy suffice, or is parenteral treatment required?

Both oral and intravenous rehydration may be given in the emergency department, which should result in the need for fewer inpatient admissions. Table 27.10 outlines the typical situations warranting admission. The schema of treatment is presented in Figure 27.1.

Outpatient Management: Mild Dehydration. Successful outpatient treatment of pediatric patients with mild dehydration entails four basic tasks: (*a*) replacing fluid and electrolyte losses; (*b*) reinstituting maintenance fluids; (*c*) stopping current losses; and (*d*) educating parents.

A change in the child's diet is the mainstay of outpatient therapy, provided renal concentrating function is present. Since these patients usually present with isotonic dehydration, emergency physicians should administer fluids that are relatively low in solute to prevent hypertonicity while providing sufficient electrolyte content to replace losses.

Proper usage of oral rehydration solutions (see Appendix 27.A) depends upon choosing the right composition and fluid volume. Table 27.11 lists the World Health Organization's Oral Rehydration Solution (ORS) and those available proprietary fluids. Recommended dosage for emergency department treatment is 50–100 ml/kg over 4 hours (it is most efficient to have parents administer the fluid), with the aim to provide 150 ml/kg/24 total intake ORS, plus water ad lib. For WHO fluid, use 2:1 dilution of ORS solution: water. Guidelines for the use of ORS are outlined Tables 27.10 and 27.11.

Oral fluid administration must take into account the rate and route of losses. For the older child with diarrhea and no vomiting, parents can provide clear, low-solute fluids on an ad lib basis. They should

Table 27.9.
Indications for Hospitalization

Clinical
- Shock
- Dehydration
- Persistent vomiting with worsening dehydration
- Infant (less than 2 months), especially with fever
- Bloody diarrhea—until diagnosis clarified
- "Decompensated" parents
- Diarrhea secondary to other conditions

Chemical
- Hypernatremia
- Hyponatremia
- Marked acidosis (pH less than 7.25/bicarbonate less than 15)
- Azotemia with increased creatinine

Table 27.10.
Management Guidelines for Oral Rehydration

Technique
- Exclusive use of WHO fluid is ill-advised; use diluted 2:1
- Monitor child daily
- Resume breast-feeding after first 8 hours
- After 24 hours, offer soy formula or "BRAT" diet
- After diarrhea stops, avoid lactose for 24–48 hours

Contraindications for oral rehydration
- Impaired circulation
- Electrolyte disturbance
- Severe nutritional deficit
- Persistent vomiting
- CNS disturbance with impaired intake
- Infant less than 2 months, especially with fever
- Social disturbance in family

WHO, World Health Organization (oral rehydration solution)
"BRAT": bananas, rice cereal, applesauce, toast

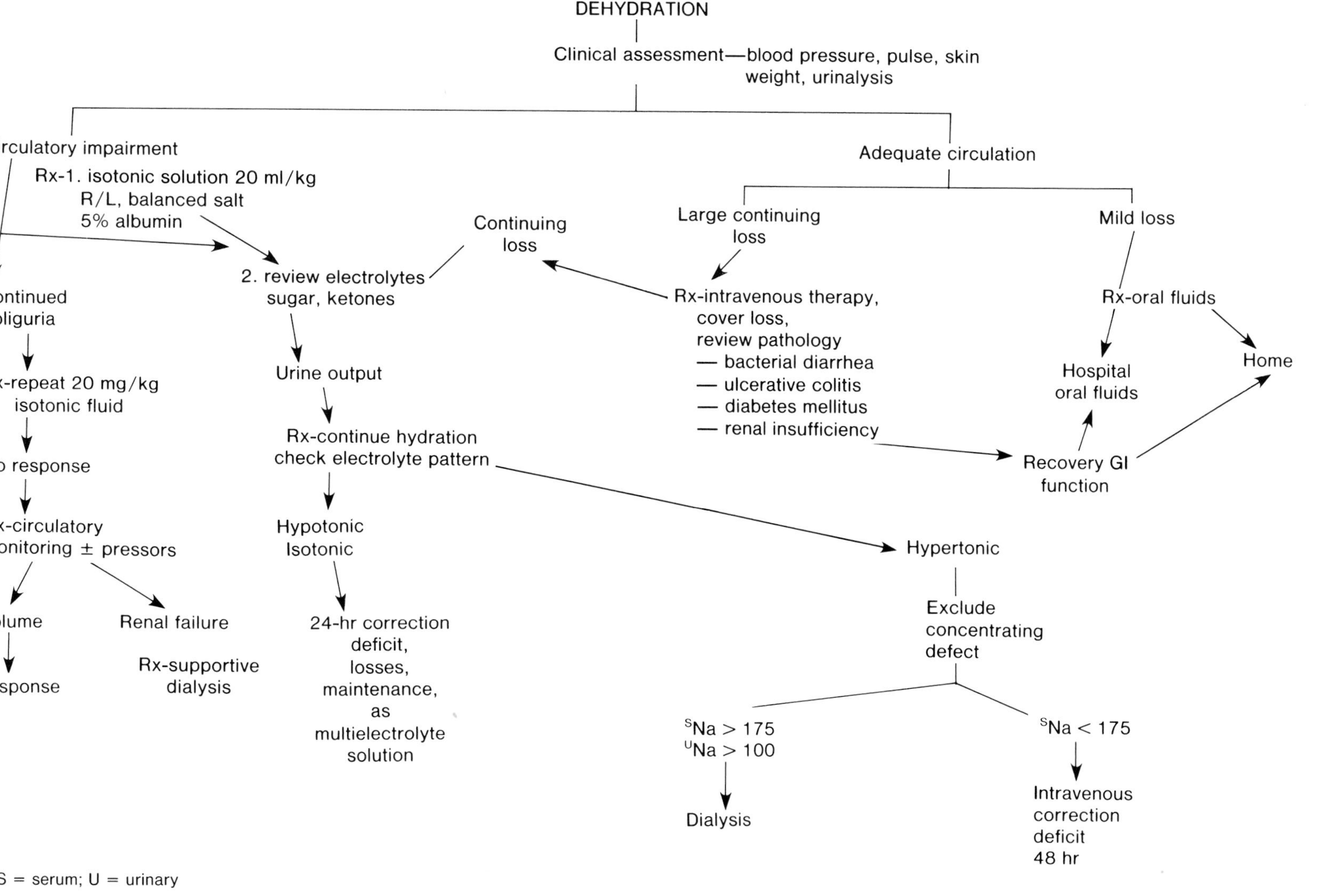

S = serum; U = urinary

Figure 27.1. Treatment scheme for dehydration.

Table 27.11.
Oral Rehydration Solution

Composition[a]	Na^+ mEq/Liter	K^+ mEq/Liter	Cl^- mEq/Liter	Base mEq/Liter	Glucose g/dl
WHO	90	20	80	30	2.0
Pedialyte RS	75	20	65	30	2.5
Infalyte	50	20	45	30	2.0
Lytren	50	25	45	30	2.0

Dose:
In Emergency Department
Mild dehydration 50 ml/kg in 4 hours
Moderate dehydration 100 ml/kg in 4 hours
Total: 150 ml/kg/d plus water ad lib
For WHO solution: dilute 2 parts ORS to 1 part water

[a] See Appendix 27.B for complete listing of various solutions.
WHO, World Health Organization; RS, Rehydration Solution; ORS, Oral rehydration solution.

encourage the child to drink as thirst dictates *and to withhold solid foods until the diarrhea stops.* In infants and younger children (under 6 months), however, low-solute fluids alone over several days may lead to catabolism. In this age group, it is thus necessary to advance to half-strength formula—preferably a nonlactose one or Nutramigen—within 24 hours and to progress as tolerated to a full diet.

For patients with vomiting, advise parents to give oral fluids more slowly to start. Initially, parents should administer only 1–2 tablespoons of room-temperature, clear, low-solute liquids every 30–60 minutes for the first 2–3 hours. This begins to replace losses, minimizes gastric distention, and tests the child's ability to tolerate oral fluids. If the child tolerates these fluids, have the parents gradually increase the volume to 1 oz/hr for the next 2–3 hours, then to 2 oz every 1–2 hours for the next 2–3 hours, and finally, to ad lib fluids every 2–3 hours thereafter if tolerated.

After the acute episodes of diarrhea and vomiting cease, return infants to their normal regimen of formula or breast milk. In older children, return to maintenance fluids or the traditional ''BRAT'' diet (bananas, rice cereal, applesauce, toast). The BRAT diet, which is high in carbohydrates and low in fat, helps absorb intestinal fluid and gives form to the stool.

If the child cannot tolerate fluids in this manner, advise parents to return with the child for reevaluation. In addition, parents should understand that children developing dry lips, a dry tongue, decreased urination, or lethargy while undergoing outpatient treatment are in potential danger and should return to the hospital for reconsideration of admission. Finally, explain that fever control with oral or rectal acetaminophen (Tylenol) is important to reduce further fluid losses from evaporation and increased metabolic rate. To ensure compliance and to check the child's progress, *emergency physicians should insist that the parents call back by phone in 12 hours.*

Inpatient Management: Moderate and Severe Dehydration. Emergency physicians initiating treatment of children with moderate or severe dehydration face entirely different problems from those encountered with outpatient therapy. For example, patients with moderate or severe dehydration may present in shock, develop significant disturbances of electrolyte and acid-base balance, or progress to acute renal failure. Therefore, physicians should be prepared to deal with these complications.

Parenteral fluid therapy can be calculated based either on the child's body surface area or on calories expended per kilogram body weight.

For patients with moderate dehydration and without circulatory or renal impairment, calculate fluid needs (Table 27.12) and begin therapy. In most cases, 5% dextrose in 0.45% normal saline or lactated Ringer's solution provide good temporary fluid resuscitation. When electrolyte values return, adjust the fluid content to meet the patient's needs. Potassium is added when urine output is established. In these less emergent cases, physicians should adjust the fluid rate to replace one-half of the deficit and maintenance fluid requirements over the first 8 hours and the other half over the subsequent 16 hours.

For all patients, assess the adequacy of the instituted treatment in 4–6 hours. A positive therapeutic response includes return of circulation, an increase in body weight (check at least daily), normal blood pressure, a urine output of at least 1.5 ml/kg/hr, and a urinary sodium of approximately 40 mEq/liter. An accurate intake and output flow chart helps physicians and nurses keep track of the rate of fluid and electrolyte replacement as well as osmolar shifts, mental status changes, and the return of renal function.

Table 27.12.
Calculation of Fluid Needs by Two Methods

	Surface Area	Calories
Maintenance	1500 ml/m²/24 hr	100 ml/100 cal Calorie requirement 3–10 kg 100 cal/kg 10–20 kg 50 cal/kg >20 kg 20 cal/kg
Example	16 kg = 0.7 m² Requires 1050 ml/24 hr	16 kg child Requires 10 × 100 cal +6 × 50 cal = 1300 cal = 1300 ml/24 hr
Dehydration	Mild 1500–2500 ml/m²/24 hr Moderate 2500–3500 ml/m²/24 hr Severe 3500–4500 ml/m²/24 hr	Maintenance + Deficit (weight loss) + Ongoing losses
Example: 16 kg child, 8% (moderate) dehydration 16 kg = 0.7 m²	Requires 0.7 m² × 2500 to 0.7 m² × 3500 = 1750–2450 ml/24 hr (+ ongoing losses)	Requires Maintenance 1300 ml + Deficit 1280 ml = 2580 ml/24 hr (+ ongoing losses)

An alternative method for calculating body fluid requirements estimating energy expended per day assigns fluid replacement based upon caloric needs (Table 27.12).

Unless one performs these electrolyte calculations regularly, it is easier, safer, and more convenient to use proprietary solutions (Appendix 27.B). Glucose, sodium, potassium, chloride, and base concentrations in proprietary multiple electrolyte solutions approximate diarrheal losses quite well; hence, in the *absence of hypertonic dehydration or underlying* adrenal or renal impairment, such solutions are appropriate and convenient.

It is important to realize that the use of proprietary multiple electrolyte solutions has drawbacks in certain clinical settings (Table 27.13). For example, such solutions provide neonates with too large a phosphate load, and in patients with renal compromise, multiple electrolyte solutions supply too much phosphate and potassium for safe administration.

The important agenda of parenteral fluid and electrolyte replacement is (*a*) to provide sufficient volume to restore circulation and renal function; and (*b*) to supply adequate electrolytes to fit the clinical and chemical profile.

In addition to electrolyte restoration, acid-base disturbance may need initial treatment. However, preoccupation with the dangers of acidosis may lead to the infusion of large amounts of sodium bicarbonate, which in turn could lead to an excess serum sodium and osmolar load. Spontaneous correction of acidosis by disposal of hydrogen ion via kidney and lung is far more efficient than disposition of a large sodium load. Formal correction of metabolic acidosis is indicated only if blood pH falls below 7.25 and serum bicarbonate is less than 15 mEq/liter. It is more important to search for underlying renal tubular acidosis or organic acidosis, e.g., an amino acid disorder in the infant or diabetes mellitus in the older child. If acidosis warrants correc-

Table 27.13.
Instances Where Multiple Electrolyte Solution Cannot be Used

Example	Reason
Infant	Excess load
Renal compromise	Excess K^+, PO^{4-}
Acute resuscitation of dehydration	Hypotonic solution, excess K^+
Hypernatremic dehydration—acute management	Same
Hypoadrenal, Addison's disease, adrenogenital syndrome	Excess K^+
Volume expansion	Hypotonic solution

Table 27.14.
Causes of Hypernatremia in Children

Loss of water in excess of sodium
- Gastroenteritis
- Inadequate fluid replacement
- Fever
- Mechanical overventilation
- Primary CNS disease limiting water access
- Renal water loss
  - Diabetic ketoacidosis
  - Diabetes insipidus
  - Osmotic diuresis (glucose, mannitol, urea, x-ray contrast media)
  - Postobstructive diuresis

Excessive salt intake
- Improper mixing of infant formula
- Sodium bicarbonate therapy
- Boiled skim milk
- Salt poisoning (accidental, malicious)

CNS, central nervous system

tion, calculate bicarbonate deficit based on a "bicarbonate space" of 40% total body weight (0.4 × body weight/kg × deficit).

For severe acidosis (pH < 7.15) give 1–2 mEq/kg $NaHCO_3$ as a bolus over 5–10 minutes. Then, correct half the remaining deficit over 8 hours, aiming for serum bicarbonate 15 mEq/liter.

Special Therapeutic Problems in Dehydration Therapy

Hypernatremia. Hypernatremic (hypertonic) dehydration (Table 27.14; see Appendix 27.C) poses a grave threat to the child. With an increased serum sodium, patients develop intracellular dehydration. If the brain cell "shrinkage" is extensive, the cerebral contents may pull away from the fixed cranial vault with resultant tearing of bridging blood vessels and central nervous system bleeding. Furthermore, prolonged intracellular brain cell dehydration may lead to permanent central nervous system deficit.

Therapy for severe hypernatremia thus needs to proceed more slowly than for severe hyponatremia to prevent cerebral or pulmonary edema. The initial step in therapy is to ensure that the patient has good circulation and urinary output. If the serum sodium remains above 175 mEq/liter, *institute peritoneal dialysis promptly.* Peritoneal dialysis should be carried out using modified dialysis fluid containing 2.5–4.25% glucose and a sodium content of 120 mEq/L. In the early phase of dialysis, it is important to monitor the patient's overall condition; follow mental status carefully, and maintain both circulation and positive fluid balance.

Table 27.15.
Summary of Treatment for Hypernatremic Dehydration

Na+ greater than 175 mEq/liter—institute *dialysis*
Shock —give 5% albumin 20 ml/kg
1st hour—give 10–20 ml/kg lactated Ringer's
4 hours —give 10 ml/kg lactated Ringer's or bicarbonate (35 mEq/liter)
4–48 hours—Aim: decrease serum sodium 10 mEq/day using multiple electrolyte solution

If the serum sodium after restoration of circulation and urine output is below 175 mEq/liter, the goal is to reduce the serum sodium concentration to 165 mEq/liter over 4 hours, to prevent changes secondary to cerebral shrinkage. Clinically, morbidity and mortality from hypernatremia are directly related to the rate of change in osmolarity; do not allow the intravenous infusion to run unchecked. Rapid decrease in serum sodium with a decrease in extracellular fluid osmolality floods the intracellular space with fluid, leading to cerebral edema and sometimes to pulmonary edema. Table 27.15 outlines a scheme aimed at smooth reduction in serum sodium.

In approximately 50% of patients with a serum sodium above 155 mEq/liter, there is hyperglycemia. This is corrected spontaneously as the hypernatremia resolves.

After initial management, monitor children closely, checking weight and electrolytes two or three times daily.

In addition, therapy should be guided by these data points to avoid acute fluid or sodium shifts. Frequent monitoring of mental status and behavior provides early warning of impending central nervous system disturbances, thereby allowing early corrective measures.

Table 27.14 lists the causes of hypernatremia. Provision of adequate free water, as previously outlined, corrects those cases of hypertonic dehydration that are secondary to water loss. Excess salt intake, whether accidental or deliberate, should be treated by prompt efforts at removal by dialysis or controlled diuresis.

Diabetic Ketoacidosis. A ketoacidotic state (see Chapter 15) may be the first sign of juvenile diabetes mellitus, or it may occur in a patient with previously diagnosed diabetes. In the latter case, it is usually associated with infection or illness if insulin requirements have not been adjusted adequately. In addition, an adolescent with known diabetes may have ketoacidosis because his insulin requirement has changed or because he has neglected insulin therapy during an emotional crisis.

Children with ketoacidosis may have varying degrees of dehydration in addition to polyuria, polyphagia, and polydipsia. The diagnosis of diabetic ketoacidosis is made by determining elevation of serum ketone and blood glucose levels with Ace-

Table 27.16.
Management of Diabetic Ketoacidosis

Fluids	
Calculate requirement—4000–4500 ml/m²/24 hr	
1st hour:	20 ml/kg NS and may repeat once
1st 8 hours:	give ½ fluid requirement as NS. Change to D5 ½ NS when blood glucose falls to 250 mg/dl.
1st 24 hours	give remainder of calculated requirement. Use ⅓–½ NS with glucose added (2½–10%) to maintain blood glucose near 200 mg/dl.
Give K^+ 40–60 mEq/liter when urine output established. Use equal amounts K^+ chloride + K^+ phosphate (to replace phosphate).	
Bicarbonate	
Give if serum bicarbonate < 10 m/Eq/liter. Infuse 1 mEq/kg as i.v. bolus; may repeat once. Then give $NaHCO_3$ at 80 mEq/liter until serum bicarbonate approaches 15 mEq/liter; then STOP.	
Insulin	
Use crystalline insulin as i.v. drip; infuse at 0.1 unit/kg/hr. Follow blood glucose every 30 minutes. When blood glucose falls to 200–250 mg/dl, stop infusion and initiate daily insulin regimen (assuming patient can tolerate a normal glucose intake).	

NS, normal saline; D5, 5% dextrose.

test tablets and Dextrostix reagent strips. The diagnosis is established if the Acetest tablets indicate ketonemia and if the blood glucose level is greater than 200–250 mg/dl. After assessment of circulatory status, a large-bore intravenous line is placed for rehydration and insulin therapy. Blood samples should be sent for a complete blood cell count and for measurement of blood glucose, ketones, electrolytes, urea nitrogen, and arterial blood gases. The urine should be tested as soon as possible for glucose and ketones. Treatment is instituted after weighing the patient and clinically assessing the degree of hydration. (Table 27.16)

One method of treating diabetic ketoacidosis consists of volume replacement and intravenous infusion of insulin with frequent monitoring of plasma glucose concentration. Such a regimen provides insulin at a constant rate, thus maintaining serum insulin levels in the therapeutic range. With this therapy, the complications of hypokalemia and hypoglycemic rebound are uncommon. One unit of insulin is administered in each millimeter of a solution of 1% albumin in physiologic saline. Such a solution is prepared by mixing 4 ml of 25% human serum albumin solution with 100 ml of physiologic saline solution, and adding 100 units of crystalline zinc insulin. The solution is infused at a rate of 0.1 ml/kg/hr to produce a steady plasma insulin level between 100 and 200 μ-units/ml. The blood glucose level is measured every 30 minutes during infusion; the level should decrease by about 10% every hour. A daily insulin dosage schedule is initiated, and insulin infusion is discontinued when the blood glucose levels reach 200–250 mg/dl, provided that acidosis has been corrected and the patient can tolerate a normal amount of glucose. Should the patient be unable to tolerate such an amount, intravenous insulin infusion may be continued at the rate of 0.1 ml/kg/hr, and a separate infusion of 5% dextrose in water given 1600–2500 ml/m²/day (50–80 ml/kg/day) to maintain plasma glucose between 200 and 250 mg/dl.

Fluid and electrolyte replacement take place concomitantly with insulin infusion. Sodium bicarbonate may be necessary in patients with severe acidosis, but is usually unnecessary after restoration of the circulatory volume. If the serum bicarbonate level is 10 mEq/l or less, sodium bicarbonate should be administered in an isotonic solution prepared by adding 20 ml of 7% sodium bicarbonate solution (20 mEq of bicarbonate) to 100 ml of 5% dextrose in water. This solution should be infused until the serum bicarbonate level is 12–15 mEq/liter, whereupon sodium bicarbonate is discontinued unless continued monitoring demonstrates increasing acidosis. An excessive dose may be dangerous because too rapid correction of metabolic acidosis may lead to respiratory alkalosis from the lag in correction of cerebrospinal fluid acidosis.

Hyponatremia. Symptoms in hyponatremia are nonspecific, and the rate of fall in serum sodium is more important than the absolute level of serum sodium in the production of symptoms. Decisions regarding therapy must be based on clinical assessment because low serum sodium levels may occur with water excess alone, salt and water excess (with water excess predominating), or sodium and water deficit.

Attempts to raise serum sodium by increasing sodium content of parenteral fluids is useful only for temporary management of symptomatic severe hyponatremia and may carry the danger of pontine myelolysis.

Water restriction is the treatment of choice in wa-

Table 27.17.
Causes of Hyponatremia

- Maternal effects
  - Diuretic therapy
  - Oxytocin antidiuretic hormone (ADH) effect
- Spurious value
  - Hyperglycemia
  - Hyperlipidemia (Intralipid treatment)
- Loss of sodium in excess of water
  - Renal loss
    - Acute tubular necrosis (secondary to shock/asphyxia)
    - Post-obstructive diuresis
    - Pyelonephritis
    - Renal hypoplasia
    - Tubular disorders: cystinosis, Fanconi syndrome, renal tubular acidosis (RTA)
    - Diuretic therapy (furosemide)
  - Adrenal loss
    - Adrenal insufficiency (disseminated intravascular coagulopathy [DIC], sepsis, hemorrhage)
    - Salt-losing adrenogenital syndrome
  - Gastrointestinal loss: diarrhea, vomiting
  - Cutaneous loss: toxic epidermal necrolysis (TEN), burn, cystic fibrosis
- Gain of water in excess of sodium
  - Acute renal failure
  - Inappropriate ADH
  - Congestive heart failure
  - Parenteral hypotonic fluid therapy

ter excess with normal sodium balance, while diuretic therapy with water replacement is more useful when both salt and water excess are present.

Assessment of volume status using weight, tissue turgor, state of the mucous membranes, blood pressure, pulse, acidosis, BUN, creatinine, hematocrit, and serum total proteins assists in the classification of the cause of hyponatremia, as follows: (*a*) decreased extracellular fluid (ECF) volume; (*b*) increased ECF volume; and (*c*) normal ECF volume. This assessment thereby guides therapy (Table 27.17).

Of paramount urgency is the symptomatic child. Usually, the serum sodium must drop below 125 mEq/liter to produce neurologic signs and symptoms, but a rapid change in serum sodium may cause similar problems despite a smaller net shift. In those patients with serum sodium below 125 mEq/liter, it is imperative that emergency physicians act quickly to avert vascular compromise and central nervous system abnormalities. If serum sodium acutely falls below 115 mEq/liter, there is a substantial chance of grand mal seizures. Judicious use of 3% NaCl (0.5 mEq/ml) prevents or terminates seizures; the usual dose of about 5 ml/kg of 3% NaCl given over 30 minutes controls seizures acutely, but one should never attempt total correction because this may provoke circulatory overload. Raising serum sodium by 5 mEq/liter, or at most by 10 mEq/liter, usually stops the acute central nervous system disturbance. Much of the sodium administered in this manner rapidly appears in the urine, so that the beneficial effect is transient. Remember: hypertonic saline is painful and caustic to veins.

Hyperkalemia. The best treatment for hyperkalemia is prevention. Most commonly, a rapidly rising serum potassium occurs as a component of acute renal compromise. Hence, the nephrologist's succinct admonition: "No P(ee), no K!" can avert major problems. False elevations of potassium are seen from heel-stick blood samples, thrombocytosis, or marked leukocytosis, as well as from hemolysis.

Rapidly rising serum potassium levels make ECG monitoring mandatory and, if changes are detected, therapy is required emergently. Meanwhile, one must identify the cause of hyperkalemia and prevent further increase in potassium concentration. Four approaches are available: (*a*) minimize the deleterious effects of hyperkalemia; (*b*) sequester the excess ion where it can do no harm; (*c*) remove K^+ from the body; and (*d*) drive K^+ into glycogen with insulin.

Steps in the treatment of acute hyperkalemia should be consonant with the danger. With serum K^+ above 7.5 mEq/liter or with ECG changes, the sequence follows: (*a*) calcium infusion, except in digitalized patients, counteracts the cardiac effects of severe hyperkalemia; (*b*) sodium bicarbonate, 2.5 mEq/kg i.v. lowers potassium about 2 mEq/liter (each increase by 0.1 pH units decreases K^+ by 1 mEq/liter within minutes); (*c*) cation exchange resins, such as Kayexalate (sodium polystyrene sulfonate) accumulate the K^+ ion in the gut, in exchange for Na^+. Kayexalate, 1 gm/kg, reduces the serum K^+ by approximately 1 mEq/liter (excessive use may produce hypocalcemia); (*d*) use of insulin-glucose has a limited role in pediatrics. This treatment is used in older children, but then, only cautiously. It produces a fall in serum potassium in 20–30 minutes. In infants, profound hypoglycemia may result. (See the later discussion of the treatment of hyperkalemia in renal failure.)

With continuing, actual, or potentially rising serum potassium, peritoneal dialysis should be initiated promptly in addition to cation exchange resins, particularly if heart failure is part of the clinical picture, because the therapy for hyperkalemia may convert impending failure to acute circulatory decompensation.

Hypokalemia. Oral therapy is usually safe and effective for chronic and irreversible causes of hypokalemia. More serious depression of serum potassium level, especially acutely or in patients on digitalis, may require intravenous treatment.

Correcting severe hypokalemia should take place as slowly as practical, since life-threatening cardiac arrythmias may occur with rapid replacement. In cases of symptomatic hypokalemia, intravenous replacement should be restricted to no more than 0.5 mEq potassium per kilogram per hour while continuously monitoring cardiac status. In extreme circumstances, when the serum potassium is less than 1.0 mEq/liter, replacement may exceed these limits, but only in the presence of a physician experienced in dealing with this problem and only with continuous electrocardiographic monitoring.

Metabolic Derangements in Reye's Syndrome

Reye's syndrome is the most common postviral neurological complication of childhood. This syndrome appears to result from a disruption in the mitochrondrial function of the brain, liver, heart, kidney, pancreas, and skeletal muscle. Cerebral edema follows cytotoxicity; early recognition and prompt management are necessary to prevent unnecessary mortality and morbidity.

In the emergency department, a high index of suspicion is necessary to allow early testing and therapy. The disorder is suspected in any child who develops vomiting and alteration in mental status, particularly lethargy or combative behavior, progressing to coma. Influenza B, chicken pox, and aspirin have been common antedating denominators.

In addition to standard metabolic tests, liver function tests, prothrombin time, serum glutamic oxalic transferase (SGOT), serum glutamic pyruvic transferase (SGPT), and serum ammonia, blood glucose, and neurological consultation, to guide potential needs for EEG, CT scan, lumbar puncture, and intracranial pressure monitoring, are necessary in patients suspected of Reye's syndrome. Liver biopsy may be necessary in patients under age 1 year, in children with lack of vomiting or prodromal illness, or in familial cases.

The differential diagnosis includes: (*a*) other causes of fulminant liver failure; (*b*) toxin or drug exposure, including aspirin, sodium valproate, acetaminophen, isopropyl alcohol; (*c*) infection of the central nervous system, such as encephalitis; and (*d*) inborn errors of metabolism: urea cycle enzyme defects, ornithine transaminase deficiency, carbamyl phosphatase deficiency, methylmalonic acidemia, propionic acidemia, congenital lactic acidosis, and glutamic acidemia.

Initial supportive management is commenced with intravenous administration of 10% dextrose in water with appropriate electrolyte supplementation. If the patient is not comatose, close observation and prophylaxis against cerebral edema are undertaken. The head is elevated to 30° in a midline position to ensure venous return, hypertonic 10–15% glucose is provided as an energy substrate and to allow water restriction if necessary. A central venous line is provided to allow monitoring of fluid volume if fluid restriction is necessary. For the comatose or deteriorating patient, the aim is to maintain cerebral perfusion and to minimize any rise in intracranial pressure. Consideration of the need for monitoring of intracranial pressure should be made early.

In this group, in addition to the positioning of the head and meticulous fluid-electrolyte monitoring and administration, standard measures for control of raised intracranial pressure are instituted. These measures include: (*a*) intubation and controlled hyperventilation aimed at maintaining $Paco_2$ at 20–25 mm Hg; (*b*) paralysis to facilitate respiration; (*c*) furosemide 0.5—1 mg/kg/day i.v. divided in 2–4 hourly doses with the frequency controlled by "bolt" intracranial pressure monitoring with direct transducing of intracranial pressure; and (*d*) osmotic agents, such as mannitol 1–2 gm/kg i.v. bolus each 2–4 hours, to maintain serum osmolality at approximately 310 mOsm. Glycerol 1–2 gm/kg may be used orally as an alternative.

Further care after immediate stabilization is undertaken in the intensive care unit where consideration is given to using dexamethasone 0.25–0.5 mg/kg/day, or to using pentobarbital-induced coma in more refractory cases.

RENAL EMERGENCIES

Renal Failure

Pathophysiology

In renal failure, the kidneys lose their ability to excrete nitrogenous wastes and to maintain water and electrolyte balance. Renal failure should be suspected in the presence of oliguria and/or azotemia. Three clinical classifications of renal failure are listed according to the mechanism or production: (*a*) *prerenal,* e.g., dehydration, sodium depletion, and protein loading; (*b*) *parenchymal,* e.g., glomerulonephritis and tubulointerstitial disease; and (*c*) *postrenal,* e.g., structural or intraluminal obstruction. Appropriate therapy requires the physician to determine which component or components are present.

Renal failure in the emergency department may be manifested as an acute episode or as acute decompensation in the presence of chronic renal failure; an emergency situation may even arise in the case of chronic progressive renal failure.

Table 27.18.
Renal Failure: General Principles of Therapy

Treatment of correctable conditions
Obstruction
Infection
Anemia or blood loss
Dehydration
Congestive heart failure
Hypokalemia
Hypercalcemia
Reduction of excretory load
Dietary restriction of protein, potassium, sodium, phosphate
Restriction of water intake to output plus insensible loss
Adjustment of drug dosage to renal function (aminoglycosides, antiobiotics, digitalis compounds, antihistamines)
Utilization of extrarenal routes of metabolism
Binding of phosphate with aluminum hydroxide gel or calcium carbonate
Binding of potassium with exchange resins
Compensation for regulatory inadequacy
Correction of acidosis with sodium bicarbonate
Administration of vitamin D supplements
Transfusion of packed cells for correction of anemia
Artificial replacement of renal function
Dialysis on acute basis (peritoneal, hemodialysis)
Transplantation on chronic basis

Symptoms of renal failure include: (*a*) change in conscious state, including somnolence, irritability, and seizures; (*b*) nausea, vomiting and diarrhea; (*c*) generalized pruritus; (*d*) muscular twitching; and (*e*) tachypnea or Kussmaul's respiration. Physical examination may reveal dehydration or fluid overload manifested by hypertension, peripheral edema, or crackling rales, signifying pulmonary edema. Urinalysis with attention to both sediment and chemistries provides further clues to the precipitating cause.

It must be remembered that oliguric renal failure is much more readily recognized than nonoliguric renal failure. Approximately one-third of patients with renal failure have a sustained urine output, particularly those with trauma, burns, crush injury with myoglobinuria, and obstructive uropathy, with or without infection.

Further confusion may follow the sustained urine flow of a moderately well-concentrated or highly concentrated urine in the syndrome of secretion of inappropriate antidiuretic hormone (SIADH), a not uncommon diagnosis in the ICU setting, or after certain drug regimens. In this instance, fluid retention may follow inappropriate fluid intake and result in decreased serum sodium, potassium, and BUN rather than the rising BUN, creatinine, and potassium seen in renal failure. Review of urinalysis, urinary sodium level, and osmolality allows differential definition.

Evaluation proceeds to exclude obstruction, restore circulation, and to consider potential causes for renal dysfunction in an orderly manner. Severe oliguria or anuria is rare; it is usually a manifestation of obstruction: bilateral renal artery, vein or ureters, or uretheral obstruction. Physical examination and ultrasonography to define/exclude a renal or bladder mass is indicated. Urinary catherization is reserved for those patients with full bladders. Pediatric urological consultation is indicated in those patients with trauma to the lower abdomen or perineum and in those patients with confirmed obstructive lesions.

Life-threatening conditions associated with renal failure include circulatory collapse, severe metabolic acidosis, hypocalcemia, hyperkalemia, sepsis, water intoxication with or without pulmonary edema, and electrolyte imbalance manifested by neurological symptoms. Hospital admission for further therapy is mandatory.

Resuscitation

Therapy for renal failure is nonspecific; the general guidelines are listed in Table 27.18. In the emergency department, circulatory collapse should first be treated and circulatory volume maintained with an isotonic balanced saline solution, such as lactated Ringer's solution or 0.45% saline with sodium bicarbonate 20–40 mEq/liter added. Once circulatory volume is reestablished, infusion is continued at a slower rate.

Acidosis must be corrected concurrently with correction of hypocalcemia, because rapid correction of acidosis may lead to painful tetany or cardiac arrythmias in the hypocalcemic patient. Acidosis is corrected by an initial infusion of 7% sodium bicarbonate solution administered over 5–10 minutes to provide a 1–2 mEg/kg of bicarbonate. This is followed by a maintenance solution of 10% dextrose in water with sodium bicarbonate added to provide 1–2 mEq/kg/day of bicarbonate. This should be administered at 750 ml/m^2/day (25 ml/kg/day). Hypocalcemia is best treated by infusion of 10–20 mg/kg of elemental calcium over 20 minutes if the patient is symptomatic, or over 6–12 hours if the patient is asymptomatic.

In a patient with hyperkalemia, an electrocardiogram should be obtained immediately. If no electrocardiographic changes are noted, acidosis should be corrected with a sodium bicarbonate solution, as outlined. An alternative initial infusion in children more than 2 years old, or in those weighing more that 15 kg, consists of infusion of 0.3 unit/kg of crystalline zinc insulin as a solution limit of insulin in 8 ml of a 50% dextrose solution, infused over 5–

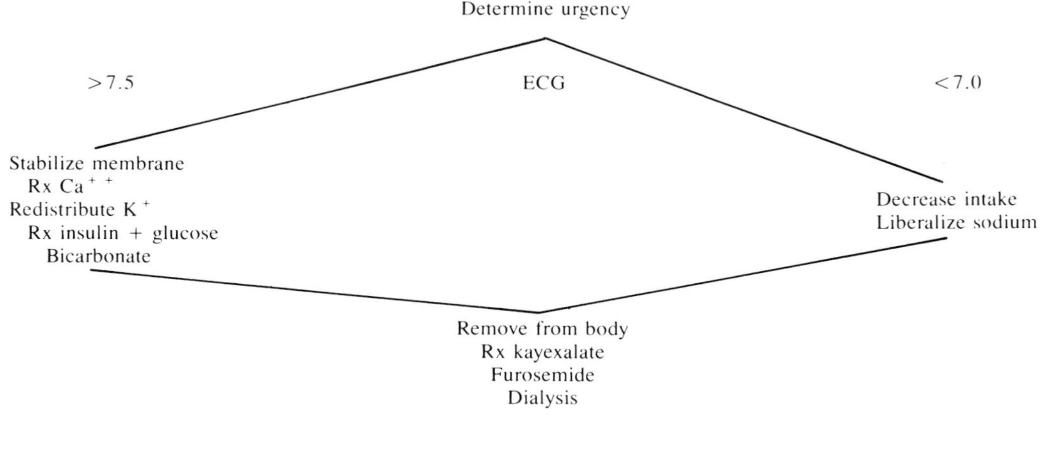

Dosages

(1) Ca^{++} – 10 mg/kg (as elemental Ca^{++})
(2) Insulin – 0.1 u/kg/hr
Glucose – 0.5 g/kg/hr (adjust PRN)
(3) Bicarbonate – 1 mEq/kg
(4) Kayexalate – 1 g/kg in 50–150 ml sorbitol
(5) Furosemide – 1 mg/kg
(6) Dialysis – 4–6 hours

Figure 27.2. Treatment of hyperkalemia.

10 minutes. Initial infusion is followed by a maintenance infusion of sodium bicarbonate until urine output is established or dialysis is instituted.

If electrocardiographic changes are noted, treatment of hyperkalemia is urgent (Fig. 27.2). First, elemental calcium, 10 mg/kg should be administered as 10% calcium gluconate over 5–10 minutes under ECG monitoring. This protective measure is followed by infusion of both the sodium bicarbonate solution and the insulin-glucose solution, then by the maintenance solution of sodium bicarbonate.

In all hyperkalemic patients, if urine flow greater than 0.5 ml/kg/hr has not occurred within 1–2 hours, ion-exchange resins such as sodium polysyrene sulfonate (Kayexelate) and/or dialysis may be required in addition to the maintenance solution. Sodium polystyrene sulfonate is administered orally or rectally, 1.0–1.5 gm/kg in 2–3 ml/kg of 10% sorbitol or 10% dextrose solution. This dose may be repeated each 2–3 hours until control is attained or dialysis instituted. Elemental calcium, 40 mg/kg/day as 10% calcium gluconate or calcium gluceptate, should be added to the maintenance infusion, but the mode of administration should be changed to oral calcium supplements, 100–200 mg/kg/day of elemental calcium as soon as practical.

Oral administration of a phosphate-binding aluminum hydroxide gel providing 150–300 mg/kg/day of aluminum assists in preventing hyperphosphatemia. For more prolonged control, a change to calcium carbonate is necessary to prevent aluminum intoxication.

Sepsis is particularly dangerous in the patient with renal failure. Prophylactic measures, such as meticulous skin and pulmonary care, ambulation or graduated exercise, and meticulous care of intravenous sites or catheters are necessary. Generalized sepsis is treated with an appropriate antibiotic, preferably one not requiring renal excretion. If a serious infection exists, administration of an aminoglycoside and a penicillin in standard loading doses is advised. Maintenance levels of these agents are calculated on the basis of the results of cultures and monitored serum antibiotic levels integrated with residual measured renal function, and the mode and frequency of dialysis.

Obstruction with pyuria and infection in an infant constitutes an emergency situation. Urethral or suprapubic catheter, or nephrostomy drainage is necessary and usually leads to rapid correction of azotemia. Postobstructive diuresis, i.e., postrelease urinary flow greater than 2 ml/kg/hr, may occur. The degree of diuresis may be forecast by preoperative measurement of the level of the blood urea nitrogen; the higher the level, the greater the diuresis. Because depletion of sodium and water may

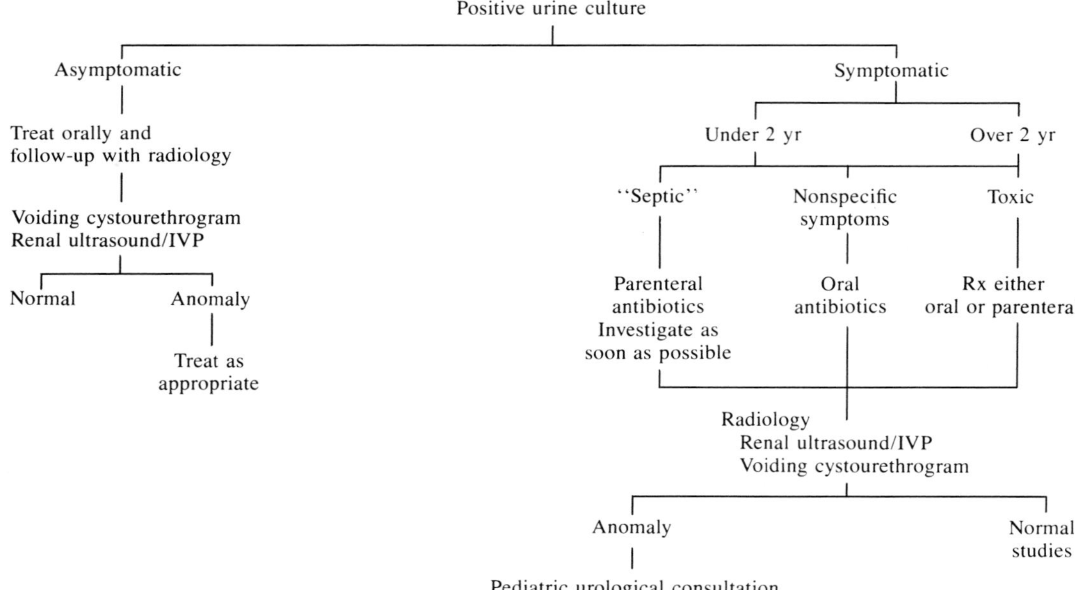

Figure 27.3. Assessment of urinary tract infection.

result from postobstructive diuresis, administration of intravenous fluid and monitoring of urinary electrolytes are necessary. A solution of 5% dextrose in 0.25% saline with added sodium bicarbonate and potassium, approximately replaces the urinary electrolyte losses of postobstructive diuresis. This solution should be initially administered at 3500 ml/m²/day (120 ml/kg/day). After 2 hours, a new hourly rate should be calculated by measuring the urinary output for the previous hour and adding 10 ml/hr to approximate insensible losses. In cases of oliguric renal failure, if there is difficulty in controlling levels of potassium or calcium, or in maintaining correction acidosis, dialysis should be instituted early.

Pulmonary edema associated with renal failure is usually secondary to salt and water overload and should be treated by dialysis. A trial of a loop diuretic, e.g., furosemide 2 mg/kg i.v., and tourniquets to three limbs, rotating every 20 minutes, may gain control until definitive dialysis and respiratory support can be instituted. Respiratory support, including positive-pressure ventilation, may be necessary in addition to, or preceding, dialysis until removal of fluid has been accomplished.

Neurological symptoms are usually associated with hyponatremia, water intoxication, or hypocalcemia. Altered consciousness, muscular twitching, or seizures require estimation of serum sodium, calcium, glucose, magnesium, urea nitrogen, and osmolality. Treatment consists of correction of the diagnosed abnormality. If hyponatremia accompanies fluid overload, and if there are acute changes in consciousness or if there are seizures, 3% saline solution should be administered intravenously, 1 ml/kg over 15 minutes. If neurological symptoms are less acute and if urine output continues or dialysis is contemplated, water should be restricted to 50 ml/m²/day (80 ml/kg/day).

Transport

If the patient is to be transferred safely to an intensive care unit, circulatory status must be adequate, as measured by blood pressure and capillary refilling after blanching. Free water administration should be restricted to the minimal amount necessary to maintain an open intravenous line, unless resuscitation is indicated. Before the patient is transported, hyperkalemia should be corrected by oral or rectal administration of sodium polystyrene sulfonate, 1 gm/kg in 2–3 ml/kg of a 10% sorbitol or 10% dextrose solution. Dialysis may be commenced before transfer by introducing the first fluid exchange and transporting the patient during the exchange period. If the time of transport will be longer than the exchange period, the patient's condition should be stabilized and 2–3 hours of peritoneal dialysis performed before transfer.

If possible, one subclavian vein and one femoral vein area should be preserved for future acute dialysis catheter access.

Urinary Tract Infection

Urinary tract infection is a common condition in children, ranking second in incidence only to upper respiratory tract infection. Findings range from bacteriuria without symptoms to troublesome symptoms including frequency, dysuria, and a mild to moderate fever. Asymptomatic bacteriuria in children lacks the long history usually found in adults. Nonspecific symptoms that herald a urinary tract infection, particularly in an infant less than 2 years old, include failure to thrive, vomiting, abdominal pain or distention, and constipation. Obvious toxemia and sepsis with pyuria may also be seen and require more urgent therapy (Fig. 27.3). If urinary tract infection is suspected, a specimen of urine should be taken for urinalysis and culture. Also, children with recurrent nonspecific febrile illnesses should be screened for urinary tract infection. A diagnostic and therapeutic protocol is presented in Table 27.19.

Obtaining a Urine Specimen

Ideally, the specimen should be obtained by a noninvasive technique, unless the child is too young to cooperate. In patients with signs of either toxemia or sepsis, urine should be obtained directly from the bladder either by suprapubic aspiration, which is preferable, or by urethral catheterization, if adequate precautions are taken to minimize the risk of introducing pathogens during the collection.

If it is possible, two clean-voided specimens of urine should be taken before treatment, especially in older children who have been toilet trained and who can void on request and who will cooperate with adequate cleansing. In uncircumcised boys, the foreskin should be retracted and the glans and sulcus should be washed with sterile distilled water. Sterilizing soap may be an irritant; its use is unnecessary if sufficient water is employed. In girls, the labia are washed, separated, and washed again to ensure that the introitus has been adequately cleansed. The labia must be spread widely and preferably held apart during voiding. The urine is caught in a sterile container. A conical flask is ideal because it is easier to hold and to manipulate than a bowl or basin. The specimen should be either cultured within a short time—less than 1 hour—or refrigerated for up to 6 hours to prevent the growth of contaminant organisms before culture.

If suprapubic aspiration is to be performed, the child should not have voided recently. The bladder should be full to percussion before this maneuver is attempted. In newborns, the bladder is almost totally an abdominal organ. In older children, the bladder is in the pelvis, but the upper margin can be percussed if the bladder is full. The younger child

Table 27.19.
Urinary Tract Infection: Diagnostic and Therapeutic Protocol for Pediatric Patients

Newborn and child of any age with toxic appearance and local tenderness
- Take blood specimen for culture and sensitivity testing
- Take urinary specimen for culture and sensitivity testing
- Institute drainage of urine
- Administer ampicillin and gentamicin intravenously
- Change to appropriate antibiotic on results of sensitivity testing
- Perform investigative studies early if symptoms persist or after 4–6 weeks if urinary sterility can be maintained
- Ultrasound does not give as clear an anatomical picture as intravenous urography
- Intravenous pyelogram
- Voiding cystourethrogram
- Cystoscopy

Child, 2 years without toxic appearance
- Take blood specimen for culture and sensitivity testing
- Take urinary specimen for culture and sensitivity testing
- Administer oral antibiotic
- Change to appropriate antibiotic on results of sensitivity testing
- Perform investigative studies early if symptoms persist or after 4–6 weeks if urinary sterility can be maintained
- Intravenous pyelogram and/or ultrasonography
- Voiding cystourethrogram
- Cystoscopy

Child, 3 years without toxic appearance
- Take blood specimen for culture and sensitivity testing
- Administer oral antibiotic after results of sensitivity tests are available
- Perform investigative studies early if symptoms persist or after 4–6 weeks if urinary sterility can be maintained
- Intravenous pyelogram and/or ultrasonography
- Voiding cystourethrogram
- Cystoscopy

Child, 4 years without toxic appearance
- Take urinary specimen for culture and sensitivity testing
- Administer oral antibiotic—single dose ampicillin 1.5–3.0 gm, depending on weight
- Repeat urinary culture in 48 hours and 2 weeks
- Treat for 6 weeks with conventional dosage if still positive at 48 hours
- No further treatment if urine sterile, or
- Administer conventional 2-week course of appropriate antibiotic determined from sensitivity testing

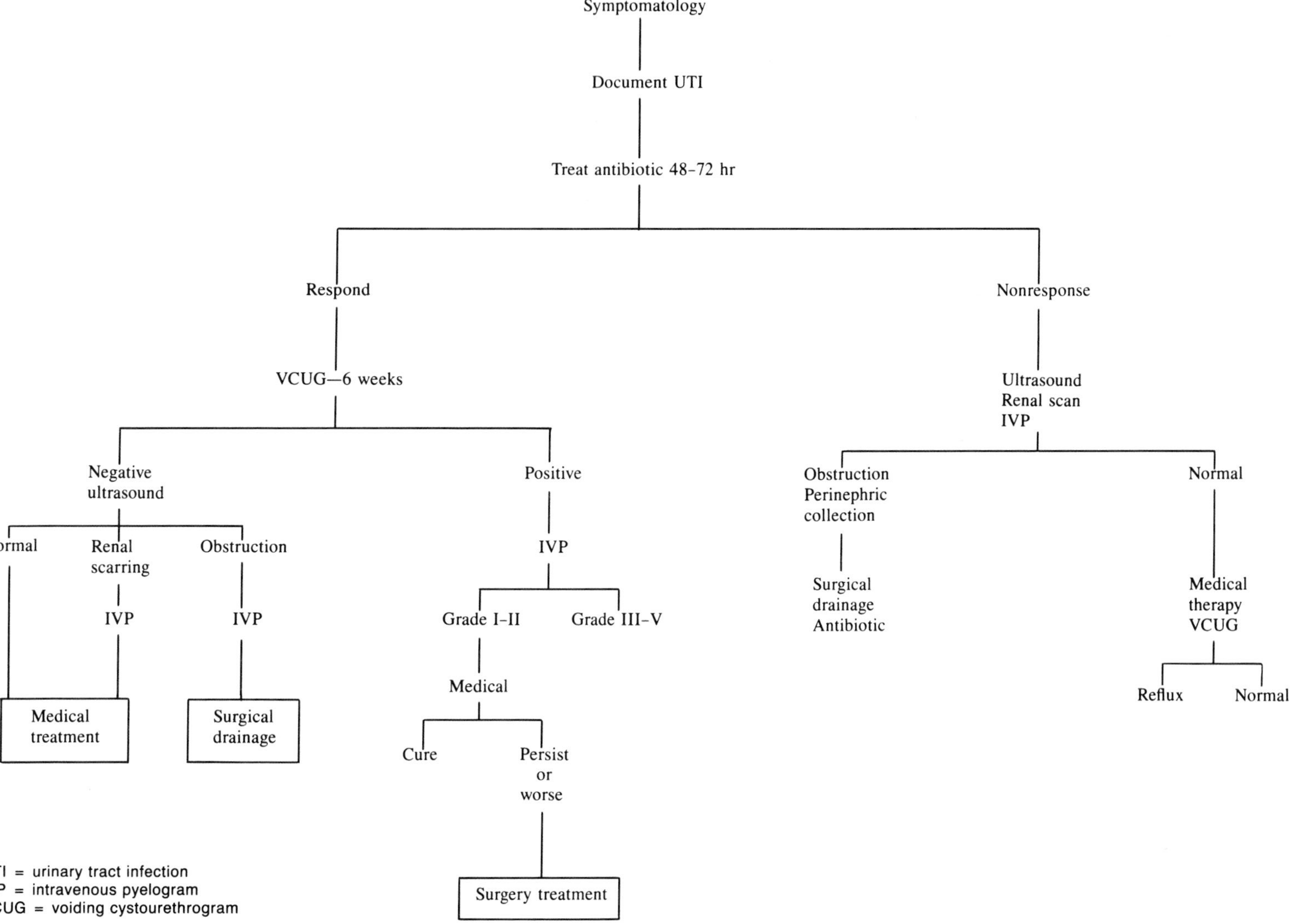

Figure 27.4. Treatment of urinary tract infection.

Table 27.20.
Pigmenturia

Antipyrine
Aniline dyes (sweets)
Anthocyanins (beets and berries)
Bile pigments
Blackberries
Congo red
Homogentisic acid
Phenolphthalein (laxatives)
Pyridium
Rhodamine B (sweets)
Serratia marcescens (red diaper syndrome)
Urates

is restrained by an assistant, and the legs are placed in a frog-leg position with firm pressure on the middle to proximal femoral shafts to stabilize the pelvis. The skin of the abdominal wall is washed with alcohol and iodine preparation solution. In girls, the assistant compresses the introital area to prevent voiding during the procedure; in boys, the urethra should be compressed. A No. 22 lumbar puncture needle, 1.5–3.0 inches long, depending on the age of the child, is inserted over the bladder, the stylet is removed, and a 6- or 12-ml syringe is attached. The needle is advanced into the bladder; in newborns, it is held perpendicular to the skin, and in older children it is held at a downward angle of 45–60°. A "give" can be felt as the needle enters the bladder. Urine is aspirated, the needle is removed, and pressure is applied over the puncture site. After the needle is disconnected from the syringe, the urine for culture is placed in a sterile container.

Treatment

Patients with toxemia or sepsis should be treated differently from those with mild to moderate symptoms (Fig. 27.3). Fever greater than 102°F (38.9°C) and a toxic appearance with pyuria signal an emergency situation, particularly in a newborn or a child less than 3 years old. In girls less than 3 years old

Table 27.21.
Hemoglobinuria

Shock
Hemolysis
Hemolytic anemia
Hemoglobinopathies
Malaria
Burns
Severe infection
Poisonings
Carbon tetrachloride
Arsenic
Paroxysmal cold hemoglobinuria
Paroxysmal nocturnal hemoglobinuria
March (exercise) hemoglobinuria

Table 27.22.
Myoglobinuria

Rhabdomyolysis
Infection
PCP (Angel dust)
Crush syndrome
Trauma
Battered child
Muscle disease
Myositis
McArdle's syndrome
Enzyme deficiencies

and in boys of all ages, an anatomic anomaly is probably the underlying cause of the infection. Therapy includes control of the infection and appropriate relief of any predisposing anomaly, including obstruction at the uretheral valves or ureteropelvic junction, megalocystis-megaloureter, or vesicoureteric reflux. In very young children, obstruction and acute infection may result in devastating damage to parenchymal tissue, which would interfere with subsequent development.

Control of infection initially requires antibiotic therapy and drainage of urine, with diagnostic evaluation as soon as possible. Pediatric dosages of commonly used antibiotics are given in Table 11.3. After a specimen for culture has been obtained, ampicillin and gentamicin should be administered. If the patient's condition has been improved with initial antibiotic therapy, one of the initial antibiotics should be discontinued and treatment should be continued with an adequate dosage of the other, with the choice guided by the culture results. If the child continues to exhibit signs of toxemia or septicemia with fever after 48 hours of antibiotic therapy, ultrasonography or an intravenous pyelogram is obtained to determine whether high-grade obstruction exists. If it does, adequate urinary drainage must be carried out before the infection can be controlled.

An asymptomatic child, or one with mild symptoms, may be treated on an outpatient basis with sulfisoxazole or ampicillin for 10 days, at which time another urinary culture is obtained. Should the child remain febrile after 24–36 hours on this regimen, urinalysis and cultures should be repeated. If infection is not controlled after 48 hours, ultrasonography or intravenous pyelography should be performed to determine whether obstruction is present. If obstruction is suspected on the basis of roentgenographic studies, the child should be admitted for definitive therapy, including further investigation by cystoscopy or retrograde pyelography, appropriate pediatric urological consultation, and, if necessary, surgical correction.

Recent studies have shown that single-dose therapy with ampicillin, gentamicin, or sulfamethoxazole-trimethaprim is as efficient as longer-term therapy for the older child or adolescent with symptoms.

Further Investigation

Following up for all children under age 10 with urinary tract infection must include radiologic studies to define their upper and lower tract anatomy (Fig. 27.4.) Children under age 10 with confirmed urinary tract infection have a 35–45% incidence of an underlying anomaly. In this regard, males have a slightly greater risk than females. Approximately 5% of children will require both medical and surgical intervention to relieve obstruction and to cure their urinary tract infection. These children are at increased risk for further renal damage and later loss of renal functional growth.

Our practice is to obtain both a voiding cystourethrogram and either a renal ultrasound study or an intravenous pyelogram to define anatomy. These studies are performed within 3–6 weeks after the infection. Further therapy or investigation, such as cystoscopy, are based on the results of these initial studies. Figure 27.3 outlines an approach based on these principles.

Long-term Prognosis

In the absence of obstruction, all children are eventually cured with medical therapy. If an anomaly is present, combined medical and surgical management will restore 60% of patients to normal function. Since some degree of renal damage occurs in as many as 40% of patients, children with documented urinary tract infection should have close clinical and bacteriological monitoring of both infection surveillance and renal functional impairment.

Table 27.23.
Renal Parenchymal Disease: Nephrological Causes of Bleeding

Primary
- Glomerulonephritis
- Interstitial nephritis—pyelonephritis
  - —drugs
- Hereditary nephritis
- Recurrent hematuria syndromes
- IgA nephropathy (Berger nephropathy)
- Exercise hematuria
- Athletic pseudonephritis
- Rapidly progressive glomerulonephritis

Secondary
- (Other systemic disease)
- Vasculitis
- Henoch-Schönlein purpura
- Subacute bacterial endocarditis
- Lupus erythematosus
- Collagen disease
- Cryoglobulinemia
- Malignant hypertension
- Hemolytic uremic syndrome

Hematuria

Although red urine or hematuria is a distressing symptom and causes real concern to the patient and parents, it constitutes a rare need for a pediatric emergency department visit; in fact, only 0.13% of admissions in one large study were related to hematuria. Because bleeding can arise from multiple causes from any level of the genitourinary tract, it is convenient to divide patients into those requiring nephrological or urological review. This allows more efficient and cost-effective testing with the least discomfort, invasion, and emotional stress.

Management

For the patient presenting with red urine, a flow sheet approach is outlined in Figure 27.5. The initial step is to bring the initial discolored urine in a sample bottle for review. If a urine sample is not available, color change is often first noted while voiding into the toilet bowl. The patient or parents should review color, presence or absence of clots, and if possible, relation to voiding, i.e., early, middle, or terminal stream, at this first abnormal voiding or the next voiding. A sample of the next voided specimen should be collected.

The urine is examined by Dipstix and microscopy. A data base may be focused from this initial urinalysis. Is bleeding macroscopic? Is bleeding painful? Is there a history of trauma, preceding in-

Table 27.24.
Nonglomerular Bleeding

Urinary Tract Conditions
- Painless
  - Anomaly
  - Tumor
  - Cystic kidney disease
  - Chronic UTI
  - Drug
- Painful
  - Calculus
  - Cystitis
  - Urethritis
  - Trauma
  - Acute UTI

Extraurinary Conditions
- Painless
  - Coagulopathy
  - Anticoagulant therapy
  - Drug
  - Platelet disorders
  - Factitious, menses
- Painful
  - Renal vascular occlusion
  - Periureteral inflammation, e.g., appendicitis, peritonitis
  - Factitious; diaper rash, balanitis, meatal ulcer

UTI, urinary tract infection.

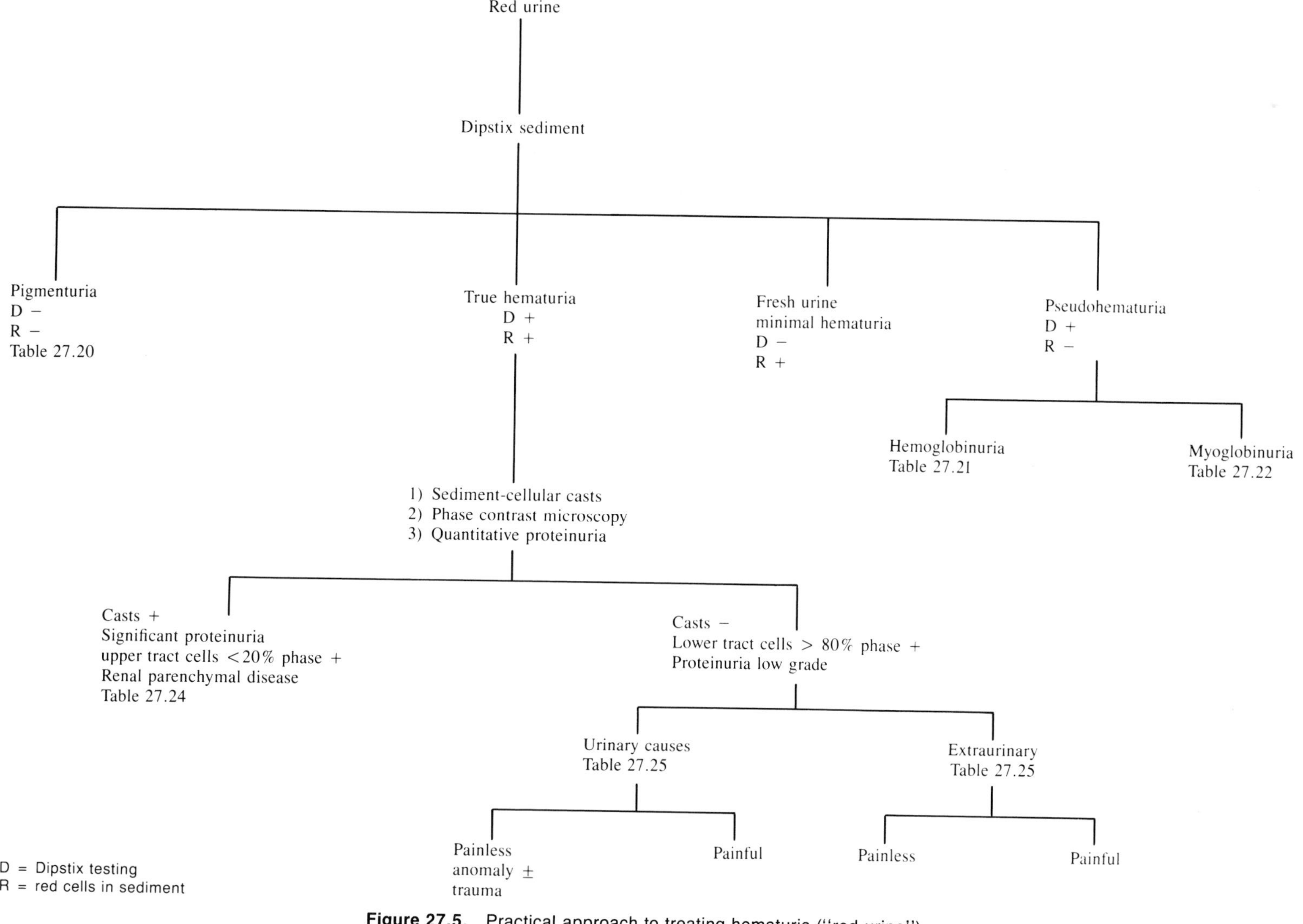

Figure 27.5. Practical approach to treating hematuria ("red urine").

fection of pharynx or skin, drug or medication ingestion? Is there a family history of renal calculi, glomerulopathy, deafness, or ocular anomalies? Is bleeding associated with exercise? In addition, timing in relation to menses should be obtained in an adolescent female.

Interpretation

The urine is examined for color and relationship to part of the stream from which it is obtained, using three-glass voiding.

This test requires the patient to clean off the urethral meatus and then to void sequentially into three separate containers: if possible, 5–10 ml of the initial specimen in container number one, the majority into container number two, and the last 5–10 ml into container number three. Interpretation is then made for:

	Container 1	Container 2	Container 3
Urethral	+	±	−
Bladder	−	−	+
Renal	+	+	+

Hematuria usually produces "cloudy" or "smoky" urine, greenish-brown, cola or tea-colored, or reddish-brown, while hemoglobinuria produces a clear, cherry wine, or cranberry-colored urine.

The presence of cellular casts or 2^+ qualitative proteinuria is suggestive of glomerular disease, and further workup can be directed to nephrological causes (Table 27.23). Baseline serum complement (CH50, C3, C4) and streptococcal antibody studies should be obtained and nephrological referral made.

Recent studies have shown that phase contrast microscopy is a simple, useful, noninvasive test. This allows discrimination of glomerular bleeding (80% red cells abnormal, 80% phase-negative). In our experience, phase contrast microscopy is a rapid and convenient screening test for recognition of glomerular bleeding and identification of cellular casts; this allows a nephrological profile (Table 27.25) to be obtained early.

If nonglomerular bleeding (Table 27.24) is suggested (85% red cells normal, intact, and phase-positive), radiological study with urological consultation are necessary. In the pediatric age group, tumors with isolated hematuria are very rare and mostly confined to ages 3–5 years. Hence, ultrasonography and/or intravenous urography is recommended in this age group and also in those patients with presumed nonglomerular bleeding (phase-contrast positive, red cells in the absence of cellular casts, with low-grade proteinuria less than 500 mg/day only.). Cystoscopy is reserved for those patients with recurrent *active* bleeding. Screening by cystoscopy defines the groups who may require retrograde pyelography or angiography (Fig. 27.6).

In patients with nonglomerular bleeding, an underlying anomaly or cystic disease may have bleeding with minimal trauma or standard aspirin doses. Bleeding from the bladder wall and dome may occur in association with exercise.

Using such a structured approach, it is possible to determine promptly the appropriate nephrological or urological consultation and further workup.

Table 27.25.
Nephrological Profile

1. Define function	Creatinine clearance
	Quantitate proteinuria
	  24 hr protein in urine
	  Urine protein/creatinine

2. Check etiology	Antistreptococcal antibodies
	  ANDB, ASO, AH
	Culture throat, skin
	Other factors, if indicated
	  Lupus erythematosus
	  Hepatitis B
	  Henoch—Schönlein purpura

3. Serum complement levels	CH50, C3, C4
4. Renal biopsy indications	Abnormal natural history Persisting hypocomplement Enuria Proteinuria greater than 1gm/day at 2 months Rapid progression Nephrotic syndrome in child greater than 6 years or not responding to steroid

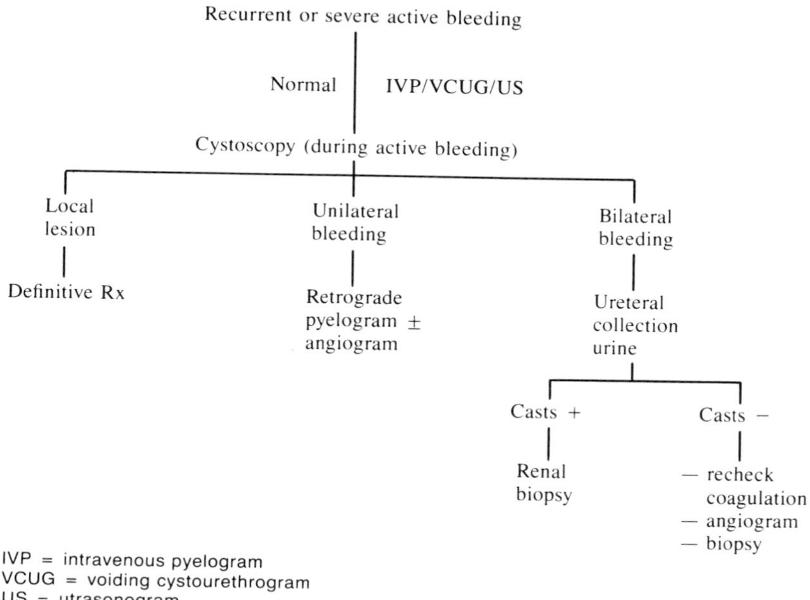

Figure 27.6. Urological investigation of patient with hematuria.

Appendix 27.A
Composition of Commonly Used Oral Rehydration Solutions

	Glucose (g/dl)	Sodium (mEq/liter)	Potassium (mEq/liter)	Chloride (mEq/liter)	Base (mEq/liter)
World Health Organization (WHO) solution	2.0	90	20	80	30
Hydra-Lyte	1.2	84	10	59	10
Pedialyte RS	2.5	75	20	65	30
Pedialyte	2.5	45	20	35	30
Lytren	2.0	50	25	45	30
Infalyte	2.0	50	20	40	30
Ginger ale	9.0	4	1		
Pepsi Cola	10.0	1	<1		
Coca Cola	10.0	1	<1		
Apple juice	12.0	2	25		
Kool-Aid	11.0	2	0.20		
Jello	15.0	13	0.20		
Chicken broth		High	?	High	

Appendix 27.B
Composition of Commonly Used Intravenous Solutions Solutions Available and Concentrations of Component (mEq/liter)

Solution	Glucose	Na^+	K^+	Cl^-	HCO_3^-	Lactate	Ca^+	NH_4^+
Multiple electrolyte solution	50	40	35	40		20	(acetate)	15
Lactated Ringer's solution		130	4	110		27	4	
Ringer's solution		147	4	156			5	

Appendix 27.B—*continued*

Solution	Glucose	Na^+	K^+	Cl^-	HCO_3^-	Lactate	Ca^+	NH_4^+
5% D/W	50							
10% D/W	100							
20% D/W	200							
0.85% saline (isotonic)		145		145				
0.9%		154		154				
3% saline		513		513				
5% saline		856		856				
⅙ M sodium lactate (1.9%)		167				167		
⅙ M NH_4Cl (0.9%)				167				167
2% NH_4Cl				374				374

Appendix 27.C
Fluid and Electrolyte Conditions Requiring Special Intravenous Therapy

System and/or Disorder	Correction
Central nervous system	
Meningitis (SIADH)	½–⅔ maintenance
Trauma	½–⅔ maintenance
Tumor	½–⅔ maintenance
Renal	
Acute renal failure (except polyuric acute tubular necrosis)	No K^+ 350 ml/m²/24 hr plus urine output
Chronic renal failure	No iv K^+ Fluid limit Na+ limit
Postobstructive diuresis (e.g., valves)	3500+ ml/m²/24 hr for at least first day. Use ½ NS plus appropriate K_+
Tubular dysfunction	Supplemental
Renal tubular acidosis	$NaHCO_3$, 2–3 mEq/kg/24 hr
Fanconi syndrome/cystinosis	Na^+, 2–5 mEq/kg/24 hr
Bartter syndrome	K^+, 2–5 mEq/kg/24 hr
Osmotic diuresis (postangiography)	Replace urine output with ½ N saline 3000–3500 ml/m²/24 hr
Endocrine	
Diabetes insipidus	4000 ml/m²/24 hr
Diabetes mellitus in ketoacidosis	Supplement K^+ after urine produced
Congenital adrenocortical (adrenogenital) with Na^+ loss	No K^+ Supplement Na^+
Addisonian crisis	No K^+ Supplement Na^+
Cardiac	
Congestive heart failure	Reduce Na^+
Gastrointestinal	
Liver compromise	Reduce Na^+ May need K^+ supplement
Respiratory	
Pneumonitis (SIADH)	⅔ maintenance
Iatrogenic	
Postanesthesia	Reduce fluids
Posthypothermia	Supplement fluids
Postextracorporeal circulation	Close attention to central venous pressure and fluids
Postangiography or IVP	Replace obligatory diuresis with ½ NS
Diuretics	May need K^+ supplement Watch for alkalosis
Accidents	
Poisoning	See Chapter 17

Appendix 27.C—*continued*

System and/or Disorder	Correction
Burns	Add to maintenance: 2 ml Lactated Ringer's × % burn surface × weight (kg) up to 50% body surface Maintenance for $AgNO_3$ surface therapy 3000 ml/m²/24 hr NS + 40 mEq/liter KCl + protein 25 gm/m²/24 hr
Drowning	½ maintenance

SUGGESTED READINGS

Fluid Electrolytes/Oral Hydration

Arieff AI, Guisada R. Effect on the central nervous system of hypernatremic and hyponatremic states. *Kidney Int,* 1976;10:104–116.

Bert T, Anderson RJ, McDonald, K, et al. Clinical disorders of water metabolism. *Kidney Int,* 1976;10:117–132.

Boineau FG, Lewy JE. Maintenance fluids and the management of diarrheal dehydration. *Pediatr Ann,* 1981; 10:280–288.

Bruck E. Fluid and electrolyte therapy. *Pediatr Clin North Am,* 1972;12:193–220.

Bruck E, Abal G, Aceto T. Pathogenesis and pathophysiology of hypertonic dehydration with diarrhea. *Am J Dis Child,* 1968;115:122–144.

Bruck E, Abal G, Aceto T. Therapy of infants with hypertonic dehydration due to diarrhea. *Am J. Dis Child,* 1968; 115:281.

Feig PV, McCurdy DK. The hypertonic state. *N Engl J. Med,* 1977;297:1444–1454.

Finberg L. Hypernatremic dehydration. *Adv Pediatr,* 1969; 16:325–344.

Finberg L. Hypernatremic (hypertonic) dehydration in infants. *N Engl J Med,* 1973;289:196–198.

Finberg L. Treatment of dehydration in infancy. *Pediatrics Rev,* 1981;3:113–120.

Friis-Hansen B. Changes in body water compartments during growth. *Acta Pediatr Search* (Suppl), 1957;46:110.

Hyman PE, Ament ME. Acute infectious gastroenteritis in children. *Pediatr Ann,* 1982;11:147–155.

Kelsh RC, Oliver, WJ. Hyponatremia in children. *Pediatrics Rev,* 1980;2:187–190.

Kleeman CR. CNS manifestations of disordered salt and water balance. *Hosp Pract,* 1979;14:59–68.

Klish W. Use of oral fluids in treatment of diarrhea. *Pediatrics Rev,* 1985;7:27–30.

Link DA. Fluid and electrolytes. In: Graef JW, Cone TG, eds. *Manual of Pediatric Therapeutics.* Boston: Little, Brown & Co, 1978:189–207.

Pizarro D, Posada G, Levine MM. Hypernatremic diarrheal dehydration treated with slow oral rehydration. *J Pediatr,* 1984;104:316–319.

Rosenfeld W, Lopez de Romana G, Kleinman R, et al. Improving the management of hypernatremic dehydration. *Clin Pediatr,* 1977;5:411–417.

Santosham M, Burns B, Nadkemi V. Oral rehydration therapy for acute diarrhea in ambulatory children in the U.S. *Pediatrics,* 1985;76:159–166.

Santosham M, Daum RS, Dillman L et al. Oral rehydration therapy of infantile diarrhea—a controlled study of well-nourished children hospitalized in the U.S. and Panama. *N Engl J Med,* 1982;306:1070–1076.

Saunders N, Balfe J, Laski B. Severe salt poisoning in an infant. *J Pediatr,* 1976;88:258–261.

Segar W. Parenteral fluid therapy. *Curr Probl Pediatr,* 1972; 3:3–40.

Segar WE, Chesney RW. Disorders of electrolyte metabolism. *Pediatr Ann,* 1981;10:286–301.

Winters R, ed. *The Body Fluids in Pediatrics.* Boston: Little, Brown & Co, 1978: 95–154.

Reye's Syndrome

Corey L, Rubin RJ, Hattwick MAW. Reye's syndrome: clinical progression and evaluation of therapy. *Pediatrics,* 1977;60:708–717.

Haller J. Intracranial monitoring in Reye's syndrome. *Hosp Pract,* 1980;15:101–108.

Renal Failure

Siegel NJ. Acute renal failure. In: Brenner BM, Stein JH, eds., *Pediatric Nephrology,* vol 12, Contemporary Issues in nephrology. New York: Churchill Livingstone, 1984: 297–320.

Hematuria

Brewer Ed, Benson GS. Hematuria: algorithms for diagnosis 1. hematuria in the child. *JAMA* 1981;246:877.

Chang B. Red cell nephrology aid to diagnosis of hematuria. *JAMA* 1984;252:1747–1749.

Emanuel B, Aronson M. Neonatal hematuria. *Am J. Dis Child,* 1974;128:204–206.

Fairley KF, Birch DF. Hematuria: a simple method for identifying glomerular bleeding. *Kidney Int,* 1982;21:105–108.

Ingelfinger JR, David AB, Grupe WE. Frequency and etiology of gross hematuria in a general pediatric setting. *Pediatrics,* 1977;59:557–561.

Kaplan MR. Hematuria in childhood. *Pediatrics Rev,* 1983; 5:99–105.

McConville J, West CD MacAdams J. Familial and nonfamilial benign hematuria. *J Pediatr,* 1966;69:207–214.

Stapleton FB, Roy S, Noe HN, et al. Hypercalcemia in children with hematuria. *N Engl J Med,* 1982;310:1345–1348.

West CD. Asymptomatic hematuria and proteinuria in children. *J Pediatr,* 1976: 89:173–182.

Urinary Tract Infection

Adelman RD. Urinary tract infections in children. In: Brenner BM, Stein JH, eds. *Pediatric Nephrology,* vol 12, Contemporary issues in nephrology. New York: Churchill Livingstone, 1984:155–190.

Caravajal HF. Kidney and bladder infections. *Adv Pediatr,* 1978;25:383–413.

Kunin CM. *Detection, Prevention and Management of Urinary Tract Infections.* Philadelphia: Lea & Febiger, 1972.

Kunin CM, Southall I, Paquin AJ. Epidemology of UTI's, a pilot study of 3057 school children. *N Engl J. Med,* 1960; 263:817–823.

Rapkin RH. Urinary tract infection. *Pediatr Rev,* 1979; 1:133–136.

CHAPTER 28

Management of Seizures in the Pediatric Patient

ELIZABETH C. DOOLING, M.D.

The emergency physician caring for a child with seizures must stabilize the medical condition, characterize the seizure, determine the appropriate diagnostic tests to evaluate etiology, and finally, choose the appropriate therapy based on this information. This chapter discusses presentation, diagnosis, and management of seizures in the pediatric patient, including status epilepticus and febrile seizures.

DEFINITIONS

Seizures are episodes that are characterized by involuntary changes in voluntary motor activity, sensation, autonomic function, behavior, and/or level of consciousness. They may be brief, lasting less than a minute, or prolonged, lasting for 30–50 minutes or more. The *focal* seizure arises from a discrete irritative locus in one cerebral hemisphere, such as encephalitis, a cortical scar, porencephalic cyst, brain abscess, tumor, vascular anomaly, vasculitis, or a thromboembolus. The *generalized* seizure is thought to arise from deeper midline cerebral structures defined as "centrencephalic." Seizures are provoked by fever, intercurrent illness, menses, and sometimes stress. There is a high incidence of seizures in childhood. It has been estimated that 5–10% of children have febrile seizures, and 5% of children from 0–18 years have afebrile seizures. There is evidence from experimental animal models that a process called "kindling" may occur in animals with poorly controlled focal seizures. Over a period of time, seizure activity may develop in adjacent or contralateral areas of brain (presumably via commissural connections). This phenomenon suggests that good seizure control, to reduce the incidence of kindling, should be a goal of treatment.

WORKUP

Initial Management

Management *precedes* diagnosis in the actively seizing or obtunded child. Securing the airway and vascular access, obtaining vital signs, performing expeditious general and neurologic examinations, and drawing blood for diagnostic studies can all take place in the first few moments while therapy directed at stopping the seizures is initiated. A complete history should be obtained after the medical condition of the child has been stabilized. It is worthwhile to spend a few extra minutes to take the history from an actual eyewitness.

Questions for the History

Answers to these questions are helpful:

1. How did the seizure start?
2. What part(s) of the body were first involved?
3. Was there loss of consciousness at the beginning, or later?
4. Was there fever before or after the seizure, with an infectious illness?
5. How long did the seizure last? (It is common to overestimate the length of a seizure, but an approximate estimate can sometimes be obtained by having the witness time what he or she thinks was the interval of seizing by the clock. If the child is found seizing, an accurate estimate cannot be made.)
6. What did the child do after the seizure stopped?
7. Was there head injury, with or without loss of consciousness?
8. Has the child ever had a seizure before, with or without fever?
9. What is the child's birth and developmental history?

10. Is there a family history of seizures, with or without fever?
11. Are there any drugs, including illicit, or other toxic agents available to the child?

Examination

The examination of the child who has had, or is having, a seizure should include the assessment of:

1. Vital signs and airway;
2. Symmetry and reactivity of pupils, arms, and legs;
3. Level of consciousness and response to voice and stimuli;
4. Skin for petechiae, needle marks, insect bites;
5. Eyes for position, deviation, disconjugate gaze, restricted range of motion, ptosis, fundi for papilledema or hemorrhages;
6. Face for symmetry of movements and reaction to pain;
7. Neck for meningismus;
8. Arms and legs for muscle tone and strength, resting posture, voluntary movement, symmetry of tendon reflexes, and plantar responses.

On neurologic examination, mental status evaluation should include notation of the level of responsiveness and ability to answer questions about name, age, place, and other age-appropriate general information. Level of cooperation should be noted. Cranial nerve evaluation should include estimate of visual fields by confrontation, especially in the child with focal seizures. Weakness of the arms should be assessed by asking the child to extend the arms at shoulder height, to observe any downward drift or overcorrection by upward drift. The child should be asked to perform simple tasks involving coordination, such as finger-to-nose, heel-to-shin, and rapid alternating movements, remembering that weakness may impair the child's ability to perform such tests. Sensation should be checked by observing symmetry of reaction time to painful stimuli. The child's gait should be observed for evidence of hemiparesis or ataxia.

In the young child who is irritable, it may be useful and necessary to include the parents in the examination procedure. The child may cooperate more for a person who is familiar. Small toys are used for checking visual fields, testing strength when trying to reach for objects out of his/her grasp, and assessing gait (crawling or walking) by placing a desirable toy at a distance on the floor. A postictal or febrile child may not be enticed by such attractions.

SPECIAL CONSIDERATIONS

Status Epilepticus

Certain seizures warrant special consideration. Status epilepticus has a mortality as high as 30%; thus, it demands urgent attention and treatment. Status epilepticus is defined as a seizure or series of seizures lasting continuously or repetitively for greater than 30 minutes without recovery of consciousness. The prolongation of seizures may be due to any of the causes listed in Table 28.1. A patient with status epilepticus is unresponsive and cannot cooperate on neurological testing. It is important to note the size and reactivity of the pupils, position of the eyes, spontaneous movements of the arms and legs, and automatisms, such as lip-smacking or purposeless, stereotyped movements.

Treatment of status epilepticus includes:

1. Assessment and establishment of adequacy of the airway;
2. Checking of blood gases and administration of oxygen;
3. Correction of electrolyte imbalance with cautious replacement of fluids to avoid cerebral edema;
4. Determination of drug levels in patient known to take anticonvulsants; and

Table 28.1.
Causes for Prolongation of Seizures

1. Accidental or nonaccidental acute trauma
2. Acute intracranial infection
   - Meningitis
   - Encephalitis
   - Brain abscess
   - Empyema, subdural or epidural
3. Metabolic
   - Hypoglycemia or hyperglycemia
   - Hyponatremia or hypernatremia
   - Hypocalcemia
   - Hypomagnesemia
   - Aminoacidopathies or organic acidemias
4. Withdrawal of anticonvulsants
5. Substance abuse, including alcohol, cocaine, stimulants, phencyclidine (PCP)
6. Accidental or nonaccidental heavy metal intoxication, such as lead
7. Hypoxia
8. Cerebral structural lesions
   - Congenital malformations such as porencephalic cysts
   - Para- or postinfectious arterial or venous infarctions
   - Arteriovenous malformations
   - Acute vasculopathy with sickle cell disease, lupus erythematosus
   - Neurocutaneous syndromes
9. Reye's syndrome
10. Burn encephalopathy

5. Saving a blood and urine sample for toxic screening tests.

The limited number of drugs available in parenteral form dictates the treatment options. The following approach is useful in an actively seizing patient:

1. Give diazepam intravenously, ≤ 1 mg/year of age, with a maximum of 10 mg/dose. Monitor pulse and respirations closely and be prepared to ventilate by Ambu bag or intubate a patient with shallow or irregular respirations or apnea; *and*
2. Give phenytoin, 10–15 mg/kg slowly, intravenously, 25–50 mg/minute, with cardiac monitoring. Do *not* give phenytoin in a 5% dextrose solution, for precipitation occurs—use a saline flush.
3. If the seizures continue for 15–20 minutes after treatment, give phenobarbital, 10–15 mg/kg slowly, intravenously. Monitor respirations.
4. An additional dose of diazepam, 1 mg/year (maximum = 10 mg) may be given intravenously if the seizures are not controlled within 15–20 minutes, and an additional 5–10 mg/kg of phenytoin intravenously.
5. If the seizures persist after 15–20 minutes, or if intravenous access has not been obtained, paraldehyde 0.3 cc/kg mixed with 1–2 equal volumes of mineral oil may be given rectally (pr). Paraldehyde pr is effective far more rapidly than phenobarbital intramuscularly.

Febrile Seizures

Febrile seizures are so common an occurrence that special attention is warranted. Simple febrile convulsions are characterized by fever and generalized seizure activity of short duration (less than, or equal to, 10 minutes), in a neurologically normal child between 6 months and 6 years of age, associated with a source of fever outside the central nervous system, and with no postictal focal deficit.

It is very important to lower the child's temperature by giving appropriate doses of antipyretics; the time-honored technique of bathing the child in tepid water may not be effective. A source for fever should be sought, and commonly will be found to be occult pneumococcal bacteremia, otitis, cystitis, or roseola. Although the yield of positive findings on lumbar puncture is quite low, unless the child has a prolonged seizure, focal deficits, a several day history of febrile illness, or physical signs of meningitis, spinal tap is nevertheless routinely performed on all children with a first-time febrile seizure. It should be performed even on the child with recurrent febrile seizures if the history or examination are suggestive of meningitis. If the conditions described above are not met, the child has had a complex febrile seizure or seizure with fever and treatment with anticonvulsants may be indicated. A first-time simple febrile seizure is not routinely treated with anticonvulsants.

Table 28.2.
International Classification of Epileptic Seizures[a]

- I. Partial seizures (seizures beginning locally)
  - A. Partial seizures with elementary symptomatology (generally without impairment of consciousness)
    - 1. With motor symptoms, e.g., Jacksonian
    - 2. With special sensory or somatosensory symptoms
    - 3. With autonomic symptoms
    - 4. Compound forms or combinations of 1–3.
  - B. Partial seizures with complex symptomatology (generally with impairment of consciousness):
    - 1. With impairment of consciousness only
    - 2. With cognitive symptomatology
    - 3. With affective symptomatology
    - 4. With "psychosensory" symptomatology
    - 5. With "psychomotor" symptomatology
    - 6. Compound forms or combinations of 1–5.
  - C. Partial seizures secondarily generalized
- II. Generalized seizures (bilaterally symmetric without local onset)
  - A. Absences (petit mal)
  - B. Bilateral massive epileptic myoclonus
  - C. Infantile spasms or myoclonic seizures of infancy
  - D. Clonic seizures
  - E. Tonic seizures
  - F. Tonic-clonic seizures (grand mal)
  - G. Atonic seizures
  - H. Akinetic seizures
- III. Unilateral seizures (predominantly)
- IV. Unclassified epileptic seizures (due to incomplete data)

[a] From Commission on Classification and Terminology of the International League Against Epilepsy. Proposal for revised clinical and electroencephalographic classification of epileptic seizures. *Epilepsia*, 1981;22:480–501.

LONG-TERM TREATMENT

The choice of anticonvulsants is based on the classification of the seizure. It is very important that the details of the seizure be described, so that appropriate therapy may be prescribed.

For simple or complex partial or generalized tonic-clonic (grand mal) seizures, one of the following drugs is usually given:

Drug	*Maintenance dose*
Phenytoin	3–8 mg/kg/d
Carbamazepine	10–20 mg/kg/d
Primidone	10–20 mg/kg/d

For absence seizures, good seizure control may be achieved with the following:

Drug	*Maintenance dose*
Ethosuximide	20–30 mg/kg/d
Valproic acid	20–60 mg/kg/d

Complex disorders (Table 28.2) such as infantile spasms and mixed seizure disorders usually require initial hospitalization and trials of special (e.g., ACTH) or combined drug therapy in consultation with a neurologist.

SUGGESTED READINGS

Anneger JF, Hauser WA, Shirts SB, et al. Factors prognostic of unprovoked seizures after febrile convulsions. *N Engl J Med,* 1987;316:493–498.

Consensus Development Panel. Febrile seizures: long-term management of children with fever-associated seizures. *Pediatr Rev,* 1981;2:209–211.

Joffe A, McCormick M, DeAngelis C. Which children with febrile seizures need lumbar puncture? A decision analysis approach. *Am J Dis Child,* 1983;137:1153–1156.

CHAPTER 29

Neglect and Physical and Sexual Abuse of the Pediatric Patient

PATRICIA J. O'MALLEY, M.D.

The emergency physician is frequently the first and sometimes the only physician to care for children who are the victims of neglect or physical and sexual abuse. It is therefore vital that emergency department personnel recognize both the overt and covert signs of these conditions and be familiar with their management and the legal responsibilities they entail. This chapter reviews the diagnosis, management, and legal aspects of child abuse and neglect and sexual maltreatment of the prepubertal child.

DEFINITIONS AND EPIDEMIOLOGY

Neglect is defined as the failure on the part of the child care giver to provide adequate food, clothing, shelter, medical care, and emotional sustenance to a dependent child. Physical abuse encompasses inflicted injuries, including drug and alcohol use forced upon the child either directly or indirectly, as with the drug-habituated newborn. Sexual assault of a child occurs when a minor refuses sex or by virtue of age cannot consent to sexual activity with an adult. Sexual maltreatment of the prepubertal child can include oral, manual, or genital contact of an offender with a child for sexual gratification, and may involve contact, exposure, fondling, insertion, or penetration.

The frequency of these problems is difficult to determine because reporting undoubtedly underestimates their actual occurrence; however, it is estimated that at least 30,000 cases of physical abuse occur each year in the United States. In children under the age of 3, 10% of all trauma, excluding motor vehicle accidents, and one-quarter of all fractures are caused by inflicted rather than accidental injury. The child identified as a victim of child abuse has a 50% chance of suffering repeated injury and a 10% risk of death from child abuse if no intervention is made. These are statistics that are found in few other childhood ''diseases.'' There are at least 2000 deaths per year from battering, and probably more than 6000 cases of mental retardation resulting from injuries inflicted on children. The American Humane Association estimates that 300,000–500,000 cases of sexual abuse in girls under the age of 14 occur annually in the United States. While the majority of sexual maltreatment victims are female, it is thought that as many as one in four victims under the age of 12 is male. Most episodes of sexual abuse in the prepubertal child are found to be chronic and recurrent, frequently not involving physical violence, as in adult rape. In up to 75% of the time, the perpetrator is someone known to the child.

PRESENTATION

Child neglect is a condition usually hidden behind a more trivial presenting complaint, and the physician caring for the infant or child with intercurrent cold or gastroenteritis should be alerted to the possibility of child neglect. The infant may show signs of poor care, poor hygiene, inadequate clothing, or failure to thrive. The neglected infant is frequently developmentally delayed and may have neurologic abnormalities, including hypotonia or spasticity. The child frequently resists cuddling or eye contact, and emergency department personnel may note that the parent seems distant, inappropriately demanding of, or overtly hostile, to the child. There is occasionally a history of parental substance abuse, emotional instability, or previous removal of a child from the home.

Child abuse should be considered with any childhood injury, and in particular: (*a*) in the child under 3; (*b*) when there has been unusual delay in seeking care; (*c*) when the described mechanism of injury does not seem to fit the physical findings or the developmental capabilities of the child (such as a 1-

Table 29.1.
Color and Approximate Age of Bruises

Age of Bruise	Appearance
24 hours	No mark, red, blue, or purple
1–3 days	Blue, blue-brown
5–7 days	Greenish
7–10 days	Yellow
Over 10 days	Brown

month-old "rolling off the changing table"); (*d*) with history of, or evidence on examination, of previous bruising at different ages. Table 29.1 describes the color and approximate age of bruises based on appearance. Although there are no findings absolutely diagnostic of child abuse, Table 29.2 lists findings suggestive of abuse with other possible differential diagnoses. Many toddlers in the course of a normal day develop bruises or scrapes on the shins, face, or chin; however, injuries on the buttocks, backs of the legs, or perineum are rarely accidental. Cigarette burns and symmetric scald burns from deliberate immersion, J-shaped welts from belt or cord whipping, and human bites are characteristic stigmata of inflicted injury. It is important to consider child abuse as the underlying cause of an acute abdomen, toxic overdose, or drug withdrawal in the young child. Because of their potentially serious nature, skull fractures in the child under 1 year of age should be carefully evaluated for the possibility of abuse, even though they are in fact frequently accidental. Table 29.3 lists the findings typical of the "shaken baby" in whom more obvious injuries may not be present.

The presentation of sexual abuse may be subtle, as in the child brought for evaluation of new onset vaginal discharge, urinary tract infection, nightmares, encopresis, enuresis, abdominal pain, or other conversion reaction symptom. On the other hand, children are increasingly brought to medical attention by their parents with the expressed concern that the child has been sexually abused. In the prepubertal child, sexual maltreatment may take the form of fondling, which the child regards as special or desirable. Less frequently, it involves physical trauma that leaves clearcut stigmata. The child with perineal bruising, rectal or vaginal tears; hymenal

Table 29.2.
Differential Diagnosis of Child Abuse[a]

Clinical Findings	Differential Diagnosis
Skin	
Bruising	Trauma Bleeding diathesis Henoch-Schönlein purpura Purpura fulminans
Erythema, blisters	Burn Impetigo Frostbite Herpes zoster/simplex Contact dermatitis
Eye	
Retinal hemorrhage	Shaking or other trauma Bleeding diathesis Neoplasm Resuscitation
Conjunctival hemorrhage	Trauma Bacterial or viral conjunctivitis Coughing
Orbital swelling	Trauma Orbital or periorbital cellulitis
Hematuria	Trauma Urinary tract infection Vasculitis Hereditary renal disorder Renal stone Sickle trait
Acute abdomen	Trauma Intrinsic gastrointestinal disease
Bone	
Fractures (multiple of various ages)	Trauma Osteogenesis imperfecta Rickets Birth trauma Leukemia Neuroblastoma Status post osteomyelitis, septic arthritis
Metaphyseal lesions	Trauma Scurvy Menke's syndrome Birth trauma
Subperiosteal ossification	Trauma Osteogenesis imperfecta Syphilis Scurvy Osteoid osteoma
Sudden infant death syndrome	Unexplained Trauma Asphyxia Occult infection Cardiac arrhythmia Metabolic abnormality

[a] Modified from Bittner S, Newberger E. Pediatric understanding of child abuse and neglect. *Pediatr Rev*, 1981;2:197–207.

Table 29.3.
Findings Characteristic of "Shaken Baby" Syndrome

Metaphyseal avulsion
Subperiosteal hematoma
Intracranial hemorrhage
Retinal hemorrhage

lacerations, especially between 3 and 9 o'clock; relaxed anal sphincter; absent gag reflex; throat, rectal, or vaginal cultures positive for gonorrhea or *Chlamydia,* is showing the stigmata of possible sexual maltreatment.

MANAGEMENT

History and Examination

When abuse, neglect, or sexual maltreatment are suspected in a child, the physician must perform and document a careful history and physical examination, including a neurodevelopmental assessment and inspection of the entire body for hygiene and skin findings, such as scars and bruises. Photographs of any physical findings may be useful. Social service personnel should be consulted, and the local child protective service should be notified. In most jurisdictions, an immediate verbal report, followed by a written report within 48 hours, is mandatory. In obtaining the history of a current injury, the physician must avoid assigning blame, but takes an attitude that reflects concern for the child and support of the family. Although it is difficult to avoid a judgmental attitude, the physician must be able to appeal to that part of the caretaker that caused him or her to bring the child to medical attention in the first place. It is important to check for the safety of other siblings who may be at similar risk for injury or neglect.

When dealing with sexual abuse, there are additional considerations. The thought or fact of sexual abuse in the prepubertal child generates a tremendous emotional burden for parents and for medical personnel alike. The younger child may in fact not understand the problem as being bad and may respond only to the sense that his parents or the hospital personnel are distressed. The older child frequently has a misplaced sense of guilt or wrongdoing that may be further aggravated by hospital staff who are unable to deal with this problem in a calm fashion. For all these reasons, it is important that the victim of possible sexual abuse be assigned a high triage priority in the emergency department, but that the workup proceed in a calm, unhurried, gentle, and empathetic fashion. When taking a history from a child, the physician should establish what names a child has for various body parts and should describe sexual acts in very simple and concrete terms to avoid confusion. Using a doll or a toy to illustrate the meaning of questions can be helpful for obtaining a history and in preparing the child for the physical examination. Children should not be challenged on their story; they are much more likely to deny an encounter than to fabricate one.

The Genital Examination

The genital examination is best performed as an integral part of a "top-to-toe" physical examination rather than as a separate, highlighted event, and as with the rest of the physical examination, should provide reassurance to the child that he or she is all right. The condition of the hymenal ring and the stage of sexual maturation of the child should be documented. The knee-chest position is often more suitable for examining young girls than the lithotomy position. Cultures of the rectum and vagina can also be obtained comfortably in this position, although some children tolerate the procedure of culturing better if they are allowed to obtain the samples themselves with guidance. Apart from obtaining cultures, an internal examination is rarely revealing of pathology unless there are signs on external examination of bruising, bleeding, discharge, or multiple hymenal scars and tags. If an internal examination is indicated, sedation or general anesthesia should be strongly considered.

Laboratory Studies

Appropriate laboratory studies vary with each case, but may include: cultures of the throat, rectum, vagina or urethra, and urine; pregnancy test in any menstruating child; venereal disease research laboratories test (VDRL). If the child has been assaulted in the past 72 hours, it is appropriate to collect forensic samples or to complete a commercial "rape kit" designed for that purpose. Suggested collection sites for culture and for checking for motile sperm include the posterior fornix or pooled vaginal secretions, between the cheek and gum back to the posterior molars and under the tongue, and in any mucoid area in the anal region. Specimens should be air-dried before sealing to prevent biodegradation, and labeled with the patient's name, hospital number, date, time, site of collection, physician's name, and chain of custody of evidence.

Prophylactic Treatment

Diseases acquired as a result of sexual abuse include gonorrhea, *Chlamydia* infection, syphilis, hepatitis, mononucleosis, AIDS, genital herpes, cytomegalic virus infection, and trichomoniasis. Prophylactic treatment for gonorrhea, *Chlamydia* infection, and syphilis should be considered, as well as for hepatitis, if the assailant is felt to be at risk of being a carrier. Several therapy regimens have been suggested:

1. Aqueous procaine penicillin 100,000 U/kg intramuscularly, to a maximum dose of 4.8 million units, divided in two sites, and preceded by oral probenecid 25 mg/kg to a maximum of 1 gm. This is effective against pharyngeal and rectal gonococcal infection, as well as pelvic disease, and probably effective against incubating syphilis.
2. Amoxicillin 50 mg/kg to a maximum of 3 gm, orally, with probenecid. Although less traumatic, it is also not effective against pharyngeal and rectal gonococcal infection.
3. Children older than 8 years of age may receive tetracycline, 40 mg/kg/day for 5 days divided 4 times per day. This may not be effective against rectal gonococcal infection, but will adequately treat chlamydial infections. Children under 8 years of age can receive erythromycin 40 mg/kg/day divided 4 times per day for *Chlamydia* infections.
4. Tetanus prophylaxis and Kwell treatment for pediculosis may need to be considered.

Although the risk of pregnancy following rape is difficult to determine, and may in fact be smaller than published estimates, prophylaxis for any molested child who has commenced menses should be offered for the child and the family to consider, if the possibility of penetration and/or ejaculation exists. If administered within 72 hours, Ovral, two tablets immediately and two tablets 12 hours later, has been an effective postcoital contraceptive treatment.

SUGGESTED READINGS

Bittner S, Newberger E. Pediatric understanding of child abuse and neglect. *Pediatr Rev,* 1981;2:197–207.

Pascoe D. Management of sexually abused children. *Pediatr Ann,* 1979;8:44–58.

Sarles RM. Sexual abuse and rape. *Pediatr Rev,* 1982;4:93–98.

Woodling BA, Kossoris PD. Sexual misuse: rape, molestation, and incest. *Pediatr Clin North Am,* 1981;28:481–499.

CHAPTER 30

Pediatric Surgical Emergencies

SAMUEL H. KIM, M.D.
DENNIS P. LUND, M.D.

PEDIATRIC TRAUMA

Trauma is the most common cause of death of children in the United States—nearly 50% of deaths in patients ages 1–14 years are due to major trauma. This is compared with one in 10 deaths in the general population that are due to trauma. Any child who has been injured in an accident requires rapid resuscitation, efficient and thorough assessment of the injuries, followed by proper assignment of treatment priorties.

Resuscitation

The ABCs of resuscitation (*A*irway, *B*reathing, and *C*irculation) apply to children just as they do to any patient requiring resuscitation. Initial management of the airway of an apneic patient should include clearing the airway, administration of oxygen, use of an Ambu bag, or even endotracheal intubation if necessary. The variability of size in children's airways can be a problem, and the appropriately sized endotracheal tubes and laryngoscopes should be available for intubation (see Tables 21.2 and 21.3 for appropriate sizes). A quick rule is that the endotracheal tube should be approximately the size of the child's little finger, and the appropriate laryngoscope blade number for intubation is the number of adult fingerbreadths from the child's chin to the hyoid bone (e.g., two fingerbreadths equals a Miller 2 blade). The child's tracheal length is variable, depending on size; the carina is about at the level of the angle of Louis. Mainstem bronchial intubation (usually right mainstem), with subsequent ineffective ventilation, is the most common complication of emergency endotracheal intubation in children.

If emergency endotracheal intubation is impossible, emergency cricothyrotomy may be necessary. The need for this should be rare. In children under the age of 12, the use of needle-catheter cricothyrotomy (see Illustrated Technique 4) is recommended for technique to avoid permanent laryngeal damage.

Once an airway is secured, the pulse and blood pressure are obtained. If neither is present, cardiopulmonary resuscitation should be initiated. External cardiac massage in the infant under 1 year of age is best performed using two hands encircling the chest with compression of the midsternum. Older children should be placed on a firm surface with massage performed on the lower portion of the sternum, as discussed in Chapter 21.

Venous access is gained using percutaneous technique with appropriately size catheters. The antecubital and saphenous veins are good sites of choice. Other access sites include the external jugular and femoral veins. The scalp veins may be cannulated in the very small infant. If percutaneous access is unsuccessful, a venous cutdown may be performed, as demonstrated in Illustrated Technique 7. Central venous lines are often difficult to place in the volume-depleted child, but once the patient has been resuscitated, a central venous catheter may be helpful for continuing management. In this case, a subclavian or internal jugular line may be placed. In children older than 4 years, the technique is the same as that used in adults, except for the use of small gauge needles and catheters. Venous cutdown over the basilic vein may also be used to thread a catheter into a central venous position. If a short subcutaneous tunnel is created and the catheter is brought through the skin at a point away from the incision, such a catheter may be used for a week or more with proper arm immobilization.

If emergency intravascular access has not been obtained after 5 minutes of attempts in the arrested child, or within a reasonable time frame in the non-arrested child, an interosseous bone marrow needle should be placed for emergency fluid resuscitation. Once the patient has been adequately resuscitated via this route, it may be easier to place a percutaneous or cutdown venous catheter. The technique for bone marrow needle placement is described in Chapter 21 (Fig. 21.6).

Initial resuscitation fluids should be warm solutions of lactated Ringer's or 0.9% saline. Rate of administration is dependent on patient size, presence of shock or dehydration, and presence of major head injury. General guidelines are provided in Chapter 21. Solutions and amounts for pediatric volume replacement are listed in Table 30.1.

Arterial blood gas determination and monitoring may be obtained by placement of a 22-gauge plastic cannula into a radial artery. This may be done after assessing adequate ulnar artery flow, either by percutaneous placement or by puncture of the artery after direct cutdown without tying off the vessel. Femoral artery puncture for blood gas determination should be avoided in children, since a significant hematoma may form after arterial puncture and go unnoticed in the groin. Arterial lines should never be used for fluid or drug administration since they may lead to arterial spasm or thrombosis.

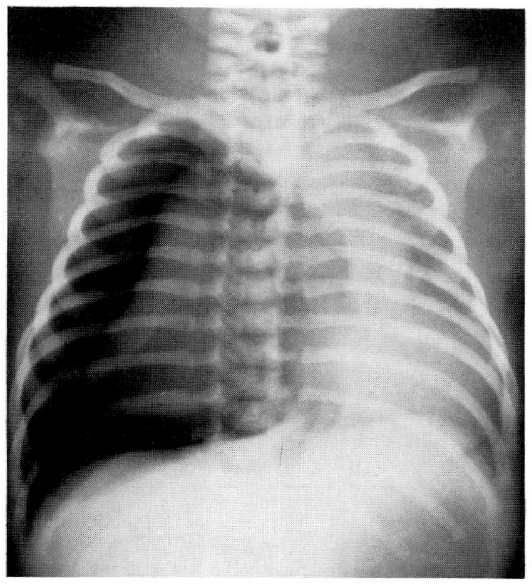

Figure 30.1. Right-sided tension pneumothorax with marked mediastinal shift.

Assessment

Once resuscitation has been initiated, the physician in charge of the traumatized child must begin a systematic, thorough evaluation of the injuries. A complete physical examination is rapidly performed, including the front and *back* of the child. Care must be taken in moving the patient until the cervical spine has been evaluated with a lateral x-ray that shows all seven cervical vertebrae. The neurologic examination should be noted, and neurosurgical consultation obtained if there is evidence of major craniocerebral or any spinal cord injury. Breath sounds are auscultated, and a chest x-ray is obtained. Absent breath sounds suggesting a pneumothorax (Fig. 30.1) may require expeditious placement of chest tube of appropriate size. A nasogastric or orogastric tube should be inserted, especially in patients with head, thoracic, or

Table 30.1.
Pediatric Volume Replacement

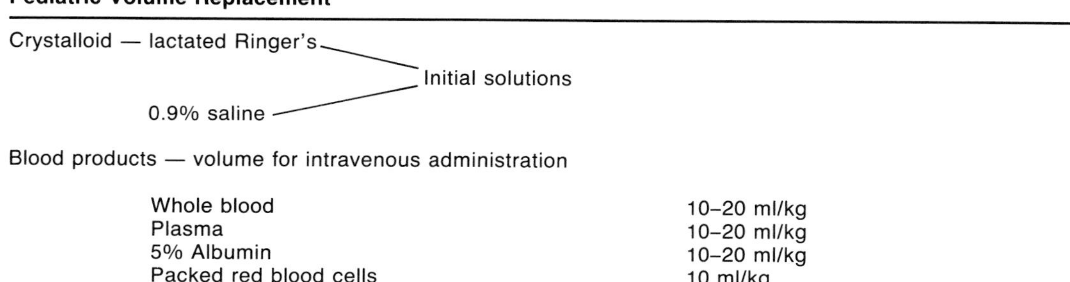

Crystalloid — lactated Ringer's	Initial solutions
0.9% saline	Initial solutions
Blood products — volume for intravenous administration	
Whole blood	10–20 ml/kg
Plasma	10–20 ml/kg
5% Albumin	10–20 ml/kg
Packed red blood cells	10 ml/kg
Platelets	1 unit = 20–35 ml

Table 30.2.
Diagnosis and Treatment of Blunt Abdominal Trauma

Diagnosis

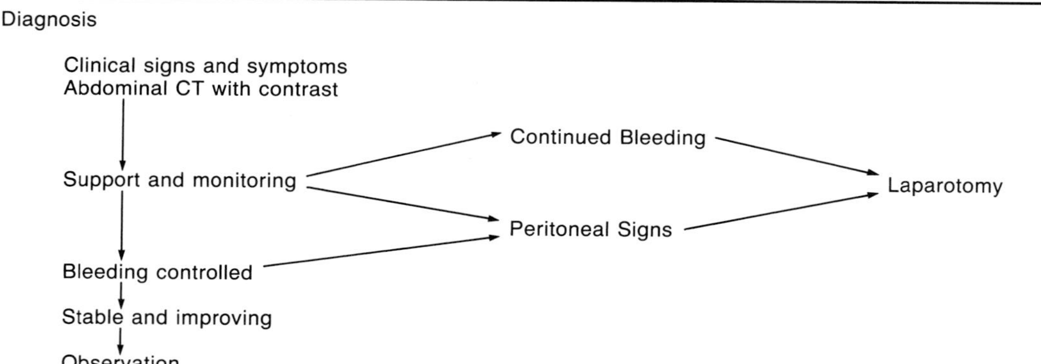

abdominal injuries. This serves to prevent vomiting and to minimize the potential for aspiration. It allows assessment of esophageal or gastric injuries, particularly in the child with gastric distension resulting from crying or from bag-and-mask ventilation. The abdomen is examined for bowel sounds and masses; the stability of the pelvis is checked. A rectal examination is performed to note the presence of guaiac-positive stool or of a floating prostate, which might indicate a urethral injury. The perineum must be inspected. Blood at the urethral meatus, a distended bladder, or an abnormal prostate suggest the possibility of urethral injury; a retrograde urethrogram should be obtained prior to Foley catheter placement. If these signs are not present, a Foley catheter is placed and the presence of hematuria noted. If bladder disruption is suspected, a retrograde cystogram is obtained. If a urethral injury is present, a suprapubic catheter should be placed (see Illustrated Technique 16).

The initial assessment of the injured child also includes the determination of hematocrit, arterial blood gases, serum electrolytes, and blood sugar. Blood is made available to the blood bank for crossmatching. Urinalysis is performed. Chest, pelvic and specific x-ray views of deformed or swollen extremities are obtained, in addition to cervical spine films, as mentioned earlier. Thoracic and lumbar spine films are indicated if there is pain or tenderness in these regions. Pediatric multiple trauma victims frequently have associated head injuries; a cranial computed tomographic (CT) scan is obtained early if there is suggestion of an abnormal neurological examination, altered mental status, or seizure activity.

Accurate clinical evaluation of the abdomen in an injured, frightened child is often difficult. A careful physical examination is crucial, since this frequently serves as a baseline for subsequent serial examinations. The indications for peritoneal lavage in children are essentially the same as those for adults, although the procedure tends to be used less frequently in children. Specific indications for peritoneal lavage include: (*a*) inability to evaluate the abdomen clinically; (*b*) hemodynamic instability without obvious source; (*c*) need for general anesthesia for operation other than for intraabdominal injury; and (*d*) penetrating injury without peritoneal signs. The technique of peritoneal lavage in children is that used for adults (see Illustrated Technique 15), with the volume instilled 10 ml/kg body weight, to a maximum of 1000 ml. Peritoneal lavage introduces air into the peritoneum and may cause peritoneal irritation, thus interfering with subsequent clinical examinations. Therefore, in the stable, injured child, contrast-enhanced CT of the abdomen is the preferred evaluation tool for intraabdominal injuries. Although not quite as sensitive as peritoneal lavage, CT has the advantage of not interfering with subsequent examinations that may be important in the nonoperative management of solid visceral injuries. An algorithm for the diagnosis and treatment of children with blunt abdominal trauma is presented in Table 30.2.

Splenic Injury

Blunt trauma is the predominant mechanism of injury in children. In blunt abdominal trauma, the most commonly injured organ is the spleen. Splenic injury may be isolated or may be a component of multiple trauma. Splenic injury should be sought whenever there is evidence of abdominal injury in a child, fractured ribs on the left, or a mechanism of trauma that could cause solid viscus injury. Physical signs of a splenic injury include ecchymosis and tenderness over the region, abdominal and left shoulder pain, and evidence of hypovolemia and blood loss (pallor, tachycardia, hypotension). Volume resuscitation is instituted, a nasogastric tube inserted, and blood typed and cross-matched, should transfusion be necessary.

A plain x-ray of the abdomen is often not of diagnostic usefulness. Young children often do not have associated lower left rib fractures. The most helpful diagnostic test for splenic injury is the contrast-enhanced CT of the abdomen. Radionuclide scanning can be helpful in diagnosing this injury, but this test has a higher incidence of false-positive results, usually due to congenital clefts in the spleen. Splenic ultrasound scanning may be used in this injury, but it is both less sensitive and less specific than CT and radionuclide imaging.

Management of the splenic injury (Table 30.3) depends on the clinical status of the patient. When possible and safe, an effort is made to save the spleen, since the incidence of overwhelming post-splenectomy sepsis has been shown to be higher in children. The stable patient with an isolated splenic injury should be admitted to the intensive care unit (ICU) for vital signs monitoring and serial hematocrats. The patient is kept at bed rest for 7–10 days, and allowed to eat as soon as he or she is stable and the ileus has resolved. Gradual ambulation can be initiated on the 7th day. These patients can usually be discharged soon thereafter. Follow-up scans are likely to show complete resolution of the injury. It is exceedingly rare for these patients to have late rebleeding from the splenic injury.

The indications for operative intervention are hemodynamic instability, persistent bleeding requiring transfusion in excess of one-half of the child's blood volume (35–40 ml/kg) and multisystem injuries requiring exploration. Detection of multiple devitalized fragments of spleen may also be an indication for surgery. When operative intervention is required, splenic salvage is attempted, if it is compatible with the overall clinical status. Splenorrhaphy and partial splenectomy are two techniques the surgeon can use in this situation.

Hepatic Injury

Although hepatic injuries result in higher mortality and have a greater urgency than splenic injuries, there is now evidence that the principles of managing splenic injuries can sometimes be applied to the injured liver as well. Clearly, the seriously injured child who is unstable and suspected of hepatic injury should be expeditiously explored. In the stable child with blunt abdominal injury, however, rapid imaging of the abdomen with contrast-enhanced CT should be performed to delineate the extent and nature of the injury. A laceration or contusion so demonstrated requires careful ICU monitoring and frequent hematocrat determination. A low threshold for operative intervention is required of the surgeon in these patients, should their clinical status change, but many such patients with liver injuries have now been successfully managed with conservative therapy alone. The pediatric surgeon must be consulted early in the emergency department; follow-up is his or her responsibility in the ICU.

Renal Injury

Kidney injury is frequent in the traumatized child, but few of these injuries require surgery. Signs and symptoms that alert the emergency department physician to a potential renal injury include flank pain, flank abrasion or mass, hematuria, or a mechanism of injury consistent with renal injury. A preexisting renal abnormality, such as hydronephrosis, pelvic or horseshoe kidney, may predispose one to a renal injury. There is a high association of other injuries with renal trauma, and one-fourth of children with left renal injuries will also have splenic injuries.

Suspicion of a renal injury should prompt a contrast-enhanced CT scan (Table 30.4) or intravenous pyelogram (IVP) to delineate the extent of injury.

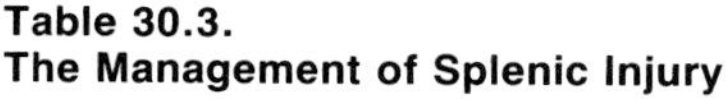
Table 30.3.
The Management of Splenic Injury

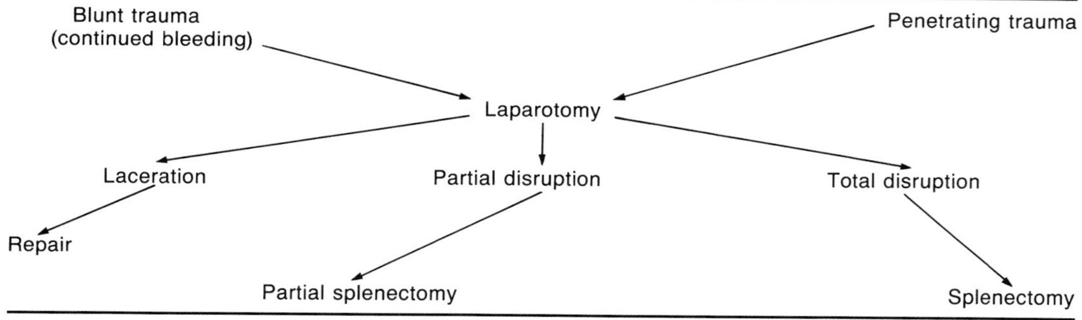

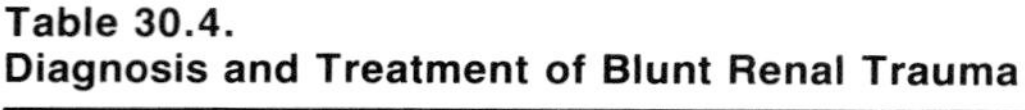

Table 30.4.
Diagnosis and Treatment of Blunt Renal Trauma

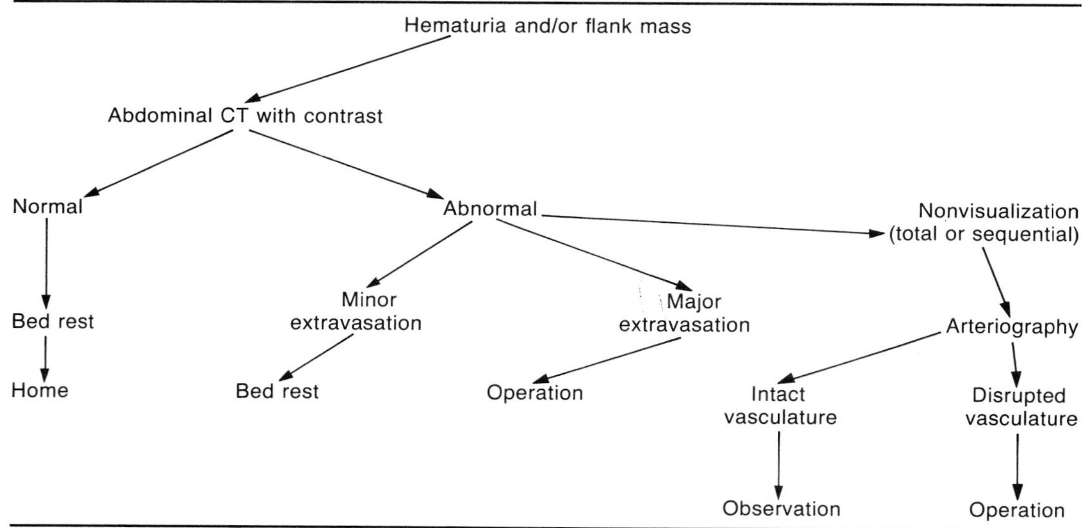

A nonfunctioning kidney requires emergency angiography and an attempt at surgical revascularization. Mild to moderate urinary extravasation and/or renal contusion can usually be managed nonoperatively, as outlined for splenic and liver trauma. Renal artery obstruction, increasing extravasation of urine or blood, or continuing bleeding require operative intervention.

Lower Urinary Tract Injuries

Particular care should be taken to look for ureteral disruption with the CT scan or IVP. Ureteral injuries are uncommon in children, most likely due to a lower incidence of penetrating trauma in children than in adults. However, the ureter can be disrupted with blunt injury; this is most likely to occur near the ureteropelvic junction. The signs of this injury are those of flank trauma and an enlarging flank mass. Extravasation of radiographic contrast material into the retroperitoneum is diagnostic. Operative repair is necessary.

Bladder and urethral injuries are also unusual in the younger child; however, they should be sought whenever a pelvic fracture is present or when the mechanism of injury involves a significant blow to the lower abdomen. If ever there is any question of such an injury, based on the physical finding of blood at the urethral meatus, an abnormal prostate, or a distended bladder, a retrograde urethrogram must be obtained prior to Foley catheter placement. If the urethrogram verifies a urethral injury, a suprapubic catheter is placed to monitor urine output and to permit further evaluation of the lower urinary tract injury. Minor extraperitoneal bladder injuries can often be managed with simple catheter drainage. Larger injuries and intraperitoneal injuries to the bladder often require repair. Urethral injuries are far more frequent in males due to the length of the urethra. This injury is often at the level of the membranous urethra. Management entails suprapubic catheter drainage with definitive repair usually taking place several months after the injury.

Pancreatic Injury

Pancreatic injury should be suspected in the child with abdominal trauma and elevated serum amylase. Serum amylase elevations can also be due to bowel or bile duct injuries. The mechanism of injury is a blow in the epigastrium compressing the pancreas against the spinal column, causing contusion or even transection of the gland. Transection usually occurs in the midbody of the pancreas, but injuries to the head or tail are also possible. Initial management of such injuries includes the administration of intravenous fluids, nasogastric suction, and bladder catheterization. Severe pancreatitis may require colloid replacement, intravenous broad-spectrum antibiotics, and even mechanical ventilation. With minor pancreatic injuries, the patient usually improves rapidly. Surgery is reserved for complications of the pancreatitis, such as abscess or pseudocyst formation, and is usually not required in the period of the acute injury. If extensive bowel rest is required due to a pancreatic injury, intravenous hyperalimentation should be instituted early in the hospital course.

Intestinal Injuries

Upper abdominal blunt trauma, as in a bicycle handlebar injury, can cause injury to the duodenum, again by compression against the spinal column. These patients present with epigastric pain and vomiting, often not until 24–48 hours after the injury. Physical examination may demonstrate an upper abdominal mass with overlying tenderness, and laboratory evaluation may demonstrate electrolyte abnormalities consistent with dehydration and protracted vomiting. In this case, an upper gastrointestinal series is the examination of choice, and is likely to show duodenal obstruction from a submucosal hematoma, the radiologic "stack of coins" sign. Treatment consists of nasogastric suction, bed rest, and intravenous fluids or hyperalimentation. The majority of these injuries resolve spontaneously, but in some cases it may be necessary for the surgeon to provide operative evacuation of the hematoma.

Clearly, any hollow viscus in the abdomen is susceptible to rupture or perforation with a given injury, blunt or sharp. Free perforation results in tenderness and signs of peritoneal irritation. An upright or left lateral decubitus x-ray examination of the abdomen usually demonstrates the presence of free air. Peritoneal lavage fluid may show an elevated amylase level, or a white blood cell count greater than 500 cells/ml. Operation is necessary whenever a perforated or lacerated viscus is suspected. Furthermore, development of peritoneal signs within the first 24 hours of abdominal trauma should alert the attending physican to the possibility of intestinal injury.

Cranial and Spinal Injuries

Central nervous system (CNS) injuries are a major cause of morbidity and mortality in trauma victims of the pediatric age group. The multiply injured child may have a head injury in addition to skeletal and visceral injuries. An initial neurologic evaluation must be made and documented by the emergency department physician as a baseline for subsequent comparative examinations. The history often provides a mechanism of injury, such as a fall, which makes one suspicious of head trauma. Once adequate resuscitation measures have been taken, the head is carefully inspected and palpated as part of the physical examination, to feel for "step-off" or depressed skull fractures. Scalp lacerations are carefully examined for evidence of open skull fracture. Otoscopy should be performed to seek hemotympanum or cerebrospinal fluid otorrhea, both signs of a basilar skull fracture. If there is concern for a cervical spine injury, the neck should be carefully immobilized pending cervical spine films. A general neurologic examination is performed with special attention to level of consciousness, arousability, evidence of seizure activity, or lateralizing neurologic signs. At the first suspicion of a CNS injury, neurosurgical consultation should be sought.

If a major intracranial CNS injury is present, intravenous fluid should be restricted to the minimum necessary to maintain vital signs, in order to minimize brain edema. Mechanical hyperventilation of the intubated patient also helps to reduce acute brain edema. Mannitol and glucocorticoids are often given to patients with major head injury, but should be done only under the supervision of a neurosurgeon.

Radiological evaluation includes anteroposterior and lateral cervical spine films. Skull films are useful in delineating skull fractures and, if there is a linear skull fracture crossing the middle meningeal groove, should arouse concern over possible injury to the middle meningeal artery, a cause of epidural hematoma. However, in the absence of loss of consciousness skull films have a low yield for demonstrating occult fractures. Computed tomography (CT) of the head is the best radiologic method for evaluation of intracranial CNS injury and also for demonstration of bony fractures.

In general, with the same degree of CNS injury, children do better than adults because of the resilience of the pediatric brain. However, the head makes up a larger proportion of the body in children, and young children may not yet have fused cranial sutures; both of these factors make children more susceptible to major CNS injury. A changing neurologic examination in a child should make the emergency physician wary that intracranial hemorrhage or swelling is occurring, and should prompt rapid neurosurgical consultation for further evaluation and therapy.

Thoracic Injuries

Injuries to the thorax are less frequent in children, again because of the lower incidence of penetrating trauma in children. Rib fractures and mediastinal injuries are less frequent with blunt trauma because of the relative elasticity of pediatric thoracic structures. When significant thoracic trauma does occur in children, it usually occurs in association with head and abdominal injuries. Despite the lower incidence of chest trauma in children, the emergency physician must keep in mind that the entire spectrum of thoracic injuries does occur in this age group. It is also worthy of note that due to the relative elasticity of the chest cage in children, significant intrathoracic injuries can occur without much associated skeletal abnormality.

The most common thoracic injury is pulmonary contusion from blunt trauma. Treatment consists of endotracheal intubation and assisted ventilation un-

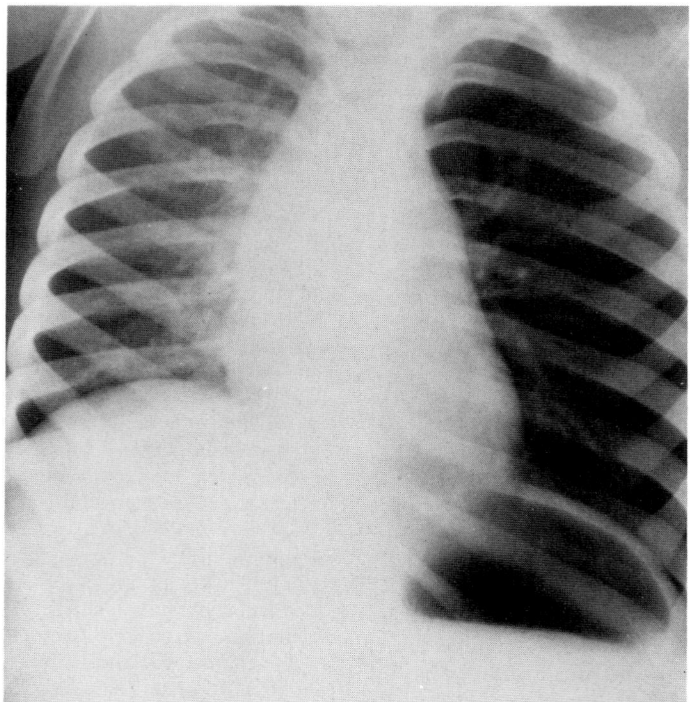

Figure 30.2. Foreign body of tracheobronchial tree with hyperlucency of left lung. The foreign body could be on either side, depending on whether there is complete obstruction or a ball-valve effect. A normal chest x-ray film does not rule out a foreign body.

til the injury begins to resolve, often quite soon. Pneumothorax or hemopneumothorax should be treated with a closed thoracostomy tube placed while the child is still in the emergency department. If an air leak persists from the chest tube and the lung fails to reexpand, a bronchial disruption should be suspected. This is an indication for prompt bronchoscopy.

Rupture of the diaphragm may result from significant blunt abdominal injury, causing herniation of abdominal contents into the chest. A ruptured diaphragm due to blunt trauma occurs most commonly on the left side. However, diaphragmatic injuries also occur with penetrating trauma; these are more evenly distributed to both sides. This diagnosis is easily overlooked because of delayed onset of symptoms. Symptoms include chest pain and shortness of breath, but may also include evidence of intestinal obstruction, if bowel is involved in the herniation. Examination may demonstrate diminished breath sounds in the affected chest, bowel sounds in the chest, and an unusually scaphoid abdomen. A plain chest radiograph often makes the diagnosis, but the presence of a nasogastric tube terminating in an intrathoracic stomach provides conclusive evidence. Immediate surgical repair is undertaken for this injury, but not before the patient has been completely evaluated, since such an injury is often not an isolated finding of trauma. Sudden herniation of abdominal contents into the thorax may cause respiratory embarrassment. The acute diaphragmatic rupture is generally repaired from the abdomen, since associated abdominal injuries are present in a high percentage of cases.

Vascular Injuries

Vascular injuries in children are usually associated with extremity trauma, and should be approached as for similar injuries in the adult. Angiography is useful in delineating the injury when time and the urgency of the situation allow for it. With smaller patients, it may be necessary to use microvascular instruments and the operating microscope for successful repair.

NONTRAUMATIC EMERGENCIES OF INFANTS AND CHILDREN

Airway and Respiratory Emergencies

The newborn presenting with respiratory distress at the time of birth or shortly thereafter most commonly suffers from prematurity, pneumonia, gen-

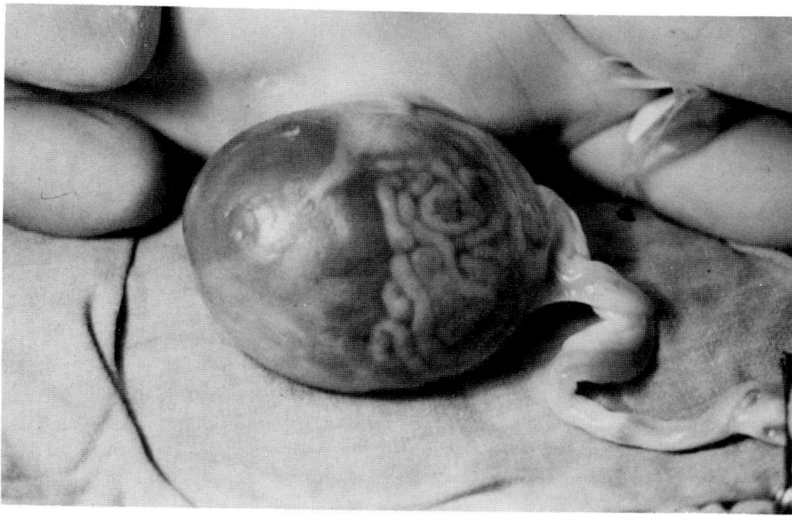

Figure 30.3. Large omphalocele with intact sac. Note umbilical cord arising from sac and not from abdominal wall. The large sacs often contain liver as well as small and large intestine. (Reproduced by permission, from *Surgical Clinics of North America,* Vol. 56, No. 2, © 1976, W. B. Saunders Co.).

eralized sepsis, or amniotic fluid or meconium aspiration. The acute stabilization of infants with these conditions generally follows the guidelines presented in Chapter 22. Conditions requiring surgical intervention are far less common and include congenital anatomic variants, such as thyroglossal duct cyst, pharyngocele or laryngocele, congenital diaphragmatic hernia, or congenital lobar emphysema. Laryngoscopy with endotracheal intubation of these infants permits stabilization and transfer to a tertiary-care neonatal facility.

Infants and children who *develop* respiratory distress most often suffer from an acquired phenomenon. Croup, epiglottitis, and bronchiolitis are discussed in Chapter 25. Aspiration of foreign bodies is common in small children, especially in their oral phase of development. Peanuts, toys (such as beads), and coins are commonly aspirated objects. Physical examination may demonstrate diminished breath sounds or wheezing. A plain chest x-ray demonstrates the object only if it is radiopaque; however, the only radiographic sign of aspiration may be hyperaeration on the affected side (Fig. 30.2). Bronchoscopic extraction of the object under general anesthesia is usually necessary. Swallowed objects that become impacted in the proximal esophagus may also cause respiratory embarrassment by compression of the trachea. Esophagoscopy is often necessary to extract the object. Extraction of a proximal esophageal foreign body can sometimes be performed using a balloon-tip catheter under fluoroscopic guidance. This should be attempted only by experienced personnel with all the equipment on hand necessary for immediate endotracheal intubation, should aspiration occur.

Congenital Anomalies (Other than Respiratory)

Certain other congenital anomalies may require some emergency management at the time of birth prior to transfer to a tertiary neonatal facility with surgical expertise. For example, *omphalocele* and *gastroschisis* should be treated by placing the baby on its side and wrapping the exposed parts in a clean plastic wrap (Fig 30.3). Nasogastric suction should be instituted, intravenous access obtained, and every effort made to keep the child warm because of the excessive evaporative heat loss from the exposed parts. Similar care should be taken with *myeloceles* and large *sacrococcygeal teratomas,* although these usually do not require nasogastric suction. For the child born with *bladder extrophy,* the exposed bladder should be covered with a sterile lubricating dressing as soon as possible. All of the above situations require prompt patient transfer to the care of a pediatric surgeon, who will most likely proceed to operative treatment as soon as possible.

Ingestion of Caustic Agents

The exploring hands of the child may often lead him into contact with potentially dangerous substances, such as household cleaners or other lye-containing agents. Because of foul taste, inadvertent ingestion of these substances is small. The child presents with redness and burns about the mouth and pharynx. These patients need immediate hospitalization for treatment. Even a strong history without any oropharyngeal signs of ingestion should prompt hospital admission and further evaluation. The patient is given nothing by mouth, and intravenous fluids are begun. Vomiting should *not* be induced. Early administration of corticosteroids and intravenous antibiotics may be of some benefit. Fiberoptic esophagoscopy is indicated within the first 24 hours to evaluate the extent of the burn injury to the esophagus. If a true burn is seen, steroids and antibiotics should be continued for 10–14 days, at the end of which time a gastrografin swallow is obtained. The majority of these injuries can be managed in such a fashion, without major surgery. If no injury is seen on early esophagoscopy, the patient is discharged. Late strictures from lye burns sometimes require dilatations. Prior to discharge, care must be taken to ensure that the accident was not due to child abuse or neglect.

Abdominal Pain

Abdominal pain is the most common complaint that the surgeon is asked to evaluate in the pediatric emergency patient. Only a small percentage of these patients ultimately need surgery since most will be diagnosed as having gastroenteritis or some other nonsurgical etiology for the pain. However, some of the causes of abdominal pain in children carry devastating consequences if overlooked, such as midgut volvulus. Therefore, it is strongly recommended that any pediatric patient with abdominal pain without obvious etiology be evaluated by a surgeon, if discharge from the emergency department is being considered.

In the child under the age of 1 year, the most common abdominal complaint requiring surgery is intussusception. Over the age of 1 year, appendicitis becomes the leading condition requiring surgery. The emergency department physician needs an accurate history of the onset and nature of the pain, whether constant or cyclic. Associated symptoms are questioned, including vomiting, drawing up of legs, diarrhea, fever, or blood per rectum. Often the parent has noted a mass or bulge in the abdomen or groin. Physical examination of a child with abdominal pain must be approached carefully to obtain the most information. Simple observation of the child prior to beginning palpation often yields important information. Potentially painful or fear-inducing maneuvers should be delayed to the end of the examination. Distracting the patient during the examination is helpful in demonstrating truly tender areas. The very uncooperative child may be given secobarbital to lend good sedation without masking tenderness. Useful ancillary study includes complete blood count, urinalysis and plain abdominal radiographs. A chest radiograph may also be of help, since pneumonia may present with a picture exactly mimicking the acute abdomen. A serum amylase determination is helpful in excluding pancreatitis.

Appendicitis

Appendicitis is the single pathologic entity requiring operation most frequently in children; it is also the most commonly misdiagnosed disease. The incidence of a "white appendix" (no pathologic change) at laparotomy approaches 20%. Near-mortality from missed appendicitis is still encountered. The combination of serious consequences (40% complications) from a missed diagnosis and lack of conclusive diagnostic tests justify the rather high rate of errors in preoperative diagnosis. Every child in the emergency department with abdominal pain should have appendicitis considered in the differential diagnosis.

Pain, vomiting, and fever constitute the symptom triad of appendicitis. The pain is usually periumbilical at onset and gradually moves to the right lower quadrant as local peritoneal irritation progresses. Vomiting, when it occurs, usually begins after the onset of pain. However, one or all of the symptom triad may be absent in a given patient; one must remember that small children often cannot give a good history of the onset of symptoms. The time from onset of symptoms to perforation is usually in the range of 24–36 hours, but accurate establishment of the time of onset can be difficult. As many as 70% of patients under the age of 2 already have perforation at the time of arrival in the emergency department. Examination of these patients may reveal signs of septic shock, such as altered mental status and hypotension, with abdominal findings being more subtle. Right lower quadrant tenderness, often with guarding or rebound tenderness, may frequently be demonstrated, but an inflamed retrocecal appendix may cause minimal peritoneal irritation. Shake or cough tenderness is often a helpful finding; a child who is willing to jump up and down on one foot is unlikely to have appendicitis. Rectal examination may demonstrate a mass or pelvic tenderness on the right.

The laboratory examination of the child with suspected appendicitis may be confusing. The white blood count and erythrocyte sedimentation rate typically are not elevated early in the disease. However, the differential smear may show an early shift of leukocytes to the left. Urinalysis is useful in excluding urinary tract infection as a cause of pain. If protracted vomiting has been part of the disease process, it is important to check the serum electrolytes as a guide to rehydration prior to operation. The plain abdominal radiograph may demonstrate lumbar scoliosis, localized ileus, a fecalith (in 10–

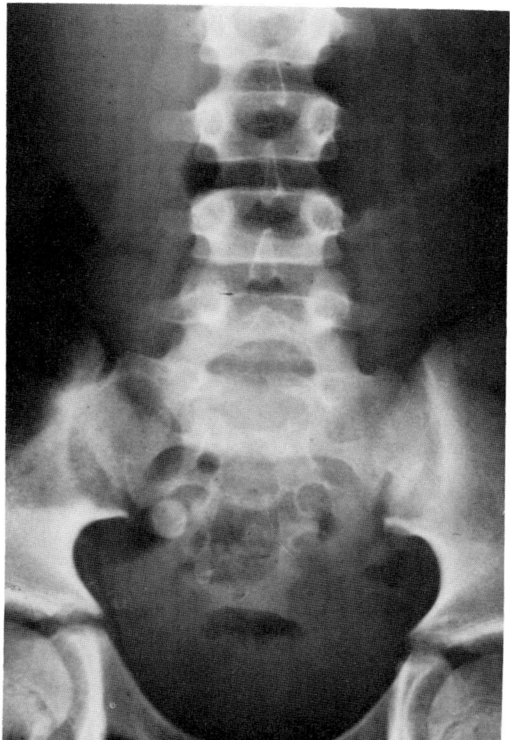

Figure 30.4. Appendicolith in child with acute appendicitis. Note the radiopaque density in right lower quadrant.

20% of appendicitis cases), or even a picture of small bowel obstruction (see Fig. 30.4). A barium enema has been thought to be of help in excluding the diagnosis if the lumen of the appendix fills, but this does not exclude inflammation in the distal portion of the appendix. This examination is not recommended (see Chapter 47).

In summary, appendicitis may be the most difficult of all diseases to diagnose accurately. Any child suspected of having this diagnosis must be seen early by a surgeon. Furthermore, if the diagnosis cannot be excluded, even if the bulk of evidence does not support it, the child should be hospitalized for serial examinations. If appendicitis is the true cause of the patient's complaint, 24 hours of observation usually reveals this fact.

Intussusception

The patient with intussusception is usually between the ages of 6 and 18 months, most often less than 1 year. The pain is crampy, the child showing periods of extreme unrest and inconsolability, frequently with drawing up of the legs, alternating with periods of relative calm. Vomiting is due to distension of bowel rather than obstruction, and it often starts early in the very young patient. These alternating periods of crampy pain may be followed by passage of loose bloody bowel movement, often described as "currant jelly" stools. This is what usually prompts the parent to bring the child to the emergency department. By this time, the patient may be listless. The examining physician may elicit a history of similar previous episodes without blood, which abated spontaneously.

On examination, the child appears lethargic and apathetic, curling up in a fetal position, except during periods of peristaltic activity when he/she is screaming and restless. The child may even be cool, clammy, and showing signs of shock. During the calm period, the abdomen is flat and soft, but often a mass—the intussusceptum—is palpable in the right upper quadrant or the epigastrium. Rectal examination sometimes demonstrates the mass. The stool is usually guaiac-positive. Fever is common; it is almost universal *after* reduction of the intussusception.

The diagnostic procedure of choice is the barium enema, because it is also therapeutic in many instances (Fig 30.5). Plain and upright radiographs of the abdomen should be obtained prior to instilling

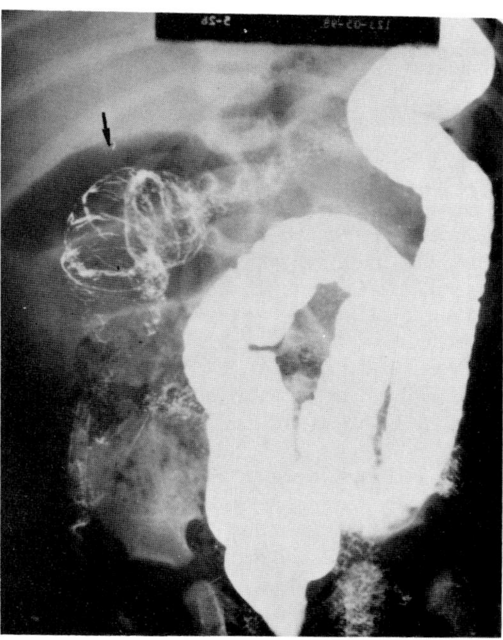

Figure 30.5. Intussusception. Barium enema reduction should be carried out if there are no signs of peritoneal inflammation. Note "coiled spring" appearance of the intussusception (*arrow*). (Reproduced by permission, from *Surgical Clinics of North America,* Vol. 54, No. 3, © 1974, W. B. Saunders Co.).

the contrast medium in order to exclude prior perforation. In most instances of uncomplicated intussusception, barium hydrostatic reduction is attempted as the initial treatment of choice. Success results in well over 50% of cases. This should be done only with a surgeon present or close at hand, prepared to proceed directly to the operating room, if necessary. The patient should have a reliable intravenous line in place prior to the start of the procedure. If this technique fails, the patient is taken to the operating room for manual reduction of the intussusceptum (see Chapter 47 on pediatric radiology for additional illustrations).

Pancreatitis

Midepigastric and midback pain, often accompanied by vomiting, are the common complaints associated with pancreatitis. This disease runs the spectrum from a mild course to a fulminant, even fatal episode. It is often recurring and relapsing, depending on its etiology. Causes include trauma and ingestion of alcohol, just as in adults, but pancreatitis in children may also be due to congenital abnormalities, such as an annular pancreas, atretic pancreatic ducts or pancreaticoduodenal duplication. These causes are rare. Just as in adults, pancreatitis in children is frequently idiopathic. Management is similar to that described for traumatic pancreatitis, including bowel rest and hyperalimentation.

Hernias

The most frequent operation performed by pediatric surgeons is inguinal herniorrhaphy. Most of these are performed under elective circumstances; however, a groin bulge is a frequent complaint with which the emergency department physician must contend. Most *inguinal hernias* present in young children, predominantly in males. Right hernias are more frequent than left; girls have a higher incidence of bilateral hernias, especially in the older age groups. There is a high incidence of inguinal hernia in the premature infant because the processus vaginalis obliterates late in gestation. There may also be a family history of hernia.

Frequently, the parent notices a groin bulge while bathing the child, and often notes that the bulge is reducible. Or, the child becomes irritable, refusing to feed or even vomiting, and the parent notes a hard groin mass and seeks medical attention. On examination, the hernia is a smooth mass lateral to the pubic tubercle emerging through the external inguinal ring, and separate from the testicle (Fig 30.6). The mass does not transilluminate. It is important to discern the position of the testicle, so as not to confuse a hernia with a hydrocele or a cryptorchid testis. If a hernia is diagnosed, a reasonable attempt is made to reduce it. This can be done with safety, although it often requires an experienced hand. The majority of incarcerated hernias occur in children under the age of 1 year, and frequently, these can be reduced. Early, but not immediate, repair is advised for reducible hernias since the risk of reincarceration is high. The *irreducible* hernia requires prompt surgical attention. These operations can be very difficult due to edema surrounding the delicate structures in the inguinal canal. Direct inguinal and femoral hernias are quite rare in children.

Umbilical hernias are common and usually do not require treatment unless incarcerated. There is a high family incidence, and in the United States, the incidence seems to be higher among black children. The majority of umbilical hernia defects close spontaneously, most by the 3rd or 4th years; small hernias close more rapidly than do large ones. However, many umbilical hernias discovered as late as 4 years of age close spontaneously by puberty. The indications for surgical intervention in umbilical hernia are pain, incarceration, ulceration, or perforation.

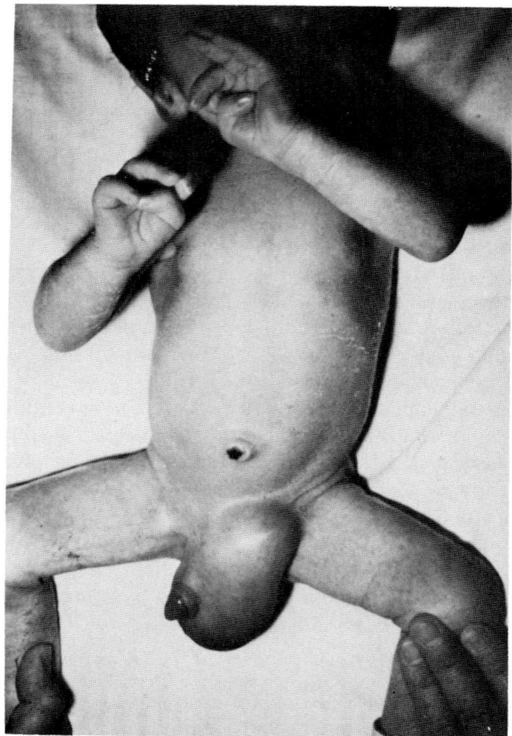

Figure 30.6. Incarcerated left inguinal hernia. Note swelling in groin as well as in scrotum. Manual reduction can usually be carried out with sedation, elevation, ice packs, and gentle compression.

Torsion of the Testis

Acute scrotal pain and swelling raise a red flag to the emergency physician that a serious condition is present. In addition to the incarcerated hernia, the major concern in this circumstance is testicular torsion. Twisting of the testis leads to occlusion of its blood supply and subsequent infarction, if not relieved. Therefore, this presentation constitutes a true surgical emergency. There is a high incidence of torsion in the newborn and in the child with a cryptorchid testis, due to the relative lack of fixation of the testis in these two situations. However, the highest incidence of testicular torsion occurs at puberty, with its peak incidence at age 14 years. Testicular torsion can actually occur at any age.

The pain is usually gradual in onset, often first noted in the morning. There may be an antecedent episode of trauma, although this is not presumed to play an etiologic role. There may also be a history of similar episodes, thought to have resolved by spontaneous detorsion. The pain gradually increases, becoming accompanied by scrotal swelling, redness, and edema. Nausea and vomiting may ensue. Physical examination reveals a swollen, erythematous hemiscrotum that is exquisitely tender. A tender, warm mass in the groin with an empty hemiscrotum should suggest torsion of a cryptorchid testis.

Torsion of the *appendix testis* may presents in similar fashion, but tends to be much less dramatic. There may simply be a tender area on the testis as opposed to involvement of the entire organ.

Management of torsion of the testis mandates a low threshold for consideration of operative exploration of the scrotum. If this diagnosis is strongly suspected, one should proceed directly to the operating room for detorsion of the testis *and* bilateral orchidopexy. If the diagnosis is in doubt, a radionuclide testicular blood flow scan or Doppler assessment of blood flow in the testis may be obtained. If detorsion is performed within 8–10 hours from onset of symptoms, the testis can be saved. It should be emphasized that a patient who has any question of torsion of the testis should at least have a testicular scan to assess blood flow prior to discharge from the emergency department.

Intestinal Obstruction

The hallmark symptom of intestinal obstruction is vomiting. In children, there are many causes of intestinal obstruction, some of which will be discussed in the following pages. In general, the history and physical examination yield clues to the etiology of the obstruction. The age, onset of the vomiting, and nature of the vomitus are important details. Associated symptoms, such as fever, pain, and bowel habits, also help the clinician to chart a clinical course that may be diagnostic. On examination, a mass may be felt, frequent high-pitched bowel sounds heard, or guaiac-positive stools discovered. A helpful test is the plain and upright radiograph of the abdomen, which not only demonstrates obstruction, but may indicate the level of the blockage (Fig 30.7).

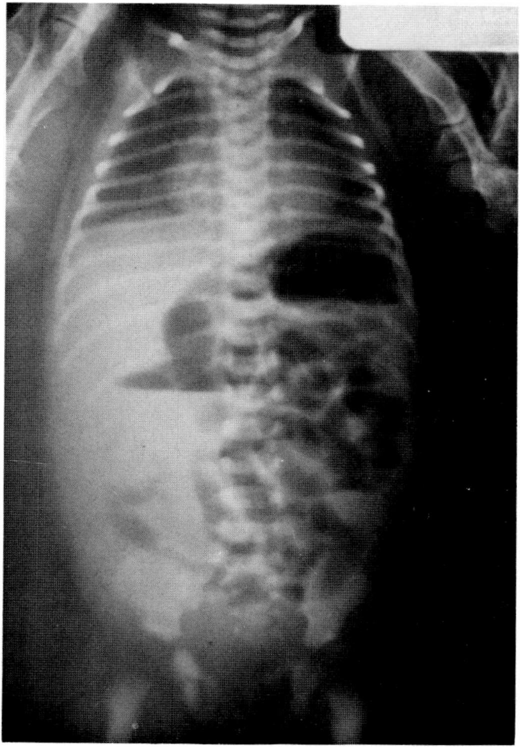

Figure 30.7. Low intestinal obstruction. Small intestine cannot be differentiated from colon on plain film in newborn. Barium enema study should be done if peritonitis is not present.

Whenever obstruction at any level is documented, an essential feature of management is the placement of a decompressing nasogastric tube. Even today, one of the major complications of intestinal obstruction in children is aspiration of vomitus, leading to aspiration pneumonitis. Often this is more life-threatening than the obstruction itself.

Hypertrophic Pyloric Stenosis

Hypertrophy of the pyloric muscle with gastric outlet obstruction leads to vomiting in infants with this problem. The usual age of onset is approximately 3 weeks, although this is variable. The child is often a first-born son, and there may be a family history of pyloric stenosis. The vomitus is described as projectile and does not contain bile. Between

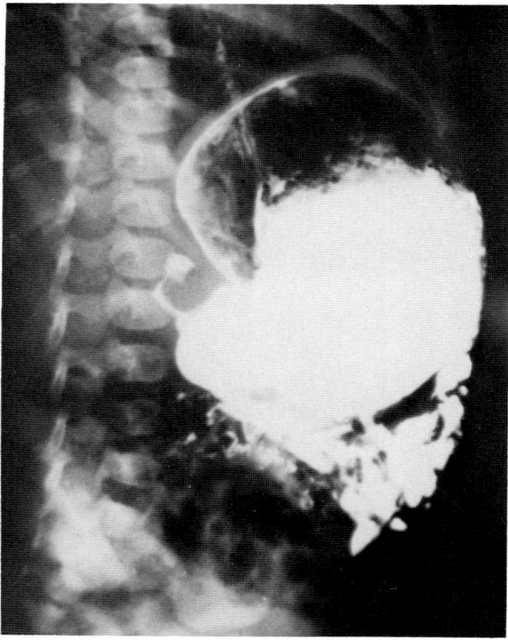

Figure 30.8. Pyloric stenosis. Delayed passage of barium through narrowed pylorus is associated with large stomach.

vomiting episodes, the child is usually calm. The male-female ratio of incidence is 4:1.

Physical examination demonstrates a right upper quadrant mass, the so-called "olive" of the pyloric tumor. However, it may be necessary to empty the stomach with a nasogastric tube in order to feel this. Useful diagnostic tests include ultrasonography, again to demonstrate the pyloric "olive," and upper gastrointestinal series, which demonstrates gastric outlet obstruction. There is a characteristic radiographic profile to the proximal pylorus (Fig 30.8).

Management of these children includes nasogastric suction and intravenous fluid replacement. Protracted vomiting creates a hypokalemic, hypochloremic metabolic alkalosis that should be corrected prior to surgery. At operation, a pyloromyotomy is performed, usually without sequelae. Hospitalization is necessary for only a few days.

Malrotation of the Intestine and Midgut Volvulus

The principal symptom of midgut volvulus is bilious vomiting. It has been said that the sun should never be allowed to set upon a patient with bilious vomiting without establishing a firm diagnosis. Midgut volvulus is due to malrotation of the intestine with malfixation or nonfixation of the mesentary. This allows the entire small intestine to rotate around the axis of the superior mesenteric artery, resulting in occlusion of the artery and subsequent infarction of the entire intestine from the ligament of Treitz to the midtransverse colon. Incomplete rotation of the intestine occurs during fetal development, with varying degrees of malrotation. The complications of anatomic variations associated with malrotation all lead to intestinal obstruction; they include midgut volvulus, duodenal obstruction due to Ladd's bands, and internal hernias.

The onset of the bilious vomiting is sudden. Severe, often colicky, abdominal pain may be present. An abdominal mass or distention may be noted. In addition, guaiac-positive stools or even gross rectal blood may be present. The patient may develop a rigid abdomen, pallor, and shock. This is truly one of the most serious surgical emergencies of children. It can occur at any age.

Plain and upright radiographs of the abdomen may show proximal small bowel obstruction or even a gasless abdomen. In an unstable patient, this should be sufficient evidence to warrant abdominal exploration. In the stable patient, one may be more thorough in the preoperative evaluation, but it must be emphasized that a casual approach is appropriate only if midgut volvulus is included in the differential diagnosis. The plain radiograph may demonstrate absent colonic gas on the right, or the classic "double-bubble" sign if duodenal obstruction is present (Fig 30.9). Barium contrast studies are helpful. The barium enema may show the abnormally fixed colon with the cecum usually in the upper abdomen. The most helpful test is the upper gastrointestinal series which shows the abnormally placed ligament of Treitz or the duodenal obstruction from Ladd's bands.

Operative repair using Ladd's technique is the treatment of choice. Every effort is made to proceed promptly with surgery for the child with midgut volvulus, since time may be essential in the viability of the intestine. The volvulus is reduced by counterclockwise rotation of the intestine, lysis of Ladd's bands across the duodenum, and placement of the entire colon on the left side of the abdomen, with the small intestine on the right. In the unfortunate circumstance of bowel infarction, extensive portions of the small intestine may require removal, with the potential consequence of the so-called short gut syndrome, with its serious nutritional problems.

Small Intestinal Atresia

Small bowel obstruction due to small bowel atresia, either duodenal or jejunoileal, usually occurs in the neonatal period. The plain abdominal radiograph may suggest the level of obstruction, and barium contrast studies may delineate the anatomy of the atresia and even the presence of a microcolon. These entities are usually often readily apparent in the nursery, and the patients are stable enough to permit transfer to a tertiary-care neonatal facility

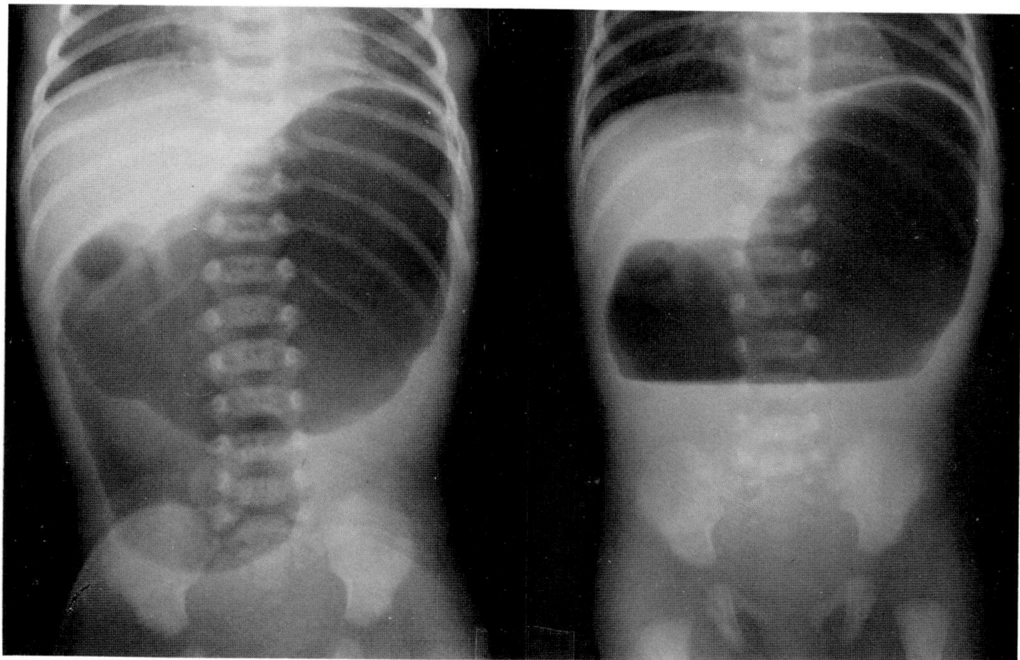

Figure 30.9. Duodenal atresia. The smaller second bubble on right side of abdomen represents dilated proximal duodenum. *Left,* kidney-ureter-bladder (KUB) film. *Right,* upright abdominal film.

for definitive therapy. The differential diagnosis includes meconium ileus and Hirschsprung's disease.

Hirschsprung's Disease

Every year, approximately 700 children are born in the United States with colonic aganglionosis, or Hirschsprung's disease. The onset of symptoms is usually in the nursery with the delayed passage of meconium, but often these children can go a long period of time without recognition. A variety of clinical presentations exist, ranging from complete obstruction in the nursery, constipation followed by obstruction at a later age, acute colitis with diarrhea, fever and distention, or simply mild constipation.

Physical examination often demonstrates abdominal distention with mild tenderness; the rectum is tight and without stool. Abdominal plain films suggest obstruction. A barium enema is diagnostic by demonstrating dilated proximal colon with a characteristic transitional zone to normal distal colon (Fig 30.10). The transitional zone is often in the sigmoid colon, and is the area where the bowel changes from normal intramural innervation proximally to the area lacking ganglion cells distally. The definitive diagnosis is made by rectal biopsy. Rectal manometric studies may be helpful.

Treatment for this entity includes supportive therapy in the acute process with intravenous fluids and antibiotics, if colitis is present. Most commonly, a proximal diverting colostomy is performed until the child is large enough to undergo a definitive anorectal pull-through procedure, usually at about 1 year of age.

Meckel's Diverticulum

Approximately 2% of the population has a Meckel's diverticulum, a remnant of the omphalomesenteric duct; the majority of them are asymptomatic. Although figures vary, it is believed that approximately 5% of people with a Meckel's diverticulum will have symptoms, and of this group 45% will develop their symptoms before the age of 2 years. The most common complications of the Meckel's diverticulum are gastrointestinal bleeding, intestinal obstruction, and diverticulitis. Hemorrhage and obstruction are more common in younger children, while diverticulitis is more common in older children.

Bleeding from a Meckel's diverticulum is episodic and painless, most often occurring in children under the age of 5 years. It is due to peptic ulceration of the base of the diverticulum from acid produced by ectopic gastric mucosa within the diverticulum. The bleeding ranges from minimal blood per rectum to massive, life-threatening lower hemorrhage. A helpful study in demonstrating the

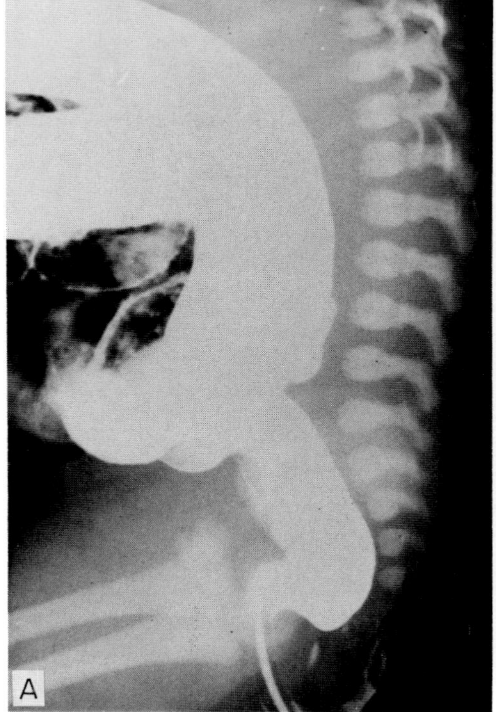

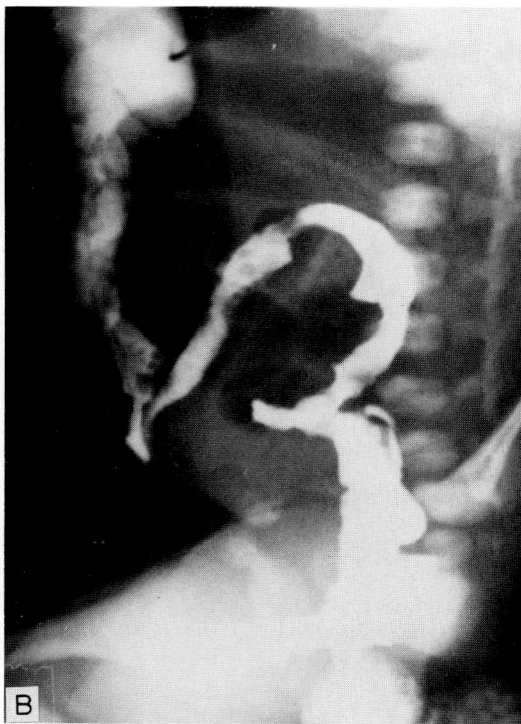

Figure 30.10. Hirschsprung's disease in newborn. *A,* Normal-appearing barium enema. *B,* Careful barium enema with only small amount of barium under fluoroscopy by experienced radiologist demonstrates clearly the abnormal, narrow, scalloped, aganglionic segment in same patient. (Reproduced by permission, from *Surgical Clinics of North America,* Vol. 54, No. 3, © 1974, W. B. Saunders Co.).

presence of a Meckel's diverticulum is a ''Meckel's scan,'' in which ^{99}Tc pertechnitate is given intravenously. This agent binds to parietal cells of gastric mucosa, identifying the diverticulum on scintiscan of the abdomen if the diverticulum contains gastric mucosa. False-positive and false-negative scans are encountered.

Intestinal obstruction due to a Meckel's diverticulum occurs from intussusception of the small bowel with the diverticulum as the leading point, or from an adhesive band to the diverticulum, creating an internal hernia with possible entrapment of the small bowel.

Meckel's diverticulitis produces a spectrum of symptoms indistinguishable because of its location from acute appendicitis. The onset of pain is usually periumbilical, and the progression of pain and tenderness may be to any location in the lower abdomen, depending on where the affected loop of small bowel lies. When exploring a patient for appendicitis, if a normal appendix is found, the terminal ileum should be examined for a distance of 3–4 feet to look for a Meckel's diverticulum.

The treatment for the symptomatic Meckel's diverticulum is excision. This can often be performed without excising the adjacent small bowel.

SUGGESTED READINGS

Barkin RM, ed. *Emergency Pediatrics.* St Louis: CV Mosby, 1984.

Fleisher G, Ludwig S, eds. *Textbook of Pediatric Trauma.* Baltimore: Williams & Wilkins, 1983.

Hendren WH, Kim SH. Trauma of the spleen and liver in children. *Pediatr Clin North Am,* 1975;22:349–364.

Holder TM, Ashcraft KW, eds: *Pediatric Surgery.* Philadelphia: WB Saunders, 1980.

Holschneider AM, ed: *Hirschsprung's Disease.* New York, Thieme-Stratton, 1982.

Mayer TA, ed. *Emergency Management of Pediatric Trauma.* Philadelphia: WB Saunders, 1984.

Raffensperger JG, ed: *Swenson's Pediatric Surgery,* ed 4. New York, Appleton-Century-Crofts, 1980.

Rickham PP, Johnston JH: *Neonatal Surgery,* ed 2. New York: Butterworths, 1978.

Ryckman FC, Noseworth J. Multisystem trauma. *Surg Clin North Am,* 1985;65:1287–1302.

Stevenson RJ, Abdominal pain unrelated to trauma. *Surg Clin North Am,* 1985;65:1181–1215.

Stevenson RJ, Non-neonatal intestinal obstruction in children. *Surg Clin North Am,* 1985;65:1217–1234.

Touloukian RJ. *Pediatric Trauma.* New York: John Wiley & Sons, 1978.

Welch KJ, Randolph JG, Ravitch MM, et al, eds. *Pediatric Surgery,* ed 4. Chicago: Year Book, 1986.

SECTION 4

Surgery

ASHBY C. MONCURE, M.D.
Associate Editor

CHAPTER 31

Cardiovascular Surgical Emergencies

ALAN D. HILGENBERG, M.D.
ASHBY C. MONCURE, M.D

TRAUMA TO THE HEART AND GREAT VESSELS

General Considerations

Motor vehicle accidents are responsible for most of the *blunt injuries* to the heart and great vessels; its victims include drivers, passengers, pedestrians, and motorcyclists. These patients often have multiple severe injuries to the head, abdominal viscera, and long bones in addition to the chest. *Penetrating thoracic wounds* are now more often caused by handguns than by knives; the result is greater visceral damage because of the larger mass and higher velocity of the bullet. Multiple wounds with injuries to organs both within and outside of the chest are increasingly common.

The general principles of emergency care of the seriously injured are followed in all cases of suspected cardiovascular trauma. The airway is evaluated and secured by intubation if necessary. Oxygen is administered, and ventilation provided as required. Vital signs are measured, and good intravenous access routes established and crystalloid infusion begun. A rapid physical examination identifies immediately life-threatening situations such as tension pneumothorax. Chest tubes are inserted without hesitation if breath sounds are diminished or absent on one or both sides of the chest, or if a penetrating wound is identified. External bleeding is controlled and fractures are splinted. Blood samples are sent, and radiographic studies and an electrocardiogram are obtained. If hemodynamic instability is present, a central venous pressure monitoring line is inserted. Careful neurologic, abdominal, and orthopaedic evaluation should proceed at the same time as the cardiovascular studies, and then a plan of treatment priorities formulated for all of the various conditions encountered. Proper attention must be paid to the entire patient, and coordination of the activities of the various surgical specialists involved in treating the patient is also essential.

Under these conditions, one physician must take charge and, as ''captain of the ship,'' coordinate all studies, interventions, and decisions.

Blunt Trauma to the Heart and Great Vessels

Cardiac Contusion

To the pathologist or laboratory investigator, cardiac contusion is an easily identified and clearly defined entity, but this is not the case for the clinician evaluating the injured patient. Experimental contusions are reliably produced by blows to the precordial chest wall, the contused myocardium is visible anatomically, and microscopically, there is intramyocardial hemorrhage, disruption of myocardial fibers, and patency of the coronary arteries. In medical practice, the incidence and clinical significance of myocardial contusion is a cloudy issue, since the diagnosis is not easily made, the findings are typically transient, the condition is usually well-tolerated by the patient, and preexisting cardiac disease may confuse the picture. The important issue facing the clinician is the decision of which trauma patients are at risk of low cardiac output as a result of the injury, and which patients are at risk of developing serious arrhythmias.

Cardiac contusions usually result from the trauma of an automobile accident, although any situation involving a blow to the chest can be the cause. The mechanisms of injury are thought to include compression of the heart between the sternum and the spine by a direct blow to the anterior aspect of the chest, and sudden deceleration of the chest, thrusting the myocardium against the anterior chest wall. The decelerative forces are directly proportional to the square of the speed of the vehicle, and inversely related to its stopping distance. This injury has been noted in automobile collision speeds of as little as 20 miles per hour.

Most patients with cardiac contusions do not have symptoms or physical findings that can be directly attributed to the cardiac injury. The complaint of chest pain and the finding of tachycardia are common, but they are totally nonspecific abnormalities. Precordial chest wall injuries arouse suspicion of this entity, but as many as one-third of the patients with a contused heart lack an obvious external chest wall injury.

Various clinical laboratory studies have been used to evaluate trauma patients in an attempt to diagnose cardiac contusion. Electrocardiograms, measurement of serum levels of CK-MB isoenzyme, echocardiograms, and invasive cardiac monitoring have all been evaluated as potential diagnostic tools. The electrocardiogram (ECG) is not specific in the diagnosis of cardiac contusion, but it is readily available in the emergency department. In fact, the ECG abnormalities most commonly lead the clinician to suspect the diagnosis. ECG changes have been described in 70–85% of patients with contusions; they include ST segment and T wave abnormalities, conduction disturbances, and arrhythmias. Nonspecific ST segment and T wave changes and sinus tachycardia account for approximately 75% of the abnormalities. Between 10–20% of the abnormal findings are intraventricular conduction disturbances, with right bundle branch block the most frequent; left bundle branch block or unifascicular block may also be noted. Partial or complete atrioventricular conduction block has been noted in about 3% of these patients. These findings have been described on initial evaluation and during the first 3 days after injury, and virtually all of them have been transient.

Arrhythmias frequently accompany clinical chest injuries and cardiac contusions in the experimental animal. When carefully followed with Holter monitoring, 73% of a series of chest trauma victims exhibited some rhythm disturbance. Premature ventricular contractions comprised the majority, and atrial fibrillation and other supraventricular arrhythmias were occasionally noted. Ventricular tachycardia and ventricular fibrillation are rarely observed in hospitalized trauma patients with cardiac contusion, but they commonly occur in the first moments following experimental contusions in animals.

Elevation of CK-MB isoenzymes may be observed during the first 48 hours after chest injuries, but as yet there is no convincing evidence to indicate that this finding discriminates the patient with myocardial contusion from other trauma victims. Although there was initial enthusiasm for technetium pyrophosphate scanning, subsequent studies have shown these scans positive in only a small percentage of patients with cardiac contusions.

Two-dimensional echocardiography appears to be a promising method of evaluating patients with suspected cardiac contusion. The findings include segmental ventricular wall motion abnormalities, mural thrombi, and dilatation of one or both ventricles. Harley and colleagues have studied radionuclide angiography in the assessment of myocardial function after blunt chest injury, and have noted abnormalities in 74% of their patients, compared with abnormal electrocardiograms in only 28% and elevated CK-MB in 12%. The abnormalities on radionuclide angiograms included depressed right ventricular ejection fraction, depressed left ventricular ejection fraction, and segmental ventricular wall motion abnormalities. A small group of patients were reevaluated 3 weeks after the injury; the abnormalities had disappeared in two-thirds.

Insertion of *pulmonary artery catheters* for direct measurement of the cardiac index can identify patients with severe functional abnormalities due to myocardial injury. The degree of ventricular dysfunction appears useful in determining the severity of the injury and in identifying patients at high risk.

For the mild forms of cardiac contusion, treatment includes bed rest, pain relief, and monitoring the cardiac rhythm for several days after the injury. The outcome is favorable in most of the patients. If a cardiac contusion is suspected in the presence of multiple severe injuries, invasive monitoring of arterial, central venous, and pulmonary wedge pressures and cardiac outputs are useful. Inotropic drugs may be required. General anesthesia must be designed to minimize myocardial depression, and surgery should be limited to repair of only the most urgent conditions until the cardiac injury has stabilized.

The prognosis for myocardial contusion appears to be directly related to the amount of ventricular dysfunction and to the severity of the associated extracardiac injuries. If invasive monitoring identifies dysfunction of either ventricle, or if the cardiac index is less than 2.9 liters/min/m^2, the risk of morbidity and mortality appears to be increased.

Traumatic Coronary Artery Occlusion

Blunt trauma can be the cause of acute occlusion of major coronary arteries with resulting myocardial infarction. Reports of such injuries are rare, but they may have been overlooked and included in the broad spectrum of cardiac contusion. The sequence of pathologic changes in this injury includes disruption of the coronary artery intima, subintimal hemorrhage, and obstructive intraluminal thrombus formation adjacent to the injured arterial wall. Automobile accidents are the most frequent cause of this injury, with assaults, sporting activities, and industrial accidents accounting for the rest. The left anterior descending coronary artery was injured in 66% of reported cases, the right coronary artery in 25%, and the circumflex artery or its branches in 8%. One patient with presumed traumatic thrombosis of a saphenous vein aortocoronary bypass graft has been described.

Electrocardiographic evidence of myocardial infarction immediately following blunt chest trauma is the clinical feature that clearly characterizes this group of patients and that separates them easily from the cardiac contusion group. Most of these patients have chest wall contusions or fractures; additional noncardiac injuries may be present. Postinfarction complications, including complete heart block, serious ventricular arrhythmias, severe left ventricular failure, ventricular aneurysm, ventricular septal defect, and pulmonary emboli, have all been described.

When this diagnosis is suspected on the basis of clinical and electrocardiographic findings, *coronary angiography* is indicated to confirm the diagnosis and to assess the extent of injury, once the patient has been stabilized. The typical angiographic finding is complete occlusion of the injured coronary artery near its origin, although subtotal obstruction has also been reported (Fig. 31.1). Left ventriculography is also indicated to identify wall motion abnormality resulting from the traumatic infarction.

The monitoring and treatment of these patients parallels that for infarction due to atherosclerotic disease. No direct approach to the acutely traumatized artery has thus far been described. Since the number of reported cases is small, the mortality rate for this injury is difficult to estimate, but it may approach 20%. Early and late deaths due to arrhythmias and pump failure have been reported. The outcome seems to depend upon the size of the infarction and the severity of the extracardiac injuries. Small areas of myocardial damage, well-developed collateral flow to the occluded vessel, and recanalization of the injured artery all appear to be favorable prognostic signs.

Intracardiac Defects

Intracardiac defects are rare but well-documented occurrences after blunt trauma to the chest. They include ventricular septal rupture, valvular damage, and ventricular aneurysm formation. A traumatic ventricular septal defect is caused by one of three distinct mechanisms: (*a*) the septum is ruptured directly by the forces of injury at the moment of im-

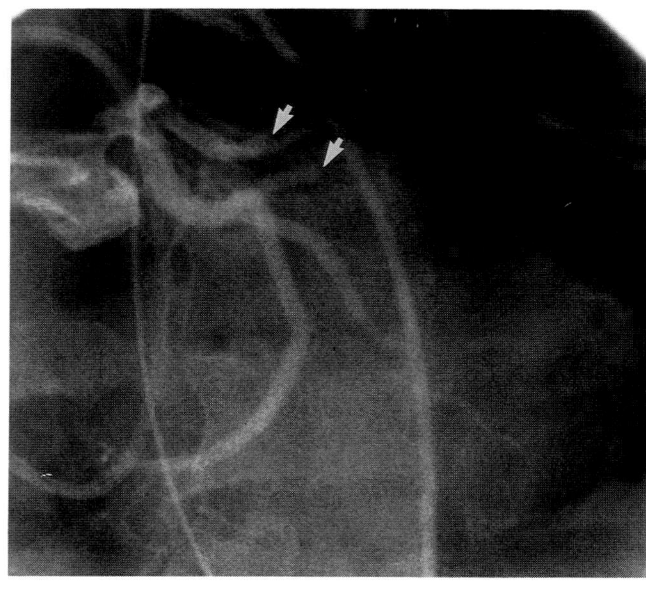

Figure 31.1. Left coronary arteriogram of a young man with blunt chest trauma from an automobile accident obtained several hours after injury. The arrows indicate the sites of occlusion of the left anterior descending and first circumflex marginal coronary arteries. He eventually expired, and autopsy revealed thrombosed traumatic pseudoaneurysms of both occluded coronary arteries and a very large myocardial infarction.

pact; (*b*) the septum is contused initially, and rupture is delayed until several hours or days after the accident; (*c*) the septum is infarcted initially as a result of traumatic coronary artery occlusion and ruptures several hours or days later. The clinical features vary, depending upon the size of the septal defect and the timing of septal rupture. When septal rupture occurs, most patients manifest acute congestive heart failure accompanied by a systolic thrill and murmur, due to the left-to-right shunt through the defect. The ECG is often abnormal but nonspecific. The chest radiograph usually shows cardiomegaly and increased pulmonary vascularity. The diagnosis is strongly suggested by two-dimensional echocardiography. At cardiac catheterization, the diagnosis is confirmed by a step-up in oxygen saturation in the right ventricle. Medical treatment of the congestive heart failure is instituted in all cases. Some patients with small shunts (less than 2:1) can be followed; an occasional defect may close spontaneously. In the symptomatic patients with larger shunts, surgical closure of the defect is required.

Valvular injuries are rare, especially in the absence of other lethal cardiac damage. The aortic valve is injured more often than the mitral and tricuspid valves. The mechanisms of injury include automobile accidents, falls from heights, and crushing chest injuries. The resulting pathophysiologic abnormality is insufficiency of the injured valve. Symptoms and findings vary, depending upon the severity of the valvular insufficiency. In some patients, abnormalities may be detected immediately after the accident, but in others, symptoms or a murmur may not appear for several weeks or months. Evaluation of patients suspected of traumatic valvular insufficiency includes two-dimensional echocardiography, Doppler examination, and cardiac catheterization. If the lesion is mild in severity, medical treatment and observation are appropriate; in cases with more severe valvular insufficiency, surgical repair or replacement of the valve is necessary, best attempted under elective circumstances.

A ventricular aneurysm does not appear until weeks or months after an injury that resulted in either a severe cardiac contusion or a traumatic coronary artery occlusion with extensive infarction. The patients may or may not be symptomatic; the ECG usually shows extensive ventricular damage; and the chest radiograph shows an abnormal cardiac contour. The diagnosis is confirmed by echocardiography and cardiac catheterization; elective surgical repair is usually advised.

Cardiac Rupture

Rupture of a cardiac chamber was noted in 64% of the cases in a large autopsy series of blunt cardiac injuries, making it a common pathologic finding. Right and left ventricular ruptures occurred with equal frequency; atrial ruptures were slightly less common than ventricular ruptures. Ninety-nine percent of the victims with ventricular ruptures died immediately, while 20% of those with atrial ruptures survived briefly. Right atrial involvement was somewhat more common than left. The pericardium was intact in most survivors. The mechanism of injury is usually a direct crushing force applied to the heart by compression between the sternum and

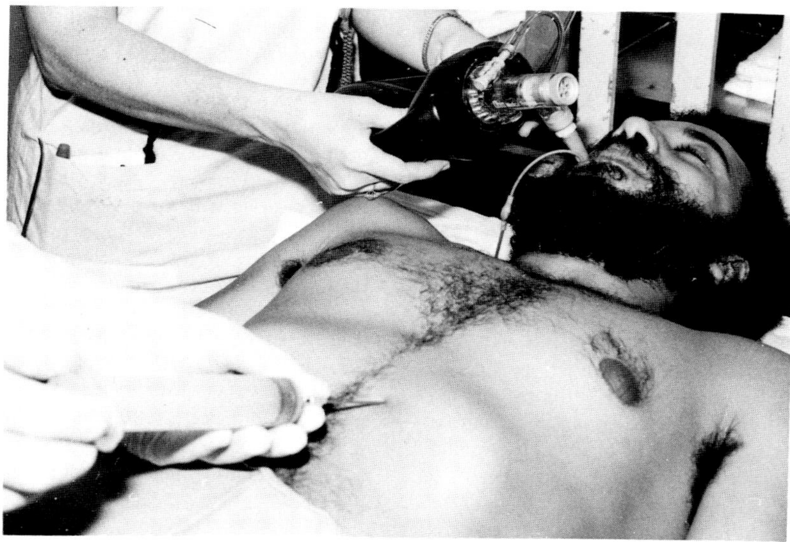

Figure 31.2. Pericardiocentesis via the subxiphoid route. A large Intracath needle is inserted just to the left of the xiphoid at a 30° angle from horizontal directed toward the left shoulder. Aspiration on the syringe is continuous. Electrocardiographic monitoring with a sterile alligator clip attached to the needle is ideal. Needle contact with the epicardium is indicated by marked ST segment elevation. If nonclotting blood is aspirated, the Intracath catheter is inserted through the needle and the needle withdrawn. Additional blood is then removed through the catheter with no danger of perforation of the heart. (See also Illustrated Technique 10).

spine; motor vehicle accidents and other crushing injuries are the usual causes.

Clinically, these patients manifest the findings of acute cardiac tamponade with evidence of blunt chest trauma. The important signs are hypotension, neck vein distention and elevated central venous pressure, and cyanosis of the upper half of the body. Most of these patients are hypotensive from blood loss as well as from cardiac tamponade; they do not respond to fluid resuscitation as readily as the usual case of hypovolemic shock without cardiac involvement. The central venous pressure may be low initially because of hypovolemia, and it may rise only after intravascular volume replacement. Elevation of the central venous pressure is the most useful emergency department finding suggestive of cardiac tamponade in the acute trauma situation. A chest radiograph usually shows a normal cardiac silhouette, since the pericardium has not had time to stretch.

When this injury is suspected, the only possibly successful therapy is prompt surgical exploration and closure of the ruptured cardiac chamber. The precarious condition of these patients precludes additional studies. Pericardiocentesis should be attempted prior to anesthesia induction; it may result in temporary hemodynamic improvement (Fig. 31.2). However, since the rapidly accumulating pericardial blood may be clotted, the pericardiocentesis may be negative. This should not prevent the surgeon from exploring the heart and pericardium if this diagnosis is strongly suspected from other findings. Ideally, this exploration should be done in the operating room via a median sternotomy incision, but if a rapidly deteriorating clinical condition precludes transfer to the operating room, an emergency department thoracotomy (described later in this chapter) may be necessary. The injury is usually found in one of the atria, and temporary control of bleeding can usually be gained with direct finger pressure or application of a vascular clamp. The defect can then usually be closed directly with sutures once the condition of the patient has been stabilized.

Traumatic Rupture of the Aorta

Aortic rupture commonly occurs as a result of an automobile collision. Death from exsanguination at the scene of the accident is the usual outcome. Most victims of aortic rupture are young men who are automobile drivers or passengers. Aortic rupture is twice as frequent in those ejected from a vehicle compared with those not ejected. The injury also occurs in pedestrians struck by automobiles, motorcycle riders, and individuals who have fallen from great heights. In only 20% is the aortic rupture sufficiently contained to allow survival to reach medical attention. In this latter group, prompt recognition and treatment of the aortic injury is of vital importance, since 33% of surviving patients die of the aortic rupture within 24 hours of the injury if untreated; 64% within 1 week; and 77% within 2 weeks.

Pathology. The upper descending thoracic aorta just distal to the origin of the left subclavian artery is the most frequent site of rupture in the patients who survive the trip to the hospitals. This location accounts for 95% of the surgically treated cases of aortic rupture. A second site of injury involves the ascending aorta just above the aortic valve; this injury is observed much more often in autopsy material than in clinical practice; these individuals usually die immediately of intrapericardial aortic rupture or of severe concomitant cardiac injuries. Uncommon sites of aortic injury include the arch, often with avulsion of one or more of its branches, the descending aorta above the diaphragm, and very rarely more than one of these sites.

When fatal, the disruption extends through the full thickness of the aortic wall and through the mediastinal pleura, allowing rapid exsanguination into the mediastinum and pleural spaces. In survivors of aortic rupture, the intima and media are disrupted, but the stronger aortic adventitia remains sufficiently intact to preserve the integrity of the circulation. The size of the intimal disruption may be only a few millimeters in length, but may extend in a transverse direction completely across the aortic circumference with separation of the two intimal and medial ends by several centimeters. The aortic adventitia, mediastinal tissues, and pleura then form the precarious wall of a false aneurysm, which is continually exposed to the pressure forces generated by each cardiac contraction.

Clinical Presentation. Many of the clinical features of aortic rupture are subtle and nonspecific, easily overshadowed by more obvious other injuries. In the Massachusetts General Hospital institutional experience with aortic rupture, associated injuries include extremity and/or pelvic fractures in 60% of the patients, rib and/or sternal fractures in 52%, and central nervous system injuries in 41%, ruptured spleen in 16%, other visceral and vascular injuries in 11%, and body burns in 7%. Therefore, in order to identify aortic trauma in these patients with other severe injuries, the index of suspicion must be high, and the threshold for obtaining additional definitive studies must be low.

Acute symptoms accompanying aortic rupture are totally nonspecific; they include interscapular or precordial chest pain and shortness of breath. The

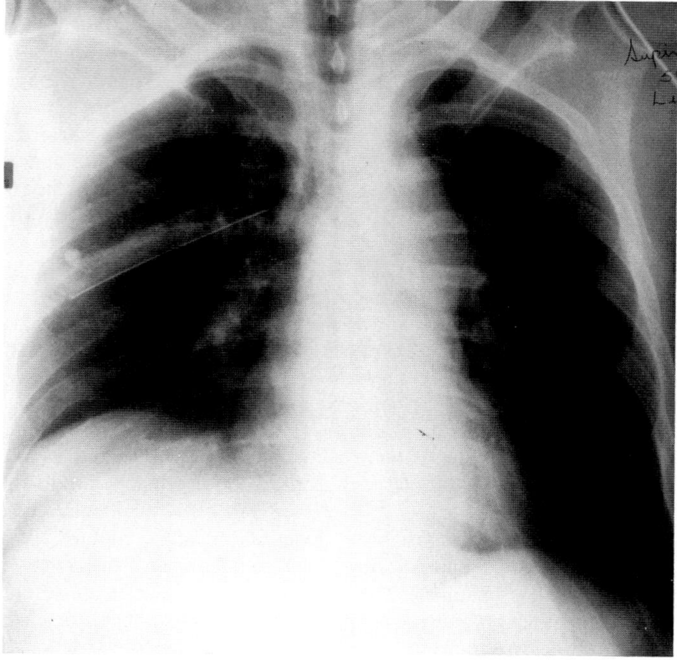

Figure 31.3. Chest radiograph from a patient with a contained disruption of the upper descending thoracic aorta. Note the widening of the superior mediastinal silhouette, obscuring of the contour of the aortic knob, deviation of the trachea to the right, depression of the left main bronchus, and the left apical extrapleural density.

most common physical finding is hypertension in the upper extremities with widening of the pulse pressure. In descending aortic injuries, as many as one-fourth of the patients will manifest the findings of an acute coarction syndrome characterized by upper extremity hypertension, diminution of femoral pulses and leg blood pressure, and a systolic murmur over the precordium or interscapular area of the back. This syndrome develops when there is sufficient infolding of the intima at the distal end of the transection to cause partial obstruction of the aortic lumen. A diastolic murmur of aortic valve insufficiency may be the clue to an ascending aortic injury with enough distortion of the aortic valve to affect its competence. No evidence of an injured chest wall is present in approximately half of the cases of aortic trauma.

Radiographic findings on the chest film are the most helpful findings suggesting this injury, and they all originate from the space-occupying effects of the mediastinal hematoma surrounding the contained aortic rupture (Fig. 31.3). In the typical injury distal to the left subclavian artery, these findings include widening of the superior mediastinum, obscuring of the aortic knob contour, deviation of the trachea to the right, depression of the left main stem bronchus, rightward displacement of the esophagus as outlined by a radiopaque nasogastric tube, a left apical extrapleural density, and at times a left pleural effusion. Rib fractures may be noted, but are absent in approximately half of these cases. The radiographic abnormalities are present at the time of the admission of the patient to the hospital in 75–90%; therefore, an occasional patient will not manifest chest radiographic abnormalities until hours or days after the injury. In a review of the radiographic findings associated with aortic rupture, the most consistently predictive observations were widening of the superior mediastinum and obscuring of the aortic knob contour. Portable films taken in the anteroposterior direction with the patient supine tend to magnify the superior mediastinum, thus making the distinction between a widened and a normal mediastinum somewhat more difficult, and emphasizing the importance of the additional findings mentioned. In ascending aortic and arch injuries, the mediastinal widening may be located predominantly to the right of the trachea, and the trachea and esophagus may be shifted to the left. The lower posterior mediastinal widening of a distal aortic injury may be particularly difficult to appreciate acutely, because it is located entirely posterior to the cardiac shadow and is easily obscured on a frontal film.

A *thoracic aortogram* is the definitive study to outline the false aneurysm occurring at the site of aortic disruption (Fig. 31.4). It can be safely accomplished by the percutaneous femoral route, and should be obtained in all trauma victims with widening of the mediastinum or any other findings suggestive of aortic rupture. In a large series of trauma patients with mediastinal widening, 40% were found to have aortic rupture on aortography. The aortogram should be obtained early in the course of the evaluation and treatment, if possible before anesthesia and operative repair of other injuries. The entire thoracic aorta from the level of the valve to the diaphragm, including the arch branches, should be visualized in anteroposterior, lateral, and oblique views. The role of enhanced computed tomographic scanning in the diagnosis of acute aortic disruption is not clearly defined. These scans will show the mediastinal hematoma, but may not be able to identify the specific site and extent of aortic disruption, particularly in the less common sites of injury. Therefore, for the cardiovascular surgeon, if aortic trauma is suspected from the clinical and plain radiographic findings, a thoracic aortogram is the next step in the evaluation of the patient.

Treatment. Treatment of the patient with an acute aortic false aneurysm includes medical measures to decrease the risk of sudden aortic rupture and surgical repair of the injured aortic segment. The medical and surgical measures are complementary, and in the timing of surgical intervention for multiple severe injuries, a plan of treatment priorities must be established. Head injuries requiring operative therapy and intraabdominal hemorrhage resulting in shock that does not respond readily to resuscitative measures usually take priority over repair of the aortic injury. However, anesthetic techniques must take the aortic injury into account, and medical measures as described later in this chapter should be instituted prior to definitive repair of the aorta. However, once the diagnosis of aortic rupture has been established, the most effective treatment of the injury is prompt surgical repair. Time is of the essence because of the constant risk of sudden rupture of the false aneurysm. In this institution, in patients with suspected or established aortic trauma, continuous radial artery pressure monitoring is begun early in the course of the evaluation, and treatment with antihypertensive agents and β-blockers is administered as needed in the preoperative period.

In the most common situation involving the proximal descending thoracic aorta, surgical repair usually consists of insertion of a tubular Dacron graft to replace the damaged segment of aorta. A posterolateral left thoracotomy incision is required for this procedure. The results of surgical repair are usually gratifying, with a 75–90% survival range. Paraplegia is a devastating operative complication occurring in 5–10% in the reported series. The unusual

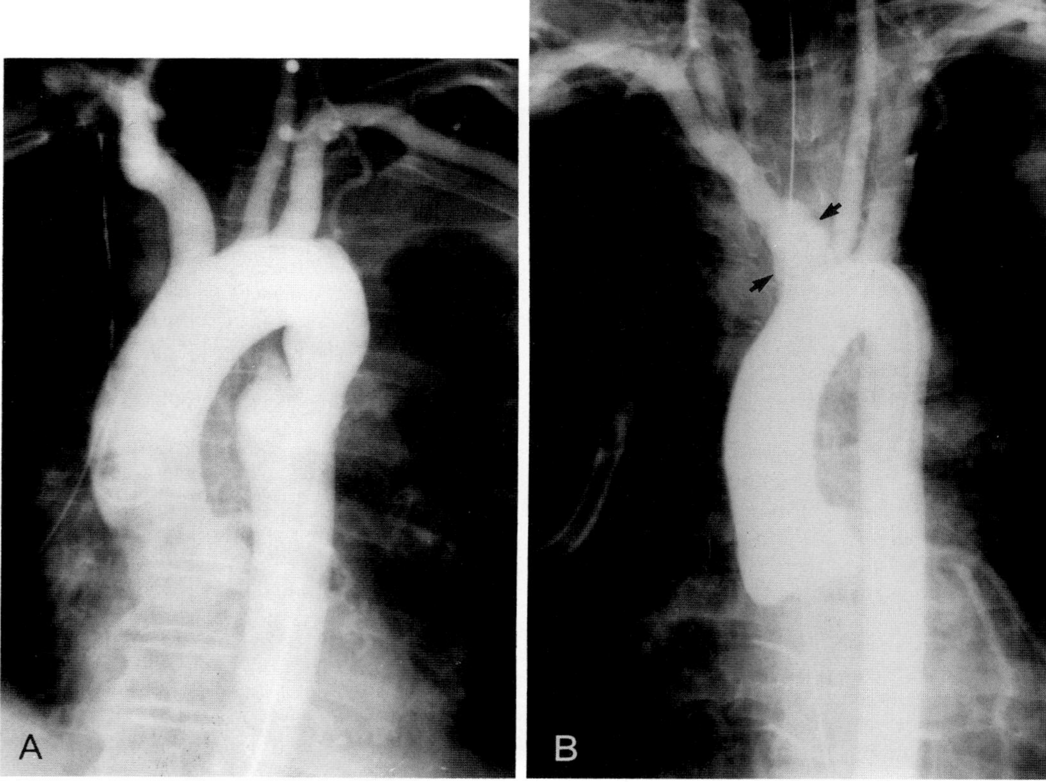

Figure 31.4. *A*, Thoracic aortogram via the femoral artery showing an acute traumatic false aneurysm of the upper descending aorta, the most frequent site of aortic injury. *B*, Thoracic aortogram showing an acute traumatic false aneurysm of the aortic arch involving the origin of the innominate artery, marked by the arrows.

ascending aortic injuries are repaired through a median sternotomy incision on total cardiopulmonary bypass. Repair of aortic arch injuries usually involve placement of bypass grafts to the involved aortic arch branches, followed by obliteration of the traumatic aneurysm.

Under certain highly selected circumstances, urgent surgical repair of aortic rupture may be inadvisable. These situations include serious central nervous system injuries with an uncertain outlook, large body burns with a likelihood of a septic course, a patient with established sepsis with its risk to a fresh aortic prosthesis, and severe respiratory failure, increasing the risks of anesthesia and thoracotomy. Medical management of the aortic injury may allow time for further evaluation and treatment of these associated problems while minimizing the risk of rupture of the false aneurysm. The medical management parallels that used for treatment of acute dissection of the aorta, and consists of administration of β-blocking drugs and antihypertensive agents. Initially, these drugs are administered intravenously with careful monitoring, and after the acute phase has passed, they can be given orally. In our experience, none of the 19 patients who received prolonged medical management prior to surgical repair experienced rupture. Five of these patients are receiving medical therapy indefinitely since they remain unsuitable surgical candidates because of extensive permanent neurological damage, and none of these patients has experienced aneurysm rupture in follow-up averaging 54 months.

Penetrating Chest Wounds Involving the Heart and Great Vessels

Cardiac Wounds

Urban violence with knives and handguns is the usual cause of penetrating cardiac wounds, and effective rapid emergency medical transportation allows at least some of these casualties to reach hospital emergency departments alive. Several centers have reported sizable experiences indicating that

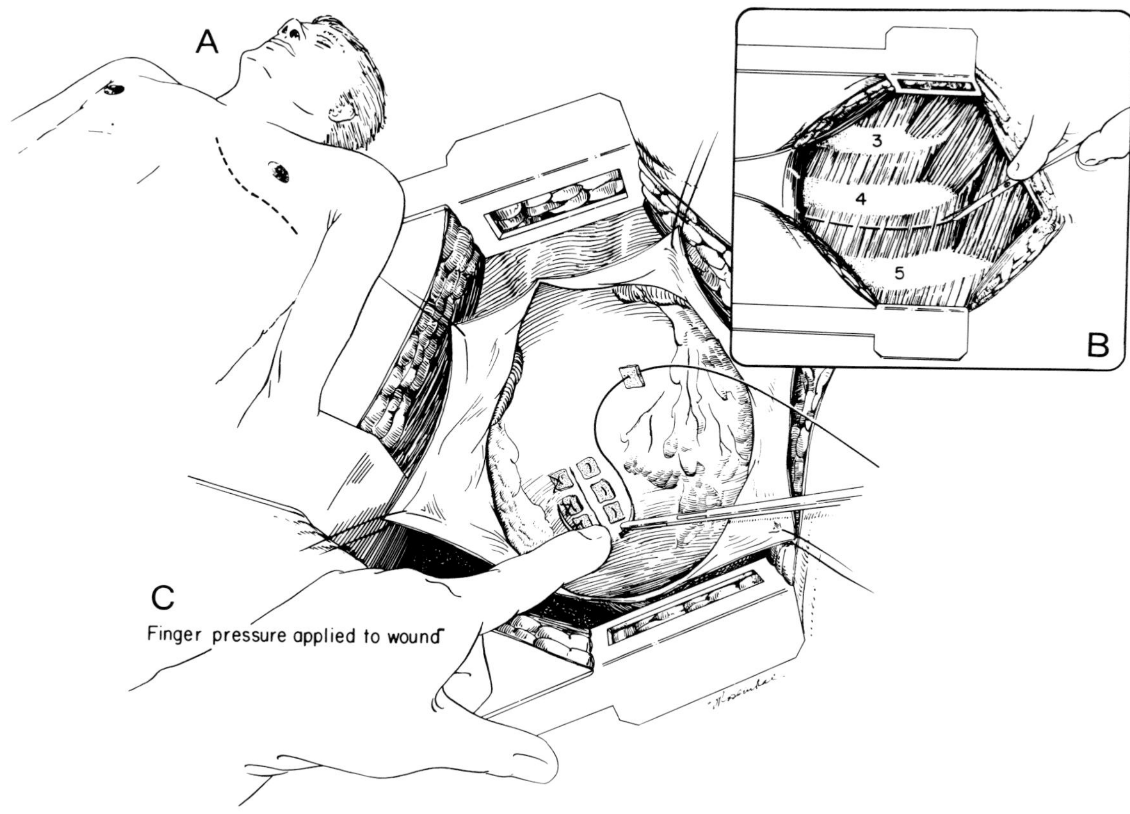

Figure 31.5. *A*, Incision for emergency department left anterolateral thoracotomy for repair of a penetrating cardiac wound. Note: An endotracheal tube and large intravenous catheter must have already been placed before the thoracotomy. *B*, The chest is opened through the fourth intercostal space. *C*, After opening the pericardium widely, finger pressure controls bleeding from a ventricular wound while buttressed sutures are placed (see also Illustrated Technique 11).

many of the victims of penetrating cardiac trauma can be salvaged by prompt recognition of the cardiac injury and aggressive surgical management. The clinical presentation of these patients depends upon the cardiac chamber injured; if the pericardium is relatively intact or widely open; whether the wound was caused by a knife or a gunshot; and the time required for transportation of the victim to the trauma center. Four distinct clinical presentations of penetrating cardiac wounds are recognizable: (*a*) cardiac arrest shortly before or shortly after hospital admission; (*b*) hemorrhagic shock; (*c*) cardiac tamponade; (*d*) initial hemodynamic instability. The evaluation and treatment differs for each group.

Cardiac Arrest and Emergency Department Thoracotomy. In the presence of a penetrating cardiac wound and circulatory arrest, closed chest resuscitative efforts will rarely be effective. This injury should immediately be suspected in the "lifeless" patient with a penetrating wound in the chest or upper abdomen, particularly if the site of penetration is in the precordial region. If the cardiac arrest occurs in the moments immediately before or after hospital admission, *thoracotomy in the emergency department* with control of the cardiac wound can result in survival of some of these patients. The treatment priorities include insertion of an oral endotracheal tube and positive pressure ventilation with 100% oxygen, insertion of large intravenous catheters with administration of crystalloid solutions, sodium bicarbonate, and vasopressors, and prompt emergency thoracotomy (Fig. 31.5). A left anterolateral thoracotomy incision is appropriate in all of these cases, and the chest can be opened in the fourth or fifth intercostal space. A chest retractor is inserted, and the pericardium is then opened widely in a vertical direction anterior to the phrenic nerve. Care must be exercised at this point to avoid injury to the phrenic nerve as well as injury to the myocardium, coronary arteries, and left atrial appendage, which are all located immediately beneath the pericardium. If additional exposure is required, the incision can be extended across the midline and the sternum divided with a Lebschke knife. Once identified, the cardiac wound can be temporarily controlled with finger pressure, and then repaired rapidly with deep mattress sutures reinforced with Teflon felt pledgets. Manual cardiac compression is then begun, and appropriate therapy for the underlying cardiac rhythm carried out, which could include direct injection of epinephrine and calcium chloride into the heart for cardiac stand-still, and direct defibrillation of the heart for ventricular fibrillation. If a cardiac rhythm can be established, but an arterial pressure cannot be maintained above 60 mm Hg, temporary cross-clamping of the middescending thoracic aorta may be considered, in order to increase the peripheral resistance in the upper body, and perhaps to improve the coronary perfusion pressure. However, this maneuver results in a marked increase in the left ventricular afterload and in ischemia of the spinal cord and kidneys; efforts at gradually removing the cross-clamp must begin when the systolic arterial pressure reaches 100 mm Hg. If the hemodynamic status can be stabilized in the emergency department, the patient is transferred to the operating room for additional assessment of the cardiac injury and its emergency repair, exploration of the remainder of the chest, exploration of other body cavities if indicated, and irrigation and closure of the chest incision. The right ventricle is the most frequently injured cardiac chamber, followed in frequency by the left ventricle, the atria, and the intrapericardial great vessels. Emergency department thoracotomy has been most valuable in the treatment of patients with penetrating cardiac wounds, and least effective in those presenting with cardiorespiratory arrest as a result of extensive nonpenetrating thoracic and abdominal trauma.

Hemorrhagic Shock. If the cardiac wound communicates freely with the mediastinum or pleural space through a large defect in the pericardium, signs of hypovolemic shock usually predominate. A cardiac wound must be suspected in the presence of a precordial penetrating chest injury, continuing major blood loss through a chest tube, and the ongoing requirement for intravascular volume replacement. This situation should lead to the rapid transfer of the patient to the operating room for thoracotomy and repair of the suspected cardiac wound. If the hemodynamics deteriorate in the emergency department despite appropriate resuscitative measures, emergency thoracotomy as described in the previous paragraphs should be performed promptly.

Cardiac Tamponade. If the pericardial defect from the penetrating agent is small, the victim may present with the clinical findings of cardiac tamponade. Initially, hypotension may be the only sign, and an elevated venous pressure may not appear until intravascular fluid replacement has been instituted. The electrocardiogram and the chest radiograph are usually not helpful. The combination of a chest wound, arterial hypotension, and elevation of the central venous pressure should lead to the prompt transfer of the patient to the operating room for a thoracotomy. If the hemodynamics are deteriorating, *pericardiocentesis* (see Illustrated Technique 10) via the subxiphoid approach should be performed; this should temporarily improve the situation. However, pericardiocentesis as a diagnostic maneuver in cardiac trauma may be misleading. False-positive taps can result from laceration of the epicardium or penetration of a cardiac chamber, and false-negatives occur when clotted intrapericardial blood does not pass into the syringe. Pericardiocentesis was once used as the primary means of treating some cardiac wounds with tamponade, but its present role is that of a temporizing procedure only, allowing some patients to be stabilized prior to definitive operation. If the hemodynamics continue to deteriorate despite resuscitation and pericardiocentesis, emergency department thoracotomy is indicated. However, if the patient is sufficiently stable, he should be transferred to the operating room for definitive therapy.

Initial Hemodynamic Stability. A few patients with cardiac wounds will present with initial hemodynamic stability. There may be time for more sophisticated evaluation, including echocardiography, but it is important to identify and repair these injuries prior to sudden deterioration of the patient. In the group with possible cardiac injury, limited intrapericardial exploration in the operating room via the subxiphoid approach may be of some value. If no abnormality is found, the patient has been subjected to a small surgical procedure. If pericardial blood is identified, the incision is extended, and cardiac repair accomplished. However, others prefer formal thoracotomy and exploration for all potentially penetrating cardiac injuries because of the improved initial control and better exposure for complete exploration of the surface of the heart.

The prognosis for patients presenting with cardiac tamponade with penetrating cardiac injuries is excellent, with approximately 90% survival; knife wounds are much more frequently encountered in this group than gunshot wounds. In the patients with hemorrhagic shock, bullet wounds predominate over stab wounds, and the outcome is less favorable, with the survival rate approximately 50%. In the cardiac arrest group, survival in 36% has been reported in patients with penetrating cardiac injuries and emergency department thoracotomy. Survival of 57% of patients with penetrating cardiac wounds undergoing emergency department thoracotomy has also been reported. Multiple injuries must also be suspected, and as many as 25% of these patients have coexisting injuries to other viscera in the chest and abdomen that require evaluation and operative repair. Among the survivors of surgical repair of acute penetrating cardiac wounds, approximately 25% will develop signs of an intracardiac defect in the postoperative period. These lesions include left-to-right shunts (ventricular septal defects are the most common), valvular insufficiency, ventricular aneurysms, and retained foreign bodies. Rare patients with an acute gunshot wound to the heart with embolization of the bullet to a peripheral site, such as a femoral artery, have been described.

Penetrating Wounds of the Great Vessels

Penetrating wounds in any part of the chest and at the base of the neck can result in injury to the great vessels within the mediastinum. Several different types of clinical presentations are possible, depending on the location of the injury, the specific vessel involved, the size of the wound, and whether the wound communicates with one of the intrathoracic cavities. Most patients with penetrating great vessel wounds present with hemorrhagic shock, and the vessel injury often communicates with the pleural space, resulting in substantial drainage of blood from the chest tube and requiring large amounts of intravascular volume replacement. In some patients with penetrating great vessel trauma, the injury is largely confined to the mediastinum, and a tamponading hematoma will temporarily limit the blood volume loss. These patients present with mild to moderate degrees of hypovolemia and a widened mediastinum on chest radiograph.

Evaluation of the unstable patient is necessarily limited, and while he or she is receiving continuing blood volume replacement, he or she should be taken to the operating room for prompt exploration. In the more stable patient with a mediastinal hematoma, an aortogram may be helpful in identifying the patient with a serious arterial injury and in precisely localizing it. Arterial injuries are always repaired surgically, but stable patients with mediastinal hematomas without aortographic abnormality may be observed. Concomitant injury to the airway and esophagus should always be suspected in patients with mediastinal great vessel injury. A survival rate of 80% has been reported for patients undergoing surgical treatment of penetrating great vessel injuries.

NONTRAUMATIC CONDITONS

Acute Aortic Dissection

Acute dissection of the aorta is a catastrophic condition characterized by separation of the layers of the aortic wall by a dissecting hematoma. Although the precise sequence of events that initiates an aortic dissection is incompletely understood, it appears that in most patients an intimal tear develops at an aortic site, which is subjected to high shearing forces; the dissection splits the layers of the media, which has been structurally weakened. The dissecting hematoma is propagated by the forces of each cardiac contraction and creates a false lumen that is separated from the true lumen by the intimal flap. The false lumen may distort the geometry of the aortic valve, may compress or occlude arterial branches of the aorta, or may rupture into the pericardium or pleural space. Predisposing factors include hypertension, Marfan's syndrome, idiopathic cystic medial necrosis, pregnancy, coarctation of the aorta, and perhaps congenital aortic stenosis.

Classifications

Two anatomic classifications of acute dissections are in use at present. The DeBakey system includes three types. In Type I, the origin is in the ascending aorta with propagation of the dissection distally to include the arch, descending aorta, and abdominal aorta in most patients. In Type II, the dissection is localized to the ascending aorta; in Type III, the dissection begins distal to the left subclavian artery. A second classification popularized by the Stanford cardiovascular surgical group is based simply upon the presence or absence of involvement of the ascending aorta. This classification readily accommodates subtypes with less frequent sites of intimal tears, yet it preserves the important prognostic and therapeutic differences between the two groups. In this classification, Type A includes all patients with involvement of the ascending aorta with varying degrees of distal dissection. It includes patients with intimal tears located in the ascending aorta and those located in the aortic arch or descending aorta with retrograde proximal dissection. Type B includes dissections in which the ascending aorta is spared, and the intimal tear is located distal to the left subclavian artery, although sites in the aortic arch and distal thoracic or abdominal aorta are also included.

Approximately 65% of all acute dissections involve the ascending aorta, and 35% are limited to the descending aorta. Dissections occur in men two to three times more frequently than in women. The average age of patients with ascending aortic dissections is 55 years, and in descending dissection, 65 years. Untreated, patients with acute aortic dissections have a mortality rate of approximately 80% within the first 2 weeks. Death is commonly due to intrapericardial rupture of the false lumen involving the ascending aorta, or congestive heart failure from acute aortic valvular insufficiency.

Clinical Presentation of Patients with Ascending Aortic Involvement

Most patients present with pain that is usually of acute onset and substernal in location. It may radiate or migrate to the back or to the abdomen. In this institution, the initial arterial blood pressure is normal in 66% of the patients, elevated in 11%, and abnormally low in 23%. A murmur of aortic valve insufficiency is audible in 66% of the patients; some of these are in overt congestive heart failure. A peripheral pulse deficit is noted in 49%. Possible neurological findings include hemiparesis or paraplegia. There is electrocardiographic evidence of either myocardial ischemia or infarction in 20% and findings of left ventricular hypertrophy in 41%. The chest radiography shows enlargement of the aorta or of the mediastinum in 40–50% of the cases. The most specific sign of dissection is displacement of aortic intimal calcification more than 6 mm from the outer margin of the aorta.

Clinical Presentation of Patients with Descending Aortic Dissection

The majority of patients experience back pain, frequently located in the back in the thoracic region; characteristically, it is migratory. Our experience with these patients includes a history of hypertension in 80%. However, elevated arterial blood pressure is noted in only 66% at the time of initial presentation. A pulse deficit in the lower extremities may be detected; paraplegia is possible. The chest radiograph is abnormal in approximately half of the patients with findings similar to those noted in the previous section.

Differential Diagnosis of Acute Aortic Dissection

Eagle and associates from the Massachusetts General Hospital reported the spectrum of conditions initially suggesting acute aortic dissection in patients who have negative aortograms. In descending order of frequency, these conditions include acute myocardial infarction, aortic insufficiency without dissection, nondissecting thoracic aortic aneurysm, musculoskeletal pain, mediastinal tumor, pericarditis, unstable angina, and cholecystitis. These investigators noted four findings that help to differentiate patients with acute dissections. Patients with dissections tend to have a history of hypertension, duration of pain less than 24 hours, migration of the pain, and left ventricular hypertrophy on the electrocardiogram.

Diagnostic Studies

Two dimensional echocardiography, computed tomographic (CT) scanning with contrast, and aor-

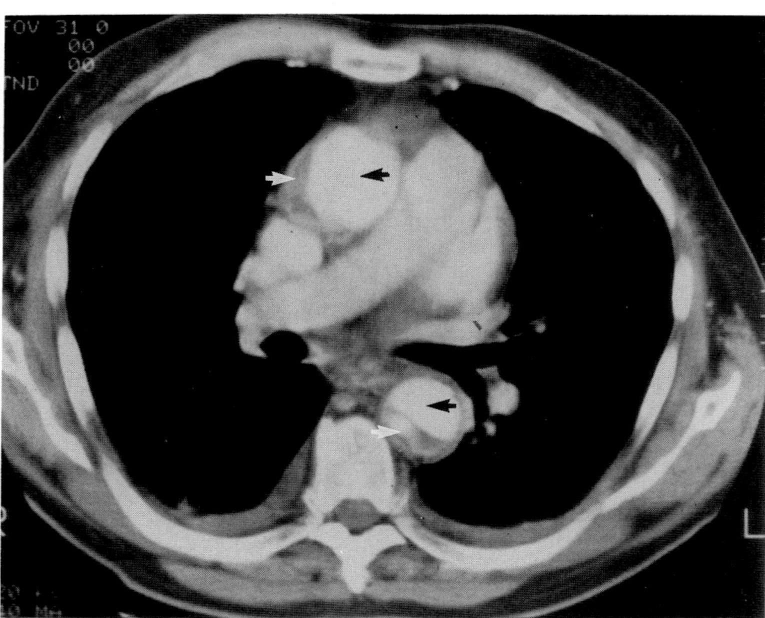

Figure 31.6. Computed tomographic scan of the chest with bolus contrast administration (dynamic scan) showing an aortic dissection with involvement of both ascending and descending thoracic aorta. The black arrows indicate the contrast filled true lumen, and the white arrows identify the false lumen, which is filled with clot and a small amount of contrast.

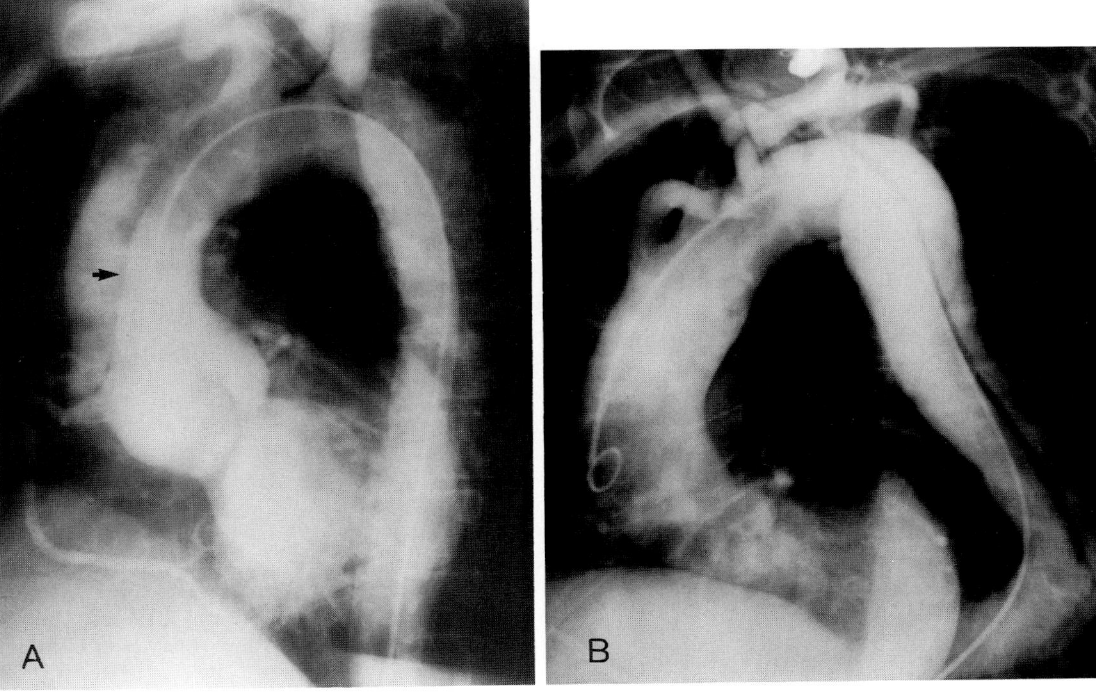

Figure 31.7. *A*, Thoracic aortogram showing an acute aortic dissection with origin in the ascending aorta. The arteriographic catheter lies within the true lumen, and the arrow marks the intimal flap. The false lumen contains less contrast than the true lumen. Both coronary arteries are visualized just proximal to the origin of the intimal flap. Moderate aortic valve insufficiency allows contrast material to opacify the left ventricle. *B*, Thoracic aortogram showing an acute aortic dissection whose origin lies immediately distal to the take-off of the left subclavian artery. The intimal flap is easily visible throughout the entire length of the descending aorta. Note the normal appearance of the ascending aorta, the aortic arch and its branches.

tography are three useful studies in the diagnosis of acute aortic dissection. They are complementary, and none is completely accurate in making or excluding the diagnosis.

Echocardiography is the least invasive but also the least reliable method of diagnosing a dissection. If an intimal flap is visualized, it is almost certain that the patient has an aortic dissection. However, in one study, echocardiography failed to identify the intimal flap in 20% of patients with dissections. Therefore, a negative echocardiogram does not reliably exclude the diagnosis of a dissection.

Computed tomography with bolus injection of contrast is an excellent study to detect the presence of an aortic dissection. Its sensitivity and specificity in the diagnosis of dissection is approximately the same as that of aortography. The usual findings are two contrast-filled channels with an intervening intimal flap (Fig. 31.6). It is usually possible to distinguish between Type A and Type B dissections. Problems arise when the false channel is thrombosed and is not filled by contrast, making the distinction between a dissection and a fusiform aneurysm of the aorta with mural thrombus difficult. Identification of the specific location of the intimal tear, identification and quantitation of aortic valvular insufficiency, and assessment of filling of aortic branches are not possible with CT scanning.

A *thoracic aortogram* identifies patients with aortic dissection; the study is usually advisable if surgical treatment is considered. In addition to identification of true and false channels and the intimal flap, additional information regarding the site of intimal disruption, degree of aortic insufficiency, and patency of aortic branches is available from the aortogram (Fig. 31.7). When the false lumen is thrombosed, contrast material may not enter it, and the diagnosis of aortic dissection is less certain.

Our policy is to use CT scanning in the patient who is stable and in whom the suspicion of dissection is only moderate. We prefer to obtain an aortogram in patients who are unstable, in those in whom the diagnosis is strongly suspected, and in patients in whom surgical treatment is being considered.

Treatment

Once the diagnosis of dissection has been confirmed, careful monitoring and medical treatment is begun in all patients. A radial artery cannula is inserted for continuous pressure monitoring, a Foley catheter inserted into the bladder, and central venous and pulmonary artery pressure monitoring instituted in those selected patients with hemodynamic instability. For hypertensive patients, systemic arterial pressure should be lowered to the normal range with intravenous agents such as nitroprusside or labetalol. Additional administration of intravenous β-blocking drugs, such as propranolol, should be considered in order to decrease the force of myocardial contraction, which tends to propagate the dissection. For those patients without involvement of the ascending aorta, continuation of medical therapy with careful monitoring usually stabilizes the situation. Long-term medical therapy is then recommended with oral antihypertensive and β-blocking drugs. The hospital survival rate is 80–90%; most patients continue to remain stable on medical therapy. If a localized aneurysm develops in the descending aorta at the site of the intimal disruption, surgical resection is recommended.

If the ascending aorta is involved, urgent surgical treatment is recommended for most patients, in order to prevent the highly lethal complication of intrapericardial rupture of the false lumen. Particularly urgent surgical therapy is required in those patients who present with evidence of cardiac tamponade or congestive heart failure from acute aortic insufficiency. Surgical treatment consists of replacement of the ascending aorta with a Dacron graft while on cardiopulmonary bypass. If the intimal tear is located in the ascending aorta, it is identified and removed. Most surgeons are prepared to locate and resect intimal tears located in the aortic arch as well. An occasional patient will have the ascending aorta involved by retrograde proximal dissection with the tear located in the descending aorta. In these patients, it appears that appropriate treatment involves graft replacement of the ascending aorta and postoperative medical treatment, since the site of intimal disruption is still present. Some patients will require concomitant aortic valve replacement, although the native valve can be resuspended and retained in the majority of cases. Reported operative survival varies betweeen 60–90%.

Thoracic Atherosclerotic Aneurysms

Atherosclerotic aneurysms of the thoracic aorta and great vessels infrequently cause acute symptoms. An insidious onset of a pressure sensation, heaviness in the chest, cough, dysphagia, or hoarseness is more common. Sudden expansion or leakage from an aneurysm of the thoracic aorta can cause catastrophic pain and shock, and on the patient's arrival at the emergency department, the symptoms may be indistinguishable from those of acute myocardial infarction. In hypertensive patients, radiologic demonstration of the aneurysm should satisfy most of the criteria for vasodilator therapy. Many patients, however, are normotensive, and intravenous propranolol may be indicated even in these patients. Angiographic demonstration of the limits of the aneurysm determines the feasibility and appropriateness of surgical therapy.

Aneurysms of the Peripheral Vascular System

Aneurysms commonly are caused by arteriosclerosis, although they may be secondary to trauma, cystic medial necrosis, or infection. The symptoms and signs of an arteriosclerotic aneurysm may be pain, shock, or a palpable mass. Pain may be caused by acute expansion of the aneurysm, by pressure of an expanding aneurysm against a nerve, or by free blood from a leak or rupture into a contained space such as the retroperitoneum or abdominal cavity. Hypovolemic shock is often a consequence of such a rupture. Rarely, hypertension caused by an increase in the afterload indicates thrombosis of an aneurysm. Acute distal arterial occlusion may result from emboli arising in laminated thrombus associated with the aneurysm. Aneurysms frequently develop near arterial bifurcations and are most commonly seen in the distal aorta, common iliac artery, common femoral artery, and popliteal artery. Aneurysms of visceral arteries are less frequently seen, the most common site being the splenic artery.

Abdominal Aortic Aneurysms

Abdominal aortic aneurysms are generally asymptomatic until they expand to 4 cm in diameter. A common symptom is abdominal pain that is usually located in the middle or lower part of the abdomen, frequently to the left of the midline. Back pain is also common. Occasionally, the patient may notice a pulsatile abdominal mass or have symptoms related to duodenal or vena caval obstruction. Thrombosis of an abdominal aortic aneurysm is rare and generally occurs to the level of the renal arteries. Symptoms include hypertension or ischemic lower extremities, or both. Ischemic digits or patchy areas of ischemic skin may be due to dissemination into endarteries of emboli from a laminated thrombus and, occasionally, cholesterol emboli from an atheroma.

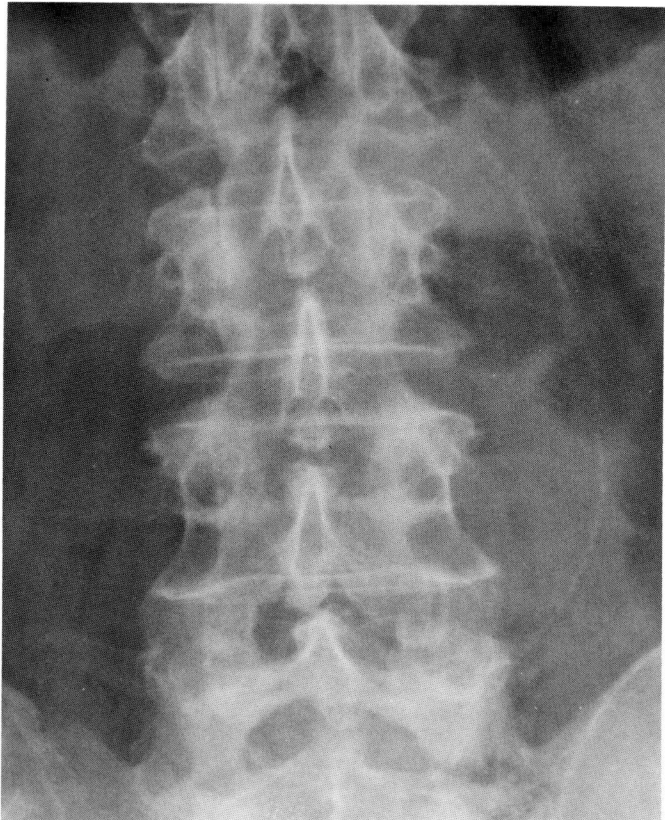

Figure 31.8. Anteroposterior roentgenogram of abdomen demonstrating calcified left lateral wall of an abdominal aortic aneurysm extending from second to fifth lumbar vertebra.

The principal physical finding in a patient with an abdominal aortic aneurysm is a palpable, pulsatile, expansile, midabdominal mass that may be tender. Since the wall of such an aneurysm frequently contains calcium, an anteroposterior roentgenogram of the abdomen and a lateral projection of the lumbosacral spine may reveal its presence (Fig. 31.8). In the absence of vessel-wall calcium, echography may be helpful in assessing the size of the aorta. In a patient whose condition is stable, aortographic examination may be helpful in demonstrating the presence of a suspected abdominal aortic aneurysm and in planning its management.

Rupture of an abdominal aortic aneurysm is usually heralded by the onset of severe pain or hypotension, in which case a palpable aneurysm may not be evident. If this diagnosis can reasonably be suspected, the patient should be transported promptly to an operating room for emergency surgery. The pneumatic antishock garment provides circumferential tamponade during transit. Blood for transfusion through large-bore central intravenous lines should be obtained immediately.

Abdominal or back pain associated with a palpable aneurysm but without hypotension should be ascribed to acute expansion of a known abdominal aortic aneurysm. Because the mortality from ruptured aneurysms compared with unruptured aneurysms is so high (50% and 3%, respectively), patients in whom aneurysmal expansion is suspected should be operated on immediately, although some other cause for the symptoms may indeed be found at operation in a few cases.

Iliac and Femoral Arterial Aneurysms

Common and external iliac arterial aneurysms present clinical findings similar to those of abdominal aortic aneurysms and must be dealt with promptly by operation. Internal iliac arterial aneurysms may produce symptoms due to compression of the colon, ureters, or bladder. Femoral arterial aneurysms do not usually rupture, but rather produce acute arterial occlusion. Laminated thrombus within the aneurysm may occlude the origin of the profunda femoris artery. In the presence of occlusion, the leg is more vulnerable to ischemia if there is embolization into the superficial femoral system. Prompt operation may be necessary to save the limb.

Pain secondary to femoral nerve compression may be the presenting symptom. Diagnosis is usually made readily by physical examination, and early operation is necessary to retrieve emboli and to reconstruct the femoral artery. Femoral arterial aneurysms are usually present bilaterally and are seen in association with aneurysms of other arteries, such as the distal abdominal aorta, iliac artery, and popliteal artery.

Popliteal Aneurysms

The symptoms of a popliteal aneurysm are usually caused by either thrombosis of the aneurysm or by distal embolization. In both cases, the symptoms are those of acute arterial occlusion, unless thrombosis has developed gradually enough to allow collateral circulation to bypass the block. In this instance, there is only mild intermittent claudication. Occasionally, pressure from the aneurysm on a nerve may produce pain, or on a vein, peripheral edema. A popliteal aneurysm rarely ruptures. On physical examination, this aneurysm is diagnosed by palpation of a mass in the popliteal fossa, which need not be pulsatile. If a popliteal mass is palpated in the other leg, the diagnosis is strongly suspected, since popliteal aneurysms occur bilaterally in approximately 60% of these patients. Arteriographic examination demonstrates the presence of a popliteal aneurysm, unless it is obscured by laminated thrombus (Fig. 31.9). Prompt operation is necessary to restore circulation by evacuating thrombus from the peripheral arterial tree and by reconstructing the popliteal artery, usually by placement of a venous graft.

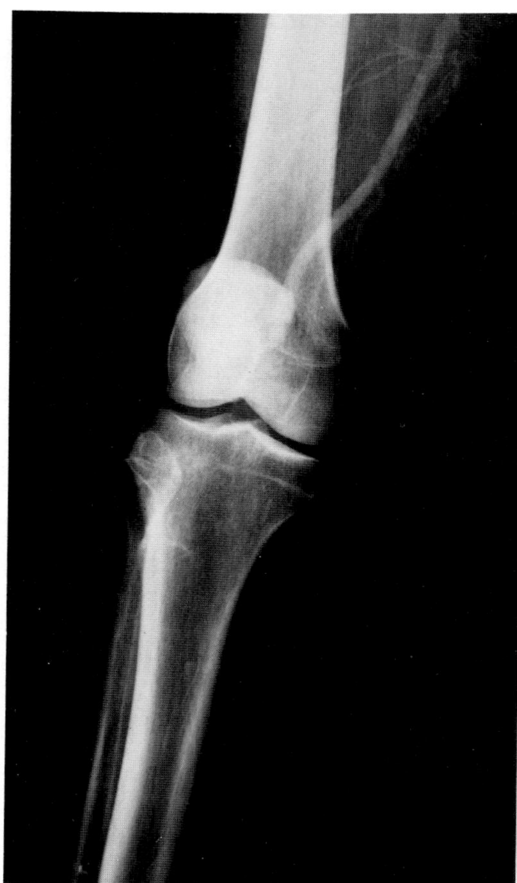

Figure 31.9. Percutaneous femoral arteriogram demonstrating occlusion of popliteal artery with absence of filling of distal vessels. Acute arterial occlusion was found to be secondary to thrombosis of a popliteal aneurysm.

Visceral and Other Arterial Aneurysms

The most common visceral arterial aneurysm is one involving the splenic artery. Since this is frequently calcified, it is evident on plain roentgenograms of the abdomen. Rupture of this aneurysm is rare, but may occur, especially during the third trimester of pregnancy. Rupture into the stomach is a rare cause of gastrointestinal hemorrhage. Renal arterial aneurysms seldom rupture, but may be associated with hypertension resulting from distal embolization of the laminated thrombus. Aneurysms of the superior mesenteric artery are unusual, and if present, frequently are infected. Other visceral arterial aneurysms may be signaled by intraabdominal or gastrointestinal hemorrhage due to rupture. Aneurysms of the arteries of the upper extremities are very rare and most commonly the result of arterial trauma.

False Aneurysms

False aneurysms from infected or disrupted arterial suture lines occur in patients who have undergone arterial reconstruction. Thus, it is critically important that the physician assessing a patient with a palpable or symptomatic aneurysm elicit a history of arterial operation and search for the operative scars of such procedures. False aneurysms may also be caused by infected arterial emboli and arterial trauma, and usually are heralded by distal ischemia produced by emboli from laminated thrombus.

PERIPHERAL VASCULAR TRAUMA

Trauma to a major artery can produce either immediate hemorrhage or arterial occlusion and eventual loss of function. Arterial hemorrhage is obvious and forces prompt action on the part of the physician. On the other hand, arterial insufficiency resulting from trauma may be difficult to recognize, and the examining physician must be highly suspicious of its presence in order to detect it promptly. Early recognition is absolutely essential to treatment, since delay may allow an irreversible ischemic injury and encourage the formation of intravascular thrombi.

Mechanism of Trauma

With *blunt trauma,* the vessel can be injured in three ways; the intima can be torn, presenting a thrombogenic surface to the blood stream; the vessel can be sheared, causing a flap of intima to roll up distally, occluding the lumen; and the vessel can be contused, causing subintimal hemorrhage and compromise of the patency of the lumen. *Penetrating trauma* is associated with hemorrhage caused by laceration, transection, or contusion of the vessel. Other later consequences of penetrating trauma are false aneurysms or arteriovenous fistulas, or both.

The initial response to traumatic interruption or occlusion of a major artery to a body area is vasoconstriction in that area, caused partly by reflex mediated through the sympathetic nervous system and partly by spasm of the affected vessel. After several hours, vasodilatation takes place as the point of occlusion in the artery is bypassed by flow through dilated collateral channels. If the patient has not suffered irreversible damage in the affected area and requires no surgical intervention, gradual hypertrophy of collateral channels occurs over the ensuing weeks to months. The degree of arterial insufficiency following arterial trauma depends on the site of arterial occlusion, being especially severe when bifurcations have been destroyed. It also depends on the ability of collateral channels to deliver an adequate blood supply to the body region.

In civilian settings, penetrating trauma is the more common source of arterial injury, but arterial injury by blunt trauma does occur in about 10% of these patients. Arterial injury most frequently is overlooked in cases of blunt trauma; careful search for distal pulses in patients with musculoskeletal trauma is essential. Peripheral pulses in the extremities should be evaluated by a Doppler ultrasonic flow detector, and segmental blood pressures in the injured extremity should be measured and compared with blood pressures in the uninjured extremity.

While examining the patient with a traumatic injury, the physician may detect persistent arterial bleeding. He may find diminished or absent pulses distal to, or at the site of, injury or a large or expanding hematoma. Proximity of the wound to a major artery indentifies the possibility of major vascular trauma. The signs of major arterial occlusion are pain and pallor in the affected area, a lack of pulses distal to the injury, and paresthesia and/or paralysis in the affected member. Tissue sensitivity

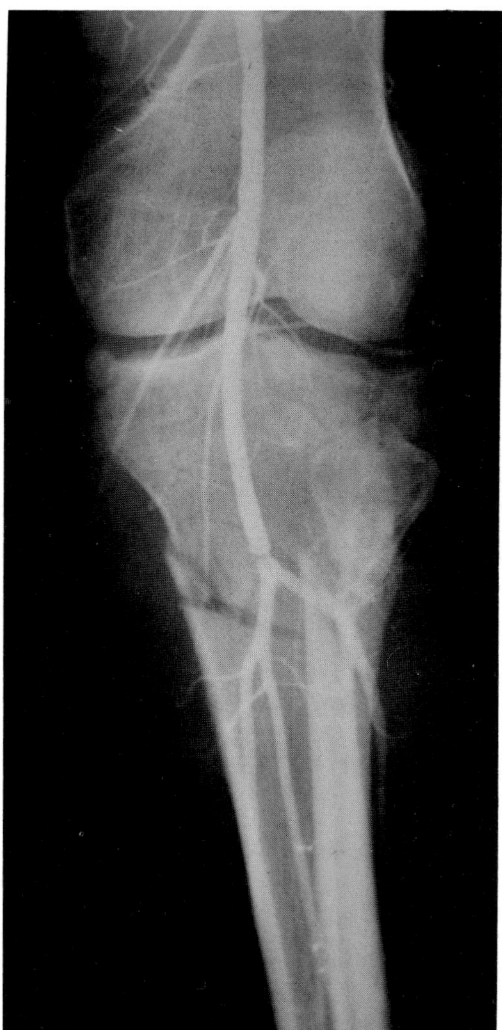

Figure 31.10. Percutaneous femoral arteriogram demonstrating intimal injury of distal popliteal artery just above its bifurcation associated with proximal tibial and fibular fractures.

to anoxia from arterial occlusion is greater in sensory and motor nerves than in skeletal muscle, bone, and tendon.

Treatment

Treatment of arterial trauma begins with management of the airway and assurance of adequate gas exchange, tamponade of hemorrhage, followed by instrumental control (not with a tourniquet), and appropriate volume replacement. If hemorrhage continues, the patient is prepared for the operating room while bleeding is controlled and transfusion is in progress. In a patient with a relatively stable condition, however, arteriographic examination should be performed to document the site of arterial injury (Fig. 31.10), but only if it can be done promptly. A critical determination of the possibility for success in the management of arterial injuries is the promptness of operative management.

Although restoration of arterial inflow is the primary concern after trauma, the consequences of venous injury must not be overlooked, and injured veins initially should be dealt with as gently as the arteries. Depending on the circumstances, it may be desirable to attempt reconstruction of veins as well as arteries.

Special emphasis is warranted concerning patients with penetrating wounds of the neck. Major vascular injury should be suspected in all such patients until the diagnosis is disproved by careful physical examination, angiography, and exploration of the wound. The tempo of the workup is dictated by the general condition of the patient. The patient with this type of injury should not be left unattended, and associated injuries to the trachea, pharynx, and esophagus must always be considered and investigated.

NONTRAUMATIC PERIPHERAL VASCULAR CONDITIONS

Acute Arterial Occlusion

Etiology

Acute arterial occlusion is usually caused by *embolism, acute arterial thrombosis,* or by *thrombosis within an aneurysm* (Fig. 31.11 *A-C*). Sudden arterial occlusion may be caused by an embolus from a central source such as the atrium (myxoma or thrombus associated with atrial fibrillation or mitral stenosis), the endocardium (mural thrombus following myocardial infarction), or a ventricle (aneurysm with thrombus). It may also originate from a source in the arterial tree proximal to the occlusion, such as an aneurysm (laminated thrombus) or a stenotic artery (fibrin or platelet aggregates). Occasionally, trauma produces acute arterial occlusion. This condition may result rarely from an inflammatory process such as granulomatous arteritis or from a hematologic disorder such as a hypercoagulable state associated with infection or with a systemic malignant condition.

Clinical Manifestations

Symptoms of acute arterial occlusion are determined largely by the suddenness of occlusion, the involvement of arterial bifurcations, the degree of collateral circulation, the presence of antecedent occlusive disease, and the presence of arterial spasm. The major symptom is pain, which occurs either abruptly or over a period of several hours. Paresthesia, coldness, and numbness also may be part of the symptom complex, and progressive loss of sensation and muscle function often ensues. If the arterial occlusion is not relieved, the symptoms persist or progress. The findings of absent pulses, cool and pallid skin, and empty superficial veins—even when an extremity is slightly dependent—suggest the diagnosis.

It may be difficult to distinguish between thrombosis superimposed on long-standing atherosclerotic occlusive disease and an embolic occlusion. A history of intermittent claudication suggests the former, although it may be difficult to ascertain whether a patient has intermittent claudication because patients frequently attribute this symptom to musculoskeletal causes and limit their activities to prevent the onset of muscular pain. Pain caused by embolism is instantaneous and severe, as opposed to that caused by thrombosis, which may develop relatively gradually and may be rather mild. If there is a recognizable source of embolism, and especially if there is a history of prior embolism, this diagnosis approaches certainty. The sudden appearance of cyanosis in one or more digits may be the first sign of ischemia in a previously asymptomatic extremity. In the presence of intact peripheral pulses, this finding represents either small-vessel thrombosis, or small-particle emboli to the digital vessels from a proximal source such as an aneurysm, ulcerated atheroma, or stenotic artery (Fig. 31.11*D*). Although symptoms produced by thrombosis of an arterial aneurysm may mimic those of embolic occlusion, the physician often makes the diagnosis by palpating a mass in the affected extremity. In addition, since they are frequently multiple, the presence of other palpable aneurysms aid in suggesting the correct diagnosis.

Partial or complete occlusion of the extracranial *internal carotid artery* leads to the possibility of transient ischemic attacks or frank strokes. After arteriographic assessment, surgery may be elected as the proper treatment. The diagnosis and treatment of this lesion are discussed in Chapter 37.

Acute occlusion of abdominal visceral vessels is a result of either emboli or of thrombosis of atherosclerotic stenotic lesions that usually occur where the visceral vessels originate from the abdominal aorta. Occlusions of arteries to the digestive system are considered in Chapter 33. Acute occlusion of a *renal* artery produces severe flank pain and may be accompanied by fever and hematuria and/or by severe hypertension. A rare condition, acute occlusion of both renal arteries is associated with severe oliguria in addition to hypertension. Although viability of the kidney is threatened by severe ischemia, enough collateral circulation may exist to

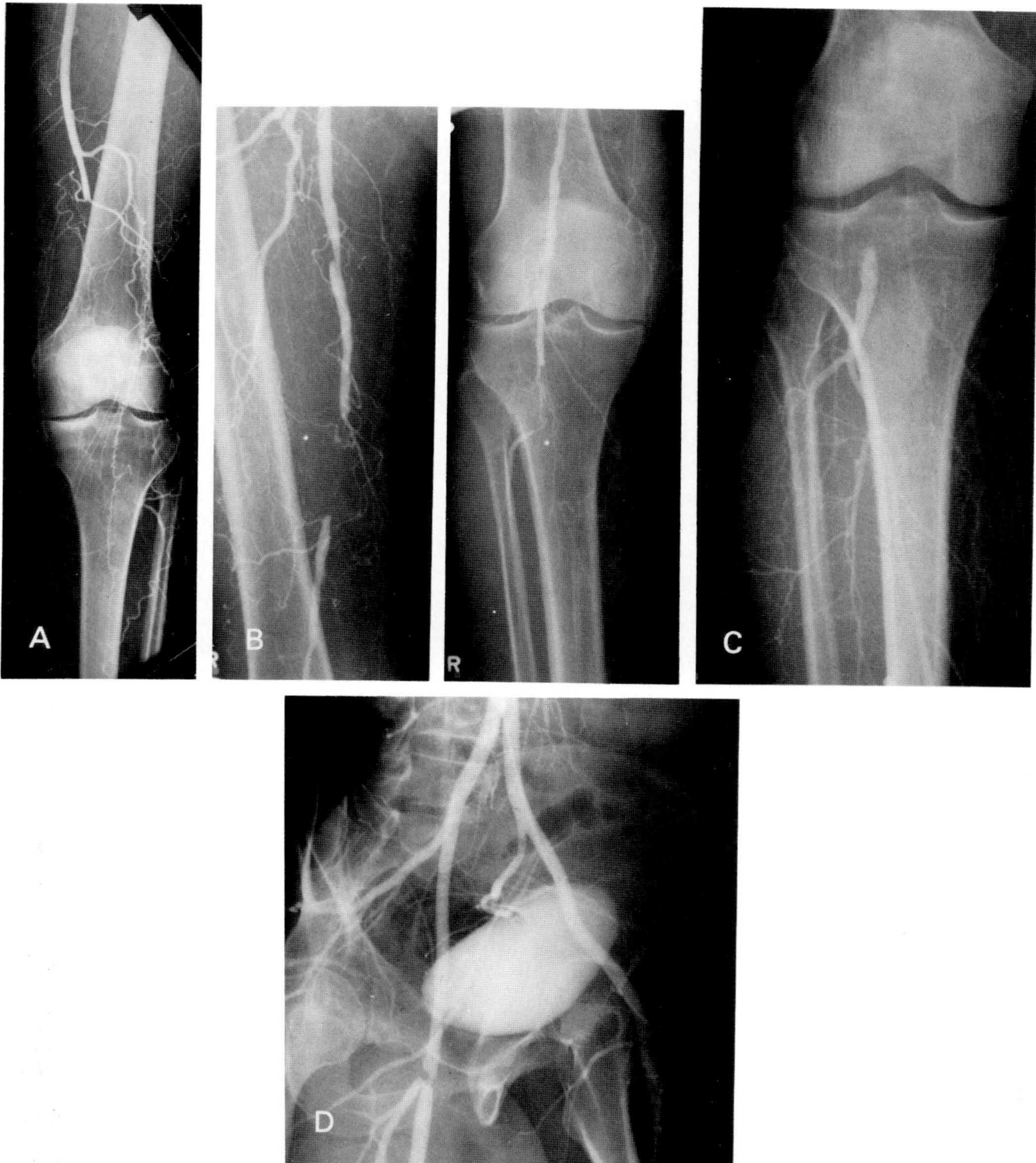

Figure 31.11. Acute arterial occlusion. *A*, Percutaneous femoral arteriogram demonstrating occlusion of popliteal and distal superficial femoral arteries proximal to point of origin of a large side branch from the femoral artery. Acute arterial occlusion was caused by a peripheral embolus. *B*, Percutaneous femoral arteriogram demonstrating superficial femoral occlusion *(left)* and thrombosis of terminal popliteal artery *(right)*. This patient had symptoms of acute arterial occlusion superimposed on longstanding symptoms of intermittent claudication in same extremity. *C*, Percutaneous femoral arteriogram demonstrating occlusion of popliteal artery in patient with a thrombosed popliteal aneurysm. *D*, Oblique runoff aortogram demonstrating high-grade stenosis of right common femoral artery just above its bifurcation produced by an atheroma. Patient had ischemic digits secondary to small-particle emboli believed to be formed at site of femoral arterial stenosis.

prevent irreversible ischemic changes, and prompt diagnosis can make successful revascularization possible. As soon as the diagnosis of renal arterial occlusion is entertained, renal perfusion should be evaluated by scintiscanning with intravenous radionuclide. If renal perfusion is not demonstrated, arteriographic assessment of the renal artery should be undertaken and a vascular surgeon should be consulted immediately.

Treatment

In cases of acute arterial occlusion, success in restoring normal function depends on the promptness of restoration of arterial blood flow. The examining physician must deal with the problem definitively and must not consign the patient to a prolonged period of observation. When the diagnosis of acute arterial occlusion is entertained, a surgeon experienced in the management of this condition should be consulted for further therapy, and arrangements should be made for angiographic examination. In the interim, intravenous administration of heparin is advisable, unless there is a specific contraindication.

Chronic Arterial Occlusion

Clinical Presentation

Less frequently, patients may come to the emergency department with chronic arterial occlusive disease, usually atherosclerotic in origin. Their primary complaint is usually intermittent claudication, but they may also have other symptoms, such as cutaneous ulceration or ischemic pain at rest. Recent progression of symptoms indicates acute thrombosis superimposed on the chronic process.

The history and physical examination usually suggest the diagnosis. The physician establishes the time of onset of discomfort and the progression of symptoms. The usual symptom, intermittent claudication, is described as a cramp, an ache, tightness, or tiredness in the affected muscle. Since the patient frequently attributes this symptom to a musculoskeletal disorder, the examiner must establish carefully what aggravates and alleviates the pain. Intermittent claudication almost always occurs with exercise and usually develops after the same amount of exercise, for example, walking a specific distance. It is relieved completely by rest. *Sudden* progression of the symptoms indicates occlusion within the affected arterial tree.

Ischemic pain at rest involves the most distal parts of the affected extremity, but may be localized to an ulcer or a gangrenous digit. It may be aggravated by cold or elevation of the limb. Pain of ischemic neuropathy, on the other hand, is generally diffuse and involves a large area of the affected extremity. It may not be aggravated by cold or elevation of the limb.

Acute deep venous thrombosis in an extremity may also cause severe pain characterized by diffuse deep aching. As in intermittent claudication, the pain may be caused by exercise. It is not relieved by rest, however, although elevation of the extremity may produce relief.

A physical abnormality elsewhere in the cardiovascular system may alert the physician to the underlying disease responsible for pain in an extremity. For example, the physician suspects an embolic occlusion, if such a patient with this type of pain is found to have atrial fibrillation or mitral stenosis.

Diagnosis

Physical examination of the patient with suspected peripheral vascular disease includes assessment of the blood pressure in *both* arms. Determination of segmental blood pressures in the affected extremity in comparison with the normal extremity is accomplished by a blood pressure cuff and a Doppler ultrasonic flow detector. In patients with leg symptoms, comparison of blood pressures in the ankle in the resting state and after a standard exercise test is also helpful. The more profound the ischemia, the greater the drop in pressure recorded after exercise. If there is no drop in pressure, other causes for symptoms must be considered, such as a musculoskeletal or neurologic disorder.

The heart, origins of the great vessels, the distal abdominal aorta, and the carotid, subclavian, iliac, and femoral arteries should be auscultated to detect bruits. Pulsations in the peripheral arteries are assessed carefully by palpation. The degree of arterial pulsation is evaluated best by someone experienced in examining for pulses in both healthy persons and those with arterial disease. Pulses are generally graded on a scale of 0–4, 0 indicating absent pulsation, and 4, normal pulsation.

The physician searches for cutaneous manifestations of vascular disease such as xanthoma, and notes the color of the skin. Cutaneous signs may be more noticeable immediately in the acute state than in chronic arterial occlusion; in the former, the skin distal to the occlusion is blue or white. The ischemic muscle is tender, and there is diminished sensation and motor function in the ischemic area.

In chronic arterial occlusion, skin and muscle atrophy may be apparent. Cutaneous ischemia can be documented by an elevation and dependency test. In a healthy person, elevation of an extremity causes mild pallor, but in a person with significant arterial occlusive disease, the degree of pallor after 1-minute elevation is more marked. When the extremity of a healthy person is returned to the dependent position, it resumes the normal skin color in roughly

10 seconds. In patients with arterial occlusive disease, significant pallor may be evident when the affected extremity is elevated about 45°, normal color returns more slowly on dependency, and the extremity eventually assumes a deep redness, termed dependent rubor. The degree of ischemia is measured both by the time prior to the appearance of rubor and by its proximal extension. In the case of acute arterial occlusion with no antecedent arterial disease, rubor does not develop until ischemia has existed for more than 10 days.

Venous filling time is the time necessary to fill the superficial veins of the foot after emptying by elevation of the leg and subsequent dependency. A venous filling time longer than 15 seconds in the absence of venous varicosities is evidence of arterial insufficiency.

Treatment

Patients with chronic arterial occlusion and ischemic ulcers should be hospitalized. If the ulcer is infected, specimens are taken for a Gram's stain and culture and the patient treated with appropriate antibiotics, elevation of the head of the bed, and saline dressings on moist, open lesions. Patients with ischemic pain at rest should also be hospitalized with elevation of the head of the bed, warm room temperature, and administration of necessary analgesics for pain. The feasibility of reconstruction is assessed by arteriographic examination (Fig. 31.12).

Venous Thrombosis

Deep Venous Thrombosis

Clinical Findings. The symptoms of venous obstruction depend on the level and degree of obstruction, the available collateral venous circulation, and the underlying cause of the obstruction. The diagnosis is sometimes obvious, as in a swollen limb that is either tender from local inflammation at the point of thrombosis or "silent," becoming evident only when a pulmonary thromboembolic event ensues. Deep venous thrombosis is more common in association with congestive heart failure, childbirth, operation, serious illness, and trauma. It may result from an obstruction to venous outflow such as pelvic tumor, or in the case of the arm, impingement on the subclavian vein by thoracic outlet compression.

Thrombotic occlusion of the inferior vena cava or either common iliac vein produces leg symptoms including edema, pain, varicosities, and/or cutaneous signs of chronic stasis with ulceration. The patient may have intermittent episodes of thrombophlebitis. This syndrome is sometimes seen after ligation of the inferior vena cava, or placement of an intracaval filter.

Treatment. Because of the risk of pulmonary embolism, it is *imperative* to hospitalize patients with deep venous thrombosis. Patients in whom this diagnosis is suspected are treated initially with bed rest and heparin, a 5000-unit bolus intravenously, followed by continuous intravenous heparin, 1000 u/hr, monitored by frequent partial thromboplastin times. Phlebography is then performed to demonstrate the accuracy of the diagnosis of deep venous thrombosis (Fig. 31.13). If no thrombus is visualized in the deep venous system, anticoagulants are discontinued and other causes considered, such as a ruptured plantaris tendon, a systemic cause for dependent edema, chronic postphlebitic state, local infection, primary lymphedema, and secondary causes of lympathic obstruction, including malignant conditions.

If deep venous thrombosis is confirmed by phlebography, the patient is hospitalized for an additional 7–10 days for continuous intravenous heparin therapy, during which time oral anticoagulant therapy with sodium warfarin (Coumadin) is started. In patients in whom anticoagulation is contraindicated, such as those with an active duodenal ulcer or acute cerebrovascular accident, either angiographic placement of an intracaval filter, or ligation or plication of the inferior vena cava is necessary. Patients with recurring episodes of thrombophlebitis in the leg are treated on an outpatient basis with long-term anticoagulant therapy, elastic support when ambulatory, and elevation of the leg at rest.

Occasionally, deep venous thrombosis progresses beyond the usual clinical phase of acute thrombophlebitis *(phlegmasia alba dolens)* to blue phlebitis *(phlegmasia cerulea dolens)*. The latter condition is manifested by engorgement of the extremity with cyanosis and tenderness. If the retrograde venous pressure increases sufficiently, arterial flow may cease, leading to ischemia and even gangrene. The diagnosis of phlegmasia cerulea dolens is made by physical examination and phlebography, excluding arterial involvement by arteriography when necessary. Most of the patients are best treated by anticoagulants and extreme elevation of the leg. If gangrene seems imminent, venous thrombectomy and long-term anticoagulation are sometimes necessary.

Superficial Venous Thrombosis

Symptoms of thrombosis of the superficial venous system include pain over the course of the thrombosed vein and occasionally erythema. If no infection seems present, this condition is managed on an outpatient basis with elastic compression and heat. If, however, involvement extends to the saphenofemoral junction, hospitalization and anticoagulation are advisable because of the threat of

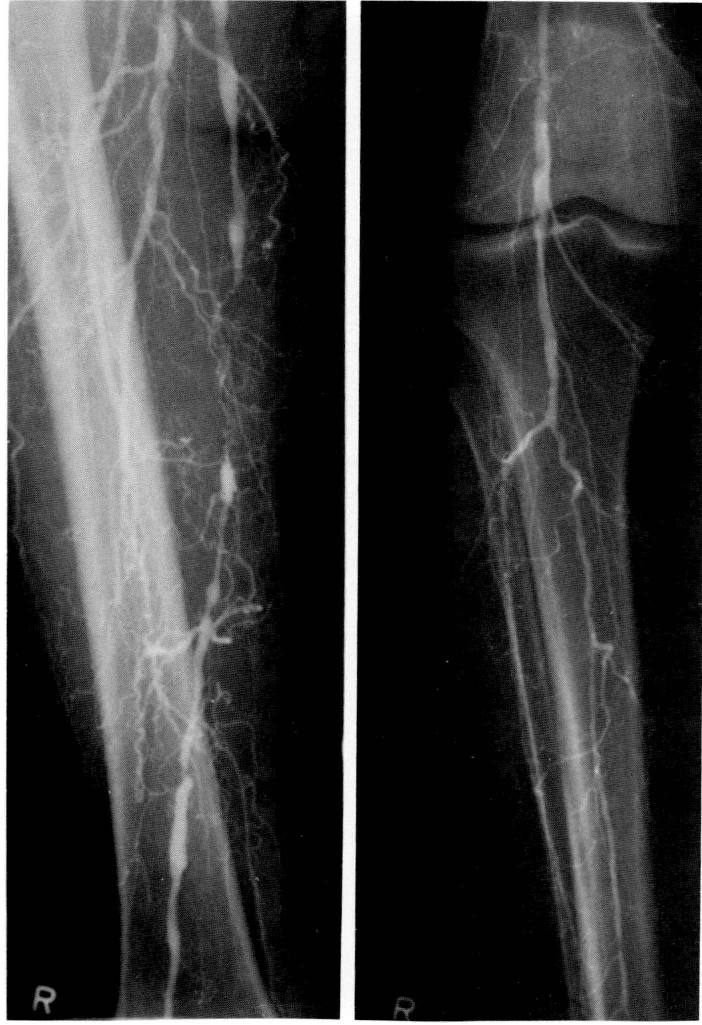

Figure 31.12. Percutaneous femoral arteriogram demonstrating extensive atheromatous occlusive changes in superficial femoral artery *(left)* and popliteal and tibial arteries *(right)*, a pattern frequently seen in patients with diabetes mellitus.

deep venous thrombosis. If infection is present, often the case at sites of recent venipuncture for intravenous therapy, the patient is hospitalized, cultures obtained, and appropriate antibiotic therapy instituted.

Cutaneous changes due to venous stasis, occurring primarily in the distal part of the lower leg, may lead to skin ulceration. If distal pulses are diminished or absent, the lesion must be regarded as an ischemic ulcer and treated with prompt hospitalization, conservative debridement of necrotic tissue, antibiotic therapy, and subsequent evaluation of the adequacy of arterial circulation. If pulses in the foot seem normal, the physician should ascertain whether there is invasive infection and whether treatment of the patient outside the hospital will be effective. In most cases, the patient should be hospitalized for treatment of the ulcer and instruction on how to care for it at home.

The Diabetic Foot

Clinical Considerations

The emergency physician frequently is called on to treat ulceration, infection, and gangrene resulting from complications of diabetes mellitus, such as obliterative arterial disease and neuropathy. In a diabetic patient, obliterative arterial disease involves both large and small arteries. Lesions may develop

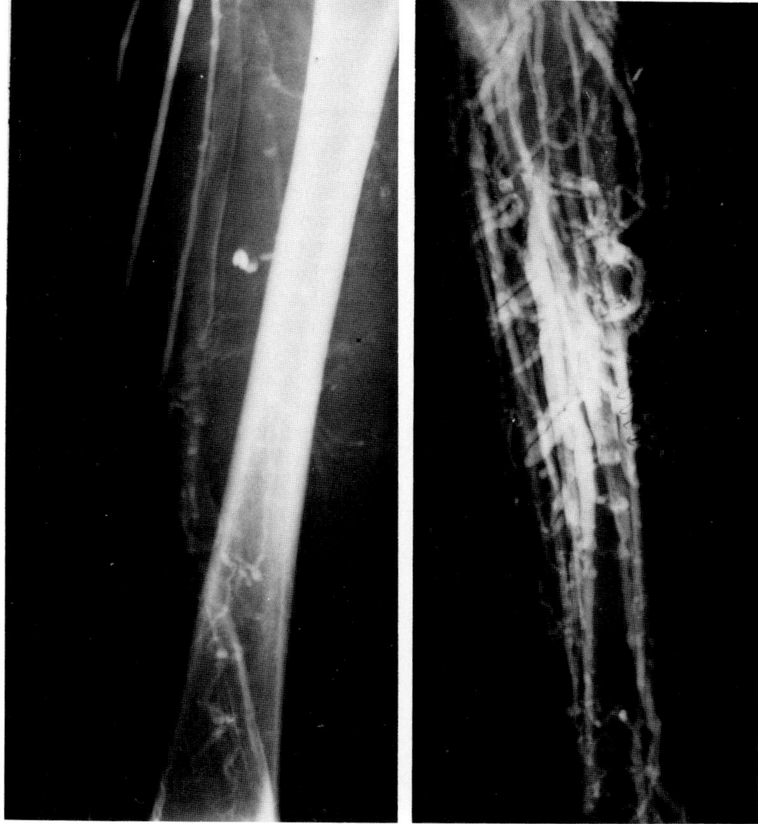

Figure 31.13. Phlebogram of a lower extremity demonstrating extensive deep venous thrombosis in superficial femoral vein *(left)* and soleal veins *(right)*.

as a consequence of occlusion of either the aortoiliac or femoropopliteal systems, or of the small arteries of the lower leg and foot. The progression of the obliterative process differs in large and small arteries, and gangrenous changes in a toe or the distal part of the foot can actually occur in the presence of bounding pedal pulses. With extensive obliterative disease of other small vessels, infection in the soft tissue of a digit may progress to cause complete thrombotic occlusion of the arterial supply, with resulting gangrene. This condition is termed *infectious gangrene of the digits*. As another complication of diabetes mellitus, neuropathy is important in that loss of sensation of pain and temperature may prevent the patient's perception of mechanical or thermal trauma with resulting ulceration and invasive infection. Lesions in the feet of diabetic patients are much more common in the presence of such neuropathy.

The portal of entry of infection is often near a toenail or through an ulcer in a callus at the site of constant friction. These calluses are usually located over the heads of the metatarsal bones. Progression of invasive infection may develop, depending on the resistance of the host, virulence of the organism, and promptness of treatment.

Treatment

All diabetic patients with foot infections should be hospitalized for bed rest. Gram's stains and cultures with sensitivity testing are obtained, and systemic antibiotic therapy started on the basis of the Gram's stain. Antibiotics should not be withheld until return of the results of cultures and sensitivity tests. The physician carefully ascertains whether the foot requires drainage of trapped pus and debridement of necrotic tissue. A diabetic foot threatened by sepsis may be saved by early, careful debridement and drainage. It is important for the emergency physician to consult a surgeon early in the treatment plan. The physician must keep in mind that metabolic management of a diabetic patient is complicated by the infection and that coexistent cardiac and renal problems may lead to further morbidity and possible death.

The presence of atherosclerotic occlusive disease in the aortoiliac or femoropopliteal system in a diabetic is suggested by the absence of pulses and confirmed by arteriographic examination, from which the feasibility of arterial reconstruction can be assessed. Early arterial reconstruction may save an extremity threatened by an ischemic lesion.

Vasospastic States

Acute vasospasm leading to severe pain, ulceration, and necrosis of the tips of digits usually occurs in the arm and is commonly termed either Raynaud's *phenomenon* when it is secondary to an underlying connective tissue disorder or Raynaud's *disease* when the underlying cause cannot be determined. This commonly occurs in young women, with a frequent history of pain and blanching of the fingers, and occasionally the toes, associated with emotion or exposure to cold. The physician should search for bruits, palpate for peripheral pulses, determine segmental blood pressures, and assess whether there is entrapment of structures within the thoracic outlet.

In the differential diagnosis, the possibilities of an atherosclerotic occlusion at the origin of the brachiocephalic vessels, compression at the thoracic outlet, arterial embolism, chronic dissecting aneurysm, and arteriosclerotic changes in the digital vasculature must all be considered. A chest roentgenogram questioning a cervical rib and angiograms are helpful diagnostic aids. If vasospasm is believed to be the primary difficulty and if these differential entities can be excluded, an active search for collagen disease is begun on an office diagnostic basis. Immediate relief may be produced by reserpine or papaverine administered intraarterially or by stellate ganglionic blockade, if there is persisting painful vasospasm. A patient with vasospasm and a digital ulcer should be hospitalized for local care, antibiotic therapy, and consideration for cervicodorsal sympathectomy.

Complications Following Arterial Reconstruction

With advances in vascular surgery leading to increasing operations for aneurysms and arterial occlusive disease, it is inevitable that both early and late complications of these procedures will be seen more frequently in an emergency department. Early complications include local wound infections and hematomas, deep venous thrombosis with the threat of pulmonary embolism, thrombosis of the reconstructed arterial tree causing distal ischemia, mechanical obstruction of the small intestine, and flare-up of antecedent illness. A late complication is proximal and/or distal progression of the atherosclerotic occlusive process, producing *thrombosis of arterial grafts* and of arteries on which endarterectomy has been performed. Symptoms resemble those of either acute or chronic arterial occlusion with increasing ischemia. A less common late complication is *aneurysm* at a suture line. These aneurysms usually increase in size, resulting in either a local mass with pain and venous obstruction, or rupture with acute hemorrhage, demanding prompt operative intervention. As with all aneurysms, laminar clot in the aneurysmal wall may break away and result in distal embolic occlusion. Thrombus formed along the wall of an arterial graft may also cause distal embolic occlusion. A rare late complication of aortic and iliac arterial grafts is formation of a *fistula* to the small intestine at a graft suture line. This results in gastrointestinal bleeding that is, surprisingly, often intermittent until a major life-threatening hemorrhage occurs. The early evidence of this complication must not be overlooked.

If patient has undergone arterial reconstruction, the records of the previous hospitalization are invaluable in the identification of details of the prior operation. Prompt assistance of the vascular surgeon who previously cared for the patient should be sought.

SUGGESTED READINGS

Akins CW, Buckley MJ, Daggett WM, et al. Acute traumatic disruption of the thoracic aorta: a 10-year experience. *Ann Thorac Surg,* 1981;31:305–309.

Anton GE, Hertzer NR, Beven EG, et al. Surgical management of popliteal aneurysms. Trends in presentation, treatment and results from 1952 to 1985. *J Vasc Surg* 1986;3:125–134.

Athanasoulis CA, Pfister RC, Greene RE, et al. Interventional Radiology. Philadelphia: WB Saunders, 1982.

Baker, CC, Thomas AN, Trunkey DD. The role of emergency room thoracotomy in trauma. *J. Trauma* 1980;20:848–854.

Beare, JP, Scribner RG, Fogarty, TJ. Arterial thromboembolism. A 20-year perspective. *Arch Surg,* 1985;120: 595–599.

Beebe, HG (ed). Complications in Vascular Surgery. Philadelphia: JP Lippincott, 1973.

Bergan JJ, Yao JST (eds). Surgery of the Aorta and Its Body Branches. New York: Grune & Stratton, 1979.

Bergan, JJ, Yao, JST (eds). Cerebrovascular Insufficiency. New York: Grune & Stratton, 1983.

Bergan, JJ, Yao JST (eds). Evaluation and Treatment of Upper and Lower Extremity Circulatory Disorders. New York: Grune & Stratton, 1984.

Bergan JJ, Yao JST (eds). Surgery of the Veins. New York: Grune & Stratton, 1985.

Bergan JJ, Yao JST (eds). Vascular Surgical Emergencies. New York: Grune & Stratton, 1987.

Blaisdell, FW, Steele M, Allen RE. Management of acute lower extremity arterial ischemia due to embolism and thrombosis. *Surgery* 1978;84:822–834.

Bondai BI, Smith JP, Ward RE, et al. Emergency thoracotomy in the management of trauma. A review. *JAMA* 1983;249:1891–1896.

Borman KR, Aurbakken CM, Weigelt JA. Treatment priorities in combined blunt abdominal and aortic trauma. *Am J Surg* 1982;144:728–732.

Breaux EP, Dupon JB, Albert HM, et al. Cardiac tamponade following penetrating mediastinal injuries: improved survival with early pericardiocentesis. *J. Trauma* 1979;19:461–466.

Bryant LR, Mobin-Uddin K, Dillon ML, et al. Cardiac valve injury with major chest trauma. *Arch Surg* 1973;107:279–283.

Case Records of the Massachusetts General Hospital. Case 20–1984. *N Engl J Med* 1984;310–1310.

Cranley JJ. Ischemic rest pain. *Arch Surg* 1969;97:187–188.

Crisler C, Bahnson HT. Aneurysms of the aorta. *Curr Probl Surg* 1972;9(Dec),1–64.

Dale WA. The swollen leg. *Curr Probl Surg* 1973;10(Sep), 1–66.

Danto LA, Fry WJ, Kraft RO. Acute aortic thrombosis. *Arch Surg* 1972;104:569–572.

Dean RH, Yao JST. Hemodynamic measurements in peripheral vascular disease. *Curr Probl Surg* 1976;13(Aug), 1–76.

Doty DB, Anderson AE, Rose EF, et al. Cardiac trauma: Clinical and experimental correlations of myocardial contusion. *Ann Surg* 1974;180:452–460.

Eagle KA, Quertermous T, Kritzer GA, et al. Spectrum of conditions initially suggesting acute aortic dissection but with negative aortograms. *Am J Cardiol* 1986;57:322–326.

Egan TJ, Neiman HL, Herman RJ, et al. Computed tomography in the diagnosis of aortic aneurysm dissection or traumatic injury. *Body Computed Tomography* 1980;136:141–149.

Ergin MA, Galla JD, Lansman S, et al. Acute dissections of the aorta. *Surg Clin North Am* 1985;65:721–741.

Evans J, Gray LA, Rayner A. et al. Principles for the management of penetrating cardiac wounds. *Ann Surg* 1979;189:777–784.

Fairbairn JF, Juergens JL, Spittell JA (eds). Peripheral Vascular Disease. Philadelphia: WB Saunders, 1980.

Godwin JD, Korobkin M. Acute disease of the aorta. Diagnosis by computed tomography and ultrasonography. *Radiol Clin North Am* 1983;21:551–574.

Graham LM, Zelenock GB, Whitehouse WN, et al. Clinical significance of arteriosclerotic femoral artery aneurysms. *Arch Surg* 1980;115:502–507.

Gray L Jr, Kirsh M. A new roentgenographic finding in acute traumatic rupture of the aorta. *J Thorac Cardiovasc Surg* 1975;70:86–88.

Gundry SR, Williams S, Burney RE, et al. Indications of aortography in blunt thoracic trauma: a reassessment. *J Trauma*, 1982;22:664–671.

Harley DP, Mena I, Narahara K, et al. Traumatic myocardial dysfunction. *J Thorac Cardiovasc Surg*, 1984;87:386–393.

Heiberg E, Wolverson MK, Sundaram M, et al. CT in aortic trauma. *Am J Roent*, 1983;140:1119–1124.

Imparato AM, Kim G, Davidson T. et al. Intermittent claudication. Its natural course. *Surgery* 1975;78:795–799.

Ivatury RR, Shah PM, Ito K, et al. Emergency room thoracotomy for the resuscitation of patients with "fatal" penetrating injuries to the heart. *Ann Thorac Surg*, 1981;32:377–385.

Killen DA, Gobbell WG Jr., France R. Post-traumatic aneurysm of the left ventricle. *Circulation* 1969;39:101–108.

King RM, Mucha R Jr, Seward JB, et al. Cardiac contusion: A new diagnostic approach utilizing two-dimensional echocardiography. *J Trauma*, 1983;23:610–614.

Kirsh MM, Sloan H. Blunt Chest Trauma. General Principles of Management. Boston: Little, Brown & Co, 1977.

Kirsh, MM, Behrendt DM, Orringer MB, et al. The treatment of acute traumatic rupture of aorta: A 10-year experience. *Ann Surg*, 1976;184:308–316.

Levin ME, O'Neal LW (eds). The Diabetic Foot. St. Louis: CV Mosby, 1983.

Liedtke AJ, Demuth WE. Nonpenetrating cardiac injuries. A collective review. *Am Heart J*, 1984;86:687–697.

Mannick JA. Current concepts in diagnostic methods. Evaluation of chronic lower extremity ischemia. *N Engl J Med*, 1983;309:841–843.

McCready RA, Pairolero PC, Gilmore JC, et al. Isolated iliac artery aneurysms. *Surgery*, 1983;93:688–693.

Miller DC, Stinson EB, Oyer PE, et al. Operative treatment of aortic dissections: Experience with 125 patients over a sixteen-year period. *J Thorac Cardiovasc Surg* 1979;78:365–382.

Miller DC, Mitchell RS, Oyer PE, et al. Independent determinants of operative mortality for patients with aortic dissection. *Circulation* 1984;70(suppl. 1):I–153.

Moore EE, Moore JB, Galloway AC, et al. Postinjury thoracotomy in the emergency department: A critical evaluation. *Surgery* 1979;86:590–598.

Oliva PB, Hilgenberg AD, McElroy D. Obstruction of the proximal right coronary artery with acute inferior infarction due to blunt chest trauma. *Ann Intern Med* 1979;91:205–207.

Pairolero PC, Walls JJ, Payne WS, et al. Subclavian axillary artery aneurysms. *Surgery*, 1981;90:757–763.

Parmley LF, Mattingly TW, Manion WC, et al. Nonpenetrating traumatic injury of the aorta. *Circulation*, 1958;17:1086–1101.

Pickard LR, Mattox KL, Beall AC, Jr. Ventricular septal defect from blunt chest injury. *J Trauma*, 1980;20:329–331.

Pifarre R, Grieco J, Garibaldi A, et al. Acute coronary artery occlusion secondary to blunt chest trauma. *J Thorac Cardiovasc Surg*, 1982;83:122–125.

Potkin RT, Werner JA, Trobaugh GB, et al. Evaluation of noninvasive tests of cardiac damage in suspected cardiac contusion. *Circulation*, 1982;66:627–631.

Rosenthal A, Parisi LE, Nadas AJ. Isolated interventricular septal defect due to nonpenetrating trauma. Report of a case with spontaneous healing. *N Engl J Med*, 1970;283:338–341.

Rutherford R. Vascular Surgery. Philadelphia: WB Saunders, 1984.

Sefczek DM, Sefczek RJ, Deeb ZL. Radiographic signs of acute traumatic rupture of the thoracic aorta. *Am J Roent*, 1983;141:1259–1262.

Slater EE, DeSanctis RW. The clinical recognition of dissecting aortic aneurysm. *Am J Med*, 1976;60:625–633.

Smith JM III, Grover FL, Marcocas JL, et al. Blunt traumatic rupture of the atria. *J Thorac Cardiovasc Surg*, 1976;71:617–620.

Stanley JC, Thompson NW, Fry WJ. Splanchnic artery aneurysms. *Arch Surg*, 1970;101:689–697.

Symbas PN. Great vessels injury. *Am Heart J*, 1977;93:518–522.

Tavares S, Hankins JR, Moulton AL, et al. Management of penetrating cardiac injuries. The role of emergency room thoracotomy. *Ann Thorac Surg*, 1984;38:183–187.

Tawes RL, Harris EJ, Brown WH, et al. Arterial thromboembolism. A 20-year perspective. *Arch Surg*, 1985;120: 595–599.

Taylor LM, Porter JM. Drug treatment of claudication: Vasodilator, hemorrhologic agents and antiserotonin drugs. *J Vasc Surg*, 1986;3:374–381.

Trinkle JK, Toon RS, Franz JL, et al. Affairs of the wounded heart: penetrating cardiac wounds. *J Trauma*, 1979;19:467-472.

Torres-Mirable P, Gruenberg JC, Brown RS. Spectrum of myocardial contusion. *Am Surg*, 1982;48:383–389.

Unger SW, Tucker WS, Mrdeza MA, et al. Carotid arterial trauma. *Surgery*, 1980;87:477–487.
Wernly JA, Campbell CD, Replogle RL. Traumatic avulsion of the innominate and left carotid arteries. *J Thorac Cardiovasc Surg*, 1982;84:392–397.
White RD, Lipton MJ, Higgins CB, et al. Noninvasive evaluation of suspected thoracic aortic disease by contrast-enhanced computed tomography. *Am J Cardiol*, 1986;57:282–290.
Wilson SE, Veith FJ, Hobson RW. Vascular Surgery. Principles and Practice. New York: McGraw-Hill, 1987.

CHAPTER **32**

General Thoracic Emergencies

DOUGLAS J. MATHISEN, M.D.
JOHN M. HEAD, M.D.

All medical personnel should be well-versed in the recognition and management of certain thoracic emergencies. Disturbances of the critical elements of ventilation make thoracic emergencies potentially life-threatening situations. Successful outcomes demand prompt recognition, awareness of principles of management, knowledge of a few fundamental procedures, and the expeditious implementation of a plan of action. Failure on any of these counts can lead to loss of life or significant morbidity for the patient. Coordinated efforts among a variety of medical professionals may be required to achieve these goals.

Only in the context of an overall plan for management can the emergency physician truly comprehend his or her role; thus, in many subjects discussed in this chapter a brief description is supplied for operative management after leaving the department.

AIRWAY OBSTRUCTION

Initial Steps

Relief of airway obstruction takes first priority in any emergency. No resuscitation attempt is successful in the presence of an inadequate airway. The following steps should be observed: *(a)* The mouth and hypopharynx should be cleared of secretions or blood by digital exploration and suction. *(b)* An obstruction at the level of the hypopharynx should be relieved by an oral airway. *(c)* An obstruction at the glottic or subglottic level requires tracheal intubation. The quickest method is usually passage of an orotracheal tube with the aid of a laryngoscope for visualization of the vocal cords. Alternately, a rigid bronchoscope may be passed and left in place until it can be replaced by a nasotracheal or tracheotomy tube. An obstruction low in the trachea can be relieved only by passage of a bronchoscope, long endotracheal tube, or tracheotomy tube to a level of just above the carina.

All indwelling tubes used for assisted ventilation should be fitted with low-pressure, high-volume cuffs to avoid the complications of tracheal erosion, stenosis, and perforation.

In a case of extreme urgency when proper equipment is unavailable, such as a patient aspirating food at a restaurant, another method for relief of acute laryngeal obstruction must be used. If food aspiration is suspected, a brief attempt should be made to clear the hypopharynx with the fingers or a curved forceps. If this is unsuccessful, the *Heimlich maneuver* is employed to dislodge the obstructing material. This is performed by standing behind the patient with arms around him/her, placing the fists one on top of the other high in the epigastrium, and forcibly squeezing. If neither of these methods is quickly effective, *emergency cricothyrotomy* must be performed. Insertion of a 15-gauge (1.5 inch) needle through the cricothyroid membrane will sustain

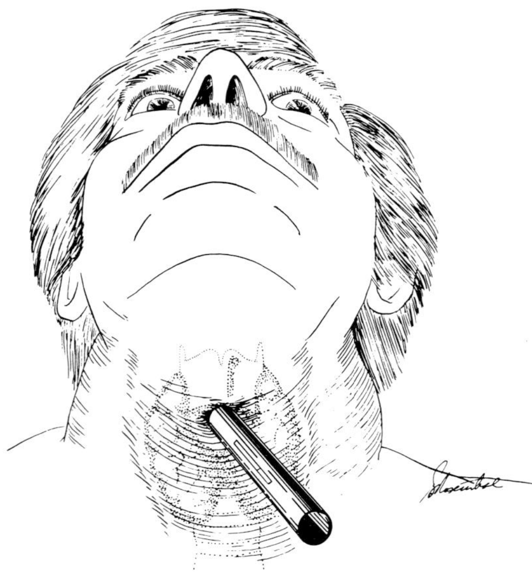

Figure 32.1. Emergency (out of the hospital) cricothyrotomy performed by rapid incision of skin with transverse stab wound of cricothyroid membrane and insertion of barrel of ballpoint pen.

life for 15–20 minutes in an otherwise healthy person (see Illustrated Technique 4). Similarly, rapid incision of the cricothyroid membrane and insertion of the empty barrel of a ballpoint pen (Fig. 32.1) is satisfactory until intubation, formal tracheotomy, or removal of the obstruction can be accomplished. As soon as an adequate airway is established, secretions and blood must be aspirated to clear the lower respiratory tree.

All physicians engaged in emergency care should obtain instruction in emergency laryngoscopy, intubation, and bronchoscopy from an anesthesiologist or thoracic surgeon or through a course of postgraduate instruction. These techniques are essential to adequate care in thoracic emergencies. A brief discussion of endotracheal intubation and bronchoscopy is presented in the following sections.

Endotracheal Intubation

Endotracheal intubation is preferred in the management of a wide variety of conditions manifested by obstruction and/or inefficient respiration. Upper airway obstruction in any patient can be relieved by intubation if passage of a tube is technically feasible. Likewise, an endotracheal tube will be necessary in any patient requiring positive-pressure assisted ventilation.

No absolute indications for intubation can be set forth. In general, it is indicated if severe obstruction due to hypopharyngeal or laryngeal edema is developing. It is also required when fatigue impairs ventilatory function or when respiration becomes too inefficient to maintain the arterial partial pressure of oxygen (Po_2) above 60 mm Hg or the partial pressure of carbon dioxide (Pco_2) below 50 mm Hg.

A nasotracheal tube is preferred to an orotracheal tube if intubation is required for more than 24 hours. It is more comfortable for the patient, and there is less motion and less possible damage of the tracheal mucosa. The caliber of the tube should be as large as possible to permit adequate aspiration of secretions and to minimize plugging. A nonreactive plastic tube with a low-pressure, high-volume cuff is preferred. It may be left in place for weeks if necessary, but if intubation is required for more than 7–10 days, tracheotomy should be performed. A tracheotomy tube is more easily kept free of crusts, allows more efficient suctioning, and eliminates dead space, which might be crucial for certain patients.

In adults, it is important to remove endotracheal tubes in favor of tracheotomy tubes when prolonged mechanical ventilation seems likely. The risks of properly performed tracheotomy are less than those of endotracheal tubes. Large tubes in a small larynx, pressure of a balloon pulled inadvertently against the cricoid or larynx, or local reaction in the larynx predispose the patient to glottic or subglottic stenosis. These may be complicated, if not impossible, problems to repair satisfactorily. When cricothyrotomy has been performed, it should be converted to a formal tracheotomy within 24 hours to avoid these same potential problems. Exception to these guidelines can be made for infants, for whom it has been shown that tracheotomy carries a greater risk than long-term endotracheal intubation.

Certain injuries make endotracheal intubation dangerous, if not impossible. Massive intraoral hemorrhage or severe facial fractures may make visualization of the airway impossible. When an urgent airway is needed in this situation, emergency cricothyrotomy is preferred. Laryngotracheal trauma ia another instance when intubation may be difficult and dangerous. Destruction of laryngeal surfaces by inhalation burns is a third situation where endotracheal intubation may not be possible.

Bronchoscopy

Emergency bronchoscopy, or perhaps more properly, tracheoscopy, to provide an airway or to aspirate the airway may be a lifesaving maneuver. It requires the services of a physician trained in its use. The following tips are helpful in performing either emergency rigid or flexible bronchoscopy. The patient is placed in the supine position, and nasal cannulae are placed to oxygenate the patient. Electrodes for electrocardiogram (ECG) monitoring are placed on the patient. Topical anesthesia can be induced by spraying the back of the pharynx with 2% lidocaine (Xylocaine). The use of a 21-gauge butterfly intravenous needle connected to a syringe with 5 ml of 2% lidocaine is then used to provide intratracheal anesthesia. The needle should penetrate the midline of the cricothyroid membrane aiming inferiorly at a 30° angle. Gentle aspiration of the syringe provides a rush of air when the needle is in the airway; the lidocaine can then be safely administered slowly to avoid excessive coughing with the risk of laceration of the airway by the needle. The patient should then be encouraged to cough after all has been given, to help spread the lidocaine and also to anesthetize the vocal cords. The tongue is grasped by an assistant with a gauze sponge to aid in visualization of the epiglottis. The bronchoscopist stands at the head of the patient. An endotracheal tube may be placed over the flexible bronchoscope and advanced over the flexible scope once it is in the trachea. This can be used to secure an airway or to provide repeated access to aspirate secretions. Additional lidocaine can be administered through the bronchoscope as needed, but the limits of toxicity should be kept in mind. When using topical anesthesia, one must be prepared to deal with the consequences of lidocaine overdosage, predominately seizures, with airway control and intravenous Valium. For rigid bronchoscopy, the same procedures are utilized. The bronchoscope is kept in the midline, the epiglottis is visualized and lifted anteriorly until the cords are seen. The bronchoscope is then turned 90° to allow its tip to pass between the vocal cords into the trachea. The most common error is passage of the instrument too far beyond the epiglottis before lifting anteriorly, causing the instrument to enter the esophagus rather than the trachea.

SPACE-OCCUPYING COLLECTIONS

Needle Aspiration

Collections of air or fluid frequently require removal. In an emergency, needle aspiration is performed first to confirm the diagnosis and to determine the appropriate site for intercostal tube drainage, should the latter be necessary. If tension pneumothorax is present, needle aspiration alone provides temporary relief; a large-bore needle (15-gauge) left open to the air until a chest tube is inserted may be lifesaving. If tension exists, prompt measures should be immediately taken to insert an intercostal chest tube. *Needle aspiration should always precede insertion of a chest tube to confirm the presence of a collection.* This procedure may cause pneumothorax on occasion, but is far less dangerous than ill-advised attempts to insert intercostal catheters into nonexistent spaces, especially in the presence of pleural symphysis, since such attempts may result in laceration of the lung or pulmonary vessels.

Thoracentesis

The technique of thoracentesis depends on the location of the intrapleural collection. If possible, preliminary chest x-ray films consisting of posteroanterior and lateral views should be obtained with the patient in the upright position. Fluid collections are poorly seen in vertical projections with the patient in the recumbent position. When the upright position is not feasible, lateral decubitus and across-the-table lateral views in the supine position are helpful. The presence of pleural effusion should be confirmed, if possible by fluoroscopic examination or by lateral decubitus films to avoid the confusion occasioned by pleural thickening. When available in the emergency department, computed tomographic (CT) scanning is very helpful in confirming a pleural effusion.

In patients with pneumothorax, the best site for thoracentesis and subsequent thoracostomy, except in women or thick-chested men, is the second intercostal space at least 2 cm lateral to the sternum. Needle aspiration and chest tube insertion should be performed near the upper border of the rib to avoid the intercostal vessels. Unless the situation is extremely urgent, preliminary local anesthesia is employed, in which each layer, including the pleura, is anesthetized sequentially.

Information gained from the infiltrating needle is useful in estimating the thickness of the chest wall and of the pleura, and air or fluid aspirated from the pleural space serves as a diagnostic aid. If no air or fluid is obtained through a fine-gauge (no. 22) needle, an alternative site must be considered. If air or fluid is obtained, a chest tube may be inserted safely at the site.

In the management of pleural effusion or hydropneumothorax, thoracentesis or tube thoracostomy should be performed via the axilla if the patient must remain supine, or posterolaterally if he/she can sit up. The common error of attempting to place a needle or tube into the lowest level of an effusion often results in injury to the diaphragm, liver, or spleen. Frequently, it is impossible to determine the level of the diaphragm by radiologic evaluation (Fig. 32.2) or by physical examination, whereas the upper limit of the fluid is determined easily by either method. Percussion and auscultation are the most reliable means of determining the site of aspiration. As pleural fluid is removed, the lung expands and the meniscus remains at the same level, permitting removal of almost all of the fluid.

Intravenous catheters may be used for thoracen-

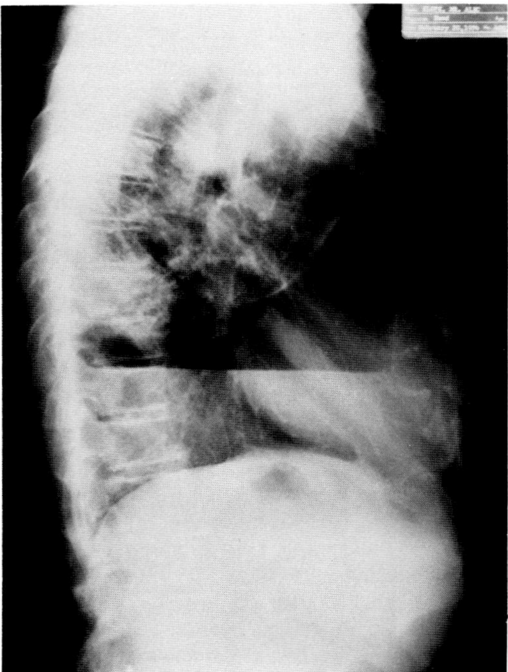

Figure 32.2. Lateral x-ray film of chest showing that diaphragm is visible only on normal left side. A large pleural effusion completely obliterates diaphragm on right side.

tesis instead of needle (see Illustrated Technique 12). Although they are less likely to injure the visceral pleura, they become plugged more easily when fibrin is present in the effusion. A large-bore (no. 14–16) needle can be used safely if a hemostat is employed as a step to prevent insertion of the needle past the minimal distance necessary to obtain fluid (Fig. 32.3). A needle can be manipulated more easily than a catheter, and it provides more tactile information about the chest wall and the consistency of the fluid. Use of uncontrolled suction is unwise because rapid evacuation of a large effusion may cause excessive or too sudden mediastinal shift, dyspnea, discomfort, and so-called "pleural shock." Although it is more laborious, use of a syringe and three-way stopcock is safe. A gentle suction system with clamping after removal of each 400–500 ml is a satisfactory technique. These methods allow appropriate expansion of the lung and equilibration of intrathoracic pressures.

Tube Thoracostomy

The two methods of chest tube placement are by trocar and by hemostat. Although fashioning a tract by blunt dissection with a hemostat (Fig. 32.4) may be slower, this technique is safer and provides the operator with more tactile information about the thickness and consistency of the pleura. Trocars are often too sharp for safe catheter placement; they may lacerate the intercostal vessels or lung too easily. Tube thoracostomy can be performed painlessly if the skin, fascia, and pleura are infiltrated with lidocaine (see Illustrated Technique 13). A heavy silk tie around the catheter at the desired skin level is helpful in determining how far to advance the tube. Proper positioning is most helpful in inserting catheters safely: lateral recumbency , with a blanket roll under the opposite chest permitting spread of the intercostal space.

In the management of pneumothorax, the use of a no. 20 Argyle catheter anteriorly is satisfactory. Especially in women, this is placed just behind the lateral border of the pectoralis major muscle. However, collections of fluid or blood should be drained by a no. 28 Argyle catheter posterolaterally or low in the axilla. The tube must be secured to the skin with heavy nonabsorbable sutures.

TRAUMA

Trauma causes many of the serious thoracic emergencies seen in civilian and military practice. As an initial consideration, the mechanism of injury and the type of physiologic impairment must be determined.

Pathophysiology

The common types of blunt trauma include:

1. Blast injuries, which are likely to produce cardiac and pulmonary contusion, or rupture of the tracheobronchial tree and/or diaphragm.
2. Crushing injuries, which are often accompanied by disruption of the chest wall, diaphragm, or tracheobronchial tree.
3. Deceleration, which causes injuries of the chest wall, lung, myocardium, trachea, bronchi, and aorta.
4. Hyperextension, which occasionally disrupts the intrathoracic portion of the thoracic duct.
5. Flexion, which produces overlapping transverse sternal fracture.

It must be remembered that patients with major blunt thoracic injuries are likely to have damage to other areas and organs. Such damage may be more serious than the thoracic disability, and its treatment may take precedence.

Penetrating chest injuries are produced by:

1. Knife wounds, which may cause insignificant surface lacerations, but which may inflict widespread internal damage to the area reached by the blade, including pulmonary and cardiovascular lacerations.

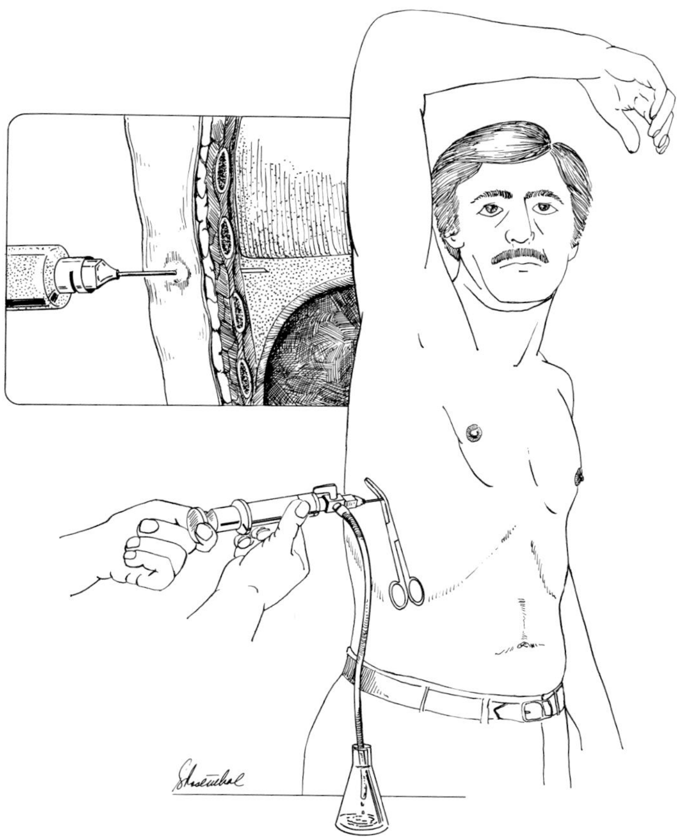

Figure 32.3. Thoracentesis: Needle is inserted just below fluid meniscus. A hemostat prevents insertion of needle more than a few millimeters past parietal pleura.

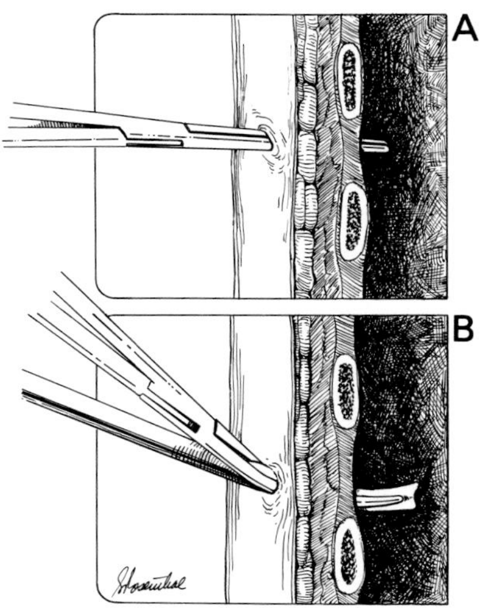

Figure 32.4. Intercostal chest tube placement. *A,* Formation of tract with hemostat. *B,* Insertion of tube with hemostat.

2. Missile wounds, which have an unpredictable path often difficult to determine and which produce tissue injury along the path of the projectile, the magnitude increasing with the velocity of the missile.

Evaluation and Initial Treatment

In the evaluation of penetrating wounds, the location of the lesion is of paramount importance. Careful recording of entrance and exit sites and of the angle of penetration is vital. Wounds of the base of the neck and of the upper part of the thorax may involve the trachea or larynx, the great vessels, the thoracic duct, the esophagus, or one or both lungs. Wounds of the midthorax are likely to damage the heart, the aorta, or a lung. Penetrating injuries lower in the chest may involve a lung, the diaphragm, the spleen, the liver, the stomach, or the colon.

The initial physical examination is crucial to the management of thoracic trauma. It is often all that is needed to make an immediate decision regarding therapy; occasionally it is all that is feasible. It should include careful observation of the wound at the entrance and exit sites and also of respiratory mechanics and skin color. Percussion and auscultation of the chest must be performed carefully and expeditiously, with the findings recorded for comparison with results of subsequent examination. Changes often reveal more about the extent of injury than does the initial evaluation. The physician should inquire briefly regarding preexisting disease. He/she should also note the characteristics of any sputum and of any material draining from the open wound and should observe the patient for the development of subcutaneous emphysema.

In any patient with major thoracic trauma, treatment must be started before diagnostic tests are completed. Lines for intravenous infusion and monitoring of central venous pressure are inserted while blood is drawn for laboratory studies and transfusion cross-matching. Central venous pressure readings are as important in the management of thoracic trauma as in the management of any other injury, because they provide vital diagnostic information concerning possible pericardial tamponade, blood volume, and circulatory dynamics. If injury of venous structures is suspected, venous access should be provided in the lower extremity. The technique of venous cutdown on the saphenous vein at the ankle (see Illustrated Technique 7) or insertion of a femoral vein line should be known to all caring for trauma patients.

In life-threatening situations, the following problems must be addressed before diagnostic evaluation is complete:

1. Upper airway obstruction must be relieved by whatever means required, and hypoxia must be treated by administration of oxygen.
2. Blood volume deficits must be replaced.
3. Major chest wall instability must be partly stabilized, either by pressure dressings, sandbags, or positive pressure-assisted ventilation.
4. Sucking wounds must be occluded by dressings.
5. Large air or fluid collections must be evacuated.
6. Pericardial tamponade must be relieved.

Once these steps are taken and the clinical state of the patient is reasonably stable, diagnostic testing can be initiated. Roentgenographic examination of the chest is the initial step including CT scanning where available, followed by chest fluoroscopy and a barium swallow, if they are indicated. If major vascular injury is suspected in a patient whose clinical condition is stable, angiographic examination should be performed early. With this radiographic information, the physician proceeds with such considerations as the need for nasogastric intubation, thoracentesis, and bronchoscopy. A Swan-Ganz pulmonary artery catheter may provide useful information in the evaluation and management of massive injuries involving multiple organs. Tetanus immunization, antibiotic therapy, and bladder catheterization complete the list of considerations. The treatment of other injuries is started.

Blunt Trauma

Most of the thoracic injuries seen in civilian practice result from blunt trauma, especially in a society oriented to contact sports and automobiles. Details of the traumatic event are important in determining the type of injury. For example, high-speed deceleration causes aortic transection, tracheobronchial disruption, and chest wall damage, whereas blast injuries cause serious cardiopulmonary contusion but little or no chest wall damage.

Chest Wall

Most thoracic trauma is accompanied by chest wall damage, ranging from localized contusion to extensive flail disruption. Chest wall damage itself is often severe enough to require vigorous treatment, and occasionally contributes to death of a patient. Central to its proper management are recognition and correction of the impaired ventilation that frequently develops.

Contusion of the chest wall results from domestic, athletic, industrial, and vehicular accidents. The diagnosis of rib fracture is usually identified by radiologic examination, but it may be impossible to exclude a fracture if the injury involves the anterior or diaphragmatic portions of the rib cage. Because local pain interferes with respiration and coughing, contusions should be treated in the same manner as simple rib fractures, with analgesic medications and chest physical therapy to assist in raising secretions. Contusions usually become asymptomatic in 1 or 2 weeks if there has been no disruption of bone or cartilage.

Simple rib fractures are usually caused by a direct blow to the chest wall. However, patients with osteoporosis are prone to rib fractures from minor trauma, or even from coughing or sneezing. Recognition of fractures is enhanced by a careful history and physical examination. The incident causing the fracture is usually known, pain develops abruptly and is aggravated by cough or motion, and the fracture site is always tender. Crepitation produced by motion of the bony fragments may be noted. A useful diagnostic maneuver is the application of pressure simultaneously on the sternum and back, avoiding pressure over the area of suspected fracture; resultant pain is a reliable indication of a rib fracture. Posteroanterior, lateral, and oblique roentgenograms are obtained when a fractured rib is suspected, as well as rib views, to exclude the possibility of intrapleural collections of blood or air.

Occasionally, collections are large enough to require evacuation even if only a single rib is fractured.

The treatment of simple rib fractures is adapted to individual needs. Patients in good health may need nothing more than a mild analgesic medication. On the other hand, an elderly patient with emphysema may require hospitalization, a narcotic analgesic, intercostal blocks, and chest physical therapy. One should not underestimate the potentially serious nature of rib fractures. Pain and splinting may lead to inadequate ventilation, atelectasis, sputum retention, pneumonia, respiratory distress, the need for assisted mechanical ventilation, or even death. A good rule of thumb in determining the potential serious nature of rib fractures is the addition of the number of rib fractures to the number of decades of the age of the patient; if this equals 10 or more, it is a potentially serious injury. Patients recovering from a fractured rib are most comfortable in a semi-upright or sitting position. Those who cannot tolerate opiates because of resultant respiratory despression may require intercostal nerve block to control pain, to permit adequate ventilation, and to allow for effective coughing. Nerve blocks are ineffective unless they involve two intercostal nerves above and two below the injured rib(s). Intercostal blocks are performed by injecting 2–3 ml of 2% lidocaine or a similar agent into the appropriate intercostal space just below the rib, 5–6 cm lateral to the posterior midline. Bupivicaine (Marcaine) 0.5% may provide longer lasting relief. The use of epinephrine in intercostal block solutions should be avoided.

First rib fractures may herald other more serious associated injuries. A great deal of force is required to fracture the first rib. The type of injury required to fracture the first rib may be associated with injuries to the cervical spine or to the aorta and its brachiocephalic branches. It is imperative to look carefully for these injuries and to utilize angiography if there is suspicion about major vascular injuries.

Sternal fracture occurs in less than 4% of major chest injuries. It rarely results from a direct blow to the sternum because the sternochondral or costochondral junctions give way instead. Sternal fractures are more often caused by acute flexion, which results in overlapping transverse disruption with or without associated fractured ribs. The upper fragment is usually displaced anteriorly over the lower fragment. (Fig. 32.5). This is a painful condition, causing severe disability. The fracture requires reduction and repair by intramedullary fixation. Injury of the internal mammary vessels may accompany sternal fracture; if so, surgical control of bleeding may be necessary. Widening of the mediastinum caused by mammary artery bleeding confuses the interpretation of chest radiographs and raises the question of aortic injury. A result of major trauma, sternal fractures are usually a component of serious anterior flail injuries and are often complicated by myocardial contusion and pulmonary laceration. The patient with a sternal fracture should be monitored for 3 days with daily full-lead ECG, cardiac isoenzymes, and continuous ECG monitoring. Thallium scanning may be used to detect suspected myocardial contusion. Sternal fractures are visible and palpable and can best be seen on lateral x-ray views or sternal computed tomography.

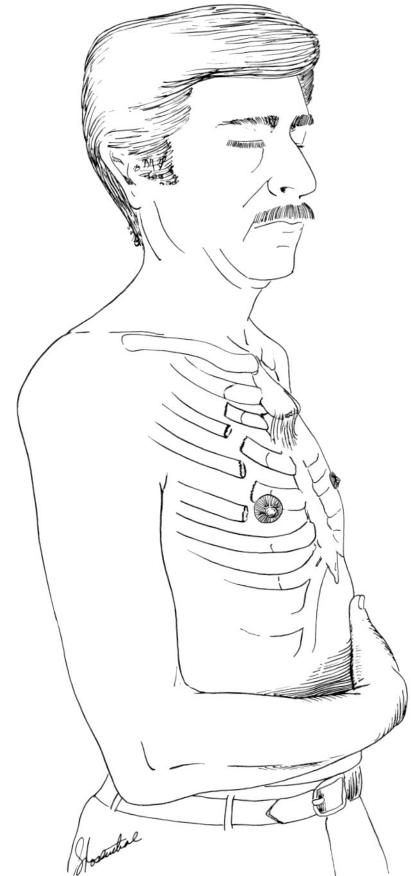

Figure 32.5. Fracture of sternum and anterior portions of ribs, showing anterior displacement of upper sternal fragment. Sternal periosteum remains intact.

Flail chest results from fracture of at least three consecutive ribs, each in two places. A fracture "plate" of this type permits paradoxical motion of the chest wall of a degree that vitiates effective ventilatory effort. Nearly 65% of such injuries result

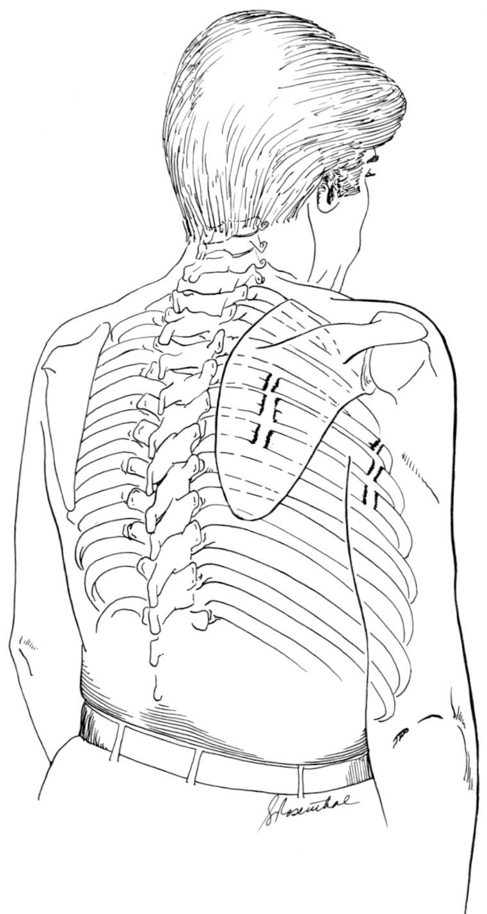

Figure 32.6. Three-rib posterolateral flail segment caused by trauma to shoulder.

from vehicular accidents, whereas about 25% are due to falls, and 10% to crushing injuries.

Posterolateral flail chest, which constitutes 55% of all flail injuries, is the result of an accident in which a force from the side is taken on the shoulder, and the scapula is momentarily driven into the chest (Fig. 32.6). Anterolateral flail injury, seen in 35% of cases, occurs after impingement on a steering wheel, although it may result from crushing. This type of injury is frequently bilateral. Other types of flail injury are combinations of: (*a*) flexion sternal fracture with rib fractures; (*b*) anterior and posterior rib fractures; and (*c*) bilateral injuries without a set pattern.

In addition to multiple rib fractures, flail chest injuries are accompanied by severe chest wall contusion, interruption of intercostal vessels and nerves, and bleeding. Contusion and laceration of the lung occur frequently, producing hemopneumothorax. The cardiovascular structures may be damaged, and rupture of the diaphragm should be considered. The injury to the chest wall itself interferes with ventilation of both lungs, since the flexibility of the chest wall and mediastinum prohibits transmission of normal inspiratory pressures to either lung on active ventilation (Fig. 32.7). Pain and pulmonary damage along with this mechanical defect make ventilation inefficient. *During the first 48 hours after injury, these consequences worsen,* with increasing displacement of rib fragments and impairment of ventilation.

Patients with flail segment generally fall into one of three categories. It may be obvious at first presentation that the patient is in respiratory distress and requires intubation and mechanical ventilation. The patient who is young and healthy may be normal initially and able to tolerate the flail segment without further intervention, except for measures aimed at pain control. The third group comprises those who initially appear to be all right. However, as time goes on, because of ineffective ventilation, pain, atelectasis, and sputum retention, the patient insidiously develops respiratory distress. These patients are difficult to identify and constitute the reason that all patients with flail chest require careful observation, serial monitoring of arterial blood gases, and chest x-rays. They require careful management of pain, vigorous chest physical therapy, flexible bronchoscopy for aspiration of retained sputum, and elective intubation before respiratory failure or pneumonia develops.

Major flail chest injuries can cause serious respiratory disability, deformity, and death. The variables of age, vigor, concomitant injuries and preexisting disease make rigid adherence to any single management approach unwise. Control of pain by intercostal blocks is effective. When significant pulmonary contusion exists, fluid restriction, salt-poor albumin administration, and diuretics should improve respiratory exchange (Table 32.1). Conventional therapy has been ''internal splinting'' by endotracheal positive-pressure ventilation until adequate chest wall stability has been reached, usually in 10–21 days. Discontent with the complications of this method, particularly tracheal damage, has led to a renewed enthusiasm for surgical stabilization of the chest wall. Intermedullary fixation of disrupted bony elements within 4 days of injury, preferably within the first 24–48 hours, is the best method of correcting deformity and achieving chest wall stability in patients who have *no other potentially lethal injuries.* This technique results in improved ventilatory mechanics, shortened hospitalization, and reduced morbidity. Tracheotomy and prolonged

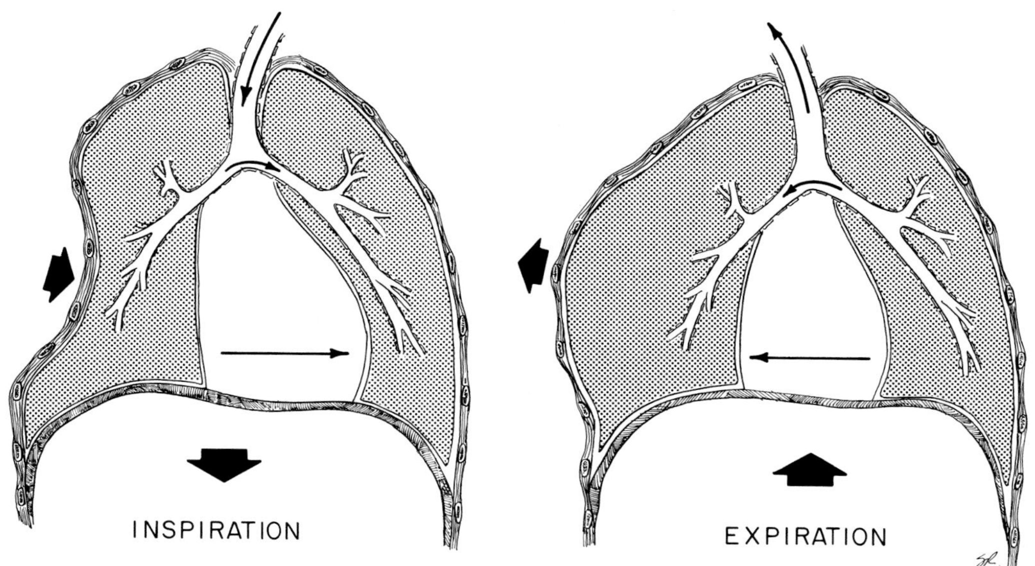

Figure 32.7. Disruption of ventilatory mechanics by flail segment on right side. Paradoxical motion of flail segment causes shift of mediastinum in same direction and affects ventilation of normal side.

ventilatory assistance are usually avoided. General thoracic surgical consultation should be sought immediately in *all* patients with flail chest.

Laryngotracheal Trauma

Laryngotracheal trauma can be life-threatening. It can occur in the busy metropolitan setting or in the most remote country setting. Injuries are related to blunt injuries, causing either direct compression of the airway against the spine, or by hyperextension of the neck and avulsion of the larynx from the trachea. Most injuries are the result of automobile accidents where passengers strike the dashboard or windshield. Motorcycle or skimobile injuries occur from the rider striking an unseen wire or chain.

Table 32.1.
Nonoperative Treatment of Pulmonary Contusion and Flail Chest[a]

1. Use lowest Fi_{O_2} possible to maintain PA_{O_2} at 60 mm Hg.
2. Maintain hematocrit between 40 and 45.
3. If transfusion needed, use freshly drawn blood or packed cells.
4. Use bronchodilators for bronchospasm.
5. Limit crystalloid solution to 50 ml/hr.
6. Administer furosemide, 40 mg intravenously immediately, and daily thereafter until no longer needed.
7. Administer albumin, 25 g immediately, and daily thereafter until no longer needed.
8. Administer methylprednisolone, 30 mg/kg of body weight intravenously immediately, and in divided doses thereafter for 3–4 days.
9. Make frequent cultures of tracheobronchial secretions.

[a]Modified from Kirsh MM, Sloan H. *Blunt Chest Trauma, General Principles of Management.* Boston: Little, Brown & Company, 1977.

The signs and symptoms range from the subtle with virtually no complaints to the obvious where the cervical structures are completely exposed. A high index of suspicion must exist to diagnose these injuries accurately and promptly. Any patient who presents following this kind of trauma with signs of respiratory distress, hoarseness, stridor, subcutaneous emphysema, hemoptysis, or localized neck pain should be suspected of laryngotracheal injury.

The evaluation of these injuries must take into account the frequent association of injuries to the cervical spine, esophagus, and major vascular structures. Cervical spine injuries dictate the appropriate management of the airway and the endoscopic evaluation of the airway and esophagus. Failure to recognize an esophageal injury will have catastrophic consequences of life-threatening mediastinitis and contamination of airway repair with increased threats of ultimate dehiscence or stenosis. Failure to evaluate the patient for pulse differentials, localized bruits, expanding hematomas, or radiographic signs of arterial injury can lead to sudden exsanguinating hemorrhage.

The critical issue in managing laryngotracheal injuries is airway control. The patient may exhibit various stages of respiratory distress, ranging from minimal hoarseness to total apnea. If there is any doubt about the status of the airway, emergency tracheotomy should be performed. A totally transected trachea may have retracted into the mediastinum. This is located by finger dissection in the area where the lower trachea should have been. Once the end is located, it is grasped with a clamp, delivered into the wound, and intubated directly through the wound with an endotracheal tube for airway control and proper ventilation.

In the less emergent situation, inspection of the airway can be carried out with a flexible bronchoscope using topical anesthesia. An endotracheal tube can be threaded over the bronchoscope once its presence in the tracheobronchial tree has been confirmed. Any attempt to intubate with either an endotracheal tube or bronchoscope should be done preferably in the operating room with complete facilities and personnel to perform emergency tracheotomy. Bronchoscopy will confirm the diagnosis of disruption by demonstrating distraction of the severed trachea, local bleeding, and a bared, offset tracheal ring (Fig. 32.8). Repeated attempts at intubation are to be avoided, and emergency tracheotomy performed at the first sign of respiratory distress.

Radiologic evaluation is not helpful in these injuries. Simple lateral neck films may reveal loss of the tracheal air column or subcutaneous emphysema. Valuable time should not be wasted in radiologic evaluation. Patients should never be sent to the radiology department until decisions about the status of the airway have been made.

Management of the injury itself is secondary to securing the airway. Careful evaluation for associated injuries are carried out, including endoscopy and direct inspection of the esophagus. Simple lacerations of the airway are repaired with interrupted absorbable suture material such as Vicryl. Complex injuries of the trachea demand conservation of the viable trachea with meticulous end-to-end repair with interrupted sutures under no tension. Concomitant injuries to the esophagus are repaired in two layers with fine silk sutures. A segment of sternohyoid or sternothyroid muscle should be interposed between the two suture lines to avoid subsequent tracheoesophageal fistula.

Special mention is made here about suspected injury to the recurrent laryngeal nerves. No attempt should be made to explore the trauma wound searching for them. It is virtually impossible to locate them; further injury may occur in the process. When injury is suspected, provisions at the completion of the repair are made to provide an airway with either a small tracheotomy tube placed at least two rings from the tracheal repair, separated from the repair by local tissue, or by a small, uncuffed endotracheal tube. If the endotracheal tube is used, the patient is taken back to the operating room 3–4

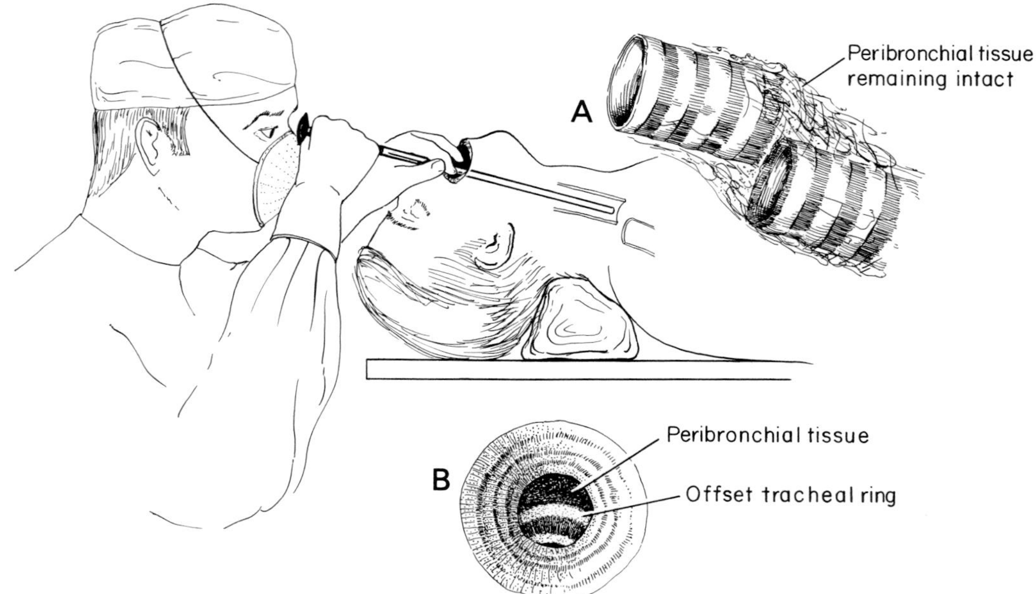

Figure 32.8. Bronchial disruption with displacement of distal fragment. *A,* Bronchial wall is frequently fractured completely, but peribronchial areolar tissue remains intact. *B,* Bronchoscopic view of bared, offset tracheal ring; usually there is a little local bleeding.

days later and assessed for airway competence. Tracheotomy is performed at that point if there is any concern.

If the surgeon is unfamiliar with the techniques of repair or if the injury is too serious, the distal trachea can be used as an end stoma and secured to the skin. The proximal end can be oversewn with a drain placed near it or brought out as a stoma as well. Reconstruction of the airway can then be performed when associated problems and inflammation and scarring have resolved. The paralyzed larynx is a useful structure and does not preclude successful reconstitution of the airway at a later date.

Tracheobronchial Injury

Injury may also occur at the tracheobronchial junction or mainstem bronchi. It is usually a result of blunt decelerating trauma. Signs and symptoms range from minimal evidence of mediastinal emphysema on chest x-ray to tension pneumothorax and respiratory distress. The classic finding is a pneumothorax that does not respond to placement of a chest tube, with incomplete reexpansion of the lung and a large persisting airleak. Concern about injury to the tracheobronchial tree is an indication for bronchoscopy to evaluate the possibility of injury.

If tracheobronchial injury is identified, it should be repaired immediately with every attempt to conserve lung parenchyma. Direct end-to-end anastomosis of the bronchus can be achieved in most cases. Surgery should be performed at the earliest time that is safe for the patient, to minimize local tissue contamination which might lessen the chance of successful primary repair.

Traumatic Asphyxia

This characteristic syndrome is caused by a sustained crushing injury of the chest. Massive venous hypertension of the upper chest, neck, face, and brain is produced during crushing, resulting in typical violaceous edema, subconjunctival hemorrhages, and varying degrees of cerebral edema. Epistaxis and visual disturbances may occur. Associated injuries of the chest wall, spine, and brain should be treated as indicated. No specific therapy for the syndrome itself is necessary.

Penetrating Injury

Pathophysiology

Penetrating injuries of the chest produce two problems: *(a)* a potentially open wound of the chest wall; and *(b)* perforation or laceration of intrathoracic or intraabdominal organs, or both. The classic sucking wound of the thorax consists of a chest wall defect that admits air on inspiration but acts as a flap valve to prevent its expulsion on expiration. The tension pneumothorax that results must be treated before management of the wound itself is considered.

The vagaries of penetrating wounds are legendary. A stab wound on one side of the neck, for example, may lacerate the jugular vein, the esophagus, and the opposite lung. Lacerations in the midline of the neck or back may involve the spinal cord. Seemingly innocuous stab wounds of the shoulder may cause hemopneumothorax. High-speed projectiles cause the most destructive penetrating injury to bones, intercostal vessels, lungs, esophagus, thoracic duct, heart and pericardium, spinal cord, diaphragm, and upper abdominal organs. It is often impossible to estimate the path of missile except by the evidence of the injury it produces. It is especially important to remember that a penetrating injury to the lower chest, i.e., below the nipple line, may have traversed the diaphragm and produced an abdominal injury.

Sucking wounds of the chest usually are obvious. Hemothorax due to vascular injury and hemopneumothorax caused by pulmonary laceration may be suspected on the basis of chest films and confirmed by thoracentesis. The recovery of chyle from the pleural space points to thoracic duct laceration, whereas if saliva or ingested dye is recovered, esophageal injury is implicated. Bile or food removed from the thoracic cavity signals injury to the diaphragm and stomach. Contrast studies and angiographic examination usually reveal the location of an esophageal or vascular defect. Mediastinal air may come from esophageal or bronchial injury; bronchoscopy and barium swallow should demonstrate the source of the injury. Fiberoptic esophagoscopy may be necessary to localize esophageal disruption.

Sucking Wound

In the emergency department, a sucking wound of the chest wall should be occluded with a dressing of petrolatum gauze and Elastoplast to prevent further entry of air, and the pneumothorax evacuated with a chest tube. If tension pneumothorax is causing acute respiratory distress, the chest tube can be inserted through the wound and left in place until definitive treatment is undertaken. After collections of blood and air have been evacuated and the condition of the patient stabilized, transfer to the operating room is planned for debridement or excision of the chest wall wound. If continued bleeding, serious leakage of air, or major visceral injury becomes evident, emergency operative repair of the implicated organs is imperative.

The chest wall wound itself may be a major problem. If a large defect exists after debridement of devitalized tissue, it may be necessary to utilize muscle flaps to achieve adequate closure.

Most penetrating thoracic wounds are complicated by hemothorax; this condition is usually managed satisfactorily by intercostal catheter drainage. There is little evidence that administration of fibrinolytic agents is effective. Only occasionally is pulmonary decortication indicated to prevent crippling fibrothorax.

Visceral Injury

Penetrating wounds are more likely to damage blood vessels, pulmonary tissue, the tracheobronchial tree, the esophagus, the thoracic duct, and the abdominal viscera. When massive bleeding indicates a serious vascular or cardiac injury, immediate thoracotomy is necessary to prevent death. A lung shattered by a high-velocity projectile may require resection, but in the treatment of most contusions and lacerations of the lung, excision of tissue should be avoided. Lacerations of the esophagus and trachea or major bronchi must be repaired without delay. Division of the thoracic duct is indicated by chylothorax and can be managed initially by insertion of a chest tube for drainage. Since persistent leakage of chyle eventually produces malnutrition, thoracotomy with ligation of the duct may be necessary. Injury to abdominal organs and the diaphragm is frequent, and surgical repair is commonly indicated.

Diaphragmatic Rupture

Blunt chest or abdominal trauma may cause diaphragmatic rupture. Left-sided injuries are three to four times more common than right-sided injuries. The injury may be silent and unrecognized, or may present with respiratory compromise and shock. Acute injury should be suspected by excessive percussional tympany or the auscultation of bowel sounds in the chest. The presence of a dilated stomach in the lower chest on x-ray is classic but must not be confused with subpneumonic pneumothorax or free subphrenic peritoneal air. The demonstration of a nasogastric tube curled in this airspace is helpful. Contrast studies determining the location of the stomach are diagnostic.

The treatment of diaphragmatic injury is surgical repair. It should be undertaken as soon as the patient is stabilized. The threat of strangulation of abdominal organs and respiratory compromise are the reasons for prompt surgical intervention. Left-sided injuries are explored transabdominally because of a high incidence of associated intraabdominal injuries. Right-sided injuries are explored transthoraci-

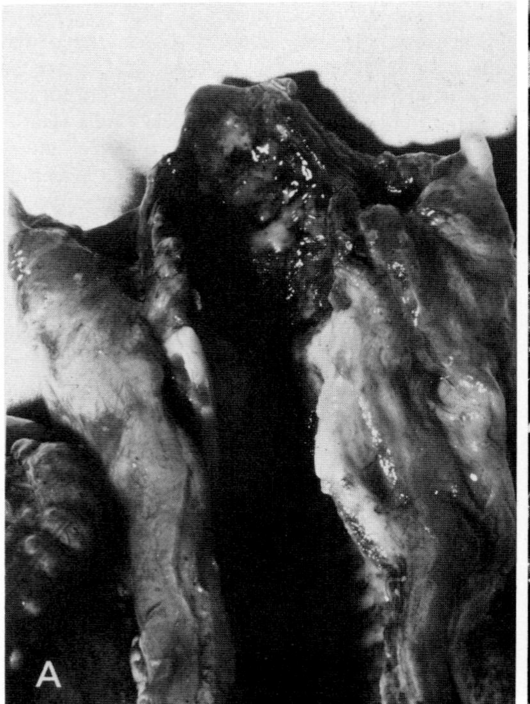

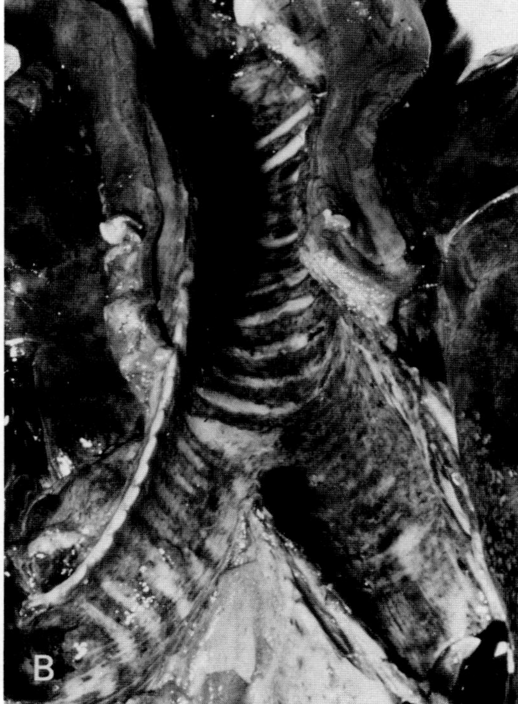

Figure 32.9. Severe thermal injury of airway. *A,* Necrosis of epiglottis and larynx. *B,* Denudation of mucosa of tracheobronchial tree in same patient.

cally because of the location of the liver. Repair consists of reduction of all abdominal viscera and suture of the diaphragmatic tear. Use of Marlex mesh, or transposition of the diaphragm to a higher level of the chest wall if it has been avulsed are other techniques.

Unrecognized injuries may present many years later on incidental chest x-rays. In this situation, abnormal bowel gas patterns are seen in the chest or a suspicion of a paralyzed diaphragm is raised. Careful history usually yields a history of previous blunt trauma. Fluoroscopy may show the diaphragm to function. Barium contrast studies confirm the location of the stomach or colon above the diaphragm. Surgery should be considered to lessen the risks of strangulation—in this case by the transthoracic approach. Early consultation should be sought by the emergency physician.

Burn Injury

A vague and poorly defined term, "smoke inhalation" refers to inspiration of a variety of gases as well as soot. The products of combustion depend on the material burned: wool releases irritating aldehydes and resins; wood produces cyanides; some plastics release phosgene. Most fires generate carbon monoxide, and exposure to it must be assumed in any fire victim. Certain combustible agents such as hydrazine are toxic and can be inhaled in gaseous form at temperatures below their ignition points. The result of smoke inhalation is direct irritation of the mucosa of the airway that causes injury ranging from edema to necrosis, with or without damage to the alveolar-capillary membranes. Systemic absorption of toxic substances can also occur.

The term respiratory or pulmonary "burn" is used even more loosely, since thermal injury of the intrathoracic airway never occurs unless the victim inhales gas containing steam or heated carbon particles or has no laryngeal protective reflexes. Laryngospasm normally prevents the passage of dry air that is hot enough to produce subglottic trauma. If a fire victim sustains injury to the respiratory tract, the damage is produced largely by the toxic products of combustion and is augmented by a thermal component only if steam or hot soot is inhaled. Severe thermal burn of the subglottic airway (Fig. 32.9) is seen in less than 5% of cases and usually occurs only in the comatose patient. The term "inhalation injury" is used to describe the results of inhalation of the products of combustion.

Inhalation Injury

Inhalation injury should be suspected in a fire victim under any of the following conditions:

1. The burn occurred in an enclosed space.
2. The fire involved toxic chemicals or plastic, including many synthetic materials used in clothing and in home furnishings.
3. The patient has an extensive facial burn.
4. There is soot in the sputum.
5. Erythema and edema of the oropharynx are noted.
6. The voice is hoarse.

In general, the diagnosis of inhalation injury is made by history and physical examination rather than by laboratory or radiologic assessment. The pulmonary interstitial tissue and the small airways are affected before radiologically visible changes develop. If inhalation injury has occurred, tachypnea and agitation heralding respiratory deterioration always develop within the first few days, preceding the appearance of abnormal arterial blood gas measurements and x-ray findings. The effects of inhalation injury are usually at their worst on the fourth or fifth day and subside within 14 days in survivors.

Erythema, edema, and soot seen on examination of the hypopharynx, larynx, and trachea reliably indicate inhalation injury. The severity of mucosal changes, however, can be either more or less than the severity of physiologic damage. Laryngoscopy and bronchoscopy can be useful in guiding treatment. Chest x-ray films almost always are normal for 24–48 hours and, therefore, are seldom helpful.

Edema of the upper portion of the airway may cause obstruction that is suggested by labored respiration and the use of accessory respiratory muscles and by sternal retraction. The clinical signs of respiratory insufficiency caused by damage to the lower airway, however, resemble those of pulmonary edema.

When inhalation injury is suspected, treatment should be started immediately. A short-term (12-hour), high-dose course of a corticosteroid compound should be instituted without delay, since these agents are ineffective unless started within a few hours of injury. They are given to reduce the tissue damage caused by toxic inhalation, although clinical and laboratory proof of their efficacy is incomplete. Intravenous administration of methylprednisolone sodium succinate, 10 mg/kg initially, is recommended with a possible repeat administration 12 hours later. Tapered doses thereafter are unnecessary.

Airway obstruction and failing respiration, with evidence by deteriorating arterial blood gas values, are managed best by orotracheal, or preferably nasotracheal intubation. Tracheotomy should be performed initially only if intubation from above is impossible. Since most of these patients have burns of the face and neck, tracheotomy is often followed by cervical wound sepsis and bacterial invasion of the tracheobronchial tree. Death from bronchopneumonia is the usual result. Tracheotomy may be performed safely at a later time, if prolonged ventilatory support is required and if there is no local burn. After intubation, a warm humidified oxygen (usually 40–50%) is administered.

Reluctance to use indwelling nasotracheal tubes for long periods is understandable. In the treatment of a potentially lethal burn injury, however, fear of laryngeal damage by a tube must not interfere with administration of lifesaving support. Plastic endotracheal tubes with low-pressure, high-volume cuffs can be used for 6–8 weeks in most patients without serious permanent laryngeal damage. After long periods of intubation, endoscopic examination of the larynx and trachea must be performed at the time of extubation to assess the adequacy of the upper airway and the need for tracheotomy or reconstruction.

In patients with deteriorating arterial blood gas values from either alveolocapillary diffusion block or inefficient ventilatory mechanics, assisted ventilation with intermittent positive-pressure breathing (IPPB) is indicated. Positive end-expiratory pressure (PEEP) may be needed as respiratory failure and interstitial pulmonary edema develop. Careful monitoring of central venous pressure during fluid replacement is essential to avoid overload and the superimposition of left heart failure and pulmonary edema on the inhalation injury.

A difficult problem frequently encountered is the management of a person brought to the hospital because of "smoke inhalation." Usually the patient recovers after receiving humidified oxygen for 1–2 hours. However, those who show visible evidence of upper airway injury and those injured in fires involving chemicals or plastics should receive corticosteroids and should be hospitalized for observation in case of exposure to a potentially lethal agent, such as phosgene. Rarely does the inhalation injury syndrome develop later than 2 days after exposure.

Recognizing that exposure to carbon monoxide occurs in most fires, the physician can manage inhalation injury as follows:

1. Humidifed oxygen (100%) should be administered on admission and for 4 hours thereafter.
2. The patient and the circumstances of the injury should be evaluated.
3. Laryngoscopic and bronchoscopic examination should be performed if the diagnosis is in doubt.
4. Corticosteroids should be given if inhalation injury is confirmed, or even strongly suspected.
5. Nasotracheal intubation should be performed for upper airway edema, with the use of IPPB and PEEP if respiratory failure develops.

Thermal Injury

In patients with thermal injury to the airway, maximal damage is to the pharynx, larynx, and trachea. Swelling of the hypopharynx and larynx may cause upper airway obstruction. Thermal damage to the tracheobronchial tree is seen occasionally as the result of inhalation of steam or of superheated air by a comatose patient. Tracheal injury that is visible on bronchoscopic examination usually terminates at the level of the carina. Most of these injuries are manifested by erythema and edema; occasionally, necrotic mucosa may slough and produce obstruction, unless it is removed endoscopically or by coughing. Severe thermal damage predisposes the airway to invasive sepsis, which is rapidly fatal if not controlled. Even mild degrees of thermal injury to the trachea lower mucosal resistance to the effects of indwelling tubes and suction catheters.

It may be difficult to determine whether tracheobronchial injury is caused by heat or by toxic gases. There is often a mixture of the two. Bronchoscopic examination is the best method of differentiation. Toxic inhalation injury produces redness and edema to all bronchial divisions, most marked in the lower lobes, whereas thermal injury causes uniform, continuous redness and swelling to a demarcated level

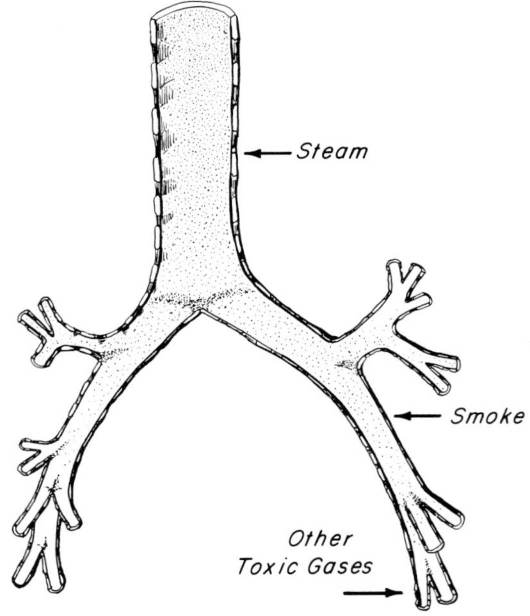

Figure 32.10. Sites of inhalation and thermal injuries. Thermal damage—by steam, for example—involves only the trachea and mainstem bronchi. Smoke damages the entire bronchial tree. Some toxic products of combustion, such as phosgene, produce injury primarily at alveolar level.

that is usually in the trachea (Fig. 32.10). Both findings may be evident in the same patient. Rarely is the treatment substantially affected by confusion between the two. If there is any evidence of toxic inhalation, corticosteroids should be given.

Management of thermal injury may be summarized as follows:

1. Administration of humidified oxygen;
2. Evaluation of the patient and the circumstances of the injury;
3. Laryngoscopic and bronchoscopic assessment, obtaining specimens for cultures;
4. Nasotracheal intubation if significant edema of the hypopharynx and larynx develops; tracheotomy only if the neck is not burned;
5. Administration of intravenous broad-spectrum antibiotics for severe injuries;
6. Repeated bronchoscopic removal of mucosal sloughs, if needed;
7. Extubation as soon as possible;
8. Later tracheal reconstruction if indicated.

Other Injuries

Three other respiratory problems can result from major burns: aspiration of vomitus, ventilatory restriction due to circumferential deep burns of the thorax, and early respiratory failure without inhalation injury.

Vomiting occurs after any major trauma; burns are no exception. In approximately 1% of patients with extensive burns, death results from aspiration of vomitus. Gastric dilatation and paralytic ileus frequently follow burns, particularly in children. Routine introduction of a nasogastric tube on admission prevents this complication.

Deep circumferential thoracic burns (en cuirasse) restrict ventilation in the same manner that circumferential burns of the extremity impair the circulation. Restricted respiratory motion is visible. Double or triple vertical escharotomies may be needed to release the constriction interfering with motion of the chest wall (Fig. 32.11). Escharotomies are always made within the burned tissue and must be carried down through the full thickness of the burn.

Rarely, early respiratory failure develops after cutaneous burns where there is no inhalation injury. The patient is usually elderly, and the burn is extensive. This phenomenon is poorly understood in humans, although alveolocapillary hyperpermeability and interstitial pulmonary edema readily develop after cutaneous wounds in experimental laboratory animals. The syndrome is similar to shock lung and may be caused by a circulating burn toxin. These patients require the same treatment as do those with inhalation injury.

Pulmonary Aspiration of Gastroesophageal Contents

Despite recognition by Hippocrates more than 2000 years ago and the classic descriptions by Hunter, Simpson, Mendelson, and Teabout during the past two centuries, and despite numerous studies during recent years, bronchopulmonary aspiration is still a vexing problem. The setting, risks, methods of prevention, and treatment are known and are not controversial for the most part. Constant attention to detail is required for success in averting aspiration; and even then, aspiration cannot always be prevented.

The precise frequency of gastropulmonary aspiration is unknown, but some generalities are well-documented. After surgery, more often with general anesthesia, some degree of gastroesophageal regurgitation occurs as much as 25% of the time, and pulmonary aspiration may occur as much as 16% of the time.

About 40% of intubated patients develop some degree of aspiration. Endotracheal cuff inflation can reduce this to 20%, but even careful use of high-volume, low-pressure cuffs on endotracheal tubes does not guarantee protection against aspiration.

Pathophysiology

Especially prone to aspiration are patients with *(a)* neurologic and seizure disorders, particularly when consciousness and cough reflex are depressed; *(b)* drug and alcohol overdose and anesthesia; and *(c)* poor gastric or esophageal emptying or induced gastric distention (i.e., use of esophageal obturator airways).

Aspiration of solid material causes an entirely different syndrome from that of inhalation of gastric juice. The former causes airway obstruction manifested by cyanosis, stridor, and labored respiration. It often follows trauma or overindulgence at meals. The bronchopulmonary response to the inhalation of gastric contents depends on the pH of the aspirate. It is estimated that 0.3 mg/kg of gastric juice with a pH below 2.5 is needed to produce serious pulmonary damage. This is a chemical injury, clinically identical to the inhalation injury associated with major burns. Massive acid aspiration causes pulmonary edema within minutes, accompanied by bloody bronchorrhea, hypotension, and low cardiac output. Atelectasis, shunting, and infiltrates visible by x-ray develop within 8 hours, the radiologic abnormalities becoming fully developed by 24 hours. The major pathology is usually in the lower lobes. Clinical deterioration and hypovolemia continue for 48 hours with a 60% mortality. Aspiration of smaller quantities of acid gastric juice produces a more leisurely, less severe course. The basic pathology is capillary endothelial injury with intersti-

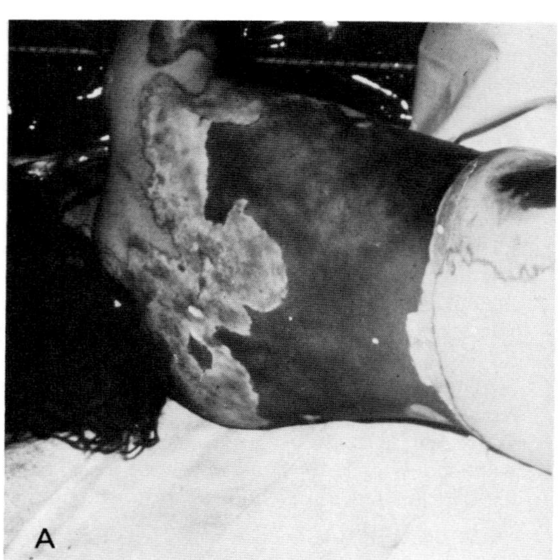

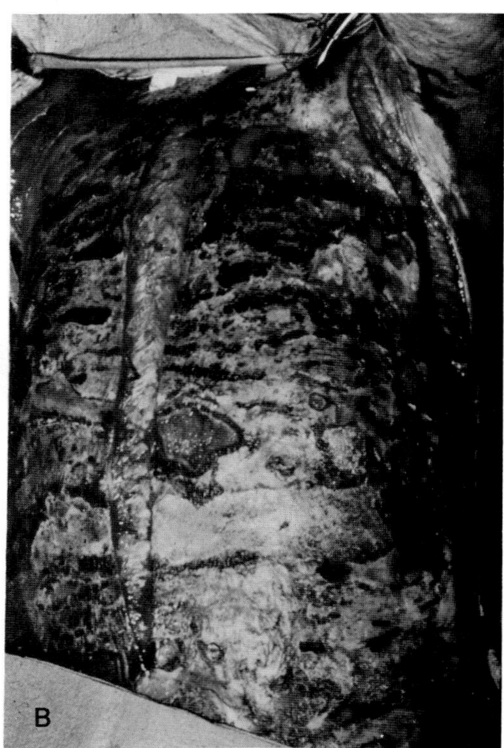

Figure 32.11. *A,* Deep, circumferential thoracic burn of type that restricts ventilatory motion. *B,* Vertical escharotomies to release constriction that has persisted after primary excision and skin grafting. These are more often necessary in the acute, deep third-degree burn.

tial edema, inhibition of surfactant, reduced compliance, elevated airway pressures, and vascular shunting. In severe cases, thrombosis of segmental pulmonary artery branches occurs. When ischemia develops in areas of damaged lung, shunting diminishes. Thus, reduction of the initial degree of shunting after serious aspiration injury actually may be an ominous sign.

The role played by bacterial invasion is variable. Acid gastric juice usually has a sparse bacterial flora. However, patients taking cimetidine or ranitidine, or who are suffering from small bowel obstruction have a rich intestinal flora in their stomachs. In this case, bacterial pneumonia frequently occurs after the initial injury.

Treatment

The emergency treatment of gastropulmonary aspiration should be keyed to the pathology. When aspiration of particulate matter causes tracheobronchial obstruction, bronchoscopic clearing of the airway is necessary. When aspiration of liquid contents occurs, thorough endotracheal suctioning should be performed, followed by intubation and intermittent positive-pressure ventilation.

Ventilator therapy probably prevents irreversible pulmonary vascular spasm and thrombosis, and thereby reduces mortality. Intravenous restoration of intravascular volume is important; albumin administration is particularly effective, as most of it is retained in the intravascular space. Ventilator therapy should be continued for at least 12 hours. Immediate administration of steroids is beneficial in the laboratory, though unproved clinically. Steroid dosage should be large and continued only for a brief period of time. Bronchopulmonary lavage may be more damaging than helpful. There is experimental evidence that prostacyclin and ibuprofen are beneficial, perhaps because they block release of capillary permeability factors. This information may point the way to future therapy for this type of pulmonary inhalation injury.

A word about prevention in the emergency department is in order. Trauma victims often have full stomachs and vomit while partially conscious or during induction for emergency surgery. Prompt insertion of a properly functioning nasogastric tube with continuous suction applied will prevent needless deaths. The current use of the esophageal obturator airway in resuscitation not only increases the risk of aspiration, but also necessitates gastric deflation afterwards. The administration of intravenous cimetidine to patients prior to emergency surgery reduces the severity of any subsequent aspiration by controlling the gastric pH.

Caustic Injuries

There are approximately 6000 chemical burns of the esophagus each year involving predominantly children under the age of 5 years. The agents are caustic in over 80% of the cases, and the remainder are attributed to acid injuries. Solid caustics cause liquefaction necrosis and thrombosis of blood vessels. The solid fragments frequently stick to the mucous membranes, causing the worst injuries in the mouth and esophagus. Liquid caustics have the same mechanism of action but cause much more extensive injuries and are more likely to involve the stomach. Factors influencing the damage of the stomach are the amount and strength of the caustic agent, duration of contact, presence of food in the stomach, and pylorospasm. Acid injuries cause coagulative necrosis. The eschar that forms may limit the depth of penetration and permit relative sparing of the esophagus. The stomach may be the primary site of involvement leading to pyloric obstruction, antral stenosis, or an ultimate hourglass gastric deformity.

The initial management of these injuries should include careful physical examination searching for signs of perforation somewhere in the gastrointestinal tract. The oral cavity should be carefully inspected for evidence of a chemical burn. Esophagoscopy should be performed within the first 6–12 hours to identify evidence of a chemical burn. The endoscopist should stop at the first sign of a burn of the esophagus to lessen any possibility of perforating the esophagus. Chemical burns are graded much as thermal burns of the skin: first degree, showing superficial mucosal hyperemia; second degree, loss of the mucosa with transmucosal ulceration; and third degree, transmucosal necrosis with penetration into the periesophageal tissue. No attempt should be made to induce vomiting; caution is advised regarding passage of a nasogastric tube for fear of perforation. Supportive measures should be instituted to correct potential fluid deficits and steroids instituted to diminish swelling and the possible subsequent formation of scar tissue. Antibiotics against oral Gram-positive organisms should also be administered. The patient must be followed carefully for perforation, which is masked by the use of steroids. Alimentation can be allowed when the acute pain subsides. Dilatations may be necessary if stenosis develops. Acute dilatation carries some potential danger of perforation and should be delayed until the pain has resolved and signs of mucosal regeneration are seen.

Each patient with a chemical burn is at risk for concomitant injury to the larynx with secondary swelling and stenosis, leading to airway obstruction. Signs of increasing airway stridor may signal the need for tracheotomy.

More serious injuries may occur, leading to peritoneal signs and shock. If peritoneal signs exist, the patient should be explored to determine whether necrosis or perforation have occurred. If necrosis is detected, resection should be undertaken with reconstruction planned for a later date. Necrosis of abdominal organs may herald the same type of problem as the thoracic esophagus. If the esophagus is found to be necrotic, it should be removed as well. Reconstruction of the gastrointestinal tract is deferred until a future occasion. Provisions should be made to feed the patient through a gastrostomy or jejunostomy.

NONTRAUMATIC EMERGENCIES

Respiratory Tract

Respiratory failure may be caused by many infectious, inflammatory, neoplastic, or neuromuscular diseases, as well as by drugs and nonspecific processes. The approach to management should be guided by the physiologic defect involved. Respiratory emergencies secondary to alveolocapillary diffusion block caused by pulmonary edema, pneumonia, or other inflammatory disease are discussed elsewhere, along with those due to obstructive airway disease and hypoventilation (see Chapter 9). If tidal volume falls too low in a patient with a neuromuscular disease such as myasthenia gravis, poliomyelitis, or acute idiopathic polyneuritis, ventilatory assistance may be required.

Airway Obstruction

Mechanical obstruction of the upper airway may be caused by a variety of diseases ranging from infections, such as diphtheria, to tracheal neoplasms. Emergency treatment depends on the level of obstruction; most patients can be managed by endotracheal intubation or by tracheotomy. Obstruction by a tumor low in the trachea (Fig. 32.12) may necessitate intubation of a mainstem bronchus for adequate ventilation. Inflammatory obstruction of the larynx can be treated successfully with humidified oxygen and racemic epinephrine inhalations in many instances, reserving endotracheal intubation or tracheotomy for severe cases.

Tumors of the trachea or major bronchi occur at any level and are manifested by a characteristic syndrome consisting of some degree of respiratory obstruction and an audible wheeze. Chest x-rays are

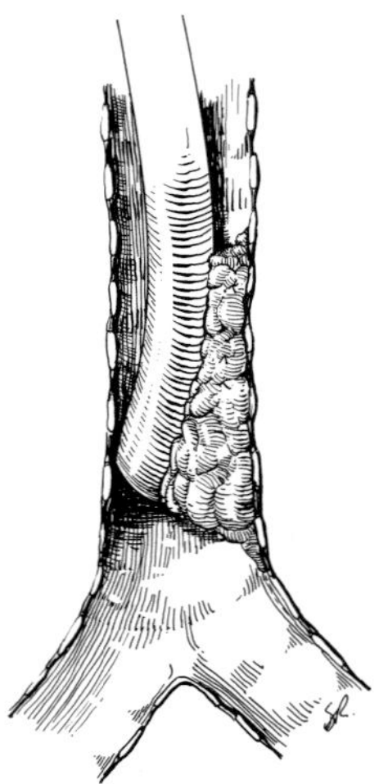

Figure 32.12. Relief of obstruction caused by tracheal tumor by passage of endotracheal tube down to or past lower limit of tumor.

usually normal. The correct diagnosis is suggested by radiologic visualization of the trachea, preferably by planar tomography. Since the airway of these patients is often marginal, any manipulation such as bronchoscopy should be performed only under full operating room conditions with an anesthesiologist available and a long endotracheal tube at hand to pass into a mainstem bronchus, should total obstruction result from bleeding and edema. Bronchoscopic removal of as much tumor as possible to restore an adequate airway is sometimes the best emergency treatment in this difficult situation, allowing time for evaluation and planning of definitive radiation or surgical therapy. This must be done carefully to avoid excessive bleeding. The tip of the rigid bronchoscope can be used to "core out" the tumor by using it in a corkscrew fashion. Biopsy forceps can be used to remove any of the remaining tumor or to retrieve fragments that have gravitated distally. Pledgets soaked in an epinephrine solution 1:10,000 are used to control any persistent oozing. Major hemorrhage has not been a problem. This is not an emergency department technique and should be carried out by the surgeon in the operating room.

There has been interest in using the laser to open such malignant strictures. While the laser is indeed an alternative to the coring technique, it is time-consuming, tedious, and more expensive. Its main indication at this time is for the unusual case where the other technique is not applicable.

Nonneoplastic stenosis of the trachea causes problems similar to those caused by neoplastic occlusion. Patients who have had tracheotomy or endotracheal intubation may return to the hospital within the year because of progressive stridor due to obstruction. A wheeze is usually audible; obstruction is frequently more severe than the physician suspects. Obstruction results early from formation of tracheal granulation tissue or late from cicatrical stenosis after damage from the cuff of the endotracheal tube. When tracheal narrowing is caused by granulations, the diagnosis is suggested by the irregular contour of the stenotic segment, which can be demonstrated by tomographic examination of the trachea and confirmed by bronchoscopy. Emergency treatment consists of bronchoscopic removal of the granulations with cauterization when this is feasible, or passage of an endotracheal tube through the obstructed zone to relieve acute obstruction, if necessary. Cicatrical stenosis of the trachea is suggested by tapered narrowing that is demonstrated by tomography and confirmed by bronchoscopy. Bronchoscopy should be attempted *only* in the operating room with inhalation anesthesia expertly achieved without intubation. If surgical resection is not planned at this time, the stenosis can be dilated with rigid bronchoscopes under direct vision. A series of gradually increased sizes of bronchoscopes should be used to lessen the risk of perforation. Dilatations give only short relief and either definitive resection planned or tracheotomy performed to provide a satisfactory airway. A tracheotomy should be placed through the area of stenotic trachea so as to conserve as much normal trachea for subsequent reconstruction as possible. Flexible bronchoscopy is *not* recommended for evaluation of this problem because of the risk of sudden airway obstruction.

Tracheal obstruction by a foreign body may be an acute emergency, whereas a foreign body in a distal bronchus often causes collapse of the lung distal to it with subacute infection. Foreign bodies should be removed endoscopically as soon as the diagnosis is suggested by history or demonstrated radiologically. After a foreign body has been lodged in a bronchus for more than a few hours, edema forms around it, atelectasis occurs distal to the obstruction, and pneumonitis quickly develops. Endoscopic removal of a chronically impacted foreign body obscured by granulations is difficult; early removal of bronchial foreign bodies avoids the need for possible thoracotomy and bronchotomy later.

Occlusion of the superior vena cava by carcinoma, lymphoma, or thrombus produces facial, neck, and upper extremity edema made worse in recumbency. In addition, a severe superior vena caval syndrome often results in ventilatory impairment, requiring immediate treatment with humidified oxygen and elevation of the head of the bed, as well as administration of diuretics, and corticosteroids. If the obstruction appears to be neoplastic, radiation treatment should begin promptly, sometimes without histologic confirmation. If these measures fail, intubation and ventilatory assistance may be necessary.

It is apparent from this discussion of respiratory emergencies that bronchoscopic instruments are essential in any emergency facility. A rigid bronchoscope saves lives in true emergencies. Most endoscopic examinations for diagnosis and therapy, however, should be performed in the operating room.

Massive Hemoptysis

Although uncommon, massive hemoptysis can be a difficult problem with serious implications. Mortality rates vary with the rapidity of bleeding and often reach 75% if blood loss exceeds 600 ml in 6 hours. Asphyxia is the usual cause of death. Tuberculosis, mycetoma, abscess, bronchiectasis, arteritis, vascular anomalies, and carcinoma are among the causes. Thus, serious bleeding may occur at any age, usually from bronchial vessels.

A poor outcome can be avoided only by prompt assessment and vigorous management, using all available techniques. Early steps in management include cross-matching of several units of blood, placement of a reliable infusion line, accurate measurement of blood loss, and close monitoring of vital signs. The patient should lie on the affected side, if known, and be encouraged to clear the airway by gently coughing. The cough reflex should not be abolished by sedation. When possible, careful radiographic study is important, because it may indicate the diagnosis and localize the source.

Early bronchoscopy is vital. A rigid bronchoscope should be used to clear the bronchial tree of blood and clots and to localize the source, if possible. The fiberoptic bronchoscope is less effective for the removal of large amounts of liquid and clotted blood, but is more likely to permit localization of the source after the clearing of the airway. If the source cannot be identified, angiography is indicated.

Control of bleeding must then be attempted. There are three available methods; the proper choice will depend on accuracy of localization, the underlying disease process, and the condition of the patient. The approaches are: (*a*) endobronchial balloon tamponade; (*b*) arterial embolization; and (*c*) surgical ligation of bronchial arteries or the resection of necessary parenchymal tissue.

Endobronchial tamponade can be performed by inserting a Fogarty catheter through either rigid or flexible bronchoscopes into the lobar or segmental bronchus from which the bleeding occurs. If this must be the primary method of treatment, as in a poor-risk patient with diffuse lung disease, the balloon is left in place, inflated for 24 hours. If there is no further bleeding in several hours after deflating, the catheter is removed. If the primary lesion is surgically resectable, preliminary Fogarty balloon tamponade or unilateral endotracheal tube intubation may be used to control bleeding during preparation for surgery.

Arterial embolization is an attractive approach in certain situations. If localization of the bleeding site is possible by bronchial or intercostal angiography, especially in the presence of diffuse pulmonary disease, therapeutic embolization may be possible. The risk is thrombosis of a spinal artery arising from the intercostal artery embolized. This technique is useful in the treatment of recurring hemoptysis in patients who have diffuse pulmonary disease, such as cystic fibrosis, or untreatable tumor.

The key to the management of severe hemoptysis is recognition of its lethal nature and prompt intervention centered on endoscopic location and/or control. The emergency physician needs the prompt consultative help of a general thoracic surgeon.

Pleural Space Problems

A common thoracic emergency, *spontaneous pneumothorax* usually results from rupture of a superficial apical bleb. This may occur at any time. It occurs in healthy young adults, but it also can be found in middle-aged or elderly patients who have chronic obstructive pulmonary disease. Pneumothorax frequently occurs without warning or predisposing incident, and is manifested by sudden chest pain with varying degrees of dyspnea. Young persons may experience relatively little disability, since the leak seals quickly as the lung deflates; older patients with asthma or emphysema are more severely disabled and often respond to treatment slowly. In either type of patient, initial treatment is the same. A small pneumothorax (less than 20%) can either be observed closely or be managed by anterior needle or catheter aspiration if there is no evidence of continuing air leakage. A larger collection of air or pneumothorax with persistent air leakage should be treated by intercostal catheter suction. Tube thoracostomy is performed easily by an anterior or axillary approach. In the long term, this procedure usually shortens the hospital stay. *Tension pneumothorax* is an urgent emergency requiring immediate pleural decompression, often prior to a confirming x-ray.

The leaking bleb usually seals with stable expansion of the lung within a few days. When there is underlying emphysema, however, it is common for air leakage to continue for 7–12 days. If a leak persists with no sign of impending closure, active measures must be taken to close it, especially if there have been previous episodes of pneumothorax. Permanent protection against recurrence is particularly necessary in patients who have had contralateral pneumothorax, because spontaneous bilateral pneumothorax can be fatal. Thoracotomy and resection of blebs, along with pleural abrasion is an effective therapeutic and preventive measure. In patients who have serious pulmonary disease, chemical pleurodesis may be better tolerated than open thoracotomy.

Large *pleural effusions* often require emergency treatment, whether caused by benign or malignant disease. Thoracentesis usually resolves the urgent problem. ''Pleural shock'' caused by mediastinal shift can be avoided if the fluid collection is withdrawn slowly. In patients with recurrent malignant pleural effusion, an intercostal thoracotomy tube should be inserted laterally or posterolaterally to permit continuing evacuation of the fluid. This may later be followed by intrapleural instillation of a sclerosing agent, such as tetracycline, to produce permanent pleural symphysis.

An uncommon emergency, *spontaneous hemothorax* may result from rupture of a bleb or may be caused by systemic disease such as uremia, hemophilia, or a connective tissue disorder, such as rheumatoid disease or lupus erythematosus. Aspiration by needle or catheter should be employed when possible, although thoracotomy may be necessary in cases of clotted and loculated hemothorax. Hemothorax in a hemophilic patient is best controlled by tube evacuation following the administration of Factor VIII (see Chapter 13).

Empyema can also result in a true emergency. Pleural space collections of purulent material may be caused by hematogenous infection of a preexistent effusion, by pleural extension of pneumonia or tuberculosis, by perforation of an organ, or by contamination due to rupture of a subphrenic abscess through the diaphragm. Regardless of the cause, acute empyema should be confirmed by needle aspiration and drained by intercostal catheter suction, concomitant with appropriate antibiotic therapy. When the physician is certain that adjacent pleural symphysis has occurred, rib resection and open drainage are the proper measures; this seldom is an emergency.

Esophagus

Obstruction

Esophageal obstruction is a common manifestation of a variety of mechanical and motor problems, such as strictures, webs, lower esophageal rings, tumors, diverticula, and achalasia. In most cases, the acute incident is precipitated by eating. In children, the more common cause of obstruction is a foreign body, such as a coin or small plastic toy, usually unaccompanied by esophageal disease. Emergency treatment depends on the nature of the obstructing object, its location as confirmed by barium swallow or chest x-ray if opaque, and the type of underlying esophageal disease. An ingested foreign body should be removed promptly. If gentle traction employing a balloon-tipped catheter under fluoroscopic control is unsuccessful, endoscopic removal is necessary. When a bolus of food is producing obstruction, dissolution should be attempted by ingestion of 5 ml of a 2.5% solution of papain, a proteolytic enzyme prepared from papaya, every half hour for a total of six doses. This can be effective only if the obstructing bolus is protein. If this fails to clear the obstruction, esophagoscopy with mechanical extraction of the bolus is necessary. When the cause of acute esophageal obstruction is unknown, radiologic and endoscopic examinations should be performed, and bougienage may be necessary. Obstruction caused by achalasia or stricture yields temporarily to the passage of a Hurst or Maloney mercury bougie. However, most patients who seek attention for obstruction caused by intrinsic esophageal disease should be admitted for intravenous hydration, diagnostic studies, and appropriate treatment. It should be stressed that obstructive dysphagia does not occur without cause, and it is the duty of the emergency physician to consider demonstration of that cause. Dilatation in the presence of an obstructed esophagus must be done very carefully because of the increased risk of perforation; it is not the task of the emergency physician.

A few patients seek emergency care because of a large esophageal diverticulcum that has progressed to severe, unremitting obstruction. This diagnosis can be suspected by the history, and is often confirmed by demonstration of gurgling in the neck on palpation. Barium contrast study is definitive. *Instrumental manipulation is never indicated.* Direct hospital admission may be necessary. Curative operation should be performed only after dehydration and malnutrition have been corrected intravenously.

Acute esophagogastric obstruction is sometimes the result of an incarcerated hiatal hernia. This emergency is discussed with other conditions related to the diaphragm later in this chapter.

Perforation

Acute perforation of the esophagus may be caused by peptic ulcer, tumor, an ingested sharp object, instrumental manipulation, or trauma. So-called spontaneous perforation of the normal esophagus occurs after retching, usually with an overfilled stomach; the likely mechanism is transmission of elevated intragastric pressure into the esophagus while the glottis and the cricopharyngeal sphincter are closed. By the same mechanism, blunt trauma to the upper part of the abdomen can tear the esophagus; this also commonly occurs proximal to the esophagogastric junction. Decelerating automobile injury with sudden seat belt pressure against a distended stomach is one such mechanism. All types of perforation cause pain, fever, and toxic malaise. Subcutaneous emphysema is a late physical finding. Some bleeding may occur. The pain may be felt in the *upper abdomen,* the back, the substernal region, or the neck, depending on the level of perforation. Pleural effusion with subsequent empyema accompanies perforation of the intrathoracic esophagus when the mediastinal pleura is penetrated. The diagnosis can be made if air is visualized in the mediastinum, the upper retroperitoneum, or the neck on x-ray films. Water-soluble contrast studies should be performed to demonstrate the site of the leak, before interventional surgery is planned.

The level of perforation is an important determinant of prognosis and treatment. Leaks in the neck have a better prognosis than those located distally in the intrathoracic esophagus. They can be treated by antibiotics and observation until a cervical collection or abscess is localized sufficiently for incision and drainage. Early cervical exploration and drainage should at least be considered in most cases. The emergency physician should consult a surgeon without delay. Oral feeding must be withheld until any fistula is closed. If perforation is noted during or immediately after instrumentation, immediate surgical closure is advisable.

Intrathoracic perforation of the esophagus still produces excessive mortality and, therefore, is a true surgical emergency. Prompt recognition and operative closure are the keys to a successful outcome. The clinical improvement seen after preliminary chest tube drainage of an esophagopleural fistula should not delay operation. Closure is best accomplished while the tissues in the region of the perforation are still reasonably healthy; so it must be done as soon as the diagnosis is confirmed. Location of the leak and the presence of underlying disease dictate the details of the surgical method. If carcinoma is associated with the perforation, emergency esophagectomy may be necessary.

The sharp distinction between the prognosis and treatment of perforations at different levels points out the need for prompt suspicion of and confirmation of the diagnosis, along with precise radiologic location of the perforation. Location by means of endoscopy is not reliable because the site of perforation often is not visible.

Occasionally, esophageal leaks become evident several days after they have occurred. Empyema in the right hemothorax, for example, may develop a week after endoscopic examination, and the barium swallow may or may not demonstrate a leak. A dye such as methylene blue, given by mouth and recovered from the pleural space, confirms the presence of a small fistula. Such a subacute situation can sometimes be managed conservatively by treatment of the empyema, if mediastinitis has not progressed and if the fistula closes spontaneously.

Hemorrhage

Esophageal hemorrhage is an uncommon complication of esophagitis, achalasia, and tumor, but is a regular result of gastroesophageal mucosal tears of the Mallory-Weiss type and of esophageal varices. A rare cause of bleeding and partial obstruction is "esophageal apoplexy," a spontaneous intramural bleeding in the presence of hypertensive arteriosclerotic disease, which may perforate through the mucosa into the esopageal lumen.

In most cases, esophageal bleeding subsides without surgical treatment. Persistent, rapid bleeding, however, requires prompt investigation and active management. Gentle nasogastric intubation and iced saline lavage to clear the stomach and esophagus of clots aids in subsequent endoscopic attempts to visualize the bleeding site. Endoscopy should be performed *before* a barium swallow; coating of the esophagus with barium obscures the mucosa for at least 24 hours. Should the cause and site of hemorrhage still be unknown after these maneuvers, angiographic demonstration is required. A bleeding site located by angiography may be treated with injection of vasospastic drugs or embolization of the feeding vessels (see Chapter 46). In patients with massive bleeding due to achalasia or esophagitis, however, resection may be lifesaving. In cases of *persistent* bleeding from Mallory-Weiss or other lacerations, early surgical repair is the treatment of choice.

Acute Esophagitis

A common condition, *reflux peptic esophagitis* is sometimes severe, causing pain, esophagospasm, and dysphagia, with occasional perforation or bleeding. In the absence of bleeding or perforation, emergency treatment consists of elevation of the head of the bed, frequent administration of antacids, cimetidine or ranitidine, and antispasmodic agents, and bougienage if there is a stricture. If the diagnosis is suspected, it should be confirmed by esophagoscopy.

Bleeding associated with this type of esophagitis usually subsides after such a conservative regimen. If it does not, a course of vasoconstrictor drugs should be administered by angiographic techniques; if this too fails, emergency esophagectomy must be performed if the bleeding is exsanguinating.

Infectious esophagitis is an uncommon condition caused by a variety of organisms. Bacteria have been the usual infecting agents, but the more common organisms at present are yeasts and fungi that multiply in the esophagus when pharyngeal and esophageal bacteria are suppressed by antibiotic therapy or when chemotherapy or immunosuppressive therapy is employed for malignant conditions. Inflammatory edema and esophagospasm produce pain and dysphagia. The diagnosis is usually evident on examination of the mouth, although esophagoscopy occasionally is necessary for confirmation. Treatment consists of oral and intravenous fluids and the frequent ingestion of antifungal solutions, such as nystatin.

The rare patient with bacterial esophagitis requires prompt diagnosis by esophagoscopy and culture and early treatment with appropriate antibiotics. Parenteral nutrition may be necessary in severe cases.

Esophagospasm

The pain of esophagospasm is a common cause of admission to an emergency facility because of its similarity to cardiac pain. The history is usually diagnostic when there is no conclusive evidence of cardiac disease. It is necessary to inquire about the relation of pain to swallowing and/or posture and about any history of gastroesophageal disease or emotional tension. Esophageal manometric studies and acid-perfusion testing may be necessary to differentiate esophagospasm from cardiac disease.

A few patients have remarkably obstructive dysphagia due to diffuse esophageal spasm. Severe motility disorders manifested by tertiary contractions occasionally may be seen in elderly patients. Presumably, these are caused by a neurologic deficit. No emergency treatment is needed. These diagnoses can be suspected after barium swallow, but must be confirmed by manometric study. No emergency treatment is necessary other than reassurance. A surgical consultation is necessary because the symptoms may be relieved only by esophagomyotomy.

Diaphragmatic Hernia

Any type of diaphragmatic herniation may cause a true emergency. Hernias at the foramina of Bochdalek and Morgagni may lead to incarceration and strangulation of upper abdominal viscera. Hiatal hernias cause several types of serious problems:

1. Paraesophageal hernias, commonly involving incarceration of the gastric fundus, cause bleeding, and occasionally strangulation.
2. Large axial hernias may admit small intestine or colon into the intrathoracic sac, where it becomes obstructed and/or strangulated.
3. Large axial hernias containing more than one-half of the stomach are prone to gastric volvulus; this produces complete obstruction and may result in bleeding or gangrene.

All large diaphragmatic hernias are first suspected if an air-fluid level is demonstrated on a chest x-ray film. In the absence of pain, fever, leukocytosis, or obstruction, satisfactory treatment may consist of elevation of the head of the bed, administration of intravenous fluids, and gastrointestinal decompression, with repair to follow within a few days. However, persistent obstruction, pain, or bleeding require early operation. In the case of the large incarcerated axial hiatal hernia, pain and obstruction may be relieved quickly by nasogastric intubation. If this fails or if there is fever, leukocytosis, or reactive pleural effusion indicating possible or impending gastric necrosis, immediate surgical intervention is mandatory to prevent ischemic perforation, pleuritis, and peritonitis. Because gastric volvulus in huge hiatal hernias usually occurs in elderly patients, it may be fatal if operative treatment is delayed.

SUGGESTED READINGS

Aspiration Pneumonia

Broe PJ, Toung TJK, Cameron JL. Aspiration pneumonia. *Surg Clin North Am,* 1980;60:1551–1564.

Strain JD, Moore EE, Markovchick VJ, et al. Cimetidine for the prophylaxis of potential gastric acid aspiration pneumonitis in trauma patients, *J Trauma,* 1981;21:49–51.

Utsunomiya T, Frausz MM, Valeri, CR, et al. Treatment of aspiration pneumonia with ibuprofen and prostacyclin. *Surgery,* 1981;90:170–176.

Caustic Injury

Kirsh MM, Ritter, F. Caustic ingestion and subsequent damage to the oropharyngeal and digestive passages. *Ann Thorac Surg,* 1976;21:74–82.

Diaphragmatic Rupture and Hernias

Symbas, PN. Blunt traumatic rupture of the diaphragm. *Ann Thorac Surg,* 1978;26:193–194.

Orringer MB, Kirsh MM, Sloan H. Congenital and traumatic diaphragmatic hernias exclusive of the hiatus. *Curr Probl Surg,* 1975;12(Mar)1–68.

Hood RM. Traumatic diaphragmatic hernia. *Ann Thorac Surg,* 1971;12:311–324.

Beauchamp G, Khalfallah A, Girard R, et al. Blunt diaphragmatic rupture. *Amer J Surg,* 1984;148:292–295.

Esophageal Perforation

Cameron JL, et al. Selective non-operative management of contained intrathoracic esophageal disruptions. *Ann Thorac Surg,* 1979;27:404–408.

Grillo HC, Wilkins EW Jr, Michel L, et al. Esophageal perforation: the syndrome and its management. In Skinner D, DeMeester, T, eds. *Esophageal Disorders—Pathophysiology and Therapy.* New York: Raven Press, 1985: 493–499.

Michel L, Grillo HC, Malt RA. Operative and nonoperative management of esophageal perforations. *Ann Surg,* 1981,194:57–63.

Flail Chest

Moore BP. Operative stabilization of nonpenetrating chest injuries. *J Thorac Cardiovasc Surg,* 1975;70:619–630.

Shackford SR, Virgilio RW, Peters RM. Selective use of ventilator therapy in flail chest injury. *J Thorac Cardiovasc Surg,* 1981;81:194–201.

Trinkle JK, Richardson JD, Franz JL, et al. Management

of flail chest without mechanical ventilation. *Ann Thorac Surg,* 1975;19:355–363.

Yee ES, Thomas AN, Goodman PC. Isolated first rib fracture: Clinical significance after blunt chest trauma. *Ann Thorac Surg,* 1981;32:278–283.

Hemothorax

Wilson JM, Boren CH Jr, Peterson SR, et al. Traumatic hemothorax: Is decortication necessary? *J Thorac Cardiovasc Surg,* 1979;77:489–494.

Laryngotracheal Trauma

Mathisen DJ, Grillo HC. Laryngotracheal trauma. *Ann Thorac Surg,* 1987;43:254–262.

Mathisen DJ, Grillo HC. Laryngotracheal trauma—acute and chronic. In Eschapasse H, Grillo HC, eds. *International Trends in General Thoracic Surgery,* vol 2. Philadelphia: WB. Saunders, 1987:117–123.

Massive Hemoptysis

Garzon AA, Guourin A. Surgical management of massive hemoptysis. *Ann Surg,* 1978;187:267–271.

Swersky RB, Chang JB, Wisoff BG, et al. Endobronchial balloon tamponade of hemoptysis in patients with cystic fibrosis. *Ann Thorac Surg,* 1979;27:262–264.

Penetrating Chest Trauma

Mattox K. Management of penetrating chest trauma. *Hospital Medicine* 1977;8–26.

Hankins JR, McAslan TC, Skin B, et al. Extensive pulmonary laceration caused by blunt trauma. *J Thorac Cardiovasc Surg,* 1977;74:519–526.

CHAPTER **33**

Abdominal Emergencies

ASHBY C. MONCURE, M.D.
LESLIE W. OTTINGER, M.D.
CHARLES J. McCABE, M.D.

INTRODUCTION

The first task of an emergency physician caring for a patient with an abdominal complaint is to arrive at a working, or tentative, diagnosis as promptly as possible. The diagnosis must then be refined on the basis of a thorough history, complete physical examination, and evaluation of specific laboratory tests and roentgenograms. Valid clinical judgment requires accurate information; inaccurate or incomplete information can be disastrously misleading. Even if an exact diagnosis is not immediately achievable, the physician should be able to ascertain whether a potentially life-threatening condition such as hemorrhage, visceral perforation, or advancing infection seems likely, and to consult with a surgeon accordingly.

The History

Since the patient with an abdominal complaint is frequently so uncomfortable and/or lethargic as to be inaccurate in responding to questions, the examiner must compensate for this with thoroughness and specific queries. If feasible, the examiner asks the patient for a chronologic narrative of his/her difficulty. Information should include the mode and site of onset of the symptom; the character of any pain, including its reference or extension; the presence or absence of nausea, vomiting, constipation, obstipation, or diarrhea; the character of vomitus or stool; the presence or absence of fever or chills, previous occurrence of the symptom as well as its constancy or intermittency; and maneuvers employed by the patient to gain relief. Accompanying relatives or friends, as well as previous medical records, can be invaluable in leading to a correct diagnosis. A detailed medical history including previous operations, medications, allergies, and diseases may provide significant information regarding the present illness.

The Examination

After the patient is *completely* disrobed, physical examination is begun with careful evaluation of the vital signs. The blood pressure, the presence or absence of fever, and the character and rate of the pulse and respiration are recorded. It may be necessary to establish an adequate airway or to start blood replacement, or both, before continuing with the examination. The general appearance of the patient is noted—whether he/she appears ill, icteric, diaphoretic, or pallid. His/her position is important—a patient lying supine with flexed knees may indicate peritoneal irritation.

After the vital signs are evaluated, the physician examines the skin, head, neck, breasts, chest, abdomen, groins, rectum, pelvis, and extremities. A physical abnormality far from the abdomen may signify the underlying disease responsible for an abdominal complaint. For example, a patient with abdominal pain who is found to have atrial fibrillation or mitral stenosis may have an embolus in a visceral artery.

During auscultation, the character of peristalsis is noted. Peristalsis may be increased in acute gastroenteritis and mechanical intestinal obstruction, and is commonly diminished or absent in the presence of peritoneal irritation. Audible, normal peristalsis does not exclude the possibility of intraabdominal inflammation.

Before palpating the abdomen, the examiner requests a cough to help locate the site of pain; thus he/she may choose to palpate this area after examining the remainder of the abdomen. The most reliable physical finding indicating peritoneal irritation is the presence of *voluntary or involuntary spasm*, or both. Spasm can be determined accurately only by gently placing the palm of the hand on an abdominal quadrant over the rectus muscle, asking the patient to breathe deeply, and gently depressing the examining hand with the other hand. Voluntary spasm of the rectus muscle disappears as the patient exhales; involuntary spasm does not. With involuntary spasm, the muscle remains tense and boardlike.

The exact area of tenderness is noted by gentle palpation with one finger. This may suggest the viscus affected by the intraabdominal process. On removal of the hand pressing near the tender area, rebound tenderness may be felt in the primary site of pain, providing further evidence of peritoneal irritation. The flanks are carefully palpated along with the lower part of the chest wall. A posterior inflammatory process adjacent to the retroperitoneum is suggested by pain elicited on extension of the iliopsoas or obturator muscle.

The patient is examined for masses, hepatosplenomegaly, and free fluid within the abdominal cavity. If dullness and tenderness coincide on gentle percussion, a mass is sought in this location. Herniation through a previous abdominal incision is sought by increasing intraabdominal pressure with a cough or raising the head.

The groins are examined carefully and gently in all patients. The scrotum is invaginated with the index finger to permit palpation of the external inguinal rings and the inguinal canals, where a mass usually indicates a hernia. An indirect inguinal hernia is palpable as an elliptical mass descending along the spermatic cord, usually descending further with cough or Valsalva's maneuver. A direct inguinal hernia is palpable as a globular mass close to the pubis. A femoral hernia is more difficult to outline because the empty space of the femoral canal, where the herniation occurs, is not distinctly palpable. The readily indentifiable structure in the femoral canal is the pulsating femoral artery as it emerges from under the inguinal ligament. Therefore, after identifying the femoral artery, the examiner searches for the hernia two fingerbreadths medial to the artery.

The inguinal region is more difficult to assess in the female because the labia cannot be invaginated. This region is examined by placing the finger in the area of the external ring and then the palm of the hand over the area of the internal ring and having the patient cough as each area is examined. The femoral region is examined as in the male. If possible, the examination is conducted with the patient in both supine and standing positions.

Pelvic and rectal examinations must be carried out for complete evaluation of patient's condition. Pelvic examination is described in Chapter 34. The anus and rectum are inspected and palpated. Endoscopic examination of the rectum is frequently necessary. Extreme pain on rectal introduction of the palpating finger usually indicates acute inflammation or stenosis of the anal canal. In this case, further efforts to examine this area are postponed.

Usually, after moderate resistance, the sphincter relaxes and the finger can be advanced to examine the rectum circumferentially. The prostate gland or the area of the pouch of Douglas are also palpated. Proctosigmoidoscopic examination may provide further information.

Acute abdominal disease in the elderly man may present in atypical fashion. Awareness of this may lead to earlier diagnosis. Advanced disease may be indicated by subtle symptoms or signs, due presumably to altered pain threshold and response to examination. In these patients, repeated abdominal examination may be necessary to diagnose a possibly life-threatening intraabdominal process.

Laboratory Evaluation

A complete blood cell count, urinalysis, examination of a stool specimen for occult blood, and determination of the blood glucose, blood urea nitrogen, and serum amylase levels are required in all abdominal emergency patients. Hematocrit determinations can be repeated easily and frequently. Although the hematocrit value cannot be employed as the sole guide to suspected blood loss or changes in plasma volume, it is frequently used in conjunction with observation of blood pressure, pulse, urinary output, and central venous pressure. A low initial hematocrit reading suggests an antecedent chronic illness, chronic gastrointestinal blood loss, or acute hemorrhage.

The white blood cell count is usually elevated in inflammatory conditions, although it is occasionally normal early in the course of acute disease. In the elderly, it may be within normal limits even in the presence of marked intraabdominal inflammation. If the white blood cell count is normal, an abnormal differential often suggests an inflammatory process. In the presence of inflammation, there is usually an increased number of polymorphonuclear leukocytes and band forms as well as toxic granulation within the leukocytes.

Determinations of the platelet count, prothrombin time, and partial thromboplastin time are necessary in patients with hemorrhage. Measurement of serum electrolyte levels is valuable in patients with gastrointestinal losses from either vomiting, diarrhea, or intraluminal fluid sequestration accompanying intestinal obstruction. In all patients with abdominal pain, even in children, the serum amylase and lipase levels are determined.

Paracentesis is considered in patients with abdominal pain or with trauma. Its findings may rapidly alert the physician to the presence of free blood, bile, or purulent material. A negative tap does not exclude the presence of abdominal fluid. Paracentesis is performed with a long, 19-gauge needle on a small syringe passed through a locally anesthetized area lateral to the rectus muscle in each abdominal quadrant. It may also be accomplished by percutaneous placement of a polethylene catheter through the midline below the umbilicus (see Illustrated Technique 14) in patients who have not un-

Table 33.1.
Upper Quadrant Pain: Causes

Gastrointestinal
- *Right:*
  - Hepatitis/hepatomegaly
  - Hepatic neoplasm
  - Biliary colic
  - Cholecystitis
  - Peptic ulcer
  - Pancreatitis
- *Left:*
  - Gastritis
  - Pancreatitis
  - Spleen (enlargement, infarct)
  - Splenic flexure carcinoma

Referred
- Retrocecal appendicitis
- Pelvic inflammatory disease
- Renal pain
- Pneumonia
- Emphysema
- Pericarditis
- Myocardial ischemia

Table 33.2.
Lower Abdominal Pain: Causes

Gastrointestinal
- *Right:*
  - Appendicitis
  - Regional enteritis
  - Perforated ulcer
  - Mesenteric adenitis
  - Right-sided diverticulitis
  - Small bowel obstruction
  - Cecal cancer
  - Psoas abscess
- *Left:*
  - Sigmoid diverticulitis
  - Intestinal obstruction
  - Sigmoid carcinoma
  - Psoas abscess

Gynecologic
- Ectopic pregnancy
- Pelvic inflammatory disease
- Mittelschmerz
- Endometriosis
- Ovarian cyst

Urologic
- Ureteral calculi
- Renal pain
- Cystitis
- Psoas abscess

Table 33.3.
Suggested Emergency Evaluation for Right Upper Quadrant (RUQ) Pain

1. History and physical examination
2. Chest x-ray/plain abdominal x-ray.
3. Liver function tests, amylase, CBC with differential count[a]
4. ? RUQ ultrasonography

[a] CBC, complete blood count.

Table 33.4.
Suggested Emergency Evaluation for Right Lower Quadrant (RLQ) Pain

Male
1. History and physical examination
2. CBC with differential count, urinalysis[a]
3. ? Intravenous pyelography (IVP)

Female
1. History and physical examination
2. CBC with differential count, urinalysis
3. Pregnancy test, β-hCG
4. ? IVP
5. ? Pelvic ultrasonography

[a] CBC, complete blood count; hCG, human chorionic gonadotropin.

dergone any previous abdominal operation. This is done after the patient has voided. Gram's staining and culture of any fluid is carried out along with examination for amylase content and red and white blood cell counts.

Since coronary thrombosis occasionally causes upper abdominal pain, an electrocardiogram should be recorded in patients more than 25 years old.

Roentgenographic Study

Roentgenographic examination of the patient with an abdominal complaint is essential. It includes abdominal films with the patient supine and upright; both diaphragms need to be shown in the erect film. If the patient cannot be upright, a left lateral decubitus film should be taken across the table. If an intravenous pyelogram is indicated, it may be accomplished while the plain films are being taken. A chest film is essential, since lower thoracic processes can cause abdominal pain. An abdominal ultrasound examination often provides information regarding the presence of masses, fluid, gallstones, and biliary ductal dilatation. Angiographic examination is used to evaluate patients with trauma and those in whom an occluded visceral vessel or a dissecting aneurysm is suspected. Radionuclide scanning may be helpful in evaluating the liver and spleen after trauma. Barium or gastrografin contrast examination of the stomach or intestine may be necessary to define disease of these viscera. Computed tomography of the abdomen with contrast enhancement may also be useful in evaluation of the abdomen, particularly following trauma.

With this pertinent information, the clinician must establish a working diagnosis by weighing probabilities. If the patient's life seems threatened, consultation with a surgeon is both necessary and wise. If a serious intraabdominal process is not suspected, a plan must be formulated for further diagnosis and for treatment. Therapy may require hospital admission or ambulatory care with follow-up evaluation. If the patient is seen later with the same complaint, he probably should be hospitalized for further diagnostic studies. *Under such circumstances, a specific reason for discharge is required.*

Table 33.5.
Suggested Emergency Evaluation for Left Lower Quadrant (LLQ) Pain

1. History and physical examination
2. CBC with differential count, urinalysis[a]
3. Chest x-ray, plain abdominal x-ray (KUB)
4. ? Intravenous pyelography
5. ? Sigmoidoscopy
6. ? Gastrografin or barium enema

[a] CBC, complete blood count; KUB, kidneys-ureter-bladder.

ACUTE ABDOMEN

A common presenting symptom of patients coming to the emergency department is that of abdominal pain (Tables 33.1–33.5). In almost all nontraumatic abdominal emergencies, the correct diagnosis can be established with a detailed history and careful physical examination alone. Laboratory tests are usually needed only for diagnostic confirmation. In many instances of acute abdominal pain, however, the patient may require supportive therapy before a diagnosis can be made. For example, as soon as the presence of diffuse purulent peritonitis is detected and before the surgeon establishes the cause at laparotomy, the physician must start intravenous antibiotic therapy, volume replacement, and supportive measures required in a given patient. The management of the patient with painful acute abdomen, therefore, requires a two-fold approach. On the one hand, the physician must protect against the hazards of the underlying pathologic process. On the other hand, he/she cannot treat the patient definitively until the diagnosis is established. Diagnostic and therapeutic procedures must proceed simultaneously, each giving way to the other under appropriate circumstances. Because of these dual considerations—diagnosis and therapy—it is important that the overall responsibility for treatment of the patient be *delegated to one person.* Transfer of responsibility to another individual must follow a formal procedure, and all those caring for the patient must know whom to consult for decisions relating to priority of therapeutic and diagnostic measures. The emergency physician transfers such responsibility to the surgeon just as soon as (*a*) admission is elected, and (*b*) the surgeon is in attendance.

The onset and character of the pain, its time of onset, the quality and site at onset, changes in site and character, whether it has interrupted or prevented sleep, and exacerbating or relieving factors are all important details. Such factors include eating, defecation, micturition, walking, coughing, and changes in truncal position. Although patients may be unable to describe pain clearly, the physician must try to determine the degree of localization of the pain, its sharpness or dullness, its periodicity, whether it has been uniform since onset, or whether it has diminished or even disappeared.

Pain: Mechanisms and Interpretation

Abdominal pain can be characterized as visceral or somatic, that is, originating from a viscus or from parietal peritoneum, abdominal wall, or retroperitoneal tissues. Although it is clear that these dissimilar types of pain result from a differing distribution of pain receptors, the neurologic pathways for transmission of each type are not fully understood.

The surfaces of abdominal viscera contain pain receptors similar to those in skin, but in the viscera these receptors are widely spaced. Thus, these organs are relatively insensitive to localized stimuli. Diffuse stimulation of nerve endings, such as that caused by forceful contraction of the smooth muscle or occlusion of blood supply, is the usual cause of visceral pain. On the other hand, tissues of somatic segments contain a higher concentration of pain receptors, and stimuli of many types evoke pain in these areas.

Visceral pain is typical of conditions such as acute obstruction of the small intestine, passage of a calculus through the urinary tract, and acute obstruction of the common bile duct. Patients sometimes have difficulty describing such visceral pain clearly. Afferent nerve fibers traverse the intestinal ganglia and enter the spinal cord in such a way that it is often impossible to discern whether the cause of pain lies on the right or the left side. Pain arising from either the right or the left colon, for example, is usually perceived in the midline of the lower abdomen. (This principle does not apply to the urinary tract.) Even though visceral pain of gastrointestinal origin is usually referred to the midline, the level in the longitudinal axis often reflects the source. Pain from the biliary tree or duodenum may be felt in the epigastrium, from the small intestine in the umbilical region, and from the colon below the umbilicus. Visceral pain often has a gripping or cramping quality because it is produced by rhythmic peristaltic spasms. It can, however, be due to severe intestinal ischemia. In this case, the precise mechanism of pain stimulation is unclear. Although severe spasm of intestine deprived of its arterial blood supply sometimes may provide the stimulus, ischemic abdominal pain can last long after the intestinal spasm. Ischemia alone may, in fact, cause the pain. Severe, diffuse, anterior abdominal distress unrelieved by narcotics is characteristic of visceral ischemia.

Somatic pain is usually differentiated easily from visceral pain. The patient can specify its location fairly accurately, and may describe it as sharp, burning, or tearing. Since somatic pain is the result of irritation or injury to a specific area of abdominal parietes, it can be exacerbated by local pressure or by a change in position.

Interpretation of referred pain is more often misleading than helpful, since visceral pain may be perceived as originating from a somatic segment because of crossover between visceral and somatic afferent nerve pathways. On the body surface, referred pain is located at the dermatome of the segment from which the viscus developed in the embryo. A striking example of referred pain is that which accompanies the passing of a renal calculus. Pain appears in the right flank, and moves obliquely across the flank into the groin, even into the labium or testis, before it is relieved by passage of the calculus into the bladder. Gallbladder discomfort can be referred to the middle and lower regions of the right scapula. Frequently, somatic pain from the diaphragm is referred to the posterior aspect of the ipsilateral shoulder down to the level of the midscapula. Referred diaphragmatic pain is particularly important in the detection of upper abdominal peritoneal irritation.

Peritoneal Irritation: Etiology

Inflammatory reactions such as perforation of the appendix, perforation of a colonic diverticulum, and cholecystitis irritate the parietal peritoneum and cause somatic pain. Local irritation from an invasive infectious process, rather than the mere presence of bacteria, seems to produce such irritation. For example, when perforation of the colon occurs and large numbers of bacteria escape into the peritoneal cavity, signs of peritoneal irritation do not appear until inflammation and invasive infection are established.

Several types of fluid may cause somatic pain when released into the peritoneal cavity. Blood may or may not. For example, in hemorrhaging ruptured ectopic pregnancy, the patient may have either signs and symptoms suggesting severe, diffuse peritonitis or a distended but otherwise normal abdomen. Fluid from a tumor can be exceedingly irritating. Such irritation occurs with ruptured ovarian cysts. These patients may have symptoms of acute, diffuse peritonitis. Bile and urine usually cause severe peritoneal irritation.

The more acid contents of the digestive organs are the most irritating. Gastric acid evokes immediate and severe symptoms, whereas intestinal con-

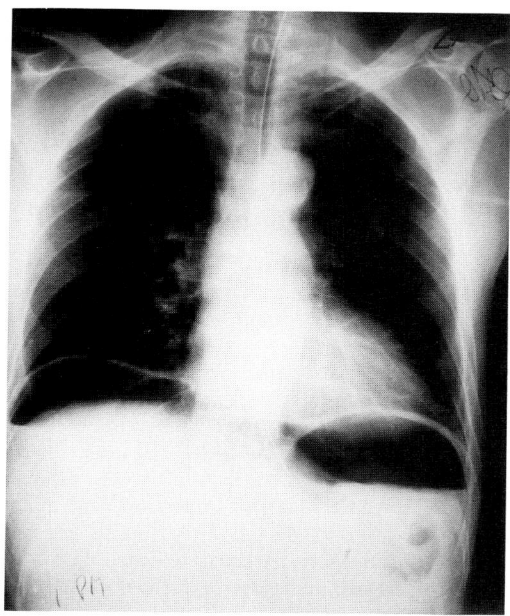

Figure 33.1. Chest x-ray demonstrating air under the right hemidiaphragm, secondary to a perforated duodenal ulcer.

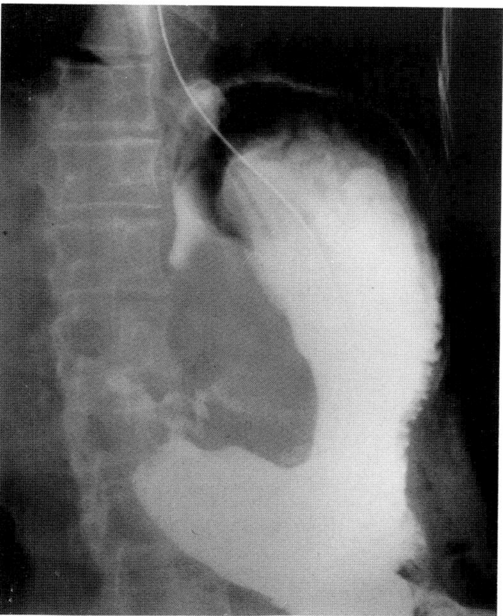

Figure 33.2. A gastrografin upper gastrointestinal series demonstrates extravasation of the gastrografin from the duodenal area. The patient is in the supine position, and the gastrografin pools along the lesser curvature at the fundus of the stomach.

tents with a more neutral pH, cause symptoms only after the onset of bacterial peritonitis. Because there are relatively few bacteria in the small intestine, such a perforation may not cause signs of peritoneal irritation for many hours.

Specific Conditions

Noninflammatory Perforations

Distal Esophageal Perforation. Spontaneous perforation of the distal portion of the esophagus is not usually associated with preceding pathologic esophageal changes. Since the perforation, which is usually a linear tear, occurs near the stomach, gastric contents and gas are released into the mediastinum and to the left or, occasionally, the right pleural space. Onset of pain is sudden, and resembles that of a perforated peptic ulcer. In some patients, perforation occurs soon after a heavy meal or forceful vomiting. Severe epigastric pain is the most typical feature. On physical examination, there is little evidence of peritoneal irritation in the upper part of the abdomen. This combination of severe pain and absent physical signs alerts the physician to the diagnosis. Thoracic symptoms related to the presence of infected pleural fluid appear later. A chest roentgenogram showing fluid and possibly gas in the pleural space adds support to the diagnosis. An early film may show only mediastinal air. If the diagnosis remains obscure, contrast studies may be employed, but a water-soluble contrast solution should be used in place of barium. Antibiotics are immediately begun and volume replacement started. It is important to diagnose this condition early; mortality increases with delay in operation.

Gastric Ulcer or Tumor. In patients with perforated gastric ulcer or tumor, symptoms often develop gradually because these lesions frequently occur in the presence of a low level of gastric acid secretion. The patient experiences epigastric pain with possible referral to the shoulders. There may be a history of the rather nonspecific symptoms of gastric ulcer and tumor: i.e., changes in tolerance for food, gnawing visceral pain in the upper abdomen, and weight loss. Except when a tumor is strongly suspected, laparotomy should take precedence over contrast studies.

Duodenal Ulcer. Because a duodenal ulcer is usually associated with normal or high levels of gastric acid secretion, its perforation is frequently accompanied by a dramatic onset of symptoms. Key information in the history includes longstanding duodenal disease or recent epigastric distress and heartburn. Upper abdominal, peritoneal, and diaphragmatic irritation is common, producing prominent tenderness and resistance on palpation. Conversely, if the amount of escaping gastric con-

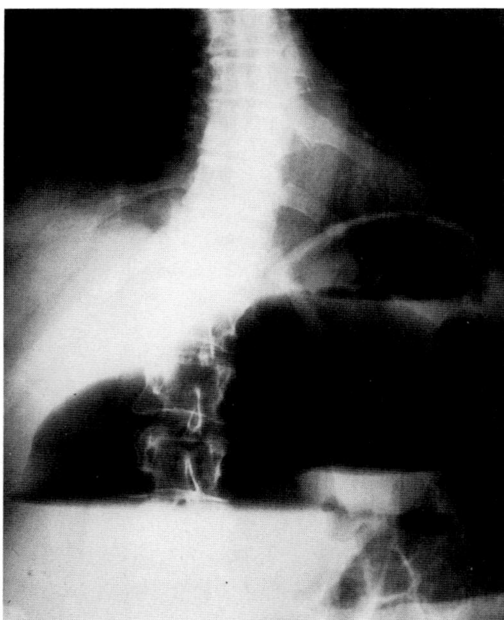

Figure 33.3. Plain abdominal film reveals large bowel obstruction.

tents and acid is small, the presentation of symptoms may be surprisingly subtle. The first strong evidence of such a perforation may be free air under the diaphragm on roentgenographic examination (Fig. 33.1). Contrast studies of the upper gastrointestinal tract may not demonstrate perforation if it has been sealed off by adjacent structures, but a gastrografin study may be helpful (Fig. 33.2). If perforation is suspected, nasogastric decompression should be started. Colloid loss from peritoneal surfaces injured by released acid may be high, and the need for replacement must be anticipated.

Meckel's Diverticulum. Perforation of a Meckel's diverticulum occurs so rarely that preoperative establishment of the diagnosis is unusual. Perforation results from ulceration related to heterotopic gastric mucosa within the diverticulum, occasionally from lodgement of a pointed foreign body.

Colonic Perforation. When unrelated to inflammatory conditions, most perforations of the colon occur in the cecum. Obstructing carcinoma in the left colon or severe impaction can cause dilatation and perforation with release of gas and colonic contents. Since these do not cause much irritation to peritoneal surfaces, signs of peritonitis develop gradually as invasive bacterial infection becomes established. Decompression of the colon is not a necessary sequel to perforation. Often, a colon dilated with gas is noted on the plain roentgenogram despite the presence of free gas. As a rule, perforation is considered imminent when the diameter of the cecum exceeds 12 cm (Fig. 33.3). Parenteral antibiotics are administered immediately. Contrast study of the left colon (Fig. 33.4) can guide the surgeon in correct management, but complicating contamination of the peritoneal cavity with barium may result. Nonobstructive colonic dilatation (Ogilvie's syndrome) must be differentiated from the

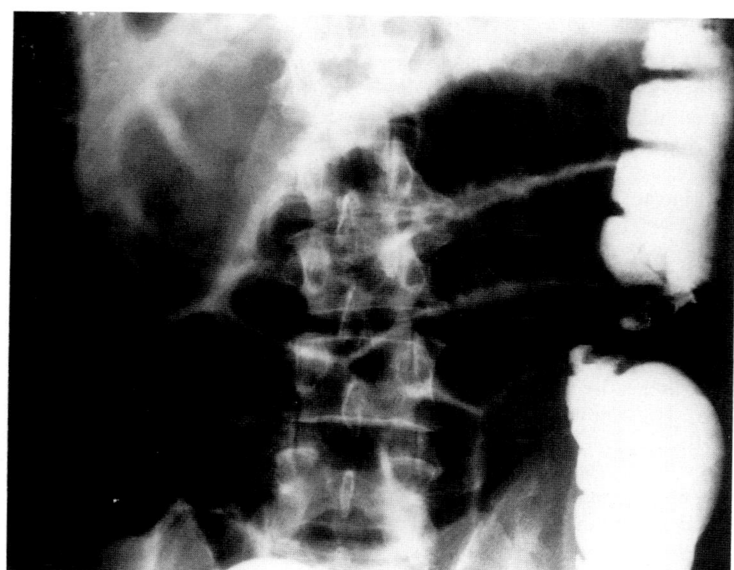

Figure 33.4. Barium enema findings, demonstrating an obstructing carcinoma of the mid-descending colon.

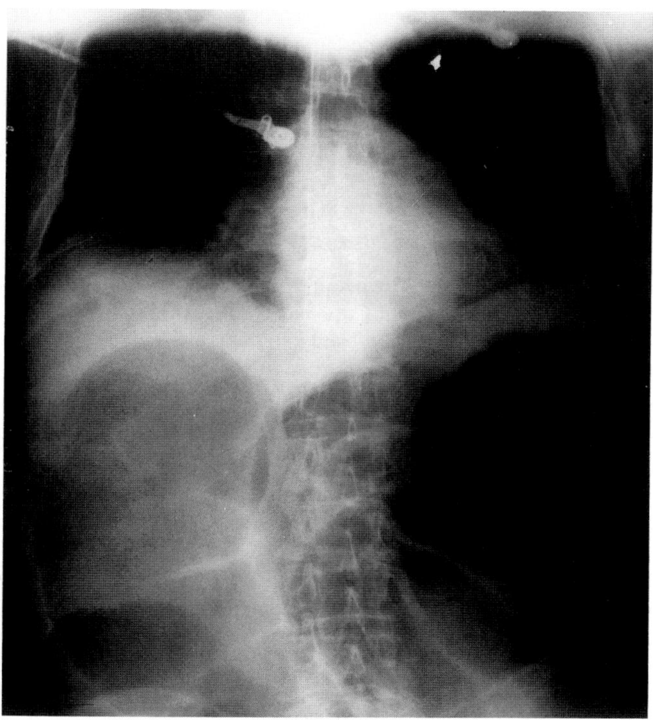

Figure 33.5. Plain abdominal film demonstrates massive large bowel distention in a chronic cathartic abuser. Barium enema revealed no evidence of colonic obstruction.

symptoms mentioned above. Frequently, this occurs in patients who are elderly, have had recurrent episodes of colonic dilatation (Fig. 33.5) and use cathartics heavily. A contrast examination reveals the lack of colonic obstruction. Therapy includes nasogastric decompression, fluid support, and the possible use of colonoscopy to decompress the colon.

Pelvic Conditions. The contents of a perforated ovarian tumor, especially of an endometrioma, may prove strongly irritating to peritoneal surfaces. Sudden onset of severe lower or diffuse abdominal pain is the first sign of such a perforation. Bleeding from an ectopic pregnancy may produce the same symptom. However, since the peritoneum is not necessarily sensitive to the presence of blood, somatic pain may be absent, and hypovolemic shock may ensue without warning. The character of preceding menstrual periods may suggest either an endometrioma or ectopic pregnancy. This is usually not true with ovarian cysts.

Inflammatory Conditions

Cholecystitis. The precise mechanism of mild attacks of cholecystitis is unclear. Obstruction of the cystic duct by a calculus may generate visceral symptoms of upper abdominal discomfort and fullness. Or, an inflammatory reaction may cause somatic pain. In severe episodes of cholecystitis, inflammation of the parietal peritoneum over the gallbladder causes characteristic sharp, burning distress in the upper right abdominal quadrant. Referral of pain to the right scapular region may occur in mild attacks and is common in severe attacks.

Mild episodes of cholecystitis may be of short duration, and the patient usually attributes them to "indigestion." An attack severe enough to cause a patient to seek emergency care is likely to be different. Often, it will have started a few hours after a meal. The pain may have wakened the patient during the night and then intensified, reflecting an increased inflammatory component with peritoneal signs. Plain roentgenograms show gallstones in only about 20% of patients. (Fig. 33.6). An unusual presentation of severe cholecystitis is emphysematous cholecystitis (Fig. 33.7 *A* and *B*) wherein the radiologic findings are diagnostic, and early operative intervention is necessary to anticipate perforation. Imaging techniques utilizing ultrasound or computed tomography can demonstrate the presence of gallstones, as well as neighborhood fluid. Ultrasonography has become the initial diagnostic procedure to look for nonopaque gallstones. The oral cholecystogram is of limited value in the diagnosis of acute cholecystitis. If normal gallbladder function is demonstrated, cholecystitis can be excluded. The converse is not true, however, since abnormal or absent function can result from several other disorders, such as pancreatitis or even acute gastroenteritis. Radioisotope scanning techniques may be utilized as well, but clinical correlation is necessary in appropriate interpretation.

An attack of cholecystitis lasting longer than a few hours can lead to complications such as empyema, gangrene, or perforation. The patient should be hospitalized and treated with parenteral antibiotics, nasogastric decompression, and timely operation. A surgeon must be consulted early in the evaluation of such a patient, both for determination of need for hospitalization and timing of surgery.

Cholangitis. This is a bacterial infection within the hepatic ducts associated with partial obstruction of the common hepatic duct by calculus, stricture, or less commonly, tumor. The gallbladder sometimes is involved in the inflammatory process. A careful history may elicit the cause of the obstruction. The patient complains of gradually increasing discomfort in the epigastrium and back. This pain has both visceral and somatic components, and may be deceptively mild. Tenderness in the right upper abdominal quadrant is a sign of accompanying inflammation of the gallbladder. Scleral icterus, a finding seldom seen with uncomplicated cholecystitis, may be detected. The physician can often demonstrate tenderness of the liver by gentle percussion with the fist along the ribs over the right hepatic lobe. Because bacteria in biliary radicles are disseminated readily into the bloodstream, a high incidence of septicemia complicates cholangitis. The emergency physician should start antibiotic therapy immediately and seek surgical consultation in preparing the patient for surgical decompression of the obstructed biliary tree.

Pancreatitis. The diagnosis of acute pancreatitis is one of the most difficult to make on the basis of history and physical findings alone. The patient with an acute attack usually can give a specific time of onset of symptoms. Pain commonly is experienced in the upper abdomen, and may extend through to the back. Nausea, anorexia, and vomiting are frequent. Upper abdominal tenderness is ordinarily deeper than that caused by a perforated peptic ulcer. The examiner may palpate a tender mass in the upper abdomen. If pancreatitis is suspected, confirmation by laboratory tests is essential. The serum amylase determination is a fairly reliable test for acute pancreatitis. Ultrasonic abdominal examination or computed tomographic evaluation of the abdomen may suggest an edematous pancreas.

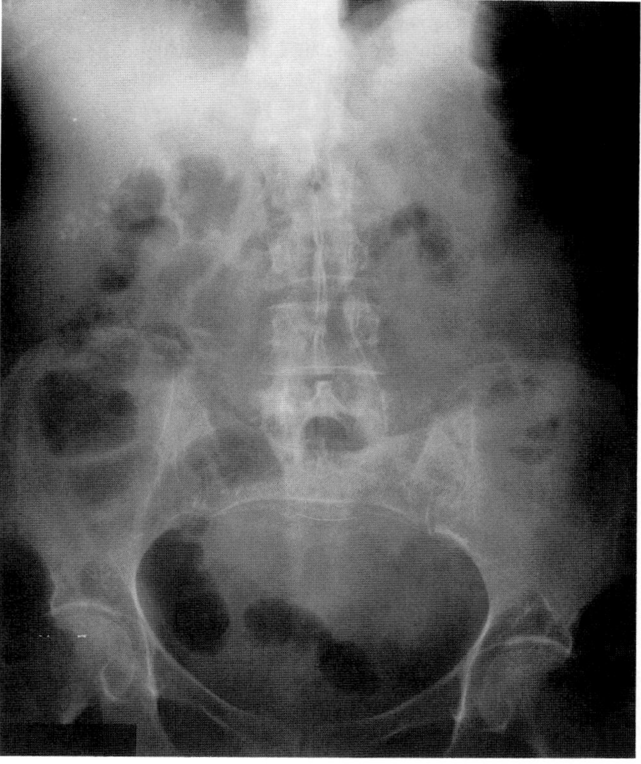

Figure 33.6. Plain abdominal film reveals gallstones in right upper quadrant.

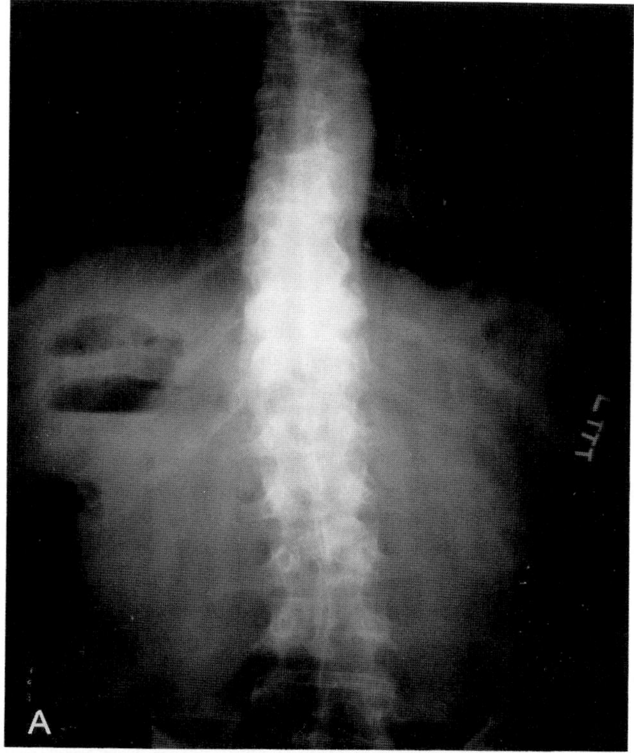

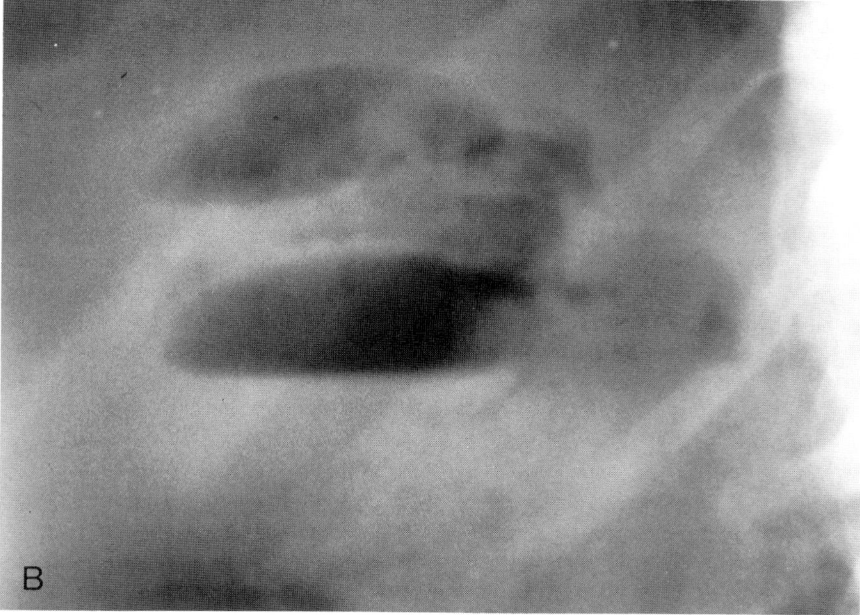

Figure 33.7. *A,* Plain abdominal film demonstrates emphysematous cholecystitis. Air is seen in the right upper quadrant and, on close inspection, a halo of air can be seen in the wall of the gallbladder. *B,* A close-up of the right upper quadrant demonstrates the halo effect of air in the wall of the gallbladder.

Early management includes nasogastric decompression, colloid replacement, and antibiotic therapy.

Patients with chronic or relapsing pancreatitis often have a history suggesting the diagnosis. Each attack may mimic acute pancreatitis, but there are usually fewer physical findings. The serum amylase level is frequently normal. Recurrent attacks sometimes may be caused by a chronic pseudocyst that may be palpable in the upper part of the abdomen. Its presence is readily confirmed by ultrasonography or especially enhanced computed tomography.

Duodenal Ulcer. Unless perforation occurs, duodenal ulcers seldom cause sufficiently intense symptoms to be abdominal emergencies. A posterior perforation may result in pancreatic inflammation that in its early stages cannot be distinguished from pancreatitis due to other causes. This type of attack, however, tends to be mild.

Regional Enteritis. This chronic disease, distinguished by long-standing symptoms of intermittent abdominal cramps, diarrhea, and weight loss, is seldom an acute condition. Occasionally, perforation of the small intestine occurs, and the resultant abscess may dissect along tissue planes and emerge at a remote location, such as the femoral area or the flank. The diagnosis is suspected from the history and the presence of these abscesses.

Some attacks involving the terminal portion of the ileum are not preceded by chronic symptoms, and may be indistinguishable from acute appendicitis, especially if the first episode. A mass in the right lower abdominal quadrant frequently is palpable; this alone does not confirm the diagnosis. Since barium studies are contraindicated in the possible presence of appendicitis, the diagnosis is usually established at surgery.

Ulcerative Colitis. Patients with ulcerative colitis are less likely to be seen initially with acute abdominal pain than those with regional enteritis. Many days of increasingly severe cramps, nausea, and diarrhea customarily precede the somatic pain caused by toxic dilatation and perforation of the intestine in ulcerative colitis patients. The usual chief complaint is bloody diarrhea. Sigmoidoscopic examination is usually diagnostic, confirming ulceration, friability, and easy bleeding of the mucosa when rubbed. If the disease has progressed to the toxic stage, fever and abdominal distention, not pain, may be the distinguishing signs.

Patients with granulomatous colitis have the same general symptoms and signs as patients with regional enteritis or ulcerative colitis, and abdominal pain without a suggestive prior history is unusual.

Appendicitis. Perhaps more has been written about acute appendicitis and its diagnosis than about any other cause of abdominal pain. The diagnosis, however, is frequently missed, especially in very young and very old patients. Typically, the patient describes recent revulsion to food and visceral pain in the middle of the abdomen as the initial symptoms. Symptoms of nonspecific gastroenteritis, such as diarrhea and vomiting, sometimes may precede appendicitis. As local peritoneal irritation develops, the patient experiences sharp somatic pain in the right lower abdominal quadrant. The local inflammatory process, particularly in the presence of an abscess, may form a palpable tender mass. It is important to remember that with acute appendicitis a completely typical presentation is the exception. In males, the differential diagnosis includes regional enteritis, mesenteric adenitis, Meckel's diverticulum, right-sided diverticulitis, and in the older patient, cecal carcinoma with perforation. Ureteral colic may masquerade as appendicitis, as well. In the female, gynecologic causes for these symptoms include ectopic pregnancy, ruptured ovarian cyst or follicle, endometriosis, and pelvic inflammatory disease (Table 33.2). Diagnostic measures include β human chorionic gonadotropin level (β-hCG), urine pregnancy test, ultrasonic or computed evaluation of the pelvis, and especially bimanual pelvic examination with speculum visualization of the cervix.

In both genders, a rectal examination is necessary in that retrocecal or low-lying appendicitis may be evident only by this examination.

Mesenteric Adenitis. An inflammation of the lymph nodes in the mesentery of the terminal portion of the ileum, mesenteric adenitis may simulate appendicitis, although the history is likely to be less precise and the physical findings are less well-localized. Unless improvement is observed within a few hours, laparotomy is necessary to establish the diagnosis and to avert the risk of appendiceal perforation. When mesenteric adenitis mimics appendicitis, removal of a normal appendix is not an unacceptable procedure. When this diagnostic dilemna is present, surgical consultation is mandatory.

Perforated Carcinoma of the Cecum. This neoplasm may result in perforation because of necrosis or because of cecal dilatation behind the tumor. A palpable mass and positive stool guaiac test may suggest the correct diagnosis, but often the signs resemble those of appendicitis. If a perforated malignant lesion of the cecum is suspected, laparotomy without roentgenographic studies other than plain films is preferable in most patients.

Perforated Colonic Diverticulum. If a diverticulum of the right colon becomes perforated, the symptoms may also mimic those of appendicitis. Diverticula of this type are more common in

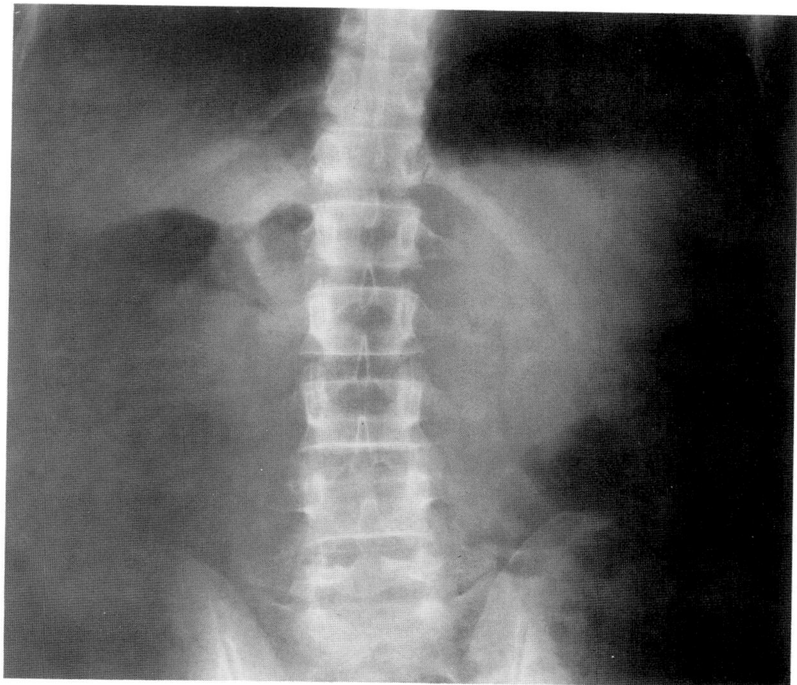

Figure 33.8. Plain abdominal film reveals air-fluid level in a distended stomach.

patients of Oriental extraction. Again, laparotomy is preferable to roentgenographic studies in establishing the diagnosis.

Perforation associated with a diverticulum is more likely to occur in the distal portion of the sigmoid colon than in the transverse or right colon. Occasionally, the perforation occurs without prior symptoms. There may be a recent history of obstipation or diarrhea, along with increasingly severe somatic pain in the left lower abdomen, the pelvis, and the perineum. Left lower abdominal and suprapubic tenderness is typical. The involved segments occasionally may lie so deep within the pelvis that only on vaginal and rectal examination can tenderness be appreciated. Edema and abscesses associated with perforated sigmoid diverticula produce a boggy and often ill-defined mass whose size and discreteness may indicate the severity of the septic process. Abscesses are usually contained by contiguous structures, but occasionally may rupture into the peritoneal cavity, causing symptoms and signs of diffuse peritonitis in the lower abdomen. In patients in whom the sigmoid colon lies to the right of the midline, signs of perforation may be confused with those of appendicitis, although the history is usually different.

Diverticulitis. Acute sigmoid diverticulitis may present with large bowel obstruction, and differentiation from obstructing sigmoid carcinoma may be difficult, even with retrograde barium contrast examination. Colonoscopic examination may be helpful if the mucosa is seen intact. Since barium studies frequently are deceptively normal in patients with perforating sigmoid diverticulosis, they should not be regarded as the decisive diagnostic procedure.

The treatment of nonperforated acute colonic diverticulitis includes nasogastric decompression, intravenous crystalloid support, and antibiotics. These patients must be admitted under a surgeon's care.

Pelvic Inflammatory Disease. Acute paracervicitis, salpingitis, and tubo-ovarian abscess with contiguous peritoneal inflammation categorized together as pelvic inflammatory disease, may simulate most inflammatory conditions of the lower abdomen. A careful history is paramount in establishing the correct diagnosis. Pelvic inflammatory disease typically occurs in young, sexually active women. The patient may report previous similar episodes. The physical findings include fever, diffuse lower abdominal tenderness, pain on motion of the cervix and often a tender mass in either pelvic vault. The white blood cell count may be higher than in other suspected diagnoses. Laparoscopic examination is sometimes of great value when the diagnosis is in doubt. Response to antibiotics may be dramatic. Surgical exploration, however, is sometimes necessary to drain an abscess or to exclude the presence of a septic process unrelated to the pelvic genital structures (see Chapter 34).

Perihepatitis (Fitz-Hugh-Curtis syndrome) is an unusual complication of gonococcal pelvic inflammatory disease characterized by upper abdominal peritonitis, especially on the right, with somatic pain. On auscultation, a rub may be heard over the liver. Unless the accompanying pelvic symptoms and signs are florid, the condition is likely to be confused with acute cholecystitis. It responds rapidly to antibiotics.

Acute Gastroenteritis. Acute gastroenteritis is common among younger patients, and may be confused with many of the conditions previously discussed. Specific causes include bacteria, enteric viruses, amoebae, and gastrointestinal irritants. Recent nausea, vomiting, diarrhea, and cramping visceral pain are typical complaints. Similar symptoms may be elicited from the patient's acquaintances. Abdominal tenderness, when present, is usually minimal and poorly localized. Observation in the emergency department is often necessary to confirm the diagnosis.

Obstruction

Gastric Obstruction. Acute gastric obstruction usually occurs at the pylorus. It is most often the result of scarring from chronic peptic ulcer disease, but may also be produced by pyloric edema and spasm. The typical history entails peptic ulcer symptoms and recent vomiting. There may be acute abdominal pain. A hugely dilated stomach is often detectable (Fig. 33.8), and the diagnosis confirmed by aspiration of gastric contents. Gastric tumors and bezoars rarely lead to acute obstruction, tending instead to produce chronic partial obstruction. An upper gastrointestinal series confirms the diagnosis (Figs. 33.9 and 33.10) of gastric outlet obstruction.

An unusual cause of acute gastric obstruction is incarceration of a large paraesophageal hiatal hernia. These hernias may not be associated with a history of esophageal reflux, although the patient may experience postprandial discomfort due to distention of the herniated portion of the stomach. Physical findings are lacking. Evidence of bleeding suggests strangulation. Diagnosis is often suggested by the chest roentgenogram, especially if a nasogastric tube identifies the incarceration. The presence of gastric obstruction requires admission to the hospital for nasogastric tube decompression. Upper gastrointestinal endoscopy may add further information concerning the cause of the obstruction. Surgical correction is often necessary.

Small Intestinal Obstruction. In its early stages, obstruction of the small intestine is associated with anorexia and intermittent visceral pain. In its acute stage, it provokes proximal forceful peristaltic contractions, which lead to intense cramping pain. As the obstructed loops dilate, peristalsis ceases. Pain may subside and be replaced by the sensation of fullness and distention.

In most patients, vomiting occurs. If the upper portion of the small intestine is obstructed, it may begin within 1 or 2 hours of the onset of pain. If

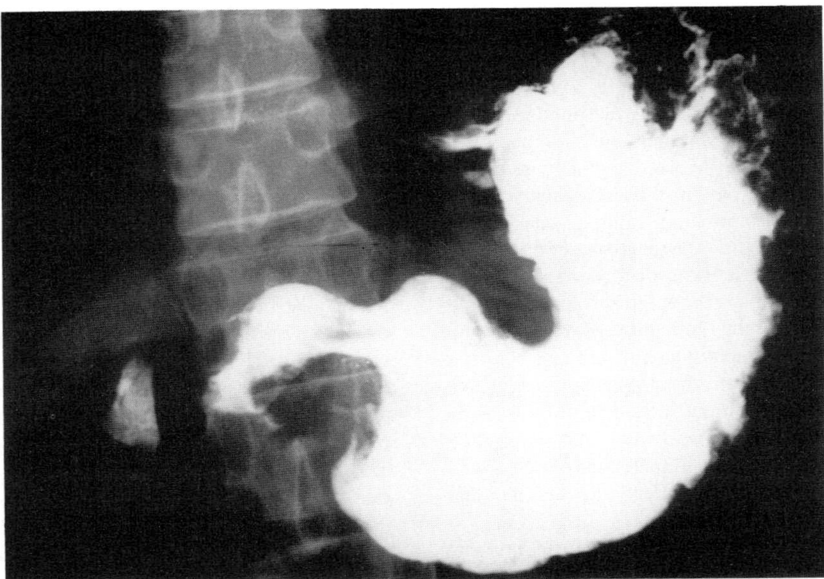

Figure 33.9. Upper gastrointestinal series reveals gastric outlet obstruction secondary to a chronic duodenal ulcer.

the site is more distal, many hours may elapse before vomiting begins. The vomitus is initially light brown and thin, being the contents of the stomach and duodenum. Later, as the contents of the small intestine reflux into the stomach, the vomitus becomes more viscid and opaque, and is often dark brown and foul-smelling. As the intestinal muscular layers proximal to the obstruction become stretched and flaccid, vomiting may cease. Distal to the obstruction there is still active peristalsis, so that it is not uncommon for defecation to occur after the onset of pain. However, obstipation eventually develops.

Physical examination in the early stages of obstruction reveals no tenderness, and bowel sounds may seem normal. Later, as loops of intestine become dilated, the tone of peristalsis becomes cavernous or high-pitched. Borborygmi, frequently described but seldom observed vigorous rushes of peristaltic sound, are probably present only during the earliest stages of obstruction.

Postoperative adhesions are the most common cause of obstruction of the small intestine in adults, and the history often includes a previous abdominal operation. Another cause of obstruction is abdominal hernia. The physical examination should include a search for a hernia in the umbilical region,

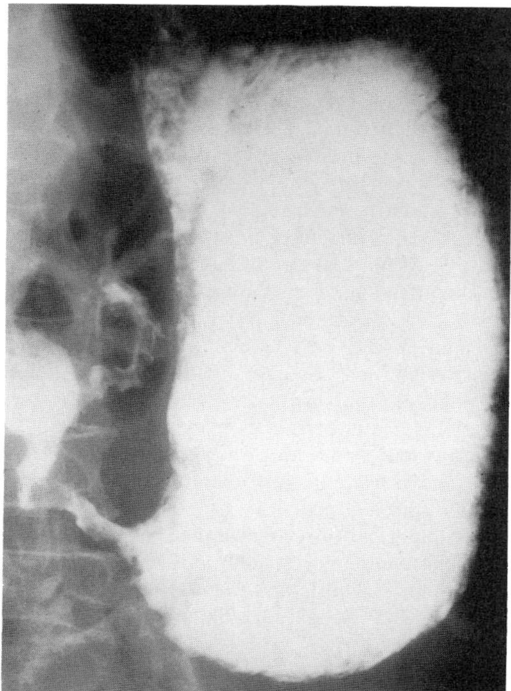

Figure 33.10. Upper gastrointestinal series reveals gastric outlet obstruction secondary to carcinoma.

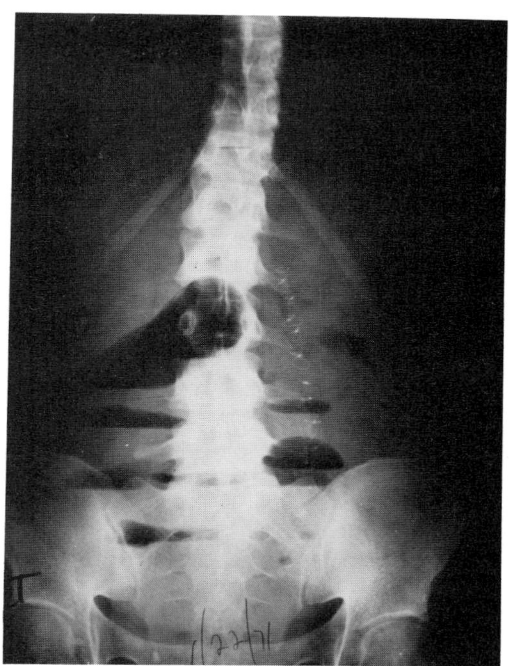

Figure 33.11. Upright film of the abdomen reveals multiple air-fluid levels consistent with small bowel obstruction.

at previous abdominal incisions, and in the inguinal and femoral regions. A femoral hernia in an obese patient may be easily overlooked. When intestine incarcerated in a hernia is the cause of obstruction, the herniated mass is almost always tender, even after long-standing incarceration. Obstruction may also be caused by intussusception of an intraluminal lesion, such as a polyp. In the case of intussusception, the resultant mass itself is sometimes palpable. Bleeding from vascular compromise of the intussuscipiens may occur.

Less common causes of obstruction of the small intestine are metastatic peritoneal implants and incarceration of intestinal loops in internal hernias. The former may be suggested by the history. Volvulus involving the cecum, the sigmoid colon, or the small intestine around an adhesion, or the midportion of the ileum about the superior mesenteric artery is another cause of mechanical obstruction. Plain abdominal roentgenograms with upright and supine views usually confirm the diagnosis of intestinal obstruction (Fig. 33.11), regardless of its cause.

The presence of severe, steady pain in a patient with intestinal obstruction suggests vascular compromise of a segment of intestine, which may occur with volvulus of any kind, intussusception, or strangulation of an incarcerated hernia. In the presence

Table 33.6.
Suggested Emergency Evaluation for Large Bowel Obstruction

1. History and physical examination
2. CBC with a differential count, urinalysis[a]
3. Serum electrolytes, liver function tests
4. Plain and upright abdominal films
5. Sigmoidoscopy, barium or gastrografin enema
6. ? Colonoscopy

[a] CBC, complete blood count.

of this type of pain, the potential for infarction dictates early surgical consultation for urgent surgical management.

Colonic Obstruction. Mechanical obstruction of the colon is a treacherous condition ordinarily caused by a left-sided carcinoma. Malignant lesions in the colon tend to spread circumferentially, narrowing the lumen so that it is readily blocked by fecal material. Fecal impaction itself without tumor can also cause colonic obstruction.

If the ileocecal valve does not permit reflux of colonic contents into the small intestine, the colon becomes greatly distended while the small intestinal pattern remains normal. In this case, there is no vomiting to indicate blockage. Perhaps because peristaltic activity in the colon is less vigorous than in the small intestine, the patient often reports very little pain. Passage of a small, watery stool at the onset of symptoms is common. This in turn is followed by obstipation. Abdominal examination may reveal minimal distention, although cavernous bowel sounds are usually detected on auscultation. It is necessary to establish an early diagnosis (Table 33.6) because spontaneous perforation may occur if the colonic contents cannot reflux into the small intestine.

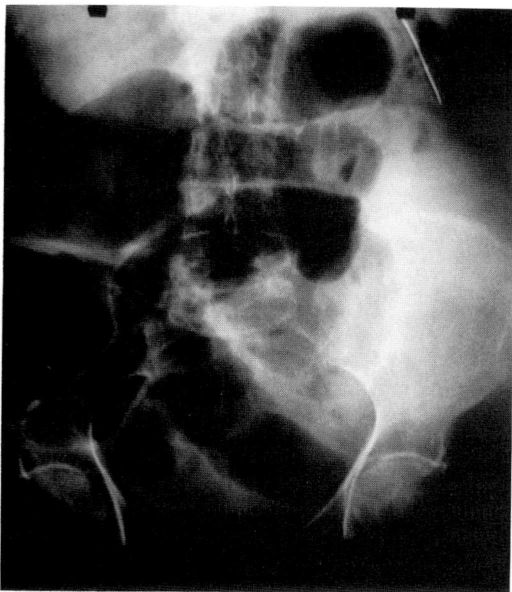

Figure 33.12. Plain abdominal film reveals both large and small bowel dilatation.

Plain roentgenograms with the patient in the supine and upright positions are a mainstay in the diagnosis of obstruction. Expert interpretation is essential, since obstructed loops may be filled with fluid rather than gas. Confirmation of the diagnosis of colonic obstruction (Fig. 33.12) may be obtained by sigmoidoscopic examination and barium studies.

Sigmoid and cecal volvulus are often easily diagnosed by plain abdominal roentgenograms (Figs. 33.13 and 33.14). A sigmoid volvulus may be decompressed through a tube placed by sigmoidoscopy. If this is not successful, a barium enema may be utilized to reduce the volvulus. If neither is successful, surgery is necessary to reduce the volvulus (Fig. 33.15), and provide tube decompression. An elective resection can be accomplished at an interval. Cecal volvulus always requires operative intervention. The emergency physician needs to be aware of these important subtleties.

Initial treatment of any patient suspected of intestinal obstruction should include the placement of a nasogastric tube to minimize the possibility of aspiration of vomitus. Anticipation of loss of large amounts of fluid, high in protein and electrolytes, into obstructed loops of intestine allows for adequate fluid replacement. Although long tubes may be used for intestinal decompression, surgical exploration is the primary form of treatment in most cases.

The operative management of large bowel obstruction secondary to colonic carcinoma or diverticulitis is dependent upon the general condition of the patient and the level of obstruction of the colon. The level is determined by barium enema (Figs. 33.4 and 33.16). Rectal, sigmoid and descending colon lesions may be initially managed by more proximal colostomy and later elective resection, but in lesions at and proximal to the splenic flexure, definitive resection with primary anastomosis may be the initial operative procedure, particularly in an otherwise healthy patient.

It is important to recognize that large bowel obstruction represents an acute surgical emergency, and prompt diagnosis and management are necessary to avoid bowel perforation and its consequences.

Ischemia

Although abdominal pain due to intestinal ischemia is seen infrequently in the emergency facility, it deserves stress for two reasons. First, the signs and symptoms are so nonspecific that the diagnosis is exceedingly elusive. Second, salvage of a sufficient length of intestine for normal long-term survival may depend on early diagnosis and operative intervention. The emergency physician, must therefore, be keenly aware of this possibility and seek early surgical consultation.

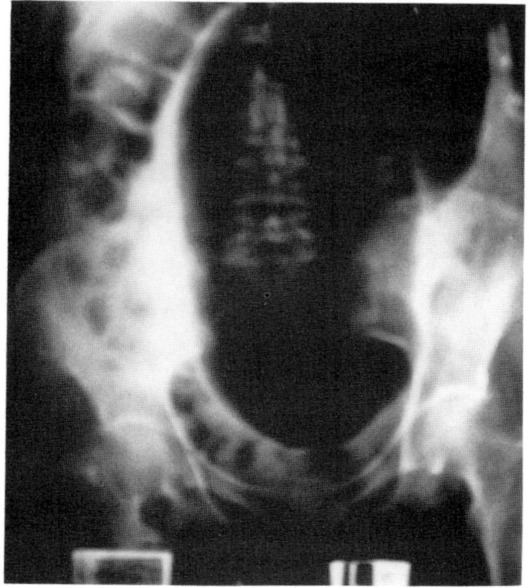

Figure 33.13. Plain abdominal film demonstrates sigmoid volvulus.

Intestinal Infarction. Regardless of the cause, intestinal infarction is a surgical emergency. The major causes are arterial thrombosis and embolization, venous occlusion, occlusion of small arteries resulting from arteritis, and occlusion of the major visceral arteries resulting from dissection of the abdominal aorta. Intestinal infarction can also develop in patients without any discoverable obstruction of a major vein or artery, particularly in low flow states.

Whatever the cause, the initial response of ischemic intestine and its symptoms are the same. Submucosal edema occurs first, followed by mucosal infarction, which produces intraluminal bleeding. The muscular layers respond initially with intense spasm and then with loss of tone and dilatation. Spasm often leads to vomiting and diarrhea. Perforation follows after a variable length of time.

As has been noted, all patients with intestinal infarction have pain as a presenting symptom. Although pain is visceral because it results from muscular spasm, it persists even after the intestine becomes dilated, tending to be intense, poorly localized, and steady rather than cramping. Onset of pain may be gradual or abrupt; sudden onset is typical of pain caused by an embolus. Intestinal infarction may develop in some patients with a history of episodic intestinal angina, which is characterized by postprandial abdominal pain and weight loss over the period of the attacks.

In the early stages of intestinal infarction, there is no abnormality on abdominal examination. Ex-

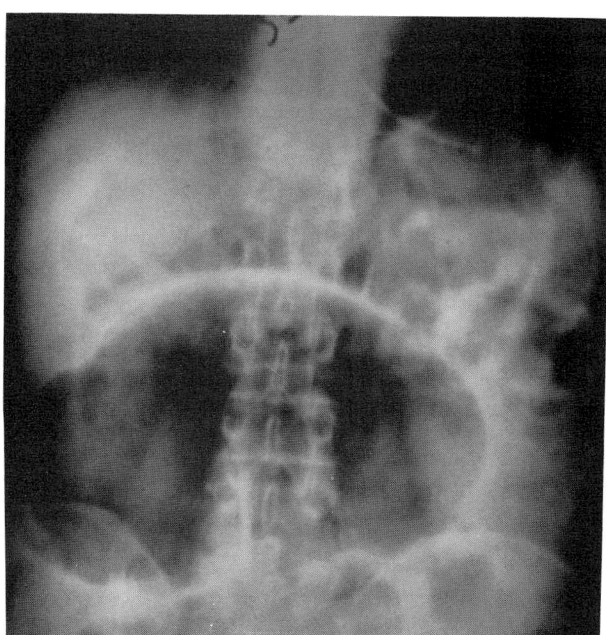

Figure 33.14. Plain abdominal film reveals the findings in a patient with cecal volvulus.

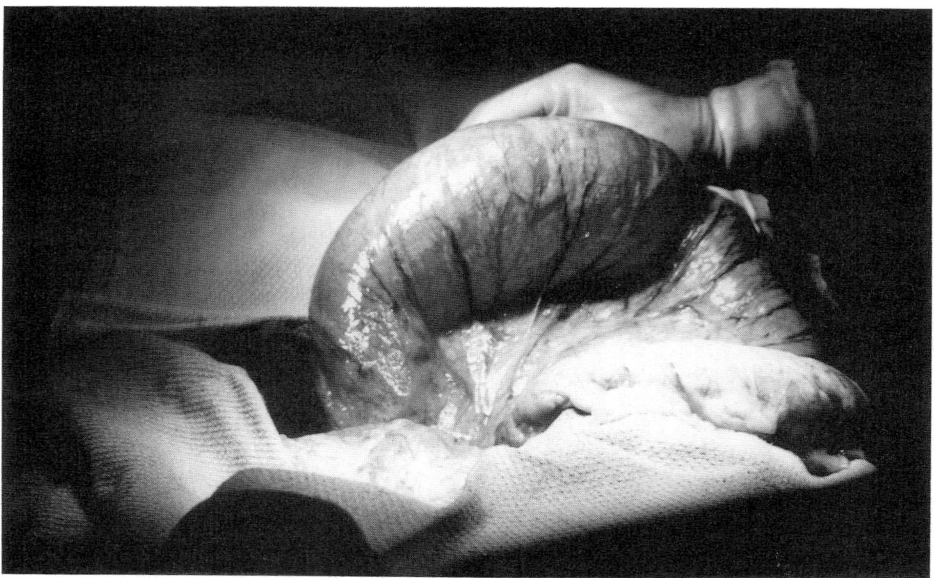

Figure 33.15. Operative findings in the patient demonstrated in Figure 33.13. The sigmoid is massively dilated, and its veins are congested.

cept for occult blood in the gastric and rectal contents, there is a puzzling absence of abnormal physical findings in these patients, who at the same time appear to be suffering from a major abdominal catastrophe.

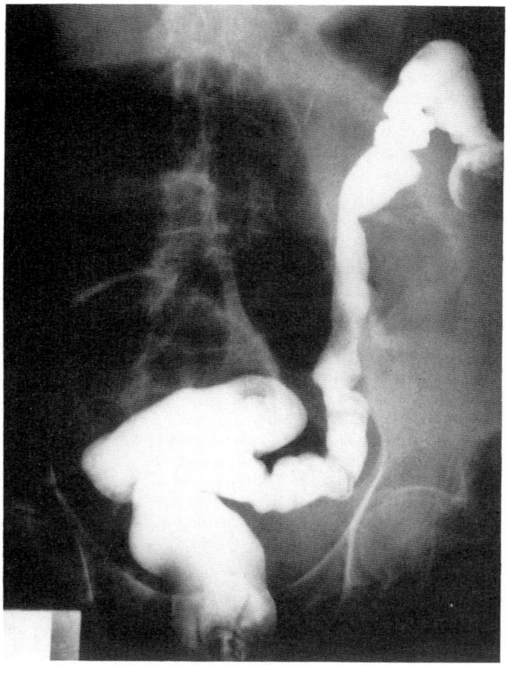

Figure 33.16. Barium enema findings reveal colonic obstruction at the level of the splenic flexure.

Leukocytosis is not an invariable sign of intestinal infarction. In many instances, the higher the white blood cell count, the more extensive the infarction. The serum amylase level usually is mildly elevated. Plain abdominal roentgenograms may show characteristic signs of infarction, edema, ''thumbprinting'' and hemorrhage, but may show no abnormality in the acute phase. Early selective angiographic examination is usually diagnostic when the infarction is caused by an arterial thrombus or embolus.

Ischemic Colitis. This process is associated with both impaired vascular supply and bacterial invasion of colonic segments, and it must be differentiated from colonic infarction resulting from major arterial or venous occlusion. The patient describes left-sided abdominal pain and bloody diarrhea without a history of previous episodes. On physical examination, there is tenderness in the region of the involved colonic segment, almost invariably the descending colon from the splenic flexure to the middle of the sigmoid. Contrast studies usually demonstrate characteristic ''thumbprinting'' indicating pseudopolyposis caused by submucosal edema and hemorrhage. Sigmoidoscopic examination does not reach the level of mucosal abnormalities, whereas in instances of infarction resulting from occlusion of the inferior mesenteric artery, the injury extends low enough to involve the rectal mucosa. Since many patients with ischemic colitis recover without surgical intervention, it is important to differentiate between this disease and infarction caused by major occlusion, usually by selective arteriography. For the emergency physician, appropriate evaluation requires the assistance of both radiologist and abdominal surgeon.

Retroperitoneal Processes

Infection, calculus, and obstruction of the urinary tract are discussed in Chapter 35. Of the other retroperitoneal causes of abdominal pain, the only one meriting emphasis is rupture of an abdominal aortic or iliac arterial aneurysm. Almost one-half of patients with ruptured aneurysms complain primarily of abdominal pain, although back pain is more characteristic of this catastrophe. The pain is sometimes one-sided. An initial step in the evaluation of any patient complaining of abdominal or back pain should be palpation of the abdominal aorta. In a few patients with ruptured aneurysms, only a mass will be palpated, but in most cases the pulsatile aneurysm is easily detected. Any patient with a previously diagnosed abdominal aortic aneurysm who complains of either abdominal pain or back pain must be considered to have retroperitoneal leakage from the aneurysm. Emergency operative intervention offers the only chance of survival. If surgery precedes the development of hypotension, ischemic renal injury, and cardiac arrest, the patient usually recovers.

Unusual Causes of Acute Abdominal Pain

Acute abdominal pain can be caused by conditions unrelated to the abdominal organs themselves. For example, when diabetes mellitus escapes control, it sometimes causes diffuse, nonspecific abdominal pain as well as elevation of the serum amylase level. Porphyria, sickle cell disease, tabes dorsalis, and spinal osteomyelitis may also produce abdominal symptoms. Patients with pulmonary tuberculosis may have a history of episodes of abdominal pain that can be associated with enteric tuberculosis. Pleural conditions such as pleurodynia or pneumonia sometimes produce pain in the adjacent somatic segments of the upper abdomen; this is a reason for a routine chest roentgenogram in patients with abdominal pain. Finally, abdominal pain is a common symptom in patients with acute myocardial infarction. In most instances it is referred pain, but in some it is caused by intestinal ischemia.

Systemic Factors Influencing Intraabdominal Emergencies

Several systemic factors may influence the occurrence, presentation, and management of some of the conditions that have been discussed. Among these is diabetes mellitus. In the diabetic patient, infection seems less well-contained by normal tissue response. Cholecystitis in the diabetic, for example, tends to progress more quickly to gangrene, empyema, and perforation.

Patients receiving long-term corticosteroid therapy or immunosuppressive therapy exhibit a less dramatic response to many of the conditions discussed. Because these drugs suppress inflammation, signs and symptoms tend to be less intense and slower to develop. For example, it is more difficult to judge the severity of peritonitis resulting from perforation in a patient receiving corticosteroids.

General obtundation, such as that which may accompany hypotension, hypoxemia, or septicemia, also tends to obscure abdominal symptoms. In such cases, the physician must consider the possibility that abdominal disease may be the underlying cause of abnormal signs and symptoms.

The patient with a neurologic lesion blocking the sensation of pain over the abdominal wall presents an especially difficult problem. The diagnosis hinges on the few findings elicited by history and physical examination, and repeated laboratory tests. In some patients, local peritoneal reflexes will persist, so muscle spasm may develop despite the fact that the abdomen is generally flaccid.

The patient who is readmitted to an emergency facility soon after being discharged following an abdominal operation deserves brief comment. By far the most frequent reason for such a readmission is the development of an abdominal wall or intraabdominal abscess, sometimes representing an impending fistula. Intelligent management begins with obtaining the details of the operative procedure. Septicemia, bleeding, or obstruction, require the usual treatment.

Finally, no better advice could be offered to those interested in this subject than to become familiar with *The Early Diagnosis of the Acute Abdomen* by Sir Zachary Cope. This small volume is the most informative source available for assistance in diagnosing abdominal emergencies.

GASTROINTESTINAL HEMORRHAGE

Emphasis in this section is on patients whose life is threatened by hypovolemia due to rapid blood loss. Most patients who are evaluated by the emergency physician are not in this category, however, having either less severe hemorrhage or chronic intestinal blood loss. All the lesions that are to be discussed can lead to either of these forms of bleeding. It should be emphasized that the initial responsibility of the emergency physician pertains to the life-threatening aspects of the hemorrhage. The earliest possible estimate of quantity and rate of blood loss, rather than the exact diagnosis, is the key to initial management of patients with massive hemorrhage.

Both the duration and the rate of blood loss affect the emergency presentation of patients with gastrointestinal bleeding. Occasionally, prolonged losses at a slow rate result in severe anemia and precipitate secondary problems, such as congestive heart failure. At the other end of the spectrum is the acutely exsanguinating hemorrhage, typically from esophageal varices or a duodenal ulcer. Site also determines the way in which bleeding presents. Esophageal bleeding, as from varices, frequently leads to vomiting of almost all the blood lost. Bleeding from the stomach may be manifest by hematemesis, but most of the blood may pass into the distal portion of the gastrointestinal tract. When the site of origin is the duodenum, all blood may pass distally in this way. When the upper gastrointestinal losses are slight or moderate, the blood is changed in its passage, and melena results. With massive bleeding, maroon stools and even unchanged blood clots are passed rectally. Likewise, lesser degrees of bleeding from the small intestine and even from the right side of the colon can be manifested by melena. Finally, blood lost from the rectum or anus is usually unchanged and obvious to the patient, even when the loss is slight.

A careful history obtained from both the patient and relatives often indicates the source of bleeding. Chronic alcoholism with attendant portal hypertension and symptoms suggesting long-standing peptic ulcer disease are both helpful in establishing the correct diagnosis. Recent use of aspirin, aspirin-containing drugs, and upper gastrointestinal irritants must be checked.

It is necessary to assess the quantity of blood lost and to determine the origin in the gastrointestinal tract. In an episode of acute hemorrhage, stabilization of the hematocrit drop may take several hours, so that an abnormal hematocrit value may not be an accurate guide to the quantity of blood lost. Vital signs provide a more valid index. The observation that tachycardia and hypotension in the seated patient disappear in the supine position serves as a warning that although the condition of the patient appears stable, vascular collapse is impending.

While bleeding persists, passage of a nasogastric tube may confirm the source of hemorrhage in the esophagus, stomach, or duodenum. In the patient with red rectal bleeding, sigmoidoscopic examination provides information to help determine if the blood originates from above the lower part of the rectum. Both of these measures should be carried out as soon as possible. Screening tests to exclude a prothrombin or platelet deficiency have early priority.

Whatever the cause of bleeding, initial management is directed toward preventing hypovolemia and its complications. This includes placement of large intravenous catheters for rapid infusion of fluids, cross-matching of whole blood, and monitoring of vital signs. Every patient with gastrointestinal bleeding should be treated as if hypovolemic shock were about to develop. Once sufficient data have accumulated to justify a less urgent approach, such emergency measures can be modified or discontinued. Unfortunately, it is all too common to treat the patient conservatively until hypotension unexpectedly signals massive hemorrhage.

Fiberoptic esophagogastroscopy and selective angiography are major contributions to the management of profuse gastrointestinal bleeding. Barium studies are less valuable, and usually should be deferred until the condition of the patient is stabilized and the bleeding controlled.

The specific sequence in which various diagnostic maneuvers are employed depends on the rapidity of blood loss, the most likely source of bleeding, and the availability of skilled endoscopists and angiographic radiologists. *One person must have responsibility* for the integration of diagnostic and therapeutic steps. Although the identity of this individual can change as the patient is transferred from the emergency facility, there should be no doubt at any time about who is responsible and in command.

Upper Gastrointestinal Hemorrhage

The management of exsanguinating hemorrhage from any source in the upper part of the gastrointestinal tract is a challenge. The surgeon must be invited early to help face this challenge. Bleeding may be exacerbated by any of the three diagnostic measures now commonly employed—barium studies, endoscopy, and angiography. The benefits of immediate operative intervention must be weighed against the increased risk of delay and diagnostic tests. The mounting availability of selective angiography, not only for diagnosis but also for therapy, has given the physician a new option, and in institutions where it is available, it has caused a shift of emphasis away from immediate surgical treatment. The recent development of endoscopic sclerotherapy for bleeding esophageal varices and endoscopic electrocoagulation of bleeding lesions in the duodenum and stomach, has also shifted emphasis from immediate surgical treatment of these entities.

Esophageal Varices. The esophagus and esophagogastric junction are seldom sources of exsanguinating hemorrhage except under two circumstances. The first of these is the presence of esophageal varices associated with portal hypertension. Because bleeding occurs directly into the esophagus, copious hematemesis is common. The patient often describes blood welling up in the mouth, rather than forceful vomiting. Many patients have a history of previous episodes of upper gastrointestinal bleeding and, most, of either heavy, prolonged alcohol usage or an episode or known hepatitis or clinical jaundice. If hemorrhage continues and varices are the suspected source, the physician should pass a Sengstaken-Blakemore tube or similar device designed to tamponade the distal portion of the esophagus. Cessation of bleeding indicates that the blood is coming from the esophagus rather than from a more distal site. In this sense, the tube is diagnostic and therapeutic. The physician must remember that a tube for tamponade will obstruct the esophagus, so that blood and secretions proximal to the balloon must be aspirated. If there is cerebral obtundation, a cuffed endotracheal tube should be placed to prevent the common complication of aspiration pneumonitis. Vitamin K and fresh-frozen plasma may help to shorten a prolonged prothrombin time when this contributes to continued bleeding.

Mallory-Weiss Tears. These short, linear mucosal lacerations at the esophagogastric junction are the other source of copious esophageal hemorrhage. They are sometimes associated with a history of forceful vomiting. The bleeding comes from lacerated small arteries. Pain is not a usual complaint. The diagnosis is established only by endoscopy, angiography, or laparotomy with proximal gastrotomy. A tube for the tamponade of varices does not always control this arterial hemorrhage. Surgical intervention is often required.

Hiatal Hernia. A large paraesophageal or axial hiatal hernia may be manifest by upper gastrointestinal hemorrhage. Endoscopic examination and barium studies of the stomach provide the diagnosis. Once established, urgent operative intervention is necessary, since bleeding may indicate incarceration with strangulation.

Esophagitis. Massive bleeding is uncommon in the patient with chronic esophagitis secondary to gastroesophageal reflux. The rare exception occurs in the presence of a deep esophageal ulcer. The history and early endoscopic examination are most important in making the diagnosis.

Gastric Conditions. Hemorrhage from the stomach may complicate gastritis or superficial stress ulceration. Gastric ulcers and ulcers in tumors are less common causes of massive gastric hemorrhage. Endoscopy and angiographic examination provide the diagnosis; barium studies frequently do not. Whatever the source, gastric bleeding is less likely to stop as long as the stomach is distended with clot. Passage of a large orogastric tube for evacuation of clots and irrigation with iced saline may be attempted to stop the bleeding, and provide a means of measuring the rate of blood loss.

Peptic Ulcer. The most common cause of severe upper gastrointestinal bleeding is peptic ulcer disease. Because of erosion of the ulcer into the gastroduodenal or pancreaticoduodenal arteries, which are large vessels, the amount of blood lost can be massive. Although most patients with a bleeding peptic ulcer have long-standing symptoms and often a previous diagnosis proved by an upper gastrointestinal series, some, particularly older patients, have no such history.

If there is a large amount of bleeding into the proximal portion of the duodenum, blood refluxes into the stomach and is vomited or recovered on aspiration of gastric contents. The blood may be lost entirely into the distal portion of the gastrointestinal tract, and is manifest by black or maroon stools and even by passage of blood clots. If bleeding persists, angiographic or esophagogastroscopic examination will either establish the diagnosis or provide sufficient information that the presence of a bleeding ulcer may be inferred. An upper gastrointestinal series almost always shows either an active ulcer or a deformity of the duodenum, but this finding does not establish it as the bleeding site. Here too, lavage of the stomach is useful in clearing blood clots and in judging the rate of blood loss. Recovery of small amounts of blood from the stomach does not, however, exclude extensive ongoing loss into the distal portion of the gastrointestinal tract. Signs of hypovolemia and increased vigor of peristaltic activity provide additional clues of continuing blood loss. The decision whether to operate, or to intervene endoscopically to sclerose varices or to electrocoagulate vessels within an ulcer, or to persist with medical management must be made quickly and in concert with a surgeon when hemorrhage is massive.

Rare Causes of Upper Gastrointestinal Hemorrhage. Other rare causes of major upper gastrointestinal bleeding are hepatic injury leading to hematobilia, duodenal tumors, and aortoenteric fistulas.

Hematobilia is associated with colicky pain, intermittent jaundice, and profuse hemorrhage. The diagnosis is established on angiographic examination.

Because of the vascularity of the duodenum, *duodenal tumors* tend to bleed if they become necrotic. The presence of such a tumor is suggested by a history of weight loss and partial obstruction of the duodenum or biliary tree. An upper gastrointestinal series supports the diagnosis. Tumors arising from adjacent retroperitoneal structures, such as the kidney, may also cause duodenal bleeding. Endoscopy confirms the diagnosis if the gastroscope can be negotiated through the pylorus into the abdomen.

Aortoenteric fistulas are almost always a complication of the graft implanted after aortic resection. The diagnosis should be considered in any patient with gastrointestinal bleeding and previous operation on the aorta or iliac vessels. Surprisingly, bleeding from such fistulas is not always profuse. Upper gastrointestinal endoscopy to include the distal duodenum, and enhanced computed tomography of the retroperitoneum are the appropriate diagnostic studies. Aortic anerusyms can give rise spontaneously, though rarely, to fistulas into the duodenum.

Definitive therapy of upper gastrointestinal bleeding is governed by the site and cause of hemorrhage. Hemorrhage from a Mallory-Weiss tear will often stop spontaneously, but may also require surgery or angiographic embolization. Bleeding from esophagitis usually responds to antacid therapy. Hemorrhage from gastritis not responding to gastric irrigation usually responds to a vasopressor infused angiographically into the left gastric artery, (see Chapter 46). This may avoid a major gastric resection.

Hemorrhage from esophageal and gastric varices can frequently be controlled temporarily by Sengstaken-Blakemore or Linton tube tamponade, followed by endoscopic sclerotherapy. Failure of these methods may lead to portosystemic shunting, transthoracic ligation of varices or devascularization of the upper stomach and lower esophagus. These are surgical decisions.

Massive hemorrhage from gastric and duodenal ulcers requires prompt operative intervention to control bleeding. More stable patients, after volume resuscitation, may have endoscopic confirmation of the diagnosis and, if possible, control of bleeding with electrocoagulation. Nonoperative treatment in patients with this entity include nasogastric decompression, antacids, and H_2 blocking agents, such as cimetidine and ranitidine.

Lower Gastrointestinal Hemorrhage

Lesions of the Small Intestine

The small intestine is rarely the source of massive bleeding. Three exceptions are bleeding from an ulcerated Meckel's diverticulum, from hamartomatous tumors in patients with Peutz-Jeghers syndrome, and from jejunal diverticula similar to that seen in patients with bleeding colonic diverticula. Rarely, arteriovenous malformations and a leiomyoma may also lead to bleeding from the small intestine. Angiographic examination is the most accurate and often the only method by which the site of bleeding can be established prior to laparotomy.

Diverticulosis

Any major bleeding in the colon leads to the passage of maroon and red stools, although slow bleeding from the right colon and right portion of the transverse colon may be manifest by melena only. Massive colonic bleeding almost always originates from diverticula. Colonic diverticula arise at sites where major blood vessels perforate the muscle wall, and bleeding is usually the result of erosion into one of these vessels. A typical history of bleeding diverticulosis includes passage of a large, bloody stool without premonitory symptoms, followed by a sensation of faintness. Angiographic examination provides the only specific means of diagnosis. If it is not available, barium studies must be performed to assist the surgeon in planning the details of possible emergency operation, despite the fact that such studies may increase the likelihood of renewed bleeding.

Other Colonic Lesions

Copious colonic bleeding may also arise from cecal ulceration and vascular malformations. Tumors of the colon, including polyps, bleed routinely, but seldom enough to provoke hypovolemia. Chronic ane mia is the more usual presentation. Ischemic and ulcerative colitis are two other causes of bleeding. They are usually suggested by characteristic histories.

Hemorrhoids

Hemorrhoidal bleeding occa sionally is profuse enough to be frightening. In this instance, sigmoidoscopic examination is of obvious importance. Portal hypertension or a blood dyscrasia is suspected in the patient whose hemorrhoidal bleeding is voluminous enough to constitute a serious, acute problem.

The initial effort in management, after volume resuscitation, is directed to determining the site and cause of the hemorrhage. Available diagnostic procedures include rigid sigmoidoscopy, flexible colonoscopy, angiography, and barium contrast examinations of the rectum and colon. Discrimination from upper gastrointestinal hemorrhage may be difficult.

Many causes of lower hemorrhage may be determined only angiographically; hence, barium contrast examination should be avoided early if angiography is available. Infusion of pressors by angiographic means may control hemorrhage and allow elective colonoscopy.

ABDOMINAL TRAUMA

Guidelines

Abdominal trauma is a surgical disease, and in many cases its therapy requires operative intervention. It is unusual for the abdomen to be injured in isolation. The principles of initial evaluation and management as described in Chapter 1 are paramount. Once the primary survey and initial resuscitation have been completed, further evaluation of the patient can occur. At times complete stabilization of the patient in the emergency department is not possible; operative intervention may be required.

The emergency physician and the surgeon must work closely in the evaluation and management of the patient with abdominal trauma. The clinical evaluation of the patient with abdominal trauma may be obscured by neurologic injuries (brain and spinal cord), drugs, and alcohol. An aggressive, at times invasive, evaluation of the abdomen is necessary to avoid missing injuries. Between 30% and 60% of patients that die of trauma suffer deaths that are "preventable." These deaths are secondary to inadequate resuscitation and to missed or delayed diagnoses. The emergency physician and the surgeon together provide the experience and technical capabilities to provide correct therapy.

Abdominal trauma is most easily divided into penetrating and blunt trauma. The frequency of presentation of patients with these injuries depends upon the location of the hospital. In metropolitan areas, penetrating injuries predominate. In rural and community hospitals, blunt trauma is more common secondary to automobile accidents. The four areas of the abdomen that require evaluation in trauma are: (*a*) the intrathoracic abdomen—that is the parenchymal organs between the nipple line and the subcostal arch; (*b*) the true abdomen—from the subcostal arch to the pubis; (*c*) pelvic abdomen—containing the bladder, rectum, and uterus and adnexae and (*d*) the retroperitoneal abdomen.

Penetrating Trauma

Penetrating injuries result from gunshot and sharp instrument wounds. A penetrating injury to the area between the nipples superiorly, the anterior axillary lines laterally, and the subcostal arch inferiorly, is more likely to cause intraabdominal than intrathoracic injuries. The abdomen is a cylinder and injuries that penetrate posteriorly may have traversed the lumbar muscles to cause an intraabdominal injury.

Since *gunshot wounds* transmit tremendous force in transit through the abdominal space and their trajectory is never totally known, their presence invariably necessitates abdominal exploration. If shock results from penetrating injuries of the abdomen (stab wounds or gunshot wounds), the cause is almost always injury to a major blood vessel. These patients require expeditious transit to the operating room for exploratory laparotomy. Occasionally, transthoracic control of the descending thoracic aorta (by cross clamping) may be necessary to allow any chance for survival.

Stab wounds of the abdomen may be handled in various ways. If a patient with a stab would of the abdomen presents with shock, evisceration, or with peritonitis, operative intervention is clearly necessary. If none of these signs is present, there are several methods that may be appropriate in evaluating these patients: (*a*) admission to the hospital: with careful reexamination in a sequential fashion, monitoring the hematocrit, and, if the patient and the hematocrits remain stable, the bowel sounds active, and abdominal examination negative, discharge within 2 or 3 days. If the patient develops peritonitis, abdominal exploration is performed. In the work of Nance, there were no complications associated with delayed exploration in these patients; (*b*) an attempt to determine if the stab wound has penetrated the peritoneum with exploration of the stab wound tract under local anesthesia. If the stab wound has not penetrated the fascia, no intraabdominal injury has occurred. The wound may be irrigated, the patient placed on antibiotics, and discharged within 24 hours. If the stab wound has penetrated the fascia, the knife may or may not have caused an intraabdominal injury. Fascial penetration may be considered an indication for abdominal exploration with the knowledge that a certain percentage of these abdominal explorations will be negative. Or, peritoneal lavage may be performed on patients with stab wounds that have penetrated the fascia. It is not clear exactly what red blood cell count should be considered a positive peritoneal lavage. Some authors have considered greater than 1000 red blood cells per mm^3 a positive peritoneal lavage, i.e., indicative of major intraabdominal injury.

In any case, all patients with peritoneal penetration by sharp instruments must either undergo abdominal exploration or be closely followed with sequential examination. Patients with penetrating injuries are started on antibiotics, including coverage for Gram-negative and anaerobic organisms. The gastrointestinal tract is decompressed with a nasogastric tube. Impaled abdominal objects are *not* removed in the emergency department. They require laparotomy and removal under direct vision.

Blunt Trauma

Evaluation of the abdomen following blunt trauma may be difficult. A negative abdominal examination is not always final. An aggressive diagnostic approach is necessary. In the unstable patient, this is best accomplished by peritoneal lavage. Using the open or semi-open technique, a peritoneal lavage catheter is placed into the peritoneal space (see Illustrated Technique 15). Aspiration of 10 ml of free blood, the presence of greater than 100,000 red blood cells mm^3, or greater than 500 white blood cells mm^3 is considered a positive lavage. Any of these findings indicates the need for abdominal exploration. It is the responsibility of the emergency physician to develop a rapport with the surgeon involved with the care of these patients. The technique of performing peritoneal lavage is not difficult and may rest within the capability of the emergency physician. However, the surgeon who will ultimately be caring for the patient should decide who performs the peritoneal lavage.

Peritoneal lavage is inadequate in evaluating the retroperitoneum. The ascending or descending colon and pancreas may be injured with peritoneal lavage totally negative. Pelvic fractures may cause a false-positive peritoneal lavage. In patients with pelvic fractures, the procedure should be performed supraumbilically to avoid the dissecting hematoma. Computed tomography may be useful in evaluating the pelvis and retroperitoneum as well as the visceral organs in the *stable* patient.

Specific Organ Injuries

Spleen

The abdominal organ most frequently injured by blunt trauma is the spleen. Splenic rupture is most commonly suffered after a fall or a motor vehicle accident. In children, it may result from a sporting injury or altercation. Penetrating injuries also cause splenic rupture. In adults, the diagnosis is suggested by a positive peritoneal lavage after blunt trauma.

Currently, there is controversy concerning the appropriate management of the ruptured spleen. It has become clear that in children every effort should be made to preserve the spleen. As a result, many children with ruptured spleens are not operated upon, and peritoneal lavage has therefore become a diagnostic technique not indicated in children. Clinical assessment with noninvasive testing methods are used to make the diagnosis (computed tomography, ultrasonogram, liver/spleen scan, and even arteriography). Adult patients commonly experience left shoulder pain (Kerr's sign).

The treatment of a ruptured spleen in an adult is exploratory laparotomy and attempt at repair of the spleen (splenorrhaphy). If this is not possible, the spleen should be removed, and the patient receive Pneumovax and instructed in the possibility of overwhelming postsplenectomy infection. Replantation of the ruptured spleen into the greater omentum has not proved beneficial. The pediatric patient is observed in the intensive care unit with careful monitoring of hematocrit, blood requirement, and abdominal examination. If he/she becomes unstable, exploration is undertaken, and the spleen is repaired, or removed if absolutely necessary. *It is to be emphasized that this policy is not recommended in adults.* Postoperative antibiotics are indicated in pediatric patients.

Liver

The liver is commonly injured in blunt abdomen trauma. It may be the most commonly lacerated organ secondary to stab wounds of the abdomen. It is commonly associated with other intraabdominal injuries. The major physiological alteration with liver trauma is massive blood loss, leading to hypotension. A positive peritoneal lavage or a positive computed tomographic scan in the emergency department often substantiate the diagnosis.

Stomach

Injuries to the stomach usually are secondary to penetrating wounds and are associated with injuries to neighboring structures. A gastric injury is suspected because of the trajectory of the penetration. Blunt injury may occur as a result of a direct force applied to the epigastrium. This may result in a "traumatic Boerhaave's syndrome." When trauma to the stomach occurs, blood will be present in the nasogastric aspirate. Prompt surgical exploration is necessary.

Duodenum

The duodenum is occasionally injured in blunt abdominal trauma. Due to its retroperitoneal position, the signs and symptoms may be subtle. Retroperitoneal air is rarely identified on a plain abdominal film. Peritoneal lavage is not highly sensitive in identifying duodenal injuries because of its largely retroperitoneal position. A gastrografin upper gastrointestinal series may reveal extravasation. Duodenal injuries are often associated with pancreatic trauma.

Uncommonly, a blunt abdominal force produces an intramural hematoma of the duodenum manifest as gastric outlet or high small bowel obstruction, even several days after the injury. The diagnosis is made by contrast examination of the upper gastrointestinal tract. It is most commonly located in the third portion of the duodenum overlying the vertebral column. Initially, management includes nasogastric decompression of the stomach and intravenous fluid therapy.

Small Intestine

Along with the liver, the small intestine is a commonly injured intraabdominal organ secondary to penetrating trauma. Blunt trauma may cause small bowel injury either by causing compression of the small intestine against the vertebral column, the mesentery being torn by acceleration/deceleration forces applied to the abdomen, or by bursting from sudden high pressure. More small bowel injuries are identified as patients now survive high-speed motor vehicle accidents by wearing seatbelts. Because of the nearly neutral pH of small bowel contents and the lower number of bacteria in the small intestine, the diagnosis may not be readily apparent but will be discovered over a period of hours as the abdomen is examined sequentially. With peritoneal lavage, the white blood cell count and the amylase are often elevated in the peritoneal effluent, rather than the red blood cell count. Operative repair is necessary.

Large Intestine

Blunt injury to the large intestine may be caused by avulsion of the mesentery in a high-speed accident or from disruption resulting from blunt forces. These commonly occur at the cecum, in the transverse colon, or in the sigmoid colon. Peritoneal lavage is not a sensitive method of determining ascending and descending colon injuries, since these are retroperitoneal structures. If this injury is suspected by the trajectory of the penetrating object, e.g., wounds to the back or flanks, a contrast-enhanced computed tomographic enema may help to define the injury. If this is not available, close clinical observation with admission to the hospital is necessary. The rectum is rarely injured in blunt abdominal trauma, but its injury should always be suspected in patients with pelvic fracture. Trauma to the rectum may result from an introduced foreign object. An effort should be made in the emergency department to remove the object. If this is not possible, the object should be removed in the operating room under spinal anesthesia. Regardless of where the object is removed, the patient should undergo full sigmoidoscopy once the foreign object has been removed. A gastrografin enema is also necessary to exclude injury to the sigmoid colon. Both the colon and rectum may be injured in penetrating trauma to the buttocks or perineum. Prompt operation is necessary in this case.

Pancreas

The pancreas may be fractured by blunt trauma over the vertebral column near the superior mesenteric artery, or it may be injured by penetrating trauma. Physical findings may be few, and peritoneal lavage is often negative. Signs usually develop over an interval of time while the patients is under observation. Computed tomographic scanning and ultrasound examination of the pancreas are occasionally helpful. Patients with pancreatic trauma require abdominal exploration.

Kidney

Renal injury is caused by blunt flank trauma and may produce gross or microscopic hematuria. A contrast-enhanced computed tomographic scan or an intravenous pyelogram may demonstrate the injury and lead to urologic consultation.

Pelvis

Pelvic fractures may be occult, and the physical examination misleading. Routinely, in patients with blunt abdominal trauma, a plain abdominal film is obtained to define the presence of a pelvic fracture. If present, an evaluation of the urethra and bladder is necessary (in the male). If the patient has blood at the urethral meatus, a scrotal hematoma, or a misplaced or "floating" prostate, a retrograde urethrogram is necessary. Likewise, a cystogram is necessary to evaluate for extravasation of dye and for the presence of a pelvic hematoma evidenced by the elevation of the bladder out of the pelvis. This allows one to estimate the amount of blood in the retroperitoneum.

Pregnancy must be considered in female patients. Bimanual examination is part of physical assessment. A rectal examination is absolutely necessary in all patients with pelvic fractures to rule out injury to the rectum. Full evaluation of pelvic contents includes a vaginal speculum examination, sigmoidoscopy, gastrografin enema, retrograde urethrogram and cystogram, and arteriography.

It is important to recognize that a pelvic fracture can result in massive retroperitoneal bleeding. The MAST (Military Anti-Shock Trousers) may be helpful in its tamponade. Venous hemorrhage may tamponade itself in the retroperitoneal tissues. In the patient requiring four or more units of blood, angiography should be done to identify a source of arterial hemorrhage. The source of bleeding may be controlled with embolization of the appropriate artery. Once hemostasis is obtained, stabilization of the bony pelvis is accomplished within 24–36 hours by use of the external fixator. Bladder disruption occurring intraperitoneally should be repaired. Urethral disruptions are best repaired at an interval after the bladder has been drained with a suprapubic tube (see Chapter 35).

Summary

The important function of the emergency physician in the evaluation and management of the patient with abdominal trauma is to determine (*a*) if an intraperitoneal injury has occurred, and (*b*) if abdominal exploration is necessary. This is far more important than to determine which specific organ has been injured.

SUGGESTED READINGS

Bailey RW, Bulkley GB, Hamilton SR, et al. Pathogenesis of nonocclusive ischemic colitis. *Ann Surg,* 1986;203:590–598.

Berry J Jr., Malt RA. Appendicitis near its centenary. *Ann Surg,* 1984;200:567–481.

Bongard F, Landers DV, Lewis F. Differential diagnosis of appendicitis and pelvic inflammatory disease. *Am J Surg,* 1985;150:90–96.

Buchman TG, Zuidema GD. Reasons for delay of the diagnosis of acute appendicitis. *Surg Gynecol Obstet,* 1984;158:260–266.

Brenner PF, Roy S, Mishell DR Jr. Ectopic pregnancy. *JAMA,* 1980;243:673–676.

Chaikof EL, Goodson JD, McCabe CJ. Postsplenectomy pneumococcemia in a healthy vaccinated adult. *Am J Emerg Med,* 1984;2:141–143.

Chaikof EL, McCabe CJ. Fatal overwhelming postsplenectomy infection. *Am J Emerg Med,* 1985;149:534–539.

Cope's Early Diagnosis of the Acute Abdomen, revised by Silen W. New York: Oxford University Press, 1979.

Deitz DM, Standage BA, Pinson CW. Improving the outcome in gallstone ileus. *Am J Surg,* 1986;151:572–576.

Fabian TC, Mangiante EC, White TJ, et al. A prospective study of 91 patients undergoing both computed tomography and peritoneal lavage following blunt abdominal trauma. *J Trauma,* 1986;26:602–608.

Feliciano DV, Bitondo CG, Mattox KL, et al. A four-year experience with splenectomy versus splenorrhaphy. *Ann Surg,* 1985;201:568–573.

Flancbaum L, Dauterive A, Cox EF. Splenic conservation after multiple trauma in adults. *Surg Gynecol Obstet,* 1986;162:469–473.

Gaston MH, Verter JI, Woods G. Prophylaxis with oral penicillin in children with sickle cell anemia. *New Eng J Med,* 1986;314:1593–1599.

Jacobs ML, Daggett WM, Civetta JM, et al. Acute pancreatitis: Analysis of factors influencing survival. *Ann Surg,* 1977;185:43–50.

Jarvinen HJ, Hastbacka J. Early cholecystectomy for acute cholecystitis. *Ann Surg,* 1980;191:501–506.

Kasahara Y, Umemura H, Shihara S. Gallstone ileus. *Am J Surg,* 1980;140:437–440.

Lutzker LG, Chung K. Radionuclide imaging in the nonsurgical treatment of liver and spleen trauma. *J Trauma,* 1981;21:382–387.

Mahon PA, Sutton JE Jr. Nonoperative management of adult splenic injury due to blunt trauma: A warning. *Am J Surg,* 1985;149:716–721.

Malangoni MA, Levine AW, Droege EA, et al. Management of injury to the spleen in adults. *Ann Surg,* 1984;200:702–705.

McCook TA, Ravin CE, Rice RP. Abdominal radiography in the emergency department: A prospective analysis. *Ann Emerg Med,* 1984;11:23–24.

Mentzer RM Jr., Golden GT, Chandler JG. A comparative appraisal of emphysematous cholecystitis. *Am J Surg,* 1975;129:10–15.

Moore FA, Moore EE, Moore GE, et al. Risk of splenic salvage after trauma. *Am J Surg,* 1984;148:800–804.

Morgenstern L, Uyeda RY. Nonoperative management of injuries of the spleen in adults. *Surg Gynecol Obstet,* 1983;157:513–518.

Moulton S, Adams M, Johansen K. Aortoenteric fistula. *Am J Surg,* 1986;151:607–611.

Nance FC, Wennar MH, Johnson LW, et al. Surgical judgment in the management of penetrating wounds in the abdomen. Experience with 2212 patients. *Ann Surg,* 1974;179:639–646.

O'Mara CS, Wilson TH Jr., Stonesifer GL, et al. Cecal volvulus. *Ann Surg,* 1979;189:724–731.

Ottinger LW. The surgical management of acute occlusion of the superior mesenteric artery. *Ann Surg,* 1978;188:721–731.

Ottinger LW. Mesenteric ischemia. *N Eng J Med,* 1982;307:535–537.

Curiel K, Schwartz S. Diverticular disease in the young patient. *Surg Gynecol Obstet,* 1983;156:1–5.

Peitzman AB, Makaroun MS, Slasky BS, et al. Prospective study of computed tomography in initial management of blunt abdominal trauma. *J Trauma,* 1986;25:585–592.

Phillips T, Sclafani SJ, Goldstein A, et al. Use of contrast-enhanced CT enema in the management of penetrating trauma to the flank and back. *J Trauma,* 1986;26:593–601.

Ranson JH, Rifkind KM, Turner JW. Prognostic signs and nonoperative peritoneal lavage in acute pancreatitis. *Surg Gynecol Obstet,* 1976;143:209–219.

Ranson JH, Spencer FC. The role of peritoneal lavage in severe acute pancreatitis. *Ann Surg,* 1984;187:565–574.

Rodkey GV, Welch CE. Changing patterns in the surgical treatment of diverticular disease. *Ann Surg,* 1984;200:466–478.

Shumacker HB Jr. Splenectomy and postsplenectomy sepsis. *Surgical Rounds,* 1986;2:57–63.

Williams GR. Presidential address: A history of appendicitis. *Ann Surg,* 1983;197:495–506.

Williamson WA, Bush RD, Williams LF Jr. Retrocecal appendicitis. *Am J Surg,* 1981;141:507–509.

Sakai L, Keltner R, Kaminski D. Spontaneous and shock-associated ischemic colitis. *Am J Surg,* 1980;140:755–760.

Smith WR, Goodwin JN. Cecal volvulus. *Am J Surg,* 1973;126:215–222.

Starling JR. Initial treatment of sigmoid volvulus by colonoscopy. *Ann Surg,* 1979;190:36–44.

Trunkey D, Federle MP. Computed tomography in perspective (editorial). *J Trauma,* 1986;26:660–661.

CHAPTER **34**

Gynecologic and Obstetric Emergencies

DONALD C. PATTERSON, M.D.
DAVID S. CHAPIN, M.D.

INTRODUCTION

Emergencies involving the female reproductive system frequently confront the emergency physician. A practical approach is presented to diagnosis and care for the common gynecologic and obstetric emergencies. It is intended for the nonobstetrician and nongynecologist in the emergency department environment. Pertinent information relative to the common gynecologic and obstetric emergency problems is detailed in this chapter.

Patient History

The emergency physician must have a quiet area to interview the female patient to decrease anxiety and to minimize the psychological trauma of the emergency department environment. A gentle, caring attitude by the physician and the nurse will improve the acquisition of pertinent history. This caring attitude eases the female physical examination and improves the precision of diagnosis, the hallmark of successful treatment. The emergency department interview should include age, gravity and parity of the patient, the date of her last normal menstrual period, contraceptive method, the presenting complaint, signs and symptoms of disease, and any associated gastrointestinal or genitourinary symptoms. In the event of pregnancy an estimate of gestational age should be made.

Physical Examination

The hallmark of the gynecologic evaluation is the pelvic examination. A grave error in diagnosis may be made if this examination is overlooked in the emergency department. A proper pelvic examination table with comfortable adjustable stirrups is essential, along with a strong spotlight, and vaginal specula of all sizes. An empty bladder facilitates an accurate bimanual examination and ensures greater patient comfort. The anxiety and discomfort of the lithotomy position may be decreased by gentleness of voice, manner, touch, and direct eye contact. Respect for modesty is both important and helpful.

The external genitalia are observed for swelling, lesions, and inflammation. Laceration and gland secretion about the hymen and introitus are visualized with the labia gently spread apart with the fingers. With gentle strain, the support of the pelvic structures, vaginal wall, cystocele, rectocele, and urinary incontinence are noted.

Speculum examination requires an instrument of appropriate size. Most sexually active women accept comfortably a medium Graves or Pedersen speculum. Virginal women require a small or virginal Pedersen speculum. A large Graves speculum should be available for the obese or large woman. Insertion of the speculum should be slow and gentle with a downward posterior tilt and slight oblique angle of the speculum. Pressure on the posterior fourchette of the vagina avoids the sensitive urethra and periosteum of the pubic bone. Surgical lubricant is avoided to minimize possible compromise of the Papanicolaou cytologic smear, Gram's stain, and cervical culture. Warm water is an appropriate substitute as a lubricant. The vaginal wall and cervix can be evaluated visually, taking care not to incorporate pubic hair in the set screw of the speculum. Smears for exocervical cytologic examination are taken by scraping the cervical os with a spatula. Swabbing the inside of the cervical canal provides endocervical cells for cytologic smear as well as culture. The cervix and its ligaments are palpated for motion tenderness.

The bimanual examination is performed with the index and middle finger of a gloved hand, lubricated, and gently inserted into the vagina, and with the other hand gently palpating the suprapubic area. Cervix, uterus and adnexae are felt between the two examining hands. Size, shape, mobility, and tenderness of the organs are noted, as well as the presence of any abnormal masses. Finally, the examiner changes gloves and places one finger in the rectum and one in the vagina to evaluate the cul-de-sac and rectovaginal septum. It is helpful at the completion of the physical examination to acknowledge to the patient that it was a difficult and perhaps uncomfortable examination for her, but necessary information was obtained.

Once a tentative diagnosis has been made, the emergency physician must take time to explain carefully to the patient what was found and how it may have developed. When appropriate, he should state clearly that the condition can be treated and that the genital organs will function normally again without permanent damage.

VULVOVAGINAL DISEASE

Fungal and Parasitic Infections

The most common cause of vaginal discharge, is *Candida albicans*. This yeast-like fungus, commonly part of the normal vaginal flora, can overgrow after a course of antibiotics, menses, or a change in diet, climate, or sexual partner. Pregnancy, diabetes, and birth control pills are predisposing factors. Infection occurs most often in the summer, when wet bathing suits and perspiration-soaked underclothes are worn for extended periods of time. The patient complains of an irritating itch, most often associated with a thick, cheesy discharge. Dysuria is common. The labia may be red and edematous, but the vagina usually appears normal except for the discharge. If a drop of discharge is placed in potassium hydroxide solution and smeared, microscopic examination reveals budding mycelia. However, the itch can be so severe and the discharge so characteristic that it is improper to withhold treatment even if mycelia are not seen. Culture on Nickerson's medium or Sabouraud agar confirms the diagnosis. Treatment consists of the insertion of nystatin vaginal suppositories twice a day for 10 days or miconazole nitrate cream (Monistat) at bedtime for 1 week. A 3-day course of miconazole or clotrimazole (Gyne-Lotrimin) has become an acceptable alternative. A nystatin corticosteroid cream may be applied to the labia to relieve symptoms.

Trichomonas vaginalis is another common cause of vaginal discharge. A protozoon that lives in the genital tracts of both men and women, it is transmitted by sexual contact, which may not necessarily have been recent. The patient complains of recent

Table 34.1. Vulvovaginitis

	Symptoms	Signs	pH	Smear
Candidiasis	Pruritus; recent antibiotics	White, cheesy clumps; vaginal erythema	4.0	KOH – spores, mycelia
Trichomoniasis	Wet, profuse discharge; ± irritation	Frothy, greenish discharge	>5.5	Wet prep-motile trichomonads
Bacterial vaginosis	Malodorous, nonirritative discharge	Absent	5.0	Wet prep-"clue" cells

onset of a copious, odorous vaginal discharge and an intermittent itch. Her sexual partner has no related physical complaints. Examination reveals red, edematous labia and a red, rough vaginal wall. The cervix often is covered with punctate red spots. The discharge is classically green and frothy; when a drop is mixed with an equal part of physiologic saline solution and examined microscopically, motile trichomonads can be seen. This flagellated protozoon is slightly smaller than the accompanying white blood cells. Treatment consists of the administration of metronidazole (Flagyl), 250 mg orally three times a day for 7 days. The sexual partner(s) must be treated with 250 mg orally twice a day for 7 days to minimize the likelihood of recurrence. As an alternative measure, treatment of both partners with 2 gm over 24 hours is equally effective. The patient must be warned that alcoholic beverages cause gastrointestinal upset while metronidazole is being taken. In cases resistant to this therapy, a vinegar douche can be used, in the proportion of 2 tablespoons of white vinegar to 1 quart of warm water, twice a day.

Bacterial Infections

Gonorrhea, caused by *Neisseria gonorrhoeae,* is the most common venereal infectious disease in the United States. Discharge, often green and unpleasant-smelling, may be the only symptom, although dysuria is often present as well. Vaginal inflammation is minimal, but the potential for involvement of the pelvic genital organs is great. The finding of Gram-negative intracellular diplococci is the key to the diagnosis of gonorrhea; the diagnosis may be suggested by a Gram's stain of the discharge and confirmed by culture on Transgrow or Thayer-Martin medium. If gonorrhea is suspected, the physician should ask the patient whether her sexual partner(s) have urethral discharge, or dysuria. Blood is drawn for serologic testing for syphilis. The patient is treated with procaine penicillin G, 4.8 million units intramuscularly, and probenecid, 1 gm orally. In the penicillin-allergic patient, tetracycline, 1.5 gm orally followed by 0.5 gm orally 4 times a day for 4 days, or spectinomycin, 2 gm intramuscularly, will suffice (see also Chapter 11). The patient should *not* be told that she has gonorrhea or be reported to public health authorities *until the culture is proven positive.*

Bacterial vaginosis (formerly Gardnerella-associated vaginal discharge, *Haemophilus vaginalis* vaginitis, or nonspecific vaginitis) appears to be a common pathogenic factor in vaginitis. The discharge is white or yellow and thick, and is more bothersome in its volume and malodor than in the irritation it causes. Microscopic examination of the discharge, when mixed with saline, reveals so-called "clue" cells, epithelial cells with dots of bacterial matter clinging to the cell membrane. The final diagnosis is established by culture on blood agar. Treatment has been controversial, but it has been suggested that metronidazole, 500 mg twice a day for 5–7 days, is the only reliable therapy. Other systemic antibiotics seem to cure less than 50% of patients with this problem. The partner(s) should also be treated for this sexually transmitted disease.

The differential diagnosis of these specific vulvovaginal infections is aided by reference to Table 34.1.

Nonspecific Vaginitis

If a patient complains of vaginal discharge and if none of these pathogens is identified, a diagnosis of nonspecific discharge is made by exclusion. It is likely that such discharge is caused by streptococci, staphylococci, or other vaginal bacterial inhabitants, but neither wet microscopic preparations, cultures, nor Gram's stains are diagnostic. This type of discharge must be treated with one of the many available nonspecific vaginal creams, liquids, or douches, and the patient should be told at the outset that more than one such medication may be tried before the condition is alleviated.

Atrophic vaginitis caused by lack of estrogen in postmenopausal or oophorectized patients may require estrogen replacement therapy. Vaginal estrogen preparations, such as conjugated estrogens, 1 gm intravaginally several times a week, or an oral estrogen supplement, are helpful. Allergic (reactive) vaginitis, secondary to new synthetic, color-dyed underclothing or chemical hygiene deodorants, may represent an occult cause of vulvovaginitis.

Herpetic Vulvovaginitis

Herpetic vulvovaginitis has increased in incidence concomitantly with other sexually transmitted diseases. Herpes simplex virus type II is the usual infecting agent, but type I is isolated in 10–15% of cases. In primary cases, herpetic vesicles form in clusters on the perineal skin and labial mucosa. They commonly rupture after 12–36 hours, leaving small grouped ulcerations. Usually, by the time the patient seeks medical attention, the ulcers are extremely painful. The patient may be unable to sit, and the ulcers burn on urination. On physical examination, the physician sees grouped ulcerations 2–3 mm in diameter on the labia and perineum and occasionally in the vagina or on the cervix. Inguinal lymph nodes are enlarged and tender on palpation. The diagnosis can be made by inspection and is confirmed by culture of the virus or by biopsy. Serum titers are rarely helpful. The differential diagnosis of this mucocutaneous lesion includes chancroid, lymphogranuloma venereum, granuloma inguinale, syphilis, trauma, hypersensitivity reactions, and bacterial or fungal infection.

Many methods of treatment, including photoinactivation, ether, acetone, corticosteroids, and antimetabolites, have been tested; they are all either unreliable or of no benefit. A new drug, acyclovir (Zovirax), has been approved. A 5% ointment and an oral preparation are available. A 200 mg oral capsule is recommended every 4 hours, five times daily, for 10 days. When used in a first episode of herpes, it reduces both severity of symptoms and the time to crusting of vesicles, but it does not prevent recurrence. Fortunately, the disease is self-limited. The first attack usually lasts 10–14 days, and the patient may be unable to work or attend school during the first week; in this case, a medical excuse is appropriate. Analgesics, Burow's solution soaks, and frequent sitz baths relieve symptoms until the process subsides. Attacks may recur months or even years later, but these episodes are usually shorter in duration and less uncomfortable. Since there may be a causal relationship between genital herpetic infection and cervical cancer, these patients should have a Papanicolaou smear every 6 months after the diagnosis is made.

Bartholin's Cyst and Abscess

A Bartholin's cyst often appears after an episode of vaginitis, especially gonorrheal vaginitis, but it also may appear without preceding infection. Located just under the skin at the lateral border of the vaginal fourchette, the swollen gland may produce mild symptoms or none at all, requiring no treatment except explanation and reassurance. If the cyst is red, tender, and fluctuant, making intercourse and even sitting impossible, incision and drainage under general anesthesia are indicated. If it is not yet fluctuant, hot sitz baths, antibiotics, and analgesics are temporizing measures. General anesthesia is advised for surgical drainage, since local anesthesia is rarely adequate. After incision and drainage of a Bartholin's gland abscess, an asymptomatic cyst remains. Elective marsupialization or excision of this lesion prevents recurrent abscess.

VAGINAL BLEEDING

Sudden severe vaginal bleeding is a most frightening occurrence to a woman. The physician is obligated not only to diagnose and to treat the cause of the bleeding, but also to meet the related emotional needs of the patient.

The physician must first assess the extent of bleeding, institute supportive measures, and begin laboratory evaluation before attempting to define the diagnosis by means of the history and physical examination. A calm, reassuring manner is essential. The physician can estimate the amount of bleeding by examining clothing and pads and by checking vital signs. Intravenous infusion for volume replacement should be started immediately, and specimens for a complete blood cell count, sedimentation rate determination, serologic test for syphilis, urinalysis, and pregnancy test should be sent to the laboratory. Blood is drawn at the same time for typing and cross-matching. While waiting for the results of laboratory tests, the physician takes additional history and performs further physical examination.

Diagnostic Procedures

The diagnostic possibilities in patients with vaginal bleeding severe enough to be classified as an emergency include complications of pregnancy, such as incomplete abortion (possibly septic), ectopic pregnancy, placenta previa, abruptio placentae, and postpartum hemorrhage. Vaginal trauma, cervical or endometrial carcinoma, and menstrual dysfunction can also cause bleeding.

Complications of Pregnancy

History

As in all gynecologic evaluations, a complete menstrual history including menarche, periodicity, duration and amount of regular flow is obtained. The date of the last period, and whether it was normal, constitute the most important data. Pregnancy should be suspected whenever a period is delayed or scanty. Spontaneous abortion can be suspected if the last period was 6–8 weeks previously; ectopic pregnancy usually results in mild bleeding after 5–6 weeks of amenorrhea.

The physician should ask the patient if she has had recent intercourse. Since patients may deny sexual activity if they think the physician will disapprove, he should ask the question in a kind, matter-of-fact way, with the same tone as other questions. He also should determine whether birth control was utilized, and if so, which method. Use of contraceptive pills makes the possibility of pregnancy unlikely, whereas an intrauterine device may suggest the possibility of an ectopic pregnancy.

If the patient is bleeding and reports symptoms of early pregnancy, such as nausea, fatigue, breast tenderness, and urinary frequency, and if the menstrual history suggests pregnancy, spontaneous abortion is likely. This condition may especially be suspected if the symptoms of pregnancy disappeared a day or two before the bleeding began.

If the patient has abdominal pain, its location, duration, mode of onset, and persistence afford diagnostic clues. Crampy midline pain beginning after onset of vaginal bleeding suggests spontaneous abortion, whereas constant pain that may precede the bleeding can signal ectopic pregnancy. If pelvic infection is present, the pain is more likely to be constant and bilateral.

If the patient is in the 26th week of pregnancy or beyond and is bleeding, two serious conditions are possible: *abruptio placentae* and *placenta previa.* In the former, the normally positioned placenta separates prematurely. Manifestations include pain, which is either rhythmic or steady, and a tense uterus. The major complications of abruptio placentae are excessive blood loss, disseminated intravascular coagulation, and fetal death, which may be seen with a toxemia (preeclampsia or eclampsia) syndrome. Placenta previa is a condition in which the abnormally positioned placenta covers the cervix below the fetus. Blood loss is usually slow and unaccompanied by pain, but hypovolemic shock occasionally occurs. Because pelvic examination of bleeding patients in the third trimester of pregnancy may precipitate sudden massive hemorrhage by dislodging the placenta, it should be performed only in the operating room or after pelvic ultrasonography has localized the placenta. Heavy bleeding after delivery or therapeutic abortion usually results from retained products of conception, as is the case in incomplete abortion.

Postpartum hemorrhage constitutes a life-threatening emergency and is a leading cause of maternal mortality. Uterine blood flow at term can be 700 ml per minute. Shock can occur within several minutes and death within 15 minutes. During the first 24 hours, early postpartum hemorrhage is due to (*a*) retained placental tissue; (*b*) cervical, vaginal, or uterine lacerations; (*c*) uterine atrophy; and (*d*) coagulopathy (abortion, abruptio placentae, amniotic fluid embolism, or fetal necrosis). Management involves examination of vaginal and cervix tissue and repair of lacerations. If tissue is visualized at the cervix, its removal allows the uterus to contract and stop bleeding. Anesthesia may be necessary to explore the uterine cavity for retained placental tissue and uterine lacerations. Bimanual massage of the uterus and administration of methylergonovine maleate, 0.2 mg intramuscularly, or pitocin, 20 units in 1000 cc lactated Ringer's solution is effective treatment for uterine atony, but only *after* lacerations and retained placental parts have been ruled out. A coagulopathy is suggested by bleeding from other sites, such as phlebotomy sites, nose, or mouth, or by the appearance of petechiae. If suspected, the prothrombin time, partial thromboplastin time, fibrinogen and platelet count should be checked.

Physical Examination

In addition to performing a general physical examination, the emergency physician should pay careful attention to the following details:

1. *Temperature.* A temperature of 100° F (37.8° C) may be present with either incomplete abortion or ectopic pregnancy; a higher fever strongly suggests infection complicating one of these conditions or pelvic inflammatory disease (PID).
2. *Abdomen.* The signs of peritonitis, such as localized tenderness, rebound tenderness, and guarding, accompany ectopic pregnancy, septic abortion, and PID, but usually do not accompany uncomplicated incomplete abortion. Bowel sounds are often normal. A mass in the midline is consistent with second-trimester abortion.
3. *Cervix.* If blood is coming from the cervical os and if no tumor is seen, the endometrium is the source of bleeding. If the cervix appears dilated on either speculum or digital examination, abortion is complete, incomplete or about to begin. The physician looks for signs of induced abortion, such as tenaculum marks or lacerations. Placental tissue in the cervical os or vagina indicates abortion; it should be removed and sent for pathologic examination. Bleeding often decreases after removal of this tissue. Pus in the cervical os or cervical tenderness points to sepsis; specimens for culture should be taken during the speculum examination, before lubricant has been introduced into the vagina.
4. *Uterus.* Enlargement usually indicates pregnancy, either aborted or intact. Tenderness on palpation suggests sepsis; crepitation signals clostridial infection. The incidence of this complication, commonly seen in criminal abortion, fortunately has declined since the legalization of therapeutic abortion.
5. *Adnexa.* Unilateral tenderness and/or enlargement suggest ectopic pregnancy, whereas bilateral tenderness or enlargement are more consistent with either PID or septic abortion.
6. *Cul-de-sac.* Bulging into the posterior part of the vaginal fornix signifies intraperitoneal hemorrhage, as in ectopic pregnancy.

Laboratory and Radiologic Findings

The hematocrit value will be low whatever the cause of bleeding, but will not reflect sudden recent blood loss. A white blood cell count of 12,000–15,000 may reflect incomplete abortion or ectopic pregnancy; a higher count indicates sepsis. A sedimentation rate more than 20 mm/hr (Wintrobe) is consistent with chronic infection. Clotting studies should be performed and fibrin split products measured if abruptio placentae is suspected.

The urine pregnancy test is positive in approximately 95% of women in whom the pregnancy is normal, but in only 50% with an ectopic pregnancy and is therefore of little diagnostic value. The serum test for the β subunit of human chorionic gonadotropin (hCG) aids greatly in the diagnosis because it is positive in normal pregnancy even before the missed period, and is also positive when there is minimal functioning trophoblastic tissue, such as ectopic pregnancy. Serial β-hCG serum testing with sensitive radioimmunoassays should show a doubled titer in a 48-hour time period. A falloff or leveling in the expected rise in titers of β-hCG suggests an abnormal pregnancy. A discriminatory zone of approximately 6500 β-hCG subunits suggests that an intrauterine pregnancy should be visualized by ultrasound examination. Ultrasonography, in practice, is probably better in the diagnosis of early intrauterine pregnancy than in early extrauterine pregnancy. However, ultrasonography is very sensitive to fluid in the cul-de-sac.

An upright x-ray film of the chest may reveal air under the diaphragm if the uterus has been perforated, and an anteroposterior x-ray film of the abdomen may show gas in the uterus if clostridia are present.

Definitive Diagnosis

The diagnosis of postpartum hemorrhage is usually obvious by the history; other serious vaginal hemorrhage, such as bleeding due to either an aborting or ectopic pregnancy, can be more difficult to diagnose.

Abortion. When patients in the first trimester of pregnancy have vaginal bleeding without pain, the diagnosis of threatened abortion can be made. This situation occurs in 20–25% of all pregnancies, but only 40–50% of these result in complete abortion. Cramps, extremely heavy blood loss, passage of tissue other than blood clot, or an effaced or dilated cervix indicate incomplete or inevitable abortion. The patient has a complete abortion if the conceptus has been expelled, the uterus has returned to normal size, and cramps and bleeding have subsided. Septic abortion is defined as any abortion, induced or spontaneous, in which infection is present; in this case, septic shock may be more life-threatening than the bleeding.

Ectopic Pregnancy. It is essential to consider the possibility of ectopic pregnancy in a reproductive age female with pelvic pain. Since it has myriad manifestations, ectopic pregnancy must be suspected in any patient with a recently irregular menstrual pattern, lower abdominal pain, signs and symptoms of recent blood loss, or a pelvic mass. Only one of these factors need be present to raise the suspicion, and neither the patient nor the physician should sleep until the diagnosis is excluded. Culdocentesis, the insertion of a 20-gauge spinal needle on a large syringe into the cul-de-sac through the posterior vaginal wall with withdrawal of peritoneal fluid, can be performed without anesthesia in the emergency department in order to determine the presence of hemoperitoneum (see Illustrated Technique 17). If positive, the diagnosis is ectopic pregnancy or ruptured ovarian cyst. Negative results do not exclude these diagnoses, however, and laparoscopy in the operating room may be necessary to make the final diagnosis. The availability of accurate sensitive serum tests for the β subunit of hCG has simplified the preoperative diagnosis of ectopic pregnancy. Fig. 34.1 presents an algorithm useful in the investigative workup and treatment for suspected ectopic pregnancy.

Therapy

Abortion. The therapy for both *spontaneous* and *induced abortion* as well as for postpartum hemorrhage is dilatation and curettage. Although curettage is not mandatory in a small percentage of apparently complete abortions, it is usually safer to perform this procedure, since curettage ensures completion. In many cases, dilatation and curettage may be performed under local anesthesia, and should be performed immediately unless bleeding is so minimal as to permit it to be done later. If the abortion is septic, intravenous broad-spectrum antibiotics should be initiated before the procedure. The drugs of choice presently are penicillin, 1–5 million units every 4 hours, and chloramphenicol, 500–750 mg every 6 hours, given in combination. Clindamycin, 600 mg every 8 hours, is an excellent alternative antibiotic because of its anaerobic spectrum. An aminoglycoside, such as gentamicin 1.5 mg/kg intravenously may be indicated. It usually is safe to operate after the second dose of intravenous penicillin has been administered. Oxytocin may be given intravenously, 10–20 units/liter, to reduce bleeding before the operative procedure, and if hypovolemic or septic shock is present, it must also be treated before surgery (see Chapter 3).

The patient needs repeated reassurance that spontaneous abortion was not brought on by anything she did or did not do and that it will have no effect on future pregnancies. Almost all patients feel guilty in such a situation and require psychologic support.

Ectopic pregnancy. The treatment of *ectopic pregnancy* is immediate laparotomy and removal of all trophoblastic tissue. If possible, the fallopian tube should be preserved by salpingostomy or segmental resection, but salpingectomy is often necessary. The ipsilateral ovary can usually be saved.

Abruptio Placentae. In patients in the third trimester of pregnancy who are bleeding and who have pain suggesting abruptio placentae, hypovolemic shock should be treated and blood clotting studies begun immediately. If there is no evidence of disseminated intravascular coagulation (normal

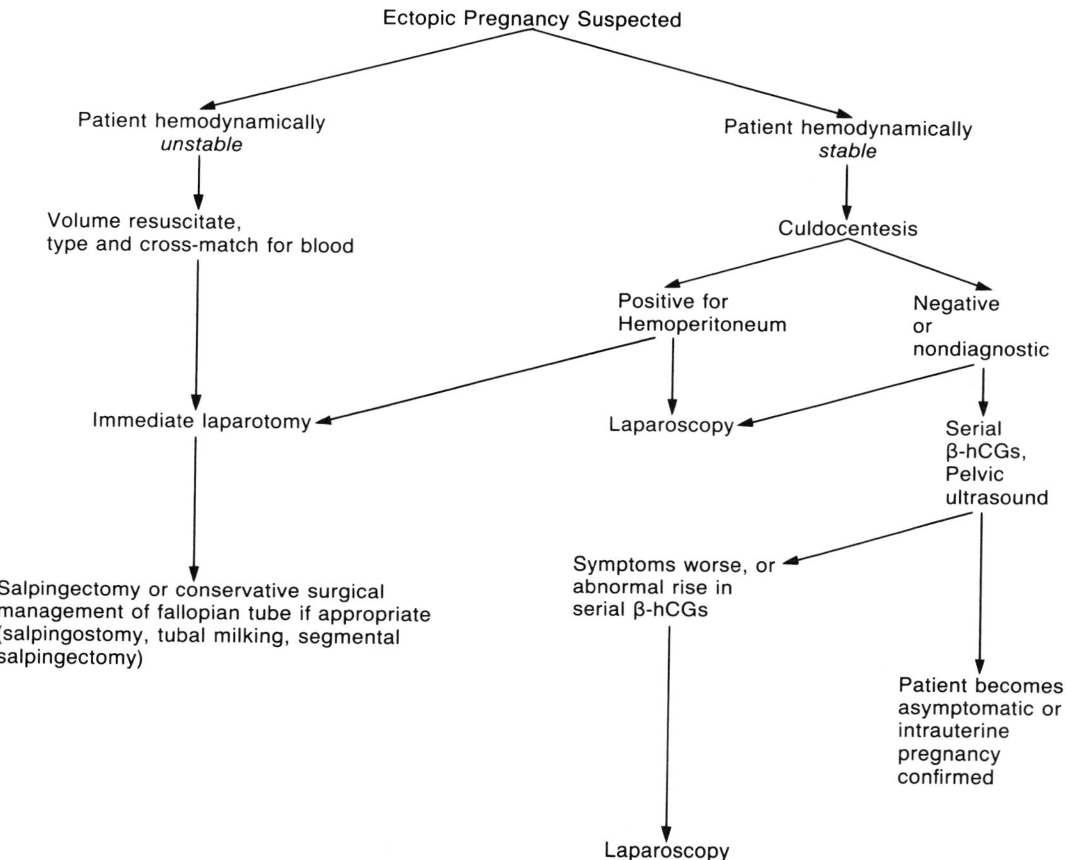

Figure 34.1. Workup for suspected ectopic pregnancy.

partial thromboplastin time, platelet count, and fibrinogen level), and if the fetus demonstrates a normal heart rate on monitoring, normal labor can be anticipated and observed, at least temporarily. If, however, the fetus is in distress or the clotting factors are depressed, whole blood, fresh-frozen plasma, or cryoprecipitate should be administered and caesarean section performed immediately. Delivery is the ultimate treatment of abruptio placentae.

Placenta Previa. In patients with painless bleeding, in whom placenta previa is more likely, ultrasonography will confirm the diagnosis. Bed rest will usually slow the bleeding, and delivery can be postponed to a more elective time. Occasionally, however, severe blood loss persists and warrants immediate caesarean delivery. *Pelvic examination in the third trimester bleeding patient should be performed only in the operating room,* or if pelvic ultrasonography has excluded the possibility of placenta previa.

Vaginal Trauma

When the history is taken, the patient should be questioned about the possibility of vaginal trauma. Accidental impalement on fences, sticks, and bicycle seats occurs in children. Chemicals, such as lye and potassium permanganate, instilled in attempts at abortion can cause multiple bleeding ulcerations. Sexual abuse of children should also be considered (see Chapter 29).

Bleeding from *traumatic lesions* of the vagina and vulva usually can be controlled by suture under local anesthesia; children require general anesthesia.

Carcinoma

If carcinoma is visualized in the cervix or if endometrial carcinoma is suspected because of postmenopausal bleeding, the diagnosis may be confirmed in the emergency department with cervical or endometrial biopsy. However, the bleeding is usually slow enough to permit admission for colposcopic biopsy and perhaps dilatation and curettage.

Since most *carcinomas* bleed slowly, admission to the hospital for exact diagnosis and a staging procedure is more important than emergency therapy. If bleeding from a cervical lesion is excessive, vaginal packing usually decreases the flow; occasionally, an endometrial lesion requires immediate admission for curettage to minimize the loss of blood.

Dysfunctional Bleeding

Dysfunctional or anovulatory uterine bleeding occurs in women ranging in age from the teens to the 40s. It consists of irregular periods that are either too frequent and/or too long. Bleeding is usually not excessive, but the patient often seeks emergency care. If the pelvic examination is normal and if abortion is ruled out, an endometrial biopsy specimen demonstrating proliferative endometrium confirms the diagnosis. Biopsy is not usually part of the emergency department workup, however, and may be postponed, provided gynecologic consultation is arranged.

Patients with *anovulatory bleeding* do not require immediate therapy. Dilatation and curettage at a later time is necessary to exclude carcinoma in patients more than 35 years of age. An injection of progestin or oral progesterone to stop the bleeding is *undesirable,* not only because of the heavy withdrawal flow a few days later, but also because it renders the results of subsequent endometrial biopsy invalid. Reassurance and short-term follow-up care constitute better emergency treatment, with planned gynecologic consultation.

PELVIC PAIN

Lower abdominal and pelvic pain in women presents a difficult diagnostic problem, requiring expertise of the general surgeon, internist, and gynecologist. It is one of the common complaints of women who present to the emergency department, along with vaginal discharge and vaginal bleeding. It may be difficult to identify accurately the origins of symptoms and signs of pelvic disease. Therefore, an understanding of the common gynecologic diseases of the pelvis is mandatory. A few general points may prove helpful:

1. Sudden or acute onset of pelvic pain suggests rupture of an ovarian cyst, endometrioma or tubal pregnancy with chemical irritation of the peritoneum. Such pain may also accompany torsian or twisting of an ovarian mass on its pedicle.
2. Gradual onset of pain suggests an inflammatory reaction, such as appendicitis or pelvic inflammatory disease, or a leaking ovarian cyst, or endometrioma. Dysmenorrhea or inevitable abortion may be associated with gradual increasing pelvic pain.
3. It is essential to rule out pregnancy or its complication in any female patient of reproductive age, that is, from menarche to menopause. In the United States, this means age 12 years to 50 years, respectively. This is important in avoiding potential pelvic disaster.

Pelvic Inflammatory Disease

Acute pelvic inflammatory disease (PID) and ectopic pregnancy are the two emergency conditions of greatest concern to the gynecologist. The classic history and physical findings of the latter have been described; the former is at least as protean in its aspects.

History

Commonly manifested by dull, continuous, worsening bilateral pain in the lower part of the abdomen, PID often begins after a menstrual period. The pain usually has been present a day or two before the patient seeks help. She complains that activity, especially running and sitting, aggravates the pain. Intercourse may be impossible because of deep dyspareunia. Bleeding and discharge may be present. Nausea, a common symptom of developing appendicitis, is not a usual feature of PID, nor is a change in bowel habit. Previous venereal disease, or a partner with urethral discharge, infertility, recent abortion or delivery, and use of an intrauterine device are factors predisposing to pelvic infection. A complete history must include these specific questions.

Physical Examination

On physical examination, the physician elicits bilateral lower abdominal tenderness, often with marked rebound tenderness and guarding. Bowel sounds are normal, neither hypoactive as in peritonitis caused by appendicitis, intestinal perforation, or pancreatitis, nor hyperactive as in gastroenteritis. Extension of the iliopsoas and obturator muscles is not painful. In severe cases, tenderness is elicited when the torso is shaken or when the patient coughs. Temperatures as high as 104–105° F (40–40.6° C) are seen, although some patients with severe infection can be afebrile.

If PID is suspected, the pelvic examination should be modified to provide the maximal amount of information with minimal discomfort. Speculum examination should be performed without lubricant, and specimens of blood and pus should be taken for cultures and Gram's stains. In the bimanual examination, slow, gentle motion of the examining fingers is essential. Tenderness of the uterine fundus on compression, and bogginess and tenderness of the adnexa on palpation, confirm the diagnosis of PID. Enlargement and tenderness of the adnexal structures are signs of tuboovarian abscess. Manipulation of the cervix stretches the intensely inflamed parametrial tissues, causing severe pain that can make the patient jump for the ceiling. This "chandelier" sign is pathognomonic of acute PID, but it also destroys all hope of further meaningful evaluation, so it should be elicited last in the bimanual examination.

If the fundus and adnexae are not tender but cervical manipulation elicits pain, a less severe episode of PID may exist. Ectopic pregnancy must always be considered when diagnosing pelvic infection. The benefits of laparoscopy for definitive diagnosis make it worth the risk, and its more frequent requested use by emergency physicians will undoubtedly result in delivery of proper treatment to more patients. The emergency physician should remember that pelvic examination often exacerbates symptoms and increases fever, and he/she should keep the number of examinations to a minimum.

Laboratory Findings

Laboratory findings consistent with the diagnosis of PID are an elevated white blood cell count (often more than 25,000), elevated sedimentation rate, normal hematocrit, and a Gram's stain revealing *N. gonorrhoeae.*

Therapy

Once PID has been diagnosed, it should be treated with bed rest and antibiotics. Intrauterine devices should be removed. If the patient is afebrile and the white blood cell count is low, outpatient therapy is justified. Offending organisms include the gonococcus, *Chlamydia,* bacteroides, enterobacteriaceae, streptococci, and mycoplasma. Antibiotic options include cefoxiten 2.0 gm, intramuscularly, plus oral probenecid, 1.0 gm, or amoxicillin 3.0 gm, by mouth, plus oral probenecid, 1.0 gm, followed by doxycycline 100 mg by mouth, twice daily for 14 days. In addition, bed rest at home, abstinence from sexual intercourse, and frequent follow-up visits are necessary. This is sufficient for patients who can be relied on to take medication regularly, but follow-up examination in 3 or 4 days is essential nonetheless.

If the patient has a temperature above 101° F (38.3° C) and/or a white blood cell count more than 15,000, hospitalization and parenteral administration of antibiotics will effect a more rapid cure and result in less permanent damage: cefoxiten 2.0 gm intravenously four times a day plus doxycycline 100 mg intravenously twice daily for 4 days, then doxycycline 100 mg orally twice daily for 10 days. An alternative is clindamycin 600 mg intravenously four times a day and gentamicin 1.5 mg/kg three times a day. Inactivity is at least as important as antibiotic therapy. Fowler's position with the pelvis as dependent as possible aids in localizing the infectious process. The patient can be discharged after she has been afebrile for 48 hours; she should be seen for follow-up in a week.

If fever persists and/or tuboovarian abscess develops, laparotomy with excision or drainage of the abscess is necessary. The treatment of tuboovarian abscess that is already present on admission is controversial. Some authorities prefer immediate laparotomy. We recommend at least 48 hours of therapy with antibiotics, reserving laparotomy for those patients whose condition either fails to respond or worsens. If laparotomy for appendicitis reveals pelvic infection instead, the physician should remove nothing, but merely drain the abscesses and rely on intravenous administration of antibiotics postoperatively.

If the diagnosis is definite and if there has been no recent pregnancy, a gonococcal infection is the most likely cause. Pending culture reports, this possibility should not be mentioned to the patient. Recent laparoscopic studies suggest that gonococci account for only 30–40% of all PID cases, with Gram-negative bacilli, anaerobes, and chlamydiae accounting for the rest. The patient should be informed of the possibility of tubal damage from gonococcal PID and of the necessity for vigorous treatment and avoidance of repeated infection. The physician should not lead the patient to believe that she is sterile; however, many unwanted pregnancies have resulted from attempts to prove the physician wrong.

Ovarian Cyst

Cysts of the ovary, both benign and malignant, rarely cause pain; they are commonly discovered during a routine pelvic examination. Occasionally, however, a corpus luteum cyst ruptures spontaneously, causing hemoperitoneum; symptoms and physical findings are similar to those of ectopic pregnancy. An uncommon condition, a twisted ovarian cyst, causes pain, leukocytosis, and fever, but rarely causes peritonitis or hemorrhage. The presence of a unilateral tender mass on pelvic examination suggests the diagnosis, but unilateral PID should also be considered. Occasionally, an asymptomatic ovarian mass is found in a patient with unrelated symptoms and signs. These lesions require no therapy or evaluation in the emergency department; if they persist, the patient will require elective laparotomy.

Laparoscopy is an excellent low-risk procedure

that allows the emergency physician to differentiate between ruptured or twisted ovarian cysts and ectopic pregnancy, or even to exclude them. If physical examination, laboratory tests, and laparoscopy are not diagnostic, the physician should reassure the patient that the pain does not represent significant disease, and should examine her again in 2 or 3 days.

HYPERTENSION AND PREGNANCY

Pregnancy-induced hypertension (toxemia of pregnancy, preeclampsia, eclampsia syndrome) is a syndrome characterized by the development of hypertension associated with proteinuria occurring in the second half of pregnancy. Pregnant women with hypertension may be separated into patients with preexisting hypertension who develop during the course of their pregnancy an increase in their blood pressure associated with proteinuria and hyperreflexia. In other women, there is no preexisting knowledge of hypertension or renal disease; they may develop pregnancy-induced hypertension and the syndrome of preeclampsia. Edema may also be associated with this syndrome. It should be noted, however, that approximately 25% of pregnant women will have dependent edema. However, edema of the face and hands may be significant in association with hypertension and proteinuria. The significance of the preeclampsia syndrome is that it may be associated with progressive hepatic and/or renal failure, disseminated intravascular coagulopathy (DIC), central nervous system disturbances, such as grand mal seizures and hemorrhagic stroke, and abruptio placentae. The patient with pregnancy-induced hypertension is at risk to develop any or all of these disorders which may ultimately lead to fetal and maternal death. Pregnancy-induced hypertension may occur in up to 25% of twin pregnancies. Along with sepsis and hemorrhage, the preeclampsia, eclampsia, toxemia syndrome is a leading cause of maternal deaths.

Preeclampsia

Pregnancy-induced hypertension associated with proteinuria, with or without edema of the hands and face (Table 34.2), occurs in approximately 5% of pregnancies after the 20th week. It is a disease of unknown etiology associated with severe arteriolar vasospasm. It may conveniently be divided into mild or severe preeclampsia. This does not suggest that mild preeclampsia is a benign process; it probably represents a progressive disorder that can lead to convulsions and maternal and fetal death if untreated. Patients with mild hypertension, no evidence of renal disorder with proteinuria, and no central nervous system irritability (hyperreflexia) need to be treated with bed rest. A 24-hour urine specimen is collected for protein determination, an ultrasound fetal survey done to establish gestational age, and a nonstress test to evaluate fetal heart and status. The patient should then have close follow-up with her obstetrician. If proteinuria or hyperreflexia develops, hospitalization is mandatory.

Severe preeclampsia requires immediate hospitalization and treatment. Delivery is generally required to correct this condition. If gestational age is less than 36 weeks, delivery is indicated if there is evidence of organ deterioration, such as renal or hepatic failure, a consumption coagulopathy, or if there is evidence of central nervous system disturbance. In addition, if there is evidence of fetal distress suggesting deterioration of the intrauterine environment, delivery is indicated. Evaluation of fetal maturity by amniocentesis with determination of the lecithin-sphingomyelin ratio is helpful in making a decision to deliver the fetus. If the patient requires intravenous or intramuscular drug therapy to depress the blood pressure, delivery must also be considered. In general, if the gestational age is greater than 36 weeks, the fetus should be delivered.

Eclampsia

Grand mal seizures associated with pregnancy-induced hypertension are the criteria defined as eclampsia. The sudden onset of a grand mal seizure disorder in pregnancy may be associated with maternal and fetal demise. Headache, visual changes with scotomata and blurring, hyperreflexia, mental irritability, and upper gastric pain herald the onset of generalized convulsions (grand mal seizures). Hydration, administration of magnesium sulfate, and delivery of the patient constitute the essential treatment. (Table 34.3). Hydralazine will lower blood pressure; if blood pressure is maintained between 100 and 110 diastolic, uteroplacental blood flow should be sufficient for the fetus. Disseminated intravascular coagulation (DIC) may develop; it is treated by delivery of the fetus and replacement of deficient clotting factors: platelets and fibrinogen. Abruptio placentae may occur, heralded by an irritable uterus with palpable tenderness between contractions. The uterus may also fail to relax completely. Vaginal bleeding may develop in association with fetal distress. Fetal mortality approaches 25% and maternal mortality 10%, if this condition is not recognized and appropriately treated. Magnesium sulfate or intravenous diazepam are used to treat convulsions in pregnancy (see Chapter 8 for the specific details and dosages of therapy).

Table 34.2.
Diagnostic Criteria for Preeclampsia

	Blood Pressure (BP)	Proteinuria	Edema
Mild Preeclampsia	Systolic BP > 140, or rise over baseline > 30 mm Hg Diastolic BP > 90 mm Hg, or rise over baseline > 15 mm Hg	300 mg–2 gm/24 hr	Hands, face
Severe Preeclampsia	BP >160/110	> 2 gm/24 hr	General

MANAGEMENT OF EMERGENCY STATES IN THE PREGNANT WOMAN

Pregnant women are seen in emergency facilities with almost all the diseases they may contract when not pregnant, from the common cold to a ruptured cerebral aneurysm. Each condition must be evaluated and treated while paying particular attention to the fetus and the altered physiologic state of the mother.

Diagnostic procedures such as physical examination, cardiograms, and blood tests are easily performed without risk. The position of the appendix moves higher as pregnancy progresses. A white blood cell count of 12,000–15,000 may be normal during pregnancy. In general, however, diagnostic tests are interpretable in their usual way.

The treatment of shock in pregnant patients differs little from standard treatment. Rapid fluid replacement is essential to restore intravascular volume and to preserve blood flow to the uterus and to the maternal kidneys and brain. The patient is placed in the left lateral position to displace the uterus to the left, since uterine pressure on the inferior vena cava accentuates the effects of hypovolemia.

Table 34.3.
Treatment of Severe Preeclampsia and Eclampsia

1. Magnesium sulfate 2–4 gm slow intravenous (i.v.) push loading dose, 1–2 gm/hr i.v. continuous infusion for maintenance.
2. Hydralazine 2–5 mg i.v. every 30 minutes.
3. Maintain urine output > 40 ml/hr.
4. Monitor respiratory rate > 12; deep tendon knee reflex must be present; keep magnesium serum level < 10 mg/100 ml but > 4 mg/100 ml. Reduce diastolic blood pressure to 100–110.
5. Monitor fetal heart rate.
6. Prepare for delivery.
7. Antidote to magnesium toxicity (respiratory depression) is 1 gm calcium gluconate i.v., slowly.

Surgical treatment for acute conditions unrelated to pregnancy, such as appendicitis, cholelithiasis, trauma, penetrating injury, intestinal obstruction, or recurrent pulmonary emboli, should be carried out as indicated. Maternal death may result from failure to perform these necessary procedures. Although surgery in the first trimester may result in abortion, the pregnancy usually is unaffected and the fetus unharmed, as long as teratogenic drugs are avoided. Surgery in the second trimester rarely interrupts the pregnancy unless sepsis is involved. Although surgery in the third trimester may trigger premature labor, it can be temporarily inhibited by β-sympathomimetic drugs, such as ritodrine hydrochloride.

Irradiation During Pregnancy

The use of diagnostic x-ray examination during pregnancy is controversial. It is best to avoid any unnecessary radiation in pregnancy. In the female of reproductive age, if pregnancy is considered, a sensitive test such as a serum β-hCG may be diagnostic. Ultrasonography may replace radiography in certain instances. Although no threshold dose of radiation has been established beyond which there is a risk to the fetus, 10 rads may produce fetal pathology. Skull series, cervical spine, chest, and extremity x-rays result in 1–10 millirads of fetal radiation exposure, even if the uterus is shielded. Abdominal radiography provides up to 300 millirad per film. Fluoroscopy exposure provides 2 rads per minute. Excessive radiation, as in radiation therapy for a malignant condition or in a nuclear accident or holocaust, is teratogenic. It is important to shield the uterus, if possible. Therefore, while unnecessary x-ray examination must be avoided, concern for safety should not prevent its proper use for necessary diagnosis in the pregnant patient. Prior consultation with a radiologist is advisable to keep exposure to a minimum. In particular, chest x-ray films when pneumonia is suspected, intravenous pyelography when a renal calculus is suspected, or a lung scan when pulmonary embolism is suspected, should not be avoided just because the patient is pregnant.

Use of Drugs in Pregnancy

The use of drugs in pregnancy presents the physician with a confusing body of knowledge and misinformation. The reader should remember that there is a difference between the lack of evidence for an association of drug use with malformation or disease and evidence for association. A few drugs are proved teratogens or are otherwise dangerous, and many presently have no defined danger. The general rules should be to avoid all drugs if possible and to use those of no proved danger when necessary.

The first trimester is the time when drugs have the greatest potential for interference with embryogenesis and organogenesis. Table 34.4 lists proved and suspected teratogens; they must be avoided unless absolutely necessary. If use is necessary, the risks must be explained to the patient. For example, a woman requiring phenytoin for epilepsy may be willing to take the 4–6% chance of bearing an infant with heart disease or cleft palate; this is approximately double the risk in the general population. Common drugs that appear to be safe in the first trimester include antibiotics of the penicillin family, analgesics including aspirin, and the decongestant Actifed.

After the first trimester, drugs still pose a threat to the fetus. Analgesics of all types can be used until the last month or two, when salicylates and prostaglandin inhibitors must be discontinued. Their anticoagulant properties pose a threat of intracranial hemorrhage to the fetus. They may also be associated with premature closure of the ductus arteriosus in the fetus and with delayed or prolonged labor. Acetaminophen and narcotics, used for acute problems, are not associated with these dangers. Antibiotics can be given readily to pregnant women when necessary, with the exceptions of tetracycline and erythromycin estolate. Sulfonamides should be avoided in the third trimester since they compete with bilirubin for binding sites in the fetal liver and can lead to increased neonatal jaundice. Psychotropic drugs, such as barbiturates and tricyclic antidepressants, can be used if absolutely necessary, but their safety is no better established than their dangers. Adrenal corticosteroids, once thought to be dangerous, now appear, in chronic use in diseases such as asthma, severe allergy, and Addison's disease, to result in no damage to the fetus. In fact, these drugs are now of proven benefit when given to the mother to help mature the fetal lungs, when premature delivery is imminent. Anticoagulants pose a special problem. Sodium warfarin crosses the placenta, causes malformations in the developing embryo, and causes anticoagulation in the fetus later in pregnancy. Heparin does not cross the placenta. Consequently, when treating a pregnant woman for thrombophlebitis or pulmonary embolus, the physician must provide long-term parenteral anticoagulation with herapin.

The common environmental hazards to the fetus in our society are tobacco, alcohol, and caffeine. Neonates born to smokers weigh an average of 200 gm less than those born to nonsmokers. The incidence of obstetric complications is higher in smokers. Intake of more than 8 cups of coffee a day is associated with decreased birth weight and an increased fetal mortality rate. Alcohol intake of more than 3 oz/day is associated with a group of anomalies termed the fetal alcohol syndrome. Minimal alcohol consumption is not associated with anomalies, but since the maximum safe level is not known, the Food and Drug Administration has recently advised pregnant women to consume no alcohol at all.

During lactation, most drugs appear in the milk in quantities equal to amounts in the plasma. Consequently, drugs that should be avoided in the third trimester should also be avoided during lactation.

Table 34.4.
Proven and Suspected Teratogenic Agents

Proved Teratogens
Synthetic progestins
Diethylstilbestrol (DES)
Androgens
Chemotherapeutic agents
Organic mercury
Sodium warfarin
Trimethadione
Hydantoins
Thalidomide
Suspected Teratogens
Antihistamines
Tetracycline
Lysergic acid diethylamide (LSD)
Marihuana
Diazepam (Valium)
Chlordiazepoxide hydrochloride (Librium)
Hexachlorophene

Precipitate Delivery in the Emergency Department

Women occasionally arrive at the emergency department in the second stage of labor, fully dilated and pushing; the receiving physician has no time in which to transfer her to the labor area or to an obstetric hospital. Delivery is imminent when the fetal scalp is showing at the introitus, the rectum is dilated, and the perineum is bulging. Once these observations are made, another contraction or two is all that is necessary for delivery. The patient is placed on an examination table or stretcher and allowed to assume either a supine or a lateral recumbent position. Her knees should be bent and the upper leg supported by an attendant if she chooses the lateral position. No attempt should be made to prevent the head from emerging. The patient should be encouraged to push gently and slowly if possible, and to concentrate on the words of instruction of the attendant. As the patient pushes the fetal head out, gentle pressure on the head by the attendant's hand toward the patient's rectum prevents periurethral injury and puts more stretch on the perineum. If the perineum is not stretching sufficiently and a crack appears in the skin, or if blood from inside the vagina is noted, episiotomy can be performed while the patient is pushing. This procedure consists of a 3- to 4-cm scissors cut posterior from the fourchette toward the rectum. The patient does not feel this if done at the height of a push; local anesthesia is unnecessary. During this entire process, it is essential to communicate to the patient what is happening and to instruct her when to push more slowly and when to stop pushing. As soon as the head emerges, she should stop pushing for a few seconds while the infant's mouth and nose is suctioned free of mucus with a bulb syringe and the umbilical cord is doubly clamped and divided if around the infant's neck. Gentle posterior pressure on the head then allows the anterior shoulder to pass under the pubic symphysis. When this stage has been completed, anterior pressure helps the posterior shoulder over the perineum or episiotomy. The remainder of the infant usually slips out quickly without pushing after delivery of the shoulders. If the head delivers and the shoulders are trapped by the maternal pelvic bones (shoulder dystocia), immediate flexion of the hips with knees flexed on the abdomen will usually release the infant's shoulders, or it permits manual rotation of the shoulders by the physician. The slower the delivery, the less tearing or episiotomy extension.

The baby is slippery and may be dropped easily. The newborn should be placed slightly downward on the bed or table and the throat and nose suctioned until clear crying is heard. The infant delivered this easily usually cries well without external stimulation. If respiration does not begin in 30 seconds, remembering that flow though the undivided umbilical cord is still oxygenating the baby, gentle stimulation by striking the soles with a finger or rubbing the back usually suffices. Do *not* strike the baby on the buttocks.

After good respiration is established, the cord is doubly clamped about 3–6 cm from the baby and cut between the clamps. The baby can then be given to the mother. The placenta will separate in 2–10 minutes and usually can be removed from the vagina by gentle traction on the cord with pressure on the uterine fundus. Once the placenta has been delivered, it is inspected for the presence of all cotyledons, and the uterine fundus massaged to minimize bleeding. The episiotomy or lacerations are then sutured under local anesthesia, with the patient supine.

Good verbal contact with the mother, with proper positioning of the staff, is more important than preparation of the skin or draping of the patient. Delivery is an imperfectly sterile procedure at best, and loss of control of the birth process by persistence in observing the formalities of sterile precautions serves no interest.

Precipitate deliveries frequently are associated with cervical tears, postpartum hemorrhage, and amniotic fluid embolism. Therefore, the vagina and cervix are inspected carefully, and an intravenous infusion containing oxytocin, 10–20 units/liter of lactated Ringer's solution is started as soon as feasible.

Quick deliveries usually proceed easily. Pursuance of these guidelines permits the emergency staff to avoid panic, minimize maternal anxiety, and allow the baby to emerge into an atmosphere of calm and tenderness.

Resuscitation of the Newborn

Upon delivery of the newborn infant, several important hemodynamic, pulmonary, and metabolic changes take place. The transition from intrauterine fetal circulation and its maintenance of acid-base balance to the neonatal circulation and pulmonary respiration requires vigilance of the emergency physician. The newborn is an obligate nasal breather; it is therefore important to suction gently the nasal pharynx and the oral pharynx for removal of amniotic fluid. It is important to keep the wet newborn dry and warm. Gentle stimulation by toweling aids in the breathing movements of the newborn. It must be remembered that evaporation lowers the infant body temperature and increases oxygen consumption allowing for increased metabolic acidosis and pulmonary vasculature constriction. If the infant heartbeat is less than 100, the extremities are blue, there is minimal flexion of the extremities, and the respiration is slow and irregular, this infant is depressed and should respond to gentle aspiration of the nose and oral pharynx, oxygen by mask, and gentle stimulation by flicking of the feet. If there is severe depression of the infant and a comatose appearance with no respiration, limp muscle tone, absent reflexes, absent heartbeat, or generalized cyanosis, the infant needs urgent, critical resuscitation. This means oral suction of the trachea with a DeLee mucus trap, followed by mask delivery of intermittent positive-pressure oxygen. If ventilation does not ensue, endotracheal ventilation is indicated. Occasionally, the hypoxic asphyxiated infant requires umbilical catheterization and the slow administration of sodium bicarbonate, 2 mEq/kg diluted with an equal volume of 10% glucose. This usually requires a pediatrician with neonatal intensive care experience.

In summary, normal newborns respond to gentle suctioning of the nasal and oropharynx, stimulation by gentle towel drying, and warmth. The satisfaction of safe obstetrical delivery in the emergency department has been shared by many emergency physicians.

Trauma in the Pregnant Patient

Trauma during pregnancy requires the expert skill of the emergency physician in the evaluation and resuscitation of not only the patient, but of the fetus. Due to physiologic and anatomic alterations of the gravid state, it is important that the management of the injury be performed with maternal well-being assured. The fetal survival is best correlated with maternal survival. The literature suggests that accidental injury occurs in approximately 6% of pregnancies and accounts for perhaps 20% of nonobstetrical maternal deaths. Maternal deaths result primarily from head, chest, and abdominal trauma. Blunt maternal injury is generally due to vehicular accidents, falls, or assaults. Major maternal injuries are associated with approximately 25% chance of maternal death and in over 50% of fetal deaths. There may be up to 25% fetal deaths, however, even in minor maternal injuries. Rupture of the pregnant uterus is rare, but must be considered in any known pregnant patient with hypovolemia or severe abdominal pain. Most experts agree that a lap seat belt worn below the gravid uterus at the iliac crest minimizes trauma to both mother and fetus in the event of a vehicular accident. As pregnancy progresses, the risk of fetal injury also increases. Physiologic alterations of pregnancy include cardiovascular, pulmonary, and gastrointestinal changes. The maternal blood volume increases approximately 50% during pregnancy. The maternal oxygen consumption increases at approximately the same rate, associated with an increase in cardiac rate. Respiratory tidal volume increases, which may lead to a mild compensation respiratory alkalosis. The normal P_{CO_2} in the third trimester of pregnancy is 30–35 mm Hg. There is delayed maternal gastric emptying during pregnancy, which may be associated with unanticipated vomiting and the possibility of aspiration following trauma. It should be remembered that the fetal response to hypoxia is bradycardia, a fetal heart rate less than 120. Fetal heart monitoring is essential to indicate either fetal well-being or distress following maternal trauma. Fetal survival is best correlated with fetal maturity. At approximately 1000 gm of fetal weight (approximately the 29th week of gestation), the fetus has a 50% chance of survival with delivery. The major risk is hyaline membrane disease. At about the 32nd week, when the fetus weighs 1250 gm, the expected survival approaches 80%. A grossly immature fetus must *not be delivered* if there is the possibility of continued safe intrauterine existence.

It is important in the triage process to recognize the injured pregnant patient. Very often, resuscitation of the injured mother involves care to avoid further potential injury to the fetus. Fluid replacement should be with lactated Ringer's solution. If hemodynamic stability is not obtained with instillation of 2000 cc of lactated Ringer's, blood transfusion should be considered. Type-specific blood should be given in an emergency situation. In general, vasopressors are contraindicated with the exception of ephedrine, so that constriction of uterine vessels is avoided. Supplemental oxygen is appropriate for all pregnant patients. Placement of the traumatized pregnant patient in the left lateral recumbent position avoids potential obstruction of the inferior vena cava by the weight of the uterus. One must rule out the possibility of spinal cord injuries.

Injured pregnant patients should be admitted to the hospital if they develop vaginal bleeding, ruptured amniotic membrane, abdominal pain, or abnormalities of fetal heart rate tracing or heart tones.

Postmortem Cesarean Section

When the mother has sustained lethal head injuries or has been declared dead, the emergency physician must be prepared to perform immediate postmortem Cesarean section. This may also be required in the event that maternal injuries make survival unlikely and a mature fetus is in distress. It has been suggested that the fetus has a good chance of survival if no more than 10 minutes has elapsed from the time of maternal death to fetal delivery. Transfer to the operating room for a sterile Cesarean section may result in delayed delivery of a viable infant and the potential development of hypoxic brain injury to the fetus. If the fetal age is undetermined and the fetus does not appear distressed with bradycardia, life support efforts may prolong fetal survival until adequate determination of the fetal age is possible. If the maternal condition stabilizes, supportive efforts for the mother until the 34th week of gestation may be feasible, and increased survival of the fetus may be anticipated.

The technique for postmortem Cesarean section is straightforward. A vertical midline incision from umbilicus to pubic symphysis is extended quickly through the abdominal wall to the peritoneum; a vertical incision is made in the uterus and the fetus delivered. Resuscitative efforts of the newborn are carried out as discussed earlier.

TOXIC SHOCK SYNDROME

Toxic shock syndrome, described in 1978 by Todd, defines a syndrome that appears to be distinct from other infectious diseases. Toxic shock syndrome was initially considered a disease of young women occurring during their menstrual cycle and associated with the use of tampons. Although the majority of cases in this clinical study were young women, it affects males also. The toxic shock syndrome is clinically characterized by fever, a diffuse macular erythroderma or rash, desquamation of this rash 1–2 weeks after the onset of illness, particularly on the palms and soles, hypotension, and diarrhea. Renal and/or liver failure, or bone marrow depression can occur. It has been estimated that at least three-fourths of patients are young women who develop this complex of symptoms during their menstrual cycle. Statistically significant is their use of tampons. It is therefore important for the physician to consider toxic shock syndrome in patients who have any or all of these symptoms. It has been estimated that there is a 30% chance of recurrence at the time of the menstrual cycle and, therefore, women who describe this recurrent symptom complex should be considered for this diagnosis. The current theory concerning cause of the syndrome involves a circulating exotoxin produced by a bacteriophage Type I *Staphylococcus aureus.*

Table 34.5.
Toxic Shock Syndrome Case Definition[a]

1. Fever (temperature > 38.9° C).
2. Rash (diffuse macular erythoderma).
3. Desquamation, 1–2 weeks after onset of illness, particularly of palms and soles.
4. Hypotension (systolic blood pressure < 90 mm Hg for adults or < 5th percentile by age for children < 16 years of age, or orthostatic syncope).
5. Involvement of 3 or more of the following organ systems:
   a. Gastrointestinal (vomiting or diarrhea at onset of illness).
   b. Muscular (severe myalgia or creatine phosphokinase level > 2 × upper limit of normal).
   c. Mucous membrane (vaginal, oropharyngeal, or conjunctival) hyperemia.
   d. Renal (BUN or creatinine upper limit of normal, or > 5 white blood cells per high power field, in the absence of a urinary tract infection).
   e. Hepatic [total bilirubin, serum glutamic oxalic transaminase (SGOT) or serum glutamic pyrrhuvic transaminase (SGPT) > twice the upper limit of normal].
   f. Hematologic (platelets < 100,000/mm).
   g. Central nervous system (disorientation or alterations in consciousness without focal neurologic signs when fever and hypotension are absent.
6. Negative results on the following tests, if obtained:
   a. Blood, throat, or cerebrospinal fluid cultures.
   b. Serologic tests for Rocky Mountain spotted fever, leptospirosis, or measles.

[a] From Centers for Disease Control. *Morbidity and Mortality Weekly Report;* Sept. 14, 1980;29:441–445.

Treatment

The prime importance in the treatment of toxic shock syndrome is the recognition of this disease process and the correction of the body response to the exotoxin insult. The possibility of bacteremia is checked with the appropriate blood, throat, cerebral, and spinal fluid cultures. Serologic tests for Rocky Mountain spotted fever, leptospirosis, and measles should be performed in the consideration of a likely differential diagnosis. Evaluation of renal, hepatic, and hematologic parameters is important to provide a baseline and to evaluate response to therapy. Hypotension is corrected with fluid replacement, and urine output maintained to avoid renal failure. Hemodialysis may be indicated if uremia has become significant. Inotropic agents, such as dopamine, are occasionally indicated to support blood pressure. Hypocalcemia must be considered. The adult respiratory distress syndrome (ARDS) has been reported.

Intravenous antibiotics are administered for antistaphylococcal coverage. A β-lactamase-resistant penicillin or cephalosporin has been recommended. Steroid therapy is controversial; if used, doses in the range of 20–30 mg/kg of methyl prednisolone are given every 12 hours. Because the recurrence rate of toxic shock syndrome may be as high as 30%, women should be warned against repeated use of tampons for 6 months to a year. Prudent alternating use of tampons and pads should be considered, in preference to extended use of tampons. It has been suggested that tampons not be utilized overnight and that they should be frequently changed. In summary, toxic shock syndrome is a specific syndrome best summarized in a report from the Centers for Disease Control (Table 34.5).

RAPE AND SEXUAL ASSAULT

History

The physician should question the patient sympathetically, openly, and respectfully. The chief complaint "I've been raped" should be accorded the same credibility as any other chief complaint. It may be difficult and painful for the patient to talk about the details of the rape, since under normal circumstances they would be considered too intimate for discussion. The patient should, however, be encouraged to discuss the assault and the events preceding it to help integrate this shocking reality. The patient usually feels guilty, but must be told that this is normal.

The physician should evaluate the emotional state of the patient, noting responses to certain topics of discussion. These notes can be helpful to the victim at a later court action and also to the psychiatrist or social worker attempting to evaluate emotional needs. While taking the history, the physician should ascertain the date of her last menstrual period, whether she has had pelvic inflammatory disease, keeping in mind that her past sexual behavior has no bearing on whether or not she was raped.

Physical Examination

The patient usually is not hysterical, contrary to common belief. Instead, she probably will be calm and inquisitive and will need to know the details of her examination to be able to differentiate it from the rape itself.

A gentle physical examination should be performed. All unusual findings are noted, such as scratches, bruises, friction burns, lacerations, disheveled appearance, and torn clothing. Most rape patients do not fight back, in order to get out of the situation alive.

The pelvic examination should focus on vaginal lacerations, secretions, cervical trauma, and uterine and adnexal tenderness. Specimens from the cervix and rectum should be cultured for gonococci. Vaginal secretions should be saved for microscopic and laboratory examination. The clothing, properly labeled, should be saved for police examination. Proper labeling includes the names of personnel who received the articles and the place of storage. Pubic hair should be combed and the products saved in a similar manner. The importance of keeping patient confidence during the examination by answering all her questions cannot be overemphasized.

Laboratory Findings

A wet preparation of vaginal secretions should be examined promptly for sperm, and the results recorded. Mucus from the cervix should be cultured on either Thayer-Martin or Transgrow media, and a Gram's stain performed in a search for Gram-negative intracellular diplococci. A specimen of vaginal secretions or a scraping from underclothing or both should be sent to the chemical laboratory for an acid phosphatase determination; this may be available only at the police laboratory. A pregnancy test using urine or serum should be performed to exclude conception previous to the rape. Blood should be drawn for a serologic test for syphilis; this test should be repeated 6 weeks after the rape.

Therapy

All rape patients should be treated as venereal disease contacts. Procaine penicillin G, 4.8 million units intramuscularly, should be administered with probenecid, 1 gm orally. In penicillin-allergic patients, tetracycline, 250 mg orally four times a day for 10 days, or spectinomycin, 2 gm intramuscularly, can be substituted.

Diethylstilbestrol (DES) has been advocated for use as a postcoital contraceptive measure. The side effects and possible long-term complications are sufficiently undesirable that its use should be restricted to those patients who are likely to be ovulating; administration should begin within 48 hours of the assault. The recommended dosage, 25 mg twice a day for 5 days, may cause enough nausea and vomiting that the patient discontinue the pills. Prochlorperazine (Compazine) rectal suppositories should be provided for this eventuality. An alternative is Premarin 25 mg intravenously, repeated in 12 hours. DES has been implicated in malignant tumors of the vagina in the female offspring of women who took it during pregnancy. The long-term effects of the recommended high dosage have not yet been established. In most large cities, therapeutic abortion is available should the patient wish to terminate a pregnancy resulting from rape. These two alternatives should be discussed with the patient so that she may make an informed choice. If she elects to take DES, she must be advised that an abortion will be recommended should pregnancy occur and also that the date of her next period cannot be predicted.

Diazepam (Valium), 5 mg four times a day for 5 days, or another tranquilizer should be offered to the patient; it is our experience that almost all rape victims require it within a short time. The physician may also prescribe a sleep medication, such as flurazepam hydrochloride (Dalmane), 30 mg, as required.

The need for emotional support should be obvious. She must deal with the crisis—not avoid it—and must be encouraged to verbalize her feelings. Resources for provision of this support vary from community to community. A rape crisis center, known to police and health care facilities, is ideal, should it exist in the area. The police department may have a rape unit. A rape crisis center provides support, counseling, and exposure to groups of other rape victims. It also helps in interactions with police, lawyers, courts, family, and friends. The center may refer her to professional groups for psychotherapy if necessary. The support of the rape crisis center should be solicited as soon as possible, preferably at the time of the initial examination.

The legal responsibilities of the physician in cases of rape are not defined clearly nor uniformly. In most states, only the physical findings are admissible as evidence in court. In some states, however, the physician testimony may be allowed for corroboration if he/she was the first person to hear the details of the assault. In any event, accurate records are of the utmost legal importance. Physician participation in legal procedures after a rape depends on willingness to help the patient's cause. The physician must learn the local statutes pertaining to rape and the locations of supporting resource facilities.

SUGGESTED READINGS

Amir M. *Patterns in Forcible Rape.* Chicago: University of Chicago Press, 1971.

Buchsbaum HJ, ed. *Trauma in Pregnancy.* Philadelphia: WB Saunders, 1979.

Davis JP, Chesney PJ, Wand PJ, et al. Toxic shock syndrome: Epidemiologic features, recurrences, risk factors, and prevention. *New Eng J. Med.* 1980;303:1429–1435.

Diagnostic x-rays are no cause for abortion—but caution is advised. *JAMA,* 1976;236:2269, 2277–2279.

Green R, ed. *Human Sexuality: A Health Practitioner's Text.* Baltimore: Williams & Wilkins, 1975.

Jones GS, Jones HW Jr. *Novak's Textbook of Gynecology.* 10th ed. Baltimore: Williams & Wilkins, 1981.

Medea A, Thompson K. *Against Rape.* New York: Farrar, Straus, Giroux, 1974.

Mole RH: Radiation effects on prenatal development and their radiological significance. *Br J Radiol,* 1979;52:89–101.

NIH Conference: Herpes simplex virus infections: biology, treatment, and prevention. *Ann Intern Med,* 1985;103:404–419.

Pritchard JW, ed. *William's Obstetrics* 7th ed. Baltimore: Williams & Wilkins, 1981.

Rein MF, Holmes KK: "Nonspecific vaginitis," vulvovaginal candidiasis, and trichomoniasis: clinical features, diagnosis, and management. In Remington JS, Swartz MR, eds. *Current Clinical Topics in Infectious Diseases.* New York: McGraw-Hill, 1983, Vol. 4.

Romero R, Copel JA, Kadar N, et al. Value of culdocentesis in the diagnosis of ectopic pregnancy. *Obstet Gynecol,* 1985;65:519–522.

Romero R, Kadar N, Jeanty P, et al. A prospective study of the value of the discriminatory human chorionic gonadotropin zone. *Obstet Gynecol,* 1985;66:357–360.

Schwarz RH, Yaffe SJ. *Drug and Chemical Risks to the Fetus and Newborn.* New York: Alan R Liss, 1980.

Weber CE. Post mortem caesarean section: review of the literature and case reports. *Am J Obstet Gynecol,* 1971;110:158–165.

Symposium: Drug Therapy and Pregnancy: Maternal, Fetal and Neonatal Considerations. *Obstet Gynecol,* 1981;58(suppl 5):1–105.

CHAPTER **35**

Urologic Emergencies

STEPHEN F. SCHIFF, M.D.
STEPHEN P. DRETLER, M.D.

The emergency physician must be fully acquainted with the various acute and chronic urologic conditions seen daily in the emergency department. This chapter is divided into major sections on traumatic injuries and nontraumatic emergencies; conditions requiring immediate surgical attention are distinguished from those necessitating more conservative treatment. The hope is that all physicians—whether surgeons, internists, or pediatricians—may identify clearly the clinical problem by the history, physical examination, radiologic evaluation, and laboratory analysis, and make the appropriate judgment for surgical consultation or medical care.

TRAUMATIC EMERGENCIES

Injury to the genitourinary tract may result from trauma to the chest, flank, abdomen, pelvis, or perineum. If the patient has gross hematuria or obvious perineal injury, the presence of genitourinary damage will be apparent. In the absence of immediately recognizable signs, however, the recognition and treatment of genitourinary injury requires knowledge of the anatomy of the structures involved, the circumstances in which damage to these organs occurs, the signs and symptoms of injury, the available methods of diagnostic evaluation, and the general principles of management.

Upper Urinary Tract

Pathophysiology

The kidneys and their vascular pedicles are located in the retroperitoneum behind the twelfth rib, overlying the transverse processes of the upper lumbar vertebrae. The left kidney and upper ureter with their enveloping fascia, Gerota's fascia, lie adjacent to the spleen, separated only by peritoneum. The kidney lies in contact with the posterolateral chest wall (the tenth, eleventh, and twelfth ribs), the diaphragm and overlying pleura, and the tail of the pancreas at its superomedial margin. It is posterior to the descending colon. The right kidney and upper ureter are 1–2 cm lower, also protected by the diaphragm and the eleventh and twelfth ribs. The right renal pelvis is adjacent to the duodenum, and its upper pole, which is separated from the liver by peritoneum, is posterior to the hepatic flexure of the colon. The fascia of each kidney includes an adrenal gland at its upper pole.

Despite the protection to the kidneys provided by their anatomic position, traumatic injuries are not uncommon and are accompanied by injury to other organs in 60–80% of cases.

Penetrating renal injuries result from gunshot and stab wounds. On the right, they may be associated with injuries to the lung, diaphragm, pleura, liver, colon, and duodenum; and on the left, the diaphragm, pleura, spleen, lung, pancreas, and colon. Any penetrating injury of these regions suggests involvement of a kidney or its pedicle. *Blunt injuries* to the chest, flank, or abdomen may cause renal damage by: (*a*) direct compression of the kidney against the vertebrae and paraspinal muscles; (*b*) laceration by a fractured rib or fractured transverse vertebral process; or (*c*) tearing or avulsion of the pedicle. Renovascular injury may result from acceleration-deceleration forces that produce partial or complete avulsion of the renal pedicle or disruption of the renal arterial intima with subsequent thrombosis. *Ureteral injury* may occur from blunt or penetrating trauma to the upper part of the abdomen or the flank. Stab and gunshot wounds commonly cause ureteral and renal pelvic lacerations, and severe hyperextension may cause ureteropelvic avulsion, especially in children. Relatively minor trauma may produce renal pelvic rupture in a congenitally deformed kidney.

Signs and Symptoms

Because other organ injuries are often associated with renal trauma and require emergent therapy, renal injuries are overlooked. A high index of suspicion must be maintained in evaluating all patients with blunt or penetrating injury. The most common sign of renal injury is hematuria; however, the degree of hematuria does not correlate directly with the degree of renal injury. Other signs and symptoms include flank pain or colic with the passage of blood clots or kidney fragments, ecchymosis, or a mass caused by blood and/or urine. The pain may be referred to the testis, groin, or shoulder. Hemorrhagic shock may be the chief finding. Transient hypertension occurs from segmental injury with ischemia or from compression by a perirenal hematoma (the so-called Page kidney). Absence of hematuria, of a mass, or of pain in the flank does not exclude the possibility of renal injury. Lacerations may occur without hematuria, especially if the ureter or renal pelvis is avulsed. Shock may decrease renal blood flow in such a way that neither hematoma nor extravasation of urine is immediately obvious. Vascular thrombosis may result in total loss of renal function without signs of flank hemorrhage, hematuria, or urinary extravasation. Hematuria is absent in 65% of patients with major renal vascular injuries. Therefore, even in the absence of obvious signs and symptoms of renal injury, trauma to the lower part of the chest, the abdomen, or the flank necessitates complete renal evaluation.

Most renal injuries are classified into one of four groups: (*a*) contusion/hematoma; (*b*) laceration/fracture without collecting system injury; (*c*) laceration/fracture with collecting system injury; and (*d*) renal pedicle injury.

Diagnostic Studies

The patient who has sustained multiple injuries without obvious perineal injury or pelvic fracture should undergo urethral catheterization with a No. 18 Fr Foley catheter unless blood at the urethral meatus suggests urethral damage. If perineal, pelvic, or lower abdominal injury has occurred, retrograde urethrography should be performed before urethral catheterization. Catheterized urine containing 5–10 red blood cells per high power field does not necessarily indicate genitourinary tract injury. If possible, the patient should void a specimen for accurate determination of hematuria. Urethral catheterization in patients with multiple injuries without proper evaluation of the lower urinary tract is condemned; it may convert partial urethral injury to complete disruption.

All patients with major blunt or penetrating injury to the lower part of the chest, the flank, or the abdomen require radiologic kidney-ureter-bladder (KUB) examination and intravenous *drip infusion nephrotomography.* The KUB film may demonstrate a fractured rib or transverse process, obliteration of the shadow outlines of the psoas margins or of the renal outline by extravasated blood or urine, scoliosis to the side of renal injury resulting from ipsilateral psoas muscle spasm, displacement of bowel loops, elevation of the diaphragm, or foreign bodies in the region of the kidney. If the KUB film is normal, however, renal injury is not excluded. Drip infusion nephrotomography with 120 ml of a 50% solution of meglumine or sodium diatrizoate (Hypaque) over 5 minutes is necessary to exclude urinary tract damage. This study is indicated for any of the following: hematuria; flank tenderness or mass; evidence of a fractured tenth, eleventh, or twelfth thoracic vertebra or transverse process; or signs of intraabdominal injury, such as radiologic evidence of air under the diaphragm or positive abdominal paracentesis.The nephrotomogram demonstrates penetrating renal injury, fracture, urinary extravasation, segmental destruction, and/or loss of function in 95% of cases. Renal *arteriography* is indicated if the patient has any of these nephrotomographic findings, or an enlarging flank mass or continued blood loss. If the nephrotomogram reveals only minor injury, arteriographic examination may be deferred until the clinical course of the trauma victim is more defined.

Renal *technetium scanning* is used to assess renal injury in patients allergic to iodine contrast media. Scanning is a good noninvasive method of monitoring the function of an injured kidney.

Retrograde pyelography is used only if extravasation is noted on a drip infusion pyelogram suggesting damage to the renal pelvis or the ureter.

Treatment

The indications for surgical exploration and repair of injury to a kidney are: (*a*) loss of function confirmed by arteriography; (*b*) massive or continuing blood loss; (*c*) major extravasation; (*d*) major laceration or fracture; and (*e*) penetrating injury. Loss of function indicates avulsion of the pedicle or arterial intimal tearing and thrombosis. If the pedicle is avulsed, bleeding is usually massive, requiring immediate surgical intervention. The presence of a contralateral kidney must be demonstrated before exploration; this may be done in the operating room with intravenous infusion of 120 ml of a 50% solution of meglumine or sodium diatrizoate and a KUB film. Thrombosis of the renal artery without avulsion also requires immediate surgical treatment, even though the salvage of such kidneys is low. Therefore, if other serious life-threatening injuries have occurred, such as multiple chest and/or head injuries, renal arterial thrombosis is treated conservatively. In the cases of continuing blood loss or of extravasation with an expanding flank mass, arteriographic examination must be performed before exploration to define the extent of injury. Failure to do this preoperatively may result in unnecessary nephrectomy. Major renal lacerations or fractures are debrided, drained, and repaired. Penetrating renal injuries are explored to debride necrotic tissue and to provide drainage for possible septic material.

Most renal injuries result from blunt trauma. Although the injuries discussed require surgical repair, 85% of renal injuries can be managed nonoperatively. Contusions and minor lacerations in kidneys shown to function during infusion pyelography are best treated by hospitalization and observation to monitor renal function, urinary extravasation, blood loss, and hematuria.

The principles of management of renal injuries in children are similar to those in adults. In children, however, the kidneys are more susceptible to injury because they are proportionally larger and have a lesser amount of protective fat. Moreover, Gerota's fascia, which provides a protective cover around the adult kidney, is poorly developed until age 10. Approximately 20% of renal injuries in children occur in the presence of preexistent disease, such as hydronephrosis or a Wilms' tumor.

Ureteral laceration is usually managed by surgical exploration after its identification by retrograde urography. When shock has occurred, renal blood flow decreases and urinary extravasation from ureteral injury may be unrecognized. Therefore, the course of the ureters should be observed carefully on the urogram and any questionable area examined with a retrograde ureteropyelogram. Renal salvage depends on early recognition of the ureteral injury and repair during the initial abdominal exploration. Delayed recognition of ureteral injuries may result in an otherwise avoidable nephrectomy.

Lower Urinary Tract

Bladder

Pathophysiology. The urinary bladder is protected anteriorly and laterally by the bony pubic arch, supported inferiorly by the pelvic musculofascial diaphragm, and covered superiorly and posteriorly by peritoneum and intraperitoneal structures. Bladder injuries are classified as: (*a*) contusion; (*b*) intraperitoneal rupture (20–40%); (*c*) extraperitoneal rupture (60–80%); and (*d*) combined intraperitoneal and extraperitoneal rupture (2–35%). Injury results from blunt or penetrating trauma to the lower abdomen or pelvis, and occurs most frequently when the bladder is distended. Blunt trauma accounts for at least 80% of all bladder injuries. Although 70% of patients with blunt injuries to the bladder have an associated pelvic fracture, only about 15% of patients with pelvic fractures have an associated bladder injury.

Long-distance runners may be seen in the emergency department with gross hematuria and suprapubic pain secondary to continuing blunt trauma of the empty bladder against the bladder base. An area of contusion at the bladder base and posterior wall at cystoscopy confirms the diagnosis.

Pressure necrosis of the bladder base with tissue slough and a vesicovaginal fistula may occur after childbirth as a result of prolonged pressure of the fetal head on the bladder base during a difficult delivery.

In children, the bladder is abdominal, not pelvic; hence, even when not distended, it is susceptible to injury from lower abdominal trauma.

Signs and Symptoms. Bladder injury may be unrecognized in the presence of other major trauma. The first sign of rupture, whether intraperitoneal or extraperitoneal, may be a nonpalpable bladder with absence of urine on placement of a Foley catheter. Intraperitoneal rupture with extravasation of blood and urine causes peritoneal irritation, tenderness, muscle guarding, and lower abdominal rigidity. Blood and urine under the diaphragm is a cause of pain referred to the shoulder. If uninfected, however, intraperitoneal urine may be well tolerated. Extraperitoneal rupture occurs on the anterolateral wall near the neck of the bladder, resulting from perforation by bony segments of a fractured symphysis or pubic arch. Lower abdominal pain, tenderness, and guarding occur, but are more localized than in patients with intraperitoneal rupture. All degrees of bladder injury may result in either gross or microscopic hematuria. Incontinence in the female raises the possibility of vesicovaginal fistula.

Diagnostic Studies. When lower abdominal or pelvic trauma has occurred, a Foley catheter is not inserted until a radiograph has established whether the pelvis is fractured. If the patient has a fractured pubic arch or symphysis, a urethrogram must be performed to exclude the possibility of urethral injury before passage of the catheter. If there is no evidence of pelvic fracture, a Foley catheter may then be placed. The presence of urine in the bladder does not rule out perforation. A gravity cystogram with anterior, posterior, and right and left oblique views is performed if rupture is suspected. The bladder is filled with 300–400 ml of radiopaque contrast material which is left in the bladder for 10 minutes; small perforations may not be visible immediately. Because a filled bladder may obscure small areas of extravasation, a post drainage film is imperative. Intraperitoneal ruptures may allow contrast material to outline loops of intestine or accumulate in the dependent portions of the peritoneal cavity, especially along the paracolic gutters (Fig. 35.1*A*). In patients with extraperitoneal rupture, the contrast material is confined to the perivesical area (Fig. 35.1*B*) After cystography is completed, an intravenous urogram is obtained to confirm the integrity of the upper urinary tract. If extravasation of

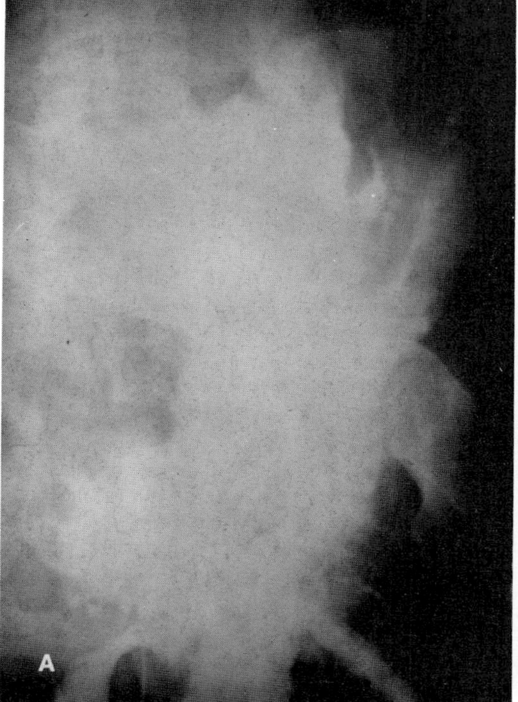

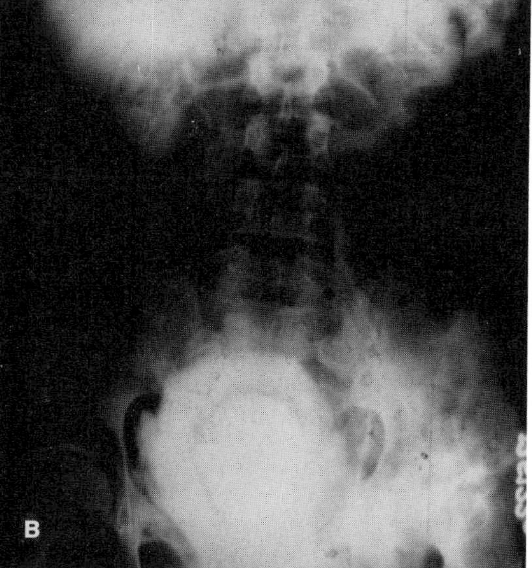

Figure 35.1. Bladder rupture. *A*, Intraperitoneal bladder rupture with total extravasation of dye causing sunburst effect. *B*, Extraperitoneal bladder rupture with extravasated dye confined to perivesical space, producing halo effect.

contrast on the cystogram is so massive as to obscure the lower portions of the ureters, retrograde ureterograms may be necessary.

Treatment. Patients with suspected bladder contusions with hematuria, but without cystographic extravasation may be treated nonoperatively with or without a Foley catheter.

In general, patients with extraperitoneal bladder injuries are subjected to surgical exploration with drainage of the perivesical space, placement of a suprapubic cystotomy catheter, and antibiotic coverage. Small extraperitoneal bladder perforations have been successfully managed by catheter drainage alone, if the injury and resulting extravasation is indeed small on cystography, is recognized within several hours of its occurrence, and if the urine is uninfected.

Patients with intraperitoneal bladder ruptures are treated by surgical exploration and primary repair. On occasion, minor perforations may be treated by catheter drainage and antibiotics. However, in the absence of other major trauma it is a better policy to explore and close the majority of these injuries. Only when the leak is small and the urine uninfected can conservative management ever be offered.

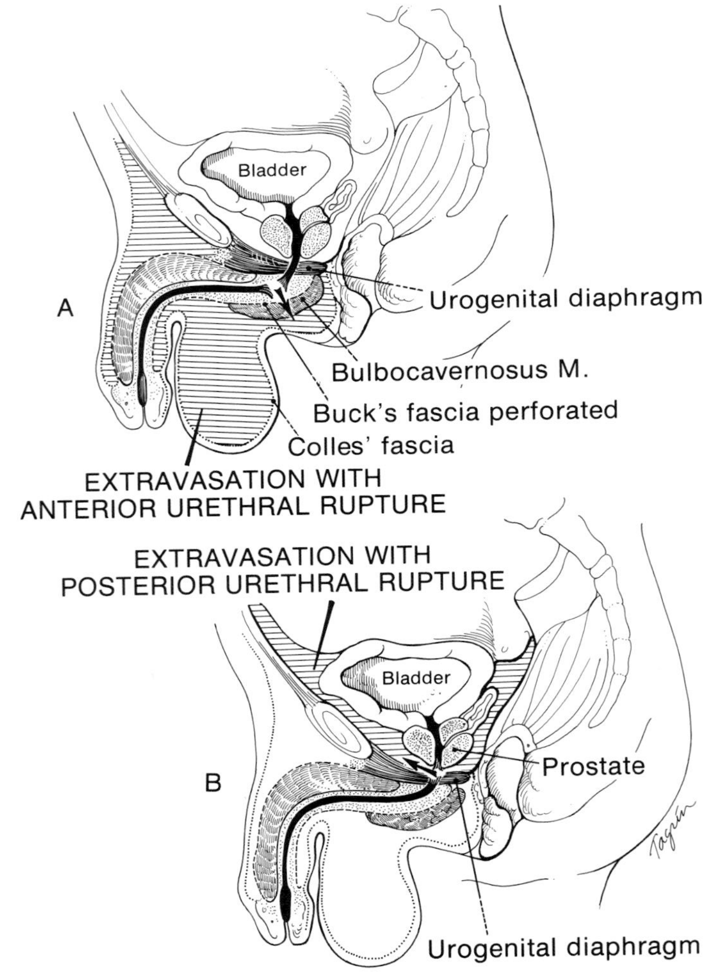

Figure 35.2. Urethral rupture. *A,* Anterior rupture of bulbar urethra distal to urogential diaphragm. Typically, there is extravasation of blood and urine through Buck's fascia into perineum, scrotum, and anterior abdominal wall. *B,* Posterior urethral rupture demonstrating prostate sheared proximal to urogenital diaphragm and elevated cephalad in pelvis. Characteristically, because of the intact fascial plane of the urogenital diaphragm, extravasated blood and urine are contained within anterior and posterior retroperitoneum of pelvis. Ecchymosis of the perineum or scrotum would not be found unless this fascial plane were torn.

Urethra

General Information. The anatomic location and extent of a urethral injury determine its presenting symptoms and its treatment. Injury may result in partial transection of the urethral mucosa or total disruption, with considerable differences in the therapy necessary and the eventual outcome.

A urethral injury must be assumed when blood is present at the meatus or in a voided posttrauma specimen, or if the patient is unable to void. Urethral injuries should be suspected in any patient with pelvic fractures, or with perineal or so-called "straddle" injury.

The key to the diagnosis of urethral injury is urethrography. A catheter must *not* be passed before urethrography in any patient suspected of having a urethral injury; partial disruption may be transformed into a complete disruption. Urethrography is performed fluoroscopically with the patient in a 45° right posterior oblique position and the hips flexed. Water-soluble nonviscous radiopaque contrast material, 10–20 ml, is instilled through a no. 12 French Foley catheter inserted only into the fossa navicularis of the penis, just inside the meatus. Partial rupture is characterized by periurethral extravasation at the site of injury with some contrast material visible in the bladder, whereas complete disruption shows only periureteral extravasation. Patients with partial disruption may have no flow of contrast material into the bladder because of edema alone obstructing the proximal urethra.

Anterior Injury. Pathophysiology. The male urethra is divided into anterior and posterior portions. The anterior urethra is located distal to the urogenital diaphragm, which surrounds the external sphincter, and includes the bulbous and pendulous segments of the urethra. It is surrounded by the corpus spongiosum and corpora cavernosa, which are enveloped by Buck's fascia. Posteriorly, Buck's fascia attaches to the urogenital diaphragm, and anteriorly, it extends to the abdominal wall. Buck's fascia must be perforated for blood and urine to extravasate into the perineum or scrotum; there it is contained by Colles' fascia. With extensive injuries, extravasation may be noted along the anterior abdominal wall all the way to the axillae, as Colles' fascia is continuous with Scarpa's fascia. (Fig. 35.2)

There are four general types of injury to the anterior urethra: (*a*) blunt trauma, seen in the classic straddle injury; (*b*) injury secondary to instrumentation or probing; (*c*) penetrating trauma; and (*d*) injury resulting from indwelling catheters. The most common is the straddle injury in which the bulbous segment is crushed against the undersurface of the pubic rami, resulting in contusion or laceration of the urethra and corpus spongiosum. Falls on the rung of a ladder, the top of a fence, or the horizontal bar of a bicycle are classic examples of straddle injury. Probing injuries usually result from self-inflicted trauma, experimentation, or attempts to pass catheters. Injuries due to instrumentation occur at fixed portions of the urethra: the meatus and the suspensory ligament. Penetrating injuries occur from gunshot or stab wounds. Trauma from indwelling catheters results from infection, scarring, and pressure necrosis with subsequent formation of fistula.

A foreign body in the urethra may cause urethral injury and produce symptoms of lower urinary tract irritation. Sometimes—not always—a history of insertion of the foreign body is obtained. Frequently, the diagnosis is made only after x-ray examination of the lower part of the abdomen. Admission and urologic evaluation by endoscopic techniques are necessary for foreign body removal.

Signs and Symptoms. The history of a blow to the perineum or of a straddle injury should alert the physician to the possibility of anterior urethral injury, especially if blood is found at the urethral meatus or if the patient is unable to void. Initially, hematuria may be present, but the urine may clear as blood is washed from the damaged urethra. Extravasation of blood and urine into the perineum or scrotum indicates urethral injury with perforation of Buck's fascia. Anterior urethral injury without dis-

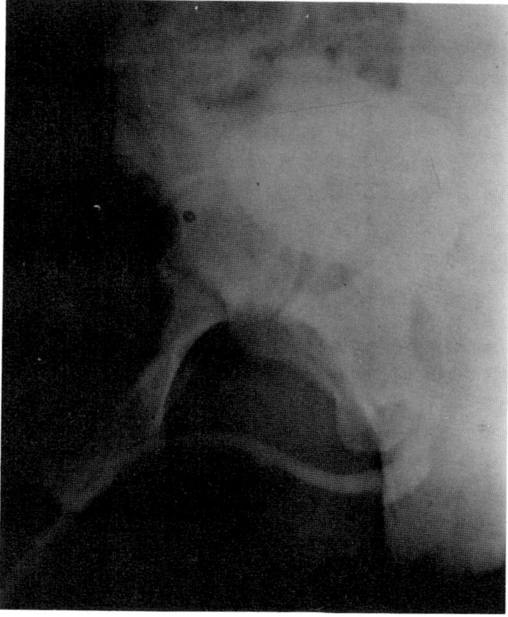

Figure 35.3. Anterior urethral rupture. Retrograde urethrogram shows extravasation of dye from bulbar urethra.

ruption of Buck's fascia confines blood and extravasated urine to the penile shaft.

Urethrography is essential to confirm the diagnosis and to define the extent of injury (Fig. 35.3).

Treatment. Partial disruptions of the anterior urethra can be treated by one of two methods, depending on the extent of injury and the degree of hematoma and extravasation. If the associated hematoma and "urinoma" are extensive, local drainage is advisable. Suprapubic urinary diversion is instituted by percutaneous cystotomy or formal operative cystotomy. One method of treatment involves initial suprapubic drainage with later assessment of urethral healing, whereas the second involves gentle passage of a urethral catheter to stent the injury during healing. Insertion of a percutaneous suprapubic catheter with drainage of any large fluid collections seems preferable. Later, a cystogram with voiding films is obtained, and 1 week after injury, urethroscopy is performed and a urethral catheter placed. Secondary repair of urethral strictures may be necessary.

Complete anterior urethral disruptions are treated similarly. Immediate repair has been advocated, but a course of delayed repair, performing formal urethroplasty after resolution of all periurethral reaction, has been accomplished without difficulties.

Posterior Injury. Pathophysiology. The posterior portion of the urethra includes the membranous segment, which traverses the urogenital diaphragm, and the prostatic segment. Ruptures of the posterior urethra are not usually associated with extravasation of blood or urine into the perineum, scrotum, or anterior abdominal wall (Fig. 35.2*B*) because of the strong fascial planes that attach the urogenital diaphragm laterally to the inferior ischiopubic rami, anteriorly to the pubic symphysis, and posteriorly to the ischial tuberosities and the perineal body. The prostate gland is held in position by the puboprostatic ligaments. Distortion of the pelvic girdle during trauma shears these ligaments, with resulting avulsion of the urethra at the prostatomembranous junction. Around the entire posterior urethra run the parasympathetic and sympathetic nerves responsible for erection and ejaculation. Injury to this area, therefore, may result in impotence, whereas injury to the urinary sphincter, which lies in the urogenital diaphragm, may result in incontinence. Shearing forces that avulse the puboprostatic ligaments produce complete detachment of the prostate gland and bladder from the urogenital diaphragm, resulting in cephalad migration of these structures. Hemorrhage results from tears of pelvic veins, fragmentation of bone, and laceration of the obturator artery.

Trauma to the membranous and prostatic portions of the urethra carries a high and often permanent morbidity, frequently resulting in obliterative scarring of the urethra, impotence, and incontinence. If unnecessary manipulation is avoided at the time of surgery, however, these complications can be minimized.

Signs and Symptoms. When pelvic trauma has occurred, possible urethral injury must be suspected. Indications include: inability to avoid, blood at the urethral meatus, and a distended bladder palpable well out of the pelvis, especially after fluid replacement. This occurs when the bladder and prostate gland are detached from the pelvic diaphragm and migrate cephalad. The internal sphincter of the bladder neck prevents urine from leaking into the retroperitoneal space. The most reliable sign of urethral disruption is the "high riding" prostate on rectal examination. This usually results from cephalad migration of the prostate and a periprostatic hematoma. Shock ensues if laceration of a pelvic vein or of the obturator artery has resulted in massive retroperitoneal bleeding. Unless the urogenital diaphragm is ruptured, blood does not appear in the scrotum or perineum.

Diagnostic Studies. A KUB film should be obtained whenever pelvic injury is suspected. If it reveals a pelvic fracture on diastasis of the pubic symphysis, or if blood is seen at the urethral meatus, retrograde urethrography is performed. If urethral laceration is apparent on the urethrogram (Fig. 35.4), suprapubic drainage of urine is necessary since introduction of a catheter into an open retropubic space may result in infection of the retroperitoneal hematoma. An enlarging hematoma elevates the bladder further out of the pelvis and compresses its sides, giving the diagnostic inverted teardrop shape in the cystographic phase of an intravenous urogram or on a cystogram performed via a cystotomy tube. Percutaneous transfemoral arteriography is the best technique to locate the source of retroperitoneal bleeding.

Treatment. Laceration of the posterior urethra is best treated with immediate suprapubic cystotomy, blood replacement, and control of pelvic hemorrhage. This is best accomplished by injection of Gelfoam or autologous clot during arteriography to occlude the bleeding site (see chapter 46). Repair may be carried out at a later time of election.

External Genitalia

Penis

Elastic bands, bottles, rings, nuts, and other constricting objects may cause severe penile edema. In some cases, swelling may be so great that the band causing the constriction is obscured, but careful examination of the penis reveals the foreign body. Removal of the object requires anesthesia by penile nerve block, sometimes requiring the combined in-

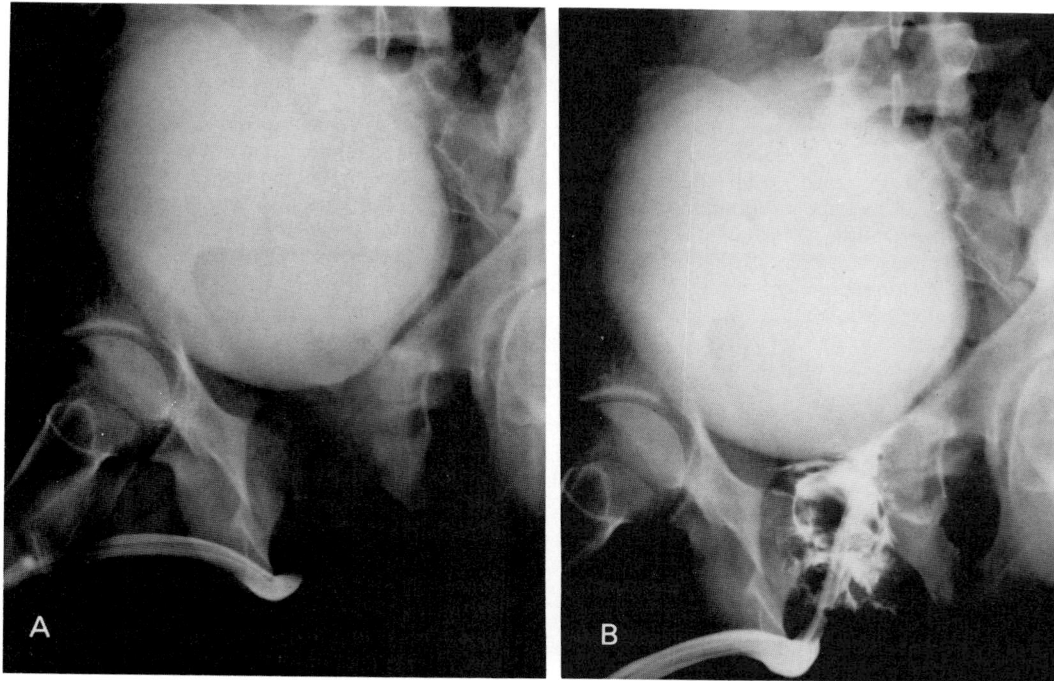

Figure 35.4. Posterior urethral rupture. *A*, Early phase of retrograde urethrogram showing cephalad elevation of bladder with retained dye from intravenous pyelogram. *B*, Later phase of retrograde urethrogram showing misplaced Foley catheter resulting from posterior urethral rupture. Note extravasation of dye into periprostatic tissue.

genuity of the emergency physician and hospital maintenance personnel, who may be called on to supply the proper tools.

Penile lacerations should be treated with the same attention to tissue preservation and function as lacerations in other areas. If the ventral surface is lacerated, the examiner must recognize the possibility of urethral injury and obtain a urethrogram. If doubt exists, endoscopic examination is definitive. Despite the apparent severity of the laceration, repair of the corpora, urethra, and the skin provide excellent functional and cosmetic results. If skin has been lost from the shaft, the injury is debrided with preservation of as much tissue as possible. Split thickness skin grafts are applied with good cosmetic results; such grafts usually do not contract. Rupture of the corpora cavernosa, often referred to as "fracture of the penis" follows vigorous sexual activity or a direct blow to the erect penis. Immediate surgical repair is indicated with a reasonable expectation for preservation of erectile potency.

Testes

Scrotal trauma results in contusion, laceration, destruction, or dislocation of a testis. Contusion of a hydrocele may cause a hematohydrocele, but hemorrhage is usually tamponaded within the hydrocele sac. Testicular laceration results in extravasation of blood into that side of the scrotum. Scrotal ultrasonography is an excellent modality to evaluate suspected testicular fracture. Immediate surgical repair with drainage of the severely lacerated testis decreases morbidity. Unless the testis is destroyed, orchiectomy is rarely necessary. When the testis is dislocated as the result of forceful trauma to the scrotum, it may be displaced upward into the inguinal canal; in this case, exploration and fixation are imperative.

Avulsion of scrotal skin, leaving exposed testes, may be seen when clothing becomes entangled in machinery or, occasionally, when suction devices are used for sexual arousal. Classically, these injuries have been treated by placement of the testes into thigh pouches; however, split thickness skin grafts may sometimes be used with good results.

Autonomic Dysreflexia

Patients with acute or stable spinal cord injuries above the sixth thoracic vertebra and intact distal spinal cords may have *autonomic dysreflexia* in response to nociceptive and proprioceptive stimuli applied below the level of the spinal cord lesion. This syndrome is characterized by severe headache, paroxysmal elevation of systolic and diastolic blood pressure, reflex bradycardia, convulsions, and even cerebral hemorrhage. Flushing and excessive sweating of the face, neck, and dermatomes above the level of the cord lesion are seen along with nasal congestion, and a pilomotor response.

The common stimuli for autonomic dysreflexia are urinary retention and rectal dilatation. The emergency physician must be careful in considering bladder catheterization or rectal examination in paraplegic patients. Treatment is directed at prompt relief of the inciting stimulus; physiologic therapy includes α-adrenergic blocking agents and/or spinal anesthesia. This is a life-threatening condition requiring prompt and thorough evaluation.

NONTRAUMATIC EMERGENCIES

Colicky Flank Pain

Flank pain of urinary tract origin, whether colicky or noncolicky, results from stretching of the renal capsule, and is referred along the eighth, ninth, and tenth thoracic nerve roots. It may be due to obstructed urinary outflow, intrarenal swelling, or alterations in renal blood flow. The character of the pain, the prior medical history, physical examination, laboratory data, and radiologic studies are all important in the differential diagnosis.

Acute, colicky flank pain suggests partial or complete obstruction of urinary outflow, usually due to one or more calculi. The colic results from smooth muscle spasm and intermittent distention of the proximal portion of the ureter and the renal pelvis that occurs with each peristaltic wave. If obstruction is at the ureteropelvic junction, the pain is referred only to the flank. Upper ureteral obstruction may cause pain referral to the testis along the eleventh and twelfth thoracic nerve roots. Obstruction in the middle of the ureter causes pain referred to the ipsilateral lower abdominal quadrant, and thus may mimic appendicitis or diverticulitis, although without localized point tenderness or muscle rigidity. Lower ureteral pain from the intravesical ureter causes the symptoms of an irritated bladder or referred pain to the scrotum.

Causes

A history of renal calculi is suggestive, but conditions other than calculi also cause colic, including blood clot from a renal or pelvic tumor or a sloughed renal papilla. Sloughing of a papilla is particularly likely in diabetic patients, patients with a history of acute or chronic urinary tract infection, and patients with a history of analgesic abuse, particularly phenacetin.

Physical Examination

The patient with colic is agitated, diaphoretic, and in excruciating pain. In contrast with the patient immobilized by peritoneal irritation, the renal colic patient thrashes about the bed, unable to find a comfortable position. Few other intraabdominal processes are as consistent in their clinical presentation. Physical examination reveals tenderness at the costovertebral angle, with little evidence of abdominal guarding and no rigidity nor rebound tenderness. Nausea and vomiting are prominent acute symptoms. Fever occurs if infection is present proximal to the site of obstruction: life-threatening Gram-negative bacteremia may accompany colic, especially if urinary tract infection was present before the onset of acute obstruction.

Diagnostic Studies

Urinalysis usually reveals red blood cells, but rarely clots. Traces of protein are present when the urine contains many red blood cells. The absence of red cells on urinalysis does not preclude renal or ureteral obstruction if complete. Pyuria is present if infection accompanies the obstruction. Urinary cultures should therefore be obtained. A urine pH of approximately 8.5 suggests urea-splitting organisms, usually of the *Proteus* species, and the presence of struvite (magnesium-ammonium-phosphate) calculi. Examination of the urine for crystals of uric acid, calcium oxalate, and cystine helps establish a diagnosis before a KUB film or an intravenous urogram is obtained. Elevation of the white blood cell count may occur during colic; more than 15,000 suggests active infection.

The KUB film may reveal radiopaque calculi, composed of calcium oxalate, cystine, calcium phosphate, or magnesium-ammonium-phosphate (struvite). Because uric acid calculi, papillae, and blood clots are radiolucent, they are not seen on the KUB film. Approximately 85% of renal calculi are radiopaque, however. Confusion may occur if calcified mesenteric lymph nodes or phleboliths in the pelvic veins are detected on X-ray. Phleboliths are spherical and have a hollow center, while calculi are usually irregularly shaped and have an eccentric depression on one surface, their site of attachment to the renal papilla. Staghorn and branched calculi may be visualized on the KUB film at the calyceal infundibulum and at the ureteropelvic junction.

Because a significant percentage of KUB films fail to confirm the diagnosis even in the presence of radiopaque calculi, the intravenous urogram is an essential emergency procedure in the patient with colic, especially if he or she has severe, unremitting pain or fever. Patients whose pain has diminished and who are afebrile may be treated with analgesics, with a urogram obtained on the following day; if x-ray facilities are available in the emergency department, however, an intravenous urogram at the time of the colicky episode is preferable. During an episode of renal colic, the urogram may show a delay in function of the ipsilateral kidney as a result of distal obstruction. This delay may be 5 or 10 minutes in the presence of acute or partial obstruction, or it may be several hours in total or chronic obstruction. The contrast medium eventually fills the ureter to the site of the obstruction; several films may be necessary before this visualization. Persistence by the radiologist taking delayed films at regular intervals, may be necessary for satisfactory anatomic detail. In acute obstruction, small amounts of urine and contrast may extravasate around the renal pelvis. This is due to the higher osmotic pressure of the dye within the obstructed urinary tract, which increases the volume in the renal pelvis and ruptures a calyceal fornix (Fig. 35.5). Such extravasation, if minor, is not an indication for surgical intervention, but is an indication for close clinical observation.

If a calculus is suspected on the KUB film, the urogram confirms its presence and position. Small, irregular calcifications in the pelvis may be suspect as calculi, but a column of contrast material must end at the calcification to confirm this initial im-

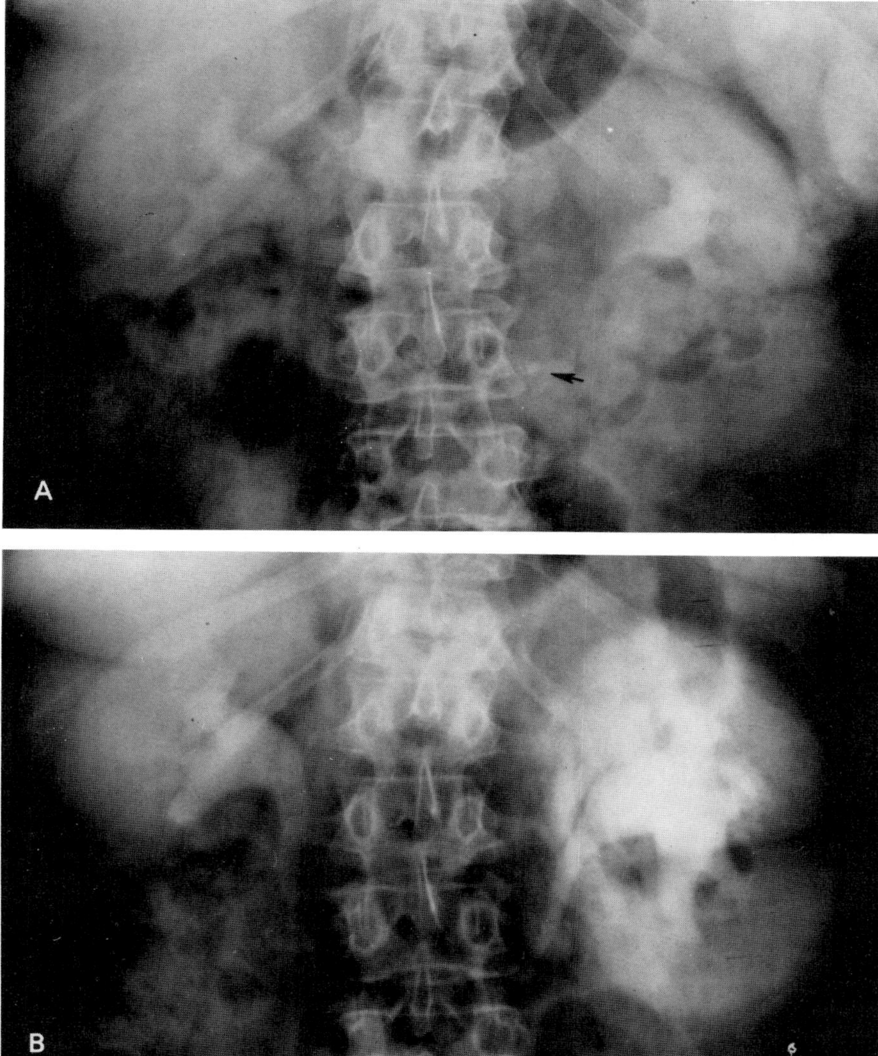

Figure 35.5. Acute renal obstruction with extravasation. *A*, Intravenous pyelogram 10 minutes after injection of dye. Note calcified stone *(arrow)* at tip of left transverse process of third lumbar vertebra and delayed function of left kidney. *B*, Forty minutes after injection, excretion of dye ends at level of calculus with peripelvic extravasation of contrast material. Note acute dilatation of calyces and general swelling of left kidney.

pression. Oblique films are necessary to demonstrate that the calcification on the KUB film remains within the contrast-filled ureter. If the patient has a calculus at the ureterovesical junction, an oblique film after the patient has voided may demonstrate the calculus at the apex of the ureter.

Treatment

The ureter progressively narrows as it courses from the renal pelvis to the bladder. Just distal to the ureteropelvic junction, the ureter assumes a diameter of approximately 10 mm. Crossing the iliac vessels, it narrows to approximately 4 mm, and in the region of the ureterovesical junction, the ureter narrows to 1–5 mm. Consequently, the three common areas for stones to obstruct and cause symptoms are at the ureteropelvic junction, where the ureter crosses the iliac vessels and at the ureterovesical junction. The emergency department physician with the consultative help of a urologist, if available, must determine whether the calculus is small enough to pass through the ureter spontaneously.

Calculi lodged at the ureteropelvic junction are usually too big (more than 8 mm in diameter) to pass spontaneously down the full length of the ureter. Symptoms often subside as the calculus becomes dislodged and floats back into the renal pelvis. Calculi smaller than 8 mm in diameter, not causing sepsis, total obstruction or both, may spontaneously pass with conservative management: hydration, administration of analgesics, and antibiotic coverage. If the calculus is larger and does not spontaneously pass, intervention is necessary. Options at that point include extracorporeal shock wave lithotripsy (ESWL), percutaneous ultrasonic lithotripsy (PUL), or pyelonephrolithotomy. In the case of uric acid calculi, medical therapy may be attempted. Since uric acid calculi usually dissolve in alkaline urine, raising the urine pH with either sodium bicarbonate or potassium citrate may be successful. However, in the presence of sepsis, some form of immediate intervention is usually necessary, regardless of the type of calculus.

In patients who have a calculus in the ureter, the indications for intervention are sepsis, persistent pain, fever, or obstruction. If a calculus is < 4 mm and is in the lower ureter, there is a 90–95% chance of spontaneous passage. If the calculus is > 6 mm, the spontaneous passage rate is $< 20\%$. Eighty percent of stones that are going to pass, do so in a 4-week period. Delay until 12 weeks increases this only to 86%. Upper ureteral stones may be removed ureteroscopically or by ESWL with prior stent placement. Lower ureteral calculi may be removed with the ureteroscope.

If colic is caused by a sloughed papilla or a blood clot, treatment must also be directed toward the primary cause, including diabetes, acute infection, neoplasm or phenacetin/analgesic abuse.

Noncolicky Flank Pain

Causes

Noncolicky flank pain of renal origin results from several conditions. Acute onset of noncolicky pain is usually caused by alteration in blood flow due to a renal arterial embolus, renal venous thrombosis, dissection of the renal artery, or rupture of a renal arterial aneurysm. The most common cause of a renal arterial embolus is atrial fibrillation; emboli may also occur in patients with a mural thrombus after myocardial infarction or in patients with an atrial or ventricular septal defect.

Nonacute, noncolicky flank pain of renal origin usually results from intrarenal changes or perinephric infection. The conditions commonly associated with this pain are acute pyelonephritis, renal abscess, perinephric abscess, bleeding into a renal tumor, and nonobstructing renal calculi.

Acute pyelonephritis is more common in women and occurs in the otherwise normal urinary tract. However, it is not unusual to find an underlying disorder, such as vesicoureteral reflux, obstruction at any level of the urinary tract, diabetes mellitus, or hematogenous embolization as precipitating factors. Urinary obstruction in association with pyelonephritis may be extrinsic or intrinsic to the urinary tract. Pyelonephritis may be unilateral or bilateral, and commonly presents with flank pain, fever, and chills. High fever is common. Associated symptoms, such as urinary frequency, urgency, and dysuria, may precede other symptoms. In severe cases, nausea and vomiting also occur.

Renal abscess may occur from intrarenal obstruction or hematogenous spread. Suppuration caused by intrarenal obstruction usually results from Gram-negative bacteria, whereas abscesses arising from hematogenous spread are often staphylococcal. The clinical signs and symptoms are indistinguishable from those of pyelonephritis.

Nonacute, noncolicky pain of renal origin must be distinguished from nonurologic conditions that cause pain in the back, including the costovertebral angle. The common nonurologic conditions include musculoskeletal and duodenal disorders, cholecystitis, pancreatitis, pneumonitis, and pulmonary infarction.

Diagnostic Studies and Treatment

In patients with a *renal arterial embolus,* urinalysis reveals albuminuria (2+ to 3+) and microscopic hematuria. An intravenous urogram may show partial or total loss of function, depending on the site at which the embolus has lodged. If confusion exists regarding whether delayed function is

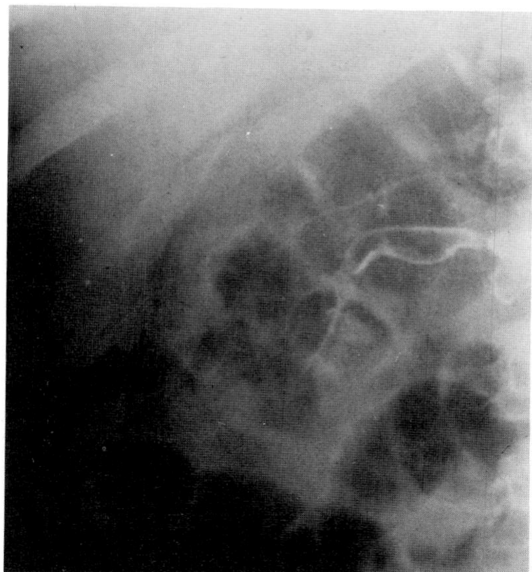

Figure 35.6. Renal artery embolus. Arteriogram shows nonfunction of right kidney with intraluminal filling defect outlined by contrast medium.

due to ureteral obstruction or vascular deficiency, renal scanning may provide clarification. If loss of function is seen on the urogram, and calculus is not the cause, a renal arteriogram is obtained as soon as possible and surgical treatment is planned. Embolization may be differentiated from renal venous thrombosis by renal arteriography. In renal venous thrombosis, the arteriogram shows a patent artery with only a nephrogram to represent function. In the presence of embolization, however, the arteriogram reveals arterial obstruction with nonfunction of the affected kidney or segment (Fig. 35.6). Renal venous thrombosis may be either unilateral or bilateral, and usually is associated with severe albuminuria. Diagnosis is confirmed by an inferior vena cavagram or by selective renal venography. Treatment requires anticoagulation with high doses of heparin and often must include management of an underlying associated disorder such as a malignancy, thrombophlebitis, or the nephrotic syndrome. Renal arterial embolectomy has been successful in selected patients with obstruction of the main renal artery or of one of its primary branches.

Patients with *aortic dissection* involving the renal arteries have pain in both the flank and the back; urography shows no function on the affected side. Therapy is directed toward the aortic dissection (see Chapter 31).

Rupture of a *renal arterial aneurysm is* rare, and is manifested by the acute onset of flank pain and hemorrhagic shock. Seldom does a patient with this condition live long enough to arrive at an emergency facility for treatment. Small leaks however, may be demonstrated on an arteriogram. Because of the significant risk of spontaneous rupture, the presence of a renal artery aneurysm is an indication for surgical correction.

In patients with *acute pyelonephritis* caused by urea-splitting bacteria, the urine pH will be more than 8.5. Mild proteinuria is common in patients with renal infection. Microscopic examination of urine reveals abundant white blood cells, and the presence of white blood cell casts indicates a renal origin. Bacteria may be identified on the Gram's stain of unspun urine. If a single organism is identified in each high power field of Gram's-stained uncentrifuged urine, culture of that specimen is usually associated with a count of more than 100,000 organisms/ml. Therapy should be started. Leukocytosis is usually present.

The treatment of patients with acute pyelonephritis is determined by the degree of sepsis and the presence of underlying disorders. Patients who do not appear severely ill and who have a temperature less than 101°F (38.3°C) should have a urine culture and then be given oral antibiotics; they may be followed as outpatients. Elderly persons, those with chills and/or a temperature of more than 101°F, and those suspected of an underlying urologic disorder should be hospitalized for parenteral antibiotics and immediate urographic examination to identify that underlying disorder. The management of Gram-negative sepsis is discussed in Chapter 11.

In patients with a *renal abscess* caused by hematogenous spread, urinalysis may show no cells. If high fever is present, the urogram is obtained immediately. The presence of a mass and fever suggest abscess. Tomographic sections of the kidney may reveal the fluid-filled cavity (Fig. 35.7), and should be obtained if available on an emergency basis. Ultrasound studies may also demonstrate a fluid-filled cavity with thickened walls, which is consistent with abscess. A gallium radionuclide scan may confirm the presence of leukocytes in an abscess cavity. Renal arteriography performed to differentiate abscess from tumor reveals a relatively avascular mass. Computed tomography differentiates renal masses quite well. If septicemia persists despite antibiotic treatment, surgical intervention is necessary.

Perinephric abscess is difficult to distinguish from pyelonephritis and renal abscess. Perinephric inflammation leads to loss of the psoas shadow on that side on the KUB film and to scoliosis, concave towards the affected side. Ultrasonography or computed tomography may demonstrate a perinephric fluid collection and confirm the diagnosis. Nephrotomography may reveal a thickened Gerota's fascia lifted away from the renal shadow. Inspiratory and expiratory films may show no movement of the kidney with respiration because of the inflammatory

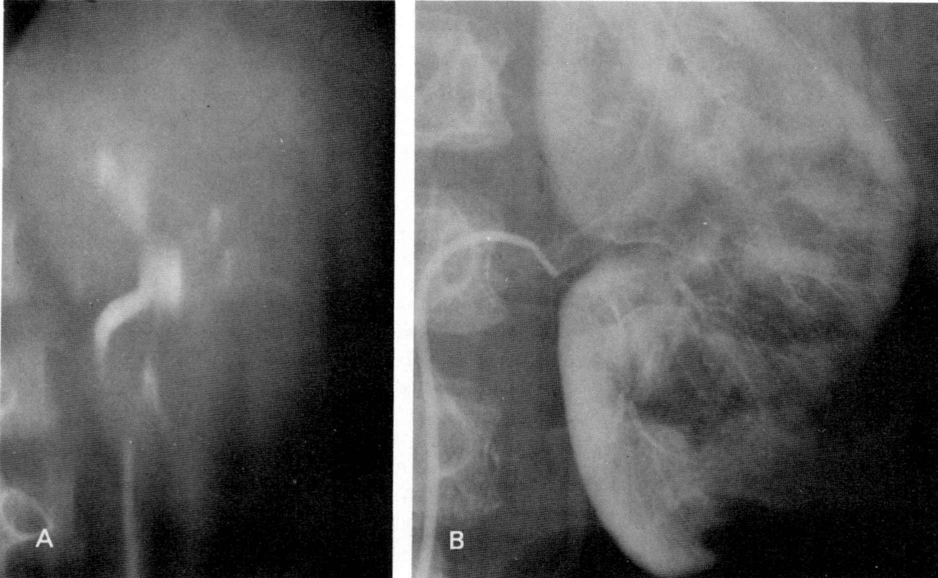

Figure 35.7. Renal abscess. *A,* Intravenous pyelogram shows calyces of left lower pole to be splayed and flattened, suggesting a mass. *B,* Arteriogram shows poor function in left lower pole with draping of tertiary vessels around abscess wall.

reaction. Chest x-ray films may show an ipsilateral pleural effusion or elevation of the ipsilateral diaphragm. The underlying source of the abscess should be sought. Treatment consists of appropriate intravenous antibiotics and incisional or percutaneous drainage.

Bleeding into a renal tumor may cause noncolicky flank pain. Flank tenderness, hematuria, and mild leukocytosis may be present, but pyuria and other indications of sepsis are absent. The intravenous urogram should suggest the diagnosis, ultrasound studies will support the presence of a solid lesion, and angiographic examination or computed tomography will best confirm a tumor of the renal parenchyma. A tumor of the renal pelvis, however, may not be well-visualized with computed tomography and may require retrograde pyelography and cytologic study of the urine for delineation.

Hematuria

Hematuria may occur as a manifestation of many primary and secondary diseases of the upper and lower portions of the urinary tract (Fig. 35.8). The character of the bleeding often suggests the site and cause.

Description

Gross hematuria refers to obviously bloody urine, whereas microscopic hematuria denotes ostensibly clear urine with red blood cells seen only with a light microscope. Hematuria noted only at the beginning of urination is termed initial and is caused by a urethral condition. Blood appears in the first portion of the urinary specimen as the clear urine from the bladder washes the bleeding area. Unless urethral bleeding is brisk, only microscopic hematuria occurs in the remainder of the specimen. Hematuria occurring only at the end of urination is termed terminal and usually comes from the prostate gland, bladder neck, or trigone, as a result of bladder neck contraction after voiding. Total hematuria, or urine that is blood-tinged throughout urination, occurs with active bleeding anywhere in the urinary tract, but usually indicates a site above the bladder neck. The passage of long, stringy, or vermiform clots suggests bleeding above the bladder as the result of formation of a ureteral cast. Large, fresh clots most often occur when bleeding is from the bladder or prostate. Painless bleeding is characteristic of tumors; it also may occur, however, in hemorrhagic disorders, benign prostatic hyperplasia, and other nonmalignant conditions. In the older male, the common etiology for painless total gross hematuria is benign prostatic hyperplasia; however, tumor must always be ruled out. Painful hematuria is common in inflammatory diseases, most notably cystitis and urinary calculus disease.

History

In addition to the descriptive character of the hematuria, other facets of the medical history may indicate the cause. Cyclophosphamide (Cytoxan) may produce hemorrhagic cystitis. Anticoagulant therapy and platelet disorders may result in hematuria, not only by causing abnormal blood clotting, but also by stimulating an asymptomatic tumor. Even if the character of the bleeding suggests a site or cause and the bleeding is self-limited, every patient with hematuria requires a thorough investigation consisting of history, physical examination, urinalysis, blood studies, urography, and cystoscopy for precise identification of the bleeding point.

Physical Examination

A patient with atrial fibrillation, flank pain, and hematuria should be suspected of having an embolic renal infarct. A palpable flank mass suggests a renal tumor. Flank tenderness indicates a ureter blocked by a calculus, clot, or tumor; glomerulonephritis; or papillary necrosis due to diabetes, acute pyelonephritis, or phenacetin therapy. In patients with cystitis, suprapubic or bladder tenderness is common. Prostatic tenderness often is elicited in the presence of acute prostatitis, and a hard, nodular prostate gland indicates carcinoma until proved otherwise. Total gross hematuria in older men may be secondary to benign prostatic hyperplasia. Urethral tumors are commonly palpable. In women, a urethral caruncle or prolapsed urethra may be the site of bleeding; and it should be easily visualized during pelvic examination. Although infiltrating carcinoma of the bladder may be palpated on bimanual examination, the absence of a palpable mass does not exclude the possibility of carcinoma as a source of bleeding.

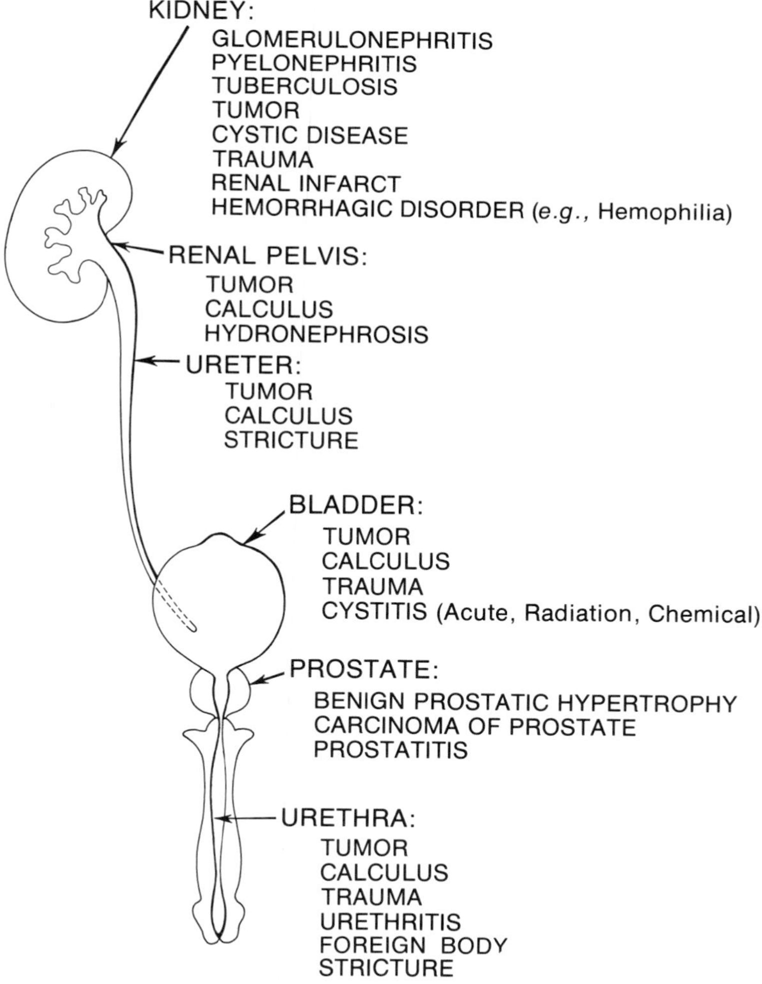

Figure 35.8. Causes of gross and microscopic hematuria.

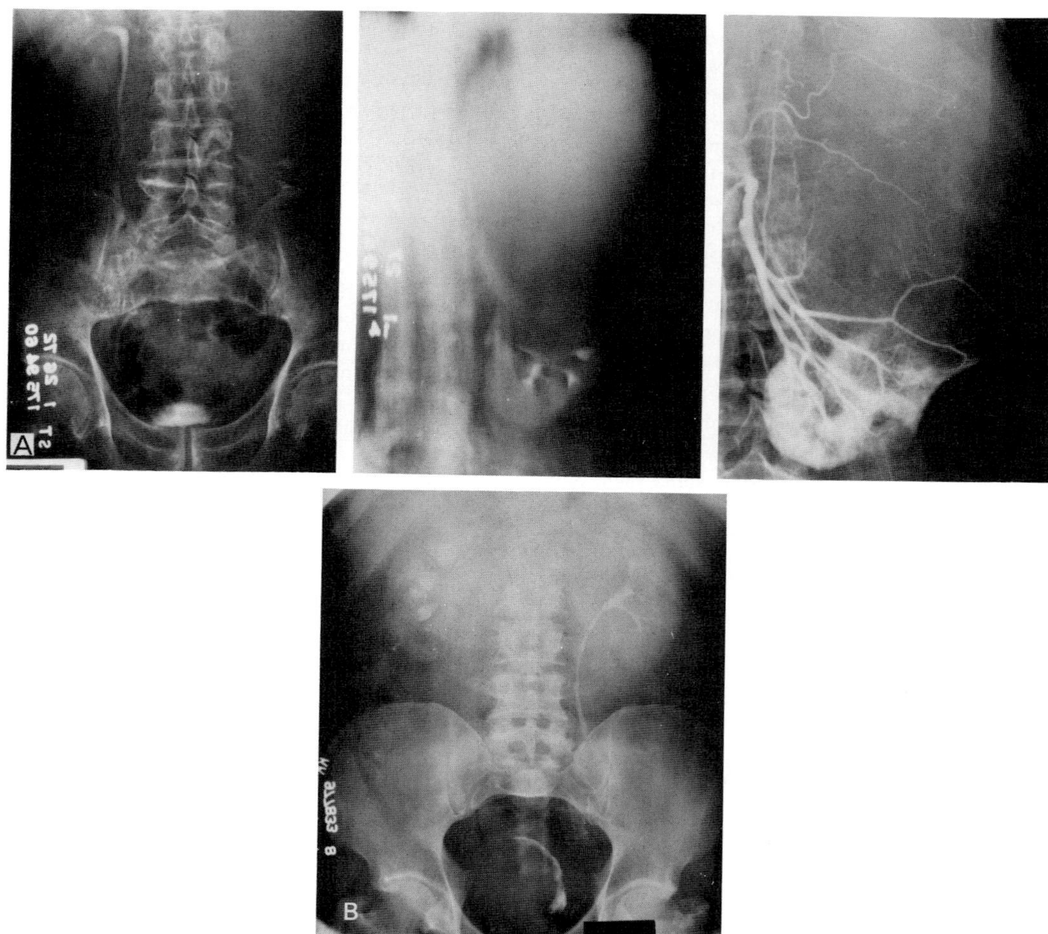

Figure 35.9. Renal cell carcinoma. *Left,* Intravenous pyelogram shows left upper pole mass compressing left lower pole with flattening of calyces and nonfunction of upper pole. *Middle,* Tomographic cut of intravenous pyelogram confirms left upper pole mass. *Right,* Arteriogram confirms huge left upper pole mass compressing hilar structures and renal parenchyma downward. *B,* Bladder tumor. Huge intravesical filling defect causing right renal obstruction and hydronephrosis.

Diagnostic Studies

Urinalysis. Even in the presence of gross hematuria, red blood cells must be identified under the microscope in all instances of apparent urinary tract bleeding. Red urine without blood cells may occur after eating beets, after ingestion of laxatives containing phenolphthalein, and in hemolytic syndromes that result in hemoglobinuria. Red cell casts may accompany red blood cells in patients with acute or focal glomerulonephritis. Obvious bacterial cystitis in women accompanied by gross hematuria should be confirmed with urinalysis and urinary culture and appropriate follow-up studies planned.

Blood Studies. The hematocrit indicates possible chronic blood loss and provides baseline information for the management of severe bleeding. The prothrombin time, partial thromboplastin time, and platelet count are necessary to exclude a coagulation defect. Immediate blood typing and crossmatching are necessary in patients with major bleeding. Serum creatinine and blood urea nitrogen levels are obtained to assess renal function; platelet function is adversely affected in azotemic patients. Since elevations of serum calcium may occur in patients with renal cell carcinoma, the serum calcium, phosphorus, and alkaline phosphatase are measured when this diagnosis is suspected. Similarly, the serum acid phosphatase is measured in patients in whom a diagnosis of prostatic carcinoma is a possibility.

Intravenous Urography. An intravenous pyelogram should be obtained in the emergency department, or as soon as possible, in all patients with gross or microscopic hematuria. Delay may be hazardous if severe bleeding starts abruptly, possibly followed by shock, Gram-negative sepsis, or acute clot retention. The urogram may be helpful in identifying renal mass (Fig. 35.9*A*), ureteral obstruction, and complete or partial loss of function resulting from emboli, or may suggest the presence of a bladder tumor (Fig. 35.9*B*). Often the cystographic phase of the intravenous pyelogram may show unsuspected bladder clot retention. In patients allergic to intravenous contrast agents, a radioisotopic scan of the kidney may be obtained to visualize and quantitate renal function.

Cystoscopy. Cystoscopic examination is necessary in all but the most obvious cases of hematuria—for example, in the presence of urethritis, or obvious cystitis. Although it is most effective in identifying the site of bleeding, if performed during an active bleeding episode, emergency cystoscopy is not always possible. Patients with recurrent bleeding from an unidentified source, however, should undergo immediate cystoscopy in an attempt to identify the bleeding site. Obvious bleeding from one of the ureteral orifices helps localize the bleeding source to that renal unit. Fulguration of bleeding points, biopsy of tumors, and retrograde studies may also be performed at the time of cystoscopic examination.

Urine Cytology. Urine specimens for cytologic examination should be obtained in all patients in whom a neoplasm is suspected. However, identification of malignant cells in the sediment is hampered by the presence of many red blood cells and more accurate cytologic examination is possible when active bleeding has ceased.

Treatment

The emergency treatment of patients with hematuria should be directed at replacing blood volume, preventing or treating clot retention, and gaining as much information as possible about the cause, so that specific therapy may be instituted promptly. If the urine is darker in color than rosé wine or if it contains clots, a whistle-tip catheter is placed into the bladder and saline solution is infused by hand with an irrigating syringe to clear the bladder of clot. Parenteral administration of analgesics may be necessary when the bladder is vigorously irrigated. The bladder should be free of clots and the urine should be almost clear before irrigation by hand is stopped; a no. 22 French three-way Foley catheter with a 5-ml balloon is inserted for continuous normal saline irrigation. When the clots have been irrigated from the bladder, bleeding often ceases. A bladder distended with clots does not allow for vessel contraction. After clot retention has been relieved, further evaluation may be carried out.

If attempts to free the bladder of clots by hand irrigation are unsuccessful or if clots plug the catheter, it may be necessary to evacuate the clots under anesthesia, utilizing a cystoscope.

If the patient has had a recent prostatectomy and if irrigation fails to keep the urine clear, or if for other reasons, bleeding is suspected from the prostatic fossa, the three-way catheter with a 30-ml balloon is placed on traction to occlude and to tamponade the bladder neck. Although a small amount of oozing may occur around the catheter, the main source of bleeding from the prostatic fossa is tamponaded by the large balloon just proximal to the fossa at the bladder neck.

In the absence of trauma, uncontrollable bleeding from the upper urinary tract rarely occurs. A blood clot usually blocks the ureter, and urine production proximal to the obstruction tamponades the bleeding. If continuous, uncontrollable hemorrhage occurs from the upper tract, emergency evaluation including intravenous urography and arteriography is necessary. In isolated instances, transarteriographic embolization of renal bleeding points may be used to stop hemorrhage. Otherwise, surgical exploration may be necessary.

In patients with massive bleeding from prostatic carcinoma, fibrinolysis may be the cause. This occurs when fibrinolysins are released from the carcinoma either locally or systemically to promote conversion of plasminogen to the proteolytic enzyme plasmin, which destroys fibrin. When this diagnosis is suspected, the levels of serum fibrinogen and fibrin split products must be determined. If the fibrinogen level is below normal and if fibrin split products are increased, intravenous therapy with ϵ-aminocaproic acid is instituted, 5 gm in 250 ml of 5% dextrose in water over 1 hour, followed by 1 gm/hr thereafter during acute bleeding.

All patients with gross hematuria and patients passing blood clots, except, perhaps, women with symptoms of acute cystitis, should undergo thorough urologic evaluation. Even if hematuria has ceased, it is essential that the patient have a complete and thorough investigation to discover the source of bleeding. Too often, patients are seen with one episode of bleeding and are discharged from the emergency department. It is the responsibility of the emergency physician to see that this does not happen.

Lower Tract Irritation and Inflammation

Symptoms

The onset of urinary frequency, urgency, or dysuria indicates either primary or secondary irritation of the lower urinary tract, that is, the bladder, prostate gland, seminal vesicles, or urethra. Voluntary voiding usually does not occur until urine volume in the bladder reaches 350–400 ml. and the stretch reflex along the second, third, and fourth sacral nerves is activated. The reflex is mediated by the cerebral cortex. When voiding is incomplete, the critical volume that initiates the voiding reflex is reached more rapidly and urinary frequency occurs. Irritation of the lower tract by infection or a foreign body also causes the bladder to contract at lower volumes, and frequent voiding and dysuria then develop. The dysuria that accompanies inflammation may be sensed as pressure in the suprapubic area, but is experienced more often as pain in the urethra.

Primary infections of the kidneys and ureters may result in secondary irritation of the lower urinary tract and symptoms of frequency and dysuria. In addition, calculi lodged in the intramural portion of the ureter may mimic lower tract inflammation. Frequency may result from reduction in bladder volume by extravesical masses or from glycosuria, diabetes insipidus, renal concentrating defects such as chronic pyelonephritis, potassium depletion nephropathy, uric acid nephropathy, and sickle cell disease. In addition, diuretics may result in frequency. Upper tract disease as a cause of urinary frequency and dysuria usually may be ruled out by: (*a*) a careful history; (*b*) the absence of glycosuria; (*c*) a urinary specific gravity greater than 1.010; and (*d*) the absence of flank pain and tenderness.

Conditions and Treatment

Cystitis. As an isolated condition, cystitis occurs almost exclusively in women. Although acute infection of the bladder may develop in men, it is almost always a secondary manifestation of upper tract disease or mechanical obstruction. In women, acute cystitis may be bacterial or nonbacterial; the symptoms of each, however, are similar: frequency, urgency, dysuria, and suprapubic discomfort. Hematuria is common, but is not always present. The symptoms of cystitis often occur after sexual intercourse, since vaginal and perirectal intestinal organisms may be introduced into the urethra, where they multiply. Although the patient may seek emergency care for the initial episode, the natural history of cystitis is one of frequent recurrences. Unless pyelonephritis is also present, flank pain, high fever, and elevation of white blood cell count usually do not occur.

Physical examination reveals urethral and suprapubic tenderness, especially during bimanual examination. Pressure on the urethra frequently causes small droplets of pus to exude from infected periurethral glands. The urethral meatus may be strictured. Meatal stenosis may be congenital in younger women, whereas in older women the urethral meatus may be pinpoint in diameter because of scarring caused by atrophic vaginitis.

Urinalysis usually reveals bacteriuria and also may show significant hematuria. If a Gram's stain of the uncentrifuged urine shows organisms, it can be assumed that culture of that specimen will reveal more than 100,000 organisms/ml. A "midstream" urinary specimen is collected for culture before antibiotic therapy is given. Intravenous urography is unnecessary as an emergency procedure unless upper tract disease is suspected. Similarly, voiding cystourethrography (VCUG) should not be performed on an emergency basis, since inflammation of the bladder may cause small amounts of ureteral reflux. Once inflammation has subsided, a VCUG may be obtained to rule out reflux as a contributing factor to infection. Lower urinary tract infections in men require thorough evaluation, including cystoscopy.

Oral administration of antibiotics should be started on an outpatient basis without waiting for urine culture results. Most intestinal tract bacteria that invade the urinary tract respond to usual antibiotics. The most common organism to cause cystitis in women is *Escherichia coli.* For uncomplicated cystitis, the sulfonamides are recommended—sulfisoxazole 2 gm initially followed by 1 gm every 6 hours for 7–10 days. Other antibiotics, including ampicillin and tetracycline, may be equally effective. Except when cystitis is associated with Gram-negative sepsis, these patients usually are treated as outpatients.

Nonbacterial cystitis may be caused by tuberculosis, schistosomiasis, or intersititial cystitis (Hunner's ulcer). Tuberculosis of the bladder may occur without a history of pulmonary disease, and typically produces pyuria sterile to routine culture. The symptoms are usually severe and unremitting, and the diagnosis frequently is made by characteristic x-ray findings and by cystoscopic examination of the bladder wall following failure of the usual antibiotic treatment for bacterial cystitis. Cultures take up to 6 weeks for positive results; rarely is this diagnosis made in the emergency department. Schistosomiasis may cause severe nonbacterial bladder symptoms; the diagnosis depends on eliciting a history of residence in an endemic area and on characteristic calcifications seen on x-ray. Interstitial cystitis is characterized by extremely painful, frequent voiding, and its onset is rarely acute. The absence of pyuria in a middle-aged female patient with severe urgency, frequency, and dysuria should lead the examiner to suspect this diagnosis. Confirmation is possible only by cystoscopic examination.

Emphysematous cystitis occurs when gas-producing bacteria colonize the bladder and infiltrate the bladder wall, causing air bubbles that are visible on radiologic examination. Patients usually have signs of Gram-negative sepsis as well as symptoms of lower tract infection. Treatment includes drainage of the bladder, administration of antibiotics, and correction of the causative factor, which is usually obstruction.

Bladder Calculi. Calculi in the bladder cause irritative symptoms manifested by frequency, urgency, and dysuria. They rarely occur spontaneously, and are usually the result of chronic infection and/or bladder outlet obstruction. The history of a neurogenic bladder, an indwelling urethral catheter, chronic urinary tract infection, or symptoms of outlet obstruction suggests this diagnosis. Physical examination is usually uninformative. Urinalysis reveals both red and white blood cells and bacteria when infection is present. A urinary pH greater than 8.5 suggests urea-splitting bacterial infection, which creates the alkaline medium necessary for precipitation of magnesium-ammonium-phosphate complexes, the most common type of "infection" calculus. Calculi associated with outlet obstruction and no infection are usually composed of uric acid, and are not visualized on the KUB film. However, if intravenous urography is performed, the uric acid calculi appear as filling defects in the bladder. Other causes of radiolucent filling defects include an enlarged median lobe of the prostate gland, bladder tumor, blood clots, a Foley catheter balloon, and ureterocele. Removal of bladder calculi may be accomplished endoscopically or by open cystolithotomy. Any underlying pathology, such as prostatic hyperplasia or infection, must be addressed.

Acute Prostatitis. This disease usually occurs in men between the ages of 20 and 40 years. In addition to urinary frequency, urgency, and dysuria, symptoms may include fever, suprapubic discomfort, perineal pain, low back pain, referred pain in the testes, initial or terminal hematuria, and hemospermia. The patient may have a urethral discharge of a thin, white, watery consistency, which increases in the morning or with a Valsalva's maneuver. Frank urinary retention occurs if prostatic swelling is severe enough to cause total outlet obstruction. A history of nonspecific urethritis or gonorrhea is common; however, neither of these is necessary for prostatitis to occur.

Physical examination may reveal suprapubic discomfort, epididymitis, and a tender boggy prostate gland. If a prostatic abscess is present, one segment of the prostate may be exquisitely tender or may feel fluctuant. Prostatic massage to obtain secretions should be avoided in patients with acute prostatitis since this manipulation may induce retrograde seeding of bacteria via the vas deferens to the epididymis, resulting in acute epididymitis or septicemia.

Urinalysis may show red blood cells and/or white blood cells. The three-glass urinary test may be used to differentiate the site responsible for the pyuria or hematuria. In this test, the patient is asked to void the first 10 ml of urine into a container. This washes the anterior urethra. He is then instructed to void most of the remaining urine into a second container and the last few milliliters into the third. If the first specimen contains the largest number of blood cells, the disease process is localized to the anterior urethra. If the largest number of cells is in the third specimen, this indicates disease of the prostate gland, bladder neck, or posterior urethra, since contraction of the bladder neck as voiding ceases forces cells into the urine. If the number of blood cells is the same in all specimens, the site of disease is usually above the bladder neck.

A Gram's stain and culture of urethral discharge should be obtained to rule out gonorrhea. Although systemic bacterial infection may be localized to the prostate gland, and although infections from common urinary pathogens, such as *E. coli*, the enterococci, and *Klebsiella* may occur, in many instances of acute prostatitis, no bacterial pathogen is identified.

If the diagnosis is established by these means, emergency urography is unnecessary. If a KUB film is obtained, prostatic calcifications may be noted; these indicate a chronic inflammatory process, but prostatitis may certainly occur in their absence.

If the gonococcus is not implicated, the most effective antibiotic for the treatment of acute prostatitis is tetracycline, 500 mg by mouth four times a day for 10 days. The other agent useful in this situation is a combination of sulfamethoxazole and trimethoprim (Bactrim), both of which act as folic acid antagonists. Trimethoprim crosses the cell barrier and enters the prostatic secretions. Nonsteroidal anti-inflammatory agents are also useful. Bed rest and hot tub baths may help to relieve symptoms. Instrumentation with a urethral catheter should be avoided, since the presence of a catheter in the prostatic fossa causes an inflammatory reaction around the orifices of the prostatic ducts, impeding drainage. Urinary retention in the presence of acute prostatitis should be treated with percutaneous suprapubic drainage.

Palpable prostatic abscesses require systemic antibiotic therapy and may need drainage by needle aspiration, transurethral unroofing, or perineal exploration.

Seminal Vesiculitis. This condition is almost impossible to distinguish from acute prostatitis unless a discrete tender mass is palpable above the prostate gland on rectal examination. Seminal vesiculitis rarely occurs as an isolated phenomenon and usually accompanies prostatitis. The treatment is identical.

Acute Urethritis. This condition is manifested by urinary frequency, dysuria, and urethral discharge. The discharge can be thick, yellow, and purulent when caused by *Neisseria gonorrhoeae* or thin, white, and watery when caused by *Trichomonas, Chlamydia*, or other nonbacterial organisms.

The symptoms of gonococcal urethritis begin 3–10 days after sexual exposure. Except for a discharge, the findings on physical examination may be normal. The rectum and oral cavity should always be examined for signs of extragenital involvement. A Gram's stain of urethral secretions reveals Gram-negative intracellular diplococci; even if the smear is negative, a specimen should be cultured. A serologic test for syphilis should always be performed before antibiotic treatment.

Acute gonococcal urethritis is best treated with penicillin, 4.8 million units intramuscularly, together with probenecid, 1 gm orally to prolong the blood level of penicillin by blocking renal tubular excretion. This treatment is successful in most patients. Persons allergic to penicillin should be given tetracycline, 500 mg four times a day for 15 days, with the expectation of a 96% success rate. Erythromycin, 500 mg by mouth, four times a day, for 15 days may also be used. Follow-up outpatient treatment is important and should be arranged before leaving the emergency department.

An alert from the Massachusetts Department of Public Health (April 1988) suggests treatment for patients with presumed gonococcal infection in Suffolk County with ceftriaxone 250 mg intramuscularly or spectinomycin 2 gm intramuscularly, this because of a prevalence of resistant gonorrhea. All culture isolates should be evaluated for β-lactamase production and for chromosomally-mediated resistance to penicillin or tetracycline.

Nonspecific urethritis shows no evidence of Gram-negative intracellular diplococci on the Gram's stain, and cultures may not reveal a urinary pathogen. Tetracycline, 500 mg four times a day for 10 days, is the most effective treatment. Recurrences are frequent.

Strains of *Chlamydia* have been associated with nonspecific urethritis. They do not grow on ordinary commercial culture media and can be cultured only under special sophisticated laboratory conditions. These strains seem to be responsive to the tetracyclines, which is probably why most cases designated as nonspecific urethritis respond well to these agents.

Urethritis caused by *Trichomonas* is distinguished from nonspecific urethritis by the presence of flagellated protozoa seen during examination of the discharge by the hanging-drop technique. Identification of these organisms is an indication for simultaneous treatment of both sexual partners with metronidazole (Flagyl) for 10 days.

Periurethral Abscess. The symptoms of periurethral abscess are those of lower urinary tract irritation. Pain and a palpable mass at the penoscrotal junction, along the course of the urethra in women, or in the perineum should alert the examiner to the possibility of this diagnosis. Communication between the urethra and the abscess cavity may result in intermittent, urethral discharge of purulent material. Another symptom suggesting this diagnosis is the complaint of postvoid dribbling. This occurs in both men and women as the abscess cavity fills and then empties after urination.

This condition at one time was most often seen as a result of gonococcal infection with subsequent urethral perforation, abscess formation, and the formation of multiple terminal fistulas (the "watering-pot perineum"). Presently, periurethral abscess is more commonly found at the penoscrotal junction as a result of pressure necrosis from an indwelling urethral catheter and at sites of urethral perforation from instrumentation or trauma.

Physical examination shows a tender, fluctant mass; pressure on the mass causes pus to exude from the urethra. Treatment is accomplished with systemic antibiotics and temporary suprapubic urinary diversion by either a percutaneous technique or by open cystotomy, depending on the period of drainage required. Local incision, drainage, and urethroplasty may be necessary. Hospital admission and urologic consultation are required.

Acute Urinary Retention

The adult patient with acute urinary retention seeks emergency care because of suprapubic discomfort, the inability to void, dribbling, or severe urinary frequency. The more common causes of acute urinary retention are listed in Table 35.1. The history and physical examination aid in determining the cause of retention and, therefore, the treatment.

History

Progressive symptoms of decrease in the force of urinary stream, nocturia, urinary frequency, or dysuria in an elderly man suggest benign prostatic hypertrophy. A history of urologic procedures, including prostatectomy, catheterization, or endoscopic examination, may indicate bladder neck contracture or urethral stricture, whereas prior prostatic carcinoma suggests obstruction at the bladder neck from growth of the neoplasm. Inflammatory diseases of the urethra, especially gonorrhea, predispose to urethral strictures. In young men with prostatitis and posterior urethritis, urethral discharge, fever, and perineal pain precede acute urinary retention. Acute episodes of herpes progenitalis may result in retention, and a history of such ulcers should be sought. Urethral bleeding (initial hematuria) suggests a urethral tumor or foreign body as the case of retention. A history of neurologic disease indicates that the patient may have an incompetent, flaccid neurogenic bladder. If the patient recently has ingested drugs, such as antihistamines, atropine compounds, or adrenergic stimulators, these may be the cause of acute retention. Sudden interruption of the urinary stream followed by inability to void implies a urethral or bladder calculus. The diagnosis of psychogenic urinary retention is a diagnosis of exclusion, but this condition commonly is encountered in young hospital-associated women who have no history to suggest another cause.

Causative Factors and Treatment

Penis. Phimosis, or adherence of the prepuce, may be found during physical examination. This causes retention by obstructing the flow of urine. Relief of obstruction in the emergency department is accomplished by instillation of a local anesthetic for either dilatation of the pinpoint meatus or a dorsal slit procedure. Paraphimosis, or the inability to pull the prepuce back over the glans penis, may cause constriction of the urethra and vascular insufficiency because of circumferential obstructing bands; it therefore requires immediate reduction. Meatal stenosis is obvious as the examiner tries to separate the glans to visualize the urethral orifice; this condition may follow circumcision, indwelling catheterization, or a urethral surgical procedure, or may occur without obvious cause. Meatotomy under local anesthesia in the emergency department provides immediate relief of obstruction (Fig. 35.10). If for any reason a dorsal split procedure or meatotomy cannot be performed by the emergency physician, a percutaneous suprapubic cystotomy should be placed to provide drainage. This allows definitive therapy to be undertaken at a later time by a urologist.

Urethra. Palpation of the urethra may reveal a tumor, foreign body, or calculus. In men, obstructing tumors of the urethra usually occur in the bulbomembranous urethra. Relief of obstruction requires proximal drainage by cystotomy or suprapubic placement of a catheter. A calculus lodged in the urethra is usually palpable at or just distal to the penoscrotal junction. Since the urethra narrows proximal to this point, the force of the urinary stream usually wedges the calculus in this area. A gentle attempt to ''milk'' the calculus along the remaining length of the urethra may be made after instillation of anesthetic jelly. However, this is usually unsuccessful because the jagged edges of the calculus snag and macerate the urethral mucosa. A calculus that is too large to be removed in this manner requires cystoscopic or operative removal.

Urethritis, whether nonspecific, trichomonal, or gonococcal, may cause copious urethral discharge or meatal swelling with associated urinary retention. Although passage of a urethral catheter may be possible, an indwelling foreign body will exac-

Table 35.1.
Causes of Acute Urinary Retention in Adults

Penis	Neurologic causes
Phimosis	Motor paralytic
Paraphimosis	Spinal shock
Meatal stenosis	Spinal cord syndromes
Foreign body constriction	Sensory paralytic
Urethra	Tabes dorsalis
Tumor	Diabetes
Foreign body	Multiple sclerosis
Calculus	Syringomyelia
Urethritis (severe)	Spinal cord syndromes
Stricture	Herpes zoster
Meatal stenosis (female)	Miscellaneous
Hematoma	Drugs
Prostate gland	Antihistamines
Benign prostatic hypertrophy	Anticholinergic agents
Carcinoma	Antispasmodic agents
Prostatitis (severe)	Tricyclic antidepressants
Bladder neck contracture	α-Adrenergic stimulators
Prostatic infarction	''Cold'' tablets
	Ephedrine derivatives
	Amphetamines
	Psychogenic problems

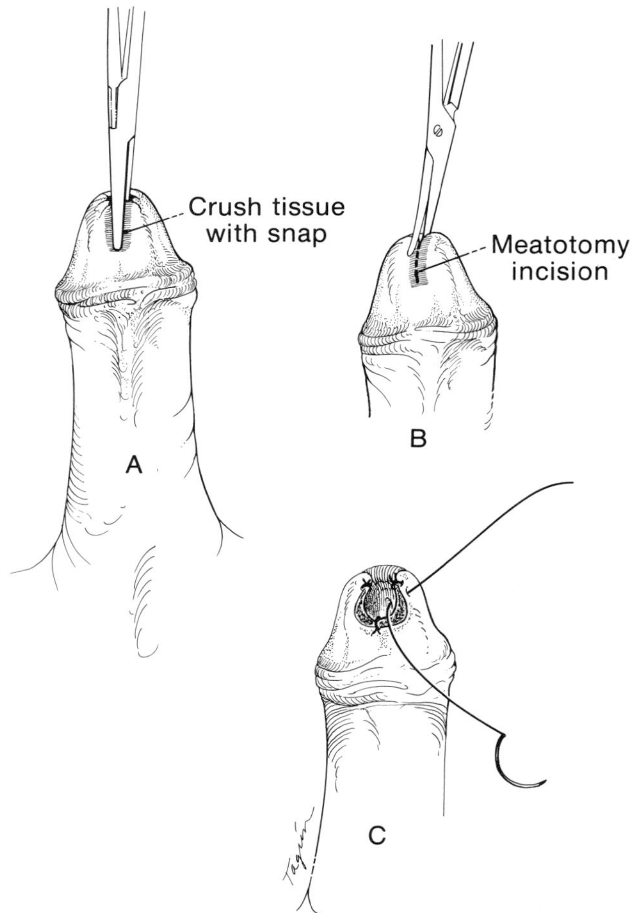

Figure 35.10. A difficult catheterization because of meatal stenosis may be simplified with meatotomy. *A,* After local anesthesia is used, a straight clamp is placed into the urethra, and meatal tissue is crushed at 6 o'clock to prevent bleeding. *B,* Meatotomy is performed with scissors along crushed tissue. *C,* Cut edges of urethra and glans penis are approximated with interrupted 4–0 chromic absorbable sutures.

erbate the urethritis. Temporary urinary diversion by means of a suprapubic catheter with appropriate antibiotic therapy is the treatment of choice.

Unless the patient has a history of urethral stricture or urethral instrumentation, a stricture may not be recognized unless the examiner has difficulty passing a catheter to the level of the prostate gland. The most common sites of stricture formation are the submeatal area (fossa navicularis) and the bulbomembranous urethra just distal to the urinary sphincter. Before urethral dilatation is attempted, the physician should try to insert a no. 12 French Foley catheter or a no. 10 straight infant feeding tube. If one of these is successfully passed through the strictured area, it should be left in place, and then, in the course of the next few days, progressively larger catheters may be passed as the stricture softens. A stricture should not be dilated progressively in the emergency department because urethral injury and sepsis too often ensue. *Under no circumstances should anyone other than a urologist attempt to dilate a stricture with urethral sounds or stylets in the emergency department.*

Failure to pass a small catheter is no longer an indication to attempt the blind passage of filiforms and followers. Urethral dilatation should be carried out under direct endoscopic vision in a cystoscopy suite if the patient is obstructed.

The preferred treatment of urethral obstruction that cannot be overcome with gentle attempts at passing a urethral catheter is the positioning of one of the many percutaneous suprapubic tubes now available. With appropriate preparation of the suprapubic skin, local anesthesia, and sterile technique, this method causes minimal discomfort and trauma, and leaves the urethra unscathed so that thorough radiologic and endoscopic evaluation may be performed later under optimal conditions (see Illustrated Technique 16).

Prostate Gland. A history of progressive urinary outlet obstruction, with hesitancy, nocturia, and diminished stream, in an elderly patient suggests prostatic disease. The most common condition is benign prostatic hyperplasia. Rectal examination reveals a prostate gland that may or may not feel enlarged; the size of the prostate bears no relation to the degree of obstruction. The anatomic difficulty in benign prostatic hypertrophy is compression of the urethral lumen by the lateral lobes of the prostate gland, or obstruction of the proximal end of the urethral lumen by an enlarged median lobe (Fig. 35.11).

When benign prostatic hyperplasia is suspected, the urethra is anesthetized with lidocaine jelly, and a no. 16 French Foley catheter with a 5-ml balloon is inserted. Larger balloons are avoided because they cause bladder spasms. If it cannot be easily passed into the bladder, a coudé catheter may be used. The deflection in the distal 3 cm of the coudé catheter allows it to be passed over an obstructing median lobe. Failure to pass a coudé catheter successfully may be due either to total obstruction of the bladder neck by median lobe elevation or to bladder neck contracture so severe that only a pinpoint orifice is present. Filiforms, followers, sounds, and stylets are avoided in this situation, because the median lobe may be perforated easily, resulting in possibly uncontrollable bleeding and sepsis. Suprapubic catheter placement is the treatment of choice.

When drainage is established successfully, the bladder is decompressed slowly, 300–400 ml initially, followed by 200 ml/hr. Rapid decompression of a chronically distended bladder sometimes leads to mucosal hemorrhage with clot retention. During the first few hours after decompression of a chronically distended bladder, postobstructive diuresis may develop. Urine is passed at a rate of up to 1000 ml/hr with resulting hypotension and shock, unless fluid is replaced. Postobstructive diuresis may be caused by one or more of the following: (*a*) an increased concentration of blood urea nitrogen secondary to obstructive renal failure, acting as an osmotic diuretic; (*b*) damage to the proximal and distal renal tubules by hydronephrosis, resulting in a renal concentrating defect; (*c*) failure of the damaged distal tubule to respond to endogenous or exogenous antidiuretic hormone; and (*d*) total body water overload. If this syndrome develops, an intravenous line is immediately placed so that fluid volume may be promptly restored. Replacement therapy is based on urinary and serum electrolyte determinations and maintenance of stable vital signs.

Once a catheter has been placed, its function is tested by instillation and withdrawal of irrigating solution to ensure that it is in the bladder and not curled in the prostatic fossa. Oral antibiotics and

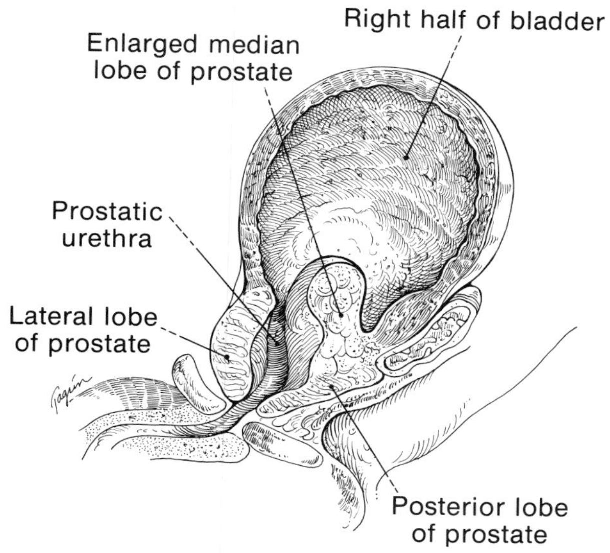

Figure 35.11. In addition to prominent lateral lobes, enlarged median lobe of prostate contributes to marked bladder outlet obstruction. In such instances, a curve-tipped coudé catheter may negotiate channel of prostatic urethra more easily than a standard straight-tipped Foley catheter.

attention to asepsis at the penile meatus reduce the incidence of catheter-induced infection. Asepsis is maintained with applications of antibiotic ointment, such as Neosporin, and frequent washings with benzalkonium chloride (Zephiran). The patient is then admitted, and further diagnostic workup performed.

Neurologic Causes. Many neurologic conditions result in acute urinary retention. Spinal shock and spinal cord syndromes are easily recognizable, as are other neurologic diseases that are accompanied by obvious neurologic signs. However, the neurogenic bladder resulting from tabes dorsalis, diabetes, multiple sclerosis and syringomyelia may be difficult to recognize when urinary retention is the primary manifestation of the disease. The emergency physician should be particularly aware of these possibilities in young patients who do not have any signs or symptoms of outlet obstruction. Patients in whom neurologic impairment is recognized as a cause of urinary retention should have a catheter passed to empty the bladder and to relieve obstruction; but it should not be left in place. Patients with neurologic bladder disease, despite adequate treatment, may continue to have residual urine after voiding. This urinary stasis predisposes to infection, which is difficult to eradicate. Therefore, these patients should be managed with straight catheterization every 6–8 hours. This reduces the incidence of infection and stone formation. Bladder function studies should be performed and a program developed for improving emptying of the bladder. This may best be accomplished by hospital admission.

Pharmacologic Causes. Medications cause acute urinary retention in patients with no history or only mild symptoms of obstructive uropathy. Drugs that cause bladder atony include antihistamines (Benadryl), anticholinergic and antispasmodic agents (Donnatal, Lomotil, and Pro-Banthine), and tricyclic antidepressants (Tofranil and Elavil). Drugs that cause bladder neck closure by their action as α-adrenergic stimulators include over-the-counter cold preparations, ephedrine derivatives, and amphetamines.

Patients with urinary retention who have taken these drugs should be catheterized to compensate for atony and to allow bladder decompression. The catheter should then be removed. Once the offending agent is discontinued, barring other underlying physiologic or anatomical abnormality, the normal voiding pattern should resume.

Psychogenic Origin. Urinary retention in young women in the absence of outlet obstruction or neurologic incompetence suggests the possibility of psychogenic cause. This rarely occurs in males. When a psychogenic origin is suspected, treatment consists of catheterization for the isolated episodes of retention without use of an indwelling Foley catheter. Follow-up psychiatric consultation is encouraged once the urologic workup has established the absence of an organic cause.

Penile Edema

Conditions and Treatment

Balanitis and Posthitis. Inflammation of the glans penis (balanitis) and inflammation of the foreskin (posthitis) commonly occur together and result from poor hygiene or phimosis. The foreskin becomes edematous and erythematous; in severe circumstances, the inflammatory response may progress proximally along the penile shaft. Bullous edema, local ulcers, and a weeping drainage may occur. In less severe cases, foreskin retraction, cleansing with soap and water, and application of an antibiotic ointment such as Neosporin may be sufficient treatment. Severe or recurrent inflammation, or inability to retract the foreskin (phimosis), necessitate circumcision after the local swelling has diminished.

Phimosis. In this condition, the meatus of the foreskin is too narrow to permit retraction over the glans. Phimosis may be congenital or acquired, the latter more common in diabetes. If the meatus of the foreskin is adherent, urinary retention may occur. In this circumstance, a small probe may not even fit into the orifice. Dilatation with a hemostat may provide immediate relief of urinary obstruction. An emergency dorsal slit procedure (Fig. 35.12) may be necessary; dilatation of the orifice, however, usually suffices in the emergency situation, after which circumcision may be carried out as an elective procedure.

Paraphimosis. Paraphimosis is the condition in which the foreskin becomes permanently retracted behind the corona of the glans penis. There is a proximal and a distal contraction ring. As a result, the tissue between the rings becomes edematous and tender, occasionally progressing to infarction. This may occur after masturbation, intercourse, or failure to reduce the foreskin following catheter insertion. This swelling should not be confused with angioneurotic edema of the foreskin, which occurs as a localized phenomenon in response to allergy, especially in children. In angioneurotic edema, the constriction bands are absent. The treatment of paraphimosis is directed toward immediate reduction of the foreskin over the glans. If gentle pressure on the glans penis with simultaneous traction on the foreskin is unsuccessful, the base of the penis may be infiltrated with a local anesthetic *without epinephrine*, the edema fluid squeezed from the foreskin between the constriction bands, and the prepuce then pulled over the glans.

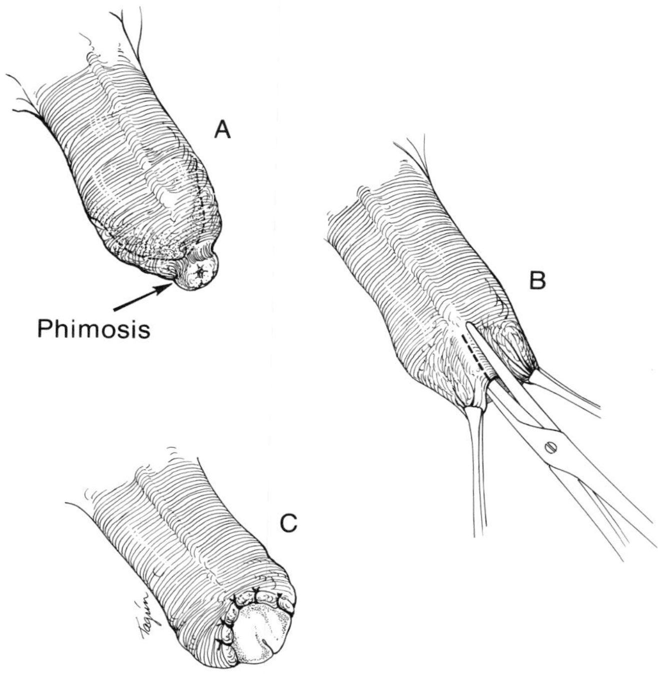

Figure 35.12. Dorsal slit procedure under local anesthesia. *A,* Phimotic foreskin. *B,* After foreskin is crushed with a straight clamp at 12 o'clock, it is incised with scissors. *C,* Cut edge of foreskin should be hemostatically sutured with interrupted 4–0 chromic absorbable sutures. Formal circumcision may be performed as an elective procedure when patient's condition has stabilized.

Both constriction rings must be reduced. Partial reduction is common, but if reduction is incomplete, total paraphimosis recurs within minutes. Failure to reduce the foreskin manually necessitates an emergency dorsal slit procedure.

Lymphedema. Penile lymphedema always almost is accompanied by scrotal swelling. The lymphatic vessels of the scrotal halves freely anastomose with those of the penis and drain into the superifical and deep inguinal lymph nodes, and then into the iliac node chains. Lymphedema of the penis and scrotum may be caused by obstruction due to tumor or by inguinal adenitis, as in filariasis or lymphogranuloma venereum. Pelvic tumors involving the iliac node chains may block the lymphatics to the genitalia, resulting in penile and scrotal lymphedema. Radiation treatment to pelvic lymph nodes may also result in this condition. Lymphedema must be differentiated from other causes of penile and scrotal swelling, such as tuberculosis, anasarca, deep pelvic venous thrombosis, a large pelvic tumor, or urinary extravasation due to trauma. The treatment of penile lymphedema should be directed toward the primary cause. Compression dressings should not be applied.

Local Infection. An abrasion or skin disorder may result in local infection and lead to penile swelling. Infection of the suture line after circumcision is a common cause of penile edema. Treatment consists of local dressings and appropriate antibiotic therapy, depending on culture sensitivities.

Priapism. In this condition, the penis becomes uncontrollably erect for a prolonged period because the venous drainage of the corpora cavernosa fails. The blood trapped in the corpora loses oxygen and accumulates carbon dioxide. Ultimately, the intracorporal pressure approximates the arterial pressure, and sludging occurs, further impairing venous drainage. It may be an isolated phenomenon (idiopathic); or it may be secondary to a variety of disorders, including sickle cell disease or trait, trauma, instrumentation, tumor, or leukemia. In many instances, the condition may be reversed spontaneously, but if priapism persists, it ultimately results in fibrosis of the corpora cavernosa and impotence. Since the advent of surgical methods for correction of priapism, this condition has been categorized as a surgical emergency.

The diagnosis of prolonged erection is recognized easily, but unfortunately, procrastination accompanying the disorder frequently results in a decreased chance of surgical success. The examiner must try to determine the primary underlying disease; examination should include a complete blood cell count with differential, a sickle cell preparation, hemoglobin electrophoresis, and careful evaluation for the possibility of an underlying malignancy.

Treatment has included several conservative measures, such as intracorporeal instillation of heparin, fibrinolytic therapy, local application of ice, ice water enemas, and drainage of the corpora. Initial attempts to irrigate the corpora free of clots should be carried out. A 35-ml syringe and 15-gauge needle are used to irrigate with a solution containing 1 ml of 1:1000 epinephrine in 1000 ml of saline. Failure to relieve the priapism by irrigation necessitates a surgical approach. If erection has persisted for more than few hours, a corpus cavernosum-corpus spongiosum shunt should be performed under local anesthesia by a urologic surgeon. Since the venous drainage of the corpora cavernosa has been impaired and since the corpus spongiosum rarely is affected, this shunt provides the easiest and more successful method of internal drainage of the obstructed corpora cavernosa. Immediate consultation and treatment are therefore essential for these patients.

Scrotal Masses

History and Physical Examination

The recognition of a scrotal mass, even in the absence of pain, may be sufficient cause for an anxious patient to seek emergency care. Most scrotal masses may be differentiated by history and physical examination; some, however, require surgical exploration for confirmation and diagnosis. A history of trauma, urinary tract infection or instrumentation, or systemic diseases, such as mumps and syphilis, aid in the differential diagnosis. The mode of onset, and the presence or absence of pain are important details. Physical examination must be performed with the patient both standing and supine, to determine the exact site of the mass and its relation to the testis, the epididymis, the spermatic cord, and the inguinal canal. Transillumination should be attempted with either flanged flashlight or with the cord from a fiberoptic light source.

Conditions and Treatment

Hydrocele. A nontender, fluid-filled mass surrounding the testis is termed a hydrocele. It results from the accumulation of fluid between the two layers of the tunica vaginalis. The diagnosis is confirmed by transillumination. Most hydroceles occur in older patients, are idiopathic and asymptomatic. An acute, symptomatic hydrocele is frequently a complication of orchitis, epididymitis, trauma, or a malignant tumor. A hydrocele in a younger patient, especially if acute, suggests the possibility of underlying disease and the need for further investigation. A patent processus vaginalis allows fluid from the peritoneal cavity, such as ascites, to pass into the scrotum and present as a scrotal mass. Careful physical examination alerts the physician to this possibility. Testicular tumor is also a cause for an acute hydrocele. Methods of investigation include ultrasonography, testicular scanning, and surgical exploration. Specific therapy is not necessary for simple, asymptomatic hydroceles.

Testicular Tumor. Although a testicular neoplasm is manifested as a painless mass in the body of the testis, acute pain due to tumor necrosis and hemorrhage may precipitate a visit to the emergency department. Except in a large tumor, the epididymis is normal and is palpable separate from the testicular mass. Pain may be elicited on palpation. The mass cannot be transilluminated, although the presence of a secondary hydrocele may cause some confusion. Physical examination may reveal gynecomastia due to chorionic gonadoptropins if the tumor is a choriocarcinoma. The absence of gynecomastia does not exclude choriocarcinoma. All intratesticular masses must be considered tumor until proven otherwise. If a testicular tumor is suspected, the patient should be advised to have transinguinal exploration as soon as feasible. There is no role for transscrotal testicular biopsy in suspected tumor.

Torsion. Torsion of the spermatic cord is common in young men and in children. It is characterized by the onset of acute testicular pain during physical activity or at rest. The involved testis immediately swells. Physical examination reveals an exquisitely tender mass in which the epididymis and the testis cannot be distinguished. A secondary hydrocele may be present, in which case transillumination may demonstrate fluid. With the examiner facing the patient, the torsion occurs counterclockwise in the left testis and clockwise in the right. The twist initiates cremasteric muscle spasm and causes the affected testis to become elevated in the scrotum. The rapid onset and the absence of pyuria aid in distinguishing torsion from epididymitis. Prehn's sign may also be helpful; elevation of the testis relieves the pain of epididymitis, but increases that of torsion. The distinction, however, is difficult, and exploration of the scrotum is often necessary to substantiate the diagnosis. Radionuclide testicular flow scanning has helped in the differentiation by showing absent blood supply in the testis that has undergone torsion. Use of a Doppler probe is helpful in distinguishing spermatic cord torsion from epididymitis and orchitis by direct assessment of arterial circulation.

Treatment of suspected torsion is immediate surgical exploration with untwisting and fixation. The opposite testis is also fixed at the same operation because of the high incidence of later torsion in that side. Emergency treatment is of utmost necessity, since failure to restore the blood supply to a testis within 4–6 hours results in a high incidence of testicular infarction. Even if several hours have passed, however, and infarction of the seminiferous cells seems to have occurred, exploration and untwisting are warranted in an attempt to preserve the more hardy testosterone-producing interstitial cells.

Epididymitis. In patients with epididymitis, the onset of pain is usually gradual; the pain peaks after several hours or days. Epididymitis is manifested initially by epididymal tenderness without a palpable mass. There is frequently an associated history of urinary tract infection, prostatitis, gonnorhea, instrumentation, or heavy straining. Retrograde passage of bacteria down the vas deferens is postulated as the means by which the epididymis is seeded with pathogens.

Physical examination shows only a slight induration or a tender nodule, usually in the most inferior and dependent portion of the epididymis. In other patients the entire epididymis is involved, and an associated hydrocele may be present. This makes the distinction between epididymitis, orchitis, tumor, and torsion difficult. Urinalysis reveals pyuria if there is an associated urinary tract infection. A urine specimen should be cultured when the diagnosis of epididymitis is suspected. The white blood cell count is often elevated. Scrotal ultrasonography is helpful in confirming the diagnosis of epididymitis.

Treatment includes bed rest, ice packs applied to the scrotum, scrotal suspensory support, anti-inflammatory agents such as indomethacin (Indocin), and antibiotics. Unless a specific pathogen is known, a broad-spectrum antibiotic suffices for initial therapy. If the patient is afebrile, antibiotics may be given orally. If the patient has a temperature greater than 101° F (38.3°C) or has a tender, fluctuant mass, hospitalization for the intravenous administration of antibiotics is necessary. Persistent fever or temperature spikes during antibiotic therapy may indicate a necessity for surgical exploration and epididymal excision.

Orchitis. Orchitis is rare, but may occur secondary to epididymitis or a viral infection. Mumps is the most common cause. Orchitis parotidea ("mumps" orchitis) is usually unilateral. The onset of pain is sudden and difficult to distinguish from that of torsion. The testis becomes enlarged, congested, and tender, probably because of infarction necrosis of the seminiferous tubules. The overlying scrotum may become erythematous and edematous. The absence of pyuria or any other urinary tract symptoms, and the associated presence of parotitis, aid in distinguishing this condition from epididymitis. In orchitis associated with mumps, microhematuria and proteinuria may be present. The virus is actually recoverable in the urine, but only by special methods.

Treatment is directed toward relief of pain. Infiltration of the spermatic cord with a local anesthetic may provide considerable relief. Bed rest, analgesics, and ice packs may be helpful. Mumps orchitis results in loss of spermatogenesis in 25–35% of patients, although androgenic function usually remains. Hospitalization may be necessary.

Varicocele. Varicosity of the left spermatic vein may result in an ill-defined scrotal mass. This is usually a chronic process associated with discomfort or heaviness in the affected side of the scrotum. Approximately 15% of men have a left varicocele to some degree, which is most often asymptomatic. The acute onset of a varicocele on the left or the right side may be the first symptom of a retroperitoneal mass.

On the right side, the testicular vein empties into the inferior vena cava. A right varicocele is always the result of obstruction of the right spermatic vein at this level. Vena caval thrombosis or compression by an extrinsic mass, such as carcinoma, lymphoma, or sarcoma, is usually the cause.

The left spermatic vein empties into the left renal vein. The acute onset of a left varicocele with pain localized to the scrotal area is most often due to renal cell carcinoma with propagation of a tumor thrombus into the left renal vein, resulting in obstruction of the left spermatic vein. Renal venous thrombosis and, rarely, lymphoma may also cause this problem.

Intravenous urography, ultrasonography, vena caval angiography with selective catheterization of the renal vein, and transfemoral arteriography are often necessary for the identification of any underlying condition. Treatment is directed toward the underlying cause, not toward the varicocele itself. A scrotal support usually relieves the symptoms. However, persistent pain and swelling despite conservative care may be relieved by inguinal exploration and ligation of the veins of the spermatic cord at the internal inguinal ring.

Other Scrotal Masses. Other than the masses discussed, the most common scrotal mass is an inguinal hernia that descends into the scrotum. Careful examination defines the limits of the hernia in the scrotum and its extension into the inguinal canal. The testis can be palpated distinct from the mass. Unless examination is conducted carefully, an incarcerated hernia may be confused with a mass of testicular or epididymal origin. Other lesions, including spermatocele, epididymal tumor, and mesenchymal tumor of the cord structures, may all be palpated as scrotal masses, but are not usually seen as acute problems.

SUGGESTED READINGS

Ahmed S, Morris LL. Renal parenchymal injuries secondary to blunt abdominal trauma in childhood: A 10-year review. *Br J Urol* 1982;54:470–477.

Althausen AF. Injuries to the genitourinary tract, In Burke JF, Boyd RJ, McCabe CJ (eds): *Trauma Management.* Chicago, Year Book, 1988, pp 126–139.

Bright et al. Significant hematuria after trauma. *J Urol* 1978;455–456.

Carroll PR, McAninch JW. Operative indications in penetrating renal trauma. *J Trauma* 1985;25:587–593.

Carroll PR, McAninch JW. Major bladder trauma: The accuracy of cystography. *J Urol* 1983;130:887–888.

Cass AS, Johnson CF, Khan AU et al. Nonoperative management of bladder rupture from external trauma. *Urology* 1983;22:27–29.

Cass AS. Immediate radiologic and surgical management of renal injuries. *J Trauma* 1982;22:361–363.

Cass AS. The multiple injured patient with bladder trauma. *J Trauma* 1984;24:731–734.

Cass AS, Luxenberg M. Unilateral nonvisualization on excretory urography after external trauma. *J Urol* 1984;132:225–227.

Federle MP, Kaiser JA, McAninch JW et al. The role of computed tomography in renal trauma. *Radiology* 1981;141:455–460.

Guice K, Oldham K, Eide B et al. Hematuria after blunt trauma: When is pyelography helpful? *J Trauma* 1983;23:305–311.

Hayes EE, Sandler CM, Gorrier JN Jr. Management of the ruptured bladder secondary to blunt abdominal trauma. *J Urol* 1983;129:946–948.

Heyns CF, Deklerk DP, Dekock MLS. Stab wounds associated with hematuria—A review of 67 cases. *J Urol* 1983;130:228–231.

Karmi SA, Young JD Jr., Soderstrom O. Classification of renal injuries as a guide to therapy. *SGO* 1979;148:161–167.

Lang EK, Sullivan J, Frentz G. Renal trauma: Radiological studies. Comparison of urography, computed tomography, angiography and radionuclide studies. *Radiology* 1985;1–6.

McAninch JW. Traumatic injuries to the urethra. *J Trauma* 1981;21:291–297.

MacMahon R, Hosking D, Ramsey EW. Management of blunt injury to the lower urinary tract. *Canad J Surg* 1983;26:415–418.

McAninch JW, Federle MP. Evaluation of renal injuries with computed tomography. *J Urol* 1982;128:456–460.

Palmer JK, Benson GS, Corriere JN Jr. Diagnosis and initial management of urological injuries associated with 200 consecutive pelvic fractures. *J Urol* 1983;130:712–714.

CHAPTER **36**

Orthopaedic Emergencies

DAVID B. LOVEJOY, M.D.
EDWIN T. WYMAN, JR., M.D.

GENERAL CONSIDERATIONS

Patients with traumatic and nontraumatic musculoskeletal conditions constitute a significant proportion of emergency department clientele. This chapter outlines the diagnosis and treatment of uncomplicated orthopaedic emergencies and the initial care of patients with more serious conditions who will be referred to the orthopaedic surgeon.

Emergency medical technicians usually are well-trained in extrication and splinting techniques, and patients should arrive in the emergency department with fractures properly splinted. Physician review of splinting techniques with nonhospital paramedical personnel will help improve early patient care. A manual such as the American Academy of Orthopaedic Surgeons' *Manual on Emergency Care and Transportation of the Sick and Injured* is most useful for this purpose.

History

The physician should question the patient about the mechanism and severity of the trauma, the mode of onset of a nontraumatic condition, and whether there had been previous injury to the affected part. The possibility of referred pain should be considered; for example, knee pain may be the only indicator of a hip problem.

Physical Examination

Physical examination should enable the physician to reach an accurate diagnosis in most cases; knowledge of topographic anatomy is essential in this regard. Early, accurate evaluation of neurovascular function is important; the examiner should document it carefully, noting motor and sensory deficits indicating partial or complete injury to peripheral nerves or nerve roots (Figs. 36.1 and 36.2). In the severely injured limb, distal pulses and capillary filling must be evaluated. If vascular injury is suspected, arteriographic examination may be indicated. Compartment syndromes may be subtle, or they may present with the classic signs of muscle ischemia, including pain, pallor, paralysis, pulselessness, and paresthesias, particularly when associated with a fracture of the tibia, radius, ulna, or distal part of the humerus. Pain on passive extension of the fingers or dorsiflexion of the ankle is the best early clinical sign of an impending compartment syndrome. Repeated readings of fascial compartment pressures or Doppler changes may be helpful. Compartment pressures may be measured early with an 18-gauge needle and saline manometer, or if available, a wick catheter and pressure transducer. Normal tissue pressure is 12–20 cm H_2O. When tissue pressure exceeds diastolic pres-

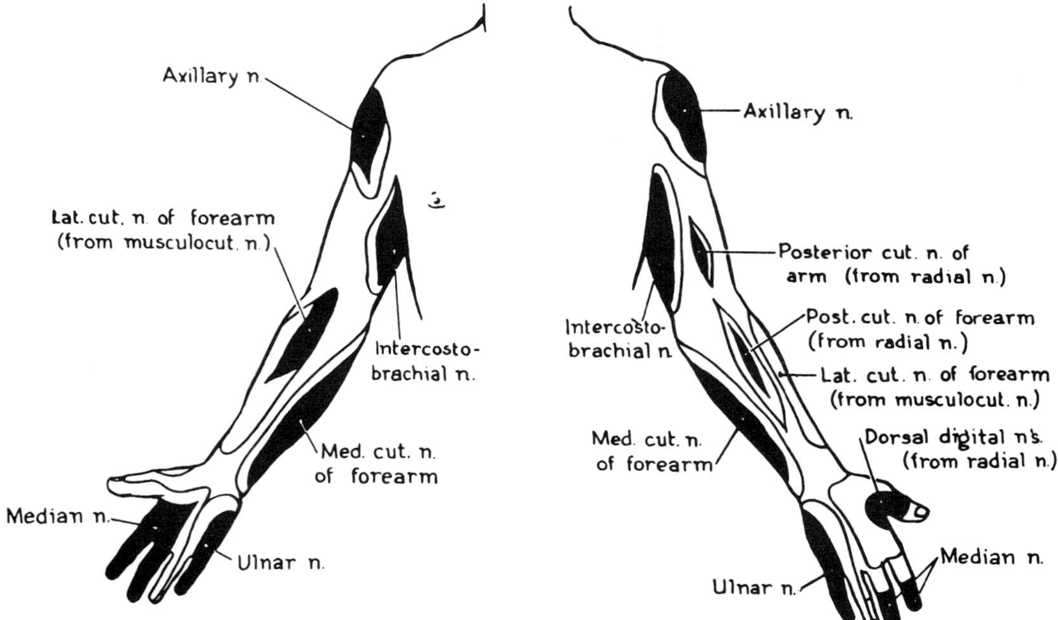

Figure 36.1. Map showing typical distribution of major peripheral nerves in upper limbs (from Foerster O. Die Symptomatologie der peripheren Nerven. In Lewandowsky MH: *Handbuch der Neurologie* [Berlin: J. Springer, 1929], Erganzungsbd. 2. Teil, pp. 975–1508).

sure (cm H_2O—mm Hg), fasciotomy should be considered immediately. Effective treatment of compartment syndromes depends totally on *early recognition,* through tissue pressure measurement and monitoring.

Splints and Dressings

After physical examination but before x-ray films are taken, fractures should be splinted for immobilization (Fig. 36.3). In general, if there is enough concern to order an x-ray film, the extremity should be splinted. Splints need not be complicated. The requirements are that they: (*a*) immobilize the part; (*b*) do no further damage, such as cause excess pressure on the skin; (*c*) are comfortable; and (*d*) are transportable. Splints prevent bone ends from doing further damage and provide more comfort than any amount of pain medication alone. They may be improvised easily, and in only one case, the Thomas' splint for a femoral shaft fracture (Fig. 36.3*B*), is a specific splint always needed. Neurovascular function distal to the fracture should be evaluated. Gentle traction and realignment of a badly displaced fracture often restore distal circulation. After specimens are taken for culture, open (compound) fractures should be cleansed of gross debris, dressed, and splinted. Loose pieces of bone and traumatized skin should *not* be discarded. Broad-spectrum antibiotics should be started and tetanus prophylaxis given as indicated (see Chapter 11). The cast or splint should be checked a day after application to assess circulation of the limb. Persistent pain, especially if in one area, requires that the part be evaluated in detail to rule out circulatory compromise or excessive skin pressure. Evaluation will involve cast adjustment or removal, and should be done by the physician responsible for the treatment of the fracture.

Orthopaedic Injuries in Multiple-Trauma Patients

In patients with multiple system injuries, life-threatening emergencies often require such immediate evaluation and treatment that significant orthopaedic injuries may be overlooked for an extended time. To avoid this, within the first half-hour that the patient is in the emergency department, a member of the emergency department team should perform a brief but complete examination of all bony parts. Examination should include observation of deformity; and palpation for edema, crepitation, or pain. Passive and active range of motion for all joints should be assessed as well as abnormal motion of joints or bones. Suspicious areas should be evaluated first for distal neurologic change and circulatory status and then splinted. Cross-table lateral x-rays of the cervical spine and x-rays of the thoracolumbar spine should also be taken prior to moving the patient because of the danger of neurologic injury. An anteroposterior x-ray of the pelvis and hip is also necessary because pelvic injuries are often missed on physical examination.

SPINAL INJURIES

Cervical Spine

Remember:

1. Unconsciousness may indicate a cervical spine injury.
2. A scalp laceration may suggest a cervical spine injury.
3. X-ray films must show the entire cervical spine.

Fracture and Dislocation

Injury to the cervical spine should be presumed, until proved otherwise, in any patient who is unresponsive and unconscious after a fall, a diving injury, or a motor vehicle accident. An adequate airway must be established and the neurologic status evaluated. Tracheal intubation may be performed if the physician is careful not to hyperextend the patient's neck. The head and neck should be immobilized temporarily with a collar, sandbags, or four-poster brace, and x-ray films should be obtained as soon as possible. Cross-table x-rays should be obtained initially to check for gross malalignment; further x-rays are then ordered, depending on the results.

In addition to anteroposterior and lateral views, oblique and open-mouth views are necessary. Facet fractures and dislocations can be seen in oblique views, whereas the open-mouth view shows the odontoid process. Since the cervicothoracic junction is difficult to visualize in muscular persons, either the patient's shoulders must be pulled down or an oblique (''swimmer's'') view taken, with one arm up and one arm down. The physician must not dismiss the possibility of a dislocation or fracture until the cervical spine has been visualized completely (Fig. 36.4).

If dislocation or fracture is diagnosed, definitive immobilization with skull tongs or a halo device is carried out. Dislocations may be reduced by either manipulation or gradually increased skull traction. Patients with undisplaced fractures, such as mild compression fractures, may wear a Thomas collar, a Philadelphia collar, or a four-poster brace until further treatment decisions are made.

Soft-Tissue Injury

Sprain. The neck frequently is injured in rear-end automobile collisions. The occupants are suddenly accelerated, which causes hyperextension of the head and neck beyond normal physiologic limits. The resultant condition has been called ''whiplash'' injury; more appropriate terms are either acute cervical sprain or acceleration-extension injury of the cervical spine. Properly adjusted head restraints on car seats minimize this injury.

Patients with acute cervical sprain may have some limitation of neck motion and muscle tenderness, although in the first hours after the injury the physical findings may be minimal. Later, conspicuous muscular spasm and tenderness may occur in all the

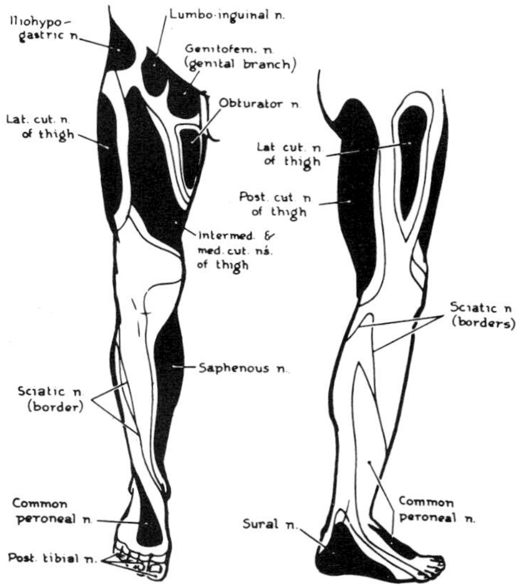

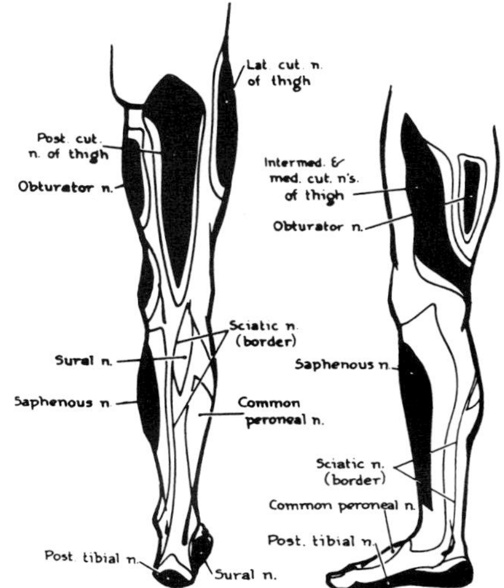

Figure 36.2. Map showing typical distribution of major peripheral nerves in lower limbs (from Foerster O. Die Symptomatologie der peripheren Nerven. In Lewandowsky MH: *Handbuch der Neurologie* Berlin, J. Springer, 1929, Erganzungsbd. 2. Teil, pp 975–1508).

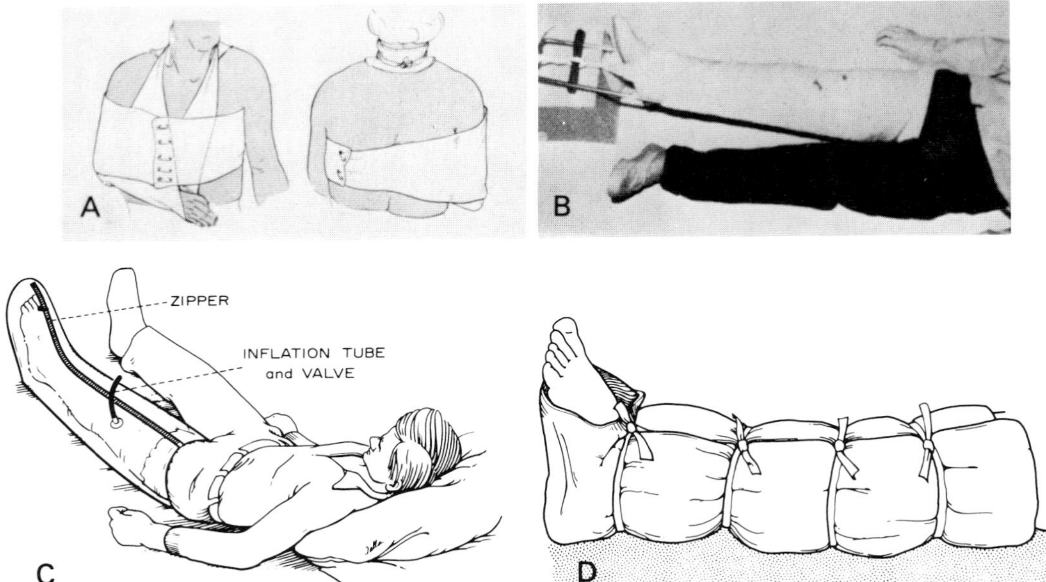

Figure 36.3. Temporary fracture immobilization. *A*, Velpeau's bandage (sling and swathe) for shoulder and humeral injuries. (Reproduced with permission, from Rowe CP. Shoulder girdle injuries. In Burke JF, Boyd RJ, McCabe CJ (eds): *Trauma Management* Chicago, Year Book, 1988, pp 277–324. *B*, Thomas splint for hip and femoral fractures. *C*, Air splint and *D*, pillow splint for tibial, ankle,and foot injuries.

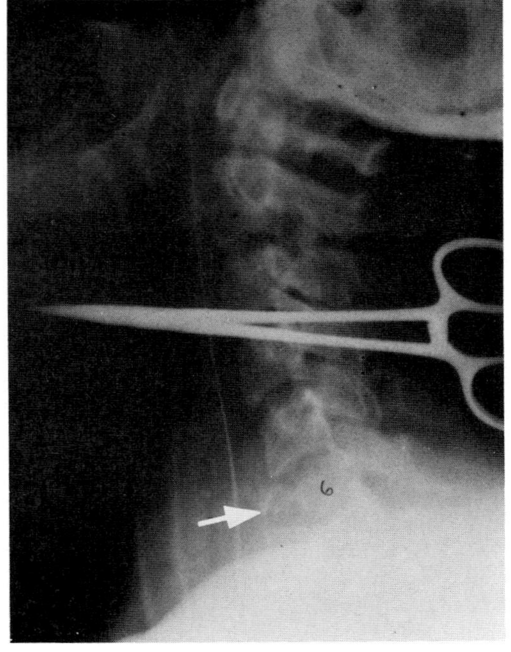

Figure 36.4. Cervical spine fracture. Bursting fracture (*arrow*) of body of sixth cervical vertebra resulting in quadriplegia (earlier radiograph only showed down to fifth vertebra).

cervical musculature. Abnormal neurologic findings are uncommon.

X-ray films of the cervical spine are usually normal in patients with acute cervical sprain, although a small chip or avulsed fragment occasionally is seen along the anterior edge of a vertebral body. The space between the spine and the larynx may be widened by retropharyngeal hematoma.

A soft collar, analgesic medications, and muscle relaxants combined with either heat or ice usually are sufficient for treatment of this injury. Commonly prescribed muscle relaxants are diazepam (Valium), methocarbamol (Robaxin), carisoprodol (Soma), and orphenadrine citrate (Norgesic). In severe cases, bed rest for several days or longer may be needed. Physical therapy utilizing massage, traction, ultrasound, or electric stimulation may be helpful.

Radicular Pain. Neck pain unrelated to traumatic injury may be caused by a number of conditions affecting nerve roots, and the onset may be sudden or gradual. The physician sometimes can establish which nerve root is involved by determining whether pain extends to the interscapular area, shoulder, arm, or fingers. During physical examination, he or she should elicit muscle or nerve tenderness and test sensation, reflexes, and muscular strength.

Anteroposterior, lateral, and oblique x-ray films

may show cervical spondylosis due to degenerative changes, with narrowing of the intervertebral spaces and osteophytes in the neural foramina. On the other hand, such films may be normal in the patient with an acute cervical disc condition.

Radicular pain may be relieved with hot packs, muscle relaxants, analgesics, and a cervical collar. Head halter traction of 3–4 kg with the neck slightly flexed is recommended, and is most effective with the patient lying down rather than sitting. Patients with severe pain should be hospitalized and may require narcotic analgesics.

Thoracic and Lumbar Spine

Remember: Fracture of the thoracic or lumbar spine may cause severe ileus.

Fracture and Dislocation

The patient with a suspected fracture or dislocation of the thoracic or lumbar spine should be transported on a spinal board or other firm surface (see Chapter 37). The physician should turn the patient with a "logrolling" technique and examine the back for bruises and tenderness to ascertain the level of injury. Spinal cord injury necessitates careful neurologic examination, with special attention to the presence or absence of sacral sparing.

Anteroposterior and lateral films are usually adequate for initial evaluation. Laminagraphy and myelography may be used in some instances to evaluate compromise of the neural canal by bone or disc fragments. Computed tomography (CT scan) has become the definitive tool for evaluation of thoracolumbar fractures, however, and should be obtained once the patient is stabilized. The patient may be placed on a turning frame, such as the Stryker, or a firm mattress. Frequent changes in position are essential, since pressure sores over bony prominences can appear within four hours. General supportive measures, including intravenous fluid administration and insertion of a Foley catheter, are carried out and the patient evaluated for other injuries. Since retroperitoneal hematoma may cause ileus lasting several days, introduction of a nasogastric tube is a wise precaution. Patients with minimal compression fractures of the thoracic or lumbar vertebrae may not require hospitalization.

Soft-Tissue Injury

A patient with pain in the lower back from a fall or from lifting a heavy object may have a lumbar soft-tissue injury; this often is superimposed on a chronic back problem. In making the diagnosis, however, the physician should also consider other nonorthopaedic possibilities such as renal calculi or infection, a gynecologic condition, a leaking aortic aneurysm, or herpes zoster.

In the orthopaedic workup, the physician should test the range of motion of the lumbar spine. Muscle spasm may cause sciatic scoliosis. The physician can evaluate the strength of the leg muscles by having the patient walk on heels and tiptoes. Limited passive straight leg raising on the affected side indicates irritation of the sciatic nerve. Palpation over the lumbar area and the sciatic nerve in the buttock and posterior part of the thigh often elicits tenderness. Weakness of the quadriceps muscle and a decreased knee reflex indicate involvement of the third and fourth lumbar nerve roots. If the fifth lumbar nerve root is involved, there may be weakness of the extensor hallucis longus, tibialis anterior, or peroneal muscles and decreased sensation over the dorsum of the foot. A lesion of the root of the first sacral nerve may cause weakness of the gastrocnemius muscle, sensory loss over the lateral aspect of the foot, or decreased ankle jerk. Differentiation between acute lumbar sprain and disc injury may be difficult on initial physical examination.

Roentgenographic findings are often normal in patients with acute back pain. Spina bifida occulta is usually an incidental finding. About 5% of the population have either spondylolysis, a defect in the pars interarticularis that is best seen on oblique views (Fig. 36.5), or spondylolisthesis, a forward slip of the fifth lumbar vertebra onto the first sacral vertebra. These conditions are often symptomatic. Narrowed interspaces, which occur as intervertebral discs degenerate, may also be visualized. Droplets of myelographic dye seen on the x-ray film testify to prior back problems.

Treatment of pain in the lower back includes analgesic medications, hot packs or ice packs, muscle relaxants, and bed rest in the lateral position or supine with pillows under the knees. A lumbar corset may be helpful. Evaluation by physical therapists to correct improper body mechanics and the teaching of proper exercises can often help in preventing further injuries.

INJURIES OF UPPER EXTREMITIES

Shoulder

Remember:

1. X-ray examination is not complete unless an axillary or tangential scapular (Neer) view is obtained.
2. Shoulder pain after a seizure may indicate posterior dislocation.
3. Shoulder pain with lack of passive external rotation may also indicate posterior dislocation.
4. An anteroposterior x-ray view of the shoulder in a patient with a posterior dislocation may appear normal.

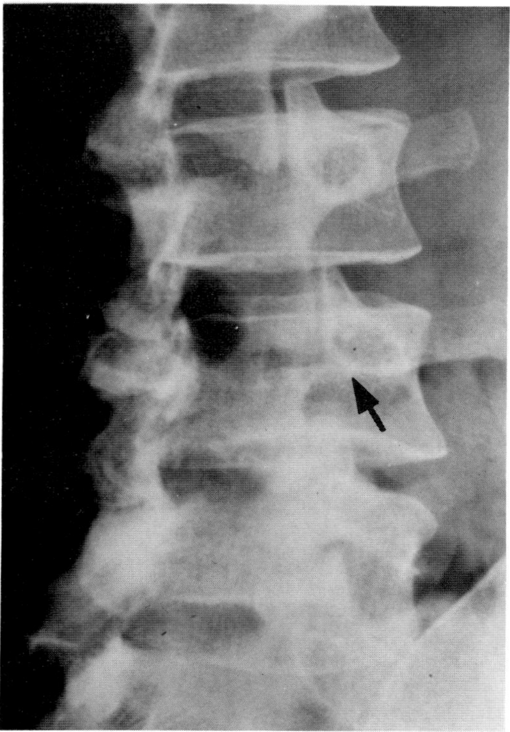

Figure 36.5. Spondylolysis. Oblique radiograph showing defect (*arrow*) in pars interarticularis of fourth lumbar vertebra.

5. Inability to initiate active abduction may indicate rotator cuff tear.
6. Shoulder pain with normal x-ray findings may indicate rotator cuff injury.

Brachial Plexus

Severe depression or hyperabduction of the shoulder girdle can stretch or tear the brachial plexus. On physical examination, the physician may palpate fullness and elicit tenderness from the hematoma in the supraclavicular fossa. Neurologic examination reveals the extent of the damage. Horner's syndrome may be evident if the cervical sympathetic chain is damaged.

Sternoclavicular Joint

The sternoclavicular joint rarely is injured, but when the shoulder is struck hard from the side, the inner end may be dislocated upward or retrosternally. Pressure on the trachea by the clavicle in a retrosternal dislocation may cause acute, life-threatening dyspnea. The diagnosis is made by physical examination. Palpation reveals the absence of the head of the clavicle just lateral to the sternal notch. Upward dislocation can be seen on anteroposterior and oblique x-ray views; laminagrams may be needed to demonstrate retrosternal dislocation.

Closed reduction of a retrosternal dislocation may be done by placing a tightly rolled towel between the shoulders and applying firm pressure backward on both shoulders. It may be possible to grasp the inner end of the clavicle and pull it up. Closed reduction usually is successful if the dislocation is recent; open reduction may be otherwise necessary, although many chronic dislocations are relatively asymptomatic. Upward dislocation is reduced easily, but is difficult to immobilize effectively.

Clavicle

Fracture of the clavicle results commonly from a fall on the extended arm or on the shoulder but may

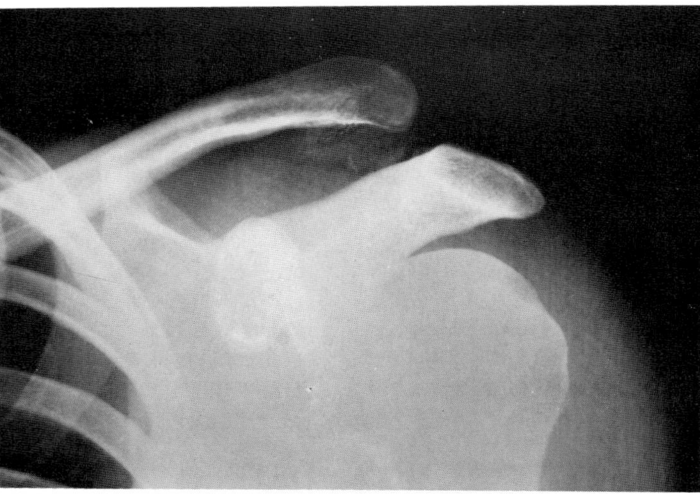

Figure 36.6. Dislocation of acromioclavicular joint. Distal clavicle is displaced upward 1 cm.

result from direct clavicular trauma. The clavicular deformity may be visible. Tenderness and crepitation over the fracture site are elicited by palpation. Anteroposterior and oblique x-rays usually demonstrate the fracture. A soft figure-of-eight bandage padded in the axillae is effective and comfortable treatment; it should be tightened every few days to keep the shoulders abducted. In older people who cannot tolerate the figure-of-eight bandage, an arm sling is often sufficient. The figure-of-eight bandage should remain in place from 4–8 weeks, depending on the rate of bony union. Nonunion is rare; therefore, open reduction is rarely necessary.

Acromioclavicular Joint

Injury to the acromioclavicular joint results from a fall on or a blow to the tip of the shoulder. Three types of injuries can be distinguished:

1. *Strain* (Grade I injury): The patient has tenderness over this joint without visible displacement on x-rays.
2. *Subluxation* (Grade II injury): Less than 1 cm of upper displacement of the distal clavicle is apparent on physical examination and x-ray film. This may be differentiated from a Grade I injury by x-ray views with the patient holding 2 kg weights in both hands while standing in the upright position (Fig. 36.6). These x-rays allow differentiation between Grades I, II, and III injuries in questionable cases, as well as permitting comparison between the involved and the uninjured shoulders.
3. *Dislocation* (Grade III): There is more than 1 cm of upward displacement, caused by the upward pull of the trapezius muscle.
4. *Grade IV Injury:* The distal clavicle is herniated through the deltopectoral and claviculopectoral fascia and lies immediately subcutaneously. This injury cannot be reduced by closed techniques.

Patients with strains and subluxations may be treated with a sling for 1–2 weeks. Reduction of a complete dislocation by downward pressure on the distal clavicle is easy to achieve but difficult to maintain by closed means. For younger, athletic patients, or patients who do manual labor using arms over the head, operative repair is indicated.

Glenohumeral Joint

Dislocation. The glenohumeral joint frequently is dislocated from a fall or from abduction of the arm. In a patient with a previous dislocation, minimal trauma may cause recurrence. It may be difficult or impossible to reduce a dislocation that is more than a few days old. The emergency physician should be aware of this, particularly in chronic alcoholic patients. In an anteroinferior dislocation, the humeral head is palpable in the anterior part of the axilla. The patient should be examined for evidence of axillary nerve injury (lack of sensation over the lateral part of the shoulder and deltoid muscle palsy). Occasionally, pressure of the humeral head on the axillary structures causes distal neurovascular compromise.

Posterior dislocations (Fig. 36.7) are uncommon and may go unrecognized. *Inability to rotate the arm externally* is the principal diagnostic sign. If the physician stands behind the seated patient, he may see that the affected shoulder is flat anteriorly and full posteriorly. In roentgenographic examination, at least two views are necessary for accurate diagnosis, an anteroposterior view and either a Neer view or an axillary view. Transthoracic views are difficult to interpret in heavy patients, and should not be obtained in these cases.

There are several techniques for reducing an anterior dislocation (Fig. 36.8), all of which depend on relaxing the shoulder muscles, particularly the subscapularis and pectoralis major. Muscle relaxation may be potentiated with intravenous analgesics or drugs such as diazepam. Occasionally, general anesthesia is necessary. Traction on the wrist with the arm somewhat abducted, together with countertraction using a sheet passed under the axilla, often is successful. The Kocher maneuver involves slowly and gently flexing the arm and applying traction to the elbow with abduction and external rotation, followed by adduction and internal rotation. The Stimson method involves use of a weight tied to the wrist of a prone patient with the arm hanging over the side of the stretcher. The elevation method uses traction to pull the arm almost directly overhead, followed by thumb pressure under the humeral head to lift it into the glenoid fossa.

A sling and swathe, or Velpeau's bandage (Fig. 36.3*A*), should be maintained for 3 weeks in the case of an anterior dislocation, to allow the articular capsule of the glenohumeral joint to heal. An x-ray film should be obtained after reduction to confirm the reduction and to ascertain that no fractures have occurred during manipulation or that were unrecognized in the original films.

Fracture. Many types of fracture and fracture-dislocation occur in the head and neck of the humerus. Proximal humeral fractures have been classified by Neer according to displacement, comminution, and anatomic location of the fracture (Fig. 36.9). Muscle pull on fracture fragments causes displacement of the fracture and leads to malunion or nonunion of the fractures. Treatment plans depend upon the radiologic appearance of the fracture.

Clinically, if the humeral head or neck is fractured, there is local pain, swelling, and ecchymosis.

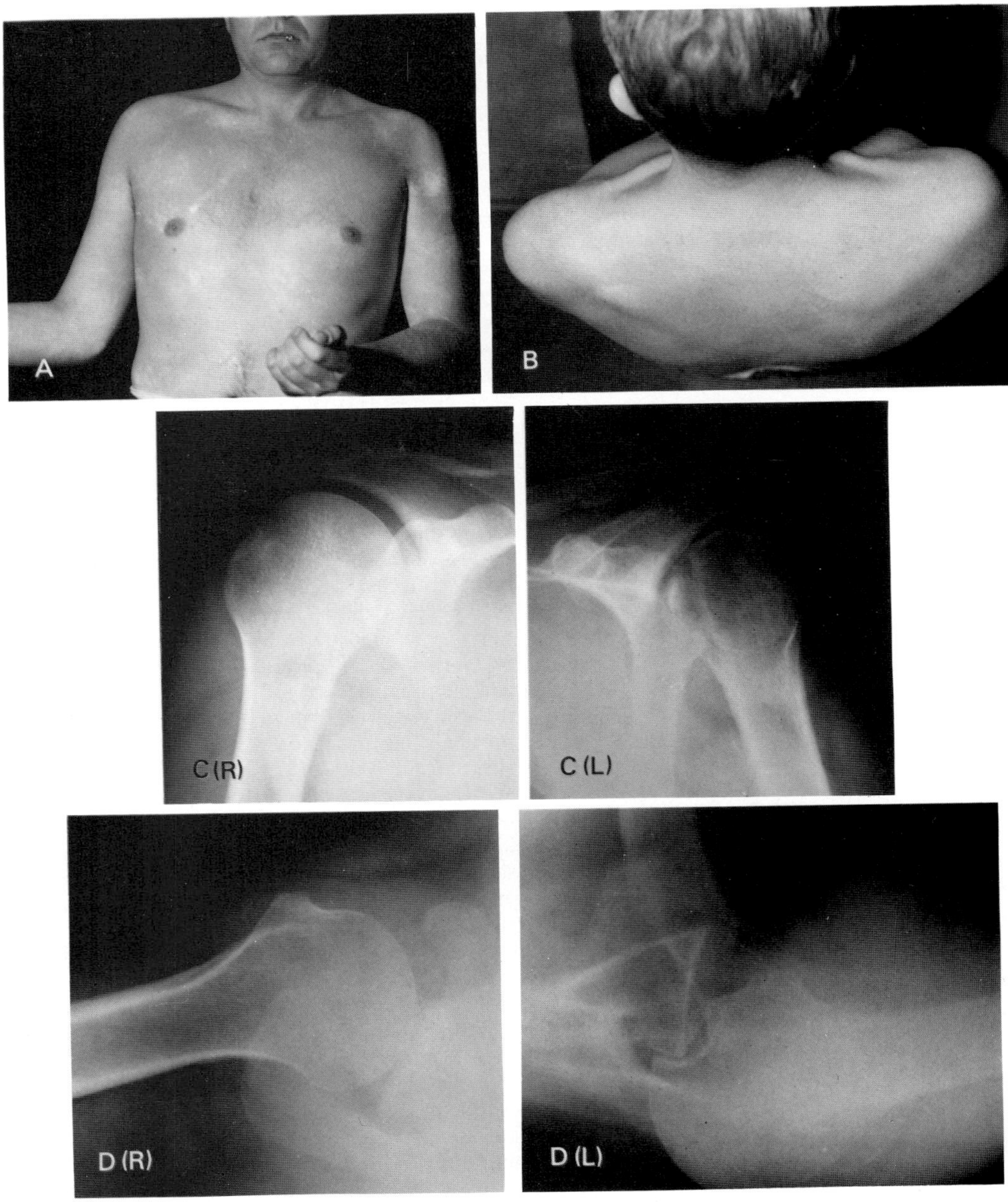

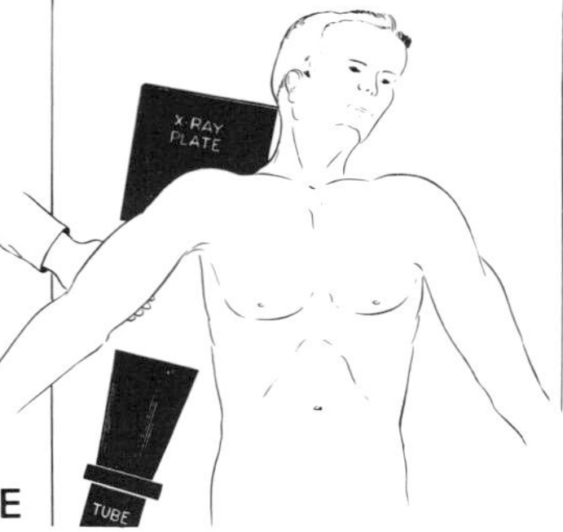

Figure 36.7. Posterior dislocation of shoulder. *A*, Patient is unable to externally rotate left shoulder that has posterior dislocation. *B*, Viewed from above, left shoulder is prominent posteriorly, *C*, Anteroposterior radiographs of right and left shoulders show some asymmetry, but diagnosis of posterior dislocation is not obvious. *D*, Axillary radiographs (right and left) show left humeral head posterior to glenoid fossa. *E*, Technique of axillary radiographic view. (Parts *A*, *B*, and *E*, all reproduced with permission, from Rowe CR. Shoulder girdle injuries. In Burke JF, Boyd RJ, McCabe CJ (eds): *Trauma Management,* Chicago, Year Book, 1988, pp 277–324.)

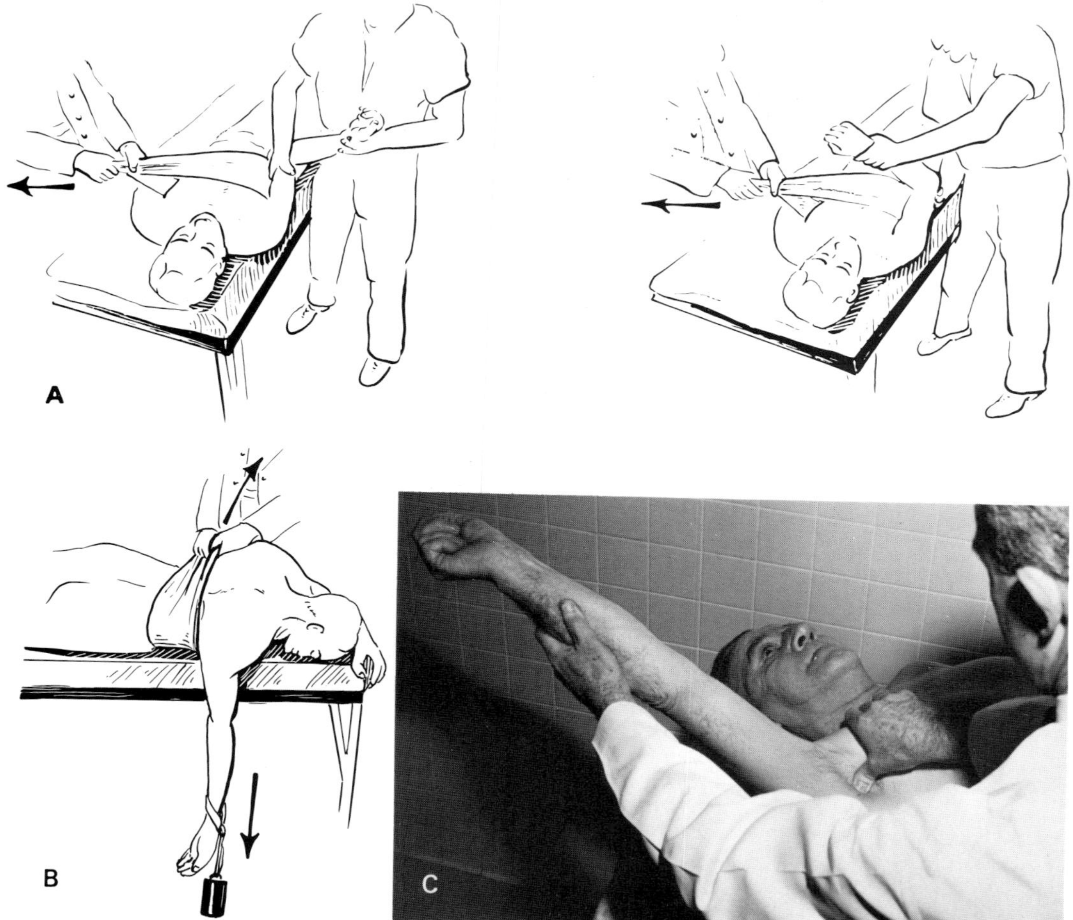

Figure 36.8. Reduction of anterior shoulder dislocation. *A*, Kocher method, *B*, Stimson method, *C*, Elevation method (*A-C* reproduced with permission from Rowe CR. Shoulder girdle injuries. In Burke JF, Boyd RJ, McCabe CJ (eds): *Trauma Management.* Chicago, Year Book, 1988, pp 277–324.

The physician can often elicit crepitation on moving the arm. Anteroposterior and axillary films are essential for diagnosis, to determine whether the humeral head is dislocated, and to help determine the fracture pattern. Most patients can be treated nonoperatively with immobilization with or without closed reduction. Severely comminuted and displaced fractures require open reduction or prosthetic replacement. All these fractures may need immobilization for 4–6 weeks. Early motion, including pendulum exercises, helps prevent the shoulder girdle stiffness that frequently occurs after these fractures.

Humeral Shaft

Remember:

1. Fracture of the humeral shaft requires checking radial nerve function before and after reduction.
2. In patients with a humeral supracondylar fracture, a compartment syndrome (Volkmann's ischemia) may develop.

Especially in the presence of a fracture of the middle or distal part of the humerus, the patient should be tested for injury to the radial nerve. Radial nerve sensation can be tested at the dorsum of the first web space, and motor function can be ascertained by asking the patient to extend the wrist *and metacarpophalangeal joints.* (The interphalangeal joints are extended by the lumbrical and interosseus muscles, which are innervated by the median and ulnar nerves.)

Anteroposterior and lateral films should be obtained to confirm the diagnosis. Gentle traction usually produces good alignment of the humeral shaft. The reduction can be maintained by coaptation plaster splints placed medially and laterally, snugly wrapped from axilla to elbow, with the forearm supported by a collar and cuff at the wrist (Fig. 36.10). A hanging plaster cast may produce distraction or angulation at the fracture site.

Elbow

Remember:

1. Elbow pain without x-ray findings may indicate radial head fracture.
2. Elbow injuries in children less than 10 years old require films of *both* elbows for comparison.
3. A line on any x-ray film of the elbow drawn through the center of the radius always meets the center of the capitellum if the radius is not dislocated.

If the physician suspects a fracture or dislocation of the elbow, he or she should palpate the bony prominences (medial and lateral epicondyles, olecranon, and radial head) for tenderness and crepitation. Neurovascular evaluation of the forearm and hand should be carefully carried out.

Anteroposterior and lateral x-ray films are obtained. If the physician suspects a fracture of the radial head, several rotational views are ordered. The radial head normally points at the capitellum in all views; if it does not, it is dislocated (Fig. 36.11). In children, the multiple secondary ossification centers are confusing, and films of the opposite normal elbow are often helpful for comparison.

Dislocation

Dislocations of the elbow are usually reduced easily and are immobilized in a posterior splint and

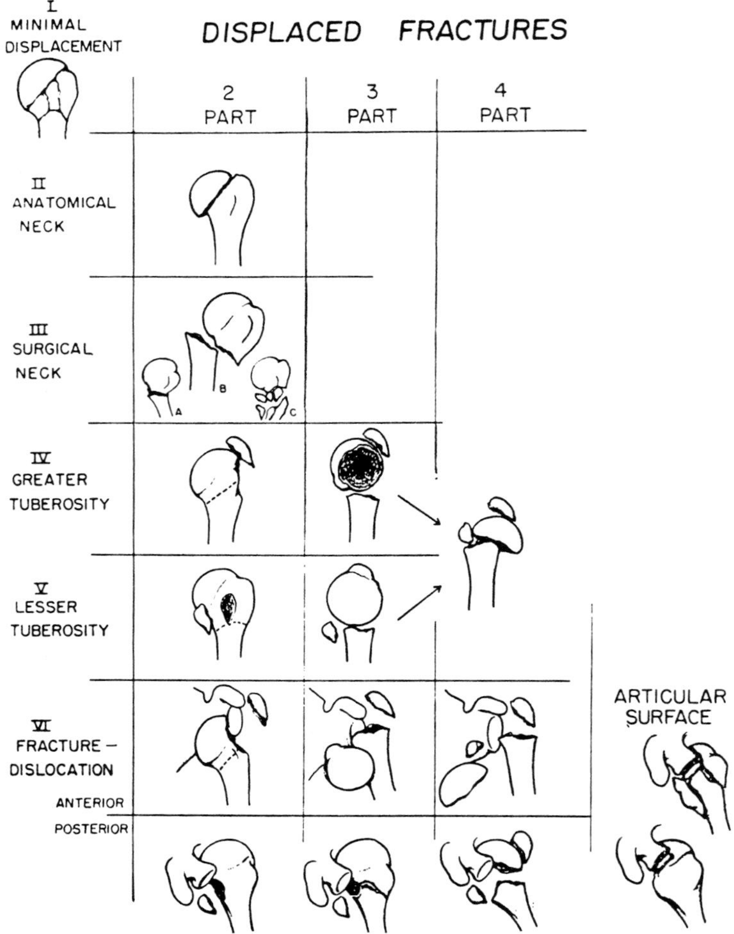

Figure 36.9. Anatomic classification of displaced fractures of the proximal humerus. (From Neer CS II. Displaced proximal humeral fractures. Part I. Classification and evaluation. *J Bone Joint Surg* 52A:1079,1970. Used by permission.)

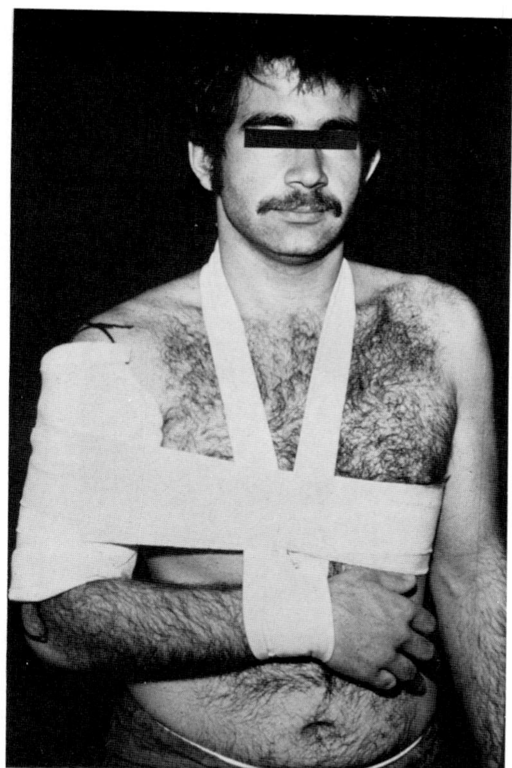

Figure 36.10. Coaptation splints with collar and cuff for humeral fracture.

sling with the elbow flexed 90°. The dislocations are usually posterior, and reduction can be accomplished by traction along the line of the humerus with forward traction on the forearm. Range of motion exercises should be started as soon as the swelling begins to subside—1–2weeks—but the elbow should be protected in the splint when the exercises are not being done. Isolated radial head dislocations do occur and must be recognized; this injury occurs more commonly, however, with a fracture of the proximal part of the ulna (a Monteggia fracture, Fig. 36.12). In a young child, a sudden pull on the arm by an older child or an adult may cause subluxation of the radial head, commonly called "pulled elbow" or "nursemaid's elbow." The patient refuses to use the arm. Physical examination reveals resistance to full supination. X-ray films are normal. Firm supination of the forearm produces a palpable click over the radial head, and the child is usually asymptomatic within a few minutes.

Fracture

In adults, displaced olecranon fractures require excision or repair of the bony fragment. Radial head fractures with minimal disruption of the articular surface respond to conservative measures, including aspiration of accompanying hemarthrosis. Gentle testing of pronation and supination is carried out. If this results in less than 60° of each motion, or if a loose body is present on x-ray examination, operation probably will be required. Adult patients with supracondylar fractures of the humerus require hospitalization for traction or operative repair. In children, since a supracondylar fracture may compromise circulation and lead to muscle ischemia and Volkmann's contracture, the radial pulse must be monitored carefully after closed reduction. If the circulatory status is uncertain, treatment with traction or cross-pinning with K-wires is the safest course.

Forearm

Remember:

1. Displaced forearm fractures in adults usually require open reduction.
2. Reduced green-stick fractures in children may angulate again, even in a cast.
3. Compartment syndromes occur in patients with forearm fractures.

Obvious angular deformity accompanies fracture of the forearm. Immediate, careful evaluation of neurovascular function is essential. X-ray films should include anteroposterior and lateral views from the wrist to the elbow.

In children, green-stick fractures of the forearm must be bent the other way to fracture the opposite cortex, or angulation will recur; surgical repair is rarely necessary. In adults, closed reduction when both the radius and the ulna are fractured often fails to produce good alignment, particularly in rotation. The usual treatment, therefore, is open reduction and fixation with rods or plates. On the other hand, isolated fractures of one bone may at times be treated with closed reduction. Compartment syndromes can occur in patients with these fractures.

Wrist

Remember:

1. Wrist pain with normal x-ray findings may indicate navicular fracture.
2. Navicular fracture or rupture of thumb abductor tendon can occur with Colles' fracture.
3. Always check the position of the lunate bone to rule out perilunate dislocation.
4. Wrist pain with negative x-ray findings may indicate intercarpal subluxation.

Injuries to the distal part of the radius and ulna are common and usually are caused by a fall on the outstretched hand. Colles' fracture, a term mistakenly used for wrist fractures in general, refers to a

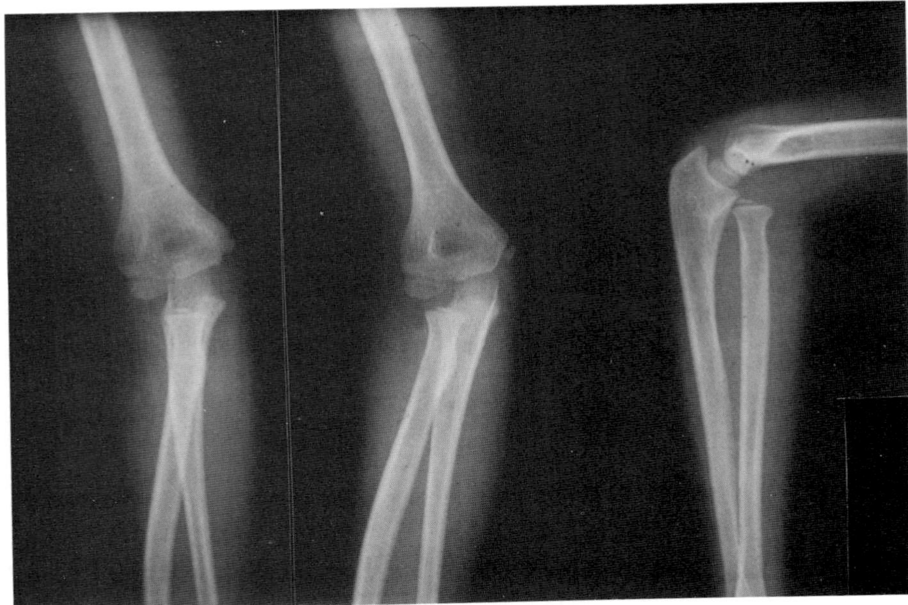

Figure 36.11. Three x-ray views of dislocated radial head in right arm of 6-year-old child (*left* to *right:* anteroposterior, oblique, and lateral). Radial head does not point to capitellum.

dorsally displaced fracture of the lower end of the radius with accompanying fracture of the ulnar styloid process (Fig. 36.13). Dorsal displacement of the hand and wrist produces the silver-fork deformity. Tenderness over the anatomical snuffbox suggests a navicular fracture.

X-ray films should include anteroposterior and lateral views, with navicular views if a navicular fracture is suspected. Comparison views of the other wrist are helpful in evaluating other carpal fractures and dislocations.

Local, regional, or general anesthesia is used in

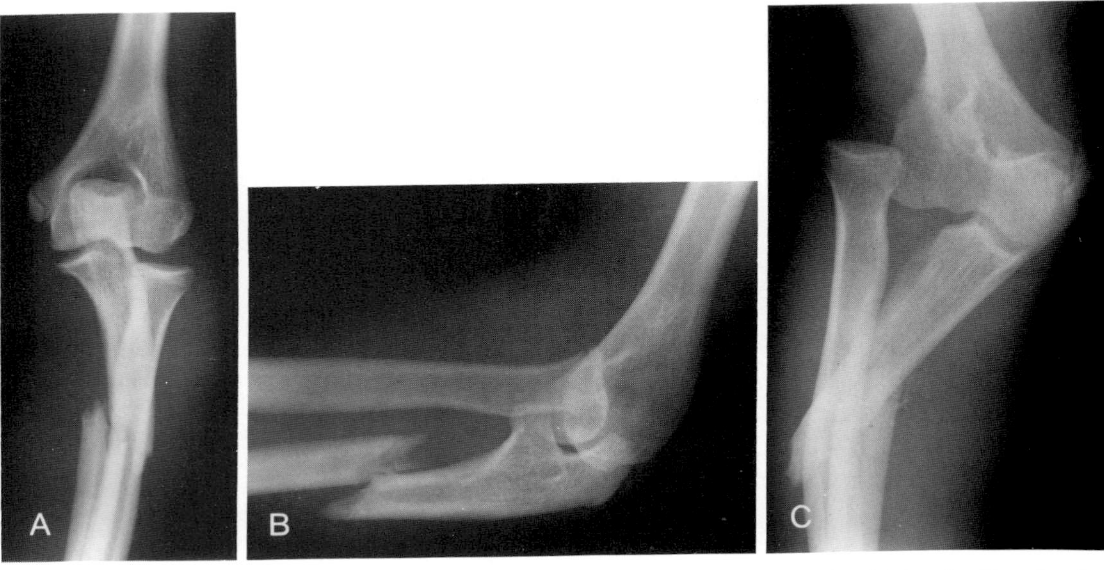

Figure 36.12. Monteggia fracture. *A*, Anteroposterior view and *B*, lateral view. Radial head subluxation is subtle, but it is apparent on both views that a line drawn up the center of the radius would not bisect the capitellum. *C*, Oblique view. On this view, dislocation is obvious.

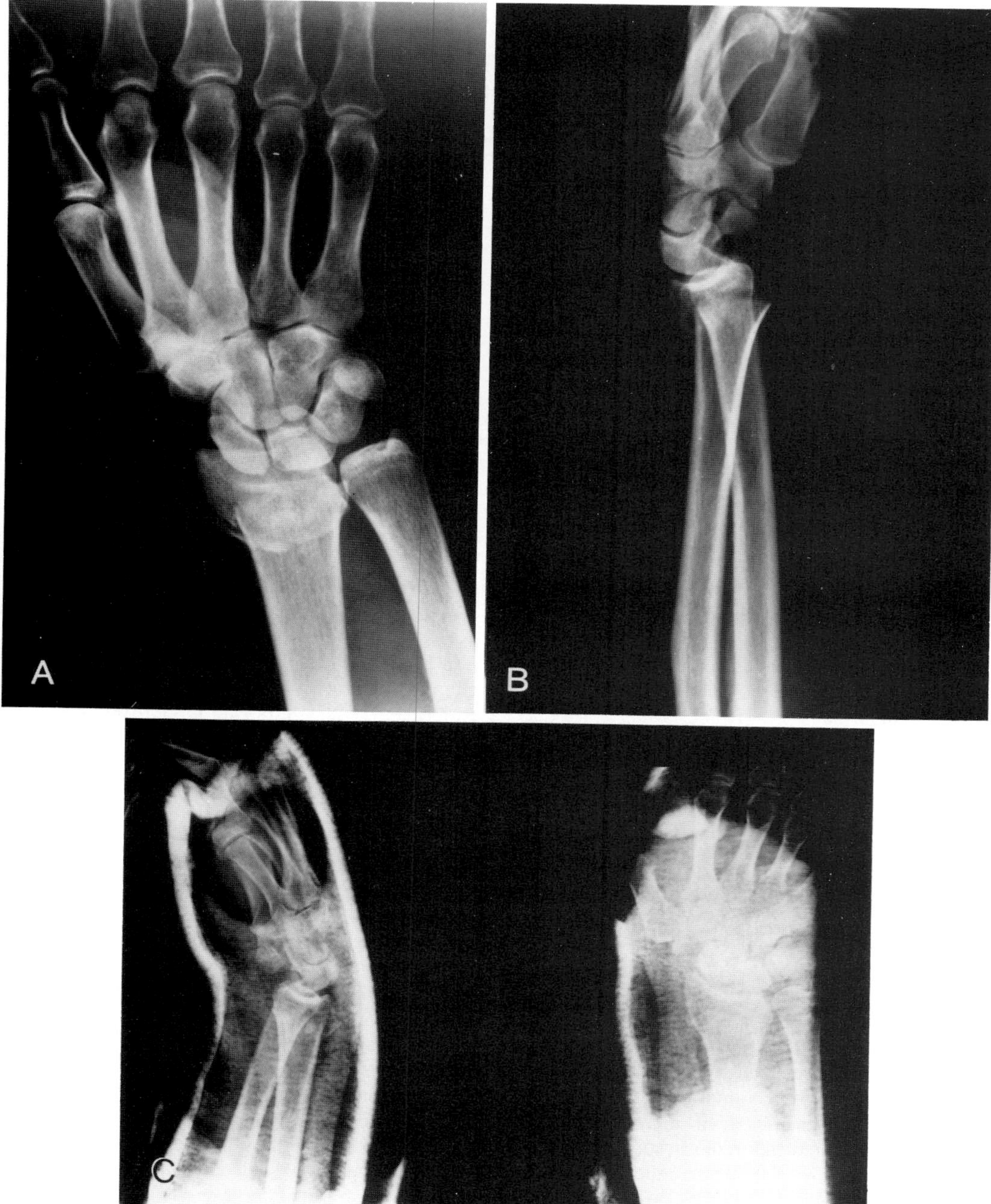

Figure 36.13. Colles' fracture. *A*, Anteroposterior view shows radial shortening and deviation of wrist. *B*, Lateral view shows dorsal angulation. *C*, Postreduction films obtained after reduction show restoration of anatomic position.

the repair of displaced fractures of the wrist. Strong traction and countertraction are applied to disengage and to disimpact the bony fragments, which are then pushed into place and maintained in a stable position. The hand and wrist (after a Colles' fracture) usually are held in pronation, with ulnar deviation and some wrist flexion. Smith's fracture, or reverse Colles' fracture, is best held in supination with slight wrist flexion. Either a gutter splint open on the ulnar side or volar and dorsal plaster splints are applied, wrapping them on carefully to avoid wrinkles. The elbow is then immobilized to prevent forearm rotation. A cast circling the wrist should be avoided because of the possibility of soft-tissue swelling, and volar plaster splints should not extend beyond the midpalmar crease, to allow full metacarpophalangeal flexion. The patient should be seen on the following day to assess the reduction and circulation, tightening or loosening the splints as indicated. Finger and shoulder exercise should be encouraged to prevent later complications, such as causalgia and Sudeck's atrophy. In elderly patients, the fracture may not be reduced in order to regain early function. This results in permanent cosmetic deformity, however. Median nerve compression is a possibility with this fracture, and nerve function should be evaluated.

In an adult patient, the diagnosis of "wrist sprain" should be made only after navicular fracture has been excluded. If there is any tenderness over the navicular bone, a cast that includes the thumb as well as the wrist should be applied even if x-ray films do not demonstrate a fracture. Films are then repeated in 2 weeks without the cast. If a navicular fracture has occurred, it will be visualized, and the cast should be replaced. If no fracture is seen, the definitive diagnosis of wrist sprain can be made, and the cast left off.

Wrist trauma may include dislocation or subluxation of the proximal or the distal carpal row. These injuries, which may be subtle and which may occur without visible fracture, require detailed study of intercarpal relationships and comparison with the normal wrist. A common injury of this type is perilunate dislocation, in which hyperextension of the wrist occurs with dislocation of the distal carpal row dorsally. Return of the hand to the neutral position then flexes the lunate bone 90°. Even though the lunate is now rotated to this degree, the x-ray film looks deceptively normal unless the examiner looks carefully at the lunate itself (Fig. 36.14). Tomographic x-rays may be helpful with carpal injuries.

In older children, displacement of the distal part of the radial epiphysis is common, and requires accurate reduction to avoid growth retardation. A torus fracture of the distal radius (buckling of the dorsal cortex), commonly seen in children, requires only a splint or a light cast for 2–3 weeks.

INJURIES OF LOWER PART OF TRUNK

Pelvis

Remember:

1. Pelvic fracture may cause fatal retroperitoneal bleeding.
2. Pelvic fracture may also cause major injury to the urethra and bladder.
3. Fractures of the acetabulum may disrupt hip function or injure the sciatic nerve.
4. Fractures through the sacral foramen may impair bowel and bladder function.
5. A catheter should not be introduced if there is blood at the penile meatus.

Patients with a pelvic fracture may have local tenderness over the pelvic or ischial rami, iliac wings, or sacrum. Diastasis of the pubic symphysis may be palpable, and compression of the ilia may cause pain in the pelvis or sacroiliac region. Hypotension and a decreased hematocrit provide evidence of blood loss; an increase in abdominal girth indicates retroperitoneal hemorrhage. Rectal examination may reveal bony tenderness, the presence of hematoma, and/or inability to palpate a prostate gland. The latter indicates a posterior urethral tear. Injuries to the femoral, obturator, or sciatic nerves may accompany pelvic fractures. Identification and early documentation of nerve injuries are important.

An anteroposterior film of the pelvis and lateral films of the sacrum and coccyx are necessary for diagnosis. Anteroposterior films with the tube tilted 30° caudad and cephalad (inlet-outlet views) allow assessment of injuries to the pelvic ring. Ipsilateral injuries to the sacrum, ischium, and pubis (Malgaigne fracture) create a highly unstable fracture pattern and require surgical immobilization in many cases. Films taken in 45° internal and external oblique projections provide additional information about displacement in complicated pelvic and acetabular fractures. The computed tomography (CT) scan, however, provides the most definitive information about fracture displacement and is useful in demonstrating fractures that are not otherwise well-visualized on plain radiographs.

The emergency physician must be aware that major or even fatal hemorrhage can follow a pelvic fracture (see Chapter 46). Surprisingly, minor fractures to the pubic rami, for example, can result in major retroperitoneal bleeding. With severe pelvic fractures, exsanguination has occurred. Intravenous fluid and blood replacement is essential. An external pressure device (G-suit or MAST trousers) may save the patient's life by providing temporary tamponade. An external skeletal frame (fixator) can also be applied to help stop venous bleeding. Angiographic embolization of the bleeding arteries may be necessary as a lifesaving measure.

Injuries to the bladder and urethra often are associated with pelvic fractures (Fig. 36.15). In the presence of such a fracture, the emergency physician should consult a urologist before performing any procedures involving these structures, particularly if there is blood at the penile meatus (see Chapter 35). Catheters must be avoided in patients with urethral perforation. A retrograde urethrogram is therefore necessary before attempts to pass a catheter. If extravasation is demonstrated, suprapubic drainage of the bladder is necessary.

Hip

Remember:

1. If the leg is flexed, adducted, and internally rotated, the hip is posteriorly dislocated.
2. If the leg is shortened and externally rotated, the hip is fractured.
3. Hip dislocation may cause sciatic nerve injury.
4. Ability to walk and move the hip does *not* prove that the femoral neck is not fractured.

Hip fractures occur primarily in elderly patients. If the patient has a displaced fracture of either the femoral neck or the intertrochanteric region, the affected leg is shortened and externally rotated; attempts to move the leg are painful. Severe trauma may cause dislocation of the hip posteriorly. In this situation, the leg is adducted, flexed, and internally rotated. Injury to the sciatic nerve occurs in about 15% of posterior dislocations, and function of the peroneal and posterior tibial divisions of the nerve should therefore be evaluated. Anterior and obturator dislocations rarely occur; in these situations the leg is externally rotated and the femoral head may be palpable.

Anteroposterior and lateral x-ray films are necessary. The examiner should remember that the farther a structure is from the film, the more it is magnified. Thus, in the anteroposterior film, the affected femoral head will appear larger than the normal femoral head if the dislocation is anterior, and smaller if it is posterior. Undisplaced fractures of the femoral neck, greater trochanter, and acetabulum may be difficult to visualize, and the films must be examined carefully. *The emergency physician examining the patient must view the films.*

Fractures of the femoral neck may be strongly impacted in a slightly valgus position (Fig. 36.16). This may result in enough stability for the patient to move the hip moderately comfortably and even to walk, although with a limp. These fractures may be hard to outline on x-ray films, and often are not diagnosed. The patient may be discharged from the emergency department with crutches, only to have the fracture become fully displaced later. Therefore, any patient with a painful hip after a fall, even if able to walk and with negative x-ray findings, should be admitted and placed on bed rest until *re-*

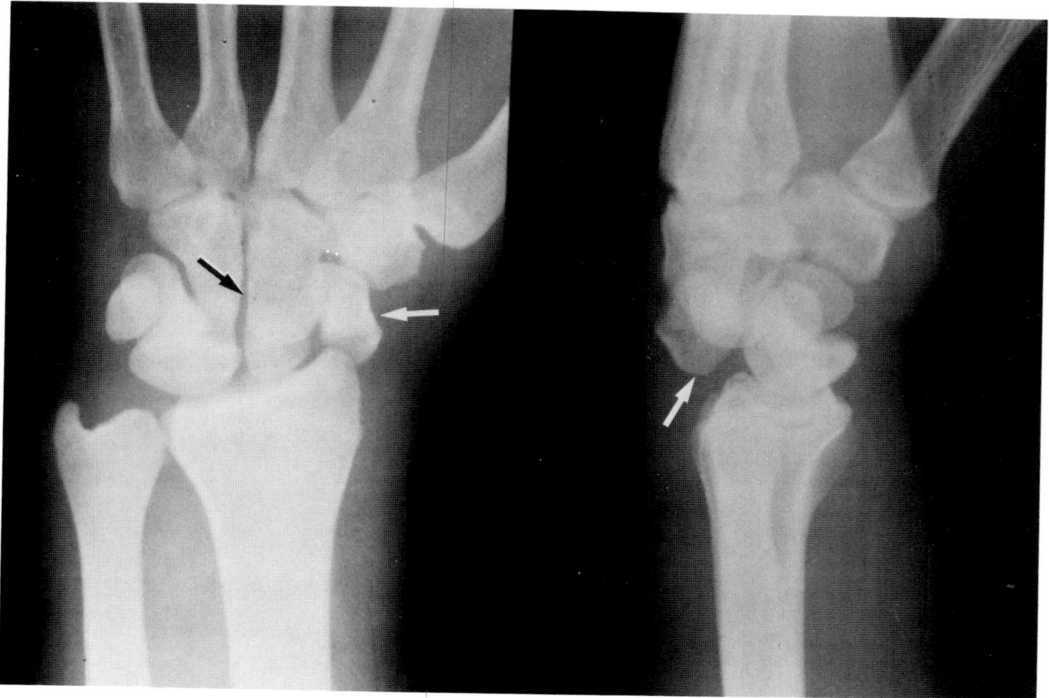

Figure 36.14. Perilunate dislocation. *Left,* Anteroposterior view. *Arrows* indicate abnormalities of navicular and lunate configurations. *Right,* Lateral view. The lunate bone does not articulate with distal carpal row (*arrow*).

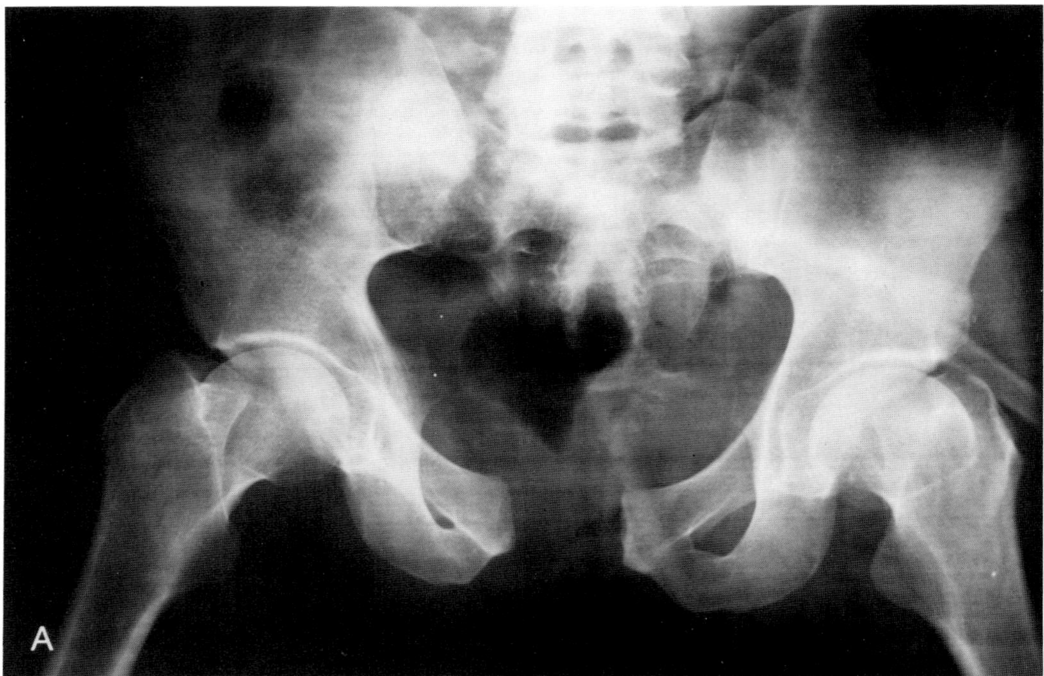

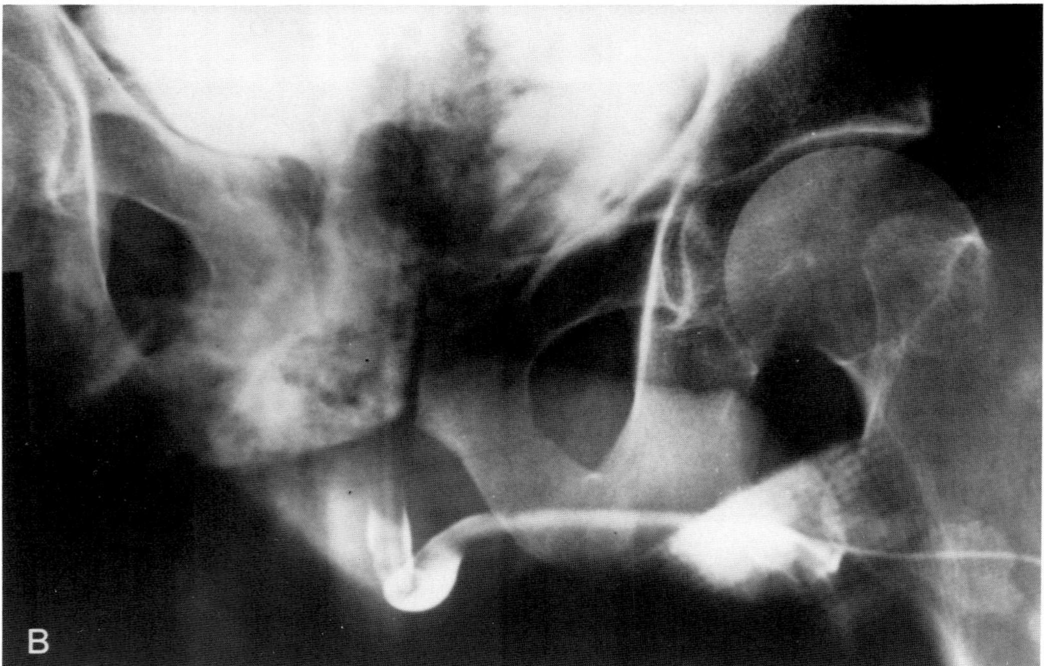

Figure 36.15. Pelvic fracture. *A*, Disruption of pubic symphysis and sacroiliac joint with wide displacement. *B*, Urethrogram confirms urethral injury.

peated x-ray films and absence of symptoms on rest prove there is no fracture.

In patients with a hip fracture, Buck's extension should be applied with traction straps below the knee, using 2 kg of weight. Hip dislocations require immediate reduction, usually under general or spi-

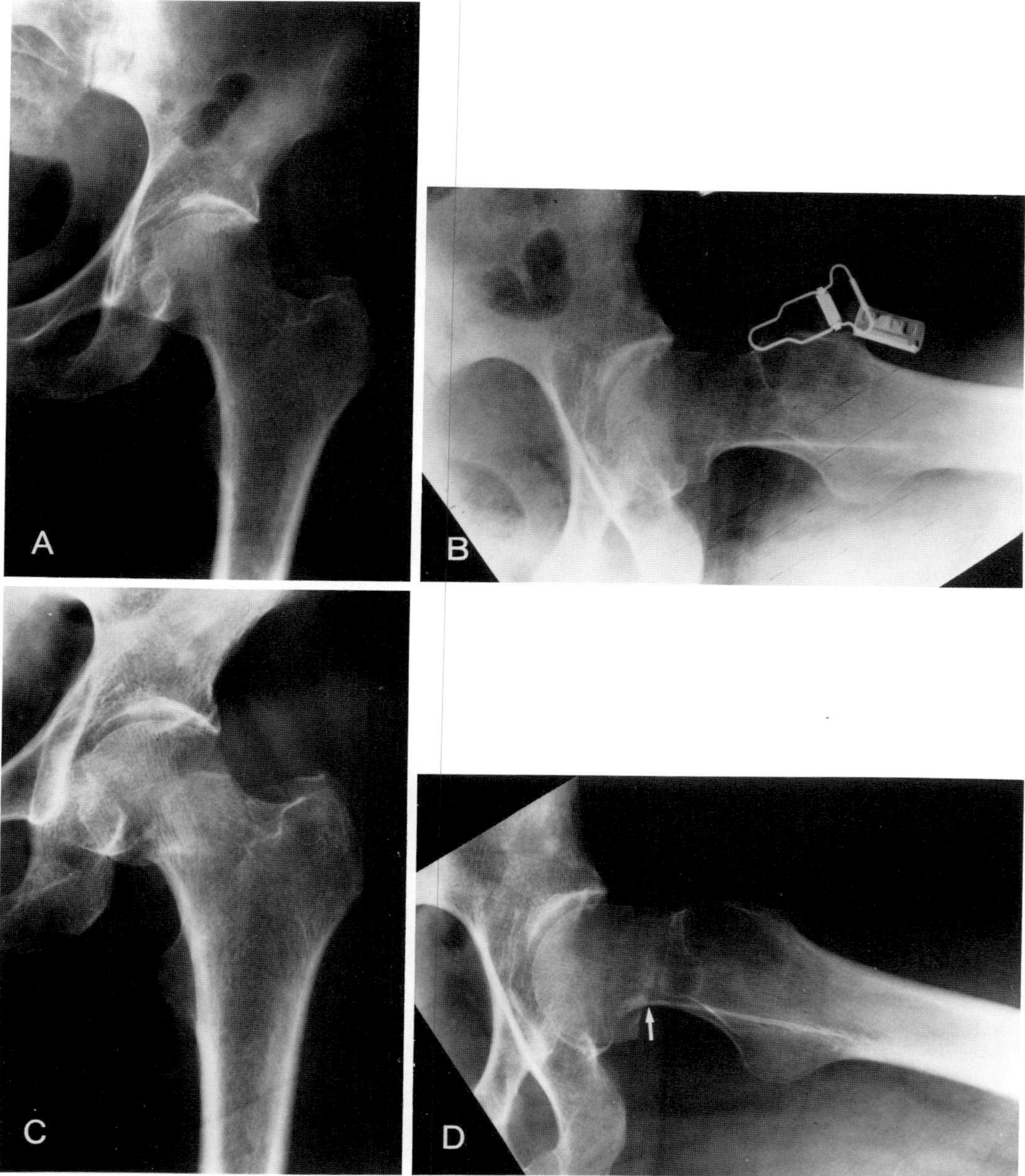

Figure 36.16. *A*, Anteroposterior view and *B*, lateral view of normal hip. *C*, Anteroposterior view of undisplaced, slightly impacted femoral neck fracture. Note appearance of fracture line at superior femoral neck and area of sclerosis (impaction) and trabecular irregularity medially just beneath femoral head. *D*, Lateral view of same fracture. Note overlap of trabecular lines (*arrow*) and cortical break posteriorly just below femoral head.

nal anesthesia. Intertrochanteric fractures and comminuted acetabular fractures may cause major hemorrhage. All patients with hip fractures and dislocations should be hospitalized for definitive treatment.

INJURIES OF LOWER EXTREMITIES

Thigh

Remember:

1. The patient may lose 4–6 units of blood into the soft tissue surrounding a femoral fracture.

2. Femoral fractures require traction with a Thomas splint in the emergency department, preferably at the scene of the accident.
3. This injury can occur with hip dislocation: x-ray films of the pelvis and hip are always necessary.

Fracture of the femur is diagnosed easily. The leg should be splinted at the scene of injury, and immobilization and traction should be applied in the emergency department with a Hare traction splint or a Thomas splint (Fig. 36.3*B*). The status of distal neurovascular structures must be ascertained. Anteroposterior and lateral x-ray films are taken, including the entire femur and hip in case an ipsilateral hip fracture or dislocation has occurred simultaneously (Fig. 36.17). Since a closed femoral fracture can cause loss of 4–6 units of blood into the tissues of the thigh, blood should be replaced as indicated. Surgical fixation is the definitive treatment for these fractures.

Knee

Remember:

1. Patellar fractures may be associated with hip dislocation.
2. Knee dislocations commonly compress, occlude, or lacerate the popliteal artery.
3. The presence of pedal pulses in a young person with knee dislocation does *not* rule out arterial injury.

Fractures of the patella often can be palpated. If the fracture is complete, it prevents active knee extension by inhibiting quadriceps activity. Fractures of the distal femur or tibial plateau can cause rapid tense, painful hemarthrosis. Aspiration of the hemarthrosis under sterile conditions relieves symptoms. If the aspirate contains fat globules floating on top of the blood, communication between the marrow canal and the joint is proved. The extremity is immobilized or placed in traction, as indicated.

Ruptures can occur within the quadriceps muscle above the patella or in the patellar tendon below. These usually can be palpated and, if complete, will not allow the patient to lift his leg with the knee extended. The patella may be seen too high or too low on the lateral x-ray film. Complete ruptures of this type require surgical repair.

Dislocation or subluxation of the patella is common, occurring frequently in obese women who

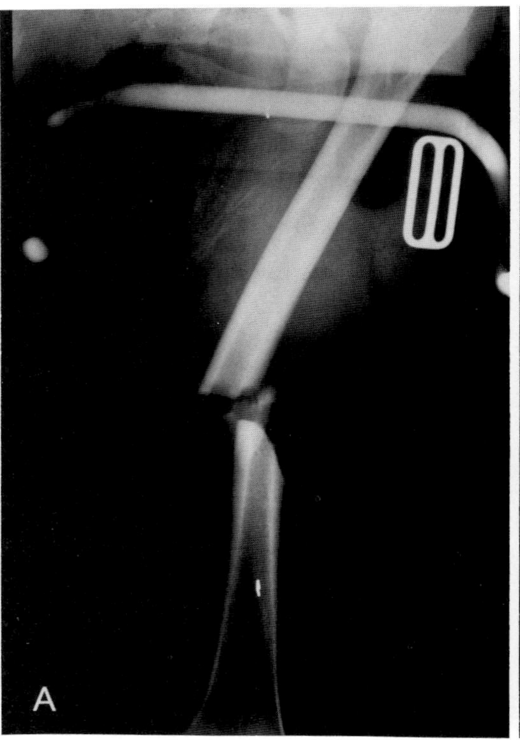

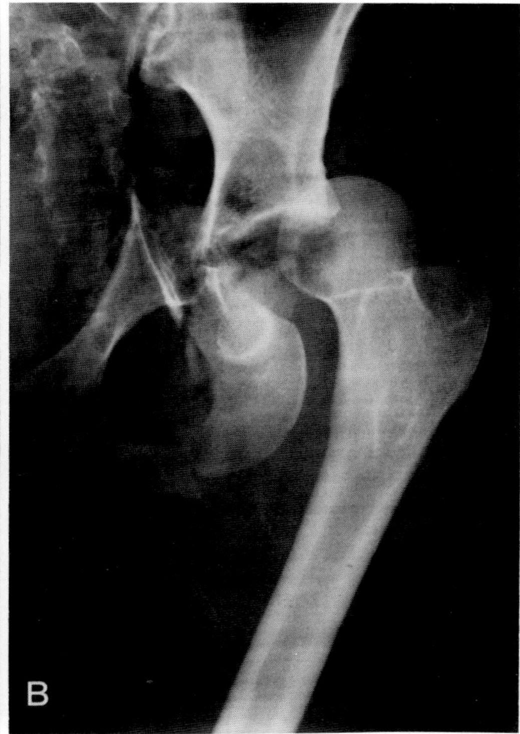

Figure 36.17. Femoral shaft fracture. *A*, Anteroposterior view reveals adducted proximal fragment. *B*, Hip film reveals concomitant posterior fracture-dislocation.

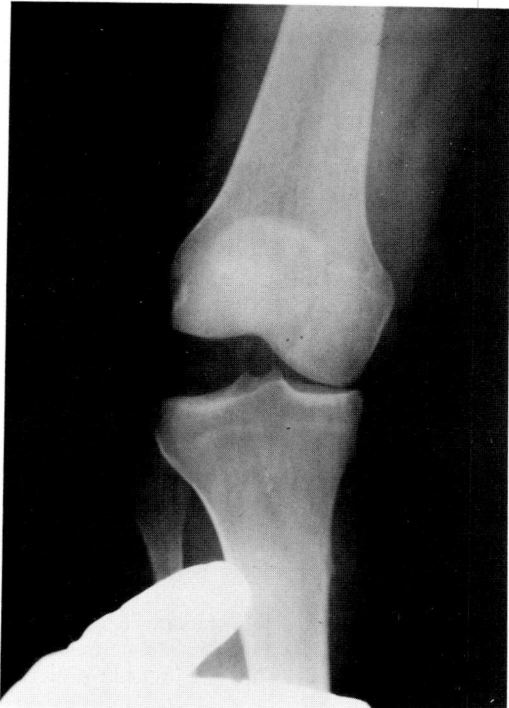

Figure 36.18. Stress radiograph of knee. Application of varus stress reveals complete disruption of lateral ligaments.

have genu valgum (knock-knee). The dislocated patella sometimes can be palpated lateral to its normal position; more often, subluxations of the patella reduce spontaneously, and the diagnosis can then be made if the patient complains of pain when the patella is pushed laterally.

Soft tissue injuries around the knee joint are common. Squatting and twisting may damage the medial or lateral meniscus. A torn meniscus can cause the knee to lock in flexion or may prevent its full extension. It is often associated with knee effusion, containing clear yellow fluid. Palpation of the joint line usually elicits tenderness over the affected meniscus. Sprains and tears of the collateral ligaments can be diagnosed by careful palpation and by stressing the knee in the anteroposterior and medial lateral planes. Minor strains of the collateral or cruciate ligaments (Grade I) are demonstrated by pain on stress testing without demonstrable instability. These are treated by immobilization with casts or a knee immobilizer. Grade II strains are characterized by instability with a painful end point to stress testing. Grade III injuries are characterized by no discernible end point to stress testing. Grade II injuries are usually treated conservatively again with casts or a knee immobilizer, while Grade III injuries often require surgical correction.

Stress testing of the medial and lateral ligaments should be done with the knee in full extension. Injury to the anterior or posterior cruciate injuries are demonstrated by stressing the knee in the slightly flexed position at approximately 20–30°.

In the case of a knee injury, anteroposterior and lateral x-ray films are ordered routinely. A tangential view is helpful in patellar injuries, and stress films should be obtained to evaluate injured ligaments and fractures of the tibial plateau (Fig. 36.18).

A result of severe trauma, true dislocation of the knee is rare. All ligaments are torn, rendering the knee completely unstable. Anterior dislocation, with tibia dislocated forward, is likely to stretch or tear the popliteal artery; the peroneal nerve is also often stretched.

A true orthopaedic emergency, the dislocated knee should be reduced immediately. Peripheral pulses should be evaluated after reduction, and if compromise of the popliteal artery is suggested, arteriographic examination should be carried out promptly. The injured vessel should be repaired, since collateral circulation in the popliteal area is insufficient to nourish the distal leg. Pedal pulses may be present because of excellent collateral circulation about the knee in a young patient. Often this is not sufficient, however, to prevent eventual distal circulatory compromise, as swelling occurs in the injured area. Therefore, arteriography is needed to define the exact status of the popliteal artery.

Dislocation of the patella can be reduced by extending the knee and flexing the hip, so-called straight leg raising, to relax the quadriceps muscle. It is treated with a compression dressing composed of multiple layers of either sheet wadding or Webril and an Ace bandage wrapped from ankle to groin. Crutches are adjusted to leave 2.5 cm between the top of the crutch and the axilla to insure that weight is borne on the hands, not on the axillae.

If the emergency physician diagnoses patellar fracture, a partial or complete ligamentous tear, or injury to a meniscus, the patient may need to be admitted to the hospital for definitive treatment.

Lower Leg

Remember:

1. Fracture of the neck of the fibula may damage the peroneal nerve.
2. Fracture of the proximal third of the tibia may cause circulatory impairment.
3. In fractures of the fibular shaft, treatment of symptoms is sufficient.

Intraarticular fractures of the proximal tibia usu-

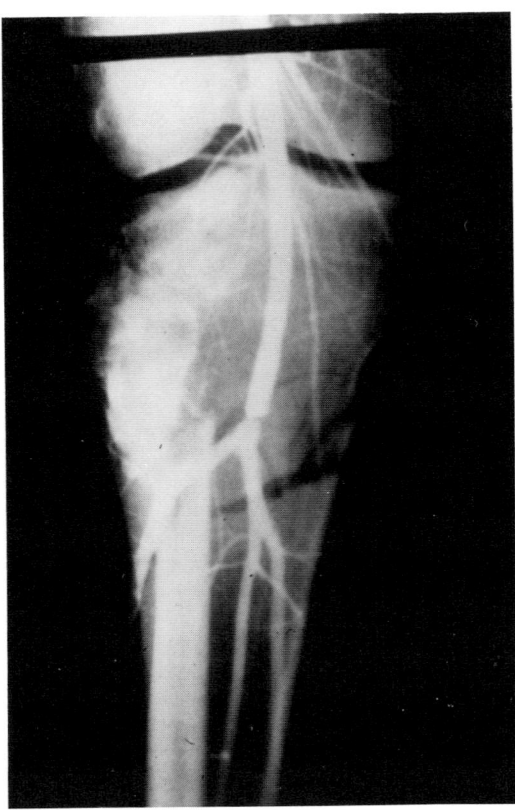

Figure 36.19. Fracture of proximal tibia with intimal tear of popliteal artery proximal to its trifurcation, where artery is tightly fixed.

ally occur on the lateral side (''plateau'' fracture) because of a valgus knee injury. Aspiration of blood from the knee showing fat globules will indicate this. Significant depression of fragments into the metaphysis of the tibia indicates the need for open reduction of the fracture. Tomograms may be helpful in differentiating fracture fragment depression in questionable cases.

Isolated fractures of the shaft of the fibula, except for those within 3 inches of the lateral malleolus, occur from direct blows and may be treated symptomatically, since this part of the fibula does not take part in weightbearing. Attention must be paid to the ankle, however, because severe ankle injuries may be associated with proximal fibular fractures (Maisonneuve).

Fractures of the proximal third of the tibia may cause vascular compromise because of their proximity to the arterial trifurcation where it is tethered (Fig. 36.19).

Because of its subcutaneous position, the tibial fractures are frequently open. The wound can range from a pinpoint opening from a small piece of bone piercing the skin from within (Grade 1) to a large area involving skin and muscles that result from severe external trauma (Grade 3). The neurovascular status distal to the wound must first be evaluated carefully; gentle traction with alignment often restores distal circulation. Open fractures are inspected, specimens taken for culture, and the wound cleansed of debris. A sterile dressing is then applied, and the limb is splinted in an air or pillow splint (Fig. 36.3*C* and *D*). Definitive surgical treatment is then necessary. If the wound is large and bleeding briskly, bleeding is best controlled with pressure dressings, since attempts to clamp the vessel under emergency conditions may damage the adjacent nerves.

Anteroposterior and lateral x-ray films, taken with the leg splinted, should include both the knee and the ankle. In open fractures, antibiotics and tetanus prophylaxis are administered, and the patient is admitted for further treatment. Most patients with closed tibial fractures should be admitted for elevation of the leg and observation of the circulation. Patients with isolated fibular fractures or, occasionally, undisplaced tibial fractures may be treated on an outpatient basis with proper immobilization of the leg in a cast.

Ankle

Remember:

1. The mortise view is the most important x-ray view.
2. A widened mortise without fracture can indicate a Maisonneuve fracture of the fibula.

Twisting injuries of the foot produce sprains and fractures of the ankle. Ligamentous injuries should be assessed as soon as possible before swelling occurs. The most commonly injured ligaments in the body are the lateral ligaments of the ankle (Fig. 36.20*A*), which are stretched or torn when the foot is inverted. Careful palpation reveals the site of damage. Stressing the foot and ankle demonstrates whether the tear is complete, since complete ligamentous tears are less painful to stress than partial tears. Injuries of the deltoid (medial) ligament are less common, but must be recognized since the deltoid ligament is important for ankle stability.

Fractures of the ankle are also evaluated by palpation and stressing. A displaced medial malleolus can often be diagnosed before x-ray examination by the presence of a palpable fracture line over the distal and medial portions of the tibia. Until definitive treatment is undertaken, the ankle should be treated with ice packs, splints, and elevation. In general, it is best to ''overtreat'' ankle sprains. Immobilization

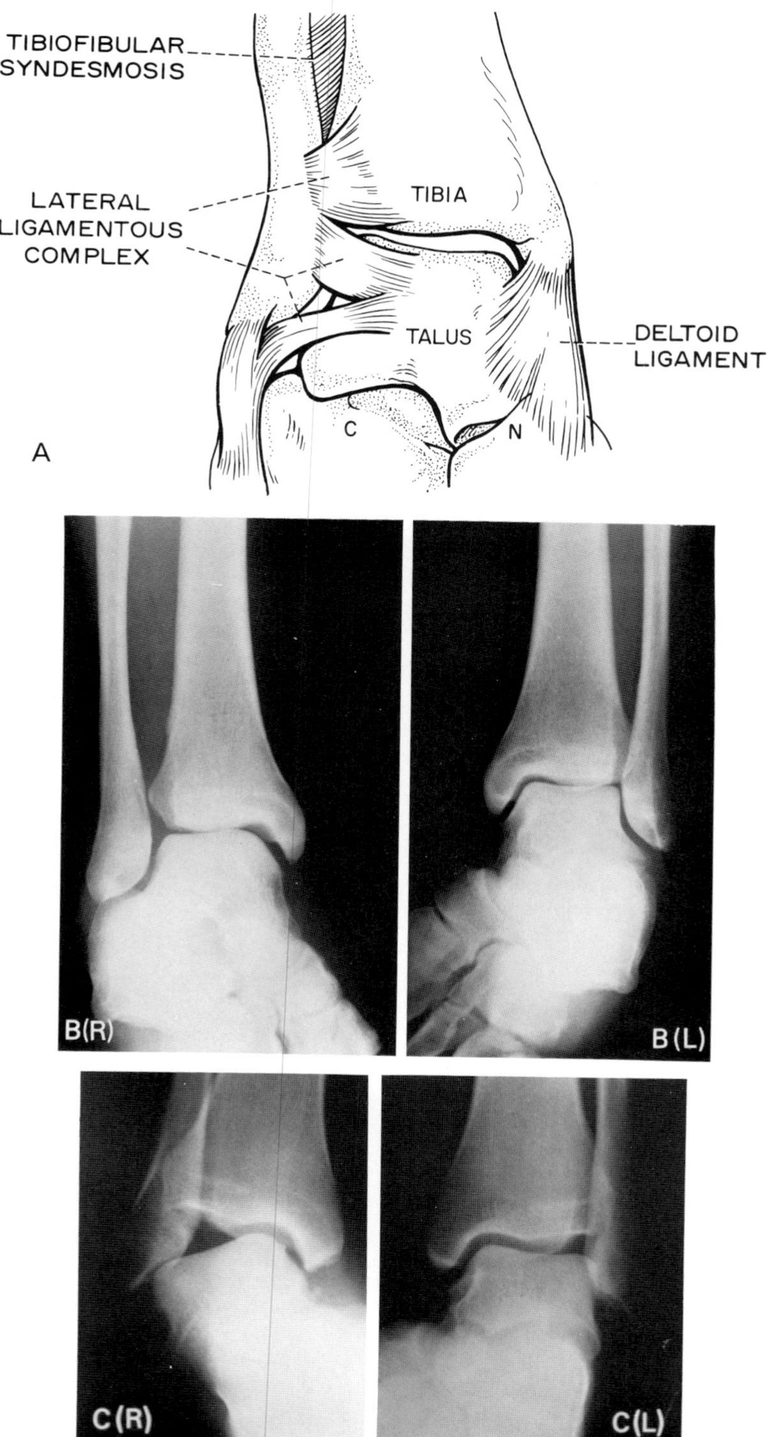

Figure 36.20. Ligamentous injuries of ankle. *A*, Major ligaments of ankle; N = navicular bone, C = calcaneous bone. *B*, Mortise views of injured (*right*) and normal (*left*) ankles; in right ankle note increased space between talus and tibia medially (torn deltoid ligament) and widening of interval between tibia and fibula (torn syndesmosis). *C*, Inversion stress views of injured (*right*) and normal (*left*) ankles in another patient; in right ankle note marked tilting of talus resulting from complete tear of lateral ligaments.

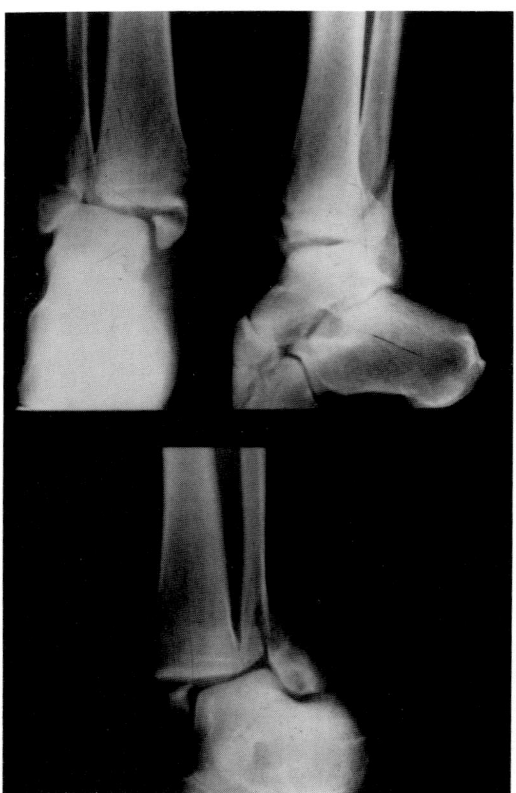

Figure 36.21. Trimalleolar fracture-dislocation of ankle. Note fractures of medial, lateral, and posterior malleoli, and disruption of ankle mortise.

in a plaster cast provides the best environment for the healing of fractures or *severe* sprains. The cast should be continued, allowing weightbearing as tolerated, until the patient has been bearing full weight without pain for 1 week. This usually takes 3–4 weeks, but can take as long as 8 weeks. An alternative to casting is aggressive treatment, using physical therapy including ice, whirlpools, electrical stimulation, active motion exercises, and nonweightbearing with crutches. This may allow more rapid return to function, but requires a cooperative patient and one who understands the necessity of adhering to a strict protocol. Minimal sprains can be treated with air splints or ace bandages and crutches. Adhesive strapping is reserved for later support, such as in athletic exercise.

Fractures of the ankle can involve the lateral malleolus alone, the lateral and medial malleoli (bimalleolar), or the lateral, medial, and posterior malleoli (trimalleolar) (Fig. 36.21). They result usually from an internal rotation force of the body on the fixed foot. Complete or partial dislocation of the talus can occur; treatment is directed at restoration of the mortise to provide stability to the ankle. Significant loss of fibular length requires correction. Widening of the mortise may be apparent on x-ray films without a visible fracture. Palpation of the side of the calf usually elicits tenderness over the middle and upper part of the fibula. The Maisonneuve fracture (Fig. 36.22) is a rupture of the deltoid ligament with a high fibular fracture, allowing lateral displacement of the talus and a widened mortise without visible x-ray fracture. It is a commonly undiagnosed injury in emergency departments.

Anteroposterior, lateral views, and a mortise view should be routinely obtained. The mortise view (Fig. 36.20*B*) is similar to the anteroposterior view, but the leg is internally rotated about 30°. A distance larger than 5 mm between the medial malleolus and the talus is evidence of injury to the deltoid ligament. In a normal ankle, the tibia and fibula overlap. If they are separated, the tibiofibular ligament has been torn (Fig. 36.23). The posterior mal-

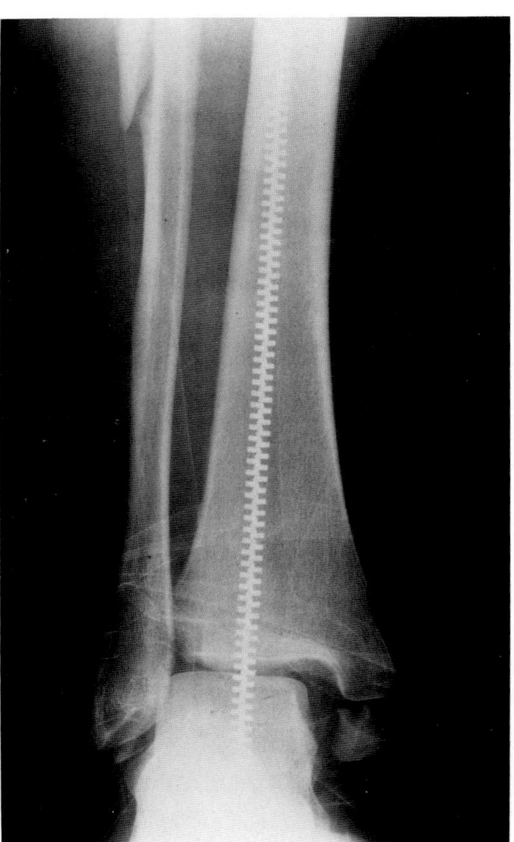

Figure 36.22. Maisonneuve fracture. Note widening of mortise and high fibula fracture that may easily be missed on films of the ankle only.

leolus of the tibia can be evaluated on the lateral view. Stress views can be taken for full evaluation of ligamentous injury and stability (Fig. 36.20*C*).

In a fracture-dislocation of the ankle, with the talus displaced laterally or posteriorly, it is often possible to reduce the talus back under the tibia without anesthesia. This should be done as quickly as possible to minimize swelling and neurovascular compromise. An undisplaced or minimally displaced fracture can be treated with a cast. X-ray films should be taken after the cast is applied to be sure that the position remains satisfactory.

Malleolar fractures can also occur in conjunction with severe shattering of the distal tibia in an intra-articular fracture. This is the so-called pilon fracture, which often results in late posttraumatic osteoarthritis.

Ankle sprains can be associated with osteochondral fractures of the talus, which may be seen as small flecks near the medial or lateral portion of the tibial articulation of the talus. These injuries are more severe than sprains and may require surgical intervention.

Foot

Remember:

1. Midfoot pain and swelling may indicate metatarsal-tarsal (Lisfranc) dislocation.
2. Metatarsal neck fractures require lateral x-ray films (plantar angulation).
3. Fractures of the neck of the talus and talar dislocations can result in avascular necrosis.
4. Os calcis fractures can be accompanied by spinal compression fractures.

Fractures of the talus usually involve the talar neck and can compromise the bony circulation, leading to avascular necrosis. Displacement of the fragment on the lateral x-ray film must be corrected accurately. Dislocations of the talus from the tibia above or the os calcis below can also occur, with or without accompanying fractures. These injuries are prone to later avascular talar necrosis. Reduction usually can be accomplished by closed methods under general or spinal anesthesia.

Fractures of the os calcis usually result from falls and commonly are work-related. The fracture may

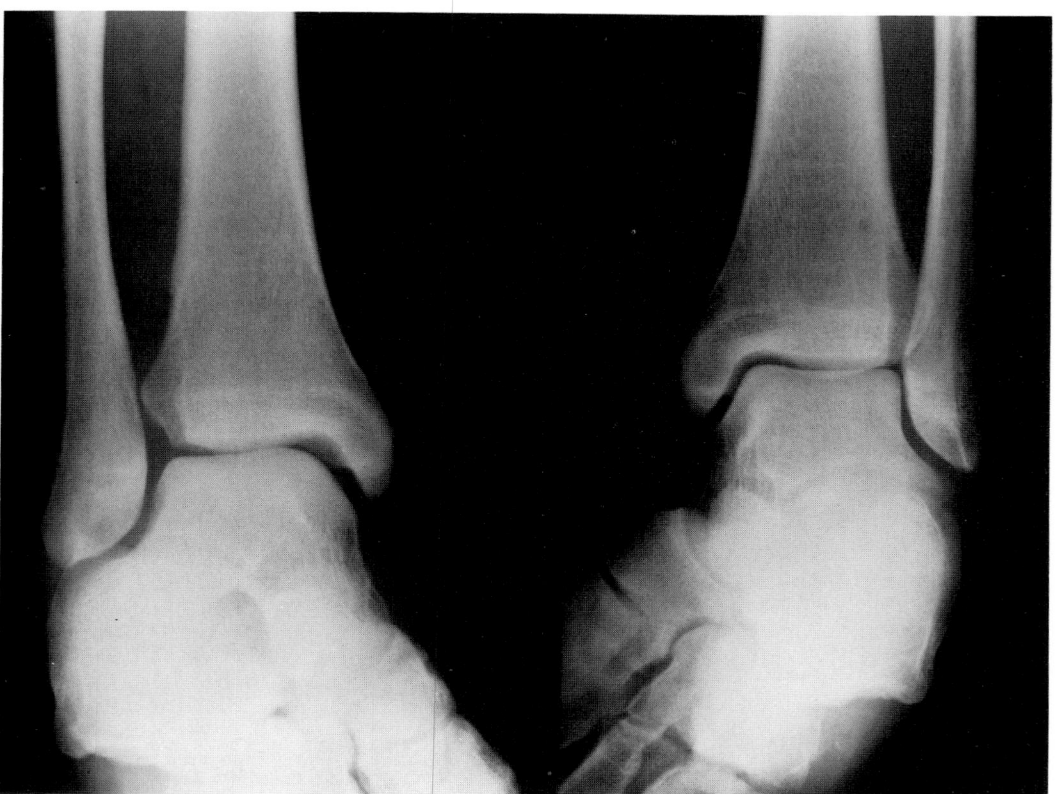

Figure 36.23. Tear of tibiofibular ligament. *Left,* Mortise view demonstrates that fibula and tibia do not overlap and that there is increased space between them. *Right,* Mortise view of normal ankle for comparison. Stress views would confirm the diagnosis.

be an avulsion of a large piece of the posterior os calcis by the gastrocnemius tendon attachment; this usually requires open reduction to restore effective lengths of the involved muscle. However, it is more often a crush injury, with a decrease in the height of the bone, lateral protrusion, and severe involvement of the subtalar joint (Fig 36.24). The injury commonly is accompanied by a lumbar compression fracture. Therefore, an os calcis fracture requires careful examination of the back. Functional recovery is long, and return to work usually is slow. Early treatment consists of splinting with a compression dressing, plaster support, and elevation. Hospital admission usually is indicated. Intraarticular fracture of the os calcis at its articulation with the cuboid bone can also occur; it is commonly undiagnosed because it is obvious only on oblique films of the foot.

The midfoot (navicular and cuneiform bones on one end, and metatarsal bases on the other) is an area of great stress at the apex of the arch of the foot. Dislocations in this area occur with or without fractures of the metatarsal bones (Lisfranc fractures), with the metatarsals usually moving as a unit on the midtarsal bones (Fig. 36.25). Closed reduction can be unstable, and surgical fixation then required. These injuries are difficult to interpret on x-ray examination, but should be suspected whenever there is considerable swelling and pain in the midfoot. Since compromised circulation is a definite danger in these fractures, admission is mandatory for close observation.

Fractures of the metatarsal shaft occur from direct blows, when not associated with Lisfranc type injuries; conservative management with a cast is sufficient. Fractures of the metatarsal neck, however, present a different problem because they often angulate in a plantar direction and present weight-bearing problems later if allowed to heal in that position. Recognition of this fracture can be difficult since lateral x-ray films are required to show the deformity, and these are not obtained routinely in most radiology departments. Simple closed manipulation to correct the plantar angulation together with cast immobilization is all that is needed. The most common metatarsal fracture is an avulsion fracture of the base of the fifth metatarsal bone by the peroneus brevis tendon, in inversion injury. Treatment of its symptoms without cast immobilization is usually sufficient. A fracture more distal in the fifth metatarsal (Jones' fracture) occurs in the proximal cortical portion of the metatarsal shaft. This fracture heals slowly and requires cast immobilization for many weeks; occasionally, operative correction.

Metatarsophalangeal dislocations occur with the

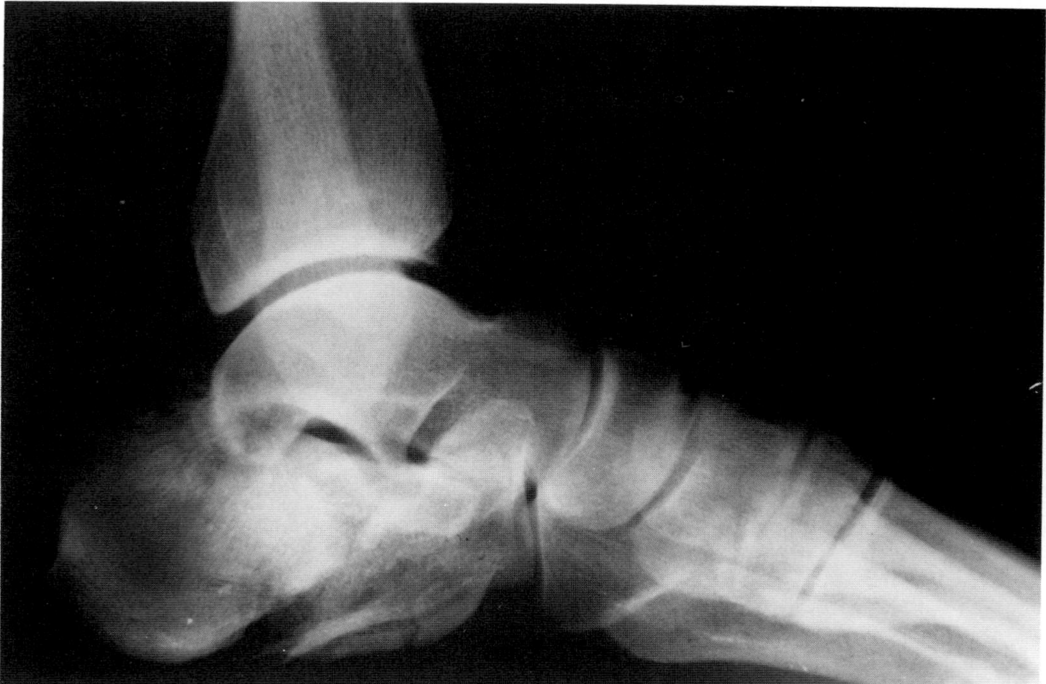

Figure 36.24. Os calcis fracture. Note decrease in height of heel, as well as comminution and disruption of subtalar joint anatomy.

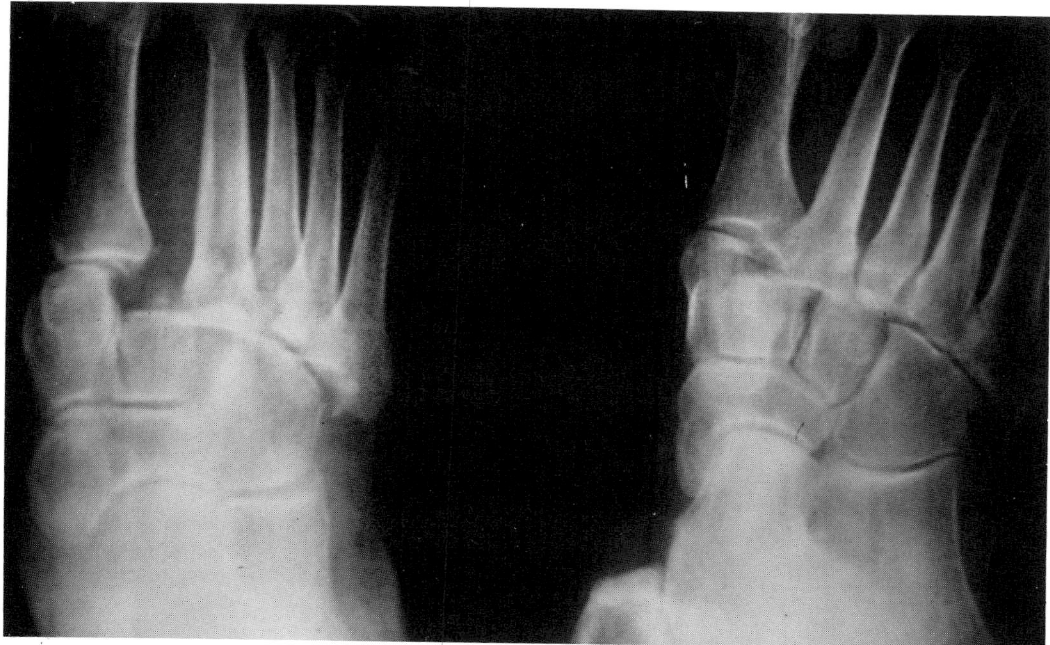

Figure 36.25. Lisfranc fracture. *Left,* Anteroposterior view; *right,* oblique view. Note lateral dislocation of second through fifth metatarsals, best seen on anteroposterior view.

phalanx dislocated dorsally. Although closed reduction usually is accomplished easily, at times the capsule or flexion tendon prevents closed reduction; open reduction is then required.

Fractures of the phalanges of the toes occasionally are angulated enough to require manipulative reduction, but more commonly they require only taping to the neighboring toe for support. The proximal phalanx of the great toe bears much greater stress, however, and often requires support by a splint or a cast.

Stress Fractures

Remember:

1. Pain without injury following prior unusual activity may indicate stress fracture.
2. Stress fracture can occur in any weightbearing long bone.
3. Stress fracture will not show on x-ray films for 2–4 weeks.

Although stress fractures most commonly occur in the second metatarsal shaft, they can occur in any weightbearing long bone, including the femoral shaft or neck. The patient has no history of injury, but usually has participated in some unusual activity such as a long walk or a stressful athletic event. There is tenderness over the involved part, but x-ray findings are negative. Only after some external callus has formed in 2–4 weeks is the diagnosis assured. Since treatment is applied according to symptoms, the emergency physician needs only to suspect the diagnosis, treat the part to protect weightbearing, and see that more x-ray films are later obtained to confirm the diagnosis (Fig. 36.26).

Avulsion Fractures

These injuries usually occur in athletic events, often in sports requiring sudden stops and starts, such as basketball, sprinting, and hockey. They are basically tendon or muscle "pulls," but instead of the muscle failing, its insertion to bone is pulled away. The diagnosis may be made on x-ray examination by observation that the location of the avulsion is the same as the location of muscle insertion. Common sites are the anterosuperior iliac spine (sartorius muscle), the anteroinferior spine (rectus femoris), the lesser trochanter (psoas), and the ischial tuberosity (adductors). Displacement can seem substantial on x-ray films, but treatment of symptoms is usually all that is needed. Symptoms can be intense, however, and brief hospitalization for control of pain is sometimes required.

PEDIATRIC INJURIES

Remember:

1. Fractures rarely are treated by open reduction.

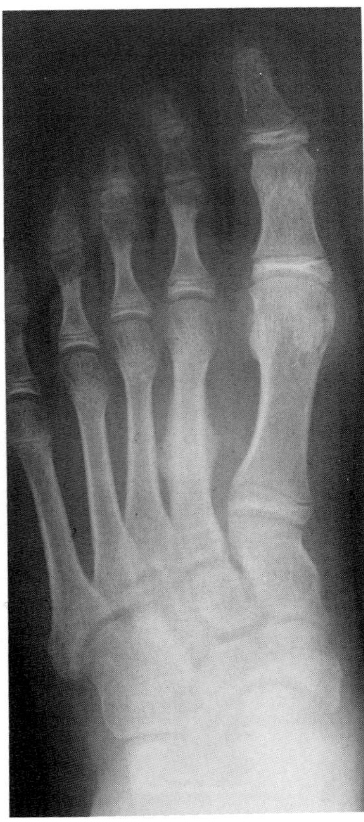

Figure 36.26. Stress fracture. Callus about second metatarsal bone in cross-country runner indicates healing stress or fatigue fracture.

2. Remodeling depends on growth potential and rotational malalignments remodel poorly.
3. Supracondylar humeral fractures are dangerous because of the frequency of compartment syndromes.
4. Lateral condylar humeral fractures in young children are difficult to recognize because of unossified epiphyses.
5. Repeated fractures or unusual mechanisms of injury suggest child abuse.
6. Anteroposterior subluxations up to 4–5 mm in the midcervical spine in young children occur normally or with upper respiratory tract infections.

Fractures in children almost always are treated conservatively. Depending on the age and potential for growth, a considerable degree of malalignment is remodeled within the first year after fracture. Angular deformities are remodeled better if they occur near a joint. Rotational deformities are remodeled poorly. Thus, in many fractures, less satisfactory reductions are accepted than would be the case in adults. Because periosteum in a child is thicker and more active, and because the growth potential is greater, healing times are shorter than in adults. However, for the same reason, the extra blood flow needed to heal the extremity fracture may cause general overgrowth of the bone for a year afterward. In the lower extremities, this may cause a significant discrepancy of leg lengths.

Green-stick fractures are common in children. These fractures splinter rather than break cleanly; they can angulate even though close contact of the fragments is maintained by the thick periosteal tube. The least significant of these fractures is the torus or ''buckle'' fracture, most common in the radius. There is no angular deformity or displacement, and x-ray films show only a small cortical buckling on one side of the bone. The injury, often unrecognized, is treated according to its symptoms. If angular deformity occurs in more extensive green-stick fractures, and if correction is carried out, it is desirable to break the opposite cortex during reduction to prevent recurring angular deformity. X-ray films should be repeated over the next 4 weeks to evaluate maintenance of the reduction.

In growing children, the *epiphyseal plate* is often the point of least resistance to the force of trauma, it may ''slip'' with or without some attached epiphyseal or metaphyseal bone. These injuries are classified by Salter (Fig. 36.27). They commonly

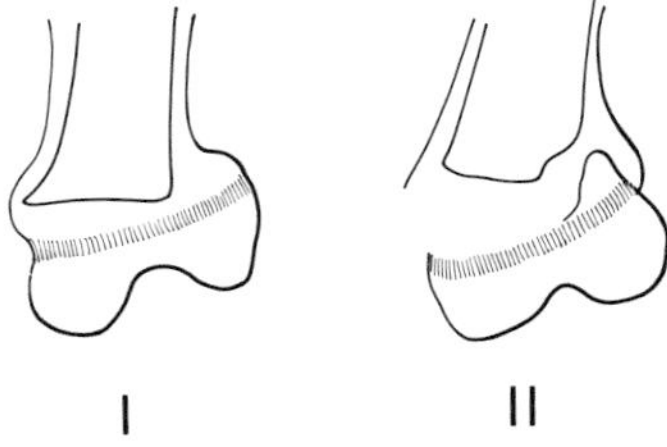

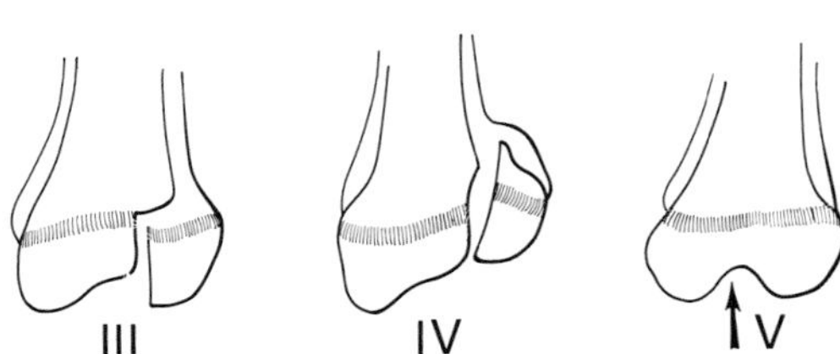

Figure 36.27. Salter classification of epiphyseal plate injuries. *I*, Injury includes epiphyseal plate only. *II*, Injury includes epiphyseal plate and metaphysis. *III*, Injury includes epiphyseal plate and epiphysis. *IV*, Injury includes epiphyseal plate, epiphysis, and metaphysis. *V*, Compression injury to epiphyseal plate only. (Since there is no displacement, x-ray findings are negative.)

occur at the wrist, shoulder, and ankle. Grade 1 injuries of the distal femur easily may be mistaken for knee ligamentous injuries in young football players. Acute epiphyseal slips usually are reduced easily by closed methods. Since the injury is essentially through soft tissue at the epiphyseal plate, healing times are less than for fractures. Reduction is difficult if delayed for even a few days. Later growth disturbance due to arrest of the injured epiphyseal plate is uncommon in grades 1, 2, and 3 injuries. It can occur, however, particularly in grades 4 and 5 injuries, and parents should be advised of this at the time of injury. All patients with epiphyseal plate injuries should have x-ray films 1 year later to evaluate the condition of growth.

Two fractures about the elbow should be mentioned specifically. *Fractures through the lateral epicondyle* of the humerus almost always extend through the capitellum, which in younger children remains largely uncalcified and therefore invisible on x-ray films. The pull of the extensor muscles can rotate this large intraarticular fragment as much as 180° *without* showing wide displacement of the ossification center of the capitellum. For this reason, it is imperative that if this injury is suspected, *both* elbows be carefully x-rayed in the same projection, for comparison of the relative position of the capitellar ossification centers on both sides. If there is any difference in position, this fracture is likely. Open reduction is usually necessary. If displacement is not recognized, permanent and irreparable damage to the elbow will occur.

Supracondylar fractures of the humerus commonly occur in falls on the outstretched arm. While these may be undisplaced and heal in 3–6 weeks with splinting only, wide displacement may be present in anteroposterior, mediolateral, and rotational planes. Closed reduction may be unstable; often the fracture is treated by traction or pinning. If rotational reduction is not well achieved, unsightly varus deformity with decreased carrying angle ensues. Proper treatment requires meticulous and constant orthopaedic judgment and care. This fracture can damage the brachial artery or cause significant swelling and ischemia within the deep volar compartment of the forearm, leading to Volkmann's contracture if unrecognized. This compartment syndrome is the most common encountered in childhood fractures, and its onset can be insidious. The earliest sign of Volkmann's contracture is increasing volar forearm pain on passive finger extension, rather than the absence of radial pulse, blueness of fingers, or motor loss. *All patients with displaced supracondylar humeral fractures must be admitted to the hospital,* and most patients with undisplaced or minimally displaced fractures should also be admitted for observation.

Cervical spine injuries occur in children, but it should be remembered that, in the young child, inflammatory conditions in the throat, even normal anatomy, allow 4–5 mm of forward subluxation of one cervical vertebra on another, particularly in the midcervical spine. If a child is seen after injury with a fixed rotatory deformity of the head, the examiner should remember that rotatory subluxation of the first cervical vertebra on the second can occur and that the deformity can be due to more than muscular spasm alone.

Avulsion fractures occur in teenagers as in young adults, and are treated in a similar manner. Some avulsion fractures, however, include part of an adjacent epiphysis, as in the case of avulsion of the tibial tubercle. If displaced, these fractures may require open reduction and fixation.

Fractures of the femoral neck, either through bone or epiphyseal plate, do occur in children and nearly always require open reduction and internal fixation. A good result is less likely than in the elderly because of the high incidence of avascular necrosis of the femoral head.

Fractures that seem to have an unusual mechanism of injury should alert the examiner to the possibility of child abuse, particularly when evidence of a prior fracture is apparent from history or x-ray findings. The examiner and other members of the emergency staff, such as pediatricians and social service personnel, must thoroughly investigate the possibility of child abuse if it is suspected (see Chapter 29).

OTHER CONDITIONS OF SOFT TISSUES AND JOINTS

Bursitis and Tendonitis

Severe discomfort can occur within a few hours of the onset of bursitis or tendonitis. Areas commonly affected include the shoulder, elbow, hip, and knee. If the shoulder is involved, glenohumeral motion may be limited or nonexistent because of pain. Gentle palpation may elicit point tenderness over the supraspinatus tendon, subacromial bursa, or bicipital groove. At the elbow, the olecranon bursa or the lateral epicondyle may be involved. Inflammation of the latter is known as "tennis elbow." Inflammation of the bursa over the greater trochanter of the hip can be painful enough to limit or prevent walking. Four bursae of the knee are affected similarly: the prepatellar, infrapatellar, Voshell's, and anserine. Voshell's bursa lies between the superficial and deep layers of the medial collateral ligament at the joint line, and the anserine bursa lies beneath the tendons of the sartorius and gracilis muscles near their insertion to the tibia. With the exception that calcification may be present in the supraspinatus tendon, subacromial bursa, or Voshell's bursa, x-ray findings are usually normal.

Treatment consists of anti-inflammatory medications given orally, locally by injection, or in combination. Local application of heat or ice is often helpful along with immobilizing with a sling, splint, or crutches. Nonsteroidal anti-inflammatory drugs are used in preference to steroidal preparations for oral use. They are *contraindicated* in patients with active ulcer disease. Temporary relief can be gained by local infiltration of the painful area with a mixture of a local anesthetic, such as Xylocaine, and a corticosteroid preparation. Corticosteroids usually quiet the inflammation within 1–2 days. Narcotic analgesics are sometimes necessary.

In olecranon and prepatellar bursitis, the emergency physician must determine whether the inflammation is sterile or septic. Fluid is aspirated from the bursa for a Gram's stain and culture; if infection is present, hospitalization for surgical drainage and antibiotic therapy is necessary.

Joint Pain

The sudden onset of pain in a joint arises from conditions such as internal derangement (loose body or torn meniscus), infection, gout, or pseudogout (chondrocalcinosis). The emergency physician examines the joint for erythema, tenderness, and effusion, and tests it for range of motion. Some infections, such as those caused by the gonococcus, may affect more than one joint. Fluid should be aspirated under sterile conditions (see Illustrated Techniques 24–25) and the following laboratory procedures performed: white blood cell count and differential, glucose determination with simultaneous blood glucose measurement, mucin test, Gram's stain, culture in aerobic and anerobic media, and examination for crystals. Under polarized light, urate crystals have strongly negative birefringence, but calcium pyrophosphate crystals have weakly positive birefringence; the former are diagnostic of gout, the latter of pseudogout. Anteroposterior and lateral x-ray films of the joint are examined for a loose body. Calcification of menisci or articular cartilage suggests pseudogout.

Infectious arthritis is treated by drainage of the joint and administration of specific antibiotics. Gout responds well to colchicine, indomethacin, or phenylbutazone. Pseudogout is best treated with phenylbutazone.

Ruptured Tendons

The shoulder, knee, and leg are the common sites of ruptured tendons; rupture often occurs during strenuous activity. At the shoulder, inability of the patient to abduct the glenohumeral joint may signal rupture of the rotator cuff. To differentiate rotator cuff tears from local bursitis, injection of the subacromial bursa with Xylocaine alleviates pain and allows the examiner to test muscle strength in a pain-free situation. Partial ruptures of the rotator cuff may be treated conservatively. Complete ruptures are often repaired surgically, depending on the age, health, and occupational requirements of the patient.

Unusual fullness of the biceps muscle when tensed suggests rupture of the tendinous attachment

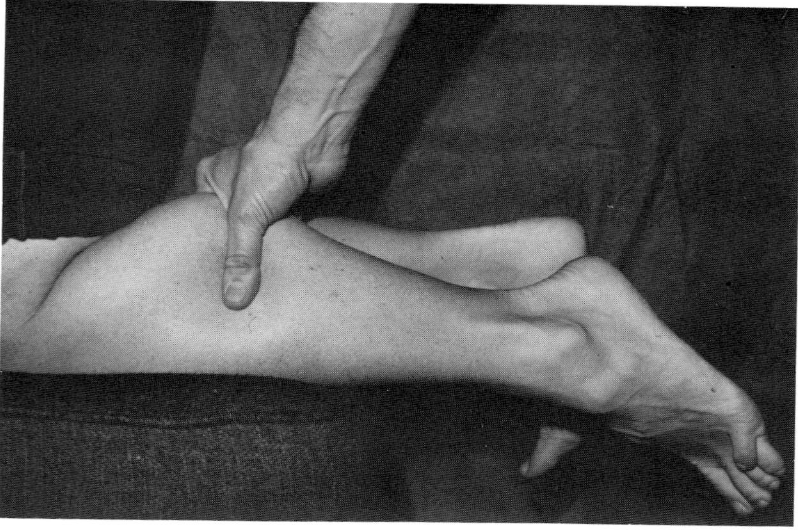

Figure 36.28. Squeeze test for Achilles tendon injury. If tendon is ruptured, plantar flexion will not occur; this tendon is intact.

of the long head. This rupture is often associated with shoulder pain, but there is little or no loss of strength in elbow flexion. Surgical repair improves the appearance of the arm by eliminating the muscle bulge, but does not necessarily improve function.

At the knee, rupture of the quadriceps or patellar tendon results in inability to fully extend the knee actively; a defect above or below the patella can usually be palpated. These ruptures are common in patients taking oral or parenteral steroids and usually require surgical repair.

In the leg, a sudden pushoff can rupture a tendon; the patient usually reports a sharp snap or a sensation as being hit in the back of the calf with a rock. In diagnosing this injury, the emergency physician should differentiate among three conditions: (*a*) rupture of the plantaris tendon, which causes tenderness and swelling, followed by ecchymosis in the upper part of the calf or at the lateral ankle; (*b*) partial tear of the musculotendinous junction of the gastrocnemius muscle, termed "tennis leg," which is diagnosed by eliciting point tenderness of the medial calf at the inferior edge of the muscle belly; and (*c*) rupture of the Achilles tendon, which is indicated by weakness of plantar flexion, a palpable gap just above the os calcis, and a positive squeeze test. For the squeeze test, the patient kneels with the feet hanging free, the calf musculature is squeezed, and plantar flexion results if the Achilles tendon is intact; there will be no motion of the ankle if it is ruptured (Fig. 36.28). X-ray findings are normal in tendon injuries.

Plantaris ruptures or partial tears of the gastrocnemius muscles are treated symptomatically with ice, crutches, and a raised-heel shoe. Achilles tendon ruptures are usually treated by open repair with cast immobilization, foot in equinus.

SUGGESTED READINGS

Angtuaco EJC, Binet EF. Radiology of thoracic and lumbar fractures. *Clin Orthop*, 1984;189:43–57.

Blount WP. *Fractures in Children.* Baltimore: Williams & Wilkins, 1954.

Burke JF, Boyd RJ, McCabe CJ, eds. *Trauma Management.* Chicago: Year Book, 1988.

Charnley, J. *The Closed Treatment of Common Fractures.* 3rd ed. Baltimore, Williams & Wilkins, 1961.

Crenshaw AH, ed. *Campbell's Operative Orthopaedics.* 5th ed. St. Louis, CV Mosby, 1971.

DePalma A. *The Management of Fractures and Dislocations: An Atlas.* Philadelphia, WB Saunders, 1970.

Emergency Care and Transportation of the Sick and Injured. Committee on Allied Health, American Academy of Orthopaedic Surgeons. Chicago, 1977.

Gulliny SF, Ward RF, Holcroft JW, et al. Immediate external fixation of pelvic fractures. *Am J Surg*, 1985;150:721–724.

Harris, JH Jr, Harris WH. *The Radiology of Emergency Medicine*, 2nd ed. Baltimore: Williams & Wilkins, 1981.

Heppenstall C (ed). *Fracture Treatment and Healing,* Philadelphia, WB Saunders, 1980.

Rang M. *Children's Fractures*. Philadelphia. JB Lippencott, 1974.

Rockwood CA Jr, Green DP, eds. *Fractures*. Philadelphia: JB Lippincott, 1975.

Watson-Jones R. *Fractures and Joint Injuries.* Baltimore. Williams & Wilkins, 1952 (vol 1), 1955 (vol 2).

Whitesides TE Jr, Haney TC, Morimoto K, et al. Tissue pressure measurements as a determinant for the need of fasciotomy. *Clin Orthop*, 1975;113:43–51.

CHAPTER 37

Neurosurgical Emergencies

LAWRENCE F. BORGES, M.D.
JAMES G. WEPSIC, M.D.

Numerous catastrophic disorders of the central nervous system may require evaluation and treatment in an emergency department. Such problems include: occlusive carotid artery disease, subarachnoid hemorrhage from aneurysm or arteriovenous malformation, spontaneous intracerebral hemorrhage, brain tumor, brain abscess, and subdural or epidural empyema. The initial management of these disorders is discussed in Chapter 15. This chapter focuses on the management of trauma to the brain and spinal cord. The management of upper limb traumatic peripheral nerve injuries is described in Chapter 41.

HEAD INJURY

Trauma to the central nervous system is common. Approximately 70% of all serious accidents involve injury to the central nervous system. Epidemiological studies have determined that the annual incidence for significant head injury is 274 per 100,000, while that for less serious head injury is 673 per 100,000. Although most serious head injuries are the result of road traffic accidents, other activities also result in significant head trauma. One study estimated that 1% of all high school football players sustained a significant head injury each year.

Head injuries are not only common problems in the emergency department; they also stress the resources of most facilities. Most serious head injuries from road traffic accidents occur late at night or on weekends. It is therefore crucial that facilities likely to receive such patients have an efficient system of management unaffected by these conditions. Such a system, the Level I trauma center, must include the ready availability of a neurosurgeon, computed axial tomographic (CAT) scan facilities, operating room, and intensive care unit. Civilian and wartime experience has demonstrated that the overall mortality and morbidity from serious head injuries is lowered substantially when the patient is transported directly to a facility that provides complete neurosurgical diagnostic studies and definitive treatment. Emergency facilities without the resources for full management of central nervous system trauma must be capable of rapid stabilization and transfer of these patients to a Level I trauma center with neurosurgical expertise. Patients to be transported with serious head injuries should be intubated, and hypoxia, hypercapnia, and hypotension should be corrected.

Management at the Accident

The first priority in treating a patient with a head injury is the maintenance of a satisfactory airway and proper ventilation during every phase of treatment. Hypoxia and hypercapnia greatly exacerbate the brain swelling seen with major intracranial trauma; prevention of these abnormalities takes precedence over other initial considerations. Insertion of a nasotracheal or endotracheal tube to guarantee a patent airway, proper ventilation, and to prevent aspiration may be lifesaving in the comatose patient and may limit subsequent neural damage from hypoxia. Such a task is performed readily by a paramedic trained in advanced life-support techniques. All patients with a significant head injury should be assumed to have a concomitant unstable cervical spine injury. Therefore, flexion and extension of the neck must be avoided during intubation. Administration of this advanced life-support care at the scene of an accident has been credited with the recent reduction in morbidity and mortality in San Diego County (Klauder et al).

When personnel with advanced life-support training are not available to perform on-scene tracheal intubation, or when the victim is not comatose, the patient should be managed by placing him on his side to allow gravity drainage of oral contents. Debris should be cleared from the mouth and any loose objects, such as dentures, should be removed. The jaw can be pulled outward to facilitate a proper airway. Patients transported in this manner should be strapped to a body board with cervical spine immobilization.

Once an airway has been established, significant bleeding or shock are next addressed, as outlined in Chapter 4. In particular, any sizable scalp laceration should be managed with a pressure bandage to control blood loss while en route to the emergency department.

Following these initial resuscitative measures, the paramedics or ambulance personnel should obtain a *succinct* history of the event and perform a *rapid* initial neurological evaluation. An accurate history concerning the mechanism of the injury is of utmost importance and is usually obtained from friends, coworkers, or passersby. Sometimes a fall is the result of a neurological catastrophe, such as a subarachnoid hemorrhage from a ruptured aneurysm. An accurate description of the events leading to the injury often guide the emergency department physicians to a correct diagnostic formulation. Other information of the medical history, such as medications, allergies, existing conditions, and drug or ethanol intoxication, may also be available at the accident scene. The neurological examination should be brief and oriented around the Glasgow Coma Scale (Table 37.1). This straightforward method of assessment is easily mastered and is seldom prone to misinterpretation. In addition, the pupils should be observed for size and degree of reactivity. Subsequent alterations in patient responses are important in guiding additional diagnostic and therapeutic intervention.

Table 37.1.
Glasgow Coma Scale

Verbal Response	
Oriented	5
Confused conversation	4
Inappropriate words	3
Incomprehensible sounds	2
None	1
Eye Opening	
Spontaneous	4
To speech	3
To pain	2
None	1
Best Motor Response	
Obeys	6
Localizes pain	5
Withdraws	4
Abnormal flexion	3
Abnormal extension	2
None	1
Maximum total:	15

Add the figure for each component. The higher the score, the better the prognosis.

Management in the Emergency Department

Airway

Initially, the emergency department should reassess the patency of the airway and the adequacy of ventilation. Nonintubated patients in coma or with significant alterations in consciousness should have an endotracheal tube placed to maintain ventilation and to prevent aspiration. Once intubated, these patients are placed on a respirator and hyperventilated to maintain the Pco_2 of 26–30 mm Hg and the Po_2 > 80 mm Hg. Initially, the average adult should be ventilated at a rate of 14 breaths/minute and a tidal volume of 800–1100 ml, using 100% oxygen. Subsequently, arterial blood gases are monitored to guide ventilation adjustments.

Circulation

The adequacy of the circulation and the causes of hypotension should be identified and corrected next. Approximately 15% of patients with head injury present in shock. Head injury is associated with the loss of cerebrovascular autoregulatory mechanisms. Therefore, brain function cannot be adequately assessed in hypotensive patients with head injury. Patients with systolic blood pressures of 60–70 mm Hg may be unresponsive, only to "awaken" when the systemic blood pressure is elevated to a level greater than 100 mm Hg. Prolonged hypotension may also lead to further neuronal damage. Cerebral perfusion pressure must be maintained above 40 mm Hg to prevent cerebral ischemia. Since increased intracranial pressure commonly accompanies brain trauma, systemic hypotension further reduces cerebral perfusion pressure and exacerbates neuronal ischemia. Patients with head injury and shock have a twofold higher mortality rate and a higher incidence of permanent neurological morbidity than do patients without shock.

Head injury, by itself, does not result in shock, except in unusual circumstances. Therefore, the cause of shock in these patients must be sought in other injury sites. Infants, with open skull sutures usually less than 1 year old, may lose enough blood into an intracranial hematoma to become hypotensive. Scalp lacerations, particularly those that transect the superficial temporal or occipital arteries, may result in the loss of a large quantity of blood and subsequent hypotension. This occurs most commonly in children. Children and adults both may develop hypotension from the blood loss that accompanies dural sinus tears. Dural sinus injuries also may result in air emboli, which themselves cause hypotension. Massive injury to the medullary cardiovascular centers is perhaps the only discrete brain lesion that produces hypotension. These patients are usually apneic and flaccid and do not survive the injury. Hypotension with warm extremities may occur following injury to the spinal cord and may be an early indication of spinal cord injury in a comatose patient.

Prior to the ultimate departure of ambulance personnel from the emergency department, the historical facts about the accident and the details of the initial neurological evaluation should be conveyed to the emergency department physicians. Additional historical details should be obtained from the relatives as soon as is practical. A thorough neurological evaluation is obtained next and recorded carefully. Along with the previous evaluations by the ambulance personnel, it represents the baseline from which subsequent neurological improvement or worsening is determined.

Level of Consciousness

The single most important factor in determining the presence of significant or worsening neurological dysfunction at any stage is the level of consciousness. Orientation and ability to speak in clear, lucid sentences are assessed easily in awake patients. Such patients should be queried about headaches, visual disturbances, hearing loss, numbness, tingling and pain in the neck, back, or elsewhere. Patients with significant facial fractures may have been intubated for airway control and be unable to respond verbally. Their level of alertness may be ascertained by asking them to hold up a specific number of fingers, to hold up the number of fingers that are left when 16 is subtracted from 20, or to perform a three-step touching task. *Repeat testing of the level of consciousness should be performed often in the emergency department.* Expanding intracranial hematomas or worsening cerebral edema cause alterations in the level of consciousness prior to affecting other parts of the neurological examination. Patients with expanding intracranial mass lesions may become noisy, boisterous, and obstreperous before becoming drowsy. Therefore, any change in the level of consciousness should be evaluated promptly with a cranial CAT scan to rule out worsening intracranial pathology.

Ocular Movements

The neural pathways that subserve pupillary and extraocular movement traverse large areas of the central nervous system. Therefore, their evaluation provides important information to help localize structural lesions. The size of the pupils and their reactivity to light are noted and checked frequently. Toxic and metabolic causes of coma do not usually cause pupillary abnormalities. Although pupillary dilatation may occur secondary to direct orbital trauma, a unilaterally dilated pupil that does not constrict to bright light implies transtentorial herniation until proven otherwise by a CAT scan. Bilaterally fixed and dilated pupils occur with rostral midbrain injuries, with bilateral transtentorial herniation, and in the terminal phase of tentorial herniation or brainstem compression. They can also occur following significant hypoxia. Pontine lesions disrupt descending sympathetic pathways, irritate parasympathetic pathways, and produce bilaterally small pupils. Lateral medullary damage causes a mild Horner's syndrome. Patients in light coma may exhibit spontaneously roving side-to-side eye movements when their eyelids are opened manually. These patients are often aroused with noxious stimuli to a state of thrashing and incomprehensible swearing, at which time the eyes fix conjugately on the examiner. When left undisturbed, they quiet down, close their eyes and again demonstrate the roving eye movements. Such eye movements are not indicative of a specific structural lesion, but rather demonstrate that the brainstem pathways between the midbrain and lower pons that subserve extraocular movements are intact. In the absence of such roving eye movements, the integrity of these pathways may be demonstrated by assessing "doll's eyes'' movements or the eye movements produced by irrigation of the ear canals with ice water (ice water caloric testing). Testing ''doll's eyes'' movements requires turning the head rapidly from side to side. Such a test is inappropriate in the comatose patient unless a cervical spine injury has been ruled out *conclusively*. Ice water caloric testing can be performed without moving the head, irrigating 50 ml of ice water into one ear canal. After five minutes, this is repeated in the opposite ear canal. *This test should not be performed if the tympanic membrane is ruptured or if blood or cerebrospinal fluid is present in the external ear canal.* The normal response following ice water irrigation into the right ear is nystagmus with the slow component toward the right ear and the fast component toward the left. The nystagmus is rhythmic, regular, lasting 2–3 minutes, and is not associated with significant deviation of the eyes from the midline. As consciousness is lost from worsening supratentorial tissue damage, the fast component is lost and the eyes tonically deviate toward the ear irrigated with the ice water. Patients with pathology that involves the brainstem itself also lose the conjugate tonic deviation. Vertical eye movements are assessed in the comatose patient by simultaneous irrigation of both auditory canals with ice water. If the oculovestibular pathways are intact, the eyes should deviate downward. Conjugate lateral deviation of the eyes is sometimes observed in the comatose patient in the absence of caloric stimulation. This indicates destruction of the ipsilateral cortical frontal eye field, an irritative lesion of the contralateral frontal eye field, or a destructive lesion in the pons in the region of the abducens nucleus.

Motor function. Motor function is evaluated by observation of the posture and tone of the extremities, and by the appraisal of voluntary movement, spontaneous movement, or movement in response to noxious stimuli. Voluntary motor power is assessed using the international scale outlined in Table 37.2. If depressed consciousness precludes voluntary muscle testing, then the response to noxious stimuli is assessed. Noxious stimuli should produce a strong attempt to move the limb away from the offending stimulus, often accompanied by a groan or grimace. Such a response implies the presence of functioning sensory pathways, as well as partially intact descending motor input from cerebral cortex to muscle. A flaccid limb that does not respond to noxious stimulation may result from damage to the brain, spinal cord, neural plexus or peripheral nerve. Abnormal posturing or movement of the limb into, rather than away from, a noxious stimulus, indicates damage to the cerebral hemispheres or brainstem. These abnormal postures have conventionally been called *decorticate* and *decerebrate* rigidity. Neither physiological studies nor human postmortem material provide a precise anatomical basis for these abnormal responses to noxious stimuli. In response to a noxious stimulus, a patient with decorticate posturing exhibits flexion of the elbow and wrist, and extension of the leg. This posture reflects more rostral and less severe supratentorial impairment than that associated with decerebrate posturing. A patient with decerebrate posturing extends both arm and leg and externally rotates the arm. This posture implies deeper, more severe supratentorial dysfunction. Extensor responses in the arms combined with flexion at the knees is seen most commonly with pontine lesions. Flexor responses in the upper extremities have been associated with a higher potential for recovery than extensor responses in the upper extremities. Diffuse muscle flaccidity, with little or no response to noxious stimulation, implies severe brainstem damage distal to the lower pontomedullary regions.

Table 37.2.
Assessment of Motor Power

Normal power	5
Active movement against gravity and some resistance	4
Active movement against gravity	3
Active movement with gravity eliminated	2
Flicker or trace of contraction	1
No contraction	0

Neurological evaluation also includes an external evaluation of the head, looking for lacerations, skull fractures, facial bone fractures, mastoid ecchymosis (Battle's sign—indicative of a basilar skull fracture), hemotympanum, periorbital ecchymosis, otorrhea, and rhinorrhea. If time permits, the ocular fundi should be evaluated with an ophthalmoscope to assess for retinal hemorrhages and the presence of venous pulsations. Papilledema does not develop for hours to days after elevation of intracranial pressure. Therefore, its absence is of no clinical significance in acute trauma.

Uncal Herniation. The syndrome of a unilaterally expanding mass lesion that produces uncal herniation, such as from an epidural hematoma, should be familiar to all emergency department physicians. As the hematoma expands, the state of alertness changes. The level of alertness varies from combativeness to near coma. The earliest consistent physical finding in these patients is the unilaterally dilating pupil. Initially, the pupils appear unequal in size. The larger pupil exhibits a more sluggish response to light. At this stage, the respirations, extraocular movements, and motor responses may be normal. A sign of Babinski is often noted contralateral to the dilated pupil. As the condition worsens, the pupil dilates widely (6–7 mm) and no longer constricts in response to a bright light. Hemiplegia contralateral to the dilated pupil appears. This may rapidly progress to decorticate and finally to decerebrate posturing, unilaterally or bilaterally. If the opposite cerebral peduncle is compressed against the medial edge of the tentorium (Kennohan's notch phenomenon), hemiplegia develops ipsilateral to the dilated pupil. In the absence of successful treatment, signs of midbrain damage appear and progress. The opposite pupil may dilate or become midpositional (5–6 mm), and be fixed to light. Respiratory abnormalities, especially hyperpnea, are common. Oculovestibular responses are lost. Motor dysfunction progresses to bilateral decerebrate ridigity.

Once the signs of uncal herniation appear, they may progress rapidly; removal or correction of the offending lesion must proceed forthwith. *Patients who arrive awake in the emergency department, only to exhibit those characteristic neurological changes, should be taken directly to the operating room.*

Adjuncts to Management

The management of patients with central nervous system injury in the emergency department is often facilitated by the use of certain adjuncts. Since many of these are used in both head and spinal cord injury, they are discussed here.

Dehydration. The cranial vault is a closed compartment; therefore, cerebral swelling secondary to head injury may cause further compromise to brain blood flow and lead to more widespread neuronal dysfunction and necrosis. *Controlled hyperventilation* helps to regulate intracranial pressure; most patients with serious head injury, however, should also be managed with *dehydrating agents.* The most commonly used is mannitol. Mannitol, the six-carbon alcohol of mannose, is a nonmetabolized hyperosmolar substance supplied in a 20% solution. It must be kept in a warming closet to prevent precipitation of the mannitol crystals. Mannitol creates an osmotic gradient that acts to dehydrate those portions of the brain that have an intact blood-brain barrier. It improves blood flow through the microcirculation. This effect may be more important in spinal cord injury. During initial management, 1–1.5 gm/kg is administered by rapid intravenous infusion. Because the mannitol solution contains 20 gm mannitol per 100 solution, the average 60–70 kg adult should receive one 500 ml bottle of mannitol initially. Additional doses of 0.25–0.5 gm/kg can be administered every 4–6 hours as needed. Reduction in intracranial pressure is usually evident within 30 minutes, the effect lasting 3–6 hours. Mannitol can be combined with furosemide to increase diuresis and to further lower intracranial pressure. Furosemide should be used with caution in the patient with depleted circulating blood volume. The use of mannitol in spinal cord trauma is currently being assessed at several spinal cord injury centers.

Other agents, such as urea, glycerol, and dimethylsulfoxide, have been used. Their use is neither as safe nor as straightforward as mannitol. The use of mannitol by paramedics at the scene of the accident is also under current study.

Corticosteroids. Corticosteroids are very effective in reducing the cerebral edema associated with brain tumors. While laboratory investigations have demonstrated that steroids reduce the formation of cerebral edema in certain defined experimental traumatic situations, several clinical studies have failed to show that steroids improve the outcome in patients with severe head injury. Some neurosurgeons believe that steroids may be more useful in patients with mild to moderate head injury, by reducing the neuropsychological impairment that follows these injuries.

The dose of steroid appropriate for the patient with head and spinal cord injury remains controversial. Proponents of steroid usage recommend high doses of corticosteroids (an initial 100 mg of dexamethasone, followed by 24–30 mg per day), tapering over 1–2 weeks.

The major short-term complications of corticosteroids include gastrointestinal bleeding, impaired wound healing, and exacerbation of preexisting diabetes mellitus. Patients on corticosteroids should also receive antacids and an H_2 blocker, such as ranitidine or cimetidine.

Anticonvulsants. Patients with structural brain injury are likely to have seizures. Therefore, all patients with serious head injury should receive prophylactic anticonvulsant medication in the emergency department. Phenytoin is the drug of choice; it is rapidly effective and does not interfere with levels of consciousness. Adults should receive 1 gm and children 10 mg/kg as initial loading doses, given intravenously at a rate of 15 mg/min. Subsequently, a maintenance dose of 100 mg every 8 hours is recommended for adults; for children it is 5 mg/kg in divided doses every 8 hours. Maintenance doses are further evaluated and monitored with serum phenytoin levels. If seizures occur despite the administration of phenytoin, phenobarbital therapy is instituted. Children may present to the emergency department in status epilepticus following head injury. In this situation, benzodiazepines are used to control the initial seizures, while the phenobarbital loading dose is completed.

Barbiturates. Despite aggressive treatment with fluid restriction, hyperventilation, and mannitol, severe intracranial hypertension can still occur. High-dose barbiturate therapy with pentobarbital, thiopental, or the newer agent, althesin, may help to control intracranial pressure in these situations. Their principal mode of action is a direct constrictor effect on cerebral vasculature with reduction of cerebral blood volume. These agents are not usually used in the emergency department, but are more common during subsequent management in the intensive care unit.

Temperature Control. Elevated body temperature increases the rate of cerebral metabolism and may increase neuronal dysfunction and cerebral edema. Disordered thermoregulation with elevated body temperatures may be seen in patients with severe head injury. Modest elevations in body temperature are controlled with acetaminophen, while high fevers require cooling blankets and the use of phenothiazines. Hypothalamic injury often presents initially with disordered thermoregulation; the accompanying diabetes insipidus does not appear for 24–48 hours.

Neuropeptides. Many peptides have been identified within the central nervous system. These substances serve as neurotransmitters or neuromodulators and have a number of physiologic and pathophysiologic roles. Endogenous opioids appear to play a pathophysiologic role in the secondary injury that follows spinal trauma, brain trauma, and cerebral ischemia. Therefore, several centers are currently involved in protocols assessing the role of opioid antagonists, such as naloxone or thyrotropin-releasing hormones, in the therapy of head and spinal cord injury. An advantage of these agents, if they prove effective, is that they could be easily administered at the accident scene by paramedics.

Diagnostic Studies

Computed Tomography

Since its clinical introduction by Hounsfield in 1973, computed axial tomographic (CAT) scanning has become the primary diagnostic imaging tool in the evaluation of patients with head trauma. CAT scanning is noninvasive; there is no need to give intravenous contrast agents for the initial evaluation of head trauma. It is also fast. A single scan slice requires an acquisition time of 3 seconds on newer scanners. Rapid scan acquisition minimizes the image degradation from patient motion and makes possible scanning of the entire brain in 10–15 minutes. A good CAT scan demonstrates hematomas anywhere within the cranium, the presence of edema or contusion, the size and position of the ventricles, displacements of the midline, the presence of foreign bodies, the air-fluid levels within paranasal sinuses, and many fractures of the skull and facial bones. CAT scanning is so superior to older imaging modalities that an emergency department without rapid access to a CAT scanner is not fully prepared for the evaluation of head trauma.

The major advantage of CAT scanning is that it allows a high resolution look at the brain tissue itself. Blood with a hematocrit of 45 has an average attenuation of 56 Hounsfield units, which is greater than that in normal brain. Therefore, areas of acute hematoma appear bright white in contrast to the surrounding neural tissue. The high attenuation values for blood are largely secondary to the protein fraction of hemoglobin, while the iron fraction contributes only 7–8% of the attenuation value. Because there is a linear relationship between hematocrit and attenuation, an intracranial hematoma occurring in a severely anemic patient may be isodense with the surrounding brain. Two other potential pitfalls in CAT scan interpretation require mention. CAT scans without intravenous contrast enhancement do not reveal the vascular anatomy of the brain, because circulating blood has the same attenuation values as normal brain. Therefore, traumatic intracranial aneurysms and carotid cavernous fistulae cannot easily be identified on routine CAT scans. Depressed skull fractures at the vertex of the skull may not be identified on routine axial images. The emergency physician seeing serious head injury patients should develop some facility with CAT scan interpretation, so that he or she can better guide the overall evaluation and therapy.

Plain x-ray films of the skull are usually obtained to determine if a skull fracture is present. Most linear and depressed fractures of the convexities will be apparent on skull x-rays. The presence of a skull fracture indicates that a severe force has been imparted to the head; it alerts the physician to the possibility of underlying structural brain damage. The actual yield of abnormalities from skull x-rays is as low as 2–3%, however. Various clinical criteria have been proposed to enhance the yield of skull x-rays, but a standard set of guidelines has not been adopted universally.

Angiography

Prior to the introduction of CAT scanning, cerebral angiography was the standard test to evaluate for the presence of a surgical lesion within the intracranial compartment. Intracranial hematomas were identified because they displaced blood vessels away from their normal positions. The widespread availability of CAT scanners has markedly reduced the use of angiography in the acute situation. However, cerebral angiography still has a role in the later evaluation of intracranial vascular trauma, as in traumatic aneurysm and carotid-cavernous fistula.

Radiological modalities, such as ventriculography, radioisotope brain scanning, and echoencephalography, have no place in the current evaluation of head trauma. Similarly, electroencephalography and lumbar puncture should not be used acutely in these patients.

Magnetic Resonance Imaging

Magnetic resonance imaging (MRI) is the newest modality and offers the promise of even higher resolution than CAT scanning, easy acquisition of sagittal images, and visualization of proximal intracranial arteries without the use of intravenous contrast agents. Despite these advantages, several features limit its practical usefulness at present: *(a)* interpretation of bony detail and fractures is not as clear as on CAT scans; *(b)* MRI scanners are more expensive and not generally available and, when available, are often physically removed from the emergency department because of space required for the magnetic fields; *(c)* the powerful magnetic fields surrounding the scanner preclude the use of metallic devices within the scan room, making special provisions necessary for ventilated patients; *(d)* the time necessary to acquire the scan is considerably longer than with CAT scanners. As MRI technology improves, and experience with it increases, it may come to have a greater role in the acute evaluation of patients with head injury.

Clinically Important Head Injuries

Scalp Lacerations

Because of its luxuriant blood supply, the scalp shares with the face the distinction of being the most rapidly healing, infection-resistant tissue in the human body. This vascularity can be a liability, however, in that extensive scalp lacerations can result in major shock-producing blood loss. Bleeding is controlled easily by digital pressure or by application of fine hemostats to the arterial bleeders with eversion of the galea aponeurotica while the initial neurologic and general medical appraisal proceeds. Repair of lacerations should await examination of skull x-ray films to determine whether a more serious injury requiring operation is present.

If the injury is limited to the scalp, the surrounding hair should be shaved, the skin antiseptically prepared, and the scalp infiltrated about the wound with 1% lidocaine, with epinephrine, injected through healthy scalp rather than through the edges of the wound. Satisfactory anesthesia can be achieved by field block if the physician is familiar with the innervation of the scalp. The area is then reprepared, drapes applied, and the wound irrigated with saline solution to remove hair and foreign material, such as road dirt or gravel. If the laceration is full thickness, the underlying skull should be inspected visually and *digitally* for fracture. Any fracture is, by definition, compound, and should be assessed by a CAT scan. If no bony depression, indriven fragments or intracranial clots are identified, the laceration may be carefully closed using full aseptic technique in the emergency department. Otherwise, the injury should be repaired in the operating room. If no fracture is found, contused devitalized skin, galea, and periosteum are trimmed to viable tissue and the wound closed without drainage. Regardless of the method, the integrity of closure rests on the strength of the galea. These wounds can be closed with either a layer of absorbable sutures in the galea plus nylon or polyester sutures in the skin, or by full-thickness sutures of wire, nylon or polyester, taking particular care to include the galea.

Lacerations involving loss of small areas of scalp often can be closed as described above if tension-free apposition of the wound edges can be obtained by undermining the surrounding scalp in the subgaleal plane. Larger areas of scalp loss may require advancement or rotational scalp flaps; plastic surgical assistance should be sought in these circumstances.

In infants, cephalohematoma may occur as a consequence of birth trauma or after minor injury. Usually subgaleal, the swelling dissects over wide areas of skull; if it is subperiosteal, expansion of the clot is limited by the joints of the skull, and the configuration of the mass conforms with the anatomy of the underlying bone. In these small patients, the mass may become alarmingly large, but the temptation to aspirate these clots should be resisted; they eventually undergo spontaneous resorption. A cephalohematoma may occasionally become calcified, but the resultant cosmetic defect is rectified later by natural remodeling.

Linear Skull Fractures

The finding of a linear skull fracture on x-ray examination serves as an indicator of the force and locus of the blow to the head, and should alert the physician to the possibility of a serious underlying brain lesion. In the cadaver skull, it has been shown that the striking force must increase to 400–800 kg/0.001 sec to produce a linear frontal bone fracture. Greater force is required to produce comminuted or depressed skull fractures. Approximately 80% of skull fractures are linear. Many simple linear fractures are unaccompanied by structural brain damage, but they may occur with any combination or degree of intrinsic brain injury or intracranial hematoma. Conversely, some patients with devastating brain injuries have no fracture. Most fractures of the convex skull are diagnosed easily on plain x-ray films, but fractures of the base of the skull, extending into the paranasal sinuses, orbits or the middle ear, are usually demonstrated only by special views or on CAT scans. Some basal fractures are manifested by the clinical signs of blood behind the tympanic membrane, i.e., fracture of the petrous pyramid, or cerebrospiral fluid (CSF) leakage, i.e., fracture into paranasal sinus or middle ear. Some are indicated by associated x-ray findings, such as, intracranial air or opacification or air-fluid levels within the sinuses.

The fracture itself requires no treatment. Most acute epidural hematomas and almost all posterior fossa hematomas, however, occur with fractures crossing the vascular grooves of the middle meningeal vessels or extending into the foramen magnum, respectively. However, 10% of these fractures may be small enough to escape detection on plain radiographs. In addition, some of the complications of linear skull fractures are delayed in appearance or in recognition. For these reasons, in-hospital observation for at least 24 hours is advisable in patients suspected of having these fractures. The indications for CAT scan evaluation of linear fractures are listed in Table 37.3.

Depressed Skull Fractures

A greater force or a more sharply focused blow is required for depressed fracture than for linear fracture; the bone is comminuted and splits in the plane of the middle table as it is driven inward. The brain may escape injury with minor degrees of depression, but dural and cortical laceration-contusion is common and may give rise to subdural or intracerebral hemorrhage in as many as 30% of cases. The extent and location of the focal brain wound and the presence of associated hematoma determine the nature of the resultant neurologic deficit. These fractures are diagnosed on plain x-ray films (Fig. 37.1), often supplemented with tangential views noting the deformity of the calvarium or the increased density in regions of bone fragment overlap. The degree of depression and comminution is usually underestimated by this method. CAT scans almost always reveal these fractures. They often are detected by visual or digital examination of scalp lacerations.

Table 37.3.
Indications for CAT Scan Evaluation of Linear Skull Fractures

1. Severe headache or vomiting
2. Worsening neurological status
3. Fracture line enters posterior fossa, especially if it enters foramen magnun
4. Fracture line crosses an obvious vascular groove in the skull, or a dural sinus
5. Any evidence of depression
6. Fracture line enters an air-containing sinus

Surgical elevation is indicated for fractures depressed by more than the thickness of the skull, particularly if they lie adjacent to the motor strip or speech cortex. Small depressions over the cerebellum do not require repair, and those over dural venous sinuses are best left undisturbed unless sinus obstruction or hemorrhage is present. Eighty percent of depressed skull fractures are compound fractures. Compound depressed skull fractures should be repaired as early as possible to lessen the risk of wound infection leading to meningitis or brain abscess. The infection rate in cases treated promptly should be under 5%, with a concomitant decrease in the incidence of posttraumatic epilepsy.

The surgical approach to these lesions is through a scalp flap placed about the circumference of the depressed area. These fractures are usually impacted tightly, and a burr hole at the perimeter is usually required to gain access to the epidural space. Sometimes the depressed fragments can be levered gently into place with a periosteal elevator; more often, portions of the depression must be removed with a ronguer before this can be done. If dura and cortex are lacerated, they are suitably debrided and hemostasis obtained before dural closure. Underlying cortical markings are usually visible through intact dura, but if they are not seen unmistakably, the dura should be opened to exclude the presence of subdural hematoma. Larger bone fragments can be wired into place, and residual gaps in the skull can be filled with bits of bone laid in as a mosaic graft; they are usually incorporated if postoperative infection is prevented. Every attempt is made to preserve bone fragments, especially those that comprise cosmetically important parts of the skull, such as the frontal bone and supraorbital ridges. If bone fragments enter an air-containing sinus, such as the frontal sinus, the mucosa of the sinus should be removed, the nasofrontal duct obliterated, and the sinus cavity filled with autologous fat. The bone fragments are then wired into place to restore a cosmetically acceptable forehead appearance.

Depressed fractures in infants, often called "ping-pong" fractures, rarely undergo spontaneous resolution and usually require elevation. The flexible bone of infants, unlike that of adults, usually can be reduced by a periosteal elevator placed through an adjacent burr hole, which is then filled with bone dust.

Complications of Skull Fractures

Carotid-Cavernous Fistula. Basal fractures of the sphenoid bone and missile injuries may result in carotid-cavernous fistulas from laceration of the internal carotid artery as it courses within the cavernous sinus. The syndrome is also produced by spontaneous rupture of an intracavernous carotid

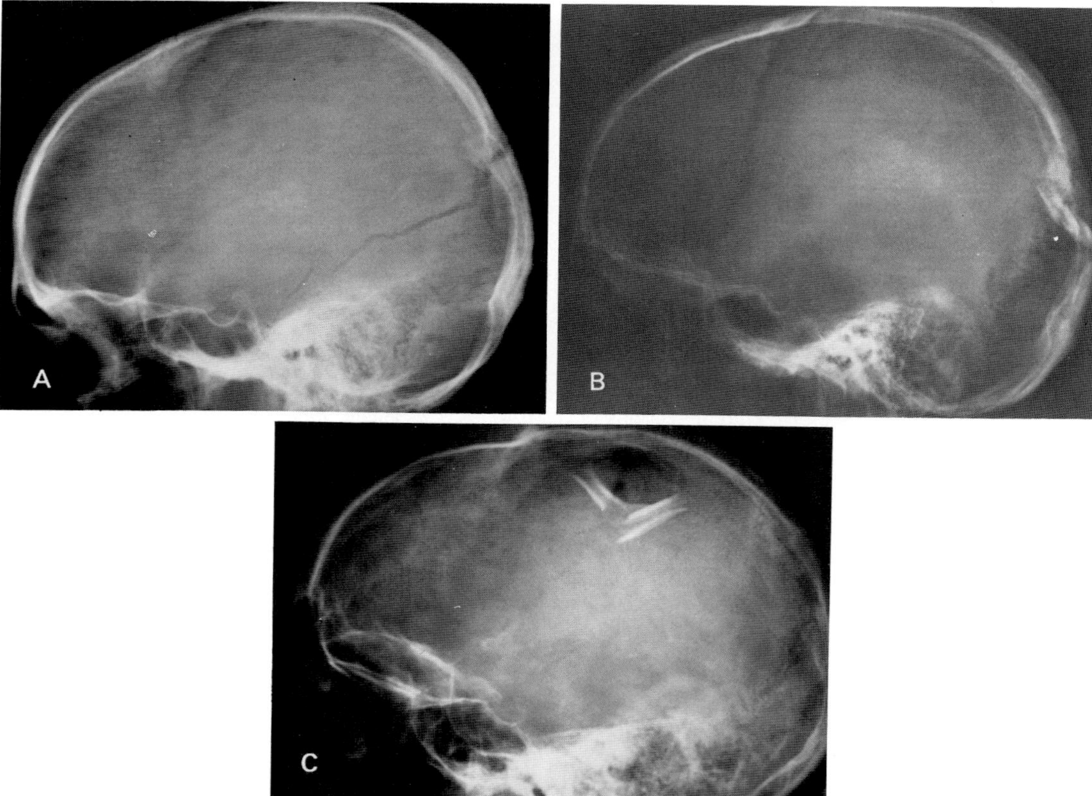

Figure 37.1. Skull fractures. *A,* Linear parietoccipital fracture that crosses midline posteriorly. Sagittal sinus laceration may occur with this fracture. *B,* Depressed occipital fracture with associated sinus laceration. *C,* Depressed parietal fracture with cerebral laceration by bony fragments.

artery aneurysm. Blood perfuses the cavernous sinus under arterial pressure, and causes extreme dilatation of tributary veins and retrograde flow into the orbits; intracranial rupture seldom occurs. Massive conjunctival injection, chemosis, scleral hemorrhage, and bilateral pulsating exophthalmos follow. A bruit may be audible over the orbits, temple, or forehead. Continued progression results in extraocular palsies and loss of vision.

Obliteration of the fistula may be accomplished by interventional neuroradiological techniques. A calibrated-leak, flow-directed balloon is guided into the fistula from a transfemoral arterial approach, and inflated. In many instances, the fistula may be closed, while normal carotid artery flow is preserved. Transient worsening of cavernous sinus symptoms may persist for 1–2 weeks after balloon inflation. The relative safety of this procedure suggests that it should be attempted before open-trapping procedures.

Cranial Nerve Injury. Injury to a cranial nerve usually results from a fracture through the foramen of its exit at the base of the skull. The *olfactory* nerve is the most frequently affected, and may be damaged either by cribriform plate fracture or by the shearing action of the brain at the moment of a blow to the occiput, which can avulse the olfactory filaments as they pass through the cribriform plate. The resultant anosmia is permanent, but rather than complaining of loss of smell, patients tend to complain more of distortion or loss of taste, since appreciation of flavor is mediated largely by olfactory perception. Injury to the *optic* nerve from fracture through the optic foramen is rare. Since this nerve develops embryologically as a fiber tract of the brain, regeneration does not occur, and surgical decompression of the optic foramen has been unsuccessful in restoring lost vision, except in unusual circumstances. Surgical decompression of an optic foramen should be performed only if visual function worsens under medical observation. Patients whose eyes are blind from the moment of impact are not candidates for decompressive surgery.

Partial or complete *oculomotor* palsy may be a result of transtentorial herniation; the nerve is compressed at the tentorial notch by the medial temporal lobe that is displaced by an expanding intracranial mass. These patients are comatose with other ominous signs of hemispheral and brainstem dysfunction. Oculomotor nerve palsy in a conscious patient, with signs of trauma to the face or front of the head, is likely to be due to injury within the orbit. The *trochlear* and *abducens* nerves may also be injured in the orbit or from fracture through the superior orbital fissure. Occasionally, isolated abducens nerve palsy occurs as a false lateralizing sign, from diffuse brain injury of any degree or simply from raised intracranial pressure.

Intracranial injury to the *trigeminal* nerve is uncommon, but sensory loss due to division of its peripheral branches is frequently encountered with facial lacerations and fractures; rarely, painful facial dysesthesias are a late sequela. Facial lacerations should be closed carefully to avoid further injury to the nerve or its inclusion in the suture. The prognosis for regeneration of the nerve with restoration of sensation is excellent.

Fractures through the petrous portion of the temporal bone may injure the *facial* nerve or the auditory or vestibular branches (or both) of the *acoustic* nerve. Peripheral facial palsies are characterized by paralysis of the ipsilateral side of the face, including the forehead, whereas central facial palsies of cortical origin spare the forehead because of the bilateral innervation of forehead muscles. Facial palsies may be immediate or may occur days after injury, the so-called tardy facial palsy. Neither type requires operation, but the chances of recovery are much better with the delayed type. Function cannot be recovered after acoustic nerve injury, but patients with posttraumatic hearing loss should undergo otologic evaluation, lest potentially treatable causes of conduction deafness, such as ossicular disruption, be overlooked.

Injuries to the lower cranial nerves are usually the result of penetrating wounds outside the skull.

Cerebrospinal Fluid Rhinorrhea and Otorrhea. About 5% of patients have cerebrospinal (CSF) rhinorrhea or otorrhea after closed-head injury. CSF leakage requires a pathway of communication from the subarachnoid space into the sinuses, nasopharynx, or middle ear through a dural tear, fractured bone, and lacerated mucosa. Fractures into the ethmoid sinus through the cribriform plate or into frontal or sphenoid sinuses are the common avenues of rhinorrhea. CSF in the middle ear results in otorrhea if the tympanic membrane is ruptured; if not, CSF may flow through the eustachian canal into the nasopharynx and give rise to an interesting variety of rhinorrhea. The fluid is identified as CSF by testing for glucose and chloride content. Saliva and nasal secretions contain negligible amounts of glucose, whereas the glucose level in CSF is about two-thirds that in blood, and the CSF chloride concentration is approximately 120 mEq/liter.

Patients with CSF leakage are treated with bed rest and the head elevated; they are instructed not to blow the nose or attempt to stem the flow of fluid, lest they cause retrograde flow of contaminated debris into the subarachnoid space. Otorrhea usually stops within 1–3 days; operative treatment seldom is required. In about 85% of patients with rhinorrhea, the leak closes spontaneously, but a small percentage of patients may return months or even years later with delayed meningitis.

The role of prophylactic antibiotics remains unsettled, but since the most common organism resulting in meningitis, secondary to rhinorrhea, is *Streptococcus pneumoniae,* some surgeons advocate antibiotic use in this group of patients and in patients with preexistent sinusitis or ear infection.

If the fracture is complex, identification of the pathway of the CSF fistula may be difficult and may require CT scanning in both axial and coronal planes, conventional tomography, and dye or radioisotope studies in conjunction with careful ear-nose-and-throat examination.

Generally accepted indications for surgical repair include persistent rhinorrhea, meningitis, and cerebral herniation into the fracture. Surgical repair is accomplished after brain swelling has subsided and after any overt infection has been eradicated.

Intrinsic Brain Injuries

Cerebral Concussion. The clinical correlates of cerebral concussion include: (*a*) amnesia—retrograde amnesia for events immediately preceding injury, and a usually longer period of antegrade amnesia for happenings after injury; and (*b*) a period of unconsciousness lasting up to 5 minutes. Longer periods of unconsciousness are likely to be related to at least minor degrees of brain contusion. Young children occasionally manifest generalized seizures or transient cortical blindness after concussion; these are alarming phenomena, but are not necessarily of unfavorable prognostic importance. Generalized seizures should be treated promptly with anticonvulsants.

These patients should be admitted for overnight observation. X-ray films of the skull should be obtained, but CAT scans or other diagnostic studies are not ordinarily required unless lethargy, vomiting, or focal neurological signs are observed.

In uncomplicated cerebral concussion, neurologic deficit is maximal at the time of injury and is followed by rapid and steady improvement. Variations from this course should alert the physician to the possibility of a more serious head injury.

Concussion or minor head injury afflicts 1.5–2 million persons in the United States each year and constitute over 50% of all head injuries. Although CAT scans are usually normal in these patients, pathological studies have revealed evidence of diffuse axonal disruption. Although these patients may have a normal neurological examination on discharge from the hospital, they may experience difficulty returning to former levels of activity or employment for 3–6 months. Most patients score lower on neuropsychological tests than the expected norms, with the principal problems being cognitive deficits in attention, concentration, memory, and judgment. Consistent support, encouragement, and recognition of this syndrome helps such patients return to gainful employment.

Cerebral Contusion. Mechanical damage to the brain at the moment of impact results from the linear and rotational forces imparted by the blow, which disrupts axons and nerve cell bodies and frequently lacerates the cerebral cortex. Coincident vascular damage may give rise to acute subdural or intracerebral hematoma, or traumatic subarachnoid hemorrhage, depending on the size and location of the injured vessel. The area of structural injury may be limited to the cortex and adjacent white matter directly beneath the blow, or in the case of contrecoup contusion, it may be limited to the opposite side of the brain, with the tips and undersurfaces of frontal and temporal lobes the sites of predilection. With larger impact forces, extensive disruption of white matter occurs deep within the cerebral hemispheres and brainstem. The clinical spectrum of patients with brain contusion ranges from those with minor damage and a neurological syndrome only slightly more severe than cerebral concussion, to those having devastating brain destruction with decerebration and irreversible coma. Brain contusions are common in the absence of either fracture or hematoma, and are a major cause of death or lasting neurologic disability.

The syndrome of *primary brainstem injury* deserves special mention because controversy has surrounded notions about its very existence. Extensive, direct brainstem trauma is so incompatible with life, that most patients are never examined in the emergency department. However, large clinical services encounter some patients with primary brainstem pathology who can survive for several days. Typical pathological findings include a pontomedullary tear, laceration at the pontomesencephalic junction, or complete separation of the cervicomedullary junction. All these lesions occur at the moment of impact and are incompatible with long-term survival.

Patients rendered comatose at the moment of impact, arriving at the emergency department with evidence of midbrain dysfunction, or other brainstem signs, more commonly have the pathological alterations of diffuse axonal injury. Severe forces of rotational acceleration are implicated in producing these lesions, which consist of diffuse small hemorrhages, areas of necrosis, and shearing of nerve fibers. These lesions occur typically in the corpus callosum and dorsolateral pons. Therapy is directed at controlling intracranial pressure, but prognosis is poor, and such patients usually remain in a persistent vegetative state.

Traumatic Intracranial Hematomas

Acute Epidural Hematoma. Rapidly evolving and often lethal, acute epidural hematomas are formed by laceration of a dural vessel, which produces a clot between the skull and the dura. Hemorrhage originates most often from a branch of the middle meningeal artery that has been lacerated by a fracture, although bleeding from meningeal veins, dural sinuses, or emissary veins can also produce less rapidly evolving clots. In 90% of adult patients with an epidural hematoma, skull fracture is demonstrated by x-ray examination, at operation, or at autopsy. Only about 50% of children, however, have skull fractures associated with this lesion. When a linear fracture crosses the grooves of the meningeal vessels or dural sinuses, the physician should suspect such a clot.

The classic history is that of an injury resulting in a brief loss of consciousness from which the patient wakens and is comparatively well—the so-called lucid interval—followed in a few hours by expansion of the clot, compression of the brain surface, cerebral edema, and an increase in the overall intracranial pressure. The increased pressure results in headache, vomiting, weakness of the contralateral limbs, and deterioration of the state of consciousness. With further enlargement of the clot, transtentorial herniation occurs. The temporal lobe is displaced inward until its most medial portion, the uncus, is forced down over the free edge of the tentorium, compressing the brainstem and the adjacent ipsilateral oculomotor nerve (Fig. 37.2 showing similar process in subdural hematoma). Unless the brainstem compression is relieved quickly, death results. As the medial portion of the temporal lobe herniates, it displaces the oculomotor nerve, first paralyzing the pupilloconstrictor fibers; the ipsilateral pupil becomes widely dilated and unreactive to light. Further displacement of the temporal lobe compromises the blood supply to the midbrain, and the midbrain itself is compressed with displacement against the contralateral tentorial edge and, finally, compression of the opposite oculomotor nerve. As these events occur, the hemiparesis becomes a hemiplegia, coma deepens, decerebrate rigidity develops, the opposite pupil becomes dilated and fixed

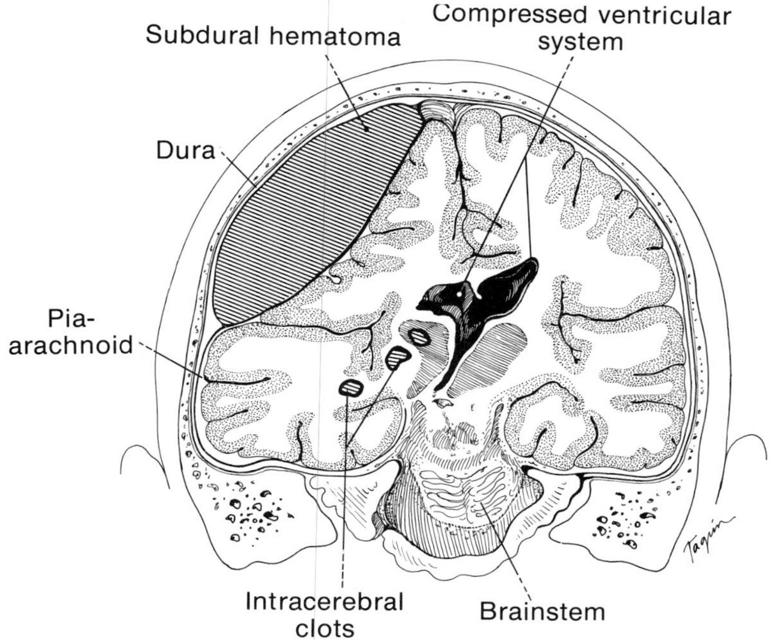

Figure 37.2. Subdural hematoma compressing temporal lobe and displacing brainstem against edge of tentorium and compressing third nerve.

to light, midbrain hemorrhages develop, the centers for cardiorespiratory regulation cease functioning, and death follows. Although this pattern is classic and occurs in most patients with a temporal extracerebral hematoma, one phase in the evolution of the midbrain compression may occur more quickly than another, and progressive neurologic worsening may be subtle. Careful observation of the level of consciousness and the neurologic status is imperative if an epidural hemorrhage is considered.

Early removal of the hematoma before transtentorial herniation is essential for a favorable outcome. In one large series, 77% of patients who were decerebrate before operation died, whereas only 1 of 74 who were conscious before operation died.

If time permits, a CAT scan should be obtained because it is confirmatory (Fig. 37.3*A*), but patients arriving in the emergency department with clear-cut signs of an evolving epidural hematoma, or in whom the signs develop after arrival, should be intubated, cross-matched for blood, and taken directly to the operating room for exploratory burr holes without further diagnostic studies. Although there are more than 2000 board-certified neurosurgeons in the United States, the urgency of these lesions occasionally requires the general surgeon to intervene while awaiting neurosurgical assistance; it therefore behooves surgeons in training to prepare themselves for this contingency. Emergency physicians should not sit by while the deadly events of transtentorial herniation unfold to a fatal conclusion, and if a neurosurgeon is not at hand, they must proceed with burr hole evacuation of clot (Fig. 37.4).

Aside from timeliness, the two essential components of a successful procedure are: *(a)* removing the clot to relieve brain compression; and *(b)* securing the source of bleeding to prevent recurrence. The initial burr hole should be placed over the laceration or fracture. If none is obvious, the burr hole is made over the temporal area on the side of the dilated pupil. A vertical scalp incision is first made 2 cm anterior to the ear and carried down to the zygoma to allow access to the temporal bone. The temporalis fascia and muscle are divided, preferably with a cautery, and the muscle is retracted and striped from the outer table of the skull. Frequently, a fracture line is noted at this stage. The burr hole is placed with a standard drill and burr, and as the blood clot extrudes, the craniectomy is enlarged with rongeurs. This relieves the pressure and allows further time for more extensive neurosurgical intervention, which may include conversion of the craniectomy to a temporal craniotomy utilizing a standard bone flap.

As the clot is removed, hemostasis is achieved by electrocoagulation *and* ligation of the main trunks of the middle meningeal vessels as they appear on the dura; occasionally, the middle meningeal artery

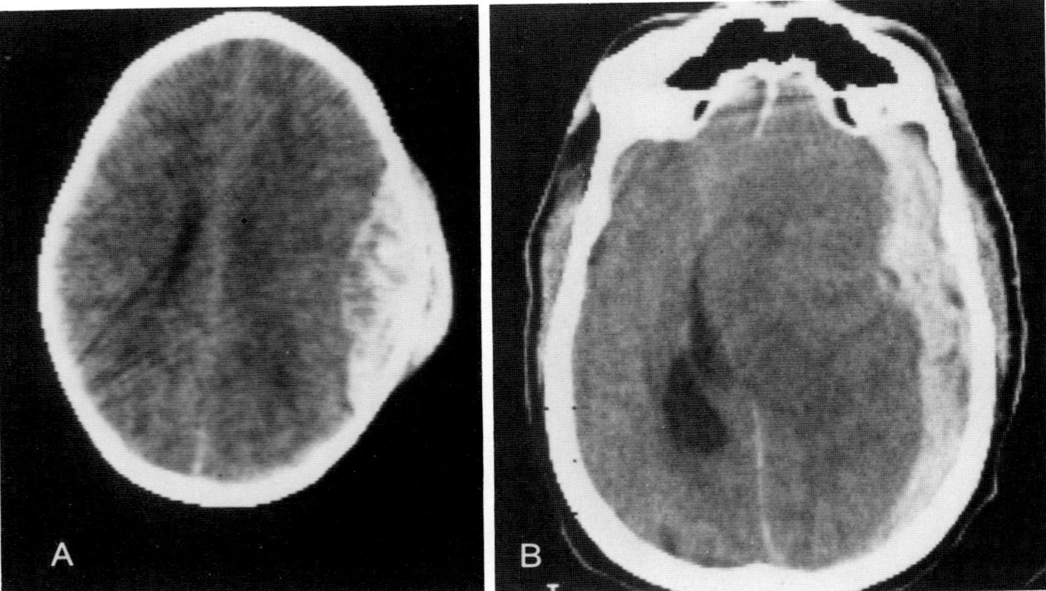

Figure 37.3. *A,* Acute epidural hematoma in 8-month-old infant who underwent scanning 30 minutes after a fall. Clot is 2 cm thick. Note swelling of overlying scalp. En route to operating room, the child showed early signs of tentorial pressure cone. Immediate evacuation of clot was followed by complete neurologic recovery within a few hours. *B,* Acute subdural hematoma with compression and displacement of ventricles. Subdural blood is free to spread over the convexity, but extension of epidural clot is restricted by attachments of dura to skull. These hematomas tend to be thick, relative to the area of brain covered.

must be dissected to its origin at the foramen spinosum and ligated there. Any obvious dural bleeding is coagulated, and dural tenting sutures are placed between the outer layer of dura and the inner layer of temporalis muscle of pericranium to control dural venous oozing. Once the clot has been removed and extradural hemostasis is absolute, the presence of a coexistent subdural hematoma can be determined by opening the dura and examining the underlying cortical surfaces. There is often little obvious brain damage. If the postoperative progress is not satisfactory, a CAT scan is in order to determine whether any other treatable lesion is present.

Acute Subdural Hematoma. Acute subdural hematoma (Fig. 37.3*B*) is over 30 times more common than epidural hematoma and is the lesion most frequently associated with death or morbidity in reported series of head injuries. Usually the result of a vehicular accident, assault, or fall, most of these lesions are accompanied by severe impact-produced intrinsic brain injuries, such as laceration-contusion, often bilateral, intracerebral hemorrhage, and diffuse axonal injury. In older persons, the cortical arteries may adhere to the inner surface of the dura and give rise to arterial subdural hematomas. For years, the reported mortality ranged from 70–90%. In one series, 89% of patients with decerebrate rigidity died; if dilated fixed pupils were also present, the mortality rose to 95%. However, Seelig in 1981 reported a remarkable reduction in mortality to 30% in patients undergoing operation within 4 hours of injury, compared with 90% in those operated on after 4 hours. Improved functional recovery also occurred in the first group. These are the best results that have been reported, and they were achieved by effective triage and CAT scan diagnosis, followed by immediate evacuation of the clot and the aggressive use, during every phase of treatment, of all medical measures to control intracranial hypertension.

Surgical removal is accomplished by a rapid subtemporal craniectomy with partial evacuation of the clot to effect at least some degree of decompression, followed by craniotomy sufficient to provide exposure to remove the rest of the clot and to secure the source of the bleeding. Intracerebral hematoma, if present, is removed and obviously devitalized brain tissue debrided. Because of the consistency of rapidly clotted blood, these lesions cannot be adequately treated by multiple burr holes alone.

Chronic Subdural Hematoma. Often the result of minor trauma that cannot be recalled, this lesion occurs mainly in those with some degree of brain atrophy due to either normal aging or the chronic cytotoxic effects of alcohol. Chronic subdural hematoma is also one of the common major complications of long-term anticoagulant therapy

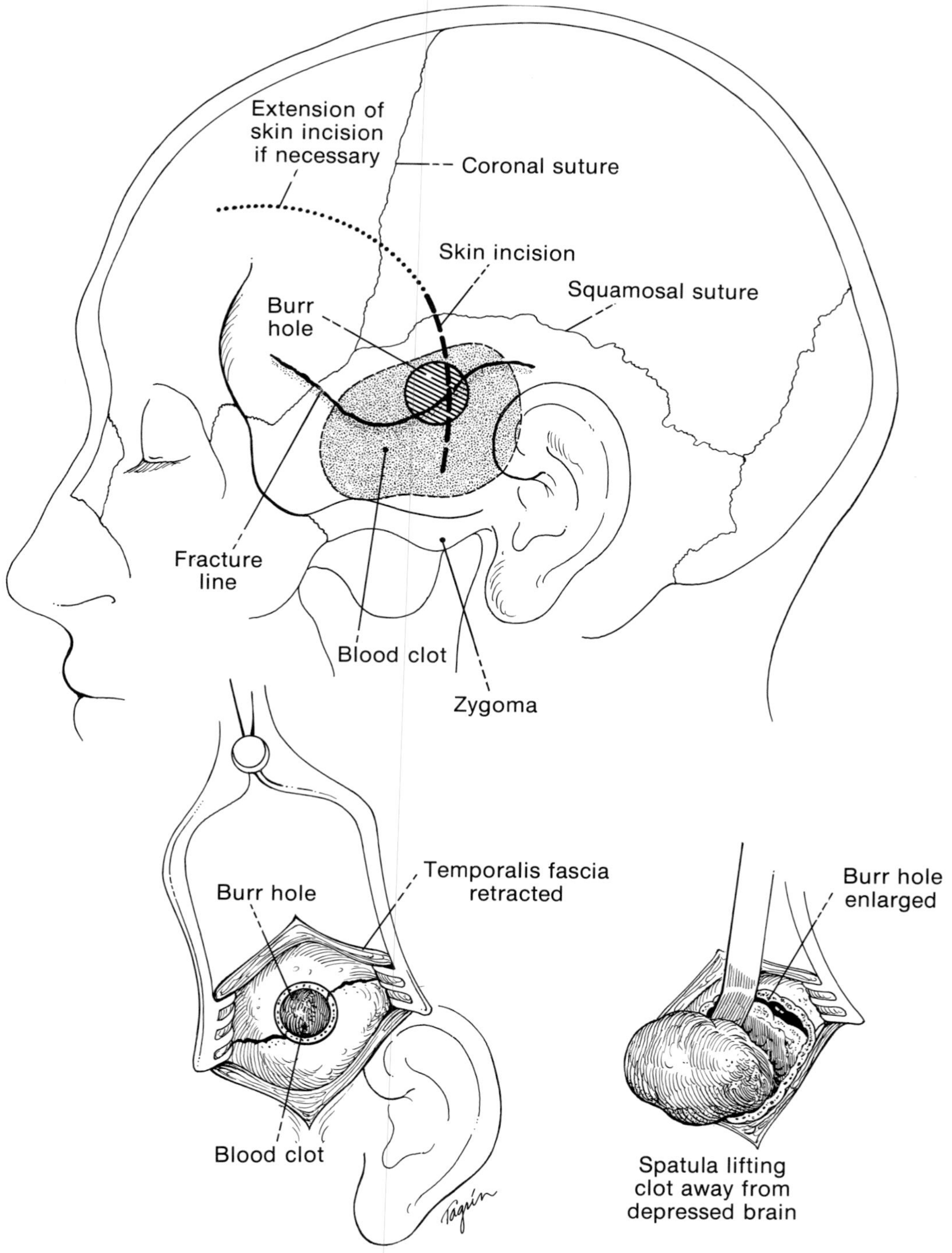

Figure 37.4. Technique of acute epidural clot evacuation.

(Fig. 37.5). The current mortality approaches 20% and reflects the difficulties in diagnosis and treatment of this disorder in an elderly population with major diseases in other body systems. Bleeding usually originates from a cortical vein that has been lacerated near its entry into the superior sagittal si-

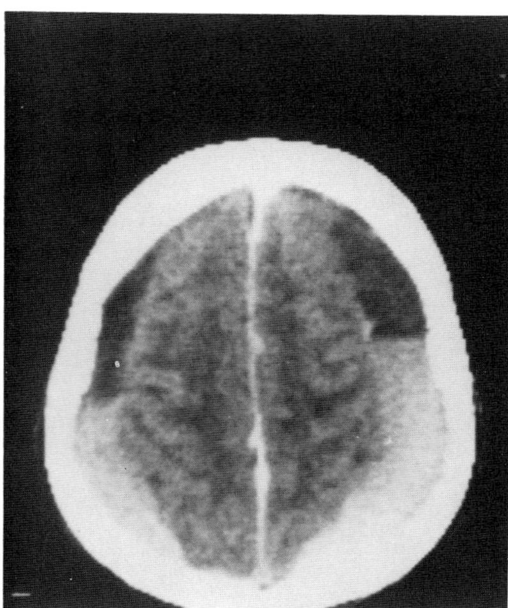

Figure 37.5. Bilateral chronic subdural hematomas in patient receiving anticoagulants. With the head in the supine position for scanning, the heavier particulate matter in this liquefied clot has settled posteriorly; the serum component of low attenuation value is layered over the more anterior convexity.

nus by shearing movement at the moment of impact. After clotting, the blood becomes sequestered by the formation of subdural membranes; as time passes, the volume of the hematoma increases. The initial gradual enlargement of the mass is well-tolerated, but when compensatory displacement of the brain and ventricular system begins to fail, clinical signs and symptoms appear. The patient may complain of headaches, and relatives note changes in mentation accompanied by psychomotor slowing. As brain compression slowly increases, the patient becomes dull, and focal neurologic changes appear. Because these presenting complaints are nonspecific, chronic subdural hematomas are often misdiagnosed as stroke, tumor, metabolic derangement, dementia, or even senility, unless a high index of suspicion is maintained in evaluating each of these illnesses.

Shift of the pineal gland on plain skull films is common unless the hematoma is bilateral, which occurs in about 20% of cases. Chronic subdural hematomas are readily diagnosed by CAT scanning, and should be surgically evacuated without delay. Some chronic subdural hematomas appear isodense with brain on the CAT scan. Their presence may be determined by an intravenous infusion of contrast (Urovist or Renagrafin). Completely liquefied hematomas can be evacuated through burr holes, but solid clot requires the wider exposure of a bone flap. The major postoperative problem in these patients with preexistent loss of brain substance is failure of the brain to reexpand and fill the cavity formerly occupied by the hematoma. Brain expansion is encouraged by the use of subdural drains, generous hydration, and nursing care with the patient in the head-down position. Despite these measures, recurrent subdural collections are common. Recurrence is suggested by the postoperative clinical course, and is confirmed by CAT scanning. The recurrent collection should be removed either by needle aspiration through the original burr holes, or by reopening the burr holes in the operating room.

Posterior Fossa Hematoma. Hematomas in the posterior fossa are 20 times less common than supratentorial hematomas; they are more often extradural than subdural, and if extradural, they may extend upward over the occipital lobes. More than 50% of these hematomas occur in children. Most cases result from a direct blow to the occiput, and a fracture extending into the foramen magnum or across the transverse sinus is nearly always present. The hematoma compresses the cerebellum and medulla, and obstructs the outflow of CSF from the fourth ventricle, producing acute hydrocephalus. Besides signs of local trauma, the clinical findings include altered consciousness, severe headaches, gaze palsies, and papilledema. Difficult to diagnose before CAT scanning, those clots were located by exploratory burr holes placed for clinical reasons. It may be that they are much more common than previously thought. Immediate suboccipital craniectomy with removal of the clot is the treatment of choice.

Intracerebral Hemorrhage. Acute intracerebral hematoma frequently occurs as an element of a high-velocity acceleration-deceleration injury in association with acute subdural hematoma and cerebral laceration-contusion. The devastating effects of an expanding clot within the white matter of the cerebral hemisphere are compounded by the compressive effects on adjacent brain tissue, with resultant edema and ischemia, intracranial hypertension, and displacement-compression of brainstem structures. The CAT scan (Fig. 37.6) provides accurate localization and permits the surgeon to approach the mass through the most expendable portion of the brain surface.

Delayed intracerebral hematoma may occur days or even weeks after injury, and is being increasingly recognized as a cause of cerebral deterioration after initial neurologic stabilization.

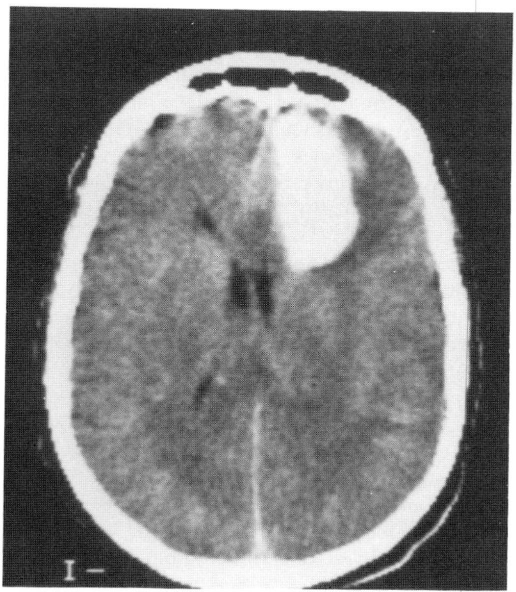

Figure 37.6. Acute intracerebral hematoma. This contrecoup lesion followed a blow to the occiput.

Penetrating Brain Injuries

The extensive experience of military neurosurgeons in Vietnam resulted in reduction in the mortality of missile-produced brain wounds to just under 10%. This figure is not usually matched in civilian practice, where most gunshot wounds are self-inflicted and the weapon is perhaps better aimed. A bullet striking the calvarium shatters the bone locally and usually fragments, driving pieces of bone and metal into the brain as secondary missiles. Sometimes, a bullet fragment traverses the brain, but lacks the energy to exit through the opposite side of the skull and ricochets back into the brain, producing even more extensive destruction (Fig. 37.7). To understand the anatomic structures traversed by the missile, the physician must first study the position of the entry and exit wounds and the trajectory of the projectile as seen on radiographs, including stereoscopic views. He or she must then correlate this information with the neurologic findings. CAT scanning may provide more precise information regarding the proximity of the track to the ventricular system and major vascular structures, as well as delineate secondary intracerebral hemorrhage.

The principles of treatment are well-known from military experience. They consist of early debridement with removal of bone fragments, hematoma, and devitalized brain tissue, followed by watertight dural closure with pericranial or fascial graft, if necessary, to lessen the probability of postoperative infection from without and to prevent CSF leakage or local cerebral herniation. The decision to search

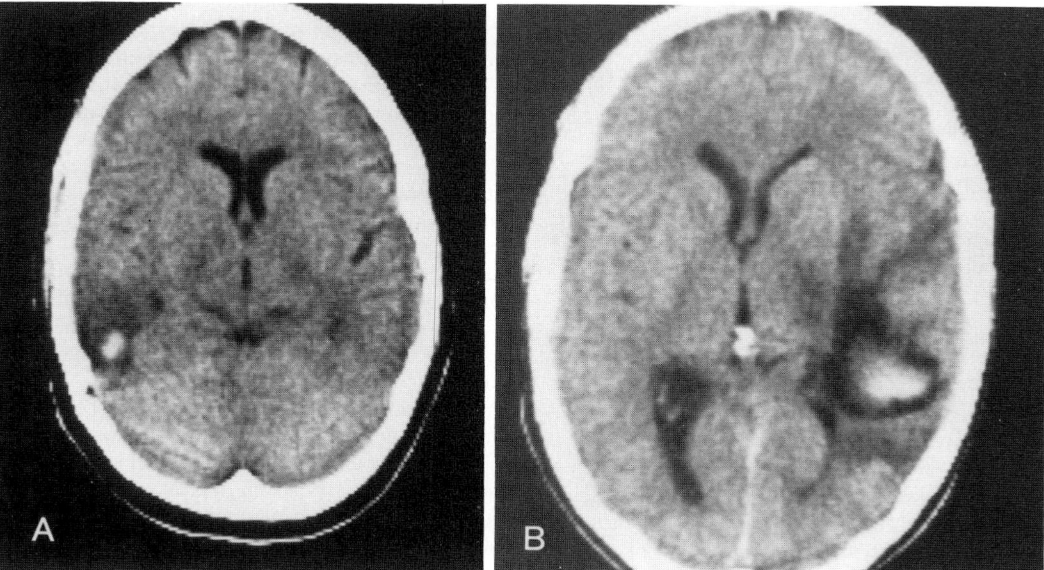

Figure 37.7. *A,* Hemorrhagic contusion of posterior left temporal lobe 8 days after injury. This lesion was not visible on initial scan. *B,* Right parietal contusion with computer-measured 6 mm shift of midline. Extensive edema of adjacent white matter and deformity of ventricle may be seen.

for an isolated piece of metal outside the main track is a difficult one, especially if it lies in an important, otherwise uninjured, sector of brain; sometimes these fragments are best left in place.

Diagnosis of Brain Death

The diagnosis of irreversible coma and brain death can seldom be made in the emergency department because most criteria specify a time interval over which the listed neurological signs must be present. There are several sets of acceptable criteria for brain death. The "Harvard Criteria" proposed in 1968 are accepted widely. However, advances in recent years have led to the proposal of new criteria, especially those of the President's Commission. This report defines death as the irreversible cessation of circulation and respiration or the irreversible cessation of all brain functions, including those of the brainstem. Cerebral unreceptivity and unresponsivity are present; i.e., the patient is in deep coma. An electroencephalogram (EEG) may be used to support this observation, but is not mandatory. All brainstem functions are absent. Pupillary light, corneal, oculocephalic, oculovestibular, oropharyngeal, and respiratory (apnea) reflexes should be tested. Adequate testing for apnea requires preoxygenation and the measuring of arterial blood gases at the conclusion of the apnea test, usually 10 minutes, to document a $Paco_2 > 60$ mm Hg. Spontaneous breathing efforts during this test indicate that part of the brainstem is functioning. Peripheral nervous system activity and spinal cord reflexes may persist after death. Seizures or true decerebrate or decorticate posturing are inconsistent with the diagnosis of death. The cause of coma should be established and the coma irreversible.

Except for patients with drug intoxication, hypothermia, young age, or shock, there have not been any reports of cases of brain function return following a 6-hour cessation, documented by clinical examination and confirmatory EEG. In the absence of a confirmatory EEG, a period of observation of at least 12 hours is recommended.

SPINAL INJURY

Transportation

Transportation of the patient with a spinal cord injury must be carefully planned and well-organized. The patient should not be moved until a sufficient number of trained persons is available to lift him as a unit, maintaining the head, neck, and thorax in the position in which the patient was found. Jostling or other motion of the neck may dislocate a fracture and produce an increase in neurologic deficit. The patient who is to be transported any distance should be placed on a firm board or stretcher with pillows or blanket rolls under the normal cervical and lumbar curvatures. If neck injury is suspected, sandbags should be placed against both sides of the head or a Mixter four-poster or Philadelphia collar applied. The patient should be treated with minimal amounts of analgesics, since these many interfere with respiratory function and neurologic evaluation.

Initial Evaluation

A thorough, detailed history of the injury should be obtained, including whether motor movement was immediately impaired. A complete general physical examination should be performed maintaining the patient in a neutral position with the head and spine aligned.

Respiratory embarrassment often accompanies spinal cord injuries. Lesions from the fifth cervical vertebra to the midthoracic region interfere with intercostal and abdominal breathing. The cell bodies for the phrenic nerves lie at about the level of the fourth cervical vertebra, and cord injury at or above this level interferes with diaphragmatic breathing too. Arterial blood gases, tidal volume, and vital capacity should be measured early. If necessary, nasotracheal intubation may be carried out to maintain adequate oxygenation, taking care not to move the neck. If intubation is not possible, tracheotomy may be performed. Adequate spontaneous respiration can often eventually be established once the acute effects of the injury subside. Therefore, early support of ventilation is essential. Hypotension may develop as a result of the functional sympathectomy produced by the spinal cord injury, and may be difficult to diagnose in the patient with multiple lesions. However, the presence of warm extremities and major neurologic deficit should alert the examiner to the possibility of sympathetic injury; treatment with vasopressor agents, fluids, and wraps of the extremities should be instituted accordingly. Injury to the autonomic fibers in the cord also causes bladder paralysis and cessation of intestinal peristalsis. Therefore, these patients should be managed initially with a bladder Foley catheter and nasogastric tube suction. Frequently, head injuries and cervical spine injuries are present together. Examination of the front and the back of the head for evidence of trauma may provide some clue as to the nature of the spinal injury, whether it be one of extension or flexion.

The motor and sensory systems should be evaluated completely. It is crucial that a sensory examination with charting of findings be carried out as soon as possible after the injury so that documentation of progression or regression of deficit can be established. This is important in deciding on surgical treatment, as well as in estimating the prognosis. The dermatome level of the sensory loss

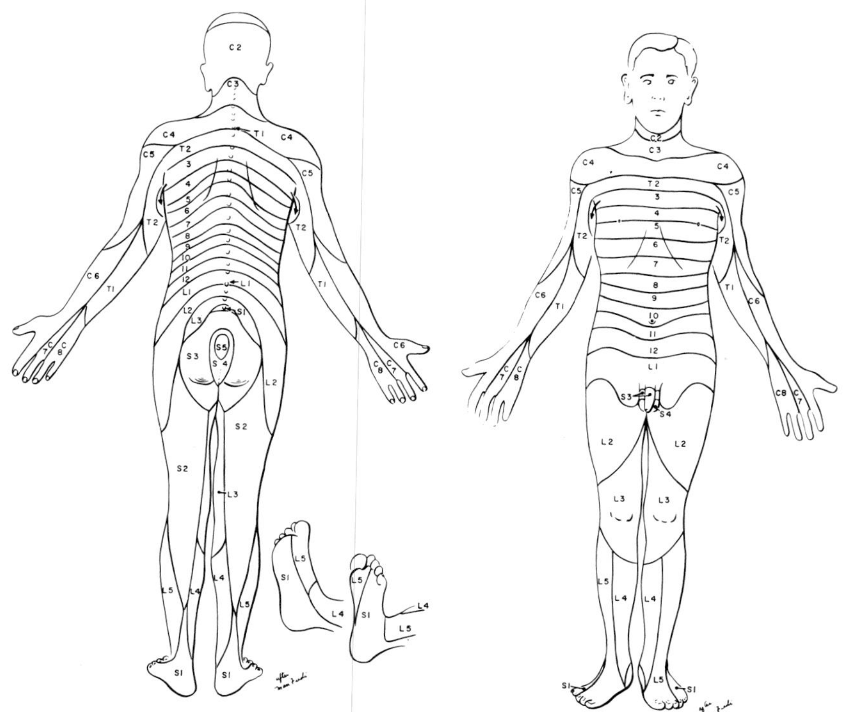

Figure 37.8. Dermatome map of human body. Note position of cervically innervated skin on anterior portion of chest and high thoracic innervation of inner aspect of arm. Reproductions of this map should be available in patient care areas so that sensory findings in patients with spinal cord injuries can be charted daily. (Reproduced with permission from Barr JS, Heros RC, Pierce DS. The treatment of spinal trauma. In Burke JF, Boyd RJ, McCabe CJ, eds. *Trauma Management.* Chicago: Year Book, 1988.)

should be estimated (Fig. 37.8). Muscle strength and tone should be evaluated carefully and the deep tendon reflexes noted. Reference to a motor function chart may be useful for those not routinely involved with the care of neurologic patients (Table 37.4).

Anatomy

In adults, the spinal cord extends from the foramen magnum to the second lumbar vertebra, suspended by the dentate ligaments, nerve roots, and supplying blood vessels within an arachnoid sac containing shock-absorbing CSF (Figs. 37.9 and 37.10). It is covered by tough, fibrous dura that is hydraulically buffered by the surrounding epidural fat and blood vessels, and it is enclosed within the bony confines of the spinal canal. This structural and buffering arrangement makes the spinal cord one of the most protected body organs. Besides having a firm bony covering, constructed to allow maximal movement, an hydraulic system within the subarachnoid space provides excellent shock absorption. The cauda equina begins approximately at the interspace of the first and second lumbar vertebrae and extends to the sacrum. The lower part of the spinal canal with its enclosed nerve roots is less sensitive to injury than the upper portion housing the cord.

The cord receives its blood supply from a network of extensive collaterals that enter the spinal canal with the nerve roots (Fig. 37.11). In most persons, one ventral radicular artery is usually considerably larger than the others; this artery originates from the aorta between the eighth thoracic and third lumbar vertebrae, and provides the blood supply for most of the thoracic section of the cord. Paraplegia can result from occlusion of this artery by traumatic or iatrogenic dissection. The arterial supply of the more rostral part of the cord is derived from the vertebral arteries. As the vessels terminate within the cord, they are endarteries that provide little collateral circulation within the gray matter of the cord itself.

The spinal cord is almost cylindrical, with its width always greater than its dorsoventral diameter. It noticeably enlarges at the region of innervation of the upper extremities and at the lumbosacral region. There are usually 31 pairs of spinal nerves.

Table 37.4.
Motor Function Chart[a]

Cord Segment	Muscles	Action to Be Tested	Nerves
	Shoulder Girdle and Upper Extremity		
C1–4	Deep neck muscles (sternomastoid and trapezius also participate)	Flexion of neck Extension of neck Rotation of neck Lateral bending of neck	Cervical
C3–4	Scaleni Diaphragm	Elevation of upper thorax Inspiration	Phrenic
C5–T1	Pectoralis major and minor	Adduction of arm from behind to front	Thoracic anterior (from medial and lateral cords of plexus)
C5–7	Serratus anterior	Forward thrust of shoulder	Long thoracic
C5(3–4)	Levator scapulae	Elevation of scapula	Dorsal scapular
C4–5	Rhomboids	Medial adduction and elevation of scapula	Dorsal scapular
C5	Supraspinatus	Abduction of arm	Suprascapular
C5–6	Infraspinatus	Lateral rotation of arm	Suprascapular
C5–8	Latissimus dorsi, teres major and subscapularis	Medial rotation of arm Adduction of arm from front to back	Subscapular (from posterior cord of plexus
C5–6	Deltoid	Abduction of arm	Axillary (from posterior cord of plexus)
C5	Teres minor	Lateral rotation of arm	Axillary (from posterior cord of plexus)
C5–6	Biceps brachii	Flexion of forearm Supination of forearm	Musculocutaneous (from lateral cord of plexus)
C6–7	Coracobrachialis	Adduction of arm Flexion of forearm	Musculocutaneous (from lateral cord of plexus)
C5–6	Brachialis	Flexion of forearm	Musculocutaneous (from lateral cord of plexus)
C6–8	Triceps brachii and anconeus	Extension of forearm	
C5–6	Brachioradialis	Flexion of forearm	
C5–7	Extensor carpi radialis	Radial extension of hand	Radial (from posterior cord of plexus)
C6–8	Extensor digitorum communis	Extension of phalanges of index finger, middle finger, ring finger, little finger	
C6–8	Extensor digiti quinti proprius	Extension of phalanges of little finger Extension of hand	
C6–8	Extensor carpi ulnaris	Ulnar extension of hand	Radial (from posterior cord of plexus)
C5–7	Supinator	Supination of forearm	
C6–7	Abductor pollicis longus	Abduction of metacarpal of thumb Radial extension of hand	
C6–7	Extensor pollicis brevis and longus	Extension of thumb	
C6–8	Extensor pollicis brevis and longus	Radial extension of hand	Radial (from posterior cord of plexus)
C6–8	Extensor indicis proprius	Extension of index finger Extension of hand	
C7–T1	Flexor carpi ulnaris	Ulnar flexion of hand	
C8–T1	Flexor digitorum profundus (ulnar portion)	Flexion of terminal phalanx of ring finger, little finger Flexion of hand	Ulnar (from medial cord of plexus)

Table 37.4—*continued*

Cord Segment	Muscles	Action to Be Tested	Nerves
C8–T1	Adductor pollicis	Adduction of metacarpal of thumb	Ulnar (from medial cord of plexus)
C8–T1	Abductor digiti quinti	Abduction of little finger	
C8–T1	Opponens digiti quinti	Opposition of little finger	
C8–T1	Flexor digiti quinti brevis	Flexion of little finger	
C8–T1	Interossei	Flexion of proximal phalanx, extension of two distal phalanges, adduction and abduction of fingers	
C6–7	Pronator teres	Pronation of forearm	
C6–7	Flexor carpi radialis	Radial flexion of hand	
C7–T1	Palmaris longus	Flexion of hand	
C7–T1	Flexor digitorum sublimis	Flexion of middle phalanx of index finger, middle finger, ring finger, little finger Flexion of hand	Median (C6–7 from lateral cord of plexus; C8–T1 from medial cord of plexus)
C6–7	Flexor pollicis longus	Flexion of terminal phalanx of thumb	
C7–T1	Flexor digitorum profundus (radial portion)	Flexion of terminal phalanx of index finger, middle finger Flexion of hand	
C6–7	Abductor pollicis brevis	Abduction of metacarpal of thumb	
C6–7	Flexor pollicis brevis	Flexion of proximal phalanx of thumb	
C6–7	Opponens pollicis	Opposition of metacarpal of thumb	Medial (C6–7 from lateral cord of plexus; C8–T1 from medial cord of plexus)
C8–T1	Lumbricals (the two lateral)	Flexion of proximal phalanx and extension of the two distal phalanges of index finger, middle finger	
C8–T1	Lumbricals (the two medial)	Flexion of proximal phalanx and extension of the two distal phalanges of ring finger, little finger	
		Trunk and Thorax	
T2–11	Thoracic, abdominal, and back	Elevation and depression of ribs	Thoracic and posterior lumbosacral branches
		Contraction of abdomen	
		Anteroflexion and lateral flexion of trunk	
		Hip Girdle and Lower Extremity	
T12–L3	Iliopsoas	Flexion of hip	Femoral
L2–L3	Sartorius	Flexion of hip and eversion of thigh	
L2–L4	Quadriceps femoris	Extension of knee	
L2–3	Pectineus	Adduction of thigh	
L2–3	Adductor longus	Adduction of thigh	
L2–4	Adductor brevis	Adduction of thigh	Obturator
L3–4	Adductor magnus	Adduction of thigh	
L2–4	Gracilis	Adduction of thigh	

Table 37.4—*continued*

Cord Segment	Muscles	Action to Be Tested	Nerves
L3–4	Obturator externus	Adduction of thigh Lateral rotation of thigh	Obturator
L4–5,S1	Gluteus medius and minimus	Extension of thigh	
L4–5,S1	Gluteus medius and minimus	Medial rotation of thigh	Superior gluteal
L4–5	Tensor fasciae latae	Flexion of thigh	
S1–2	Piriformis	Lateral rotation of thigh	
L4–S1	Gluteus maximus	Abduction of thigh	Inferior gluteal
L5–S2	Obturator internus	Lateral rotation of thigh	Muscular branches from sacral plexus
L4–S2	Gemelli	Lateral rotation of thigh	Muscular branches from sacral plexus
L4–S1	Quadratus femoris	Lateral rotation of thigh	Muscular branches from sacral plexus
L4–S2	Biceps femoris	Flexion of leg (assists in extension of thigh)	
L4–S1	Semitendinosus	Flexion of leg (assists in extension of thigh)	Sciatic (trunk)
L4–S1	Semimembranosus	Flexion of leg (assists in extension of thigh)	
L4–5	Tibialis anterior	Dorsal flexion of foot Supination of foot	
L4–S1	Extensor digitorum longus	Extension of toes II–V Dorsal flexion of foot	
L4–S1	Extensor hallucis longus	Extension of great toe Dorsal flexion of foot	Deep peroneal
L4–S1	Extensor digitorum brevis	Extension of great toe and the three medial toes	
L5–S1	Peronei	Plantar flexion of foot in pronation	Superficial peroneal
L5–S2	Tibialis posterior and triceps surae	Plantar flexion of foot in supination	
L5–S2	Flexor digitorum longus	Plantar flexion of foot in supination Flexion of terminal phalanx, toes II–V	Tibial
L5–S2	Flexor hallucis longus	Plantar flexion of foot in supination Flexion of terminal phalanx of great toe	
L5–S1	Flexor digitorum brevis	Flexion of middle phalanx toes II–V	
L5–S2	Flexor hallucis brevis	Flexion of proximal phalanx of great toe	
S1–2	Small muscles of foot	Spreading and closing of toes Flexion of proximal phalanx of toes	Tibial
S2–4	Perineal and sphincters	Voluntary control of pelvic floor	Pudendal

[a] Reproduced by permission, from Wepsic JG. Injuries to the spinal cord and cauda equina. In Cave EF, Burke JF, Boyd RJ, eds. *Trauma Management.* Copyright © 1974, by Year Book Medical Publishers, Inc., Chicago.

The first pair originates from the vertebral column between the first cervical vertebra and the skull, with each of the remaining pairs of cervical nerves leaving above the vertebra of the corresponding number. Since there are eight pairs of cervical nerves and only seven cervical vertebrae, the eighth

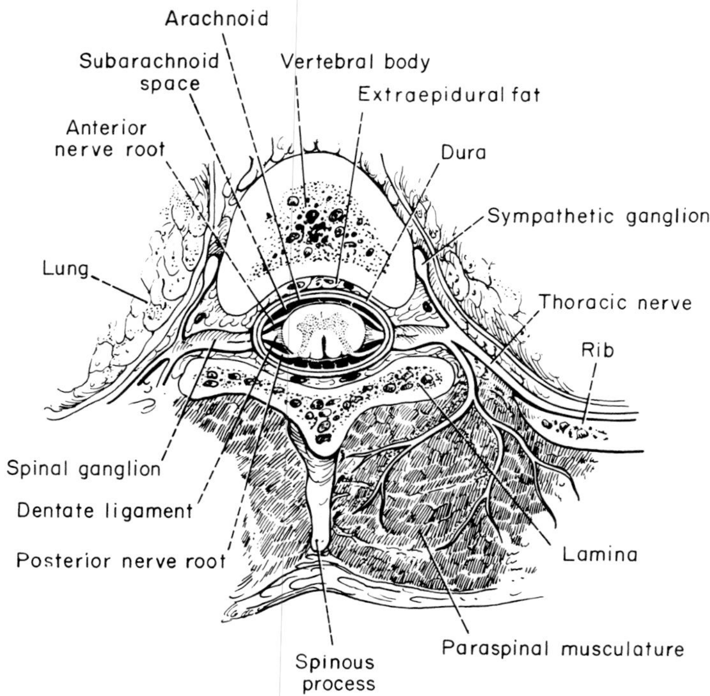

Figure 37.9. Transverse section through a thoracic vertebra and the spinal cord. Excellent protection of cord is apparent when relationships of surrounding musculature, bony canal, epidural fat, and cerebrospinal fluid are considered. Relation of dorsal root to spinal cord is shown. (Reproduced with permission from Wepsic JG. Injuries to the spinal cord and cauda equina. In Cave EF, Burke JF, Boyd RJ, eds. *Trauma Management.* Chicago: Year Book, 1974.)

cervical nerve leaves the spinal column between the seventh cervical and first thoracic vertebrae. Beginning with the first thoracic nerve, all the remaining spinal nerves pass from the vertebral column below the vertebra of the corresponding number (Fig. 37.12).

The effects of spinal cord trauma are expressed as motor, sensory, and visceral deficits distal to the site of injury. Usually, the major effect is interruption of the descending or ascending white matter tracts; although gray matter lesions are extremely important in the midcervical region in patients with "central cord injury," the vital motor and sensory deficits noted on first examination are due to tract interruption (Fig. 37.13).

Motor impulses descend in three corticospinal tracts: the crossed lateral tract, the uncrossed lateral tract, and the ventral tract. These originate mainly in the precentral gyrus and descend from the cortex via the internal capsule and cerebral peduncle, crossing to the opposite side along the ventral aspect of the medulla. The fibers terminate on cells in posterior, intermedullary, and ventral gray matter; their interruption produces voluntary motor paralysis. The reticulospinal tracts originate in the pontine and medullary reticular formations. Interruption of, or injury to, these fibers in the upper cervical region may result in apnea while the patient sleeps. Visceral activity is modulated by the reticulospinal fibers, and by other multisynaptic chains of neurons that terminate on both preganglionic autonomic and somatic efferent neurons. "Automatic" visceral activity is eventually possible in the absence of descending impulses if the relevant nerve roots and segmental cord levels are preserved in the presence of higher transection of the cord.

Ascending pathways carry information about distal visceral and cutaneous sensibilities. The spinothalamic tracts related to pain and temperature sensibilities arise from cells in the dorsal gray matter, cross the midline via the ventral commissure, and ascend in the lateral portion of the anterior quadrant to terminate in the medullary and thalamic nuclei. Touch and vibration sensibilities are served by the posterior columns. The more lateral group of fibers, the fasciculus cuneatus, originates from dorsal horn cells of the first cervical vertebra to the sixth thoracic vertebra, whereas the more medial group, the fasciculus gracilis, originates from cells below the sixth thoracic vertebra. They terminate in

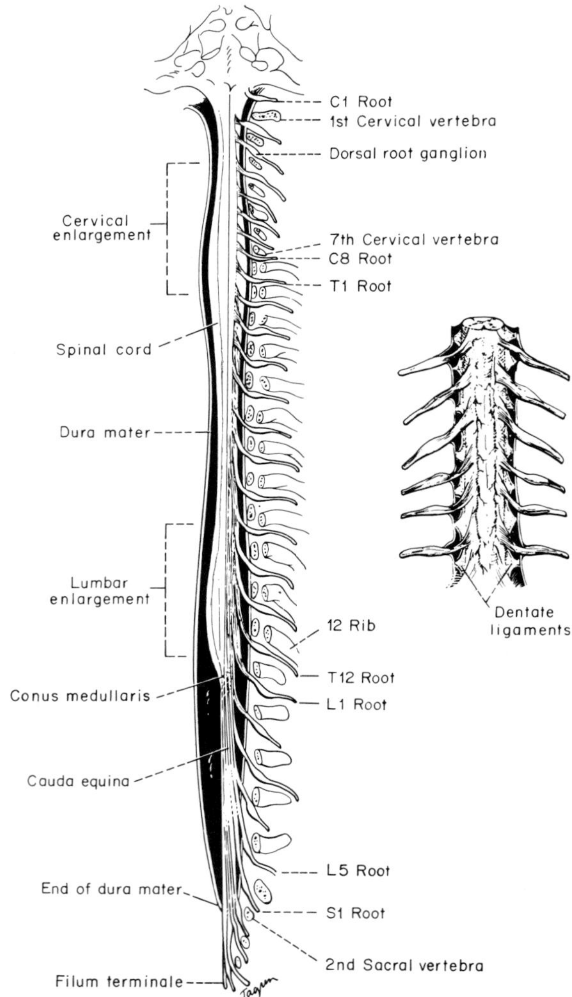

Figure 37.10. Spinal cord and surrounding structures. Note position of first, seventh, and eighth cervical roots with respect to vertebral level at which they emerge. Cervical and lumbar enlargements are depicted with relationship of dentate ligaments to the cord, posterior rootlets, and dura mater. (Reproduced with permission from Wepsic JG. Injuries to the spinal cord and cauda equina. In Cave EF, Burke JF, Boyd RJ, eds. *Trauma Management.* Chicago: Year Book, 1974.)

the nucleus cuneatus and nucleus gracilis and then project rostrally via the medial lemniscus.

Management in the Emergency Department

Cervical spine fractures are the most dreaded of all spinal fractures because of the devastating neurological injury they can produce. They are also the most common spinal fractures. This discussion will emphasize these cervical spinal injuries.

Upon arrival in the emergency department, all patients with suspected cervical spine trauma and all patients in coma must have a lateral cervical spine x-ray performed that demonstrates the cervical spine to the top of T1. It may be necessary to pull the shoulders downward while the x-ray is taken, or place the arms in the "swimmer's position" to visualize adequately the lower cervical spine. The lateral projection should be supplemented by anteroposterior and open-mouth x-rays. While cervical spine x-rays usually identify fractures or dislocations, they may not portray accurately how unstable the spine is. In addition, *neural damage may be severe even when x-ray findings do not indicate serious injury.* This is especially true in children and older patients.

If any misalignment of the bony spine is identified, restoration of normal bony alignment is the next priority. A halo ring or Gardner-Wells tongs should be placed and 5–10 lbs of traction applied. Additional weights should be added every 5 minutes, depending upon the level and type of injury until the normal alignment is restored. Experienced neurosurgeons may begin with greater amounts of weights for low cervical fractures. Frequent repeat lateral spine x-rays should be obtained to document the progress of realignment and to ascertain that the spine is not being distracted by the weights. Realignment should be accomplished within 30–60 minutes rather than gradually. Some neurosurgeons have advocated closed manipulative reduction of dislocations that fail to reduce with weights alone. Bilateral and unilateral facet dislocations may fall into this category. Closed manipulation of a fractured cervical spine seems a risky procedure. Our practice has been to proceed with open reduction and stabilization when weights fail to restore the bony alignment. Once traction restores bony alignment, the amount of weight is reduced to just that necessary to maintain alignment, usually 10–15 lbs. If alignment is maintained for several hours, a halo vest may be applied. Once a halo vest is applied, these patients may be managed in a regular hospital bed in a variety of positions, rather than on a Stryker frame; this facilitates skin care. Repeat cervical spine x-rays should be obtained several hours after halo vest placement, and on the following day, to document that adequate alignment is maintained.

Fractures and fracture-dislocation in the thoracic, thoracolumbar, and lumbar regions may also be reduced by gravity techniques. However, this requires a prolonged period of subsequent bed rest, often 9–13 weeks. Therefore, many neurosurgeons favor open decompression, internal stabilization, and fusion for these injuries. The precise operative ap-

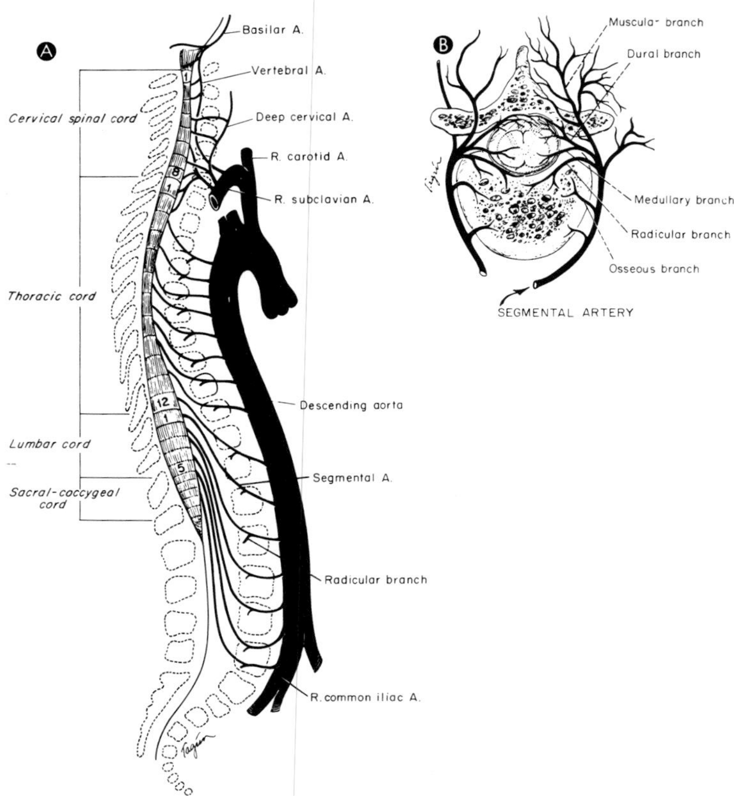

Figure 37.11. *A,* Blood supply of fetal spinal cord arising from subclavian artery, iliac artery, and aorta. Note that the vertebral artery supplies segmental arteries in upper cervical region, whereas more direct branches from the deep cervical artery supply mid and lower cervical cord. Variability in this supply is great, and the most consistent feature of detailed examination of the blood supply to the cervical cord, in particular, is its variability. The number of important large radicular branches varies, as does the level of entry or position of the vessel with respect to anterior or posterior roots. In general, a large radicular branch arising from the aorta between the eighth thoracic and third lumbar vertebrae provides largest amount of blood to thoracic cord. This is the artery of Adamkiewicz. *B,* Spinal anatomy of a large segmental and radicular artery. Supply to dura mater, muscles, and bone arises from these vessels. Entry of medullary arteries through the intervertebral foramen is variable. Microscopic dissection during operation on posterior or anterior roots is often necessary to preserve this important blood supply. (Reproduced with permission from Wepsic JG. Injuries to the spinal cord and cauda equina. In Cave EF, Burke JF, Boyd RJ, eds. *Trauma Management.* Chicago: Year Book, 1974.)

proach is based upon the geometry of the fracture. Surgical intervention may be undertaken as part of the initial management, although some surgeons prefer to delay surgery for several days.

Following the restoration of bony alignment, additional radiographic studies are indicated to document that no bone or disc continues to compress the spinal cord. A high resolution CAT scan through the level of injury often provides this documentation. Sagittal MRI scans, especially those using surface coil technique, are excellent in demonstrating the relationships between the spinal cord and bony spine. As this technique becomes more widely available, it will have an important role in evaluating spine trauma and will replace myelography.

Myelography, using Pantopaque, gas, or a water-soluble contrast agent, is reserved for patients who demonstrate deterioration of neurological function or who fail to improve clinically from a partial lesion after 5–7 days. Patients with a complete loss of neurological function below the level of injury are not usually candidates for myelography, although a more aggressive approach to these patients is being investigated currently at several spinal cord injury centers.

Operative Indications

The indications for operative intervention in spinal cord injury continue to evolve. Not many years ago, neurosurgeons advocated aggressive decom-

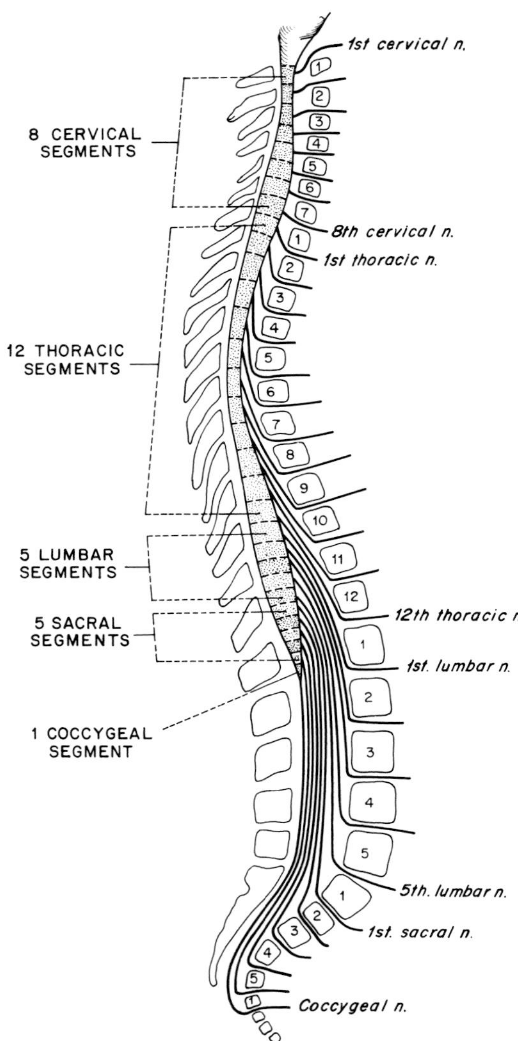

Figure 37.12. Relation of bony vertebral level to spinal cord level and nerve root exit. (Reproduced with permission from Wepsic JG. Injuries to the spinal cord and cauda equina. In Cave EF, Burke JF, Boyd RJ, eds. *Trauma Management.* Chicago: Year Book, 1974.)

pression of the cervical spinal cord, and some even advocated ice water lavage of the injured spinal cord. The emergence of more accurate diagnostic radiographic techniques, coupled with studies that failed to demonstrate a benefit from such aggressive surgical approaches, have reduced the indications for operative intervention. Currently, the most frequent indication for surgical intervention is the restoration of bony alignment, when closed reduction with weights does not yield satisfactory alignment. Worsening neurological signs and lack of improvement in partial neurological syndromes often lead to surgical intervention when diagnostic studies suggest a surgically remediable lesion. Additional indications for surgical intervention include: complete myelographic block, penetrating wound of the spine, and the presence of a foreign body, bone, or disc within the spinal canal. Surgical decompression or realignment may then be followed by internal stabilization and fusion.

The operative approach is based on the geometry of the offending lesion. That geometry is best seen on CAT scans. Centrally herniated discs are removed from an anterior approach, while facet dislocations are reduced via a posterior operation.

Clinically Important Fractures and Spinal Syndromes

Fractures and Dislocations

Figure 37.14 shows spinal fracture-dislocations. *Linear fractures* without dislocation are relatively mild injuries and may involve only the transverse or spinous processes. If no neurologic deficit or spinal instability is present, the patient may be treated with collar immobilization in cervical level injuries; there is usually no lasting disability.

Compression fractures usually result from hyperflexion injuries. The anterior surface of the vertebra is pinched, the centrum giving way laterally or posteriorly into the spinal cord. This type of fracture occurs frequently in the cervical region as the result of a diving accident, but is most common at the thoracolumbar junction in patients who have fallen onto the buttocks or feet. An immediate profound deficit often results.

Atlantooccipital dislocations are rare and usually result in immediate death. *Atlantoaxial dislocations* are caused by a sudden backward jerk of the head and neck and are associated with fracture of the odontoid process and rupture of the cruciate ligaments. In patients who do not die immediately, this lesion is usually not accompanied by a neurologic deficit. Treatment consists of halo immobilization, with stabilization developing over a 6–8-week period. At that point, fluoroscopic examination of head motion should cautiously be carried out to see whether surgical fusion of the first and second cervical vertebrae and the occiput is necessary.

''Hangman's fracture'' is a bilateral avulsion fracture through the arch of the axis, without injury to the odontoid process, resulting from sudden severe hyperextension of the head and neck. This type of injury may be seen in victims of motor vehicle accidents. If the patient survives, there is usually no associated neurologic deficit. This is probably due to increased space in the upper cervical canal

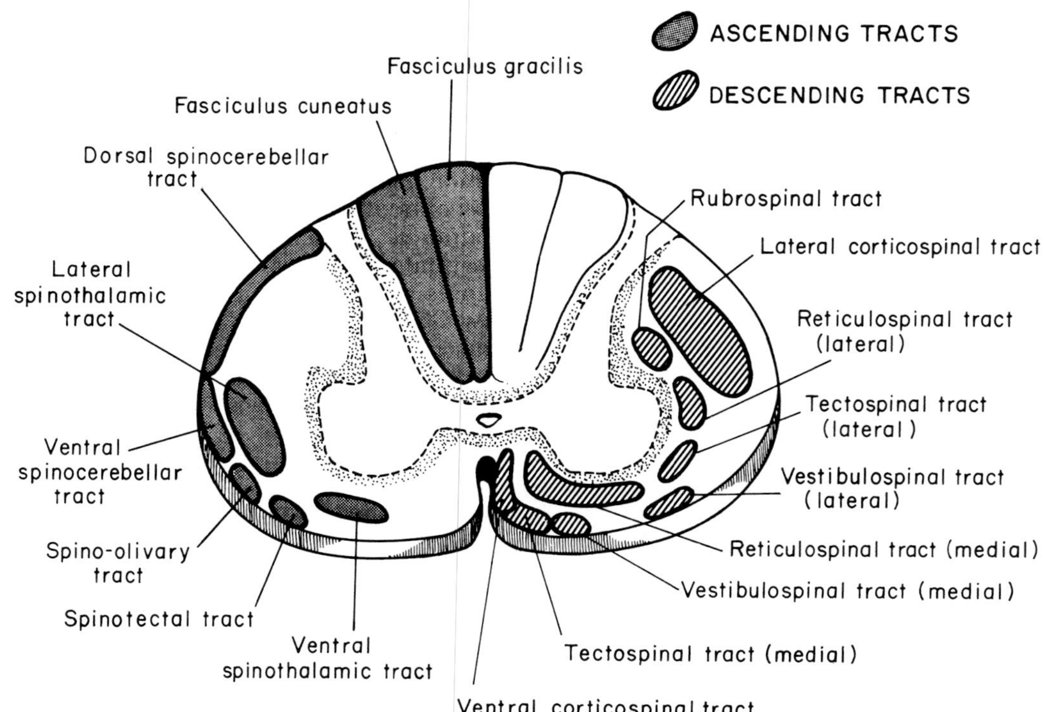

Figure 37.13. Cross-section of low cervical spinal cord showing ascending and descending tracts. (Reproduced with permission from Wepsic JG. Injuries to the spinal cord and cauda equina. In Cave EF, Burke JF, Boyd RJ, eds. *Trauma Management.* Chicago: Year Book, 1974.)

compared with the size of the cord and because decompression occurs during the injury by avulsion of the neural arches. These fractures heal spontaneously and are usually best treated by halo immobilization.

Teardrop fractures are cervical fractures produced when extreme flexion causes the involved vertebral body to be compressed with the anteroinferior fragment displaced downward and forward and the posteroinferior portion projected into the spinal canal. The posteroinferior portion may thus injure the anterior portion of the spinal cord.

Spinal Cord Injury

Anterior spinal cord injury results from acute impingement of bone or herniated disc fragments on the anterior portion of the cord. Corticospinal and spinothalamic functions are immediately interrupted, with some preservation of touch, position, and vibration sense. Myelographic definition and surgery may be indicated.

Central cervical spinal cord injury may result from hyperextension of the cervical spine in patients with significant cervical spondylosis. It is characterized by considerable impairment of motor movement in the upper extremities and frequently less severe impairment of the lower extremities. Sensory loss and bladder dysfunction occur as well. The mechanism of this injury remains unclear; some believe it is due to contusion, whereas others believe it is caused by ischemia. Such a lesion does not require operation, and patients experience a variable degree of recovery, although residual impairment of hand function is common.

Brown-Séquard's syndrome with loss of motor function on one side and loss of sensory function on the other is not commonly seen in spinal fracture-dislocations because it requires the presence of a unilateral cord injury that completely spares the opposite side. This syndrome is produced by interruption of the corticospinal tracts supplying the ipsilateral musculature and the spinothalamic tracts receiving sensibility impulses from the contralateral side. A traumatic lateral disc herniation or epidural clot may produce such a finding; surgical decompression may be necessary if myelographic examination demonstrates such a lesion.

Acute Back Pain

The emergency department is often the place where patients with sudden back pain associated with exertion seek treatment. Many patients state

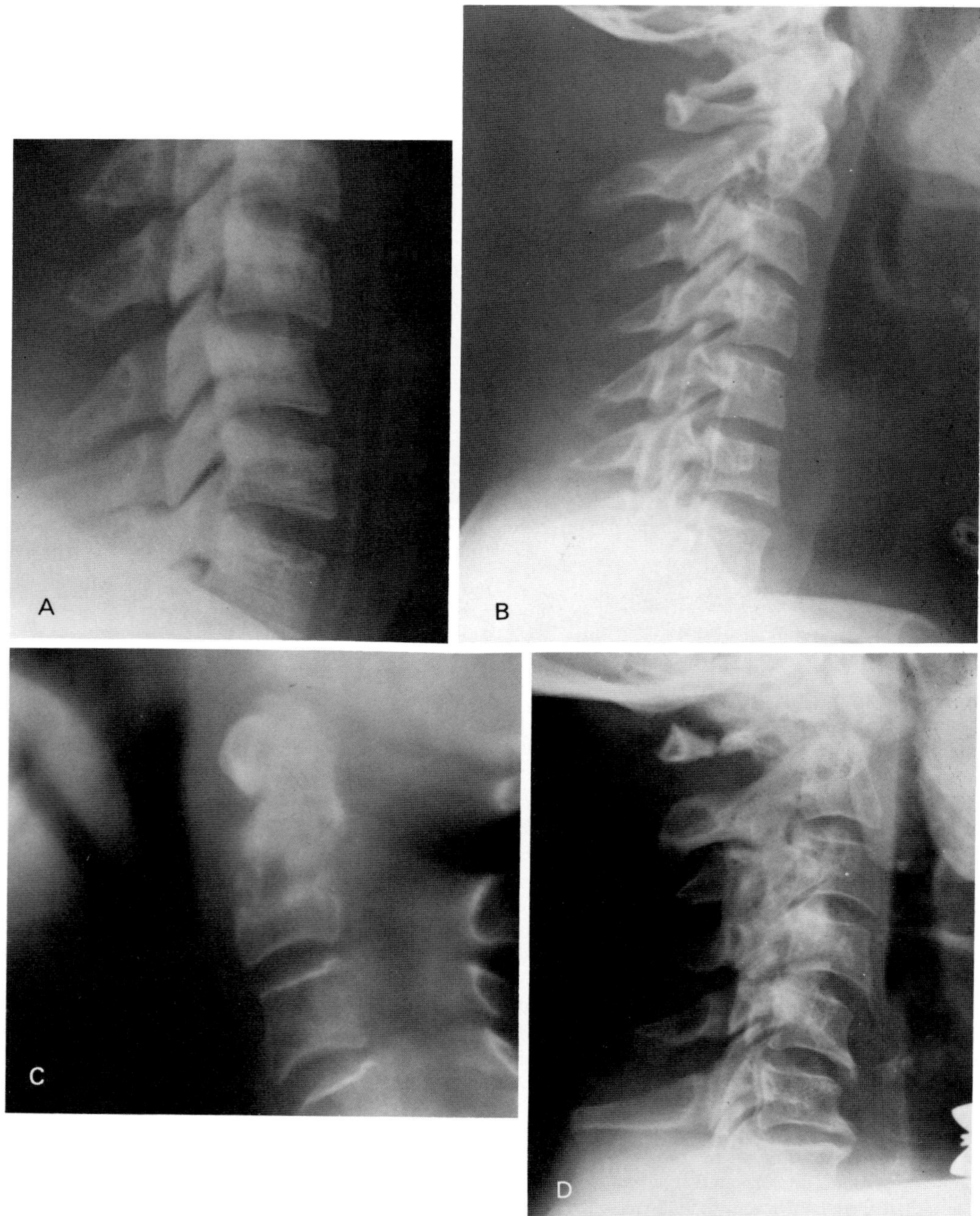

Figure 37.14. Spinal fracture-dislocations. *A,* Posterior dislocation of sixth cervical vertebra producing quadriplegia. *B,* Fracture-dislocation of second and third cervical vertebrae without neurologic deficit. *C,* Fractured odontoid process (tomogram). *D,* Fractured arch of first cervical vertebra.

that they had sudden, severe, incapacitating back pain on lifting an object, with muscle spasm and varying amounts of pain extending into the lower extremities; in addition, they were unable to straighten up. The differential diagnosis includes possibilities from simple muscle spasm and strain to acute ruptured intervertebral disc. Although most patients have a minor condition treatable with mus-

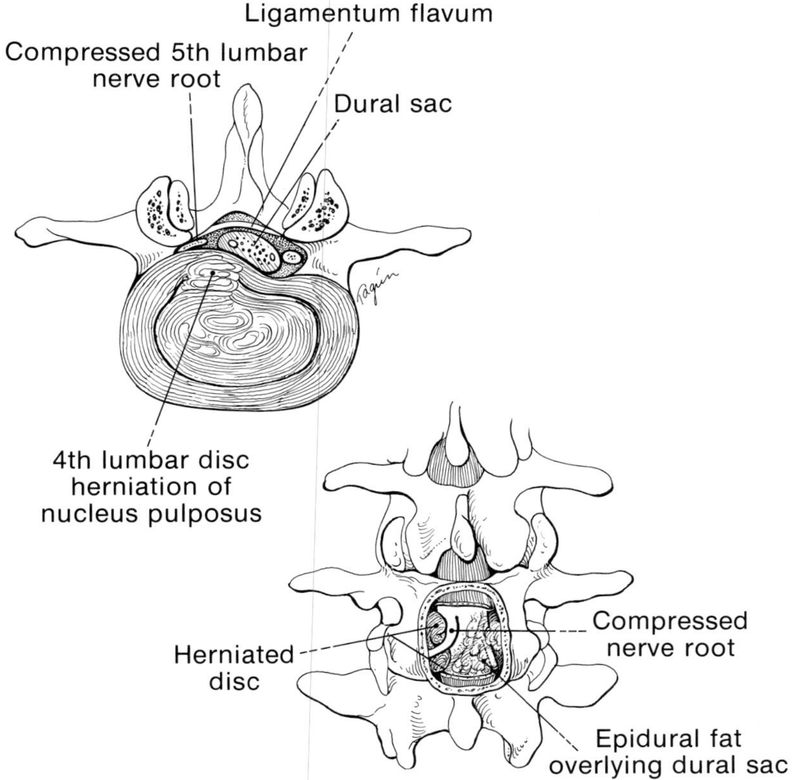

Figure 37.15. Lumbar disc fragment compressing exiting nerve root.

cle relaxants and bed rest, patients with reflex changes, sensory loss, motor weakness, or difficulties with bowel or bladder function require special attention.

The presentation of patients with acute neurologic loss associated with motion-induced back pain is usually due to posterior protrusion of the herniated or ruptured nucleus pulposus into the intervertebral foramen, causing compression of the exiting nerve roots (Fig. 37.15). The first sacral nerve root between the fifth lumbar vertebra and the sacrum is compressed most frequently, producing loss of the ankle jerk, sensory loss on the lateral aspect of the foot and on the sole, and weakness of the gastrocnemius and soleus muscles. Less frequently, disc protrusion occurs between the fourth and fifth lumbar vertebrae with compression of the fifth lumbar nerve root, resulting in no reflex changes but loss of sensation over the dorsum of the foot and great toe, with weakness of the foot and dorsiflexion muscles of the toes. Large midline disc protrusions that may initially fill the spinal canal are occasionally seen between the fifth lumbar and first sacral vertebrae and between the fourth and fifth lumbar vertebrae. These protrusions may result in compression of the entire cauda equina below this level, producing sacral sensory loss and urinary retention. They are neurosurgical emergencies that require immediate operation.

After neurologic examination has established the degree of neural involvement, lumbosacral spine films are obtained to document the presence of bony abnormalities. Narrowing of the relevant interspace is often observed.

Complete bed rest for 2 weeks often results in significant alleviation of low back pain and muscle spasm, and sometimes even reversal of neurologic deficit. CAT scan or myelographic examination (Fig. 37.16) is recommended only after such a regimen; it should be followed by surgical correction of the nerve root compression if one is demonstrated. All too often, patients with a slight neurologic deficit and minimal symptoms are subjected to myelographic examination and operation when a more progressive conservative approach could yield favorable long-term results. To facilitate bed rest, adequate analgesia and sedation must be provided; nonsteroidal anti-inflammatory medications are very effective in decreasing muscle spasm and radicular discomfort.

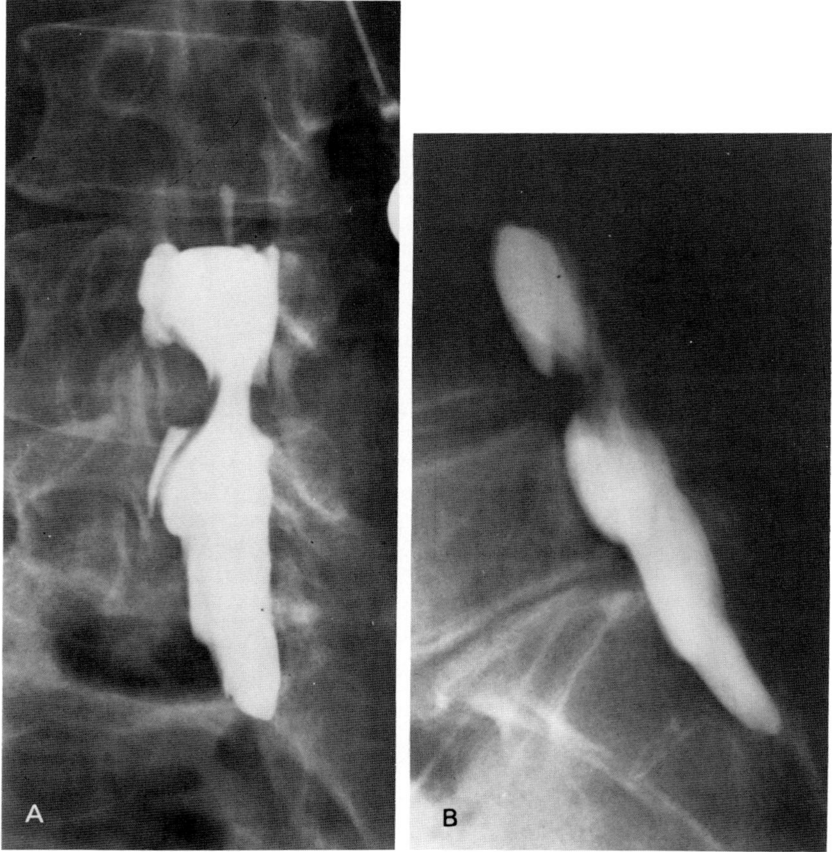

Figure 37.16. Myelograms demonstrating herniated lumbar disc. *A,* Oblique view showing large defect with compression of exiting root. *B,* Lateral view showing posterior dislocation of dural sac by disc fragment.

Neck pain is a frequent complaint of patients who suffer an acceleration-deceleration injury. The extent of injury may range from muscle spasm and pain, the "whiplash" syndrome, to severe fracture-dislocation that may not have an associated neurologic deficit. Caution should be exercised in evaluating this type of condition in the emergency department. Fracture-dislocation should be assumed until disproved. Only then is it reasonable to treat the patient conservatively with a cervical collar and muscle relaxants. A period of immobilization with adequate analgesics and nonsteroidal anti-inflammatory medications usually results in a decrease in the muscle spasm. Persistent neck and occipital pain after accidents of this type are difficult to treat; patients may complain of pain for several months or even years. A conclusive pathologic study of this entity has never been done; patients rarely have a neurologic deficit and seldom undergo special diagnostic studies. When neurologic loss is present, hospitalization should be considered; if improvement does not occur, a myelogram is required to demonstrate the presence of cervical disc herniation. When large disc herniation is present, spinal cord compression may result with quadriparesis and other long tract signs. These signs are indications for immediate surgical intervention.

Thoracic disc rupture, although extremely rare, can be manifested by paraplegia, and immediate attention to the patient with a history of heavy lifting, sudden pain in the middle of the back, and bilateral lower extremity paresthesias, or weakness is essential. Emergency myelographic examination should be carried out and surgical decompression performed when the myelogram reveals spinal cord compression. Delay may result in an irreversible neurologic deficit.

SUGGESTED READINGS

Adams JH, Mitchell DE, Graham DI, et al. Diffuse brain damage of immediate impact type: Its relationship to "primary brain stem damage" in head injury. *Brain,* 1977;100:489–502.

Braughler JM, Hall ED. Current application of "high-dose" steroid therapy for CNS injury. *J Neurosurg*, 1985;62:806–810.

Bruce DA, Alavi A, Bilanink L, et al. Diffuse cerebral swelling following head injuries in children: The syndrome of "malignant brain edema." *J Neurosurg*, 1981;54:170–178.

Davies WE, Morris JH, Hill V. An analysis of conservative (nonsurgical) management of thoracolumbar fractures and fracture-dislocations with neural damage. *J Bone Joint Surg* 1980;62A:1324–1328.

Dearden NM, McDowell DG. Comparison of etomidate and althesin in the reduction of increased intracranial pressure after head injury. *Br J Anaesth*, 1985;57:361–368.

Debrun G, Lacour P, Vinuela F, et al. Treatment of 54 traumatic carotid-cavernous fistulas. *J Neurosurg*, 1981;55:678-692.

Faden AI. Neuropeptides and central nervous system injury. *Arch Neurol*, 1986;43:501–504.

Faden AI, Jacobs TP, Holaday JW. Thyrotropin-releasing hormone improves neurologic recovery after spinal trauma in cats. *N Engl J Med*, 1981;305:1063–1067.

Geberich SC, Priest JD, Boen JR, et al. Concussion incidences and severity in secondary school varsity football players. *Am J Public Health,* 1983;73:1370–1375.

Grabow JD, Offord KP, Rieder ME. The cost of head trauma in Olmsted Country, Minnesota, 1970–74. *Am J Public Health*, 1984;74:710–712.

Guidelines for the determination of death: Report of the medical consultants on the diagnosis of death to the President's Commission for the Study of Ethical Problems in Medicine and Biomedical and Behavioral Research. *JAMA*, 1981;246:2184–2186.

Han JS. Head trauma evaluated by magnetic resonance and computed tomography: a comparison. *Radiology*, 1984;150:71–77.

Ignelzi RJ. Cerebral edema: Present perspectives. *Neurosurgery*, 1979;4:338–342.

Jane JA, Steward O, Gennarelli T. Axonal degeneration induced by minor experimental head injury. *J Neurosurg*, 1985;62:96–100.

Jennett WB, Teasdale G. Aspects of coma after severe head injury. *Lancet*, 1977;1:878–881.

Jennett WB, Teasdale G. *Management of Head Injuries.* Philadelphia, FA Davis, 1981.

Klauder MR, Marshall LF, Toole BM, et al. Cause of decline in head injury mortality rate in San Diego County, California. *J Neurosurg*, 1985;62:528–531.

Marshall LF, Smith RW, Shapiro HM. The outcome with aggressive treatment in severe head injuries. *J Neurosurg,* 1979;50:26–30.

McGraw CP, Alexander E, Howard G. Effect of dose and dose schedule on the response of intracranial pressure to mannitol. *Surg Neurol*, 1978;10:127–130.

Mendelow AD, Teasdale G, Jennett, B, et al. Risks of intracranial hematoma in head injured adults. *Br Med J*, 1983;287:1173–1176.

Miller JD, Jones PA. The work of a regional head injury service. *Lancet*, 1985;1:1141–1144.

Miller JD, Sweet RC, Narayan R, et al. Early insults to the injured brain. *JAMA*, 1978;240:439–442.

New PFJ, Aronow S. Attenuation measurements of whole blood and blood fractions in computed tomography. *Radiology*, 1976;121:635–640.

Odom GL. Central nervous system trauma research status report. National Institutes of Health, 1979.

Plum F, Posner JB. *The Diagnosis of Stupor and Coma,* ed 3. Philadelphia: FA Davis, 1980.

Reiss SJ, Raque GH, Shields CB, et al. Cervical spine fractures with major associated trauma. *Neurosurgery*, 1986;18:327–330.

Rimel RW, Giordani B, Barth JT, et al. Disability caused by minor head injury. *Neurosurgery*, 1981;9:221–228.

Rosenbaum WI, Greenberg RP, Seelig JM, et al. Midbrain lesions: frequent and significant prognostic feature in closed head injury. *Neurosurgery*, 1981;9:613–620.

Sainsbury CPQ, Sibert JR. How long do we need to observe head injuries in hospital? *Arch Dis Child*, 1984;59:856–859.

Schecter WP, Pepper E, Tuatoo V. Can general surgery improve the outcome of the head injury victim in rural America? *Arch Surg*, 1985;120:1163–1166.

Schmidek HH, Gomes FB, Seligson D, et al. Management of acute unstable thoracolumbar fractures with and without neurological deficit. *Neurosurgery*, 1980;7:30–35.

Seelig, JM, Becker DP, Miller JD, et al. Traumatic acute subdural hematoma: major mortality reduction in comatose patients treated within four hours. *N Engl J Med,* 1981;304:1511–1518.

Strich SJ. Shearing of nerve fibres as a cause of brain damage due to head injury. *Lancet*, 1961;2:443–448.

Youmans JR. Causes of shock with head injury. *J Trauma*, 1964;4:204–209.

CHAPTER 38

Thermal Injuries

NICHOLAS E. O'CONNOR, M.D.
MICHAEL B. LEWIS, M.D.

More than 100,000 burned patients are admitted to hospitals in the United States each year. Although the figure is unknown, a greater number of burned patients are seen in the emergency department, treated, and released. These patients together constitute a large group who by the very nature of their injury are first seen by the emergency physician. The severity of the burn injury varies from a mild sunburn requiring no treatment to a major full-thickness burn whose treatment requires the extensive resources of modern medicine. Although many factors determine the final outcome, proper emergency care is the first step toward satisfactory recovery.

As with any injured patient, the first priority is to ensure an adequate airway and to stop hemorrhage. Some respiratory problems unique to the burned patient are discussed.

An initial responsibility of the physician is to stop the burning process. Burning has usually stopped before arrival in the emergency department, but occasionally, bits of smouldering clothing are still attached to the skin. A glowing fiber is extremely hot and must be removed to prevent further injury.

The emergency care of the burned patient has been divided into the following topics:

1. Determination of the cause of the burn;
2. Determination of the extent and depth of the burn;
3. Evaluation of the general health status of the burn victim and the presence or absence of coexistent injuries;
4. Initiation of the necessary resuscitative measures, including fluid replacement, respiratory care, and treatment;
5. Initiation of burn wound care;
6. Determination of the need for hospitalization.

By no means should the order of presentation of this material be interpreted as implying priorities. In fact, in the actual care of the burned patient, the different aspects of management are carried out simultaneously.

Electrical burns, chemical burns, and frostbite are discussed separately at the end of the chapter.

PATHOPHYSIOLOGY

Etiology

Many agents can cause burns. These include ultraviolet light, scalding liquids and steam, flash explosives, flame, electricity, and certain chemicals. Most burns necessitating hospital admission result from flash or flame injury, whereas many of the more minor burns not requiring admission result from contact with scalding material or hot metal.

Determination of the causative agent is important because it may suggest the depth of the burn and the presence of coexistent injuries. For instance, a scald due to a hot liquid is usually a partial-thickness burn that is not associated with other lesions. On the other hand, a flame injury sustained in a closed space most likely is a full-thickness burn that is probably accompanied by respiratory injury.

As many details as possible about the accident should be obtained. The time that the burn occurred and any previous treatment should be noted.

Table 38.1.
Rule of Nines: Rapid Means of Estimating Body Surface Area Burned in Adult Patients

Area	Percent
Head and neck	9
Arm	
Right	9
Left	9
Torso	
Front	18
Back	18
Leg	
Right	18
Left	18
Genitals and perineum	1
Total	100

Extent and Depth of the Burn

Knowledge of the extent of the body surface involved and the depth of the burn is necessary to determine the prognosis, the need for hospitalization, the resuscitative measures indicated, and the proper treatment of the burn wound.

The "rule of nines" (Table 38.1), which is probably the simplest method for determining body surface area burned in an adult patient, divides the surfaces of the body into units that are multiples of nine. By determining the portion of each unit involved, the examiner quickly estimates the body surface area burned. Because the percentage of body surface area represented by the different anatomic units varies with age, a different system is needed for infants and children. The "rule of fives" (Table 38.2) is a reasonably accurate system similar to the rule of nines in design and use, except that each of the body units is a multiple of five.

In discussions of the burn wound, the terms first-, second-, and third-degree burn are used to indicate the depth of injury to the skin. The terms partial-thickness burn and full-thickness burn are used interchangeably with second-degree burn and third-degree burn, respectively. All full-thickness burns and some partial-thickness burns require skin grafting for definitive wound closure. Although no completely reliable method exists for determining the depth of a burn when first seen in the emergency department, there are many clues. The most helpful diagnostic considerations are the type of burning agent, the appearance of the burn wound, and the presence or absence of sensation. The relationships of these factors to the depth of the burn are outlined in Table 38.3.

All this information should be recorded accurately and completely. This is most readily done and the information most easily interpreted at a later time if a diagram is used (Fig. 38.1).

Table 38.2.
Rules of Fives: Rapid Means of Estimating Body Surface Area Burned in Infants and Children

Area	Infant, %	Child, %
Head and neck	20	15
Arm		
Right	10	10
Left	10	10
Torso		
Front	20	20
Back	20	20
Leg		
Right	10	15
Left	10	15
Total	100	105

EVALUATION

History

All pertinent information should be gathered, including the patient's age and weight, allergies to drugs, medications being taken, tetanus immunization status, and acute or chronic medical illnesses. A rapid but thorough physical examination should include the recording of pulse rate, blood pressure, respiration rate, temperature, and level of consciousness. Examination of the internal nares for singed vibrissae and the posterior oropharynx for soot may suggest an inhalation respiratory injury. The judicious use of a laryngoscope is helpful in examining the pharynx.

Examination

The emergency physician should examine the patient carefully for other trauma sustained at the time of the burn injury; coexistent injuries are not uncommon, but often are missed. Respiratory damage and long bone fractures occur frequently, but central nervous system, chest, and abdominal trauma may also occur. These injuries must be sought and given appropriate priority in treatment.

Laboratory Study

In the more seriously burned patient requiring hospitalization, the following laboratory and x-ray studies are necessary: complete blood cell count; urinalysis; measurement of serum electrolytes, blood urea nitrogen, and serum proteins; prothrombin time; typing and cross-matching of blood; and chest x-ray films.

When the history and physical examination suggest the presence of concomitant disease or injury, the following tests may be indicated: liver chemistries; measurement of serum creatinine and blood

Table 38.3.
Depth of Burn Injury

Depth or Classification	Structural Damage	Causal Agent	Clinical Appearance	Sensation
First-degree	Only superficial layers of epidermis devitalized; dilatation of intradermal vessels.	Ultraviolet exposure Very short flash	Erythema; blanches with pressure	Present
Second-degree (partial-thickness)	Destruction of epidermis to basal layer; deeper skin appendages preserved in dermal layer; clefting of epidermis with fluid collection	Spillage of scalding material Flash Some chemicals	Blister formation, erythema, weeping; superficial skin can be wiped away; erythematous areas should blanch with pressure	Present
Third-degree (full-thickness)	Destruction of all skin elements, epidermal and dermal; coagulation of subdermal blood vessels	Flame Immersion Some chemicals	Dry, pale white, charred, leathery, inelastic, visible thrombosed vessels; sometimes red from fixed hemoglobin and will not blanch	Absent
Fourth-degree (involvement of muscle, bone, and other deep structures)	Destruction of all skin elements along with necrosis of deeper structures	Electricity Flame occasionally	Deeply charred, shrunken, often with exposed bones; explosive-appearing	Absent

glucose; stool guaiac test; urine hemoglobin and myoglobin; arterial blood-gas analysis; skull, facial, long bone and abdominal x-ray films; and an electrocardiogram.

Need for Hospitalization

The decision to hospitalize a patient is based on many factors, including age, concomitant disease or injury, and most importantly, on the extent, depth, and location of the burn. Although each case differs, certain guidelines for admission have been found helpful (Table 38.4). In addition, all patients suspected of having an inhalation injury and patients with small burns associated with other severe injuries should be admitted.

RESUSCITATIVE MEASURES

Prevention of Shock

In patients requiring hospitalization because of the extent of the burn injury, the accumulation of edema fluid with water, electrolytes, and protein in the burn wound is of such magnitude that hypovolemic shock will occur if it goes untreated. Burn wound edema has been thought to develop progressively during the first 48 hours after injury, but recent evidence suggests that the accumulation of edema fluid is complete within 24 hours. Fluid replacement should begin immediately. Most methods of determining the initial fluid requirement are based on body weight and percent of body surface area burned. The commonly used formulas for fluid replacement are the Brooke, Evans, and Baxter formulas (Table 38.5). It is standard not to use a figure greater than 50% body surface area in these formulas, even though the actual percentage is higher.

These formulas should be used only as a guide to begin fluid replacement. Alterations in the rate of fluid administration must be made frequently, depending on the adequacy of treatment and response as determined by monitoring of the following signs: (*a*) urinary output (40–60 ml/hr in the adult) and specific gravity; (*b*) vital signs (blood pressure, pulse rate, and respiration rate); (*c*) central venous pressure; and (*d*) hematocrit (a minor degree of hemoconcentration is acceptable). Two intravenous catheters should be placed, one with its tip centrally located so that central venous pressure can be determined. No indwelling venous catheters should be inserted in lower extremity veins because of the high incidence of resulting thrombophlebitis. An indwelling urinary catheter should be inserted to allow recording of urine output. These variables are easily monitored and should be recorded carefully every 30–60 minutes. Changes suggest the need for altering the rate of fluid administration. The use of

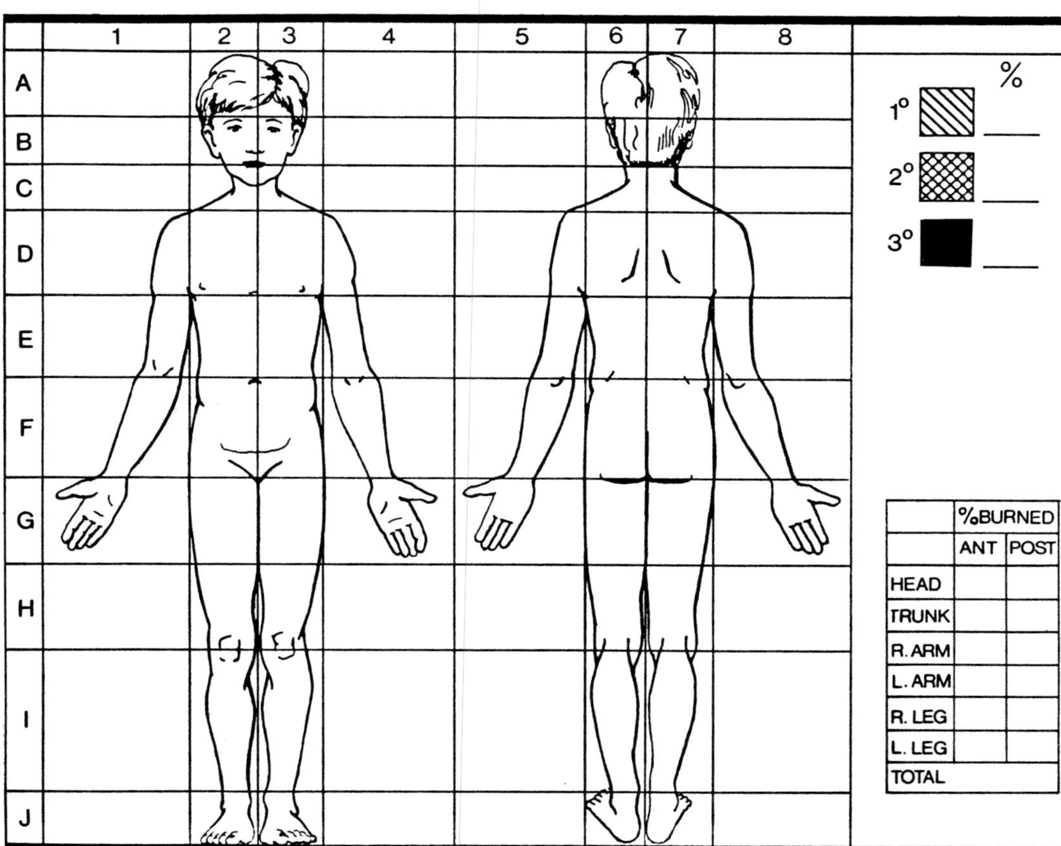

Figure 38.1. Burn diagram. This allows quick, accurate, and reproducible recording of surface area and depth of burn; it should become a permanent part of the patient's record.

flow sheets (Figs. 38.2 and 38.3) allows these decisions to be made rapidly and accurately. In patients with even more serious burns and in those with coexistent cardiac or pulmonary disease or injury, monitoring of the arterial blood gases (Po_2, Pco_2, and pH) is helpful (Fig. 38.2).

Inhalation Injury

Injury to the respiratory tract is one of the most frequent and dangerous complications of burns and is the leading cause of death in fire victims (see also Chapter 32). More than one-half of the 6000 annual fire deaths in the United States are caused by inhalation injury. There are three kinds of inhalation injury: upper airway damage, pulmonary parenchymal injury, and carbon monoxide poisoning.

Upper airway and laryngeal edema result from the inhalation of hot gases and the irritating chemicals in smoke. The tissue damage caused by these agents leads to upper airway edema and laryngeal spasm and edema, usually within 3–6 hours of injury. Increasing hoarseness, inability to swallow secretions, and an increased respiration rate are signs of impending upper airway obstruction.

On examination, burns of the face or neck, singed nasal hairs, inflamed or swollen posterior pharyngeal mucosa, and edema of the glottis suggest potential airway difficulty. These patients should be

Table 38.4.
Admission Guidelines for Burned Patients

Age	Burn Depth	Body Surface
<10 yr >65 yr	Second-degree	10% or more
10–65 yr	Second-degree	20% or more
All ages	Third-degree	>5%[a]
All ages	Deep second- or third-degree	Face, perineum, hands, or feet

[a] In many cases, these patients are best treated with primary excision and grafting of the burn wound.

considered for immediate endotracheal intubation. If the airway edema has progressed too far, intubation may be impossible, and tracheotomy will be necessary. Humidified air should be provided through the endotracheal tube.

Pulmonary parenchymal injury is always suspected with a history of fire in a closed space—a fire being associated with copious smoke production—or if other victims of the same fire have inhalation injury. The same irritating chemicals, such as aldehydes and nitrates in wood smoke, cyanides, ammonia, chlorine, and phosgene in smoke from synthetic materials that cause airway damage, are toxic to the pulmonary parenchyma; they may lead to necrotizing bronchiolitis, intraalveolar edema, and hyaline membrane formation. Soot particles in the sputum and an elevated blood carboxyhemoglobin concentration warn of pulmonary injury. The injury produces the pathophysiologic changes seen with bronchopneumonia. These changes usually are not manifest for 12–24, or as long as 48 hours. The patient may then have an increased respiration rate, auscultatory signs of bronchospasm, a chest x-ray appearance compatible with congestion and edema or bronchopneumonia, and a falling arterial Po_2. The chest x-ray signs usually lag behind the clinical signs. Early fiberoptic bronchoscopic examination is helpful in determining the extent of damage to the lower part of the airway. Patients with this injury are treated for hypoxemia and infection. Endotracheal intubation and mechanical ventilation with positive end-expiratory pressure is the treatment of choice for severe injuries. The addition of corticosteroids to the treatment regimen has now been shown ineffective, and may accentuate the risk of infection. Prophylactic antibiotics are not thought to be effective; however, careful monitoring of fluid administration to prevent pulmonary overload is important.

Carbon monoxide poisoning, the most common single cause of death in burn victims, is distinct from upper airway or pulmonary injury in its pathophysiology. Carbon monoxide is a colorless, odorless, tasteless, nonirritating gas liberated from incomplete combustion of carbon compounds. Carbon monoxide combines with hemoglobin to form carboxyhemoglobin. The affinity of hemoglobin for carbon monoxide is approximately 250 times greater than its affinity for oxygen and, therefore, even a small amount of carbon monoxide in the atmosphere competes successfully with oxygen for the binding sites of hemoglobin. The resulting carboxyhemoglobin, besides rendering the patient functionally anemic, shifts the oxyhemoglobin dissociation curve to the left, making the patient even more hypoxic. Death is due to hypoxia, hypercapnia, and acidosis.

Carbon monoxide poisoning is suggested by any of the signs associated with inhalation injury, but is confirmed by determining the level of carboxyhemoglobin in an arterial or venous blood sample. A carboxyhemoglobin level from 15–25% suggests mild carbon monoxide poisoning. A level greater than 25% suggests serious poisoning, especially if the injury occurred more than 1 hour before testing. Patients with mild poisoning are treated with oxygen administered by face mask. Those with serious poisoning are intubated and placed on assisted ventilation with 100% oxygen. Administration of 100%

Table 38.5.
Fluid Replacement Formulas for First 24 Hours

Source	Colloid	Electrolyte Solution	Water	Rate
Brooke[a]	0.5 ml/kg/% BSA burned	1.5 ml/kg/% BSA burned	2000 ml	1/2 first 8 hr 1/4 second 8 hr 1/4 third 8 hr
Evans[a]	1 ml/kg/% BSA burned	1 ml/kg/% BSA burned	2000 ml	1/2 first 8 hr 1/4 second 8 hr 1/4 third 8 hr
Baxter[b]		4 ml/kg/% BSA burned		1/2 first 8 hr 1/4 second 8 hr 1/4 third 8 hr

BSA, body surface area.
[a] Approximately one-half the amount estimated for the first 24 hours is given the second 24 hours.
[b] Only maintenance fluids are given the second 24 hours; colloid is given as necessary.

PERMANENT RECORD COPY
MASSACHUSETTS GENERAL HOSPITAL

CRITICAL CARE DATA SHEET

#	Time	Conditions (spont/Vent type/O_2 Flow)	FiO_2	pO_2	pCO_2	pH	Na	K	Hct.	TP	OSM	C.I.	O_2 Cont.	VENTILATION			
														TV	RR	IP	PEEP
1																	
2																	
3																	
4																	
5																	
6																	
7																	
8																	
9																	
10																	
11																	
12																	
13																	
14																	
15																	
16																	
17																	
18																	

BLEEDING STUDIES					
Time	PT	PTT	Plats.	Fibrin	Other

RENAL							
Time	Na	K	OSM	BUN	Creat.	pH	Analysis/ Other

X-Rays Results
Time

Miscellaneous	
Time	Result

Figure 38.2. Critical care data sheet. A flow sheet to record electrolytes, arterial blood gases, and hematocrit in early resuscitative phase facilitates interpretation of data. This should be readily available at bedside.

NAME

DATE OF BURN:
HOUR OF BURN (H.B.):

DATE OF ENTRY:
HOUR OF ENTRY:

UNIT NO.

		FLUID INTAKE							OUTPUT					
DATE	HOUR INTERVAL	TOTAL	PLASMA	WHOLE BLOOD	SALINE SOLS. IV	SALINE SOLS. PO*	OTHER FLUIDS IV	OTHER FLUIDS PO*	TOTAL	URINE Vol.	URINE S.G.	VOM-ITUS	DIARRHEA	EXUDATE
	m to m													
	m to m													
	m to m													
	m to m													
	m to m													
	m to m													
	m to m													
	m to m													
	m to m													
	m to m													
	m to m													
	m to m													
12 hour total														
24 hour total														

* SALINE SOLS. = any fluid containing salt.
* OTHER FLUIDS = fluids which do not contain salt, such as milk, fruit juices, broth not containing salt, bottled beverages, tea, coffee.

Figure 38.3. Fluid balance sheet. Knowledge of exact intake and output is critical to management of the acutely burned patient. A flow sheet should be used and be readily available at bedside.

oxygen is continued for several hours until the carboxyhemoglobin level is below 10%.

General Treatment

Most burned patients requiring hospitalization have some degree of reflex ileus. Oral feedings of both liquids and solids should be withheld until proper function of the gastrointestinal tract has returned. This could take only 1 or 2 hours, or as long as 24 hours or more.

In severely burned patients and in patients with an altered level of consciousness, insertion of an indwelling nasogastric tube for immediate gastric emptying and constant suction drainage is indicated to prevent regurgitation and/or vomiting with possible aspiration. This is especially important if the patient is to be transported to another hospital or to a different area in the same hospital.

Most burned patient have enough discomfort and apprehension to require analgesia and sedation. Agitation may be a sign of cerebral hypoxia, not of discomfort; medication might only aggravate the situation. When sedation and analgesia are necessary in the hospitalized patient, a small dose of morphine sulfate, 1–3 mg intravenously, is usually sufficient. Oral, subcutaneous, or intramuscular routes should not be used, because the degree of absorption cannot be predicted. For outpatients, oral analgesics and sedatives can be given safely.

A standard set of admission orders should be established for burned patients requiring hospitalization (Table 38.6).

Table 38.6.
Typical Admission Orders for Burned Patients Requiring Hospitalization

Nothing by mouth
Intake and output every hour (record)
Vital signs every hour (record)
Urinary output and specific gravity every hour (record)
Central venous pressure every hour (record)
Fluid orders (Brooke, Evans, or Baxter formula)
Wound care specifics
Nasogastric tube, gravity or low suction (record output)
Humidified oxygen by face mask
Aqueous penicillin, 600,000 units intravenously twice a day for 48 hours
Morphine sulfate, 1 mg/15 kg body weight intravenously every 3 hours as needed
Wound care
Daily weight

BURN WOUND CARE

Cleansing and Debridement

Most burns require little cleansing or debridement. Blisters should be left intact. Adherent clothing, dirt, and other foreign material should be removed. A mild nondetergent soap and warm water rinse may be helpful; strong detergent soaps, especially those containing hexachlorophene should be avoided.

Sterile precautions should be taken when burn wounds are handled. A cap, mask, sterile gown, and sterile gloves should be worn. Wound specimens for culture should be taken before initiating topical treatment. The burned areas should be elevated several centimeters above heart level if possible.

Specific Wound Care and Topical Agents

First-degree Burns

Most of these injuries result from excessive exposure to the ultraviolet rays of the sun or a sunlamp. Topical and oral analgesics are usually all the treatment necessary. Patients with very extensive sunburn may occasionally develop significant edema with malaise, fatigability, anorexia, and nausea. Except in very young or very old patients, this situation can still safely be managed on an outpatient basis.

Sunburn patients must be examined carefully for ocular injuries, and ophthalmologic consultation should be obtained, if indicated.

Second-degree Burns

Most isolated partial-thickness or second-degree burns result from scalding. Although immediate immersion of the burn in cold water is effective in limiting the depth of the injury and in controlling edema, immersion is of little benefit after the first few minutes except to relieve pain. Since most patients arrive in the emergency department several minutes to several hours after injury, immersion is probably not helpful.

Both open and closed methods of treatment are acceptable, but for reasons of comfort and convenience, the closed method is preferable. This is especially true for outpatients. Dressings should be applied under sterile conditions. A single layer of nonadherent fine-mesh gauze placed immediately next to the wound is covered by several layers of multiple-ply, coarse-mesh gauze without cotton filling. This is secured by an elastic wrap or bias stockinette applied firmly, but not tightly. The dressing should be changed under sterile conditions every 4–5 days. Temperature elevation above 100.4–101.3°F (38–38.5°C), purulent drainage, and other signs of infections are reasons for more frequent dressing changes.

The burned parts should be immobilized and kept elevated, if possible, with bed rest for lower-extremity burns, an arm sling for upper-extremity burns, and elevation of the head of the bed for head and neck burns. If the hand is burned, it should be splinted with the wrist extended, the metacarpophalangeal joints flexed, and the interphalangeal joints extended. After the dressing has been applied, a plaster or isoprene splint should be molded and secured to the burned hand (Fig. 38.4). At each dressing change, the joints of the hand should be put through active and passive range-of-motion exercises. As soon as the wound is healed, usually in less than 2 weeks, the splint is discarded.

Partial-thickness burns of the face and neck often are treated more easily by the open technique, bulky dressings are difficult to manage around the eyes, nose, and mouth. In the open method, the wound should be rinsed gently twice a day with sterile physiologic saline solution, followed by application of an antibiotic ointment such as bacitracin, neomycin, or polymyxin B.

Partial-thickness burns should heal spontaneously. Depending on the depth of the burn, it may take from 5 days to 3 weeks for a complete epithelial cover to develop. Dressing should be continued throughout this period. Table 38.7 summarizes the outpatient management of partial-thickness scalds.

Patients with partial-thickness burns in combination with full-thickness burns are best treated with the technique used for the latter.

Third-degree Burns

Most full-thickness burns result from flame injury or immersion in hot liquid. Unless the wound is very small, these patients require hospitalization. The emergency department treatment of such patients is summarized in Table 38.8.

Several topical agents have been developed that decrease bacterial proliferation in the burn wound and thereby prevent some secondary septic complications. These agents have been most beneficial in increasing survival in those patients with full-thickness burns covering 40–80% of the body surface area, but they are routinely used in all full-thickness burn injuries. The four most commonly utilized agents are 0.5% silver nitrate solution, 10% mafenide acetate cream (Sulfamylon), 1% silver sulfadiazine cream (Silvadine), and povidone-iodine ointment (Betadine). Techniques of application, advantages, and disadvantages of these four agents are given in Table 38.9. No one agent is clearly superior to the others; the one used should be determined by familiarity and availability. The agents should be applied as soon as possible after

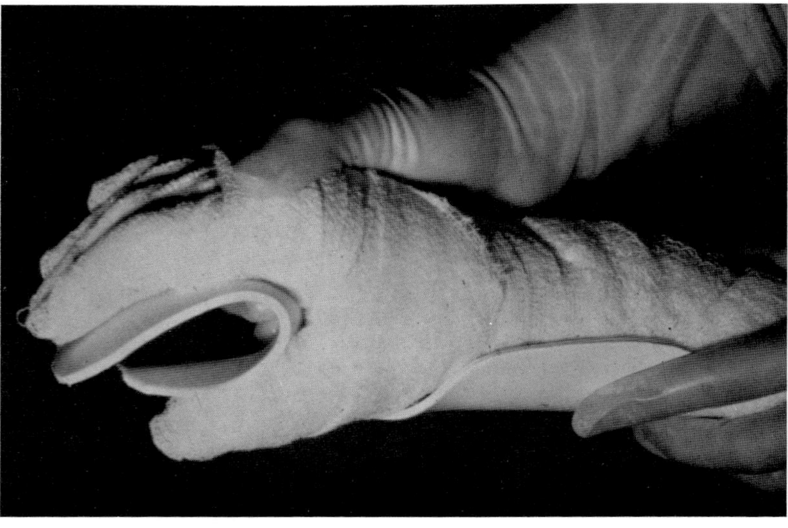

Figure 38.4. Isoprene splint for hand and forearm is depicted with wrist extended, metacarpophalangeal joints flexed, and interphalangeal joints extended. This facilitates return of good function.

cleansing the wound. The patient should be covered with sterile sheets to maintain sterility and to provide warmth.

The concept of early or primary burn wound excision that is applied to the management of small, full-thickness burns has been expanded to include more extensive full-thickness burns as well. Reports indicate that this can decrease morbidity, mortality, and length of hospitalization. This does not change the initial wound care necessary in the emergency department, however.

Table 38.7.
Outpatient Management of Partial-thickness Scald

- Historical and physical findings related to burn injury
  - Cause
  - Time
  - Pictorial description of extent and depth of burn
  - Related injuries
- Pertinent past medical history
  - Chronic illnesses
  - Medications
  - Allergies
  - Status of tetanus prophylaxis
- Sterile burn wound care
  - Minimal cleansing and debridement; blisters are left intact
  - Application of dressing
  - Elevation of burned parts; splints
  - Dressing change in 4–5 days
- Tetanus prophylaxis
- Low-dose penicillin therapy for 5 days

Escharotomy

In circumferential full-thickness burns of the extremities or torso, escharotomy may become an ur-

Table 38.8.
Emergency Department Treatment of Partial-thickness and Full-thickness Flame Burns Requiring Hospitalization

- Initiate any emergency airway measures necessary
  - Administer humidified oxygen
  - Be alert for respiratory distress and treat appropriately
- Elicit historical and physical findings related to burn injury
  - Cause
  - Time
  - Prior treatment
  - Pictorial description of extent and depth of burn
  - Related injuries
- Elicit pertinent past medical history
  - Chronic illnesses
  - Medications
  - Allergies
  - Status of tetanus prophylaxis
- Obtain necessary laboratory and radiologic studies
- Insert the following catheters:
  - Intravenous
  - Central venous pressure
  - Indwelling urinary
  - Nasogastric
- Initiate fluid replacement with electrolyte-containing solution
- Calculate expected fluid requirements
- Start flow sheet of vital data
- Begin local wound care
- Administer tetanus prophylaxis
- Give first dose in penicillin therapy

Table 38.9.
Comparison of Available Topical Agents for Burn Management

Agent	Technique of Application	Advantages	Disadvantages
0.5% silver nitrate solution	2.5 cm thick coarse-mesh gauze dressing soaked every 2 hr with solution; dressing changed ever 12 hr	Only minimal pain with application; occlusive dressing comfortable; decreased evaporative losses; easily used in grafted and ungrafted areas	Delays eschar separation; electrolyte abnormalities—hyponatremia, hypokalemia, hypocalcemia; discolors everything; does not penetrate eschar
10% mafenide acetate cream (Sulfamylon)	Apply every 24 hr and replenish as needed; dressing usually not used	Penetrates eschar; easy to apply; nonstaining	Acidosis; burning pain with application; delays eschar separation; sensitivity reactions (10–15%); inhibits epithelialization
1% silver sulfadiazine cream (Silvadene)	Apply every 12 hr and replenish as needed; dressing of fine-mesh gauze may be used	Easy to apply; nonstaining; minimal pain; no electrolyte or acid-base problems	Does not penetrate eschar well; delays eschar separation; occasional suppression of white blood cell count
Povidone-iodine ointment (Betadine)	Apply every 8 hr; dressing of fine-mesh gauze usually used	Easy to apply; minimal pain	Increases serum iodine levels; occasional burning pain; delays eschar separation

gent necessity. The constriction resulting from this type of burn injury can lead to circulatory compromise in the extremities, manifested by peripheral cyanosis, edema, and later ischemic changes that are limb-threatening, if not treated adequately and promptly. Circulation in the hands and feet should be assessed every few hours: feeling for peripheral pulses, observing capillary refill, and if possible, checking arterial pulse volumes and flows with Doppler recorders.

A circumferential burn of the thorax associated with an inelastic eschar can seriously limit respiratory motion, increase the work of breathing, and lead to respiratory failure, manifested by rapid and labored respirations, cyanosis, irritability, and inability to ventilate even after intubation and ventilatory support. Although escharotomy rarely requires anesthesia, since the eschar is insensate, it is best performed in the operating room where adequate sterility, lighting, instruments, and assistance are available. The escharotomy incision is always placed in the burn eschar, never in normal or lesser burned tissue.

Tetanus Prophylaxis

All partial-thickness and complete-thickness burns result in necrotic tissue. Under these conditions, the possibility of tetanus exists; although this disease is rare, adequate prophylaxis should be carried out (Table 11.6), since tetanus in the burned patient is almost always fatal. Toxoid booster injections should be given to those already immunized; injections for passive immunization must be given to those without a previous history of active immunization, and must be repeated during the course of treatment.

Systemic Antibiotic Therapy

Although the common cause of morbidity and mortality in burned patients is infection, the intensive use of systemic antibiotic prophylaxis has been ineffective in decreasing the incidence of invasive sepsis. During the first few days after a burn injury, the eschar seems to be a barrier to invasive organisms, except for the virulent β-hemolytic streptococcus. Since this organism is so common in the upper part of the respiratory tract, especially in children, routine low-dose penicillin prophylaxis is indicated. Usually, 600,000 units of penicillin G twice a day for 2 days is sufficient, particularly if primary excision is planned.

ELECTRICAL BURNS

Electrical burns are also thermal injuries. They result from direct damage to cell membranes from the passage of current and from the conversion of electrical energy to thermal energy. They often differ in presentation and treatment sufficiently to require separate consideration. For descriptive and clinical purposes, these injuries are usually divided into those of high voltage (more than 1000 volts) and low voltage (fewer than 1000 volts) and into flash injuries and actual contact or arc injuries.

Flash burns result from the heat generated by a nearby electrical flash or "explosion." The current of electricity does not contact or arc to the body surface. In low-voltage flash burns, the injury is usually a first- or second-degree burn. The skin surface appears charred, but this blackening of the epidermis usually is cleansed away easily. High-voltage flash burns can lead to more extensive second- and third-degree burns, which should be managed as any other second- or third-degree burn.

It is the actual contact or arc electrical burn that results in a different type of injury. The lesion is almost always full-thickness, and in high-voltage injuries, damage to muscle, blood vessels, nerves, tendons, fat, and bone commonly occurs. The proportions of the deep wound and necrosis in high-voltage injuries are often much more extensive than the surface necrosis indicates; this is suggested by ischemia, cyanosis, edema, and anesthesia in a limb. Whereas high-voltage contact or arc injuries are extensive, low-voltage burns are usually localized. A common low-voltage arc injury in small children is the full-thickness lesion of the oral commissure or lip sustained when a child chews through an electrical cord or sucks on an extension cord outlet (110-volt household current). This injury is discussed more fully in Chapter 39.

Much of the discussion on the emergency evaluation and treatment of the more usual thermal burns applies to electrical burns as well. In addition, the following points should be noted:

1. The voltage of the current contacted and the points of entrance and exit should be determined. These two areas are usually the most extensively damaged, since the current accumulates at these points. If these two points are known, the approximate pathway of most of the current can be established.
2. Early fasciotomy of the extremities is often necessary, since intense muscular swelling in confined fascial compartments occurs. This is an operating room procedure, but impending ischemia of the limb should be sought carefully in the emergency department.
3. Because these burn injuries are often deep, the usual topical methods of treatment are inadequate. Surgical debridement is necessary. However, these wounds can be dressed temporarily in the emergency department under sterile conditions with one of the topical agents mentioned earlier.
4. Myoglobinemia and severe acidosis often occur as a result of extensive muscle damage. If these are inadequately treated, renal failure quickly results. Treatment depends on recognition and careful monitoring. Myoglobin is manifested by a port-wine color to the urine. Laboratory tests are available for confirmation, but are rarely necessary. Acidosis is best diagnosed and monitored by means of arterial blood-gas determinations. For this, an indwelling arterial line is helpful. Treatment is based on adequate hydration to maintain a good urine output and on alkalization of the serum and urine. Vital signs should be monitored to prevent overhydration and pulmonary edema. Enough electrolyte solution should be given to maintain a urine output of 100 ml/hr or greater. Sodium bicarbonate should be added to the intravenous solutions in sufficient amounts to keep the urine alkaline and the serum pH within the normal range. Myoglobin casts do not precipitate so readily if the urine output through the renal tubules is rapid and alkaline.
5. Damage to internal organs has been reported; when the entrance and exit points suggest a pathway through the thoracic or abdominal cavity, the area must be evaluated carefully to rule out the possibility of internal injuries.
6. Myocardial damage can result from high-voltage electrical injuries. In its most severe form, immediate ventricular fibrillation and death occur. An electrocardiogram should be obtained immediately on arrival in the emergency department. The myocardial injury can be an infarct or arrhythmia, and should be treated accordingly.
7. Late development of cataracts and neurologic sequelae has been reported; initial examination should note the status of the eyes and nervous system. Proper consultation should be obtained as indicated.
8. Because of the violent muscle contractions that occur with high-voltage contact and the frequency of an associated fall, long bones are sometimes fractured.
9. Damage to the spinal cord may occur and may not be apparent on initial examination. A demyelinating lesion may develop. Since this injury can be progressive, daily neurologic assessment is necessary.

CHEMICAL BURNS

These infrequent injuries result from contact with a wide variety of chemical agents. The degree of injury depends on the chemical, its concentration, duration of contact, and the natural penetrability and resistance of the tissues involved. Chemicals do not usually "burn," in that they do not cause destruction by hyperthermic activity. Rather, they damage tissue by coagulation of protein by one of several processes: reduction, oxidation, desiccation, corrosion, or vesication.

The causative chemical agent should be carefully determined; treatment varies with the chemical (Table 38.10). The immediate treatment for most chemical burns is irrigation of the surface with copious amounts of water to dilute and to remove the residual offending agent. Standing in a shower or holding the injured part under a water spigot is the easiest means. If the eyes are involved, they should be irrigated with copious amounts of sterile physiologic saline solution or water and ophthalmologic consultation promptly obtained.

In injuries resulting from some chemical agents, water lavage is contraindicated, because it causes additional ionization, heat, and further damage. In these few cases, neutralization with the appropriate agent is proper (Table 28.10).

Of special interest are those injuries caused by hydrofluoric acid, commonly used in the semiconductor industry, in rust-removing agents, and for etching glass. The fluoride ion is more harmful than the hydrogen ion and tends to penetrate deeply, causing necrosis and painful ulceration unless neutralized. The best method of neutralization is direct injection of 10% calcium gluconate solution into the involved areas. This often immediately relieves the pain.

Once the initial stage of treatment is completed, be it irrigation, neutralization, or other means, further wound management depends on the degree of injury and does not differ from the management of burns caused by other more common agents.

COLD INJURY

There are two kinds of cold injury: systemic hypothermia and cold-induced tissue injury. The three categories of tissue injury are frostbite, trench foot, and immersion foot. Hypothermia may be associated with local tissue injury, and vice versa. Hypothermia is also discussed in Chapter 10.

Hypothermia

Accidental hypothermia, whether from exposure to cold air or cold water, reflects an imbalance between the heat produced by the body and the heat loss from it. By adjusting rates of heat production and heat loss, humans maintain a stable core body temperature range for optimal enzyme functioning. For example, for each centigrade degree of temperature drop, biochemical activity decreases about 10%. The normal core body temperature is in a nar-

Table 38.10.
Methods of Treatment for "Burns" from Chemical Agents[a]

Employ water lavage	*Cover with oil*	*Avoid oils*
Chromic acid	Na metal	Cantharides
Potassium permanganate	Phenol (cresol)	*Avoid water lavage*
Cantharides	White phosphorus	Na metal
Dimethyl sulfoxide	Mustard gas	H_2SO_4
Lyes		HCL (muriatic acid)
KOH		
NaOH		
NH_4OH		
LiOH		
$Ba(OH)_2$		
$Ca(OH)_2$		
Chlorox		
Phenol (cresol)		
Dichromate salts		
Tungstic acid		
Picric acid		
Tannic acid		
Sulfosalicylic acid		
Trichloroacetic acid		
Cresylic acid		
Acetic acid		
Formic acid		
Give calcium salts		
Oxalic acid		
Hydrofluoric acid		

Special methods	
Na metal	—excision
Lyes	—weak acid lavage
Hydrofluoric acid	—boric acid or $NaHCO_3$ wash
Chromic acid	—dilute Na hyposulfite wash
Chlorox	—milk, eggwhite, starch paste, or 1% Na thiosulfate
Phenol (cresol)	—avoid alcohol
White phosphorus	—1:5000 $KMNO_4$ or 2% $CuSO_4$
Dichromate salts	—(a) 2% hyposulfite wash (b) monobasic/dibasic K-Na HPO_4 solution 7%/18% in water buffer wash
Alkyl mercury agents	—debride and remove blister fluid
Lewisite	—British anti-Lewisite (BAL)
H_2SO_4,HCL (muriatic acid)	—soda lime, soap as magnesium hydroxide washers

[a] Reprinted by permisson from Jelenko C III: Chemicals that "burn." *J Trauma,* 1974;14:65–72.

row range from 97.5–99.5°F (36.4–37.5°C). Heat may be convected, conducted, and radiated from the body surface and released by evaporation of sweat. Control of the environment and use of protective clothing are the major defenses against heat loss. Physiologic adjustments to protect against decreased body heat include exercise, shivering, basal thermogenesis under the control of the hypothalamus, and peripheral vasoconstriction. For example, shivering can increase the basal metabolic rate 4–5 times that of normal.

Accidental hypothermia is classified as acute, subacute, and chronic. An individual who is plunged into cold water that causes his core body temperature to decrease, swiftly experiences acute immersion hypothermia. A person exposed much of the night to snow or rain in the cold with insufficient clothing or shelter to maintain body core temperature may suffer from subacute hypothermia. Chronic hypothermia, in which cooling occurs over several days, is usually the result of drugs, disease, or failure of the temperature-regulating mechanism, perhaps combined with age, that causes a slow but nonetheless potentially lethal cooling. This may occur indoors without the individual's leaving his or her living quarters if room temperatures are lower than the person can safely tolerate. Patients with chronic hypothermia almost always have some associated serious disease.

Accidental hypothermia is defined as the pathologic state occurring after core body temperature is reduced below 95°F (35°C) as a result of accidental cold stress. With continued stress, the condition may be progressive and fatal unless body temperature is restored and concomitant metabolic aberrations are corrected. The diagnosis is made by taking a rectal temperature with a low-reading thermometer. Axillary and oral temperatures are misleading. With the rectal temperature below 95°F (35°C), shivering and vasoconstriction become intense, and the patient loses manual dexterity but is still oriented. At this stage, hypothermia is easily reversible. Below 89.6°F (32°C), hypothermia becomes severe; shivering is replaced by marked muscular rigidity and stiff movement. The patient is obtunded and is progressing to full stupor. The blood pressure may not be detectable, but a strong carotid or femoral pulse can be palpated. Breathing becomes shallow and irregular, and the heart rate begins to slow. Below 80.6°F (27°C), hypothermia is profound with deep coma and rigidity. Pulmonary edema can occur. There is a great risk of ventricular arrhythmia.

The most devastating effect of hypothermia occurs when the core temperature drops below 77°F (25°C). Below this temperature, ventricular fibrillation usually develops, and as the temperature gets below 68°F (20°C), asystole occurs. If hypothermia is acute, there may be only relatively mild associated acidosis. If it is chronic, more serious acidosis may accompany cardiac arrest.

As soon as hypothermia is recognized, action must be taken to prevent further cooling. Wet clothing is removed, and the patient is placed in a dry blanket. Rewarming should begin as soon as possible, but only in facilities where medical resources are available to deal with resulting complications. This is especially true for patients with severe and profound hypothermia. Individuals with mild hypothermia can have external heat sources applied, (such as the bodies of warm companions), can be given hot drinks, and can be encouraged to do isometric exercises.

In the rewarming of patients with severe or profound hypothermia, it is important, if possible, to warm the core of the body before the periphery. If the periphery of the body is warmed first, as when a patient is immersed in warm water, peripheral vasodilatation quickly occurs, allowing the previously trapped cool blood to return centrally and causing the core body temperature to decrease further. This leads to rewarming shock, in which the supercooled heart cannot return the amount of blood that the rewarmed skin demands. The most effective way of rewarming the patient's body core is to use peritoneal, gastric, or colonic lavage. Peritoneal lavage is carried out by insertion of a catheter and use of isotonic peritoneal dialysate heated by a blood-warming coil to 95–98.6°F (35–37°C). Every 20–30 minutes, 2 liters of dialysate are exchanged with the object of raising the rectal temperature above 86°F (30°C) as soon as possible to avoid refractory ventricular fibrillation. At the same time, an endotracheal tube should be inserted to protect the airway since vomiting may ensue with central rewarming. Once the rectal temperature exceeds 86°F (30°C), a hypothermia pad or warm-water bath can be used to raise the temperature more slowly. The patient will require an infusion of saline solution to support blood pressure as the periphery becomes rewarmed. Furthermore, any associated acidosis should be avoided. There are many case reports of patients with profound hypothermia and cardiac arrest who have been successfully treated with prolonged cardiopulmonary resuscitation and rewarming.

Frostbite

In the United States, most cases of frostbite occur in persons who have become comatose from injury or alcohol. Except in rare instances, frostbite is restricted to the extremities of the body or to areas such as the chin, cheeks, nose,and ears. The severity of injury is influenced by the intensity of the initial exposure, i.e., type and duration of contact, and the length of time before adequate circulation is restored.

Two types of reaction occur when tissue comes in contact with cold. First, the superficial tissue at the site of contact freezes to a depth dependent on the degree of cold and the duration of contact. With freezing, ice crystals grow between cells, and if the source of cold is not removed, the crystals continue to grow, dehydrating and severely damaging the adjacent cells. Intense freezing causes crystals to form within the cells, damaging them immediately. Second, arteriolar vasoconstriction occurs in the tissue adjacent to the frozen layer, rapidly reducing the blood flow in this zone. With arteriolar constriction, shunts occur that allow blood to bypass the affected capillary bed. If the source of cold is not removed, the whole area begins to freeze.

The following retrospective classification designed by the United States Army during the Korean War divides frostbite injury into four stages: (*a*) erythema and edema with no blister formation; (*b*) erythema and edema with blisters; (*c*) full-thickness injury with gangrene and no loss of part; and (*d*) complete necrosis with loss of part. This classification is useful in reporting frostbite injuries, but it is more helpful to the clinician to divide frostbite injuries into superficial and deep, that is, before the injured part has been thawed.

Superficial frostbite involves only the skin or the tissues immediately beneath it. The frozen part is white and firm on the exterior, but soft and resilient below the surface when depressed gently and firmly. After rewarming, the frostbitten area first becomes numb and mottled blue or purple; it then swells, stings, and burns. In more severe cases, blisters will occur beneath the epidermis in 24–36 hours. These slowly dry and become hard and black in about 2 weeks. General swelling of the injured area occurs and subsides in the same period. After edema subsides, the skin peels and remains red, tender, and extremely sensitive even to mild cold. It may also perspire abnormally for a long time.

In *deep*, unthawed frostbite, a much more serious injury, the injured part is hard and solid and the soft tissue cannot be depressed. Damage not only involves the skin and subcutaneous tissue but also goes deep into tissue, even to bone. Deep frostbite is usually accompanied by huge blisters that may take from 3 days to 1 week to develop. Swelling of the entire hand or foot takes place and lasts for 1 month or more. After rewarming the frostbitten area becomes blue, violet, or gray, and throbbing pains may occur that last up to 8 weeks. The blisters eventually dry, blacken, and slough, leaving beneath an exceptionally sensitive, thin, red layer of new skin that takes months to return to its normal state.

In extreme cases of deep frostbite, the frostbitten part turns gray and remains cold when thawed. If edema and blisters develop, they appear along the line of demarcation between the severely frostbitten area and the remainder of the limb. From 1–2 weeks after injury, the tissue becomes black, dry, and shriveled to the beginning of the healthy tissue. Eventually, it falls off. If the dead tissue becomes infected, it becomes painful and swollen; the eventual amount of tissue loss increases.

The first and most important principle in the treatment of frostbite is rapid rewarming of the injured part. It should be immersed in water kept between 98.6–104°F (37–40°C); warmer water can be harmful. Rewarming at this temperature usually takes only 20 minutes; longer periods are not thought to be helpful. Rewarming is painful, and if the patient's condition is otherwise good, he or she may be given an analgesic. After the injured part is warmed, it should be covered with sterile bandages carefully to minimize friction or trauma. It is critically important to protect the injured tissue at all times. A frozen part should *never be rubbed* before, during, or after rewarming.

Other measures in the treatment of frostbite are similar to those use for patients with burn injuries. The patient is given tetanus prophylaxis, placed on a penicillin regimen for several days, and given intravenous fluids if needed.

Administration of low-molecular-weight dextran to help improve circulation to the injured part and heparin to prevent further thrombosis of small vessels in the injured area is sometimes carried out and depends on the condition of the patient. Once the patient is admitted to the hospital, the use of α-adrenergic blocking agents and sympathectomy may be considered. Finally, the physician should never debride or amputate any tissue because it is very difficult in the early stages of frostbite to determine eventual viability of the injured part.

Trench foot and *immersion foot* are the subacute and chronic variations of frostbite. The eventual tissue injury can be as severe as with frostbite, and therefore, these injuries should be treated in the same way. Trench foot and immersion foot are rare in civilian life.

SUGGESTED READINGS

Arturson MG. The pathophysiology of severe thermal injury. *J Burn Care Rehabil*, 1985;6:129–146.

Boss WK, Brand DA, Acampora D, et al. Effectiveness of prophylactic antibiotics in the outpatient treatment of burns. *J Trauma*, 1985;25:224–227.

Housinger TA, et al. A prospective study of myocardial damage in electrical injuries. *J Trauma*, 1985;25:122–124.

Hunt JL, Mason AD Jr., Masterson TS, et al. The pathophysiology of acute electric injuries. *J Trauma*, 1976;16:335–340.

Hunt JL, Sato RM, Baxter CR. Acute electric burns. Current diagnostic and therapeutic approaches to management. *Arch Surg*, 1980;115:434–438.

Jackson D MacG. The diagnosis of the depth of burning. *Br J Surg,* 1953;40:588–597

Jelenko C III. Chemicals that "burn". *J Trauma*, 1974;14:65–72.

Lund T, Goodwin CW, McManus WF, et al. Upper airway sequelae in burn patients requiring endotracheal intubation or tracheostomy. *Ann Surg,* 1985;201:374–382.

Merrel SW, Saffle JR, Sullivan JJ, et al. Fluid resuscitation in thermally injured children. *Am J Surg*, 1986;152:664–669.

Mortiz AR, Henriques FC Jr. Studies of thermal injury. II. The relative importance of time and surface temperature in the causation of cutaneous burns. *Am J Pathol*, 1947;23:695–706.

Navar PD, Saffle JR, Warden GD. Effect of inhalation injury on fluid resuscitation requirements after thermal injury. *Am J Surg*, 1985;150:716–720.

Purdue GF, Hunt JL. Electrocardiographic monitoring after electrical injury: Necessity or luxury? *J Trauma*, 1986;26:166–167.

Rubin WD, Mani MM, Hiebert JM. Fluid resuscitation of the thermally injured patient. Current concepts with definition of clinical subsets and their specialized treatment. *Clin Plast Surg*, 1986;13:9–21.

Sykes RA, Mani MM, Hiebert JM. Chemical burns: Retrospective review. *J Burn Care Rehabil*, 1986;7:343–347.

Thompson PB, Herndon DN, Traber DL, et al. Effect on mortality of inhalation injury. *J Trauma*, 1986;26:163–165.

CHAPTER 39

Maxillofacial and Soft-tissue Injuries

MICHAEL B. LEWIS, M.D.

Editor's note: There is a broad overlap in the specialties of plastic surgery, oral and maxillofacial surgery, and otolaryngologic surgery. The reader or researcher is therefore advised to consult chapters 39, 40, and 42 when inquiring about the face.

Injuries to maxillofacial structures and soft tissues occur frequently, constituting the largest group of injuries seen in many emergency departments. These injuries result from a variety of causes, including motor vehicle and home accidents, athletic and occupational accidents, animal bites, and intentional trauma. They are discussed in one chapter because of their many similarities, but they are separated into maxillofacial and soft-tissue injuries because of some important differences.

MAXILLOFACIAL INJURIES

The face is an individual's most important physical characteristic, and as such, great emphasis has been placed on it by society. When the face is injured, the goals of treatment must include not only return of function, but also restoration of appearance. This requires a thorough understanding of the anatomy and function of the tissues involved and an absolute insistence on excellence of work. The specialty of plastic and reconstructive surgery was founded and developed on these principles.

Maxillofacial trauma can be classified as (*a*) soft-tissue injury, or (*b*) facial bone fractures. It is important to classify all facial trauma for statistical and medicolegal reasons in addition to proper treatment, which depends on differentiating the types and locations of these injuries.

The mechanism of injury should be determined, because it often suggests the presence of other injuries or the need for special treatment. For example, the patient with facial trauma resulting from an automobile accident is more likely to have associated serious injuries and to require immediate emergency measures.

Many of these injuries have medicolegal sequelae, and the attending physician, who is often asked to provide information, must be able to supply factual data regarding the injury, treatment, and prognosis. It is mandatory, therefore, that accurate, complete records be kept. Diagrams and photographs are excellent means of recording the injury.

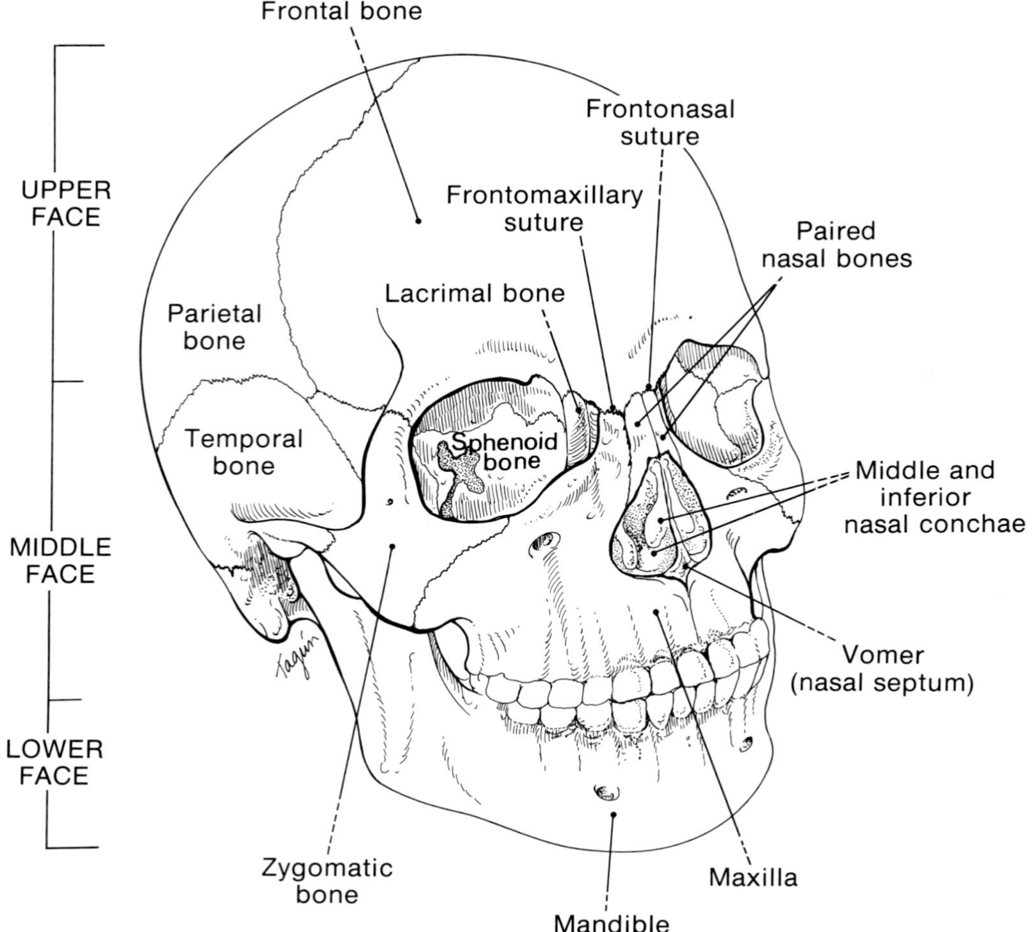

Figure 39.1. Facial bones. For descriptive purposes, the face is divided into upper, middle, and lower regions.

Anatomy

Before attempting to treat facial injuries, basic facial anatomy must be understood. A textbook of anatomy should be available in every emergency department. An understanding of the relations of the facial bones to the skull bones is particularly important (Fig. 39.1), as is knowledge of the facial and trigeminal nerves.

The facial nerve (cranial nerve VII) exits from the stylomastoid foramen at the base of the skull and turns immediately downward and laterally to enter the parotid gland, where it divides into multiple branches that supply the muscles of facial expression in the ipsilateral half of the face (Fig. 39.2). Because it is relatively deep throughout most of its course, especially the proximal portion, it is not often injured. Deep lacerations in the region of the parotid gland, however, may injure the facial nerve and the parotid duct. The parotid (Stenson's) duct usually lies deep to the middle third of an imaginary line extending from the middle of the upper lip to the tragus, and is closely accompanied by the buccal branch of the facial nerve (Fig. 39.2).

Most of the sensation on the face is provided by the sensory branches of the trigeminal nerve (cranial nerve V). Injury to the arborizing branches of this nerve rarely result in permanent anesthesia because of regeneration of the nerve and the overlapping sensory pattern. It is not necessary to repair these small sensory nerves. Knowledge of the pertinent anatomy (Fig. 39.3) is helpful, however, because specific patterns of decreased sensation often result from specific facial fractures.

The arterial blood supply to the face is derived

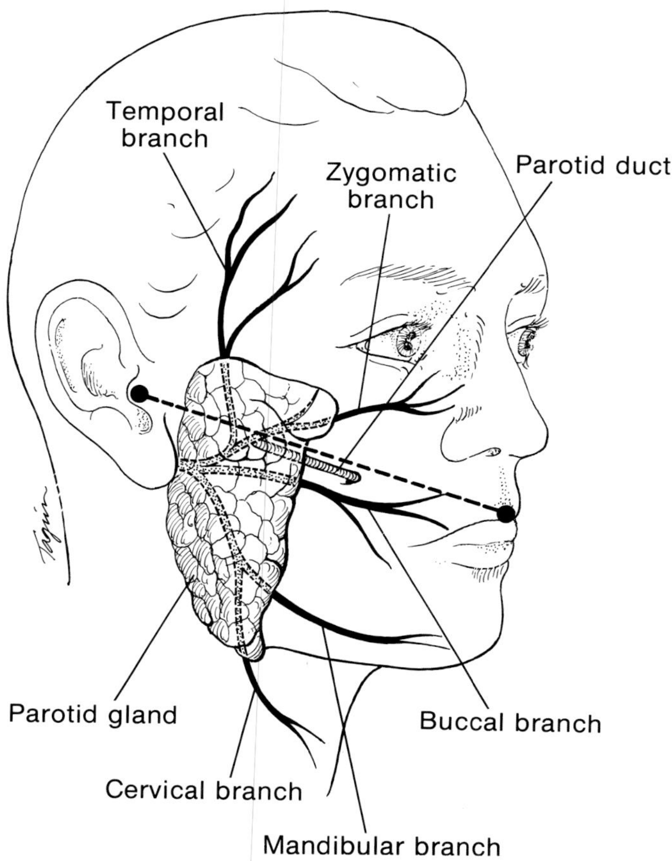

Figure 39.2. Facial nerve and its branches in relation to parotid gland and duct. Facial nerve lies deep in gland substance.

from branches of the external carotid arteries, and venous drainage is accomplished through the internal and external jugular systems. Rarely, massive hemorrhage occurs when one or more of the major branches are injured.

Immediate Treatment

Airway

As with any injured patient, establishment of an adequate airway is the first priority. An obstructed airway is manifested by rapid and labored respirations, tachycardia, cyanosis, lethargy, and, often, extreme agitation. Breath sounds are decreased, and rhonchi are present. The possible causes of airway obstruction in maxillofacial injuries are multiple. Facial fractures (maxilla and mandible) can result in posterior displacement of these bones and their attached soft tissues, obstructing the upper part of the airway. In addition, hemorrhage into the soft tissues can lead to progressive swelling and airway obstruction. Foreign bodies, such as teeth, dentures, glass, and clothing can also become lodged in the airway. Or, hemorrhage sufficient to "drown" the patient can occur. Finally, direct laryngeal or tracheal injury can collapse and obstruct that portion of the airway.

Emergency tracheotomy is rarely needed in cases of airway obstruction accompanying maxillofacial injuries, except in the unusual instance of direct laryngeal injury. If the airway appears obstructed, a quick digital search for a foreign body lodged in the upper airway should be carried out. If the airway is obstructed by intraoral and pharyngeal bleeding, the patient usually struggles to sit up if he or she is conscious, because it is easier to expectorate the blood and to clear the airway in the upright position. The patient should be helped in this effort and should be provided with a suctioning device.

Obstruction caused by displacement of soft tissues posteriorly in mandibular and maxillary fractures is alleviated immediately by grasping the tongue or jaw and pulling it forward. Placing the patient on his or her side to prevent posterior displacement is often sufficient to maintain an airway if the patient is conscious and alert. In the unconscious or semiconscious patient with an obstructed airway, oral endotracheal intubation is necessary. This is preferable to emergency tracheotomy for several reasons. It is quicker, it makes tracheotomy unnecessary, and it is safer. In emergency tracheotomies there is a high incidence of inadvertent injury to important neighboring structures.

Hemorrhage

Because of the rich blood supply to the face from the external carotid arteries, a certain amount of bleeding accompanies most injuries. Massive bleeding, however, is rare. Most external bleeding can be controlled with pressure. When this is inadequate, the lacerated vessels must be clamped and ligated, being careful to avoid injury to branches of the facial nerve. Excessive bleeding from lacerations of the oral mucosa is best controlled by closing the lacerations with sutures. Intranasal hemorrhage from branches of the internal maxillary artery, when it is persistent, must be controlled by packing. Positioning a postnasal pack against which the anterior packing is placed is necessary to control this type of hemorrhage (see Chapter 42).

Shock

Hemorrhagic shock from maxillofacial injuries alone is rare. When shock is present, even when the patient has a severe maxillofacial injury, some other cause must be sought and is often found.

Associated Injuries

Most major maxillofacial injuries result from motor vehicle accidents and are frequently accompanied by other major injuries. Fractures of the skull, cervical portion of the spine, and long bones are

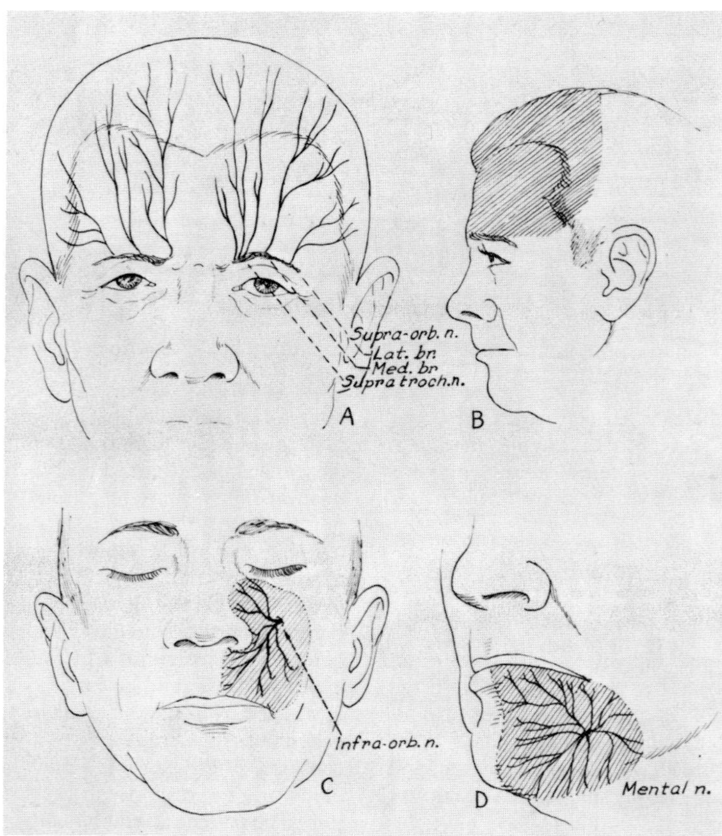

Figure 39.3. Sensory nerves of facial region (trigeminal origin). *A*, Sensory nerves of forehead often injured in frontal sinus-supraorbital rim fractures. *B*, Resultant area of anesthesia. *C*, Area of anesthesia resulting from injury to infraorbital nerve common in zygomatic fractures. *D*, Area of anesthesia resulting from injury to inferior alveolar nerve common in fractures of mandibular body. (Reproduced by permission, from Converse JM. *Kazanjian & Converse's Surgical Treatment of Facial Injuries,* 3rd ed. Baltimore: Williams & Wilkins, 1974.)

common; thoracic and abdominal organs may also be injured. A quick but thorough examination is mandatory to establish treatment priorities. Special care is necessary in handling patients who may have a cervical spinal injury, because improper handling of such an individual may result in quadriplegia (see Chapter 37).

Wound

Although definitive treatment of soft-tissue injuries can be delayed, it is important to unravel all distorted flaps of skin, tacking them in place with a single stitch, when necessary, to avoid vascular compromise. A dry sterile dressing can be placed temporarily over the wound to prevent further contamination.

Diagnosis

The three techniques used in diagnosing facial injuries are inspection, palpation, and x-ray examination.

Inspection

Soft-tissue injuries are usually readily visible. The type of injury should be noted and foreign bodies sought. The eyelids should be separated, and the globe examined. If ocular injury is suspected, ophthalmologic consultation should be obtained. The mouth should be opened, and the mucosal surface examined for laceration and hematoma. Missing teeth should be noted and accounted for. Function of the facial musculature should be determined.

Inspection alone often suggests facial fractures. Facial asymmetry, localized hematoma or ecchymosis, disturbances in ocular movement, diplopia, anesthesia of areas innervated by the terminal branches of the trigeminal nerve, epistaxis, malocclusion, sublingual hematoma, limitation of mandibular excursion, and buccal sulcus lacerations all suggest underlying fracture. The details are given later with discussion of specific injuries.

Palpation

Palpation of known bony prominences on both sides often suggests asymmetry when swelling and ecchymosis prevent this determination from inspection alone. Tenderness, crepitation, sharp "step-offs," angulations, and abnormal movement are further signs of facial fractures.

X-ray Examination

For confirmation of suspected facial fractures and delineation of unrecognized fractures, x-ray examination is necessary. X-ray films of the cervical spine, including C7 vertebra, and of the skull should also be obtained in all cases of severe facial fracture. The most useful views for the facial bones are (*a*) Waters' view (occipitomental)—for fractures of the middle of the face involving the maxilla, the zygomatic bones, the nasal, and orbital regions; (*b*) posteroanterior view—for mandibular, frontal, and zygomatic fractures; (*c*) Towne projection view—for fractures of the mandibular rami and condyles; (*d*) lateral oblique views of the mandible—for fractures of the mandibular body, angles, and rami; (*e*) submental vertex or jug-handle view—for fractures of the zygomatic arches; and (*f*) nasal views, both lateral and occlusal.

Computed tomography can be extremely helpful in delineating complex fractures in the frontal, orbital, ethmoidal, and maxillary areas.

Preliminary Considerations

Priorities

Except for the emergency measures described, the treatment of facial injuries is not lifesaving and should be deferred until more immediately threatening injuries have been treated. Although soft-tissue closure can be postponed up to 24 hours with the use of sterile dressings and antibiotics, it should be delayed this long only when absolutely necessary. With coordination between specialists, soft-tissue damage can be repaired simultaneously with surgical treatment of damage in other regions.

Except for nasal fractures, the treatment of facial fractures can be delayed several days without affecting the final result. In fact, this is often preferred, because the early swelling and ecchymosis make accurate fracture reduction and placement of cosmetic incisions more difficult.

Transportation

Before the patient with severe facial injuries is transported to another hospital or to another area within the same hospital, several precautionary measures should be taken. A good airway must be present. The stomach should be emptied by means of an indwelling nasogastric tube. If there has been an associated cervical spine injury, the head and neck must be stabilized with sandbags or a four-poster brace. An intravenous line should be placed, and basic laboratory studies, such as a complete blood cell count and typing and cross-matching of blood, should be performed.

Tetanus Prophylaxis

Patients with facial injuries should receive tetanus prophylaxis (see Table 11.6). The removal of all devitalized tissues is equally important in preventing tetanus, which has an extremely high mortality.

Anesthesia

General anesthesia is necessary when repair is extensive and complicated, when severe intraoral lacerations have occurred, especially in children, and in most facial fractures. If general anesthesia is being used for the correction of other conditions, it may be convenient to repair the facial injuries concomitantly.

Most minor soft-tissue injuries can be repaired under local anesthesia. The preferred anesthetic is a 1% solution of lidocaine with epinephrine (1:100,000). In small lacerations, local infiltration of these agents through the wound edges minimizes the pain and the amount of agent required. Although anesthesia occurs rapidly after infiltration, the beneficial vasoconstrictive effect of epinephrine takes approximately 10 minutes, and debridement and suturing should be delayed for this period.

In infants and children, sedation and restraint are often necessary. The following combination is effective: meperidine hydrochloride, 25 mg/ml; promethazine hydrochloride, 8 mg/ml; and chlorpromazine hydrochloride, 5 mg/ml. The dosage is 1 ml/25 lb to a maximum of 2 ml. Morphine, 0.1 mg/kg is an alternative, but should not be given to infants less than 6–8 months old. These agents must be given adequate time to take effect, i.e., 45 minutes, before restraining the patient and repairing the injury.

Wound Preparation, Healing, and Postoperative Care

Except for superficial abrasions that heal by epithelialization alone—leaving no scar—wounds heal by one of the following methods: (*a*) primary intention—direct approximation of wound edges; (*b*) delayed primary intention—wound closure by approximation of wound edges or grafting after the wound has been allowed to develop early granulation tissue; (*c*) secondary intention—wound closure by granulation, contraction, and epithelialization. Since skin is an organ, unable to regenerate completely, all these methods of wound healing leave scars that are composed primarily of collagen.

In general, the most aesthetically acceptable scars result from healing by primary intention. Anything that interferes with primary healing, even in a portion of the wound, causes additional scarring and a less acceptable result. Proper wound preparation, debridement, suturing, and postoperative management are the prerequisites for primary healing.

The skin around the wound should be prepared with a bland nondetergent soap, and the wound itself irrigated with sterile physiologic saline solution, and all foreign material removed. Devitalized tissue should be debrided. Excision of large amounts of questionably viable tissues is not recommended; later revisional operation is preferable to the unnecessary sacrifice of viable tissue. Repair should be carried out meticulously and skillfully with minimal and delicate handling of tissue. Postoperatively, wounds should be protected by occlusive dressings that provide some pressure and immobilization. Pressure helps to prevent hematoma and excessive swelling, both of which interfere with primary wound healing. Constant and excessive motion of a wound after repair causes additional inflammation, promotes "suture marks," and leads to unnecessary scar tissue.

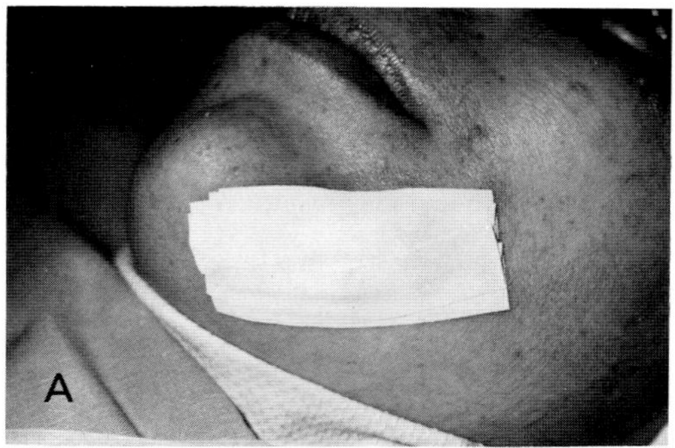

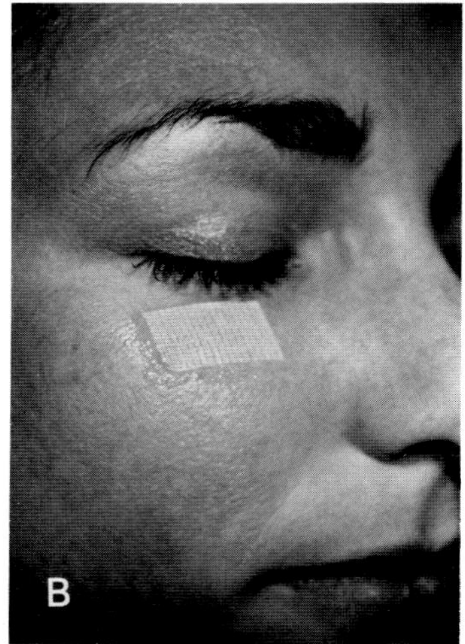

Figure 39.4. *A*, Cocoon dressing. *B*, Fine-mesh gauze/collodion dressing.

An effective means of providing pressure and immobilization for smaller wounds is the cocoon tape dressing (Fig. 39.4*A*). A single layer of fine-mesh gauze is placed next to the wound, reinforced by several layers of coarse gauze, all held in place by multiple layers of 0.5-inch adhesive tape. In areas where this type of dressing is difficult to place, a dressing of fine-mesh gauze and collodion is a good substitute (Fig. 39.4*B*). Larger or multiple wounds are best protected with a circumferential head dressing. Excessive talking and chewing are discouraged to avoid unnecessary motion at the wound site. The head should be kept elevated. Sutures should be removed within 3–5 days and the wound dressed again for an additional 7–10 days.

The final aesthetic result in wound healing depends on many factors, some of which are beyond the control of the surgeon. The relation of the final scar to the relaxed skin tension lines is extremely important (Fig. 39.5). Scars that are parallel or nearly parallel to these lines usually look better. The degree of crush and contusion plays an important role, as does the age of the patient and the location of the injury. In discussing the prognosis with the patient or his/her family, the physician must point out these factors.

Treatment

General Management of the Soft-tissue Injury

Most soft-tissue injuries result from relatively minor trauma and can effectively be treated in the emergency department. Extensive injuries and those involving specialized areas of the face, however, require special expertise, time, and assistance not usually available in the emergency facility. These patients should be referred to the plastic surgeon for care; they often require hospitalization and surgical repair in the operating room.

Simple Laceration. This is probably the most common facial injury. Repair should be carried out under local anesthesia. After the surrounding skin is prepared and the wound irrigated, devitalized tissue is very conservatively debrided. Ragged and contused wound edges should be excised to provide healthy, perpendicular skin margins. When necessary, hemostasis should be achieved by fine catgut ligatures or cautery. Slight undermining of the wound margins at the subdermal plane allows more accurate suture placement and relieves some tension from the wound margins.

Interrupted loop sutures are probably the most accurate means of closing a laceration (Figs. 39.6 and 39.7). If correctly placed, the sutures provide good approximation with just the proper amount of wound edge eversion without leaving any dead space. Equal "bites" with a perpendicular course of the needle ensure level wound edges. Any fine adjustments can be made by knot placement. Suture material should be 5–0 and 6–0 monofilament nylon swaged on a cutting needle; sutures should be placed every 2–3 mm. It is important to tie the sutures just tightly enough to approximate the wound edges. Some postoperative wound edema should be anticipated when determining the tightness of each suture.

In deeper lacerations, multilayered closure is required to eliminate dead space, to ensure proper alignment of deeper structures, and to prevent a depressed, widened scar. Muscle should be approximated with interrupted absorbable sutures of either 4–0 chromic catgut or polyglycolic acid (Dexon). Subcutaneous or subcuticular suturing should be performed with interrupted sutures of polyglycolic acid or 5–0 plain catgut (Fig. 39.8).

Intraoral lacerations of the tongue or mucous membranes should be closed with interrupted 4–0

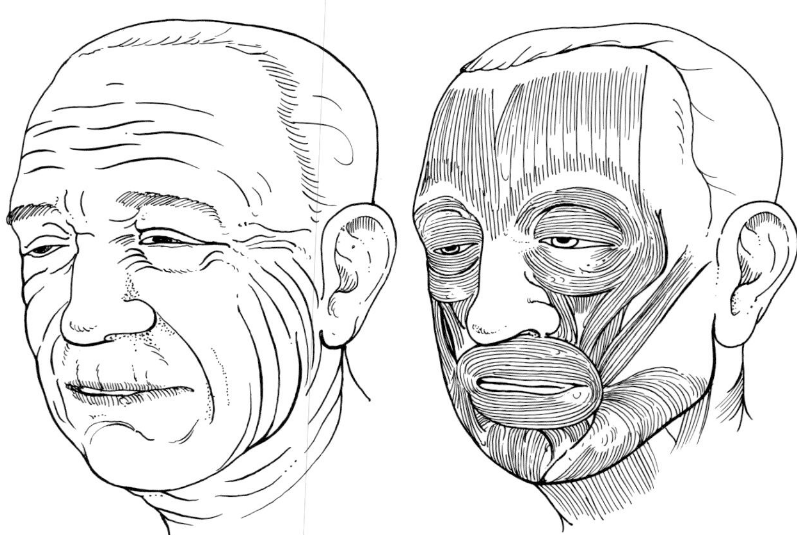

Figure 39.5. Relaxed skin tension lines (wrinkle lines) and underlying facial muscles. (Reproduced by permission, from McGregor IA. *Fundamental Techniques of Plastic Surgery and Their Surgical Applications*, 6th ed. Edinburgh: Churchill Livingstone, 1975.)

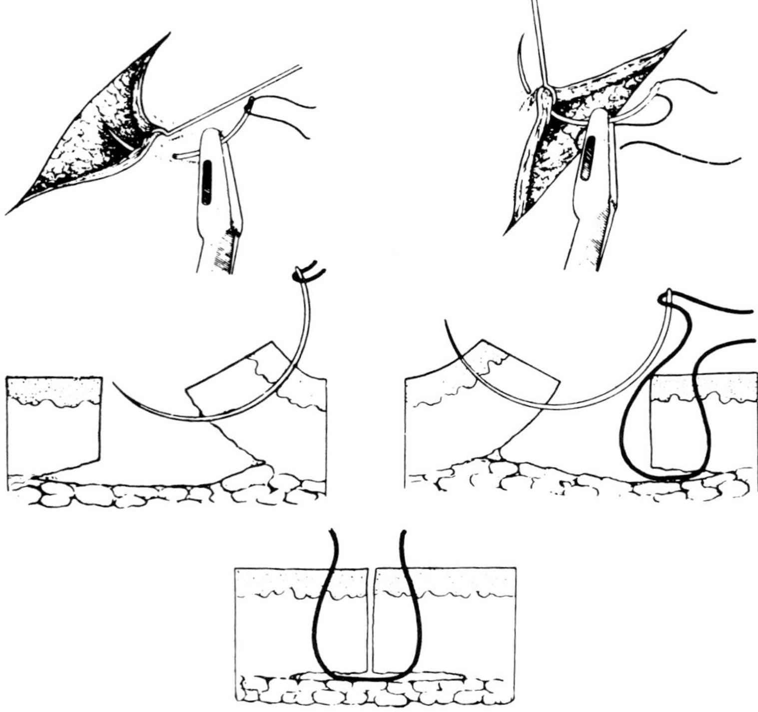

Figure 39.6. Simple loop suture, with perpendicular course of needle through everted skin edge. (Reprcduced by permission, from McGregor IA. *Fundamental Techniques of Plastic Surgery and Their Surgical Applications,* 6th ed. Edinburgh: Churchill Livingstone, 1975.)

chromic catgut or black silk sutures. Catgut has the advantage of not needing removal, but its knot-holding capacity is less than that of silk.

A number of other suture techniques are available (Fig. 39.8). The vertical mattress suture is helpful in everting wound edges when this is a problem. Continuous sutures save time, but offer less edge and tension control. A continuous subcuticular, intradermal suture has the advantage of not leaving suture marks even when left in place for 10–12 days. Accurate skin apposition is more difficult, however.

Complicated Laceration. Included are those lacerations that are irregular or stellate or that contain partly avulsed tissue (flaps). These injuries are generally more difficult to treat and result in less than ideal scar deformity. If the wound is small enough that it can be completely excised and the resulting defect closed primarily without distortion, this should be done. Otherwise, a conservative approach to debridement should be taken. Distorted tissue should be returned to its appropriate place. Where several lacerations meet, a single buried stitch is helpful in bringing the points together. Severely beveled skin edges, which are frequently seen in partial avulsion injuries, should be excised sharply.

Avulsion Injury. When a significant amount of tissue has been lost, some form of local flap or free skin graft is often necessary for closure. This requires the skill of a specialist and is best performed in the operating room. However, if the area of tissue loss is small and primary closure can be obtained without undue tension, the wound should be converted to a lenticular shape with freshened, undermined edges and closed primarily.

Human and Animal Bites. Puncture wounds of the face resulting from human or animal bites should *not* be closed. After they are carefully cleaned, irrigated, and debrided, *no* suturing should be undertaken. Lacerations resulting from animal bites, however, may be sutured. Special attention to irrigation, debridement, and tetanus prophylaxis is required, and antirabies precautions should be taken (see Chapter 10, p 200). Broad-spectrum antibiotics are administered for 1 week. When substantial tissue has been avulsed, more complicated reconstruction is necessary, and a plastic surgeon should be consulted.

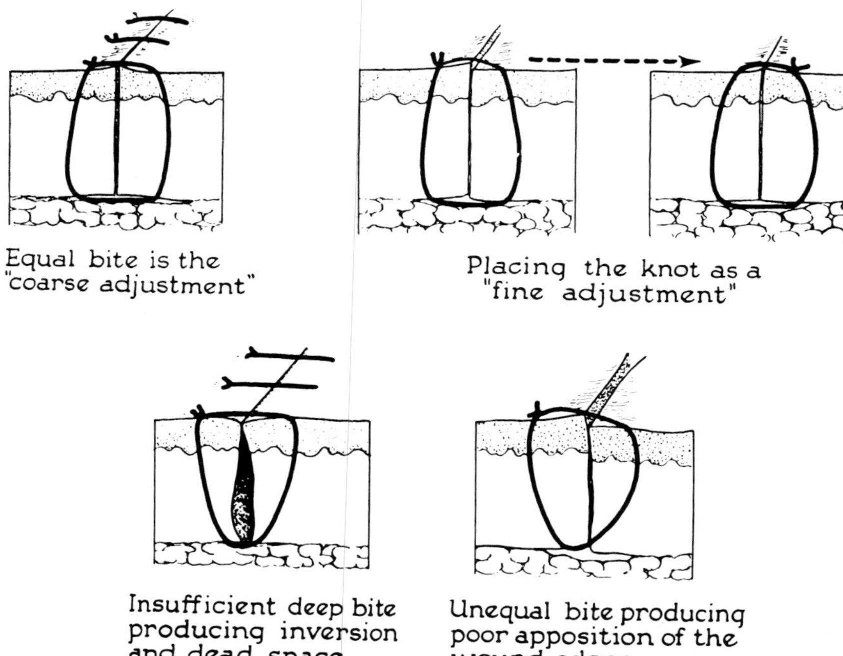

Figure 39.7. Correct adjustments and possible errors in placement of simple loop sutures. (Reproduced by permission, from McGregor IA. *Fundamental Techniques of Plastic Surgery and Their Surgical Applications,* 6th ed. Edinburgh: Churchill Livingstone, 1975).

Human bites are potentially more dangerous because of the introduction of many types of pathogenic bacteria. Admission to the hospital for systemic antibiotic administration and wet dressings is often necessary. The wound should be cleansed and debrided thoroughly when first seen and closed a few days later with nylon sutures loosely approximating the skin. Deep sutures should be avoided. Later scar revision may be necessary. Tetanus prophylaxis should be carried out.

Abrasion. This injury, which implies partial thickness damage, heals spontaneously by epithelialization. The wound should be cleansed with a bland soap and water solution and protected by frequent applications of an antibiotic ointment, or covered with a single layer of a nonadherent petrolatum-impregnated gauze.

Accidental Tattoo. In certain types of injuries, small foreign particles become imbedded in the dermis. The particles are usually obvious because of the color they impart to the area after cleansing and irrigation have removed all the loose foreign material. If left untreated, accidental tattoo results in permanent discoloration of the area.

These particles are best removed within the first 12 hours before they become fixed in the tissue. Scrubbing with a stiff, sterile brush is the best method for doing this. Grease or oil in a wound can usually be dissolved and removed with small amounts of ether or acetone. The treated areas are dressed with an antibiotic ointment or covered with a single layer of petrolatum-impregnated gauze.

Only small, easily accessible areas are amenable to this treatment under local anesthesia. General anesthesia is usually necessary to treat larger areas.

Foreign Bodies. In general, all foreign bodies should be removed at the time of initial treatment. Despite meticulous attempts to remove completely very small foreign bodies, such as multiple glass splinters, these patients often require later removal of foreign bodies.

Small metal fragments of missiles that are located deeply in noncritical locations are often best left alone. More harm can be done by attempting removal than by leaving them.

Specific Soft-tissue Injuries

Eyelids. Eye examination for corneal abrasion, anterior chamber hemorrhage, laceration of the globe, and visual disturbance should precede any repair in this area. Simple lacerations of the eyelid skin present no special problem, especially if oriented transversely. Careful suturing usually results in an inconspicuous scar. If the eyebrow is involved, it should be cleansed, but *never* shaved. If the laceration traverses it, the eyebrow must be

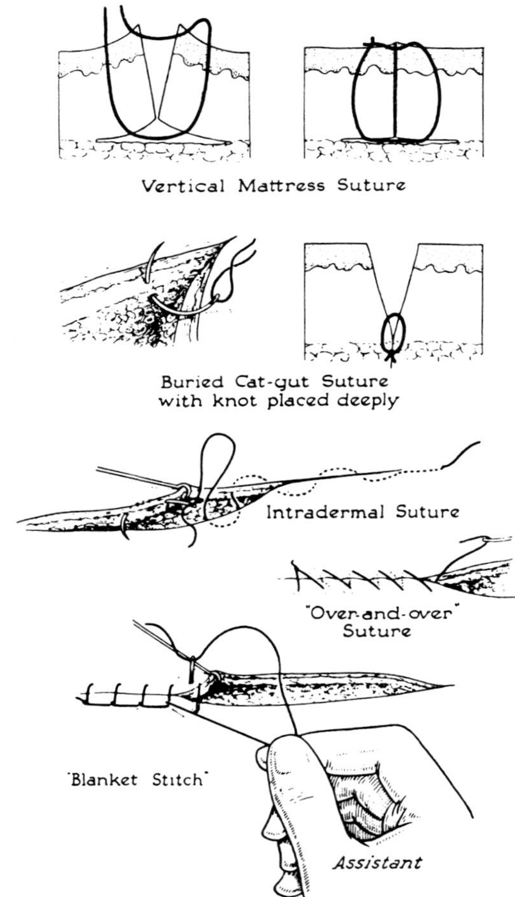

Figure 39.8. Other commonly used skin suture techniques. (Reproduced by permission, from McGregor IA. *Fundamental Techniques of Plastic Surgery and Their Surgical Applications,* 6th ed. Edinburgh: Churchill Livingstone, 1975.)

aligned properly during suturing. In more complicated lacerations of eyelid skin in which small flaps have resulted, minimal debridement should be carried out. Careful salvage and placement of each flap can produce an excellent result in many cases. Lacerations in this region are often associated with multiple imbedded foreign particles, and care should be taken to remove these before suturing. Lacerations involving the full thickness of the eyelid, the medial canthal region with its nasolacrimal apparatus, or the lateral canthus require repair by a plastic specialist.

Nose. Full-thickness nasal lacerations that enter the vestibule require layered closure. Because of the bony character of the upper part of the nose, these lacerations usually occur in the lower half (Fig. 39.9). The nasal mucosa or vestibular lining is closed with 5–0 catgut interrupted sutures, placing the knots to face into the nasal cavity. It is usually unnecessary to suture the nasal cartilage, but if alignment is difficult, a few very fine catgut sutures can be placed in the perichondrium. The skin of the nose is ideal for the continuous subcuticular, intradermal suture technique. A 5–0 nylon suture material is recommended. This relieves tension on the 6–0 nylon interrupted simple loop cutaneous sutures that are then placed, and allows their early removal. In the fleshy tip of the nose, with its numerous sebaceous glands and pores, cutaneous sutures tend to cut in and to leave marks; their early removal is important.

Avulsion injuries of the nose require grafting; this patient should be referred to a plastic surgical specialist.

Lip. Lacerations of the lip that cross the vermilion-cutaneous junction or "white roll" (Fig. 39.10*A*) require accurate alignment of this anatomic landmark (Fig. 39.10*B*). Full-thickness lip lacerations should be closed in three layers. The mucosal layer should be closed with interrupted sutures of 5–0 catgut with the knots placed on the mucosal surface. Since these knots tend to untie, two or three extra "throws" should be placed and the ends cut long. The muscular layer of the lip should be approximated carefully with interrupted 4–0 chromic catgut or polyglycolic acid sutures. The skin should be closed with 6–0 nylon, taking care to align the vermilion-cutaneous junction accurately.

Avulsion injuries of the lip, which result most frequently from dog bites, require complicated reconstruction, either immediately or later; the patient should be seen by a plastic surgeon as early as possible. This also applies to electrical burns involving the lip. This injury is common in toddlers who inadvertently place a live extension plug into the mouth or chew through a "hot" cord. As the current arcs through the saliva at the corner of the mouth, extremely high temperatures develop, destroying the full thickness of the lip and commissure (Fig. 39.11). The need for early debridement of this necrotic tissue is controversial. Many surgeons prefer to allow the tissue to slough spontaneously. This may result in late hemorrhage from the labial artery. If this course is chosen, the parents and nursing staff should be so cautioned. Tetanus immunization and a clear liquid diet are recommended.

Intraoral Injury. Lacerations of the mucous membranes and the tongue should be closed primarily with interrupted 4–0 chromic catgut or black silk sutures.

Parotid Duct and Facial Nerve. Deep laceration in the cheek may injure the parotid duct and facial nerve; this happens infrequently because of their relatively deep location (see p 776 and Fig.

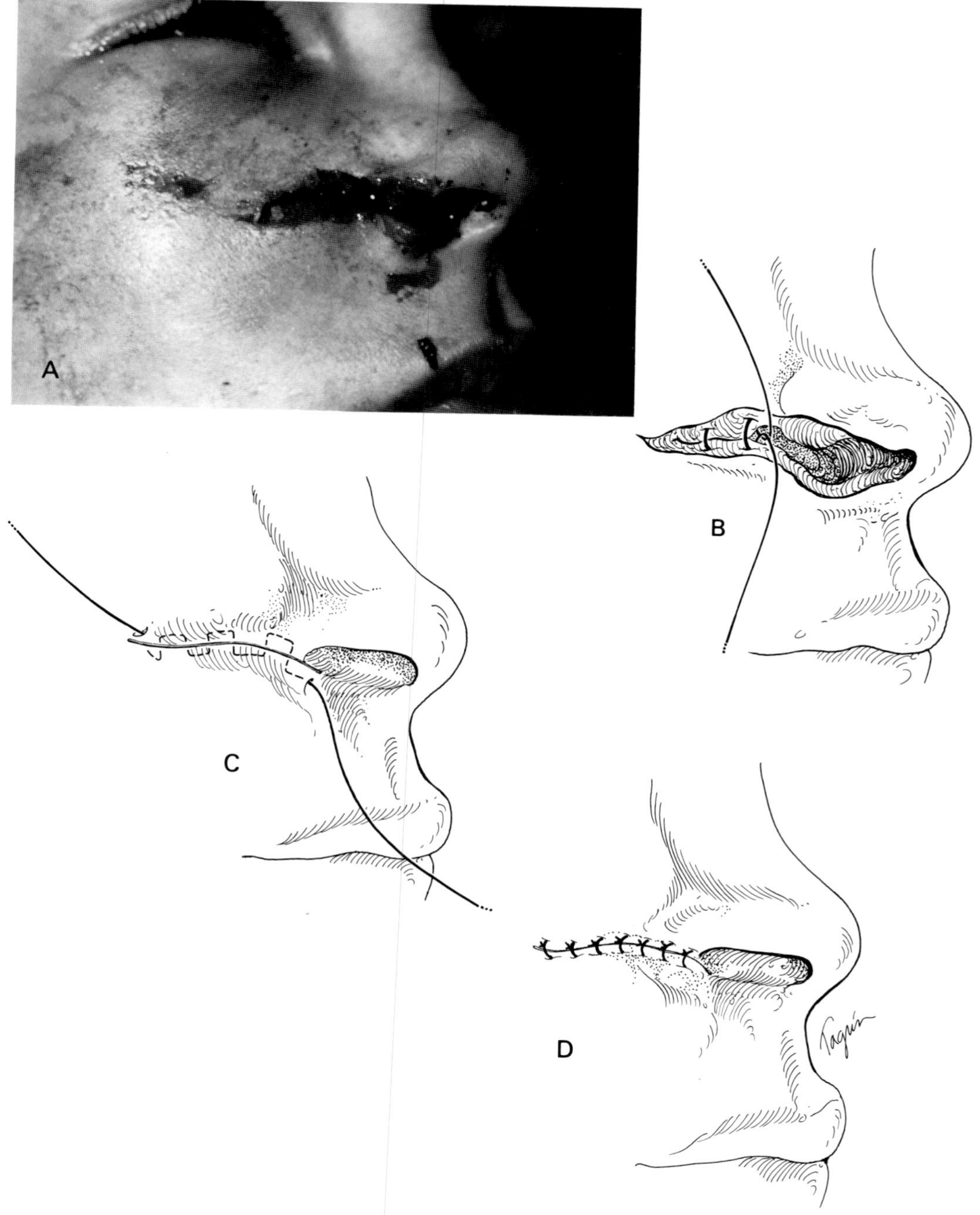

Figure 39.9. *A*, Full-thickness nasal laceration, *B*, Closure of vestibular lining with 5–0 catgut interrupted sutures, followed by *C*, a 5–0 nylon continuous subcuticular suture, followed by *D*, 6–0 nylon interrupted simple loop skin sutures.

39.2). A high index of suspicion is necessary to diagnose injuries to these structures. Weakness of some or all of the ipsilateral facial musculature indicates injury to the facial nerve. Leakage of clear fluid from a laceration of the cheek suggests injury to the parotid duct or the gland substance. If a fine polyethylene catheter or lacrimal probe passed into the oral opening of the parotid duct, opposite the upper second molar, emerges in the cheek wound, there is division of the duct.

The small peripheral branches of the facial nerve, those anterior to an imaginary vertical line from the lateral canthus of the eye, do not require neurorrhaphy. However, the divided deep soft tissue must be approximated accurately. This usually results in restoration of function after a period during which nerves regenerate. Injury to the more proximal portions of the facial nerve or parotid duct requires more sophisticated, exact repair by a plastic surgical specialist.

Ear. Injuries to the ear often result in jagged lacerations and partial avulsions. The ear is extremely vascular, and flaps based on very small pedicles often survive; they should not be excised during debridement. Because of its vascularity, precise hemostasis is necessary if hematomas are to be avoided.

Lacerations involving only the skin of the ear can be managed satisfactorily in the emergency department. Field block anesthesia is easily obtained by the injection of 1% lidocaine solution with epinephrine (1:100,000) around the ear at its attachment to the head. This avoids the need for difficult, painful injection of the anesthetic agent into the ear itself. Fine 6–0 nylon interrupted sutures should be used.

If the cartilaginous framework of the ear has been lacerated, it is usually necessary to trim the cartilage along the wound so that the skin can be approximated over it without tension and without buckling of the cartilage. A few absorbable 5–0 interrupted sutures in the perichondrium are used to hold the cartilage together.

Subperichondral hematoma resulting from blunt trauma can cause "cauliflower" ear if not immediately and adequately treated. Needle aspiration of all blood should be carried out after preparing the skin with an antiseptic solution. If this is impossible, or if hematoma recurs, hospitalization and surgical intervention will be required.

After repair of these injuries, a conforming com-

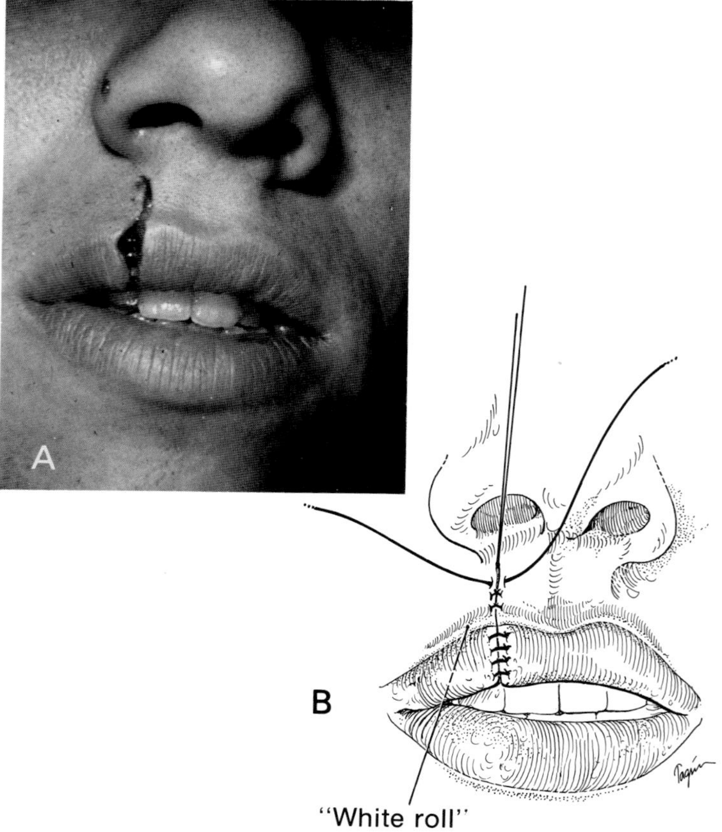

Figure 39.10. *A*, Lip laceration through vermilion-cutaneous junction ("white roll"). *B*, Repair of lip laceration demonstrating accurate placement of suture to align "white roll."

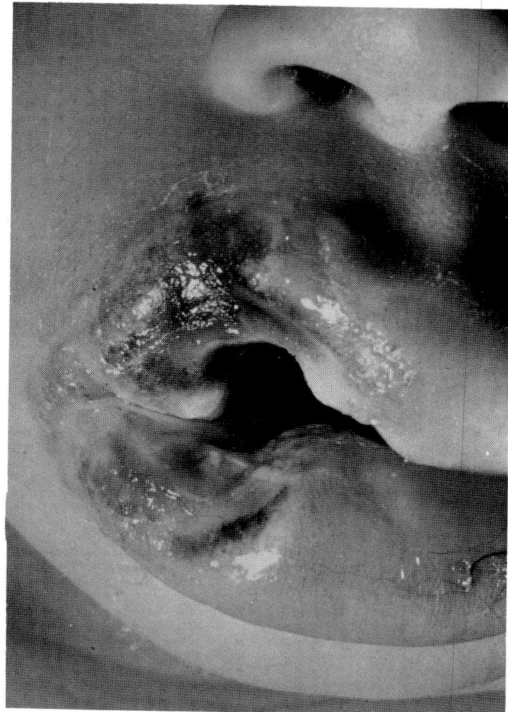

Figure 39.11. Severe full-thickness electrical burn involving oral commissure and upper and lower lips.

pression dressing is necessary. Slightly moistened pieces of cotton are placed behind the ear and within the contour of the anterolateral surface. The ear is then covered with fluffed gauze, and a circular head dressing applied.

In more severe avulsion injuries, every effort must be made to save all exposed cartilage; later reconstructive duplication of this intricate structure is impossible. The remaining portion of the ear can be buried in the adjacent mastoid or temporal skin, followed later by reconstructive surgery by a plastic surgeon. Early referral is recommended.

Facial Fractures

Most facial fractures require reduction and fixation under general anesthesia. Because of this and the frequency of associated injuries, hospitalization is necessary. The emergency measures have already been discussed. In open fractures communicating with the oral, nasal, or sinus cavities or to the skin surface, broad-spectrum antibiotic prophylaxis is preferred. This is especially important when a dural tear has occurred, resulting in cerebrospinal fluid rhinorrhea. Definitive treatment of all but simple nasal fractures requires specialized training. The emergency physician must be able to recognize all facial fractures.

The most commonly fractured facial bones are the nasal bones, the zygomatic bones, and the mandible. Their relative prominence on the face and the lesser force required to cause fracturing are factors. Facial fractures are less common in children because the relatively greater size and prominence of the cranium affords protection to the smaller facial bones.

Nasal Fractures. Isolated nasal fracture is common, frequently resulting from intentional or athletic trauma. The diagnosis of nasal fracture is made clinically, the signs including (*a*) epistaxis; (*b*) depression or deviation of the nasal pyramid; (*c*) periorbital ecchymosis and edema; (*d*) tenderness; (*e*) crepitation and abnormal motion of the nasal bones on palpation; and (*f*) obstruction of the airway by a buckled or deviated septum.

X-ray films of the nasal bones should be obtained to document the injury and for medicolegal purposes, but should not dictate treatment. Treatment should be undertaken on the basis of the clinical appearance of the nose (Fig. 39.12). Undisplaced nasal fractures diagnosed by x-ray findings alone do not need treatment, except for splinting. In children, a seemingly insignificant nasal injury or undisplaced fracture can result in later deformity due to altered growth, and parents should be cautioned about this possibility.

The results of treatment of nasal fractures are frequently poor. It is a difficult problem to deal with, even for experienced physicians. If possible, nasal fractures should be treated by surgeons familiar with

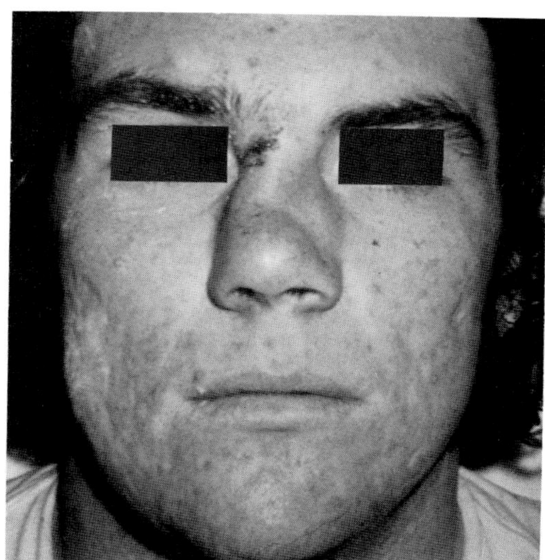

Figure 39.12. Nasal fracture with obvious deformity.

nasal surgery and corrective rhinoplasty. Treatment is best undertaken early, before swelling and fixation of a buckled septum take place.

Since many nasal fractures are managed in the emergency department, a detailed description of the technique follows:

The first step is the determination of the exact deformity present, namely, depression, angulation, or septal distortion. Then, after the face is washed with soap and water, local anesthesia is attained. Cotton applicators soaked in a 10% cocaine solution provide topical anesthesia to the mucous membranes. The infraorbital nerves (Fig. 39.3) are blocked with a 1% lidocaine solution with epinephrine (1:100,000) and field block anesthesia is accomplished by infiltration of the same agent across the glabellar region and the base of the columella. It takes 10–15 minutes for anesthesia to be complete, and reductions should not be carried out until this time has passed.

A closed Kelly clamp covered with a thin piece of rubber tubing is effective for disimpacting, mobilizing, and reducing the nasal fracture if the other hand simultaneously palpates and molds the nose. Walsham forceps are also used for this maneuver. An Asch forceps is the best instrument available to reposition and to mold the deviated nasal septum (Fig. 39.13).

An external splint of plaster of Paris is used to protect the nose and to control edema. Internal packing is rarely necessary; when it is used, it should not block the airway or be placed so that it displaces the nasal bones laterally.

Nasal fractures in children require general anesthesia for reduction, and brief hospitalization is therefore necessary.

Nasoorbitoethmoidal Fracture. These fractures occur in conjunction with other fractures of the middle of the face. In addition to the signs in simple nasal fractures, lateral displacement of the medial canthi is noted (traumatic telecanthus). The Waters' view is a helpful x-ray film in confirming this injury. Treatment is complex and often involves open reduction and internal fixation.

Zygomatic Fracture. There are usually three points of fracture and some degree of separation in fractures of the zygomatic bone—along the inferior orbital rim, at the frontozygomatic suture region, and at the junction with the temporal bone in the arch (Fig. 39.14). The following clinical signs may be present: (*a*) periorbital ecchymosis and edema; (*b*) anesthesia in the distribution of the infraorbital nerve (Fig. 39.3); (*c*) flattening of the "cheekbone" eminence; (*d*) angulation and tenderness of the infraorbital rim; and (*e*) trismus. Diplopia, limitation of external ocular movements due to involvement of the orbital floor, and muscle entrapment are less frequently seen.

The Waters' x-ray view is best for demonstrating the fractures, and often shows clouding of the maxillary antrum. The submental vertex (jug-handle) view demonstrates the fracture line in the zygomatic arch.

Several different procedures have been described to reduce and to immobilize the depressed zygomatic bone. Many fractures can be reduced by the semi-open technique described by Gillies and colleagues without internal fixation. Experience is necessary to know which fractures are correctable by this approach. The remainder must be repaired by direct open reduction with internal interosseous wire fixation. General anesthesia is necessary for these operations.

Isolated fracture of the zygomatic arch results from a direct blow with a narrow object. Fractures usually occur simultaneously in three places along the arch, and depression results. The clinical signs for diagnosis include: (*a*) swelling and tenderness in the region of the zygomatic arch; (*b*) interference with mandibular movements from impingement on the coronoid process; and (*c*) periorbital ecchymosis and edema.

The submental vertex x-ray view best demonstrates this fracture. It can usually be elevated by the semi-open technique described by Gillies and colleagues (1927). Only rarely is internal fixation necessary.

Maxillary Fracture. These fractures result from a direct force applied to the middle of the face or from beneath the lower jaw. When severe, they are often associated with mandibular fractures, nasoorbital ethmoidal fractures, basilar skull fractures, and cerebrospinal fluid rhinorrhea. It is this group of patients that is most likely to have problems with hemorrhage and airway obstruction. LeFort classified maxillary fractures into three groups (Fig. 39.15): I (transverse), II (pyramidal), and III (craniofacial dysjunction.). Fractures of the maxilla are not always so isolated as LeFort implied, but this classification is a useful aid in thinking about these injuries. Clinical and x-ray findings depend on the location of the fracture, but the following clinical findings are often present: (*a*) malocclusion; (*b*) elongation of the middle of the face; (*c*) periorbital ecchymosis and edema; (*d*) abnormal mobility of the maxilla when grasped between the thumb and forefinger and forceful motion attempted, causing pain with the abnormal motion; and (*e*) mucosal lacerations in the upper buccal sulcus.

The Waters' view is the most helpful x-ray film. Treatment of these complex fractures is based on

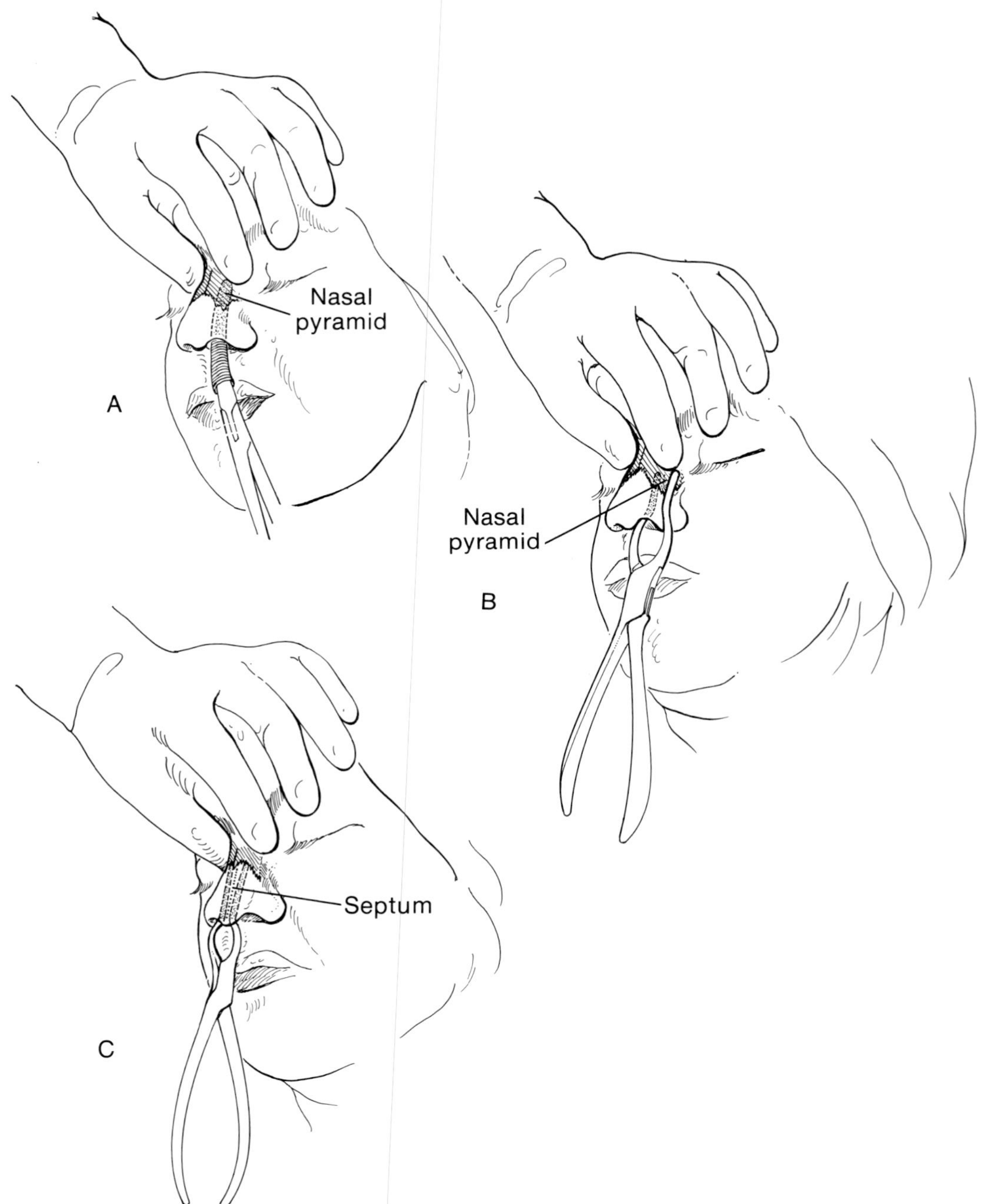

Figure 39.13. Instruments and techniques used in treating nasal fractures. *A*, Kelly clamp. *B*, Walsham forceps. *C*, Asch forceps.

the objectives of restoration of normal occlusion, cephalad fixation to a stable foundation, and the use of aesthetically acceptable incisions.

Orbital Floor (Blow-out) Fracture. The pure blow-out fracture involves only the thin orbital floor, sparing the orbital rim; it usually results from a direct force applied to the globe itself. Without injury to the globe, the force is transmitted to the

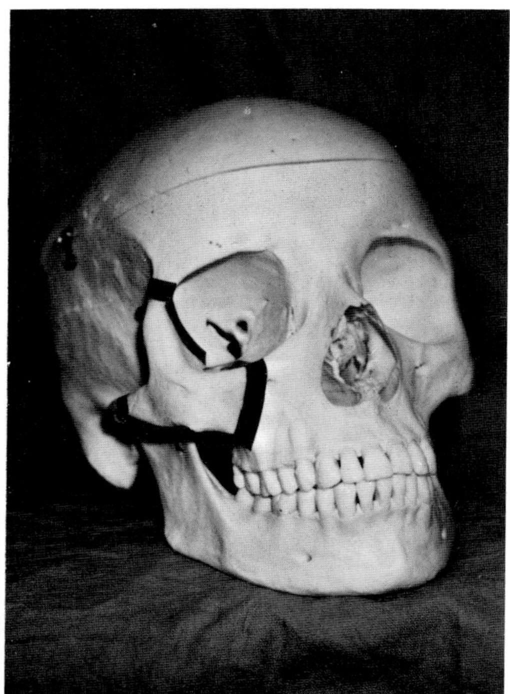

Figure 39.14. Lines of usual zygomatic fracture.

orbital floor, which fractures into the maxillary sinus. The findings may include: (*a*) periorbital ecchymosis and edema; (*b*) limitation of external ocular movements because of muscle entrapment; (*c*) enophthalmos and diplopia (before swelling compensates for the displacement of the orbital contents into the maxillary sinus); (*d*) discrepancy of eye level; and/or (*e*) hypersthesia over the distribution of the infraorbital nerve.

The examiner must be alert to this possible injury. Waters' view usually shows only clouding of the maxillary antrum. Tomograms of the orbital floor are necessary to confirm the diagnosis.

Muscle entrapment, enophthalmos, and persistent diplopia are indications for surgical correction to free the muscles and to replace the intraorbital contents. Blepharoplasty or a conjunctival incision is used; often a small disc of autologous tissue or silicone is required to reconstruct the floor of the orbit.

Mandibular Fracture. The mandible is the most frequently fractured facial bone in children, but mandibular fracture is seen much more commonly in adults. Fracture results from a direct blow to the mandible, often occurring in more than one site. The common clinical findings include: (*a*) malocclusion; (*b*) limitation of mandibular movement; (*c*) abnormal motion; (*d*) ecchymosis, swelling, and tenderness near the fracture site; (*e*) mucosal lacerations of the lower buccal sulcus; (*f*) missing or loose teeth; (*g*) anesthesia of the ipsilateral region of the lower lip because of injury to the inferior alveolar nerve (Fig. 39.3); and (*h*) sublingual hematoma.

Fractures of the mandible are best demonstrated by posteroanterior, lateral oblique, and occlusal views. The Towne projection view is helpful in demonstrating fractures of the mandibular rami and condyles. Treatment almost always requires intermaxillary fixation, often augmented by open reduction and internal fixation.

Frontal Sinus-Supraorbital Rim Fracture. This is an unusual fracture resulting from a direct blow, and is frequently associated with skull fracture. Possible signs include (*a*) periorbital ecchymosis and edema; (*b*) local tenderness and depression; (*c*) anesthesia of the forehead (Fig. 39.3); (*d*) commonly a bursting type of laceration over the fracture; and (*e*) epistaxis.

The x-ray examination that demonstrates these fractures best are the Waters' and posteroanterior and lateral views of the skull.

SOFT-TISSUE INJURIES

The types of soft-tissue injury that occur elsewhere on the body are, in general, similar to those that occur in the facial region, and in many respects, the treatment is similar. However, because of less abundant blood supply, differences in function, and differences in time required for the healing wound to attain adequate strength, the specific management of lesions varies. This is especially true with soft-tissue injuries of the lower extremities. Discussions of electrical burns and frostbite are found in Chapter 38.

Minor Injuries

Minor abrasions, contusions, and lacerations are managed under local anesthesia in the emergency department. The skin should be prepared with bland soap and water, and the wound irrigated with sterile physiologic saline solution. All foreign bodies should be removed, and necrotic tissue debrided. Tissues are handled atraumatically with delicate forceps and skin hooks. Needless crushing of tissue delays healing and increases both the chance of infection and the amount of scar tissue. Hemostasis is accomplished with catgut ligatures. The subcutaneous tissues should be approximated with absorbable sutures of 3–0 or 4–0 catgut, depending on the strength required. The skin is closed with 4–0 or 5–0 nylon sutures spaced at 3–5 mm intervals and at equal distances from the wound margin. The wound is then protected with a dressing that applies

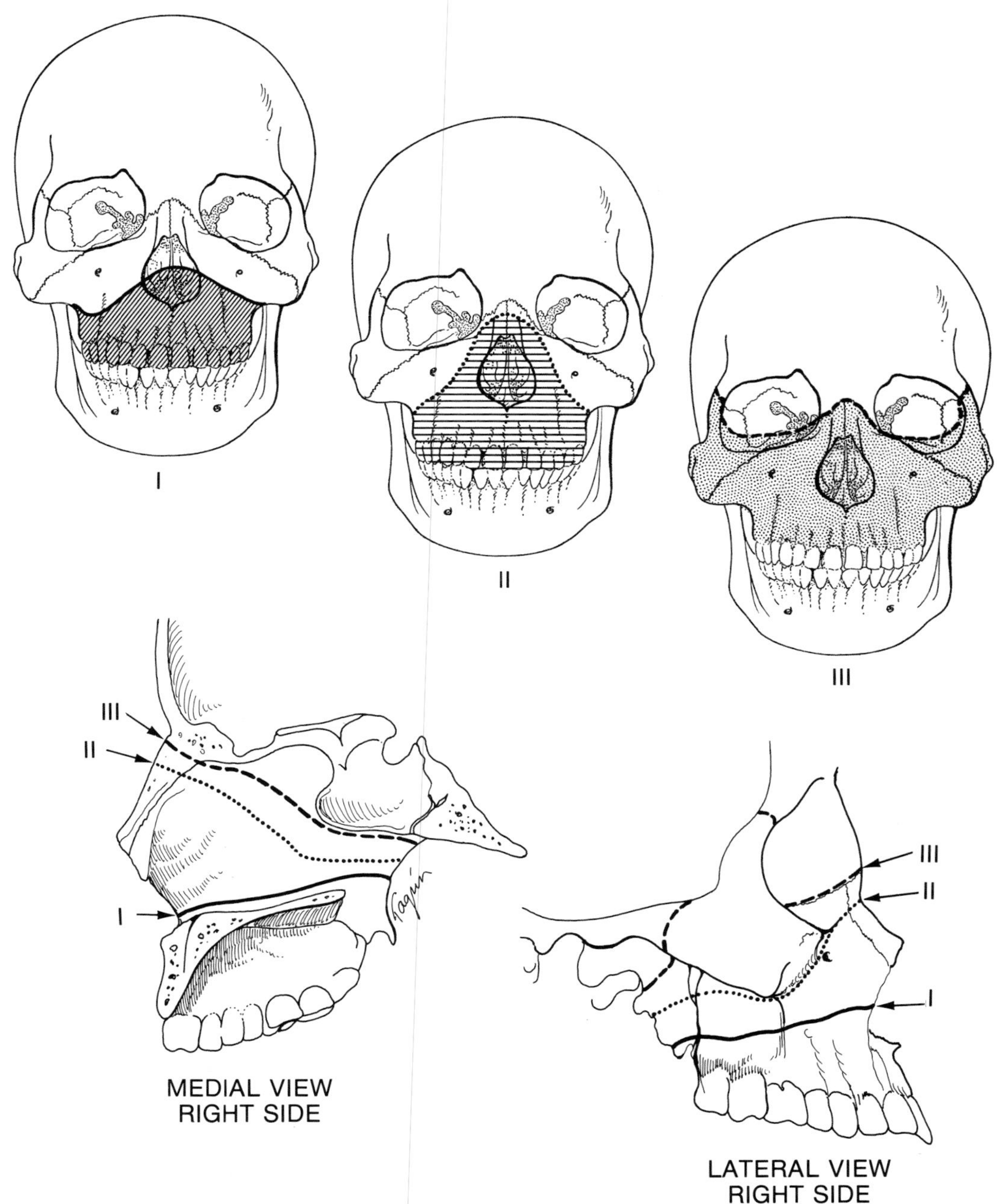

Figure 39.15. LeFort classification of maxillary fractures. *I*, transverse; *II*, pyramidal; and *III*, craniofacial dysjunction.

light pressure and offers some immobilization. Excessive motion at the wound site increases inflammatory response, causes unnecessary oozing of blood, increases the possibility of infection, and affects the final cosmetic result. The injured areas are best kept elevated. The need for tetanus prophylaxis is considered. Antibiotics are not routinely administered for minor lacerations or abrasions.

Clean lacerations may be closed safely up to 8 hours after injury. After this time and in extremely untidy wounds, a delayed primary technique should be considered.

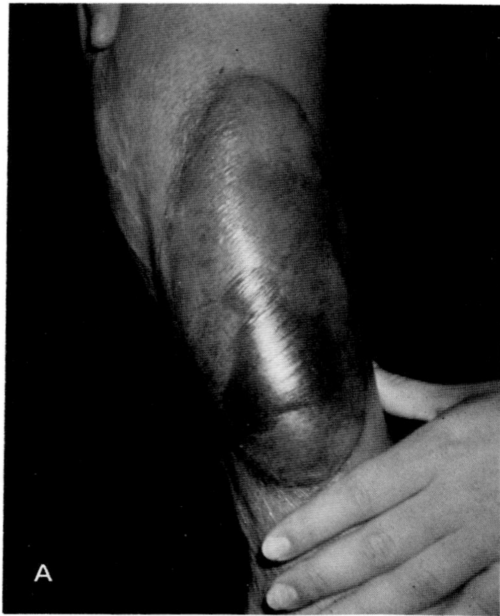

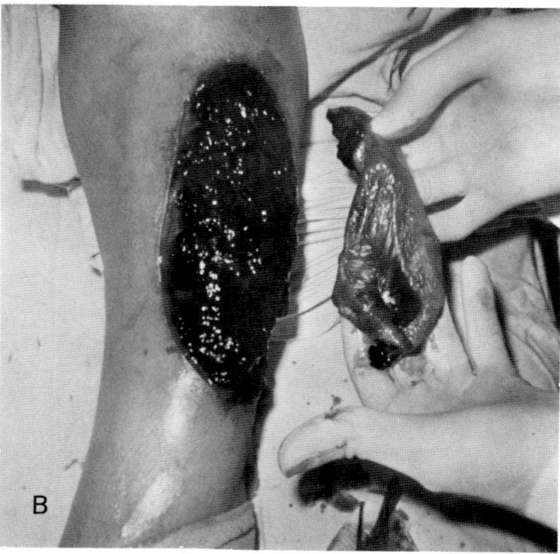

Figure 39.16. *A*, Large hematoma in pretibial region. *B*, Necrosis of overlying skin.

Major Injuries

Most severe soft-tissue injuries are associated with other critical injuries, including fractures and intrathoracic, intraabdominal, and/or head injuries. Initial care includes the resuscitative measures necessary to establish an airway, stop hemorrhage, and treat shock. Hemorrhage from major soft-tissue wounds can be controlled by local pressure or by a properly placed tourniquet when an extremity is involved. This allows time for evaluation and resuscitative measures to be carried out before transfer to the operating room, where these wounds are treated in conjunction with other emergency surgical procedures.

Tetanus prophylaxis is extremely important, and systemic administration of broad-spectrum antibiotics should be started before operation.

Lower Extremity Soft-tissue Injuries

Because of unique position and function in weight-bearing and because of a relative lack of anastomosing blood vessels in the skin, the lower extremities are vulnerable to unusual manifestations of soft-tissue injuries. All the injuries described require hospitalization and general anesthesia for definitive treatment. Bed rest with elevation is necessary to aid healing.

Contusion. Blunt trauma that does not disrupt the skin can injure blood vessels of all sizes. If only smaller, superficial vessels are damaged, a relatively innocuous ecchymosis (bruise) results. However, if one or more larger blood vessels is damaged, a large collection of blood (hematoma) results. Smaller hematomas resolve spontaneously, but rest, elevation, and mild compression of the area may be necessary. An enlarging hematoma requires incision, evacuation of the blood, and ligation of the bleeding vessel(s).

Hematoma between the muscular fascia and overlying subcutaneous fat usually occurs as a result of a shearing or degloving force, and often results in necrosis of the overlying skin and subcutaneous tissue. This is common in the pretibial region (Fig. 39.16). Excision of necrotic skin, evacuation of the blood, and skin grafting are required.

Laceration. Deep lacerations extending beneath the skin and superficial subcutaneous tissue require that distal motor and sensory function be examined thoroughly; the possibility of injury to a major vessel must be considered. Thorough knowledge of the regional anatomy is necessary to evaluate these injuries properly. Because repair is often complicated, surgical and orthopaedic consultations are required.

An unusual type of injury is the pretibial laceration. Because the cortex of the tibia is so close to the skin surface and because the subcutaneous fat is minimal, injuries that appear to be only lacerations are often partly avulsing or degloving. Suturing alone does not suffice, since necrosis of all the degloved or partly avulsed tissue often occurs (Fig. 39.17).

Although this type of injury may appear innocuous, skin grafting is usually required, and patients often must be hospitalized for several weeks for complete healing.

Degloving Injury. In this common injury, the skin and subcutaneous tissue are separated from the underlying fascia. This occurs as a result of a shearing force, and is most often seen when a leg has been run over by the wheels of a motor vehicle. Degloving of a large portion of the leg can occur without any disruption of the skin, although there are usually breaks in the skin with flaps of avulsed tissue. Because of the poor circulation and the associated crush injury, much of the degloved skin and subcutaneous tissue will not survive; and proper treatment may include debridement and skin grafting.

Crush Injury. Fractures of the long bones of the leg and foot are commonly associated with crush injuries. In addition, if a leg has been crushed under a considerable weight for a relatively long period, serious closed injury, primarily to muscle, is likely. After the pressure has been removed, the leg swells because of extravasation of red blood cells and plasma through damaged vessels and capillaries. Myoglobin and other products of damaged tissue leak into the general circulation. The combination of these events can cause the crush syndrome, which, if untreated, leads to shock and renal insufficiency.

Treatment includes the prompt restoration of blood volume with blood, plasma, and electrolyte solution sufficient to maintain a good urine output (75–100 ml/hr). The urine may have a port-wine color from the pigments of myoglobin and hemoglobin. Alkalinization of the urine with intravenous solutions containing sodium bicarbonate is important to prevent precipitation of the pigment in the renal tubules. The legs should be immobilized, slightly elevated, and left uncovered. Because of possible circulatory impairment from the swelling, careful and frequent evaluation is necessary. Extensive fasciotomy of all muscle compartments is often required and, if needed, should be carried out early. Early surgical consultation is in order.

The crush syndrome is an extremely serious injury; early resuscitation and treatment are similar to that required for the patient with a major electrical burn (see Chapter 38).

Stab Wounds

Deep injury to nerves, major blood vessels, and tendons can result from a stab wound. Careful neuromuscular and vascular examination is required. Excessive bleeding from the wound or an unusually large hematoma suggest injury to a major vessel. A surgeon must see these patients in the emergency department.

Missile Wounds

Bullets or shotgun blasts are the causes of missile wounds seen in civilian hospitals. The degree of injury depends on the caliber, the velocity, and the distance that the missile traveled. Emergency measures include controlling hemorrhage by direct pressure or a tourniquet, treating shock if present, covering the wounds with a sterile dressing, and evaluating the extent of the deep injury. All but the

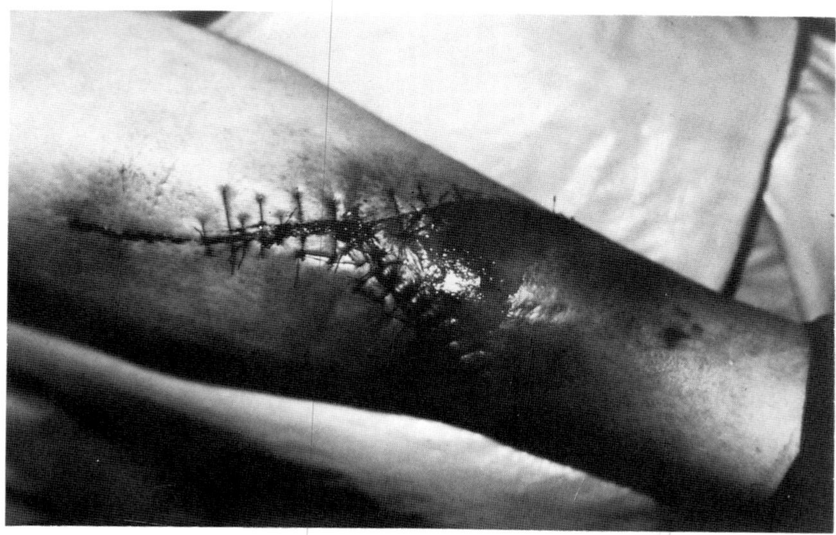

Figure 39.17. Impending necrosis of skin flaps around unwisely sutured pretibial laceration. Suturing under tension actually increases amount of tissue loss.

most superficial wounds require operative debridement. When a major vessel is injured, immediate reconstruction is necessary. Nerve repair may be delayed. The wounds are closed by a delayed primary technique or are allowed to close by secondary intention. It is unnecessary to remove all metal fragments; attempted removal may, at times, do more harm than good.

SUGGESTED READINGS

Converse JM. *Reconstructive Plastic Surgery,* 2nd ed. Philadelphia: WB Saunders, 1977, vol. 2.

Mathog RH. *Maxillofacial Trauma.* Baltimore: Williams & Wilkins, 1984.

McGregor IA. *Fundamental Techniques of Plastic Surgery and Their Surgical Applications,* 6th ed, Edinburgh: Churchill Livingstone, 1975.

Rowe NL, Williams JLI. *Maxillofacial Injuries.* Edinburgh: Churchill Livingstone, 1985.

Schultz RC. *Facial Injuries.* Chicago: Year Book, 1970.

CHAPTER **40**

Oral Surgical Emergencies

WALTER GURALNICK, D.M.D.
R. BRUCE DONOFF, D.M.D., M.D.
JOHN P. KELLY, D.M.D., M.D.

Oral surgical emergencies range from toothache to severe facial bone fractures. Within this broad spectrum are a variety of problems commonly seen in the emergency department, such as postextraction hemorrhage, salivary gland afflictions, acute dental infection with accompanying cellulitis, dislocated jaws, and avulsed teeth. Since the emergency department serves as the primary care facility for a large number of patients, diagnosis and management of oral surgical emergencies is important to all emergency physicians.

DENTAL EMERGENCIES

Postextraction Hemorrhage

Bleeding from a tooth socket is not usually a serious problem, but it is frightening for the patient, and it can be frustrating and difficult to control. It is therefore a common reason for seeking emergency treatment. Bleeding results most frequently from lack of compression of the clot, which appears as a protruding gelatinous mass extending from the socket over the adjacent teeth. As long as the clot remains, bleeding will continue. The clot should be removed with a sponge or suction tip, and a tight gauze wad large enough to create pressure should be placed over the socket. If pressure for 20–30 minutes does not stop the bleeding, other measures should be taken. Bleeding most frequently occurs from either of two sites—the edges of the socket or the interdental papilla. Therefore, if bleeding persists, sutures of 3–0 catgut on a cutting needle should be placed across the socket after injection of a local anesthetic agent. Profound anesthesia is easily obtained in the mouth by proper use of a local anesthetic. As a general rule, the upper jaw is anesthetized by infiltration, the lower jaw by blocking the appropriate inferior alveolar nerve. For those unacquainted with intraoral injection techniques, several texts are available, such as *Pain Control* by Trieger (1974). If bleeding is still uncontrolled, an absorbable hemostatic agent, such as Gelfoam or Surgicel, can be put in the socket after debriding the clot, and sutures can then be placed again.

If bleeding continues, the possibility of a hemorrhagic disorder should be considered. Persistent unexplained bleeding may be a symptom of a severe hemorrhagic condition, such as hemophilia, or it may be the initial indication of acute leukemia. Also, in patients receiving anticoagulants, bleeding may persist after an extraction if the prothrombin time is greater than 1½ times the control value. In such cases, appropriate laboratory studies are necessary before effective treatment can be given.

Fractured and Avulsed Teeth

Another common problem in the emergency department is a fractured tooth or avulsion of one or more teeth. If the crown of the tooth is fractured without exposure of the pulp, immediate treatment is unnecessary. The patient is advised to see a dentist as soon as possible, preferably within a few days. If the fracture transects the pulpal tissue, however, pain is intense, and emergency treatment consisting of extirpation of the pulp should be rendered. If a dentist is not available within the hospital, the patient should be referred to one immediately. Local dental societies usually maintain an on-call list of practitioners available for emergency needs.

In cases of avulsion, the patient is frequently a

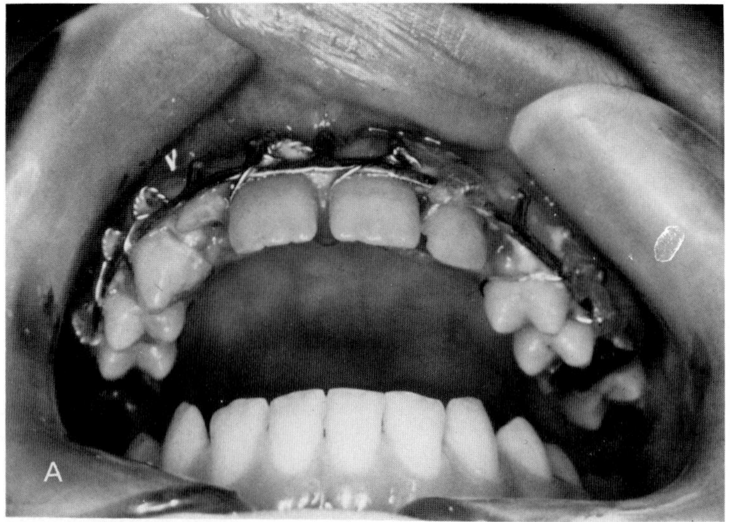

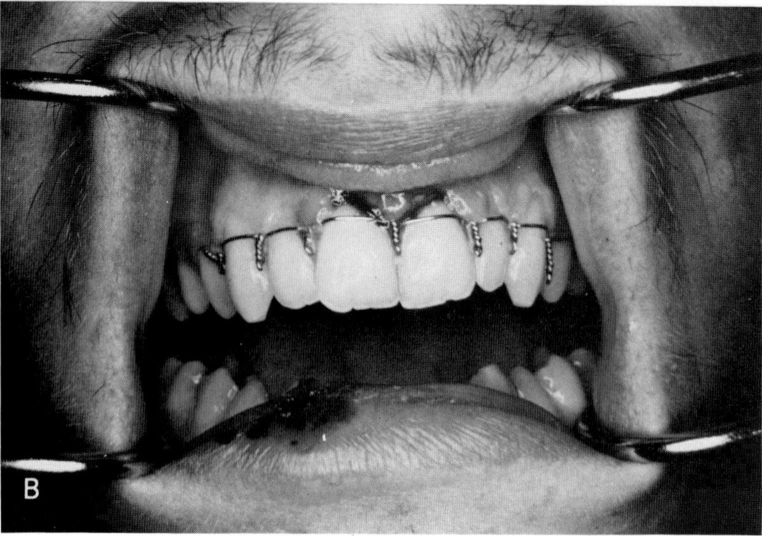

Figure 40.1. Stabilization of avulsed teeth. *A,* Arch bar technique. *B,* Wiring.

child who has fallen and knocked out an incisor. A tooth that has been avulsed and brought with the patient usually survives if it is replanted within a few hours. It should be washed with sterile saline, and inserted into the socket under local anesthesia. The tooth may be stabilized after replantation by suturing medially and distally to it or by using periodontal packing as a cementing device. Another technique is to wire or bond the replaced tooth to firm adjacent teeth; this is a quick, simple way of effecting good stabilization (Fig. 40.1.). The patient should take antibiotics, usually penicillin, for 7–10 days and should be restricted to a soft diet. In about 3 weeks, the replanted tooth should be firm. Replantation should always be attempted if the tooth is available, although the prognosis becomes poorer the longer the tooth has been out of the mouth. Lacerations of the mucosa and through-and-through lacerations should be closed with sutures as carefully as the skin surface.

Occasionally, a group of teeth with attached alveolar bone is dislodged. In such cases, reduction to proper anatomic position is accomplished by manual manipulation under local anesthesia. The prognosis for both bone and teeth is surprisingly good after such manipulation. As with avulsed teeth, some form of immobilization must be provided for several weeks.

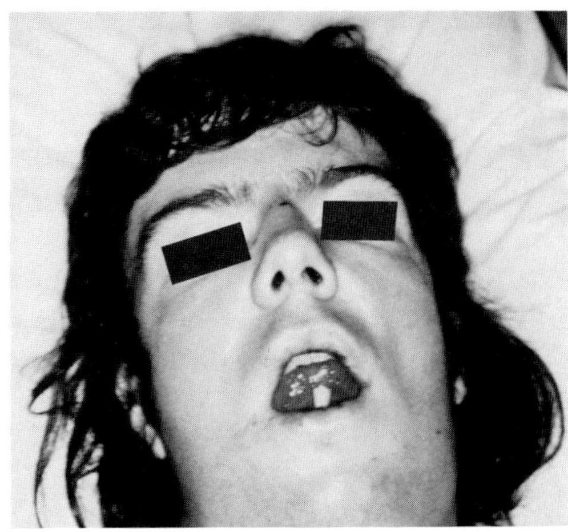

Figure 40.2. Ludwig's angina. Note protrusion of tongue resulting from elevation of floor of mouth.

ORAL INFECTIONS

Acute Alveolar Abscess

Patients with an acute alveolar abscess, with or without cellulitis, are frequently seen in the emergency department. Such patients are in severe pain, and if the infection is severe, as in Ludwig's angina (Fig. 40.2), the patient may be in serious trouble. As with any other abscess, the treatment is drainage if there is fluctuation, removal of the offending agent (a tooth, in this instance) if it is necessary and if it can be done atraumatically, and finally, antibiotic therapy and supportive care. If either intraoral or extraoral fluctuation exists (Fig. 40.3 and 40.4), incision and drainage should be accomplished with appropriate anesthesia. In some cases, the procedure can be performed on an outpatient basis, but in many instances, admission is warranted. The choice of antibiotic depends on the patient's history of drug sensitivity and the fact that the predominant organism in odontogenic infections is a penicillin-sensitive streptococcus. Nonallergic patients with severe cellulitis should be given 10 million units/ day of aqueous penicillin in divided doses via an open intravenous line. For less severe infections, particularly in ambulatory patients, oral penicillin should be prescribed; 500 mg of penicillin V four times a day is a suggested regimen.For penicillin-allergic patients, erythromycin and clindamycin, are possible alternatives. In all cases of acute odontogenic infection, the possibility of admission should seriously be considered.

Pericoronitis

A common odontogenic infection is pericoronitis, inflammation of the gingiva surrounding an impacted wisdom tooth. Facial swelling, painful swollen gingiva in the mandibular retromolar area, submandibular adenopathy, and trismus are typical findings. Emergency treatment consists of application of heat to the face, warm saline rinses, antibiotics, and analgesics. Penicillin V, 250 mg orally four times a day, is the drug of choice if not contraindicted by allergic or idiosyncratic reaction. Symptoms usually resolve significantly in 48 hours, and definitive treatment—removal of the impacted tooth—can be undertaken thereafter.

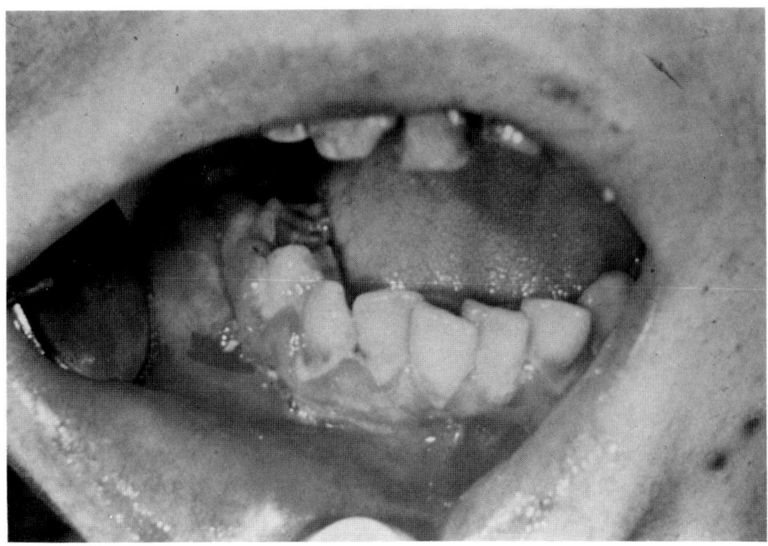

Figure 40.3. Fluctuation in buccal sulcus.

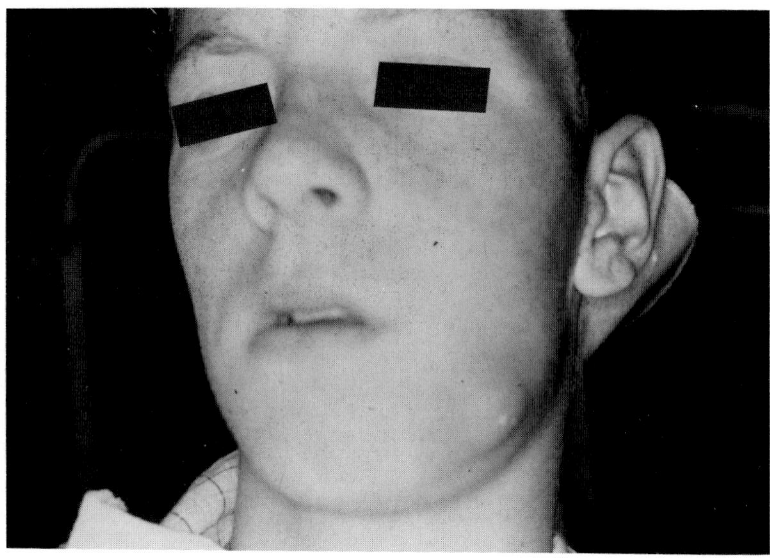

Figure 40.4. Extraoral fluctuation.

Salivary Gland Infection

The differential diagnosis of facial swellings must include infections of the parotid and submandibular glands. These conditions are usually manifested by tender preauricular or submandibular swellings. Diagnosis is often made by intraoral examination of the parotid (Stensen's) or submandibular (Wharton's) duct. The opening of the parotid duct is on the buccal mucosa adjacent to the maxillary molar teeth; the opening of the submandibular duct is in the anterior floor of the mouth. The area of the opening is dried with a gauze sponge, and pressure is then applied repeatedly from back to front along the course of the duct. The examiner may find diminished salivary flow, inspissated saliva, or pus, all of which suggest a pathologic process. Palpation may reveal the presence of a calculus, which can be confirmed by radiologic examination, using an occlusal view for the submaxillary gland (Fig. 40.5) and a lateral jaw film or panoramic view for the parotid duct and gland.

The condition of patients with parotitis, particularly older patients, may be extremely toxic. Fever, dehydration, and an elevated white blood cell count are usual. Hospitalization with supportive care, in-

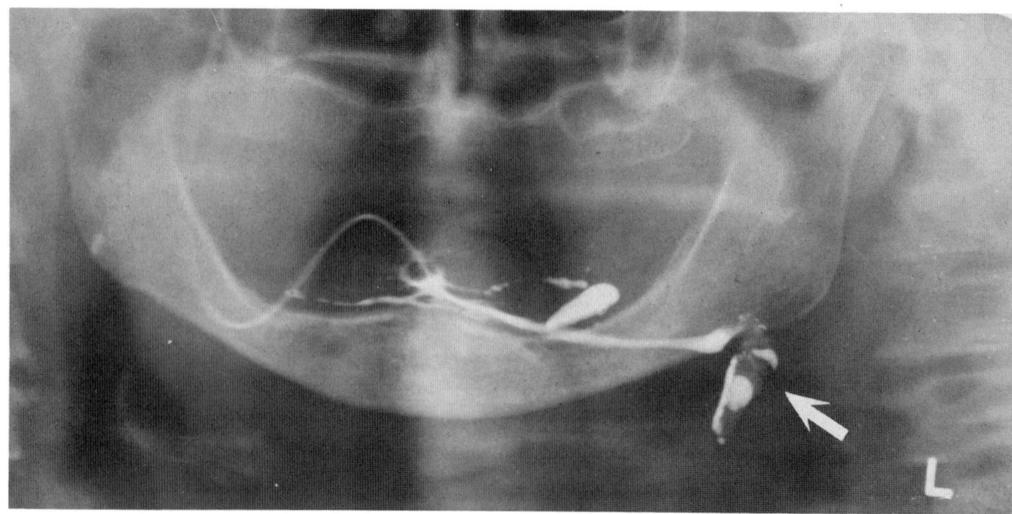

Figure 40.5. Stone in submaxillary gland (*arrow*).

travenous fluids, and antibiotics is required. In contrast with other oral infections, *Staphylococcus aureus* is the usual pathogen. Intravenous oxacillin, 6–8 gm/day, is the drug of choice in the nonallergic patient. Ampicillin, clindamycin and cephalothin are alternatives. Stimulation with heat and lemon drops is a useful adjunct. If present, pus should be cultured; failure to respond to treatment within 48 hours raises the possibility of an abscess requiring surgical drainage. Fortunately, this is uncommon, and resolution usually occurs with conservative but vigorous measures.

Submandibular glands more commonly become infected because of calculus formation or duct stricture. Calculi should be removed intraorally if possible, preferably after infection has been controlled. Calculi in the gland, however, necessitate excision of the gland. Sialography is useful in both parotid and submandibular gland infections. Irregularities of the main duct system or calculi may be revealed, and the procedure has a useful dilating effect. Sialography should not be performed until the infection has been controlled.

If salivary gland infection due to obstruction is eliminated in the differential diagnosis of such facial swellings, other possibilities must be considered, including mumps, drug-induced "mumps," mononucleosis, cat-scratch fever, and cellulitis of the external auditory canal. Parotid tumors are usually not tender. Systemic lupus erythematosus and sarcoidosis may cause unilateral enlargement of the parotid gland; Sjögren's syndrome is usually bilateral. Tuberculosis and some fungal diseases may also mimic salivary gland infections.

Acute Mucous Membrane Disease

Patients with acute Vincent's disease (trench mouth, Vincent's infection, Vincent's angina) or other lesions of the mucous membranes such as herpes or aphthobullous stomatitis are often seen in the emergency department. All these mucosal diseases cause considerable pain, bleeding gums, and occasionally an elevated temperature and generalized malaise. They also produce understandable anxiety. They may be symptomatic of underlying disease ranging from benign mononucleosis to such serious conditions as leukemia and pemphigus. Treatment in the emergency department is primarily directed at alleviating pain. This can be accomplished by prescribing topical anesthetics such as lidocaine (Xylocaine Viscous) or diclonine hydrochloride (Dyclone), as well as analgesics. A complete blood cell count may be advisable as a preliminary screening test, and, in all instances, follow-up treatment should be advised, and appropriate arrangements made for such care.

FACIAL FRACTURES AND DISLOCATIONS

Traumatic lesions constitute a large percentage of the conditions seen in the emergency department. The patient's survival may depend on initial evaluation and treatment, long before a specialist or team of specialists is called on for definitive repair of injuries. Although it is preferable to repair facial fractures promptly, definitive treatment need not be compromised if it is deferred for as long as 7–10 days because of a concomitant life-threatening condition. Initial attention is focused on patency of the airway, control of hemorrhage, neurologic abnormalities, and internal injuries. The cervical spine must be immobilized until fracture has been ruled out.

Respiratory embarrassment is common in patients with mandibular and midface fractures. It may be caused by mechanical obstruction if the tongue has fallen back into the oropharynx because of fracture at the symphysis with resultant release of the genial attachments. In such cases, bringing the tongue forward with a ligature tied extraorally relieves the obstruction promptly. Occasionally, foreign bodies such as fragments of dentures or teeth may also mechanically occlude the airway. Suspicion of such obstruction calls for rapid but careful inspection of the mouth and throat. Dentures are constructed of acrylic and are not radiopaque; missing fragments should carefully be sought. Respiratory embarrassment may also be caused by severe hemorrhage from a lacerated tongue or other lacerations, nasal bleeding, and through-and-through wounds that have severed large vessels. Control of bleeding sites must be accomplished quickly or an alternate airway provided by either endotracheal intubation or emergency tracheotomy.

After an airway is established and hemorrhage is arrested, the patient's neurologic status should be assessed. If it is indicated by the history and the examination, neurosurgical consultation takes precedence over treatment of facial fractures. At the same time, possible thoracic and abdominal injuries must be considered before proceeding with extensive examination of facial injuries.

Mandible

In the management of facial fractures, the findings derived from careful clinical examination are confirmed by certain specific x-ray views. It is important to understand the value of each type of view that may be ordered. Diagnosis of a mandibular fracture usually requires several views. A panoramic film is an excellent initial screening view and may occasionally be all that is necessary. Other views include the lateral oblique, which is particu-

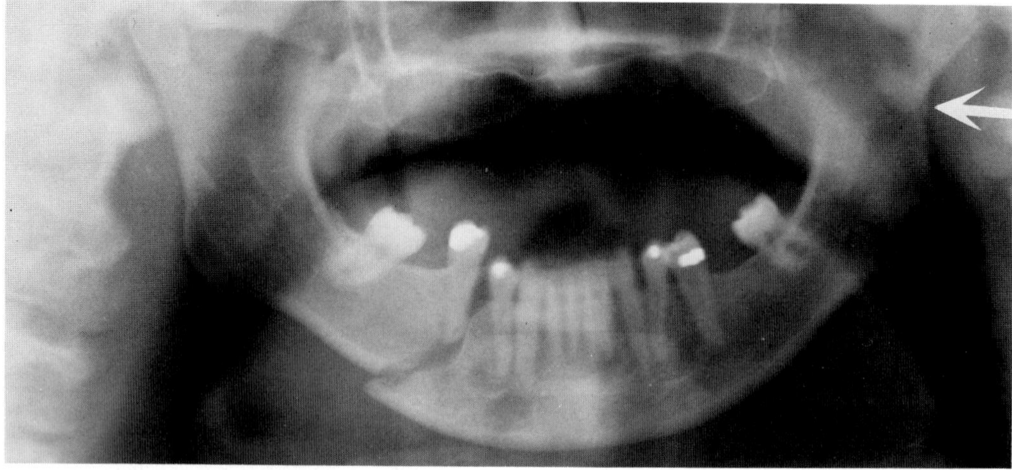

Figure 40.6. Typical fracture of body of mandible and contralateral condylar fracture (*arrow*).

larly useful in visualizing the body of the mandible, and the posteroanterior, which is helpful in assessing the condition of the symphysis and the condyles, as well as in visualizing lateral displacement of the body and fractures of the rami. In addition, an occlusal view is helpful in elucidating a suspected fracture of the symphysis. Condylar fractures that are not readily seen are best diagnosed by means of the Towne's projection view or a panoramic film (Fig. 40.6).

Emergency treatment of mandibular fractures is usually definitive except in the presence of hemorrhage or an airway blocked by a posteriorly displaced fractured lower jaw. If definitive closed or open reduction must await treatment of other injuries or neurologic clearance, the mandible should be stabilized temporarily with circumfrontal wire, either alone or in conjuction with an arch bar.

Since condylar fractures often present a problem in management, recognition is important. A blow on the chin often produces no injury other than fracture of a mandibular condyle. Clues to diagnosis include (*a*) malocclusion because of premature molar contact resulting from a decrease in the height of the mandibular ramus; (*b*) inability to palpate the condylar head as the patient opens and closes his mouth (palpation can be attempted either anterior to the ear or with a finger in the external auditory meatus); (*c*) pain in the preauricular area on opening the mouth; and (*d*) deviation to the fractured side when the mouth is opened. Careful radiologic assessment is imperative since condylar fractures are often subtle and can be overlooked because of more obvious injuries. The Towne's projection view and the panoramic view offer the best means for radiologic diagnosis.

Diagnostic failure can lead to disturbing symptoms of pain and deviation of the jaw. In children, the condylar region is extremely vascular until the age of about 6, and, during these years, injury may cause extensive hematoma, ankylosis, and growth impairment. Treatment is therefore directed to early mobilization. If necessary, short-term intermaxillary fixation is employed to establish occlusion; if occlusion is normal, fixation is not used.

Although a condylar fracture in a patient with massive maxillofacial injury such as a LeFort III fracture (see Fig. 39.15) may seem trivial, ability to restore the normal appearance of the face rests on alignment of the maxilla against an intact mandible. This is difficult to achieve if there are no posterior teeth or if the mandible has ''gagged open'' because of collapse on the side of the condylar fracture. In the management of these fractures in adults, basic principles include the following: (*a*) if there is malocclusion, intermaxillary fixation for 10–21 days is required to establish proper occlusion in either unilateral or bilateral fractures; (*b*) if there is no malocclusion, a soft diet and limited jaw motion are recommended; and (*c*) if an open bite exists and particularly if the patient has no posterior teeth, open reduction (Fig. 40.7) of at least one side in bilateral fractures should be considered.

Zygomaticomaxillary Complex

Assessment of the zygomaticomaxillary complex is somewhat more complicated than assessment of the mandible. Extensive edema occurs rapidly and makes it difficult to diagnose the underlying skeletal injuries. Careful physical and radiologic examination provides accurate diagnosis from which appropriate surgical treatment can be planned.

On inspection, an elongated face and bilateral circumorbital ecchymosis are noted in midface fractures—the result of dropping of the maxilla. At the same time, in LeFort II and III fractures, the posterior teeth often cause "gagging" of the occlusion, preventing closure, and the patient appears to have an open bite. If the patient is seen shortly after injury, flattening of the upper part of the cheek indicates a zygomatic fracture; this can be observed by standing behind the patient and sighting the superior orbital margin from above. Bleeding from the nose or ears or both should be sought, particularly to determine whether there is cerebrospinal fluid leakage—a finding that is sometimes difficult to confirm, but that suggests a LeFort II or III fracture.

Other important findings may be noted from inspection of the eyes. Discrepancy of ocular levels, as determined by a line projected between the pupils, may result from a blow-out fracture with herniation of the orbital contents through the fractured floor into the antrum. Subconjunctival ecchymosis may indicate fracture of the lateral orbital wall, part of a typical tripod fracture of the zygomaticomaxillary complex. Restriction of ocular movements is diagnostic of muscle entrapment in orbital floor in-

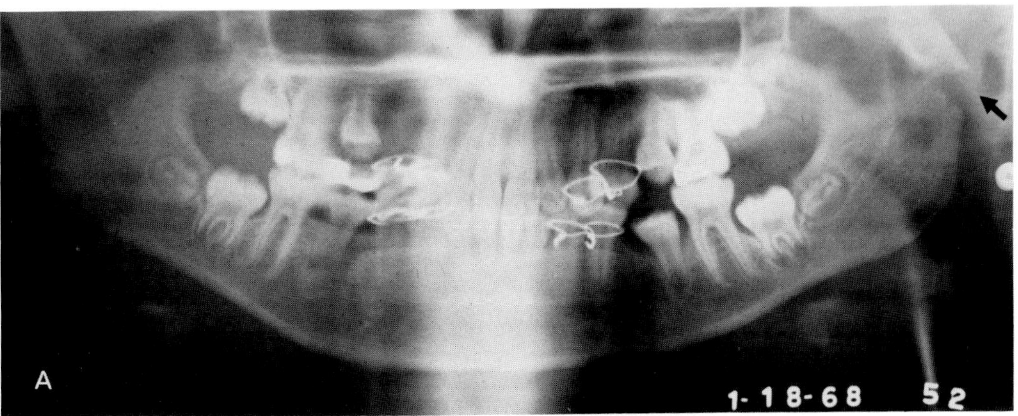

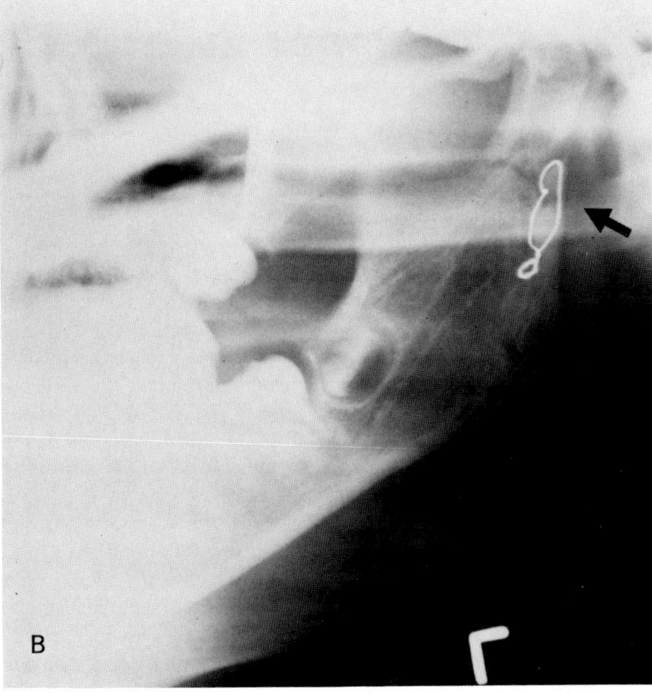

Figure 40.7. *A,* Fractured (totally distracted) condyle (*arrow*). *B,* Open reduction and interosseous wiring of condyle (*arrow*).

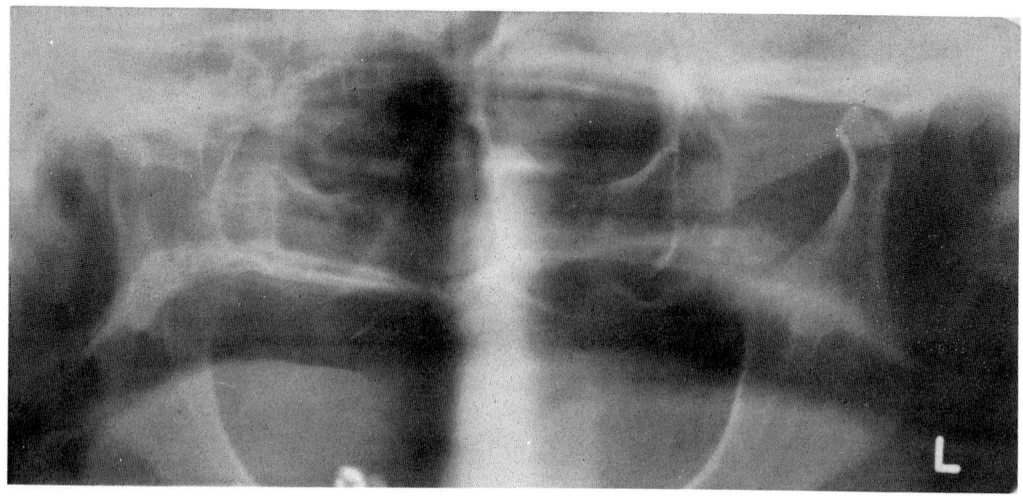

Figure 40.8. Temporomandibular joint dislocation.

jury, and diplopia suggests disruption of the orbit by a zygomaticomaxillary fracture.

Visual inspection should be followed by palpation. The index finger should be moved over the entire orbital rim to note both tenderness and step defects. Particular attention should be given to the zygomaticofrontal and zygomaticomaxillary sutures. In addition to step defects, crepitation is often detected. If the patient is conscious and responsive, anesthesia of the cheek, nose, and lips should be investigated, its existence being very suggestive of a fracture through the infraorbital foramen.

Intraoral examination follows manual inspection of the face. First, mobility of the maxilla should be tested by holding the bridge of the nose with one hand while grasping the upper anterior teeth with the other hand. Movement can be seen and felt as it is transmitted to the firmly grasped nasal bones. There may be ecchymosis of the upper buccal sulcus, as well as anesthesia of the gingiva and teeth in the area. Fractures of the lateral antral wall and zygomatic buttress can sometimes be palpated. At the same examination, gagging due to displacement of the maxilla may be observed; limitation of mandibular movement may result from impingement of a fractured zygomatic arch on the coronoid process of the mandible.

On the basis of clinical findings, certain x-ray views are indicated. The Waters' view (also known as the occipitomental projection) is the most useful film for demonstrating fractures of the zygomaticomaxillary complex. The orbital rims, zygomatic arches, and antra are all visualized. In addition, a submental vertex (jug-handle) view will demonstrate fractures of the zygomatic arch that other films might not. No radiologic examination of a patient with multiple facial fractures is complete without posteroanterior and lateral skull films to investigate possible cranial injury. The usefulness of computed tomography is addressed in Chapter 45.

Temporomandibular Joint

Another distressing jaw problem seen in the emergency department is dislocation of the temporomandibular joint (Fig. 40.8). It demands prompt reduction and careful explanation and follow-up care. In this type of dislocation, which may result from trauma or sudden stretching of masticatory muscles as in excessive yawning; the condylar head is held anterior to or on the articular eminence by myospasm. The dislocation is treated by simple manual reduction, although spontaneous reduction may occur if the patient is sufficiently relaxed. The use of meperidine hydrochloride (Demerol) or a muscle relaxant such as diazepam (Valium) can facilitate either spontaneous or manual reduction. Reduction is performed by standing in front of the patient and placing the index fingers in the buccal mandibular sulci, applying pressure inferiorly and posteriorly over the retromolar pads; at the same time, thumb pressure is directed superiorly at the symphysis. Firm pressure is applied gradually and consistently until the condyle is repositioned in the glenoid fossa. A sponge is useful as a finger cushion. To prevent recurrent dislocation, it is necessary to restrict opening of the mouth for several hours and to restrict mandibular movement for 2–3 weeks.

Occasionally, a dislocation cannot be reduced without general anesthesia and muscle relaxants. Repeated injection of a local anesthetic into the masseter muscle or joint space is usually unsuccessful and unpleasant for the patient; it is not ordinarily an alternative to general anesthesia. If dislocation occurs frequently, intermaxillary fixation may be necessary until definitive treatment can be given, but only for a short period. Patients with habitual dislocation may have to be told to bury the chin in the chest during yawning.

The extrapyramidal neuromuscular effects of phenothiazine derivatives such as prochlorperazine maleate (Compazine) are well known. Diagnosis is based on the history and clinical findings. Symptoms may include agitation, spasm of neck muscles sometimes progressing to torticolis, carpopedal spasm, trismus, and pseudo-dislocation of the jaw. Treatment includes reassurance and discontinuance of the drug. Diphenhydramine hydrochloride (Benadryl), 50 mg intramuscularly, is helpful in reversing the muscular spasm and ''dislocation''; additional oral doses may be required.

INJURY TO PAROTID GLAND AND DUCT

Soft-tissue injuries are dealt with in Chapter 39. However, injury to the parotid gland and duct, a significant and unique injury occasionally found accompanying facial trauma, deserves emphasis. Primary recognition and treatment of this class of injury prevents complications of fistula, sialocele, and infection. Careful clinical examination should be conducted in cases of laceration of the cheek. Although hemostasis must be obtained for direct visualization into the wound, blind clamping in this region is inadvisable, and definitive examination may be better carried out in the operating room.

If parotid duct injury is suspected and the duct cannot be visualized within the wound or if a severed end is not visible, the duct should be probed. A lacrimal duct probe can usually be passed via the oral opening of the parotid duct. This makes it easier to locate the duct in the wound to determine if it has been transected or lacerated; in such a case the probe will emerge in the wound. If the probe does not exit into the wound, it can be palpated through the wound, and the location of the duct in relation to the injury can be ascertained. If there is still a question as to duct injury after probing, two choices exist: methylene blue can be injected into the duct and its presence in the wound observed, or a sialogram can be obtained. These studies are useful to determine whether the parotid gland has been injured and its capsule violated. Facial nerve function must also be carefully evaluated.

The lacerated parotid duct is best treated by direct anastomosis, using 6–0 silk sutures over a plastic catheter; No. 16 or No. 18 Intracath tubing works well. The catheter is left sutured to the buccal mucosa for 10–14 days. Antibiotics should be administered prophylactically; penicillin is recommended if the patient is not allergic to it. Gland stimulation with lemon drops and dilatation of the duct are useful.

If the damage to the duct prevents direct anastomosis, the proximal portion of the duct must be found and ligated. Gland atrophy will ensue. Direct damage to the capsule and gland demands meticulous closure of the capsule and closure of the wound in layers. This is of paramount importance to recovery of distal facial nerve function as well. Usually, facial nerve injuries distal to a line projected from the outer canthus of the eye to the gonial notch of the mandible (about 2 cm from the angle of the jaw) do not require anastomosis.

SUGGESTED READINGS

Donoff RB, ed. *Manual of Oral and Maxillofacial Surgery.* St Louis: CV Mosby, 1987.

Epker, BN, Burnette JC. Trauma to the parotid gland and duct: Primary treatment and management of complications. *J Oral Surg,* 1970;28:657–670.

Foster CA, Sherman JE. *Surgery of Facial Bone Fractures.* New York: Churchill Livingstone, 1987.

Guralnick WC, ed. *Textbook of Oral Surgery.* Boston: Little, Brown, 1968.

Hötte HH. *Orbital Fractures.* Springfield, Illinois: Charles C Thomas, 1970.

Irby WB, ed. *Facial Trauma and Concomitant Problems: Evaluation and Treatment.* St Louis, CV Mosby, 1974.

Kelly JF, ed. *Management of War Injuries to the Jaws and Related Structures.* Department of the Navy, 1978.

McCarthy PL, Shklar G. *Diseases of the Oral Mucosa: Diagnosis, Management, Therapy.* New York: McGraw-Hill, 1964.

Pozatek ZW, Kaban LB, Guralnick WC. Fractures of the zygomatic complex: An evaluation of surgical management with special emphasis on the eyebrow approach. *J Oral Surg,* 1973;31:141–148.

Rowe NL, Williams JL. *Maxillofacial Injuries.* New York: Churchill Livingstone, 1985.

Trieger N. *Pain Control.* Lombard IL: Quintessence Publishing, 1974.

CHAPTER **41**

Emergency Care of the Injured Hand

RICHARD J. SMITH, M.D.†

Editors note: Gratitude is expressed to Jesse B. Jupiter, M.D. for his review of this chapter.

The initial treatment of an injured hand often determines the nature of further reconstructive surgical procedures, the duration and severity of disability, and the ultimate function of the entire limb. The goal is to restore versatility and strength, by providing smoothly gliding muscle-tendon units and a stable skeletal framework, minimizing contractures and adhesions of skin, tendons, and joints, and preserving sensation. Complications, such as subcutaneous hematoma, edema, and superficial infection, which often resolve without sequelae if they occur elsewhere, may result in permanent restriction of motion if they occur in the hand. The appearance of the hand is of great importance; a self-conscious patient may not use a limb that is badly scarred or mutilated. Although hand injuries are common in busy emergency departments, this in no way lessens their importance or the responsibilities of the physician treating them. Therefore, it is important for the thorough emergency physician undertaking initial therapy to appreciate fully the later considerations and details of management.

GENERAL CONSIDERATIONS

History

The proper evaluation and treatment of the patient with a wounded hand requires adequate knowledge of both the injury and previous medical history. The history should include the occupation and dominant hand of the patient, since the prognosis is often influenced by these factors. Details of the mechanism of injury are crucial to treatment. If the hand has been cut by glass, the type of glass is important, since tinted bottles and fine glassware frequently contain lead that may be visible on x-ray examination. A hand injured in a press may have a thermal injury as well as a crush injury. Although machine oil at the edges of a wound may make the wound look dirty, it may be innocuous. Air bubbles deep in a wound appear ominous on x-ray examination, but may merely be the result of irrigation with hydrogen peroxide solution before arrival at

† Deceased.

the emergency department. Small, seemingly harmless lacerations, however, may harbor spirochetes, streptococci, and clostridia if they are the result of a human bite.

If an amputated portion of the hand has been retrieved, its history must also be noted. Where was it found? Was it subjected to heat or repeated trauma? Was it washed, cooled, or treated with antiseptics? These questions must be asked as part of the complete history before the patient is anesthetized; surgical decisions may depend on responses.

A standard hand injury history form is often valuable in rapidly obtaining a complete, relevant record that is useful in evaluating the injury and in planning treatment. This form should be brief but comprehensive.

Emergency Examination and Evaluation

In isolated hand injuries pain relief should be accomplished early. Before the injured hand is examined, the entire limb should be inspected. The patient, a coworker, or a family member may have applied a tourniquet to stop the bleeding and the sleeve then rebuttoned, concealing it. All bracelets, rings, and other jewelry must be removed, regardless of sentiments, since such objects may act as tourniquets as the limb swells.

X-ray Examinations

Except for minor lacerations, all wounds of the hand should be examined radiologically. If the film is taken without delay and if the general condition of the patient is stable, it is advisable to perform x-ray examination first. With more serious injuries, however, excessive delay in rendering primary wound care should be avoided.

Removing the Dressing

Severe crush and explosion injuries and burns need not be inspected in the emergency department; such examination is painful and causes unnecessary contamination. Less severe wounds may be examined in the emergency department under aseptic conditions. The patient should be calmed and placed preferably in the supine position. The examiner should wear a mask and sterile gloves. After the injured hand is placed on a sterile field, all dressing are cut down to the bottom layer, which is soaked loose in a pan of sterile saline if adherent. The wound should not be probed. Coagulated blood is gently removed with a sponge soaked in diluted hydrogen peroxide solution. Superficial foreign material should be cleansed from the wound. It is not necessary to remove all ingrained dirt or grease from the surface of the skin. Benzene is an excellent, painless solvent for many types of grease, ink, and paint. The wound is then gently lavaged with sterile saline or lactated Ringer's solution, and a sterile sponge is applied until definitive care can be rendered.

Inspection

Inspection of the cleansed hand at rest is the most valuable part of the examination. With the wrist in mild dorsiflexion, any irregularity in the normal curve of the semi-flexed fingertips is immediately apparent, calling attention to a flexor tendon injury. With the forearm in pronation and the wrist in palmar flexion, a lag of extension at a metacarpophalangeal joint signals an extensor tendon injury. Malrotation of a fingernail usually indicates a rotated fracture of a tubular bone, either phalanx or metacarpal. Depression of a metacarpal head suggests a fracture of the metacarpal neck. If the thumb is supinated and adducted against the index finger, injury to the median nerve should be suspected.

The color, temperature, and moisture of the fingertips are noted. Laceration of a sensory nerve causes normal perspiration in the corresponding part of the finger to stop at once. A finger in which both neurovascular bundles are lacerated is likely to be pale and cool; its viability is precarious.

Function

Test of tendon and nerve function are performed simply and painlessly. Alternate flexion and extension of the fingers, thumb, and wrist, active adduction and abduction of the thumb and index finger, and a brief sensory examination provide most of the information required for neuromuscular evaluation (Tables 41.1 and 41.2, Fig. 41.1). Nothing distresses an alarmed child more than use of a pin or needle for pinprick evaluation. To test sharp-dull discrimination, the examiner should touch, but not jab, the skin with a pinpoint, and the patient should be allowed to watch. A more sensitive test is to ask a patient to differentiate between the milled edge of a quarter coin and the smooth edge of a nickle. To diagnose major nerve injuries, the physician should test the *autonomous zones* of the radial, median, and ulnar nerves at the *dorsum of the first web, the tip of the thumb,* and *the tip of the little finger,* respectively.

The anatomic diagnosis and the extent of all injuries are recorded, preferably with a sketch of the hand wounds. Photographs may be useful. The physician then decides if a specialist is necesary and whether to treat the injury in the emergency department or in the operating room. The limb is splinted and elevated until definitive treatment is given. The patient and his family are told of the general plan of treatment and the expected prognosis.

Table 41.1.
Intrinsic Muscle Innervation and Function of the Hand

Muscle	Function	Innervation	Test or Observation
Thenar muscles (abductor pollicis brevis, flexor pollicis brevis, opponens pollicis)	Abduction, pronation, flexion—first metacarpal; abduction, flexion—proximal phalanx of thumb; extension—distal phalanx of thumb	Median nerve, with occasional ulnar nerve contribution	Compare abduction of both thumbs from palmar plane; have patient oppose thumb tip to tip of little finger; with paralysis, thenar atrophy, poor thumb abduction from palm, poor thumb rotation
Adductor pollicis	Adduction—first metacarpal and proximal phalanx of thumb in palmar plane; flexion—proximal phalanx of thumb; extension—distal phalanx of thumb	Ulnar nerve	Have patient pull sheet of paper from examiner—interphalangeal joint of thumb will acutely flex (Froment's sign) if adductor is weak
Hypothenar muscles (abductor digiti quinti, flexor digiti quinti, opponens digiti quinti)	Flexion, pronation—fifth metacarpal; flexion—metacarpophalangeal joint of little finger; extension—interphalangeal joints of little finger	Ulnar nerve	Have patient oppose tip of little finger to thumb tip (little finger abduction possible through extensor digiti quinti proprius)
All interosseus muscles	Flexion—metacarpophalangeal joints; extension—interphalangeal joints	Ulnar nerve	No active abduction or adduction of involved fingers; ring and little fingers clawed (lumbricals of index and middle fingers, supplied by median nerve, prevent clawing)
Dorsal interossei	Abduction of fingers from middle finger		
Palmar interossei	Adduction of fingers to middle finger		
Lumbrical muscles	Flexion—metacarpophalangeal joints; extension—interphalangeal joints	Median nerve—index and middle fingers Ulnar nerve—ring and little fingers	Difficult to test if interossei are intact; if interossei are paralyzed, lack of metacarpophalangeal flexion with interphalangeal extension of index and middle fingers indicates lumbrical paralysis

Debridement and Cleansing of Complex Injuries

Thorough cleansing of the wound is most important in the treatment of an injured hand. The uninjured portion of the hand may be washed and shaved in the emergency department to permit proper examination. Complex wounds should not be cleansed deeply without regional or general anesthesia. Cleansing must be done in a sterile field. Most bleeding can be controlled with gentle pressure. It is unnecessary to attempt total hemostasis before debridement and lavage.

Complex injuries should be managed in the operating room. A pneumatic tourniquet, padded with sheet cotton, is applied to the upper arm. The limb is exsanguinated by elevation and the tourniquet cuff inflated to a pressure of 100–150 mm Hg above systolic pressure. A rubber band tourniquet around the

Table 41.2.
Extrinsic Muscle Innervation and Function of Hand

Muscle	Function	Innervation
Flexor carpi ulnaris	Flexion, ulnar deviation—wrist	Ulnar nerve
Palmaris longus	Flexion—wrist (weak)	Median nerve
Flexor carpi radialis	Flexion, radial deviation—wrist	Median nerve
Flexor pollicis longus	Flexion—distal phalanx of thumb	Median nerve (anterior interosseous branch)
Flexor digitorum profundus	Flexion—distal phalanges of fingers	Median nerve (anterior interosseous branch)—index and middle fingers Ulnar nerve—ring and little fingers
Flexor digitorum superficialis (sublimis)	Flexion—middle phalanges	Median nerve
Abductor pollicis longus	Extension—first metacarpal	Radial nerve (dorsal interosseous branch)
Extensor pollicis brevis	Extension—proximal phalanx of thumb	Radial nerve (dorsal interosseous branch)
Extensor pollicis longus	Extension—distal phalanx of thumb	Radial nerve (dorsal interosseus branch)
Extensor carpi radialis longus	Extension, radial deviation—wrist	Radial nerve
Extensor carpi radialis brevis	Extension—wrist	Radial nerve (dorsal interosseous branch)
Extensor digitorum communis, extensor indicis proprius, extensor digiti quinti proprius	Extension—proximal phalanges of fingers	Radial nerve (dorsal interosseous branch)
Extensor carpi ulnaris	Extension, ulnar deviation—wrist	Radial nerve (dorsal interosseous branch)

base of a finger or a catheter tourniquet wrapped around the wrist or forearm may cause damage to nerves or blood vessels because the pressure is unchecked. Even without anesthesia, almost all patients tolerate a properly applied pneumatic tourniquet for 20–30 minutes if the arm has been exsanguinated.

With sterile technique, the skin around the wound is washed thoroughly and the hand is sponged gently with soapy water. Coagulated blood is removed. The wound is lavaged with 4 liters of sterile saline or Ringer's lactated solution, and the hand placed on a sterile towel. The surgeon then puts on new gloves, cleanses the wound with an antiseptic solution, such as povidone-iodine and drapes the limb for operation.

The depths of the wound are now explored, and foreign bodies are extracted. The edges of the wound are held back by blunt rakes for thorough exposure and debridement. Splinters of bone not attached to soft tissue are removed. Muscle that is dark, not contractile, and obviously not viable is excised. Lacerated tendons and nerves are identified and tagged with sutures.

After the operation is completed, the wound is again copiously irrigated, the arm is elevated, and the tourniquet is released and removed. Gentle pressure is applied to the wound for 4–5 minutes. Hemostasis is usually obtained more quickly and less traumatically with cautery than with large numbers of ligatures. The edges of skin and subcutaneous tissue should be excised if they are ragged, necrotic, or crushed.

Dressings

Hand dressings that are properly applied serve several purposes. They protect the wound from contamination, absorb drainage, provide even pressure, and close potential dead spaces. Many dressings also serve as splints. A hand dressing must be comfortable, and should not cause maceration or strangulation of tissue. Tight compression dressings are *never* indicated for hand wounds.

While dressings are applied to the hand, an assistant holds the hand by the tips of the index and middle fingers to preserve the width and concavity of the palm and to prevent squeezing or flattening the first, fourth, and fifth metacarpal bones. One layer of petrolatum gauze covers the wound to prevent adherence of skin to the dressing. Loosely packed fluffs of gauze that do not contain cotton are then placed in the natural concavities of the hand, with one or two thicknesses of gauze between each finger. Volar and dorsal strips of sheet cotton are placed on the hand and forearm and the wrist supported with a plaster splint. A layer of springy gauze

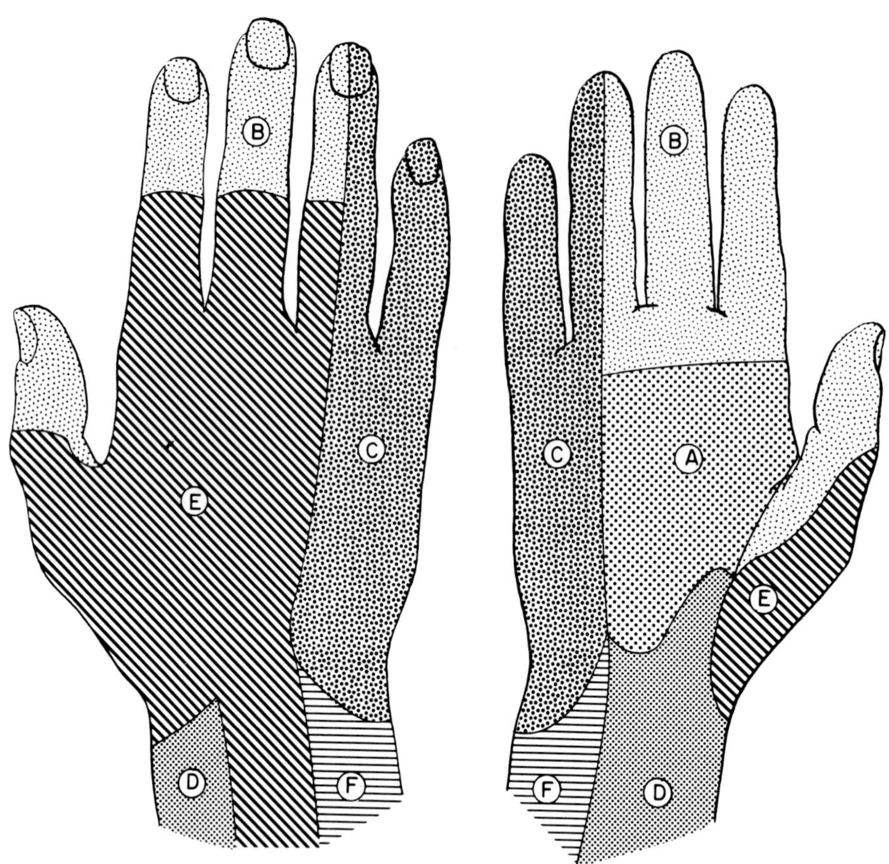

Figure 41.1. Diagram of normal sensory distribution of the hand indicates areas supplied by *A*, palmar cutaneous branch of the median nerve, *B*, digital branches of the median nerve, *C*, superficial branches of the ulnar nerve, *D*, lateral antebrachial cutaneous branch of the musculocutaneous nerve, *E*, superficial branches of the radial nerve, and *F*, medial antebrachial cutaneous nerve.

and a nonrubberized elastic bandage complete the dressing. If the fingers do not need immobilization, the dressing should end at the distal palmar crease, to allow full mobility of the metacarpophalangeal joints. If the thumb does not need immobilization, it is freed to the carpometacarpal joint. After the dressing is completed, the arm is elevated with the fingers higher than the level of the heart. A stockinette that is cut to expose the fingers and thumb may be applied over the dressing and attached to an intravenous pole. If the patient is discharged, he or she is instructed to suspend the arm by tying the stockinette to a bedpost or a high-backed chair. With infants and young children, hand dressings are always extended above the elbow, and the elbow is flexed to 70° to prevent slipping the dressing off the arm.

Postoperative Care

After operation, a severely crushed hand may exhibit borderline viability because of edema, capillary sludging, and poor venous blood flow. The fingers may remain cool and blue. Oral or parenteral enzymes are not effective in preventing or decreasing edema. Sluggish circulation may be improved with plasma expanders, anticoagulants, or cervical sympathetic blockade. The application of such treatment, is influenced by the general condition of the patient and the presence of associated injuries. In a healthy patient, 500–1000 ml of dextran 40, given at a rate of 30–50 ml/min, expand plasma volume and decrease platelet aggregation and fluid transudation into soft tissues. If the hand remains dusky, intravenous heparin or oral salicylates are administered for anticoagulation unless there are severe wounds elsewhere. If hematuria, hematoma, ecchymosis, or petechiae develop, anticoagulants are discontinued.

Continuous sympathetic blockade frequently relieves pain in the limb, and may help prevent small-vessel shutdown due to arteriolar spasm in the injured, edematous hand. Under local anesthesia a 16-gauge polyethylene catheter approximately 12.5

cm long is inserted into the region of the cervical sympathetic chain at the level of the cricoid cartilage. A 10-ml syringe is attached to the tube and taped to the neck. Every 8–12 hours, 10 ml of a 0.5% bupivacaine hydrochloride solution with epinephrine (1:200,000) is injected into the catheter. The sympathetic blockade is continued for about 5 days.

Antibiotic and Tetanus Prophylaxis

Antibiotics are administered routinely to patients with severely contaminated, deep, or contused open wounds. A history of allergy to antibiotics influences the choice of medication. Oxacillin or a cephalosporin are preferred, and administered intravenously for 3 or 4 days. If the patient is afebrile after this time and if the wound appears to be healing normally, intravenous administration is discontinued, and the patient is given oral antibiotics for another week. Outpatients with dirty or edematous wounds are treated with oral oxacillin or cephalexin. Local irrigation with a bacitracin-neomycin solution is employed for severe wounds and for wounds entering a joint. A tetanus toxoid booster dose is given unless the patient has had a full course of tetanus immunization including a booster within five years. Immune globulin is unnecessary in the treatment of clean, minor wounds if the patient has had complete tetanus immunization.

SOFT-TISSUE INJURIES: OPERATIVE MANAGEMENT

Primary or Secondary Wound Closure

Whether a wound should be closed primarily or secondarily is a serious decision. Inappropriate primary wound closure may jeopardize the function of the hand if edema, necrosis, and infection supervene. However, appropriate primary closure prevents continuing contamination, desiccation, and drainage of the deep tissues. The decision for or against primary closure depends on the following factors.

1. *Degree and type of contamination* at the time of injury. Hand wounds in persons working in bacteriology and autopsy laboratories or in dirty areas, such as barnyards, and injuries from human and animal bites, are notorious for the virulence of the bacterial contaminants. Rarely should such wounds be closed.

2. *Time since injury.* Because the bacterial count increases geometrically within hours after injury, primary closure of a badly contaminated wound more than 24 hours old is not justified.

3. *Type of wound.* Rank and Wakefield have differentiated between "tidy" and "untidy" wounds. In tidy wounds, such as those caused by a knife, glass edge, or razor blade, foreign material is not ground into the deeper tissues or pushed through fascial or synovial planes. Only the local tissues are injured, tissue viability is determined easily, and edema is minimal. In untidy wounds, tissues are crushed, torn, burned, or ripped, and it is often impossible to assess the extent of venous thrombosis, edema, deep tendon injury, necrosis, and contamination on initial examination. If an untidy wound is treated late, it may be wiser to debride and to lavage the wound, closing it secondarily, in order to minimize the possibility of necrosis or infection.

4. *Other factors.* There are many types of injuries, including snakebites, injection injuries, close-range gunshot wounds, and thermal injuries that require special treatment. These wounds are often best left open.

If careful evaluation of the degree and type of contamination, the time since injury, the tidiness of the wound, and the other factors raise doubt about the wisdom of primary closure, the physician should leave the wound open for delayed closure, applying wet dressings in the interim.

The following repairs generally require a hand surgeon and are performed in the operating room.

Skin Grafts

Split-thickness Skin Grafts

A thin split-thickness skin graft has an excellent chance of "taking" over virtually any tissue bed on the surface of the hand, with the exception of cortical bone and bared tendon. At the dorsum of the hand, loss of skin and subcutaneous tissue is preferentially treated with split-thickness skin grafting. Small fingertip losses with intact subcutaneous pulp may also be managed with a split-thickness graft. These grafts should not be used to treat a partly amputated finger with exposed bone, since dysesthesia and a tender fingertip frequently result.

Split-thickness skin grafts often contract, as much as 75%. To prevent joint contracture, the surgeon should design the edges of the recipient area so that the edges of the graft are not perpendicular to skin creases. Since thin split-thickness grafts are friable, they are not recommended in the gripping areas of the hand, such as the palm and the volar aspects of the fingers and thumb. Either a thick split-thickness graft or a full-thickness graft is preferable in these areas.

Small split-thickness skin grafts may be removed from the medial aspect of the arm several centimeters above the elbow, or from the thigh or buttock. Since grafts from the volar aspect of the forearm may cause a hyperpigmented, readily visible scar, this region is not a preferred donor site. Multiple postage-stamp-sized grafts leave unsightly donor and recipient sites and are not used.

In adult patients, the graft is taken 0.018 inch thick, and is held to the recipient site with interrupted sutures of 5–0 nylon. In children, a graft 0.014-inch thick is used and may be sutured in place with absorbable catgut. Opening numerous drainage holes by means of small incisions in the graft, known as "piecrusting," is of little value. The graft is covered with a single thickness of petrolatum gauze, held snugly to the graft with interrupted catgut sutures. The gauze must not be applied circumferentially. This technique is preferable to a stent for holding the graft evenly over the convex areas of the hand. Several thicknesses of wet sheet cotton are placed over the gauze and held in place with dry dressings. The recipient area is splinted. Unless drainage, pain, or signs of infection develop, the dressing is not disturbed for 5 days.

Full-thickness Skin Grafts

A full-thickness skin graft contracts less than a split-thickness graft, and resists friction and pressure better. Thus, these grafts are preferred to split-thickness grafts for the gripping surfaces of the hand, when the patient has a good graft bed of viable and vascular tissue. Full-thickness skin grafts should not be placed over bone or tendon sheath; without a good vascular bed, these grafts may fail to become revascularized fast enough to maintain viability. As with split-thickness grafts, the recipient site is designed so that the edges of the graft are not perpendicular to flexion creases.

Small grafts may be removed from the medial aspect of the upper arm. In patients with dark skin, grafts to the fingertips may be taken from the arch of the foot, or from the area adjacent to the medial malleolus, to minimize hyperpigmentation of the graft. Larger grafts are removed from the inguinal crease. No subcutaneous tissue is transferred with the full-thickness graft. The thickness of the donor skin is carefully trimmed so that it has an "orange-peel" appearance. Like the split-thickness graft, after the full-thickness graft is sutured to the donor site, it is held in place with a sutured petrolatum gauze dressing.

Flaps

If skin with subcutaneous tissue is transferred to a recipient area with its viability maintained through a vascular stalk, the transfer is considered a flap. Frequently, flaps of skin and subcutaneous tissue may be advanced, transposed, or rotated in such a manner that the vascular pedicle remains permanently undisturbed. These one-stage *local flaps* retain sensation, contract little, and do not become hyperpigmented as do many split-thickness and full-thickness skin grafts. Pedicle flaps may be transferred to any clean tissue bed, and thus provide ideal coverage for exposed bone and tendon.

Frequently, large areas cannot be covered by shifting adjacent skin, and pedicle flaps must be constructed from a more remote region such as the opposite arm, the chest, the inguinal region, or the abdomen. *Remote flaps* must be detached from the donor site after they have become revascularized from the recipient area. Although they provide excellent coverage, such flaps do not retain sensation because nerves and vessels are transected when the flap is detached. Remote flaps shrink little, but do become hyperpigmented. Pedicle flaps from the abdomen tend to become more adipose when the patient gains weight, and may appear bulky. For these reasons, local flaps are preferred when possible.

Free vascularized tissue transfers may be used to cover relatively large skin defects in one stage. These *free flaps* may be removed from any one of several regions where the skin and subcutaneous tissue are well-perfused by a vascular stalk. The vein and artery of the flap are joined to the recipient vessels.

Local Flaps

Amputated fingertips with several millimeters of distal phalanx exposed are best treated with a *V-Y advancement flap* (Fig. 41.2). Use of a lateral V-Y flap (Kutler flap) results in a longitudinal scar at the fingertip, which may be tender and dysesthetic. The volar V-Y advancement is therefore preferred. A V-shaped incision is made *through the skin only*, with its apex at the level of the distal flexion crease of the finger. Incisions are *not* made through the subcutaneous tissue. A triangle is formed with the amputation site as the base. The scalpel blade is then inserted through the amputation site adjacent and parallel to the volar cortex of the remaining portion of the distal phalanx. The subcutaneous tissue is separated from the phalanx and from the insertion of the flexor digitorum profundus tendon. The flap is then advanced distally to cover the defect. The base of the V is sutured to the nailbed and to the dorsal skin of the fingertip. The defect left at the apex of the triangle by advancing the flap is closed side to side, forming the stem of the Y. Contour, padding, and excellent sensation are usually restored with this flap.

With avulsion of the skin of the thumb tip, a *quadrangular volar advancement flap* (Fig. 41.3) has proved to be safe and versatile. Longitudinal midaxial (dorsolateral) incisions are made through the skin and subcutaneous tissue on both sides of the thumb from the wound to the proximal flexion crease. The skin, subcutaneous tissue, and both

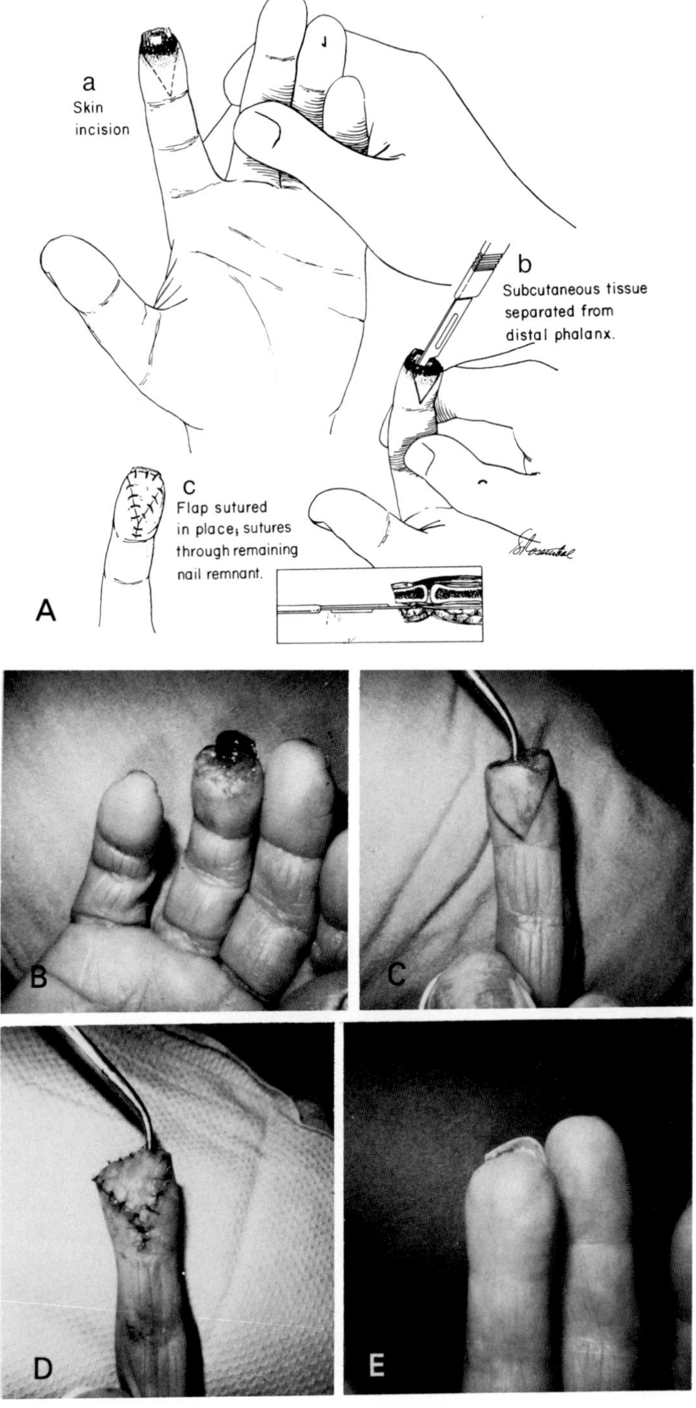

Figure 41.2. Volar V-Y advancement flap. *A,* Technique. *(a)* Skin incision extends to defect. Its apex lies at level of distal flexion crease. *(b)* Subcutaneous tissue is separated from distal phalanx by transecting longitudinal septa just superficial to the periosteum. Care should be taken not to detach the insertion of the flexor digitorum profundus tendon. *(c)* The triangular flap is advanced distally and sutured to the dorsal skin or nail. This leaves a proximal defect that is closed, side to side. In the dissection, subcutaneous tissue is not incised, but is drawn distally with the skin flap. *B,* Avulsion of ring fingertip has left 1.5 cm of distal phalanx protruding from site of injury. *C,* Outline of skin incision is drawn. *D,* After the skin has been incised and subcutaneous tissue freed from the volar aspect of the distal phalanx, the flap is advanced distally and sutured in place. *E,* Four weeks later, appearance of fingertip is good. Sensibility and circulation to the flap have remained intact.

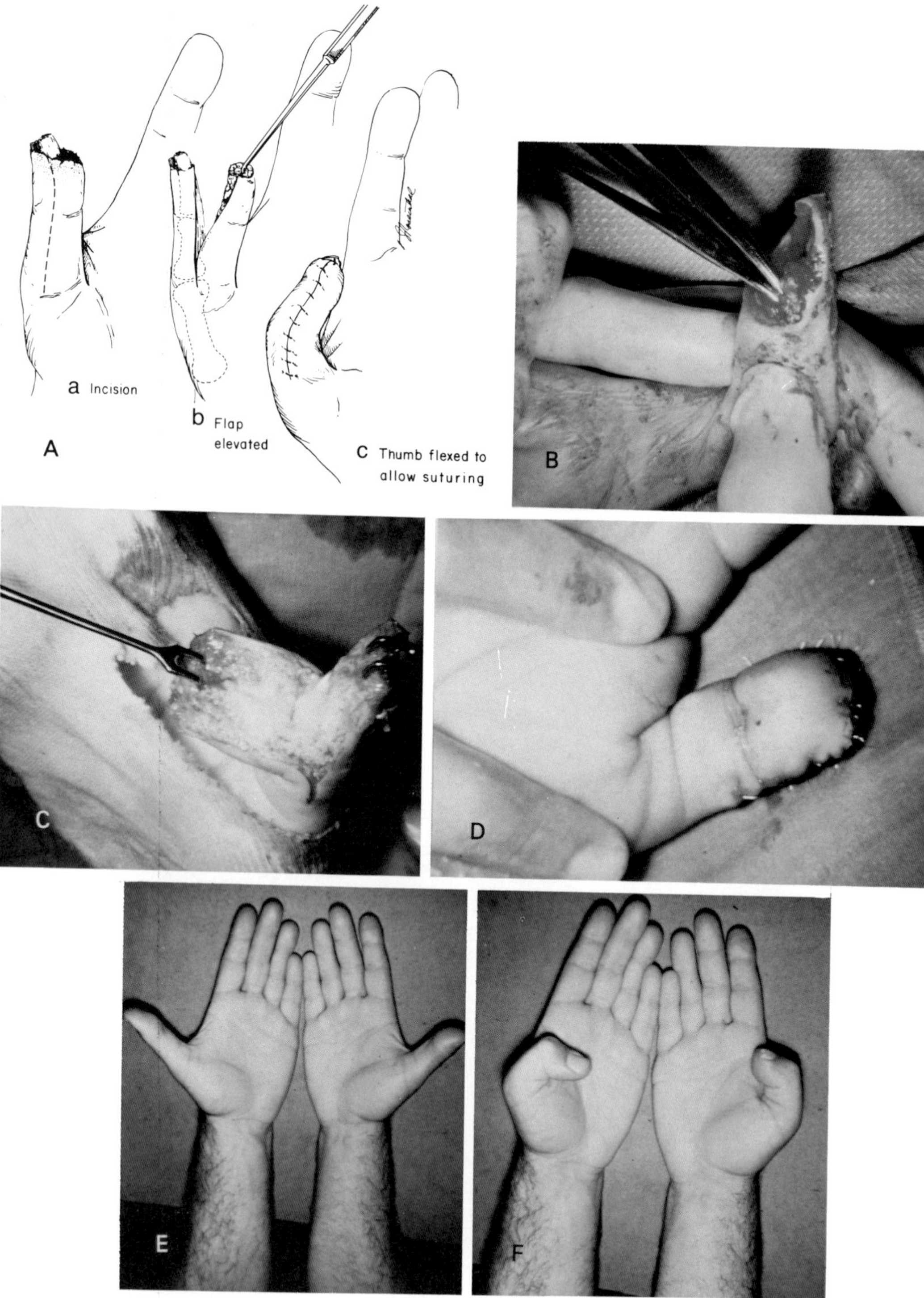

Figure 41.3. Quadrangular volar advancement flap. This should only be used for the thumb and not for the fingers. *A,* Technique. *(a)* Longitudinal midaxial incisions are made on either side of thumb to proximal flexion crease. *(b)* Skin, subcutaneous tissues, and neurovascular bundles are elevated. *(c)* Interphalangeal joint of thumb is flexed and flap is advanced distally. *B,* Volar avulsion injury of thumb tip sustained an hour previously. *C,* Volar flap is developed with subcutaneous tissues and neurovascular bundles freed with flap from phalanx. *D,* Flap is advanced and sutured in place. *E,* Two months postoperatively, there is complete extension of thumb tip and good thumb tip padding with skin of normal sensibility. *F,* There is mild loss of interphalangeal flexion of thumb because of initial injury.

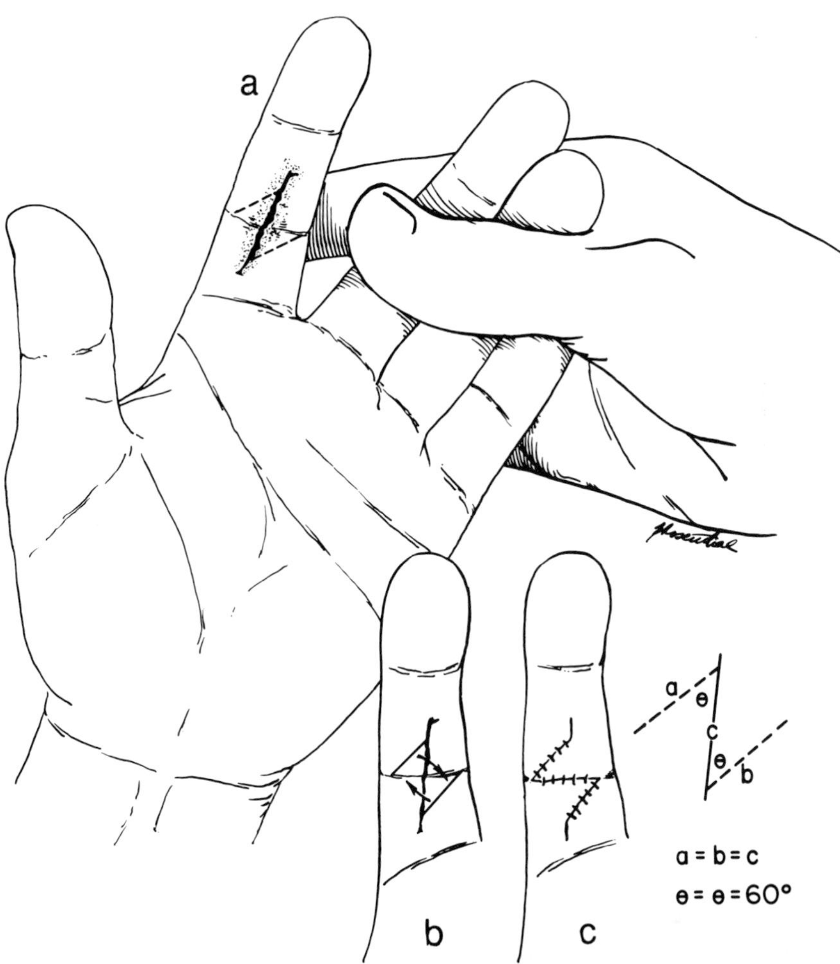

Figure 41.4. Z-plasty may be used to transpose a longitudinal scar so that it does not cross a flexion crease. If a scar is perpendicular to a flexion crease, it is likely to cause flexion contracture. *(a)* Oblique limbs, usually drawn 60° to the longitudinal scar, are placed equidistant from the flexion crease. Each limb should equal the length of the longitudinal scar between them. *(b)* The triangular flaps are transposed. *(c)* The transposed flaps are sutured in place. This increases the length of the injured skin by about 50%, but may cause some narrowing in the area of flap transposition. For large wounds, multiple Z-plasties are therefore recommended.

neurovascular bundles are elevated with the flap from the underlying bone and from the pulleys and sheath of the flexor pollicis longus tendon. The thumb tip is flexed and the flap is advanced distally to be sutured to the nailbed and dorsal skin. Such flaps can be advanced up to 2.0 cm. The thumb tip is kept partly flexed for 3 weeks while the advanced skin heals in its new position. Although the ability to hyperextend the interphalangeal joint of the thumb may be lost after this procedure, flexion contracture is rare. An excellent aesthetic and functional result is usually achieved. This procedure should be used only for the thumb and should *not* be used to cover defects in the fingers. Quadrangular advancement flaps in the fingers often cause flexion contracture of the interphalangeal joints and may jeopardize both the venous drainage and arterial supply of the dorsal skin. These problems are rarely encountered in the thumb.

Z-plasty (Fig. 41.4) may be used to prevent flexion contractures in fingers with a longitudinal volar wound that crosses flexion creases. Oblique incisions are made at 60° angles to the skin laceration to form the letter Z. Each of the three limbs of the Z should be equal. The midpoint of the longitudinal limb of the Z (the laceration) should fall at a flexion crease. With the two flaps transposed, the longitudinal incision is rotated 90° so that the scar lies in the line of the flexion crease. Skin length is increased about 50%. To prevent excessive tension on the apex of each flap, sutures should be inserted obliquely to advance each flap toward its apex.

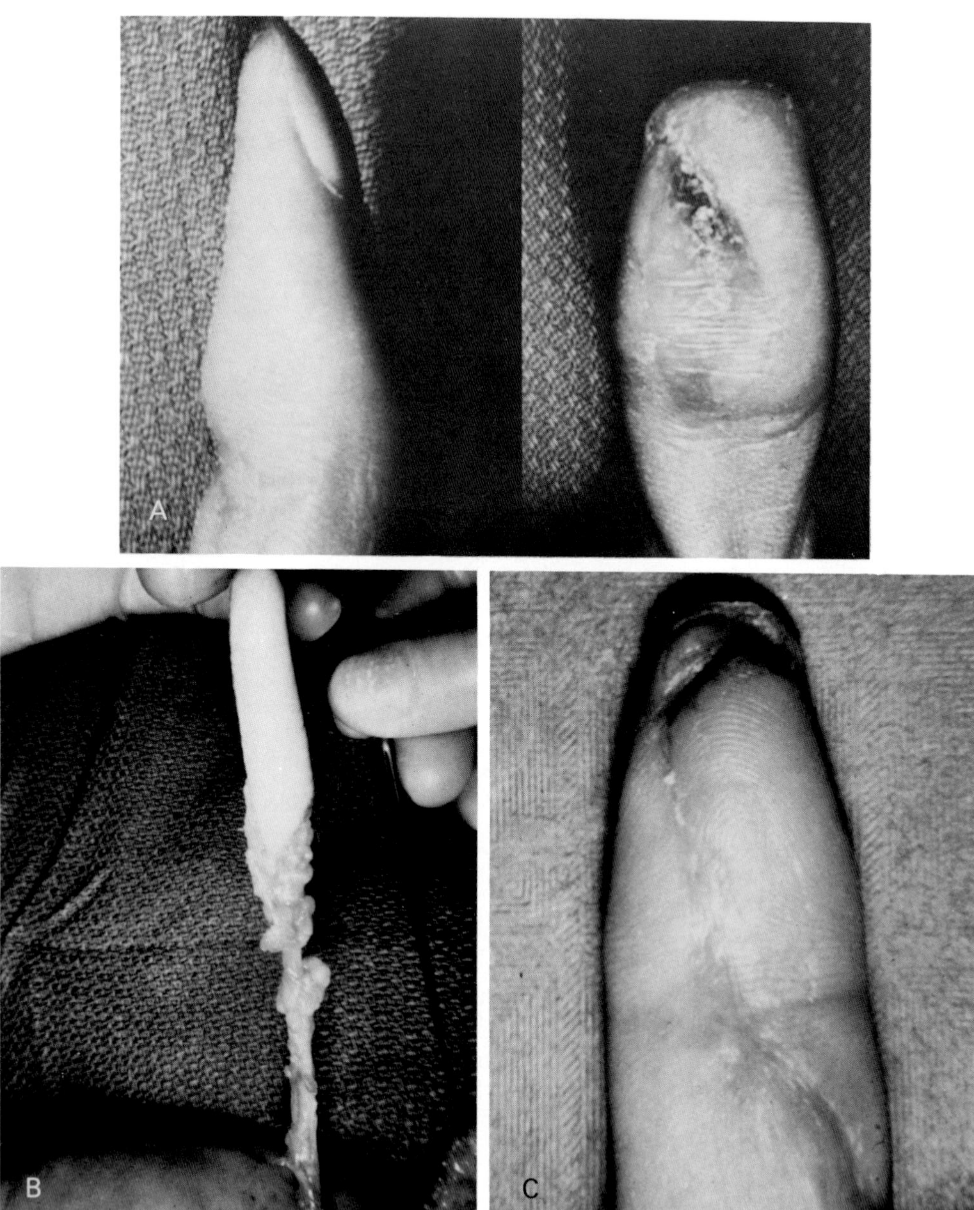

Figure 41.5. Neurovascular island pedicle flap. *A,* Planing injury to volar aspect of thumb tip covered with split-thickness skin graft. Without padding, the thumb tip is tender and dysesthetic. Subcutaneous tissue, blood supply, and sensibility are required. *B,* Skin and subcutaneous tissue have been transposed with neurovascular bundles from middle finger to thumb tip. Donor site was covered with full-thickness skin graft. *C,* Two months after transposition of neurovascular island pedicle flap, there is excellent two-point discrimination and good padding to thumb tip. The patient was able to return to his job as a carpenter.

The *neurovascular island pedicle flap* (Fig. 41.5) is rarely used in emergency operations. Occasionally, if there is extensive soft-tissue loss on the volar side of the thumb and associated severe injury to an adjacent finger requiring amputation, use of a primary neurovascular island pedicle flap is indicated. The volar skin and subcutaneous tissue of the donor finger are elevated with its neurovascular bundle. The neurovascular bundle is carefully traced proximally into the palm. The proper digital nerve to the adjacent finger is identified, and its fibers are preserved and separated from the donor nerve in the

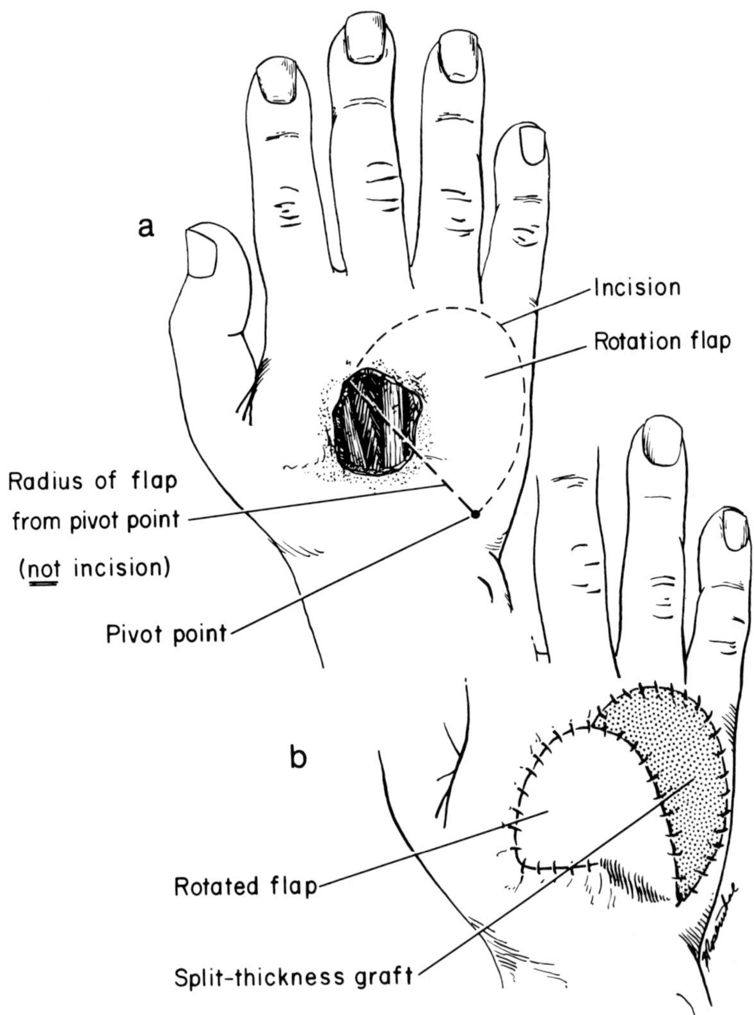

Figure 41.6. With an avulsion injury to the dorsum of the hand, skin with subcutaneous tissue and excellent blood supply can be provided over tendons and bones by means of a rotation flap. *(a)* The pivot from which the flap is rotated should be selected so as to leave a wide base to the flap and to provide sufficient skin to cover the defect. *(b)* Flap is rotated to cover defect. Donor site is covered with split-thickness skin graft.

common digital nerve stem. Communicating and perforating branches of the donor digital artery and vein are ligated distal to the superficial palmar arch. The donor flap is then transferred with its neurovascular pedicle by tunneling it to the recipient site at the thumb tip. Although excellent sensation and circulation are restored to the thumb by this procedure, the patient usually continues to perceive the thumb as the donor finger. It is best to transfer this flap as a secondary procedure.

Rotation and transposition flaps may be swung from the dorsum of the finger to cover a volar defect. The donor area is covered by a split-thickness skin graft. Occasionally, large defects in the skin and subcutaneous tissue at the dorsum of the hand overlying the tendons or joints may also be covered by rotation or transposition flaps (Fig. 41.6). If properly designed, the donor tissue should move readily, without tension, to fill the defect. The surgeon should cut a pattern of the proposed flap from a rubber glove or sponge and plan the design of the flap carefully before making any incision.

Remote Pedicle Flaps

A large soft-tissue defect on the volar side of the finger or thumb can often be covered with a *cross-finger pedicle flap* (Fig. 41.7). This is particularly useful when the flexor tendons are exposed. The margins of the recipient area are enlarged, if necessary, so that the borders of the flap are not perpendicular to finger flexion creases. An appropriately shaped flap of skin and subcutaneous tissue is elevated from an adjacent finger with its uncut base at the side of the recipient finger. The donor flap is made approximately 15% larger than the measured recipient area to ensure adequate skin coverage. The flap is elevated to include the soft tissue over the dorsal tendon aponeurosis of the donor finger. As the flap is freed, it is brought to the volar side of the recipient finger as if one was turning the pages of a book. Lateral skin ligaments (Cleland's ligaments) at the hinge ("bridge") side of the flap anchor the skin to the deep fascia in the region of the proximal interphalangeal joint, and must be divided to ensure adequate freedom of the flap with transfer. The donor site and the flap bridge are covered with a split-thickness skin graft that is covered with petrolatum gauze and a sterile dressing. A sponge is placed between the bridge and the web of the involved fingers, and the fingers are held together with soft dressings of sheet cotton and springy gauze. Plaster of Paris is rarely necessary. The cross-finger flap is detached after 3 weeks. The donor site will appear depressed, but gradually fills in. Within 3–6 months, normal flexion creases appear within the flap at the recipient site. The donor site usually becomes hyperpigmented. With circumferential loss of skin from a thumb or finger, the volar side may be covered with a cross-finger flap, and the dorsum of both the recipient and donor fingers may be covered with a split-thickness skin graft.

The *thenar flap* (Fig. 41.8) is useful for covering a large avulsion injury of the fingertip with bone exposed in a young patient in whom a V-Y advancement flap would not provide sufficient tissue for coverage. The immobilization that is necessary after a thenar flap is applied risks flexion contracture in the recipient finger. This operation should be

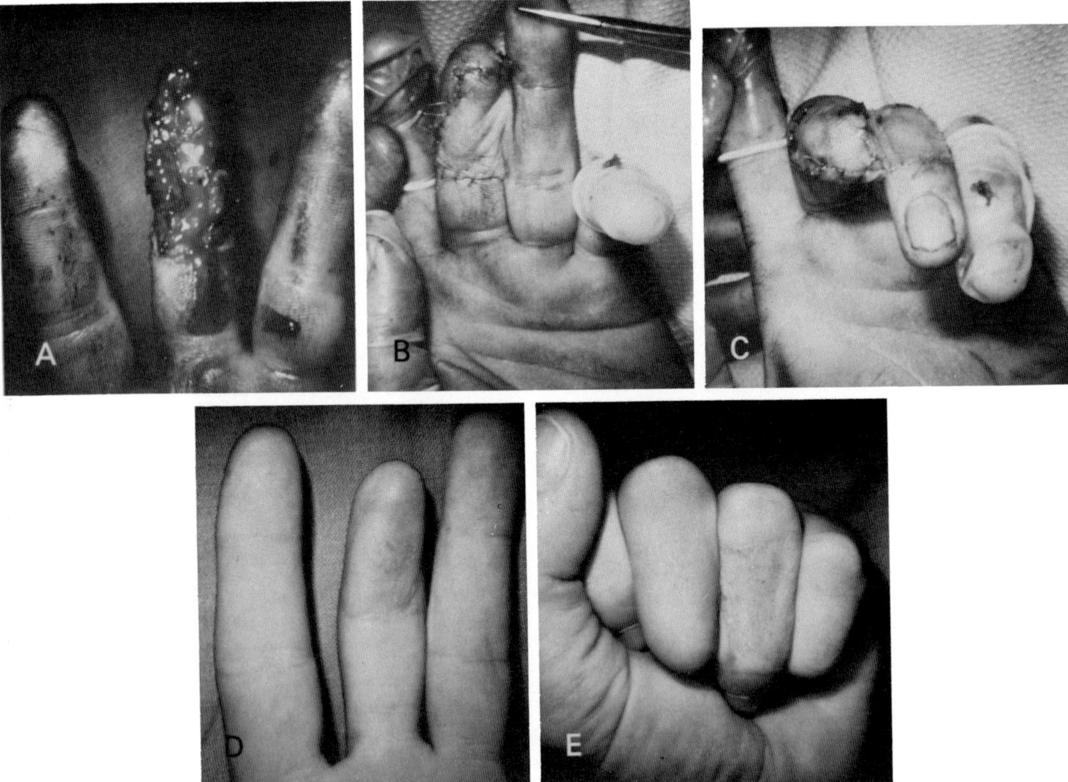

Figure 41.7. Cross-finger pedicle flap. *A,* Volar aspect of middle finger was severely injured in a press machine. The distal phalanx was amputated, and flexor tendons were exposed throughout the remaining stump. Skin with subcutaneous tissue is required. *B,* A cross-finger flap is elevated from dorsum of ring finger. The flap is freed volar to skin ligaments (Cleland's ligaments) to radial side of ring finger. The flap is made 15% larger than the defect so that it can be sutured without tension. *C,* Donor site of cross-finger flap is covered with split-thickness graft. *D,* Six months later, durable skin covers recipient site of middle finger. *E,* Donor site has healed with slight discoloration but no functional disability.

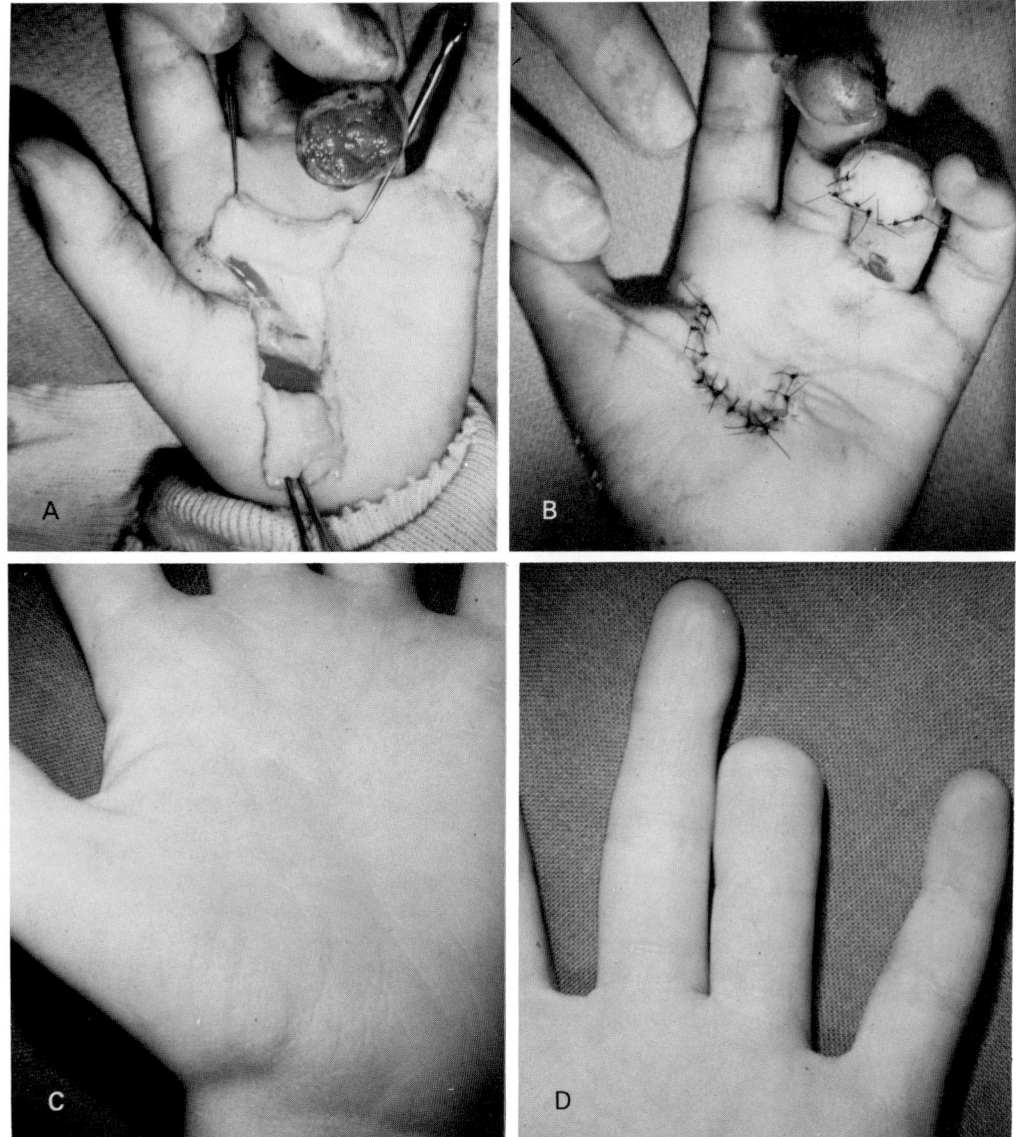

Figure 41.8. Thenar flap. *A,* This child sustained an amputation at the tip of the ring finger. Bone is protruding. An H-flap is elevated from the thenar eminence. The distal thenar flap is sutured to the volar aspect of the fingertip and the proximal thenar flap to its dorsum. This creates a closed system. *B,* The finger is detached from the palm 17 days later. The distal thenar flap is used to close the donor site. The proximal thenar flap remains attached to the finger and is sutured to close the defect. *C,* Six months later, the donor site is virtually invisible. *D,* Recipient site is healed with well-vascularized, well-padded skin.

avoided in patients with small-joint arthritis or stiffness. Two quadrangular flaps are elevated from the thenar eminence in the form of the letter H. The proximal flap is sutured to the dorsum of the recipient finger: the distal flap, to the volar side of the fingertip. The bases of the two flaps are then advanced and sutured to each other, creating a completely closed system. At 17 days, one flap—usually the distal one—is detached from the finger, and the other—usually the proximal flap—from the thenar eminence. The donor and recipient sites are closed by advancing each of the flaps. The finger is held in complete extension for several days with an aluminum splint padded with foam rubber, after which range-of-motion exercises are begun.

Major loss of skin and subcutaneous tissue, such

as a severe avulsion or explosion injury, is best treated in the operating room with coverage by a *remote flap. Axial pattern flaps* derive their circulation from a vascular pedicle that provides robust circulation through a narrow base. *Random flaps*, such as the cross-finger pedicle, cross-arm, and abdominal flaps, are perfused diffusely and must be elevated on a broad base if they are to survive. The *groin tube flap* is one of several versatile axial pattern flaps that may be used to replace major skin defects in acutely injured patients. The groin tube is elevated from the inguinal region and is based on the superficial circumflex iliac vessels as they exit from the femoral vessels. Because of the excellent blood supply, relatively long tubes may be raised and applied in one stage. This permits considerable mobility of the recipient limb, and generous amounts of skin and subcutaneous tissue are available for soft-tissue cover.

If the volar skin has been lost from several digits, the *cross-arm flap* should be considered. Immobilization of the hand to the medial aspect of the opposite arm for 3 weeks allows complete mobility of the elbow and hand on the donor side and is relatively comfortable. The skin is of good quality and less fatty than skin from the abdomen or groin.

Abdominal flaps provide excellent coverage of broad areas. They should be defatted at the time of application, and they should be based on a broad pedicle, preferably no smaller than the length of the flap.

NERVE INJURIES

Major Types

These injuries must be recognized, and repair considered. A hand surgeon should be consulted. Peripheral nerve injuries are of three major types: neurapraxia, axonotmesis, and neurotmesis. *Neurapraxia* results from contusion, ischemia, or local pressure on a nerve, and causes functional interference with impulse transmission. As the effects of contusion subside or the source of pressure is relieved, the nerve recovers spontaneously and often quite rapidly. For example, neurapraxia of the radial nerve may result from sleeping with the head resting on the arm. The hand is numb and has ''fallen asleep.'' The extensors of the fingers and wrist are weak. Speed of recovery depends on the duration and severity of the injury. With mild neurapraxia, the patient may recover completely within a few minutes. In other cases, recovery may take days or weeks. Return of sensibility and muscle function occurs diffusely and not proximally to distally.

If a nerve has been damaged more severely as the result of a traction injury, or prolonged or severe compression or contusion, anatomic interruption of the axons or *axonotmesis* can occur. The supporting structures of the nerve, including the Schwann cells, endoneurium, perineurium, and epineurium, remain intact. If the cause of axonotmesis is eliminated, the nerve recovers as the axons regenerate at the rate of 1–2 mm/day. *Neurotmesis* represents complete anatomic interruption of axons and supporting neural structures, either as a result of division of the nerve or severe traction or compression. Patients with neurotmesis require operation for restoration of function.

Differentiation

If a hand has been severely injured, it may be difficult to determine whether the abnormality of nerve function is due to neurapraxia, axonotmesis, or neurotmesis. Neurotmesis may be suspected if the patient has total anesthesia in the autonomous sensory distribution of the nerve, an open wound over the suspected area of nerve injury, or Tinel's sign (paresthesia in the sensory distribution of the injured nerve on percussion at the site of injury). Irregular distribution of hypesthesia, rapid improvement of the sensory deficit, or continued perspiration in the sensory areas supplied by the involved nerve suggests neurapraxia or axonotmesis, and operation may often be deferred or may prove unnecessary.

Repair

Following World War II, many surgeons advocated secondary repair of nerve lacerations. After reviewing the long-term results of battle injuries, they concluded that better restoration of function and sensation was achieved if nerve repair was delayed for 3–4 weeks. Several factors may have influenced the results: a less hurried and better equipped operating staff at the time of elective reconstruction, clearer visualization of the extent of nerve injury, a thicker epineurium better able to hold sutures, and a lower incidence of wound infection. In the case of a cleanly lacerated wound, however, with relatively little contusion, traction, or tearing, primary neurorrhaphy performed by a competent, well-equipped staff is preferred to delayed nerve repair. Primary repair is the treatment of choice in cleanly incised wounds treated within 24 hours because the nerve ends are more easily oriented, nerves and tendons can be repaired during one operation, and the patient usually recovers more quickly. If the nerve cannot be repaired primarily, the ends of the lacerated nerve should be sutured side to side to prevent retraction and to facilitate secondary repair.

Group fascicular repair is often used for the larger nerves, and is performed in the operating room. Under magnification, the cut ends of the nerve are oriented by matching the location of the vasa nervorum on either cut end and by matching groups of fascicles according to their size and shape. Each group of fascicles is then repaired with 10-0 nylon sutures. With small nerves, 8-0 or 9-0 interrupted nylon epineurial sutures provide neat approximation.

VASCULAR INJURIES

Diagnosis and treatment of major arterial injuries to the upper limb are discussed in Chapter 31. The viability of the hand is endangered only rarely by ligation of either the radial artery or the ulnar artery, and the viability of a finger is seldom threatened by ligation of one or even both digital arteries. It has been suggested, however, that the high incidence of sensitivity to cold in previously injured limbs may be lessened by primary vascular repair of injured arteries in the fingers or wrist. The emergency physician should recognize the injury and consult the hand surgeon. Although it is not always necessary to repair these vessels if the hand is pink and clearly viable, such repairs should be considered by surgeons familiar with microvascular techniques.

Volkmann's Contracture

Ischemic contracture of the muscles of the forearm or the intrinsic muscles of the hand is an alarming sequel to many injuries of the upper limb. The muscles of the forearm are subdivided into anterior and posterior compartments by the radius, ulna, and interosseous membrane and are encased by circumferential investing fascia. Fractures about the elbow and forearm, direct trauma to the forearm, and constrictive dressings and pressure to the limb each may cause edema of the volar compartment of the forearm. As the muscles swell, venous outflow is further impeded and edema increases. Since the anterior compartment is a closed space, any pressure on the arterioles and capillaries will result in ischemia with necrosis of muscle cells. Within a few hours, tissue pressure in the anterior compartment can rise dramatically. The patient complains of severe, increasing pain exacerbated by any attempt to extend the wrist or fingers passively. The hand becomes pale and cyanotic. As the pressure within the forearm builds, compressive neuropathy develops, first affecting the median nerve and then the ulnar nerve. The deepest muscles of the forearm are affected earliest and most severely. The flexor digitorum profundus, flexor pollicis longus, and later the flexor superficialis and the wrist flexors gradually lose their power to contract. Ulnar and radial pulses may disappear.

If the compression is not released promptly, irreversible changes may occur in these muscles and nerves. As the muscle cells become necrotic, they are replaced by yellow fibrous tissue. The nerves are enveloped by a thickened constricting epineurium. The contracted joints become fibrotic and resist any attempt at passive motion. An established Volkmann's contracture (Fig. 41.9) causes severe deformity and disability. The forearm is thin, and atrophic, the wrist is held in acute palmar flexion, the palm is flattened, and the fingers are clawed. There is atrophy of the thenar and interosseus muscles and hypesthesia of the entire palm. Active flexion of the interphalangeal joints is markedly limited because of loss of muscle substance. Passive correction of joint contraction may be impossible.

If this tragic progression is to be avoided, an impending Volkmann's contracture must be recognized and treated promptly and vigorously. A flexed elbow must be extended even if it jeopardizes fracture reduction. All tight restrictive bandages should be released. The limb should be elevated. Measuring intracompartmental tissue pressure by means of a needle attached to a manometer or a wick catheter has been useful in evaluating the severity of the deep edema. When intracompartmental pressure exceeds 40 mm Hg, operation is usually indicated. Clinical signs, however, are often more useful in evaluating whether conservative measures are effective in stopping the increasing edema. If any of the signs of impending Volkmann's contracture persist, such as sluggish capillary refill, absent radial or ulnar pulses, continuing or increasing pain about the forearm, persistent hypesthesia in the median and ulnar nerve distribution, and pain on passive extension of the fingers, the investing fascia of the forearm should be surgically incised and the pressure released.

Fasciotomy should be performed promptly, before muscle necrosis has begun. The lacertus fibrosus is transected when the volar antebrachial fascia is released. Each of the muscle compartments of the volar side of the forearm must be freed. Once the muscles are freed, they often bulge volarly well past the level of the skin. In these cases, the skin should be allowed to remain open, and secondary closure should be performed several days later. If a serpiginous skin incision has been made, portions of the wound may be closed after the primary operation.

Use of intraarterial tolazoline (Priscoline), sympathetic nerve block, anticoagulants, and plasma expanders has been suggested for the treatment of impending Volkmann's contracture. However, since the penalties of delay are irreversible changes in muscles, joints, and nerves, if there is any serious doubt regarding the vascular status of a limb 30–60 minutes after all external pressure has been removed, this is sufficient indication for operation.

Occasionally, ischemic contracture of the dorsal

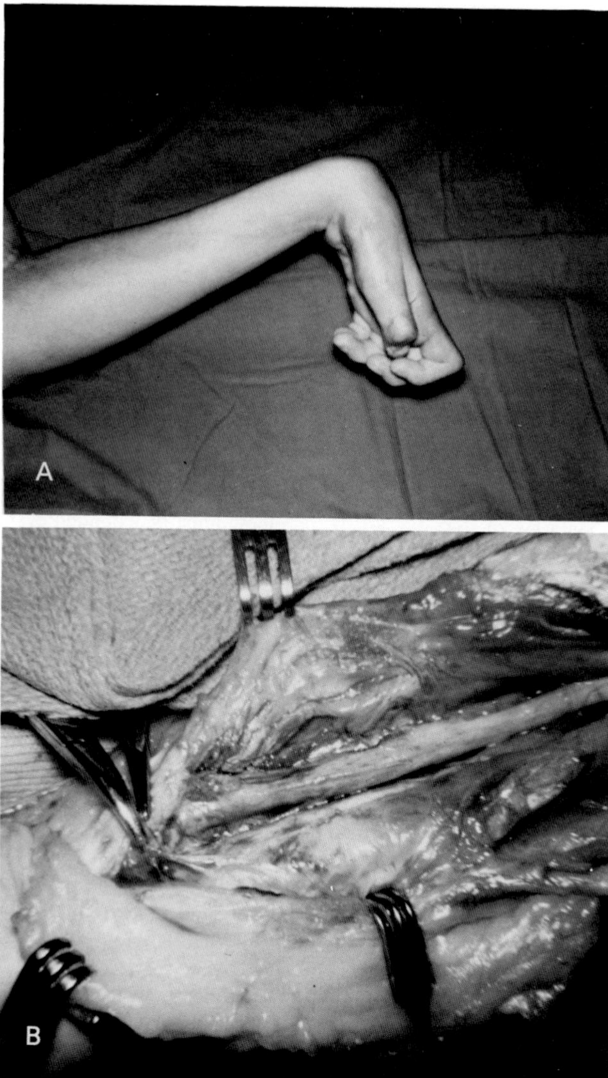

Figure 41.9. Volkmann's contracture. *A,* Supracondylar fracture resulted in severe vascular compromise of the forearm. Fascial release had not been performed and Volkmann's contracture developed. The wrist is acutely palmar-flexed, the fingers are in the claw position, and the thumb is flexed at the interphalangeal joint. This deformity can be avoided by prompt fascial release and revascularization of the forearm. *B,* Exploration of forearm reveals fatty necrosis of muscle and compression of ulnar nerve (seen here) and median nerve with constricting scar. Nerve function can usually be restored if neurolysis is performed promptly.

compartment of the forearm may occur after a serious injury to the forearm. These patients have pain with attempts at passive flexion of the metacarpophalangeal joints. Under these circumstances the dorsal compartment should be released down to the interosseous fascia.

Late treatment of Volkmann's contracture consists of excision of the infarcted tissue, neurolysis of the involved nerves, and occasionally tendon transfers and nerve grafts.

Ischemic Contracture of Intrinsic Hand Muscles

The interosseus muscles of the hand lie in a closed compartment bounded by the volar and dorsal interosseous fascia and the four metacarpals. Rapidly increasing edema may initiate a cycle of ischemia, muscle necrosis, and further edema. Any attempt to flex the interphalangeal joints while the metacarpophalangeal joints are held in extension is painful and limited. If untreated, ischemic contrac-

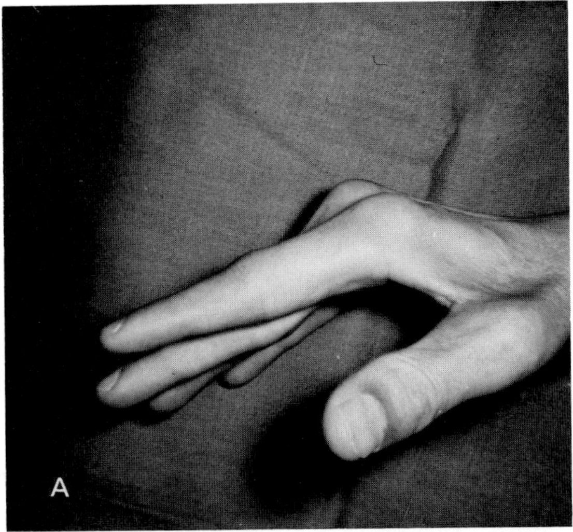

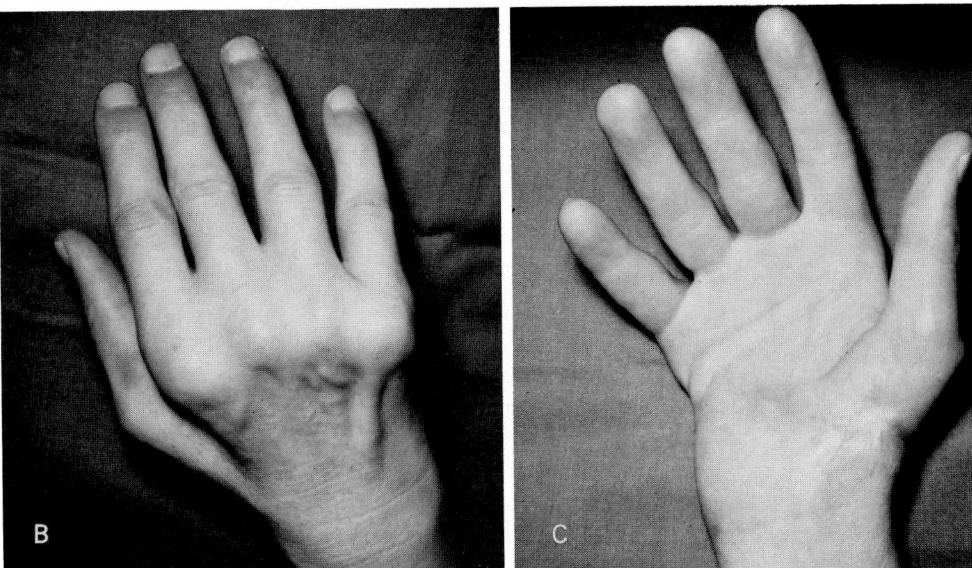

Figure 41.10. Ischemic contracture of intrinsic muscles caused by cast compression. *A,* Ischemic contracture of intrinsic muscles of the hand will occur if there is severe vascular embarrassment of the hand subsequent to injury. In this case, a tight cast had been applied to treat a fracture of both bones of the forearm. This led to severe venous engorgement and intrinsic muscle contracture. The metacarpophalangeal joints were acutely flexed and interphalangeal joints extended. This deformity can be prevented in most cases by release of tight constricting casts and dressings. If there is severe edema of the hand after injury, the intrinsic muscles should be decompressed by interosseous fasciotomy before necrosis has occurred. *B,* Interosseus muscle atrophy may be associated with intrinsic contracture if there is muscle necrosis. *C,* Severity of cast compression is suggested by scarring secondary to cutaneous necrosis at thumb base.

tures of the interosseus muscles (Fig. 41.10) cause an ''intrinsic-plus'' deformity. The fingers stiffen in flexion at the metacarpophalangeal joints and in extension at the interphalangeal joints. Although the pathologic process that causes ischemic contracture of the interosseus muscles is identical to that of Volkmann's contracture of the forearm, the resultant deformity is the reverse. The deformities of Volkmann's contracture are due to fibrosis of the extrinsic flexor muscles combined with ulnar and median nerve palsy; this causes clawhand. The metacarpophalangeal joints are hyperextended and the interphalangeal joints are flexed. With ischemic contracture of the interossei, however, imbalance is due to excessive intrinsic muscle tone.

With signs of impending ischemic contracture of the interossei, all interosseus muscle compartments should be released. Through a dorsal transverse incision, the dorsal interosseous fascia proximal to each of the four web spaces is divided. The muscles are permitted to expand freely. If necessary, skin closure may be delayed. If the adductor pollicis appears tight, its fascia may be released through a dorsal or palmar skin incision. If edema has caused interosseus muscle compartment syndrome, it may well have caused constriction. Postoperatively, the hand should be immobilized with the thumb in abduction and the metacarpophalangeal joints in extension for 1–2 weeks. Active and passive flexion exercises of the interphalangeal joints are begun immediately after operation.

TENDON INJURIES

Flexor Tendons

It is recommended that these be repaired in the operating room.

Laceration

No topic causes more controversy among hand surgeons than the treatment of flexor tendon lacerations. Because of the tight area in which the tendons must glide and the restricted tendon excursion caused by peritendinous adhesions, loss of mobility is common after primary tendon repair. The results of surgery depend on *(a)* which tendon is injured; *(b)* when, where, and how the tendon was injured; *(c)* the age of the patient; and *(d)* the operative technique. The plan of primary care of cleanly lacerated flexor tendons is given in Table 41.3; sites of injury are illustrated in Figure 41.11.

Table 41.3.
Evaluation and Primary Care of Flexor Tendon Lacerations

Tendon	Site of Injury[a]	Other Considerations	Treatment
FDP and FPL	1		Advancement
FDP	Between 1 and 2		Suture; advancement if 0.5 cm or less
FDP	2	Fracture, contused tissues, untidy injury	Tenodesis at distal interphalangeal joint
		No bone injury; clean, sharp wound	Suture; early motion with rubber band flexion splint
FDP and FDS	2	Comminuted fracture, badly contused tissue, untidy injury	Close wound; secondary tendon graft
		No bone injury; clean, sharp wound	Suture FDP; may suture FDS or excise proximal cut end; early controlled motion with rubber band flexion splint
FPL	2, 6	Clean, sharp wound	Suture primarily
FDP and FDS	3	1 finger involved	Suture both tendons
		>1 finger involved	Suture both tendons to index finger; suture FDP only, to other fingers in untidy wounds
FDS	3	Child, or 1 or 2 tendons in adult	Suture
		3 or 4 tendons in adult	Suture index only
FDP and FDS	4	Median nerve almost always injured	Suture FDP and nerve; excise segment of FDS of ulnar fingers; close carpal canal if "bowstringing"
FDP and FDS	5	Nerves usually involved, FCU and FCR frequently involved	Suture all structures in tidy injuries; in adults with untidy wounds, do not suture FDS of ulnar 3 fingers; ? suture of FCU if ulnar nerve injured
FCU or FCR	5		Repair
PL	5		None

FDP, flexor digitorum profundus; FPL, flexor pollicis longus; FDS, flexor digitorum superficialis; FCU, flexor carpi ulnaris; FCR, flexor carpi radialis; PL, palmaris longus.
[a] See Figure 41.11.

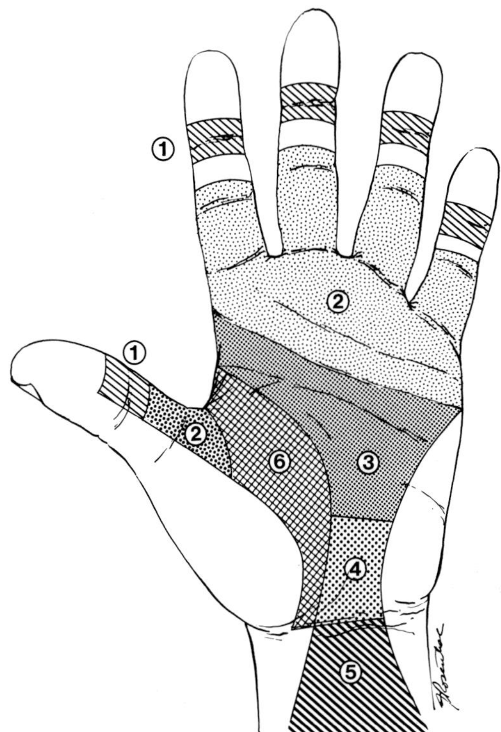

Figure 41.11. Diagram of zones of potential tendon injuries to the hand.

The treatment of flexor tendon injuries varies with the surgeon. Some prefer primary repair of both the flexor digitorum profundus and the flexor digitorum superficialis, regardless of the site of injury; others, never repair flexor tendons in zone 2 primarily, because tendons repaired in this area have the highest risk of failure due to adhesions. If the wound is grossly contaminated or if there are signs of severe contusion, tendon avulsion, severe joint injury, or a badly comminuted fracture adjacent to the tendon injury, the tendons are not repaired primarily. An early secondary flexor tendon graft is utilized instead.

It has been contended that with laceration of both flexor tendons in "no-man's-land" (zone 2) the risks of tendon rupture and peritendinous adhesions are lessened if the superficialis and profundus tendons are both repaired. The theoretical advantages of repairing the superficialis tendon are that *(a)* repair preserves the blood supply of the profundus tendon through the vinculum longus and *(b)* the superficialis provides a good sliding bed for the repaired profundus. When two tendons are repaired, there is twice the tendon bulk and twice the amount of suture material; this increases the mass of collagen that must glide through the tight digital canal. Profundus tendon blood supply through the vinculum longus and the flattened insertion of superficialis can be preserved without suturing both tendons. With laceration of both flexor tendons in zone 2, if the nature of the wound suggests a high risk of postoperative adhesions, 2 cm of the proximal cut end of the superficalis are resected, leaving the distal end undisturbed.

Motion is achieved early after operating, without tension to the repaired profundus tendon, by protecting the hand with a dorsal plaster splint that maintains the wrist and metacarpophalangeal joints in 30° of palmar flexion. The repaired finger is flexed further by rubber band traction to a small hook cemented to the fingernail or to a suture placed through the fingernail (Fig. 41.12, *B* and *C*.) The patient is encouraged to extend the finger actively to the limits of the splint after the first day. Flexor tendon lacerations in "no-man's-land" in infants and children up to 4 years of age are difficult to treat by this method. The fingers should be immobilized in moderate flexion for 4 weeks after injury.

Avulsion

Closed avulsions of the flexor digitorum profundus are most common in the ring finger, and they frequently result from a football injury when a finger is caught on the jersey of an opponent. There is swelling of the proximal segment of the finger with inability to flex the distal joint. There is often limited flexion of the proximal interphalangeal joint too, because of both incarceration of the ruptured profundus tendon at the insertion of the superficialis tendon and retraction of the lumbrical muscle with the ruptured profundus. Proximal retraction of the lumbrical origin on the flexor digitorum profundus causes increased tension on the lumbrical tendon. This results in hyperextension of the middle phalanx known as "lumbrical-plus" deformity. If the profundus tendon is to be repaired, treatment must be prompt because a delay of more than 1–2 days is likely to cause irreparable contraction of the end of the tendon. X-ray examination usually reveals a small avulsed fragment of the volar lip of the distal phalanx near the neck of the proximal phalanx. At operation the tendon is threaded back to its insertion and held there with a pullout suture. The hand is immobilized in mild flexion for 4 weeks.

Extensor Tendons

Laceration

Most extensor tendon lacerations may be repaired primarily, regardless of the site of injury. The flexor tendons lie within synovial sheaths in the fingers and palm, but the extensor tendons are surrounded by a specialized connective tissue called paratenon

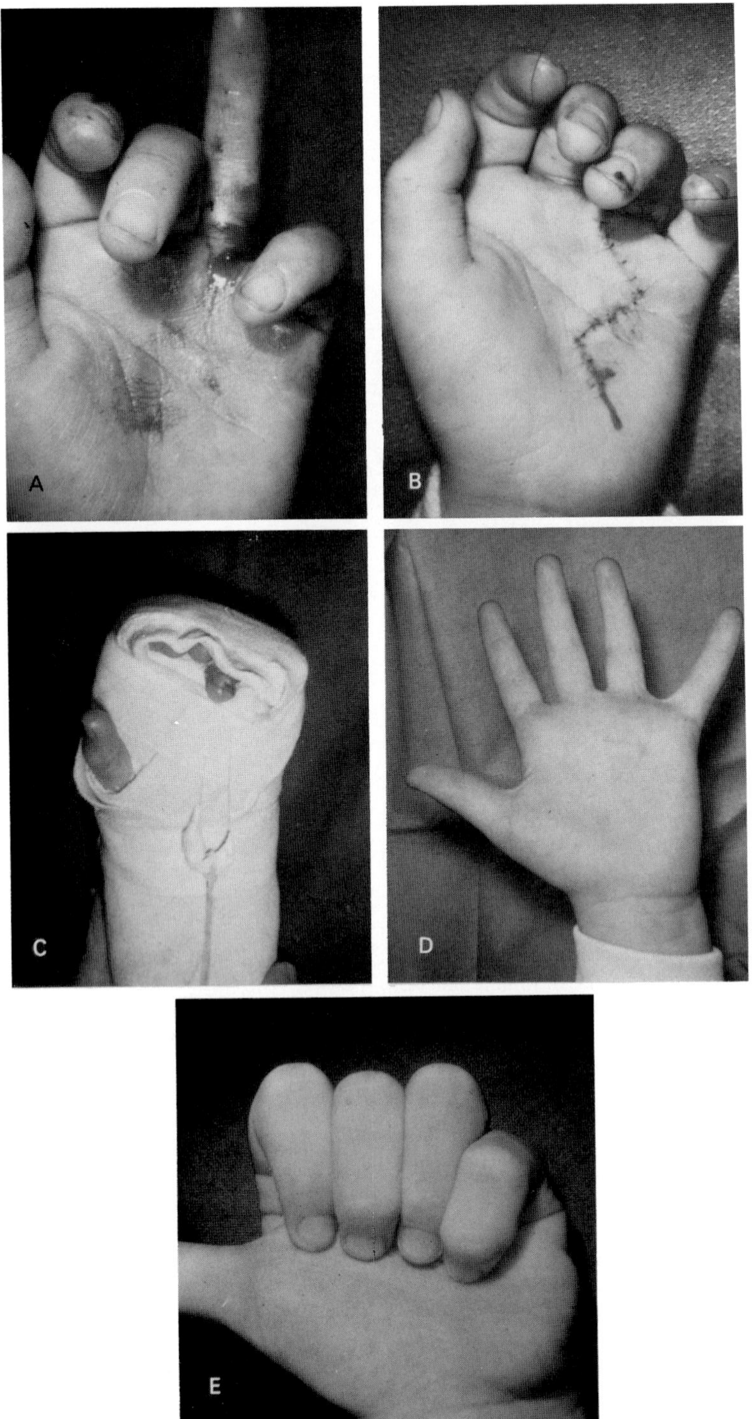

Figure 41.12. Repair of lacerated flexor tendons in "no man's land." *A,* Laceration of flexor digitorum profundus and flexor digitorum superficialis in zone 2 of ring finger by a piece of glass several hours previously. *B,* Primary repair of flexor digitorum profundus was performed. Three cm of proximal cut end of flexor digitorum superficialis was excised. A suture is passed through nail to be attached to rubber band flexion device. A small hook can be cemented to fingernail for rubber band flexion rather than placing a nail suture. *C,* A dorsal plaster splint is applied to the wrist and finger in mild flexion. The finger is further flexed with rubber band traction attached to a safety pin in the dressings. *D,* Two months after operation, there is full extension. *E,* Excellent flexion has been restored.

at the dorsum of the metacarpal bones and fingers. Thus, repair is less likely to be complicated by restrictive adhesions. Although flexor tendon repairs should be performed in the operating room, a well-equipped emergency department may be suitable for repair of a cleanly lacerated extensor tendon. The lacerated ends are approximated with either a buried figure-of-8 suture or a horizontal mattress suture of 4-0 nylon. Several 7-0 nylon interrupted sutures may be used to smooth the juncture site. After repair, a volar plaster splint is applied to support the wrist in 30° of dorsiflexion with the metacarpophalangeal and interphalangeal joints in about 15° of flexion. *All four fingers are immobilized even if only one has been repaired.* If an extensor tendon of the thumb has been repaired, a splint is applied to hold the thumb abducted from the plane of the palm with the metacarpophalangeal and interphalangeal joints in 15° of flexion. The emergency physician should avoid splinting the metacarpophalangeal joints in full extension or hyperextension because of the risk of extension contractures. Immobilization should be continued for 4 weeks.

Rupture

Closed avulsion of the extensor tendon at its insertion on the distal phalanx produces a *mallet* finger. Operation is infrequently indicated. The finger should be immobilized for at least 5 weeks in full extension at the distal joint and in mild flexion at the proximal interphalangeal joint. Premade plastic splints are available to hold this position. A circular plaster cast may be applied around a layer of tubed gauze held to the finger with tincture of benzoin. Some physicians insert a Kirschner wire through the distal joint to maintain the immobilization; however, this is not recommended because the distal joint may become infected or stiff.

Rupture of the central slip of the extensor tendon and of the triangular ligament that holds the lateral bands dorsally results in volar subluxation of the lateral bands and retraction of the central slip proximally. This produces the *boutonnière* deformity, in which the distal interphalangeal joint gradually becomes hyperextended and the proximal interphalangeal joint is swollen and flexed. *Surgical repair is not the proper primary treatment for such injuries.* A volar splint or circular cast is applied to the finger while the proximal interphalangeal joint is held in full extension. Active and passive flexion of the distal joint are encouraged. Immobilization must be continued for 5 weeks. If active extension of the proximal interphalangeal joint is not regained by this treatment, operation is then required.

FRACTURES

Most fractures of the hand can be treated by simple reduction and immobilization. Open reduction and internal fixation are required for phalangeal and metacarpal fractures with rotational deformity or excessive angulation, for irreducible Bennett's fractures, and occasionally for fractures of the carpal bones. *Use of pulp traction, skeletal traction, or banjo splints is contraindicated* because such methods of reduction and immobilization are more hazardous to the skin and joints than open reduction and internal fixation.

Phalanges

The only treatment required in fractures of the tuft of the distal phalanx is treatment of symptoms, such as drilling holes in the base of the fingernail to relieve pain by decompression of a subungual hematoma. Nondisplaced fractures at the interphalangeal joints may be immobilized for 3 weeks with a volar splint. A nondisplaced fracture of the volar lip of the middle phalanx should be treated with a dorsal splint in 30° of flexion. Active proximal interphalangeal flexion is encouraged. Extension past 30° is prevented for 3 weeks. If a large articular fracture is displaced, it is treated with open reduction and fixation with a Kirschner wire. Angulated fractures of the proximal and middle phalanges are usually reduced by gentle traction under local anesthesia and immobilized in semiflexion over a plaster or aluminum splint. Persistent angulation of up to 30° is acceptable in children, and usually causes little disability or deformity. Indeed, in children up to the age of 10 years, open reduction of such fractures is rarely necessary, except in cases of rotational malalignment.

Metacarpals

Fracture of the metacarpal neck is one of the most common fractures in the hand, often the result of a fight. If the volar angulation of the distal fragment is more than 30°, closed reduction may be attempted under local anesthesia by flexing the entire finger acutely and pushing the proximal phalanx dorsally to extend the metacarpal head. Once the fracture is reduced, the finger must not be immobilized in this acutely flexed position. If the deformity recurs with relaxation of the pressure and extension of the finger, open reduction and internal fixation should be performed if there is more than 20° of volar angulation of the second or third metacarpal bone (these bones are relatively immobile at their bases), or if there is more than 40° of angulation of the fourth or fifth metacarpal bone, (these are quite mobile at the carpometacarpal joints).

Compound fractures should be surgically explored, debrided, and lavaged. If necessary, they should be fixed with nonthreaded crossed Kirschner wires passed through the fracture site in a retrograde, oblique direction. The wires are removed in 6–8 weeks. Cerclage bands or wires are rarely employed. Compression plates and screws may be needed to maintain reduction of unstable fractures and to permit early active motion.

To manage metacarpal bone loss following a machine accident or gunshot wound, the fractured metacarpal bones are aligned with longitudinal Kirschner wires and their length is maintained with transverse wires holding them to adjacent uninjured metacarpal shafts. After operation the metacarpophalangeal joints are held in 70° of flexion to prevent joint contracture, and the thumb is held abducted from the palm.

A *Bennett's fracture* is a fracture of the ulnar base of the first metacarpal bone. It is usually associated with subluxation or dislocation of the metacarpal on the trapezium. To reduce this fracture, the thumb is placed in traction and immobilized in opposition. If the dislocation is reducible but the metacarpal tends to slip out of position, percutaneous Kirschner wires are passed through the trapeziometacarpal joint and between the first and second metacarpals. If reduction cannot be achieved by closed methods, open reduction and internal fixation of both the fracture and the dislocated bone are indicated. The fracture site is exposed by a J-shaped incision at the dorsal base of the first metacarpal bone curving volarly across the thenar eminence. Care is taken not to injure the superficial nerves of the thenar eminence. The origins of the thenar muscles are retracted distally, and Kirschner wires are drilled retrograde through the metacarpal and across the fracture site. The fracture is reduced, the wire is drilled proximally, and a second wire is used to maintain reduction of the dislocation, passing from the first to the second metacarpal bone.

Carpus

Fractures of the carpal bones are usually reduced and held in a plaster cast without difficulty. A scaphoid fracture should be suspected after a fall on the outstretched hand with resulting tenderness in the anatomical snuff-box, even if x-ray findings are normal. If suspected, immobilization of the thumb and wrist for 2 weeks with a plaster splint is wise. A second x-ray film is obtained in 2 weeks, and the splint removed if no fracture seen. Scaphoid fractures usually require prolonged immobilization of 3 months or more for healing. When the plaster cast is applied, the thumb tip only is left free, with the thumb placed in opposition and the wrist immobilized in 20° of palmar flexion and radial deviation. With vertical scaphoid fractures and fractures of the proximal pole of the scaphoid bone, immobilization of the elbow is included for the first 3 weeks to prevent forearm rotation. These fractures are particularly slow to heal.

JOINT INJURIES

Phalangeal Dislocations

Dislocations of the interphalangeal joints usually are reducible by traction; in fact, patients report spontaneous reduction immediately after the injury. In all cases, the joint is immobilized for 3 weeks; active and passive exercises are encouraged thereafter. These injuries should always be x-rayed. With dorsal subluxation or dislocation of the middle phalanx, a small avulsed fragment of the volar lip is frequently seen on x-ray examination. In these patients, a dorsal splint preventing extension past 30° is applied after reduction. The patient is allowed to flex his fingers actively, but hyperextension is prevented; this maintains the mobility of the joint while allowing the fracture and avulsion to heal.

Occasionally, dorsal dislocation of the metacarpophalangeal joint may not be reducible by closed means; this is especially true in the index finger. In this instance, the head of the second metacarpal bone is trapped between the lumbrical muscle, the flexor tendons, the volar plate, and the superficial palmar ligaments. Dorsal dislocations of the proximal phalanx of both the thumb and the little finger may also not be reducible by closed means because of interposition of the volar plate or entrapment of the metacarpal head by the flexor tendons. In all such cases, open reduction is required promptly to free the incarcerated tendons or ligaments.

Gamekeeper's Thumb

Gamekeeper's thumb refers to a deformity caused by gradual stretching of the ulnar collateral ligament of the metacarpophalangeal joint of the thumb, although the term has been extended to include acute ruptures of this ligament. These injuries heal poorly if there is extreme instability of the proximal phalanx to passive radial stress. If deviation of more than 45° is produced, if the proximal phalanx is subluxated volarly, or if there is a grossly displaced fracture fragment, primary operation is indicated; the avulsed ligament and any associated fragment of bone are repaired with imbrication of the adductor tendon. The reverse deformity, rupture of the radial collateral ligament, is also repaired by operation if the joint exhibits extreme instability. A sprained thumb with less than 45° of lateral instability rarely requires operation, and is usually treated with immobilization in plaster for 3 weeks.

Carpal Dislocations

Dislocation of one or more carpal bones is frequent after severe injuries to the wrist. X-ray films should always be examined carefully to determine whether the capitate bone fits well into the distal concavity of the lunate bone; anterior dislocation of

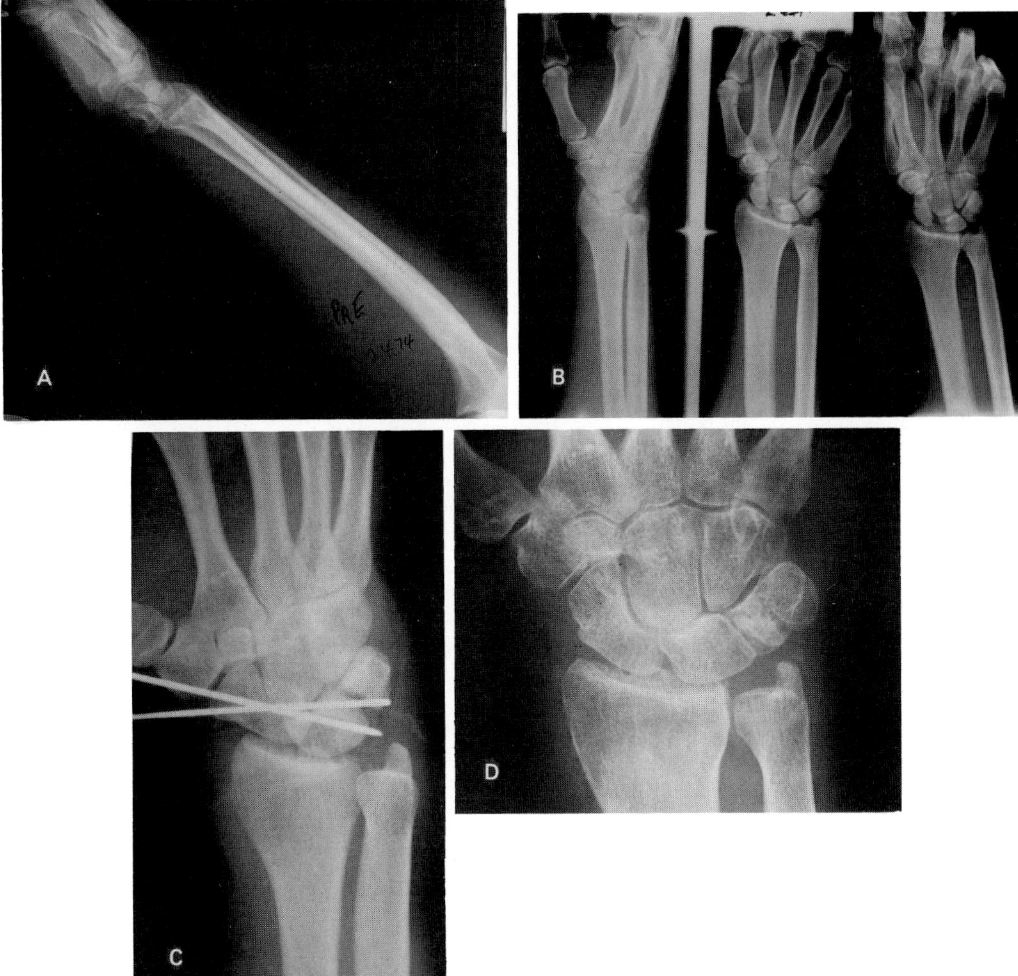

Figure 41.13. Volar dislocation of lunate resulting from a fall on the outstretched hand. *A,* X-ray film of injury. *B,* After closed manipulation, the lunate dislocation is completely reduced. There remains, however, rotatory subluxation of scaphoid. This is best demonstrated by widening between proximal pole of scaphoid and radial side of lunate. *Left,* oblique view; *center,* posteroanterior view in pronation; *right,* anteroposterior view in supination. *C,* Open reduction and internal fixation are usually required for rotatory subluxation of scaphoid. In this case, transverse Kirschner wires are placed between the scaphoid and the lunate. The dorsal wrist capsule had been avulsed from the radius and was reattached. The wrist was immobilized in a plaster cast for 6 weeks. Occasionally, rotatory subluxation may be reduced without operation by positioning the hand with the wrist in neutral flexion-extension and mild radial deviation. *D,* One year after operation, intercarpal and radiocarpal alignment is maintained.

the lunate and perilunar dislocation are frequently overlooked. On an anteroposterior x-ray film of the wrist, the lunate should appear quadrangular. If it is triangular and overlaps the capitate, intercarpal dislocation should be suspected. These dislocations require immediate closed reduction, which is usually achieved by traction, flexion, and digital pressure on the lunate bone, followed by restoration of the neutral position. After reduction, another x-ray film should be obtained and examined carefully for widening between the scaphoid and lunate bones; an abnormally large space signals probable rotatory subluxation of the scaphoid bone. This injury usually requires open reduction, repair of the torn intercarpal ligaments, and internal fixation (Fig. 41.13).

TRAUMATIC AMPUTATIONS

Stump Closures

The treatment of amputated fingertips has been discussed (see pp 810–813). In the case of a more proximal amputation of a finger, primary closure is preferred after a clean injury. If disarticulation through the proximal or distal interphalangeal joint has occurred, the tendons should be advanced distally, severed, and allowed to retract. Tendons *should not be sutured to each other over the end of the bone.* Nerves should be cleanly transected so that they do not lie adjacent to the amputation stump. When there is disarticulation at the distal interphalangeal joint, the lumbrical tendon is transsected proximal to the proximal interphalangeal joint to prevent development of a lumbrical-plus deformity. The end of the amputated bone is rounded to avoid bony "dog ears"; it is not necessary to remove the articular cartilage.

The amputation stump should be left as long as possible with adequate coverage of skin. There are two exceptions to this. First, for both aesthetic and functional reasons, amputation through the proximal phalanx of either the index finger or the little finger is best treated by resection at the base of the corresponding metacarpal bone (ray resection). The age and occupation of the patient must be considered in making the decision whether to amputate the entire finger. Second, in ring avulsion injuries, amputation is the preferred procedure, although exceptions may be made for children, particularly if the ring finger of the left hand is involved. We believe that better functional and aesthetic results are achieved in adults if the finger is amputated at the site of injury as a primary procedure, followed by ray resection and transfer of the fifth metacarpal to the fourth metacarpal base (Fig. 41.14). This is not an emergency procedure, and may be performed at the patient's convenience.

Replantation

Few events in reconstructive surgery related to the hand have received more public attention than the replantation of limbs. Following the success in 1962 in replantation of an arm severed at the middle of the humerus, replantation of limbs, and digits has been performed successfully in many centers throughout the world, aided by recent advances both in microsurgical techniques and in materials.

Contraindications

An amputated arm, hand, or portion of the hand should not be replanted if it has been severely crushed, subjected to severe heat or cold, or torn from its attachment with avulsion of major nerves and blood vessels. Replantation is also contraindicated if there has been mishandling of the amputated part or excessive delay in transit.

Immediate Care

The amputated part should be wrapped in sterile saline sponges or towels and placed in a plastic bag. The wrapped unit is then transported cooled in a bucket of ice. The amputation stump should be covered with sterile or clean dressings. Limbs have successfully been replanted many hours after injury. Thus, although speed is desirable, a delay of several hours that is spent transporting a patient to a hospital prepared to perform replantation surgery is preferable to prompt replantation where the staff is inexperienced in microvascular techniques.

Considerations

Whether a portion of a hand should be replanted even under optimal conditions depends to a great extent on patient needs and the extent of the injuries. A hand with an amputation of either the index finger or the little finger has such good appearance and function that the value of replantation of either of these fingers is questionable. The emergency physician should consider whether it is advisable to replant the tip of a finger or thumb or to shorten the digit and to cover it with skin of normal sensation. In patients with amputations of more than one finger or clean amputation of the hand at the wrist, replantation should be attempted if the condition of both the patient and the amputated part is satisfactory.

The patient, his or her family, and medical personnel should understand that the success of a replantation does not depend solely on the viability of the replanted part. If a replanted limb or digit remains relatively insensitive, stiff, or immobile, it may ultimately require reamputation. In these circumstances, the patient may find a prosthesis more functional. Nonetheless, a cleanly amputated part in a suitable patient should usually be replanted (Fig. 41.15). The potential advantages of a successful replantation justify the risk and large expenditure of time. The emergency physician is not the person to make this decision.

SPECIAL WOUNDS

Human Bites

Certain wounds of the hand require particular attention by the emergency physician. A laceration over a metacarpophalangeal joint should lead the physician to suspect a human bite. These bites are highly contaminated and should be left open. Antibiotic and tetanus prophylaxis should be considered, and the wound well irrigated and allowed to heal by secondary intention.

Pressure-Gun Injuries

Injuries due to injection of a foreign substance under pressure, such as injuries from paint guns and grease guns, may appear innocuous on first examination, but can result in extensive contamination, vascular spasm, and ultimately necrosis. All such

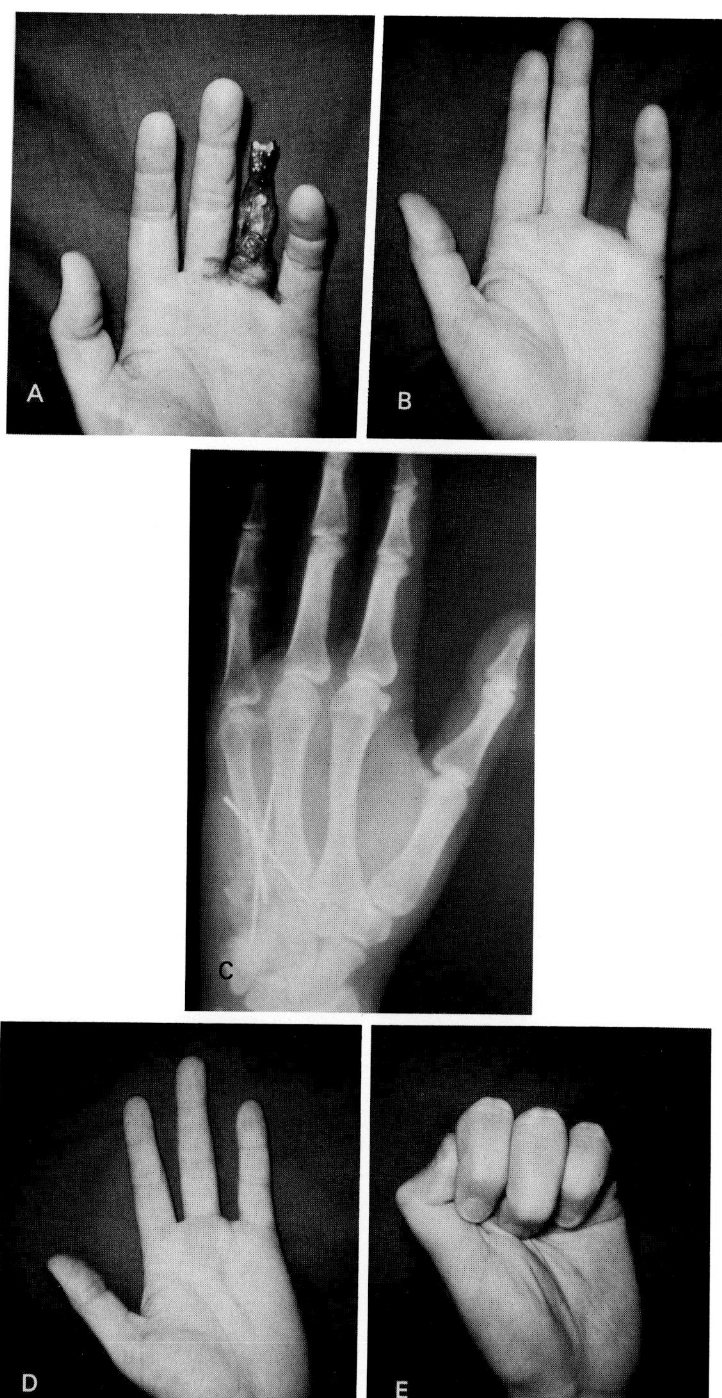

Figure 41.14. Treatment of ring avulsion injury. *A,* Two hours previously, this patient caught his ring on a hook and sustained an avulsion injury of the ring finger with amputation of the tip. *B,* Primary treatment consisted of amputation of finger at site of avulsion. *C,* Two months later, digital ray transfer was performed. The fourth metacarpal was removed to its base. Osteotomy of the fifth metacarpal was performed, and it was transferred radially. Transferred metacarpal is held in place with multiple Kirschner wires. *D,* After healing of metacarpal osteotomy and ray transfer, appearance of hand is considerably improved. *E,* Ray transfer also closes the gap between middle and little fingers, resulting in improved hand function.

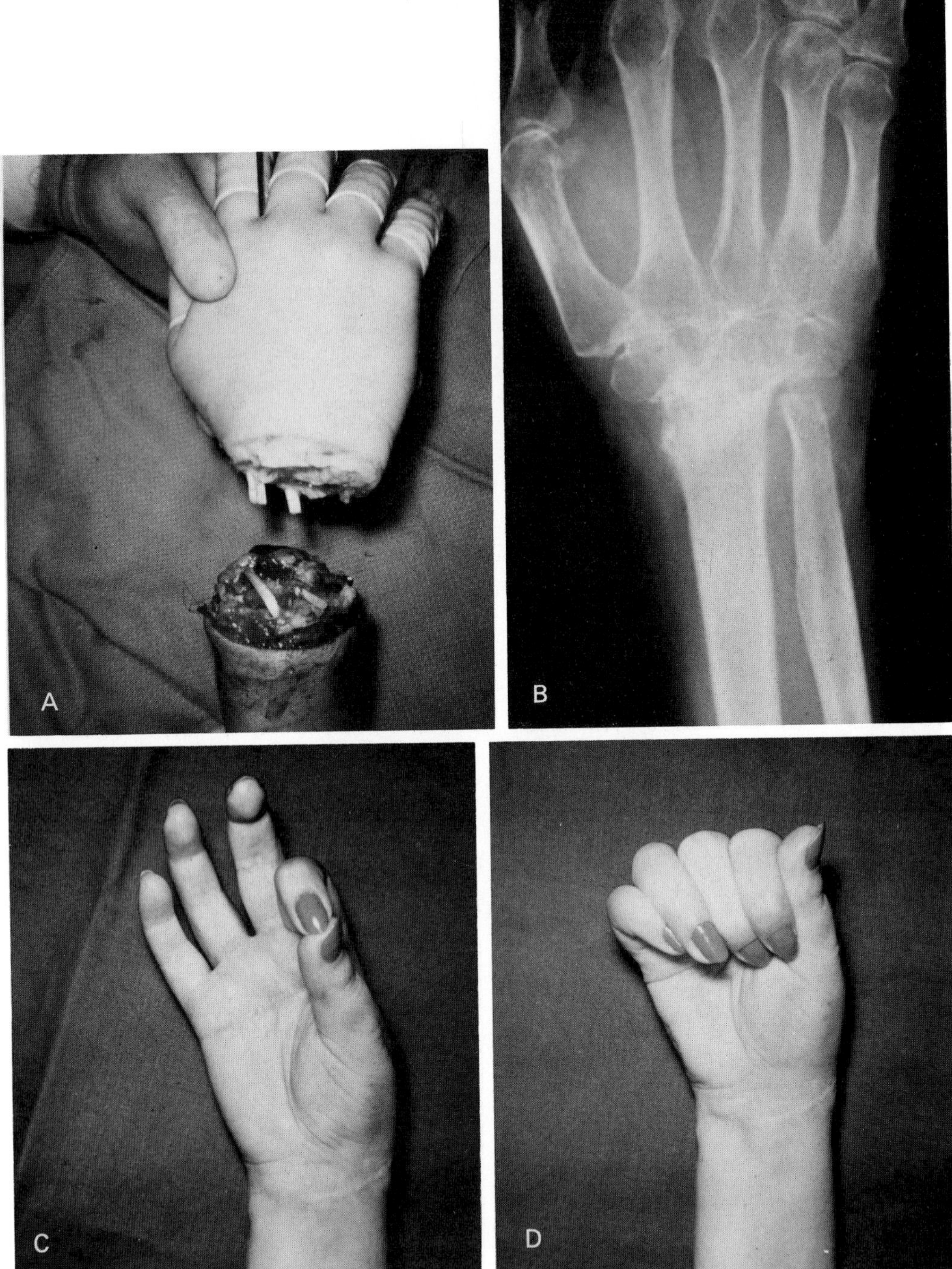

Figure 41.15. Replantation of amputated hand. *A,* Two hours previously, the hand had been amputated in a machine accident. It was transported in a plastic bag placed in an ice bucket. Replantation was performed with primary repair of nerves and tendons and resection of the proximal row of carpal bones. Two arteries and four veins were repaired. *B,* Secondary reconstructive procedures included wrist arthrodesis, volar metacarpophalangeal capsulorrhaphy, intrinsic muscle release, and arthrodesis of metacarpophalangeal joint of thumb. *C,* The patient regained good return of thenar muscle function and fair return of intrinsic muscles. Pinprick sensibility was restored about entire hand, and two-point discrimination of 5 mm was present in several fingertips. *D,* Extension and flexion of fingers and thumb permitted return to her occupation as hairdresser.

injuries should receive emergency treatment, consisting of wide excision and thorough debridement. These patients should be admitted to the hospital for immediate surgical care; the foreign material may extensively dissect soft-tissue planes, causing severe chemical irritation. If the injured finger appears blanched after extensive debridement, anticoagulants and cervical sympathetic blockade may restore the circulation to the contracted vessels.

Wringer Injuries

Wringer injuries have become less common since the advent of the electric clothes dryer. A wringer injury may result in extensive deep soft-tissue damage that is not apparent on initial examination. Skin and subcutaneous tissue may be ripped from underlying fascia with resultant deep ecchymosis and thrombosis. The limb must be elevated and observed. Necrotic tissue is promptly debrided and appropriate skin grafts applied.

Burns

Thermal burns due to either excessively low or high temperature or passage of electrical current require special treatment and close observation. These are discussed in detail in Chapter 38.

Snakebites

After a poisonous snakebite to the hand, the snake venom is activated by the body temperature and tissue pH. The activated venom hydrolyzes and destroys local tissues, and causes local bleeding due to rupture of vessel walls. Within a short time, venom and partly hydrolyzed tissue circulate throughout the vascular system, causing hypotension, nausea, tachycardia, and eventually anuria. Hemoglobin, hematocrit, and platelet levels fall because of both massive cellular exudation in the area of the bite and intravascular cell destruction. Intravascular venom causes a rapid decrease in fibrinogen levels. As local tissues are destroyed by hydrolysis, the osmotic pressure in the area of the bite rises. This causes increasing edema and results in progressive cyanosis and pain in the region of the bite.

One of the more popular methods of treating poisonous snakebites has included the use of crosscuts over the wound, local suction, and administration of antivenin. The value of this method of treatment has been questioned. The use of crosscuts over a snakebite has frequently caused considerable unnecessary damage to tendons and nerves lying beneath the site of injury. Suction has added bacteria from the mouth to an open and edematous wound. Antivenin must be used in large quantities to be effective. Many patients are allergic to the horse serum from which the antivenin is derived, and may have a severe allergic reaction. All too often, this regimen of crosscuts, suction, and antivenin has been used with tragic consequences in patients who had been bitten by a nonpoisonous snake. For these reasons, many emergency departments now recommend the following treatment for snakebites to the hand:

1. Apply ice bags to the bite site.
2. Compression dressings may be applied above and below the bite site to minimize spread of the venom in the soft tissues. Dressings should *not* be venous or arterial tourniquets.
3. Closely monitor hemoglobin, hematocrit, platelet count, prothrombin time, plasma fibrinogen, and vital signs. Central venous pressure and urinary output should be carefully checked and appropriately treated if abnormal.
4. Administer intravenous fluids to maintain normal central venous pressure and 24-hour urinary output of 50 ml/hr.
5. Give intravenous antibiotics, tetanus toxoid, and analgesics.
6. Administer hydrocortisone sodium succinate, 1 gm intravenously, before operation.

Surgical treatment consists of total debridement of the wound and fasciotomy. The wound should not be closed primarily. It may be closed after 5–7 days with a skin graft if necessary.

Many physicians now believe that antivenin is unnecessary and dangerous. They advise that neither antivenin nor crosscuts be used as first aid. Since definitive care of the poisonous snakebite may be performed only in the hospital, the best treatment as first aid is the application of ice about the wound and transportation to the hospital as rapidly as possible.

INFECTIONS

Specific treatment of the infected hand depends on the causative organism and the location and extent of the infection. Considerable information is obtained from a meticulous history. For example, an infection at the dorsum of the hand after a fight is likely due to the mouth streptococci and spirochetes of the opponent. A puncture wound from a barnyard nail may harbor clostridia. An infected finger lacerated in a hospital ward should arouse suspicion of penicillin-resistant staphylococci. In each case, the selection of antibiotics would vary (see Chapter 11). Persons with superficial skin infections, cellulitis without underlying abscess, paronychia, and intradermal abscesses may be treated as outpatients. If the patient has tender or enlarged axillary or epitrochlear nodes, the red streaks characteristic of lymphangitis, fever, or leukocytosis resulting from purulent tenosynovitis, deep space abscesses, joint infection, and osteomyelitis often require prompt admission and operation.

The position of the fingers and the location of swelling and redness must be accurately noted. Palpation must be gentle and slow, because the entire hand may be painful and the area of maximal tenderness may be masked by rough examination. The pattern of tenderness, redness, and heat may reveal the dome of an abscess better than the swollen area. For example, lymphedema at the dorsum of the hand may be more striking than palmar swelling in a midpalmar abscess. A thenar space infection may cause more puffiness of the loose dorsal skin of the first web than of the firm structures that border the abscess. The examiner must not mistake the swelling of the loose dorsal areolar tissue for the site of infection. Paronychia and small subcutaneous and intradermal abscesses may be opened and drained in the emergency department with anesthesia by ethyl chloride spray. Deeper infections require general anesthesia or regional block. A tourniquet, without rubber bandage exsanguination, is used during operation for all deep infections.

Common pyogenic infections of the hand include the following:

1. *Intradermal abscess* or infected blister. Symptoms include localized swelling and tenderness that often occur at the fingertip. Motion of the fingers is painless, and there is no proximal edema. The area should be anesthetized with ethyl chloride spray and the abscess incised in the emergency department; the patient should then soak the area periodically at home.

2. *Subcutaneous abscess.* Patients with a subcutaneous abscess have diffuse redness and tenderness of the hand, and motion is usually relatively painless at noncontiguous joints. The abscess is usually limited by fascial attachments. If the abscess occurs at the dorsum, there may be a large area of undermined skin requiring drainage.

3. *Collar-button abscess.* This is a subcutaneous abscess of the distal part of the palm that points both in the web and more proximally between the pretendinous bands. When these lesions are drained, pus must be evacuated from the dorsal web and proximal to the natatory ligaments of the palmar fascia into the distal palm.

4. *Paronychia.* Early in its development, paronychia is a superficial abscess between the nail and the eponychium. If untreated, the infection may extend into deeper tissues and "run around" the nail margins deep to the nailbed. In early cases, the eponychium should be elevated from the nail with a no. 11 scalpel blade (see Illustrated Technique 19). A skin incision is rarely necessary. Petrolatum gauze is inserted between the nail and the eponychium for several days. In later cases with more severe infection around the entire nail margin, the entire eponychium should be elevated with parallel longitudinal incisions. If it is necessary, the nailbed should be elevated.

5. *Felon.* A felon is an abscess in the pulp space of the fingertip. The tip is hot, exquisitely tender, and firm, and the finger relatively unaffected more proximally. The fascial septa hold the pus in the fingertip under pressure, and osteomyelitis of the distal phalanx may result. A J-shaped incision at the dorsolateral side of the distal segment of the finger just anterior to the fingernail is adequate for exposure and drainage. All septa must be divided. The wound should be packed with gauze until it closes from below (see Illustrated Technique 20).

6. *Tendon sheath infection.* If the index, middle, or ring finger is involved, infection extends from the base of the distal phalanx to the distal palmar flexion crease. Infections of the thumb and little finger may extend into the radial or ulnar bursa and into the wrist. The four cardinal signs of tenosynovitis, according to Kanavel, include: *(a) tenderness* over the course of the sheath, limited to the sheath; *(b) symmetrical enlargement* of the volar side of the finger; *(c) pain on extension* of the fingertip; and *(d) partial flexion* of the finger at rest.

In patients with purulent flexor tenosynovitis, drainage should be performed in the operating room. A dorsolateral incision is made at the side of the finger, and a second incision is usually necessary in the palm. At least two of the flexor tendon pulleys should be left intact during incision and drainage of the tendon sheath. The wound is occasionally closed around a plastic catheter that is used for intermittent antibiotic irrigation for 3 or 4 days. With mild early flexor tenosynovitis, an initial 12-hour trial of splinting and intravenous antibiotics may be warranted.

7. *Infections of the radial and ulnar bursae.* The radial and ulnar bursae are the proximal prolongations of the flexor tendon sheaths of the thumb and little fingers, respectively. A tendon sheath infection of either of these two digits may drain proximally and into the opposite side of the hand, forming a "horseshoe" abscess. Infections of the ulnar bursa may be drained through an ulnar incision. Those of the radial bursa frequently require an incision adjacent to the thenar eminence. In either case, an incision within the wrist is usually mandatory to drain the cul-de-sac of these bursae.

8. *Thenar space infection.* The borders of the thenar space include the thenar muscles radially, the adductor pollicis deeply, flexor tendons of the index and middle fingers superficially, and a septum extending deep to the flexor tendons of the middle finger ulnarly. Distally, the infection may involve

the first and second lumbrical canals and may extend to the dorsum of the first web. Fullness and tenderness of the radial half of the palm are noted.

Incision for drainage should *not* parallel the first web. A dorsal longitudinal incision radial to the second metacarpal bone usually provides sufficient exposure to permit adequate irrigation and drainage of the thenar space. This incision allows access to the radial half of the palm over the first dorsal interosseus and adductor muscles. If necessary, a second incision may be made in the palm.

9. *Midpalmar space infection.* The midpalmar space extends from the hypothenar muscles ulnarly to the septum of the flexor tendon of the middle finger radially. Deeply, it is bound by the third, fourth, and fifth metacarpal bones and the palmar interosseus muscles and superficially by the tendons to the middle, ring, and little fingers and the third and fourth lumbrical muscles. Distally, midpalmar abscesses may extend into the fourth and fifth lumbrical canals. The infection causes fullness and tenderness of the ulnar side of the palm.

A curved midpalmar incision paralleling the flexion creases of the palm allows ready access to the midpalmar space. Care should be taken to avoid injury to the flexor tendons and neurovascular bundles to the third and fourth webs.

10. *Joint infection.* The most frequent joint infection in the hand involves the metacarpophalangeal joint after a bite received in a fight. Any small laceration over the metacarpophalangeal joint should be suspected of a tooth injury, particularly on Saturday nights. If the extensor tendon is lacerated, contamination of the joint should be assumed. The wound should be lavaged and left open. If an infection develops in the untreated patient, the joint should be opened, lavaged, and allowed to drain.

All hand infections require splinting. Gentle active or passive motion may be instituted 2–3 days after treatment, depending on the nature of the infection and extent of the injury. Complete range-of-motion exercises once a day may be sufficient to prevent joint contractures.

THE STIFF AND SWOLLEN HAND

A stiff hand has little function. Stiffness often may be prevented by judicious and meticulous primary care of hand wounds, strict attention to surgical principles, careful application of dressings, and appropriate exercises after operation.

Treatment of the swollen hand should be directed toward maintaining joint mobility and the rapid resolution of the edema. All constrictive dressings should be loosened. Circular casts should be either removed and bivalved or replaced with splints. A crushed or swollen hand in which there are neither fractures nor injured tendons should be immobilized with the wrist in mild dorsiflexion, the thumb in maximal abduction,the metacarpophalangeal joints in approximately 70° of flexion, and the proximal interphalangeal joints in almost full extension. Although this is not the position of function, it is the position in which joint contractures are least likely to develop. When considerable edema and stiffness are feared after severe injuries, Kirschner wires may be used to fix the metacarpophalangeal joints of the fingers in flexion and the thumb in abduction.

The arm should be elevated several inches higher than the level of the heart. If there is no arterial insufficiency, the arm is suspended from an intravenous pole. A well-padded volar splint supports the wrist. A stockinette, with appropriate openings cut for the fingers and thumb, is placed over the splint and suspended from the pole. The role of oral enzymes in decreasing edema has not been substantiated.

Elastic bandages are not used in the treatment of edema of the hand. These bandages may cause more harm than good because they interfere with venous drainage. Elastic bandages are difficult to apply properly; they are dangerous when applied by the patient. The rubberized elastic bandage has little place in the treatment of any injury of the hand.

Occasionally, severe intermittent edema may result from self-induced injury. The patient may apply a tourniquet around the wrist or forearm, for example. Such patients may not be malingerers, but rather may be suffering from behavioral psychiatric disorders. This diagnosis must always be suspected when severe, otherwise inexplicable edema is limited proximally by a circumferential sulcus about the wrist or forearm. Edema often subsides rapidly if a heavily padded dressing is applied from the fingertips to the upper arm. Such a dressing prevents access of the patient to the limb. If the diagnosis of factitious lymphedema is established, the patient should be referred for psychiatric evaluation.

Any severe injury of the hand or forearm may result in edema of the soft tissues. Without prompt treatment, irreversible changes may develop rapidly about the median nerve and within the adductor pollicis and interosseus muscles of the fingers.

If the patient with a potentially stiff or swollen hand is treated and allowed to return home, he/she should be urged to return to the emergency department or to telephone if pain becomes more severe or if the fingers become pale or cold. Physician's responsibility for patient care extends beyond the time that emergency treatment is rendered; the patient must be aware that a physician is available and eager to be called if any problem develops.

CARPAL TUNNEL SYNDROME

The median nerve lies directly beneath the transverse carpal ligament and overlies the flexor tendons of the fingers and thumb. The carpal tunnel is bound deeply by the carpal bones and the volar wrist ligaments. As edema develops, the synovium surrounding the flexor tendons swells and presses the median nerve tightly against the volar ligament; an acute carpal tunnel syndrome develops. The patient has paresthesia and hypesthesia in the thumb, index and middle fingers, and radial side of the ring finger. There is tenderness proximal to the carpal canal. Percussion in this area elicits a positive Tinel's sign in the sensory distribution of the nerve. Palmar flexion of the wrist for 1 minute only adds to the compression of the median nerve and increase the paresthesia. This is known as Phalen's sign.

In these patients, carpal tunnel release is an emergency procedure that should be performed as soon as possible, but only in the operating room. A curved incision is made in the thenar crease and extended proximally to the ulnar side of the midline of the wrist and to the distal forearm. All dissection is performed ulnar to the midline to avoid injury to the palmar cutaneous branch of the median nerve. The median nerve is identified proximal to the carpal canal. With the nerve visualized, the transverse carpal ligament is transected. Epineurectomy is rarely necessary.

SUGGESTED READINGS

Beasley RB. *Hand Injuries.* Philadelphia: WB Saunders, 1981.

Boyes JH, ed. *Bunnell's Surgery of the Hand,* 5th ed. Philadelphia: JB Lippincott, 1970.

Buck-Gramcko D, Hoffman R, Neumann R, ed. *Hand Trauma: A Practical Guide.* New York: Thieme, 1986.

Flatt AE. Minor hand injuries. *J Bone Joint Surg,* 1955;37-B:117–125.

Flatt AE. *The Care of Minor Hand Injuries*, 4th ed. St. Louis: CV Mosby, 1979.

Flynn JE. *Hand Surgery,* 3rd ed. Baltimore: Williams & Wilkins, 1982.

Frykman GK, Wolf A, Coyle T. An algorithm for management of peripheral nerve injuries. *Orthop Clin North Am,* 1981;12:239–244.

Gelberman RH, Zakaib GS, Mubarak SJ, et al. Decompression of forearm compartment syndrome, *Clin Orthop,* 1978;134:225–229.

Gelberman RG, Blasingame JP, Fronek A, et al. Forearm arterial injuries, *J Hand Surg,* 1979;4:401–408.

Grabb WE, Myers MB, eds. *Skin Flaps.* Boston: Little, Brown & Co., 1975.

Halpern AA, Greene R, Nichols T, et al. Compartment syndrome of the interosseous muscles; early recognition and treatment, *Clin Orthop,* 1979; 140:23–25.

Harris C Jr, Riordan DC. Intrinsic contracture in the hand and its surgical treatment, *J Bone Joint Surg,* 1954;36:10–20.

Kleinert HE, Schepel S, Gill T. Flexor tendon injuries, *Surg Clin North Am,* 1981;G1:267–286.

Kleinert HE, Gropper PT, Van Beck A. Trauma of the hand, *Curr Probl Surg,* 1978;15:18.

Lister G. *The Hand, Diagnosis and Indications,* 2nd ed. London: Churchill Livingstone, 1984.

Milford L. The hand. In Crenshaw AH, ed. *Campbell's Operative Orthopaedics,* 7th ed. St. Louis: CV Mosby, 1987, pp 111–506.

Omer GE Jr. Physical diagnosis of peripheral nerve injuries, *Orthop Clin North Am,* 1981;12:207.

Rank BK, Wakefield AR, Hueston JT. *Surgery of Repair as Applied to Hand Injuries,* 4th ed. Baltimore, Williams & Wilkins, 1973.

Reid DAC, Tubiana R, ed. *Mutilating Injuries of the Hand,* 2nd ed, New York: Churchill Livingstone, 1984.

Schneider LH. *Flexor Tendon Injuries.* Boston: Little Brown, 1985.

Seddon H. *Surgical Disorders of the Peripheral Nerves,* 2nd ed. Baltimore: Williams & Wilkins, 1975.

Smith RJ. Intrinsic muscles of the fingers: Function, dysfunction, and surgical reconstruction. In American Academy of Orthopaedic Surgeons. Instructional Course Lectures, vol 24. St. Louis: CV Mosby, 1975, pp 200–220.

Symposium on Tendon Surgery in the Hand, Philadelphia, 1974. St. Louis: CV Mosby, 1975.

Weber ER, Davis J. Rehabilitation following hand surgery, *Orthop Clin North Am,* 1978;9:259–272.

Wynn Parry CB. *Rehabilitation of the Hand,* 3rd ed. London, Butterworths, 1973.

CHAPTER 42

Emergencies of the Ear, Facial Structures, and Upper Airway

ERNEST A. WEYMULLER, JR., M.D.
THOMAS J. MULVANEY, M.D.
RUFUS C. PARTLOW, JR., M.D.

THE EAR

Terminology and Examination Technique

Hearing loss may be divided into two basic types—conductive and sensorineural. Conductive hearing loss is caused by lesions of the sound conduction mechanism, including the ear canal, eardrum, middle-ear space, and ossicular chain (Fig. 42.1). Sensorineural hearing loss results from defects of the cochlea, eighth nerve, or the central auditory pathways.

Simple clinical tests for the degree and type of hearing loss include the voice test, Rinne's test, and Weber's test.

In the *voice test,* each ear is tested separately for the minimal level of audible hearing while a noise box creates a masking noise in the untested ear. If a noise box is unavailable, the examiner can occlude the nontested ear canal with his finger, moving it gently to generate sufficient masking noise for testing at low voice levels. Hearing is roughly normal if the patient can hear a soft whisper in the tested ear. If the patient cannot hear the examiner's voice close to the ear at normal conversational levels, there is a significant hearing loss.

Rinne's test is performed with a tuning fork with a frequency of 512 Hz. The fork is struck, and the patient is asked to compare the degree of loudness with the fork in two positions. First, the base of the fork is placed on the mastoid cortex behind the ear (bone conduction), and then the vibrating tines are placed 2–3 inches away from the ear (air conduction). In a person with normal hearing, air conduction is better than bone conduction (positive Rinne's test). A patient with sensorineural hearing loss also has a positive test. In the patient with a significant conductive hearing loss, bone conduction is greater than air conduction (negative Rinne's test). Rinne's test by itself is unreliable in a patient with total neural deafness in one ear. Such a patient will report conduction through bone as louder than conduction through air when the deaf ear is tested (false-negative Rinne's test). In this instance, when the base of the fork is on the bone, sound vibrations are transmitted through the skull and are heard in the opposite ear; the patient hears nothing in the deaf ear through air conduction, however. The examiner can distinguish this condition from conductive hearing loss by performing Weber's test.

Weber's test is performed by placing the vibrating tuning fork in the midline of the skull, usually on the forehead, nose, or on the middle incisor teeth. The patient is asked to which side of the head the sound travels. In a patient with normal hearing, or when hearing loss is symmetrical, sound is heard in the middle of the head. In a patient with unilateral conductive hearing loss, the sound is louder in the abnormal ear. In a patient with unilateral neural deafness, the sound is heard in the better-hearing ear.

Other tests used in examination of the ear include the fistula test and the position test.

The *fistula test* is performed by placing an olive-tipped rubber-bulb syringe in the ear canal of the affected ear. Sufficient pressure must be applied to prevent air leakage around the olive tip. The rubber bulb is squeezed, increasing air pressure in the ear canal. When a rubber bulb is not available, the examiner may occlude the ear canal with his or her finger and firmly pump the air column. In a positive fistula test, the patient's eyes deviate away from the affected ear; sometimes his or her body sways in that direction; and he or she feels dizzy. A positive fistula test suggests that inner ear membranes have been exposed by erosion of the bony wall.

In any patient with positional dizziness, the *position test* should be performed. The patient should be asked to sit on an examining table and then, in succession, to lie back with the head hanging straight over the edge, with the head to the right, and then with the head to the left. The patient's eyes are observed, and the direction, duration, and character of any nystagmus (rotatory, horizontal, or vertical) are recorded. It is also important to note any delay in onset and whether nystagmus can be fatigued to the point of disappearing on repeated testing.

Trauma

External Ear

Traumatic injury to the external ear usually results from being hit, torn, or bitten. On physical examination, a hematoma, laceration, or avulsion may be present. Abnormal contour of the external ear with a fluctuant swelling that may be discolored indicates hematoma. A laceration may be partial thickness or full thickness, and auricular cartilage may be exposed. All or part of the external ear may be avulsed.

Hematoma. If a hematoma is present, the ear canal and eardrum should be carefully examined. A clinical estimate of hearing should be established. After the surface of the ear is cleansed and the hair shaved 1 inch around the ear, the hematoma may be aspirated with a large-bore needle (no. 15) using sterile technique. If this measure fails to eliminate the hematoma, a stab incision is made in the area of greatest fluctuance to evacuate the clot, and a small rubber drain is placed through the stab incision. A soft dressing of sterile cotton should be applied. The cotton, moistened with povidone-iodine (Betadine) solution, is applied in small enough portions to conform to all the convolutions of the ex-

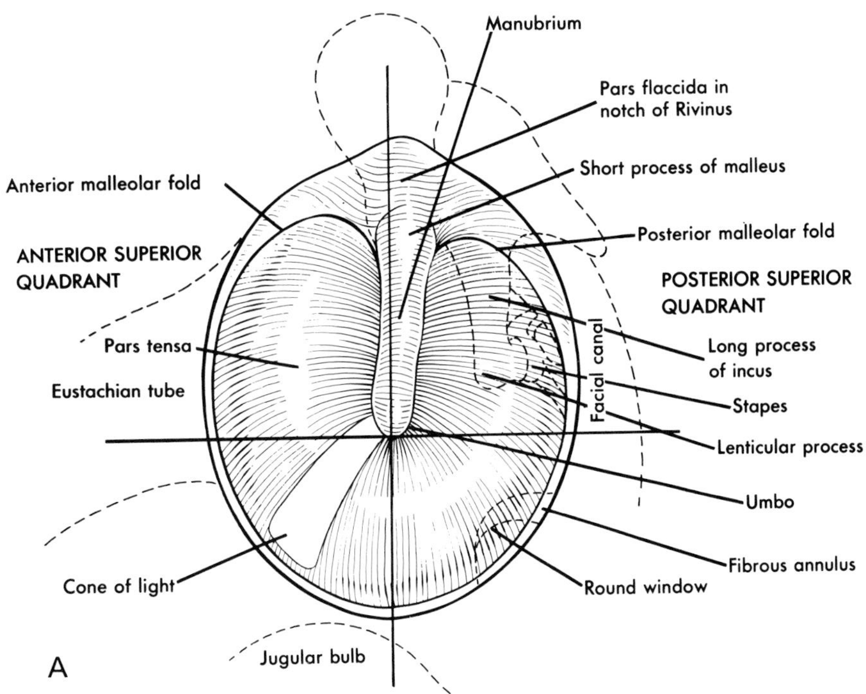

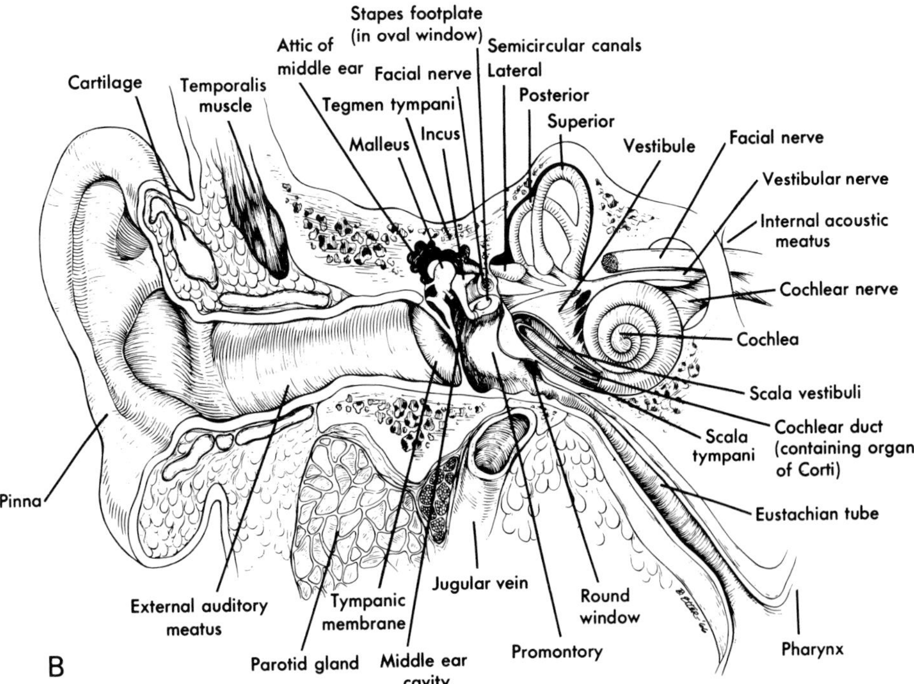

Figure 42.1. *A,* Major landmarks of eardrum (left ear). Long process of incus may be visualized through normal eardrum. *B,* Basic anatomy of the ear. (Reproduced by permission, from Miglets, Andrew W., Paparella, Michael M., and Saunders, William, H.: *Atlas of Ear Surgery,* 4th ed. St. Louis, 1986, The C.V. Mosby Co.)

ternal ear; the dressing is held in place with a wraparound gauze head bandage. Dressings should be changed daily until the hematoma no longer reaccumulates. The hematoma should be reaspirated if necessary. It is advisable to refer the patient to an otolaryngologist. Some controversy exits over the efficacy of systemic antibiotics. We recommend erythromycin, 250 mg every 6 hours for 5 days or longer if the hematoma persists, or recurs.

Laceration and Avulsion. Careful closure of a laceration with standard soft-tissue techniques (see Chapter 39) should be sufficient treatment; cartilage does not hold sutures, and the edges should be apposed by sutures in the perichondrium. Sutures should be removed in 5–7 days. In the case of a patient with total or partial avulsion of the external ear, an otolaryngologist, plastic surgeon, or general surgeon should immediately be consulted. Any fragments of the ear should be placed in iced sterile saline solution as soon as possible. Small avulsed pieces up to 2 cm maximal diameter, may be débrided and reattached, or the small defect may be closed primarily by advancing the freshened edges of the ear wound. Total avulsion of the ear may be treated by various methods, including immediate reattachment or burying the ear cartilage in the postauricular soft tissues after it is dermabraded, with plans for later reconstruction. If the latter technique is used, the raw surface left by the avulsion should be covered with a sterile dressing.

Thermal Injuries. Thermal injuries of the external ear resulting from exposure to extreme heat or cold are usually obvious from the history. In a patient with a frostbitten ear, the pinna is cold and pale; erythema and vesicles appear when the ear is warmed. Most patients with significant facial burns have associated auricular burns. Depending on the depth of burn, there may be erythema, vesicles, or charring of the external ear.

A frostbitten ear should be rapidly rewarmed with sterile cotton soaked in water at a temperature of 100–108°F (37.8–42.2°C). Systemic analgesics, such as meperidine hydrochloride (Demerol), may be administered for pain as the ear is warmed. Hair around the ear should be trimmed, but débridement with attendant rupturing of vesicles should be avoided. A topical antibacterial agent such as povidone-iodine should be applied. Silver nitrate solution (0.5%) is also an effective antiseptic agent. Oral antibiotics are indicated only if infection develops. The patient should be advised not to smoke because of the vasospastic effects of nicotine. When the ear is thawed, the patient should be hospitalized to allow continued sterile care for the ear.

First- to third-degree burns should be treated by the open method with mafenide acetate (Sulfamylon) cream. A doughnut pillow prevents pressure on the ear. A major complication is perichondritis, which may occur from 2–5 weeks after the burn. The ear must be watched carefully during convalescence. Severe charring of the ear results in autoamputation.

Ear Canal

Laceration of the ear canal usually occurs in conjunction with other traumatic injuries of the ear. Any laceration involving cartilage or skin around the external acoustic meatus should be treated in the following manner. Blood should be suctioned from the ear canal, and the eardrum should be carefully inspected. Hearing should be tested with a tuning fork and whispered voice. In cases of major trauma, x-ray views should be obtained if fracture of the temporal bone is suspected.

The laceration should be treated by open packing with 0.5-inch iodoform gauze saturated with an antibiotic ointment such as aureomycin or bacitracin. The packing not only controls the bleeding but also averts such potential complications as stenosis of the ear canal and perichondritis. After emergency treatment, the patient should be referred to an otolaryngologist. The packing should be left in for 2–3 weeks or until healing is complete.

Eardrum

Traumatic perforation of the eardrum usually occurs when a cotton-tipped applicator, bobby pin, or small stick inadvertently penetrates deeply into the ear canal and lacerates the drum. A slap to the ear and slag burns in welders also cause traumatic perforation. The patient should be questioned about hearing loss, pain, and vertigo. All debris and blood should be removed from the ear canal with a small metal suction tip. Irrigation with water is contraindicated. When the eardrum is inspected, an irregular tear is usually visible; it may be actively bleeding. The hearing should be tested with tuning fork and voice tests. A patient with a perforated eardrum may have conductive or sensorineural hearing loss or both. The eyes should be observed for nystagmus, and the fistula test performed. The patient's balance should be tested by heel-toe walking and the station test (Romberg's test).

Emergency referral to an otolaryngologist is indicated in the case of vertigo, major hearing loss, or a positive fistula test. Ear drops should not be instilled. The patient can be treated with intramuscular prochlorperazine maleate (Compazine) for nausea and vomiting.

Most perforations heal spontaneously.

Temporal Bone

Temporal bone fracture may be an isolated injury, but is more often one of many fractures present in a person with severe multiple injuries. A conscious patient with only a fractured temporal bone may complain of pain, bloody discharge from the ear, decreased hearing, and vertigo. On physical examination, ecchymoses behind the ear and over the mastoid tip (Battle's sign) may be noted, as well as laceration of the ear canal or eardrum, nystagmus, and weakness or complete paralysis of the facial muscles. The patient may complain of vertigo, nausea, and vomiting. Tests may reveal conductive or sensorineural hearing loss or both.

Before treatment of temporal bone fracture is begun, the physician should first exclude other serious injuries, including fracture of the cervical spine, obstruction of the airway, or major trauma to the chest and abdomen. A patient with cerebrospinal fluid (CSF) otorrhea should be hospitalized and treated with application of a gauze dressing to absorb drainage and with administration of systemic antibiotics. An otolaryngologist should be consulted as soon as possible after injury to complete the evaluation of such a patient.

Pain or Discharge

Local Pain

External Otitis. This condition is manifested by 1–3 days of progressive itch, pain, and discharge, sometimes with diminished hearing. The patient should be questioned about trauma to, or a foreign body in, the ear canal. On physical examination, pressure on the tragus or auricular cartilage produces pain. The ear canal is erythematous and swollen; it may be filled with debris, obscuring the eardrum. In more advanced cases, periauricular cellulitis and regional lymphadenopathy occurs. Conductive hearing loss may develop. Often, both ears are involved.

The keystone of therapy is removal of debris from the ear canal by means of a suction apparatus and a narrow metal suction tip. Examiners unfamiliar with the use of the head mirror (Fig. 42.2) can utilize a hand otoscope, suctioning through the speculum. If a foreign body is encountered, it should be removed by means of suction, a wire loop curette, or ear forceps. Any abscess in the ear canal should be incised for drainage. If the ear canal is of normal diameter, the patient may be treated with antibiotic drops, 3–4 drops four times a day for 10 days. If the ear canal is narrowed, a wick should be inserted to ensure adequate distribution of the antibiotic drops. A simple method is to insert a 2-inch strip of 0.25 inch iodoform gauze saturated with antibiotic drops by means of a small bayonet forceps. Systemic antibiotics are not indicated unless the patient has periauricular cellulitis or regional lymphadenitis; penicillin is the usual drug of choice for an outpatient. A patient with severe perichondritis of the pinna should be hospitalized and treated with intravenous antibiotics. Since external otitis can be extremely painful, a moderately strong analgesic should be prescribed for 48–72 hours. For at least 1 month after treatment, the patient should keep the affected ear protected from water during showering or hair washing by means of a cotton ball saturated with petrolatum. Simple external otitis with minimal edema of the ear canal usually does not require

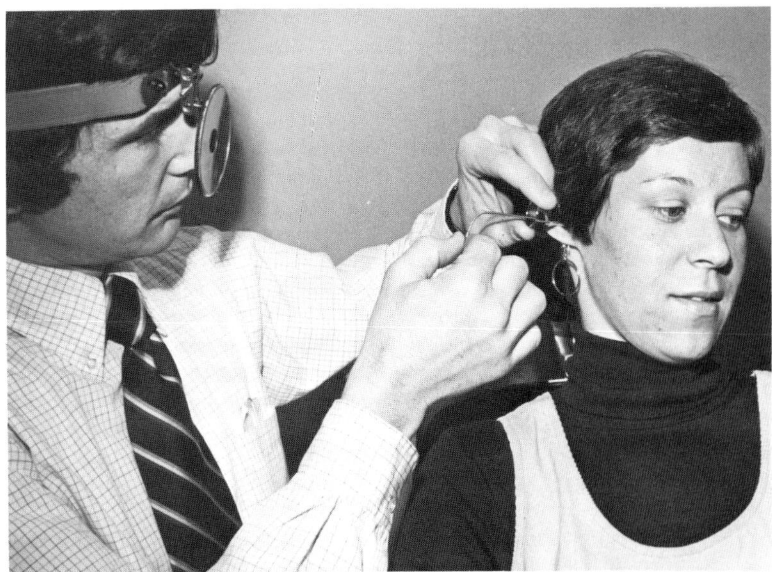

Figure 42.2. Use of ear speculum and suction for examination and cleansing of ear canal. A head mirror or head light may be used.

follow-up care. If a wick has been placed in the ear, the patient should remove it after 48 hours and continue using drops for a total of 10 days, at which time he should be seen by an otolaryngologist.

In diabetic patients, external otitis may be more severe. A well-recognized entity, *malignant external otitis* must be considered if external otitis has failed to resolve after 1–2 weeks of routine care. The patient with malignant external otitis experiences severe pain below the ear canal and in the parotid region anterior to the tragus. Granulation tissue may be evident, usually in the inferior or anterior portion of the ear canal. Malignant external otitis is life-threatening, requiring immediate hospitalization and intensive antibiotic therapy with gentamicin and carbenicillin, or their equivalent, since *Pseudomonas* is the usual infecting organism. Débridement is often needed.

Otitis Media. Usually, an upper respiratory tract infection precedes otitis media, but it may arise without previous illness. This disease occurs at any age, but is most common in children. Pain is usually constant, lasting from hours to days, and may be exacerbated by lying down. The pain may clear after a sudden discharge of purulent material from the ear canal, signifying spontaneous rupture of the tympanic membrane.

A special form of otitis media, aerotitis occurs after sudden barometric pressure changes, especially in persons with nasal congestion from a cold, allergy, or upper respiratory tract infection. Usually the patient experiences severe pain on descent either in an airplane or during deep-sea diving.

In *acute otitis media,* the landmarks of the eardrum are frequently distorted by erythema, thickening, and bulging of the drum. The skin of the ear canal may appear macerated. Conductive hearing loss is usually present. If the tympanic membrane has perforated, a pulsating discharge may be seen.

The eardrum in a patient with *aerotitis* may be red, purple, or almost black if hemotympanum exists. As in acute otitis media, conductive hearing loss may or may not be significant. The appearance of red or yellowish bullous eruptions on the surface of the eardrum signifies *bullous myringitis.* When the bullae are ruptured, clear fluid is noted. *In serous otitis,* the eardrum may vary in color from gray to blue to yellow. The drum may be retracted, and air-fluid levels (bubbles) may be visualized behind it. Blood vessels on its surface may be dilated, giving the appearance of erythema.

In children less than 6 years old, the antibiotic of choice is amoxicillin, 125–250 mg every 8 hours orally for 10 days. In the penicillin-allergic patient, a combination of erythromycin and sulfisoxazole should be used. In older children and in adults, penicillin, 400,000 units four times a day orally for 10 days, is the drug of choice; in penicillin-allergic patients, erythromycin alone should be sufficient. Nasal decongestant agents in liquid or tablet form should be used for 2 weeks. Moderately strong systemic analgesic medications are often indicated for the first 2 or 3 days until infection subsides. There is some disagreement concerning the value of myringotomy in acute otitis media. Myringotomy of a bulging eardrum can relieve severe pain; a patient with only mild to moderate pain may not require this procedure. When myringotomy is necessary, the incision should be made in the anterior inferior quadrant of the eardrum to avoid the ossicles and the facial nerve (Fig. 42.3).

Chronic otitis media may be difficult to diagnose. Some patients have an intermittent foul-smelling discharge from the affected ear, vertigo, a progressive conductive hearing loss, or facial paralysis. Others are asymptomatic. The eardrum may be intact; the only evidence for the disease may be squamous debris or cholesteatoma in the pars flaccida of the eardrum. The diagnosis is made easier when there is a chronic drainage perforation of the drum. The patient with uncomplicated chronic otitis media should be referred to an otolaryngologist.

Complications of Otitis Media. *Mastoiditis* may occur 1–2 weeks after acute otitis media. The most common symptom is persistent discharge from the affected ear. Ordinarily, pain is not significant; when it is present, abscess formation should be suspected. On physical examination of a patient with mastoiditis secondary to acute otitis, a small perforation in the eardrum with purulent discharge can often be seen. Tenderness is elicited on palpation in the postauricular region and commonly over the mastoid tip, where the skin may be thickened. The patient may have a slightly elevated temperature, but frequently does not seem extremely ill. Severe pain and tenderness or systemic toxemia suggest any one of the complications of mastoiditis. In a patient with manifestations of chronic otitis media, such as chronic perforation, chronic drainage, or cholesteatoma, mastoiditis can occur at any time and can develop into any of several conditions mentioned in the following paragraph. In a patient with mastoiditis complicating chronic otitis media, a large perforation or a cholesteatoma may be apparent. There may or may not be foul-smelling drainage from the ear. Tenderness of the mastoid tip and hearing loss are sometimes present. The emergency physician should consult an otolaryngologist immediately. In the interim, x-ray views of the mastoid bone may be obtained.

Further complications of otitis media result from extension of the disease process to involve adjacent structures. All require immediate evaluation by an otolaryngologist. *Subperiosteal abscess,* an exten-

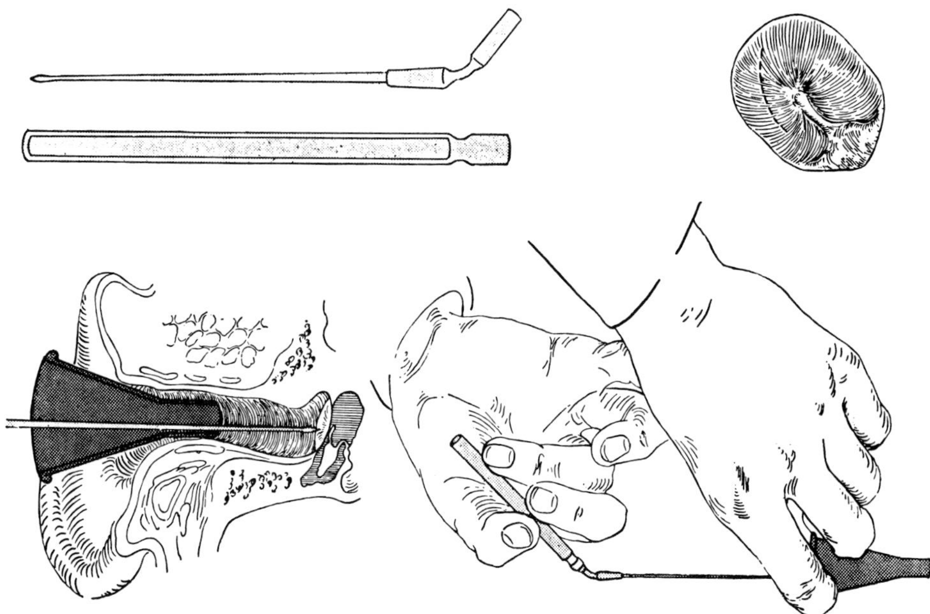

Figure 42.3. Myringotomy. Illumination is provided by head light or mirror, and an anterior inferior incision is made in eardrum with sharp myringotomy knife. (Reproduced by permission, from Boies LR. *Fundamentals of Otolaryngology: A Textbook of Ear, Nose and Throat Diseases*, 5th ed. Philadelphia: WB Saunders, 1978).

sion of infection within the mastoid bone to the mastoid tip (Bezold's abscess) or to the root of the zygomatic bone, produces pain, swelling, and tenderness in these areas. An *epidural abscess* occurring in either the middle or the posterior cranial fossa produces symptoms of localized headache, fever, and meningismus. Signs of increased intracranial pressure may also be present. *Cerebellar* or *temporal lobe abscess* may develop following otitis media and may produce the typical signs of mass lesions in these areas. *Gradenigo's syndrome* is the result of an abscess or osteomyelitis at the apex of the petrous portion of the temporal bone, and consists of a chronically draining ear with ipsilateral abducens nerve palsy and pain behind the ipsilateral orbit. In *meningitis* following acute otitis media, the usual infecting organism is either a Gram-positive coccus or *Haemophilus influenzae*. Meningitis is a rare complication of chronic otitis media; when it occurs, the agent is usually a gram-negative organism. Initial management should be directed at identifying the organism and treating the meningitis (see Chapter 11). Once the meningitis is under control, the otologic disease should be treated. *Cavernous sinus thrombosis* is typified by spiking fever, obtundation, and increased intracranial pressure occurring in the course of acute or chronic otitis media. Treatment consists of controlling the septic process with intravenous antibiotics. An otolaryngologist should be consulted regarding early operation to drain the infected thrombus.

Tumor. Aural tumors may produce pain; usually a mass is noted on examination. After the diagnosis is made, the patient should be referred to an otolaryngologist.

Referred Pain

Pain resulting from a distant pathologic process may be felt in the ear. The source of the pain may be a lesion of a tooth, the temporomandibular joint, the pharynx, the larynx, or the neck; the pain of sinus conditions may likewise be felt in the ear. Uncommon sources of referred pain to the ear include lesions in the distribution of cranial nerves IX and X, such as those of the thyroid gland, chest, and abdomen. Some of the conditions in which pain is referred to the ear are detailed below; the remainder are treated in other sections of this chapter.

In the case of a *dental lesion,* the affected tooth may often be asymptomatic; yet, constant pain may be felt deep in the ear for days or weeks. Physical examination reveals a normal ear with no hearing loss; examination of the mouth often demonstrates a decaying tooth that is tender to pressure or percussion. Gingivitis or a dental abscess may be visible. These patients should be referred to a dentist.

The chief symptom of the *temporomandibular joint syndrome* is a sharp pain related to chewing. The patient may have a history of recent injury to the jaw, recent dental work, or long-standing malocclusion. Most patients with this syndrome are women between the ages of 20 and 40. Often the problem is a manifestation of emotional stress and is the result of constant clenching of the jaw muscles. On physical examination, malocclusion may be obvious. The physician may elicit tenderness over the temporomandibular joint, especially when the mouth is open, and swelling may be noted. Limited motion of the temporomandibular joint and crepitation may be demonstrated. Complications of this syndrome include chronic disability from pain and the development of arthritic changes. The patient should be instructed to eat soft foods, apply heat locally, and take buffered aspirin, two tablets four times a day. If the symptoms are unrelieved, the patient should be referred to an oral surgeon or a dentist.

Acute Hearing Loss

Conductive Loss

Table 42.1 outlines the differential diagnosis of conductive and sensorineural hearing loss. Ear canal obstruction causing acute conductive hearing loss is discussed in the following section; other causes such as penetrating trauma and acute or chronic otitis media are discussed elsewhere in this chapter.

Obstruction of Ear Canal. A patient with obstruction of the ear by cerumen or a foreign body has diminished hearing and a sensation of fullness or pain in the affected ear. There may be discharge from the ear with associated external otitis. The physical examination reveals the obstruction or external otitis or both. A foreign body may be obscured by infection. Treatment consists of removal of the obstruction and management of external otitis. Liquid dioctyl sodium sulfosuccinate (Colace), 10–20 drops in the ear canal for 15 minutes, often softens hardened cerumen. If the first few attempts to remove the obstruction are unsuccessful or if edema of the ear canal and hemorrhage are already present, the patient should be referred to an otolaryngologist.

Sensorineural Loss

Exertional Loss. An otologic emergency, the sudden onset of significant hearing loss after exertion is associated with a sensation of fullness in the

Table 42.1.
Acute Hearing Loss: Differential Diagnosis Aid

	Conductive	Sensorineural
Symptoms		
Hearing abnormality	Sudden sensation of blockage Hollow feeling in ear	Loss of hearing Fullness in ear Tinnitus Abnormal sensitivity to loud sounds
Pain	Often present	Uncommon
Vertigo	Infrequent	Often present
Related problems	Acute infection Trauma Obstruction of eustachian tube Upper respiratory tract infection Allergy Trauma (penetrating or blunt) Skull fracture	Diabetes Arteriosclerotic occlusive disease Hyperlipidemia Ménière's disease Hypercoagulable state Trauma (labyrinthine concussion or temporal bone fracture)
Physical examination		
Ear canal	Occluded or infected	Normal
Ear drum	Infected or perforated	Normal
Hearing tests		
Voice test	Slight or moderate hearing loss	Decreased hearing or total hearing loss
Rinne's test	Negative in affected ear	Positive in affected ear or false-negative
Weber's test	Sound heard in affected ear	Sound may be heard in unaffected ear or midline
Laboratory tests to be ordered if indicated	Culture discharge if present Temporal bone x-ray film if blunt trauma Audiometric examination	Fasting blood glucose test Fluorescent treponemal antibody-absorption test for syphilis (FTA-ABS) Serum cholesterol test Partial thromboplastin time Platelet count Temporal bone x-ray film if blunt trauma Bárány's caloric test Audiometric examination

ear and tinnitus, transient or persistent vertigo, nausea, and vomiting. Frequently, the exertion involves activities, such as lifting, pushing, or straining in such a way as to create an increase in CSF pressure that is transmitted through the cochlear aqueduct, causing rupture of the inner ear membranes or the oval and round windows. On physical examination, the patient may have obvious dysequilibrium with nystagmus. On testing of hearing, a partial or total sensorineural hearing loss with a normal eardrum may be noted. The major complication is permanent total hearing loss in the affected ear. Patients with this condition should be evaluated by an otolaryngologist immediately for consideration of an urgent exploratory operation. Some advocate nonoperative treatment with hospitalization and 4–5 days of total bed rest.

Postoperative Loss. Any patient with recent operation on the ear who has a loss of hearing or vertigo should be referred immediately to his aural surgeon. Exploratory reoperation may be necessary, especially in a patient with a recent stapedectomy.

Other Causes. Patients with some or all of the typical signs and symptoms of sensorineural impairment described in Table 42.1 require early evaluation, including audiometric study by an otolaryngologist. Mechanisms of this hearing loss include trauma, infection, tumor, systemic disease, and ototoxic drugs; occasionally no mechanism is identified.

Noise trauma resulting from any sound in excess of 100 decibels, especially explosive noise such as gunfire, may cause a temporary or permanent hearing loss. There is no treatment available. Prevention should be practiced by employing adequate sound protection.

Infectious processes can cause acute sensorineural hearing loss, such as that occurring during or after a viral upper respiratory tract infection. In children, unilateral deafness may be caused by the mumps virus. Another specific viral illness, herpes zoster oticus is manifested by painful herpetic lesions of the external ear, with occasional associated facial paralysis. Hearing loss and facial paralysis caused by herpesvirus are untreatable at present, although an involved eye should be protected. Sudden unilateral sensorineural hearing loss accompanied by severe vertigo may occur during bacterial acute otitis media and signifies invasion of the labyrinth. Since the labyrinthine fluid is in direct communication with the subarachnoid space, meningitis is a potential complication. Intensive antibiotic therapy is necessary, and myringotomy is also indicated.

Tumors of the temporal bone are an uncommon cause of sensorineural hearing loss. Tumors in this group include vestibular schwannoma, congenital cholesteatoma, glomus jugulare tumor, and other rare tumors including leukemic infiltrates and metastatic lesions from the breast, kidney, and lung.

Sensorineural hearing loss may be one of the symptoms of *Ménière's disease;* others include tinnitus, aural pressure, and vertigo. These symptoms fluctuate in intensity and degree. There may be a hiatus of many years between attacks, or they may recur often. Vertigo may be mild to severe; attacks usually last from 1–4 hours. Droperidol has been effective in the management of the severe nausea and vertigo of Ménière's disease; the dosage is 2.5 mg every 4–6 hours administered intramuscularly.

Sudden sensorineural hearing loss associated with *diabetes mellitus* probably reflects occlusion of small vessels (diabetic microangiopathy); anticoagulation with heparin may be considered, and the underlying disease should be treated. *Degenerative diseases,* such as multiple sclerosis, syphilis (tertiary and congenital), and collagen disease may cause sudden hearing loss. If syphilis is suspected, serologic studies including the fluorescent treponemal antibody-absorption test (FTA-ABS) should be performed. This is one of the few forms of sensorineural hearing loss that responds to treatment. When the diagnosis is made, treatment with corticosteroids and penicillin are initiated.

Toxic substances also cause sensorineural hearing loss. The most common toxins are antibiotic and diuretic medications, listed in Table 42.2. Sudden hearing loss may also occur in adults without obvious cause. The emergency physician should exclude all the previously mentioned conditions, and an otolaryngologist should be consulted. At present, there is no well-defined treatment for this entity; vasodilators, anticoagulants, and high-dose corticosteroids have been used without statistically proved benefit.

Table 42.2.
Toxic Agents Causing Hearing Loss

Antibiotics (mostly aminoglycosides)
Streptomycin
Gentamicin
Neomycin sulfate
Kanamycin sulfate
Viomycin
Chloramphenicol
Diuretics
Ethacrynic acid
Furosemide
Others
Quinine
Salicylates
Nitrogen mustard
Phenylbutazone
Tetanus antitoxin (serum sickness—rare)

Acute Vertigo

The diagnostic evaluation of patients with vertigo is challenging. The differential diagnosis between peripheral vertigo (caused within the temporal bone) and central vertigo (caused within the central nervous system or cardiovascular system) is found in Table 42.3. Differentiation between the two major sources of vertigo often rests on the subtle differences in history, clinical examination, and ancillary studies. If no diagnosis is readily apparent, the patient's symptoms should be treated and he or she should be referred for further evaluation to an internist, an otolaryngologist, or a neurologist, depending on the general impression of the diagnosis.

Peripheral Vertigo

Peripheral vertigo can be caused by several conditions that have been mentioned, such as external otitis, otitis media, serous otitis, Ménière's disease, and trauma. It may also occur following an ear operation, in which case the surgeon should be immediately consulted. Other conditions involving peripheral vertigo are discussed in the following sections.

Complications of Chronic Otitis Media. A patient with *labyrinthitis* usually has a sensation of light-headedness or vertigo. If labyrinthitis is severe, vertigo may be constant. On examination, the affected ear may have an obvious foul-smelling discharge or a dry cholesteatoma. The patient may be nauseated and vomiting; nystagmus that is usually directed toward the affected ear may also be present.

Symptoms may be relieved by meclizine hydrochloride, 25 mg orally every 4–6 hours, or prochlorperazine maleate, 10–15 mg orally every 4–6 hours or 5–10 mg intramuscularly every 4–6 hours. If the ear is draining, antibiotic ear drops are indicated, 4 drops four times a day. Systemic antibiotics are probably not beneficial. The patient should be referred without delay to an otolaryngologist.

Erosion due to chronic infection or cholesteatoma that gradually exposes the membranes of the semicircular canal gives rise to a *labyrinthine fistula.* The patient may state that he or she becomes dizzy when placing a finger in the ear canal of the affected ear, and he or she may demonstrate dysequilibrium and nystagmus. The fistula test is often positive, and conductive hearing loss is frequently present. These patients should be referred immediately to an otolaryngologist.

A patient with *cerebellar abscess* related to chronic or acute otitis media has signs of a cerebellar lesion, such as dysarthria, headache, and loss of coordinated movement on the side of the affected ear. Physical examination demonstrates ipsilateral muscular incoordination and increased ipsilateral tendon reflexes. Signs of increased intracranial pressure may be noted as well as abnormal patterns of nystagmus. These patients should be referred immediately for otologic and neurosurgical consultation.

Benign Positional Vertigo. A patient with this condition usually experiences 1- to 3-minute episodes of severe spinning vertigo commonly precipitated by movement of the head either to the side or backward. Occasionally, the patient has had an infection of the upper respiratory tract or trauma to the head; more often these symptoms occur without prior illness. Physical examination reveals normal findings with the exception of rotatory nystagmus on position testing. The diagnosis of benign positional vertigo is based on the position test and includes the following findings:

1. Delay in the onset of nystagmus (5–10 seconds) when the patient is placed in the head-hanging position.
2. Rotatory nystagmus, reproduced whenever the patient is placed in the stimulating position.
3. Reverse of direction of nystagmus when the patient is brought upright.
4. Fatigability of nystagmus after three or four repetitions of the position test.

The patient should be instructed to avoid positions that cause vertigo and situations in which a vertiginous attack would cause danger, such as driving, working on scaffolding, or in other elevated areas. A trial course of meclizine hydrochloride, 25 mg every 6 hours, may be given; this occasionally provides symptomatic relief. The patient should be told that benign positional vertigo generally clears within 2–6 months. Patients with this problem should be referred to an otolaryngologist for complete evaluation.

Other Causes. A patient with *vestibular neuritis* usually has been unsteady and dizzy for a few days to several weeks with no change in hearing. This type of vertigo may appear in epidemic form, and in this form is usually of viral origin. Physical examination reveals normal hearing and normal aural structures with occasional spontaneous nystagmus. Treatment is directed toward relief of symptoms, since this is a self-limiting disease.

In general, drugs that cause acute hearing loss (Table 42.2) can also cause *acute toxic vertigo* that is also manifested by ataxia. In the case of gentamicin, a vestibular toxic reaction usually occurs before hearing loss. Physical examination may reveal a hearing deficit, spontaneous nystagmus, Romberg's sign, and sometimes ataxia.The causative drug should be discontinued as soon as possible,

Table 42.3.
Peripheral and Central Vertigo: Differential Diagnosis Aid

Manifestation	Peripheral	Central
Hearing loss	Common, often unilateral, lasting minutes to hours (fluctuating)	Rare, may be unilateral, lasting days or weeks
Tinnitus	Common	Rare
Aural pressure or sense of fullness	Common	Rare
Ear pain	Possible	Rare
Nausea and vomiting	Common	Possible, degree of dizziness may not correlate with degree of nausea and vomiting
Spontaneous nystagmus	Common, usually horizontal and away from affected ear	Common, usually bizarre (direction changing, up-beating)
Other cranial neuropathy	Rare	Common
Papilledema	None	Possible
Change in consciousness	None	Possible
Decrease in vision	None (subjective blurring)	Possible, especially with basilar arterial insufficiency
Headache	Rare	Possible
Positional nystagmus	Common (rotatory or horizontal)	Possible (may be bizarre with vertical component)
Recurrence	Common	Possible, especially with basilar arterial insufficiency

since permanent hearing loss and ataxia may result. On the other hand, any of these drugs are used for life-threatening illnesses, and a decision to discontinue them must be based on the clinical status of the patient.

Vertigo may be caused by *acute syphilitic labyrinthitis* of secondary syphilis or by inflammation of the osseous labyrinth from congenital syphilis. The diagnosis is made by means of a positive serum test for syphilis. Treatment includes administration of penicillin and corticosteroids.

Central Vertigo

Central vertigo, as manifested by signs and symptoms listed in Table 42.3, may be caused by several neurovascular lesions or states. Some of these, such as epilepsy and migraine headache, are discussed elsewhere (see Chapter 15); the remainder are treated as described in the following paragraphs.

Vertebrobasilar arterial insufficiency is often manifested by episodic attacks of vertigo. These attacks are usually associated with other symptoms, including visual "blackouts," dysarthria, headache, and muscular weakness; the patient may become unconscious. On physical examination the ear appears normal, and there may be variable nystagmus. The patient may exhibit the stigmata of peripheral arterial disease. The diagnosis is usually made from the history and the general appearance of the patient, who should be referred to an internist or a neurologist.

In the *subclavian steal syndrome,* the patient has a history of episodic vertigo and other symptoms of basilar arterial insufficiency, associated with cramping and tiredness in one arm. The patient may have a bruit over the subclavian artery and an occasional pulse deficit in the radial artery, especially with elevation of the affected arm. Patients with this syndrome should be referred to a vascular surgeon.

Usually, a patient with a *cerebrovascular accident* has experienced a catastrophic onset of acute vertigo with nausea and vomiting, cerebellar ataxia, dysarthria, and dysphagia. Physical examination reveals cerebellar ataxia, bizarre nystagmus, and lower cranial nerve palsies. The patient should be hospitalized with supportive measures, and a neurologist should be immediately consulted (see Chapter 15).

A *tumor of the cerebellopontine angle* causes unilateral sensorineural hearing loss with episodic or constant dizziness and sometimes an associated unilateral facial palsy. Physical examination may confirm all these findings, and an absent corneal reflex on the side of the lesion may be noted. These patients should be referred to an otolaryngologist.

A patient with *acute demyelinating disease* may have vertigo associated with other symptoms of neurologic disorder, such as diplopia, dysarthria, muscular weakness, and loss of bladder and bowel control. Bizarre nystagmus may be seen on physical examination. Such patients should be referred to a neurologist.

A *lowered effective blood volume* can cause dizziness. This is not true vertigo, but rather a light-

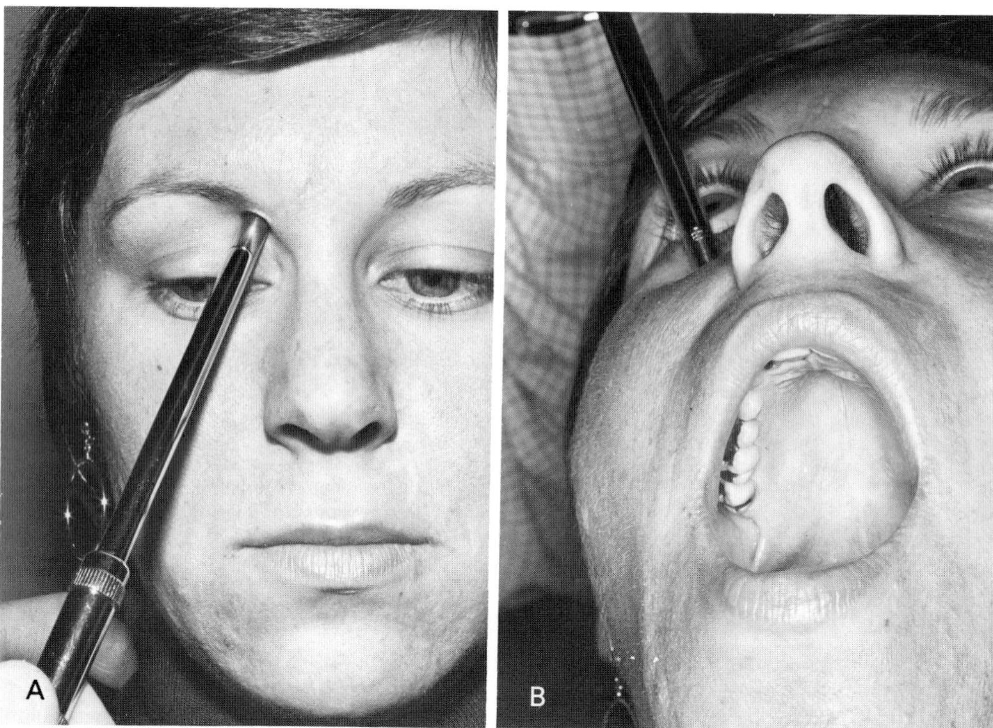

Figure 42.4. *A,* Transillumination of frontal sinus. Light source is placed deep to supraorbital rim. *B,* Transillumination of maxillary sinus. Light source is placed deep to infraorbital rim and light is viewed through palate. Totally darkened room is used.

headed feeling. Among conditions causing this symptom are cardiac arrhythmias, anemia, vasovagal attacks, and dehydration.

THE SINUSES AND FACE

Examination Technique

If a sinus condition is suspected, the physician should perform the following maneuvers. *Sinus transillumination* is performed in a darkened room with a narrow-beam light source, such as a penlight. The penlight is placed under each supraorbital rim to evaluate the frontal sinuses and over the infraorbital rims to evaluate the maxillary sinuses. Light transmitted through the palate is viewed through the open mouth. One side is compared with the other for the amount of light transmitted (Fig. 42.4). If the pattern of light transmission is asymmetric, the test is considered positive. Although this test is helpful in diagnosis and in follow-up evaluation, sinus x-ray views provide more accurate information (Fig. 42.5).

Keeping in mind the exquisite tenderness of acute sinus disease, the examiner should gently *palpate the sinuses.* The maxillary antrum is best evaluated by palpation over the canine fossa (Fig. 42.6*A*); the frontal sinus is examined by placing the finger just deep to the suproaorbital rim (Fig. 42.6*B*).

Facial Pain

Sinusitis

Sinusitis may occur as a complication of an acute upper respiratory tract infection or of allergic rhinitis. The pain is often described as steady pressure, or throbbing, and it may be severe. It may be experienced in the anterior part of the face, behind the orbits, or in the vertex or occiput of the skull. Typically, the pain is exacerbated by hanging the head down and is most pronounced in the afternoon or evening. Purulent nasal discharge may be present.

Acute aerosinusitis occurs during flight in persons with an upper respiratory tract infection or allergic diathesis. Preexistent local edema obstructs the sinus ostia, and painful hemorrhage into the sinus mucosa results from rapid pressure changes during descent.

The patient with sinusitis may have only a mildly elevated temperature. Localized swelling over the involved sinus may be visualized, and palpation of the anterior aspect of the maxillary antrum or of the floor of the frontal sinus may elicit tenderness. Intranasal examination may reveal purulent mucus drainage from the sinus ostium, but the absence of discharge does not exclude sinusitis. During the intranasal examination the examiner should search for nasal polyps, a foreign body, or tumor as a possible cause for sinusitis. Because infection in the upper teeth can cause symptoms similar to those of maxillary sinusitis, the mouth should be carefully examined and each tooth palpated. Transillumination of the sinuses may demonstrate a unilateral opacification, further aiding in diagnosis. Sinus x-ray films are indicated to determine the extent of disease and to establish a baseline for follow-up care.

Complications of Sinusitis. Occasionally seen in the emergency department, these conditions all require immediate hospitalization under the care of an otolaryngologist. During the course of sinusitis, usually ethmoid, *orbital cellulitis* may develop. This complication is suggested by worsening pain in and behind the eye, with erythema and swelling of the upper and lower lids, proptosis, chemosis, and decreasing ocular mobility. Vision may deteriorate. The end stage of orbital cellulitis, an *orbital abscess* is suggested by a fixed eye and rapidly deteriorating vision. A patient with this condition should be referred to an otolaryngologist and an ophthalmologist for consideration of urgent decompression of the orbit via a transethmoidal approach. Uncommon in the antibiotic era, *osteomyelitis of the skull* usually occurs as a complication of frontal sinusitis. Typically, the patient has puffy swelling of the brow over the frontal sinus and a localized fron-

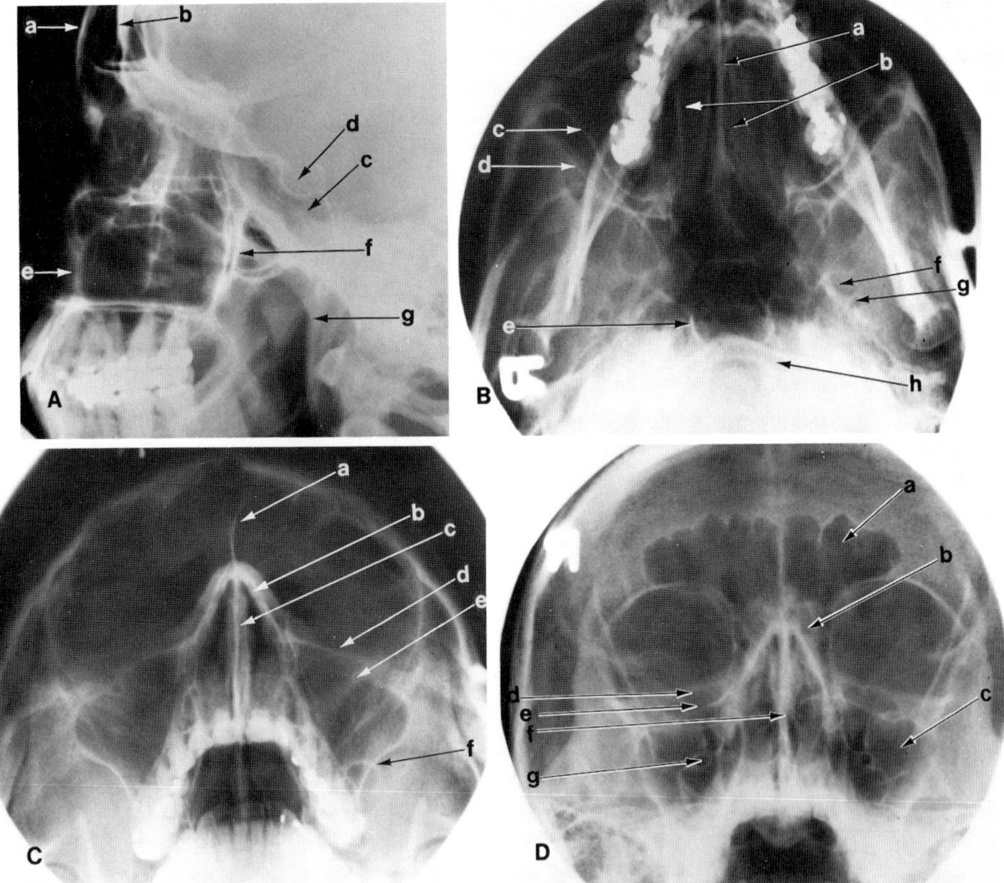

Figure 42.5. *A,* Lateral x-ray view of normal sinuses. *a,* Frontal sinus—anterior wall; *b,* frontal sinus—posterior wall; *c,* sphenoid sinus; *d,* pituitary fossa; *e,* maxillary antrum—anterior wall; *f,* maxillary antrum—posterior wall; *g,* nasopharynx—posterior wall. *B,* Basal x-ray view of normal sinuses. *a,* Nasal septum; *b,* nasal turbinates; *c,* antrum—posterior wall; *d,* orbit—lateral wall; *e,* wall of sphenoid sinus; *f,* foramen ovale; *g,* foramen spinosum; *h,* first cervical vertebra. *C,* Waters' x-ray view of normal sinuses. *a,* Frontal sinus; *b,* nasal arch; *c,* nasal septum; *d,* orbital rim; *e,* infraorbital foramen; *f,* antrum—lateral wall. *D,* Caldwell x-ray view of normal sinuses. *a,* Frontal sinus; *b,* ethmoid sinus; *c,* antral sinus; *d,* orbital rim; *e,* orbital floor; *f,* nasal septum; *g,* foramen rotundum.

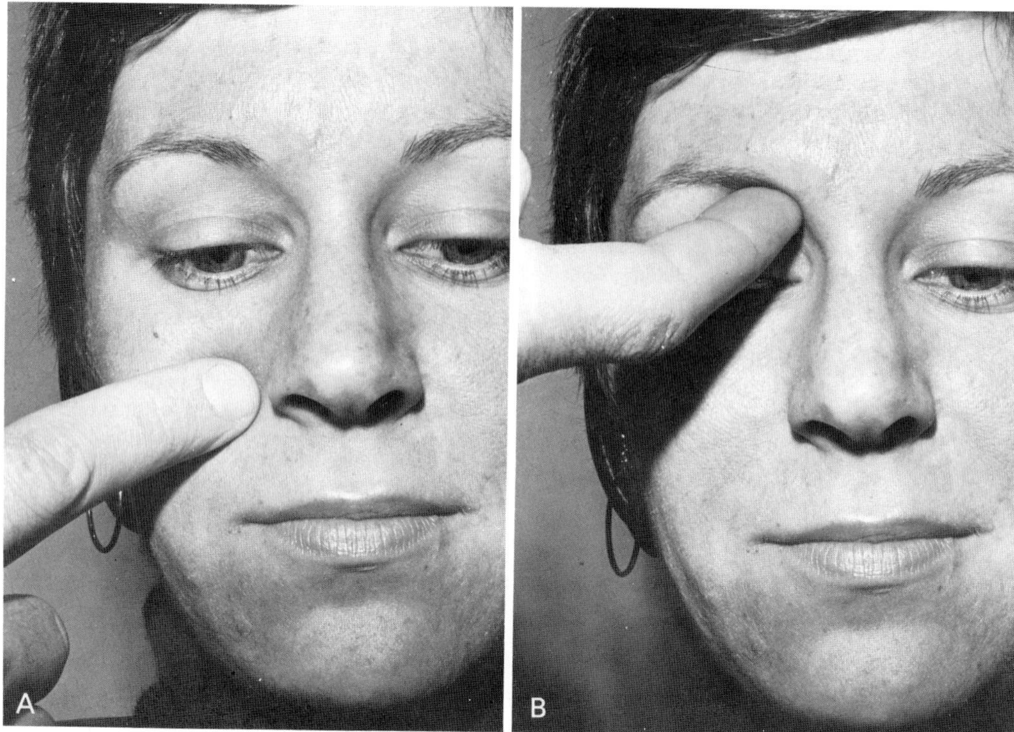

Figure 42.6. *A,* Palpation of maxillary antrum. *B,* Palpation deep to supraorbital rim to demonstrate tenderness of frontal sinus.

tal headache. Treatment includes hospitalization with intensive antibiotic therapy. Operative drainage of the sinus and débridement of dead bone may also be necessary. When uncontrolled sinus disease extends to the central nervous system, *meningitis, epidural abscess, brain abscess,* and *cavernous sinus thrombosis* can all occur.

In cases of uncomplicated sinusitis, emergency care consists of the following measures. If obvious purulent mucus is apparent in the nose, specimens for culture and sensitivity testing should be obtained. Sinus x-ray films should be ordered, and if a complication involving the eye is suggested, an ophthalmologist should be consulted. Local heat should be applied, and medications should be administered as follows:

1. *Antibiotics.* In an adult, penicillin or erythromycin should be administered orally, 250 mg four times a day for 10 days. In a child who weighs less than 20 kg, oral amoxicillin should be prescribed, 20 mg/kg/day divided into 8-hour doses for 10 days. In a penicillin-allergic child, erythromycin and sulfisoxazole are administered in combination in appropriate doses for weight for 10 days.
2. *Decongestants.* In an adult, any long-acting combination of antihistamines and decongestants is administered for 10–20 days. For a child, a similar medication in liquid form for 10–20 days is usually adequate.
3. *Nasal drops or spray.* For an adult, oxymetazoline hydrochloride (Afrin) or phenylephrine hydrochloride (Neo-Synephrine) spray is prescribed, to be applied in each nostril three times a day for a week. Phenylephrine hydrochloride (Neo-Synephrine) nasal drops (0.125% or 0.25%), 3 drops/day for a week, is sufficient for a child. The patient or the parents should be warned that use of nasal drops for more than 1 week may cause rebound nasal swelling.
4. *Analgesics.* Both adults and children may need moderately high doses of analgesic medications for the first few days of treatment.

Other Causes of Facial Pain

Acute unilateral facial pain in the absence of sinusitis suggests a pathologic process involving cranial nerve V. Neurologic disease such as tic douloureux or herpes zoster must be considered. If anesthesia is present in the area of pain, an exhaustive workup is indicated to search for an occult neoplasm involving the affected branch of the trigeminal nerve.

Facial Swelling

Facial swelling may be produced by several conditions. Swelling caused by sinus disease has been discussed. The following sections detail other conditions that give rise to the symptom.

Allergic Reactions

A patient with facial swelling may have been exposed to a known allergen or may have been bitten by an insect. Facial swelling occurring with a generalized allergic reaction may involve varying degrees of edema of the eyelids, the conjunctivae, the oropharynx, and occasionally the larynx. The eyes may sometimes close completely, and the upper airway may become obstructed. In addition to airway obstruction, another potential complication of a generalized allergic reaction is anaphylactic shock.

If the swelling is due to an insect bite, the site will itch, but there are usually no systemic symptoms. In a child with swelling of one or both eyelids, sinusitis with periorbital cellulitis rather than an insect bite should be suspected.

Treatment depends on whether the swelling is due to a local bite or a generalized allergic reaction. In the former case, 1% hydrocortisone cream and an ice pack should be applied to the bite. Diphenhydramine hydrochloride (Benadryl) may be given intramuscularly or orally, adjusting the dosage for the patient's age. The adult dosage is 50 mg every 8 hours until the reaction subsides.

In the case of a systemic allergic reaction, initial treatment consists of administration of epinephrine (1:1000) intramuscularly or subcutaneously, 0.5 ml in an adult and an appropriate smaller dose in a child. In patients with anaphylactic shock, diphenhydramine hydrochloride and intravenous corticosteroids are suggested with ventilatory assistance and cardiac support as needed.

Angioneurotic Edema

A patient with this condition usually has had recurrent edema of the face, pharynx, and larynx developing over a few hours and sometimes progressing to cause respiratory obstruction. Endotracheal intubation may be necessary until resolution of the edema, which occurs as a rule in 24–72 hours, thus obviating tracheotomy. The condition is related to a deficiency in the complement system. Some centers are experimentally treating it with androgens, fresh frozen plasma, and ϵ-aminocaproic acid. Definitive medical treatment is not yet available.

Tumors and Chronic Conditions

In the patient who has experienced progressive localized facial swelling over a period of weeks or months, a chronic infectious process or tumor must be suspected. If swelling is in the supraorbital region, frontal sinus mucocele is the most common causative lesion, but a malignant condition of the frontal or ethmoid sinus must be considered. In the infraorbital region and the cheek, fibrous dysplasia and malignant tumors of the maxilla are the two most common neoplasms. In the mandible, neoplastic swelling is usually related to a dental cyst or an odontogenic tumor, but fibrous dysplasia and malignant lesions may also occur.

Swelling of the entire face and neck suggest the possibility of venous obstruction, as by mediastinal tumor.

Lesions in the Newborn

An infant up to 2 months old who exhibits swelling, erythema, and tenderness over the maxilla, and a high temperature may have osteomyelitis of the maxilla. On examination, swelling may extend to the medial canthus. In an advanced case, an abscess may be seen on the face, in the nose, or even on the palate, and pressure on the affected cheek may produce purulent discharge from the nose. Purulent material should be obtained for a Gram's stain, culture, and sensitivity testing. High-dose intravenous antibiotics should be instituted and later adjusted according to the culture and sensitivity reports; the usual causative organism is a staphylococcus. The patient should be hospitalized under the care of a pediatrician and an otolaryngologist.

Congenital facial lesions in a newborn may appear in several sites. A midline swelling of the nasal dorsum with or without a sinus tract suggests a dermoid cyst. Patients should be referred to an otolaryngologist for evaluation. Swelling in the region of the medial canthus suggests an encephalocele, a hemangioma, or a tumor of the lacrimal apparatus or sinuses. These infants should be evaluated by both an otolaryngologist and an ophthalmologist. Swelling in the parotid region may represent hemangioma or branchial cyst.

Facial Paralysis

Terminology and Testing

Any lesion of the facial nerve (Fig. 42.7) from its nucleus in the brainstem to the motor endplate is considered *peripheral.* A peripheral lesion usually causes total unilateral facial paralysis, except when the lesion is distal to the branching of the nerve within the parotid gland. A lesion proximal to the facial nerve nucleus in the brainstem is considered *central,* and causes ipsilateral weakness in the lower two-thirds of the face. The forehead is usually unaffected because of its bilateral crossed motor innervation.

There are numerous methods of testing the function of the facial nerve, but they are usually not

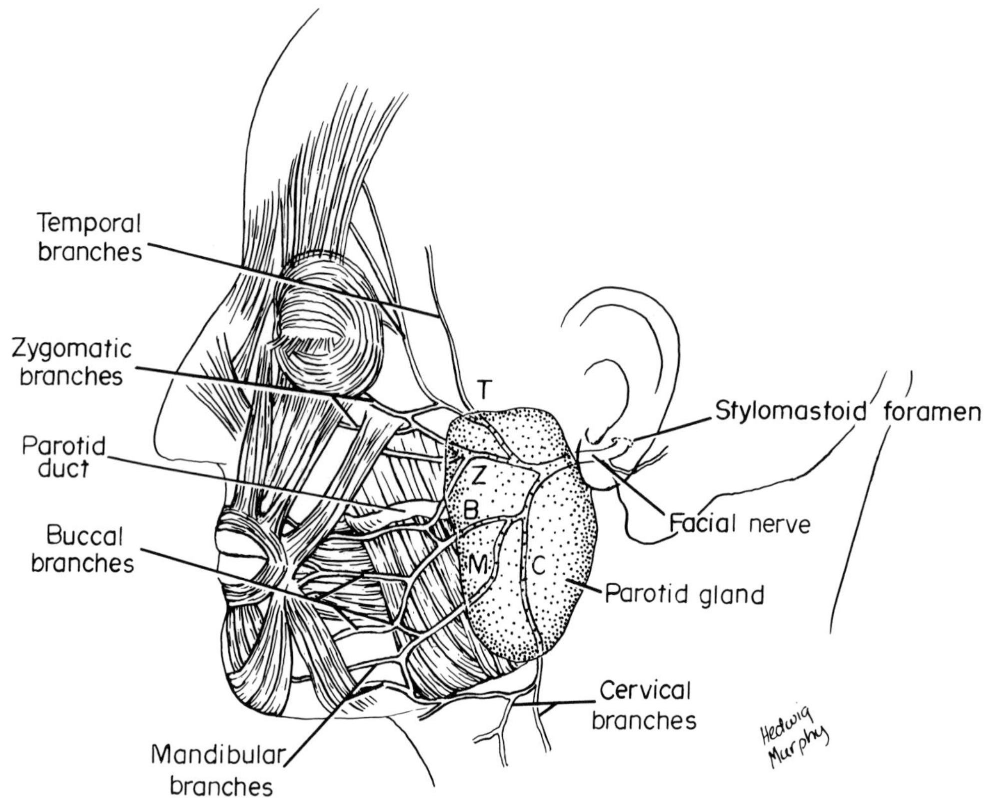

Figure 42.7. Extratemporal portion of facial nerve. Note exit at stylomastoid foramen, course through parotid gland, and relation to parotid duct.

performed by the emergency physician. In the emergency department, facial nerve weakness should be noted; the examiner should specify whether weakness is partial or complete, and whether it is evident in the upper, middle, or lower third of the face.

Common Disorders

Bell's Palsy. This condition is diagnosed by exclusion after the treatable causes of facial weakness discussed in this section are excluded. The patient experiences progression of unilateral facial weakness over 1–3 days, often associated with facial numbness and pain around the tip of the mastoid process. The patient may also experience ipsilateral facial pain. This condition may recur, and may involve both sides of the face. On examination, varying degrees of facial paralysis ranging from partial to complete are present. In a case of complete paralysis, Bell's phenomenon will occur: when the patient is asked to close the eye on the affected side, it closes incompletely and the globe rotates upward. In addition, the patient cannot elevate the eyebrow, wiggle the nose, whistle, or smile on the affected side. The ear should be examined to exclude lesions that might explain the facial paralysis.

The affected eye should be protected from the drying effects of constant corneal exposure by placing methylcellulose drops in the eye every 2–4 hours and taping down the eyelid during sleep. The patient should be referred to an otolaryngologist for complete evaluation. Controversy exists regarding the benefits of corticosteroid therapy and of surgical decompression. At present, we believe that surgical decompression for acute Bell's palsy is unwarranted, and we recommend a short course of oral corticosteroids.

Trauma. Crushing injury or sharp penetrating trauma distal to the stylomastoid foramen may involve the main trunk or the branches of the facial nerve, depending on the location of the injury. When evaluating a patient with midfacial penetrating trauma, the examiner should also consider laceration of the parotid duct and parotid gland. A patient with acute penetrating midfacial trauma with associated facial paralysis is a candidate for immediate operative exploration with suture of the nerve ends and repair of the parotid duct if necessary. Vigorous bleeding should be controlled preoperatively by pressure rather than by blind clamping, since the latter may result in damage to the facial nerve.

Temporal bone fracture may cause paralysis of cranial nerve VII. If immediate facial paralysis results from a temporal bone fracture, operative decompression of the nerve should be considered in patients whose condition is stable enough to permit anesthesia. An otolaryngologist should assist in any decision involving operation, since the timing of operation depends on the results of facial nerve testing by electrical stimulation and salivary flow tests.

Other Causes. Partial or complete facial paralysis may develop during *acute otitis media.* A patient with this complication should undergo immediate myringotomy. Facial paralysis should lessen as the ear infection resolves after antibiotic therapy. Facial paralysis in a patient with *chronic otitis media* usually progresses slowly over a few days. It may be partial or complete when the patient comes to the emergency department. The patient must be referred to an otolaryngologist for consideration of urgent operative decompression of the involved portion of the facial nerve. *Tuberculosis of the ear* causing chronic otitis media may produce facial paralysis and should be treated medically.

When *birth injury* resulting from prolonged labor or use of forceps causes complete facial paralysis, the infant should undergo surgical decompression of the nerve as soon as possible. Newborns are considered reasonable candidates for operation when they reach a weight of 4 kg. Other sources for neonatal facial paralysis include thalidomide injury and Treacher Collins' syndrome.

A patient with *herpes zoster oticus* (Ramsay Hunt's syndrome) has painful herpetic eruptions of the ear canal and auricle. Associated facial paralysis and occasional sensorineural hearing loss imply herpetic involvement of the ganglia of cranial nerves VII and VIII. There is no direct therapy for this problem; the only treatment is local skin care to prevent secondary infection, analgesia as indicated, and protection of the involved eye. The possible efficacy of acyclovir for this condition is yet to be determined. The patient should be referred to an otolaryngologist for follow-up care. Facial paralysis associated with facial pain is also consistent with a *malignant parotid tumor.* Frequently, this tumor can be palpated on physical examination. Patients should be referred to a head and neck surgeon.

Uncommon Disorders

Benign and malignant tumors of the temporal bone may cause paralysis of the facial nerve. A benign tumor of the vestibular nerve, *vestibular schwannoma,* may be manifested initially by facial paralysis, but the usual primary complaints are vertigo and sensorineural hearing loss. Patients in whom this lesion is suspected should be referred to an otolaryngologist for evaluation. Pulsatile tinnitus is the most prominent symptom in patients with a *glomus jugulare tumor.* Conductive hearing loss may be present, and facial paralysis may be a late symptom. Physical examination reveals a pulsatile reddish mass behind the eardrum. Cranial nerves IX, X, and XII may be involved; referral to an otolaryngologist is necessary. Other rare tumors of the temporal bone causing facial paralysis include *cholesteatoma, eosinophilic granuloma,* and *metastatic tumors,* most commonly from the breast, kidney, and lung. Radiologic examination reveals a lytic or blastic lesion of the temporal bone in this instance.

Disorders of the central nervous system, such as multiple sclerosis and other demyelinating diseases, stroke, and arachnoiditis may be manifested by facial paralysis, but usually other signs and symptoms make the diagnosis apparent.

Melkersson-Rosenthal syndrome is a rare condition beginning with swelling of the lip or palate or both, followed by bilateral facial paralysis. A markedly fissured tongue may be noted. This condition is typified by spontaneous regression and recurrence; it may respond to a short course of corticosteroids tapered over 1 week.

SALIVARY GLANDS AND FLOOR OF MOUTH

Trauma

Parotid Gland

In the case of blunt injury to the parotid gland (Fig. 42.8), hematoma, swelling, and abrasions are obvious. The examiner should bimanually palpate the cheek and mandible for possible associated fractures (Fig. 42.9*A*), and facial nerve function should be evaluated.

In an open injury, continuity of the parotid duct should be established. This duct is located along an imaginary line drawn from the tragus of the ear to the nasal vestibule. Continuity is examined by introducing a lacrimal probe into the oral opening of the parotid duct, which is adjacent to the second maxillary molar (Fig. 42.9*B*). Additional search should be made for associated facial fractures, dental injuries, and injuries to the major vessels of the upper neck.

In a victim of blunt trauma, the abraded skin should be thoroughly cleansed, débrided, and covered with antibiotic ointment and a sterile dressing. Cold compresses may reduce the swelling. Immediate total facial nerve paralysis suggests facial nerve avulsion at the stylomastoid foramen; an exploratory operation should be performed. If delayed facial paralysis develops, the patient should be

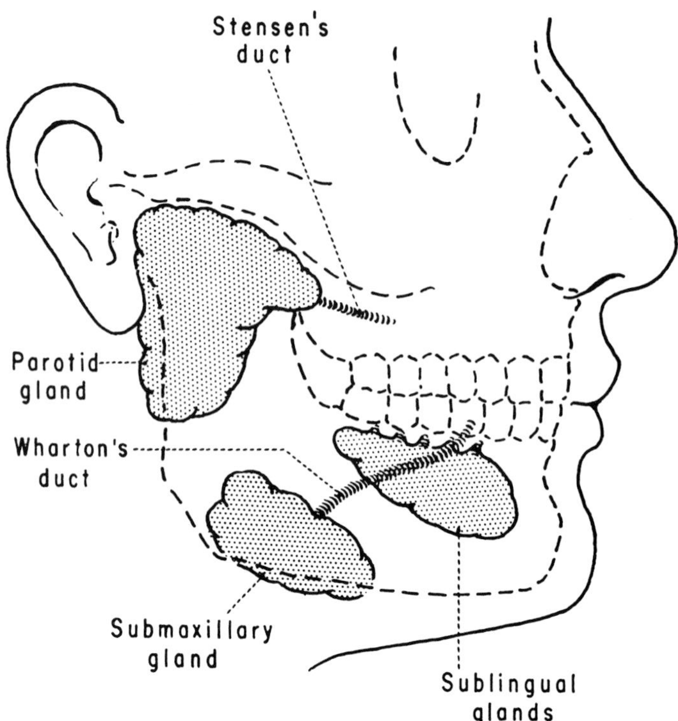

Figure 42.8. Location of major salivary glands and their ducts. (Reproduced by permission, from DeWeese, David D., and Saunders, William H.: *Textbook of Otolaryngology,* 6th ed. St. Louis, 1982, The C.V. Mosby Co.)

observed by an otolaryngologist, but operative exploration is not immediately indicated. Associated facial fractures should be managed as discussed in Chapter 39.

An open injury involving the parotid gland requires hospitalization for careful cleansing of the wound and meticulous operative closure including suture of the parotid duct and facial nerve if these structures are injured.

Submaxillary Gland

Although this gland is rarely involved in trauma because of its protected location, its duct may be lacerated by intraoral trauma or by extensive dislocation fractures of the jaw. Physical examination reveals the traumatic injury; anesthesia of the distal tongue resulting from lingual nerve injury may be associated.

An isolated laceration of the submaxillary duct may be treated expectantly since an intraoral fistula from the duct will probably develop spontaneously. In extensive injuries, the entire gland may be removed without significant loss of salivary function.

Pain and Swelling

Obstruction of Salivary Ducts

Patients with infection associated with a salivary calculus experience acute pain and swelling of the involved gland; previous episodes may be reported. On physical examination, the gland is swollen and tender, and erythema of the overlying skin may be seen. Bimanual palpation sometimes demonstrates a calculus in the duct of the affected gland. By introducing a lacrimal probe into the punctum of the duct (Fig. 42.9*B* and *D*), the physician may experience the gritty sensation of a calculus. Probing may also produce either clear secretions or purulent secretions; the latter should be cultured.

Patients with an infection should be treated with high doses of penicillin or erythromycin, analgesic medications, and hot packs over the affected gland. Any obviously fluctuant area along the duct should be drained intraorally either by probing the duct or by direct incision and drainage. If the calculus is readily approachable intraorally, it should be excised under local anesthesia and the duct should be left open as a permanent fistula. Calculi deeper in the salivary ducts require more extensive operative procedures under the care of an otolaryngologist or oral surgeon.

Infection

Mumps. Acute painful swelling of one or more salivary glands associated with a low-grade fever and malaise is typical of mumps. Viral involvement of the pancreas, gonads, and rarely the brain or heart can occur. Usually the patient is 5–12 years old and has a classic ''chipmunk'' appearance due to bilateral parotid and sometimes submaxillary swelling. In an adult, the gonads may be tender; signs of central nervous system involvement are rare. Treatment for mumps includes hydration and analgesic medications.

Acute Suppurative Parotitis. This condition usually occurs in elderly patients with severe general debility due to uncontrolled diabetes, dehydration, or cardiovascular disease. Progressive pain and swelling of the affected parotid gland occur over 1–3 days. On examination, the parotid gland is swollen and tender. The patient is often dehydrated and exhibits signs of septicemia. Poor dental hygiene and dehydration of the mouth are the usual underlying factors in this ascending infection of the parotid gland. Any discharge from the duct should be evaluated by Gram's stain, cultures, and sensitivity testing, and the patient should be hospitalized with general supportive therapy, including rehydration and control of any systemic condition, such as cardiovascular instability or diabetes. Specific treatment of acute parotitis includes intravenous administration of an antibiotic, such as a penicillinase-resistant penicillin. Incision and drainage of the infected parotid gland may be necessary. Acute suppurative parotitis signals a marked diminution of host defense mechanisms; this illness is often associated with terminal malignant disease.

Ludwig's Angina. Patients with this condition have a history of progressive pain and swelling in the tongue and floor of the mouth with dysphagia and respiratory obstruction. The tongue and floor

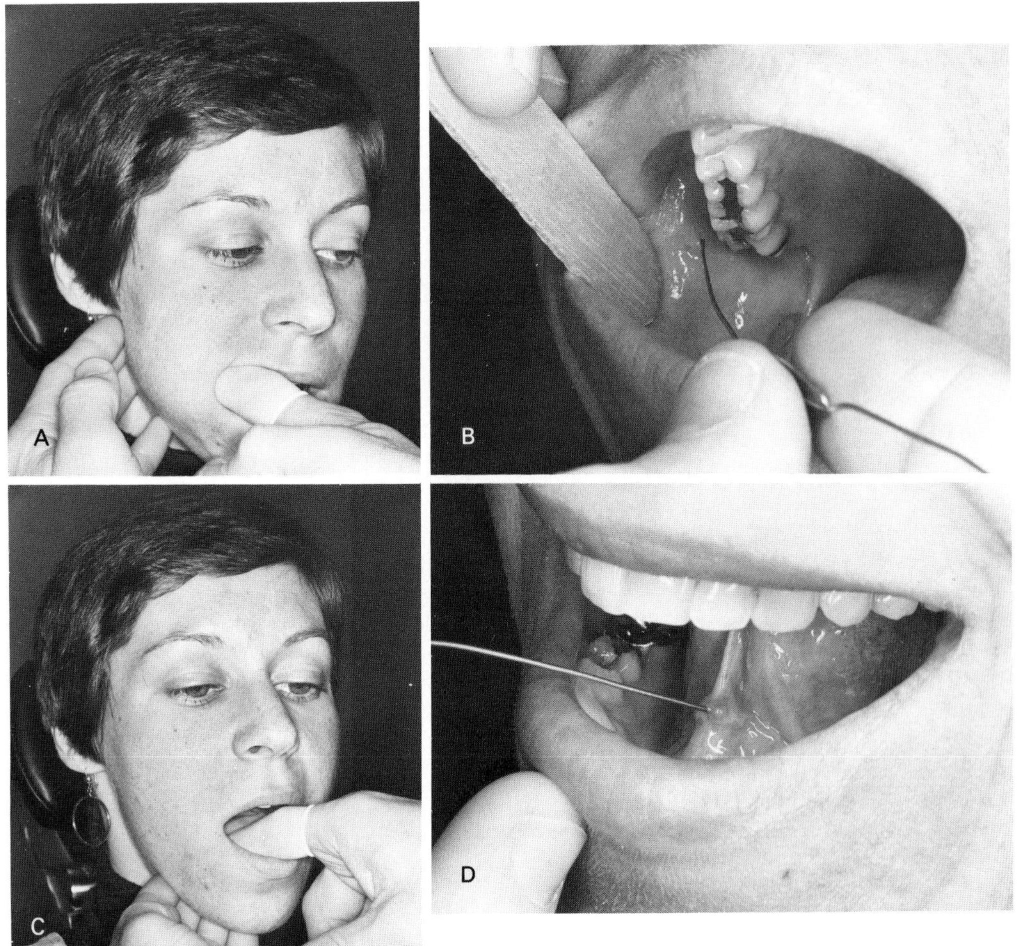

Figure 42.9 *A,* Bimanual examination of parotid region. *B,* Lacrimal probe in parotid (Stensen's) duct. *C,* Bimanual examination of floor of mouth and submaxillary region. *D,* Lacrimal probe in right submaxillary (Wharton's) duct.

of the mouth have a "woody" feeling and are extremely tender. Often this condition develops after a dental infection or dental extraction. On inspection, the tongue is swollen and displaced posteriorly and superiorly, sometimes obstructing the airway. An infected tooth or site of recent extraction may be noted. Lymphadenopathy is minimal, but the patient may have signs of sepsis.

This is a life-threatening illness because of potential airway obstruction, extension of the infection to the deep neck spaces and to the mediastinum, and generalized sepsis. The patient should be hospitalized, and specimens of oral secretions and blood should be cultured immediately. High-dose broad-spectrum antibiotics and high-dose corticosteroids should be administered intravenously. Tracheotomy is indicated in the presence of significant airway obstruction. Incision and drainage should be performed either intraorally or externally, as needed.

Dental Abscess. The patient complains of progressive pain localized to one tooth. The tooth is tender, and there may be associated edema of the gums and overlying facial tissues. The infection is treated by oral penicillin, analgesic medications, and local heat. A dentist should be consulted.

Tumors

Benign and malignant tumors may be manifested by salivary gland swelling. A discrete mass is usually palpable. Facial paralysis in association with a parotid neoplasm suggests an aggressive malignant process, and in this instance, early consultation should be obtained from a head and neck surgeon.

Rare Disorders

Salivary gland swelling may be related to tuberculosis, sarcoidosis, and Sjögren's syndrome. Another causative factor is toxic inflammation from ingestion of a heavy metal such as lead, copper, or mercury, or of a halogen such as bromide or iodide.

THE NOSE

Epistaxis

Causes

Epistaxis in children is almost invariably caused either by crusting and mucosal irritation during upper respiratory tract infection or by direct trauma. Some adults have recurrent epistaxis, usually from a small blood vessel or group of blood vessels located in the anterior portion of the septum.

Common causes of epistaxis include the following:

1. *Trauma.* Epistaxis is due either to intranasal trauma from "nose picking" or to external trauma.
2. *Hypertension.* Epistaxis may be difficult to manage until the hypertension is controlled.
3. *Upper respiratory tract infection.* Bleeding is due to mucosal engorgement and subsequent crusting and irritation of the nasal mucosa.
4. *Foreign body.* This is most commonly seen in children.
5. *Nasal polyps.* Polyps may bleed in association with an acute allergic or infectious episode.
6. *Iatrogenic induction.* Epistaxis may be precipitated by manipulation of the nose after fracture or after intranasal operation. In the latter case, the emergency physician should contact the operating surgeon immediately.
7. *Abnormality of hemostasis.* This condition is usually related to therapeutic use of sodium warfarin (Coumadin) and is more rarely associated with hemophilia, leukemic disorders, and hepatic or renal disease. The emergency physician should control bleeding with the most atraumatic method available. Treatment consists of gentle packing of the nose with either cotton soaked with epinephrine or petrolatum gauze saturated with antibiotic ointment. Cautery is contraindicated, since it usually forms an eschar, which, if it is detached, enlarges the area of bleeding.

Some rare causes of epistaxis include the following conditions and lesions. Benign *nasal tumors* infrequently bleed, but malignant tumors may cause unilateral bleeding. A tumor most commonly found in adolescent males, *nasopharyngeal angiofibroma* may be manifested by epistaxis and nasal obstruction; it should be kept in mind in the differential diagnosis of nosebleed in these patients. *Hereditary telangiectasia* (Rendu-Osler-Weber syndrome) is an autosomal dominant trait causing dilated thin-walled capillaries and venules throughout the body. This syndrome is characterized by recurrent nasal bleeding and telangiectasias of the lips and oral mucosa. Chronic diseases such as *Wegener's granulomatosis, lethal midline granuloma, tuberculosis,* and *syphilis* are also causes of epistaxis.

Treatment

In the management of epistaxis (Fig. 42.10), location of the specific bleeding point is of utmost importance. Adequate illumination and suction equipment are essential for precise management. The patient with active epistaxis is usually anxious and often needs reassurance. Sometimes mild sedation with an intramuscular narcotic or tranquilizer is helpful before examination and treatment. The blood pressure and pulse should be checked and recorded, and a blood sample should be drawn for hematocrit determination. If the history suggests a

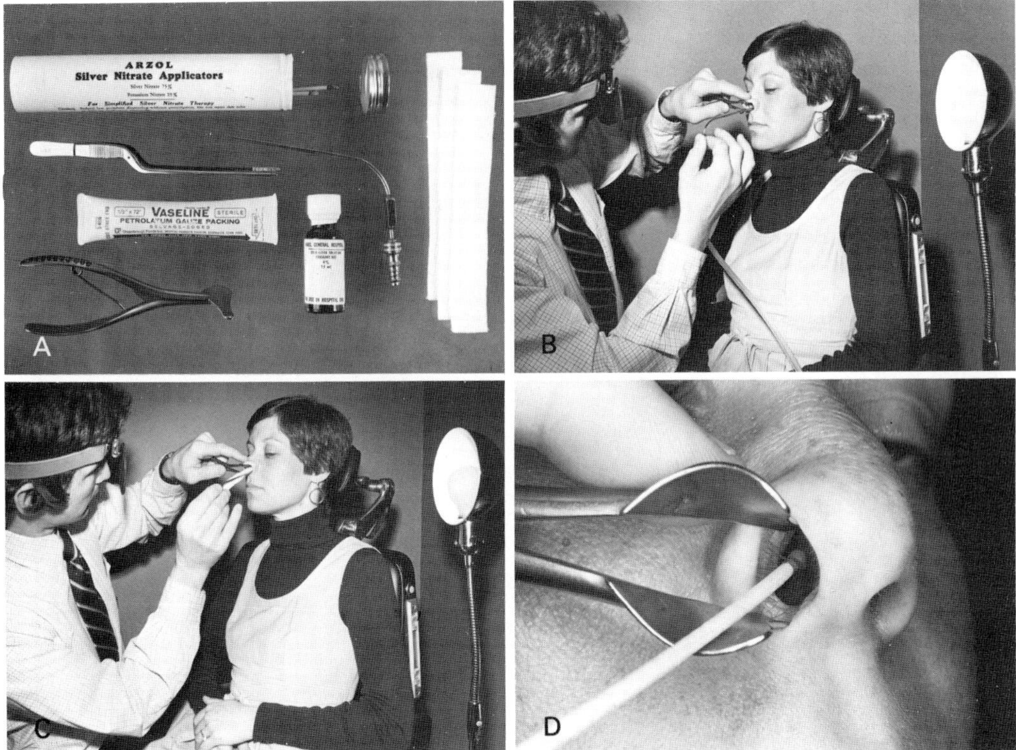

Figure 42.10. *A,* Basic equipment for management of anterior epistaxis. *Counterclockwise from top left:* silver nitrate sticks, bayonet forceps, petrolatum gauze, nasal speculum, anesthetic solution, Frazier suction tip, compressed cotton strips for initial anesthesia. *B,* Position of patient for nasal examination. Note position of nasal speculum. Suction apparatus may be used to remove mucus, foreign body, or blood. *C,* Placement of compressed cotton packing for initial control of epistaxis, vasoconstriction, and anesthesia. Note position of bayonet forceps. *D,* Application of silver nitrate to anterior nasal septum.

blood dyscrasia, the emergency physician should order the following tests: prothrombin time, partial thromboplastin time, platelet count, and bleeding time. The patient should be seated in a comfortable chair with a headrest, and should be given a basin to catch the blood.

The emergency physician and an assistant then evacuate clots with a metal suction tip and examine the nose by means of a nasal speculum and a head light or head mirror. The nasal examination should be orderly, and the nasal septum and the middle and inferior turbinates should be identified (Fig. 42.11). If the bleeding point is anterior, it can be cauterized. If it is posterior, it is important to decide which side of the nose is bleeding and whether the bleeding point is above or below the level of the middle turbinate.

Packing. After identification of an anterior bleeding point, the nose should be packed for 10 minutes with cotton gauze saturated with 4% cocaine or 2% tetracaine hydrochloride (Pontocaine). After removal of the packs, the nose will be moderately anesthetized, and a silver nitrate stick can be employed for cauterization. If point cauterization fails to stop the bleeding, the nose should be packed with 0.5-inch petrolatum gauze saturated in antibiotic ointment. The packing is placed in the nose with a bayonet forceps (Fig. 42.12*A*) while the naris is held open with a nasal speculum. As it is inserted, the packing should be watched to ensure that it has passed posterior to the visualized bleeding point. The packing is then built up from the floor to the roof of the nose to fill the anterior chamber tightly (Fig. 42.12*B*), and is supported by a strip of tape underneath the nares. The patient should be given analgesics and may be discharged. The packing is routinely removed after 3 days.

Posterior epistaxis is usually more severe and more difficult to control. The physician should note whether bleeding is from the upper or lower half of the nose, since specific arterial ligation may be necessary if posterior packing fails to control bleeding. Occasionally, a well-placed full-depth anterior pack stops epistaxis from the posterior half of the nose, but it is often necessary to place a complete antero-posterior pack. The purpose of a posterior pack is to allow placement of an extensive anterior pack that will not fall out through the posterior aspect of the nose and down the throat.

Placement of a posterior pack is an uncomfortable experience for both patient and physician. If the patient has a normal blood pressure and pulse, meperidine hydrochloride or a similar narcotic analgesic should be administered and the nose should be anesthetized by means of packs of cotton gauze saturated with 4% cocaine or 2% tetracaine hydrochloride placed in the appropriate nostril and left in place for 10–15 minutes if feasible. Additional anesthesia may be obtained by performing a bilateral sphenopalatine ganglion block by injecting 1 ml of lidocaine (Xylocaine) with epinephrine (1:100,000) with a no. 21 needle (1.5-inch length) into the greater palatine foramen, which is located in the posterolateral aspect of the hard palate approximately 1 cm anterior to the posterior rim. One of the dangers of this procedure is insertion of the needle too deep into this area, thus penetrating the orbit. This complication can be avoided if the needle

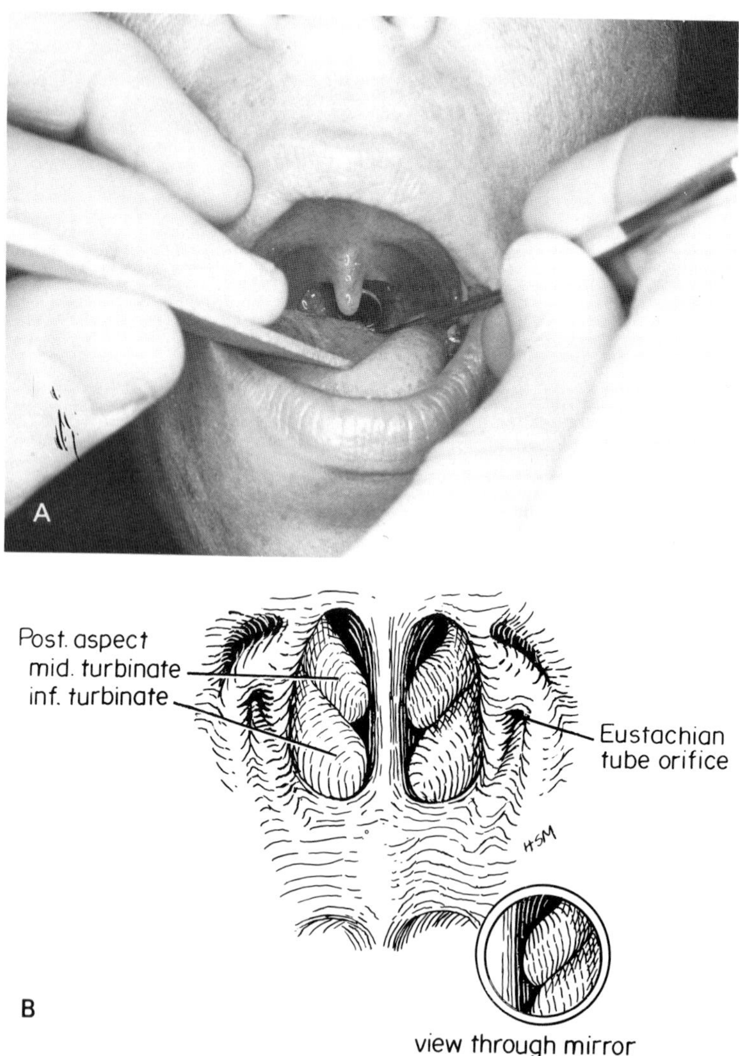

Figure 42.11. *A,* Mirror examination of nasopharynx. Mirror must be warmed with water or alcohol lamp to prevent fogging. Tongue is depressed firmly and gently with tongue blade, and mirror is inserted behind and below free margin of soft palate; the patient is requested to breathe steadily and to say "uhn . . . uhn" to drop palate down. *B,* Anatomy of nasopharynx. The posterior nasal septum is virtually always straight and is the best initial landmark. *Inset* demonstrates restricted field of view from nasopharyngeal mirror; the examiner must angle the mirror to visualize all areas.

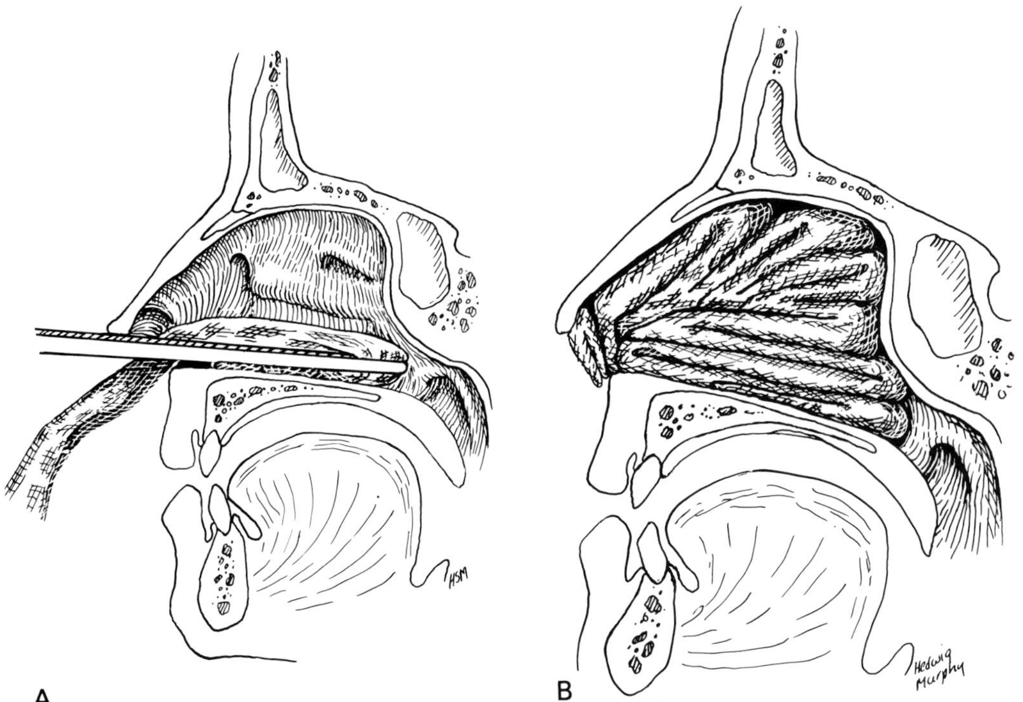

Figure 42.12. *A.,* Insertion of anterior nasal pack. *B,* Gauze is grasped with forceps 2–3 inches from end to prevent tip of gauze from slipping posteriorly. *B.,* Anterior nasal pack in place. Leading tip of pack does not protrude from choana. Pack is built up from floor of nose, then posterosuperiorly, and finally anterosuperiorly.

is prevented from passing any deeper than 2.5 cm by bending it to a 45° angle at this distance from its tip. Bilateral block provides much better anesthesia of the nasopharynx. Bleeding often stops on injection because of temporary tamponade of the internal maxillary artery, but it almost always resumes when the block wears off. Even with these efforts at anesthesia, the patient experiences pain while the pack is placed.

A conventional posterior nasal pack consists of one or two pads of cotton gauze (4 × 4 inch) saturated with antibiotic ointment, rolled into a ball, and tightly tied in the middle with two pieces of 0 silk suture, each approximately 2 feet long. This pack is placed by passing a soft rubber catheter through the nostril on the affected side, retrieving the catheter tip from the pharynx by means of a Kelly clamp and tying two strands of the suture to it, and withdrawing the catheter through the nose, bringing out the two silk sutures. The physician should tell the patient to keep the mouth wide open and to pant with deep breaths during placement of the pack. Grasping the two nasal strands with a Kelly clamp, the physician steadily pulls them with the right hand and guides the pack behind the palate and into the nasopharynx (Fig. 42.13), employing moderate pressure with the index finger of the left hand. The uvula should be pushed free of the pack; otherwise it will become necrotic. When the posterior pack is in place, an anterior pack can be built up in the nose; a tight pack usually requires 3–6 feet of 0.5-inch petrolatum gauze. An assistant must maintain constant tension on the strings holding the posterior pack in place while the anterior pack is inserted. After the anterior pack is in place, the two free ends of the silk suture coming out the naris are tied over a dental roll. The ends dangling out the mouth should be taped loosely to the cheek, and are used to retrieve the pack after it has been in place for 4 days.

The patient with a posterior pack in place should be hospitalized with modified bed rest and a semisolid or liquid diet. Moderate doses of analgesics and barbiturates can be administered; obtundation should be avoided since hypoxia can occur. Antibiotics should be administered to prevent sinusitis.

Arterial Ligation. When epistaxis is uncontrolled by cauterization or packing, arterial ligation is necessary. Bleeding in the upper portion of the nose can derive from the anterior and posterior ethmoid arteries that are part of the internal carotid system. These arteries usually bleed because of na-

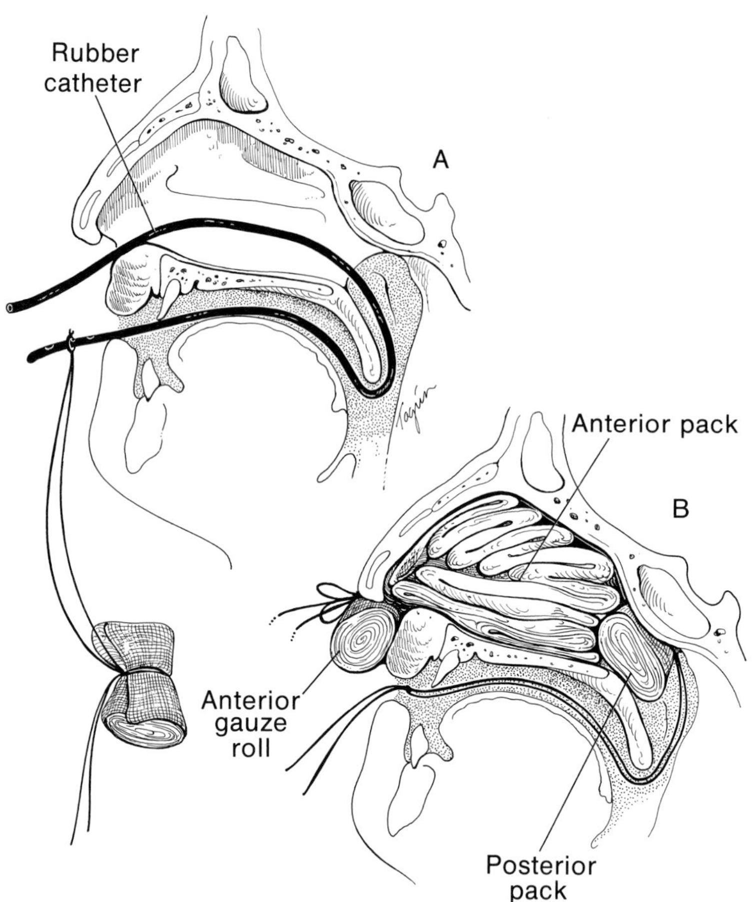

Figure 42.13. Insertion of posterior nasal pack. *A,* Soft rubber catheter is in place with pack attached to it by silk suture material. *B,* Pack has been guided into nasopharynx by means of digital manipulation and traction on suture material. Anterior pack is placed, and suture material from the naris is tied in a bow around a gauze roll.

sal trauma or hypertension. The main contributor to the blood supply of the lower half of the nose is the sphenopalatine branch of the internal maxillary artery and anteriorly, the facial artery. Both these arteries are part of the external carotid system. The internal and external carotid systems are depicted in Figure 42.14. Ligation of the external carotid artery has always been popular. Recent techniques for ligation of the internal maxillary artery through the Caldwell-Luc approach and the anterior ethmoid artery through an external approach are more effective. A decision to perform arterial ligation should be made only by an otolaryngologist.

Pain

Furuncle

This diagnosis can be suspected in a patient with a short history of inflammation and tenderness around the nasal tip with no specific causative factors. The physician may detect erythema, swelling, and tenderness in this area, and may see an obvious furuncle sometimes covered with dried pus within the nostril.

Treatment includes warm moist packs, frequently applied, and intranasal antibiotic ointment. Systemic antibiotics specifically directed at resistant staphylococci should also be given. No attempt should be made at surgical drainage; since the facial veins that drain this area are valveless and communicate directly to the cavernous sinus, excessive manipulation of the infected area should be avoided to prevent septic thrombosis of the cavernous sinus.

Nasal Vestibulitis

A chronic recurrent problem, this may be a reflection of poor nasal hygiene, sinus infection, adenoid infection, or diabetes mellitus. On

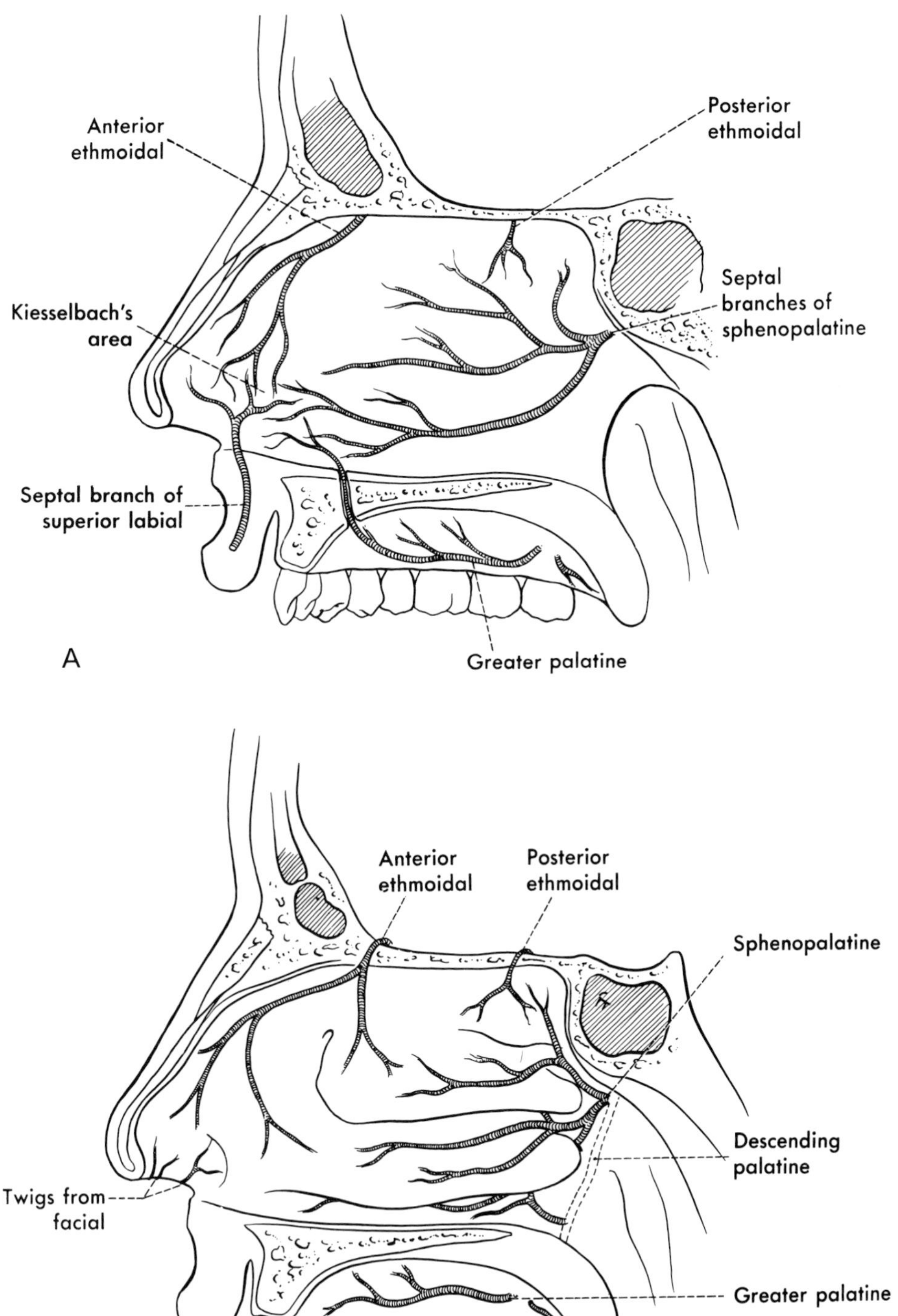

Figure 42.14. *A,* Blood supply to nasal septum. Kiesselbach's area is most common site of epistaxis. Bleeding in this area can be controlled with cautery or nasal packing or both. *B,* Blood supply to lateral nasal wall. The ethmoidal arteries are branches of internal carotid system; the others are branches of external carotid system. (Reproduced by permission, from Hollinshead WH: *Anatomy for Surgeons,* vol. 1. Hagerstown, Md: Harper & Row, 1982.)

examination, the tip of the nose is usually tender and sometimes inflamed. Folliculitis of the vibrissae can be visualized. Treatment consists of frequent cleansing of the nose with a dilute solution of hydrogen peroxide or soap and water with application of a local antibiotic ointment two or three times a day. The patient should be advised that this can be a chronic problem, and can be somewhat resistant to therapy. In a patient with no apparent underlying disease, a screening test for diabetes is recommended.

Uncommon Causes

Nasal pain may be caused by a herpes simplex infection or by herpes zoster of the maxillary nerve. Lupus vulgaris may produce pain, as may the gumma of tertiary syphilis. Primary syphilitic chancre of the nose is rare.

Trauma

Simple Fracture

The traumatic event causing fracture is usually obvious. All varieties of depression and lateral displacement of the nose can be seen with simple nasal fractures. In a more severe fracture, immediate swelling and ecchymosis are obvious, but in a milder fracture, displacement of the nose may occur without significant swelling. Fracture may be accompanied by epistaxis and deviation of the nasal septum. Careful examination of the nasal septum should be performed to exclude a septal hematoma, which is typified by soft, fluctuant swelling. Deviation of the nasal septum without hematoma should also be noted. The examiner should always search for cerebrospinal fluid (CSF) rhinorrhea and significant injury to the cervical spine or airway. Radiologic evaluation is not helpful in the management of a patient with a minor fracture. In the case of severe trauma, x-ray views should be taken to exclude accompanying fractures of other facial bones.

In the case of minor fractures with minimal swelling, reduction of the fracture may be immediate or it may be deferred from 4–7 days. Reduction should be deferred if there is significant soft-tissue edema. This procedure is indicated only for cosmetic reasons and for functional improvement of the airway.

Nasal reduction is performed under local anesthesia in the emergency department. The patient with stable vital signs should be sedated with intramuscular or intravenous meperidine hydrochloride. Both sides of the nose should be packed with gauze soaked in a 4% cocaine or a 2% tetracaine hydrochloride solution for 15–20 minutes. Since it is difficult to obtain anesthesia high in the nose, it is sometimes helpful to remove the initial anesthesia packs after 10 minutes and to replace them with a second set high in the vault of the nose. This may be supplemented with bilateral submucosal infiltration of lidocaine high in the nasal septum. An infraorbital nerve block (see Fig. 39.3) is accomplished by infiltration of 1% lidocaine with epinephrine (1:100,000), a field block anesthesia is gained by infiltration of these agents across the glabellar region and the base of the columella. When anesthesia is complete, reduction may be accomplished by means of a straight blunt elevator placed no further up in the nose than a line drawn between the medial canthi of the eyes. The level can be ascertained by laying the elevator on the side of the nose with the tip next to the medial canthus and grasping it at the level of the nares. If the grip is maintained at this point throughout the procedure, the elevator will not be inserted too far and will not endanger the cribriform plate. The fracture is then reduced by placing the elevator within the nasal cavity, gently raising the nasal framework anteriorly to disimpact the fragments, and manipulating the fractured nasal bone back into the midline. If significant epistaxis occurs, the nose may have to be packed, although epistaxis will often cease after approximately 10 minutes. Splinting a nasal fracture with plaster or a disposable nasal splint is helpful for the first week.

Septal Hematoma and Abscess

Hematoma of the septum is uncommon. It will be overlooked if intranasal examination is not performed in all cases of nasal fracture. A soft widening of the nasal septum, septal hematoma should be treated after 1% lidocaine anesthesia by making a 1 cm incision in the inferior aspect of the hematoma for drainage. A small Penrose drain can be placed in the hematoma. An anterior pack of petrolatum gauze should be inserted in the nostril to compress the flaps of the hematoma, and the patient should be referred to an otolaryngologist.

An untreated septal hematoma may become infected, and painful swelling of the nose may appear several days after a nasal fracture. Since infection can destroy the nasal septal cartilage, producing a nasal saddle deformity, and since it can progress to septic thrombosis of the cavernous sinus, it should be treated by immediate incision and drainage with culture of the abscess. Until culture reports are available, penicillinase-resistant antistaphylococcal antibiotics are administered.

Acute Cerebrospinal Fluid Rhinorrhea

This condition is usually related to facial trauma, although it may be spontaneous. Trauma to the middle of the face that appears to have caused only a simple nasal fracture may have also caused a fracture of the cribriform plate that is signaled by CSF rhinorrhea. Massive trauma to the middle and upper face should make the emergency physician suspect CSF leakage, even though it may not be readily apparent because of bleeding. CSF rhinorrhea can also occur via the eustachian tube after a temporal bone fracture. In spontaneous rhinorrhea, the patient is aware of discharge of clear watery fluid with a salty taste usually from one nostril, but sometimes from both. Leakage may be associated with the dependent head position.

On inspection, spontaneous rhinorrhea is evident as a clear, watery nasal discharge. In a patient with midfacial trauma, subcutaneous emphysema of the eyelids implies fracture of the ethmoid complex and should heighten suspicion of cribriform plate injury and associated CSF leakage. Bloody nasal drainage can be tested by placing a drop on a white cloth; if CSF is mixed with the blood, a double ring will develop, a paler outer ring and a darker inner ring, since CSF diffuses more rapidly than blood and serum. The clear drainage from the nose should be tested for glucose content.

Patients with spontaneous CSF rhinorrhea should be hospitalized for thorough radiologic evaluation of the facial bones and fluorescein dye studies of the CSF to determine the location of the leak. Prophylactic administration of antibiotics is recommended, along with constant elevation of the head. Traumatic CSF rhinorrhea often ceases when the fractures are reduced; this should be accomplished when the general condition permits. An otolaryngologist and a neurosurgeon should be consulted.

Acutely Deviated Nasal Septum

The nasal septum may be displaced by blunt trauma from below or in front of the nose. While reducing a nasal fracture under local anesthesia, the emergency physician may be able to shift the septum back into a midline position, but this is usually difficult. Consulting an otolaryngologist is recommended for consideration of an immediate operative procedure to repair this injury.

Discharge and Obstruction

Common Cold

Ordinarily, a cold has the following four stages:

1. *Prodrome.* This is characterized by a hot, dry, or tickling intranasal sensation with a widely patent nose, which lasts a few hours.
2. *Initiative.* As the viral infection spreads from the portal of entry to affect the adjacent mucous membranes, the nose becomes obstructed, with associated sneezing and watery rhinorrhea. The patient may have a sore throat with a low-grade fever. This persists for 2–5 days.
3. *Secondary infection.* After 3–5 days, bacterial superinfection may take place, heralded by increased mucopurulent nasal discharge and signs of systemic illness.
4. *Resolution.* A mild cold clears in a few days; when bacterial superinfection occurs, resolution may take 5–10 days, depending on the effectiveness of therapy.

A patient with the first stages of a cold usually has a nasal discharge and a low-grade fever, with minimal clinical findings. Bacterial superinfection causes a rise in temperature, sinus tenderness, mucopurulent nasal discharge, erythema of the throat, and regional lymphadenopathy. The symptoms of allergic rhinitis, vasomotor rhinitis, and rhinitis medicamentosa may all be confused with those of the initial stages of a cold. These conditions are discussed in the following sections.

There is no specific therapy for a cold; symptomatic treatment should be adjusted to the age and general medical condition of the patient. Bed rest aids the resolution of systemic symptoms, and humidification of inspired air (50%) at 65°F (18.3°C) is recommended. Antihistamines and vasoconstrictive agents aid in relief of symptoms and may prevent the complications of sinusitis and otitis media. Nasal drops containing phenylephrine hydrochloride or oxymetazoline hydrochloride may be employed, but the patient should be warned not to use them beyond 1 week. Salicylates help reduce fever and associated malaise. Antibiotics should not be administered in the initial stages of a cold. If bacterial superinfection occurs, however, administration of penicillin or erythromycin for 7 days speeds recovery. Ascorbic acid has been recommended in the treatment of colds, but its value is debatable.

Allergic and Vasomotor Rhinitis

It is sometimes difficult to differentiate between these two forms of irritative nasal reaction.

Allergy. In the classic situation, a patient with this condition has nasal irritation, itch, and obstruction, with paroxysmal sneezing and copious watery rhinorrhea. Episodes are usually seasonal, being exacerbated in the spring or fall or both, whenever the pollen of allergenic plants is prevalent. The patient may have a strong family history of hay fever or asthma. On examination, the patient may have a watery nasal discharge and pale, swollen nasal mucosa. Often the conjunctivae are red, associated with increased lacrimation. Auscultation of the chest may disclose wheezing breath sounds.

Similar, usually milder, symptoms may be due to perennial allergens, most commonly foods in children and inhalants, such as dust and molds, in adults. Common food allergens are milk, wheat, chocolate, eggs, fish, and citrus fruits. Common drugs that may produce an allergic reaction include salicylates, iodides, quinidine, sulfonamide compounds, and penicillins. Bacterial allergens include staphylococci, pneumococci, and streptococci.

In a patient with acute allergic rhinitis, the systemic antihistamine chlorpheniramine maleate, 4 mg every 6 hours, and a corticosteroid nasal spray, one or two sprays three times a day, usually controls symptoms. The patient should be referred to an allergist or otolaryngologist for evaluation.

Vasomotor Rhinitis. The patient may complain of any combination of nasal obstruction, discharge, postnasal drip, sneezing, facial pain, malaise, and fatigue. Physical examination may reveal massive engorgement of the turbinates with water discharge, or the nasal passages may be widely patent. In treating this condition, the physician must remember that many factors may alter the patency of the nasal airway. One major factor is excessive tone of the parasympathetic nervous system caused by the following agents or states:

1. Psychologic disturbance, usually depression;
2. Endocrine disorder, which may be related to menstruation, pregnancy, or the use of oral contraceptives;
3. Hypotensive drugs, such as methyldopa, reserpine, guanethidine sulfate, and rauwolfia, which prevent peripheral release of adrenalin;
4. Physical changes, such as temperature and humidity fluctuations.

This condition is nonemergent, and the patient should be so informed and referred to an otolaryngologist for further workup. The emergency physician should question the patient regarding hypertensive medications and psychologic history, since referral to an internist or a psychiatrist might be more appropriate.

Rhinitis Medicamentosa

One of the most common causes of severe nasal obstruction is habitual use of nasal drops. Since the drops are effective for only a few minutes or hours with habitual use, they are applied more frequently. It is virtually impossible for the examiner to see beyond the tips of the inferior turbinates in these patients because of swelling. A patient with this condition should be referred to an otolaryngologist for a thorough nasal examination to exclude any underlying nasal problems and for therapy, including topical and systemic corticosteroid agents.

Foreign Bodies

A foreign body in the nose is a common problem among young children. Ordinarily, the child is brought in immediately after placing a foreign body in the nose. A child with a foul-smelling discharge from one nostril should be suspected of having a chronically impacted foreign body. In the acute case, the foreign body can usually be seen when the nose is inspected with a speculum and head light. If the examiner is unfamiliar with the use of these instruments and is uncomfortable performing intranasal manipulations, the patient should be referred to an otolaryngologist.

Most foreign bodies can be removed in the emergency department, but if previous manipulations have caused swelling and bleeding, removal becomes more difficult, sometimes requiring general anesthesia. Solid objects may be removed in the emergency department with a bayonet forceps or a metal (Frazier) suction tip shod with rubber tubing over the tip. Before removal, 0.5% or 1.0% phenylephrine hydrochloride drops should be instilled to shrink the nasal mucosa, and the patient should be instructed to blow out the foreign body if possible. The physician must avoid posterior displacement of the foreign body into the nasopharynx and thence into the upper part of the airway, causing obstruction.

Other Causes

Patients with *chronic granulomatous disease* may have a history of blood-tinged or clear nasal discharge, unilateral or bilateral nasal obstruction, and symptoms of sinusitis. Physical examination reveals granulomatous lesions in the nasal cavity and sometimes perforation of the nasal septum. In the advanced case, total destruction of the nose may take place, along with involvement of the palate and ear. The diseases included in this group are Wegener's granulomatosis (a triad involving the respiratory tract, the genitourinary tract, and generalized vasculitis) and lethal midline granuloma, a neoplasm of lymphoreticular cells that generally has a better prognosis than Wegener's granulomatosis. Clinical evaluations should include x-ray films of the nasal cavities, sinuses, and chest and renal function tests. A biopsy of the intranasal tissue aids in diagnosis. Wegener's granulomatosis is usually treated with corticosteroids, cytotoxics, and immunosuppressive drugs. Lethal midline granuloma is sometimes treated with local irradiation.

In a chronically ill and debilitated patient, especially one with uncontrolled diabetes, *fungal infections of the nose and sinuses,* such as mucormycosis may cause nasal obstruction. Treatment consists of identification of the fungus and administration of appropriate systemic antifungal drugs, along with débridement of the nose and sinuses.

Syphilitic lesions rarely cause nasal discharge. Although acquired syphilis rarely affects the nose, gummata can occur in this area. Congenital syphilis also can cause nasal obstruction and discharge.

Obstruction

Nasal obstruction can result from swollen membranes due to such previously described conditions as the common cold, allergy, rhinitis medicamentosa, and chronic granulomatous disease. Traumatic events causing obstruction, such as acutely deviated septum, septal hematoma or abscess, and foreign body, have been discussed. Anatomic defects causing obstruction include deviated septum, intranasal scars, adenoid hypertrophy, nasal polyps, and tumors. Patients with the first two conditions should be referred to an otolaryngologist for repair of the septum or lysis of scar tissue.

Adenoid hypertrophy is probably the most common cause of nasal obstruction in children. The patient should be evaluated by an otolaryngologist. *Nasal polyps* resulting from allergic rhinosinusitis appear as boggy, grape-like intranasal masses and are almost always bilateral. In a child with nasal polyps, a workup for cystic fibrosis should be carried out. If nasal ''polyps'' are unilateral, the diagnosis of encephalocele should be considered. Dexamethasone sodium phosphate is often effective in shrinking polyps; two sprays are administered three times a day for 2–3 weeks. The patient should be referred to an otolaryngologist. Any form of epithelial or mesenchymal *tumor* can obstruct the nose. The tumors typically found in the nose include juvenile angiofibroma, olfactory neuroblastoma, lymphoepithelioma, and squamous cell carcinoma.

An unusual atrophic change of the nasal mucosa, *atrophic rhinitis* causes the patient to feel that he cannot breathe through the nose, although the nasal airway is widely patent. Physical examination reveals intranasal crusting and marked atrophy of the nasal mucosa. The patient may gain symptomatic relief by means of nasal irrigation with physiologic saline solution twice a day using a soft rubber bulb syringe. The patient should be referred to an otolaryngologist.

THE THROAT

Trauma

Oropharynx

Laceration. Treatment of lacerations of the lip and cheek is discussed in Chapter 39. Most lacerations of the *tongue* can be closed loosely in one or two layers with absorbable suture material. Since the tongue is very vascular, questionably viable flaps of tissue should be preserved in hope that they will survive. Lacerations in the *floor of the mouth* may involve the lingual nerve or the submaxillary duct or both. The integrity of the submaxillary duct can be established by a lacrimal probe. Since the lingual nerve supplies sensation to the anterior portion of the tongue, simple testing of sensation can establish its continuity. Most of these lacerations, unless they are extensive, should not be sutured, because they will close better by granulation with less likelihood of abscess formation. If a laceration of the floor of the mouth is sutured, however, care should be taken not to suture through or around the duct or the nerve; tight closure is contraindicated.

Most injuries of the *hard palate* occur in children who fall with a stick in the mouth. Small tears and flaps close well without operative intervention. The patient and family should be instructed to wash the mouth out with warm water or dilute hydrogen peroxide solution after each meal, and the wound should be closely observed until it has healed. Large tears and flaps should be closed under general anesthesia with absorbable suture material in a loose fashion to prevent abscess formation. Any penetrating wound in the region of the *tonsillar fossa* is potentially dangerous. There have been reports of internal carotid arterial thrombosis with hemiplegia and death following blunt trauma in this area. Optimal treatment for these patients is hospitalization for 48–72 hours. Careful neurologic evaluation and observation for the development of unilateral pupil dilation, hemiplegia, or obtundation is necessary. Signs of unilateral neurologic deterioration warrant arteriographic evaluation and appropriate vascular operation.

Burns. Thermal and chemical burns of the oropharynx, upper airway, and esophagus are discussed in Chapter 32.

Larynx and Trachea

A moderate injury may result from a blow by a fist or hockey stick. Use of motorcycles, minibikes, and snowmobiles account for increasing numbers of ''clothesline'' injuries—direct trauma to the laryngotracheal complex caused by striking an unseen wire clothesline or fence. Symptoms include varying degrees of hoarseness, airway obstruction, dysphonia, dysphagia, and localized pain and swelling. Laryngeal trauma is often overlooked in a patient with severe multiple injuries who has undergone early tracheotomy because of airway obstruction and whose other problems demand immediate attention.

On physical examination (Fig. 42.15*A*), a patient with a minor laryngeal injury is hoarse with no stridor and with moderate pain on swallowing or speaking. Examination of the neck may reveal either a normal laryngeal contour or perhaps a palpable fracture of the laryngeal cartilage. There may be tenderness and subcutaneous emphysema in the neck. Anteroposterior and lateral x-ray films of the neck should be requested (Fig. 42.15 *B* and *C*), and an otolaryngologist should be consulted. Signs of

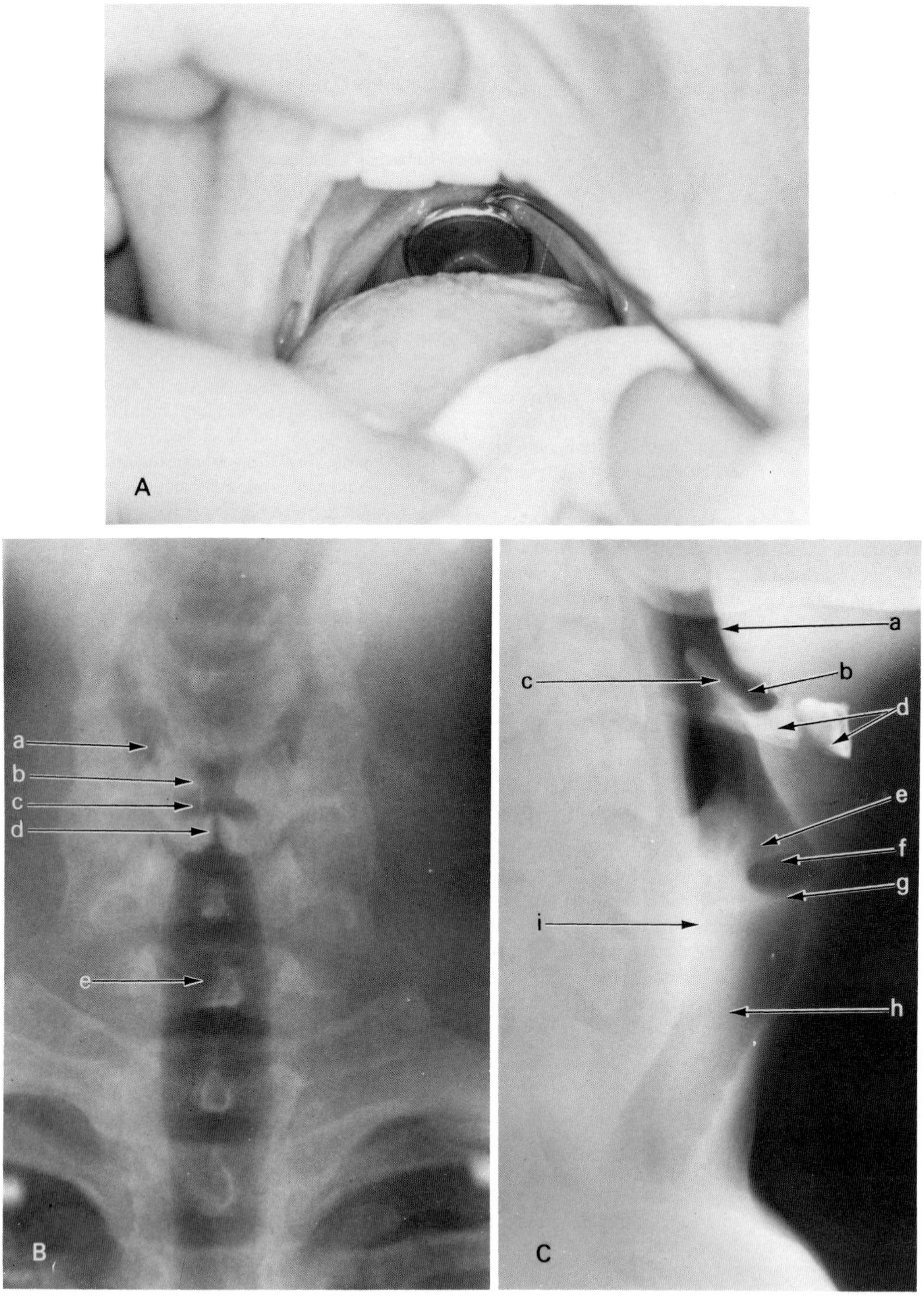

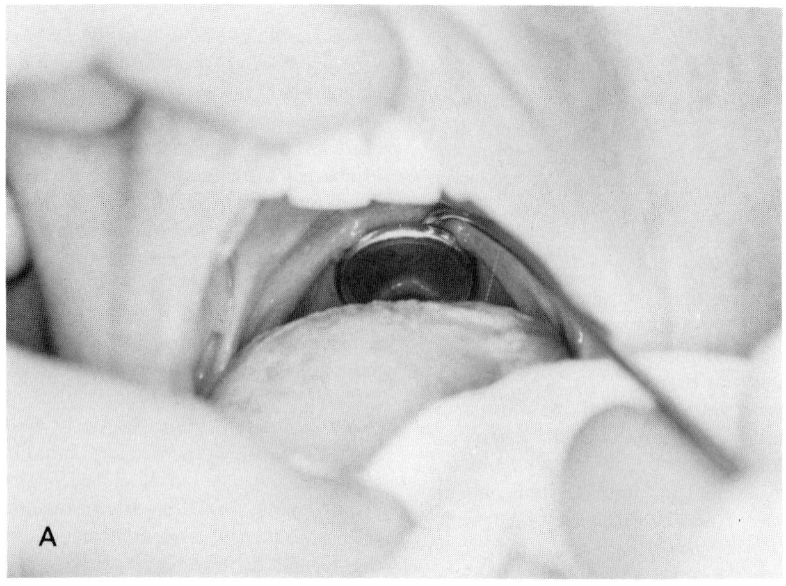

Figure 42.15. *A*, Mirror examination of larynx. Mirror must be warmed with water or alcohol lamp to prevent fogging. Patient's tongue is held gently with gauze sponge and palate is depressed in posterosuperior direction by mirror (note that epiglottis is seen in mirror). *B*, Anteroposterior soft-tissue x-ray view of normal airway during phonation (not a tomogram). *a*, Pyriform sinus; *b*, false cords; *c*, laryngeal ventricle; *d*, true cords; *e*, trachea. *C*, Lateral soft-tissue x-ray view of normal airway. *a*, Base of tongue; *b*, vallecula; *c*, epiglottis; *d*, hyoid bone; *e*, area of false vocal cord; *f*, laryngeal ventricle; *g*, area of true vocal cord; *h*, trachea; *i*, retrocricoid area.

more significant injury include contusions or open lacerations of the neck, subcutaneous emphysema, progressive airway obstruction, loss of voice, and loss of laryngeal contour. Subcutaneous emphysema signifies air leakage, implying rupture of the laryngeal or tracheal cartilage and mucosal tears. Complete laryngotracheal transection can occur without an open wound on the neck.

A patient with a history of severe laryngotracheal trauma should be evaluated for the possibility of cervical spine injury and cervical esophageal tears. In an unconscious patient with multiple injuries including airway obstruction, careful evaluation of possible laryngeal injury is essential. At the time of initial tracheotomy, the thyroid cartilage and cricoid cartilage should be closely examined. If there is any suggestion of laryngeal injury, an otolaryngologist should be consulted regarding the timing of endoscopy to assess the extent of injury and to determine whether it requires operative repair. The endoscopist should proceed with extreme caution so that loose fragments of cartilage are not detached from their blood supply.

In minor to moderate injuries, the patient must be observed 48 hours for progressive airway obstruction. Hematoma, mucosal edema, vocal cord paralysis, and anatomic derangement all contribute to this complication. During observation, systemic corticosteroids should be administered, 20 mg of prednisone every 8 hours. The patient should be in a high-humidity atmosphere, and heavy sedation should be avoided. Progressive hoarseness and stridor warrant tracheotomy, performed preferably under local anesthesia, because endotracheal intubation may further traumatize the larynx. In severe laryngotracheal trauma, early tracheotomy is essential. Long-term complications of laryngotracheal injuries include total aphonia, permanent obstruction of the airway, aspiration pneumonia, and laryngotracheoesophageal fistula. Many of these difficult sequelae may be minimized or prevented by early recognition and proper management of these injuries.

In summary, emergency management of a patient with laryngotracheal trauma consists of the following measures:

1. Assure the patency of the airway, with tracheotomy if necessary.
2. Protect the cervical spine.
3. Request radiologic studies of the cervical spine and lateral and anteroposterior x-ray films of the neck.
4. Consult an otolaryngologist as soon as possible.
5. Administer antibiotics and corticosteroids.
6. Avoid endoscopy or endotracheal intubation, pending otolaryngologic advice.
7. Prescribe parenteral rather than oral nutrition.
8. Perform corrective operation for laryngotracheal damage as early as the general status of the patient permits.

Cervical Esophagus

A patient with either a penetrating neck injury or a blunt neck injury may have a tear of the cervical esophagus. In cases of penetrating trauma, leakage of saliva into the wound suggests a hypopharyngeal or esophageal tear. If the patient is awake, this diagnosis may be confirmed by having him swallow water colored with methylene blue and observing the wound. A barium swallow with a small amount of barium can be performed to evaluate the possibility of a tracheoesophageal fistula. Endoscopic examination should be considered if the condition is stable.

A patient with a suspected tear of the cervical esophagus should be hospitalized, and oral alimentation discontinued. The wound should be treated with absorbent gauze dressing, and prophylactic antibiotics instituted. If no other major structures of the neck are injured, and if a small tear less than 0.5 cm in length is noted on endoscopic examination, the lesion can be treated expectantly; it will probably close spontaneously. Larger tears should be sutured during a transcervical exploratory operation, especially if the wound must be explored so that other structures can be repaired.

Acute Obstruction of the Airway

In most cases of acute obstruction, there is a clear history suggesting foreign body, infection, or trauma. It is important to determine whether the patient has experienced stridor or hoarseness for a long period, since this implies a chronic infection, tumor, or other long-standing laryngeal problem.

In general, a patient with upper airway obstruction has stridor on inspiration. As obstruction progresses, suprasternal retraction, tachycardia, a panicky expression, and pallor develop. The immediate problem is hypoxia; a major complication is sudden cardiac arrest when hypoxia becomes extreme.

Tracheotomy

The emergency physician treating a patient with acute upper airway obstruction should make every effort possible to secure an airway short of tracheotomy. A true emergency tracheotomy is a difficult and dangerous procedure, and endotracheal intubation is preferred if it is at all feasible. Three operative procedures can be utilized to obtain an airway: emergency cricothyrotomy, urgent tracheotomy, and elective tracheotomy.

Emergency Cricothyrotomy. This procedure is the fastest approach to the airway. It is the procedure of choice when total and complete respiratory obstruction exists and if endotracheal intubation is impossible. Common indications for this procedure include foreign body obstruction; facial or laryngotracheal trauma; inhalation, thermal, or caustic injury of the upper airway; angioneurotic edema; upper airway hemorrhage; epiglottitis; and croup.

The patient is placed supine with support under the shoulders and hyperextension of the neck. Anesthesia is usually either unnecessary or unavailable. The neck is palpated and the space between the thyroid and cricoid cartilages is identified. A skin incision, either vertical or horizontal, is made over the cricothyroid membrane, and the subcutaneous tissues are bluntly dissected to this level. A 1-cm horizontal incision is made between the cricoid and thyroid cartilages. Any flat instrument, such as the scalpel handle, is inserted in the incision and turned 90° to hold the incision open. The incision can be kept open by the introduction of a small tube. As soon as the patient's condition is stable, this temporary airway should be replaced by a standard tracheotomy between the second and third tracheal rings.

Cricothyrotomy is an excellent method of securing an airway rapidly with minimal blood loss, but it risks significant damage to the laryngeal structures, the cricoid cartilage, the thyroid cartilage, and the vocal cords. This damage can result in chronic laryngeal stenosis with airway obstruction and hoarseness.

Needle cricothyrotomy is described in Illustrated Technique 4.

Emergency Tracheotomy. Emergency tracheotomy (Fig. 42.16) is performed on a patient with progressive airway obstruction in imminent danger of total obstruction. The emergency physician must first consider endotracheal intubation; a decision for tracheotomy may be made if endotracheal intubation equipment is unavailable or if distortion of the upper airway makes intubation unlikely to succeed. This procedure is often indicated in patients with obstructing tumors, traumatic injury, or infectious disease.

An experienced assistant facilitates this operation. The patient is placed supine with support under the shoulders if possible. Often, the patient with respiratory obstruction is extremely apprehensive, agitated, and uncooperative; the operation may have to be performed with the patient in a semi-sitting position because total obstruction occurs when he or she lies down. This position increases the likelihood of an improperly high placement of the tracheotomy. In an acutely obstructed infant, placement of an endotracheal tube or bronchoscope is essential before tracheotomy, because the trachea of an infant is extremely small and mobile, making it difficult to manage, especially during respiratory stridor.

The neck is cleansed with an antiseptic solution, and sterile drapes are applied. The skin and subcutaneous tissues are infiltrated with 1% lidocaine with epinephrine (1:100,000). The surgeon palpates the thyroid and cricoid cartilages to avoid incision of the latter, and makes a vertical skin incision from just below the cricoid cartilage extending approximately 5 cm distally. A vertical incision is preferred since it directs dissection to the midline. The physician performs blunt dissection through the subcutaneous tissue and between the strap muscles, retracting them laterally and avoiding blood vessels wherever possible. Dissection should be performed beneath the full length of the incision so that a funnel-shaped wound is not created. The isthmus of the thyroid gland lies immediately beneath the strap muscles and is usually invested with numerous vessels. Although the thyroid gland can be retracted inferiorly or superiorly without dividing it at the isthmus, division is necessary if the isthmus is large, obstructing access to the trachea. The thyroid isthmus is divided by dissecting through the pretracheal fascia just above and below and tunneling with a clamp in the anterior midline space between the thyroid and the trachea. The isthmus is then divided

Figure 42.16. *A,* Sites of incision for relief of airway obstruction. Major palpable landmarks are hyoid bone, notch of thyroid cartilage, and cricoid cartilage. Cricothyrotomy is performed by incision directly over cricothyroid membrane; vertical incision for emergency tracheotomy begins at or below cricoid cartilage. Potential for venous bleeding increases as dissection proceeds inferiorly, especially below thyroid isthmus. *B,* Emergency tracheotomy. *a,* Skin and platysma are incised and the midline raphe is identified and incised. *b,* Thyroid gland is identified as strap muscles are retracted, tracheal fascia above and below thyroid isthmus is exposed if isthmus must be divided, and clamp is tunneled in midline between thyroid and trachea. *c,* Gland is divided between clamps. *d,* Free ends of thyroid gland are sutured and appropriate tracheal interspaces are infiltrated with local anesthetic. *e,* Tracheal hook is inserted to stabilize trachea, and cruciate incision is made. *f,* Circular opening is made just large enough to accommodate appropriate tracheotomy tube. *g,* Silk suture (2–0) with long ends is placed around lower tracheal ring to identify tracheal lumen should decannulation occur accidentally. *h,* Tracheotomy tube is inserted with obturator that is then replaced by inner cannula. *i,* Tube is secured, wound is loosely closed, and sterile dressing is applied. (Modified by permission, from Applebaum EL, Bruce DL. *Tracheal Intubation.* Philadelphia: WB Saunders, 1976.)

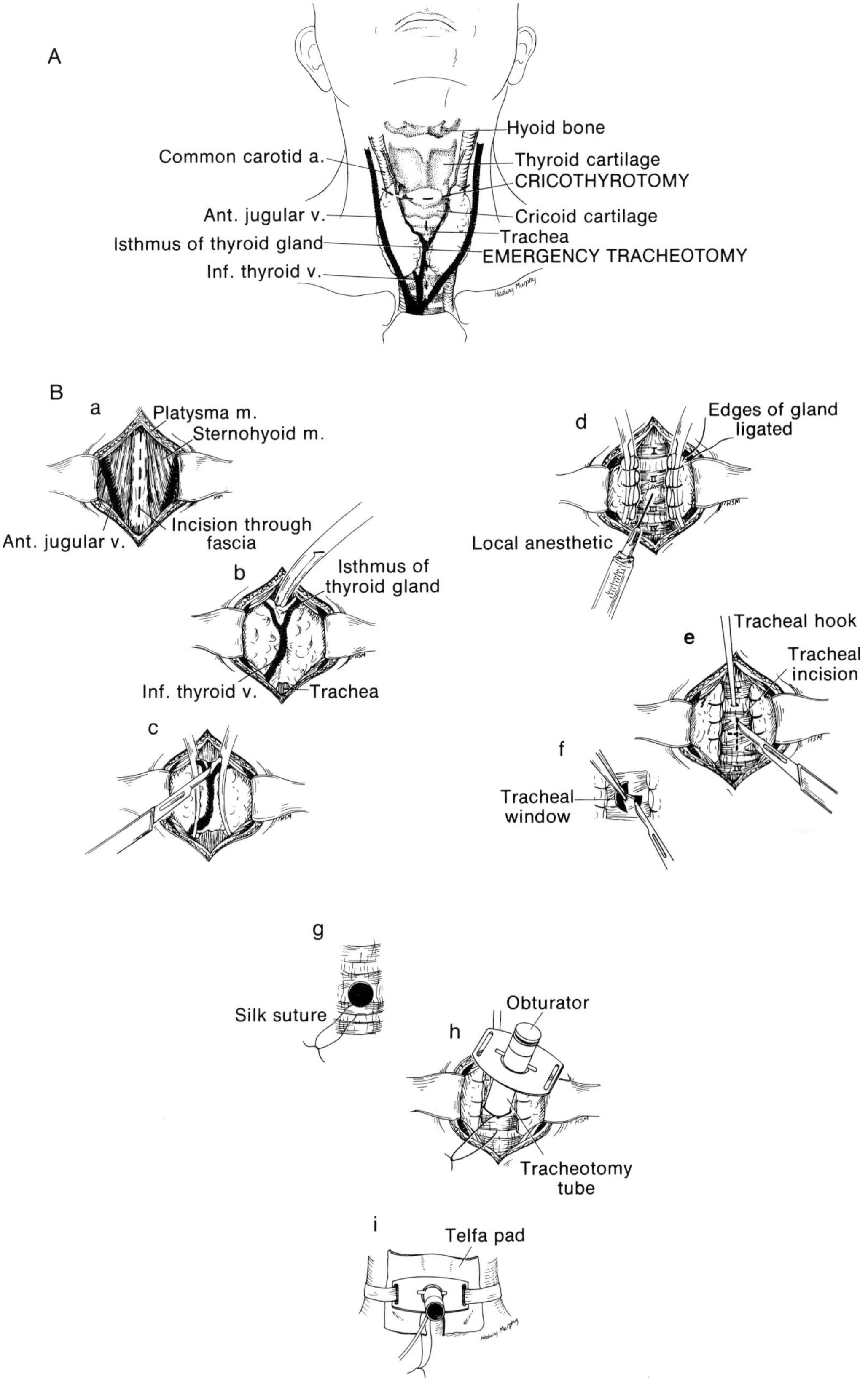

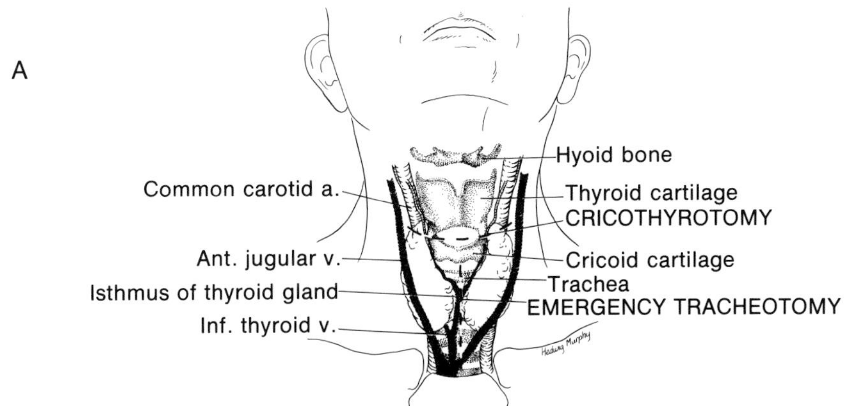

A
Hyoid bone
Common carotid a.
Thyroid cartilage
CRICOTHYROTOMY
Ant. jugular v.
Cricoid cartilage
Isthmus of thyroid gland
Trachea
EMERGENCY TRACHEOTOMY
Inf. thyroid v.
B
a
Platysma m.
Sternohyoid m.
Ant. jugular v.
Incision through fascia
b
Isthmus of thyroid gland
Inf. thyroid v.
Trachea
c
d
Edges of gland ligated
Local anesthetic
e
Tracheal hook
Tracheal incision
f
Tracheal window
g
Silk suture
h
Obturator
Tracheotomy tube
i
Telfa pad

between clamps. The two edges of the isthmus are sutured with a 2–0 chromic catgut mattress suture, once the tracheotomy tube is in place.

The second and third tracheal rings are identified, and the tracheotomy performed through this area. Injection of 1–2 ml of 1% lidocaine into the tracheal lumen with a no. 25 needle minimizes coughing. The preferred method of fenestrating the trachea is partial excision of the anterior portions of the second and third tracheal rings. The trachea is retracted superiorly by means of a tracheal hook inserted into the second interspace, a cruciate incision is made with a no. 15 knife blade with the intersection of the cuts at the interspace between the selected rings, and the resultant four corners of tracheal tissue are removed by ring punch-biopsy forceps or by sharp excision. Care must be taken to prevent aspiration of the small cartilaginous fragments. To minimize the danger of subsequent tracheal stenosis, only enough tracheal ring to permit tube placement is excised.

A tracheotomy tube with a low-pressure cuff is then inserted with an obturator that is immediately removed after tube placement. The extremes of the incision are loosely closed around the tube with skin sutures. The tracheotomy tube is carefully secured with tapes tied around the neck, and a sterile dressing is applied about the tube.

A postoperative lateral x-ray film of the neck ensures proper positioning of the tracheotomy tube. Because pneumothorax can complicate an emergency tracheotomy, especially in children in whom the apical pleura lies close to the trachea proximal to the clavicle, a postoperative chest x-ray film is also recommended.

Elective Tracheotomy. Elective tracheotomy is performed in the same fashion as emergency tracheotomy except that a transverse incision may be employed and an endotracheal tube is in place. There is also time for endoscopic examination to obtain specimens for culture and biopsy, if indicated.

Postoperative Complications. Both immediate and late complications may arise after tracheotomy, as detailed below:

1. Reflex apnea may occur as the patient's ventilatory status improves, since the central respiratory mechanism has been responding to hypoxia. Reflex apnea can be managed by mechanical ventilation until normal respiratory drive returns.
2. Immediate surgical complications of tracheotomy include pneumothorax, bleeding, and subcutaneous emphysema. Pneumothorax is corrected by insertion of a chest tube (see Chapter 32). Bleeding can usually be controlled by local pressure; if this fails, the wound should be explored to ligate the bleeding vessel.
3. The tracheotomy tube may become dislodged, if it is not well secured. If this happens in the first 48–72 hours, urgent reintubation or repeated tracheotomy may be required. After 3–4 days, the tube can be easily reinserted through the tracheotomy opening. The obturator should be taped to the patient's bed in case of this emergency.
4. The tube may become occluded. To prevent accumulation of dried mucus crusts, the inner cannula is removed and cleansed with a pipe cleaner every 6 hours, after soaking in hydrogen peroxide solution. Inspired air should be humidified, since this also minimizes crusting and obstruction of the tube.
5. Many of the long-term complications of tracheotomy can be prevented by an accurate and careful initial procedure. Postoperative stenosis of the trachea results from excessive removal of cartilage, flaps of tracheal cartilage that fall into the lumen after the tube is removed, insertion of improperly sized tracheotomy tubes that curve into the anterior tracheal wall, and high-pressure tracheotomy cuffs. Infection at the tracheotomy site may result in late stenosis.

Infectious Disease

In general, management of the patient with acute infectious obstruction of the airway begins with evaluation of the cause of obstruction. One of the major diagnostic aids is the lateral x-ray view of the neck (Fig. 42.15*C*), which demonstrates epiglottitis, retropharyngeal abscess, narrowing of the trachea from tracheitis, and laryngopyocele. The examiner should avoid instrumentation of the upper airway; gagging during introduction of a mirror may produce a sudden respiratory arrest, which may be fatal.

Acute Epiglottitis. This inflammatory condition is most common in children from 3–6 years old, but may occur at any age. Symptoms include a rapidly progressing sore throat, painful swallowing, and dysphagia. Respiratory obstruction may arise within a few hours after the onset of symptoms. The patient leans forward to improve breathing, respirations are slow and stridorous, and the voice is muffled but not hoarse. The patient may be drooling because of painful swallowing.

Any effort to examine the intraoral structures may precipitate acute respiratory obstruction and should be avoided. A lateral x-ray film of the neck (Fig. 42.17) confirms the diagnosis of acute epiglottitis without the need for intraoral examination.

Treatment consists of administration of high-dose corticosteroids, humidified oxygen, and antibiotics; ampicillin or chloramphenicol is preferred because

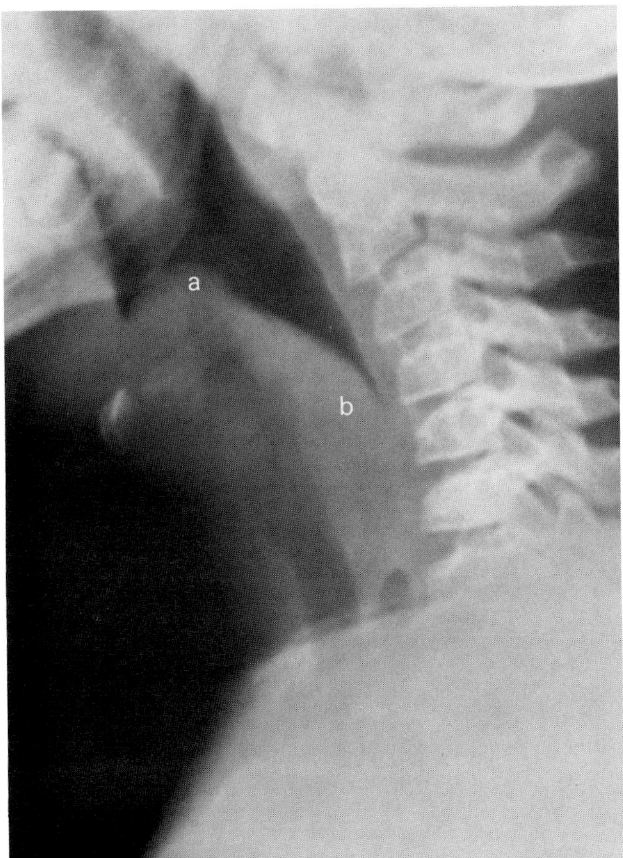

Figure 42.17. Lateral soft-tissue x-ray view of neck demonstrating epiglottitis. *a,* Edema of epiglottis; *b,* edema of arytenoid region and retrocricoid area.

of the possibility that *Haemophilus influenzae* is the infecting organism. In approximately 50% of cases, the disease is caused by a virus. Common bacterial organisms causing this problem include *H. influenzae,* staphylococcus, streptococcus, and pneumococcus. The patient should be closely observed; endotracheal intubation is indicated in any patient with signs of progressive obstruction or hypoxia.

Considerable debate exists over the necessity for tracheotomy in this situation. At present, most physicians prefer intensive medical therapy and intubation rather than tracheotomy. In the young child, treatment should be more aggressive, and intubation should be performed at an earlier stage, preferably in the operating room under general anesthesia. The tube must be firmly secured in the young child to prevent accidental extubation. If tracheotomy is necessary, it should be performed with an endotracheal tube in place and with resection of minimal cartilage.

Croup. Formally termed acute laryngotracheobronchitis, croup is characterized by a barking cough and inspiratory-expiratory (biphasic) stridor. In temperate climates, attacks usually occur at night in the winter and spring. The typical patient is 6 months to 3 years old, who has had a mild upper respiratory tract infection for 1–3 days, often with a barking cough. Physical examination reveals retractions, cyanosis, and tachycardia if obstruction has progressed.

In milder cases, the child is placed in a high-humidity atmosphere with oxygen, the so-called croup tent. Therapy also includes administration of ampicillin and corticosteroids, such as dexamethasone, 1 mg/kg/day in four divided doses. In severe cases, 2.5% racemic epinephrine (microNEFRIN) has proved effective. This substance is diluted in sterile saline solution (1:4 or 1:8) and delivered by means of the nebulizer of an intermittent positive-pressure breathing apparatus. The treatment is repeated every 15 minutes for 1 hour; if this fails to reverse the progress of obstruction, intubation and tracheotomy are advised.

Peritonsillar Abscess. Peritonsillar abscess usually occurs after a sore throat that has lasted 5–10 days. In many cases, the patient has been treated with ineffective doses of penicillin or other antibiotic and begins to complain of increasing unilateral throat pain, dysphagia, trismus, and fever. The patient appears to be in acute pain, and has difficulty swallowing even saliva. Trismus may make examination of the mouth difficult, but once the patient opens his mouth, the physician may note a bulge in the superior pole of the tonsillar fossa, with displacement of the entire tonsil toward the midline. Edema of the tonsillar pillars and soft palate with displacement of the uvula away from the peritonsillar abscess may be present. Cervical lymphadenopathy and fever are often associated. This condition is frequently confused with peritonsillar cellulitis; the examiner should determine whether there is true fluctuance in the superior pole of the tonsil, signifying an abscess. Aspiration with a large-bore needle should be performed prior to incision and drainage to prove the presence of purulent material, since aneurysmal swelling of the internal carotid artery can occur in this area.

If purulent material is present, incision across the superior pole drains it. Penicillin should be administered intravenously, and the patient should be observed for development of respiratory obstruction. Untreated peritonsillar abscess often drains spontaneously, but the condition should be treated since deep neck infection, septic thrombosis of the internal jugular vein, and mediastinitis are potential complications. The patient should undergo tonsillectomy after the acute infection has resolved. We favor immediate tonsillectomy as definitive treatment for acute peritonsillar abscess, although not all otolaryngologists agree on this matter. Consultation with an otolaryngologist should be sought if a peritonsillar abscess is suspected or diagnosed. If the treatment advice is for the patient to have a tonsillectomy in the acute phase of the abscess, a "quinsy tonsillectomy," incision and drainage may then be delayed until the patient is in the operating room under anesthesia. At operation, the entire abscess cavity is unroofed by tonsillectomy.

Retropharyngeal Abscess. Unlike peritonsillar abscess, which is usually found in adults, retropharyngeal abscess most often occurs in children aged 3 years or younger. There is usually a history of an upper respiratory tract infection that has worsened, with fever, tachycardia, drooling, dyspnea, stiff neck, and marked irritability. The patient appears ill on examination, holding the head rigidly and complaining of pain on moving the neck. Stridor is present in varying degrees. Oral examination demonstrates a bulge on the posterior pharyngeal wall, which should be confirmed by a lateral x-ray film of the neck (Fig. 42.18). In an adult, this condition results from a break in the mucosal surface of the pharynx caused by trauma, a foreign body, or rarely, osteomyelitis of the cervical spine.

The patient should be hospitalized for monitoring of respiratory status and for administration of antibiotics. A drainage procedure should be performed under general anesthesia with the head in a dependent position to prevent pooling of purulent material in the lower airway. An adenoidectomy is usually indicated at operation.

Laryngopyocele. Laryngocele, a herniation

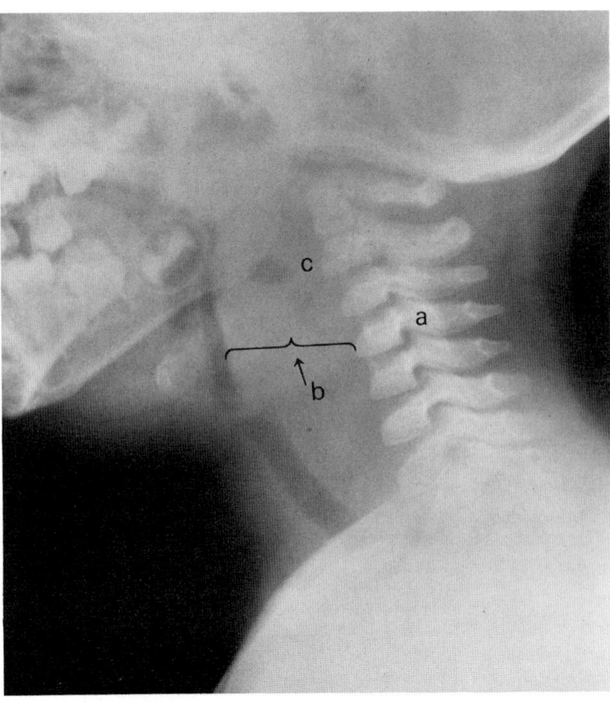

Figure 42.18. Lateral soft-tissue x-ray view of neck demonstrating retropharyngeal abscess. *a*, Straightening of cervical spine; *b*, increase in distance between posterior pharyngeal wall and vertebral column; *c*, gas pocket within abscess.

of the laryngeal ventricle, usually arises in patients whose profession involves creation of intensive pressures within the upper airway, for example, glassblowing or playing a wind instrument. A laryngocele can become infected during an upper respiratory tract infection, producing progressive hoarseness, thickening of the voice, and stridor. Speech and swallowing are painful. Indirect examination of the larynx with a mirror demonstrates unilateral edema and inflammatory changes. Anteroposterior and lateral x-ray views of the neck assist in making the diagnosis (Fig. 42.19).

Tracheotomy is mandatory, and is best performed with an endotracheal tube in place. If intubation is impossible, tracheotomy under local anesthesia may be extremely difficult; the patient is reluctant to lie down to allow the procedure because of air hunger. After tracheotomy, the laryngopyocele should be drained externally by an otolaryngologist, and appropriate antibiotics given.

Foreign Bodies

Aspiration of a foreign body occurs most frequently in young children. Symptoms of respiratory obstruction caused by a foreign body are wheezing, coughing, stridor, salivation, and inability to swallow; the parents may or may not be aware of the cause. On examination, the child may have signs of acute respiratory obstruction or may be sitting quietly with wheezing audible only on auscultation. Examination includes inspection of the oral cavity and evaluation of the hypopharynx and larynx with a mirror if possible. Auscultation of the chest may demonstrate localized consolidation or obstruction. Anteroposterior and lateral x-ray views of the neck and chest may reveal a foreign body; fluoroscopic pulmonary examination may show mediastinal shift or air trapped in one lung, and bronchograms or computed tomography (CT) may be helpful.

The adult with a foreign body in the upper part of the airway often describes it and identifies its level reasonably accurately. Common lodging sites include the tonsil, the base of the tongue, the posterior pharyngeal wall, the vallecula, the larynx, and the cricopharyngeus muscle. A foreign body at the tonsil or at the base of the tongue can be seen on direct inspection; pharyngeal and laryngeal foreign bodies can be seen on examination with a mirror or can be located by means of anteroposterior and lateral films of the neck. A tracheobronchial foreign body may be outlined by chest x-ray film or fluoroscopic study.

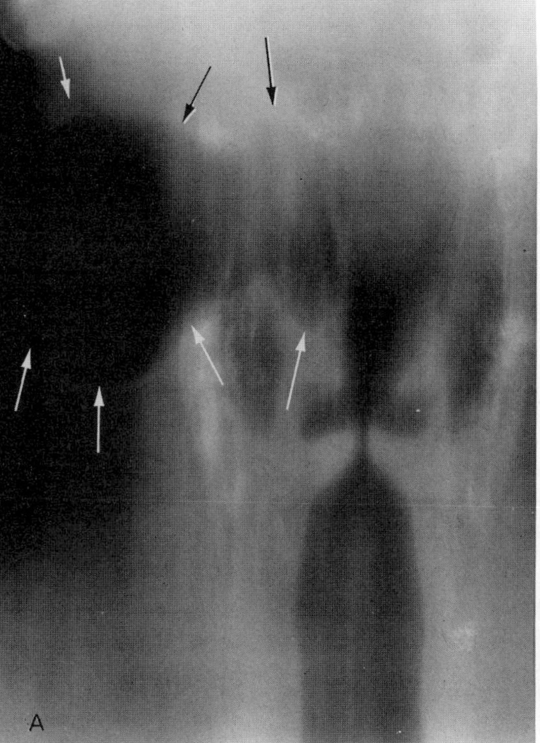

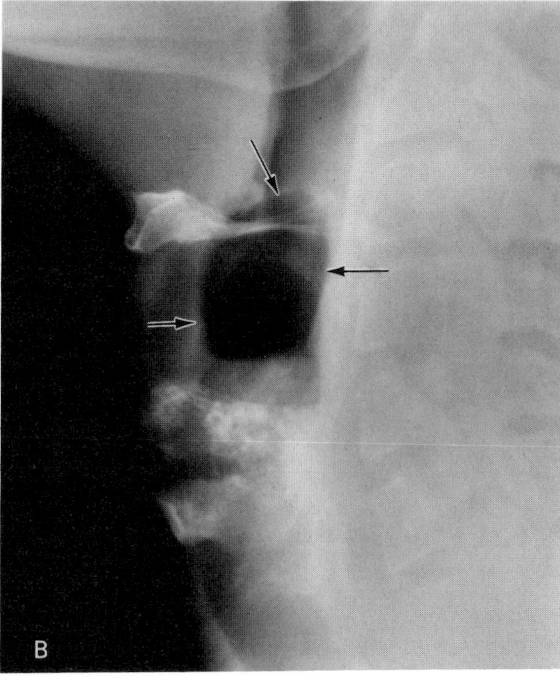

Figure 42.19. Laryngocele. *A,* Anterior tomographic view of neck. *Arrows* indicate margins of sac. *B,* Lateral soft-tissue x-ray view. *Arrows* demarcate border of sac.

Acute total obstruction of the airway may be managed by performing the Heimlich maneuver, as detailed in Chapter 32. Cricothyrotomy is necessary if this fails to dislodge the object. A patient with acute obstruction may die before arrival at the emergency department; if he has survived, there is usually time for an orderly evaluation. No attempts should be made to remove a foreign body with the fingertips, since this may move it distally. Once the object is located by history or radiologic evaluation, endoscopic removal is indicated. Occasionally, an object at the tonsil or base of the tongue may be removed directly with forceps.

Tumor

A patient with a laryngeal tumor has progressive respiratory obstruction over weeks to months, with associated symptoms of dysphagia, hoarseness, and pain in the throat and the ear. Respiratory stridor may be evident, and the tumor may be visible on direct or mirror examination. Cervical lymphadenopathy may be apparent if the tumor has metastasized. Lateral x-ray views of the neck may show soft-tissue shadows in the airway. The patient should be referred to an otolaryngologist for urgent evaluation and for consideration of immediate tracheotomy if severe dyspnea exists.

Conditions in the Newborn

Incomplete development of the laryngeal cartilaginous framework (laryngomalacia) is the most common cause of noninfectious respiratory stridor in the neonatal period. The infant usually has no stridor when he or she is upright or prone, but it develops when the infant is supine. This phenomenon results from collapse of the supraglottic airway with negative inspiratory pressure. Since the condition disappears by the time the child is 1–2 years old as the cartilaginous structures harden, it is treated expectantly.

Many rare conditions cause stridor in the newborn. These include laryngeal papillomatosis, massive enlargement of the adenoids of tonsils, craniofacial anomalies, abnormalities of the aortic arch, and hemangiomas of the subglottic region. They all require the attention of respective specialists.

Acute Sore Throat

Many of the conditions discussed in the following sections are indistinguishable on clinical grounds. In general, the more severe the symptoms and physical findings—erythema, edema, and exudate, for example—the more likely it is that the infecting organism is group A β-hemolytic streptococcus. Milder symptoms and findings suggest viral disease, although the possibility of streptococcal infection still exists.

Viral Infection. *Coxsackie virus A, adenoviruses,* and *the influenza and parainfluenza viruses* cause rhinitis, cough, and a mild sore throat with hoarseness and malaise. On physical examination the throat is mildly inflamed and erythematous, without exudate, although Coxsackie virus A may cause herpangina with pharyngeal vesicles or ulcers. There is a low-grade fever. Laboratory findings are consistent with viral infection. Treatment is directed toward symptomatic relief.

Patients with *herpetic infections of the oral mucosa* have severe pain. On physical examination, mucosal vesicles with an erythematous base and regional lymphadenopathy can be seen. Treatment includes narcotic analgesics if necessary and use of a dilute hydrogen peroxide (3%) mouthwash to maintain oral hygiene. Viscous lidocaine or triamcinolone acetonide in emollient dental paste (Kenalog in Orabase) may be applied to the lesions every 4 hours.

One of the manifestations of *infectious mononucleosis* is a sore throat. Others include fatigue, malaise, fever, dysphagia, and a diffuse rash. On physical examination the patient may exhibit pharyngotonsillitis with a gray exudate, marked cervical lymphadenopathy, fever, an enlarged liver or spleen, and rash. Laboratory findings include lymphocytosis with many atypical lymphocytes (up to 70%) and a positive heterophil test for mononucleosis. A culture of the throat exudate may show concomitant streptococcal infection. Emergency care consists of bed rest with a short course of corticosteroids, such as prednisone, administered over 3 days in decreasing doses (60, 40, 20 mg). Penicillin should be given intravenously or intramuscularly along with analgesics and fluids.

Aphthous stomatitis, a condition of unknown cause, is manifested by a localized area of severe throat pain, and tends to recur. The patient will have a flat, well-demarcated mucosal ulcer up to 2 cm in diameter in the mouth or the pharynx without purulent exudate. The patient is afebrile, and laboratory findings are normal. The condition is treated in the same manner as herpetic lesions, with follow-up care until the lesion clears. If the lesion persists longer than 2–3 weeks, the physician should consider a diagnosis of chronic granulomatous disease, syphilis, or carcinoma.

Bacterial Infection. *"Strep throat"* caused by group A β-hemolytic streptococci is characterized by a rapid onset of sore throat and fever. Generalized rash, headache, nausea, and vomiting may be associated. Upon arriving in the emergency department, the patient may have a fever, pharyngitis, or tonsillitis with exudate and regional lymphadenopathy. In the case of scarlet fever, the patient has circumoral pallor, a strawberry-colored tongue, cutaneous rash, petechial rash of the palate, and accentuated flexor creases of the elbows. Laboratory findings include granulocytosis and a throat culture positive for β-hemolytic streptococci. Therapy includes oral penicillin, 250 mg (400,000 units) four times a day for 10 days, or one injection of intramuscular benzathine penicillin G, 1.2 million units in adults, 600,000 units in children less than 6 years old, and 900,000 units in children from 6–9 years old.

Now reported only sporadically, *diphtheria* is typified by a mild to moderate, slowly progressing sore throat, a mildly elevated temperature, anterior cervical lymphadenopathy, and progressive toxemia with nausea, vomiting, and headache. Physical examination discloses marked tachycardia, a temperature to 101°F (38.3°C), and an adherent gray membrane over the tonsils and the pharynx. The pharyngeal mucosa characteristically bleeds when it is rubbed with a culture swab and has a musty odor. Laboratory tests should include an immediate sputum smear for *Corynebacterium diphtheriae.* When the emergency physician suspects diphtheria, he should isolate the patient and administer a skin test with diphtheria antitoxin to elicit an allergic reaction. If the skin test is negative, 20,000–30,000 units of diphtheria antitoxin should be administered intramuscularly as soon as possible. After all laboratory studies are done, penicillin should be administered.

The symptoms of *Vincent's angina* are a sore throat, painful gums, enlargement of the submaxillary and cervical lymph nodes, and a foul breath. The emergency physician detects a shaggy grayish membrane on the tonsils, palate, and gingivae that rubs off easily, with underlying bloody, granular, ulcerated tissue. The temperature is usually only minimally elevated. Gram's stain reveals a mixed infection with fusiform bacilli and spirochetes. Therapy includes gargling with a 3% hydrogen peroxide solution and a 10-day course of penicillin, 250 mg four times a day.

Other Conditions. A *monilial pharyngeal inflammation* may be secondary to immunosuppression, leukemia, or an overgrowth after recent antibiotic or corticosteroid therapy. The pharyngeal mucosa exhibits erythema and white patches similar to curds of milk. Emergency care consists of nystatin (Mycostatin) oral suspension, 5 ml to be gargled and swallowed every 6 hours until 2 days after the last lesions disappear.

Bullous erythema multiforme is typified by a massive bullous eruption of the lips and the mucous membrane and the cutaneous lesions of erythema multiforme. The condition may be due either to an upper respiratory tract infection or to an allergic reaction to drugs. Although the illness is self-limited, systemic corticosteroids seem to hasten healing of the lesions.

Agranulocytosis and *acute leukemia* can both be manifested by acute sore throat and fever with pharyngeal exudate or membrane. The diagnosis is made by complete blood cell count and other signs of generalized disease, such as petechiae, ecchymoses, hepatosplenomegaly, and lymphadenopathy.

Thyroiditis may result in pain and tightness of the lower portion of the throat lasting for days to weeks. The pain may extend up the neck to the ear, and the patient has fatigue and malaise. On examination, the thyroid gland is tender and sometimes swollen. Laboratory findings include an elevated sedimentation rate and normal or elevated levels of serum triiodothyronine and thyroxine. The patient is treated with salicylates, 600 mg every 4 hours, local heat, and bed rest. He or she should be referred to an endocrinologist for the possibility of corticosteroid therapy.

THE NECK

Masses

For the purpose of differential diagnosis of neck masses, three areas may be defined (Fig. 42.20). Possible diagnoses for each area, divided into pediatric and adult age groups, are presented in Table 42.4. Any patient with a mass in the neck should be referred for thorough examination, including indirect laryngoscopy and nasopharyngoscopy. Acutely infected lesions must be treated on an emergency basis.

Deep Infection

A deep neck infection is usually secondary to infection in one of three areas: a tooth, the pharynx, and the parotid gland. The patient may have been taking antibiotics for tonsillitis or an infected dental extraction site. Signs of progression to deep infection include a high temperature, swelling and tenderness of the neck or the submaxillary space, trismus, pain on motion of the neck or tongue, and stridor. The physician should search for an obvious primary site of infection, such as tonsillitis, peritonsillar abscess, infected tooth, dental extraction site, or parotitis. Antibiotics often mask obvious signs of sepsis.

In the submaxillary region, Ludwig's angina is the most common deep neck infection. Infection of the pharyngomaxillary space is commonly seen in children as an extension of tonsillitis or mastoid infection. Signs include trismus and swelling of the parotid region or the lateral pharyngeal wall or both.

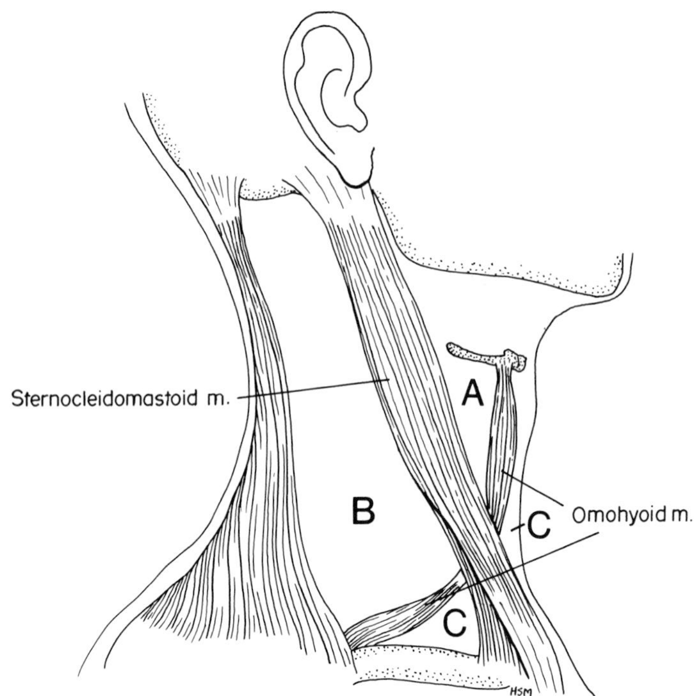

Figure 42.20. Division of neck into three areas for differential diagnosis of neck masses (see Table 42.4).

In the parotid space, signs of infection are swelling and marked tenderness over the parotid gland without trismus. The anterior part of the neck is usually infected after esophageal or hypopharyngeal trauma. Signs include tenderness along the sulcus between the sternocleidomastoid muscle and larynx, hoarseness, stridor, and dysphagia.

If the airway is compromised, intubation or emergency tracheotomy may be necessary. Anteroposterior and lateral x-ray films of the neck may aid in evaluation of the airway. Specimens should be taken from the primary site of infection for culture and from the blood if septicemia is apparent. Administration of fluid and high-dose antibiotics should

Figure 42.4.
Neck Masses: Possible Diagnoses

Zone[a]	Child	Adult
A	Branchial cyst Dermoid cyst Thyroglossal cyst Nonspecific lymphadenopathy Lymphoma Infectious disease (pharyngitis, dental abscess, tuberculosis, cat-scratch disease) Metastatic disease (rare)	Metastatic carcinoma from upper aerodigestive tract Primary tumor of parotid or submaxillary gland Inflammatory node (acute or chronic, including tuberculous) Zenker's diverticulum (rare) Laryngocele (rare) Carotid arterial aneurysm (rare) Chemodectoma (rare)
B	Infectious lymphadenopathy (pharynx, adenoids, scalp) Lymphoma Neurofibroma	Lymphoma Nasopharyngeal tumor Local skin infection Neurofibroma
C	Cystic hygroma Thyroid lesion Branchial cyst or sinus Lymphoma	Thyroid lesion Metastatic carcinoma (laryngeal, pulmonary, gastrointestinal) Aneurysm of the aorta or great vessels

[a] See Figure 42.20.

begin, and the patient should be hospitalized for intensive therapy and possible operative drainage. Antibiotics should be selected to cover a wide range of pathogens, including penicillinase-producing staphylococcus and Gram-negative organisms. The antibiotic regimen may be modified after results of culture and sensitivity tests. A short course of high-dose corticosteroids, such as prednisone, 60–80 mg/day for 3 days in an adult, may hasten the resolution of edema.

Trauma

Blunt Injury

Blunt trauma to the neck, especially the "clothesline" injury, can cause extensive damage to internal structures without breaking the skin. Potential injuries include complete laryngotracheal transection or lesser laryngeal fractures, esophageal tears, thrombotic occlusion of major vessels, contusion or stretching of the brachial plexus, and fracture or dislocation of the cervical spine.

On physical examination, abrasions and edema of the skin may make evaluation of the deeper structures more difficult. The contour of the laryngeal cartilage should be carefully palpated, and signs of disruption of the airway, such as hoarseness, stridor, hemoptysis, and subcutaneous emphysema, should be sought. Paraplegia or quadriplegia with sensory defects means trauma to the spinal cord, whereas hemiplegia, obtundation, or expanding hematoma suggests carotid injury.

Penetrating Injury

High-velocity missiles and knives may cause extensive tissue destruction. The wound is usually contaminated from foreign material such as particles of clothing, wadding, and shrapnel. If the patient survives until arrival at the emergency department, his life can probably be saved if hemorrhage can be controlled.

On examination, the emergency physician may observe either an ooze of dark blood, suggesting venous laceration, or a pulsatile flow of blood from a transected artery. A hematoma may be noted, which should be carefully observed for expansion. The patient may be in hemorrhagic shock. Isolated neurologic defects may occur, reflecting injury to one or more nerves in the neck. Pulses should be palpated at the superficial temporal and carotid arteries to assist in diagnosis of major vascular injury; the presence of pulses does not necessarily exclude the possibility of such an injury, however. An audible bruit suggests significant vascular trauma.

As many as one-third of patients with a major vascular injury have no clinical evidence of it. Some physicians advise exploration of all transplatysmal injuries that are near vascular structures; we recommend this approach for injuries above the cricoid cartilage. However, we believe that injuries of the lower neck should be initially evaluated by means of arteriography. Patients with normal arteriographic results should be observed, and those with an obvious vascular lesion should undergo exploration with transthoracic proximal control of the bleeding vessels if necessary.

The first priority in the treatment of a penetrating injury is control of hemorrhage by compression of vessels against the cervical spine. Integrity of the airway must be assured, and the cervical spine should be immobilized until significant injury to it is excluded. Intravascular volume should be replaced by means of large-bore intravenous lines.

SUGGESTED READINGS

Ballenger, JJ, ed. *Diseases of the Nose, Throat, Ear, Head and Neck,* 13th ed. Philadelphia: Lea & Febinger, 1985.

Becker W, Buckingham RA, Holinger PH, et al. *Atlas of Ear, Nose, and Throat Diseases, including Broncho-esophagology,* 2nd ed. Stuttgart: Georg Thieme, 1984.

Boies LR. *Fundamentals of Otolaryngology,* 5th ed. Philadelphia: WB Saunders, 1978.

Bossy J. *Atlas of Neuroanatomy and Special Sense Organs.* Philadelphia: WB Saunders, 1970.

DeWeese DD, Saunders WH. *Textbook of Otolaryngology,* 6th ed. St Louis: CV Mosby, 1982.

Gates GA, Folbre TW. Indications for adenotonsillectomy. *Arch Otolaryngol Head Neck Surg,* 1986;112:501–502.

Kendig EL Jr, Chernick V, eds. *Disorders of the Respiratory Tract in Children,* 4th ed. Philadelphia: WB Saunders, 1983.

Montgomery WW. *Surgery of the Upper Respiratory System.* Philadelphia: Lea & Febinger, 1971 (vol 1), 1973 (vol 2).

Schuknecht HF. *Pathology of the Ear.* Cambridge: Harvard University Press, 1974.

Shambaugh GE Jr, Glasscock ME. *Surgery of the Ear,* 2nd ed. Philadelphia: WB Saunders, 1980.

Symposium on Trauma to the Head and Neck. The Otolaryngologic Clinics of North America. Vol 16(3), Philadelphia: WB Saunders, August 1983.

Wilson WR, Byl FM, Laird N. The efficacy of steroids in the treatment of idiopathic sudden hearing loss. a double-blind study. *Arch Otolaryngol Head Neck Surg,* 1980;106:772–776.

CHAPTER **43**

Ocular Emergencies

BRADFORD J. SHINGLETON, M.D.
ALBERT R. FREDERICK, JR., M.D.
B. THOMAS HUTCHINSON, M.D.

Emergency ocular care may not always be optimal or definitive. With injuries involving multiple sites and organ injury, there may be a confluence of serious problems competing for attention. In establishing priorities, it is important to realize that prompt, knowledgeable ocular evaluation and treatment can drastically affect a patient's visual outcome. In both acute ocular disease and injuries, effective triage and treatment must differentiate between the potentially blinding eye problem and lesser pathology. The emergency department physician must identify the true ocular emergency and initiate appropriate care and consultation.

EVALUATION OF EYE EMERGENCIES

History

As with other medical problems, an accurate history is useful in evaluating medical and traumatic eye emergencies. The chief complaint should be amplified by characterizing any symptoms of altered vision, eye pain, redness, swelling, or ocular discharge. A change in vision should be pursued further to determine the presence or absence of diminished central acuity, visual field loss, diplopia, halos around lights, flashes, floaters, and metamorphopsia.

Examination Techniques

Examination in an eye emergency requires a careful and systematic approach. In particular, when the possibility of ocular rupture exists after trauma, examination must be performed under controlled conditions and with utmost care if further harm is to be avoided. Uncooperative patients and children may need to be examined under general anesthesia. The examination must provide adequate exposure without pressure on the globe; this can result in disruption of intraocular contents. To avoid overlooking important pathology, one should consider at least six points in the eye examination of every patient: (*a*) vision; (*b*) lids/orbit; (*c*) anterior segment; (*d*) pupils/extraocular movement; (*e*) ophthalmoscopy, and (*f*) intraocular pressure.

Vision

Initial examination should include the determination of visual acuity for each eye. Vision measurement is crucial for diagnosis, management, and medical/legal documentation. The *only* exception for delaying visual acuity measurement is the case of a chemical burn where vision should be tested after completion of emergency eye irrigation. A standard Snellen eye chart is recommended for determining visual acuity, with the patient wearing distance glasses. For patients who cannot read the largest character on a vision chart, record the distance at which the patient can count fingers. If the patient is unable to count fingers, record the distance at which the patient can detect hand movement in any field. If the patient cannot detect hand movement, determine whether he or she can perceive light, and, if so, in what quadrant. Accurate differentiation between light perception and hand movement has diagnostic and therapeutic implications. In cases of altered vision, neuromedical disease, or head trauma, it is important to test the patient's peripheral vision by the confrontation method.

Lids/Orbit

Examine the lids to be sure that they open and close completely. Ensure integrity of the lid margin and characterize any swelling, color change, or discharge. In cases of periorbital trauma, palpate for subcutaneous emphysema and defects in the orbital rim. Test facial cutaneous sensation, and assess globe position (exophthalmos or enophthalmos). Orbital radiographs may be indicated if orbital fracture is included in the differential diagnosis.

Ocular foreign bodies are often hidden under the inner surface of the upper lid or in the cul-de-sac formed by the reflection of upper lid and bulbar conjunctiva. Eversion of the lids is required to detect these foreign bodies. However, the lid should not be everted when perforating injury is suspected.

Single eversion exposes the under surface of the upper eyelid. It is performed as follows:

1. Instill topical anesthetic;
2. Place cotton applicator stick at the upper edge of tarsal plate of the lid;
3. Grasp eyelashes with other hand, and pull down and slightly forward, everting the lid as it is raised and folded back over the applicator;
4. Pull the lid up, and "flip" the eyelid over, using the cotton applicator stick as a fulcrum; and
5. Keep the lid everted with slight pressure on the lashes; use the moistened applicator, when removed from the fulcrum position, to remove foreign bodies.

Double eversion of the eyelids exposes the upper cul-de-sac. It is performed as follows:

1. Place the patient supine, and instill topical anesthetic;
2. Place a lid retractor on the lid 1 cm above the lid margin, grasp the eyelid, and pull the lid over the retractor; and
3. Rotate the retractor to expose the upper cul-de-sac.

Anterior Segment

The anterior segment examination consists of careful inspection of the sclera/conjunctiva, cornea, anterior chamber, iris, and lens.

Sclera/Conjunctiva. Inspect sclera/conjunctiva for vascular injection, hemorrhage, swelling (chemosis), discharge, foreign bodies, and lacerations. Retractors may aid this examination.

Cornea. The cornea is the transparent dome-shaped anterior portion of the eye. Corneal clarity may be determined with a penlight; the light reflex from the corneal surface should be crisp and sharp without irregular reflection. Topical anesthetics may facilitate the examination in cases of discomfort due to corneal abrasions or foreign bodies. Topical fluorescein stains the basement membrane in abrasions, producing an epithelial defect, and fluoresces green when illuminated by cobalt blue light. Magnification offered by loupes or slit lamp biomicroscopy greatly enhances detailed examination.

Anterior Chamber. The anterior chamber is the fluid-filled space between the cornea and iris. Examine for gross blood (hyphema) or pus (hypopyon) as well as depth.

Iris. In the setting of trauma, the iris should be examined for defects, distortion, or incarceration in full-thickness ocular lacerations. Color change is best determined by careful comparison with the fellow eye.

Lens. The lens is normally optically clear. Loss of transparency is evidence for cataract formation. An increasing number of patients having had cataract surgery may have an intraocular lens in place anterior to the iris, in the plane of the pupil, or behind the iris. As pupillary plane lenses may be dislocated with mydriasis, *patients with lens implants should not have the pupils dilated* in the emergency center without ophthalmologic assessment.

Pupils/Extraocular Movement

Examination of pupillary signs and extraocular movement are important components of the neuro-ophthalmic examination, as well as the anterior segment evaluation.

The *pupils* should be black, round, equal in size, and reactive to light. Previous ocular surgery, injury, or the use of topical medications may affect the pupils; variation in any of these parameters requires further evaluation. In cases of trauma, decreased vision, or eye pain, test for an afferent pupillary defect (Marcus Gunn pupil) utilizing the "swinging flashlight" test. In this test, a bright light shone in each normal eye of a patient causes the pupils to constrict briskly and symmetrically. In the presence of an afferent pupillary defect, the pupil constricts less and redilates faster in the eye harboring a retinal or optic nerve lesion than in the normal eye.

To assess *extraocular movement,* check each eye for fullness of excursion in four positions of gaze—up, down, right, and left. Subtle, unilateral limitation of movement of one eye may be detected by comparing range of movement of the two eyes together.

Ophthalmoscopy

Use the direct ophthalmoscope to examine the clarity of the ocular media (cornea, anterior chamber, lens, vitreous), the optic nerve, and the retina and its vessels. If the ocular media are clear, the examiner should observe a brilliant red light reflex through the ophthalmoscope when the light fills the pupil. Evaluate the optic nerve for atrophy, cupping, edema, or hemorrhages. Follow each of the vessel arcades into the periphery; examine the macular region last by having the patient look directly at the ophthalmoscope light.

Dilation of the pupils facilitates examination and can be accomplished by topical application of tropicamide 1% or phenylephrine 2.5% eyedrops. The risk of precipitating angle closure glaucoma is small with dilating drops and should not prevent the use of mydriatic drops if important information may be gained by their use. Even in an eye with a shallow anterior chamber and the small risk of angle closure, the pupil may need to be dilated for adequate posterior segment evaluation.

Intraocular Pressure

Measurement of the intraocular pressure should be performed in suspected cases of acute glaucoma or if the optic nerve is cupped and/or atrophic. Tonometry should not be attempted if there is a possibility of a ruptured globe. In the absence of a tonometer, intraocular pressure assessment can be obtained by comparing the two eyes through digital pressure on the globe through closed lids. This technique may assist the examiner in confirming the presence of unilateral acute glaucoma. However, Schötz tonometry is more accurate, relatively easy to perform, and thus better suited than digital pressure for emergency center evaluation where intraocular pressure assessment is important.

Radiology of the Orbit

Radiographic evaluation may be helpful in the assessment of fractures, intraorbital or intraocular foreign bodies, orbital hemorrhage, orbital abscess, and exophthalmos. Standard x-ray views include posteroanterior (PA), lateral, Caldwell, Waters, and base projections. Optic canal projections may supplement this standard series. In trauma and acute orbital disease, computed tomography (CT) of the orbit is often more helpful than orbital radiographs.

DIAGNOSIS AND TREATMENT OF EYE EMERGENCIES

Nonpenetrating Ocular Trauma

Injury to the eye from blunt, nonpenetrating trauma or chemical exposure may result in transient blurring of vision with minimal discomfort, or may lead to permanent, irreversible loss of vision with disorganization of the globe. It is far too easy for the nonophthalmic physician to miss significant pathologic findings, since not all injuries are detectable on routine external examination and ophthalmoscopy. Hemorrhage, glaucoma, and rupture of the globe should be treated immediately by an ophthalmologist. Most other defects may be treated at the initial examination, with less immediate need for ophthalmic consultation. The following injuries may occur alone, or frequently in combination, when trauma of moderate to severe force occurs.

Chemical Burns

Chemical burns represent a vision-threatening emergency and require *immediate* treatment in the emergency department. Prompt irrigation is the treatment of choice. The transparency of the cornea, integrity, and survival of the eye after chemical injury may be directly related to the immediacy of treatment. Alkaline burns tend to be more severe than acidic burns because of more rapid penetration through the cornea and other ocular tissues. Common sources of alkali include drain cleaners, industrial solvents, plaster, fertilizer, and lime.

The entire emergency department staff should be instructed in the emergency care of a chemical eye burn. Patients calling by phone should be instructed to initiate irrigation immediately with the nearest source of water available (cup, sink, etc.). Effective treatment in the emergency department requires that the patient be seen immediately. Defer visual acuity measurement until irrigation has been completed. To ensure complete removal of the chemical substance, apply topical anesthesia and retract the lids, using single or double eversion as necessary, removing any particulate chemical matter. Direct a continuous flow of normal saline across the exposed globe for 10 minutes, regardless of irrigation performed elsewhere. An intravenous set may serve as an effective irrigation delivery system. *Neutralizing solutions are not recommended for use.* After irrigation and the removal of particulate matter, instill a topical cycloplegic in order to reduce ciliary body spasm, a topical antibiotic drop, and a sterile patch. Systemic analgesia may be required. Prompt ophthalmologic consultation is recommended; patients with severe burns may require hospitalization for medical and/or surgical management.

Thermal Burns

Thermal injuries to the eyes and adnexae are more commonly confined to the lids than are chemical injuries because of the rapid blink reflex that protects the globe. Treatment should be directed toward minimizing scarring, as subsequent cicatricial defects of the lid often cause ocular exposure and may even be responsible for permanent visual loss. If a thermal burn of the ocular surface occurs, apply topical antibiotics and cycloplegics. A moist chamber may be required to protect the exposed cornea in cases of incomplete lid closure. To achieve this, apply sterile vaseline to the surrounding skin, and place a sterile polyethylene (Saran Wrap) sheet over the orbital area. Skin grafting and lid tarsorraphy may be needed later to establish proper lid position and adequate globe protection.

Corneal Abrasions

Corneal abrasions cause blurring of vision, foreign body sensation, photophobia, and tearing. Careful flashlight examination reveals an altered light reflection from the corneal surface in areas of abrasion. Topical fluorescein aids diagnosis; a corneal abrasion is revealed as a zone of blue-green staining when viewed with cobalt blue illumination.

Treat corneal abrasions with a topical antibiotic, cycloplegia, and a firm pressure patch that should be left in place for 24 hours to ensure complete lid closure and permit corneal reepithelialization. Large abrasions may require systemic analgesia and reexamination the next day. If the epithelial defect has not healed, or if a white infiltrate has developed, refer the patient to an ophthalmologist. *Never prescribe topical anesthetics;* chronic, unsupervised use may retard healing and predispose the eye to infection.

Recurrent corneal erosion is a possible sequela of corneal abrasion and may occur weeks or months after injury, especially after abrasions caused by fingernails, paper cuts, or tree branches. Characterized by sudden, sharp foreign body sensation similar to the original injury, recurrent corneal erosion is classically noted on awakening in the morning. Examination soon after symptoms occur reveals an irregular corneal epithelium that has been detached by movement of the lid. In some cases, the diagnosis is made by history alone, as the cornea may appear normal in a few hours. Treat recurrent corneal erosion the same as for the initial injury, but in addition, instruct the patient to apply hypertonic (5%) sodium chloride ointment to the lower conjunctival cul-de-sac at night for a period of several months.

Ultraviolet Keratitis—(Welder's Flash)

Ultraviolet energy from a sunlamp or a welder's arc may produce transient, painful corneal irritation several hours after exposure. The intense foreign body sensation, tearing, and blepharospasm often requires topical anesthesia to permit examination. Examination of the cornea with fluorescein reveals diffuse corneal stippling, indicating multiple epithelial defects. Treatment is the same as for corneal abrasion. Again, never prescribe topical anesthesia for home use.

Surface Foreign Bodies

A foreign body on the surface of the eye is the most common eye complaint in an emergency department. Since multiple foreign bodies may be present, the entire anterior segment of the eye must be examined and should include double eversion of the lids. Ocular penetration must be ruled out. Apply topical anesthesia to the eye prior to removal of the foreign body; remove loose foreign bodies on the lids or conjunctiva with a moistened cotton tip applicator or squeeze-bottle irrigation.

Corneal foreign bodies are best removed with a hypodermic needle or spud under the magnified view provided by loupe or slit lamp biomicroscopy. Metallic foreign bodies present only for a few hours may leave a rust ring on the cornea and simulate retained foreign material. A small rust ring outside the visual axis may be left untreated. Deep foreign bodies or rust rings in the visual axis should be removed by an ophthalmologist. After the foreign body has been removed, treat the eye in the same manner as for corneal abrasions.

Contact Lens Problems

The emergency department staff is often asked to treat corneal abrasions due to overwearing of lenses. Treatment for contact lens-induced abrasions include removal of the offending lens, verification that no corneal infection is present, instillation of topical cycloplegia, antibiotics, and pressure patching. Ophthalmologic follow-up is recommended. Sterile saline solution without chemical preservative is recommended for storage of hard and soft contact lenses. Topical fluorescein stains soft contact lenses and should be avoided.

Hyphema

Trauma to the eye may tear peripheral iris vessels, resulting in bleeding into the anterior chamber. This hyphema often layers inferiorly, but may be only diffusely present in the form of circulating red blood cells. In addition to the possibility of globe rupture, concomitant forms of nonperforating damage include tearing of the sphincter muscles of the pupil, traumatic pupillary dilation, lens dislocation, vitreous hemorrhage, retinal hemorrhage, or edema and detachment of the retina. Most of these problems may be identified by careful penlight and ophthalmoscopic examination.

Treat the hyphema patient as one with a possible ruptured globe. Restrict activity, elevate the patient's head to allow gravitational settling of the blood, and provide a shield for protection. Many of these patients are admitted to the hospital and treated with topical cycloplegia, topical steroids, or systemic antifibrinolytic agents. Efforts should be made to reduce the risk of rebleeding, which may result in glaucoma, cataract formation, and corneal blood staining.

Vitreous Hemorrhage

Vitreous hemorrhage may occur after contusion injuries of the globe and usually results from torn retinal capillaries. It is important to rule out a retinal tear that may result in transection of larger vessels, causing considerable intravitreal bleeding, dimming the red reflex, and obscuring details of the fundus. Early ophthalmologic consultation should be sought; there may be concurrent retinal pathology.

Retinal Damage and Detachment

Commotio retinae, or Berlin's edema, refers to retinal whitening after nonpenetrating trauma. This patchy pallor, which may last for hours or days, occurs not only at the site of impact, but also posteriorly. Variable loss of vision occurs, which may be transient or permanent. In some patients, macular holes develop. Crescentic ruptures of the choroid deep to the retina and concentric with the nerve head may also be seen after nonpenetrating traumatic injury; visual loss in this case is associated with serious exudation or hemorrhagic disorganization of the macular photoreceptors.

Contusion of the globe may result in a variety of retinal tears, the most typical of which—dialyses—occur at the retinal periphery. An eye so injured often has findings that can be seen only by indirect ophthalmoscopy. Retinal detachment due to trauma usually develops soon after injury; however, the patient initially may not be aware of any change in vision. Indirect ophthalmoscopy is advised for all contused eyes soon after trauma to detect retinal breaks before detachment, if present, extends posteriorly.

Optic Nerve Damage

A direct blow to the eye can result in hemorrhage into the optic nerve or, occasionally, in complete avulsion of the nerve. Visual loss, up to no light perception, can occur and is associated with afferent pupillary signs. In injuries in which bleeding into the optic canal or nerve sheath is suspected, pressure necrosis of the nerve may be minimized by high-dose systemic steroids or prompt surgical optic nerve decompression, provided that vision was not entirely lost initially. The decision to operate requires immediate ophthalmologic and neurosurgical consultations.

Causes of posttraumatic visual loss are listed in Table 43.1.

Perforating Ocular Trauma

Ruptured Globe/Intraocular Foreign Body

A corneal or scleral laceration is a surgical emergency. It must be identified promptly and treated appropriately in order to protect the eye from further compromise. External pressure on the eye must be avoided.

Accurate diagnosis of small lacerations or perforating foreign bodies requires a high index of suspicion and skillful evaluation because a perforated eye may not have visual blurring. Gentle separation of the lids with lid retractors may be useful. Clues to the diagnosis of a ruptured globe include the following:

Table 43.1.
Differential Diagnosis of Posttraumatic Loss of Vision[a]

Lid swelling, blood, or foreign material covering cornea; corneal damage
Hyphema; vitreous hemorrhage
Traumatic cataract; luxation of lens
Central retinal arterial or venous occlusion (from markedly increased orbital pressure or embolus)
Traumatic retinal edema and hemorrhages of retina from direct or contrecoup blows
Retinal detachment
Avulsion of optic nerve by lateral orbital wall trauma or contrecoup blow to head
Indirect trauma to optic nerves or chiasm or both
Intracranial interruption of visual pathways (hemorrhage, foreign body)
Cortical blindness from hematoma, ischemia, or anoxia (patient may be unaware of blindness)
Acute congestive (angle-closure) glaucoma precipitated by emotional trauma of recent accident or from intumescent lens or other cause
Hysteria
Malingering

[a] From Paton D, Goldberg MF. *Injuries to the Eye, the Lids, and the Orbit.* Philadelphia: WB Saunders, 1968.

1. History of severe blunt or penetrating trauma, projectile injury or contact with a sharp object. A history of previous activity involving the striking of metal-on-metal should especially alert the examining physician to the possibility of an intraocular foreign body;
2. Subconjunctival hemorrhage or laceration;
3. Uveal prolapse—indicated by dark tissue, either iris or ciliary body, on the surface of the globe or deep to the conjunctiva;
4. Irregular or pear-shaped pupil;
5. Gross blood in the anterior chamber (hyphema) or blood in the vitreous which diminishes the ophthalmoscopic red reflex;
6. Asymmetrical anterior chamber depth; and
7. Lens opacification, altering the normal black appearance of the pupil.

If a ruptured globe is suspected, place a protective shield over the eye to avoid external pressure. If premade metal shields are not available, one may be fashioned out of a plastic cup, cardboard, or firm plastic. Do not patch the eye, as the pressure of the patch may cause extrusion of the contents of the globe. Do not apply topical ointments or drops or proceed with further periocular surgery, compresses, or manipulation. Assure stability of the patient, consider tetanus prophylaxis, and refer the patient immediately to an ophthalmologist. Radiographic studies to search for a possible intraocular foreign body are best deferred until after an examination by the ophthalmologist.

Confirmation of a ruptured globe may require surgical exploration. The visual prognosis depends on the ocular tissues that are damaged. In those eyes with irretrievable visual loss after severe trauma, enucleation may be indicated. Prompt ophthalmologic evaluation and enucleation when appropriate minimizes the risk of sympathetic ophthalmia, a bilateral granulomatous ocular inflammation that develops rarely after unilateral penetrating trauma.

Conjunctival Laceration

An opening in the conjunctiva may result from an eye struck by a wire, branch, or other object. Its chief significance is that it may indicate a deeper laceration with entry into the globe itself. Because of bleeding within or beneath the conjunctiva, it may be difficult to determine whether the eye has been perforated. If a scleral laceration cannot be excluded, an ophthalmologist should surgically explore the globe. Most superficial conjunctival lacerations are small and do not require repair, but if the laceration is large, and underlying sclera and Tenon's capsule are exposed, surgical repair may be necessary.

Orbital Trauma

Nonpenetrating Blunt Trauma

Blunt trauma to the orbit may result in lid swelling, ecchymosis, subconjunctival hemorrhage, retrobulbar hemorrhage, globe rupture, and orbital fracture. Because the "harmless black eye" may be a sign of diverse, less conspicuous, but much more serious injuries, always maintain a high index of suspicion during evaluation of these injuries.

Treatment of mild lid swelling and ecchymosis includes cold compresses and pain relief as needed. Subconjunctival hemorrhages may occur with little or no trauma and require no treatment. Rarely, bleeding may occur in the retrobulbar space, resulting in proptosis, decreased vision, corneal exposure, and elevated intraocular pressure. Prompt ophthalmologic consultation is recommended because these patients may require emergency surgical intervention to reduce orbital pressure.

Orbital Fractures

Fractures of the orbit commonly involve the floor and/or medial wall. Unstable facial fractures may occur with severe trauma. Signs and symptoms of orbital blowout fracture include: diplopia, epistaxis, infraorbital nerve hypesthesia, palpable step-offs of the bony rim, and orbital emphysema. If any of these signs or symptoms is noted on presentation, emergency department radiographs are warranted. CT scanning may be required for detailed assessment.

Blowout fractures are usually not an indication for emergency surgery. Elective surgical repair is based on persistent diplopia or cosmetic needs and is best performed when soft tissue swelling has abated. However, unstable periorbital fracture may require urgent surgery. All patients with orbital and periorbital fractures should be seen by an ophthalmologist.

Lid Lacerations

The evaluation of lid lacerations should include both the functional and cosmetic features of the injury. Care must be taken to avoid missing deeper bulbar injury, such as ocular lacerations. In many cases, diagnosis and treatment of this occult injury takes precedence over the readily apparent lid laceration.

The majority of the superficial lid lacerations can be repaired by the emergency department physician. Careful reapposition of the tissues is mandatory if functional or cosmetic compromise is to be avoided. Superficial foreign bodies must be removed; tetanus prophylaxis is often appropriate.

Six types of lid lacerations merit ophthalmologic

consultation: 1. Full-thickenss lid lacerations with lid margin discontinuity must be repaired in layers. Improper closure may result in lid notching and impaired lid function. A technique for lid marginal repair is illustrated in Figure 43.1. 2. Any laceration involving the medial third of the upper and lower lid may disrupt the lacrimal drainage system. These lacerations are best repaired primarily under microscopic observation with reapproximation of the severed canaliculi. 3. Medial lacerations may also disrupt the canthal support tendons of the lids. This results in shortening of the horizontal dimension of the lid fissure and increased lid laxity. Proper canthal tendon anchoring is required during repair. 4. Deep upper lid lacerations may involve the levator aponeurosis or lid elevator. Lack of recognition may result in permanent ptosis. 5. Avulsion injuries often require repair based on mobilization of skin flaps or grafts. Preserve avulsed lid tissue for possible free grafting at the time of surgical repair. 6. Deep lacerations with fat prolapse are associated with an increased incidence of occult globe penetration and functional lid compromise.

Orbital Foreign Bodies

Orbital foreign bodies are less common than surface or intraocular foreign bodies. Protruding foreign bodies should be stabilized to prevent further migration and should not be removed until ophthalmologic consultation and radiologic evaluation have been obtained. Computed tomography is particularly helpful for detailed assessment of foreign body position. Many foreign bodies require removal in the controlled environment of the operating room.

Nontraumatic Red Eye

It is important to remember that the lids, conjunctiva, sclera, and uveal tract may become inflamed from diverse causes—physical and chemical factors, trauma, viral and bacterial infections, iritis, glaucoma, and allergic reactions. In most patients, a provisional diagnosis is made that eliminates other pathologic processes for which the therapy would be ineffectual or even harmful. As signs and symptoms of different diseases often overlap and may persist, with or without the correct diagnosis or

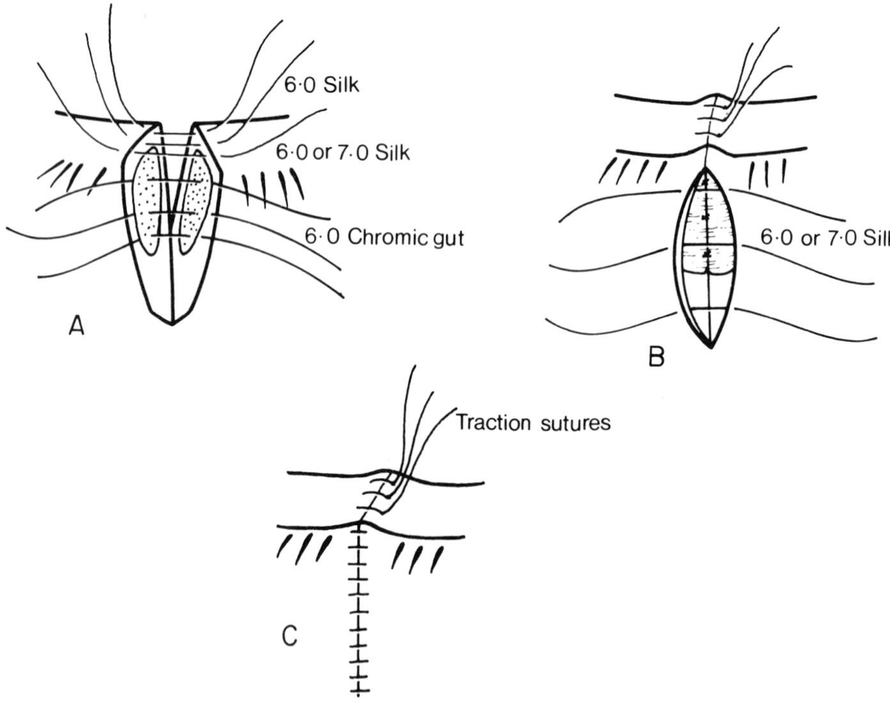

Figure 43.1. Method of closure of eyelid laceration involving margin. *A,* Tarsus should be approximated by three 6–0 chromic catgut sutures after closure of lid margin with three 6–0 silk sutures, one in gray line and one each anteriorly and posteriorly. *B,* Muscle and fascia anterior to tarsus are closed with interrupted 6–0 chromic catgut sutures to minimize wound tension, followed by skin closure with 6–0 or 7–0 silk sutures. *C,* Sutures in lid margin are left long, as traction sutures. They are taped to brow or cheek opposite injured lid for 3 days to produce puckering of margin. (Modified from Beyer CK, Reeh MJ. Lid trauma. *Int Ophthalmol Clin,* 1974; 14:11–21.)

therapy, patients with a red eye unresponsive to treatment should be referred to an ophthalmologist. Table 43.2 has been prepared to aid in the differential diagnosis.

Conjunctivitis

Conjunctivitis or "pink eye" is a frequent presenting complaint to the emergency department. Tearing and mild discomfort are common symptoms of all types of conjunctivitis. Vision is usually normal, and the cornea is clear. If there is any alteration in the corneal light reflex, the possibility of more serious eye disease, such as corneal ulceration, should be considered.

Bacterial conjunctivitis is characterized by mucopurulent exudate, lid crusting, and conjunctival injection; it is best treated with topical antibiotics and moist compresses. The patient usually improves in 7–14 days. *Neisseria* organisms may penetrate an intact cornea quickly and gonococcal conjunctivitis should be suspected in any case where marked purulent discharge is present in the neonatal period. Management of suspected gonococcal conjunctivitis includes Gram's stain, culture, hospitalization, parenteral and topical antibiotic therapy, and ophthalmologic consultation.

Viral conjunctivitis is often associated with an upper respiratory infection and may present with preauricular lymphadenopathy, watery discharge, and conjunctival injection.

Topical antibiotics may be considered if bacterial involvement is suspected. Cold compresses may reduce symptoms. Because viral conjunctivitis is easily transmitted from eye to eye and person to person, patients should be instructed to minimize eye-hand contact with others and to observe sound handwashing techniques. Epidemic keratoconjunctivitis is an especially contagious and virulent form of conjunctivitis caused by an adenovirus. Seasonal outbreaks are not uncommon, and institutional epidemics may occur; proper emphasis must be given to hygiene so that the emergency department does not become a source for transmission of the disease.

Allergic conjunctivitis is often seasonal, with itching the most prominent symptom. Tearing, injection, and swelling of the conjunctiva are commonly present. Treatment includes cold compresses and topical vasoconstrictors.

Iritis

In iritis, a sterile, intraocular inflammation, photophobia, pain, and blurring of vision are common symptoms. Vasodilation in the anterior segment of the eye, sometimes confused with conjunctivitis, is manifested by a faint, deep pink to violent flush of the sclera adjacent to the cornea. The pupil is usually small, sometimes irregular, and the cornea clear. Although iritis may be associated with glaucoma, the intracular pressure in acute iritis is usually low. Slit lamp examination, revealing circulating white blood cells and protein in the anterior chamber, is required for accurate diagnosis and management. Initial treatment usually involves topical cycloplegia and steroids, but may be more complex in difficult cases. Recurrence is common and may be complicated by cataract formation and glaucoma. General medical assessment may be warranted as this type of sterile intraocular inflammation can be an ocular manifestation of systemic disease.

Glaucoma

Glaucoma is characterized by elevation of intraocular pressure sufficient to damage the optic nerve. The diagnosis is established by tonometer determination of elevated intraocular pressure in an eye with a nerve head that is either normal or cupped and atrophic.

In open-angle glaucoma, the trabecular meshwork is anatomically open to the flow of aqueous but has a reduced capacity for aqueous outflow. Rise of intraocular pressure in chronic open-angle glaucoma is usually slow, occurring over months or years; it causes no symptoms. This type of glaucoma may be detected with relative frequency in the emergency department, since it is present in more than 2% of the population over 40 years of age.

Figure 43.2 depicts the normal eye, and Figure (43.3, *A*) shows the eye with angle-closure glaucoma. In this latter condition, the iris balloons forward into apposition with the trabeculum, and obstruction to aqueous flow develops abruptly, often causing symptoms that prompt the patient to seek emergency care. Generally a disease of the fifth and later decades, acute angle-closure glaucoma can also occur in younger persons with shallow anterior chambers. Physiologic mydriasis, caused, for example, by a darkened environment or psychic stress, and pharmacologic mydriasis, caused by belladonna-like drugs, may result in sudden obstruction to aqueous outflow. Only in the small or farsighted eye, or in the eye in which the lens begins to swell, is the space between the iris and the trabecular meshwork narrow enough to be occluded by mydriasis.

The patient with angle-closure glaucoma may not recognize that symptoms originate from the eye, and may come to an emergency department with "tension headache," "sinusitis," or even "the flu." Acute angle-closure glaucoma may be either missed or easily diagnosed, depending on the astuteness of the emergency physician. The patient usually doc-

Table 43.2.
Symptoms and Signs in Differential Diagnosis of the Red Eye

Symptom or Sign	Bulbar Perforation	Foreign Body	Conjunctivitis: Bacterial	Conjunctivitis: Viral	Conjunctivitis: Allergic	Iritis	Acute Glaucoma	Corneal Ulcer: Bacterial	Corneal Ulcer: Herpes Simplex	Spontaneous Subconjunctival Hemorrhage
Foreign-body sensation	+	+ + + +	+ +	+ +	+	±		+ + +	+ + +	
Tearing	+	+ + +	+ +	+ + +	+ + +	+ +	+	+ + +	+ + +	
Sticky or matting lids			+ + +					+ +		
Photophobia	+	±		±		+ + + +	+ to + + +	+ + +	+ + +	
Pain	±	+ + +				+ +	+ + to + + + +	+ to + +	+	
Blurring of vision	+ to + + + +	±	+			+ +	+ + +	Variable	Depends on location	
Halos							+ + + +			
Rapid onset	+ + + +	+ + + +	±	±	+ to + + + +	±	+ + +		+	±
Conjunctival injection	±	+ +	+ to + + + +	+ +	±	+ +	+ to + + +	+ + +	+ + +	
Ciliary flush						+ to + + + +	+ +	+ +		
Corneal defect	Variable	Variable					+	+ + + +	+ + + +	
Exudate		±	+ to + + + +		±			+ + +		
Pupil	Variable	Normal	Normal	Normal	Normal	Small	4–5 mm, fixed	Normal	Normal	Normal
Red reflex	Variable	Normal	Normal	Normal	Normal	↓	↓↓	Variable	Normal	Normal
Intraocular pressure	↓	Normal	Normal	Normal	Normal	Usually ↓ may be ↑	↑↑↑	Normal	Normal	Normal
Blepharospasm or squinting	±	+		Normal	Normal	+ + +	+ +	+ +	+ +	
Anterior chamber	Variable	Normal	Normal	Normal	Normal	Normal	Shallow	Normal	Normal	Normal
Lid edema		±	±		+ to + + + +			+ +		

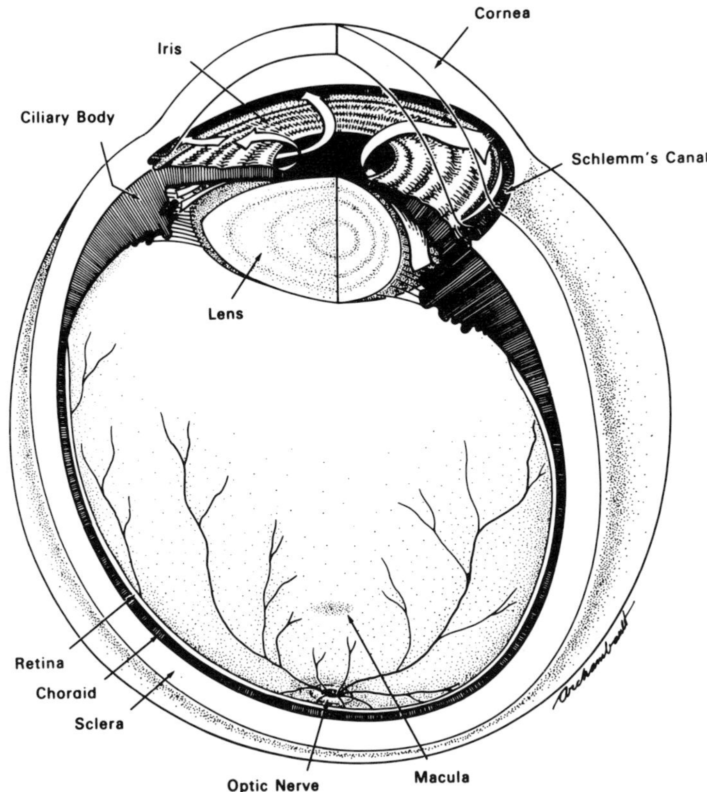

Figure 43.2. Normal eye; path of aqueous flow is indicated by white arrows.

uments the onset of symptoms, which include deep aching within the globe, a decrease in visual acuity that is sometimes described as smoky or misty vision, and the classic symptom of colored halos around point sources of light. In addition, the patient may be debilitated by the attack, and may experience nausea and vomiting.

Examination of the eye in acute glaucoma reveals a variably injected anterior segment, hazy cornea, shallow anterior chamber, and a mid-dilated, nonreactive pupil. Although the unilateral elevation of intraocular pressure may usually be appreciated by tactile comparison of the globe pressures, tonometry remains the preferred and more accurate diagnostic technique.

Initial therapy for acute angle-closure glaucoma includes the topical application of 4% pilocarpine every 15 minutes, and a topical β-blocker. Systemic medications, if no medical contraindications exist, may include acetazolamide 500 mg intravenously or orally, and an osmotically active agent—either mannitol (1.0 gm/kg) intravenously or glycerol (1.0 gm/kg) orally. A decrease in intraocular pressure to a normal level, miosis, and clearing of the cornea indicate successful therapy. The patient should be referred immediately to an ophthalmologist. After being treated for the acute intraocular pressure elevation, most patients will require laser iridectomy or surgical peripheral iridectomy (Figure 43.3,*B*) to prevent recurrence. Neglected cases with permanent synechia of the iris to the trabeculum may require more extensive filtration surgery to produce an alternative pathway for aqueous humor outflow.

Other types of acute glaucoma may simulate angle-closure. A common acute secondary angle-closure type characterized by neovascularization of the anterior surface of the iris may occur in patients with diabetes and in patients whose ocular function is seriously compromised by central retinal artery occlusion, central retinal vein occlusion, tumor, or long-standing retinal detachment. This and other forms of acute glaucoma usually require an ophthalmologist for definitive diagnosis. However, almost without exception, the aforementioned therapy causes no harm and may be utilized as initial treatment by the emergency physician in managing an acute elevation of intraocular pressure.

Corneal Ulcer/Keratitis

Inflammation or infection of the cornea is a serious vision-threatening disorder presenting with uniocular foreign body sensation, photophobia, blurred vision, and tearing. The surface light reflex is irregular, and the cornea often stains with topical fluorescein. Active infections may appear as white infiltrates. Treatment should not be instituted until diagnostic culture studies, including corneal scraping, have been performed. Since the etiological pathogens may be bacterial, viral or fungal, prompt and specific treatment should be directed by the ophthalmologist.

Herpes simplex keratitis may demonstrate a characteristic dendritic staining pattern with fluorescein. Topical steroids in any form during emergency care are absolutely contraindicated since they may potentiate viral activity and result in corneal perforation or scarring with even brief usage. Topical antiviral treatment may be initiated in the emergency department, but the ophthalmologist should provide continuing care.

Even though extended wear contact lenses enjoy greater popularity for the correction of refractive errors, these lenses may produce serious ocular disease. Emergency physicians must be especially alert to red eye problems in these patients with such lenses; they may present with few symptoms due to the bandage effect of the contact lens. Detailed inspection of the cornea is crucial, as hidden bacterial ulcers can soon develop into permanent scarring.

Blepharitis/Chalazion

Many patients are predisposed to inflammation of the lid margins either as an acute or chronic condition. Lid marginal erythema, crusting, and scaling are more prominent than injection of the globe. An inflammatory mass may develop from obstruction of one of several types of oil glands of the eyelid. These inflammatory lesions present as a chalazion, hordeolum, or stye, depending on the nature of the gland or duct obstructed. Staphylococci are the most common causative organisms.

Local therapy for blepharitis consists of hot compresses, lid hygiene to remove scaly debris, and topical antibiotics providing adequate staphylococcal protection. A persistent chalazion or stye may require incision and curettage.

Dacryocystitis

Acute inflammation of the lacrimal sac usually produces pain and local swelling, tenderness, and inflammatory reaction around the inner canthus of the eye. Gentle pressure over the sac may express pus from the lacrimal punctae. If symptoms suggest inflammation in the sinuses, radiographs are indicated as well as otolaryngological consultation. The most frequent bacterial agents are: *Streptococcus pneumoniae* and *Staphylococcus aureus.*

Treatment includes topical and systemic antibiotics after appropriate culture. Hot compresses are effective; incision and drainage are reserved for fluctuant or pointing abscesses. Recurrent infections or total lacrimal obstruction resulting in persistent tearing may require a dacryocystorhinostomy.

Periorbital Cellulitis

This urgent and potentially vision-threatening disease requires immediate treatment if serious extension is to be avoided. Preseptal cellulitis implies a lesser inflammation of only anterior orbital structures. Patients may present with fever, lid swelling, and erythema; vision and extraocular motility remain normal. Treatment of preseptal cellulitis includes warm compresses and oral antibiotics. Topical antibiotics are warranted if blepharoconjunctivitis is present. X-rays may help to evaluate contiguous sinus disease. Preseptal cellulitis in children ages 6–36 months is frequently due to *Haemophilus influenzae.* Herpes zoster (shingles) involvement of the fifth cranial nerve may be associated with preseptal cellulitis in adults and can also produce intraocular inflammation (uveitis); these patients require ophthalmic consultation.

Orbital cellulitis implies deep extension of infection, and is heralded by pain, decreased vision, impaired ocular motility, afferent pupillary defect, proptosis, and/or optic nerve swelling. Cavernous sinus thrombosis may develop if the process advances further. Evaluation includes ophthalmologic, radiologic, and otolaryngologic consultation; treatment; intravenous antibiotics; and potential surgical drain-

Figure 43.3. Angle-closure glaucoma. *A,* Aqueous, secreted into posterior chamber behind iris, flows through pupil into anterior chamber, gaining access to outflow channels of Schlemm's canal. The pressure behind the iris is slightly higher than in the anterior chamber—the difference being sufficient to lift iris off anterior surface of lens. In an anatomically predisposed eye, this small pressure difference can cause iris to bow forward to block aqueous flow into Schlemm's canal, especially if iris becomes lax, as occurs when pupil dilates. Pressure elevation depends on amount of angle closure in circumference of drainage system. *Inset* shows anatomic closure of drainage system with iris bowed forward. *B,* Effect of iridectomy. Aqueous can flow freely from posterior to anterior chamber via the iridectomy opening. The pressure differential is eliminated. The iris assumes flat contour on lens surface, and the threat of angle closure is minimal. *Inset* shows how iris drops away from outflow channels in absence of adhesions. Pupil may now be dilated without risk.

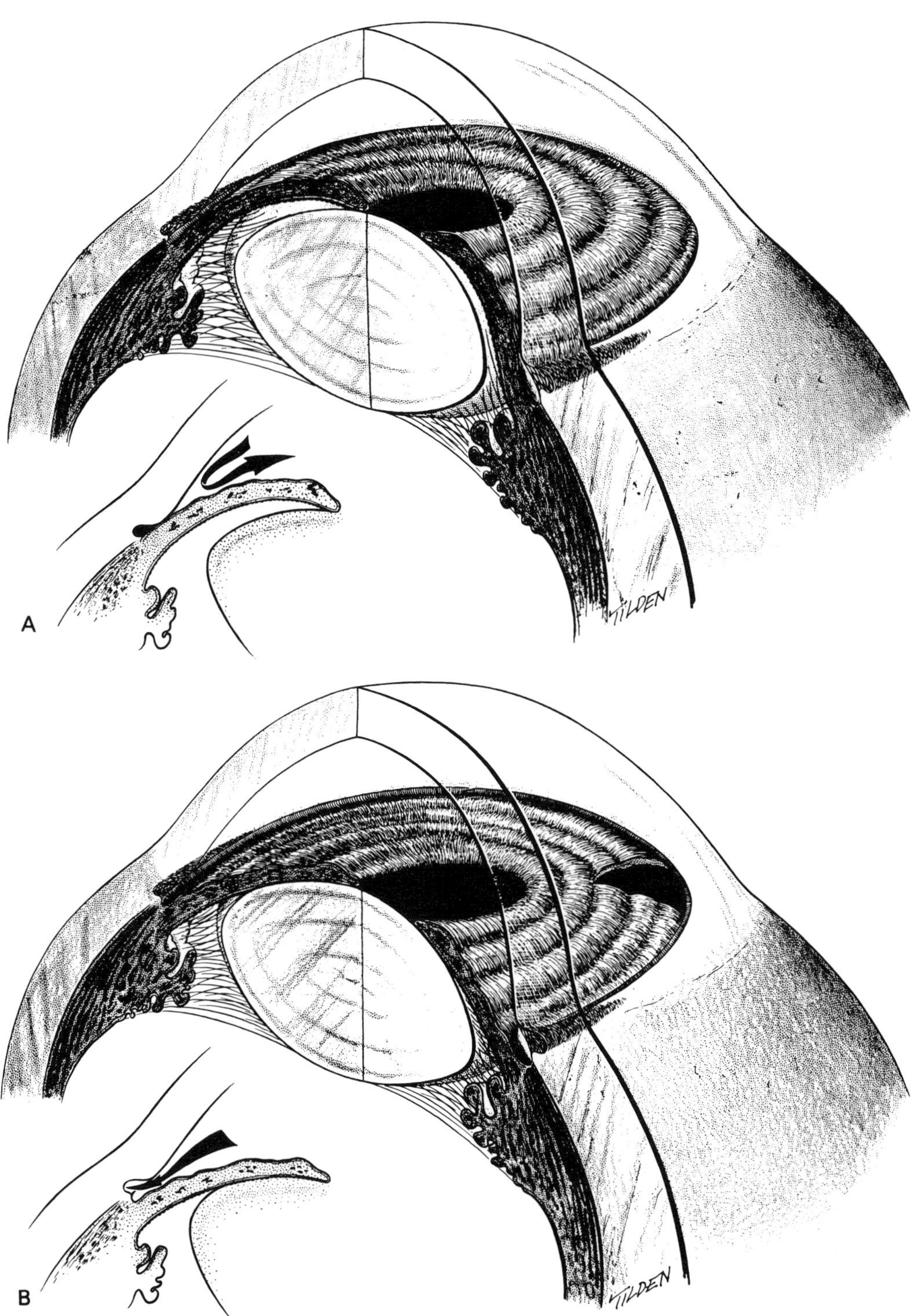

age. Chronically immunosuppressed or diabetic patients are at particular risk in that they may harbor a rapidly progressive fungal infection (phycomycosis). Such infections may be life-threatening.

Rapid Visual Loss

Rapid visual loss is usually due to pathology involving the retina, vitreous, or optic nerve. Assessment of visual loss requires evaluation for an afferent pupillary defect with careful ophthalmoscopic examination. Apparent lack of light perception can be confirmed by absence of a consensual pupillary response when the suspected blind eye is stimulated with a bright light. Except in patients with suspected intracranial injury or history of angle-closure glaucoma, there is seldom reason not to dilate the pupils for adequate examination of the fundi. Table 43.3 lists etiologies of visual loss most often encountered. Two of these diagnoses deserve special mention because they both represent ocular emergencies requiring urgent treatment: central retinal artery occlusion and temporal arteritis.

Central Retinal Artery Occlusion

Central retinal artery occlusion produces a unilateral sudden and profound loss of vision. There may be a prior history of transient ischemic attacks (amaurosis fugax). Examination confirms reduction of vision to the counting fingers or light perception level. An afferent pupillary defect is present with funduscopic evidence of a pale disk and a retinal change characterized by "milkiness" or loss of retinal transparency, due to retinal edema. This diffuse retinal edema surrounding the reddish foveal region may give the appearance of a "cherry red spot." Retinal arterioles are often narrowed with segmentation of blood columns. Occasionally at the bifurcation of a vessel or at the disk, an occluding embolic fragment can be identified. An ipsilateral carotid bruit may be present.

To be effective, treatment must enhance perfusion of the retinal arterioles immediately by decreasing intraocular pressure and/or increasing the systemic arteriolar pressure. Intermittent digital pressure, or ballottement of the globe through closed lids softens the eye and may dislodge an obstructing embolus at an arteriole bifurcation. Breathing oxygen with 5% CO_2 or rebreathing in a paper bag may encourage retinal arteriolar dilatation. The intraocular pressure may be reduced with timolol 0.5% drops, intravenous acetazolamide 500 mg, and intravenous mannitol 1.0 gm/kg. Lowering of acute intraocular pressure may also be accomplished by paracentesis of the anterior chamber with a beveled needle knife incision through the cornea. All patients with central retinal artery occlusion deserve further neuroophthalmological evaluation to determine the source of the vascular occlusion.

Table 43.3.
Common Causes of Rapid Painless Visual Loss

Vascular occlusion
Central retinal artery
Branch retinal artery (if macula is involved)
Central or branch retinal vein
Optic neuritis
Vitreous hemorrhage
Retinal detachment
Macular hemorrhage or exudative macular detachment
Macular hole
Uveitis
Hysteria and malingering

Temporal Arteritis

This potentially devastating disease may be a blinding disorder of *both* eyes and tends to occur in patients over 60 years of age. Patients often present with ipsilateral decreased vision, tenderness over the forehead and scalp, an afferent pupillary defect, and hemorrhagic optic nerve swelling. Symptoms of polymyalgia rheumatica may be present. If temporal arteritis is suspected, an erythrocyte sedimentation rate (ESR) must be obtained, and, if elevated, systemic steroid therapy should be initiated immediately. Temporal artery biopsy should be performed to confirm the diagnosis. Involvement of the second eye may rapidly follow the first if systemic steroids are not promptly utilized. Therefore, *initiation of steroid treatment should not be delayed pending performance of the biopsy.*

Retinal Vein Occlusion

In central retinal vein occlusion, vision may become blurred less rapidly than in arteriolar occlusion; visual loss may be less profound. The disk margins are blurred, the veins are distended, and retinal hemorrhages are present throughout the fundus.

Treatment is controversial. Anticoagulation has been recommended, but its usefulness is unproven. No emergency department treatment is indicated, but concurrent open-angle glaucoma, hypertension, and hyperviscosity should be ruled out. Ophthalmologic evaluation is necessary because vein occlusion has an increased incidence in the chronic open-angle glaucoma population, and up to one-third of occlusion patients may develop a serious secondary form of neovascular glaucoma.

Vitreous Hemorrhage and Retinal Detachment

These conditions are properly considered together. A patient who reports light flashes followed by black spots, strands, "film," or becomes aware of a "shadow" or "curtain" type of field defect must be examined to determine whether vitreous hemorrhage and/or retinal detachment are present.

The most common ocular causes of vitreous hemorrhage are retinal tears, possibly with retinal detachment, posterior vitreous detachment, neovascularization secondary to diabetes mellitus, or old retinal venous occlusion. Early referral of patients with vitreous hemorrhage is advised because of the high frequency of associated retinal pathology.

An increased incidence of retinal detachment is present in patients with myopia (nearsightedness) and in patients in whom cataracts have been removed; detachment resulting from trauma constitutes a small percentage of cases. In a patient with a retinal tear or peripheral retinal detachment, subjective visual acuity and visual fields may remain normal until the detachment extends more centrally toward the macula. It is therefore necessary to perform careful ophthalmoscopic examination with the pupil dilated to establish whether this occult, progressive, and treatable condition exists. If retinal detachment is present, the fundus appears gray, with the retina rippled and elevated. The retinal vessels appear abnormally tortuous, and there is loss of the underlying choroidal pattern. If the macula is still attached, an ophthalmic emergency exists, since its function and sharp central vision may not be regained, even after the retina is successfully reattached by operation. Prompt referral for admission and bed rest are indicated until an operation can be performed.

Since the entire retina can be scrutinized only by indirect ophthalmoscopic examination with scleral depression, and since significant pathologic conditions may exist in an eye considered normal after direct ophthalmoscopy, any patient with symptoms of unknown cause related to the posterior segment should be referred for ophthalmic evaluation.

Macular Disease

Painless, rapid, central visual loss, particularly in patients over 50 years, may be due to hemorrhagic or serous (exudative) macular disease. Usually, however, a more insidious loss of vision occurs, often with the development of metamorphopsia or a relatively central scotoma in this age-related degenerative process. Ophthalmoscopic examination reveals abnormal macular anatomy. In serious lesions, the foveal light reflex is lost and the macular region of the retina is elevated. Yellow, drusen-like deposits are frequently seen in the opposite eye. Although in the past these patients could not be treated, patients with abnormal maculae with reduction of central vision should be referred to an ophthalmologist, because many types of macular lesions can now be successfully managed by laser photocoagulation. Nontraumatic macular hemorrhage may be seen in younger patients with myopia, hemorrhagic diathesis, or angioid streaks.

Posterior Uveitis

Inflammatory reaction of the posterior uveal tissues may result in hazy vision due to opacification of the vitreous by cells and proteinaceous outpouring. If the process is severe and if it directly affects the macula, useful central vision may be rapidly and irreparably lost. Because the fundus may be difficult to visualize, the condition may be confused with vitreous hemorrhage. Yellowish-white patches in the choroid and retina are common. The cause of posterior uveitis often remains obscure, even after exhaustive evaluation. Among the more common etiologies are toxoplasmosis, sarcoidosis, and histoplasmosis. High dose systemic steroid therapy, often in conjunction with antibiotics or antimetabolites, is occasionally indicated.

Optic Neuritis

Loss of central acuity with a swollen, often hemorrhagic optic disk and retrobulbar pain on movement of the globe suggests optic neuritis or papillitis. If the inflammation involves the optic nerve but not the nerve-head, the diagnosis is retrobulbar neuritis. Vision may be reduced only a few lines (20/30–20/40), or it may be profoundly depressed. It is important to assess pupillary light reactivity because an afferent pupillary defect is present with optic neuritis or retrobulbar neuritis, but it is not generally present with the optic nerve swelling or papilledema secondary to increased intracranial pressure. Multiple sclerosis may be the cause in patients from 20–40 years of age; one should attempt to elicit a history of episodic neurologic defects in such patients. The attacks are self-limited, and vision usually improves. Although no proved therapy exists, some neuroophthalmologists recommend systemic administration of corticosteroids or adrenocorticotropic hormone. Toxic agents and intracranial lesions must be ruled out.

Table 43.4 has been prepared to indicate the urgency of evaluation and treatment of a variety of ocular problems. The question "which patients with eye signs or symptoms should be referred for ophthalmologic consultation?" is frequently asked. In each case, the answer relates to the severity of the problem and the interest and experience of the examining physician. It is the responsibility of the individual emergency department physician to know the limits of his or her competency.

A guide to ophthalmic equipment and medications for the emergency department follows, in Appendix 43.A.

Table 43.4.
Priority for Evaluation and Treatment

	Emergency Department Treatment by Nonophthalmic Physician		Referral to Ophthalmologist		
Condition	Immediate	Routine	Hours	1–2 Days	Within 1 Week
Central retinal arterial occlusion	×		×		
Chemical burn	×		×		
Bulbar laceration	×		×		
Acute glaucoma		×	×		
Nonpenetrating foreign body		×		×	
Penetrating foreign body	×		×		
Iritis		×		×	
Corneal ulcer		×	×		
Conjunctivitis		×			×
Herpes simplex keratitis		×		×	
Traumatic hyphema	×		×		
Orbital cellulitis		×	×		
Retinal detachment, macula attached		×	×		
Retinal detachment, macula detached		×		×	
Intraocular (vitreous) hemorrhage		×		×	
Subconjunctival hemorrhage with trauma		×		×	
Optic neuritis		×		×	
Infected hordeolum and chalazion		×			×
Dacryocystitis		×			×

Appendix 43.A
Ophthalmic Equipment and Medications for the Emergency Department

Eye Equipment

1. Vision charts for visual acuity
2. Near vision cards
3. Metal shields
4. Eye patches
5. Tape
6. Scissors
7. Polyethylene sheets (Saran Wrap)
8. Sterile irrigation fluid
9. IV tubing
10. Squeeze bottle
11. Cotton tip applicators
12. pH paper
13. Fluorescein paper strips
14. Lid retractors
15. Paper clip retractors
16. Contact lens remover
17. Contact lens case
18. 25-gauge needle with syringe
19. Foreign body removal spud
20. Focal illuminator or penlight
21. Blue filter for illuminator/penlight
22. Direct ophthalmoscope
23. Schiötz tonometer
24. Magnifying loupe lenses or slit lamp for magnified anterior segment examination

Ophthalmic Medications

Topical Anesthetics

Proparacaine hydrochloride 0.5% has a rapid onset of action, and its duration of action is approximately 20 minutes. It provides adequate topical anesthesia for permitting complete examination in patients with abrasions and for removal of surface foreign bodies. Never prescribe topical anesthetics for home use because chronic use may devitalize the corneal epithelium, retard healing, and predispose the eye to infection.

Dilating Drops (Mydriasis/Cycloplegia)

Mydriasis is best achieved with a combination of Tropicamide (Mydriacyl 1%) and phenylephrine (Neo-Synephrine 2½%) applied topically. Dilation will be achieved in approximately 15 minutes with accommodation/pupillary reaction usually returning to normal within 8 hours.

Cyclopentolate 1% drops provide more prolonged dilation (12–24 hours) and also serve as a much stronger cycloplegic agent for relaxation of the ciliary body. *Atropine should be avoided* because of its prolonged effect on pupillary action and accommodation (up to 2 weeks).

Appendix 43.A—*continued*

Constricting Drops (Miosis)

Miotics are used for constricting the pupil and in the treatment of glaucoma. Pilocarpine is most commonly used in 1%–4% concentrations.

Topical β-Blockers

Timolol, 0.25%, and 0.5%, betaxolol 0.5%, and levobunolol 0.5% are topical β-blockers used in the treatment of glaucoma. Betaxolol is more selective and may be preferable for patients with cardiac or asthmatic conditions.

Carbonic Anhydrase Inhibitors

Acetazolamide (250 mg tablets, or 500 mg capsules and intravenous preparations—500 mg) reduces aqueous humor production. Its principal emergency department use is in the treatment of acute angle-closure glaucoma.

Oral Osmotic Agents

Glycerol or isosorbide (1 gm/kg) act as hyperosmotic agents to lower intraocular pressure. They are unpalatably sweet and are best served with juice and poured over ice. Their principal use is in the treatment of acute angle-closure glaucoma.

Intravenous Osmotic Agents

Mannitol (1.0 gm/kg) serves as an intravenous osmotic agent to reduce intraocular pressure in some cases of acute glaucoma and central retinal artery occlusion.

Topical Antibiotics

Sulfacetamide, 10% solution and ointment, serves as an effective broad-spectrum antibiotic.

Erythromycin is an effective nonirritating bacteriostatic ointment for Gram-positive organism coverage.

Bacitracin ointment serves as a bacteriocidal Gram-positive directed antibiotic.

Gentamycin drops and ointment are useful in the treatment of Gram-negative ocular infections.

Topical Antivirals

Idoxuridine 0.5% ointment 5 times/day, *vidarabine* 3% (Vira-A) ointment 5 times/day and *trifluridine* (Viroptic) drops every 2 hours while awake are used for treatment of active herpes simplex keratitis.

Topical Vasoconstrictors

Naphazoline hydrochloride is an effective vasoconstrictor for reducing ocular irritation and injection characteristically associated with ocular allergies. Drops should be used 2–3 times/day and for a short interval of time (approximately 1 week) because of a potential rebound phenomenon and increasing symptoms.

Topical Steroids

Steroids may exacerbate acute herpetic ocular infection, and prolonged use may result in glaucoma or cataract formation. For these reasons, *topical steroids should not be used alone or in combination with an antibiotic by the emergency physician* except in consultation with an ophthalmologist.

SUGGESTED READINGS

Beyer CK, Reeh MJ. Lid Trauma. *Int Ophthalmol Clin,* 1974;14:11–21.

Deutsch TA, Feller DB. *Paton and Goldberg's Management of Ocular Injuries.* Philadelphia: WB Saunders, 1985.

Gombos GM: *Handbook of Ophthalmic Emergencies: A Guide for Emergencies in Ophthalmology.* Flushing, NY: Medical Examinations Publishing Co., 1973.

Grant WM. *Toxicology of the Eye,* 2nd ed. Springfield, IL: Charles C Thomas, 1974.

Paton D, Goldberg MF. *Management of Ocular Injuries.* Philadelphia, WB Saunders, 1976.

Paton D, Goldberg MF. *Injuries of the Eye, the Lids, and the Orbit.* Philadelphia: WB Saunders, 1968.

Shingleton, BJ: *Eye Trauma and Emergencies. A Slide-Script Program.* San Francisco: American Academy of Ophthalmology, 1985.

SECTION 5

Radiology

EARLE W. WILKINS, JR., M.D.
Editor

CHAPTER 44

Recommended Imaging Procedures for Common Emergency Conditions

RICHARD SACKNOFF, M.D.
ROBERT A. NOVELLINE, M.D.

A wide variety of imaging modalities is now available for the evaluation of the emergency patient. In addition to routine plain film series, conventional tomography, computed tomography (CT), ultrasonography, angiography, and radionuclide scanning may be indicated as the initial imaging examination or fit later into the diagnostic algorithm. This chapter describes recommended imaging procedures in an anatomic format for the more common traumatic and nontraumatic emergencies.

HEAD EMERGENCIES

Head Trauma

Prior to moving the traumatized patient, a lateral cervical film is usually performed to exclude an unstable cervical spine injury. Computed tomography (CT) is the examination of choice in patients requiring imaging for head trauma. A skull x-ray series is not required prior to CT. Indications for CT include an abnormal neurological exam, stupor or coma, severe injury, or deterioration in neurological status during observation. If a skull series is obtained instead of CT, certain findings are indications for a CT examination. These include a fracture crossing the middle meningeal artery groove, often associated with an epidural hemorrhage, a depressed fracture, an air-fluid level in the sphenoid sinuses suggesting a basilar skull fracture, a calcified pineal gland shifted from midline, and pneumocephalus.

The CT examination should be performed without intravenous contrast material for maximal demonstration of hemorrhage. CT may show intracranial hemorrhage, edema, contusion, and secondary midline shift. If a change in neurological status occurs, a repeat CT is helpful to exclude development of a subdural hematoma. In penetrating injury, CT localizes intracranial foreign bodies. If bone windows are reviewed, skull fractures are visualized.

A skull series is not generally considered useful in the workup of patients with head trauma because it is an insensitive indicator of intracranial injury. The majority of patients with intracranial injury after trauma have a normal skull series. When a skull fracture is detected by plain films, this finding does not often change the treatment plan. Furthermore, the low yield of fracture detection in skull films makes this study economically undesirable.

Facial Trauma

Facial examinations are tailored to the site of suspected injury. The examination for a suspected nasal fracture includes a nasal series with both lateral projections of the nose, an upright Waters' view, and an occlusal view. Maxillary and orbital fractures are evaluated with a facial series, including an upright Waters', lateral, Caldwell, and submentovertex views. Patients with suspected mandibular fracture are evaluated with a mandible series consisting of a posterior-anterior, left and right angle, and lateral Towne's views. Panorex views are preferred by some physicians but may not be possible because the patient must be upright.

Careful review of facial films is paramount for detection of subtle fractures. Helpful secondary signs of fracture include adjacent soft tissue swelling and air-fluid levels within paranasal sinuses. In patients with complex facial fractures, CT shows abnormalities that are inadequately demonstrated on plain films by better delineating the degree of fragmentation and orientation of fragments. Patients in whom a fracture is clinically suspected but in whom the plain films are normal are particular candidates for CT. CT may also identify soft tissue injuries of the face, not seen on plain films.

Acute Nontraumatic Intracranial Events

CT is indicated in any patient with suspected infarct, transient ischemic attack, intracranial hemorrhage, or intracranial infection. Initially, the CT examination is performed without intravenous contrast material to maximize detectability of intracranial hemorrhage. This may be followed by a contrast-enhanced CT scan to better visualize mass lesions and sites of infection that enhance with contrast due to disruption of the blood-brain barrier. CT may show findings of cerebritis, abscess, meningitis, or empyema, either subdural or epidural. Selective cerebral arteriography demonstrates arteriosclerotic occlusions, ulcerated plaques, thrombi, and aneurysms.

Paranasal and Nasal Conditions

The signs and symptoms of sinusitis may be nonspecific, including headache, sinus pain, congestion, discharge, and fever. Sinus films are helpful in confirming the diagnosis and excluding other entities that mimic sinusitis.

A paranasal sinus series includes a Waters' projection, Caldwell, base, and lateral views, all obtained in the upright position. With sinusitis, the films may demonstrate increased opacification of the normally air-filled sinuses, representing fluid or mucosal thickening. An air-fluid level confirms the presence of acute sinusitis. Occasionally, complications of sinusitis may be identified, including retention cysts and mucoceles. Bone destruction is usually not seen acutely. CT and conventional tomography better delineate paranasal sinus pathology and may be indicated for evaluation of patients with sinus neoplasm and other conditions requiring surgical intervention.

SPINE EMERGENCIES

Cervical Spine Trauma

A cervical spine series is indicated in all patients with suspected cervical spine trauma. It is also indicated in patients with multiple system trauma and in patients in whom initial clinical evaluation is limited by coma or neurological deficit.

A complete cervical spine series, consisting of a lateral, anteroposterior, oblique, and odontoid views, is sufficient screening for abnormality in the majority of patients with cervical spine trauma. CT or conventional tomography may be performed to resolve a questionable or abnormal finding on the plain film cervical spine series. CT is also utilized for patients with cervical spine fractures and a neurological deficit. CT may be helpful when the seventh cervical vertebra is not completely seen on the lateral x-ray examination.

All patients with suspected cervical spine trauma should be initially examined with a screening lateral film. Only after this view has been reviewed and no abnormalities identified, should the immobilizing cervical collar be removed for completion of the examination. The screening lateral film must permit evaluation of all vertebrae C1–C7. If C7 is not seen, a repeat lateral view—a swimmer's view—should be obtained prior to removal of the collar. If a fracture is suspected on the initial lateral view, the remaining films may be taken with the collar in place *without turning the head or neck.* Flexion and extension views are needed for demonstration of a ligamentous injury in patients without fracture. They should not be performed until a complete cervical spine series and CT have ruled out unstable fractures.

Cervical spine fractures have diverse appearances, depending on the mechanism of injury. Indirect indicators of injury visible on the lateral cervical spine film include: (*a*) soft tissue swelling greater than 3 mm anterior to the C3 vertebral body; and (*b*) disruption of the normal lordotic curvature by either subluxation or abrupt rotation at a single level. In the child under 8 years old, mild physiologic subluxation of C2 on C3 as well as of C3 on C4 may occur as a normal finding. This results from normal ligamentous laxity and should not be mistaken for an unstable injury.

Thoracic and Lumbar Spine Trauma

The initial screening examinations for suspected thoracic and lumbar spine trauma are anteroposterior and lateral plain films. The lateral film may be taken with a cross-table technique, if an unstable fracture is suspected. When a fracture is identified and neurological signs are present, or if a complex fracture is identified, then CT is performed at the level of abnormality. If CT is not available, conventional laminagraphy may be performed.

The initial anteroposterior chest and abdomen films of a patient with multiple trauma may show fractures of the thoracic or lumbar spine, or may demonstrate nonspecific secondary signs, such as bilateral apical pleural capping or paraspinal hematoma. These increase suspicion for thoracolumbar spine injury. Magnetic resonance imaging (MRI), myelography, or CT with intrathecal contrast are options for the assessment of suspected spinal cord injury. Up to 20% of thoracolumbar spine fractures are associated with extremity fractures, most commonly calcaneal fractures in patients who fall and land on their feet.

Simple wedge compression fractures of the vertebral body are usually stable injuries. However, CT distinguishes a compression fracture from a burst fracture with retropulsion of vertebral fragments in the neural canal. Fractures that involve the neural arch are often unstable; CT or laminagraphy is indicated in these fractures.

Acute Herniated Lumbar Disc

Patients complaining of back pain with sciatic radiation, particularly with focal neurological signs, may be evaluated with plain films or more sophisticated techniques. CT, myelography, and MRI are reserved for patients in whom conservative management has failed, and in whom a surgical or other invasive procedure is indicated for treatment.

Plain films of the lumbar spine may show narrowing of the intervertebral disc spaces. The majority of acutely herniated lumbar discs occur at the L3-4, L4-5, and L5-S1 levels. Patients with chronic herniation of lumbar discs may have secondary osteophytes. Occasionally, a vacuum disc phenomenon may be seen when disc degeneration has taken place and gas is present in the disc space. In most hospitals, CT has replaced myelography in the diagnosis of herniated lumbar disc. At CT, the herniated disc appears as a discrete nodule or bulge of soft tissue density extending into the vertebral canal. Myelography is the traditional method for diagnosing lumbar disc herniation. In recent years, water-soluble contrast materials, such as metrizamide, have replaced oil-based pantopaque. When available, MRI has become the preferred noninvasive method for diagnosing herniated lumbar discs. No ionizing radiation is utilized. This examination accurately diagnoses lumbar disc abnormality.

THORACIC EMERGENCIES

Trauma

In patients with chest trauma, posteroanterior (PA) and lateral plain film examination, which requires the patient to be upright, is obtained whenever possible. However, thoracic trauma is often a manifestation of multiple trauma, and an anteroposterior (AP) supine chest film may be the only possibility. In this situation, the mediastinum and heart appear widened, making it difficult to differentiate a normal patient from one with injuries of the heart and great blood vessels.

The most common pulmonary abnormality with blunt chest trauma is lung contusion. Edema and blood in lung parenchyma produce patchy nonsegmental regions of increased density, often with air bronchograms. Contusion characteristically appears within 6 hours of injury and clears within 3–10 days. Pulmonary laceration may result from blunt or penetrating injury. Such a laceration may fill with air, producing a traumatic pneumatocele, which appears as a thin-walled oval cavity. The laceration may fill with blood, resulting in a pulmonary hematoma, and may persist for 3–7 weeks. After clearing of surrounding contusion, the hematoma may appear as an ovoid or spheroid nodule, often simulating neoplasm. Care must also be taken not to mistake a traumatic pneumatocele for a loculated pneumothorax.

Rib Fractures

Rib fractures are often not visible on chest films; a rib film series should be requested for their detection. However, complications of rib fractures may be identified on chest films, including hemothorax, lung contusion, and pneumothorax. Occasionally, nondisplaced rib fractures are not visible, even on the initial rib series. Consequently, patients with persisting symptoms should be reexamined with a repeat rib series in 10–14 days to demonstrate bone resorption and callus formation, both of which improve detectability. Fractures of the first three ribs indicate severe trauma and are often associated with injury to the great vessels and/or tracheobronchial tree. Fractures of the ninth–twelfth ribs are frequently associated with injuries to the adjacent diaphragm, liver, or spleen.

Pneumothorax

A pneumothorax may occur spontaneously, the result of rupture of an apical bleb, or may result from penetrating or blunt thoracic trauma. A diagnosis of pneumothorax is easily made on an upright PA chest examination by visualizing a medially displaced visceral pleural line. The space between the visceral pleural line and chest wall, which is the pleural space, contains gas, but no lung markings. A small pneumothorax appears larger, and therefore more readily visible, on an expiration film. On a supine AP film, a large pneumothorax may be overlooked because the air in the pleural space floats anteriorly over the lungs. One may see gas within the anterior costophrenic angle appearing as an abnormal curvilinear lucency projected over the upper abdomen. When a patient cannot be positioned upright, a lateral decubitus film of the chest, with the suspected side of pneumothorax away from the table, may be substituted to visualize better the pneumothorax.

Tension pneumothorax is a life-threatening complication distinguished from simple pneumothorax by shift of the trachea and mediastinum away from the side of the pneumothorax. The hemidiaphragm on the side of the tension pneumothorax appears flattened or reversed in its curvature, in comparison with the opposite side.

CT may show a smaller pneumothorax than is seen on plain films, especially in the supine patient. CT is not routinely performed for the identification of pneumothorax; upright or lateral decubitus examinations are most cost-effective. However, if a CT is performed for chest trauma, or if CT images of the lower chest are obtained during an abdominal CT for trauma, lung windows are viewed to demonstrate any pneumothorax, located anteriorly in the supine patient. In the patient with multiple trauma, an abdominal CT is frequently the first study that shows a pneumothorax not visualized on the supine chest examination.

Pneumomediastinum

Pneumomediastinum, gas within the mediastinal soft tissue spaces, may be seen after trauma and indicates possible rupture of the esophagus or tracheobronchial tree. Pneumomediastinum may occur spontaneously, secondary to rupture of adjacent lung alveolae in asthmatics, during athletic competition, in neonates with hyaline membrane disease, and in cocaine users.

As with spontaneous pneumothorax, patients with pneumomediastinum may present with abrupt chest pain. In pneumomediastinum, the pain is often retrosternal, radiating to the shoulders and down both arms and is often preceded by a paroxysm of coughing, sneezing, or vomiting. Subcutaneous emphysema may be detected on physical examination of the neck and chest wall.

A frequent finding on the chest film is a small thin opaque line over the aortic arch and along the left heart border with a medial lucency corresponding to the mediastinal gas. The opaque line represents the displaced mediastinal pleura. Care must be taken not to confuse pneumomediastinum with a similarly appearing pneumopericardium in which the gas is confined only to the pericardial space. When the findings on chest film are questionable, a lateral plain film of the neck may show gas in the subcutaneous soft tissues, a frequent occurrence in these patients. If esophageal rupture is suspected, an esophagogram with water-soluble contrast is indicated to demonstrate the site of injury. In contrast, bronchoscopy is recommended for evaluation of a suspected tracheobronchial injury, rather than an imaging radiographic procedure.

Foreign Body Aspiration

Foreign body aspiration usually occurs in children under 3 years of age. Peanuts are the single most common offending object. Either partial obstruction with a check valve mechanism or complete obstruction of a bronchus may occur. The high oily content of aspirated vegetable matter may cause an associated pneumonia. Patients present with respiratory distress, coughing, or wheezing.

PA chest films should be requested in both inspiration and expiration. In cases of check-valve obstruction, the inspiration examination may be entirely normal. However, the partially obstructed side remains overinflated during expiration and causes a shift of the mediastinal structures to the uninvolved side. With complete bronchial obstruction, the chest films may show atelectasis and collapse of the involved segment of the lobe. Occasionally, a radiopaque foreign body may actually be visualized within a bronchus. Fluoroscopy is helpful in showing diminished diaphragmatic motion on the affected side in check-valve obstruction. CT may show a nonopaque foreign body in a bronchus that cannot be seen on plain films.

Empyema

An empyema is a collection of purulent fluid in the pleural space resulting from underlying pneumonia, lung abscess, penetrating injury, or extension of subphrenic abscess. It is often loculated, making diagnosis and specific treatment difficult. On chest films, an empyema appears as either a pleural effusion or pleural-based mass. A loculated empyema may not layer out on lateral decubitus examination. In this situation, ultrasound imaging is useful in identifying the abnormal fluid collection and facilitates appropriate placement of a chest tube for drainage. CT may also identify empyema pockets, as well as differentiate a loculated empyema from a similarly appearing peripheral lung process, such as abscess.

CARDIOVASCULAR EMERGENCIES

Pericardial Effusion

In patients with a pericardial effusion, the PA chest film usually shows a flask-like enlargement of the cardiac silhouette. Occasionally, a specific diagnosis of pericardial effusion may be made on the lateral radiograph by demonstration of a fluid-density stripe between the lucent epicardial fat and lucent fat of the adjacent anterior chest wall. When cardiac tamponade occurs, the PA chest film may demonstrate abnormally lucent lungs with normal or diminished pulmonary vasculature, despite enlargement of the cardiac silhouette.

Echocardiography is the imaging examination of choice for diagnosing pericardial effusion. In a quickly performed, accurate test that does not require ionizing radiation, pericardial fluid is shown as a sonolucent space anterior and posterior to the heart. CT is not required for diagnosing a suspected pericardial effusion; however, if performed for other indications, it readily demonstrates the pericardial effusion.

Pulmonary Embolus

Patients with suspected pulmonary embolus are examined with plain chest films, a ventilation/perfusion lung scan, and pulmonary arteriography. It is important to consider a diagnosis of pulmonary embolus in symptomatic patients with predisposing risk factors, including recent surgery, trauma, or postpartum states, as well as patients with deep venous thrombosis, diabetes, obesity, heart disease, lung disease, and those taking birth control pills. The common presenting clinical findings include pleuritic chest pain, shortness of breath, cough, hemoptysis, tachycardia, tachypnea, fever, cyanosis, and hypotension.

The PA and lateral chest examination is most often entirely normal. The most common abnormality is diminished lung volume, including an elevated hemidiaphragm and nonspecific subsegmental atelectasis. If pulmonary infarction occurs, a hemorrhagic pleural effusion may be present. Later, a pleural-based consolidative process (Hampton's hump) may be seen. Occasionally, sufficient pulmonary oligemia is present to appear as a relative lucency in the lung periphery with increase in size of hilar pulmonary arteries (Westermark's sign).

The ventilation/perfusion radioisotope lung scan is an accurate screening examination for pulmonary embolus if the chest x-ray is normal and there is no underlying lung disease. A high probability scan for pulmonary embolus shows two or more lung segments with absent perfusion but normal ventilation. The findings are often bilateral. A low probability lung scan demonstrates minor, nonsegmental perfusion defects, or perfusion defects with matching ventilation defects. The most accurate lung scan is one that shows absolutely normal perfusion; this scan is nearly 100% accurate in ruling out pulmonary embolism. No confirmatory arteriography is required. Lung scans should be performed temporally near the onset of the symptoms for greatest sensitivity.

A pulmonary arteriogram is the most accurate technique for detection of pulmonary emboli. Selective arteriography requires right-heart catheterization and is, therefore, a more invasive test than the lung scan. Pulmonary arteriography is indicated when the lung scan diagnosis is indeterminate, when the scan is interpreted as high probability in a patient at risk for anticoagulation, and when the scan is interpreted as low probability in a patient with an overwhelmingly suggestive clinical history. Also, pulmonary arteriography is performed as the primary study in patients with underlying chest x-ray abnormalities, which make the lung scan nondiagnostic for pulmonary embolus. Other candidates for pulmonary arteriography are those requiring inferior vena cava filter placement or clipping if pulmonary emboli are found. At pulmonary arteriography, pulmonary emboli appear as arterial intraluminal filling defects, or as sharp arterial cutoffs with an absence of normal arterial branching patterns.

Aortic Dissection

Patients with aortic dissection usually present with acute severe chest pain radiating into the back. The pain may be associated with the onset of hypertension, stroke, acute myocardial infarction, intestinal ischemia, hematuria, diminished or absent limb pulses, or new neurological deficits. Risk factors for aortic dissection include Marfan's syndrome, hypertension, and pregnancy. Pathologically, there is separation of the layers of the aortic wall with formation of a new false lumen that may be filled with freely flowing blood or with hematoma. The symptoms are produced by occlusion of aortic branches by the intimal flap.

Aortic dissections are classified by location. Type I involves the entire aorta, originating from just above the aortic valve and extending through the arch and beyond. Type II is limited to the ascending aorta. Type III, originates distal to the left subclavian artery and extends down the thoracic aorta, often into the abdominal aorta.

Plain chest films may show widening of the mediastinum and thoracic aorta due to increase in its overall caliber. There may be a secondary shift of the trachea to the right. A specific sign on the PA chest film is the finding of increased soft tissue density between the calcified intima and the outer wall of the aorta at the level of the aortic arch.

CT with intravenous contrast is currently the procedure of choice for diagnosing suspected aortic dissection. Following bolus injections of the contrast medium, CT at specified levels demonstrates the intimal flap and identifies the true and false lumens.

Although more invasive than contrast-enhanced CT, aortography is necessary when a surgical repair is planned; aortography is the superior examination for determining the actual extent of a dissection. The site of the original intimal tear, the distal extent of the dissection, and the patency of aortic branches are all readily shown.

Traumatic Rupture of the Thoracic Aorta

The thoracic aorta is especially prone to trauma during deceleration injuries with the usual site of injury just distal to the left subclavian artery. The degree of aortic damage varies from a simple intimal tear or laceration with false aneurysm formation to transection of the aorta. Traumatic rupture of the aorta most commonly occurs in victims of high speed motor vehicle crashes or falls from heights. For those patients who survive long enough for transportation to a hospital (only 15–20%), rapid diagnosis and treatment are mandatory.

The initial chest radiograph may show only widening of the upper mediastinum. The outline of the aorta may be ill-defined due to false aneurysm formation and adjacent hemorrhage. If possible, an upright PA film is often needed to distinguish between widening of the mediastinum after trauma and physiological widening often normally seen on AP supine chest films. Other radiographic signs of traumatic aortic rupture (in the normally positioned aorta) include a left apical pleural cap, displacement of the trachea and nasogastric tube to the right, depression of the left mainstem bronchus, and a left pleural fluid collection. When any of these findings are seen on the chest film of a patient who has suffered a deceleration injury, an aortogram should be performed.

Abdominal Aortic Aneurysm

Abdominal aortic aneurysms usually involve the infrarenal aorta. They often present as a pulsatile abdominal mass on physical examination. Back pain and hypotension are signs of aneurysmal leak or rupture. When rupture occurs, there may be no time for imaging studies; however, in hemodynamically stable patients, emergency CT quickly and accurately establishes or excludes the diagnosis.

Calcification of the intimal layer of the aortic wall may allow a plain film diagnosis of an abdominal aortic aneurysm. A measurement of 4 cm or greater diameter is usually abnormal. In an asymptomatic patient with a newly diagnosed pulsatile abdominal mass, ultrasound imaging is considered the procedure of choice in making a diagnosis of aortic aneurysm and in estimating its size. Occasionally, obesity or overlying bowel gas interferes with an aortic ultrasonic examination.

CT is the procedure of choice for imaging the abdominal aortic aneurysm suspected of leaking. It is performed without oral or intravenous contrast material; its accuracy approaches 100%. The diagnostic finding at CT is hemorrhage adjacent to the aneurysm in retroperitoneal tissues and less commonly in the peritoneum. The presence of leak is not so readily detected with ultrasonography and angiography.

Aortography is indicated in patients undergoing preoperation evaluation. It is useful for determination of the extent of aneurysm and specific involvement of aortic branches. In certain patients with simple infrarenal aneurysms not extending into the iliac arteries, CT may provide sufficient information for surgical planning.

GASTROINTESTINAL EMERGENCIES

Ruptured Abdominal Viscus

The most common cause of nontraumatic abdominal viscus rupture is perforation of a peptic ulcer of the stomach or duodenum. Perforation of a colonic diverticulum or tumor is not uncommon.

Small amounts of free intraperitoneal gas are best demonstrated on upright plain films of the abdomen or chest. If an upright film cannot be obtained, a left lateral decubitus abdominal film is substituted. To maximize sensitivity, the patient is placed in the upright or decubitus position for several minutes prior to the film. Free intraperitoneal air is identified as a curvilinear collection of gas under the right or left hemidiaphragm on the upright chest or abdomen film. On the lateral decubitus film the abnormal curvilinear lucency of gas is seen between the liver and right abdominal wall.

To find the site of perforation, an upper gastrointestinal (UGI) series with water-soluble contrast material is indicated; this examination may demonstrate the gastric or duodenal ulcer with associated extravasation of contrast material into the peritoneum or retroperitoneum. Similarly, an enema with water-soluble contrast material may show extravasation from a perforated colonic diverticulitis or tumor.

CT is not usually indicated in the evaluation of suspected free intraperitoneal air, but readily demonstrates its presence. Because patients are routinely scanned in the supine position, the gas collects anteriorly and is identified adjacent to the anterior abdominal wall. The same CT window and level settings used to evaluate the lung parenchyma provide the maximal sensitivity for showing small amounts of intraperitoneal gas.

Intraabdominal Abscess

Patients with intraabdominal abscesses typically present with fever, leukocytosis, abdominal pain, anorexia, and malaise. Many are recovering from recent abdominal surgery. Ultrasonography and CT have greatly facilitated detection and treatment planning of abdominal abscesses. The ultrasound examination is particularly useful in evaluating the subphrenic regions, the right upper quadrant, and the pelvis. CT diagnoses abscesses with high accuracy and is the preferred technique for areas of the abdomen that may be obscured by bowel gas during ultrasonography. Less popular are radionuclide scans with gallium-67 (^{67}Ga) or other isotopes; these lack anatomical detail and often require 24–72 hours before imaging takes place. Plain films of the abdomen are often nonspecific but may show an abnormal collection of gas outside the bowel, or displacement of normal abdominal structures by a mass or an abscess.

At ultrasound examination, an abdominal abscess appears as a rounded or ovoid mass or collection of fluid. Unlike simple cysts, there usually are internal echoes within abscess fluid collections. Flecks of highly echogenic gas may be visible within the mass or fluid collection.

At CT, an abdominal abscess appears as a rounded or ovoid heterogeneous extraluminal mass, with a well-defined wall and lower density center. A specific CT sign of abscess is extraluminal gas within the mass. Confirmation of an abscess may be performed with a percutaneous 20- or 22-gauge needle aspiration using local anesthesia and CT or ultrasound guidance. Fluid or pus aspirated from abscesses typically show white blood cells and usually bacteria on Gram's stain.

In selected cases, percutaneous abdominal abscess drainage may be performed in the radiology department for emergency department patients. If an abdominal abscess is thought to be a consequence of a perforated viscus, an UGI series or barium enema should be performed to demonstrate the underlying lesion.

Intestinal Obstruction

Colon

Colonic obstruction is most frequently caused by carcinoma of the colon. Less commonly, diverticulitis, benign tumors, volvulus, hernias, or extrinsic compressions may cause obstruction. Prompt diagnosis of volvulus or closed loop obstruction is required to prevent colonic ischemia and infarction.

Plain films of the abdomen show a dilated gas-filled colon proximal to the level of the obstruction. The cecum may be markedly dilated, and air-fluid levels may be present in the colon or small bowel. If the ileocecal valve is patent, gas may reflux into the small bowel, resulting in dilatation of the distal small bowel with air-fluid levels mimicking the findings in small bowel obstruction.

Barium enema is the diagnostic procedure of choice and usually provides a specific diagnosis. A single contrast barium enema is preferred to an air-contrast examination. Routine preparation of the bowel with enemas or oral cathartics is contraindicated in suspected colonic obstruction.

Small Bowel

Small bowel obstruction is commonly caused by adhesions from prior abdominal surgery. The usual symptoms include crampy midepigastric pain and vomiting. These are often episodic. Plain abdomen films demonstrate multiple dilated air- and fluid-filled loops of small bowel. The small bowel loops may be distinguished from colon by their position in the abdomen and the presence of valvulae conniventes. These mucosal markings extend entirely across the lumen of dilated small bowel loops and are closer than colonic haustral indentations. The upright film usually shows multiple air-fluid levels in a stepladder configuration. A distinguishing feature of small bowel obstruction is the lack of distention of the cecum and remainder of the colon. Mechanical small bowel obstruction may cause increased bowel motility, resulting in evacuation of colon contents. However, it is difficult to distinguish an adynamic bowel ileus from mechanical small bowel obstruction when the colon has not been evacuated of gas and stool. Follow-up radiographs are helpful.

Before a barium upper gastrointestinal series is undertaken, it is important to exclude proximal colonic obstruction, which may mimic small bowel obstruction. If colonic obstruction is suspected, a barium enema should be performed first. A barium UGI series is contraindicated in colonic obstruction because barium hardens with colonic water absorption if it remains in the colon proximal to an obstructing lesion.

An UGI series with small bowel examination demonstrates delayed transit and dilatation of small bowel loops to the level of the obstruction. Water-soluble contrast material is not suitable for small bowel contrast examinations because dilution with small bowel fluid renders the contrast material insufficiently concentrated for diagnosis. The high osmolarity of water-soluble contrast material tends to draw fluid into the small bowel, further aggravating fluid and electrolyte imbalance.

Acute Cholecystitis

Acute cholecystitis is usually caused by a gallstone lodged in and obstructing the cystic duct. Patients with acute cholecystitis present with right upper quadrant pain, often referred to the shoulder or back. The pain may be episodic, and fever may be present. Tenderness to right upper quadrant palpation may be noted on physical examination. Abdominal ultrasonographic and radioisotopic scanning with iminodiacetic acid (IDA) labelled with technetium 99M (^{99m}Tc) are the two common techniques for diagnostic imaging. Many physicians prefer ultrasonography as the initial examination because it is performed more quickly with superior anatomic resolution. Oral cholecystography and intravenous cholangiography are no longer recommended for diagnosing acute cholecystitis.

An abdominal plain film may demonstrate calcified gallstones. However, most gallstones are not radiopaque. Gas within the gallbladder wall or lumen (emphysematous cholecystitis) may be visualized if there is infection with gas-producing organisms. A localized intestinal ileus with dilatation of adjacent bowel loops is a common but nonspecific finding.

In patients with acute cholecystitis, abdominal ultrasound examination may demonstrate gallstones as discrete bright echoes, dependent within the gallbladder, which cause acoustic shadowing of the ultrasound beam. Specific ultrasonographic signs of cholecystitis are abnormal thickening of a distended gallbladder wall and fluid surrounding the gallbladder. However, a pericholecystic fluid collection is a nonspecific finding, also seen in patients with ascites. Another reliable sign is the presence of focal tenderness when the transducer is depressed directly over the gallbladder; this tenderness represents the ultrasonic equivalent of Murphy's sign.

In normal patients a radionuclide scan with ^{99m}Tc-labelled IDA shows activity in the gallbladder and biliary tree with subsequent activity visible in the common bile duct and bowel. A gallbladder failing to take up the isotope (a positive scan) within 30–60 minutes suggests cholecystitis. False-positive radionuclide examination may be seen in chronic cholecystitis, prior cholecystectomy, or jaundice.

Acute Pancreatitis

Acute pancreatitis is often difficult to diagnose clinically because its signs and symptoms are nonspecific and often confused with biliary tract or peptic ulcer disease. Ultrasonic study and CT are the recommended procedures of choice today to confirm a diagnosis of pancreatitis and to exclude its complications.

Plain films of the abdomen may be helpful in excluding other acute abdominal conditions that may mimic pancreatitis. They may also show the nonspecific findings of pancreatitis, such as a single dilated loop of small bowel (the sentinel loop) representing a response of the bowel to adjacent inflammation. A specific sign of pancreatic disease is calcification within the pancreas, seen in chronic pancreatitis.

With acute pancreatitis, abdominal ultrasonography may demonstrate an enlarged or sonolucent pancreas. Often, excessive bowel gas or the habitus of the patient may result in inadequate ultrasonic visualization of the pancreas. In those patients and in patients considered sufficiently ill to warrant surgery, CT is indicated.

CT may show an enlarged low density pancreas due to the edema of acute pancreatitis. Pancreatic calcifications from chronic pancreatitis may be seen with CT even where there is insufficient calcification for detection on plain films. CT is particularly helpful in identifying the complications of pancreatitis, including pseudocysts, phlegmon, abscesses, and necrosis.

Acute Appendicitis

Diagnostic imaging is usually not contributory in the diagnosis of acute appendicitis. The patient is usually treated on the basis of clinical and laboratory findings. A plain film of the abdomen is often uninformative; it may show nonspecific generalized adynamic ileus with dilated loops of small bowel and colon. An appendicolith—a round or ovoid calcification in the right lower quadrant—may be seen. Occasionally, a right lower quadrant mass is present, indicating an appendiceal abscess. A nonspecific sign of appendicitis is scoliosis of the lumbar spine convex to the left, caused by contraction of the right psoas muscles from adjacent inflammation. When gas is identified in the appendix, it may represent a normal finding due to communication of the appendix with the GI tract, or it may represent the presence of gas-producing organisms within an inflamed appendix. Barium enema or CT are not usually performed for appendicitis, although both may show the presence of an appendiceal abscess or periappendiceal inflammation. Ultrasonic examination of the appendix with graded compression has been described. It should not be widely adapted for diagnosing appendicitis.

Upper Acute Gastrointestinal Hemorrhage

Imaging examinations recommended for the diagnosis of patients with upper gastrointestinal (GI) bleeding include plain films of the abdomen and arteriography. The UGI series is not recommended in the acute setting because the barium interferes with subsequent angiography if indicated. An upper GI series may be indicated in the clinical setting where angiography is not available.

The abdominal plain films often demonstrate no specific abnormality. They may occasionally demonstrate blood clot in the stomach appearing as a speckled air and soft tissue density in the left upper quadrant or enlargement of the spleen in patients with portal hypertension and gastroesophageal varices. Plain films are more commonly performed to exclude the presence of free intraperitoneal air.

Selective arteriography of the UGI tract is utilized to determine the bleeding site in patients with unremitting hemorrhage. Esophagogastroduodenoscopy is recommended prior to this examination. Bleeding must be active for angiographic demonstration; this determination is made by observation of the nasogastric tube aspirate. In patients with arterial bleeding, extravasation of contrast material from arteries supplying the bleeding site may be demonstrated. Angiographic treatment with intra-arterial vasopressin infusion or embolization may be utilized in an effort to control the hemorrhage (see Chapter 46). With gastroesophageal variceal hemorrhage, no extravasation is seen at angiography, but the varices themselves are well-shown.

Lower Acute Gastrointestinal Tract Hemorrhage

With lower GI tract hemorrhage, abdominal plain films, radioisotope bleeding scans, and selective arteriography are indicated, usually in that sequence.

Again, the goal of imaging is identification of the site of hemorrhage. Barium enema in an unprepared bowel is not only uninformative, but contraindicated in acute bleeding because the retained barium interferes with needed imaging studies, such as angiography. However, a barium enema may be performed at a later date if the etiology of lower GI hemorrhage is not immediately diagnosed.

The abdominal plain films may be helpful in screening for the presence of intraperitoneal gas, a mass, or signs of intestinal obstruction. It is not helpful for localization of hemorrhage. The radioisotope bleeding examination is indicated as a screening device before arteriography in patients in whom it is uncertain whether active bleeding is taking place. A ^{99m}Tc radioisotope tag is applied to a sample of the patient's red blood cells, which are then reinjected for subsequent imaging of the abdomen. Accumulation of radioisotope overlying the lower small bowel or colon may not only confirm active bleeding, but indicate the approximate site of hemorrhage.

Selective arteriography (Chapter 46) is indicated in patients who are actively bleeding from the lower GI tract and fail to stop with conservative management. Bleeding sites are identified by contrast extravasation into the bowel lumen. Intraarterial vasopressin infusion usually controls the acute bleeding. When surgery is required, angiography helps localize the abnormal segment of bowel that needs to be resected.

Jaundice

Jaundice may be caused by hepatocellular disease or biliary obstruction. In the latter case, imaging examinations help confirm biliary obstruction and identify the anatomic level and cause of obstruction. Plain films of the abdomen are usually uninformative but may show a right upper quadrant mass or calcified gallstones.

Abdominal ultrasonography is considered the most useful initial imaging test for patients with jaundice because it differentiates between the obstructive and nonobstructive jaundice of hepatocellular disease. At ultrasonography, intrahepatic dilatation of bile ducts appears as prominent and supernumerary tubular structures within the liver. The common hepatic bile duct at the level of the portal vein and hepatic artery may be measured; a diameter of 0.6 cm or greater suggests dilatation due to obstruction. A dilated common bile duct may be followed to the level of the obstruction where a neoplastic mass may be identified. In patients with jaundice due to an obstructing common bile duct stone, the level of obstruction may be shown, but ultrasonography may not detect the calculus itself. Also, ultrasonic study may not detect small ampullary tumors. Specific causes of obstructive jaundice that may be identified by ultrasonography include hepatic or pancreatic neoplasms and periportal adenopathy.

CT offers better anatomical detail in cases where biliary obstruction is identified and no clear etiology demonstrated by ultrasonography. Intravenous contrast material is used to enhance visualization of liver masses or dilated bile ducts. Retroperitoneal and periportal adenopathy is better shown by CT than by ultrasonography. Thin contiguous CT slices through the common bile duct may show a common bile duct stone. Ampullary stenosis or tumors often present with common bile duct dilatation without an identifiable stone or mass.

Endoscopic retrograde cholangiography and pancreatography (ERCP) are often performed for suspected periampullary obstruction of bile ducts. X-ray images are obtained after the cannulated common bile and pancreatic ducts are injected with contrast material. Biopsy of an ampullary tumor or removal of an obstructing common bile duct stone are possible during ERCP. An ampullary stenosis may be treated with papillotomy.

Percutaneous transhepatic cholangiography is reserved for patients requiring direct visualization of the biliary system after biliary obstruction has been demonstrated by ultrasonography or CT. It is performed by injecting contrast material through a long 22-gauge needle inserted percutaneously into a peripheral bile duct. It is helpful for identifying sites of biliary obstruction not clearly shown by other studies; it clearly demonstrates the stricture formation that occurs in sclerosing cholangitis. A therapeutic percutaneous biliary drainage procedure may be indicated to alleviate the symptoms of obstructive jaundice in patients either not requiring or not candidates for immediate surgery.

ABDOMINAL TRAUMA

Spleen

Injuries of the spleen are common life-threatening sequelae of abdominal trauma. The signs and symptoms are nonspecific and include left upper quadrant pain, referred pain to the left shoulder from diaphragmatic irritation, and hypotension if substantial bleeding has occurred. In addition to major injuries causing immediate splenic rupture, minor splenic injuries may occur, resulting in lacerations and subcapsular hemorrhage which subsequently may increase and rupture hours or days after the traumatic event. Consequently, patients with a suspected splenic injury should undergo immediate diagnostic imaging, preferably with contrast-enhanced CT.

Occasionally, indirect signs of splenic trauma may be apparent on plain films of the chest or abdomen. Findings associated with splenic injury include fractures of the left 9th–12th ribs, a left pleural effusion, elevation of the left hemidiaphragm, and a left upper quadrant mass with medial displacement of the stomach air bubble, or of the nasogastric tube if the air bubble has been aspirated. The presence of free peritoneal fluid on a plain film suggests intraperitoneal hemorrhage. Normal plain films of the chest and abdomen do not rule out the possibility of splenic rupture; in fact, one-half of patients with splenic rupture do have normal plain films.

CT has very high accuracy in the detection of splenic trauma and has been adapted as the examination of choice in many emergency centers. Ultrasonic examination is less accurate and may be limited or suboptimal because associated rib fractures interfere with the examination. In addition, sonographic findings of splenic injury are subtle, easily overlooked, or indeterminate. Radionuclide splenic scans are less accurate than CT with less anatomic resolution, although they may be useful screening examinations if CT is not available, especially when normal. Splenic arteriography is an invasive procedure, that is less accurate than CT. It cannot be done as quickly as CT and provides information about other potentially injured abdominal organs, such as the liver, pancreas, or mesentery, only with additional manipulation. Splenic angiography is now recommended when a splenic scan is abnormal and CT is unavailable.

Duodenum

The duodenum is prone to shearing injuries following blunt abdominal trauma because it is partially fixed in the retroperitoneum. Often, the related symptoms of progressive nausea, vomiting, or abdominal pain are not initially evident, but become increasingly severe hours or days after the patient may have been discharged.

An UGI series is the recommended examination for the diagnosis of duodenal hematoma. The usual findings include irregular thickening of duodenal folds by submucosal hemorrhage, often in a characteristic stacked-coin appearance. The hematoma may resolve spontaneously or result in delayed perforation, gastric outlet obstruction, or bleeding into the retroperitoneum. Duodenal hematoma is not as reliably diagnosed by CT, although CT may show a small amount of free or retroperitoneal air with perforation not detectable on plain films. CT is recommended if a coexisting pancreatic injury is suspected.

GENITOURINARY EMERGENCIES

Trauma

The intravenous pyelourogram (IVP) is commonly used for the evaluation of patients with renal trauma, but it may overlook minor trauma that is better detected with CT. Nephrotomography should be included as a part of urography for trauma patients, to improve diagnostic quality. Today, CT is recommended when available for evaluation of all patients with suspected renal trauma. However, the IVP is often the initial screening examination because of its general availability. When performed, the IVP should be evaluated for bilateral symmetry of contrast material excretion. If complete absence of excretion is identified, renal pedicle injury should be considered. In these cases, arteriography is recommended to detail the injured renal vessels. Minor renal injuries produce contusions, which appear as irregular lucencies in the kidneys, representing areas of hemorrhage and edema. Although the urogram is relatively insensitive to small perirenal hematomas, large amounts of retroperitoneal hemorrhage may displace the kidney. Filling defects within the renal collecting system usually represent blood clots; the calyceal system may be distorted by either edema or hemorrhage. Extravasation of contrast material occurs when lacerations are sufficiently deep to disrupt the collecting system.

CT is both more sensitive and specific in the diagnosis of renal injuries than the IVP. In addition, CT may demonstrate associated injuries to the liver, spleen, bladder, or pelvis. Compared with plain films and ultrasonography, CT is unaffected by overlying bowel gas. It more accurately delineates parenchymal injuries in order to differentiate those patients with minor injuries who can be treated conservatively from those with major injuries who will require surgery.

Bladder injuries may be visualized by intravenous urography, cystoscopy, or CT. There may be elevation of the bladder or a mass effect compressing the bladder walls from adjacent pelvic hemorrhage. Occasionally, intravesical filling defects due to blood clot may be identified. Bladder perforation may be demonstrated by extravasation of contrast-enhanced urine. If trauma to the male urethra is suspected, a retrograde urethrogram with water-soluble contrast material should be performed prior to bladder catheterization.

Urinary Tract Calculi

The most frequent cause of acute obstructive uropathy is a urinary tract calculus. A calculus less than 5 mm in diameter nearly always passes spontaneously. However, a calculus greater than 1 cm often obstructs and requires intervention. Occasionally, other conditions, such as renal artery occlusion or renal vein thrombosis, may simulate the symptoms of renal calculi. A plain abdominal film often shows a radiopaque calculus projected over the kidneys, ureter, or bladder. A urinary calculus cannot always be distinguished from a phlebolith without contrast examination.

Intravenous urography is the procedure of choice for examining patients with suspected renal calculi, and is indicated for a first episode, diagnostic uncertainty, suspected coexisting urinary tract infection, or when surgical intervention may be required. In addition to confirming the presence of a lucent or opaque urinary tract calculus, the IVP may also show the exact site of the calculus and the degree of obstruction.

Ultrasonic examination is not usually recommended because it may fail to demonstrate the calculus in the ureter or bladder. In addition, patients with acute obstruction may not have sufficient dilatation of the collecting system to demonstrate hydronephrosis on ultrasonography. When apparent on ultrasonic examination, a renal or bladder calculus is seen as a discrete bright focus with acoustic shadowing.

In instances when an intravenous urogram cannot be performed, such as oliguria or severe prior contrast reaction, a noncontrast-enhanced CT scan may demonstrate the renal calculus by its characteristic high density. Even nonopaque renal calculi may be detected because they have a higher CT density than the surrounding soft tissues.

Obstructed Uropathy Hydronephrosis

Urinary tract obstruction is often manifest radiologically as secondary dilatation of an intrarenal collecting system, easily identified by an ultrasonic study. Consequently, ultrasonography is a sensitive noninvasive examination for patients with suspected hydronephrosis. False-positive diagnoses may be due to dilatation of an intrarenal collecting system that is not the result of urinary obstruction, as in physiological fullness of the intrarenal collecting system, associated with a filled bladder or vesicoureteral reflux of urine. If obstruction occurs in the context of urinary tract infection, prompt drainage of the infected, stagnant urine is required. Ultrasonography is indicated in patients with unexplained renal failure suggested by elevation of the blood urea nitrogen and serum creatinine, or by unexplained oliguria. The ultrasonic appearance of hydronephrosis is a fluid-filled dilatation of the renal pelvis displacing the normally bright echoes of renal pelvic fat. In moderate or severe hydronephrosis, contiguous sonolucent fluid-filled calyces may be visualized. Peripelvic renal cysts are usually distinguishable from hydronephrosis.

On the IVP, renal obstruction results in a delayed and hyperdense nephrogram. The kidney silhouette is usually enlarged. Subsequently, dilatation of the renal pelvis and calyces may be visualized. When the obstruction is in the ureter, columnation and dilatation of the ureter proximal to the obstruction often occurs. An IVP is recommended in cases of acute obstruction, such as by urinary calculi.

CT is helpful in the evaluation of hydronephrosis due to extrinsic mass. In patients with renal failure or other contraindication to the use of intravenous contrast, the diagnosis may usually be established without intravenous contrast. Retrograde pyelography may be used to opacify the ureter and collecting system that is sufficiently obstructed not to be seen on the IVP. Retrograde pyelography is often performed in conjunction with stent placement or ureteral stone removal.

Antegrade pyelography may be used to demonstrate the intrarenal collecting system and ureter proximal to obstructing lesions. A Whitaker test may be performed to measure the pressure gradient between the renal pelvis and bladder during stimulated urine flow, to offer a quantitative measure of obstruction. Nephrostomy tube placement may be performed percutaneously, if necessary, to decompress an obstructed kidney.

Acute Pyelonephritis

Patients with acute pyelonephritis may benefit from imaging to exclude predisposing factors, such as vesicoureteral reflux, and to exclude complications such as obstructive uropathy and abscess formation. Renal ultrasonic examination is usually normal in uncomplicated pyelonephritis, although small scattered zones of edema may be seen within the kidneys. Similarly, the urogram is also most often normal. Voiding cystoureterography (VCUG) may be helpful in excluding vesicoureteral reflux. For this test, the bladder is filled in retrograde fashion with water-soluble contrast material through a small catheter. Fluoroscopic visualization during voiding is performed to assess the reflux of contrast material from the bladder into the ureter and up into the renal pelvis. CT is indicated when complications of acute pyelonephritis are suspected, such as renal abscess or perinepheric fluid collections. Edema of the kidney or intrarenal gas are well-shown with CT.

Ruptured Ectopic Pregnancy

If untreated, ruptured ectopic pregnancy is often fatal due to hemorrhage into the maternal abdomen. Without a high degree of clinical suspicion, the diagnosis is often overlooked or delayed. The majority of patients with ruptured ectopic pregnancy do not have the classic triad of pain, vaginal bleeding, and palpable mass. Because ruptured ectopic pregnancy often occurs in the first trimester, many women do not realize they are pregnant. Therefore, serum human chorionic gonadotropin (hCG) determination and ultrasonic scanning are recommended to establish the diagnosis when ectopic pregnancy is a possibility.

A well-defined ectopic fetus is demonstrable by ultrasonography in less than 10% of cases. Consequently, other less specific ultrasonic findings must be used to establish the likelihood of this diagnosis. The first assessment is to determine whether there is an intrauterine pregnancy. Ultrasonography demonstrates an intrauterine pregnancy of at least 4–6 weeks gestational age. If an intrauterine pregnancy is present, the likelihood of a coexisting ectopic pregnancy is extremely rare (1:20,000). If a patient is accurately known to be greater than 6 weeks from the last menstrual period or has a diagnostic quantitative β-hCG level, then an ectopic pregnancy must be considered in the absence of an intrauterine pregnancy on ultrasonography. Ectopic pregnancy is most often visualized as a nonspecific adnexal or cul-de-sac mass. If rupture of an ectopic pregnancy has occurred, blood may be identified in the cul-de-sac or upper abdomen. Often, there is an amorphous collection in the uterine endometrium representing decidual reaction secondary to hormonal stimulation from the ectopic pregnancy.

Because ultrasonography does not reliably demonstrate an intrauterine pregnancy of less than 6 weeks, an early intrauterine pregnancy is often in the differential diagnosis of ectopic pregnancy. In those patients where both ultrasonic and other findings are nonspecific, either laparoscopy or careful observation may be elected. If the latter, a follow-up ultrasonic examination in 7–10 days should distinguish an early intrauterine pregnancy by visualization of the fetus at this time.

Acute Pelvic Inflammatory Disease

Acute pelvic inflammatory disease (PID) may be imaged by ultrasonography to exclude complications, such as tuboovarian abscess or pyosalpinx.

Pelvic ultrasonography is usually normal in uncomplicated PID, although the uterus may appear edematous. There is often focal tenderness to placement of the ultrasound transducer over the inflamed pelvic. A tuboovarian abscess appears as a complex sonolucent septated mass containing internal echoes. Ultrasonography does not reliably distinguish between a mass due to tuboovarian abscess and a mass related to neoplasm. Consequently, a follow-up examination by ultrasonography in those patients is usually performed to document resolution of the abscess.

Testicular Torsion

Early diagnosis of testicular torsion is critical in preventing the irreparable ischemia that rapidly follows. Twelve hours after the initial symptoms, only 20% of patients have viability of the affected testis. A radionuclide testicular scan is the imaging procedure of choice in patients with suspected torsion, and must be performed expeditiously to be of value.

Testicular scanning is performed after an intravenous injection of ^{99m}Tc-labeled pertechnetate. An initial flow study is obtained immediately after intravenous injection. Subsequently, static images are collected over a longer period of time. In early torsion, within 0–7 hours, there is homogeneous symmetrical flow of radioisotope. However, the later static images show a characteristic area of diminished activity corresponding to the torsed testis. Surrounding scrotal activity on the static images may be normal or slightly increased due to inflammation.

In midphase torsion (7–24 hours) there is increased scrotal activity surrounding the affected testis on the flow study, due to increased perfusion. This results in a halo of increased activity in the scrotum. Static images again demonstrate a halo of increased scrotal activity surrounding the testis that has diminished activity. As torsion progresses to the late phase (''missed'' torsion) of greater than 24 hours, the flow study again shows early scrotal perfusion. The static images reveal a cold testis surrounded by an even more intense halo of scrotal activity.

SKELETAL TRAUMA

Pelvic Fractures

A plain film examination is usually a sufficient screening examination for pelvic fracture and should include AP and angled views (inlet-outlet views) for evaluation of the pelvic brim and sacrum. Oblique views may be required for evaluation of possible acetabular fractures; if CT is available, it should be requested instead, to eliminate turning of the patient required for oblique views. Pelvic fractures may be classified as stable if a single break is present without disruption of the pelvic ring. If the pelvic ring is not intact, the fracture is considered unstable.

CT is indicated when further evaluation of pelvic fractures is required, especially those involving the acetabulum and sacrum. CT is superior to plain films for the depiction of fragment position, as well as for evaluating soft tissue injury and hemorrhage. Because patients with pelvic fractures have a high incidence of associated urinary tract injury, urethrography or cystography may be indicated. For patients with pelvic fractures and unremitting bleeding, pelvic angiography may demonstrate the bleeding source, and embolization of the actively bleeding branches may control the hemorrhage.

Hip Fractures

The hip is usually examined with an AP and true lateral view. The AP view should include the entire pelvis. Additional oblique views, tomography, or CT may be required if the initial films are equivocal or if an acetabular fracture is suspected. These studies are useful for patients with strong clinical suspicion of hip fractures, in whom the plain films do not demonstrate a fracture.

Suspected Acromioclavicular Dislocation

Patients with suspected acromioclavicular (AC) dislocation are examined with an AP upright view, including both AC joints. In addition, a stress view is recommended with the patient carrying weights. If the width of the AC joint is 9 mm or greater, it is considered abnormal. If the distance between the inferior margin of the clavicle and superior coracoid process is greater than 1.4 cm, then coracoclavicular ligamentous injury is suggested.

Shoulder Trauma

For suspected shoulder trauma, a neutral AP view should be obtained and supplemented with an axillary view, Neer (Y) view, or transthoracic view. The axillary or Y views are required to evaluate for dislocation of the humeral head. Anterior dislocation is by far the most common and is readily identified as anterior-inferior displacement of the humeral head with respect to the glenoid. Posterior dislocation is relatively uncommon and often overlooked. An initial clue is fixation of the humerus in internal rotation. The AP view may show lateral displacement of the humeral head with respect to the glenoid rim. Anterior dislocations may cause a Hill-Sachs deformity, a fracture of the superolateral aspect of the humeral head. An anterior glenoid rim

(Bankhart) fracture may also occur. Posterior dislocations may be associated with vertical compression fractures of the humeral head, as well as fractures of the lesser tuberosity.

Fractures of the Extremities

Extremity fractures require evaluation with two views at 90° to one another and are usually studied with AP and lateral plain x-ray views. Oblique views are included when joints are involved. Occasionally, additional coned and special views may be required. In addition to tomography or CT, arthrography may be indicated to demonstrate soft tissue joint injuries. In this instance, the orthopaedic surgeon may prefer direct arthroscopy.

ries. In this instance, the orthopaedic surgeon may prefer direct arthroscopy.

SUGGESTED READINGS

Grossman ZD, Ellis DA, Brigham SC. *The Clinician's Guide to Diagnostic Imaging.* New York: Raven Press, 1983.

Harris JH Jr, Harris WH. *The Radiology of Emergency Medicine,* 2nd ed. Baltimore: Williams & Wilkins, 1981.

Rogers LF. *Radiology of Skeletal Trauma.* New York: Churchill Livingstone, 1982.

Sacknoff R, Novelline RA. Radiology of nontraumatic surgical emergencies. In Gardner B, ed. *Quick Reference to Surgical Emergencies,* 2nd ed. Philadelphia: JB Lippincott, 1986.

Straub WH, ed. *Manual of Diagnostic Imaging.* Boston: Little, Brown & Co., 1984.

CHAPTER **45**

Imaging Trauma with Computed Tomography

ROBERT A. NOVELLINE, M.D.
RICHARD SACKNOFF, M.D.

Of the currently available newer imaging procedures, computed tomography (CT) has had the greatest impact on trauma diagnosis. It has replaced many standard radiologic examinations completely; for certain traumatic conditions, it is the initial imaging procedure. CT can be performed quickly and safely with minimal patient manipulation. Its superior contrast resolution allows excellent visualization of soft tissue structures, accurately identifying organ injuries and hematomas. CT displays transaxial and cross-sectional anatomy; it allows reconstruction of images in a wide variety of other planes. With altered technical settings, CT provides a clear depiction of bony and soft tissue injuries. In recent years, improvements in CT technology have offered faster scanning times, images with diminished artifacts, higher resolution thin sections for improved detail, and three-dimensional representation of complex anatomic structures, such as the face, pelvis, and spine. And, as compared with selective angiography and radioisotope scanning, CT provides visualization of multiple organs simultaneously in the same examination.

As with any diagnostic procedure for the injured, patient selection and procedural timing are paramount. Unstable patients are not candidates for CT examination. In fact, should the patient's condition deteriorate during CT examination, the test must be terminated so that the patient can be taken directly to the operating room. It is accepted practice that the multiple-trauma patient be initially screened during the primary survey in the trauma room with portable lateral cervical spine, anteroposterior (AP) chest and AP pelvis films. These anatomic areas are often clinically "silent," and early detection of major injuries is facilitated by these studies. Especially when the patient is unconscious, intoxicated, or unreliable in history, no signs of neck trauma may be obvious when an unstable cervical spine fracture is actually present. If the clinical findings warrant, the multiple-trauma patient may also be examined during the initial survey with additional portable screening films of the skull, abdomen, and extremities. All initial screening films are scrutinized for signs of an unstable spine fracture. Following initial resuscitative measures, and after stabilization, the patient is taken to the radiology department for definitive diagnostic imaging studies. These may include plain films, CT, contrast studies, conventional tomography, ultrasonography, radioisotopic and magnetic resonance examinations.

CT, similar to other diagnostic x-ray examinations, allows close monitoring of the acutely injured patient. This is not true for magnetic resonance imaging (MRI), where the patient cannot be carefully observed inside the magnet core. Furthermore, ferromagnetic materials, which may be required for patient monitoring and support, cannot be used during MRI. For trauma work, the CT scanner suite should incorporate all the necessary monitoring and support equipment required to sustain the acutely injured patient. The gantry room must be equipped with suction, oxygen, cardiopulmonary resuscitation cart, electrocardiogram (ECG), blood pressure, and respiratory monitors, with sufficient space for ventilators, traction devices, stretchers and personnel. The technologist/physician control area is designed to afford an optimal view of the patient.

In this chapter, the current role of CT is reviewed for injuries of head, face, spine, larynx, chest, abdomen, pelvis, and extremities. Indications for CT examination, its techniques, and the CT appearance of common injuries are discussed for each of these anatomic segments.

HEAD TRAUMA

CT has had a dramatic impact on the diagnostic workup of the patient with head trauma. When intracranial injury is suspected, CT permits diagnosis of intracranial hemorrhage, contusion, pneumocephalus, foreign bodies, and skull fractures in a quickly and easily performed examination. In addition, CT identifies the secondary effects of trauma, such as edema, ischemia, infarction, brain shift, and hydrocephalus. With acute head trauma, intracerebral and extracerebral blood collections are diagnosed with nearly 100% accuracy. Its noninvasive nature allows serial scanning without risk, providing accurate follow-up of patients after trauma. And, because of its high diagnostic accuracy, CT may even eliminate an unnecessary craniotomy.

Indications

CT is indicated in any patient who has sustained head trauma and presents with signs of neurological dysfunction. It is not necessary to obtain plain skull film series prior to CT. Routinely contiguous 10 mm-thick sections are obtained from the skull vertex to the skull base. Thinner sections may be indicated for evaluation of the posterior fossa and skull base. No intravenous contrast material is required; in fact, it is contraindicated in the initial scan series because contrast enhancement of the cortical vessels may mask a subarachnoid hemorrhage. The images are photographed at both brain (soft tissue) and bone windows (Fig. 45.1). Extravasated blood has a high protein concentration and appears white on the brain window images, when compared with the surrounding brain tissue. The bone window images show the configuration of any skull fractures, and aid in the differentiation of thin subdural and epidural hematomas from the surrounding bony calvarium.

Care should always be taken when transporting a patient with head trauma to the CT couch because of the high incidence of associated cervical spine injuries. The screening lateral cervical spine film should always be carefully scrutinized for signs of an unstable cervical spine fracture prior to CT. In the multiple-trauma patient, head CT should be performed first, and other indicated CT examinations, especially those requiring intravenous contrast material, performed after. In addition, head CT should be performed before other radiologic examinations requiring intravenous contrast, such as urography and angiography.

Depressed and Basilar Fractures

CT depicts depressed and basilar skull fractures better than plain films; however, a horizontal, nondisplaced linear fracture in the axial plane of section may be overlooked by transaxial CT. Plain skull films are always scrutinized for findings indicating the need for CT examination. These include displacement of a calcified pineal gland, pneumocephalus, an air-fluid level in the sphenoid or frontal sinuses, a depressed skull fracture, and a linear fracture crossing a meningeal artery groove or major venous sinus. Today, most patients with skull fracture on plain films are referred for CT examination.

Subdural Hematoma

At CT, subdural hematomas (Fig. 45.2) are seen as semilunar (concave-convex) collections of blood overlying the cerebral hemispheres immediately beneath the bony calvarium. Bilateral collections are common. They may also be identified in the interhemispheric fissure, along the floor of the middle cranial fossa, in the posterior fossa, or on the tentorium. Their CT appearance varies, depending upon size, the time interval since injury, the hemoglobin level, the presence of membranous compartmentalization, and the occurrence of rebleeding. The CT density of a hematoma decreases with time as the hemoglobin is metabolized.

Epidural Hematoma

Epidural hematomas result from injuries of meningeal arteries or dural venous sinuses. They nearly always appear at CT as lenticular (biconvex), extracerebral collections of blood (Fig. 45.3). Bilateral epidural hematomas are rare. The epidural hematoma is frequently associated with fractures adjacent to the site of hemorrhage.

Subarachnoid Hemorrhage

Subarachnoid hemorrhages usually result from disruption of small piaarachnoid vessels and straight bridging veins that cross the subarachnoid space. CT shows curvilinear areas of increased density

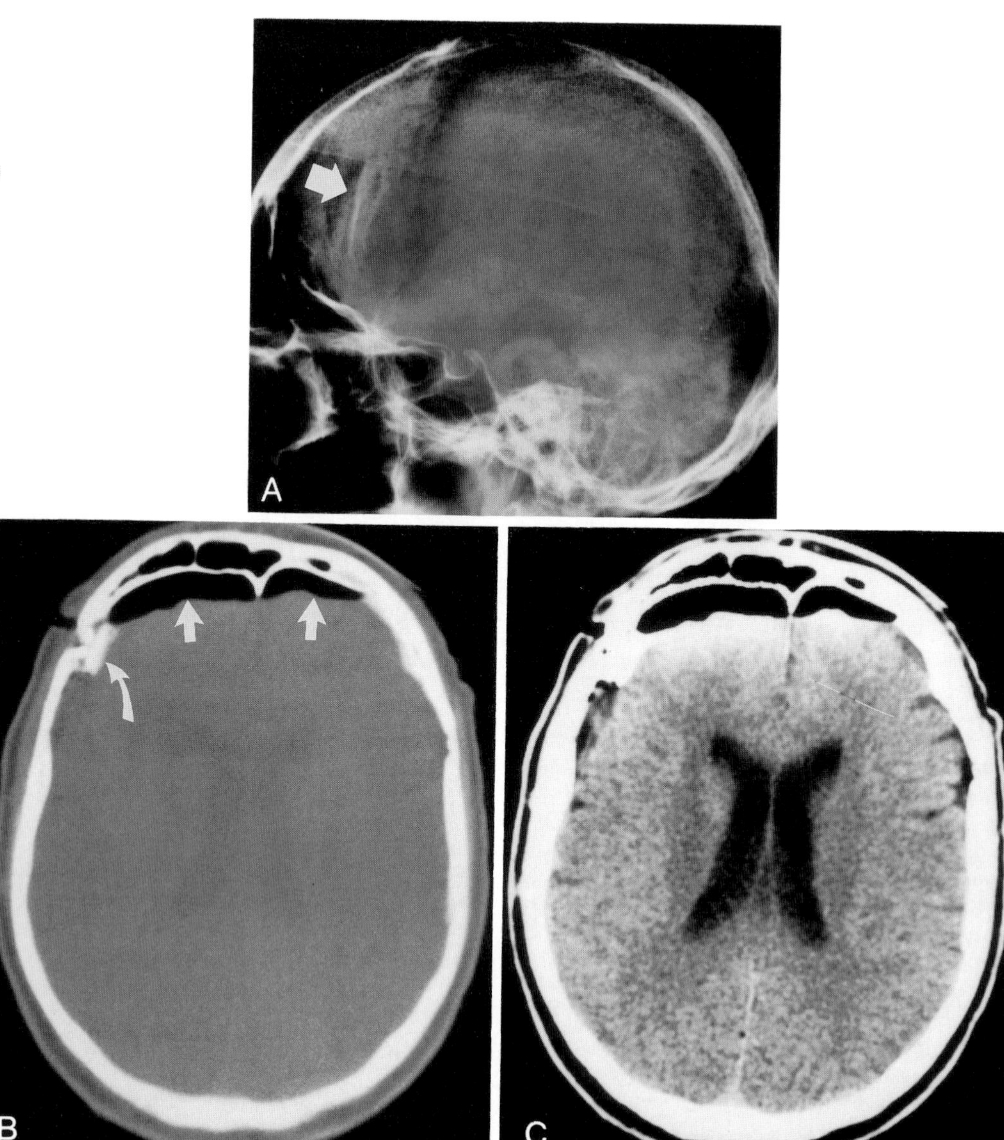

Figure 45.1. Depressed skull fracture. *A*, Lateral skull film shows a crescent-shaped area of increased density in the frontal bone *(arrow)* adjacent to a similarly shaped area of lucency; the findings indicate a depressed skull fracture. *B*, CT scan through the frontal sinuses, photographed at a bone window setting, confirm the fracture (*curved arrow*). Note the pneumocephalus (*straight arrows*), air within the calvarium and over the frontal lobes. *C*, CT scan, at the same level as *B* and photographed at a brain window, shows increased density (*whiteness*) in the frontal lobes consistent with contusion.

(hemorrhage) overlying the convexity sulci, in the interhemispheric fissure, within the basal cisterns, and overlying the tentorium.

Brain Contusion

Brain contusion usually involves the superficial brain cortex. This injury represents a bruise consisting of macerated and hemorrhagic brain tissue. The CT appearance immediately after injury is an inhomogeneous area of both high and low attenuation associated with a mass effect. The high attenuation areas represent hemorrhage, and the low attenuation areas, brain swelling. The CT appearance again varies with the time interval from injury.

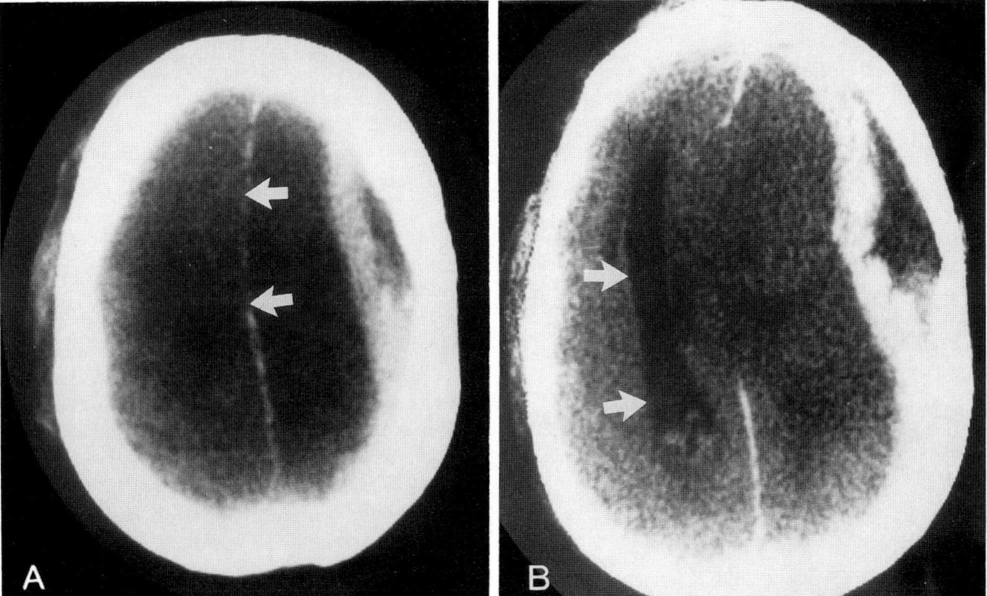

Figure 45.2. Subdural hematoma. *A*, CT scan, just below the vertex and photographed with a bone window, demonstrates a long crescent-shaped left subdural hematoma beneath the calvarium which compresses the left cerebral hemisphere and displaces it and the falx cerebri (*arrows*) to the right. *B*, A lower section also shows displacement and compression of the left hemisphere by the hematoma, with obliteration of the left lateral ventricle. Arrows point to the right lateral ventricle. (Editor's note: CT scans are always depicted with patient's right on the left of the print.)

Intracerebral Hematoma

An acute intracerebral hematoma appears as a homogeneous, somewhat round collection of increased density within the brain parenchyma, often the frontal and temporal lobes. It is generally surrounded by a zone of low attenuation representing edema and macerated tissue. The size and density of the hematoma decreases with time.

Ventricular Hemorrhage

Intraventricular hemorrhage is shown at CT as collections of increased density within the ventricular system. This diagnosis was thought to indicate a grave prognosis prior to the availability of CT, because it was made only at surgery or autopsy, or by direct ventricular tap. CT has revealed that intraventricular hemorrhage is far more common than previously appreciated and that the mortality rate is lower than previously expected. Brain swelling describes an increase in the volume of the cerebral cortex at the expense of the ventricular and subarachnoid spaces. It may result from edema or post-traumatic vascular engorgement. Generalized swelling may appear grossly normal at CT except for compression of the ventricles, cisterns, and convexity sulci. Pneumocephalus may result from open head trauma (Fig. 45.1) with a tear in the dura, or closed head trauma with fractures involving the paranasal sinuses or mastoid air cells. CT shows free air within the calvarium.

FACIAL TRAUMA

The facial bones comprise one of the most complex arrangements of curving bony surfaces in the body. This three-dimensional array is difficult to evaluate with plain films. CT's ability to display complex anatomy in a variety of imaging planes makes this modality especially suited for imaging facial injuries. Facial CT is performed quickly and easily. It may be combined with CT examinations of other injured parts. It is possible with CT to diagnose facial fractures more accurately than with plain films or conventional tomography, and to depict better the degree of fragmentation and orientation of fragments. And, importantly, the radiation dose of CT is less than for conventional tomography.

Indications

CT is not recommended as the initial screening procedure in patients with suspected facial injuries. The exception is the multiple-trauma patient who goes directly for CT after the initial evaluation, for suspected acute injuries of the head and abdomen.

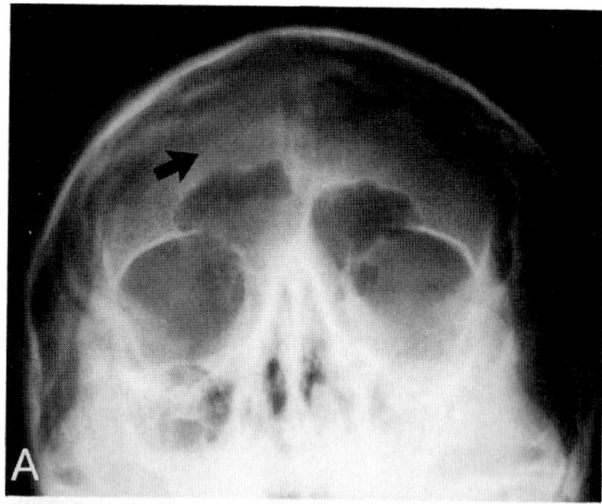

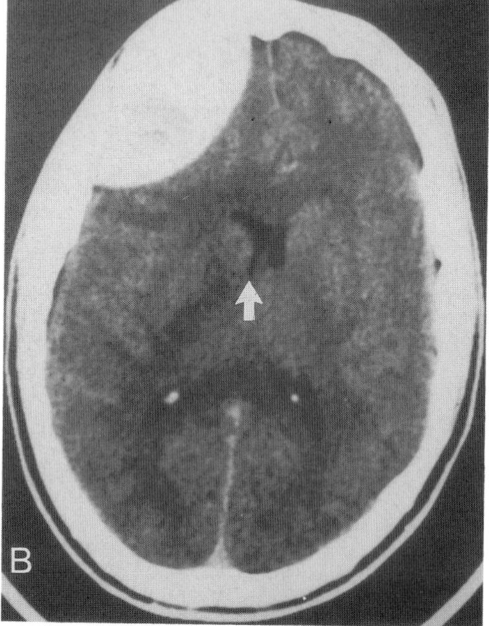

Figure 45.3. Epidural hematoma. *A*, PA upright skull film of a patient struck in the right forehead. Note the vertically oriented right frontal bone fracture (*arrow*), which runs into the right frontal sinus. An air-fluid level in the sinus indicates fresh bleeding. *B*, Axial CT scan photographed at a brain window reveals a lens-shaped epidural hematoma compressing the right frontal lobe and causing midline shift. The right lateral ventricle (*arrow*) is compressed and displaced across the midline.

In stable patients, a plain film facial series is obtained first, including upright Waters, upright Caldwell, upright lateral, and base views. If a multiple-trauma patient cannot be placed upright, the Waters and Caldwell views are taken AP with the patient supine, and the lateral film taken with a cross-table lateral technique to allow identification of sinus air-fluid levels. CT is then indicated when the plain films show complex fractures requiring further evaluation, when the plain films show only secondary signs of fracture, such as a sinus air-fluid level or orbital emphysema, or when the plain films are unremarkable but the clinical findings highly suggestive of fracture, or when soft tissue injury is suspected (Fig. 45.4).

Facial CT should be performed in two planes with the patient positioned for both direct coronal and axial sections. CT shows fractures best in planes other than the plane of section. If only axial sections are obtained, it may be possible to overlook nondisplaced fractures of structures parallel to the axial plane, such as the orbital roofs, cribriform plate, orbital floors, and hard palate. Contiguous, 5 mm-thick slices are obtained in the axial plane from above the orbital roofs through the hard palate, and in the coronal plane from the nasal bones through the sphenoid sinuses. Thinner 1.5 mm slices are indicated for areas of special interest. Axial slices are easily obtained in the multiple-trauma patient in the supine position. If the injured patient cannot be positioned for primary coronal slices that require extension of the neck, then two alternatives are possible. Either thinner and/or overlapping axial slices are obtained to allow optimal computer reformation of coronal images, or the coronal plane can be viewed with conventional tomography. Thinner axial CT slices show fractures better in the plane of section. CT images of the face are photographed with both bone and soft tissue windows to visualize optimally each of these tissues (Fig. 45.5).

The Orbit

With orbital trauma, CT delineates the extent of fracture better than other imaging techniques and depicts soft tissue injuries such as extraocular muscle entrapment and impingement, orbital hematoma, globe rupture, lens dislocation, and injuries to the optic nerve. When herniation of orbital soft tissue contents into the roof of a maxillary sinus is identified on plain films, CT may determine whether the herniated tissue contains inferior rectus muscle or only orbital fat. With fractures of the medial orbital wall, CT depicts the extent of fracture, the presence of ethmoid hematoma, and entrapment of medial rectus muscle. Coronal CT shows fractures of the orbital roofs and floors best; axial CT shows fractures of the medial and posterolateral orbital walls best. Because of its high contrast sensitivity and its ability to pinpoint objects in three dimensions, CT is the preferred technique for studying patients with suspected orbital foreign bodies.

Zygoma

When the zygoma is fractured, it is usually separated from its articulations with the maxillary,

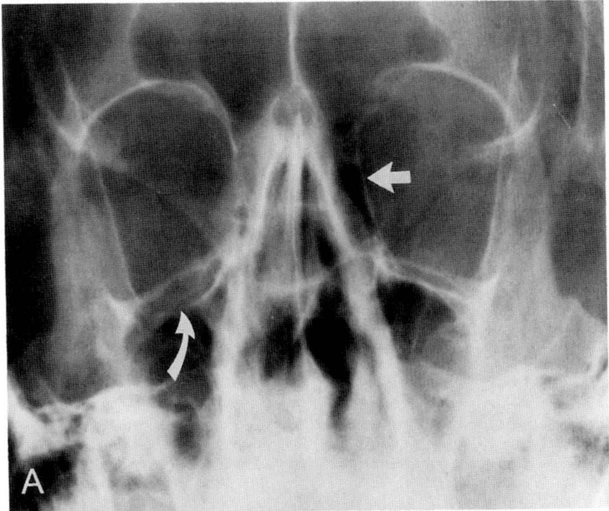

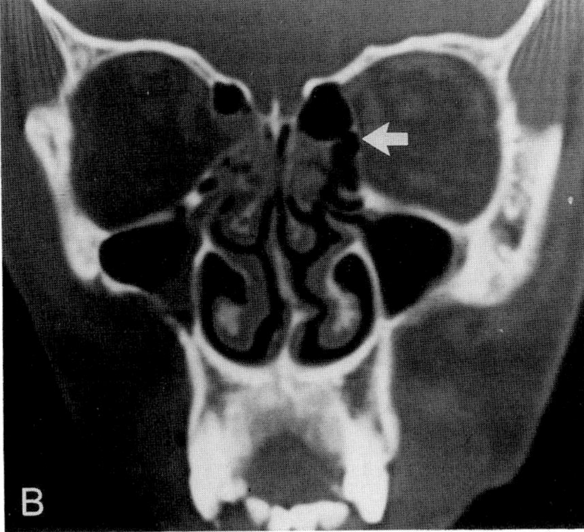

Figure 45.4. Orbital fracture. *A*, Waters' view of a patient struck in the the right eye. Loss of the right lamina papyracea (medial orbital wall) and opacification of the right ethmoid sinus are consistent with a right medial wall blowout fracture. The straight arrow points to the normal left lamina papyracea seen overyling normally aerated left ethmoid sinus. In addition, the right orbital floor (*curved arrow*) is slightly lower than the left. *B*, Coronal CT at the level of orbits, maxillary sinuses, and nasal fossa confirms a medially displaced fracture of the right lamina papyracea; the right ethmoid air cells are irregularly opacified with blood. Arrow points to the normal left lamina papyracea. CT ruled out a right orbital floor fracture; the lower position of the right orbital floor is due to slight hypoplasia of the right maxillary sinus.

frontal, and temporal bones, with varying degrees of displacement and rotation. The fractures that do occur at the articular processes of the zygoma are often comminuted. Coronal and axial CT not only depict the displacement and rotation of the body of the zygoma, but accurately delineate the degree of fragmentation and orientation of fragments of the articular process fractures. Zygomaticotemporal arch fractures, which result from blows to the sides of the face, may be difficult to demonstrate in patients who cannot be positioned for base (jug-handle) views of the face; these fractures are easily shown with CT (Fig. 45.5).

Nasal Bones

Fractures of the nasal bones are well-shown on plain films; more sophisticated imaging examinations are not usually required for diagnosis. However, the patient with severe nasal trauma may benefit from a CT examination, thus identifying associated fractures of the lateral margins of the nasal fossa (frontal processes of the maxillae), the bony nasal septum, the ethmoid sinuses, and the anterior walls of the maxillary sinuses. When a plain nasal film series shows air-fluid levels in, or opacification of, the maxillary or ethmoid sinuses, fractures of these structures should be suspected and CT then performed. Hypertelorism after trauma may indicate a nasoorbitoethmoidal fracture involving the medial orbital rims, lacrimal bones, lamina papyracea, cribriform plate, and/or orbital roofs. These complex fractures result from a severe blow to the top of the nose and are well-shown with CT.

Frontal Sinuses

Frontal sinus fractures may involve only the anterior sinus wall, or in cases of severe trauma, the posterior wall may also be fractured. In the latter

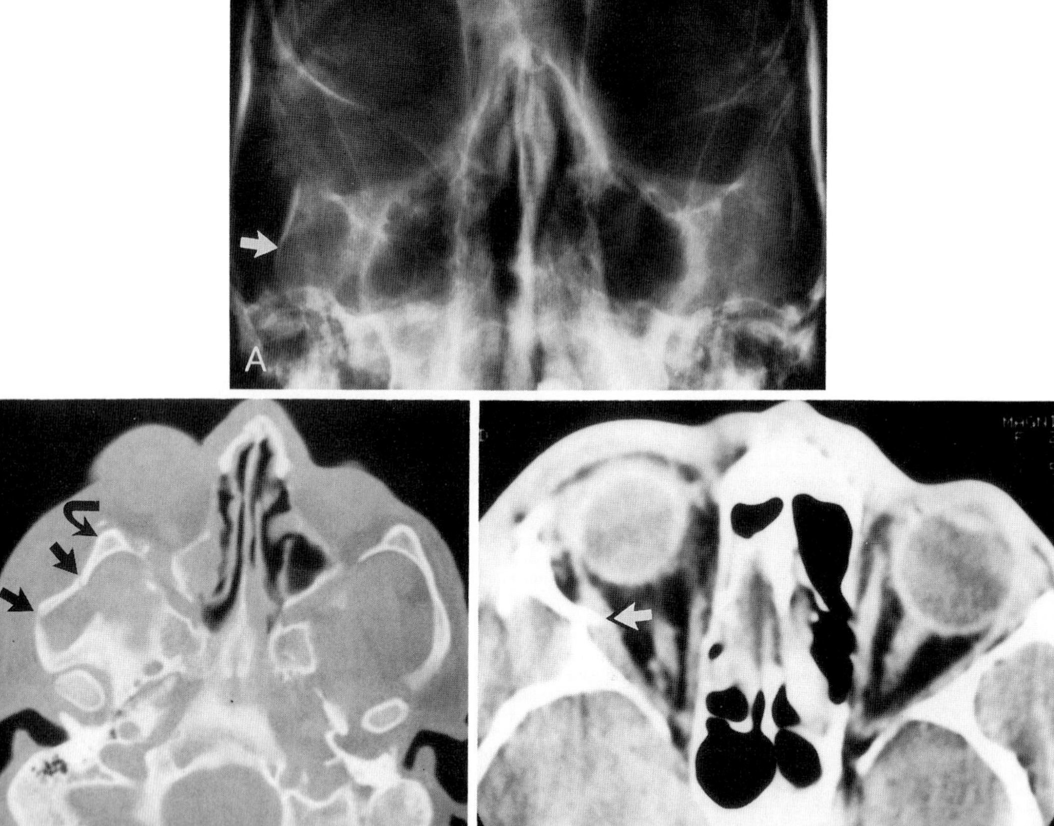

Figure 45.5. Right zygoma fracture. *A*, Waters' view shows slight medial displacement of a fractured right zygoma bone (*arrow*). Further evaluation of fracture fragments requested. *B*, Axial CT scan photographed at a bone window. The straight arrows point to two fractures of the right zygomaticotemporal arch. The mass of the right zygoma bone is displaced medially (*curved arrow*). *C*, Soft tissue window CT scan through midorbits reveal impingement of the right lateral rectus muscle by a bone fragment (*arrow*).

case, intracranial injury is especially common. Axial CT shows both sinus walls better than any other method of examination. Consequently, CT is indicated whenever the clinical or plain film findings suggest frontal sinus fracture in order not to overlook a posterior wall fracture with associated intracranial injury.

Maxilla

LeFort fractures involve the middle of the face and produce freely movable segments of bone. Three types are described (see Chapter 39). The LeFort I fracture results in a horizontal splitting of the maxillae, just above the maxillary teeth. The LeFort II fracture, referred to as the pyramidal fracture because of its shape, separates a midface segment consisting of the nose and maxillae, from the cranium and lateral aspects of the face. The LeFort III fracture separates the facial bones from the cranium. The widespread bony and soft tissue injuries occurring with all three LeFort fractures are well-delineated with CT.

Mandible

Mandible fractures are identified on plain films and/or panoramic radiography. CT is usually not needed for diagnosis. However, mandible fractures are well-shown at CT (Fig. 45.6) and should be sought in the multiple-trauma patient undergoing CT for other injuries.

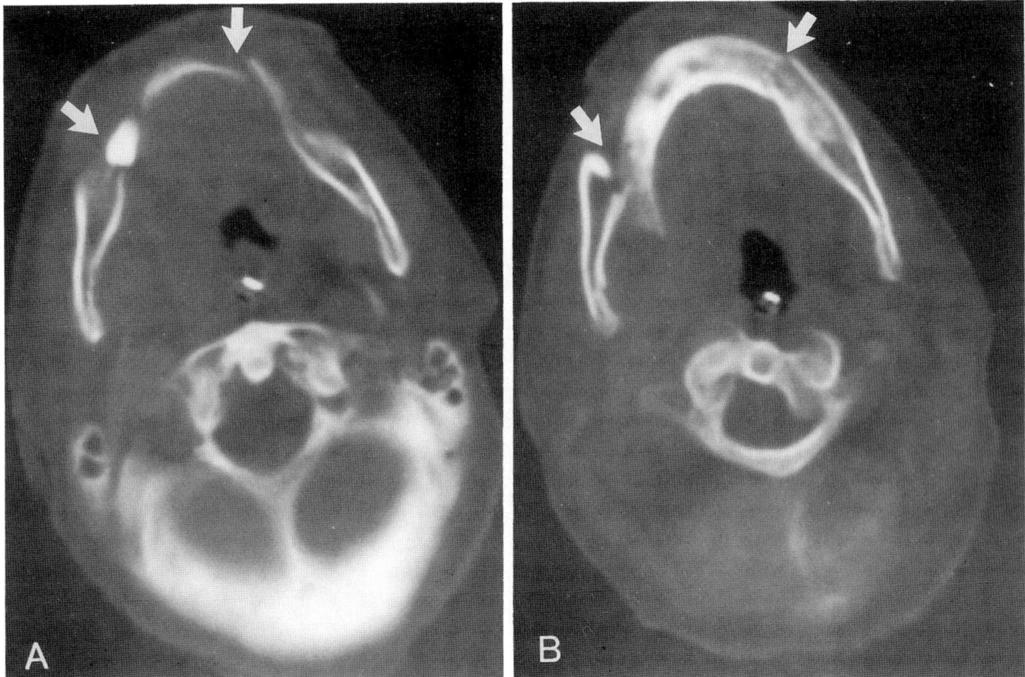

Figure 45.6. Mandible fracture. *A*, CT scan of an unconscious multiple-trauma patient shows multiple mandible fractures (*arrows*). This patient was taken to CT for a head examination; because of a clinically suspected mandible fracture, the study was extended inferiorly to include the entire face. *B*, Slightly lower section of the same patient.

SPINE TRAUMA

Indications

CT is particularly well-suited for unraveling the complex anatomy of the spine, especially after trauma. Cross-sectional, axial CT images of individual vertebrae clearly show fractures of bodies, pedicles, laminae, transverse processes, and the spinous process. Computer-reconstructed coronal and sagittal images depict the interrelationships between adjacent vertebrae to show alignment abnormalities, increased or decreased distances between vertebrae, and the status of the facet joints. CT actually depicts the degree of fragmentation, location and orientation of fragments, integrity of the bony vertebral canal, and effects of bony fragments on adjacent soft tissue structures far better than plain films or conventional tomography. Less radiation is required for CT than for conventional tomography. With soft-tissue windows and intrathecal contrast material, CT demonstrates injuries of the spinal cord and the spinal nerves, and identifies disc material and hematoma within the vertebral canal. CT images of the spine are also easier to interpret than plain films and conventional tomography. CT is particularly helpful in identifying fractures in patients with underlying chronic spine conditions, such as degenerative arthritis, or in portions of the spine, such as the seventh cervical vertebra, which are difficult to visualize.

Spine CT may be performed quickly, safely, and easily without hazardous movement or positioning of the patient. Traction may be maintained during CT examination of the spine. Unless the multiple-trauma patient is taken directly to CT for acute injuries of the head and abdomen, clinically suspicious areas of the spine are initially viewed with AP and lateral plain films. These are taken with portable units if necessary; the lateral films are taken with a cross-table technique to eliminate the turning of a patient with a potentially unstable spine fracture. All films taken during the initial evaluation of the multiple-trauma patient, including the portable skull, chest, abdomen, and pelvis films, are scrutinized for signs of spine fracture, especially in the unconscious or intoxicated patient. Plain spine films provide an overall assessment of the entire spine, or the entire length of one spine segment; the length of investigation with spine CT is more limited. In addition, subtle subluxation and increases in intervertebral distances, which may be overlooked on

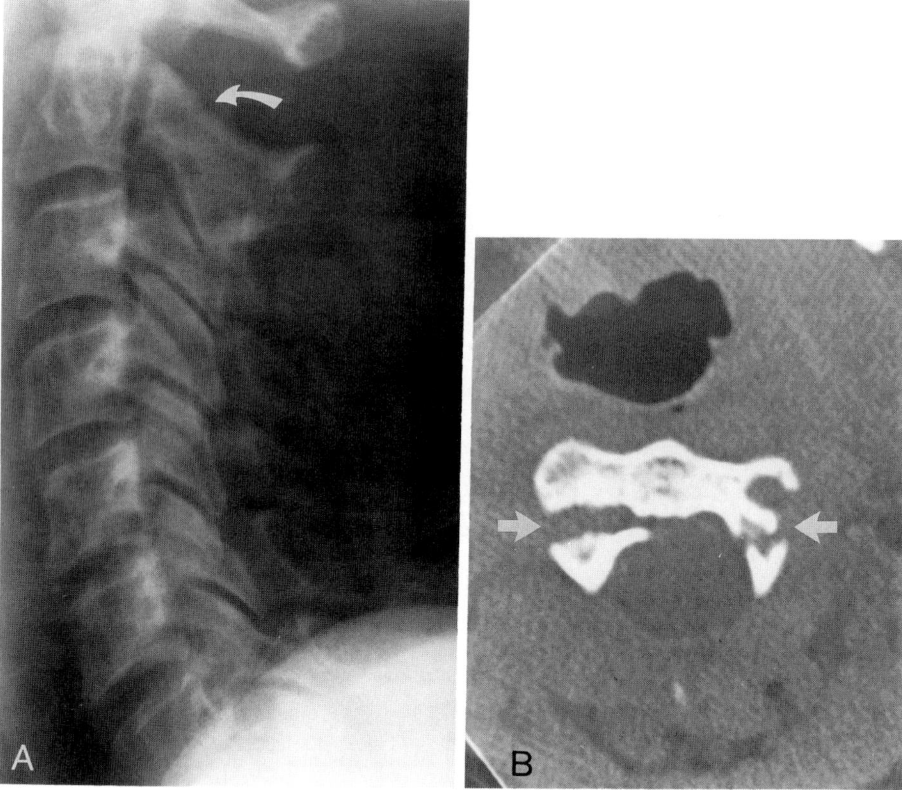

Figure 45.7. Hangman's fracture. *A*, Initial screening cross-table lateral cervical spine film was suspicious for a nondisplaced hangman's fracture. Barely perceptible is a diagonal lucency crossing the pars interarticularus of C-2 (*arrow*). *B*, Axial CT scan thorugh C-2 confirms a hangman's fracture (*arrows*).

axial CT scans, may be easily detected on plain films.

Spine CT is indicated when the plain film findings are equivocal for trauma (Fig. 45.7), when they show secondary signs of trauma such as a widened thoracic paraspinal stripe without fracture, when they show a complex fracture requiring further delineation, when neurologic findings are associated with a spine fracture (Fig. 45.8), and when there are clinical signs of a spine injury not apparent on the plain films. Slice thicknesses for spine CT should not be greater than 5 mm; overlapping slices or contiguous thinner slices (1.5 mm) are utilized if reformation is required in other planes of view. Thin slices are desirable in areas of special interest or in segments of the spine with complex anatomy, such as the craniocervical junction. One may overlook horizontal fractures in the plane of section with only thick axial slices. This is a particular problem with odontoid fractures. For evaluation of this injury, conventional tomography is preferable. CT images of the spine must be viewed at both bone and soft tissue windows; magnification algorithms may be helpful.

Cervical Spine Fractures

The cervical spine CT clearly shows the bony ring disruption of the atlas in a *Jefferson* fracture. Bilateral disruption of the pars interarticularis of the axis in *hangman's* fracture is well shown. CT is helpful in diagnosing rotational subluxation at the cervicocranial junction because the relationship of the superior articulating facets of the atlas with the occipital condyles is well shown. At all levels of the spine, CT differentiates *burst fractures* from simple compression fractures and identifies retropulsed fragments within the neural canal. *Facet dislocation* is shown at CT by a reversal in the relationship between the superior and inferior facets comprising a facet joint. Normally, the superior facets of a vertebra are anterior to the inferior facets of the vertebra above; this relationship is reversed with facet dislocation. Magnetic resonance imaging (MRI) produces a primary sagittal image of the spine, showing the vertebral canal and spinal cord in excellent detail. In stable patients, it is very helpful in the evaluation of spine trauma with associated neurologic sequelae.

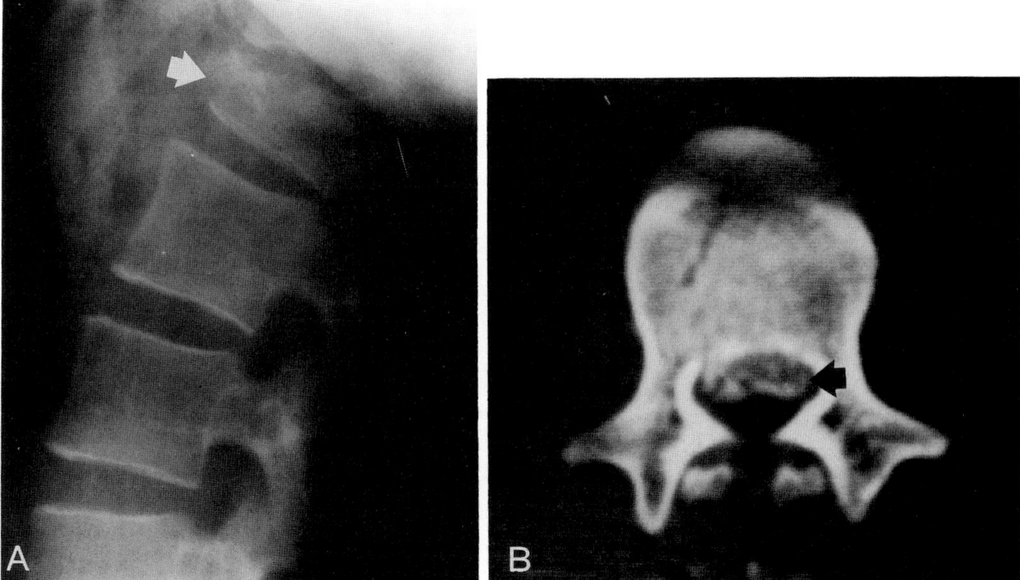

Figure 45.8. Lumbar spine burst fracture. *A*, Lateral lumbar spine film shows a compression fracture of L1 (*arrow*). Because the patient complained of perineal numbness, a CT scan was performed. Neurologic examination was normal. *B*, Axial CT scan revealed a burst fracture of L1 rather than a simple compression fracture. Note the retropulsed fragments (*arrow*) that have been displaced posteriorly into the vertebral canal.

LARYNGEAL TRAUMA

CT and laryngoscopy are complementary diagnostic procedures in the evaluation of patients with suspected laryngeal trauma. Direct laryngoscopy provides visualization of the laryngeal mucosal surfaces and detects functional impairment of the vocal cords; CT demonstrates injuries of the laryngeal cartilages and the deeper soft tissues not seen at laryngoscopy. Cross-sectional CT images of the larynx and trachea allow excellent visualization of the airway, which may be encroached upon by cartilagenous fracture fragments, hematoma, or edema. At times, marked supraglottic soft tissue swelling may preclude adequate examination by direct laryngoscopy. Consequently, CT may be utilized as the initial screening procedure to help direct the laryngoscopist in his or her examination. CT may also aid in the therapeutic decision to perform intubation or tracheotomy.

CT is indicated whenever laryngeal trauma is suspected. Preliminary plain films of the larynx are *not* required. No intravenous or oral contrast medium is required. Five mm-thick contiguous axial images are obtained from the level of the hyoid bone to the subglottic trachea. The extent of scanning may be increased, depending upon the clinical findings. CT is used in diagnosing a wide range of injuries of the trachea and larynx, although laryngoscopy is necessary to diagnose mucosal lacerations. Among the traumatic conditions easily identified at CT are soft tissue edema and hematoma, subcutaneous emphysema, cartilagenous fractures, arytenoid dislocation, and injuries to tracheal rings (Fig. 45.9).

CHEST TRAUMA

The majority of injuries resulting from chest trauma are identifiable on plain film radiographs of the chest which depict injuries of the bony structures, lungs, and pleura. The likelihood of mediastinal injury may be implied by findings on the plain film, mediastinal widening or pneumomediastinum. CT is helpful in chest trauma in resolving confusing or ambiguous findings on plain films. However, CT may also reveal additional findings important to patient management, not shown on the plain films. Toombs has reported a series of 20 thoracic trauma patients studied with both CT and plain films. The CT scans showed 50 traumatic lesions, only 12 of which could be identified on the plain films. These diagnoses included pleural fluid collection, pneumothorax, extrapleural hematoma, atelectasis, pulmonary consolidation or laceration, mediastinal hematoma, pericardial effusion, pneumomediastinum, and diaphragmatic rupture. Four instances of pneumothorax not seen on chest films

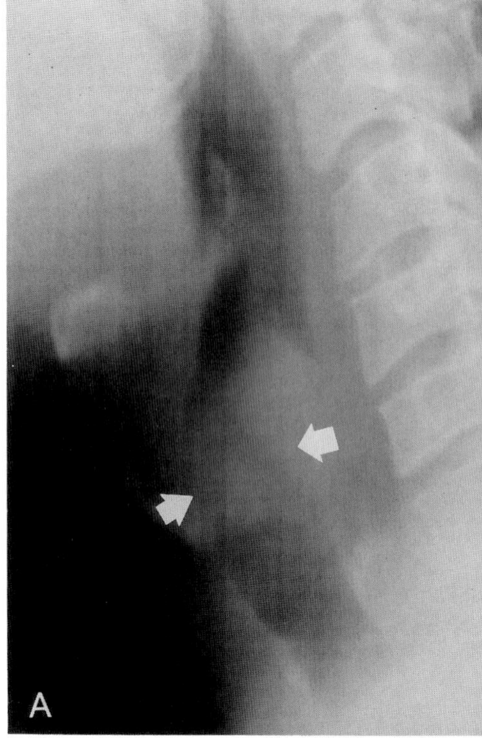

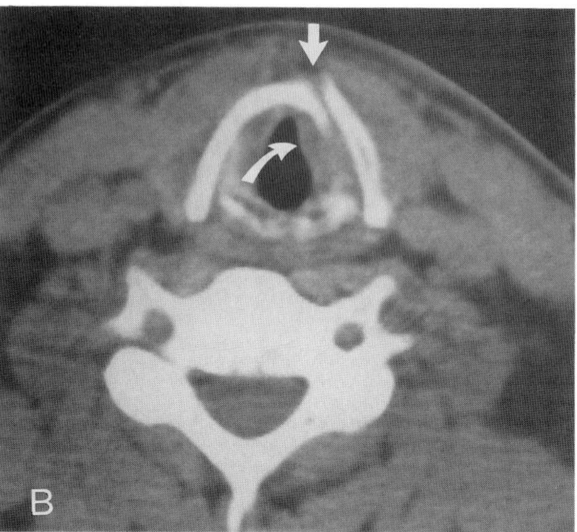

Figure 45.9. Fracture of the larynx. *A*, Lateral cervical spine film of a patient injured while driving; the steering wheel struck the anterior neck. The patient complained of laryngeal pain and hoarseness. Lateral spine film shows swelling of the laryngeal soft tissues (*arrows*) with absence of a normal horizontal lucency of air within the laryngeal ventricle. *B*, CT scan at the level of the vocal cords shows a fracture of the left anterior thyroid cartilage (*straight arrow*) and edema of the left vocal cord (*curved arrow*).

were seen on CT (Fig. 45.10). Many of these CT findings required no treatment. Consequently, CT is also recommended when the clinical findings suggest trauma not apparent on the chest films. Other authors have reported the benefits of CT in diagnosing unsuspected pneumothoraces, esophageal perforation, and diaphragmatic rupture. CT has been helpful in identifying unsuspected fractures of the bony thorax, not apparent on the initial chest film, and also fractures difficult to assess with plain films alone (Fig. 45.11).

ABDOMINAL TRAUMA

CT has improved the diagnostic workup of both adults and children with blunt abdominal trauma.

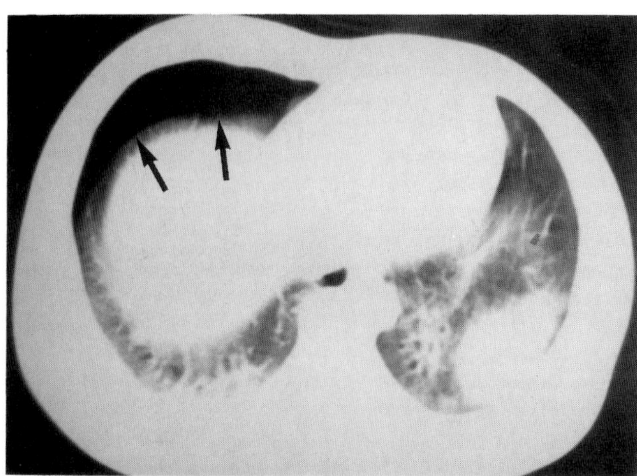

Figure 45.10. Unsuspected pneumothorax. Lung window CT scan of the lower chest of an abdominal trauma patient. Note the right pneumothorax (*black arrows*), which was not suspected clinically and could not be identified even retrospectively on the admission AP supine chest film. This scan also shows evidence of a left lower lobe contusion.

In a quickly performed, single examination, CT accurately identifies hemoperitoneum, and injuries of the liver, spleen, pancreas, mesentery, kidneys, retroperitoneum, and abdominal wall. When emergency CT is available, those patients requiring emergency surgery may be quickly identified, and the extent of their injuries more accurately assessed. Those patients whose injuries can be treated conservatively, on the other hand, may be spared an unnecessary laparotomy.

CT is indicated when any abdominal injury is clinically suspected after blunt trauma. Patients who are too hemodynamically unstable to tolerate a 30-minute abdominal CT scan should be examined with peritoneal lavage and/or proceed directly to surgery. In the stable patient, CT should always be performed prior to peritoneal lavage, if peritoneal lavage is to be performed at all. In some trauma centers, emergency CT has replaced peritoneal lavage. Even in patients with penetrating abdominal injuries, a CT scan prior to surgery may prove helpful in pinpointing the location and extent of injuries. Two distinct advantages of CT over peritoneal lavage are its capability to evaluate the retroperitoneum and to diagnose intracapsular parenchymal organ injuries that occur without hemoperitoneum.

The following CT techniques are usually followed for patients with abdominal trauma. One-cm thick contiguous scans are taken from the dome of the diaphragm to the bottom of the kidneys, in order

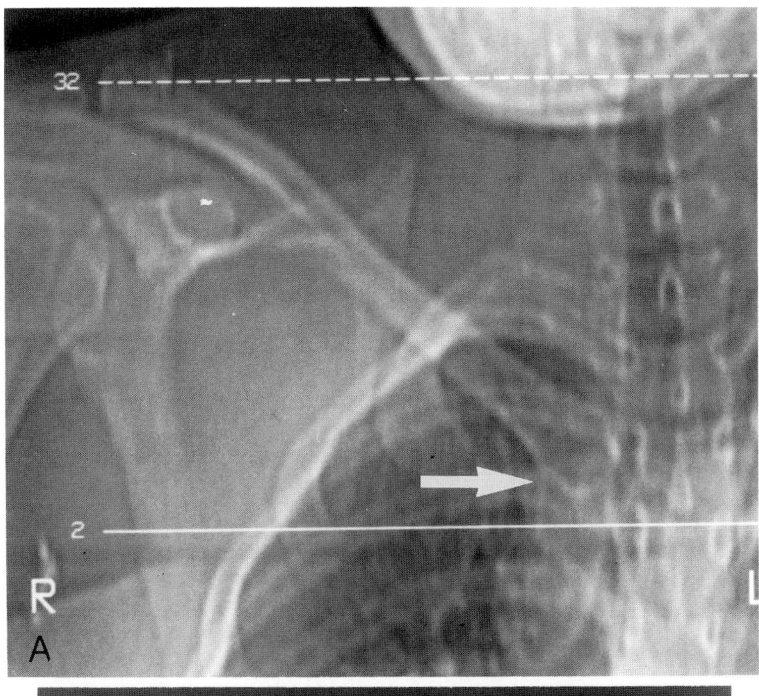

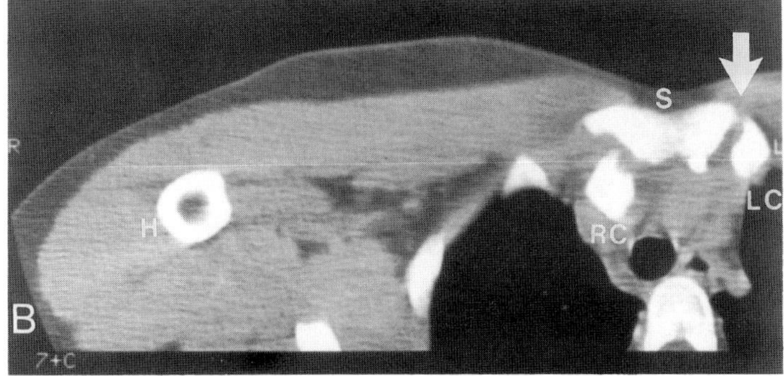

Figure 45.11. Sternoclavicular dislocation. *A*, CT scout view shows slight inferior position of medial head of right clavicle (*arrow*). *B*, CT shows posterior dislocation of the right clavicle head compared with the left. Arrow points to the normal left sternoclavicular joint. *H*—humerus; *S*—sternum; *RC*—right clavicle; *LC*—left clavicle.

not to overlook small lacerations of the liver, spleen, pancreas, and kidneys. Scans through the remainder of the abdomen and pelvis are obtained at 2-cm intervals. Intravenous contrast material is given immediately prior to scanning for improved visualization of injuries of the parenchymal organs, blood vessels, and urinary tract. The differentiation of laceration and hematoma from normal organ parenchyma is accentuated after intravenous (i.v.) contrast material. Consequently, if a multiple-trauma patient requires both head and abdominal CT exams, the head study, done without i.v. contrast medium, should be performed first. Very dilute oral contrast material is also administered prior to abdominal CT scanning, often by nasogastric tube injection, in order that fluid-filled loops of normal bowel may be opacified and differentiated from hemoperitoneum or organ hematomas. Any volume of oral contrast material remaining in the stomach may be removed by nasogastric tube aspiration prior to institution of general anesthesia. To diminish artifacts, the nasogastric tube is pulled back to the level of midesophagus, and lines and monitor leads overlying the abdomen are moved prior to scanning. The shortest scan times are used to minimize motion artifact. In addition to routine soft tissue windows, bone windows are viewed to rule out fractures, and lung windows of the upper abdomen are viewed to exclude unsuspected pneumothorax or free subphrenic air.

CT not only accurately diagnoses hemoperitoneum, but estimates the volume of bleeding. In addition, the location of small hemorrhages can be identified; this may be helpful because early collections of blood are often found adjacent to sites of organ injury. Free hemoperitoneum is usually seen as fluid in the subphrenic space, in Morison's pouch between the liver and right kidney, in the paracolic gutters, and in the pelvis (Fig. 45.12). Although this distribution is similar to that of nontraumatic ascites, it may be possible to differentiate acute hemorrhage from ascites by the higher CT density coefficient of blood. This CT differentiation may not be possible after peritoneal lavage. The appearance of blood in the abdomen depends on the CT technical settings. In comparison with head CT, intraabdominal hemorrhage may appear less white than adjacent organ parenchyma, especially following opacification with intravenous contrast material.

Spleen

The most commonly injured abdominal organ following blunt abdominal trauma is the spleen. CT is a highly sensitive procedure for detecting splenic trauma, and just as importantly, a normal CT scan is very accurate in excluding splenic injury. Federle has reported a series of 55 surgically proved splenic injuries examined preoperatively with CT; in 54 cases, splenic trauma was correctly diagnosed. Out of 1500 CT scans performed for suspected abdominal trauma, there were three false-positive diagnoses of splenic trauma. The common CT findings with splenic trauma are hemoperitoneum, perisplenic clot, splenic laceration, and subcapsular hematoma. Hematomas within splenic lacerations (Fig. 45.12) appear as linear or mottled, irregular regions of lower density than the contrast-enhanced adjacent splenic tissue. A subcapsular hematoma of the spleen appears as a crescentic fluid collection immediately beneath the capsule, effacing the lateral or medial margins of the splenic parenchyma (Fig. 45.13). The finding of a normal spleen at CT without evidence of hemoperitoneum provides reassurance that a significant injury is not being overlooked. In addition to greater anatomic resolution and higher accuracy, CT is preferred to radionuclide spleen scanning, splenic angiography, and splenic ultrasonography because other abdominal and retroperitoneal structures may be viewed during the same examination.

Liver

Lacerations and hematomas of the liver are not only important diagnoses, but an estimation of their extent is paramount in planning appropriate treatment. Because minor liver injuries, such as small parenchymal lacerations with absence of hemoperitoneum, may be managed nonoperatively, less severely injured patients are saved an unnecessary laparotomy. The presence and size of hepatic parenchymal lacerations and the amount of bleeding into the peritoneal cavity may be accurately identified by CT. Lacerations account for the majority of liver injuries following blunt trauma. They tend to appear as linear, round, or branching areas of different CT density, most often of lower density than the surrounding contrast-enhanced liver tissue. Not infrequently, they have a stellate configuration (Fig. 45.14). As with splenic injury, a subcapsular liver hematoma appears as a crescentic or ovoid fluid collection immediately beneath the liver capsule (Fig. 45.15). Isolated subcapsular hematomas are infrequent results of blunt trauma; more commonly, they are seen after penetrating trauma or interventional procedures, such as liver biopsies.

Pancreas

Trauma to the pancreas is difficult to diagnose, even with CT, but is fortunately quite uncommon with blunt abdominal trauma. Hematomas within pancreatic lacerations present a particular problem, appearing very similar to normal pancreatic parenchyma. In a series of 13 surgically proved pancreatic injuries reported by Jeffrey, CT correctly

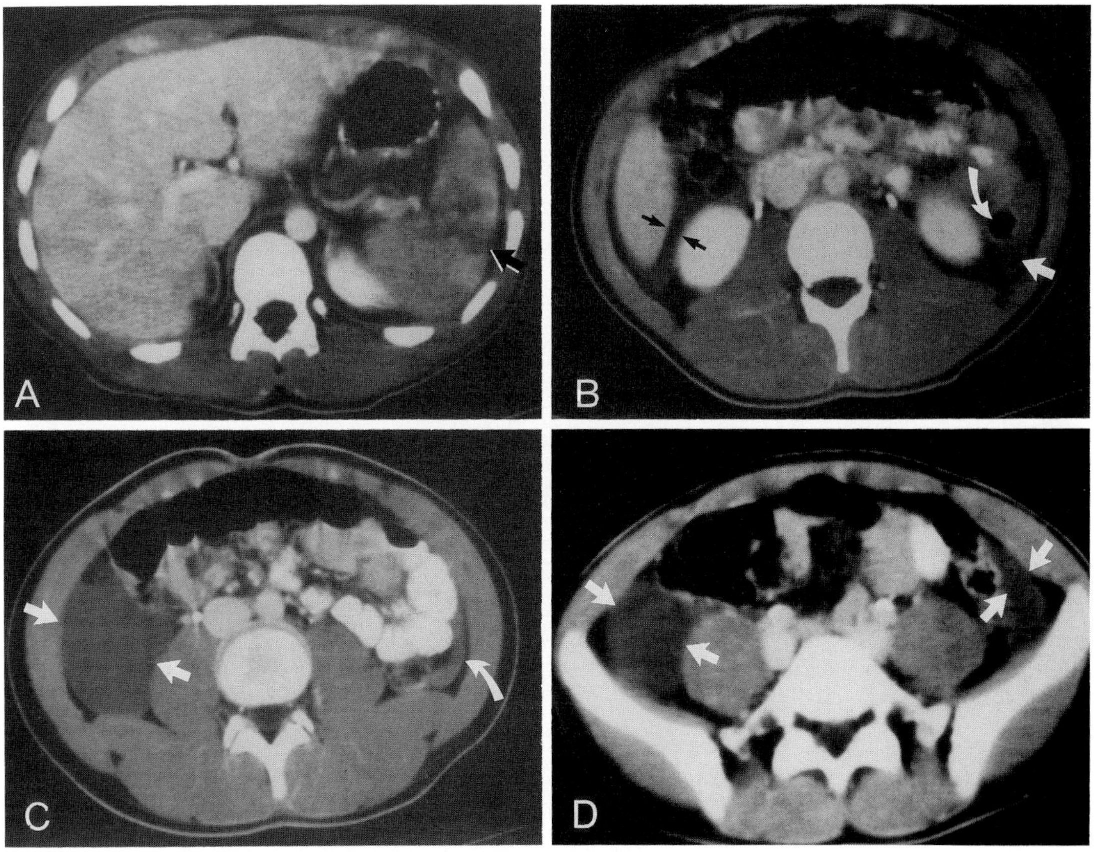

Figure 45.12. Spleen fracture with hemoperitoneum. *A*, CT scan through the liver and at midspleen shows a splenic fracture (*arrow*). *B*, Scan at the level of kidneys and inferior portion of right liver lobe reveals hemoperitoneum. Note the blood in Morison's pouch (*black arrows*) and blood in the left paracolic gutter (*straight white arrow*) lateral to the descending colon (*curved white arrow*). *C*, Scan below the kidneys shows a larger volume of blood in the right paracolic gutter (*straight arrows*) than the left (*curved arrow*). *D*, Scan at the iliac wings shows hemoperitoneum in both paracolic gutters (*arrows*).

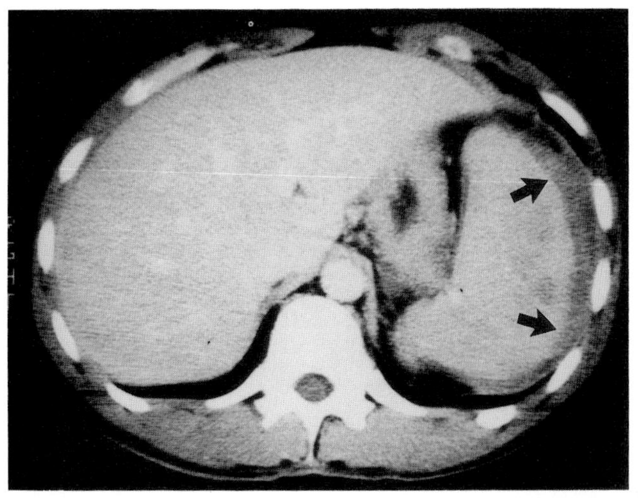

Figure 45.13. Subcapsular hematoma of the spleen. The arrows indicate a low attenuation, semilunar-shaped collection of blood overlying the splenic parenchyma, but beneath its capsule, consistent with a subcapsular hematoma. Small low-density hematomas can be seen within the spleen itself.

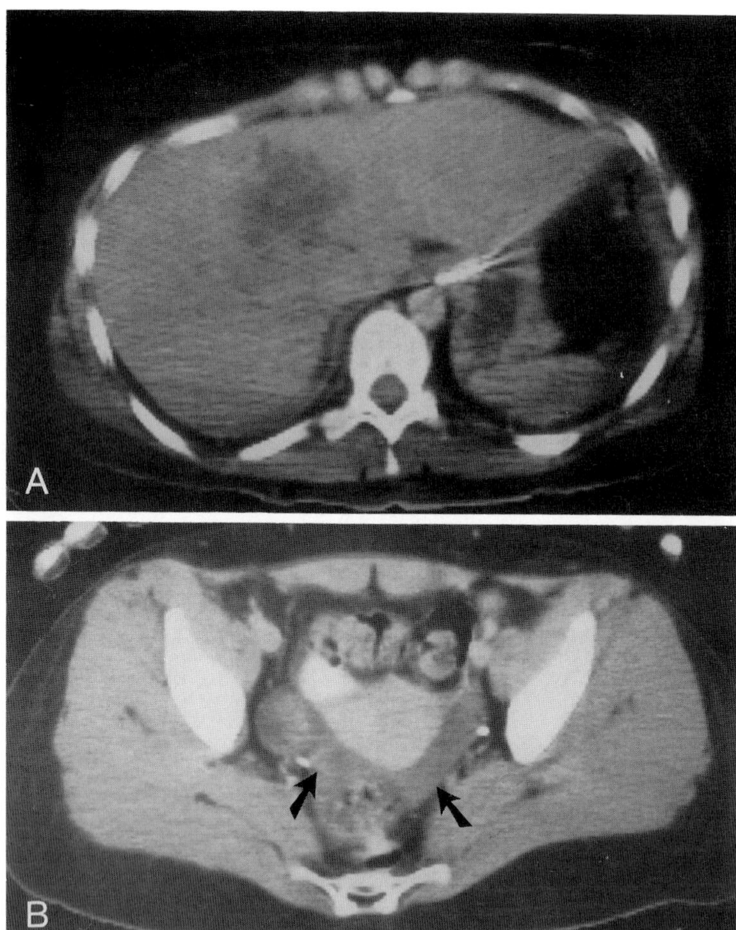

Figure 45.14. Liver laceration with hemoperitoneum. *A*, CT scan taken through the liver shows a stellate, low-density area within the liver consistent with an intrahepatic laceration and hematoma. *B*, CT scan through the pelvis of the same patient reveals free blood (*arrows*) posterior to the bladder and anterior to the rectum—evidence that the liver laceration was bleeding into the peritoneal cavity.

Figure 45.15. Subcapsular hepatic hematoma. The ovoid low-density area at the lateral margin of the right liver lobe represents a subcapsular hematoma; it resulted from a liver biopsy.

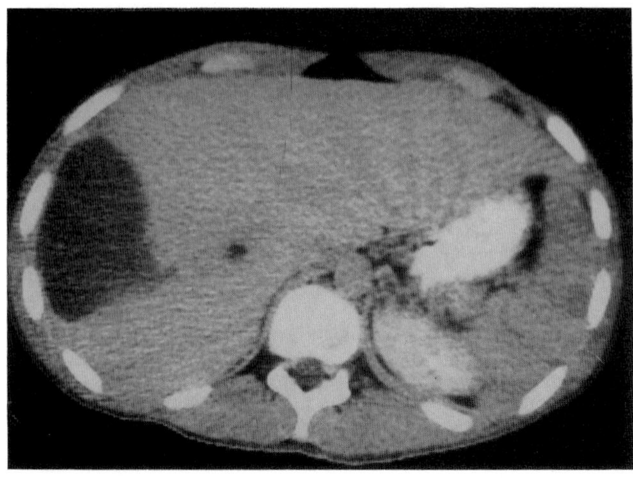

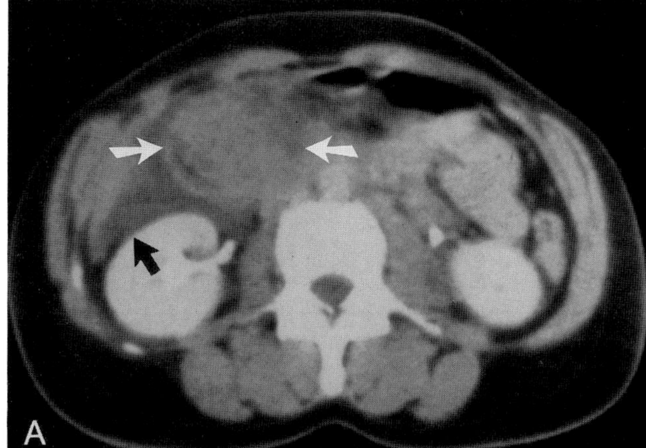

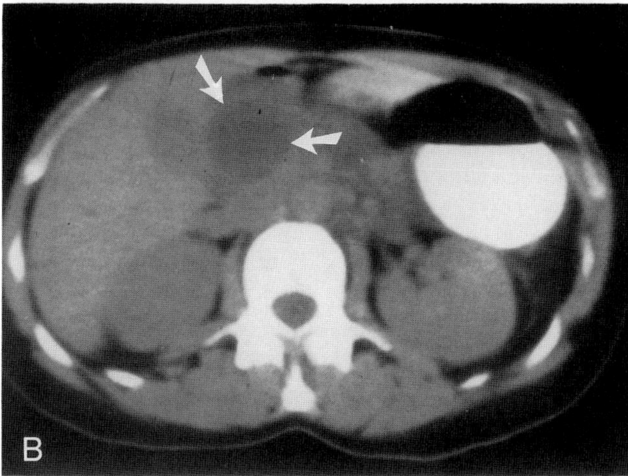

Figure 45.16. Pancreatic trauma. *A*, Initial CT scan with intravenous contrast medium shows a hematoma (*white arrows*) in the pancreatic head. Hemorrhage is seen anterior to the right kidney (*black arrow*), within the anterior retroperitoneum (*anterior pararenal space*). The patient responded to conservative therapy. *B*, A follow-up scan 1 month later, with oral but no intravenous contrast, shows a pseudocyst (*white arrows*) in the areas of the pancreatic injury.

diagnosed the injury in 11; in the two false-*negative* cases, pancreatic fractures were found at surgery. In addition, there were two false-*positive* diagnoses of pancreatic trauma in their series of 300 CT scans on patients with abdominal trauma. When positive, CT may demonstrate pancreatic lacerations, contusions, hemorrhages, or pseudocysts (Fig. 45.16). Other abdominal viscera are frequently injured with trauma to the pancreas.

Mesentery

CT has proved helpful in diagnosing mesenteric hematomas, although less so in bowel wall injuries except when a major hematoma is present. Large hematomas of the small bowel mesentery or transverse mesocolon are readily apparent at CT as high-density collections of blood within these structures (Fig. 45.17).

Intestine

An intramural hematoma of the bowel itself appears as a mass or thickening of the wall (Fig. 45.18); this may be easy or difficult to identify, depending upon the location of the injury. Most difficult in CT diagnosis are bowel lacerations or transections. Free peritoneal air may be the only sign. In the case of duodenal rupture, retroperitoneal or paraduodenal air and fluid may be present.

Urinary Tract

CT is superior to the intravenous pyelogram (IVP) in the detection of renal injuries. It may be performed after an abnormal urogram for better detail of an injury, or may be performed instead of the urogram in instances when other abdominal injuries are also suspected. With CT it is possible to differentiate major injuries of the kidney and renal pedicle requiring immediate surgery (Fig. 45.19), from minor cortical lacerations that may be treated conservatively (Fig. 45.20). Renal hematomas and lacerations appear on CT as low-density areas within the contrast-enhanced kidney. Hemorrhage around the kidney appears as a high-density fluid collection in the perirenal space. Extravasation of contrast-en-

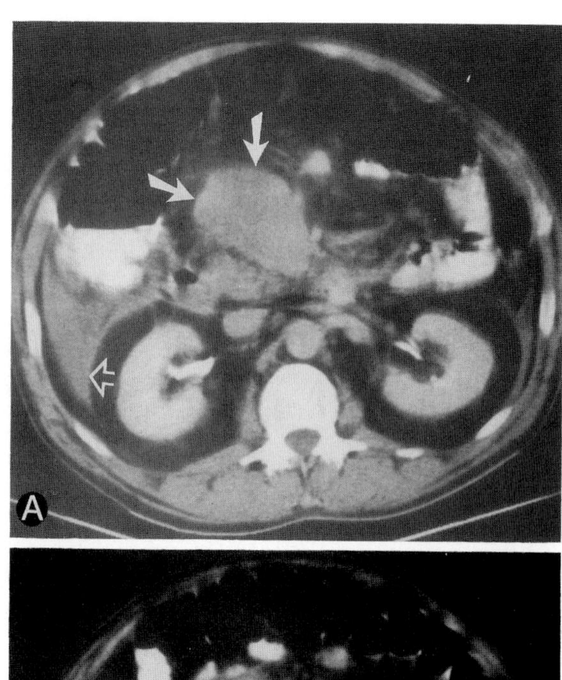

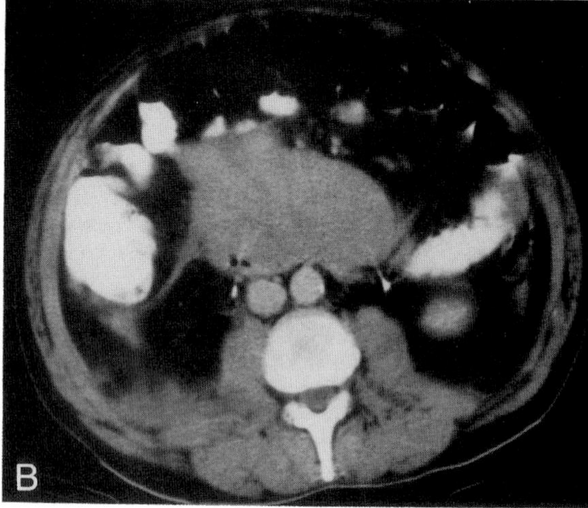

Figure 45.17. Mesenteric hematoma. *A*, CT scan at the midkidney level shows a hematoma in the root of the mesentery (*solid white arrows*) with free blood (*open arrow*) in the right paracolic gutter. A small amount of blood is seen in the left paracolic gutter. The patient was injured in an automobile accident when his abdomen struck the steering wheel. *B*, A lower scan shows the maximum diameter of the mesenteric hematoma. It required surgical drainage.

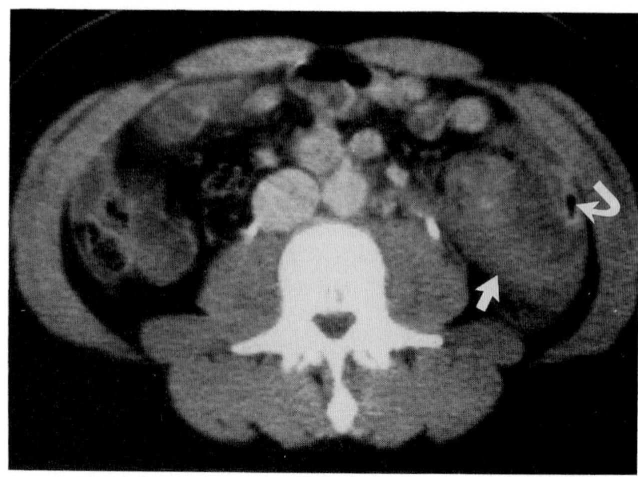

Figure 45.18. Colonic intramural hematoma. This young man suffered an injury to the left flank when he fell over a railing. The curved arrow points to the lumen of descending colon. The straight arrow indicates a hematoma within the wall of descending colon. He was managed conservatively and did well.

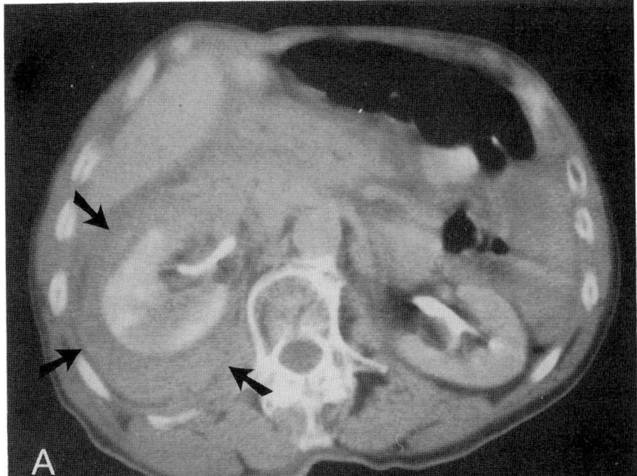

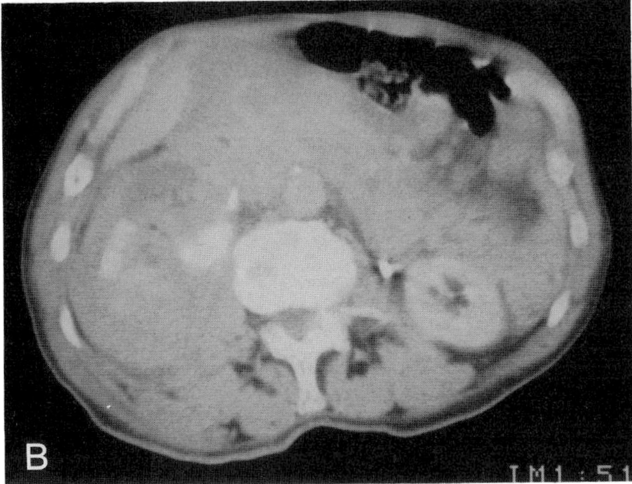

Figure 45.19. Major renal trauma requiring surgical management. *A*, CT scan through midkidneys shows a large perirenal hematoma (*arrows*) surrounding the right kidney, displacing it anteriorly. The low-density (*dark gray*) area diagonally across the renal parenchyma represents a fracture plane. *B*, CT scan taken through the lower pole of right kidney reveals that the pole was fractured. A large perirenal hematoma is again seen.

hanced urine from the kidneys, ureters, or bladder is easily identified at CT (Fig. 45.21). Renal pedicle injuries are detected at CT by absence of contrast opacification of the injured kidney; this is an indication for an emergency angiographic examination for detailed evaluation of the specific vascular injury. Often, unsuspected renal trauma is identified on CT in patients examined for injuries of other abdominal viscera.

Parietal Injury

Retroperitoneal and *abdominal wall* hemorrhage may result from blunt or penetrating trauma. Hematomas in both locations are demonstrable by CT; their identification is helpful in interpreting clinical findings and blood replacement requirements of the patient when hemoperitoneum and abdominal parenchymal organ injury have been excluded (Fig. 45.22). In the retroperitoneum, CT may show the hematoma itself by diminution of normal retroperitoneal fat planes or by diffuse enlargement of the iliopsoas muscle. Aortic injuries after penetrating trauma are usually associated with retroperitoneal hemorrhage.

PELVIC TRAUMA

CT is a superb modality for depicting the complex arrangement of the curving bony surfaces of the pelvis. Consequently, CT has become the popular technique for evaluating pelvic fractures that are difficult to characterize completely on two-dimensional plain film images. Pelvic fractures have been traditionally examined with oblique and special plain film views, which are not only inferior to CT, but require potentially hazardous rotation of the patient. With CT, once the patient has been placed on the CT couch, no other manipulation is required. In addition, CT is faster than conventional pelvic tomography with less radiation exposure. Soft

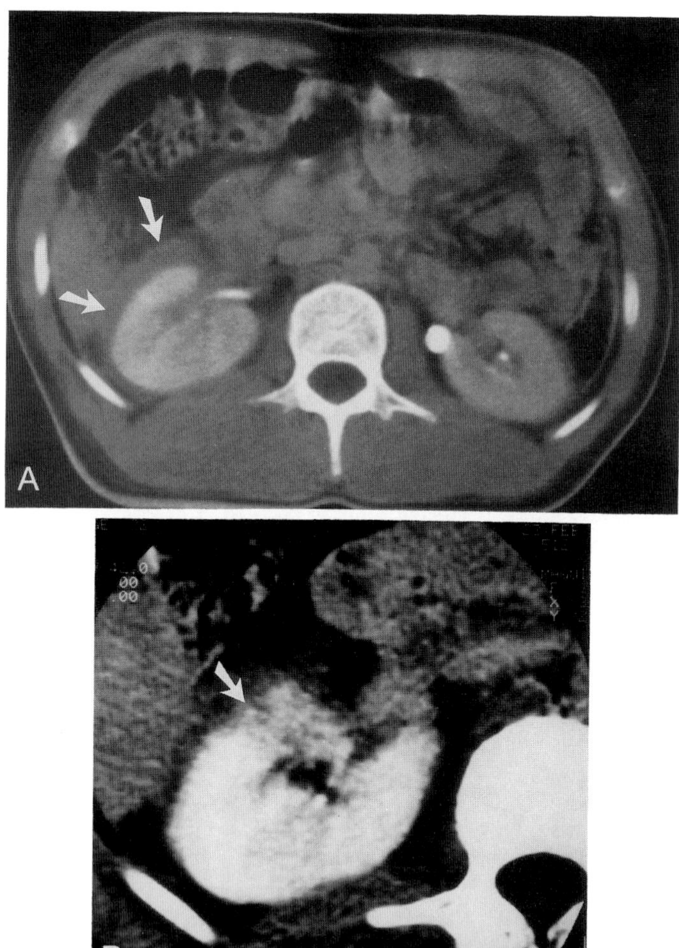

Figure 45.20. Minor renal trauma treated conservatively. *A*, Contrast-enhanced CT scan through the mid-kidneys shows a small right perirenal hematoma (*arrows*). *B*, Magnification view of the right kidney identifies the small cortical laceration (*arrow*) responsible for the hematoma. No surgery was required.

tissue CT images may identify pelvic soft tissue injuries, not apparent on plain films or conventional tomography. Computed reformation of axial images allows accurate depiction of complex acetabular and hip fractures in both coronal and sagittal planes.

With suspected pelvic trauma, an AP plain film of the pelvis is obtained first. In the unconscious multiple-trauma patient, it is prudent to obtain a screening AP pelvic film in every case. If CT is available, there is no need to risk additional injury by turning a patient with an unstable fracture for oblique plain film views, although inlet and outlet plain views may be useful, requiring only tilting of the x-ray tube. Pelvic CT is indicated for better assessment of complex pelvic and acetabular fractures, when the plain film findings are suspicious for fracture but not definitive, when the complaints or clinical findings are suspicious for fracture but none seen on the plain films, or when pelvic soft tissue injuries are clinically suspected. In many hospitals, all pelvic and acetabular fractures are examined with CT.

In the multiple-trauma patient, pelvic CT may be performed either as a part of abdominal CT or as a separate examination. The pelvis is always included as part of a routine abdominal CT examination for trauma, although when pelvic trauma is also suspected, contiguous and thinner CT sections may be indicated, particularly for the acetabulum. When only pelvic CT is necessary, the following technique is recommended. Contiguous 10 mm-thick scans are taken from the top of the iliac wings to the inferior aspect of the ischial rami. If acetabular fractures are seen on these scans, on the initial plain

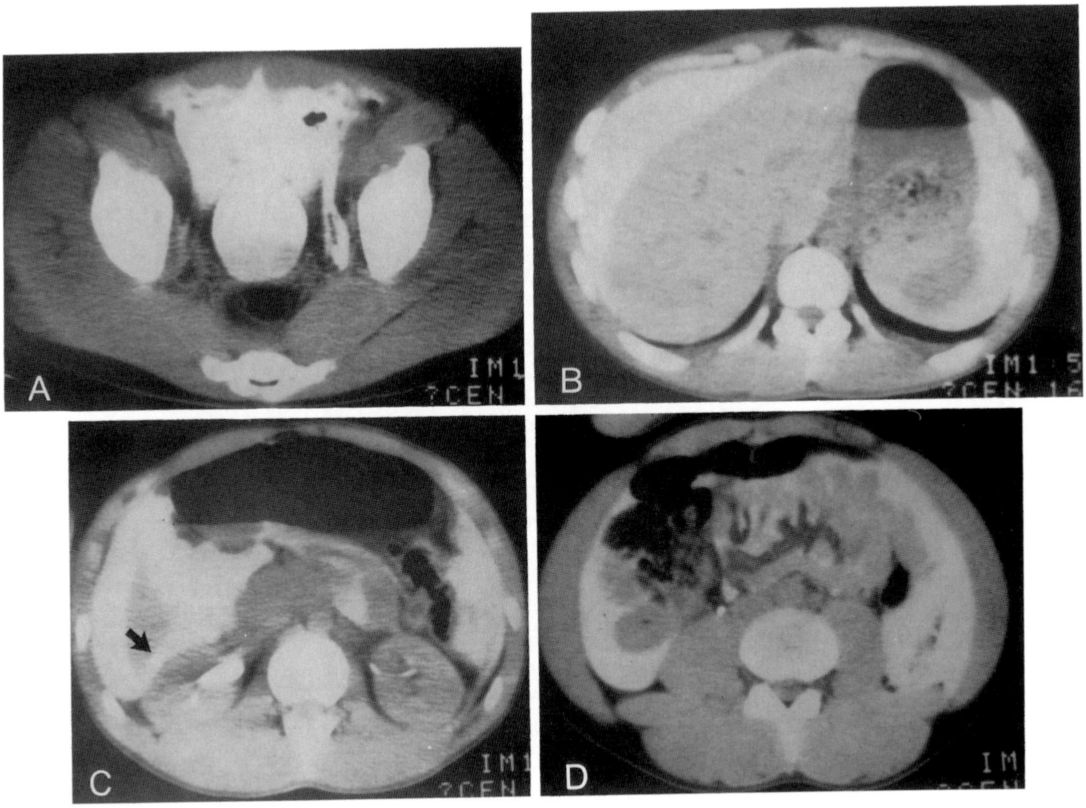

Figure 45.21. Bladder rupture into the peritoneal cavity. *A*, CT scan through the pelvis shows an anterior rupture of the bladder with extravasation of intravenous contrast medium into the pelvic soft tissues and peritoneal cavity. *B*, Scan at the level of the liver and spleen shows contrast-enhanced urine high within the peritoneal cavity. *C*, Scan through the midkidneys shows contrast-enhanced urine within Morison's pouch (*arrow*). *D*, Scan just below the kidneys shows contrast-enhanced fluid within both paracolic gutters.

films, or suspected clinically, then thinner overlapping 5 mm- or contiguous 1.5 mm-thick sections of the acetabular area are also obtained. These allow computed reformation of acetabular images into coronal and sagittal planes. No contrast material is necessary if evaluation of only bony structures is

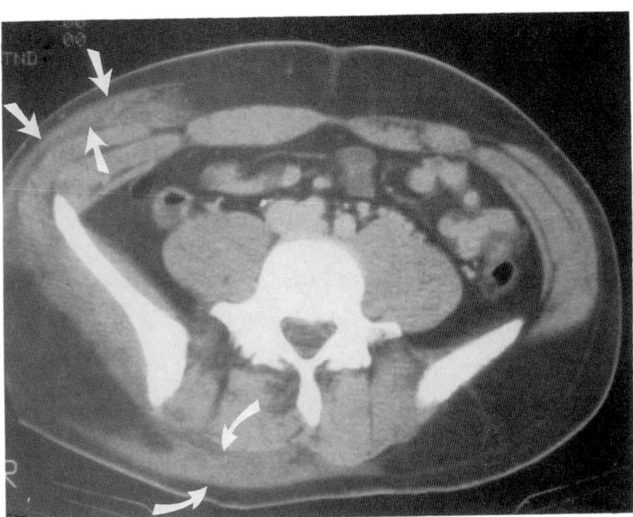

Figure 45.22. Abdominal wall hematoma. CT scan at the top of the pelvis shows hematoma within the right abdominal wall, just outside the external oblique muscle (*straight arrows*) and posterior to the spinal muscles (*curved arrows*). The patient was injured in a motorcycle accident, complained of right flank pain, and right flank hematoma was noted on clinical examination. No peritoneal or retroperitoneal organ injuries were seen at CT. The abdominal wall hematoma explained the patient's clinical findings.

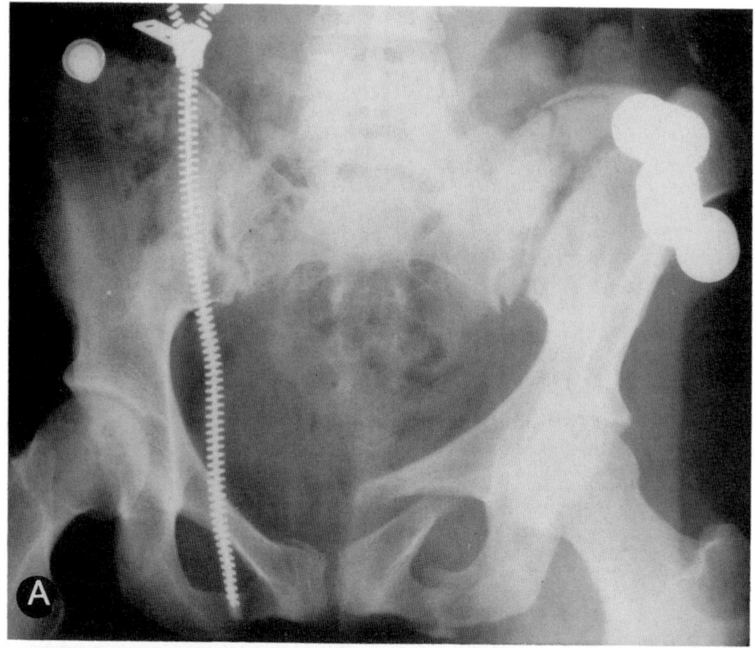

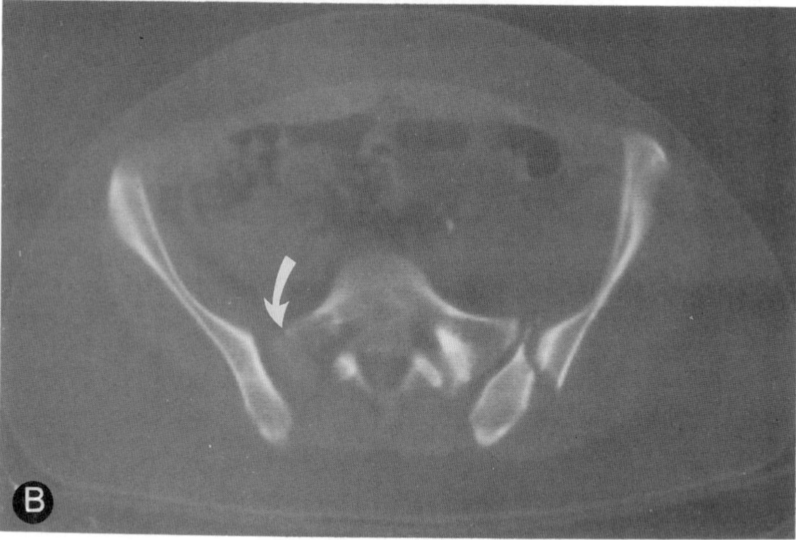

Figure 45.23. Pelvic trauma. *A*, The initial plain pelvic film shows a comminuted fracture of the left iliac wing with disruption of the left sacroiliac joint, plus fractures of the superior and inferior pubic rami. *B*, CT also demonstrates an unsuspected fracture of the right sacral wing (*arrow*).

required. If bladder or ureteral injuries are suspected, then intravenous contrast material is recommended. Rectal contrast medium aids in the diagnosis of distal bowel and/or rectal injuries.

CT differentiates stable from unstable pelvic fractures better than plain films. Stable fractures are those that do not disrupt the pelvic ring and or break it in only one place. Unstable fractures break the pelvic ring in two or more places (Fig. 45.23). Frequently, the AP plain film is difficult to evaluate in the trauma patient because of lucencies and densities overlying the pelvic bones caused by air and feces in the bowel, by fat planes, by air in superficial injuries, and by clothing and bandage artifacts. These are not problems with CT. Fractures of the sacrum are more accurately diagnosed and evaluated with CT than with plain films. Isolated fractures and fracture-dislocations of the hip and acetabulum are common in automobile accidents in which the knee strikes the dashboard, causing a posterior hip dislocation with fracture of the posterior column of the acetabulum. These injuries are accurately shown with CT (Fig. 45.24). In fact, CT depicts fractures of the anterior and posterior acetabular columns, the acetabular roofs, and the quadrilateral surface better than any other imaging examination. CT may also identify the presence of loose bodies in the hip joint space and infarctions of the femoral head. Consequently, CT is the procedure of choice for assessing acetabular fractures.

EXTREMITY TRAUMA

CT has proved helpful in evaluating a variety of extremity injuries. Thin-section multiplanar CT images produced with bone algorithms display beautifully the elaborate three-dimensional anatomy of curving bony surfaces and articulations difficult to visualize with plain films or conventional tomography. With complex fractures and fracture dislocations of the shoulder girdle, wrist, hand, knee, and foot, CT shows the degree of fragmentation, follows the course of fracture lines, and displays the distribution and orientation of fracture fragments with excellent detail. In addition, the adjacent soft tissue structures are visualized.

Conventional plain film series should be obtained first with suspected extremity trauma. CT is indicated when complex fractures identified on plain films require further radiologic evaluation or when fractures involve structures with complex anatomy. CT techniques for extremity injuries are custom-tailored to image optimally the area of interest. Comminuted fractures of the calcaneus, talus, and scapula are especially well-delineated with CT. In the hand and foot, CT has been helpful in distinguishing avulsion fractures from accessory ossicles, or congenital/developmental variations of the carpal and tarsal bones (Fig. 45.25).

With calcaneal fractures, CT provides information about the size and number of fragments, the

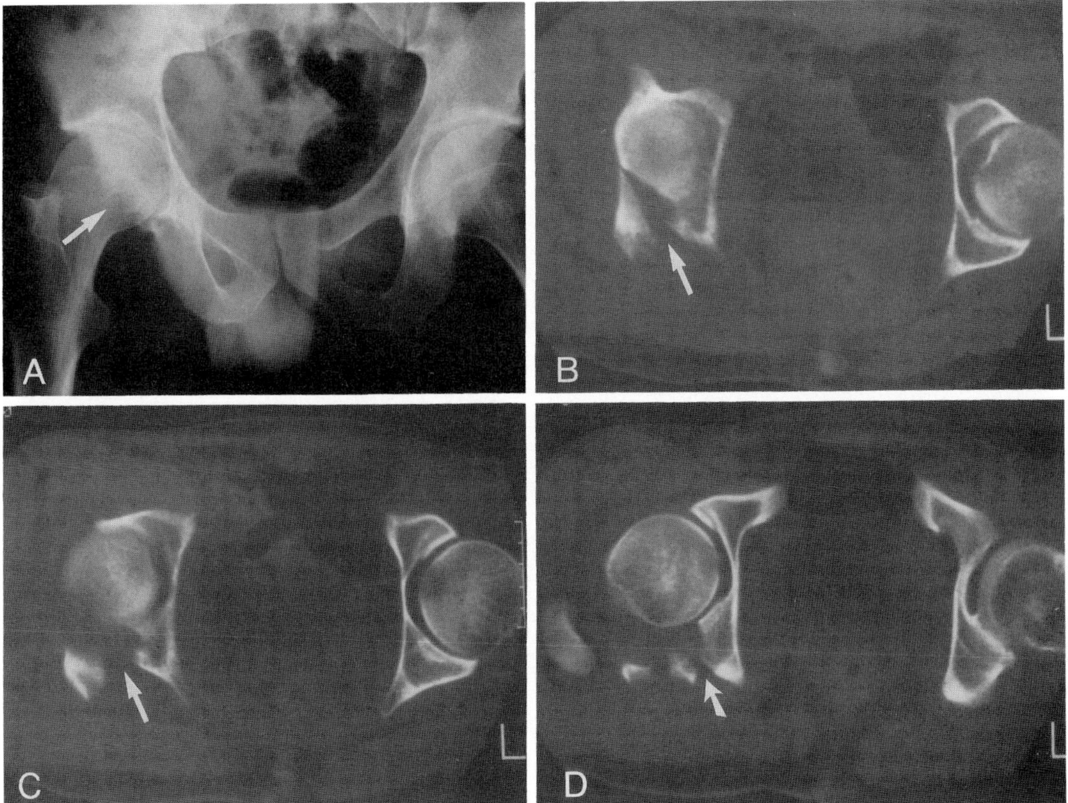

Figure 45.24. Acetabular fracture. *A*, Plain film of the hips is suspicious for right acetabular fracture (*arrow*) in this automobile driver whose right knee struck the dashboard. *B*, CT scan shows a fracture of the posterior portion of the right acetabular roof (*arrow*). *C*, and *D*, Sections through the upper and and midfemoral heads show a comminuted fracture (*arrows*) of the posterior column of the right acetabulum, which required surgical stabilization.

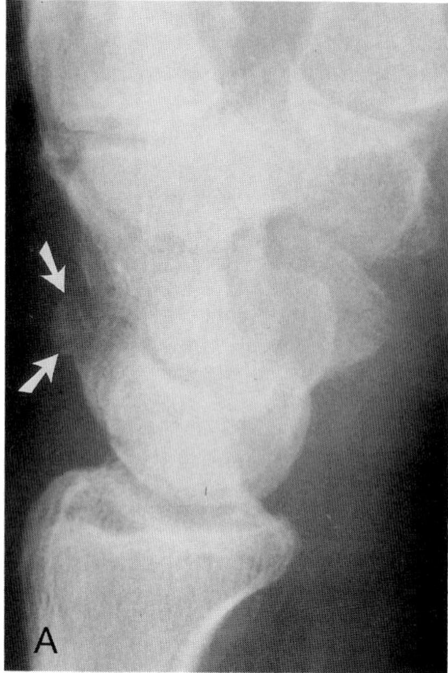

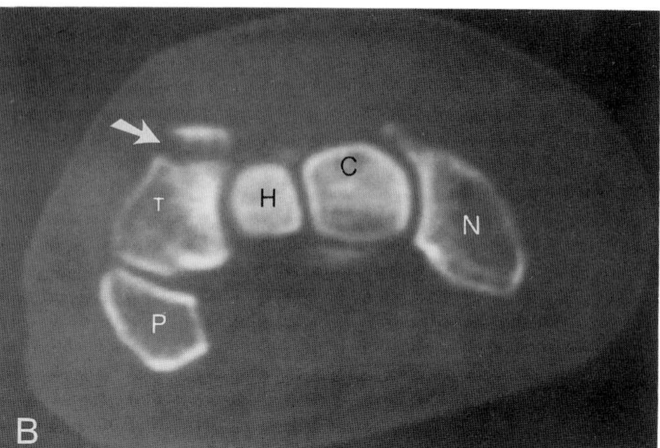

Figure 45.25. Triquetral fracture. *A*, Lateral view of the wrist shows an osseous element (*arrows*) suspicious for but not confirmatory of an avulsion fracture. Also in the differential is an accessory wrist ossicle, such as the os epitriquetrum. *B*, CT scan through the carpals confirms an avulsion fracture of the dorsal cortex of triquetrum (*T*). The white arrow indicates the fracture line and elevated compact bone. The other visualized carpals are completely surrounded with a ring of compact bone. *P*—pisiform; *H*—hamate; *C*—capitate; and *N*—navicular.

size and displacement of the sustentacular fragment, the presence of step and/or diastasis in the posterior facet, and impingement of the fibular malleolus on the tuberosity of the calcaneus due to lateral and cranial displacement of the tuberosity. CT helps the surgeon determine which calcaneal fractures might benefit from surgical intervention.

The orientation of tibial plateau fracture fragments are shown in detail on cross-section with CT. CT not only permits the diagnosis of medial and lateral meniscus lesions; it also illustrates associated lesions of the articular and extraarticular structures, including meniscus detachment, rupture, fragmentation, and displacement.

Certain dislocations, better defined with cross-sectional imaging, such as at the radioulnar joint, are also shown with CT. Both anterior and posterior sternoclavicular dislocations are easily identified with CT in a shorter time and with less patient discomfort than conventional tomography. In the shoulder, CT double-contrast arthrography has been helpful in identifying postdislocation injuries of the glenoid labrum. Myositis ossificans and posttraumatic hematoma within the soft tissues are shown in detail with CT.

SUGGESTED READINGS

Berger PE, Kuhn JP. CT of blunt abdominal trauma in childhood. *AJR,* 1981;136:105–110.

Blumberg ML. Computerized tomography and acetabular trauma. *Computed Tomography,* 1980;4:47–53.

Brant-Zawadzki M, Miller EM, Federle MP. CT in the evaluation of spine trauma. *AJR,* 1981;136:369–375.

Brant-Zawadzki M, Minagi H, Federle MP, et al. High resolution CT with image reformation in maxillofacial pathology. *AJNR,* 1982;3:31–37.

Brown BM, Brant-Zawadzki M, Cann CE. Dynamic CT scanning of spinal column trauma. *AJR,* 1982;139:1177–1181.

Destouet JM, Gilula LA, Murphy WA, et al. Computed tomography of the sternoclavicular joint and sternum. *Radiology,* 1981;138:123–128.

Dublin AB, French BN, Rennick JM. Computed tomography in head trauma. *Radiology,* 1977;122:365–369.

Dunn EL, Berry PH, Connally JD. Computed tomography of the pelvis in patients with multiple injuries. *J Trauma,* 1983;23:378–383.

Faling LJ, Pugatch RD, Robbins AH. The diagnosis of unsuspected esophageal perforation by computed tomography. *Am J Med Sci,* 1981;281:31–34.

Federle MP. Computed tomography of blunt abdominal trauma. *Radiol Clin North Am,* 1983;21:461–475.

Federle MP, Griffiths B, Minagi H, et al. Splenic trauma: Evaluation with CT. *Radiology,* 1987;162:69–71.

Federle MP, Goldberg HI, Kaiser JA, et al: Evaluation of abdominal trauma by computed tomography. *Radiology,* 1981;138:637–644.

Federle MP, Jeffrey RB. Hemoperitoneum studied by computed tomography. *Radiology,* 1983;148:187–192.

Federle MP, Kaiser JA, McAninch JW, et al: The role of computed tomography in renal trauma. *Radiology,* 1981;141:455–460.

French BN, Dublin AB. The value of computerized tomography in 1000 consecutive head injuries. *Surg Neurol,* 1977;7:171–178.

Gentry LR, Manor WF, Turski PA, et al. High-resolution CT analysis of facial struts in trauma: 1. Normal anatomy. *AJR,* 1983;140:523–532.

Gentry LR, Manor WF, Turski PA, et al. High-resolution CT analysis of facial struts in trauma: 2. Osseous and soft tissue complications. *AJR,* 1983;140:533–541.

Glazer GM, Berg JN, Moss AA, et al. CT detection of duodenal perforation. *AJR,* 1981;137:333–336.

Guerra J, Garfin SR, Resnick D. Vertebral burst fractures: CT analysis of the retropulsed fragment. *Radiology,* 1984;153.769–772.

Guyer BH, Levinsohn EM, Fredrickson BE, et al. Computed tomography of calcaneal fractures: anatomy, pathology, dosimetry, and clinical relevance. *AJR,* 1985;145:911–919.

Handel SF, Lee Y. Computed tomography of spinal fractures. *Radiol Clin North Am,* 1981;19:69–89.

Harley JD, Mack LA, Winquist RA. CT of acetabular fractures: Comparison with conventional radiography. *AJR,* 1982;138:413–417.

Healy JR, Crudale AS. Computed tomographic evaluation of depressed skull fractures and associated intracranial injury. *Comput Radiol,* 1982;6:323–330.

Heger L, Wulf K, Seddig MSA. Computed tomography of calcaneal fractures. *AJR,* 1985;145:131–137.

Heiberg E, Wolverson MK, Hurd RN, et al. CT recognition of traumatic rupture of the diaphragm. *AJR,* 1980;135:369–372.

Jeffrey RB. CT of laryngeal trauma. In Federle MP, Brant-Zawadzki MB, eds. *Computed Tomography in the Evaluation of Trauma.* Baltimore: Williams & Wilkins, 1986, p. 108.

Jeffrey RB, Federle MP, Crass RA. Computed tomography of pancreatic trauma. *Radiology,* 1983;147:491–494.

Johnson DH Jr, Colman M, Larsson S, et al. Computed tomography in maxillo-orbital fractures. *J Comput Assist Tomog,* 1984;8:416–419.

Karnayl GC, Sheedy PF, Stephens DH, et al. Computed tomography in duodenal rupture due to blunt abdominal trauma. *J Comput Assist Tomogr,* 1981;5:267–269.

Kishore PRS, Lipper MH, Becker DP, et al. Significance of CT in head injury, correlation with intracranial pressure. *AJR,* 1981;137:829–833.

Koo AH, LaRoque RL. Evaluation of head trauma by computed tomography. *Radiology,* 1977;123:345–350.

Kuhn JP, Berger PE. Computed tomography in the evaluation of blunt abdominal trauma in children. *Radiol Clin North Am,* 1981;19:503–513.

Levinsohn EM, Bunnell WP, Yuan HA. Computed tomography in the diagnosis of dislocation of the sternoclavicular joint. *Clin Orthop,* 1979;140:12–16.

Mack LA, Harley JD, Winquist RA. CT of acetabular fractures: Analysis of fracture patterns. *AJR,* 1982;138:407–417.

Mall JC, Kaiser JA. CT diagnosis of splenic laceration. *AJR,* 1980;134:265–269.

Mancuso AA, Hanafee WN. Computed tomography of the injured larynx. *Radiology,* 1979;133:139–144.

Mancuso AA, Hanafee WN. A comparative evaluation of computed tomography and laryngography. *Radiology,* 1979;133:131–138.

Merino-de Villasante J, Taveras JM. Computerized tomography (CT) in acute head trauma. *AJR,* 1976;126:765–778.

Montana MA, Richardson ML, Kilcoyne RF, et al. CT of sacral injury. *Radiology,* 1986;161:499–503.

Moon KL Jr, Federle MP. Computed tomography in hepatic trauma. *AJR,* 1983;141:309–314.

Passariello R, Trecco F, dePaulis F, et al. Meniscal lesions of the knee joint: CT diagnosis. *Radiology,* 1985;157:29–34.

Peyster RG, Hoover ED. CT in head trauma. *J Trauma,* 1982;22:25–38.

Rowe LD, Miller E, Brant-Zawadzki M. Computed tomography in maxillofacial trauma. *Laryngoscope,* 1981;91:745–757.

Sandler CM, Toombs BD. Computed tomographic evaluation of blunt renal injuries. *Radiology,* 1981;141:461–466.

Sauser DD, Billimoria PE, Rouse GA, et al. CT evaluation of hip trauma. *AJR,* 1980;135:269–274.

Schaefer SD, Brown OE. Selective application of CT in the management of laryngeal trauma. *Laryngoscope,* 1983;93:1473–1475.

Schaner EG, Balow JE, Doppman JL. Computed tomography in the diagnosis of subcapsular and perirenal hematoma. *AJR,* 1977;129:83–88.

Shirkhoda A, Brashear HR, Staab EV. Computed tomography of acetabular fractures. *Radiology,* 1980;134:683–688.

Shuman WP, Kilcoyne RF, Matsen FA, et al. Double-contrast computed tomography of the glenoid labrum. *AJR,* 1983;141:581–584.

Toombs BD, Lester RG, Ben-Menachem V, et al. Computed tomography in blunt trauma. *Radiol Clin North Am,* 1981;19:17–35.

Toombs BD, Sandler CM, Lester RG. Computed tomography of chest trauma. *Radiology,* 1981;140:733–738.

Toombs, BD, Sandler CM, Rauschkolb EN, et al. Assessment of hepatic injuries with computed tomography. *J Comput Assist Tomogr,* 1982;6:72–75.

Wall S, Federle MF, Jeffrey RB, et al. CT diagnosis of unsuspected pneumothorax after blunt abdominal trauma. *AJR,* 1983;141:919–921.

Zilkha A. Computed tomography in facial trauma. *Radiology,* 1982;144:545–548.

Zimmerman RA, Bilaniuk LT, Gennerall T, et al. Cranial computed tomography in diagnosis and management of acute head trauma. *AJR,* 1978;131:27–34.

Zimmerman RA, Bilaniuk LT, Bruce D, et al. Computed tomography of pediatric head trauma. Acute general cerebral swelling. *Radiology,* 1978;126:403–408.

CHAPTER **46**

Angiography: A Diagnostic and Therapeutic Aid in Emergencies

CHRISTOS A. ATHANASOULIS, M.D.
ARTHUR C. WALTMAN, M.D.
STUART C. GELLER, M.D.

Emergency angiography is performed on the acutely ill or injured patient for diagnosis, therapy, or both. Diagnostic angiography provides information about the nature of illness and the extent of injury. Therapeutic angiography provides the means for nonsurgical control of hemorrhage and for the treatment of ischemia.

GENERAL CONSIDERATIONS

Emergency Angiography Team

Emergency angiographic procedures call for utmost skill in performance, and expertise in interpretation of the findings. Around-the-clock availability of an expert angiography team is essential. At the Massachusetts General Hospital, such a team comprises a senior radiologist-angiographer, an assistant (fellow in training), a radiology technologist with special training in angiographic procedures, and a registered nurse. For emergencies during nonworking hours, the team can be alerted through a paging system and can be at the hospital within 30 minutes of the initial call. The call should be made as soon as information reaches the emergency department about a patient with an illness or injury that might require emergency angiography. Early notification allows the vascular radiologist to become familiar with the patient and the nature of the problem. This early involvement and consultation with the physician in charge helps to optimize the radiological workup and to determine the best type and time for an angiographic procedure.

Angiography Suite

Once the decision is reached to perform an emergency angiographic procedure, the patient is transferred to the angiography suite. Incomplete or "single-film" angiography, attempted in the emergency department by inexperienced personnel or in the emergency radiology department without appropriate equipment, is more hazardous than no angiography at all. For the entire time that the patient is in the angiography suite, intensive care continues with the assistance of medical or nursing staff who have escorted the patient. It is essential that the angiography room contain the appropriate x-ray equipment, including 1000 mA 3/phase generators, television fluoroscopy, and serial film changers with biplane filming capability. Multiplanar rotational fluoroscopic units offer the advantage of multiple projection without patient movement. Digital subtraction capabilities and/or 105 mm cine cameras are valuable for rapid imaging of vessels in acutely injured patients. In addition to the x-ray apparatus, the angiography rooms are equipped with appropriate accessories and supplies for patient monitoring and resuscitation.

Methods of Angiography

General anesthesia is not required. Mild sedation, however, may be necessary in some patients. Arteriography is carried out with catheters introduced percutaneously via either femoral artery. If femoral arterial pulses are absent, access is gained percutaneously either from an axillary artery approach or through translumbar puncture of the abdominal aorta. Access to the larger veins of the abdomen and chest is also achieved percutaneously, from either a femoral vein or an antecubital vein and, less commonly, a jugular vein. Thin wall needles, flexible guide wires, and straight or preshaped angiographic catheters are available for these procedures.

Digital subtraction angiography (DSA) offers rapid imaging of blood vessels electronically. This modality combines angiographic x-ray equipment and computers. The signal emanating from the image intensifier is digitized and fed into the computer. Manipulation of the digitized signal is then possible. With the use of electronic temporal subtraction and electronic enhancement of the subtracted image, blood vessels containing relatively dilute amounts of radiographic contrast can be imaged. Digital imaging of arteries is accomplished with either intraarterial (IADSA) or intravenous (IVDSA) injections. In emergent situations, IADSA is the preferred technique, allowing for more rapid imaging than standard film angiography with reduced contrast loads and smaller diameter catheters (Fig. 46.1). However, if very small vessel detail is required, if fields of view larger than the image intensifier are needed, or if motion artifacts become a problem, then standard film angiography can be pursued. IVDSA offers the advantage of avoiding arterial puncture, but requires larger volumes of contrast material; it may result in suboptimal imaging in up to 25% of cases due to motion artifacts. Fewer motion artifacts are observed with IADSA.

The mortality directly related to angiography is negligible; the incidence of thrombosis at the site of catheter insertion is 0.2%.

Contraindications

Contraindications to emergency angiography are profound shock and uncontrollable torrential hemorrhage. In the first instance, angiography must be postponed until the patient is resuscitated out of shock. In the second instance, the patient is taken directly to the operating room. However, immediate exploration does not preclude postoperative angiography if the surgical findings warrant. For example, a patient with massive trauma to the abdomen and pelvis on exploration may be found, after control of abdominal organ injuries, to have retroperitoneal hemorrhage from fractures of the bony pelvis. Angiography in this instance would follow exploration to determine the bleeding site and to control hemorrhage by nonsurgical means.

Known sensitivity to contrast media is only a relative contraindication, provided that emergency resuscitation equipment is available.

Clinical Conditions That May Require Emergency Angiography

An emergency diagnostic or therapeutic angiographic procedure should be considered when any of the conditions detailed below is suspected. Conditions pertaining to the heart, the head, and the central nervous system are dealt with in Chapters 31 and 37.

TRAUMA

The indications for angiography and the type of vascular procedure depend on the nature and the location of the traumatic injury.

With penetrating trauma and clinical symptoms limited to one organ or system, emergency angiography includes selective arteriography or venography, or both, of the particular organ. This is exemplified by the patient with a knife wound in the right upper quadrant of the abdomen or a penetrating wound in the flank associated with hematuria. In the first instance, abdominal aortography is complemented with selective hepatic arteriography, whereas in the second instance, selective renal arteriography or venography, or both, are performed.

Blunt traumatic and deceleration injuries due to a motor vehicle accident or a fall are usually multiple, and the clinical symptoms may be obscured by associated head injuries. Angiography in these patients can be particularly helpful, because many anatomic areas or organs can be evaluated rapidly, and multiple injuries of varying severity may be diagnosed.

Trauma to the Great Vessels

Traumatic disruption of the thoracic aorta is the most important injury in this area. It is usually the

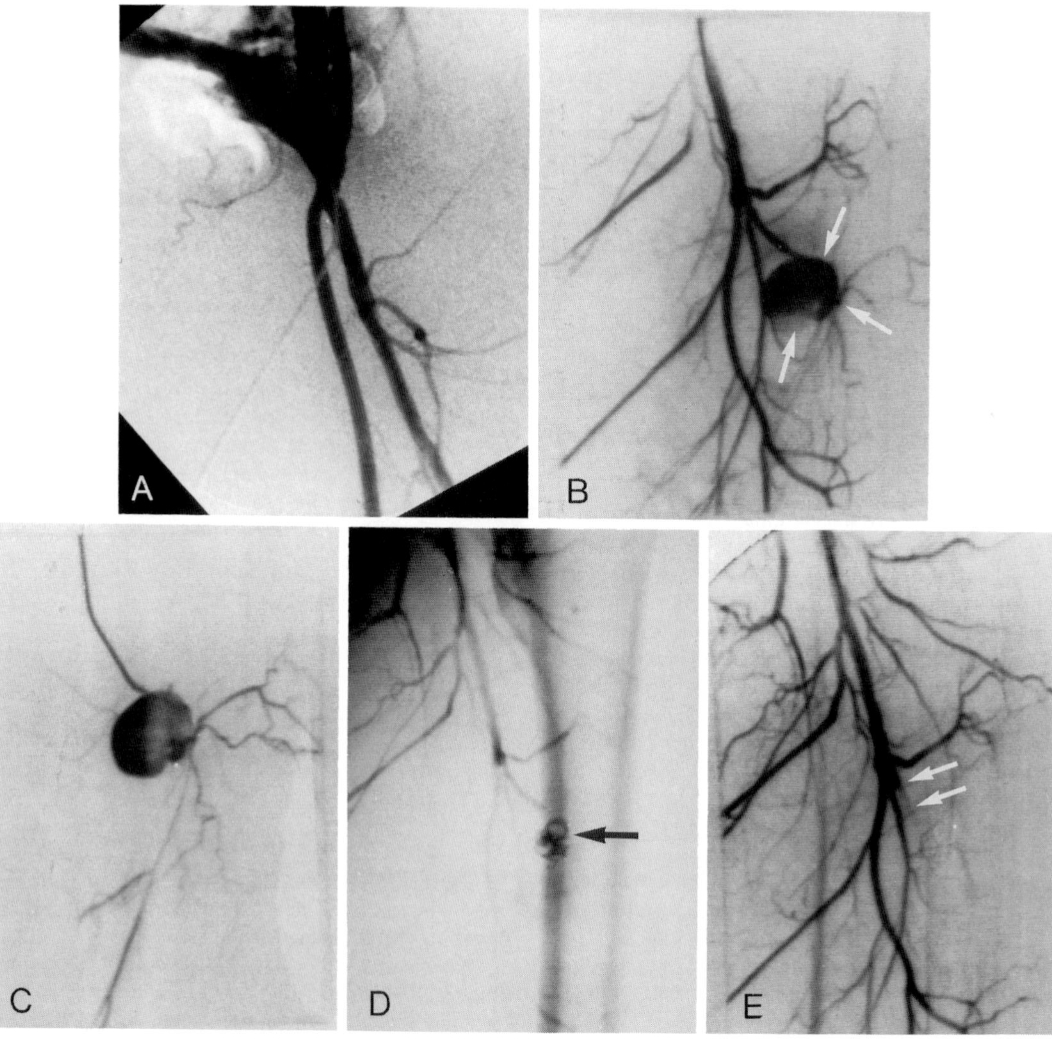

Figure 46.1. Intraarterial digital subtraction angiography (IADSA) for rapid imaging in patients with vascular trauma. Bleeding into the thigh from penetrating wound. *A*, Previous aortofemoral and femorofemoral bypass graft surgery makes percutaneous approach complex. DSA imaging of left groin defines anatomy. *B*, Catheterization of profunda femoris artery shows false aneurysm (*arrows*). *C*, Superselective catheterization of small branch giving origin to false aneurysm. *D*, Coils (*arrows*) deposited in small vessel and in aneurysm. *E*, Posttranscatheter occlusion arteriogram. Arrows point at vessel occlusion. False aneurysm no longer opacifies. Other branches of profunda femoris artery remain patent.

result of vehicular accidents. Rapid deceleration exerts a shearing force on the aortic wall at points of fixation. The thoracic aorta is fixed at the aortic valve, at the ligamentum arteriosum, and at the origins of the intercostal arteries. The aortic segment just distal to the origin of the left subclavian artery is most commonly involved. Rupture of the thoracic aorta is found in 16% of victims of fatal automobile accidents. About 20% of those who sustain aortic rupture survive for more than 1 hour. If the entity is not properly diagnosed and treated, 60% of those patients die within 2 weeks of injury.

Early diagnosis of a thoracic aortic tear is of paramount importance. A variety of plain film chest findings have been described in connection with thoracic aortic and great vessel tears. These findings include a widened or widening mediastinum, displacement of mediastinal structures such as the esophagus, defined by a nasogastric tube or the left mainstem bronchus, the presence of apical pleural caps, pleural effusion, first and second rib fractures, and sternal fractures. In the appropriate clinical setting, if one or more of the radiographic findings is present, thoracic aortography should be performed immediately. A wide field of view encompassing the entire thoracic aorta and the proximal great vessels in two views is recommended. This is best accomplished with standard film aortography in two planes.

The value of computed tomography remains to be proven. Although computed tomography may detect mediastinal hematoma, pulmonary, and chest wall abnormalities, and has occasionally detected a thoracic aortic tear, the technique is inadequate to delineate the full extent of a tear and its relationship to branch vessels. In addition, a "negative" computed tomogram does not exclude a tear. Thus, thoracic aortography is still the "gold standard" radiographic examination. Although magnetic resonance imaging holds promise for the future, the technical obstacles of imaging acutely ill patients in a high strength magnetic field make this modality impractical for the evaluation of patients who have sustained multisystem trauma. The angiographic appearance of aortic and great vessel injury may vary from irregularity of the aortic wall to a false aneurysm. (Fig. 46.2)

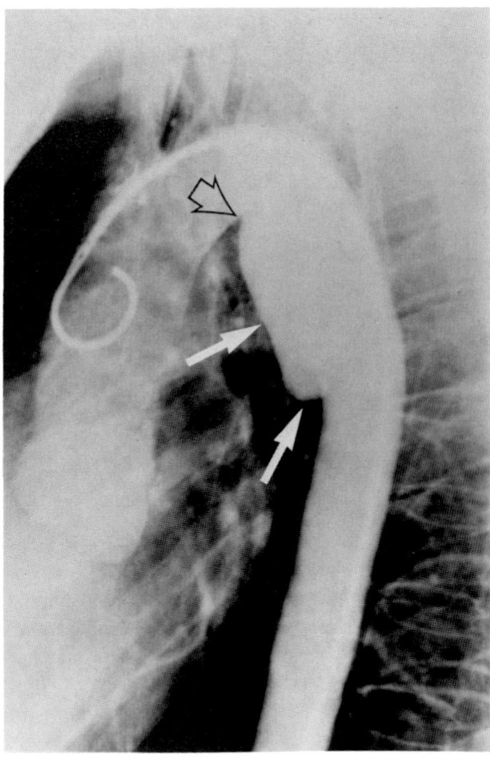

Figure 46.2. Traumatic tear of the thoracic aorta. *Arrows* point to disruption of the aortic wall and false aneurysm formation in patient with sudden deceleration injury to chest.

Abdominal Trauma

The clinical status of the patient (vital signs, physical examination, blood requirements, results of abdominal tap) and findings on other radiographic studies, such as computed tomographic and radionuclide scans, are the major factors in deciding if emergency angiography should be performed in patients with penetrating or blunt abdominal trauma. The availability of high quality, rapid computed tomography and a shift towards a more conservative approach in the management of splenic and renal trauma have resulted in a diminishing frequency of emergent abdominal angiography for diagnostic purposes only in these conditions. However, angiography in cases of hepatic, splenic, and renal trauma is still performed in more difficult diagnostic circumstances, particularly for therapeutic considerations.

Hepatic Trauma

Major avulsing lacerations of the liver are often associated with hypovolemia and profound shock, requiring immediate surgical exploration; if bleeding continues after operation, hepatic angiography should be considered. In most patients, there is ample time for the angiographic procedure.

The purposes of angiography in patients with suspected hepatic injury are:

1. To confirm or exclude a major laceration or hematoma of the liver; computed tomography usually serves as a better screening tool in this regard, but if abnormal, may not fully answer all questions relating to subsequent management; angiography may then become necessary;
2. To determine precisely the segment or segments of the liver and the arterial branches involved in the injury;
3. To diagnose underlying benign or malignant tumors that may be the cause of major bleeding incidental to minor trauma or that may aggravate hemorrhage initiated by trauma;
4. To demonstrate the arterial anatomy and also normal variations and to establish a vascular map before operation. The left hepatic artery arises from the left gastric artery 15–25% of the time. The right hepatic artery originates from the superior mesenteric artery 15% of the time. Cross-clamping of the portal trunk, therefore, in these patients does not control all vascular inflow to the liver;
5. To follow the course of an angiographically demonstrated lesion if the patient is not operated on. Radionuclide studies and computed tomography may also be helpful in this instance;
6. To diagnose and to locate complications of he-

patic trauma, such as traumatic aneurysms and hematobilia, after medical or surgical management;

7. To evaluate the presence of associated injuries in adjoining organs, such as the right kidney; again, computed tomography usually resolves this issue;
8. To control hemorrhage with transcatheter embolization of hepatic arterial branches.

Depending on the nature and extent of hepatic injury, the angiographic findings may include any of the following:

1. *Contusion*: (*a*) straightening and elongation of the arterial branches; (*b*) delayed progress of the contrast medium column; (*c*) multiple punctate areas of contrast medium extravasation; (*d*) irregular heterogeneous hepatogram of one or more segments.
2. *Intrahepatic hematoma*: (*a*) arterial displacement; (*b*) small artery occlusions; (*c*) extravasation of contrast medium; (*d*) defects during the capillary and venous phases of the hepatogram.
3. *Capsular or deep tear of the liver*: (*a*) subcapsular hematoma with hepatic displacement (Fig. 46.3); (*b*) extravasation of contrast medium; (*c*) false aneurysm; (*d*) arterioportal fistula; (*e*) arteriobiliary fistula.
4. *Hematobilia*: one or several sites of contrast medium extravasation and opacification of adjoining biliary ducts (Fig. 46.4).

Tumor vascularity, arteriovenous shunting, and tumor stain are seen at angiography in patients with either minor or major trauma *and* a coexistent tumor.

Splenic Trauma

Radiographically, the spleen can be evaluated with ultrasonography, radionuclide scanning, computed tomography, and splenic arteriography. In the acute situation, although ultrasound scanning may be helpful in the detection of large subcapsular hematomas, overlying gas and bone shadows can obscure pathology, making it less than optimal imaging. Radionuclide scanning, at one time, served as an excellent screening tool, but in most institutions has been supplanted by high quality rapid computed tomography.

If splenic injury is suspected in a hemodynamically stable patient, with single or minor injury to the left upper abdominal quadrant, with or without fractures of the lower left ribs, a computed tomogram would be the initial radiographic examination of choice. If the scan is unequivocally normal, further radiographic studies are usually unnecessary. If findings are equivocal, the patient should undergo splenic arteriography. If the scan detects a splenic injury, depending upon the nature of the injury, the patient is followed conservatively with sequential scans, undergoes immediate surgical exploration, or possibly undergoes splenic arteriography with the potential for an angiographic intervention that may

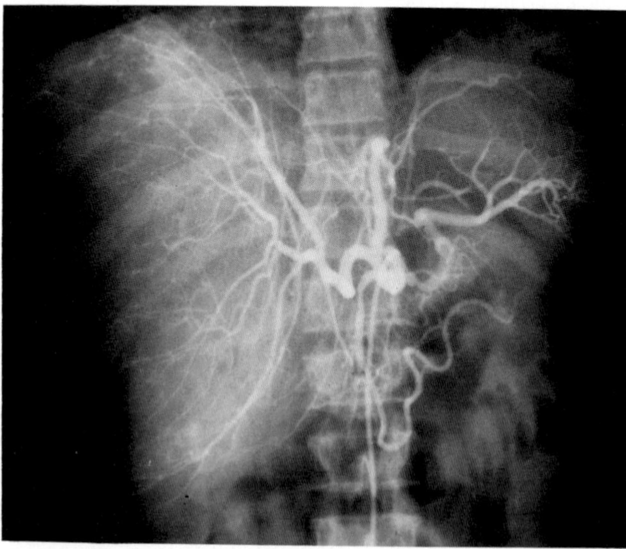

Figure 46.3. Subcapsular hematoma of liver secondary to rupture of hepatocellular adenoma. Celiac axis arteriogram in a 29-year-old man with acute abdominal pain and decreasing hematocrit. The patient had been receiving long-term replacement therapy with anabolic corticosteroids following irradiation of a pituitary adenoma. Arteriogram shows splaying of branches of hepatic artery and medial displacement of opacified liver by large subcapsular hematoma. At operation, it was found that the subcapsular hematoma was the result of a ruptured hepatocellular adenoma and carcinoma.

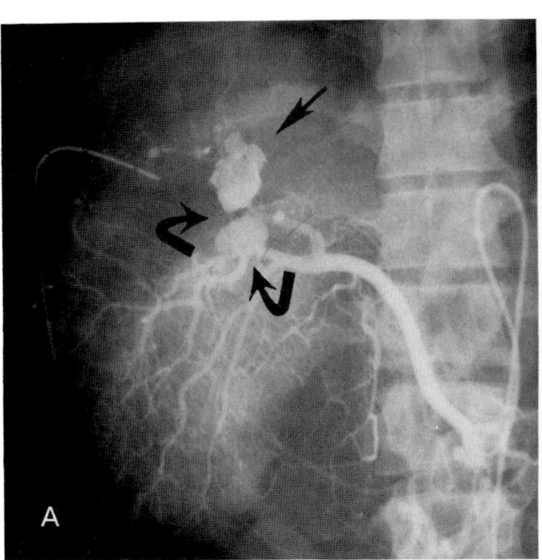

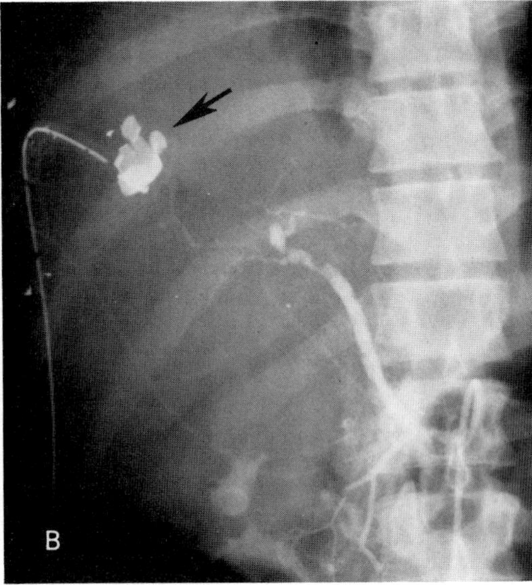

Figure 46.4. Traumatic hematobilia treated with transcatheter embolization of right hepatic artery. Traumatic hematobilia in a 35-year-old man was the result of a bullet wound in the right upper abdominal quadrant. *A*, Right hepatic arteriogram. Right hepatic artery originates from superior mesenteric artery. *Straight arrow* points to fragment of bullet. *Curved arrows* point to extravasation of contrast medium and a false aneurysm in right lobe of liver. *B*, Right hepatic arteriogram with patient in oblique position following transcatheter embolization of hepatic artery with surgical gelatin. *Straight arrow* points to bullet fragment. There is no opacification of the false aneurysm. Blood supply to left lobe of liver was not compromised. The patient was discharged 8 days after the procedure. He has remained asymptomatic for a follow-up period of 6 months.

achieve splenic salvage without need for laparotomy.

In patients with multiple injuries that otherwise require angiographic studies for diagnosis or therapy, splenic arteriography can confirm or exclude splenic rupture, and additional studies may not be necessary.

The definitive angiographic findings of splenic rupture include:

1. Gross or multifocal extravasation of contrast medium persisting into the capillary phase (Fig. 46.5). Visualization of small amounts of extravasated medium may be enhanced if arteriography is repeated after injection of 6–10 μg of epinephrine into the splenic artery;
2. Direct intrasplenic arteriovenous communication;
3. Subcapsular hematoma;
4. A wedge-shaped defect during the capillary phase with arterial displacement or occlusions secondary to a tear and intraparenchymal hemorrhage.

Displacement of the opacified spleen away from the lateral abdominal wall or the diaphragm, an irregular or mottled splenogram, and stretching of the splenic arterial branches, the so-called indirect signs of splenic rupture, are unreliable and should not be considered in the interpretation of the angiogram. A fluid- or gas-distended stomach may also produce such stretching of splenic arterial branches, especially those of the upper pole.

Renal Trauma

In 86% of renal injuries managed medically, recovery is complete and the intravenous pyelogram is normal at 6 or more months after injury. As a result, the surgical approach to renal trauma has become less aggressive, as has renal angiography.

In all patients with hematuria after trauma or without hematuria but with suspected renal injury, an infusion intravenous pyelogram or dynamic computed tomogram should be obtained. Emergency abdominal aortography and selective renal arteriography are performed if a nonfunctioning kidney is demonstrated. Arteriography is also performed when hematuria is massive or when it does not subside after several hours of bed rest and sedation (Fig. 46.6).

In patients with suspected renal injury, the goal of angiography is to reveal any of the following conditions for appropriate management:

1. Thrombotic occlusion of the renal artery;

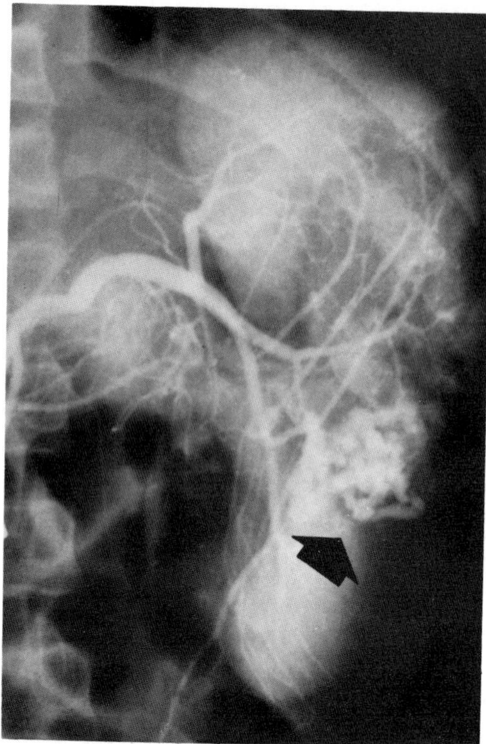

Figure 46.5. Splenic rupture. Splenic arteriogram in a 12-year-old boy who sustained severe injuries to the left upper abdominal quadrant during a fall. *Arrow* points to contrast medium extravasation within spleen. Splenic salvage is then the challenge for the operating surgeon.

2. False aneurysm;
3. Arteriovenous fistula;
4. Thrombosis of the renal vein; and
5. Underlying renal disease such as tumor, hydronephrosis, ectopia, hypoplasia, or agenesis.

Control of Traumatic Abdominal Bleeding with Transcatheter Embolization

In patients with multiple injuries and bleeding from the liver, spleen, or kidney, it may be desirable to avoid immediate surgical intervention for control of bleeding either because of the patient's poor general condition or because of associated severe neurologic injuries. If angiographic examination in such patients shows discrete extravasation of contrast medium, immediate control of bleeding can be achieved by positioning the angiographic catheter in the bleeding artery and obstructing blood flow with mechanical means. Blood flow can be obstructed either temporarily with balloon-tipped catheters or for a prolonged period by using particulate matter (surgical gelatin) for embolization of the bleeding artery. Therefore, splenectomy or nephrectomy for uncontrollable bleeding need not be performed on an emergency basis, and attention can be directed to the management of associated injuries. Further, transcatheter embolization can be selective with the tip of the angiographic catheter positioned in the bleeding branch.

In patients with trauma and bleeding into the kidney, selective embolization often obviates nephrectomy. Proximal splenic artery embolization can also result in splenic salvage without need for laparotomy in cases of splenic trauma. Massive bleeding into the liver, hematobilia, traumatic arteriovenous fistula, and retroperitoneal hemorrhage are other conditions that can be managed with angiographic methods.

Fractures of the Bony Pelvis with Hemorrhage

The mortality among patients with major pelvic fractures varies from 9–27%. As many as 60% of these deaths result from massive extraperitoneal hemorrhage. Associated genitourinary and colorectal injuries are other serious complications, but hemorrhage that is usually concealed and that may become massive is the most difficult problem to manage.

The source of bleeding can be a transected iliac vein. In such patients, rapid recognition followed by surgical ligation is lifesaving. In most patients, however, bleeding arises from the arteries and venous plexuses lining the walls of the pelvis.

Control of bleeding has been attempted with ligation of both hypogastric arteries. However, most reports indicate that this procedure does not control hemorrhage because of the presence of collateral vessels. In addition, during surgical exploration, the rate of bleeding may increase considerably, since the tamponading effect of the peritoneum and of the hematoma itself is no longer present.

Angiographic methods have been employed to determine the site of arterial bleeding and to control hemorrhage in patients with pelvic fractures. Arteriography in patients with fractures of the bony pelvis and an obvious large or increasing retroperitoneal hematoma displacing the urinary bladder, the ureters, or the kidneys reveals the bleeding site by demonstrating contrast medium extravasation from branches of the hypogastric arteries, usually the obturator arteries. The internal pudendal, superior gluteal, and iliolumbar arteries have also been shown to be sources of hemorrhage, depending on the site of the major bony injury. Venography has been of limited value in the evaluation of venous bleeding because there is no good method for visualization of all the pelvic veins.

Once the bleeding sites have been identified, hemorrhage can be controlled with selective cathe-

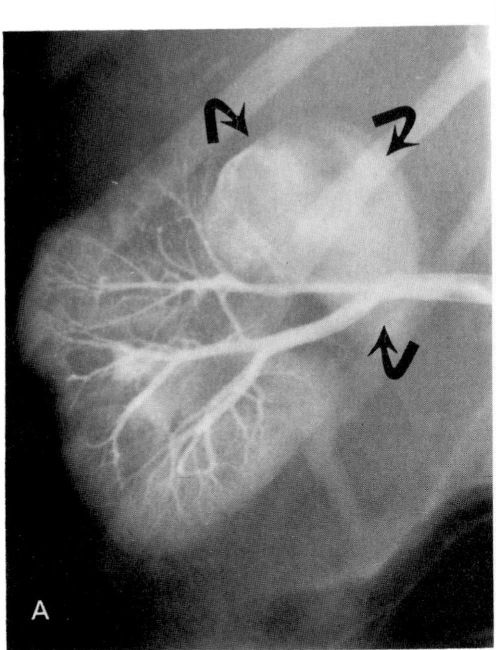

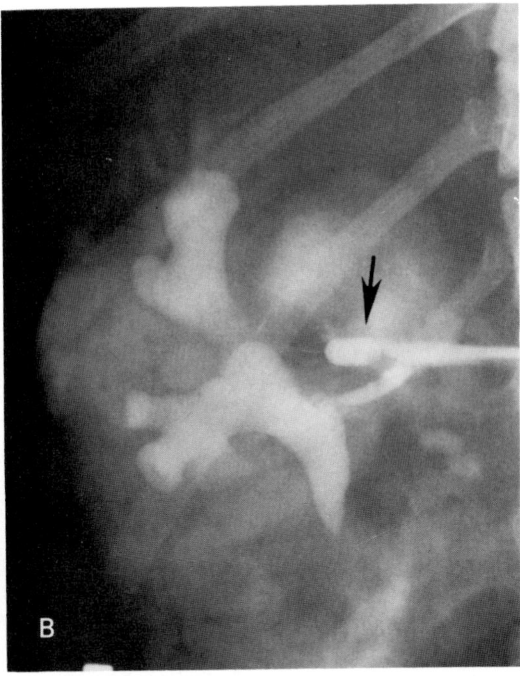

Figure 46.6. Kidney rupture with intrarenal hemorrhage. A 21-year-old woman had massive hematuria following an automobile injury. *A*, Renal arteriogram shows contrast medium extravasation into large false aneurysm occupying upper pole of kidney (*arrows*). *B*, Balloon catheter (*arrow*) has been percutaneously introduced into renal artery and inflated with radiopaque contrast medium. Injection of contrast medium proximal to balloon shows effective obstruction of blood flow and no opacification of false aneurysm. This allowed stabilization of patient's condition before transferral to the operating room for exploration and partial nephrectomy.

terization of the bleeding arterial branches of the hypogastric arteries and obstruction of blood flow to these vessels. This has been achieved with balloon catheter occlusion and embolization with a wide variety of materials, including autologous blood clots, surgical gelatin (Gelfoam) pledgets, polyvinyl alcohol (Ivalon) particles, and metallic coils (Fig. 46.7). Surgical gelatin (Gelfoam) introduced in the form of small (1 × 1 mm) plugs through the angiographic catheter is usually the material of choice. Gelfoam is considered to be a "temporary" occluding agent, with the potential for recanalization in 10–14 days. If a more "permanent" occlusion is required, Ivalon particles or metallic coils may be utilized.

Embolization of bleeding branches of the hypogastric arteries has two main advantages over surgical ligation. It produces more distal rather than proximal occlusion, and it does not interfere with the tamponading effect of the intact peritoneum and already existing hematoma. In most patients treated with embolization, bleeding ceases. No serious complications are associated with this method.

When emergency angiography is performed for the diagnosis and control of bleeding from pelvic trauma, it can be extended to evaluate the abdominal organs as well. As mentioned, if emergency operation is performed for suspected intraabdominal injury and if a retroperitoneal hematoma is found originating from the pelvis, angiography can still be performed immediately after operation for embolization of the bleeding arteries.

Trauma to Extremities

Traumatic arterial injury is manifested by either hemorrhage or arterial insufficiency. In both instances, the therapeutic goal is to restore normal vascular anatomy. Early recognition and knowledge of the exact level of vascular injury are important.

Major limb ischemia may be concealed by generalized shock or vasoconstriction, or both. If ischemia is suspected, the point of arterial obstruction may be difficult to determine clinically or with oscillometry. Further, major arteries can suffer lacerations that need repair, with no clinical evidence of arterial insufficiency. Thus, the indications for angiography are as follows:

1. Pulse deficit, if the exact site of obstruction cannot be established clinically or with other laboratory techniques;

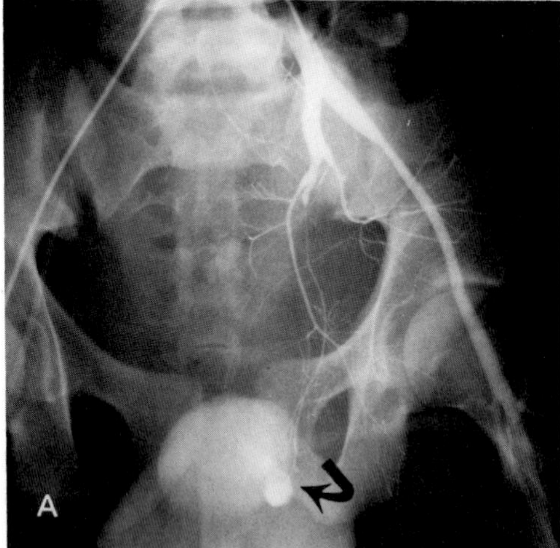

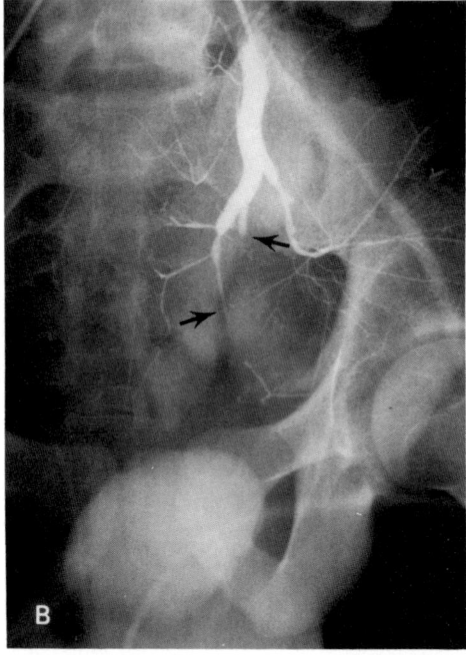

Figure 46.7. Pelvic fracture with hemorrhage—control of bleeding with embolization of branches of hypogastric artery. A patient with injuries to the bony pelvis following an automobile accident had a decreasing hematocrit. *A*, Left hypogastric arteriogram. *Arrow* points to contrast medium extravasation from branches of left hypogastric artery. *B*, Plugs of surgical gelatin were introduced through angiographic catheter, and branches of hypogastric artery were occluded (*arrows*). Repeated arteriogram shows no contrast medium extravasation. The patient's condition became stabilized following the procedure. There was no evidence of subsequent hemorrhage, and the patient was discharged several days later.

2. Large or enlarging hematoma of the wound site (Fig. 46.8);
3. Suspected false aneurysm or arteriovenous fistula;
4. Suspected vascular injury because of proximity of the vessel to a wound or fracture in the absence of clinical evidence of arterial insufficiency. An arterial injury requiring intervention is uncovered by arteriography in 5–20% of patients studied for "proximity only" injuries.

If no specific structural arterial lesion is seen during the course of arteriography, but diffuse arterial spasm of the examined limb is demonstrated, vasodilators are injected intraarterially through the angiographic needle or catheter to combat the vasoconstriction. 1–2 mg of papaverine or 100–200 μg of aqueous nitroglycerin are used for this purpose. If necessary, this may be followed with intraarterial infusion of papaverine, 0.1 mg/min for 8–12 hours.

Peripheral phlebography is considered in patients with large or enlarging soft-tissue hematomas and normal arterial studies.

NONTRAUMATIC VASCULAR CONDITIONS

Patients with conditions other than trauma affecting the aorta and its major branches may benefit from emergency angiography. In this chapter, discussion is limited to acute aortic dissection and ruptured aortic aneurysm.

Acute Aortic Dissection

In patients with clinical symptoms or signs raising the suspicion of acute aortic dissection, emergency aortography is indispensable for the following reasons:

1. If acute aortic dissection is not diagnosed and not treated, it is fatal in 75–90% of patients.
2. Angiography remains the "gold standard" radiographic examination to establish and stage or exclude the presence of aortic dissection.
3. The surgical approach and prognosis for each of the three types of dissection (DeBakey I, II, III) are different, and angiography identifies each type.
4. Opacification of the false lumen during aortography or lack of opacification is significant in selecting patients for medical vs. surgical treatment.
5. Aortography provides information about extension of the dissection into the branches of the aorta. This information is important during subsequent management, whether the treatment is surgical or medical.

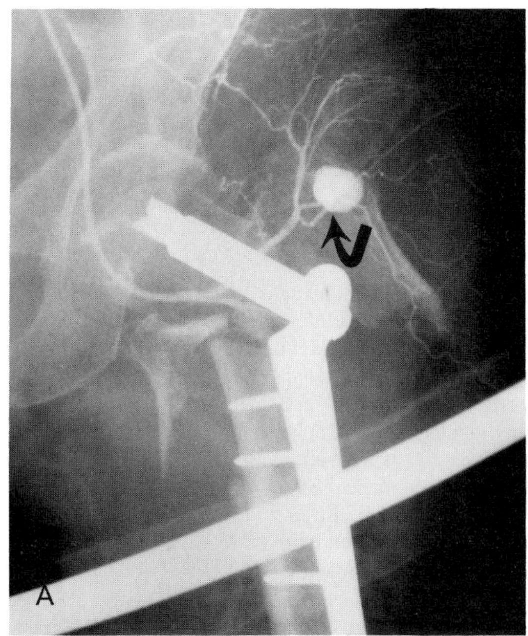

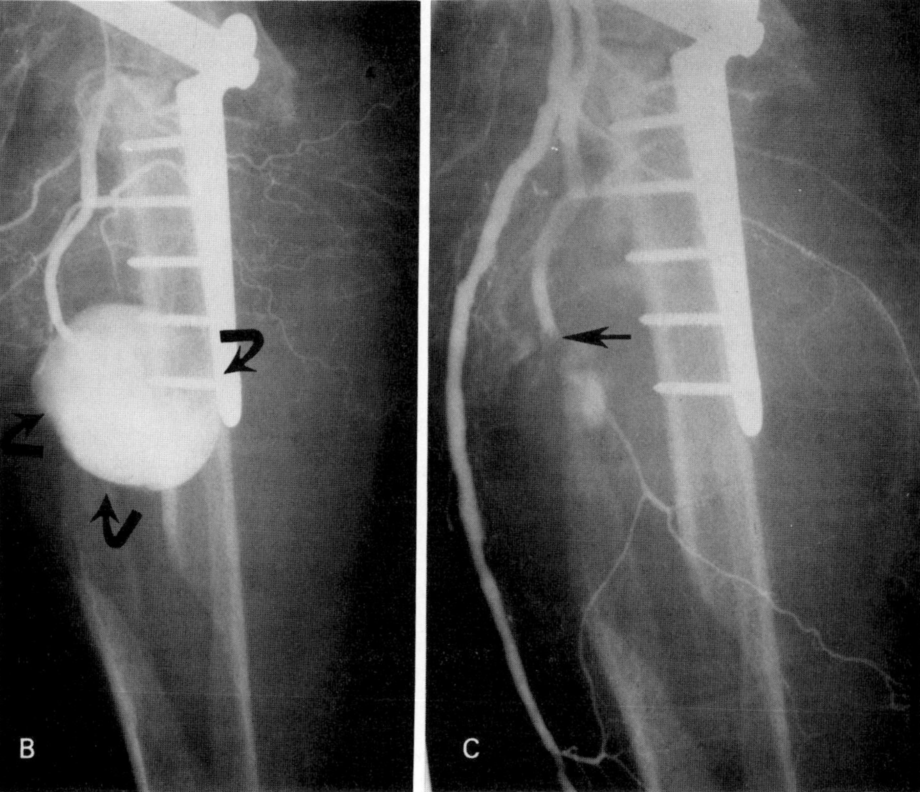

Figure 46.8. Hemorrhage resulting from fractures of a hip and femur—control of bleeding with transcatheter vessel occlusion. A 70-year-old woman sustained an intertrochanteric fracture of the femur. Following fixation, the patient had an enlarging hematoma at the operative site and a decreasing hematocrit. *A*, *Arrow* points to contrast medium extravasation from branch of lateral femoral circumflex artery. Embolization with surgical gelatin controlled the bleeding. The patient was discharged.
Nine months later, the patient sustained a fracture of the femoral shaft with an associated enlarging soft-tissue mass. *B*, Arteriogram of profunda femoris artery. *Arrows* point to large false aneurysm, the result of a tear of this artery. *C*, The false aneurysm has been obliterated following embolization of distal segment of profunda femoris artery (*arrow*) with surgical gelatin.

Computed tomography (CT), magnetic resonance imaging (MRI), and real time ultrasonography have also been used in the evaluation of patients wth aortic dissection. Their less invasive nature makes them somewhat appealing, but these modalities have proven significantly less accurate than aortography in the acute dissection. In addition, even if the detection of an aortic dissection is made by one of these cross-sectional imaging modalities, important clinical information regarding the extent of the dissection, the entry and exit points, branch artery involvement, aortic valve involvement, and false lumen patency is often lacking. Aortography can answer all of these questions and is still often necessary to make clinical management decisions concerning medical vs. surgical treatment. In addition, the results of the aortogram very often help to determine surgical approaches. There may be a limited role for CT and MRI in the long-term follow-up of those patients with aortic dissections already diagnosed, who are undergoing medical therapy.

Aortography should be rapidly and meticulously performed. Accurate diagnosis requires excellent film quality. The study should include the thoracic and abdominal aorta, and radiographs should be obtained in two planes at 90°; therefore, biplane filming capability is essential. IADSA is a very useful adjunct to standard film studies.

The approach from either femoral artery has proven safe when the procedure is performed by an experienced angiographer. Use of an axillary or brachial artery is necessary if both femoral arterial pulses are absent. A combined approach via femoral and axillary arteries may be necessary if the catheter cannot be advanced into the ascending aorta from the retrograde femoral route. The venous approach to the study of dissections does not provide optimal opacification of the aorta, and results are unreliable.

The angiographic signs of aortic dissection are direct and indirect. The direct signs include:

1. Linear radiolucency coursing longitudinally along varying lengths of the opacified aorta, representing the torn or separated intima (Fig. 46.9);
2. Opacification of two channels;
3. Demonstration of points of entry or reentry.

The indirect signs include:

1. Compression of the true aortic lumen by the nonopacified false lumen;
2. Abnormal catheter position, with the catheter in the aortic arch lying along the inner wall rather than resting against the lateral wall;
3. Thickening of the aortic wall more than 6 mm;
4. Ulcer-like projection from the aortic lumen.

Extension of the dissection to involve major branches such as the celiac, superior mesenteric, renal, or iliac arteries is common in types I and III. The lumen of an aortic branch may be compressed or occluded by the false lumen of the dissected aorta. A branch may be supplied by both the true lumen and the false lumen or by the false lumen only.

Ruptured Aortic Aneurysm

Intraperitoneal rupture of an abdominal aortic aneurysm is usually rapidly fatal, not allowing for diagnostic procedures. Fortunately, it is less common than rupture into the retroperitoneum, which initially is manifested by slow leakage. If available, computed tomography is helpful in delineating the hematoma around the aneurysm. Use of angiography in the preoperative evaluation of these patients is controversial. It appears that, if it is performed with expedience and safety, it may prove beneficial for the following reasons:

1. Rupture may be into the intestine, the inferior vena cava, or the ureter, making the diagnosis difficult without aortography (Fig. 46.10).
2. Preoperative knowledge of suprarenal extension of the aneurysm or involvement of the renal arteries is useful in planning the operative procedure.
3. Associated aneurysms or occlusive disease of the outflow vessels to the lower extremities can be demonstrated by angiography.

Ischemia

Acute Peripheral Arterial Occlusion

Sudden cessation of major arterial flow to an extremity can be caused by thrombosis, embolism, trauma, or compression secondary to dissection. Trauma and dissections have been discussed. As in trauma patients, the goal of therapy in patients with an acute peripheral arterial occlusion is not only preservation of life and the limb, but also restoration of blood flow and return of function.

Acute thrombosis of a major peripheral artery is commonly superimposed on atherosclerosis. Acute ischemia can also result from extrinsic compression, such as compression of the subclavian artery by a cervical rib or a fibrous band, and from hypotension of any cause in patients with underlying peripheral vascular disease. It can also be a complication of an arterial puncture performed for coronary, cerebral, or visceral arteriography, or for physiologic monitoring. Preoperative arteriography

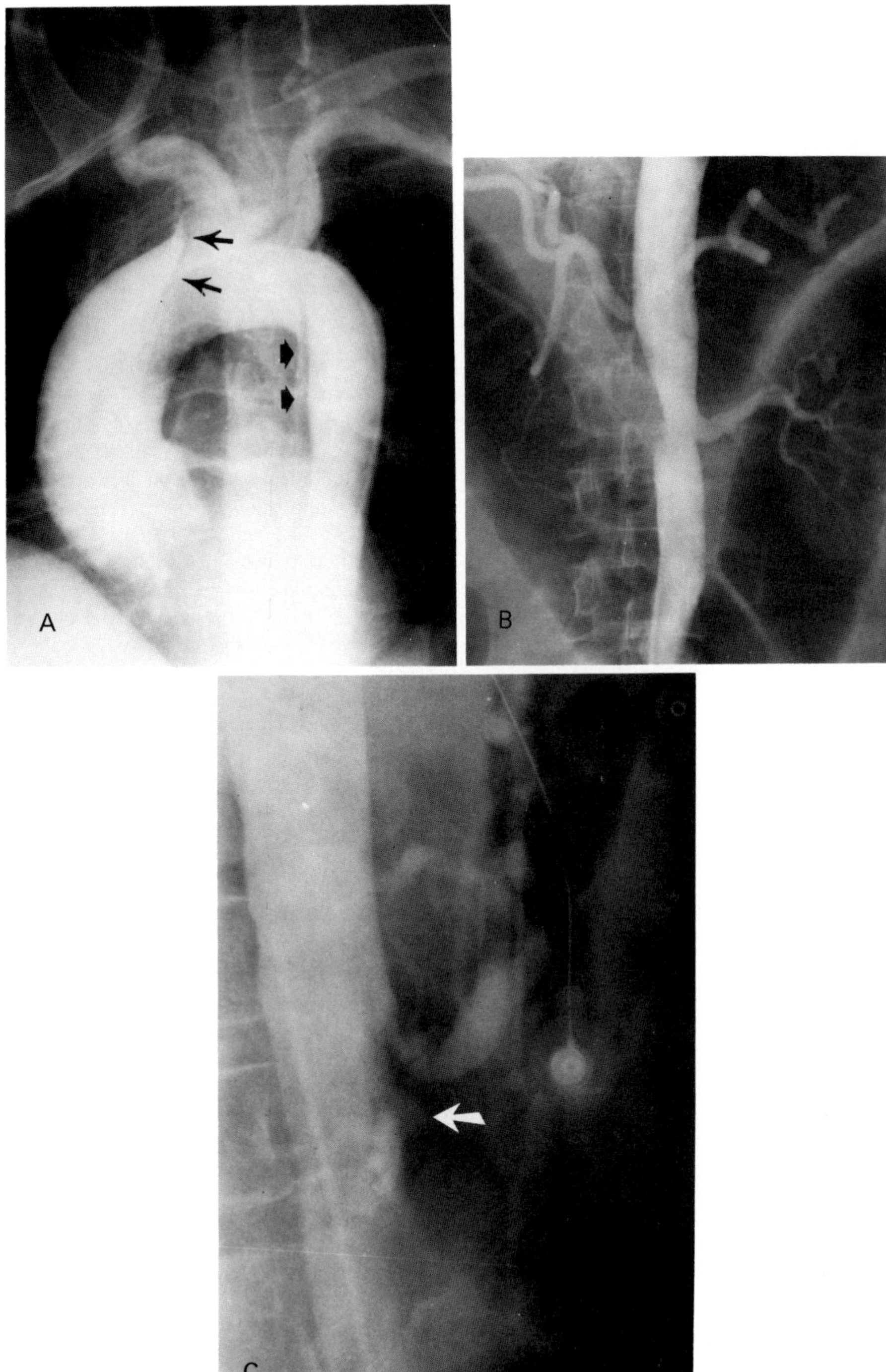

Figure 46.9. Aortic dissection extending into abdominal aorta. A 65-year-old hypertensive man was seen with acute chest pain radiating both anteriorly and posteriorly. *A*, Thoracic aortogram. Dissection extends into ascending and descending thoracic aorta (*arrows*). *B*, Abdominal aortogram, anteroposterior projection. Dissection has extended into abdominal aorta. There is no opacification of superior mesenteric and right renal arteries. *C*, Abdominal aortogram, lateral projection. *Arrow* points to stump of superior mesenteric artery, which was occluded as result of extension of dissection in the abdominal aorta.

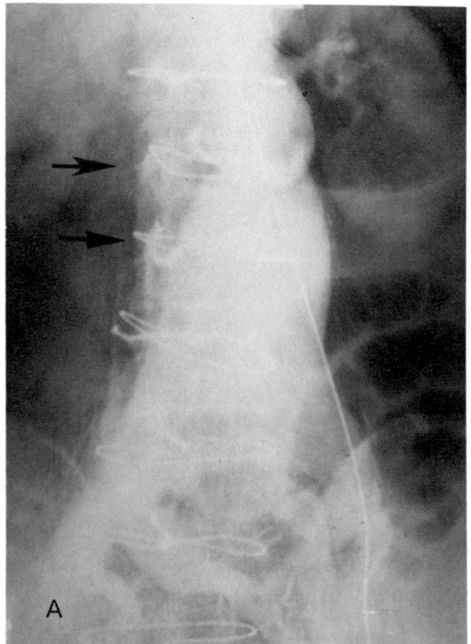

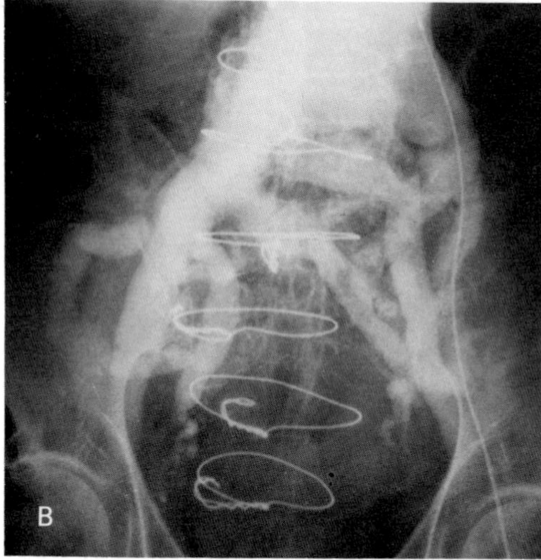

Figure 46.10. Abdominal aortic aneurysm with rupture into inferior vena cava. A 70-year-old man had a pulsatile abdominal mass and hematuria. *A*, Abdominal aortogram shows large aneurysm of abdominal aorta with simultaneous opacification of inferior vena cava (*arrows*). *B*, Pelvic arteriogram. Contrast medium was injected at aortic bifurcation. There is opacification of iliac veins and of multiple venous tributaries. At exploration, rupture of the aortic aneurysm was found with communication with the inferior vena cava.

in such patients is necessary to determine the extent of the thrombotic process and the adequacy of distal runoff.

The clinical diagnosis of arterial embolism is usually inferred from a history of myocardial infarction, atrial fibrillation, proximal aneurysm, a recent cardiac or vascular operation, or endocarditis. Arteriography in patients with suspected embolic arterial occlusion establishes the site and extent of the occlusion, the degree of collateral circulation, and the distal vessel reconstitution. When embolism results in complete occlusion of an artery, the arteriographic appearance is fairly typical, the proximal end of the embolus forming a convex margin. (Fig. 46.11)

Regional Thrombolysis

Regional thrombolysis involves infusion of a thrombolytic enzyme intraarterially, directly into the thrombus. Streptokinase and urokinase have been used, and clinical trials are underway to investigate tissue plasminogen activator. These thrombolytic agents have been infused successfully through angiographic catheters for resolution of acute arterial thrombus in the coronary, renal, and peripheral vascular beds. Acutely or subacutely occluded bypass grafts have also been successfully recanalized in this fashion. The advantages of regional over systemic thrombolysis are the avoidance of systemic complications, such as bleeding, by using a lower dose of the agent and the potential for more rapid lysis. (Fig. 46.12) Preliminary successes with low-dose streptokinase (5000 units/hour) infusions led to more widespread use of this agent, but subsequent failures led to disillusionment. The high incidence of endogenous antibodies to streptokinase, as well as factors relating to its indirect mechanism of action, resulted in unpredictable outcomes with this drug. Therefore, urokinase (40,000–100,000 units/hour) has become the current thrombolytic agent of choice. Urokinase is nonantigenic and is a direct activator of plasminogen. It is therefore a much more reliable drug. Success factors relate to patient selection, the time of the thrombosis, the nature of the underlying pathology leading to the thrombosis, the severity of the ischemia, the anatomical location of the occlusion, and the skill of the angiographer. Regional urokinase infusions for acute arterial occlusive disease result in successful lysis in approximately 80% of cases within 12–24 hours, with a major complication (usually bleeding) rate of 5–10%. This therapy is often not definitive, but adjunctive to a subsequent angioplasty or a surgical procedure.

Renal Ischemia—Acute Renal Failure

Sudden development of impaired renal function may be due to prerenal (circulatory inadequacy), postrenal (obstruction), or primary renal injury. An important step in the management of these patients

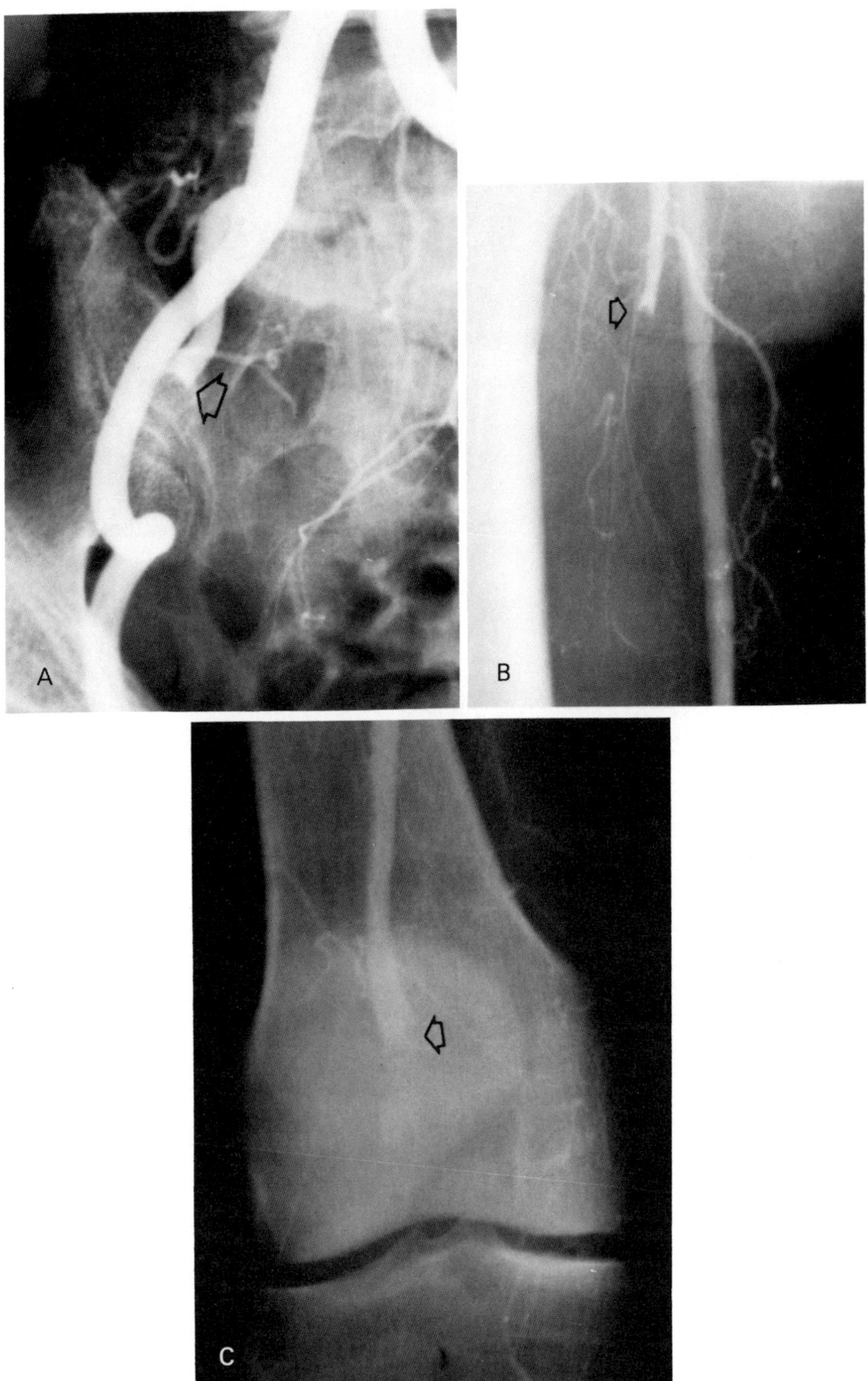

Figure 46.11. Multiple arterial embolic occlusions in patient with atrial fibrillation. Embolic occlusions of *A*, the hypogastric artery, *B*, the profunda femoris artery, and *C*, the popliteal artery are indicated with *arrows*. The curvilinear defect of meniscus is characteristic of arterial emboli.

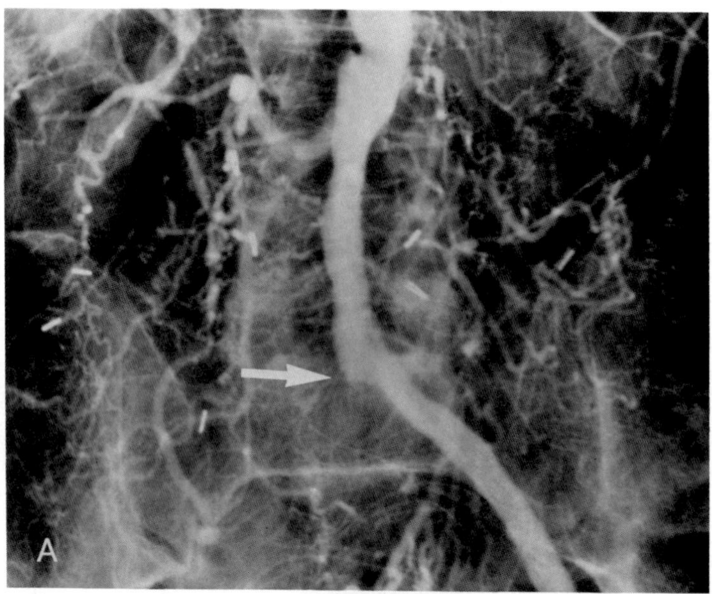

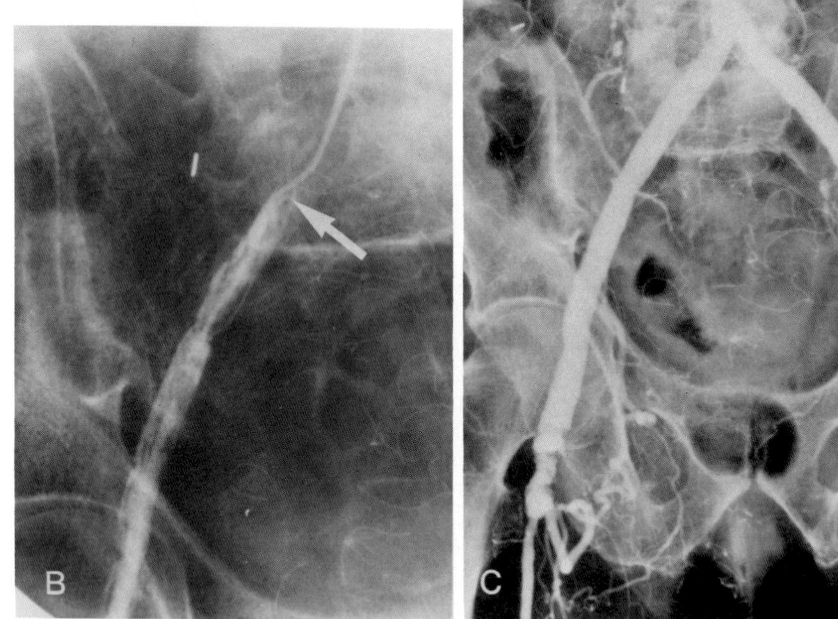

Figure 46.12. Regional thrombolysis with streptokinase. *A*, *Arrow* points to occluded right limb of an aortobifemoral bypass graft. The occlusion was acute by clinical history. *B*, A catheter has been positioned with the tip (*arrow*) in the occluded graft. Contrast injection shows partial resolution of thrombus after infusion of streptokinase through the arterial catheter at 2000 IU per minute for 40 minutes. *C*, Thrombus completely resolved after additional intraarterial infusion of streptokinase at 5000 IU per hour for 12 hours.

is to diagnose reversible or specifically treatable causes of acute renal failure. In patients with primary renal injury, aortography and renal arteriography provide the means for early diagnosis in the following situations:

1. *Renal arterial embolism*. Approximately 10% of arterial emboli involve visceral organs, including the kidneys. Although the radionuclide flow study establishes the presence or absence of blood flow into the kidney, aortography and se-

lective renal arteriography reveal proximal and distal occlusions, allowing clearer assessment.

2. *Renal arterial thrombosis.* Whether thrombosis is due to trauma, operation, or extension of a thrombotic process from the abdominal aorta, aortography has similar value and indications as in cases of renal arterial embolism.
3. *Renal failure in the immediate period after renal transplantation.* This may be due to hyperacute rejection or thrombosis at the site of the vessel anastomosis. Simple lumbar aortography or ipsilateral iliac arteriography can confirm or exclude the latter diagnosis.
4. *Atypical course for acute vasomotor nephropathy.* If acute renal parenchymal disease, vasculitis, cortical necrosis, or undiagnosed chronic renal parenchymal disease is suspected on clinical grounds, renal arteriography is helpful in conjunction with renal biopsy to avoid "sampling errors" of the biopsy if the disease process is not uniformly distributed throughout the kidney.

Bowel Ischemia

In the diagnosis and management of patients with suspected acute, extensive bowel ischemia, keep in mind that early diagnosis on the basis of physical findings alone is difficult and often impossible. A high index of suspicion and emergency angiography are essential to confirm or to exclude its presence. In addition, organic occlusions of the mesenteric artery must be differentiated from low-flow states (nonocclusive ischemia) because the treatment is different. This differentiation can be made only with angiography. No complex "superselective" arteriography is necessary to evaluate these patients. Abdominal aortography with superior mesenteric arteriography are sufficient for diagnostic and therapeutic purposes.

Figure 46.13 shows a classification of bowel is-

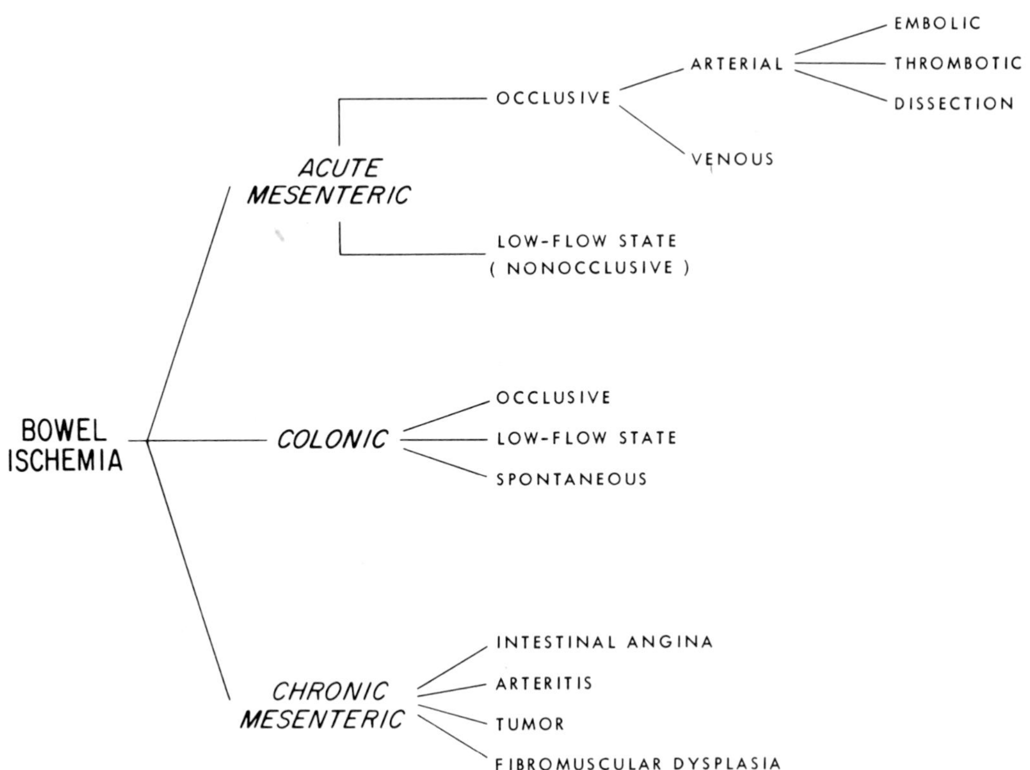

Figure 46.13. Classification of bowel ischemia.

chemia based on pathophysiology and clinical manifestations. The signs and symptoms that alert the clinician to the possibility of acute bowel ischemia are described in Chapter 33. This discussion is limited to the application of emergency angiography.

Occlusive Disease. Obstruction of the superior mesenteric artery resulting in acute bowel ischemia is evenly divided between acute thrombosis due to atheroma and due to embolism. Occasionally, dissection of the abdominal aorta involving the mesenteric artery is the underlying cause. Intestinal infarction secondary to mesenteric venous obstruction accounts for less than 10% of acute occlusive ischemia.

As soon as the diagnosis of bowel ischemia is suspected and while initial measures for fluid replacement and restoration of normal cardiac function are being taken, plain films of the abdomen should be obtained, followed by mesenteric angiography. The plain films are useful in providing baseline information concerning the intestinal gas pattern and in excluding the presence of free intraperitoneal air from a perforated viscus. Angiography must be performed on an emergency basis. It takes approximately 6 hours from the onset of ischemia to infarction.

Biplane abdominal aortography must be performed first, to evaluate the origin of the mesenteric arteries in the lateral projection. If the diagnosis is not made at aortography, superior mesenteric arteriography is then performed to establish the level of the occlusion, the presence of additional distal arterial occlusions, the degree and extent of collateral vessel development, and the patency of the mesenteric veins (Fig. 46.14).

Thrombosis more often involves the origin or proximal segment of the superior mesenteric artery, whereas emboli usually lodge at bifurcations, most often at the takeoff of the middle colic artery. Atheromatous lesions of the origins of the mesenteric arteries are common in patients without symptoms of bowel ischemia. The clinical presentation and the presence or absence of large collateral vessels during selective mesenteric arteriography should help determine the significance of a superior mesenteric arterial stenosis or occlusion. Midstream abdominal aortography can also demonstrate aortic dissection when this is the underlying cause for bowel ischemia.

Low-flow State. In this condition, otherwise referred to as nonocclusive bowel ischemia, ischemia may proceed to infarction without occlusion of

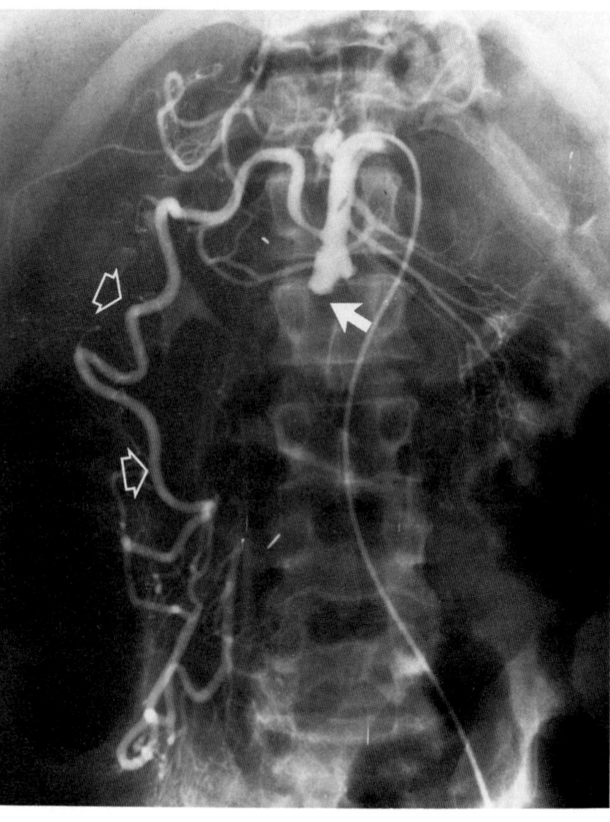

Figure 46.14. Embolic occlusion of superior mesenteric artery in patient with myocardial infarction and mural thrombus. Superior mesenteric arteriogram shows complete occlusion of superior mesenteric artery distal to origin of first jejunal and middle colic arteries (*solid arrow*). The *open arrows* point to dilated middle and right colic arteries that serve as collateral pathways to the distal ileum and right colon.

major mesenteric arteries or veins. Experimental investigations and clinical observations suggest that profound mesenteric vasoconstriction occurs because of diminished cardiac output. Hypovolemia is a prominent factor in the development of ischemic symptoms in these patients. Thus, the entity is seen in patients with recent myocardial infarction and congestive heart failure and in patients who have undergone a major thoracic or abdominal operation. Digitalis, which is a potent mesenteric vasoconstrictive agent, has been implicated as a contributing factor. The consistent process in all of these clinical situations is decreased mesenteric blood flow.

Abdominal aortography in the anteroposterior and lateral projections shows that the origins and main trunks of the mesenteric arteries are patent. Mesenteric arteriography demonstrates vasoconstriction characterized by narrowing at the origins of the branches of the superior mesenteric artery, irregularities and spasm of the arcades, and incomplete filling of intramural vessels. These changes may reverse after intraarterial infusion of vasodilator drugs into the superior mesentric artery; if they do not, the implication is that intestinal infarction has already occurred.

In view of the extremely high mortality and the increasing frequency of bowel ischemia secondary to low-flow states, a diagnostic and therapeutic approach has been developed consisting of mesenteric angiography as soon as the diagnosis of acute bowel ischemia is strongly suspected (Fig. 46.15). In the absence of organic large-vessel occlusion and in the presence of local or generalized mesenteric vasoconstriction, drug infusion into the mesenteric artery is started in an attempt to reverse vasoconstriction, promote bowel perfusion, and prevent further extension of the ischemic process to infarction.

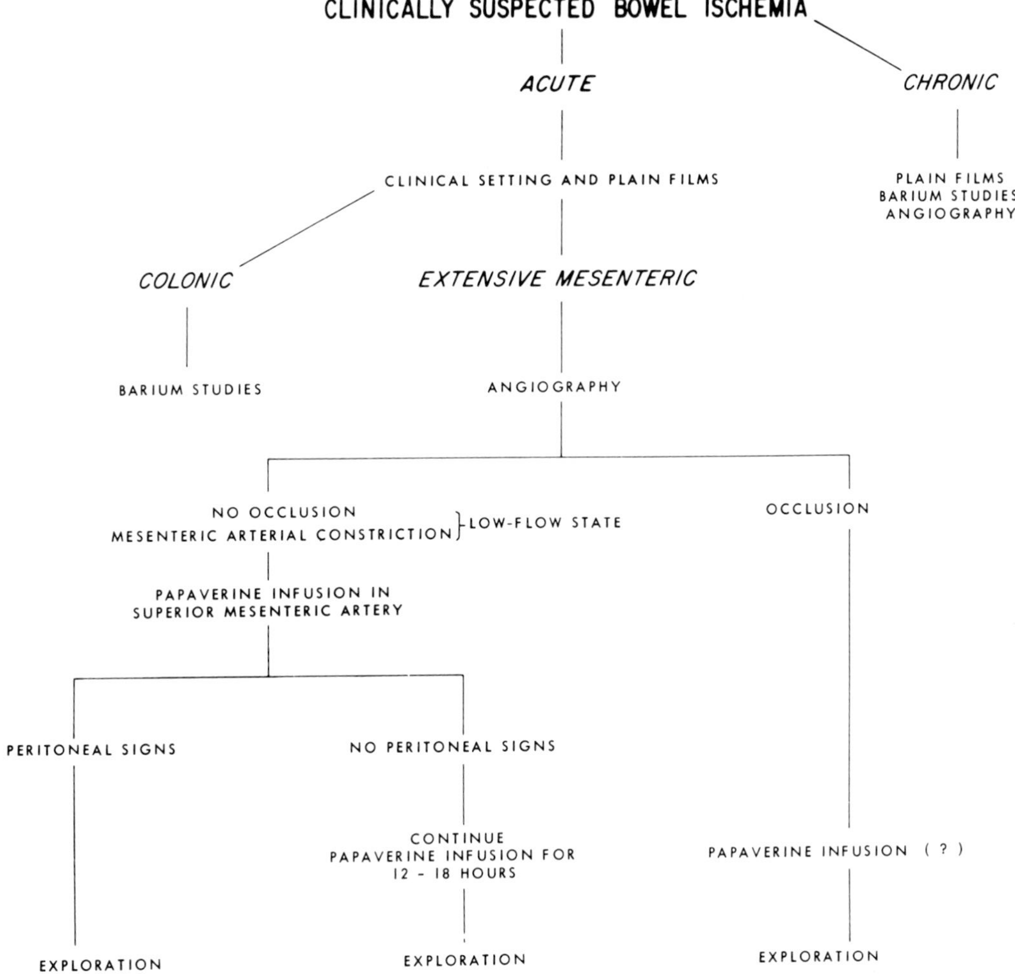

Figure 46.15. Sequence of radiologic procedures with clinically suspected bowel ischemia.

Most clinical experience has been with papaverine, 30–60 mg/hr for 12–18 hours. In the absence of peritoneal signs, this is a reasonable alternative to abdominal exploration. During infusion, measures are taken for adequate volume support, improvement of cardiac function, and control of sepsis. At the end of the infusion, abdominal exploration is commonly undertaken for resection of persisting ischemic bowel segments.

HEMORRHAGE

The objectives of emergency angiography in the hemorrhaging patient are to determine the source of bleeding and to control the hemorrhage with nonsurgical means. The latter is accomplished with infusions of vasoconstrictive drugs or with transcatheter embolization of the bleeding vessels.

Hemorrhage resulting from trauma and its angiographic control have already been discussed. The following sections focus on the application of angiography in gastrointestinal hemorrhage and in bleeding caused by neoplasia and inflammation.

Gastrointestinal Hemorrhage

Emergency angiography cannot and should not be applied to every patient with acute gastrointestinal hemorrhage. It should be reserved for those patients who continue to bleed despite conservative measures and in whom intervention is considered for control of the hemorrhage. Again, angiographic examination for such patients can provide accurate localization of the bleeding site with possible determination of etiology. It can also control the bleeding site angiographically, thus avoiding a surgical intervention.

Upper Gastrointestinal Bleeding

Determination of Bleeding Site. The sources of massive gastrointestinal bleeding are equally distributed among peptic ulcerations, gastric mucosal lesions, and ruptured esophageal varices. Gastric mucosal conditions include stress bleeding associated with major trauma, operation, or sepsis.

After initial measures are taken for volume repletion, determination of the bleeding site is the next important step in patient management. Endoscopy is the method of choice. Angiography is performed only when endoscopy is difficult to perform or is inconclusive. Timing the arteriogram to coincide with active bleeding is essential because extravasation is very often the only angiographic finding. This makes a functioning nasogastric tube an essential component of any study. Midstream abdominal aortography is performed in patients with a history of an abdominal aortic reconstructive procedure or a clinically apparent abdominal aortic aneurysm. The purpose is to detect an aortoenteric fistula. If there is no such history or suspicion, celiac axis arteriography is performed. If findings are normal, left gastric, gastroduodenal, splenic, and/or superior mesenteric arteriography follows. In 80–95% of patients with persistent red gastric aspirate on irrigation, arteriography demonstrates contrast medium extravasation at the bleeding site (Fig. 46.16).

In approximately 70% of patients with gastric mucosal hemorrhage, bleeding is shown at angiography to originate from the left gastric artery. It is therefore essential that this vessel be opacified during an emergency angiographic examination. Celiac axis arteriography would not suffice if the catheter tip were placed and the contrast medium injected distal to the origin of the left gastric artery or if the left gastric artery did not originate from the celiac axis. The supraduodenal branch of the gastroduodenal artery is the site of extravasation in most patients with bleeding duodenal ulcers (Fig. 46.17).

If no arterial extravasation site from any potential arterial feeder is identified, but gastroesophageal varices are demonstrated during the venous phase, and if gastric aspirate continues to be pink or red, ruptured gastroesophageal varices are assumed to be the source of hemorrhage. Therefore, the diagnosis of variceal bleeding by angiographic means is a diagnosis of exclusion. Contrast medium extravasation is rarely seen from a ruptured varix because, by the time the medium reaches the veins, it is diluted, and it cannot be visualized on serial radiographs unless bleeding is massive.

Control of Hemorrhage with Angiographic Methods. When the bleeding site has been determined with endoscopy or angiography, angiographic methods may be applied for the control of hemorrhage in those patients who continue to bleed despite conservative measures. The purpose is to avoid emergency operative intervention. Angiographic methods for the control of bleeding include infusion of vasopressin and occlusion of the bleeding vessel by embolization.

The best results from the infusion of vasopressin for control of bleeding from an arterial source are obtained with vasopressin infused directly into the bleeding artery. This is the left gastric artery in most patients with gastric mucosal hemorrhage and the gastroduodenal artery in patients with bleeding pyloroduodenal ulcers.

The step-by-step procedure follows:

1. A baseline arteriogram is obtained to show contrast medium extravasation.
2. Vasopressin, 0.2 unit/min, is infused for 20 minutes into the left gastric or the gastroduodenal artery with a constant infusion pump.
3. The arteriogram is repeated. If extravasation

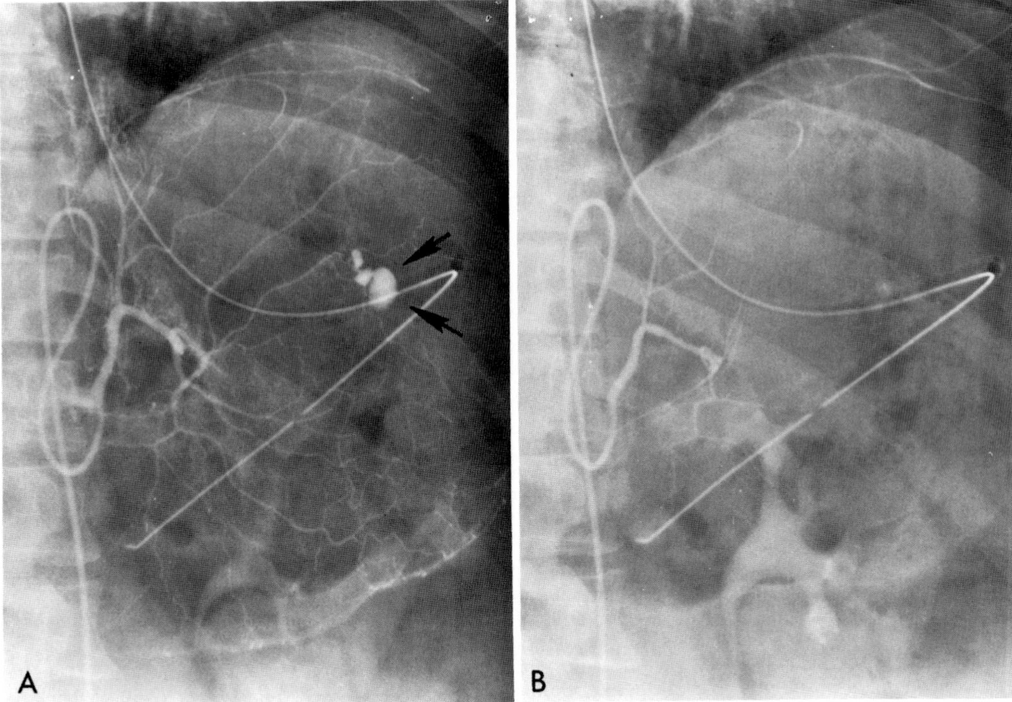

Figure 46.16. Stress bleeding in stomach controlled with infusion of vasopressin into left gastric artery. Upper gastrointestinal bleeding occurred in a patient with massive trauma and sepsis. *A*, Left gastric arteriogram shows extravasation of contrast medium at bleeding site in stomach (*arrows*). *B*, Left gastric arteriogram repeated 20 minutes after infusion of vasopressin at 0.2 unit/min shows constriction of branches of left gastric artery and no extravasation. Infusion was continued for 48 hours, and bleeding was controlled. (Reproduced by permission, from Athanasoulis CA, Waltman AC, Novelline RA, et al. *Radiol Clin North Am*, 1976;14:265–280, WB Saunders.)

persists, the infusion rate is increased to 0.4 unit/min and the arteriogram repeated 20 minutes later. If bleeding continues to persist, chances are that it will not be controlled pharmacologically. Further increase of the infusion rate is not recommended.

4. When the optimal infusion rate is established, the patient is transferred to an intensive care unit, for monitoring, with the catheter in place, and infusion is continued.
5. If there is no further clinical evidence of bleeding, the patient is weaned from the vasopressin by slowly decreasing the infusion rate over the next 12–36 hours. At this point, 5% dextrose in water is substituted for vasopressin and the catheter removed a few hours later.
6. If bleeding occurs at any time during infusion, the position of the catheter tip needs to be confirmed. Although this can be done with a portable radiograph, the patient is preferably transported to the angiographic suite for repeated arteriography.

When catheterization of the celiac axis branches is technically difficult or impossible, vasopressin can be infused into the celiac axis itself. Clinical, biochemical, and experimental data have shown that such infusions are not associated with hepatic ischemia.

With intraarterial infusion of vasopressin, bleeding is controlled in 80% of patients with gastric mucosal hemorrhage and in 50% of patients with bleeding duodenal ulcers. Recurrent bleeding occurs in 16% of patients with gastric mucosal hemorrhage. Angiography and vasopressin infusion may be repeated when bleeding recurs.

Complications of vasopressin infusion include reduction of urinary output (antidiuretic hormone effect), water retention, and possible severe hyponatremia. Occasionally, bradycardia and hypertension occur. Bowel ischemia and infarction should not occur as a result of vasopressin infusion, if arteriography is performed to assess the degree of vasoconstriction produced with a given infusion rate.

Transcatheter arterial embolization is considered in patients in whom intraarterial infusion of vasopressin fails to control gastroduodenal hemorrhage from arterial sources. For this purpose, it is essential that the tip of the catheter be positioned in the vessel supplying the extravasation point. Absorba-

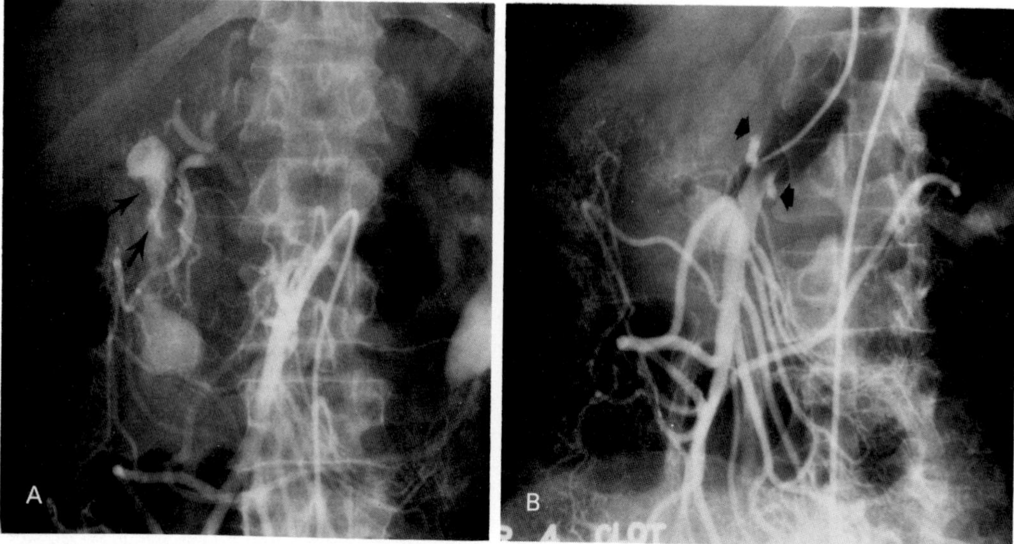

Figure 46.17. Bleeding from duodenal ulcer controlled with transcatheter embolization. A 60-year-old man had carcinoma of the colon metastatic to the liver and porta hepatis with upper gastrointestinal bleeding. Endoscopy showed a duodenal ulcer. An operative procedure with ligation of the right hepatic artery did not control the bleeding. *A*, Superior mesenteric arteriogram shows extravasation in duodenum (*arrows*) from branches of gastroduodenal artery. *B*, Following embolization of anterior and posterior branches of inferior pancreaticoduodenal artery, a repeated arteriogram shows no extravasation. *Arrows* point to occluded branches of inferior pancreaticoduodenal artery. There was no recurrent bleeding at 6 months after embolization.

ble surgical gelatin (Gelfoam), in the form of small plugs (1 mm × 1 mm) or polyvinyl alcohol (Ivalon), in the form of multiple 500–1000 μm granules, are the materials currently used (Fig. 46.18).

The following guidelines are observed during transcatheter arterial embolization in the gastrointestinal tract:

1. Diffuse gastric mucosal hemorrhage is best treated with intraarterial vasopressin and not with transcatheter embolization.
2. A discrete bleeding point in the stomach supplied by a single arterial branch is amenable to control with embolization, if superselective catheterization is possible.
3. For bleeding duodenal ulcers, embolization may be considered as the primary mode of angiographic therapy. Collateral bleeding from the pancreaticoduodenal branches of the superior mesenteric artery must be considered and excluded after embolization of the gastroduodenal artery.
4. Intense inflammatory reaction surrounding a bleeding site associated with penetrating peptic ulcer or pancreatic abscess may prevent the arteries from constricting in response to vasopressin. Embolization should be considered as an alternative.
5. Skill, experience, and good judgment are important in the application of embolization for bleeding control. Bleeding from pyloroduodenal sites is not as well-controlled angiographically as are those from esophagogastric sites; surgical treatment alternatives should be discussed fully before undertaking attempts at embolization.

Vasopressin infusion may be used for control of bleeding esophageal varices. Vasopressin infused in the superior mesenteric artery reduces portal venous pressure and may arrest bleeding from gastroesophageal varices. The infusion rate is 0.2 unit/min for 24–36 hours, followed by 0.1 unit/min for an additional 24 hours.

This form of therapy has been replaced by low-dose intravenous administration of vasopressin. Similarities exist between mesenteric arterial and intravenous infusions of vasopressin in regard to the effect on mesenteric blood flow and portal venous pressure reduction. Cardiac output reduction is no greater with intravenous administration than with mesenteric infusion of vasopressin (10–15% with both modes). The regimen for intravenous infusion of vasopressin is 0.3 unit/min for 24 hours, followed by 0.2 unit/min for 24 hours, followed by 0.1 unit/min for an additional 24 hours.

The efficacy of vasopressin infusion in controlling bleeding from ruptured varices depends on the patient's clinical status and the severity of the un-

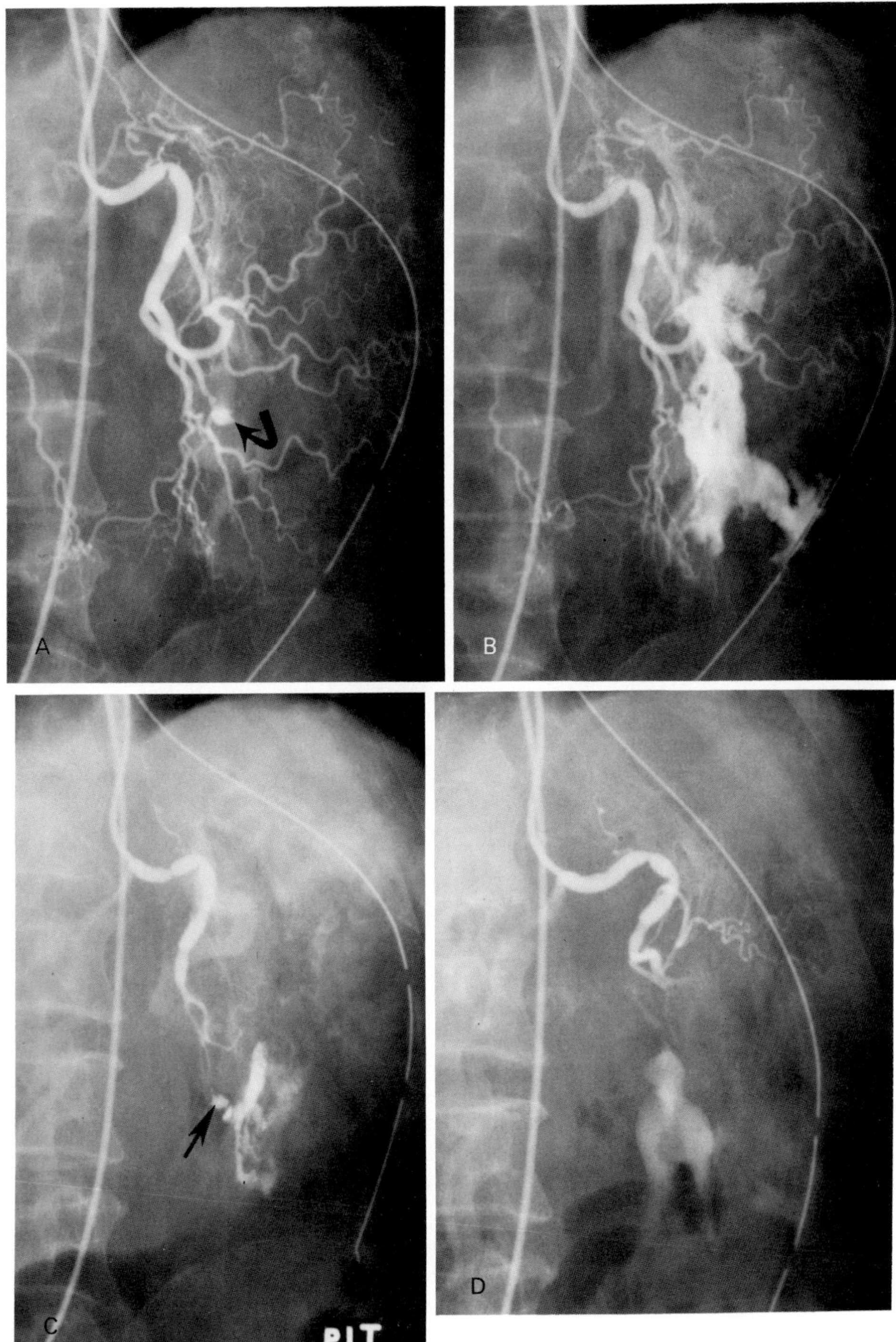

Figure 46.18. Bleeding gastric ulcer controlled with left gastric artery embolization. A 54-year-old woman, an alcoholic, had massive upper gastrointestinal bleeding. Endoscopy showed a bleeding ulcer of the lesser curvature. *A*, Left gastric arteriogram shows contrast medium extravasation at bleeding site (*arrow*). *B*, Massive extravasation of contrast medium is noted during late phase. *C*, Left gastric arteriogram following infusion of vasopressin at 0.2 unit/min for 20 minutes in left gastric artery shows constriction of branches of left gastric artery and persistent extravasation (*arrow*). *D*, The bleeding branch of left gastric artery was embolized with surgical gelatin. Repeated arteriogram shows no extravasation. The bleeding was clinically controlled, and the patient was discharged.

derlying hepatic disease. Bleeding is controlled in 90–95% of patients in Child's group A; 75% in group B; and 55% in group C.

An alternative angiographic method to control variceal bleeding is transhepatic occlusion of the coronary vein. In this technique, the portal venous system is entered and the coronary vein selectively catheterized via a percutaneous transhepatic route. The method is simple, and the risk of intraperitoneal hemorrhage from the point of entry in the liver is negligible. The coronary vein may be occluded with balloon catheters, blood clots, or surgical gelatin.

The utilization of this procedure is controversial and, at present, seems best reserved for those patients with bleeding varices who fail endoscopic sclerotherapy, vasopressin infusion, and/or balloon tamponade. Transhepatic occlusion of the coronary vein and varices serve as an alternative to emergency transthoracic ligation of varices for the acute control of hemorrhage, thereby allowing adequate preparation of the patient before an elective decompression shunt procedure (Fig. 46.19).

Lower Gastrointestinal Bleeding

It was mentioned earlier that in patients with upper gastrointestinal bleeding, endoscopy should be performed to establish the source. However, in patients bleeding from a source distal to the ligament of Treitz, endoscopy is of limited value. Angiography is the procedure of choice for determination of the bleeding site. For best results, mesenteric arteriography, to include the superior and inferior mesenteric and celiac arteries, should be performed on an emergency basis, at the time of active bleeding, so that the source can be identified with the demonstration of contrast medium extravasation.

Diverticular Hemorrhage. Colonic diverticulosis is the most common cause of massive lower gastrointestinal hemorrhage. The only reliable angiographic finding of a bleeding diverticulum is that of contrast medium extravasation. Thus, correct timing of the arteriogram with the occurrence of active bleeding is essential to the localization and diagnosis. If there is marked hemodynamic instability with obvious brisk hematochezia, the chances of a positive arteriographic study, if performed expeditiously, are good. However, the colon is a retentive organ, and often the diverticular bleeding is intermittent; the clinical assessment of moment-to-moment activity of the bleeding can be poor. In these instances, radionuclide bleeding studies with either ^{99m}Tc-in vivo-labeled red blood cells or ^{99m}Tc sulfur colloid may be helpful in the timing of a diagnostic arteriographic study.

Originally, bleeding diverticula were presumed more common in the right colon. More recent experience has suggested that there is an equal distribution of bleeding diverticula between the right and the left colon. Both superior and inferior mesenteric artery injections must therefore be carried out and, if negative, a celiac axis injection performed. On occasion, either an upper gastrointestinal hemorrhage is missed clinically and mistaken for lower gastrointestinal, or anomalous supply to the colon arising from the celiac axis, or pathologic process supplied by the celiac axis, can result in colonic bleeding.

If extravasation is demonstrated from a bleeding diverticulum, it very often pools within the diverticulum, outlining it, thereby making the diagnosis. Vasopressin may be infused in the proximal superior or inferior mesenteric artery to control the bleeding (Fig. 46.20). The infusion schedule is comparable to that described for upper gastrointestinal hemorrhage. With mesenteric arterial infusion of vasopressin, bleeding from colonic diverticulosis is controlled in approximately 80% of patients. The management of patients subsequent to the acute control of hemorrhage is debated. Approximately one-half of these patients have recurrent hemorrhage, at which time segmental colonic resection is carried out on the basis of the previous angiographic findings. Patients who do not bleed again and who do not undergo operation require a barium enema examination or colonoscopy, or both, to exclude neoplasm or other lesion.

Colonic Angiodysplasia. Angiodysplasia of the cecum and ascending colon is a potential source of massive rectal bleeding, particularly in elderly patients. The lesion is diagnosed by angiography based on the following findings (Fig. 46.21):

1. Clusters of small arteries are seen during the arterial phase adjacent to the ileocecal valve or in the ascending colon;
2. Contrast medium accumulates in vascular spaces;
3. Early opacification of the veins draining the cecum or the ascending colon, or both;
4. Intense opacification of the draining veins persists late in the venous phase.

Contrast medium extravasation may be seen if bleeding is active at the time of arteriography. Hemorrhage may be temporarily arrested with infusion of vasopressin. The definitive therapy, however, is right colectomy.

Angiodysplasia is neither seen nor palpated by the surgeon, and the pathologist has difficulty in grossly identifying the lesion in resected specimens. Injection of the vessels of the specimen with silicone rubber and examination of the clear specimen under the dissecting microscope have made it possible to identify angiodysplasia in patients in

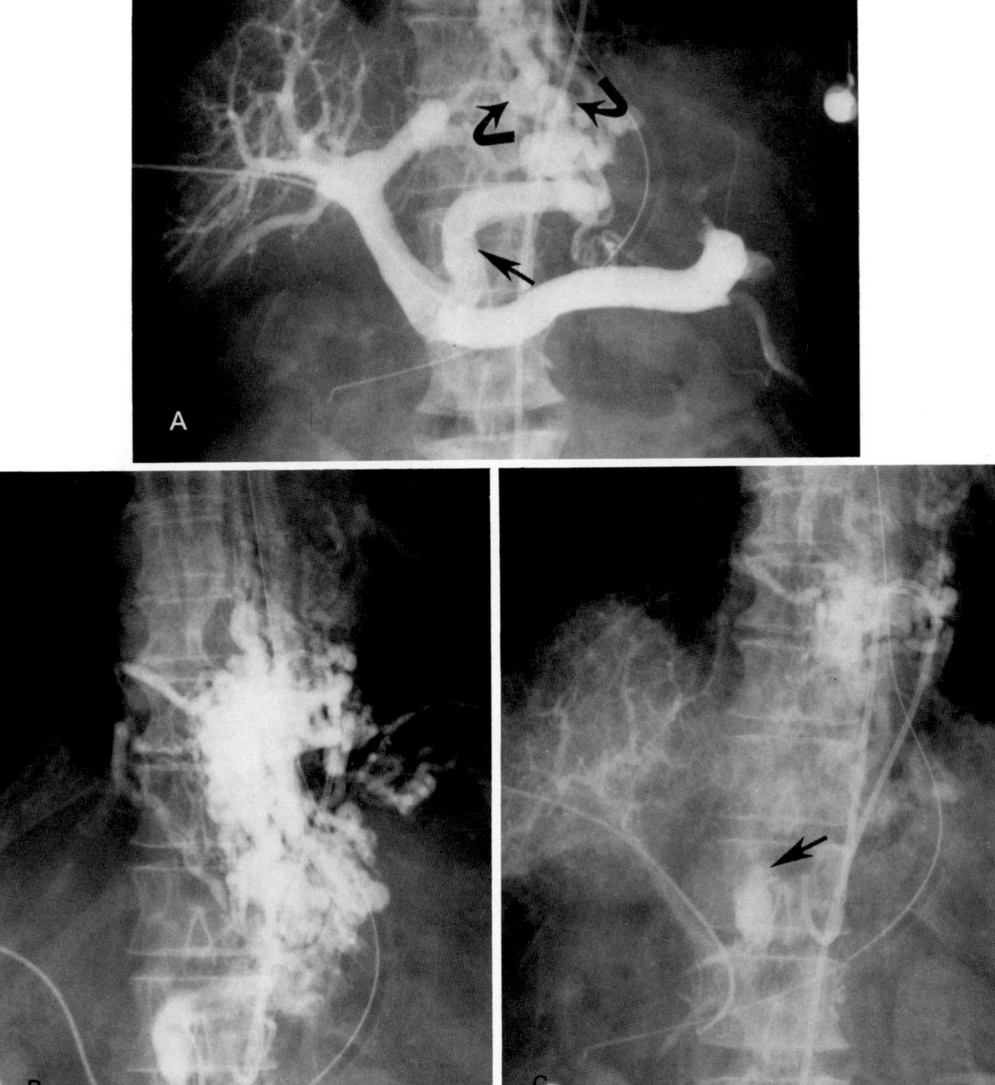

Figure 46.19. Transhepatic obliteration of coronary vein and gastroesophageal varices for control of variceal bleeding. A 65-year-old man had cirrhosis of the liver, portal hypertension, and bleeding gastroesophageal varices. Conservative measures including intravenous infusions of vasopressin and placement of a Sengstaken-Blakemore tube had failed to control bleeding. *A*, Transhepatic catheterization of portal vein. Contrast medium was injected with tip of catheter in splenic vein. There is hepatofugal flow through an enlarged coronary vein (*straight arrow*). The coronary vein drains into massive gastroesophageal varices (*curved arrows*). *B*, Selective coronary vein injection shows extent of gastric and esophageal varices. *C*, Coronary vein was obliterated with injection of several plugs of surgical gelatin. Repeated study following embolization shows stump of coronary vein (*arrow*).

whom the lesions were diagnosed by angiographic examination. Histologic study reveals dilated vascular spaces corresponding to thin-walled channels in the submucosa.

A higher incidence of bleeding from colonic angiodysplasia occurs among patients with aortic stenosis; however, a cause-and-effect relationship between these entities has not been established.

Intraabdominal Hemorrhage. Hemorrhage into the peritoneal cavity or retroperitoneum unre-

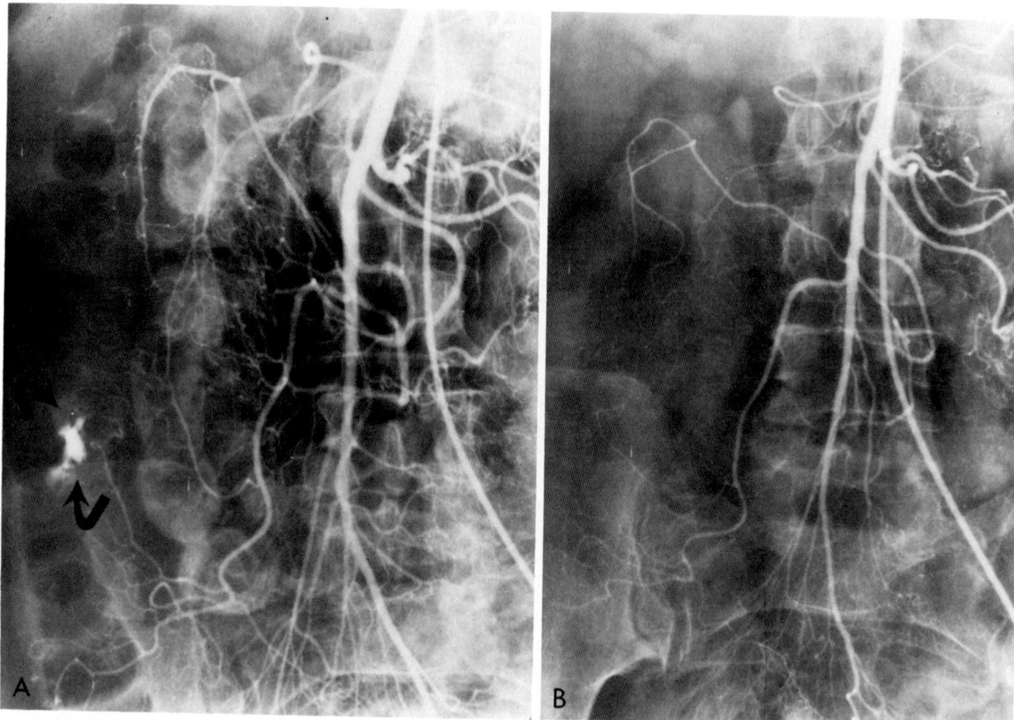

Figure 46.20. Bleeding from diverticulum of ascending colon controlled with intraarterial infusion of vasopressin. A 59-year-old woman had massive rectal bleeding. *A*, Superior mesenteric arteriogram shows extravasation of contrast medium (*arrows*) in ascending colon. *B*, Superior mesenteric arteriogram following 20-minute infusion of vasopressin at 0.2 unit/min into superior mesenteric artery. There is constriction of branches of superior mesenteric artery and no extravasation. Infusion was continued for 48 hours, and bleeding was clinically controlled. Subsequent barium enema showed diverticula of right and left colon. (Reproduced by permission, from Athanasoulis CA, Waltman AC, Novelline RA, et al. *Radiol Clin North Am*, 1976;14:265–280. WB Saunders).

lated to trauma may be due to a neoplasm, inflammation, or other condition affecting the vessels. If hemorrhage is massive, there is little time for diagnostic procedures before exploration. If, on the other hand, vital signs are maintained and the condition is stable after the initial episode, the patient may be evaluated with angiography so that the optimal operative procedure can be planned.

Tumors of the kidneys, liver, and retroperitoneum manifested by hemorrhage can be diagnosed with angiography, their local extent established, and the vascular supply defined. Hemorrhage is controlled with balloon-tipped catheters or embolization so that the definitive surgical procedure can be performed under more favorable conditions than as an emergency.

Pancreatitis may at times be complicated by retroperitoneal hemorrhage from erosion into surrounding vessels. The same diagnostic and therapeutic possibilities of angiography are applicable as with hemorrhage from tumors (Fig. 46.22).

Ruptured or ''leaking'' abdominal aortic aneurysms have been discussed. Aneurysms of the splenic, hepatic, and renal arteries also rupture. When they do, they may be diagnosed and their location determined with abdominal aortography. Transcatheter occlusion with embolization may be attempted either preoperatively or as definitive therapy.

Postoperative Bleeding

Hemorrhage into the abdominal cavity or gastrointestinal tract directly related to an operative procedure is uncommon. When it does not subside with conservative management, it may be controlled with infusion of vasopressin or transcatheter embolization. A second exploration can thus be prevented. In most instances, bleeding into the gastrointestinal tract secondary to a slipped ligature, biopsy, or polypectomy via the colonoscope can best be controlled with selective infusion of vasopressin into the bleeding artery. Embolization, on the other hand, is the method of choice for control of bleeding from the uterus, cervix, prostate gland, or blad-

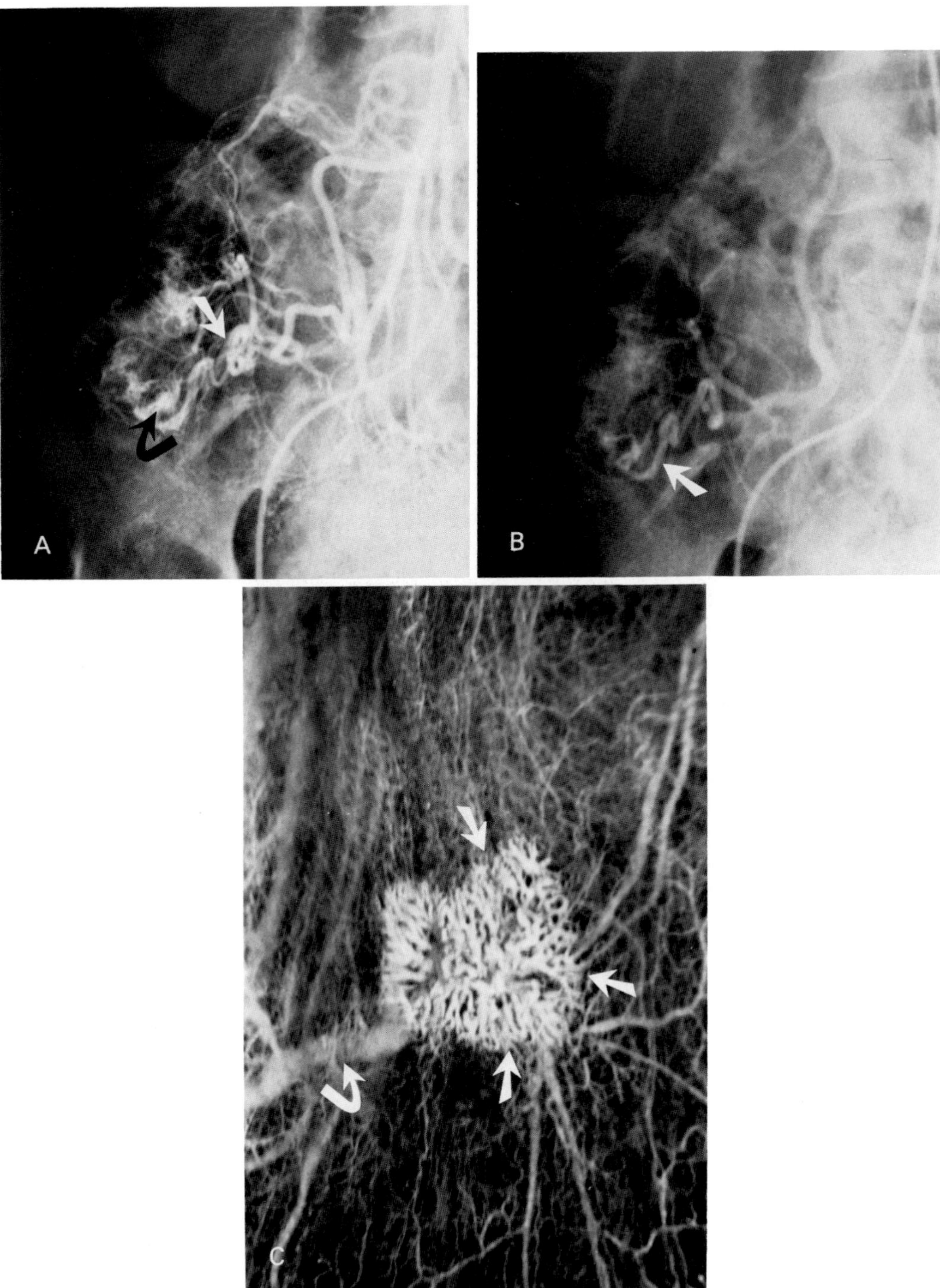

Figure 46.21. Angiodysplasia of cecum as source of rectal bleeding. A 60-year-old man had multiple episodes of rectal bleeding. Repeated barium studies and colonoscopy were unrevealing. *A*, Detailed view of cecum in superior mesenteric arteriogram. During arterial phase, there is simultaneous opacification of an artery and a vein. *Curved arrow* points to vascular tuft in antemesenteric border of cecum. *Straight arrow* points to early draining vein. *B*, In late phase of superior mesenteric arteriogram, there is intense, persistent opacification of vein draining the lesion in the cecum (*arrow*). *C*, Angiodysplasia of colon (resected specimen) as seen under the dissecting miscroscope. Vessels have been injected with silicone rubber, and tissues have been cleared with dehydration of specimen and immersion in methyl salicylate. *Straight arrows* point to several dilated vascular structures—mostly veins—that have assumed the typical appearance of angiodysplasia resembling a coral. *Curved arrow* points to a large draining vein in the submucosa.

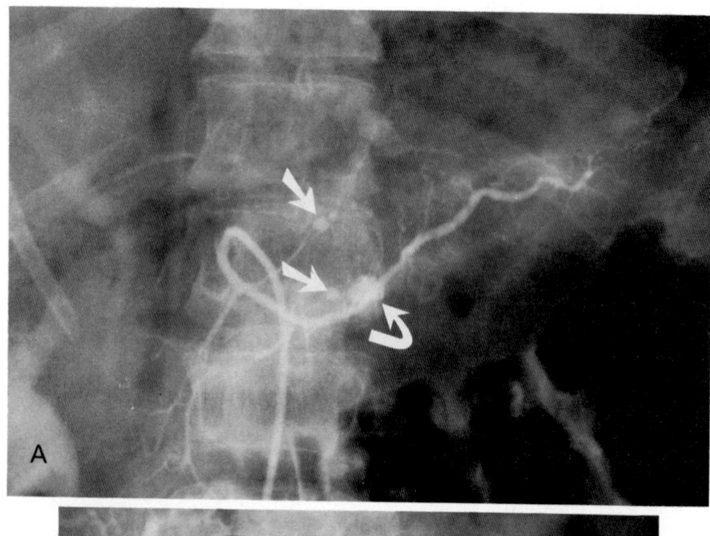

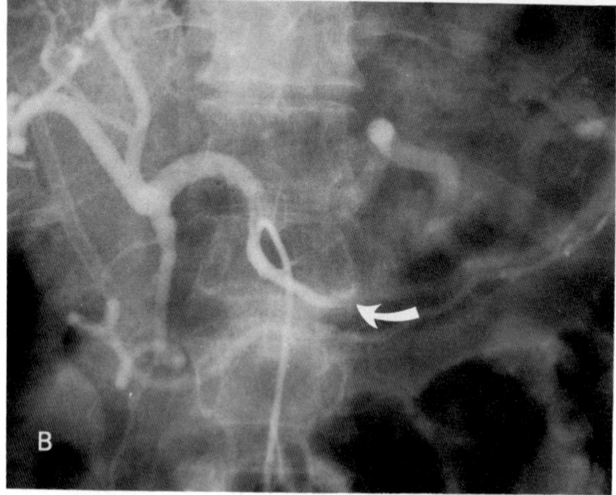

Figure 46.22. Retroperitoneal bleeding from ruptured aneurysm of transverse pancreatic artery—bleeding controlled with transcatheter embolization. A 57-year-old man had recurrent pancreatitis and a decreasing hematocrit. *A*, Selective catheterization of dorsal pancreatic artery shows multiple small aneurysms (*straight arrows*), the result of pancreatitis, *Curved arrow* points to contrast medium extravasation secondary to rupture of one of these aneurysms. *B*, The dorsal pancreatic artery was occluded with introduction through the angiographic catheter of surgical gelatin plugs. Repeated arteriogram shows occlusion (*arrow*) and no extravasation. Clinically, the bleeding was controlled.

der after a pelvic operation (Fig. 46.23). The results are good with the exception of retroperitoneal bleeding after operation on the pancreas.

ACUTE PULMONARY EMBOLISM

Thromboembolic disease is a common problem that frequently complicates other diseases and other therapy. As diagnostic modalities have increased, the algorithms to evaluate patients suspected of having thromboembolic disease have become more complex and controversial. Pulmonary arteriography is still the "gold standard" examination in the detection and diagnosis of acute pulmonary embolism.

The need to establish the diagnosis of pulmonary embolism is stressed by an approximately 30% mortality rate in the untreated patient with symptomatic pulmonary emboli. The clinical symptoms (dyspnea, pain, and cough), physical examination, and laboratory tests are nonspecific and can be found with many common disease processes of the lungs and chest. Prompt radioiogic evaluation becomes essential to establish the diagnosis and to provide an estimate of the extent of the process.

The chest radiograph is helpful in revealing other

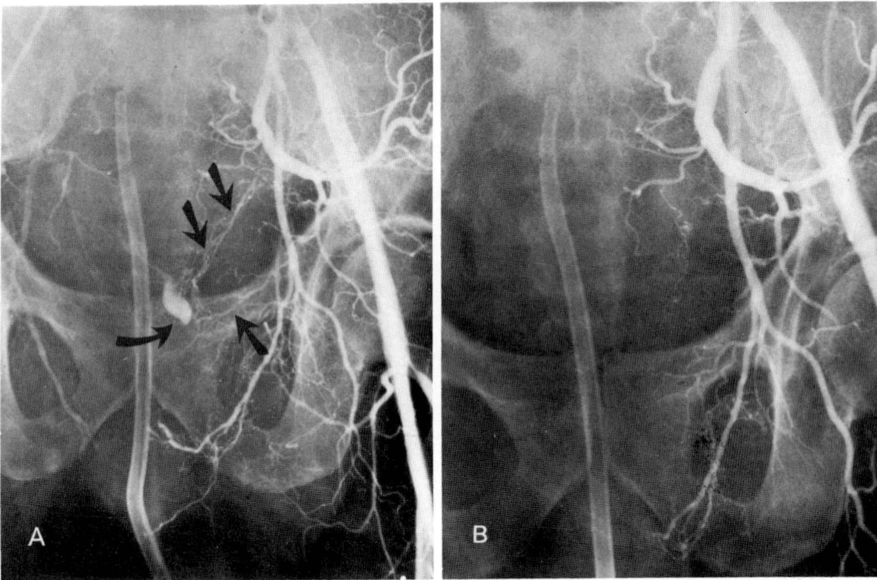

Figure 46.23. Bleeding in prostatic bed following transperineal biopsy controlled with transcatheter vessel occlusion. A 65-year-old man had an enlarged prostate gland. Transperineal biopsy was performed, followed by massive bleeding. *A*, Left common iliac arteriogram. *Curved arrow* points to extravasated contrast medium at bleeding site in prostatic bed. *Straight arrows* point to middle and superior vesical branches arising from left hypogastric artery. *B*, Left hypogastric arteriogram following embolization of vesical branches with surgical gelatin. There is no extravasation. Hematuria subsided subsequent to the procedure.

diagnoses that may have a similar clinical presentation and to help in the interpretation of ventilation and perfusion lung scans.

Perfusion lung scanning is helpful if normal. If the lung scan is normal, the chance of a pulmonary embolus is small. Unfortunately, less than 5% of lung scanning will yield normal results. Various patterns of abnormality have been described, allowing classifications of scans into either a low probability, indeterminate probability, or high probability classification for the presence of an embolus. Although clinical management decisions can occasionally be made based on these scans, these "probability" schema allow for an interpretation that is neither accurate nor certain in approximately 50% of patients submitted to lung scanning.

Pulmonary Arteriography

Pulmonary arteriography is specific in detecting pulmonary emboli.

Urgent pulmonary arteriography should be obtained in:

1. Patients with an indeterminate lung scan;
2. Patients with a mismatch of interpretation and clinical findings (e.g., strong clinical symptoms and low probability lung scan);
3. Patients at risk for anticoagulation with a high probability lung scan;
4. Prior to intervention (caval ligation, caval filter placement, systemic thrombolysis, or pulmonary embolectomy) to confirm the diagnosis;
5. Patients too ill to undergo or complete ventilation and perfusion lung scans.

Access to pulmonary arteriography is from the femoral vein. Injections of contrast material into the iliac veins and inferior vena cava are initially made. This provides information on the presence of thrombi in the inferior vena cava itself, and allows anatomic delineation of the inferior vena cava and its branches, in case of a contemplated caval interruption procedure. If there has been a caval ligation, or proven caval or iliofemoral thrombosis, the antecubital or jugular approaches are possible. If no thrombi are encountered, the right heart chambers are usually easily catheterized and bilateral selective pulmonary injections performed. Pulmonary arterial pressures should be taken prior to injections.

Single plane filming in anteroposterior and ipsilateral posterior oblique projections are usually adequate to diagnose or exclude pulmonary emboli; in rare circumstances, additional projections or the use of balloon occlusion catheters are required. Magnification permits enlarging and separating of the vessels under study.

The diagnosis is established with the demonstration of an intraluminal filling defect or an abrupt

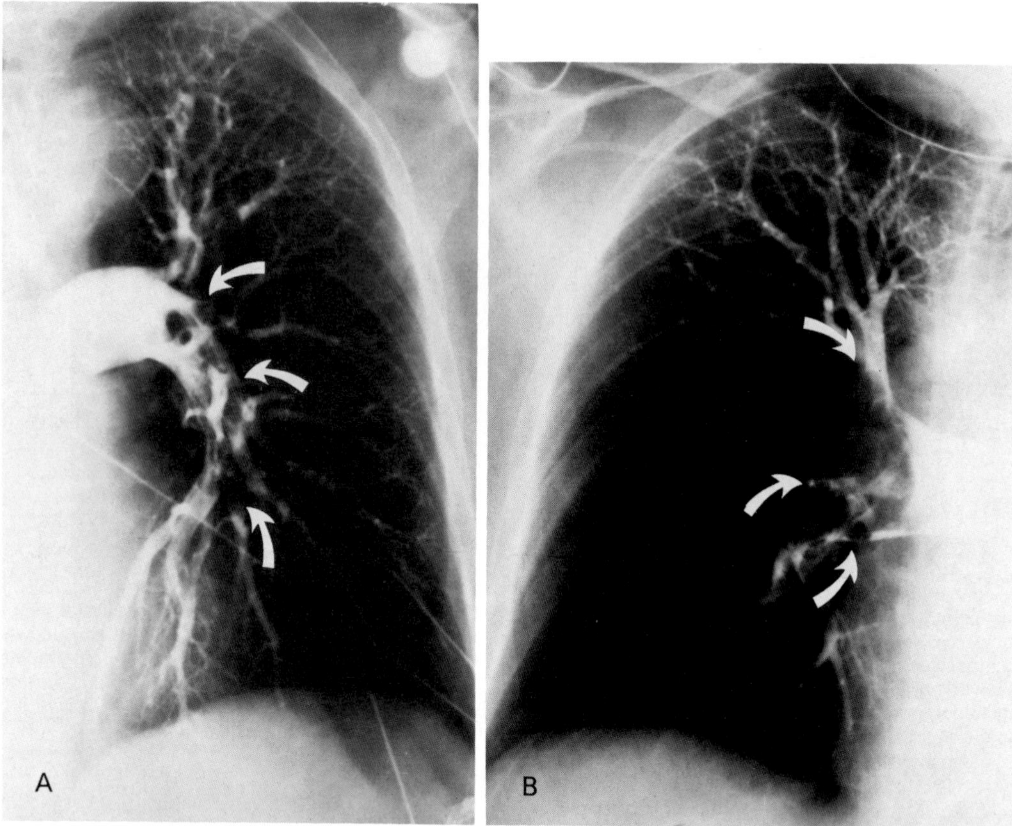

Figure 46.24. Angiography in diagnosis of pulmonary embolism. A 55-year-old woman had chest pain and shortness of breath after a pelvic operation. The lung scan showed perfusion defects. There had been a history of peptic ulcer with bleeding, and confirmation of pulmonary emboli became necessary. *A*, Left pulmonary arteriogram shows multiple intraluminal filling defects representing pulmonary emboli (*arrows*). *B*, Right pulmonary arteriogram shows obstruction of branches to middle and lower lobes by large embolus (*arrows*).

occlusion (''cutoff'') of an artery (Fig. 46.24). Poor flow to an area is insufficient evidence for this diagnosis; more selective injection and proper filming will demonstrate patency or abnormality.

Complications include small hematomas at the puncture site and occasional extrasystoles during catheter manipulation within the right heart. If the patient has left bundle branch block, the placement of a temporary pacing wire prior to the right heart catheterization is a wise precaution. Patients with marginal cardiac compensation may be forced into frank pulmonary edema and require appropriate therapy. Acute cardiopulmonary decompensation and arrest are the most feared, and fortunately uncommon, events (1–3/2000 patients). Patients with evidence of right heart failure or severe pulmonary hypertension (PA mean pressure $>$ 45 mm Hg) should have modifications in the performance of the examination. If severe pulmonary arterial hypertension is present, selective catheter positioning, reduced flow rates of injections, and the use of new low osmolar contrast media can help to reduce the potential for hemodynamic instability.

Transvenous Filter Interruption of the Inferior Vena Cava

Anticoagulation is the primary mode of therapy for patients with thromboembolic disease. However, there is a subset of patients who have either arteriographic or venographic documented thromboembolic disease, who either cannot receive anticoagulants or need additional protection against further pulmonary emboli. These patients usually fall into the following categories:

1. Have absolute contraindications to anticoagulation, such as active gastrointestinal, genitourinary, or intraabdominal bleeding;
2. Have severe relative contraindications to anti-

coagulation, such as a recent major surgical procedure or neurological lesion that may bleed;
3. Have had a complication of anticoagulation;
4. Have a documented recurrent pulmonary embolus while on adequate anticoagulation therapy;
5. Have severe pulmonary arterial hypertension and decompensation and can be anticoagulated, but need additional prophylaxis against further emboli.

These patients are candidates for interruption of the inferior vena cava.

The inferior vena cava can be interrupted either with a clip placed surgically or with a filter placed transvenously. The ease of placement and the avoidance of general anesthesia have made the filter method popular, especially among older patients with accompanying cancer, heart disease, or other problems. The Greenfield filter (Meditech, Inc., Watertown, MA) is currently most commonly used for transvenous interruption of the inferior vena cava. Although originally designed to be introduced via a surgically exposed venotomy, in either the right internal jugular or right femoral vein, angiographic techniques have now been developed to introduce these filters percutaneously. The right femoral vein and right jugular vein are still the approaches of choice, but a formal cut-down is occasionally required. Several new experimental percutaneous filter designs, including the Birdsnest filter, Amplatz filter, Gunther filter and Simon nitinol filter, are currently undergoing laboratory and clinical investigation to allow easier placement, more effective filtering, reduced caval thrombosis, and possible retrievability. It is best to perform these procedures in the angiography suite because fluoroscopy is necessary for accurate positioning of the filter in the infrarenal segment of the inferior vena cava. The diagnosis of the thromboembolic process is often made there, and now the filters can be placed through the same access routes as the diagnostic study.

With the Greenfield filter, the incidence of recurrent pulmonary embolism is 2%, and of inferior vena cava thrombosis distal to the filter, approximately 10%.

SUGGESTED READINGS

Athanasoulis CA, Pfister RC, Greene RE, et al., eds. *Interventional Radiology.* Philadelphia: WB Saunders 1982.

Athanasoulis CA, Baum S. Vascular disorders of the gut. Part III. Angiography. In Bockus HL, Berk JE, Haubrich WS, et al., eds. *Gastroenterology,* vol 4. 3rd ed. Philadelphia: WB Saunders, 1976, pp 329–358.

Athanasoulis, CA, Waltman AC, Baum S: Angiography of trauma. In Burke JF, Boyd RJ, McCabe CJ (eds): *Trauma Management.* Chicago: Year Book, 1988.

Athanasoulis CA, Baum S, Rosch J, et al. Mesenteric arterial infusions of vasopressin for hemorrhage from colonic diverticulosis. *Am J Surg,* 1975;129:212–216.

Athanasoulis CA, Waltman AC, Novelline RA, et al. Angiography: Its contribution to the emergency management of gastrointestinal hemorrhage. *Radiol Clin North Am,* 1976;14:265–280.

Baum S, Athanasoulis CA. Diagnostic studies in colonic afflictions. Part V. Angiography. In Bockus HL, Berk JR, Haubrich WS, et al., eds. *Gastroenterology,* vol 2. 3rd ed. Philadelphia: WB Saunders, 1976, pp 866–886.

Baum S, Athanasoulis CA, Waltman AC, et al. Gastrointestinal hemorrhage. II. Angiographic diagnosis and control. *Adv Surg,* 1973;7:149–198.

Ben-Menachem Y, ed. Angiography and interventional procedures in the traumatized patient. *Semin Interventional Radiol,* 1985;2:105–196.

Ben-Menachem Y. *Angiography in Trauma: A Work Atlas.* Philadelphia: WB Saunders, 1981.

Eckstein MR, Kelemouridis V, Athanasoulis CA et al. Gastric bleeding: therapy with intraarterial vasopressin and transcatheter embolization. *Radiology* 1984;152:643–646.

Freeark RJ. Role of angiography in the management of multiple injuries. *Surg Gynecol Obstet,* 1969;128:761–771.

Hauashi K, Meaney TF, Zelch JV, et al. Aortographic analysis of aortic dissection. *Am J Roentgenol Radium Ther Nucl Med,* 1974;122:769–782.

Hollenberg NK, Adams DF, Merrill JP, et al. Renal angiography in oliguria. In Abrams HL, ed. *Angiography,* vol 2. 2nd ed. Boston: Little, Brown & Co., 1971, pp 887–914.

Kadir S. *Diagnostic Angiography.* Philadelphia: WB Saunders, 1986.

Kelemouridis V, Eckstein MR, Geller SC, et al. Bleeding from the large bowel: results of therapy with pitressin or embolization. Presented at the 71st Scientific Assembly and Annual Meeting of the Radiological Society of America, Chicago, IL, November 17–22, 1985.

Lunderquist A, Vang J. Transhepatic catheterization and obliteration of the coronary vein in patients with portal hypertension and esophageal varices. *N Engl J Med,* 1974;291:646–649.

Meaney TF, Lalli AF, Alfidi RJ. *Complications and Legal Implications of Radiologic Special Procedures.* St Louis: CV Mosby, 1973.

Ring EJ, Athanasoulis C, Waltman AC, et al. Arteriographic management of hemorrhage following pelvic fracture. *Radiology,* 1973;109:65–70.

CHAPTER 47

Pediatric Radiography in the Emergency Department

THOMAS E. HERMAN, M.D.
ROBERT H. CLEVELAND, M.D.

Editor's note: This chapter contains the special radiographic features related to the special problems encountered in infants and children. A new chapter in Edition 3, it could equally have been placed in the new Section III.

The emergency physician is often called upon to interpret pediatric x-rays without the benefit of immediate radiologic consultation. This chapter reviews the common pitfalls, positive aspects, and protocols in pediatric radiography.

SKELETAL RADIOGRAPHY

Normal developmental variants confound the interpretation of skeletal films in children. The most frequent problems involve the epiphyses and apophyses, especially of the elbow and hip, pseudosubluxation of the cervical spine, and synchondroses of the pelvis. Comparison views of the opposite side are helpful. Standard radiology textbooks (Keats in Suggested Readings) feature the various developmental norms.

Trauma

Skeletal trauma in childhood presents distinctively different radiographic manifestations from trauma in adults. Because of the nature of the growing skeleton, sprains and joint dislocations are uncommon; fractures are relatively more common, especially through the growth plate or epiphysis, e.g., the Salter-Harris fracture (Fig. 47.1).

Salter-Harris Fractures

These account for approximately 20% of childhood fractures. Salter I fractures should be suspected in the child with an open epiphysiseal plate and the clinical features of a sprain, tenderness and swelling on examination localized on the x-ray to the open epiphysiseal plate. An apparent dislocation on the x-ray may be a Salter I fracture with an unossified epiphysis. Salter I fractures are most frequently seen in: (*a*) young infants, often as a result of abuse; (*b*) through a phalangeal epiphysiseal plate; or (*c*) through an abnormal epiphysiseal plate, as in leukemia or rickets. Salter II fractures are the most common type, frequently associated with a large triangular metaphyseal fragment. Salter III and IV fractures increase in frequency in adolescence as the epiphysiseal plate begins to close. The rare Salter V fractures, like the Salter I, may be difficult to spot radiographically; clinical suspicion with localized soft tissue swelling at the epiphysiseal plate, comparison views of the opposite side, and appropriate follow-up help to establish the diagnosis.

Cervical Spine

Cervical spine injuries are uncommon in childhood. Radiographic interpretation of the cervical spine series is complicated by the developmental norm of pseudosubluxation. Anterior displacement of C2 on C3 vertebra is seen in as many as 20% of children younger than 7 years (Fig. 47.2). This occurs less frequently at C3 on C4 vertebra. If there

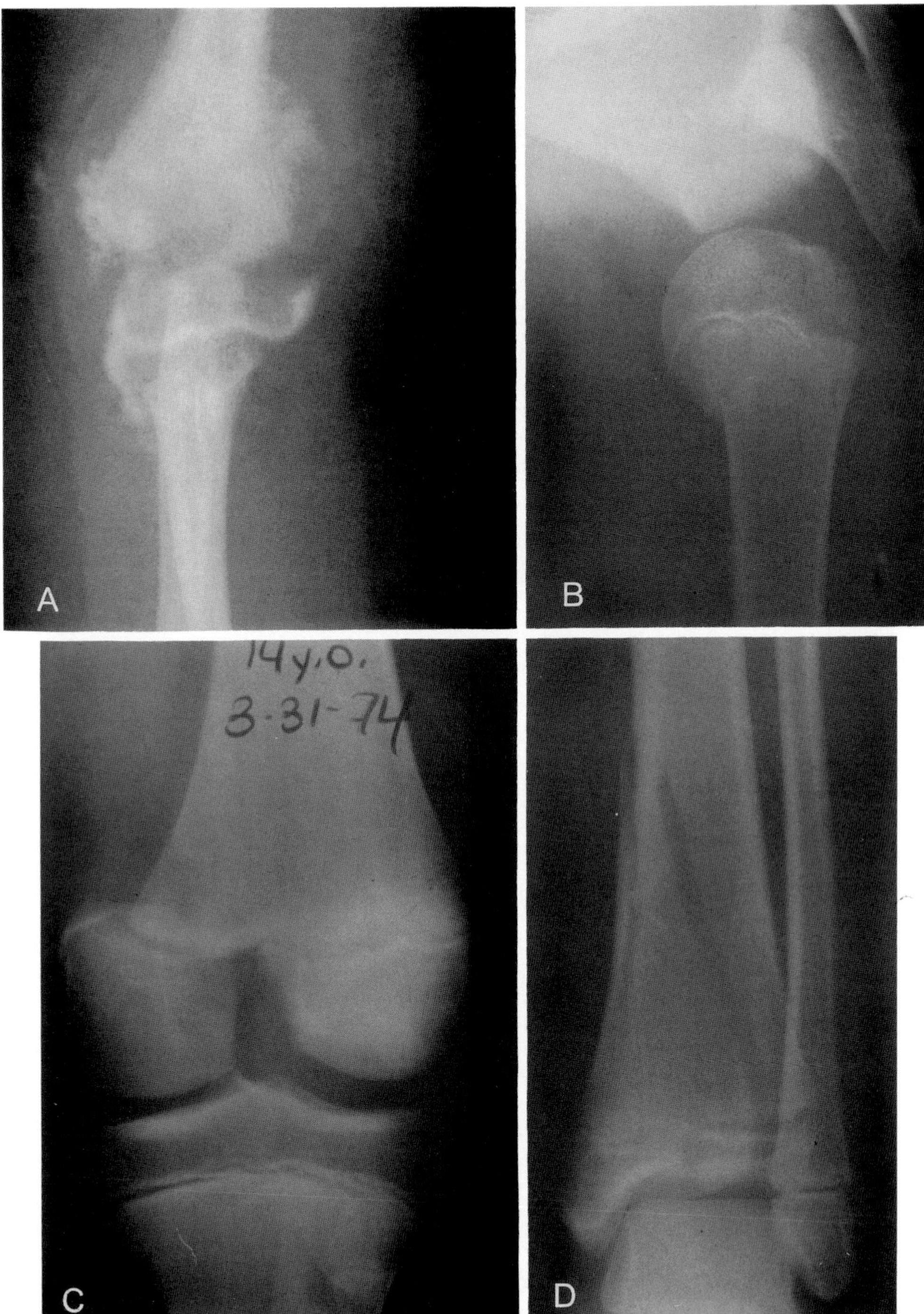

Figure 47.1. Typical Salter-Harris fractures. *A*, Elbow arthrogram of a healing Salter I fracture of the distal humerus. The unossified cartilaginous epiphysis, displaced medially, is identified by the intraarticular contrast material. *B*, Salter II fracture of the proximal humerus with a large triangular metaphyseal fracture. *C*, Salter III fracture of the distal femur with medial displacement of the epiphyseal fragment. *D*, Salter IV fracture of the distal tibia with the fracture line passing vertically through the epiphysis and obliquely through the metaphysis.

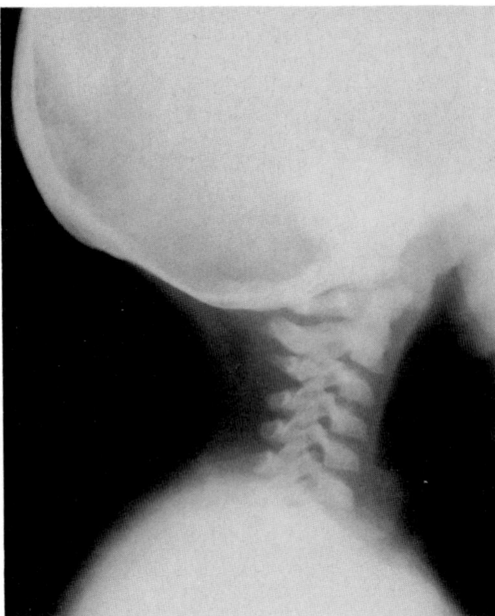

Figure 47.2. C2 vertebral pseudosubluxation. Lateral cervical spine demonstrating the normal displacement of C2 anteriorly on C3 vertebra seen in children.

is a question of an unstable injury, the child must be kept immobilized and a computed tomographic (CT) scan of the cervical spine obtained.

The Elbow

"Nursemaid's elbow" is a protrusion of the radial head through a torn annular ligament that normally surrounds the radial neck. This ligament is easily torn in children younger than 5 years, when the arm is subjected to traction stress. X-rays of the injured elbow are usually normal because the radial head returns to its normal position with supination of the arm, necessary to obtain the radiographs. However, x-rays are useful to rule out any associated fracture or to confirm reduction in the child who does not quickly resume use of the arm after attempted reduction. The reduction technique is described in Chapter 36.

The Abused Child

Skeletal trauma in the child in whom there is a clinical suspicion of abuse requires evaluation by high quality radiographs described in Table 47.1. These are not usually obtainable in a busy emergency department, particularly at night.

The radiographic findings that suggest child abuse need to be recognized, in order to specify which children need further evaluation. Skeletal trauma that suggests child abuse, particularly in the child younger than 2 years, include: (*a*) skull fractures, especially if multiple, stellate, or depressed; (*b*) rib fractures, uncommon in usual childhood trauma; (*c*) metaphyseal corner fractures; (*d*) displaced Salter I fractures; (*e*) fractures of varying ages; and (*f*) angulated long bone shaft fractures in small infants. Common injuries resulting from usual trauma include clavicular fractures, torus fractures of the distal radius, spiral fractures of the tibia (ages 9 months–4 years), and nursemaid's elbow.

Table 47.1.
Skeletal Survey for Suspected Abuse (usually in children younger than 2 years)

1. Anteroposterior (AP) and lateral skull films
2. Computed tomogram of the head—if CNS signs or symptoms present
3. AP films of chest to show ribs
4. AP extremity films, including all long bones
5. AP pelvis films
6. AP films of hands and feet
7. Lateral films of entire spine

The Septic Joint

The radiographic recognition of a septic joint, particularly of the hip in infants and small children, is of great importance. A widened hip joint space can be demonstrated on a properly positioned AP film of the pelvis. The so-called teardrop or Waldenstrom's distance (Fig. 47.3) is equal on each side. If there is greater than a 2-mm discrepancy, the joint space is definitely widened (Fig. 47.4). In the infant or child who resists "logrolling" of the hip and who may have fever and/or an elevated sedimentation rate, a widened teardrop space suggests a septic hip, dictating the need for further evaluation and treatment. This includes joint aspiration and the initiation of intravenous antibiotics. A radionuclide bone scan is helpful if the teardrop distance is not widened, but clinical signs nevertheless point to inflammation of the hip joint.

Idiopathic

A slipped capital femoral epiphysis occurs in the obese adolescent, causing subacute hip pain. If the displacement or slippage is not great, the frog leg lateral film is helpful in showing the posterior aspect of the proximal femur (Fig. 47.5). Because the risk of aseptic necrosis of the femoral head in the slipped capital femoral epiphysis increases with delay in diagnosis, any complaint of hip or knee pain representing possible reference of pain in the child undergoing a growth spurt should be investigated.

In the younger child with similar symptoms, *Legg-Perthes disease* produces avascular necrosis of the femoral head. The earliest and most subtle x-ray changes are slight lateral displacement, an antero-

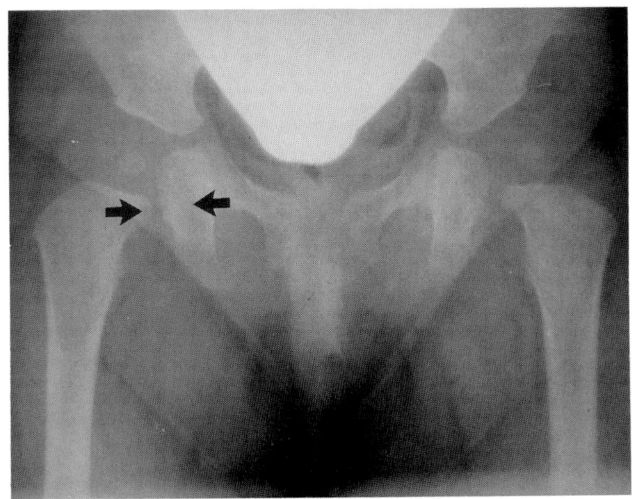

Figure 47.3. Tear-drop distance. Radiograph demonstrating the teardrop distance (marked by arrowheads) between the medial femoral metaphysis and the lateral border of the teardrop (the overlap of the pubis and ischium)

superior cleft, and increased density of the femoral head. Flattening and irregularity of the ossification center of the femoral head, broadening of the femoral neck, and the presence of metaphyseal lucent lesions are more obvious findings.

ABDOMINAL EMERGENCIES

Trauma

The imaging of children suffering abdominal trauma is similar to that for adults: CT, ultrasonography, radionuclide scanning, and angiography. Each has its specific indications. Certain traumatic conditions of childhood merit emphasis. *Duodenal intramural hematoma* resulting from blunt abdominal trauma, particularly that from a forward fall onto bicycle handlebars, should be suspected in the child who vomits following such an injury. An upper gastrointestinal (UGI) barium study is the quickest, most available method to make this diagnosis. CT may be helpful in excluding other retroperitoneal injuries, especially to the pancreas, or injuries to the liver, kidney, and/or spleen. If emergency CT is not available, a radionuclide liver-

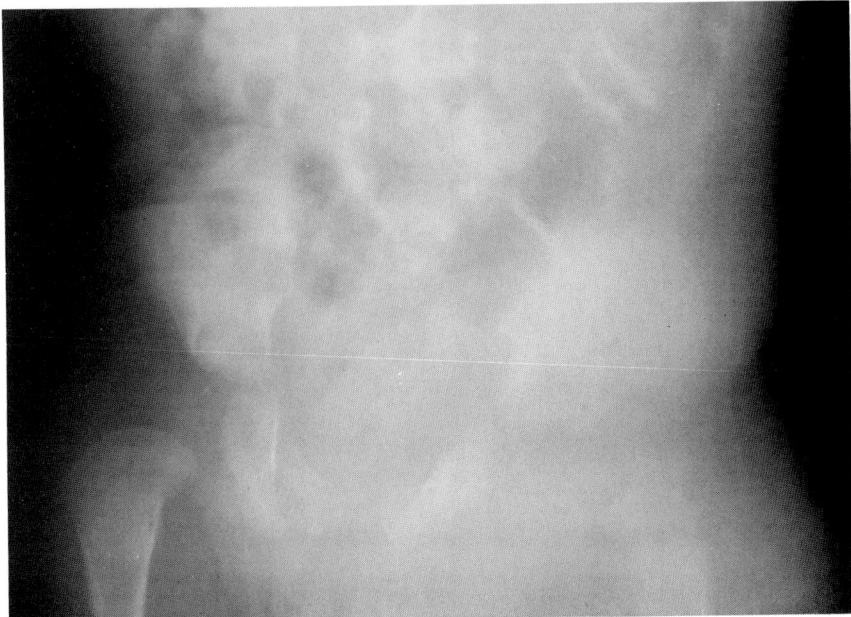

Figure 47.4. Septic hip. Markedly widened tear drop distance in an infant with a septic joint of the left hip.

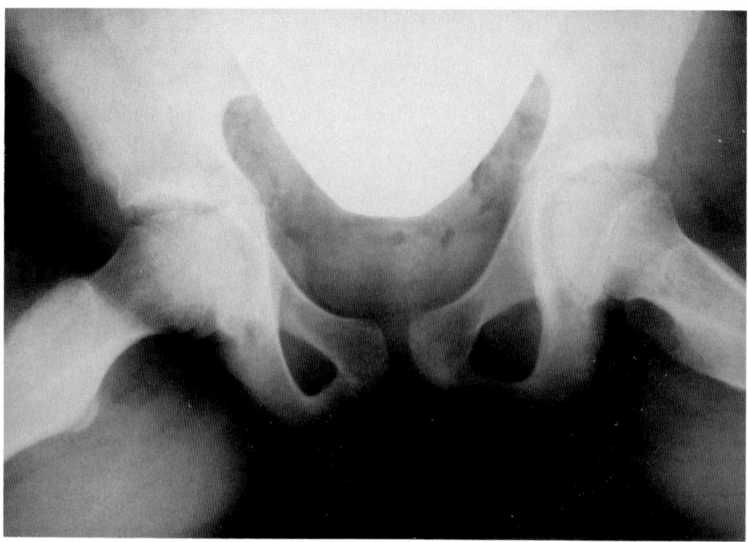

Figure 47.5. Slipped capital femoral epiphyses. Subtle bilateral slipped capital femoral epiphyses seen on the frog leg lateral hip film. Note the slight offset between the margins of the femoral capital epiphyses and the femoral metaphyses posteriorly.

spleen scan and intravenous pyelogram may be required. *The emergency physician should be aware of the possibility of child abuse in the small child with pancreatic or duodenal trauma.*

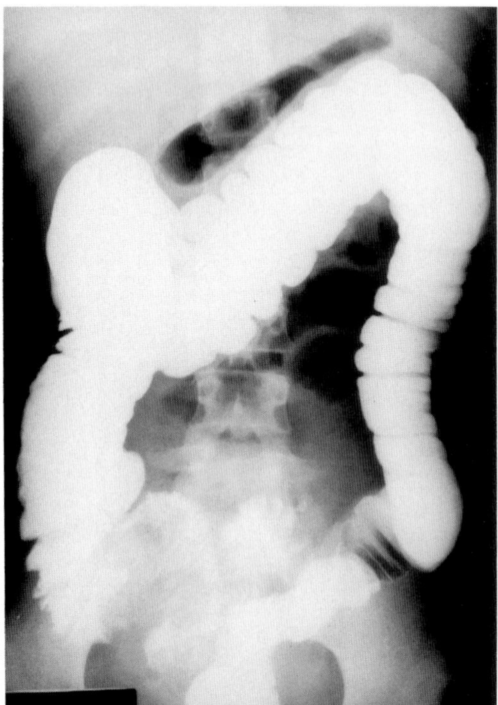

Figure 47.6. Appendicitis. A barium enema reveals a large appendiceal abscess compressing the cecum and the terminal ileum.

The possibility of a *congenital renal anomaly,* such as ureteropelvic junction obstruction, should be considered when hematuria follows apparently mild flank trauma, especially in children. The indications for urinary tract evaluation in patients with hematuria following trauma are reviewed in Chapter 35.

Appendicitis

In the evaluation of the child with abdominal pain and possible appendicitis, plain and upright films of the abdomen are often obtained in the emergency department. The findings on the plain film are usually nonspecific. A right lower quadrant mass effect and a calcified appendicolith may occasionally be found. The suggestive signs of splinting to the right, the loss of the preperitoneal fat line, the loss of the psoas margin on the right, and ileus localized in the right lower quadrant, should be interpreted as consistent with appendicitis. This condition is most difficult to confirm in the young child. The left lateral decubitus film is more helpful than the upright film in the child with possible appendicitis, because it makes use of air in the ileocecal region to outline certain abnormalities in the right lower quadrant. It is uncommon to need a barium enema to visualize further the right lower quadrant. However, if carefully performed, a barium study can be helpful in identifying an appendical abscess (Figure 47.6).

Intussusception

Idiopathic ileocolic or ileo-ileocolic intussusceptions are encountered in children from about 3

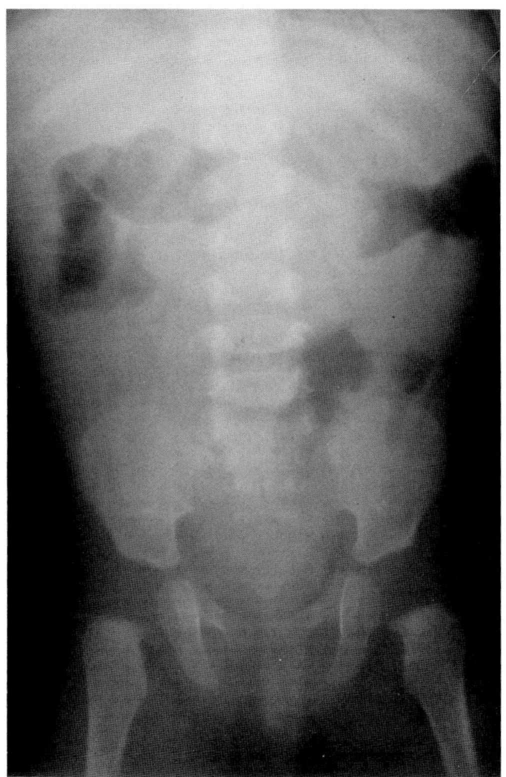

Figure 47.7. Intussusception. Five-month-old infant with an ileocolic intussusception. A mass corresponding to the palpable "sausage" is seen inferior to the stomach.

months to 3 years of age. Plain radiographs in idiopathic intussusception are very variable, ranging from normal to complete small bowel obstruction. Occasionally, the intussusceptum itself is outlined by air in the intussuscipiens (Fig. 47.7). A soft tissue mass may be appreciated in the right flank. As in appendicitis, left lateral decubitus films are more helpful than erect films in evaluating the right lower quadrant, the most common site of intussusception. However, because no plain film finding excludes intussusception, a barium enema or water-soluble contrast study should be performed for diagnosis and possible reduction. The absolute contraindications to attempted retrograde hydrostatic reduction are peritonitis and shock. This technique should be attempted only by a person trained and experienced in its use. Once the diagnosis has been confirmed, reduction may be facilitated by appropriate sedation of the child. When ileocolic intussusception is reduced, the small bowel should be filled with the contrast medium back to the jejunum to exclude an associated ileoileal intussusception.

Pyloric Stenosis

Ultrasonographic study and barium UGI study (Fig. 47.8) are both reliable and accurate methods in diagnosing hypertrophic pyloric stenosis. The barium UGI series offers the potential advantage of helping to exclude other obstructing lesions, should the child not have pyloric stenosis. It is usually quick and accurate if done with adequate distention of the antrum to outline the mass obstructing the pyloric channel. Care must be taken to empty the stomach of barium in the child with pyloric stenosis after the study is completed, in order to prevent possible barium aspiration during induction of anesthesia.

Midgut Volvulus

An important abdominal emergency of infancy is intestinal malrotation with midgut volvulus. These infants usually present at less than 2 years of age with bilious vomiting and a palpable abdominal mass. Because the obstruction in these infants is at the duodenal level, the bowel gas pattern may be normal; duodenal and gastric dilatation are sometimes noted. Ascites and ischemic bowel accompany a delay in diagnosis of midgut volvulus. The direct way to make this diagnosis is by a barium UGI series

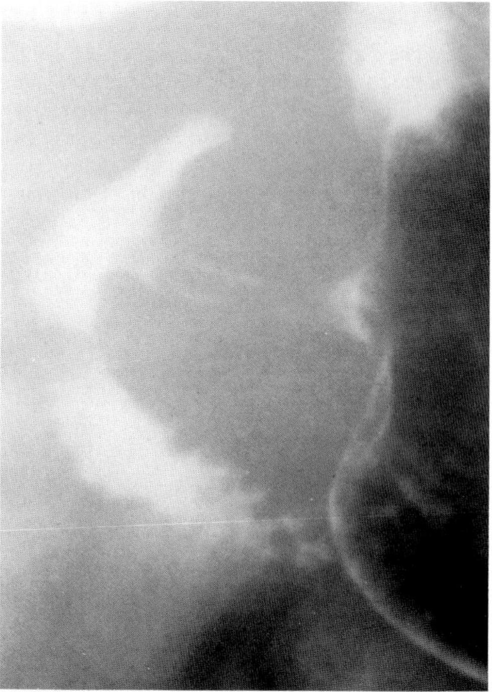

Figure 47.8. Pyloric stenosis. Elongated pyloric channel and a muscle mass indenting the gastric antrum are seen on a spot view during upper gastrointestinal series.

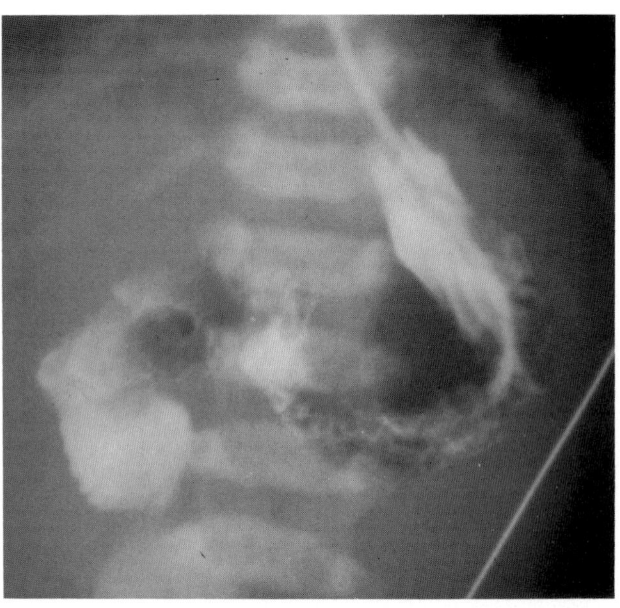

Figure 47.9. Midgut volvulus. Upper gastrointestinal series in an infant with bilious vomiting, demonstrating obstruction of the duodenum due to midgut volvulus.

(Fig. 47.9). Proximal obstruction of the duodenum resulting from the malrotation is readily apparent.

CHEST AND AIRWAY EMERGENCIES

Pneumonia

The chest x-ray is a standard part of the evaluation of the patient with cough, fever, and tachypnea, but the interpretation of the pediatric chest x-ray, particularly in the child less than 18 months of age, is often difficult. Because of the more rapid resting respiratory rate and rare cooperation of the young child in holding his or her breath, the normal chest x-ray in this age group is a midinspiratory or expiratory poorly aerated film. The radiographic differentiation of pulmonary infiltrates into those due to bacterial pneumonia and those due to viral lower respiratory infection is difficult at any age. Correlation with clinical data is mandatory in deciding to prescribe antibiotic therapy. Bacterial pneumonia produces either lobar or sublobar alveolar infiltrates, although the pneumococcus may produce a spherical or ''round'' pneumonia, which can appear alarmingly like a pulmonary mass (Fig. 47.10). Viral lower respiratory tract infections most com-

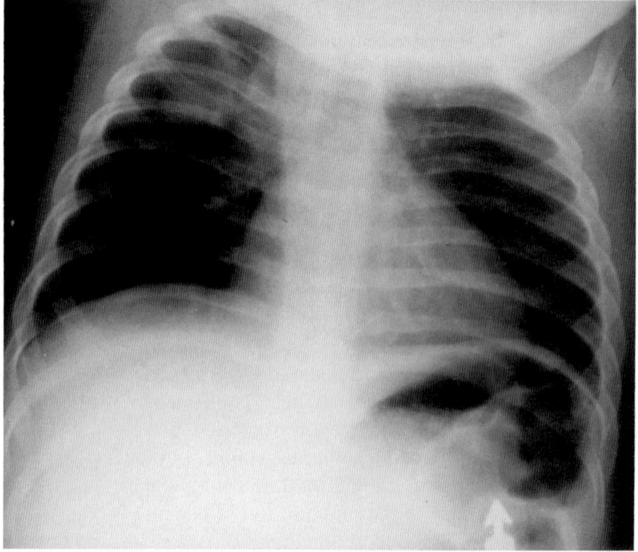

Figure 47.10. Round pneumonia. A 6-month-old infant with a right aortic arch and a round (or spherical) right upper lobe pneumonia.

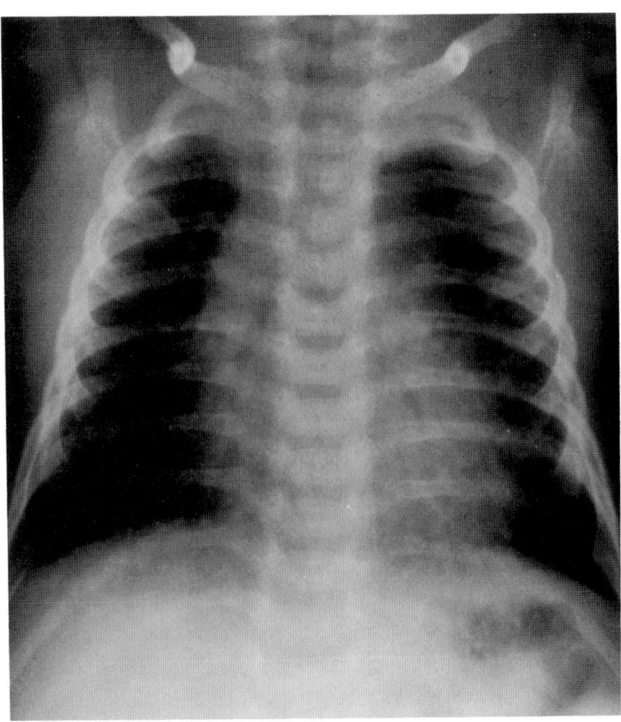

Figure 47.11. *Chlamydia* pneumonia. Ten-week-old infant with pulmonary hyperexpansion and diffuse reticular nodular infiltrates.

monly affect the airways, causing hyperexpansion, bronchial wall thickening, and focal areas of atelectasis. Differentiating a focal area of atelectasis from an alveolar infiltrate may be quite difficult. Clinical correlation is always necessary. One typical clinical syndrome, that of *Chlamydia* pneumonia, is seen in neonates from 2–12 weeks of life; it includes spasmodic cough, eosinophilia, and a chest x-ray demonstrating a hyperexpanded lung with patchy densities (Fig. 47.11).

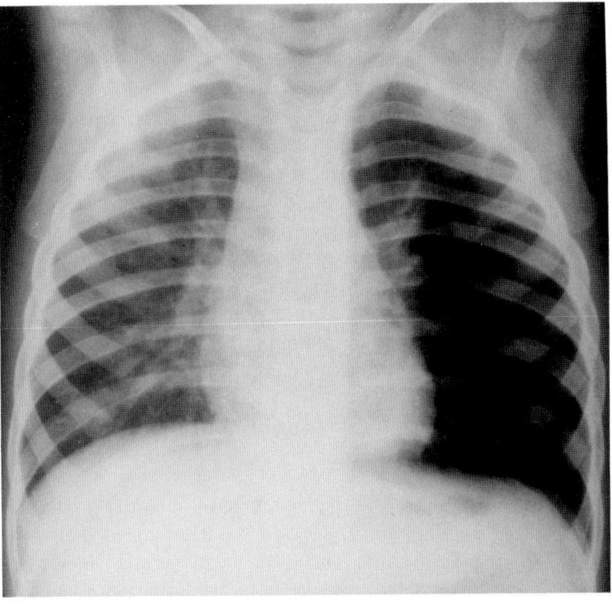

Figure 47.12. Intrabronchial foreign body. AP radiograph of a 3-year-old with intrabronchial foreign body in the left mainstem bronchus, causing air trapping of that lung.

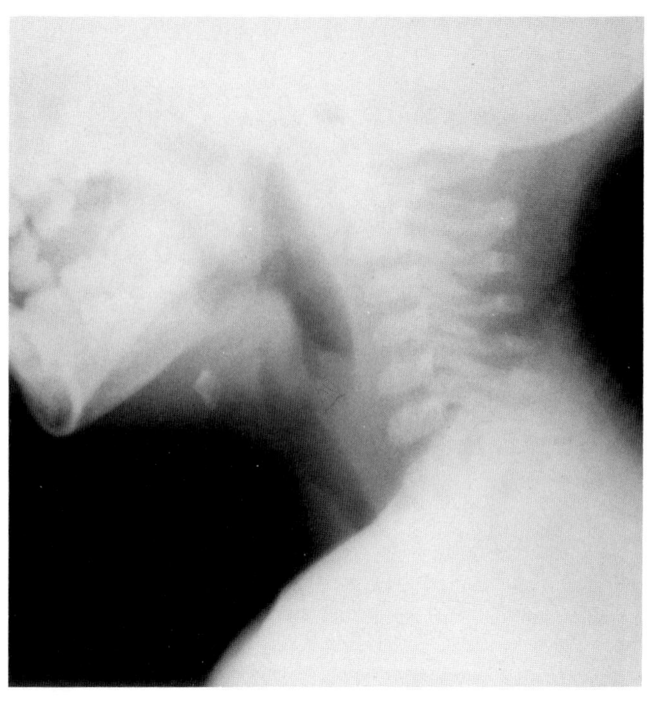

Figure 47.13. Epiglottitis. Enlarged epiglottis and aryepiglottic folds.

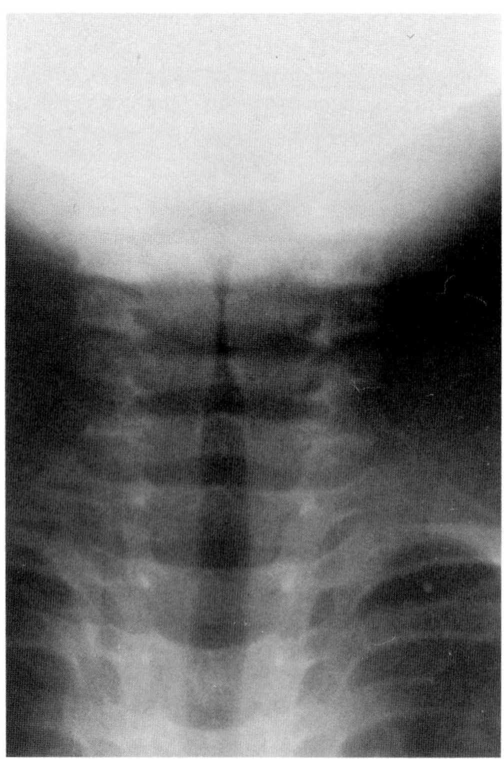

Figure 47.14. Croup. Subglottic tapering seen in croup.

Intrabronchial Foreign Bodies

An aspirated bronchial foreign body is suggested by history and the presence of localized wheezing. To document a ball-valve effect of the foreign body, decubitus films, fluoroscopy, and forced expiratory films can all be helpful. All of these techniques are aimed at demonstrating that the volume of the lung distal to the intrabronchial foreign body does not decrease with expiration (Fig. 47.12).

Epiglottitis

If the diagnosis of epiglottitis is clear on clinical grounds, or if the child is distressed enough to require urgent intubation, the lateral neck x-ray may represent an unnecessary and dangerous stress on the way to safe and expeditious laryngoscopy and intubation. Nevertheless, the radiographic recognition of epiglottitis is absolutely necessary. The airway anatomy seen in epiglottitis is shown in Fig. 47.13. The most important radiographic feature is the large thickened aryepiglottic folds extending from the epiglottis to the arytenoid cartilage, surrounding the laryngeal vestibule.

Croup

Croup or laryngotracheobronchitis produces a circumferential subglottic narrowing of the trachea (Fig. 47.14). This is a characteristic change best appreciated on an inspiratory anteroposterior (AP)

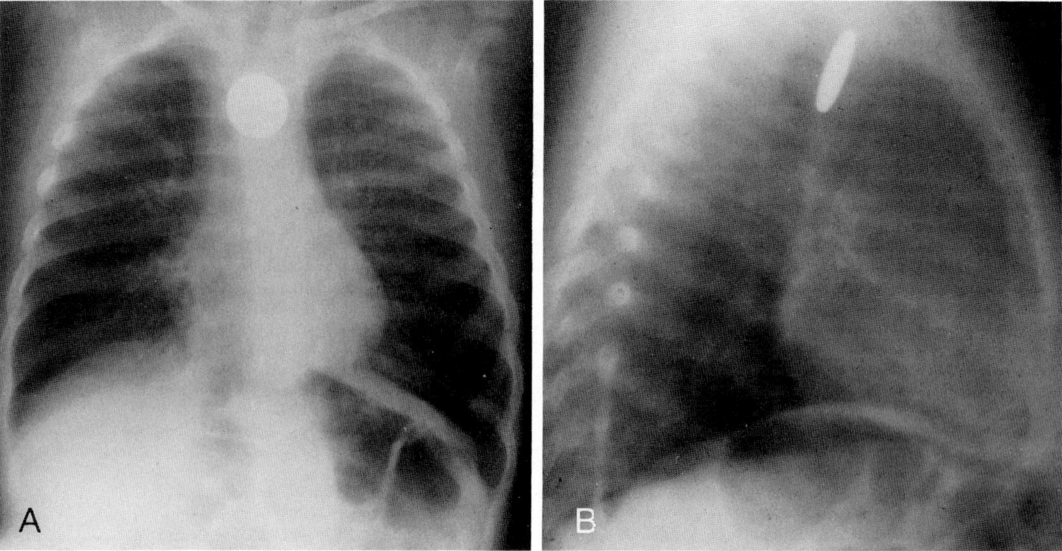

Figure 47.15. Esophageal foreign body. It is associated in this case with marked hyperexpansion and parahilar infiltrate due to aspiration.

view of the neck. Because 10–20% of patients with epiglottitis also have subglottic narrowing, a lateral film is necessary to exclude completely epiglottitis.

Esophageal Foreign Body

In addition to epiglottitis and croup, acute upper airway obstruction can also occur from an esophageal foreign body that may externally compress the relatively soft trachea of a child (Fig. 47.15). Swelling in the prevertebral tissues of the neck must be interpreted with caution. It may represent the normal buckling of soft tissue during swallowing or breathing, but that determination should be confirmed by fluoroscopy.

SUGGESTED READINGS

Keats TE. *An Atlas of Normal Roentgen Variants.* Chicago: Year Book, 1984.

Kleinman P: Avulsion of the spinous processes caused by infant abuse. *Radiology,* 1984;151:389–391.

Kohler A. *Borderlands of the Normal and Early Pathologic in Skeletal Radiography.* Grune & Stratton, Orlando, 1968.

Ogden JA. *Skeletal Injury in the Child.* Lea & Febiger, Philadelphia, 1982.

Radkowski MA: The abused child. Criteria for diagnosis. *RadioGraphics,* 1983;3:262–298.

Salter R, Zaltz C: Anatomic investigations of the mechanism of injury and pathologic anatomy of "pulled elbow" in young children. *Clin Orthop,* 1971;77:134–143.

Schwischuk L: Anterior displacement of C2 in children. *Radiology,* 1977;122:759–763.

SECTION 6

Supporting Services

PETER L. GROSS, M.D., F.A.C.E.P.
Associate Editor

CHAPTER 48

Emergency Department Nursing

VIRGINIA TRITSCHLER, R.N., B.S.

This chapter will cover some of the ways to help insure that your emergency department delivers quality nursing care. The goal is to provide a general overview, with some specific information, which emergency nurses will be able to use in developing guidelines for their individual departments.

ROLE OF THE EMERGENCY NURSE

Emergency nursing is a speciality in acute and general nursing care. Emergency nurses care for patients with all types of diseases and injuries, in acute and nonacute situations. They perform patient teaching and crisis intervention, and are a resource for both new and experienced physicians. Emergency nursing is one of the most challenging, demanding, and rewarding specialties in nursing.

One unique aspect of emergency nursing is the brevity and episodic nature of the care that is delivered. The nurse must possess refined assessment skills and the ability to make rapid and sound decisions in a broad range of clinical problems. Specifically, these skills include: knowing how to perform triage, establishing and maintaining an effective airway, participating as a member of a trauma team, initiating intravenous therapy, monitoring patients with arterial and/or pulmonary artery lines, recognizing and initiating appropriate care in patients with cardiac arrythmias and administering as well as recognizing adverse effects of numerous medications. Moreover, the emergency department (ED) nurse must possess the psychosocial skills to manage crisis intervention and counseling to rape and other trauma victims, to psychiatric patients, and to family and friends of dying or critically ill patients.

Most important, and often unrecognized, the nurse must be able to "shift gears" from the acute cases to the less acute ones. Since approximately 70% of ED visits are nonacute, the nurse must be able to care for these patients with the same efficiency and concern as for the emergent patient. The nonacute patients require those same assessment skills. The nurse must be able to teach patients of varied backgrounds, to deliver first-aid measures, to provide wound care, and to make appropriate referrals.

The ED nurse must likewise be able to interact in a positive manner with physicians, patients, anxious families, prehospital personnel, the media, outside agencies, and personnel from various hospital departments. This nurse may also participate in the communication network to receive information from prehospital personnel and, in some areas of the country, directs (under physician supervision) paramedics in the field. Leadership skills to supervise support staff, regulate patient flow, manage chaotic situations, and plan for the unexpected are requisite for the ED nurse.

Possessing the aforementioned knowledge, skills, and qualities is only the first step in the nursing process. The emergency nurse must then be able to translate those skills into expedient quality care that is delivered in an empathic and nonjudgmental manner, part of the challenge that makes this field so special.

STANDARDS

There are several different types of ED nursing standards: those imposed by external agencies (Joint Commission on Accreditation of Hospitals), those specific to emergency nursing practice, such as the ones developed by the Emergency Nurses Association, and standardized care plans. Written standards provide criteria which can then be used to evaluate practice and to demonstrate accountability for the care we deliver.

Joint Commission on Accreditation of Hospitals (JCAH)

The JCAH has developed specific standards for emergency services that must be met in order to be accredited as an emergency department. A copy of these standards should be available in all emergency departments and staff, especially leadership personnel, should be familiar with them. These standards are a useful resource in developing policies and procedures, orientation plans, and supply and equipment requirements. Standards should be developed to meet regulations, but they must also answer the needs of the individual. Table 48.1 illustrates the JCAH requirements for supplies and equipment, and Tables 48.2 and 48.3 illustrate standards developed for a specific emergency department.

Table 48.1.
Joint Commission on Accreditation of Hospitals (JCAH): Equipment and supply

Standard VI. The emergency department/service shall be designed and equipped to facilitate the safe and effective care of patients.

Equipment and supplies—at least the following shall be readily available for use . . .

- Oxygen and means of administration;
- Mechanical ventilatory assistance equipment, including airways, manual breathing bag, and ventilator;
- Cardiac defibrillator with synchronization capability;
- Respiratory and cardiac monitoring equipment;
- Thoracentesis and closed thoracostomy sets;
- Tracheotomy set;
- Tourniquets;
- Vascular cutdown sets;
- Laryngoscopes and endotracheal tubes;
- Tracheobronchial and gastric suction equipment;
- Urinary catheters with closed volume urinary systems;
- Pleural and pericardial drainage sets;
- Minor surgical instruments;
- Splinting devices;
- Emergency obstetrical pack;
- Standard drugs, antivenin (areas where indicated), common poison antidotes, syringes and needles, parenteral fluids and infusion sets, plasma substitutes and blood administration sets, and surgical supplies must be available for immediate use.

From Standards for Emergency Services. In *Standards for Accreditation of Hospitals,* JCAH, 1985.

Standards of Emergency Nursing Association (ENA)

In 1983, the Emergency Nurses Association (ENA) developed and published their *Standards of Emergency Nursing Pracıice.* These national standards cover four components of emergency nursing: practice, education, professionalism, and research. Having been developed by a professional specialty organization, these standards are likely to become an accepted standard of care by regulating agencies. As with the JCAH standards, the ENA's should be adapted to the individual facility.

Table 48.2.
Basic Equipment in All Adult Treatment Rooms

Outlets (one set for each bed):
- Oxygen (2), one with bubble-jet, one with adapter for venturi mask, respirator, or positive-pressure mask
- Suction (2), one with catheter for nasopharyngeal suction, one adaptable for gastric or chest tube suction
- Holder for catheters (1)—a cylindrical metal container (4- to 6-inch diameter, 12- to 15-inch length) attached to wall to hold 14- and 16-gauge suction catheters and tonsil-tip suction device

Sphygmomanometer

Dextrose in water solution (5%), 3 bottles (500 ml)

Intravenous supplies:
- Administration sets (3)
- Microdrip administration sets (3)
- Arm boards (3)

Bedpan (1), urinals (3 or 4), emesis basins (4 to 6), with metal holder behind door for both bedpan and urinals to save shelf space

Cups for dentures and for specimens of stool and sputum

Guaiac kits

Blood specimen kits (8) placed in an emesis basin and tied with a tourniquet:
- Tubes—for specific blood chemistry and hematology tests (6)
- Needles (15- and 20-gauge)
- Intravenous catheters (14-, 16-, and 18-gauge)
- Syringe (50-ml Luer-lok)
- Vacutainer for blood samples
- Alcohol preparation pads
- Povidone-iodine (Efodine, Betadine) ointment

Blood culture bottles (4)

Pegboard:
- Central venous pressure catheters (24-inch, 16-inch, 8-inch)
- Arterial blood-gas set (plastic bag containing alcohol sponge, needles, glass syringe with cap and heparin, which becomes unit in which ice is placed and specimen is sent to laboratory)
- Airways
- Sputum traps
- Y-connectors (sterile)
- Stopcocks (3-way) with catheter plugs
- Scalp-vein needles (19-, 21-, and 23-gauge)
- Oxygen supplies (mask and nasal prongs)

Urinary catheterization tray with no. 16 Foley catheter (5 ml) and urinometer

Gloves (sterile and rectal)

Adapters (Y-adapters, 5-in-1 adapters)

Clamps (Hunt, Hoffman, butterfly)

Bandages and applicators:
- Tongue blades
- Cotton-tip applicators
- Gauze pads
- Tape
- Band-Aids
- Lubricating gel (Lubafax)

Antiseptic supplies:
- Alcohol preparation (solution and pads)
- Iodine solution
- Povidone-iodine (spray and ointment)

Bed linen, pads (incontinence and sanitary)

Shopping bags for patient clothing, with adhesive labels

Standarized Care Plans

New to emergency nursing, although not to the nursing profession, is the development of standardized care plans. Emergency nurses in the past avoided standardized care plans because of the number of varied illnesses treated in emergency departments. Many ED nurses felt such plans were not necessary or useful in emergencies. This thinking has changed, and many more emergency nurses now realize the advantages to instituting standardized care plans, which include uniformity in orienting new nurses and some uniformity in delivering care. These plans allow for quality assurance review and provide an accepted standard of care for risk management.

Developing and implementing standardized care plans is a major task, requiring advanced planning, time, and the support and participation of the staff. Realistic and attainable goals should be set. Staff quickly loses interest and enthusiasm if care plans are written so idealistically that it is impossible for any reasonable nurse to deliver that care. Realistic time frames for completion of the task must be adopted. It is best to implement the care plans as they are developed and to avoid presenting multiple plans at one time.

NURSING MANAGEMENT

Staffing

The ED nurse manager must determine the needs of the department in recruiting and selecting staff members. Factors to consider in determining the ED's nursing staffing needs include:

1. Care capability level of emergency department and any designations such as trauma center, burn center, referral center, etc.;
2. Regulating agencies' requirements;
3. Legal requirements set by the federal, state, or city governments;
4. Physical layout of the department;
5. Availability and quality of ancillary services;
6. Teaching responsibilities of the hospital and/or department;
7. Department and hospital objectives;

Table 48.3.
Major Trauma Room Equipment

Basic equipment as in all treatment rooms on wall-mounted pegboard, in mobile cabinets, or within easy reach.
Specific equipment and supplies:
- Intubation equipment (adult and pediatric):
  - Ambu (100% oyxgen)
  - Emergency drugs (sodium bicarbonate, epinephrine, atropine, calcium chloride, isoproterenol)
- Bronchoscopy equipment (adult and pediatric)
- Tracheotomy sets—with tubes—all sizes
- Closed thoracostomy sets (3) with all sizes of chest tubes, suction sets
- Open thoracotomy set
- Antishock trousers (adult, pediatric)
- Burr-hole set
- Ventricular tap set
- Obstetric kit
- Esophageal varices set with 2 types of tubes (Sangstaken-Blakemore, Linton)
- Cervical immobilization equipment:
  - Sandbags
  - Collars: soft felt, four-poster, Philadelphia
- Intravenous solutions:
  - Mannitol
  - Lactated Ringer's
  - 5% dextrose in normal saline
  - Normal (physiologic) saline
- Suture kits with all common types of suture materials
- Surgical preparation kits with razor and sponges in tray
- Subclavian vein line insertion sets
- Cardiac monitoring units
- Defibrillators with internal paddles
- Autotransfusion kits (2)
- Burn equipment:
  - Sterile sheets and towels
  - Bandages (Kerlix)
  - Sterile basins with sponges
  - Antibacterial soapless skin cleaner (pHisohex)
  - Sterile physiologic saline solution
  - Silver nitrate solution
  - Silver sulfadiazine (Silvadene) cream
  - Xeroform gauze
- Heat lamps
- Blood warmers—Hemokinetitherm
- Volume ventilator
- Crafoord clamps (2)
- Blood infusion pumps
- Gastric tubes (assorted)

8. Community demands and needs for services;
9. Goals set for timeliness of instituting care.

Presently, there are emergency departments that have developed or are in the process of developing patient classification systems (PCS) in order to determine their staffing needs. Information that is necessary to determine staffing numbers, whether by using a PCS or other method, includes:

1. Number of patients seen per 24 hours, by shift, by time of day;
2. Type of patients seen by service and severity;
3. Number of hospital admissions;
4. Patient census by day of the week, month, seasonal trends;
5. Review of the length of stay and how this affects the next shift with carryovers.

With this information, the ED nursing staff must decide what types of skills and level of experience will be needed in staffing the department. Criteria must be developed for level educational requirements and selection standards, and decisions made for internal and external recruitment.

Experience

Again, emergency nursing is a specialty that requires a mature professional who has the knowledge and experience to make quick informative decisions. In addition, he or she must be self-directed, organized, even in a sometimes chaotic environment, able to adapt to a constantly changing pace and accompanying stress. Staff in the ED must also be able to interact with the public in a positive way. Many ED managers have found that experienced nurses are more likely to possess these characteristics than are new graduates. In hiring experienced nurses, the ED manager may also find that the turnover rate is less, since these nurses have tried other areas and generally know that emergency nursing is what they want. How much experience should be required depends on the individual ED, but 2 years of clinical nursing experience, including 1 year in an intensive care unit or another ED is a desirable background.

Staffing Mix

Careful evaluation of departmental needs must be done before determining the staffing mix. An all registered nursing (RN) staff provides flexibility in staffing and assignments, but may not be cost-effective if the RNs are being used to stock rooms, do routine patient transports, or clean equipment. The ED may be better served by having a nursing or unit assistant position.

Recruitment

Both internal and outside recruiting have their advantages. Selection of internal candidates provides a staff member who is knowledgeable about the hospital, its policies and procedures, and the roles of various personnel. With internal recruitment, the ED manager can usually make a more informed assessment of the candidate's abilities. It also strengthens morale since it shows a willingness to meet staff needs by providing more employment opportunities. Outside recruitment, however, may result in obtaining people with fresh ideas, and new or improved perspectives. It is also less costly for the institution as a whole (a cost of one orientation as opposed to two). In general, it is best to select staff by their qualifications and by department overall needs.

Applicant Interviews

The interview has always been very important, but is even more so now that employers are releasing less information in references. It is important to find the person with the right qualifications, but it is also important that the person fits in with the other staff members and with long-range plans. Interviewing is a skill, and like all skills, must be learned and practiced before one becomes proficient. Workshops, articles, books, observing others, and talking with experienced interviewers are ways to improve this skill. Preparation is an important step in the interviewing process. The following recommendations have proved helpful in conducting interviews:

1. Review the application/résumé before setting up the appointment;
2. Schedule interviews at the time of day that one functions best and not at the end of a very busy day;
3. Conduct the interview in a comfortable environment;
4. Avoid interruptions;
5. Start the interview with small talk to put the applicant at ease;
6. Know what questions one legally can and cannot ask;
7. Decide before the interview what one wants to learn about the person;
8. Let the candidate do most of the talking;
9. Experiment with different questions until one is found that provides the information needed to make a decision (Table 48.4 provides some suggestions);
10. Take notes—by the time one finishes interviewing multiple candidates, help is necessary in recalling the earlier ones;
11. Do not make a final decision at the end of the interview: allow both the candidate and the interviewer time to consider all that has been learned;
12. Give the candidates an idea when they may expect to hear and how they can make contact in case they have any more questions.

Staff Involvement

Many managers favor staff participation in the selection process. This involvement can improve morale by allowing the staff to voice individual opinions. At the same time, it truly helps the nursing manager to hear other points of view. It also gives the ED manager an opportunity to train future leaders and gives the staff member a chance to practice leadership skills under supervision. When involving staff, there should be careful planning and an educational process that includes matters such as confidentiality, legal aspects, and the interviewing process prior to their participation. However the selection is accomplished, recognize that the process can be enjoyable and less stressful if one is well-prepared and if one views the process as an opportunity to meet different people, help some, learn from others, and recruit the top candidates available.

Orientation

General Orientation

An effective orientation program will help reduce turnover, increase motivation and productivity, and contribute to a cohesive team. Whether orientation is performed by a clinical specialist, a staff member, or a nurse manager, it is important that time be taken to develop, organize, and put the plan in writing. The orientation program should be flexible enough that it is adaptable to different levels of experience and individual learning speeds. Many hospitals and EDs have adopted a staff preceptor

Table 48.4.
Suggested Interview Questions

What made you select this hospital?
What do you like best about emergency nursing/ What attracts you to emergency nursing?
Why are you leaving your present position?
What do you like least about your present job? Best?
What do you consider your strong points? Weak ones?
What frustrates or angers you at work? How do you deal with it?
What are your long-term goals?
What continuing education programs have you attended in the past 6–12 mos. and why did you choose them?
What professional and/or civic organizations do you belong to?
What have you accomplished that you are most proud of?
What type of patients does your present ED care for and how many patients are seen in a 24-hour period?
If hired, what area of emergency nursing do you feel least comfortable with, for which we should provide additional orientation?
Describe a problem area in your present department and tell me how you would go about solving it?
What traits do you like/dislike in coworkers? Immediate supervisor?
What would you like to ask me?

orientation program. This system utilizes individual staff member's strengths and expertise, and allows the trainee to become an accepted member of the team. The preceptor should be selected on the basis of expertise, performance, ability to teach, and willingness to participate in such a program.

A written orientation plan ensures uniformity and prevents omission of important material. The length and content of the program depends on the ED size, patient mix, and experience required of the new staff member. It is helpful to have staff input in the development of the program, even if they are not performing the orientation. Do not presume levels of knowledge simply on the basis of background. Orientees should be expected to demonstrate their skills under supervision until the ED leadership is comfortable that they meet the departmental standards. It is not unusual to require all orientees to be certified or tested in some or all of the following areas: initiating intravenous therapy, blind endotracheal suctioning, application of antishock trousers, use of autotransfusion, commonly used emergency medications and dosages, and knowledge of cardiac arrythmias and cardiopulmonary resuscitation (CPR). Nurses new to emergency nursing need to be taught the areas unique to this speciality, i.e., trauma and burn care and prehospital care. Arranging a day with emergency medical technicians/paramedics on an ambulance provides the new nurse with an understanding of prehospital care and the prehospital care providers, and enhances working relationships.

Orientation to Triage

Orientation to triage may not be desirable initially, depending on the size of the ED, experience of the nurse, and type of triage performed (basic or advanced). In a large ED, the new staff member has many new systems to learn and absorb, and waiting 3–6 months before orientation to triage may well result in the nurse becoming a better overall performer. In smaller EDs, or where a basic triage is used, this period of waiting may not be as necessary. Triage orientation should follow a carefully planned and written program. Again, assumptions as to skill level should be avoided. Do not, for example, assume all nurses know how to interview patients.

In the triage orientation, for the first day or more if needed, plan to be away from patient activity. During this time, have the orientee review triage policies and procedures with the preceptor and have them role-play triage situations. Practicing interviewing and decision making prior to an actual patient situation allows the orientee a chance to organize thoughts, decreasing some anxiety, and gives a perspective on the role while in a less stressful environment. The orientee should review anatomy, physiology, and disease entities prior to the start of the orientation. Providing the nurse with a reference list for additional reading on triage and emergency care is also helpful.

The length of orientation depends on the ED, but may be as long as 2 weeks. Included in triage orientation are:

1. Explanation of emergency medical services systems in the area;
2. Use and practice with all communication systems;
3. External resources available for patient referrals, i.e., detoxification facilities, social service agencies, overnight accommodations for relatives, free clinics, places for homeless people, runaways, etc.;
4. City and hospital disaster plans and the role of the triage nurse;
5. First aid (splinting, pressure dressings, etc.);
6. Rape protocol;
7. Classes on x-ray views, what to order, when;
8. Laboratory tests;
9. What to do in potentially volatile situations;
10. How to diffuse situations;
11. Dealing with the media, police, etc.;
12. Resources in the hospital, i.e., social service, security, patient care representatives;
13. Triage documentation (see section on Triage and Table 48.5).

In-service Education

Health care and emergency nursing are constantly changing with new technology, new drugs, and new methods of treating diseases and injuries. Therefore, frequent in-service education is essential to keep staff current and to help retain staff. Prior to planning formal and informal educational conferences, it is necessary to perform a needs analysis. Job descriptions, hospital and departmental objectives for the coming year, staff performance evaluations, and staff input obtained through questionnaires and meetings all help in planning meaningful conferences to answer the needs of the staff and department. Conferences do not need to be long or formal. Much can be learned in 15–30 minutes from a coworker. All EDs have lull periods that may allow time to have fire drills, mock "code" procedures, or a review of equipment that is seldom used. Even in large EDs, nurses may have a long lapse between caring for burn patients or using autotransfusion because of days off, shift changes, and different assignments. Practice conferences are useful, interesting, and can fulfill regulating agencies requirements, e.g., JCAH requires fire drills to be held quarterly on all three shifts.

Educational opportunities are also offered through

Table 48.5.
Triage Documentation Using the Subjective Objective Assessment Plan (SOAP) Format[a]

S: 17 yo M c/o being kicked in the head during karate 2 hrs. PTA. Has frontal HA, no relief with ASA, no LOC, no N&V, sl. visual blurriness. PMH none, NKA
O: Pupils equal and react, nl VS, no deformity noted, steady gait
A: Possible concussion
P: Skull x-rays, then minor surg.

S: UWM
GSW to chest
P: Trauma service
Trauma rm stat

S: 48 yo obese F c/o chest pressure × 4 hrs. PTA, no relief with NG × 5. Pain developed after exertion—climbed 2 flights of stairs. Hx angina, HBP, s/p MI, meds: Aldomet, Lasix, NG, ALLERGIC to PENICILLIN
O: Dyspneic, color—ashen, skin—diaphoretic, Pulse—irregular
A: R/O MI
P: Cardiac room, major medicine

S: 30 yo M c/o chest pain × 2 hrs. PTA, pain stabbing in nature, no dyspnea, no N&V, pain developed after being fired from job, no previous episodes, PMH and meds none, NKA
O: No acute distress, Pulse regular, EKG—nl
A: R/O anxiety
P: EKG; then medical walk-in clinic

[a] HA, headache; VS, vital signs; GSW, gunshot wound; LOC, loss of consciousness; NKA, no known allergies; PTA, prior to admission; UWM, unknown white male; ASA, aspirin; N&V, nausea and vomiting; PMH, past medical history; NG, nitroglycerine; HBP, high blood pressure; R/O, rule out; MI, myocardial infarction.

emergency medical services offices and through ENA. Attending ENA conferences on the local, state, or national level provides emergency nurses with an opportunity to attend conferences designed specifically to meet their needs and a forum in which to share ideas, problems, and solutions with other nurses who understand and share many of the same concerns. There are many other ways to provide staff with educational opportunities. The key for managers is to provide an environment that encourages growth and learning.

Communication

There are many ways for nurse managers to enhance communication and to promote an atmosphere in which people can work together. Some basic principles and methods to implement them follow:

1. Routinely schedule staff meetings that allow staff to offer suggestions, and constructive criticisms, participate in solving problems, vent frustrations, and assist in planning for the future;
2. Provide minutes to staff meetings and various committee meetings so that those who cannot attend or who are not on the committee can stay current;
3. Provide a "what's new book" or "daily log" that everyone can write in and note small changes in the department, new information pertaining to certain treatments, equipment, patients, etc.;
4. Never reprimand someone in the presence of others;
5. Allow individuals to explain reasons for carrying out a particular action;
6. Provide feedback to those who have made suggestions, requests, or criticisms;
7. Never take corrective action on rumors;
8. Clarify one's standards, goals, and expectations with the staff;
9. Provide a mechanism for staff input through interviews, meetings, or questionnaires;
10. Provide frequent positive feedback.

Verbal communication is the easiest and probably the most frequently used method of communication in an ED. However, written documentation is extremely important, especially as it relates to patient care. Written documentation by nurses is essential for good patient care and risk management, and provides a way to evaluate the care delivered. Many ED history forms lack the space for nurses to record assessments, plans, and interventions. This may result in little or no documentation, beyond basic triage information. Providing a separate nursing flow sheet is one way to improve the frequency and quality of documentation. Flow sheets should be designed by nurses to meet nursing needs. The flow sheet should be designed so that it can be used on all patients and should provide adequate space for serial vital signs, fluid resuscitation documentation, medications, and procedures. Flow sheets frequently incorporate the Glasgow coma scale, the trauma score, respiratory therapy data, and pertinent laboratory studies in addition to providing space for freehand text and other information deemed necessary for the specific emergency department (see Fig. 48.1*A* and *B*). Figure 48.2 illustrates a flow sheet that is used during arrest situations, but is not part of the permanent record. Information is transferred to the record after the emergency is over. Written documentation may be more time-consuming, but it avoids distortion, is available to more members of the team, and is permanent.

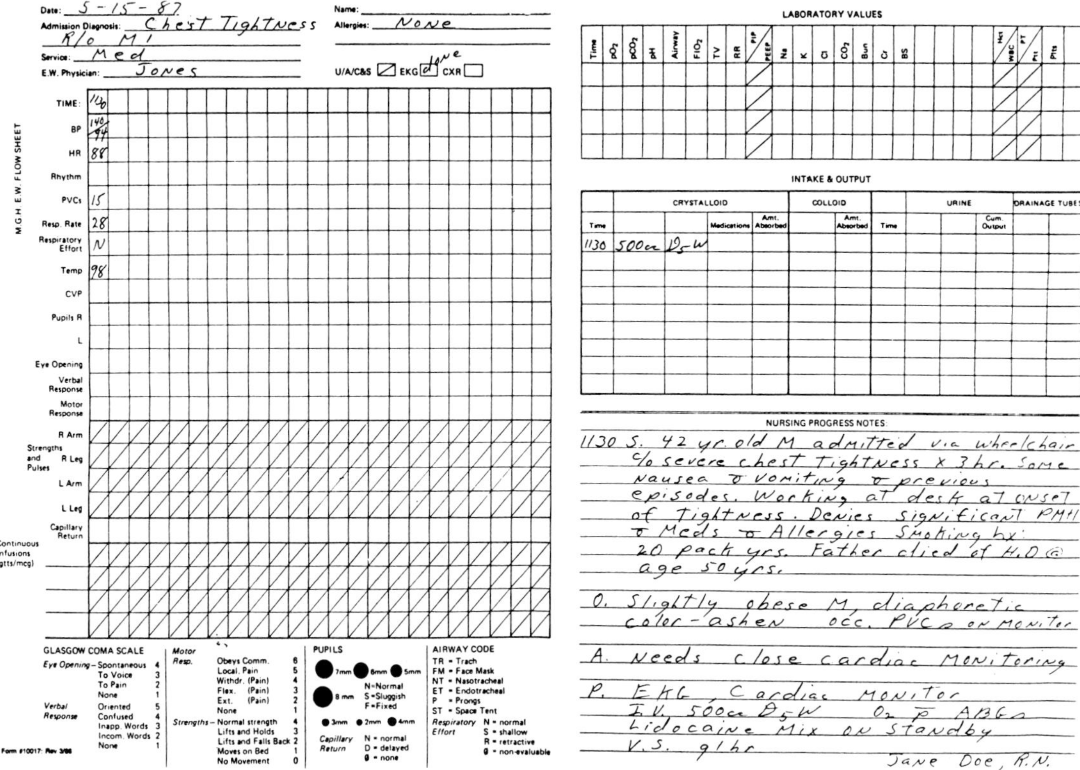

M.G.H. E.W. FLOW SHEET

Date: 5-15-87
Admission Diagnosis: Chest Tightness R/o MI
Service: Med
E.W. Physician: Jones

Name:
Allergies: None

U/A/C&S ☐ EKG ☑ done CXR ☐

TIME:	1130
BP	140/94
HR	88
Rhythm	
PVCs	15
Resp. Rate	28
Respiratory Effort	N
Temp	98
CVP	
Pupils R	
L	
Eye Opening	
Verbal Response	
Motor Response	
Strengths and Pulses R Arm	
R Leg	
L Arm	
L Leg	
Capillary Return	
Continuous Infusions (gtts/mcg)	

GLASGOW COMA SCALE

Eye Opening – Spontaneous 4, To Voice 3, To Pain 2, None 1

Verbal Response – Oriented 5, Confused 4, Inapp. Words 3, Incom. Words 2, None 1

Motor Resp. – Obeys Comm. 6, Local. Pain 5, Withdr. (Pain) 4, Flex. (Pain) 3, Ext. (Pain) 2, None 1

Strengths – Normal strength 4, Lifts and Holds 3, Lifts and Falls Back 2, Moves on Bed 1, No Movement 0

PUPILS

7mm 6mm 5mm 8 mm 3mm 2mm 4mm

N=Normal, S=Sluggish, F=Fixed

Capillary Return N = normal, D = delayed, Ø = none

AIRWAY CODE

TR = Trach, FM = Face Mask, NT = Nasotracheal, ET = Endotracheal, P = Prongs, ST = Space Tent

Respiratory Effort N = normal, S = shallow, R = retractive, Ø = non-evaluable

Form #10017: Rev 3/86

LABORATORY VALUES

Time	pO_2	pCO_2	pH	Airway	FIO_2	TV	RR	PIP/PEEP	Na	K	Cl	CO_2	Bun	Cr	BS					Hct/WBC	PT/Ptt	Plts	

INTAKE & OUTPUT

	CRYSTALLOID				COLLOID			URINE			DRAINAGE TUBES	
Time			Medications	Amt. Absorbed		Amt. Absorbed	Time			Cum. Output		
1130	500cc	D_5W										

NURSING PROGRESS NOTES:

1130 S. 42 yr. old M admitted via wheelchair c/o severe chest tightness x 3 hr. Some nausea ō vomiting ō previous episodes. Working at desk at onset of tightness. Denies significant PMH ō Meds ō Allergies. Smoking hx: 20 pack yrs. Father died of H.D @ age 50 yrs.

O. Slightly obese M, diaphoretic color – ashen occ. PVCs on monitor

A. Needs close cardiac monitoring

P. EKG, Cardiac monitor
I.V. 500cc D_5W O_2 p̄ ABGs
Lidocaine Mix on Standby
V.S. q1hr

Jane Doe, R.N.

Figure 48.1. *A*, Emergency flow sheet in use at the Massachusetts General Hospital. *B*, The Weed problem-oriented method of charting provides an organized, uniform, and concise method of documentation.

TRIAGE

The word *triage* is derived from the French *trier,* which means "to sort out." The military in World War II developed a triage system in order to effect disposition of the injured and later triage was used during civilian disasters to sort out those who needed immediate attention, those who could wait, and those who could not be helped. Over the past 25 years, most hospital emergency departments have instituted some form of triage to determine patient priority, and today, most are staffed by nurses.

The main function of a triage system is to have patients assessed and assigned to designated treatment areas as expeditiously as possible. It is also most important to classify patients according to priority. Patients are usually classified as emergent, acute, or nonacute. *Emergent* patients are those with life-threatening conditions, such as obstructive airway, uncontrollable bleeding, or multiple trauma. *Acute* conditions include those problems that must be treated within a few hours, such as extremity injuries and lacerations. *Nonacute* conditions are those that can be treated in an outpatient facility or for which delay in treatment will not cause an adverse effect on the patient, e.g., colds, hernia, chronic complaints.

Types

There are several types of triage:

Nonprofessional Triage

This system is usually performed by a receptionist or clerk who obtains patient demographic information and chief complaints. The obvious patient care and liability issues with regard to this system are that there is no medical assessment or determination of needs. Patients with acute conditions may languish in the waiting room while their condition becomes emergent.

Basic Triage

This system utilizes licensed practical nurses or registered nurses to quickly assess, list the patient's immediate needs and assign the patients to treatment areas.

Advanced Triage

This system employs registered nurses to assess the patient, initiate diagnostic procedures and first-

Onset Time ______________ Name: ______________

Unit No. __________ Age: __________

	Time/Dosage					
1. Defibrillation						
2. Medications						
Sodium bicarbonate						
Epinephrine						
Lidocaine						
Calcium chloride						
Atropine						
Bretylium tosylate						
Procainamide						
Dextrose 50						
Naloxone						
3. IV mixes						
Lidocaine, 2 gm/250 ml D_5W						
Isoproterenol, 2 mg/250 ml D_5W						
Levarterenol, 4 mg/250 ml D_5W						
Bretylium, 2 gm/250 ml D_5W						
Procainamide, 2 gm/250 ml D_5W						
Dopamine, 500 mg/250 ml D_5W						
Sodium nitroprusside, 50 mg/500 ml D_5W						
Epinephrine, 2 mg/250 ml D_5W						
CVP mix, 250 ml D_5W						
4. Other						
Blood gases						
Pacemaker (type)						
Open cardiac massage						

Figure 48.2. Cardiac arrest flow sheet.

aid measures, perform limited physical examinations, and develop a plan of action.

Physician Triage

In this system, a physician triages all patients and may treat patients at the triage area. This system may be less efficient and more costly than a nurse triage system.

Team Triage

This system employs a physician and nurse working together to triage all patients.

Emergency departments that have long waits do well using the advanced triage system. Studies have shown that patient waiting and treatment times are decreased, and that nurses have a high accuracy rate in appropriateness of diagnostic procedures ordered. Any triage system should meet the needs of the individual emergency department, be efficient, cost-effective, and periodically reviewed by quality-assurance assessment to be sure it continues to meet patient and departmental needs.

Role of the Advanced Triage Nurse

Clearly, this triage role is one of the most responsible, challenging, and stressful roles in an ED. The nurse in this role can set the tone for all other staff in the department and for the patient's hospital stay. Some of the duties of the nurse in this role are:

1. To expedite the patient's care;
2. To perform a patient assessment;
3. To establish priority of patient needs;
4. To assign patients to the appropriate treatment areas while considering the present patient load, staffing, and physical layout of the area;
5. To initiate appropriate diagnostic tests in order to expedite the patient's care;
6. To initiate appropriate first-aid measures;
7. To communicate necessary information to the appropriate people;
8. To provide information on referrals when necessary;
9. To supervise assisting personnel;
10. To be responsible for responding to prehospital communications;
11. To act as a positive public relations force with patients, visitors, prehospital personnel, and families;
12. To provide health care teaching when necessary;
13. To perform necessary crisis intervention;
14. To document prehospital treatment, triage findings, and plan of action;
15. To be able to initiate resources available to patients for social problems.

This role is frequently too stressful and busy to be made a permanent assignment. Daily reassignment in all areas of an E.D. provides the staff with changes in pace and interest while maintaining all their skills. At the same time, it provides the manager with flexibility and efficiency in staffing. Nurses who find triage especially stressful may be better off reassigned. They should receive assistance before the stress interferes with their ability to perform.

Triage nurses need experience and a formal orientation as noted earlier in this chapter. In addition the triage nurse must be able to communicate with people of varying educational and cultural backgrounds, be nonjudgmental, and understand medicolegal issues in emergency care.

Triage Process

The advanced system of triage is the most cost-effective, efficient, and safest type of triage. It is less costly than a physician triage system and less prone to error than a clerk-oriented system. The advanced system decreases waiting time, ensures that the more seriously ill are treated first, enhances patient flow and organization, utilizes resources in the most effective way, and improves patient satisfaction and the public image of the emergency department. Nurse morale is often improved by using this system since they feel that they can utilize all of their knowledge and skills and are able to make independent decisions. The role is a very responsible one, appreciated by physicians, patients and their families. Only registered nurses should perform advanced triage since it requires advanced assessment skills and the initiation of diagnostic procedures.

The components of this system include obtaining a brief history, performing a limited physical examination, identifying the problem, and formulating an initial plan of action. An explanation of these components as they relate to the problem-oriented method of documentation is provided in Table 48.5.

In busy times of the day advanced triage of this type may require assignment of two triage nurses.

Subjective Data

The subjective data includes all the information obtained from the patient or from those who accompany the patient. The data should include all the necessary information pertaining to the present complaint, pertinent past medial history, medications, and known allergies. It is important for the nurse to make the patient feel at ease, eliminate as many barriers as possible, and direct the interview. Keeping the interview on track may not always be easy, but it is important in order to obtain the needed information and to avoid wasting time. Less time should be spent interviewing the more acutely ill patient. *A patient with multiple trauma is not interviewed at all, but is assigned to a treatment area immediately.* It is also true that patients with minor injuries and illnesses frequently need only a short interview and quick assessment. Treatment received prior to the E.D. visit should be documented. Tables 48.6, 48.7, and 48.8 illustrate questions that are asked patients according to their complaints.

Objective Data

The objective data includes all that the nurse sees, feels, smells, hears, or interprets as a result of tests

Table 48.6.
Suggested Triage Questions for Trauma Patients[a]

General
- Where did the accident occur?
- When did the accident take place?
- Where are you injured?
- Has any treatment been given to you? If so, what?
- Date of your last tetanus toxoid?

Motor Vehicle Accident
- Which seat were you in?
- Were you wearing a seatbelt?
- Was the car moving or standing still?
- Was your car struck from behind? Side? Front?
- Did you strike your head, chest, etc? If so, on what?
- Any LOC?

Lacerations
- Note size and location, bleeding, pulses proximal and distal.
- What caused the cut (glass, knife, metal)?
- What time did the accident occur?
- Crush type of injury?

Fractures, Sprains, Strains
- What caused your fall (faintness, dizziness, tripped, slipped on ice)?
- Can you bear weight?
- When you fell, what part of your body did you land on? What type of surface?
- Did you turn your ankle inwards?
- Is the pain worse with respiration? Coughing? Movement?
- How much did the object weigh (lifted or fell on patient)?
- What increases the pain?
- Have you injured this area before?
- Note ROM, pulses, swelling, and color.

[a] LOC, loss of consciousness; ROM, range of motion.

obtained. Pertinent vital signs are included here. Laying a hand on the patient helps to make the patient more comfortable, and allows one to assess the patient's skin for temperature, texture, and moisture. Listen and watch the patients as they speak. Do they appear more uncomfortable than they verbalize? Do you sense that they are holding back information because fear or embarrassment prevents them from talking about the real problem? Examine the injured area to confirm which x-rays to order and, more importantly, to ensure that a patient with compromised blood flow to an injured extremity is identified and treated expeditiously.

Assessment

After obtaining the subjective and objective data, the nurse must evaluate all the information and make a decision as to the patient's problem. The trend in nursing is toward the use of nursing diagnosis, but in the triage situation, nurses should continue to make a medical assessment, i.e., if the patient is dyspneic, check for pneumothorax. It is less important that the nurse correctly diagnose patients 100% of the time. More importantly, the nurse must recognize the severity of the illness and its priority.

Table 48.7.
Suggested Triage Questions for Patients with Chest Complaints

Chest Pain
- Was there an injury?
- What is the pain like (pressure, stabbing, tightness, dull)?
- How often does the pain occur and how long does it last?
- What brings on the pain? What relieves the pain?
- Does the pain radiate to any other area, that is, down your arm?
- Are you having any nausea and vomiting, fever, cough, shortness of breath?
- Any previous episodes of this pain or similar pain?
- Do you smoke? How long? How much?

Upper Respiratory Infections
- When did it start?
- Is the cough productive or nonproductive? What color is the sputum? What is the character of cough?
- Any fever? Sore throat?
- History of pulmonary diseases?
- What treatment has been done so far?

Table 48.8.
Suggested Triage Questions for Patients with Gastrointestinal Complaints[a]

Abdominal Pain
- Where is the pain? Can you point to the pain with one finger?
- How long have you had the pain?
- What makes it better? Worse?
- Describe the pain (dull, stabbing, burning)?
- What did you eat at your last meal and when was that? Does anything affect the pain?
- Have you been nauseated or had any vomiting?
- When was your last bowel movement? Normal?
- Date of your LMP? Normal?
- Have you had any burning or pain on urination? Frequency?
- Do you have any vaginal/penile discharge?
- Have you lost weight? How much? Over how long a period of time?
- Any previous history of this type of pain?

Nausea, Vomiting, Diarrhea
- How many days/hours have you had this?
- How frequently does it occur?
- Have you noticed any blood or bile?
- Are you experiencing any pain with this?
- Have you had any recent injury?
- Have you had fever?
- Have you had any weight loss? How much? During what time span?

[a] LMP, last menstrual period.

Plan

Formulating and following through on a plan of action is the final step in the triage process. This step includes establishing patient priority, assigning the patient to a treatment area, assigning a health care provider, ordering and obtaining diagnostic procedures, and initiating any necessary first-aid measures.

Vital signs should be obtained on all patients at triage, with the exception of acutely ill emergent patients, whose signs will be obtained in the treatment area. The standard can be written for the specific ED, but it is prudent to make sure that no patient leaves an emergency department without having had vital signs taken. If a patient decides to leave without treatment, then the nurse's documentation should reflect this.

Telephone Triage or Advice Calls

This practice raises some potential risk management problems. The best and safest policy is not to allow triaging or the giving of advice over the telephone unless it is a life-threatening situation and you are guiding the caller through first-aid measures, such as CPR. If, however, established protocol allows telephone triage, written policies should be developed in consultation with hospital attorneys. These written policies should delineate responsibility and restrictions for those who perform this task. Some form of documentation to show what the caller asked and what advice was given is essential.

SUGGESTED READINGS

Blansfield J, Fackler C, Bergereron K. Developing standardized care plans: One emergency department's experience. *J Emerg Nurs,* 1985;11:304–309.

Bolles RN. *What Color Is Your Parachute?* 7th ed. Berkeley: Ten Speed Press, 1981.

Budassi SA, Barber JM. *Emergency Nursing: Principles and Practice.* St Louis: CV Mosby, 1981.

Emergency Nurses Association: *Standards of Emergency Nursing Practice.* St Louis: CV Mosby, 1983.

Estrada EG. Symposium on emergency nursing: Triage systems. *Nurs Clin North Am,* 1981;16:13–24.

Flint, LS, Hammett, WH, Martens, K. Quality assurance in the emergency department. *Ann Emerg Med,* 1985;14: 134–138.

Georg JE. Emergency nursing: Standards of care. *J Emerg Nurs,* 1984;10:52–53.

Heister K, Johnson B, Trimberger L. E.D. standards and audit criteria. *J Emerg Nurs,* 1982;8:83–87.

Joint Commission on Accreditation of Hospitals. Standards for emergency services. In *Standards for Accreditation of Hospitals.* 1985. Chicago: JCAH.

Liebler JG. *Managing Health Records: Administrative Principles,* Rockville: Aspen Systems, 1980.

Phaneuf MC, Wandelt, MA. Quality assurance in nursing. *Nurs Forum,* 1974;13:328–345.

Rakich JS, Longest BB, Darr K. *Managing Health Services Organizations,* Philadelphia: WB Saunders, 1985.

Rund DA, Rausch TA: *Triage.* St Louis: CV Mosby, 1981.

Schuler RS. *Effective Personnel Management.* St Paul: West Publishing, 1983.

Walts L, Blair F. Making quality assurance work in the emergency department. *J Emerg Nurs,* 1983;9:59–60.

CHAPTER **49**

Legal Aspects of Emergency Medical Care

ERNEST M. HADDAD, Esq.
MICHAEL BROAD, Esq.

Legal aspects of medical care have become so prominent, and in some situations so complex, that it is easy to overstate their effect on the day-to-day practice of medicine. Despite this growing prominence of legal issues, the basic standards of traditional medical care still apply to medical practice, including practice in the emergency department. Because these basic standards generally arise from state law, the rules themselves will often vary from state to state. Practitioners of emergency medicine and the institutions in which they practice should consult counsel for information on local law as necessary.

BASIC LEGAL DUTIES OF EMERGENCY MEDICINE PRACTITIONERS

Acute Emergency Care

Duty to Treat

The law expects emergency departments and emergency medical practitioners to perform the function they have assumed within the health care community: provision of acute emergency care to those in need. Although special rules apply to the treatment of nonconsenting patients, the vast majority of patients seen in emergency situations are either actively seeking care or would be doing so if they were mentally and physically able. The general rule is to treat.

Uninsured Patients

In most states, hospitals cannot withhold lifesaving or critical care because of a patient's inability to pay. Those hospitals that do not take all patients who present should have clearly delineated emergency department intake procedures for acute patients without personal funds or insurance. At the very least, these patients must be adequately stabilized before being referred or transported to another facility. The courts will look with appropriate disfavor on a hospital that allows an indigent or uninsured patient to die or suffer serious injury as a result of delay in treatment or referral to another hospital.

Good Samaritan Situations

Even outside the emergency department, physicians may be required or encouraged to provide emergency care to acutely ill or injured persons even if no physician-patient relationship exists. In some states, for example, licensure laws require that physicians render lifesaving emergency care to the extent of their professional ability. In other states, "Good Samaritan" laws exempt physicians from malpractice liability for emergency care when provided in good faith without expectation of remuneration. Even without such protection, the professional duty to save a life outweighs the risk of malpractice liability in these cases.

Quality of Medical Care

Performance Standard—The Average Qualified Physician

The law expects the physician to perform at the level of an average qualified physician or, if the physician claims a medical specialty, at the level of an average physician in that specialty. Care that falls below this level, and that injures a patient, is malpractice.

Obligations for Specialty Consultation

This performance standard includes the obligation to refer the patient for specialty consultation or treatment if the indicated medical services are beyond the physician's experience and ability. In an emergency, of course, the physician's initial obligation is to stabilize the patient before or while additional medical services are being arranged.

Informed Consent for Treatment

Definition

An essential part of overall medical care, and a precondition to actual treatment, is obtaining the patient's informed consent. For consent to be truly "informed," the physician must explain to the patient his/her condition in general terms, the proposed treatment and its associated risks and benefits, and the potential alternatives and their related risks and benefits. In addition to respecting the patient's personal integrity and satisfying legal requirements, this process has the virtues of educating and involving the patient in the treatment, and of setting appropriate expectations for the potential outcomes.

Patients Unable to Participate in Informed Consent

Obviously, emergencies restrict opportunities for extended discourse, and the amount of communication must be tailored to the patient's particular circumstances. Hospitals should develop and carefully follow internal procedures, consistent with specific requirements that may be mandated by state law, for patients unable to participate in the consent process because of trauma, mental illness or incapacity, youth, or severely limited intelligence. While these procedures may, depending on the state law, require the ultimate consent of family members, a hospital consent committee, or a court, in the emergency department the presumption should be that the patient will receive necessary emergency treatment regardless of ability to consent.

Documentation

Hospitals should also develop, and physicians should carefully follow, procedures for documentation of informed consent. Some states not only regulate the information that must be provided to a patient prior to performing significant procedures, but also insist that a particular consent form be used. In most jurisdictions, however, the manner in which informed consent is documented is left to the discretion of the physician or the hospital. It is important that the system adopted provide for documentation of the patient's inability to give informed consent, when that is the case, and of the emergency conditions that warrant the proposed treatment in those circumstances.

The physician has an additional opportunity to document special aspects of consent (as well as complications of diagnosis or treatment) in the medical record. Careful notes made at the time care is provided can be invaluable for showing the basis for a particular course of action, and for discouraging a lawsuit in the event of an undesired result.

Special Problems in Informed Consent

Refusal of Blood Products. A few commonly encountered situations present special consent problems in the emergency department. The hospital should have procedures for providing care to Jehovah's Witnesses and others who, for religious reasons, may refuse to receive blood or blood products. The general rule, of course, is that adult patients who are mentally competent may decline any proposed therapy, even if the result will be certain death. Some states have created an exception, allowing medical care providers to obtain a judicial order authorizing treatment if the patient would leave minor children (especially young children who might become wards of the state) and if the proposed treatment is relatively noninvasive and has a high likelihood of successful outcome.

Parental Refusal of Care to Children. The states more consistently intervene on behalf of children whose parents refuse to consent on behalf of their children to transfusion (or other relatively low-risk, high-benefit treatment). If the proposed treatment is medically necessary, and the child too young to express any principled objection, the court will issue an order permitting or directing the hospital or physician to proceed. If the child is close to the age of majority, and is joining the parents in actively opposing treatment, the court is less likely to order treatment.

Medical Examiner Autopsy Jurisdiction. Consent of the patient or the family may be sought to perform a postmortem examination, except in cases of serious trauma or unexplained injury when the medical examiner must be contacted. In these latter cases, consent of the family is not necessary and should not be sought; the family should be told that by law the medical examiner must be notified and will decide whether or not to do an autopsy.

Confidentiality

General Rules. The general legal rule concerning confidentiality is that communications between a patient and a physician in the course of professional consultation for diagnosis or treatment are confidential, and are not to be disclosed to outsiders by the physician. Many states elevate this confidentiality to a testimonial privilege: the patient has the privilege to prevent the physician from testifying about the communication in court or at a deposition.

Exceptions. Sometimes, however, the physician is permitted or required to disclose patient information that would normally be confidential. The typical privilege statute contains exceptions for certain types of suits (e.g., malpractice actions), and for other cases (such as those involving child custody) if the judge determines that the value of the testimony would outweigh the importance of the privilege. As discussed below, the physician must report instances of abuse or neglect of children (and sometimes also of elderly patients), and under certain circumstances must warn the potential victims of threats by the patient.

Confidentiality also does not prevent the communication of medical or pyschiatric information in connection with an involuntary commitment. In addition, certain medical conditions by law must be reported: serious communicable diseases must be reported to local public health authorities; certain serious injuries, such as gunshot wounds, must be reported to the police; and unexplained, violent or accidental deaths must be reported to the medical examiner.

LEGAL ISSUES IN EMERGENCY TREATMENT

Patients Incompetent to Give Informed Consent

Complications arise when the emergency department patient lacks mental competence. Two situations commonly arise: (*a*) the medical/surgical emergency patient who is unable to participate rationally in the treatment process (and may even be refusing to consent to necessary care); and (*b*) the emergency psychiatric patient, with few or no medical problems, who needs (and also may be refusing) treatment for mental illness. Some cases, such as the unsuccessful suicide, present elements of both.

Substituted Consent for Incompetent Patients

The concept of informed consent presumes that the patient has the mental competence to give or withhold consent. When competence is lacking—when the patient lacks the ability to understand the relevant information and make a judgment based upon that understanding—the consent procedure becomes more complicated.

Nonjudicial Resolution. The law of all states provides a mechanism for obtaining *substituted* consent when the patient is incapable of giving direct consent. In some jurisdictions, the law expressly allows nonjudicial resolution of these issues by, for example, the family and physicians, or a hospital ethics committee.

Judicial Resolution. In other states, the formal process for obtaining substituted consent involves going to court, usually in a guardianship proceeding, and presenting the relevant information to a judge or a court-appointed investigator. In these states, the court will first consider the patient's competence and, if it finds the patient incompetent to consent, the court will then apply either the ''substituted judgment'' test (a subjective analysis in which the judge determines or purports to determine what the patient would have decided under these circumstances if competent) or the ''best interests'' test (an objective test in which the judge finds and follows the patient's best interests, and whether or not the patient would have done so if competent).

Typically, the evidence presented to the judge in a ''best interests'' state will include: the patient's inability to participate in the informed consent process and to give consent; the reasons for that inability; the need for or desirability of the proposed procedure; the risks and benefits of the procedure; the alternatives (including doing nothing) and the corresponding risks and benefits; and the long-term prognosis. In a ''substituted judgment'' state, the judge will look to statements of the patient while competent, and sometimes to the patient's overall life-style as well, in order to determine or infer what the patient's preference would be in light of the risks, benefits, and prognosis.

Emergency Department Strategies

Again, hospital or emergency department personnel are well-advised to develop guidelines for these common situations. One approach to treatment of incompetent patients would be to require judicial approval whenever the delay would not significantly compromise the patient's condition. Another less legally rigorous but probably more practical approach would call for formal substituted consent only when the patient or the patient's family actively resist the proposed treatment. It is also useful to have available designated medical staff members experienced in the determination of competency for consultation in difficult cases.

Psychiatric Patients Dangerous to Self or Others

Commitment

Similar issues arise in the treatment of the emergency psychiatric patient, except that here the law provides an additional mechanism—commitment—for dealing with the patient who presents a serious danger to self or others as a result of mental condition. All states have a mechanism for involuntary commitment for a period of initial evaluation upon certification by a physician that the legal standards for commitment have been met. Typically, these standards involve a likelihood of serious harm to self or others, generally as manifested by suicidal or violent behavior.

Because the commitment is involuntary, no consent is needed from the patient or family. Typically, however, the patient has the opportunity to sign in to the psychiatric facility as a voluntary admission rather than be committed involuntarily. In such cases, the facility customarily retains the right to hold the patient for a limited period of time while seeking a court order if the patient subsequently decides to sign out.

Use of Restraints

Psychiatric patients in the emergency department can present difficult management problems. Because most acute care general hospitals are not licensed to care for involuntary patients, patients dangerous to themselves or others are generally committed to another institution specializing in mental health. During the time necessary to locate an appropriate facility and arrange transportation, emergency department personnel are responsible for ensuring the safety of the committed patient, of other patients, and of the emergency department staff as well. As required by the particular situation, it may be necessary to supervise closely or to restrain the patient. The guiding principle should be to suit the degree of restraint to the needs of the patient, using in each case the least amount of restraint reasonably necessary to prevent harm and to keep the patient from leaving.

Advising Potential Victims of Threats

The last decade has seen substantial development of a limited duty to warn potential victims of a patient's threats, even though doing so would violate traditional notions of confidentiality. Although not all states have faced the question, the clear direction of the evolving law is to require notice when: (*a*) the threat is directed to an individual or group that is sufficiently specific to make them a direct target and to make notification feasible; (*b*) the threat is sufficiently serious that, if carried through, would pose a significant danger; and (*c*) the physician has reason to believe there is a likelihood the patient will carry out the threat.

Dealing with Victims of Crime or Alleged Perpetrators

Emergency department personnel have frequent contact with both the victims of crime and the alleged perpetrators. This interaction carries with it questions about the role of the hospital and the physicians in criminal matters.

Duty to Disclose Information

Emergency patients will sometimes disclose to hospital staff their involvement in criminal activity. As a general matter, there is no legal obligation to report that a patient has confessed to the commission of a crime. In states with a strict physician-patient privilege, such disclosure might itself be a breach of legal duty. In other states, statutory privileges for communications to psychiatrists, social workers, rape counselors, or other therapists have the same effect for a smaller category of health care providers.

Even in the absence of strict confidentiality requirements, it is generally better practice for the hospital to confine its role to the rendering of medical care, leaving issues of criminal enforcement to the police and the district attorney. Exceptions, however, include situations where reporting is required by law (e.g., child abuse, gunshot wound) or where the failure to report would contravene strong public policy. In addition, the hospital (generally through its security department) may confiscate and destroy, or turn in to the police drugs or other contraband brought into the hospital by patients.

Victims of Rape or Assault

Where the patient is the victim, rather than the alleged perpetrator, different considerations apply. Although the hospital has no independent obligation to undertake criminal action, and should generally not initiate contact with criminal authorities without the consent of the patient/victim, hospital personnel should be prepared to cooperate with the patient in any action the patient elects. For the hospital, this cooperation could include calling the police at the patient's request, providing a private and quiet place for the patient to meet with police, and taking and preserving whatever medical evidence may be relevant in a future criminal prosecution. The hospital should establish procedures for gathering and retaining medical evidence in these situations. In many jurisdictions, the police or district attorney will be pleased to work with hospital personnel in setting up appropriate systems.

Often a patient/victim may be unsure whether to involve the police, or may initially state an intention not to press charges. This situation is particularly likely to arise in cases of rape or other injury with high psychological trauma. The hospital should still treat these as potential court cases, so the patient does not lose the opportunity to change the decision later.

Drug and Alcohol Testing

The police, district attorney, or registry of motor vehicles personnel may ask the hospital to draw blood to test for drug or alcohol content. As with any other medical procedure, this should not be done without the consent of the patient or a court order authorizing the test. On occasion, a person may present in the emergency department with the request that the hospital perform a drug or blood-alcohol test, usually in hopes of establishing sobriety or contradicting a test administered by the police. The hospital may establish policies for whether to perform such tests in the absence of medical necessity.

Dangerous Patients

The hospital will want to establish guidelines for dealing with dangerous patients to ensure the safety of staff and of other patients. In addition to committable psychiatric patients, discussed above, emergency department staff are likely to encounter three types of safety problems.

Weapons. Patients known to be carrying weapons should be asked to leave the weapons with the hospital security department while they are receiving medical care. If the patient is thought to be potentially dangerous, it is advisable to have security present when the request is made.

Patients in Police Custody. Patients arriving under police custody—typically, criminal suspects injured during the course of apprehension—should normally be guarded by police as needed to prevent elopement and to protect the safety of others.

Violent Patients. Dangerous patients whose violence does not result from mental illness, and who are thus not committable, often repeat patients well-known to staff, and who may threaten or attack hospital personnel, must be addressed. A common approach in these cases is to set limits for the patient, e.g., that care will be provided only if the patient arrives unarmed, comes only at scheduled times, does not threaten staff, etc. Of course, in serious emergencies, the hospital will be obliged to provide necessary medical care even if these criteria are not fully satisfied. With difficult cases, security should be present.

Autopsies and Transplantation

Dying or dead-on-arrival patients present different consent problems for the emergency department staff. If medically appropriate, physicians may seek consent to harvest organs for transplantation. Several states have considered adopting a requirement that physicians seek such consent whenever the organs would be medically appropriate for transplantation. The Uniform Anatomical Gifts Act, adopted in some form in all 50 states, allows the patient (or, after the patient's death, the family) to give such consent.

Reports of Abuse and Neglect

All states have some mechanism for notifying state child welfare officials of children suffering abuse or neglect. Most jurisdictions *require* physicians and other professionals who deal with children to make these reports if there is reasonable cause to believe a child has been abused or neglected, and failure to do so can subject the nonreporter to statutory penalties. Absolute certainty is not required: a report should generally be filed whenever there is a significant possibility of abuse or neglect that cannot be ruled out. (For further discussion, see Chapter 29.)

In some cases of serious abuse, such as when the death of a child results, state law may also require a report to be made directly to the district attorney.

Recently, some states have extended the abuse and neglect reporting requirements to include situations where older persons, less able to care for themselves, have been abused or neglected by family, nursing home personnel, or other caregivers. Standards and procedures for reporting elderly abuse are modeled after the comparable child abuse provisions.

CONCLUSION

Sensitivity to legal concerns in the emergency department is an important element in the successful delivery of high quality emergency medical care. Many common, recurring legal issues can be anticipated, and hospitals and physicians should establish policies and protocols for dealing with them. This preparation is particularly important in the emergency department, where a prompt response is often essential.

SUGGESTED READINGS

Annas GJ, Glantz LH, Katz BF. *The Rights of Doctors, Nurses, and Allied Health Professionals: A Health Law Printer.* New York, NY: Avon Books, 1981.

SECTION **7**

Illustrated Techniques

EDITH TAGRIN

Medical Artist

CHARLES J. McCABE, M.D.

Associate Editor

This section, "Illustrated Techniques," is designed to provide a visual and instructive aid to the placement of the more common "invasive" devices, including lifesaving airway tubes, monitoring lines, and diagnostic or therapeutic catheters. Some of these techniques may differ from written accounts in previous chapters; when they do, it is to offer an alternative method or to emphasize recognized differences in styles of management. The following 27 emergency procedures are illustrated:

1. Orotracheal Intubation
2. Nasoendotracheal Intubation
3. Cricothyrotomy
4. Needle Cricothyrotomy
5. Subclavian Vein Catheter Placement
6. Internal Jugular Vein Catheterization
7. Saphenous Vein Cutdown
8. Insertion of Transvenous Ventricular Pacing Electrode
9. Radial Arterial Puncture
10. Pericardiocentesis
11. Emergency Thoracotomy
12. Thoracentesis
13. Chest Tube Insertion
14. Lumbar Puncture
15. Peritoneal Lavage
16. Percutaneous Suprapubic Cystotomy
17. Culdocentesis
18. Metacarpal Nerve Block
19. Drainage of a Paronychia
20. Drainage of a Felon
21. Evacuation of a Subungual Hematoma
22. Suturing Techniques
23. Injection for Bursitis—Shoulder
24. Arthrocentesis—Knee
25. Arthrocentesis—Ankle
26. Evacuation of a Thrombosed Hemorrhoid
27. Drainage of a Perianal Abscess

1. OROTRACHEAL INTUBATION

DAVID J. CULLEN, M.D.

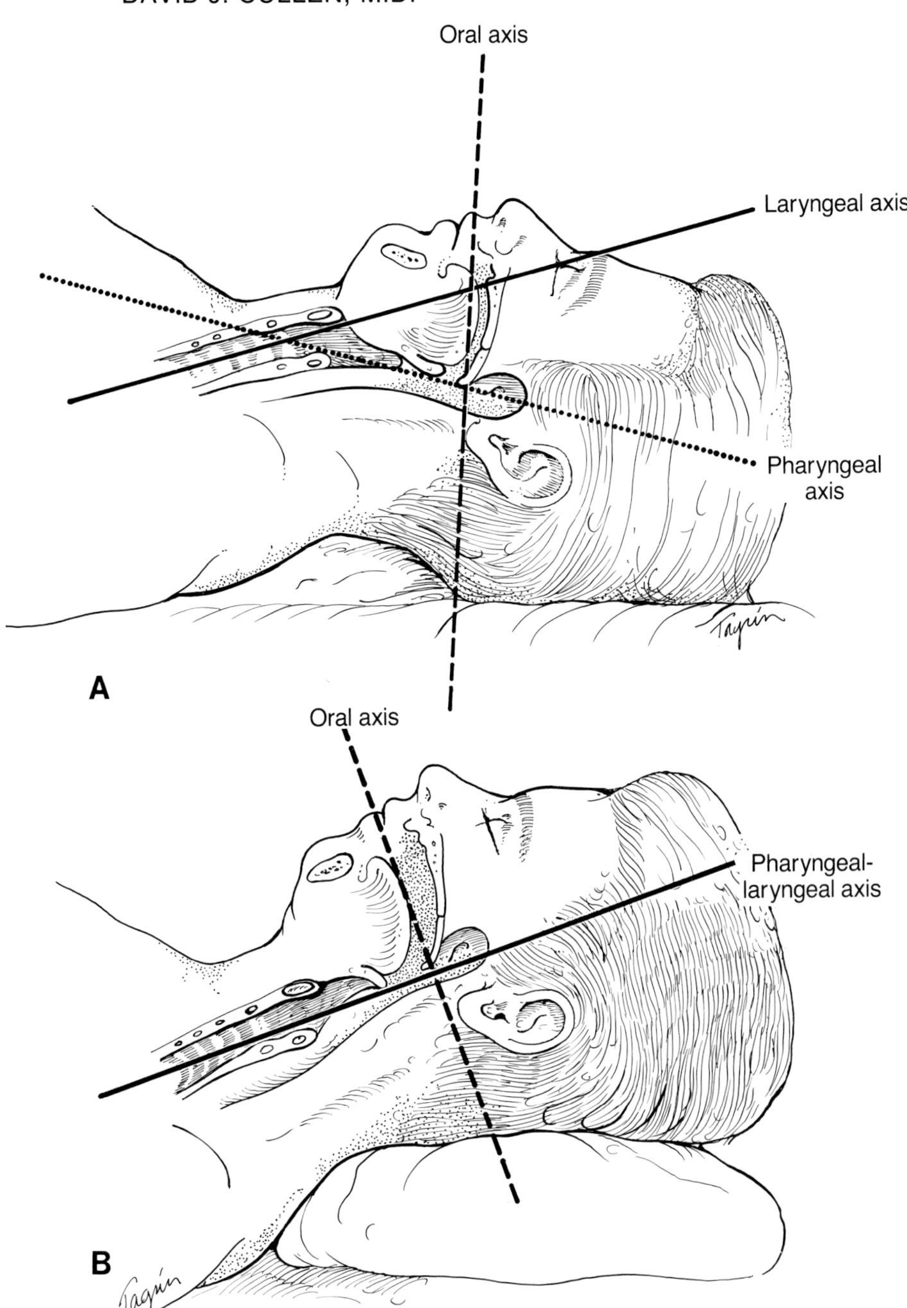

A–C, When the head is supported by a pillow or blanket and is placed in the "sniff" position, the oral, pharyngeal, and laryngeal axes merge toward one plane. Deviations from this position cause the axes to diverge, which makes intubation more difficult.

The sniff position with the head hyperextended affords a straight-line view to the vocal cords. A curved-blade (Macintosh) laryngoscope is placed in the mouth from the right side, sweeping the tongue to the left. The blade is inserted anteriorly into the vallecula; anterior force lifts the epiglottis and opens the view to the vocal cords. If a straight blade (Miller or Foregger) is used, it is inserted to just beyond the tip of the epiglottis. With lifting of the epiglottis, the cords can be seen directly.

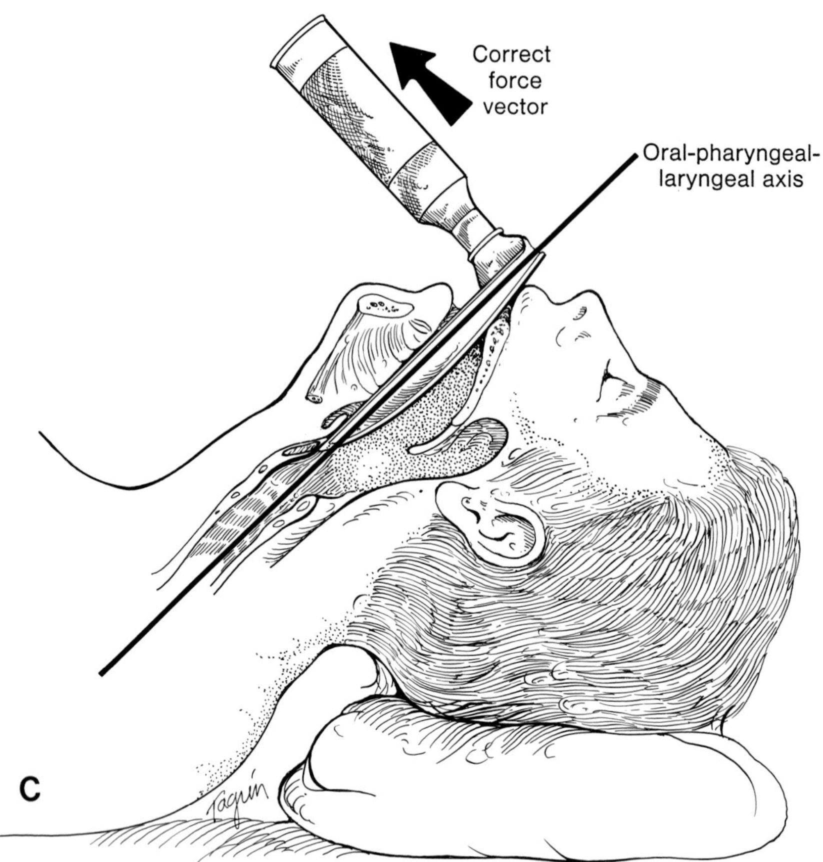

D–E, Technical considerations: (1) The laryngoscope is not to be used as a level to pry the glottis open. After insertion, the entire blade and handle are lifted anteriorly to pull the jaw in a vector toward the operator's eyes. (2) Tubes with a slight curve at the tip are easier to direct into the trachea, particularly when a curved blade is used. Some tracheas angle anteriorly, and a curved tube fits the angulation well. (3) For emergency intubation, a stiff tube will best resist kinking or bending as the tube is inserted into the trachea. (4) Use of a stylet will result in a fixed curve and a stiff tube at the tube's entry into the trachea. Once the tip of the tube is just beyond the vocal cords, the stylet should be removed to prevent trauma to the larynx and trachea. (5) On viewing the glottis, the physician usually sees a dark hole bordered by the two vocal cords, which appear pearl-gray. (6) Once the tube tip is through the cords, the tube should be inserted until the proximal end of the cuff is just beyond the cords. This will locate the tip of the tube in the middle part of the trachea. Since the trachea in adults is approximately 11 cm long, and since the proximal end of the cuff is about 5 cm from the tip of the tube, intubation of the right mainstem bronchus can be avoided. (7) The two most serious errors in intubation are: (*a*) intubating the esophagus instead of the trachea, and (*b*) inserting the endotracheal tube into the right mainstem bronchus. When the esophagus has been intubated, a characteristic gurgling sound is emitted with each positive-pressure breath, the chest wall does not rise, and the abdomen increases in size. If any doubt exists, the patient should be auscultated over the stomach while being ventilated. If the right mainstem bronchus has been intubated, breath sounds may be absent on the left side, but this is not always reliable. Pulmonary compliance will be low, but in a patient requiring emergency intubation, compliance may be decreased already. The tube's location should be ensured either by chest x-ray examination or by direct visualization of the cuff just beyond the vocal cords.

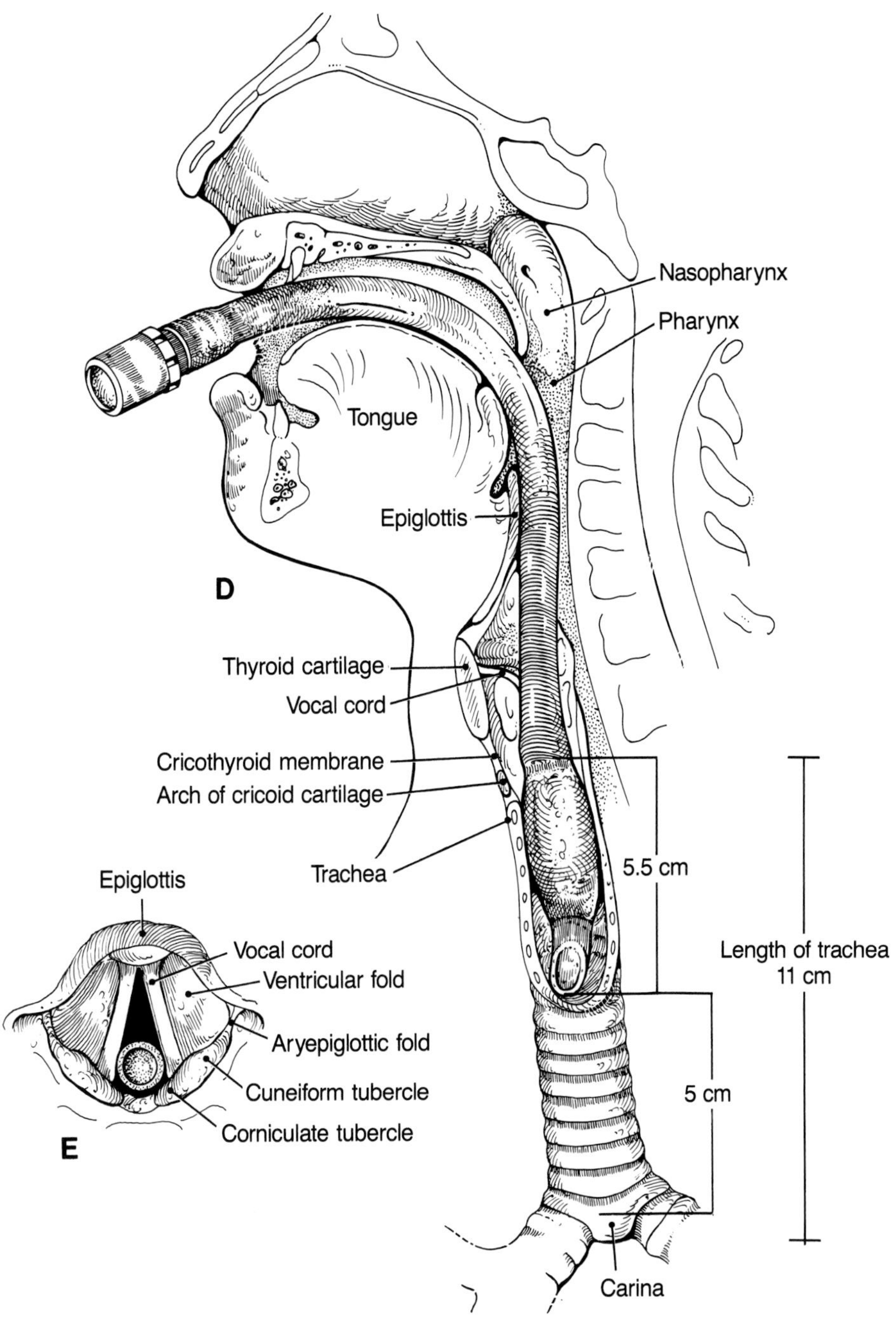
Nasopharynx
Pharynx
Tongue
Epiglottis
D
Thyroid cartilage
Vocal cord
Cricothyroid membrane
Arch of cricoid cartilage
Trachea
5.5 cm
Length of trachea
11 cm
5 cm
Carina
Epiglottis
Vocal cord
Ventricular fold
Aryepiglottic fold
Cuneiform tubercle
Corniculate tubercle
E

2. NASOENDOTRACHEAL INTUBATION

DAVID J. CULLEN, M.D.

PREINTUBATION ASSESSMENT

Determine whether nasotracheal intubation is even possible or desirable when compared with the need for orotracheal intubation. Check for patency of the nares and, if possible, obtain information from the patient concerning previous difficulties in breathing through the nose.

If movement of the neck is not contraindicated (due to possible cervical spine injury), check for neck mobility by flexing and extending the head in order to determine optimal position for intubation.

INDICATIONS FOR NASOTRACHEAL INTUBATION

Nasotracheal intubation is indicated:

1. When airway obstruction actually is present or is likely to occur;
2. When airway protection from aspiration cannot be guaranteed;
3. When full exposure of the mouth for repair of intraoral injuries or restorative work is needed;
4. When anatomic abnormalities, trauma, diseases of the upper airway, or inexperience of the operator make direct laryngoscopy difficult, dangerous, or impossible;
5. When, in the opinion of some observers, long-term intubation and ventilation are anticipated, a nasotracheal tube is usually more stable and fixed, there is less chance of the tube kinking, and there is greater comfort to the awake patient.

AWAKE VS. ANESTHETIZED NASOTRACHEAL INTUBATION

When direct laryngoscopy or positive pressure ventilation after induction of anesthesia may be hazardous, awake nasotracheal intubation is particularly valuable. Otherwise, when anesthesia can be induced safely by mask, direct nasotracheal intubation can proceed blindly after induction of anesthesia or under direct vision after proper intubating conditions have been achieved. However, *in the emergency department, awake blind nasal intubation is the most useful approach to securing the airway.*

PROCEDURE

Topically anesthetize the nasal mucosa with no more than 5 ml of 4% cocaine. This provides local anesthesia to the nose and nasopharynx and minimizes the possibility of epistaxis. If the patient does not have a full stomach (unlikely in an emergency department), complete topical anesthesia of the tongue, pharynx, glottis, and vocal cords may be accomplished with topical lidocaine. However, most patients must be assumed to have a full stomach or will be unconscious enough so that additional anesthesia to areas other than just the nasal mucosa is contraindicated.

The nostril chosen for intubation usually depends on anatomic and pathologic considerations. Check which nostril is more patent.

Obviously, the nasotracheal tube size will depend on the size and sex of the patient. A 7-mm internal diameter tube for most women and an 8-mm tube for most men, each with a large-volume, low-pressure cuff, is usually appropriate.

A–B, After introducing a well-lubricated nasotracheal tube into the chosen nostril using gentle but persistent pressure, place the head in the sniff position to align the epiglottis with the pharynx and trachea. Of greatest importance in the spontaneously breathing patient is the character of breath sounds that are used to guide the tube toward the glottis. If these sounds diminish, the tube is deviating away from the glottis; if the breath sounds increase in loudness and clarity, the tube is moving closer to the glottic opening.

When the tube is well-positioned near the glottis, wait until inspiration, then quickly advance the tube with the incoming breath, since the vocal cord opening is widest during that time. If airway reflexes are still present, the cords will attempt to close when the tube touches the glottis, hence the need for swift insertion while the cords are patent. Patients frequently cough violently once the tube is actually in the trachea, and confirmation of tube location begins by hearing tubular breath sounds and feeling air movement with each exhalation through the tube. Further confirmation of the tube location can be made by listening for bilateral breath sounds.

Obtain a portable chest x-ray to confirm intratracheal location definitely and to ensure that the tube has not been inserted beyond the trachea into the right mainstem bronchus.

PROBLEMS OF AWAKE NASOTRACHEAL INTUBATION

C–D, If the tube impinges the neck anteriorly because the tube's curvature is excessive, inspection of the neck will demonstrate this. The tube needs to be more posterior in relation to the glottis, which

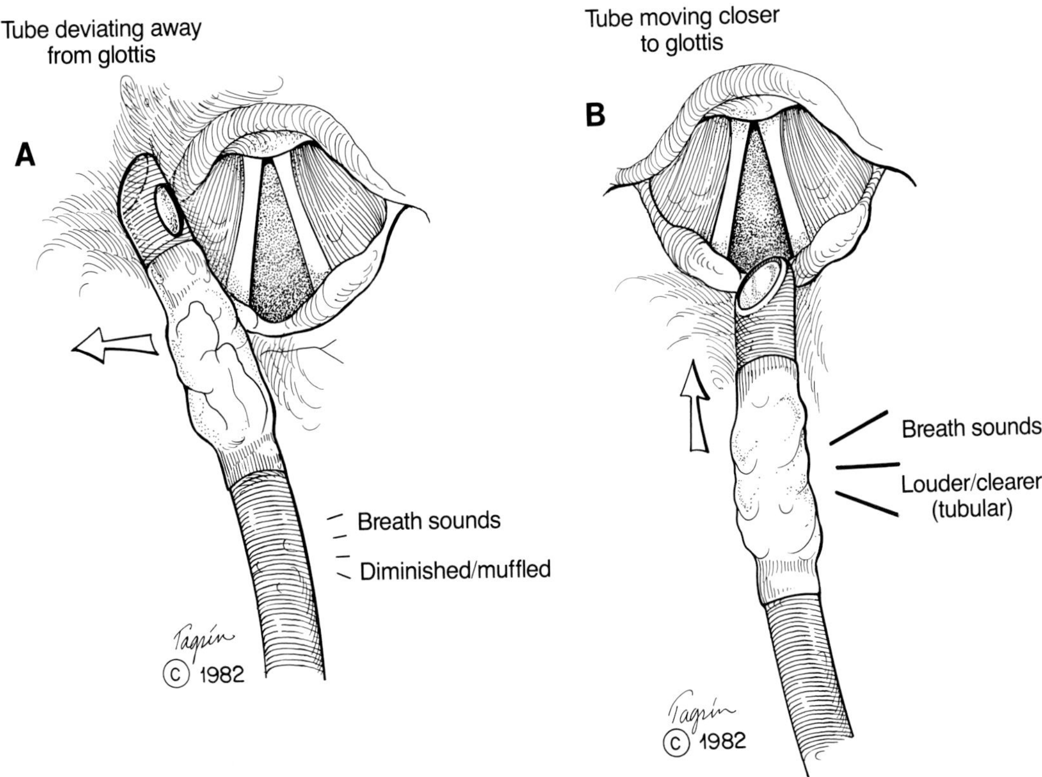

can be accomplished by further flexing the head and gently pushing the glottis posteriorly.

E–F, If the tube passes posteriorly into the esophagus because the tube curvature is insufficient to move anteriorly into the glottic opening, hyperextend the head.

G–I, If the tube is laterally displaced into the pyriform sinus, which can be detected by seeing the neck bulge with movement of the tube, withdraw slightly and turn the tube toward the midline.

A variety of other techniques may be necessary to ensure placement of a nasotracheal tube in particularly difficult subjects, usually requiring an experienced operator. However, one can try tubes with greater or lesser curvatures, or attempt to insert a smaller tube than expected if the glottic opening is also smaller than anticipated. Obviously, a stylet, useful in orotracheal intubation, cannot be used to obtain the desired tube curvature when the endotracheal tube is passed nasally.

If the patient is hypoxic, oxygen can be administered temporarily through the nasotracheal tube during the intubation process, even though the tube still resides in the posterior pharynx. In the comatose patient with some degree of airway obstruction, the tube usually relieves such obstruction and allows oxygenation with spontaneous ventilation before placing the tube in the trachea.

COMPLICATIONS

Certain complications are specific to nasotracheal intubation (in addition to many of the same complications common to oral tracheal intubation).

Nasotracheal intubation may cause epistaxis, which can be a severe problem, particularly in the anticoagulated patient or the patient who developes a coagulopathy. Anterior and even posterior packing may be necessary, as much blood may be lost.

The nasopharyngeal mucosa may be perforated to create a false passage, particularly if excessive force is used to advance the tube through the nasal pharynx. This usually can be detected if breath sounds are lost before the tube is inserted into the pharynx and further passage of the tube must cease.

Damage to the adenoids and/or tonsils may oc-

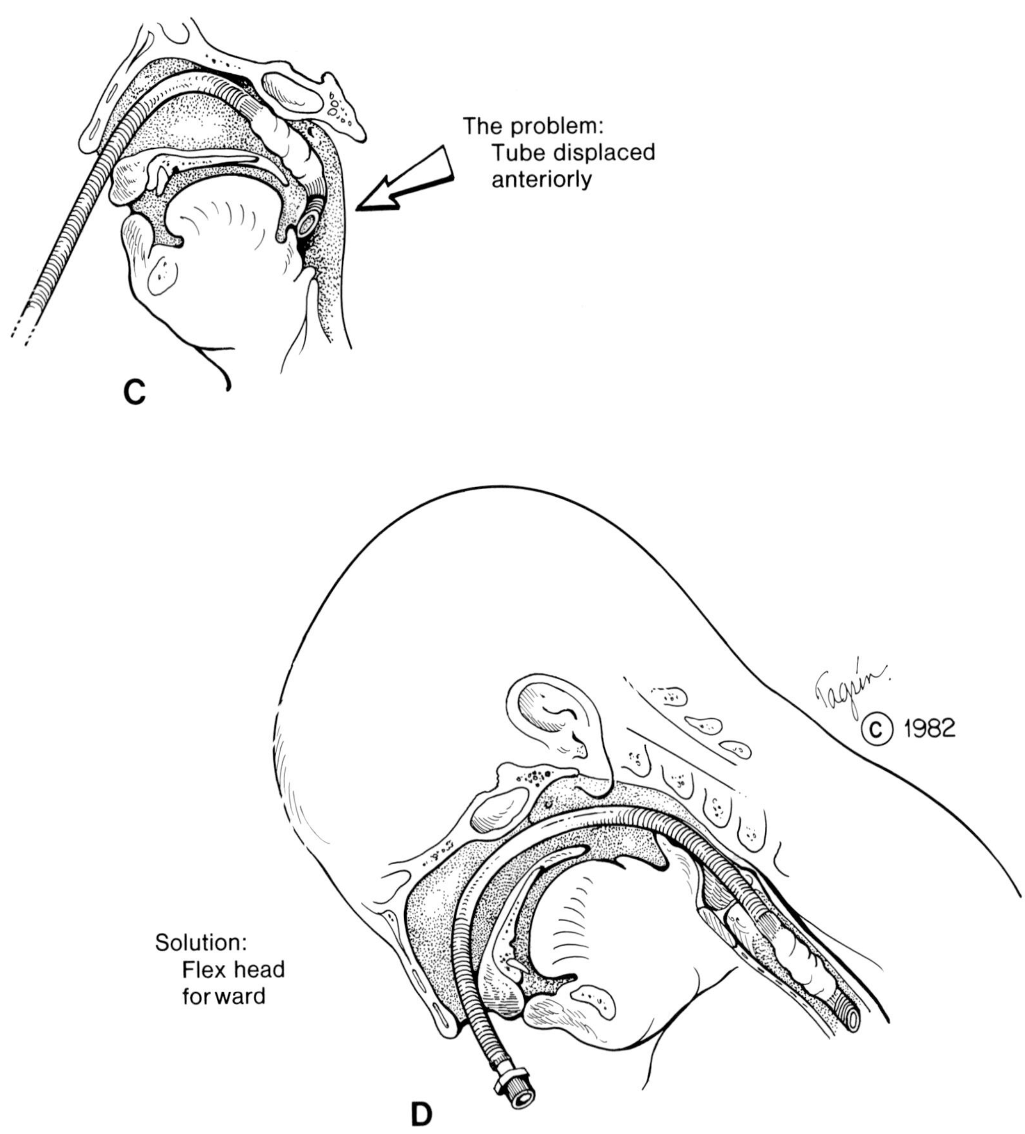

cur, particularly in children, even if care is used to advance the tube. A well-lubricated tube passed gently usually avoids this problem.

Long-term complications include:

1. Necrosis of the nasal cartilage if the tube is incorrectly fixed in position;
2. Obstruction of the eustachian tube, which may impair hearing;
3. Maxillary sinusitis because drainage of the sinus is prevented by the presence of the tube;
4. Meningitis in patients with a cerebrospinal fluid leak via a fracture of the cribriform plate.

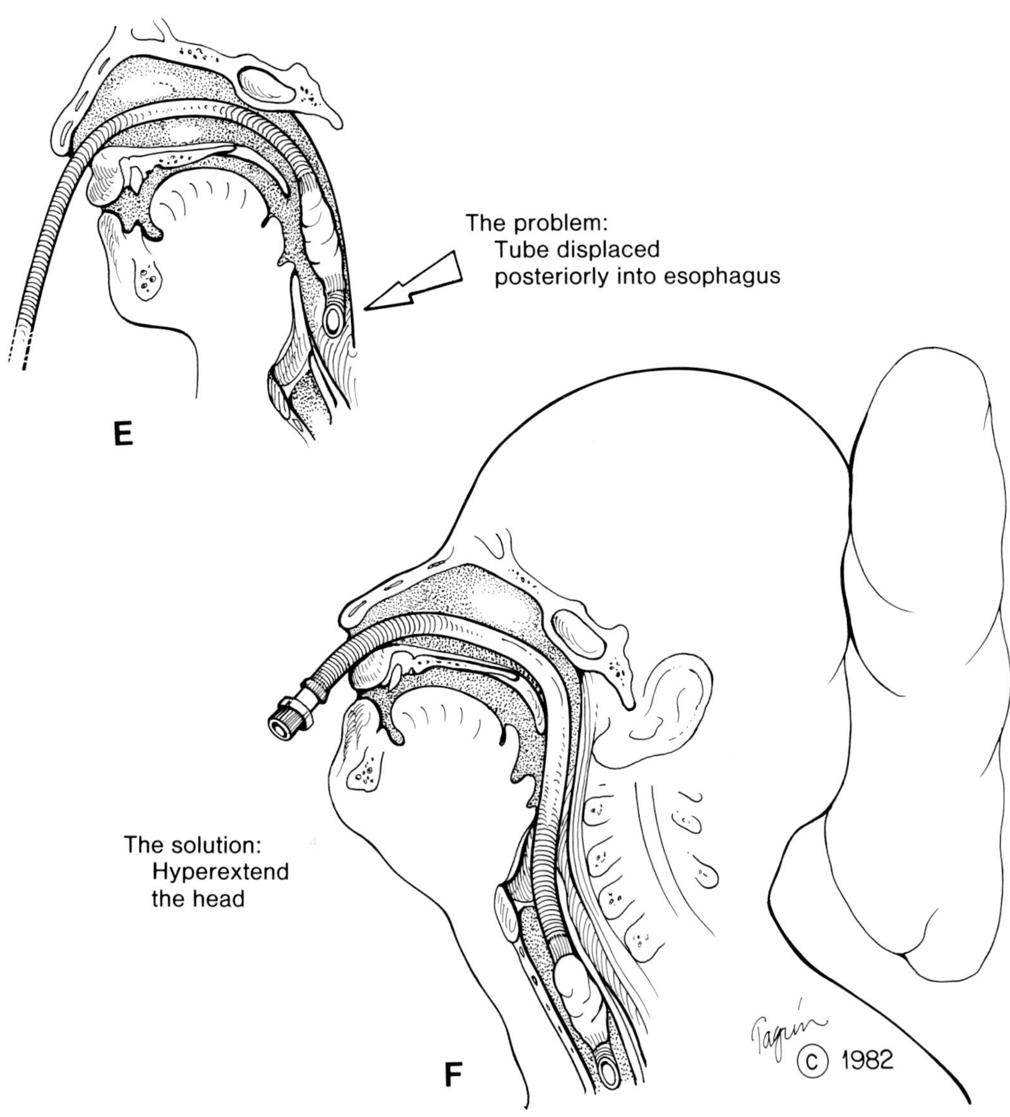
The problem:
Tube displaced
posteriorly into esophagus
E
The solution:
Hyperextend
the head
F
Taquin
© 1982

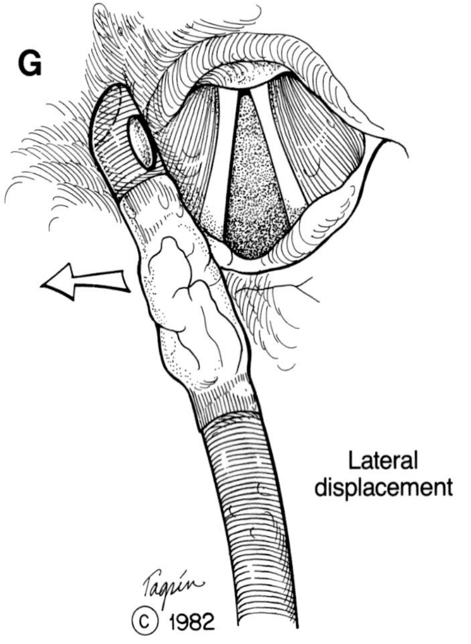
G
Lateral displacement
Tagrín
© 1982

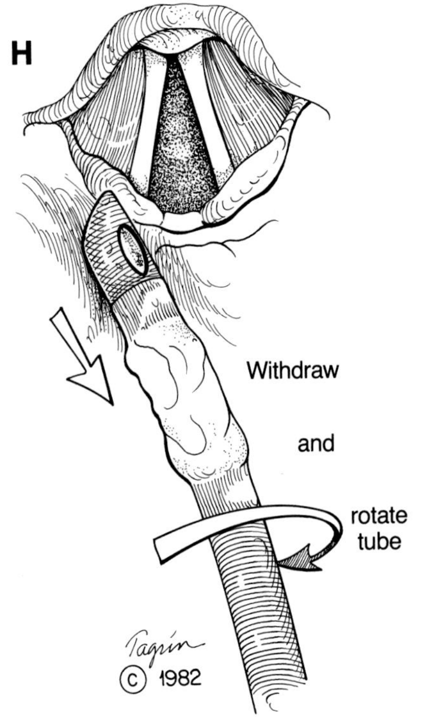
H
Withdraw
and
rotate tube
Tagrín
© 1982

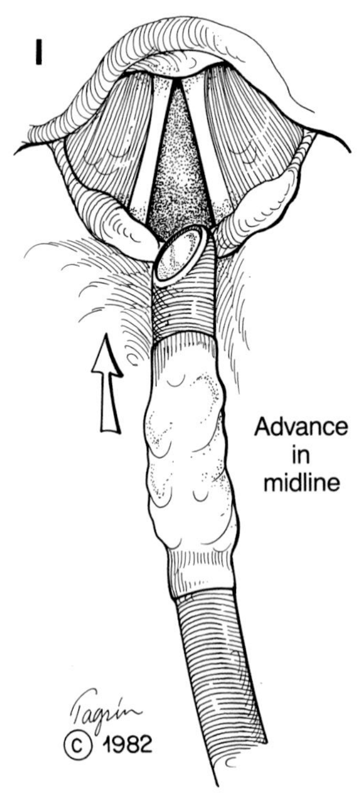
I
Advance in midline
Tagrín
© 1982

3. CRICOTHYROTOMY

ASHBY C. MONCURE, M.D.

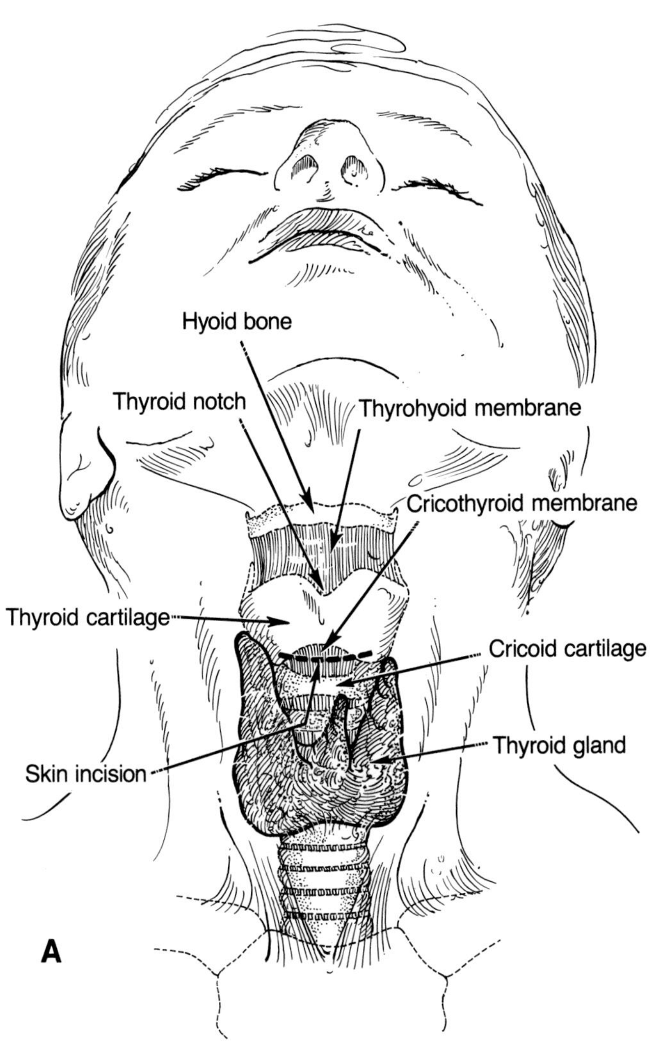

Control of the airway can usually be gained by insertion of an endotracheal tube via the oropharynx or nasopharynx. Occasionally, a bronchoscope can be utilized to achieve control quickly. If neither of these methods can be accomplished promptly, the obstructed airway is best managed by an incision through the cricothyroid membrane.

A, With the patient's neck extended, the depression between the thyroid cartilage and the cricoid cartilage in the anterior midline is identified, and a 2-cm transverse incision is made, centered in the anterior midline. The thumb and index finger are used to spread the wound apart in order to identify the cricothyroid membrane, which in incised horizontally on the cephalad edge of the cricoid cartilage.

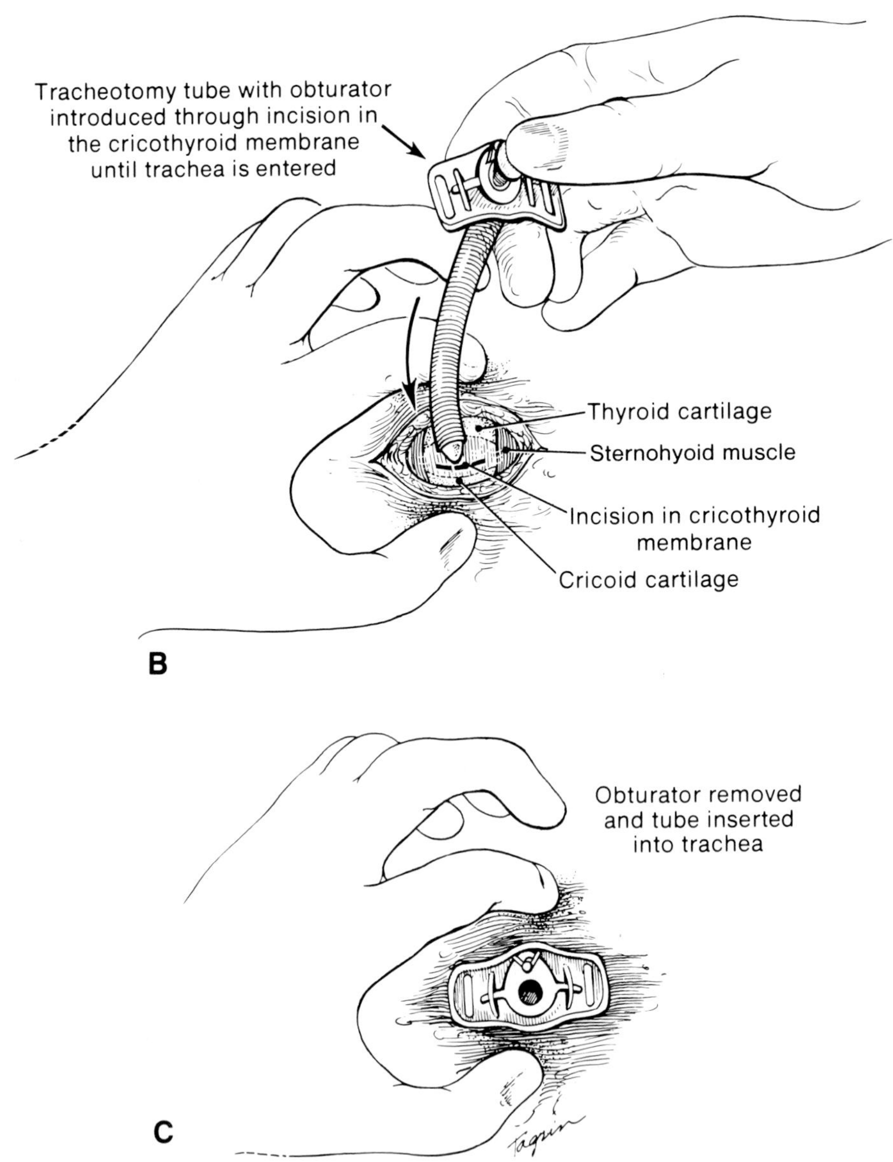

B, A no. 3 or no. 4 silver tracheotomy tube with an indwelling obturator is inserted into the trachea. *C*, The obturator is removed, and endotracheal ventilation and suction are carried out without use of an inner cannula. Thereafter, tracheal intubation via the oropharynx can again be attempted, and if efforts are unsuccessful, conventional tracheotomy can be carried out.

4. NEEDLE CRICOTHYROTOMY

CHARLES J. McCABE, M.D.

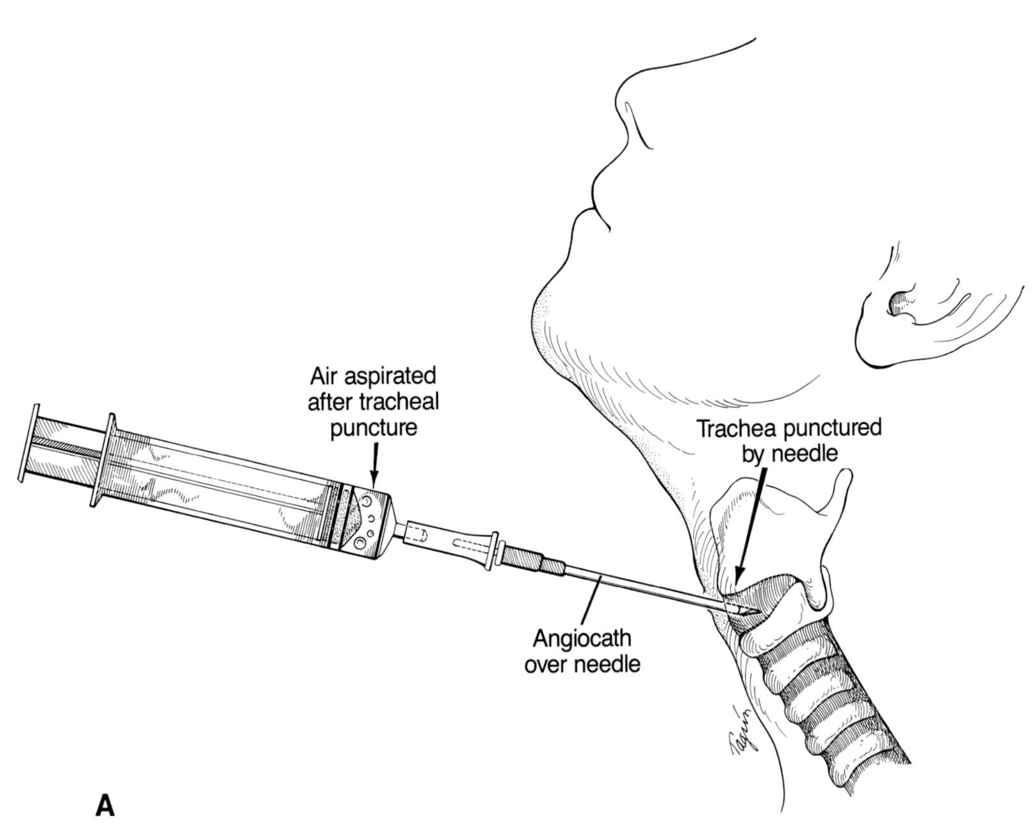

This procedure is a reasonable alternative to Number 3.

For this procedure, a 14-gauge angiocatheter, a no. 3 pediatric endotracheal tube adaptor, two pieces of oxygen extension tubing (approximately 6 feet long), and a Y-connector are necessary. Oxygen can usually be supplied by an oxygen jet, which will deliver 100% oxygen at 50 pounds per square inch (PSI) pressure.

A, The syringe is connected to the hub of the 14-gauge angiocatheter. The trachea is stabilized with the nondominant hand, and the needle is directed perpendicularly into the cricothyroid membrane. Once puncture of the trachea occurs, air can easily be aspirated from the lumen. Care must be used to prevent perforation of the posterior trachea wall. The bevel is placed inferiorly.

B, Once the trachea is entered and air is freely

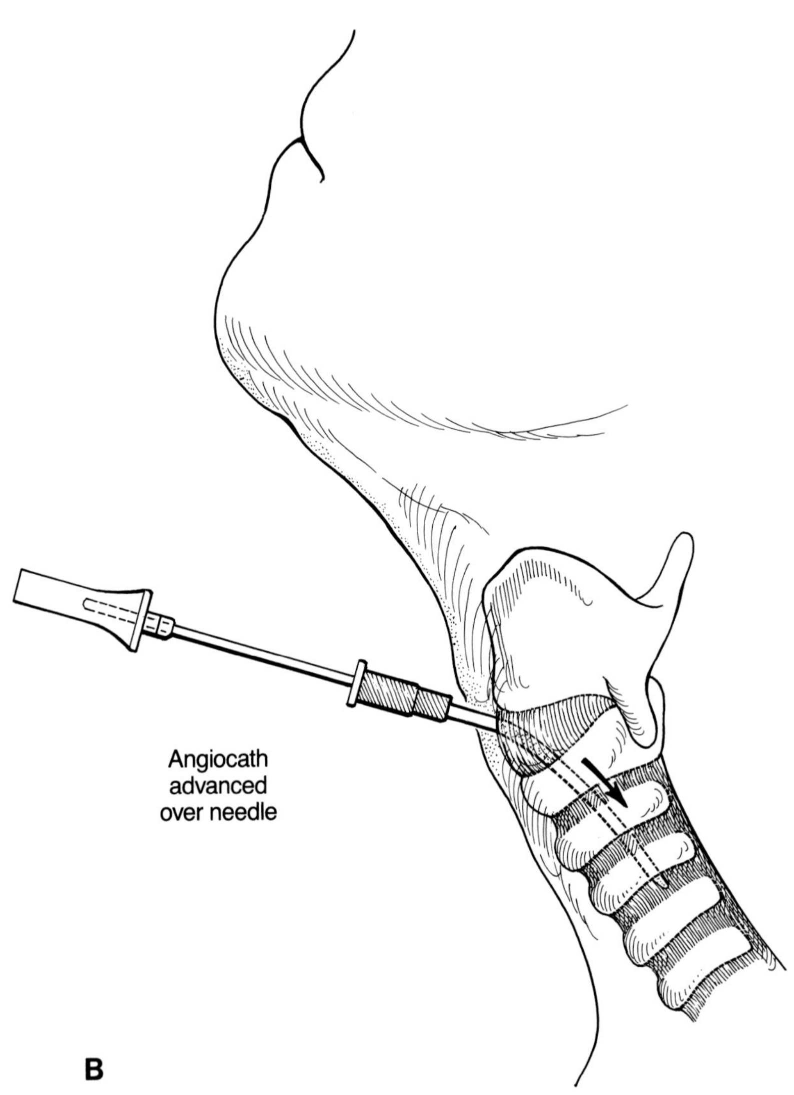

aspirated, the catheter is advanced into the tracheal lumen.

C, After satisfactory placement of the catheter, it is connected via a no. 3 pediatric endotracheal tube adaptor to the oxygen extension tubing and then to the oxygen jet at the wall. The lungs can be inflated with oxygen by occluding the arm of the Y-piece. Exhalation occurs passively through what remains of the patency of the tracheobronchial tree.

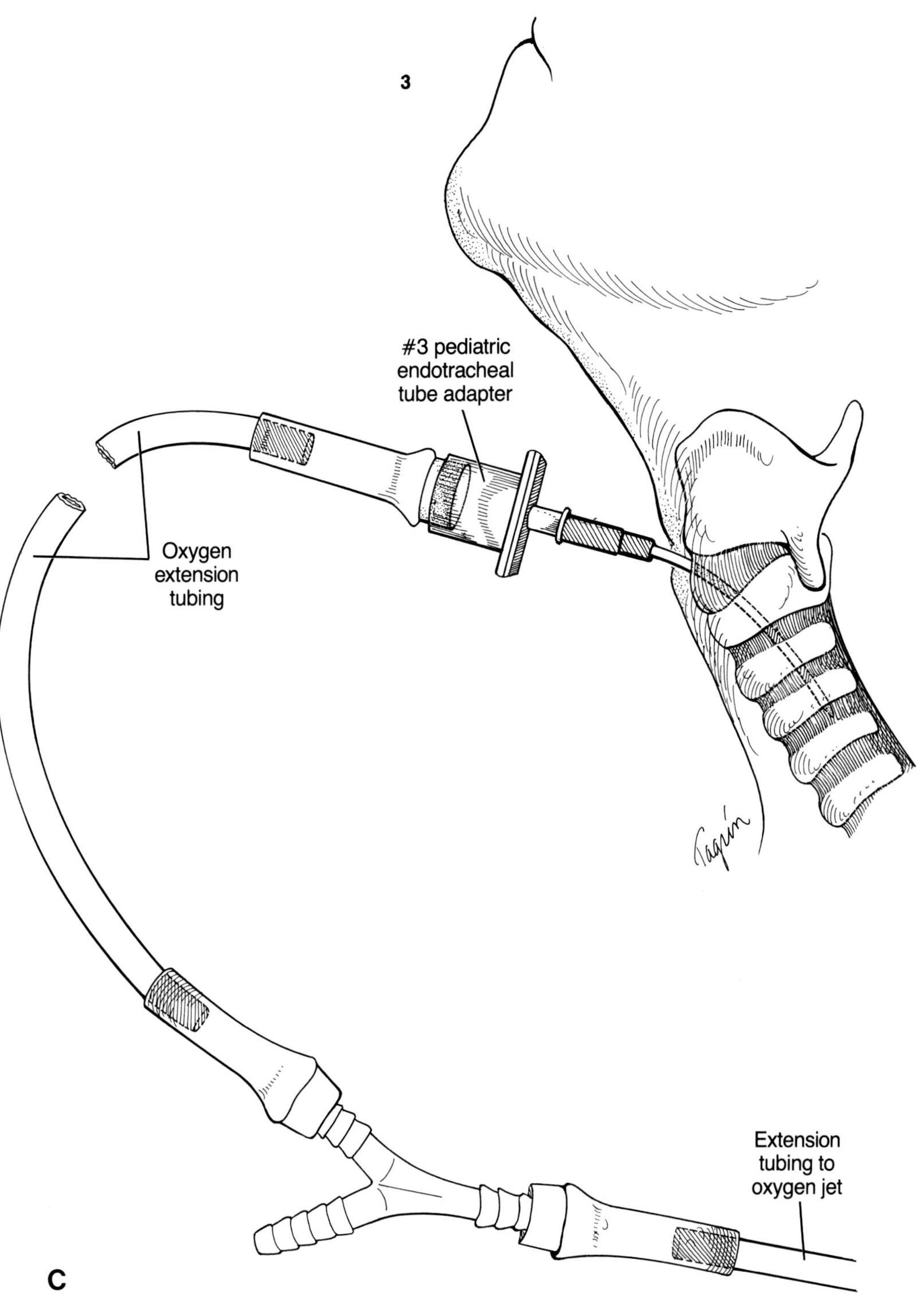
3
#3 pediatric
endotracheal
tube adapter
Oxygen
extension
tubing
Extension
tubing to
oxygen jet
C

5. SUBCLAVIAN VEIN CATHETER PLACEMENT

RITA COLLEY, R.N.
HERBERT FREUND, M.D.
JOSEF E. FISCHER, M.D.

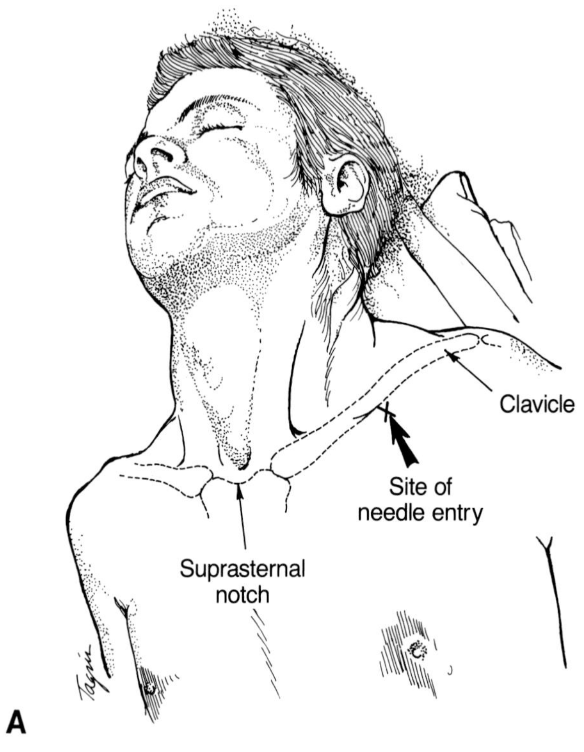

A, The patient is placed in Trendelenburg's position to increase venous pressure. A towel roll under the cervicothoracic vertebrae allows the patient's shoulders to drop back and the clavicles to rise.

B, After the skin surface is prepared with acetone and scrubbed with 2% iodine solution, the skin and underlying tissue are infiltrated with 1% lidocaine (Xylocaine). Lidocaine is infiltrated along the needle track, and the subclavian vein is located with the 22-gauge needle used for infiltration of the local anesthetic. The skin is then punctured with a 14-gauge needle along the middle third of the clavicle beneath the bony prominence. After puncture, aspiration should be constant to determine venous entry. *C*, The needle is advanced to enter the subclavian vein. Entry is verified by aspiration of free-flowing blood into the syringe. *D*, The bevel of the needle is turned caudad. The patient is told to take a deep breath and to hold it. After 2–3 seconds, the syringe is removed and a 16-gauge Intracath is inserted through the needle and advanced into the superior vena cava. The patient may then breathe normally again. The purpose of having the patient hold his or her breath is to prevent air embolism.

E, The needle is pulled back over the catheter and locked into the catheter hub with a twisting motion. A needle guard is then clipped over the needle. After a single suture is placed at the insertion site to immobilize the catheter, the stylet is withdrawn, again with maintenance of the Valsalva maneuver while the catheter is open to air.

F, Intravenous tubing is joined to the catheter hub and locked in with a twisting motion. Iodophor ointment is then placed on the catheter insertion site, and the site is covered with small gauze sponges. *G*, After the larger area of skin around the puncture site and the needle are treated with tincture of benzoin, occlusive dressing (Elastoplast) is applied. The bandage comes *halfway* down the catheter hub; this

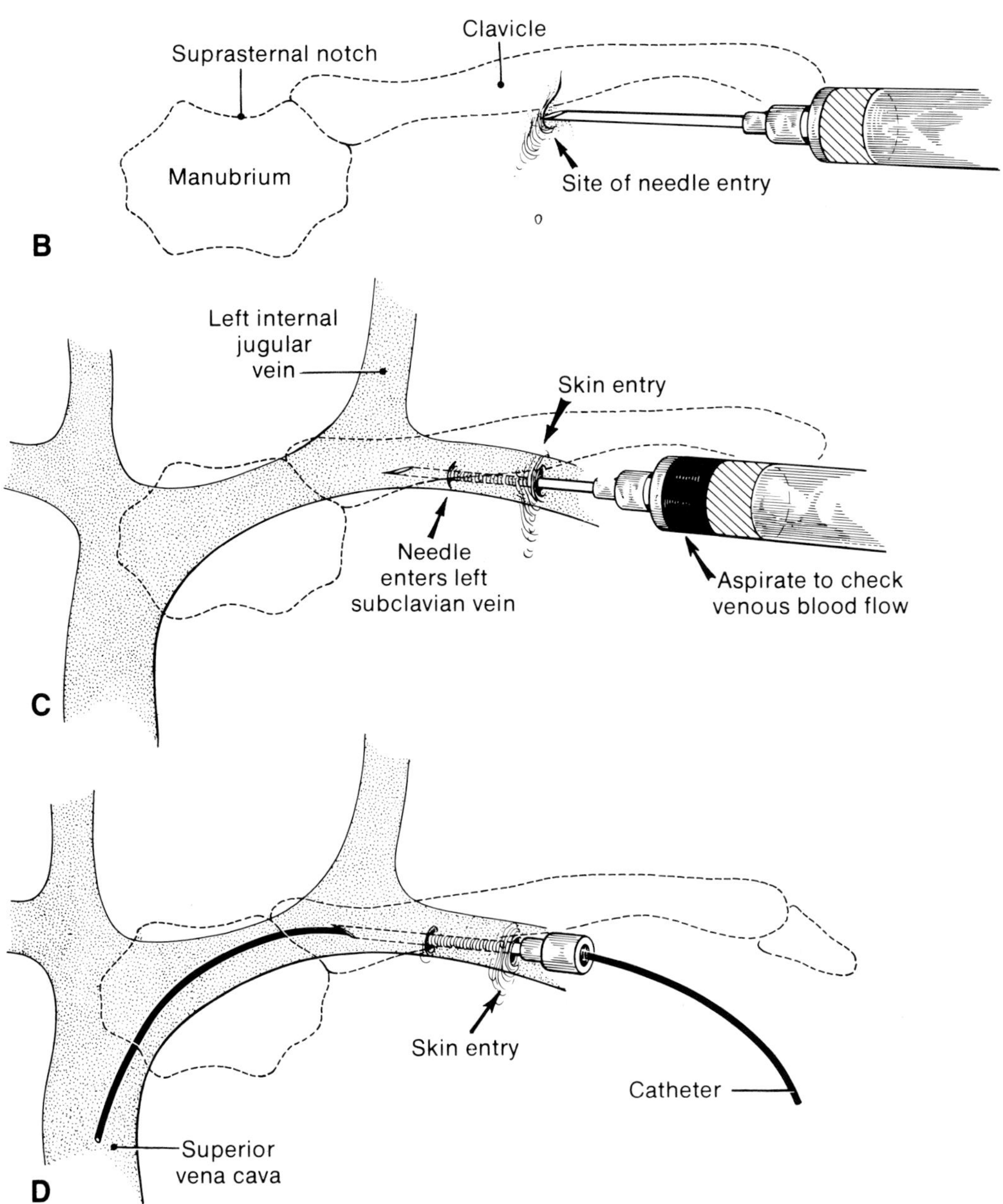

allows the intravenous tubing to be changed without destroying the occlusive quality of the dressing. *H*, One-inch adhesive tape secures all sides of the dressing and all intravenous tubing junctions. It also anchors the intravenous tubing to the dressing.

Beware of possible complications from subclavian catheter placement: pneumothorax, hemothorax, hydrothorax, inadvertent arterial puncture, air embolus, catheter embolus, brachial plexus injury, hemorrhage, and cardiac irritability. To avoid complications, obtain a chest x-ray film after placement, withdraw the catheter tip from the atrium if necessary, apply appropriate direct pressure if an artery has been entered, have the patient perform the Valsalva maneuver when the catheter is open to air, give transfusions or vitamin K if necessary before catheterization, and observe the patient carefully for signs and symptoms of clinical deterioration.

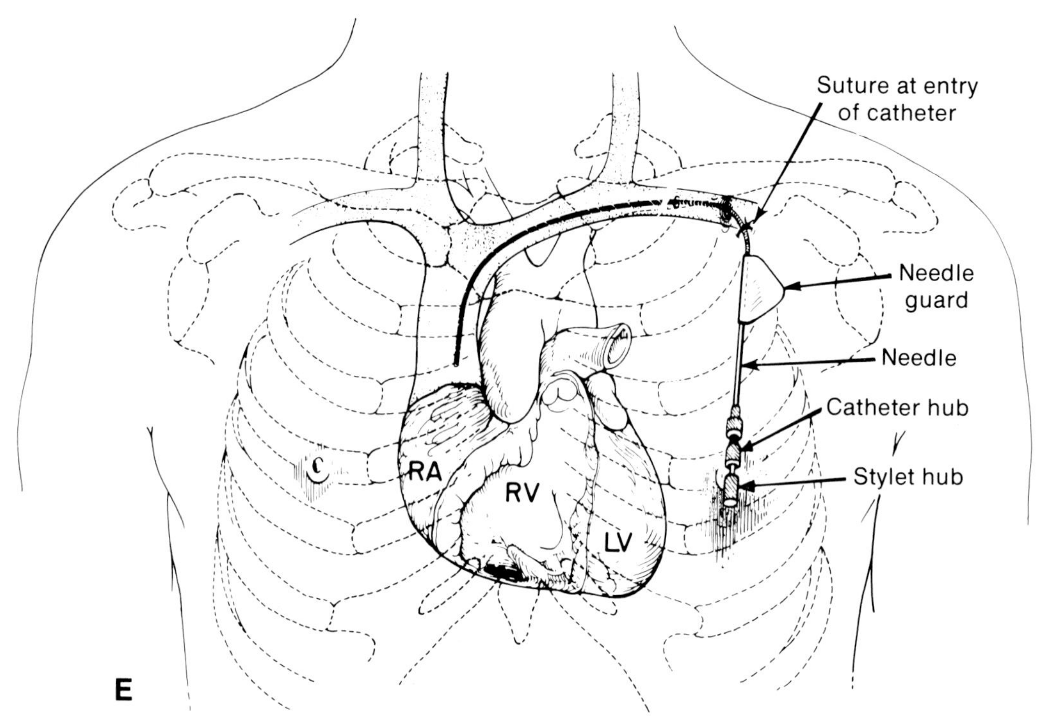
Suture at entry of catheter
Needle guard
Needle
Catheter hub
Stylet hub
RA
RV
LV
E

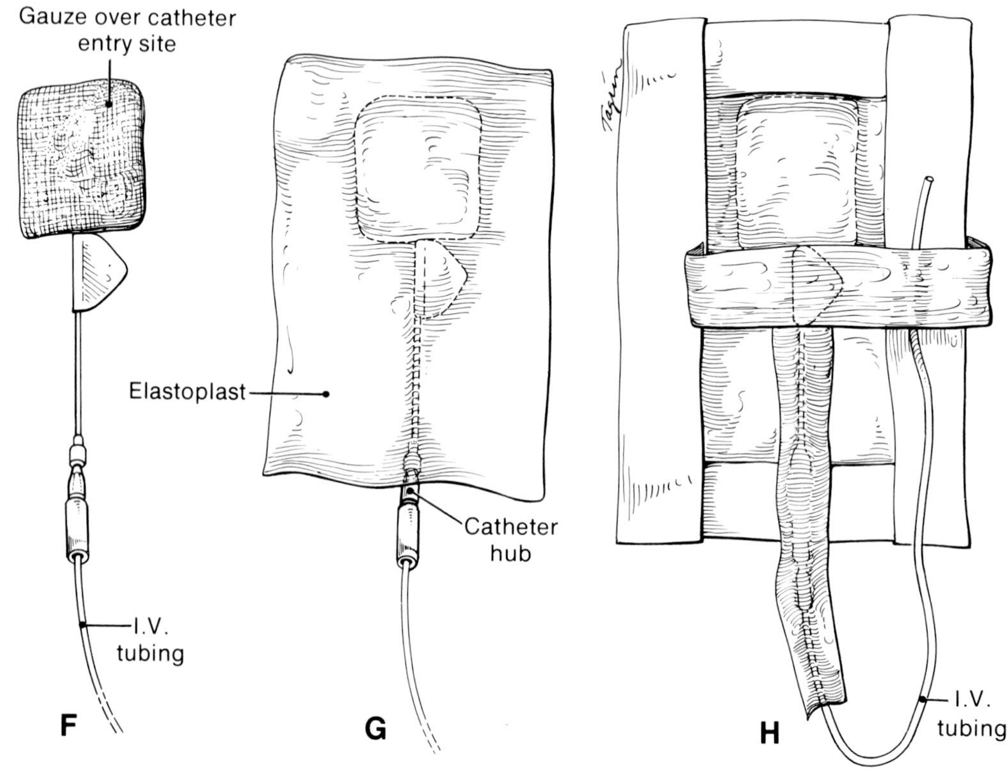
Gauze over catheter entry site
Elastoplast
Catheter hub
I.V. tubing
I.V. tubing
F
G
H

6. INTERNAL JUGULAR VEIN CATHETERIZATION

CHARLES J. McCABE, M.D.

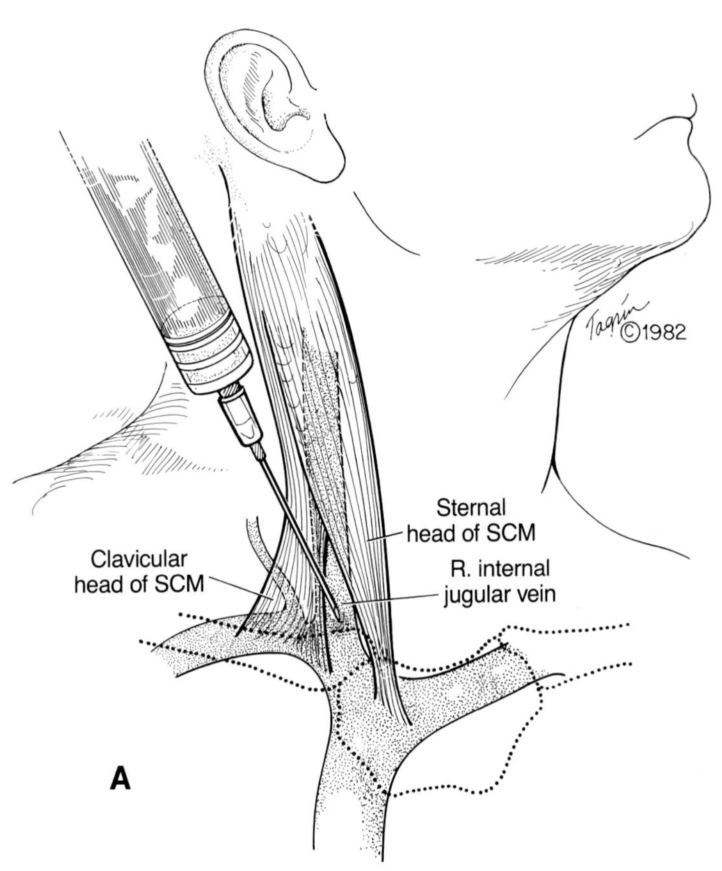

A, The approach to the internal jugular vein is between the sternal and clavicular heads of the sternocleidomastoid muscle. The patient is placed in 30° of Trendelenburg's position in order to distend the vein. Sterile preparing and draping of the area are performed. The apex of the triangle between the two heads of the sternocleidomastoid muscle is used for the insertion of the needle. Local anesthesia is accomplished with 1% lidocaine (Xylocaine). The carotid pulse is palpated and the head turned to the opposite side. The needle is directed lateral to the pulse, aiming at the ipsilateral nipple at a 30° angle to the horizontal. The initial location of the vein is done with an 18-gauge needle.

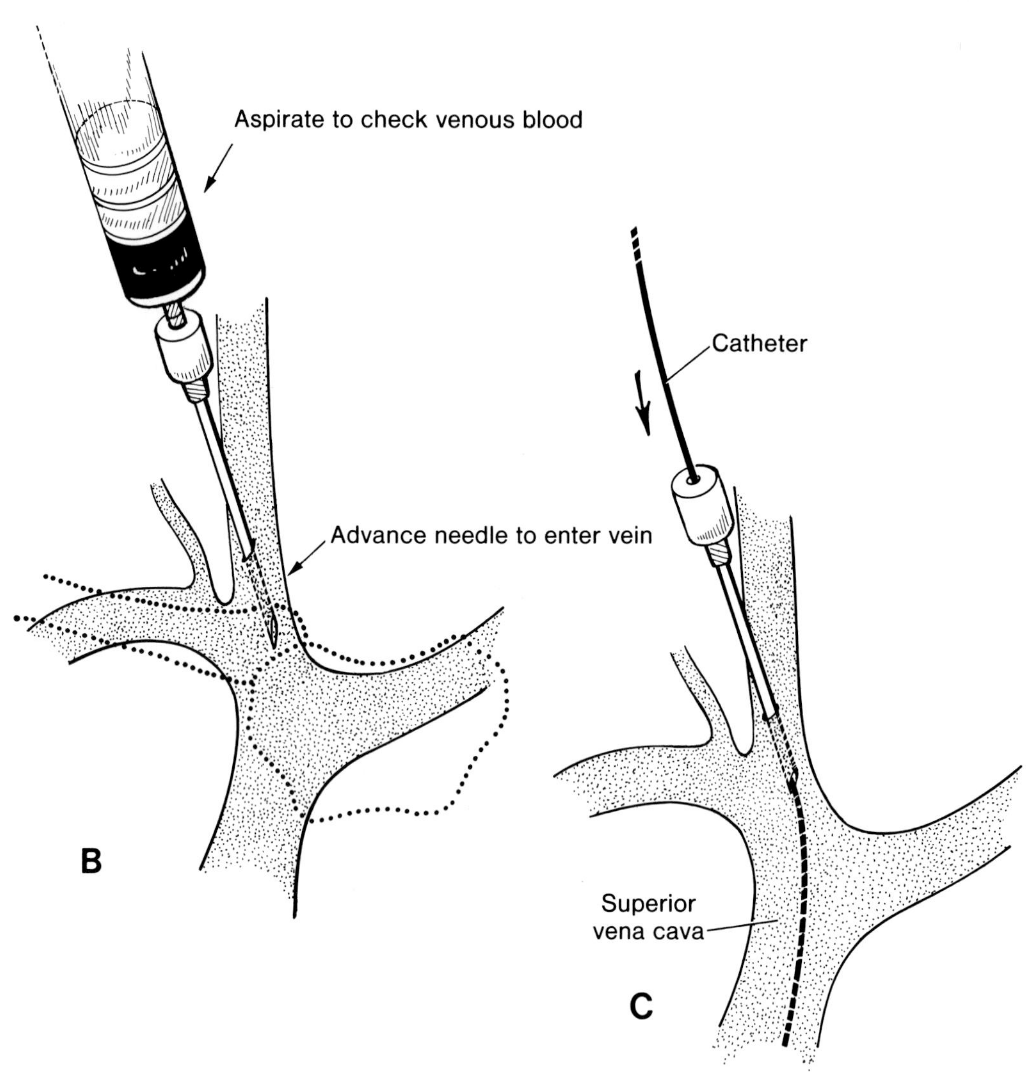

B, Once the vein is located, the larger gauge needle is then inserted in the same direction as the smaller needle. The vein is entered, and the venous blood is aspirated.

C, Once good flow of venous blood is obtained, the syringe is removed, and the patient is instructed to hold his/her breath. The catheter is inserted through the needle into the superior vena cava. If the catheter does not thread easily, the entire needle and catheter is removed as one piece to prevent sheering of the catheter. Another attempt is made.

7. SAPHENOUS VEIN CUTDOWN

CHARLES J. McCABE, M.D.

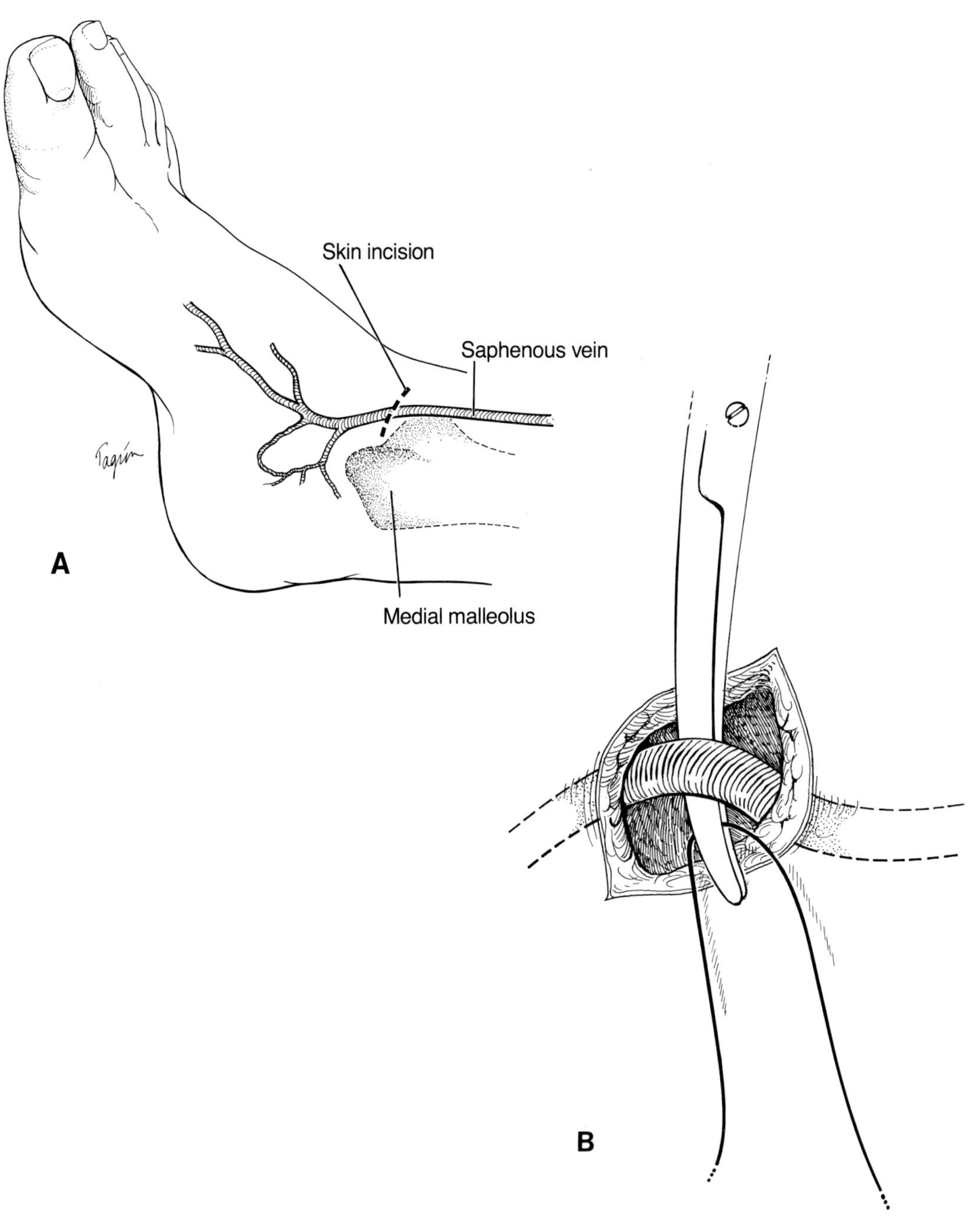

A, The saphenous vein is located anteriorly and superiorly to the medial malleolus. After anesthetizing the skin with 1% lidocaine (Xylocaine), a 1½–2-cm transverse incision is made.

B, The saphenous vein is exposed using blunt dissection with a curved hemostat. The vein is isolated by passing silk ligatures proximally and distally.

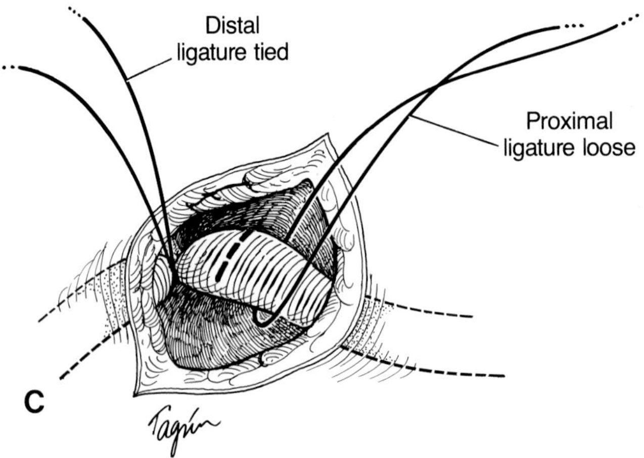

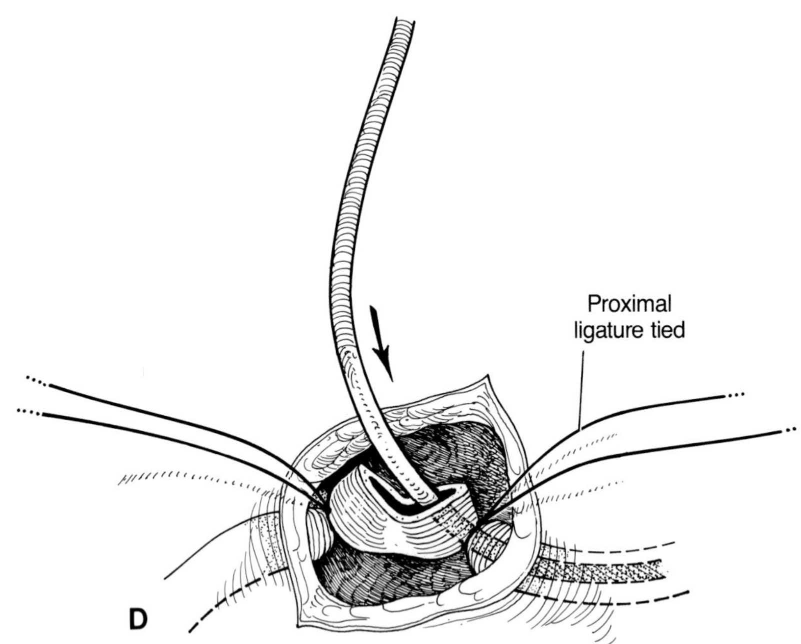

C, The distal ligature is tied. A small transverse incision is made in the anterior wall of the vein, and the proximal ligature is used to control venous bleeding.

D, The catheter is inserted through the incision in the vein. The proximal ligature is tied, and the catheter is connected to the intravenous tubing and solution. The skin incision is closed and a sterile dressing applied. (Note: Proper skin care is similar to that described in *G*, Illustrated Technique 5).

8. INSERTION OF TRANSVENOUS VENTRICULAR PACING ELECTRODE

PETER C. BLOCK, M.D.

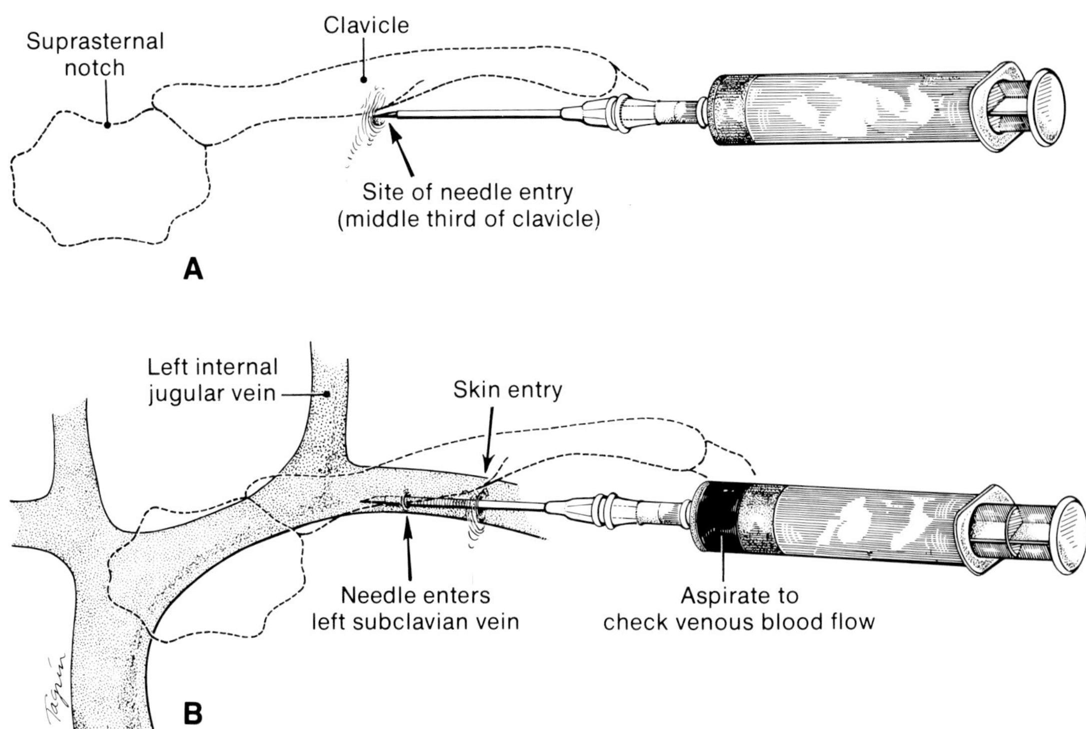

The skin over the left subclavian vein should be prepared and draped with standard surgical technique. The left subclavian vein is preferred because of the natural "loop" of the pacing electrode, which facilitates passage across the tricuspid valve.

A, With a no. 14 Angiocath after 1% lidocaine (Xylocaine) infiltration, subclavian puncture is performed where the vein passes near the inferior clavicular surface along the middle third of the clavicle. *B*, Venous blood should be aspirated to ensure proper placement of the cannula tip in the subclavian vein.

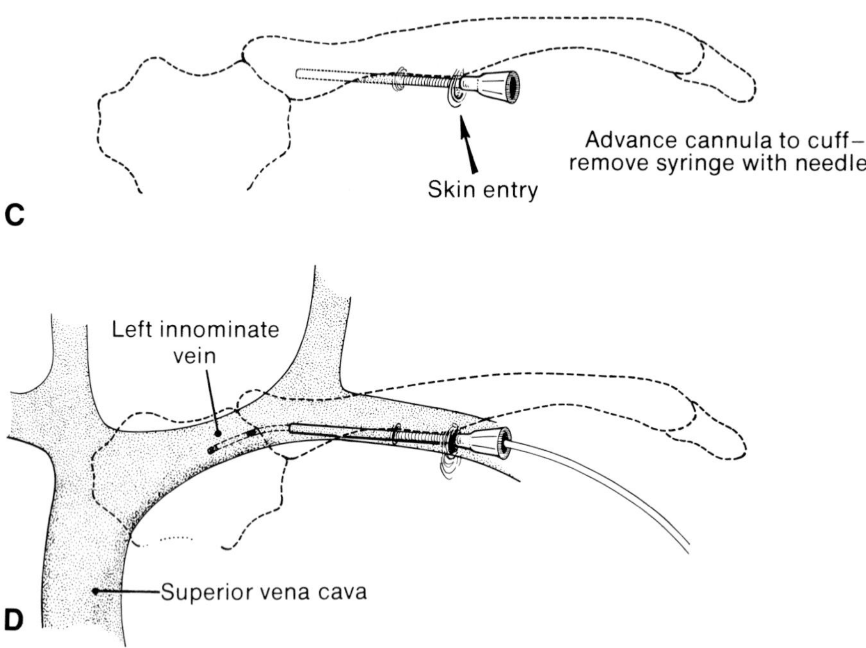

C, The cannula is advanced slightly to maintain proper intravascular position, and the needle is removed. *D*, The temporary pacing electrode is introduced through the cannula into the subclavian vein. Insertion of the electrode with the curved tip directed *inferiorly* facilitates passage into the left innominate vein and avoids cephalad passage into the internal jugular vein, which may occur if the tip is directed superiorly. The electrode is advanced approximately 15 cm. Electrocardiographic monitoring is then begun by attaching connected alligator clips to the proximal electrode terminal and to the V lead of the electrocardiograph.

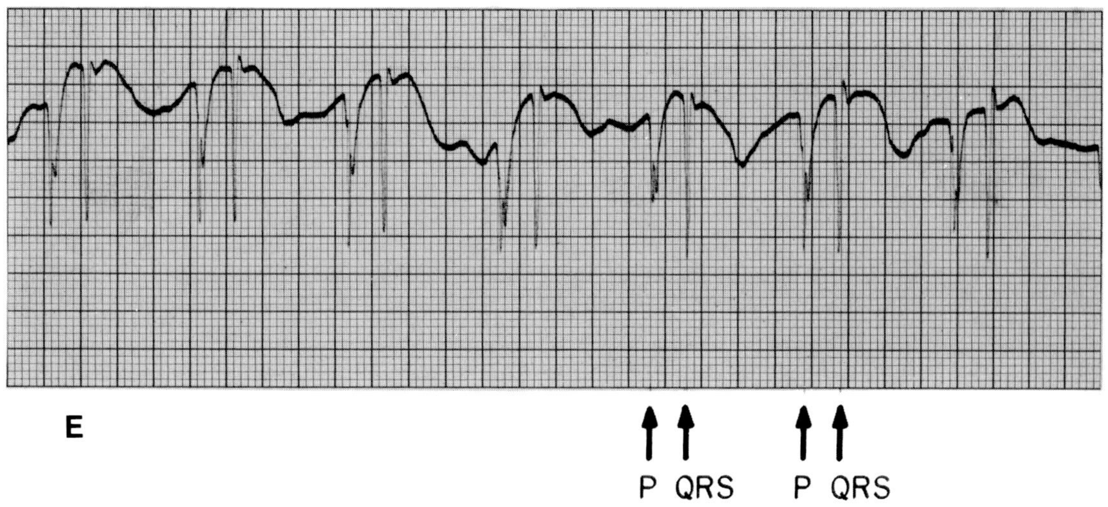

E

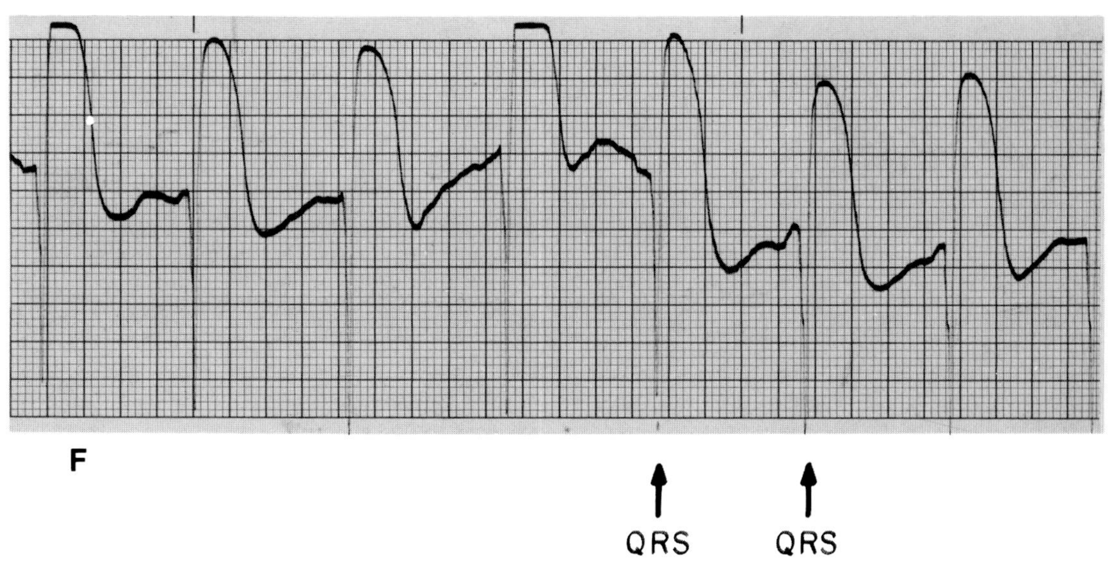

F

E, The V lead is monitored as the electrode is advanced into the right atrium, where the intraatrial recording shows large spiked P waves.

F, The electrode then is advanced across the tricuspid valve into the right ventricle, where the intraventricular recording shows its characteristic wide stylus displacement. One or two ventricular premature beats usually occur when the electrode tip first touches the right ventricular endocardium.

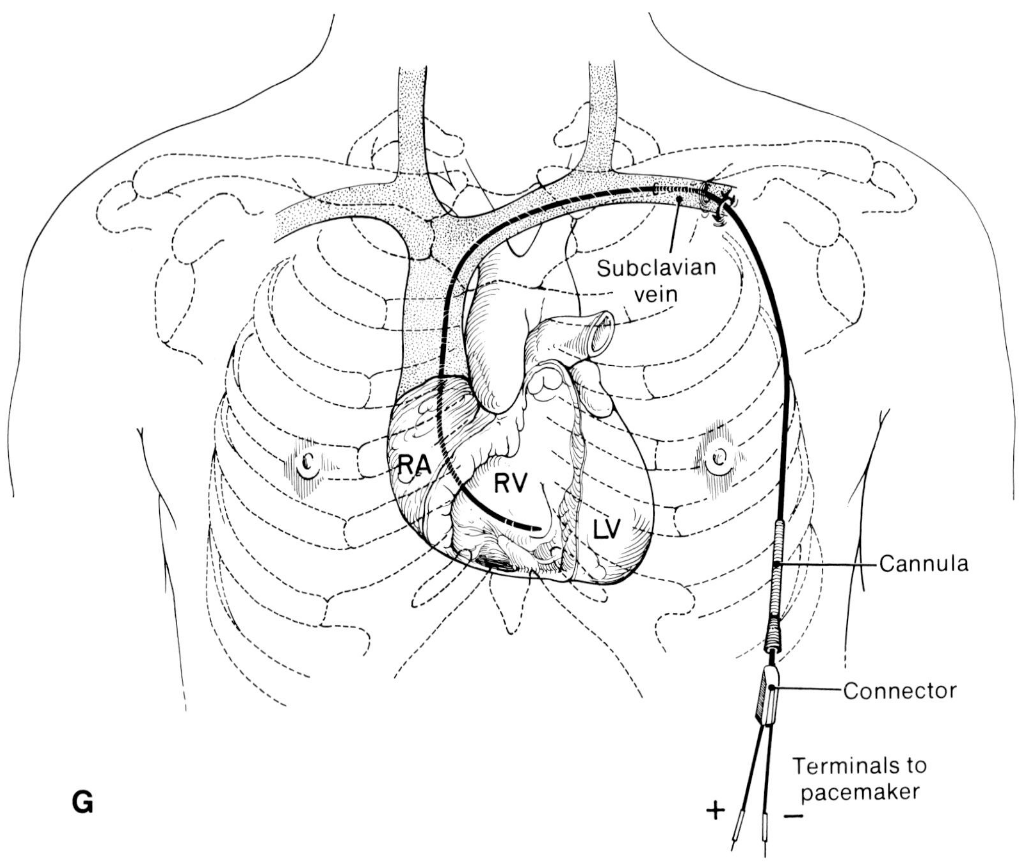

G, At this point, the alligator clips are removed, and the connector to the pacemaker is attached at the proximal end of the electrode. Pacing is begun, and the threshold for pacing is determined. The threshold should preferably be less than 2 mA, but in emergency situations, higher thresholds are acceptable. An ideal threshold is less than 1 mA. The cannula in the subclavian vein is carefully removed over the electrode without dislodging the electrode tip from the right ventricle, and the electrode anchored to the skin at the insertion site with a 3–0 silk suture.

The entire procedure must be performed under sterile conditions so that the electrode is not contaminated during insertion. A sterile dressing is applied at the end of the procedure to maintain sterility as long as possible. (See technique under *G*, Technique 5.)

9. RADIAL ARTERIAL PUNCTURE

CHARLES J. McCABE, M.D.

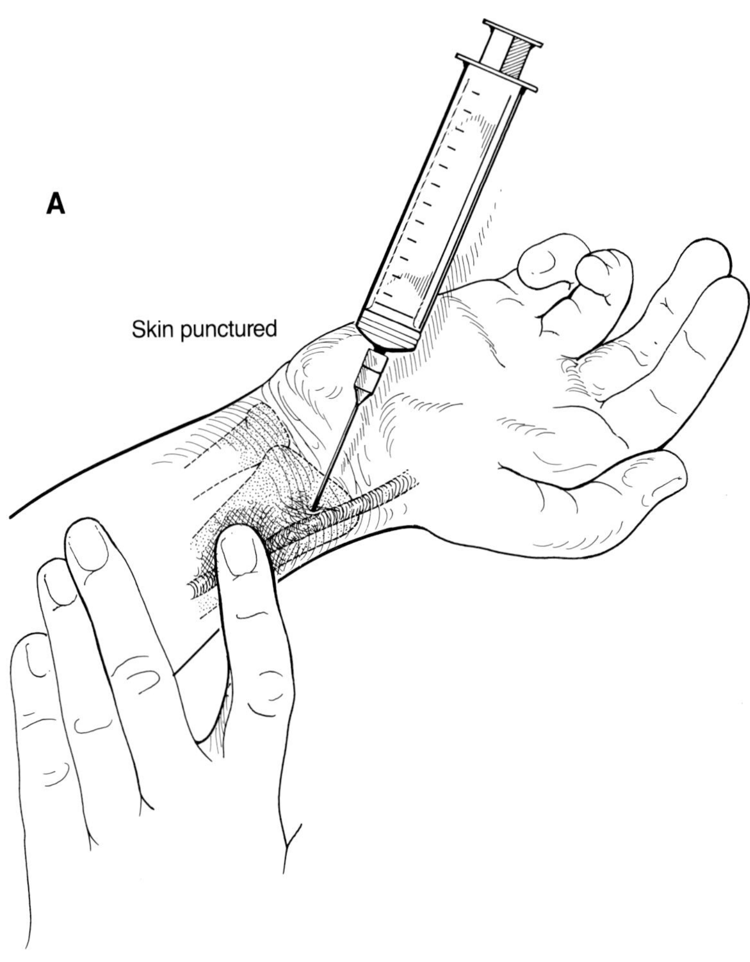

It is always wise to perform an Allen's test, which assesses radial and ulnar artery adequacy, before performing radial arterial puncture or inserting the arterial line. If this test suggests discontinuity of the palmar arch between radial and ulnar arteries, the opposite radial artery is used.

A, The hand is placed in the supinated position as illustrated, and the radial artery palpated. With the index finger palpating the pulse continuously, the artery is punctured with a no. 21–23 gauge needle.

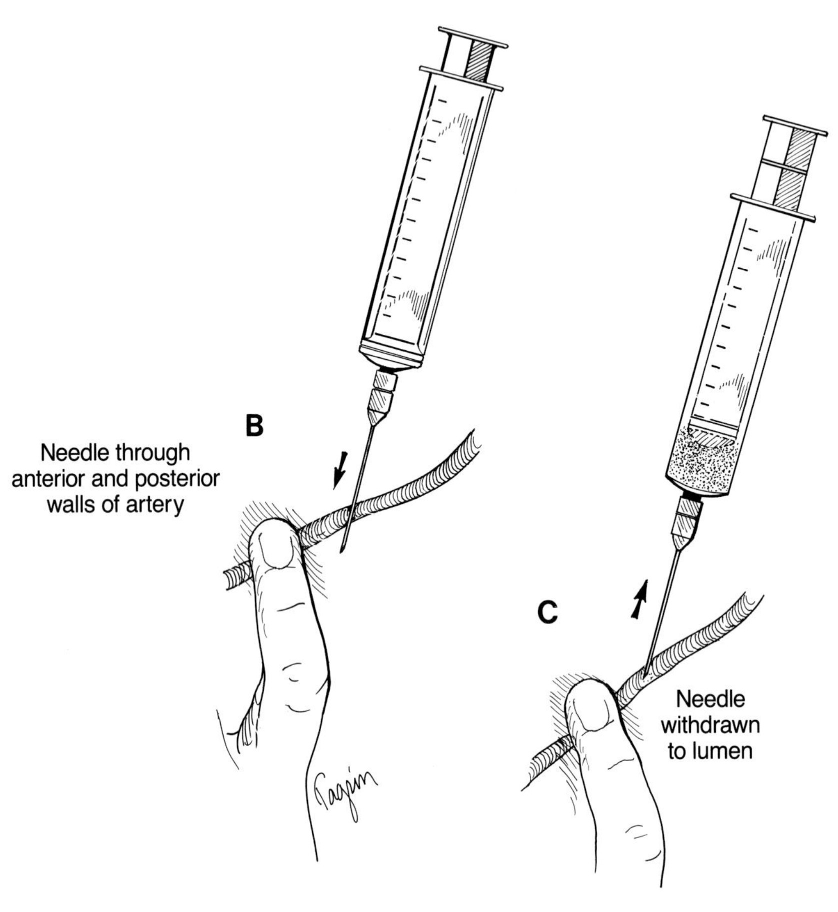

B–C, The needle is penetrated through both the anterior and the posterior wall. The syringe and needle are withdrawn, and as the lumen of the artery is entered, arterial flow occurs into the syringe. A sample of 2–3 cc of arterial blood is removed. Digital compression of the puncture site is maintained for 5 minutes.

10. PERICARDIOCENTESIS

A. JOHN ERDMAN III, M.D.†

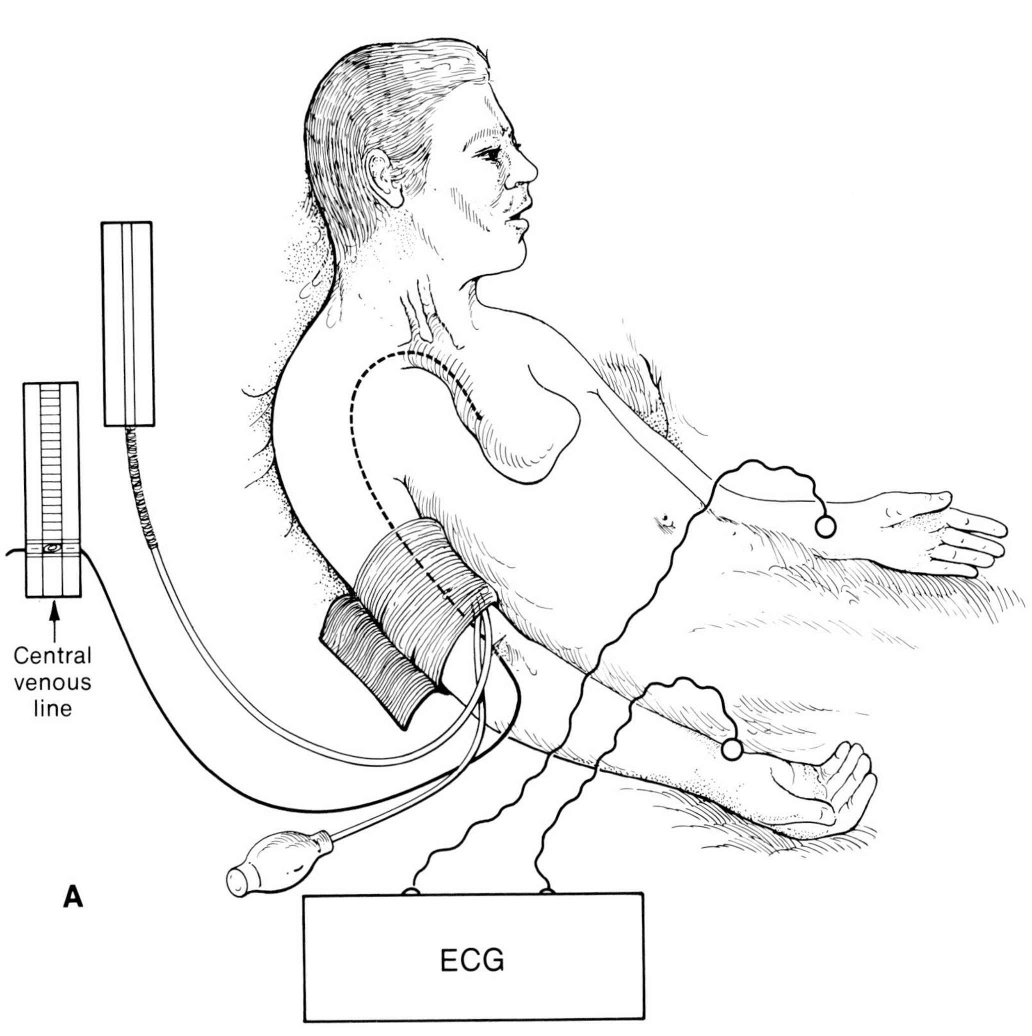

A, The patient should be semirecumbent. The electrocardiogram, systemic blood pressure, and central venous pressure are followed. Continuous intraarterial monitoring is extremely helpful.

† Deceased.

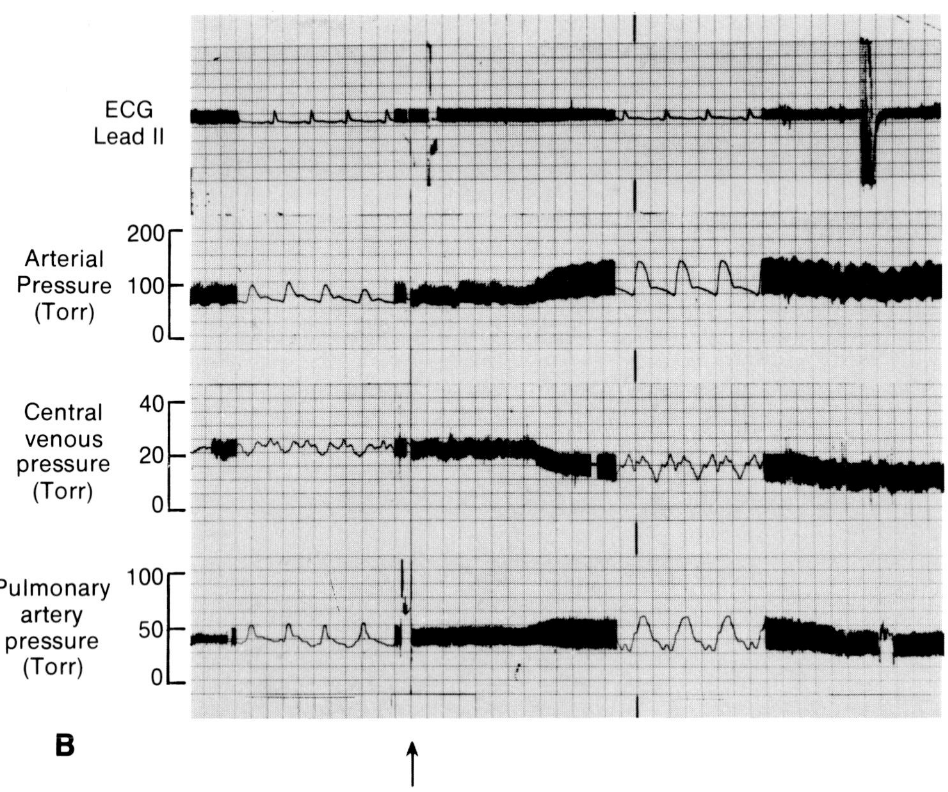

B, Hemodynamic tracings of a patient with acute pericardial tamponade. Before drainage, the central venous pressure is 25 mm Hg and the aortic pressure is 100/70 with marked pulsus paradoxus. At the *arrow*, the needle is inserted into the pericardial space. A brief current of injury is obtained on the electrocardiogram, but fluid is then withdrawn. First the venous pressure falls, and then the arterial pressure begins to rise. Simultaneously, the pulmonary arterial (PA) pressure falls, the pulsus paradoxus disappears, and hemodynamic stability is restored. (The PA tracing shown herein is to illustrate the physiologic response to pericardial decompression. It is not a routine monitoring for pericardiocentesis.)

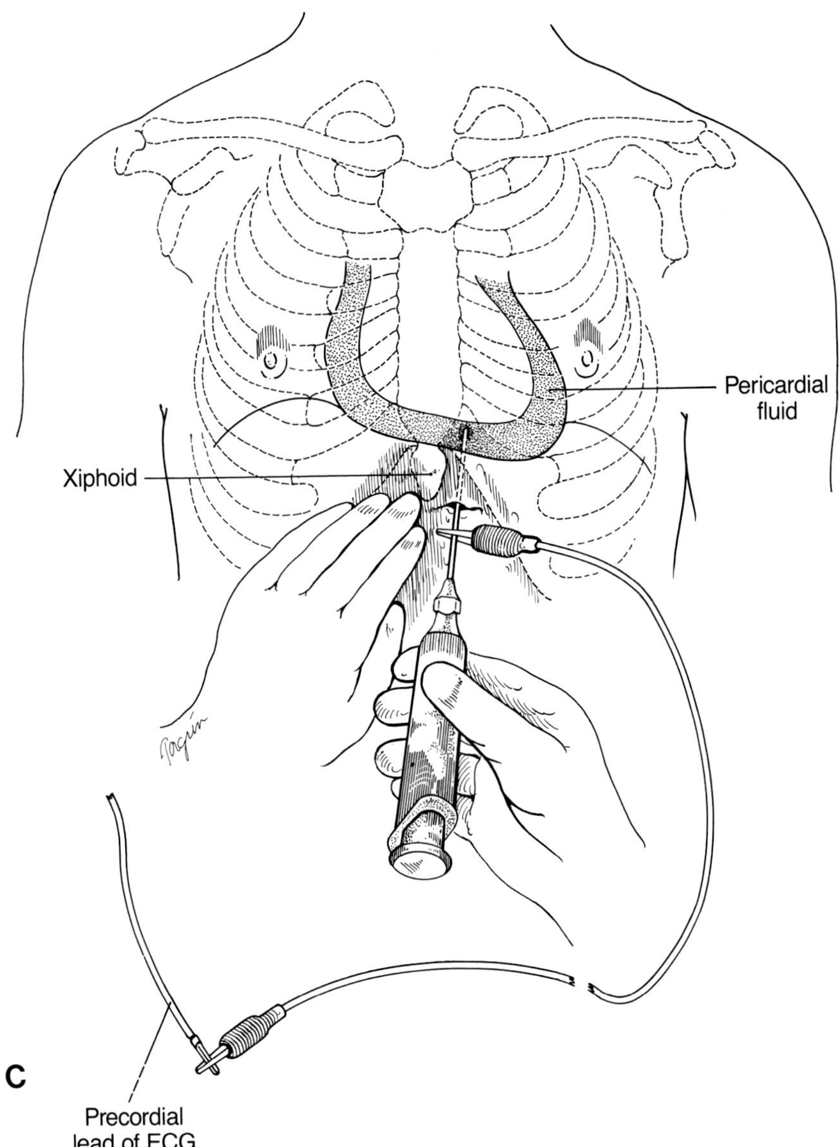

C, Local anesthesia is obtained with 1% lidocaine (Xylocaine). General anesthesia should not be used in a patient with pericardial tamponade because it may precipitate profound hypotension. An 18-gauge spinal needle is insinuated beneath the xiphoid process, with continuous monitoring of the electrocardiogram through sterile alligator clips attached to the needle and to the precordial lead. The needle is advanced almost parallel with the skin and directed cephalad until either a current of injury is obtained on the tracing or blood or other fluid is aspirated with the syringe.

11. EMERGENCY THORACOTOMY

CHARLES J. McCABE, M.D.

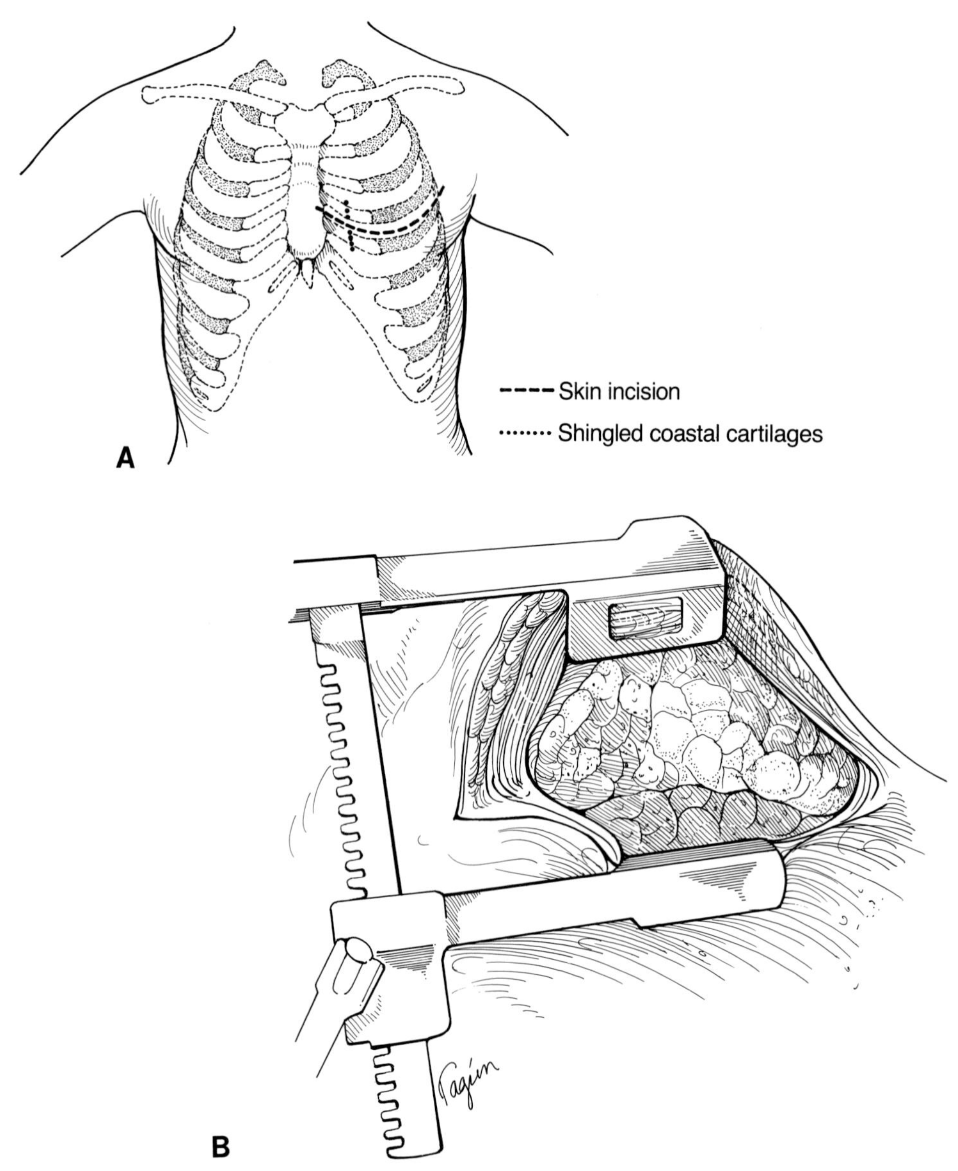

A, An incision is made from the lateral edge of the sternum as far laterally as can be reached in the fourth intercostal space. In a female, the incision is made in the skin crease below the breast. Muscles are transsected until the intercostal space is identified. The intercostal muscles are divided between the fourth and fifth ribs.

B, A chest wall spreader is placed in the interspace and opened. To gain greater access, the costal cartilages can be "shingled" (divided) in order to allow full opening of the chest (*dotted line* in *A*).

C, Upon entering the chest, the lungs bellow out. The heart lies anteriorly and medially. The phrenic nerve is identified along the lateral aspect of the pericardial sac. The pericardium should be grasped with a forceps or clamp and opened anterior to the nerve. This allows evacuation of any pericardial hematoma. Open cardiopulmonary resuscitation may

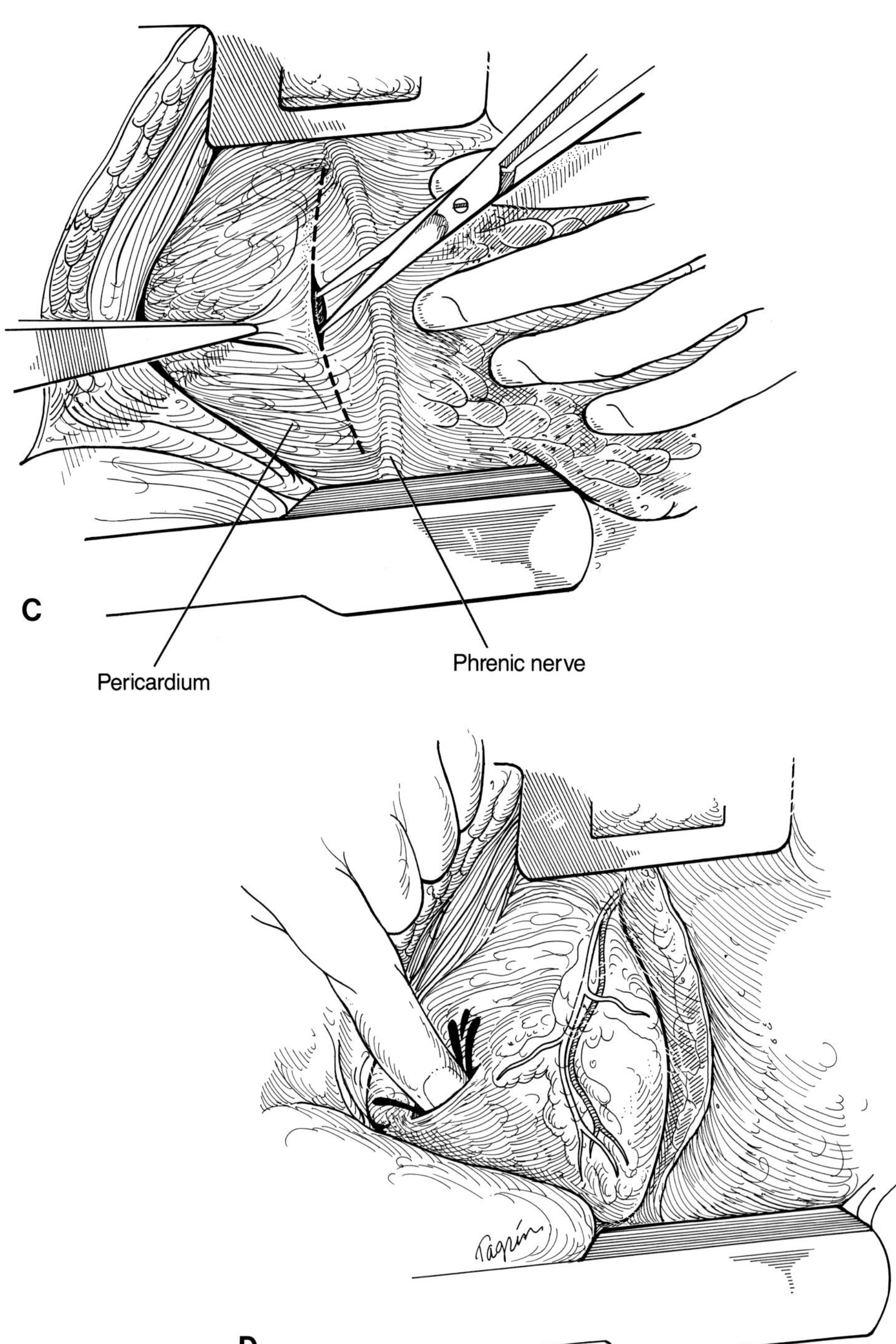

be performed by compressing the heart forward against the sternum. The intrathoracic aorta may be compressed against the vertebral column, or a vascular clamp may be applied for occlusion.

D, Any bleeding from the myocardium is controlled by placing the thumb or index finger over or into the hole.

E, A horizontal mattress suture of 2–0 silk with

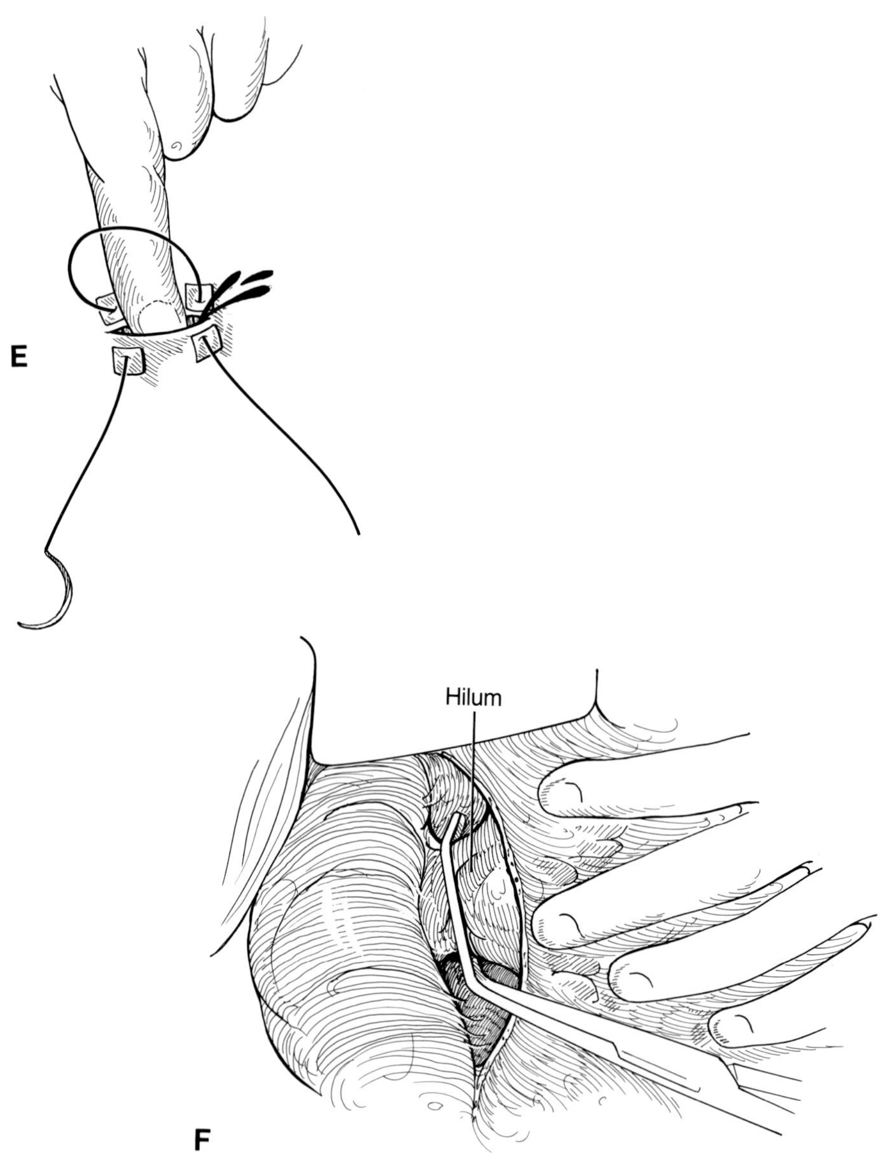

vascular needle, using Teflon felt pledgets, is placed to close the myocardial defect.

F, Bleeding from the hilar vessels or from the parenchyma of the lung is controlled by clamping the hilus of the lung with an appropriate vascular clamp. (A Satinsky clamp is shown.)

12. THORACENTESIS

EARLE W. WILKINS, JR., M.D.

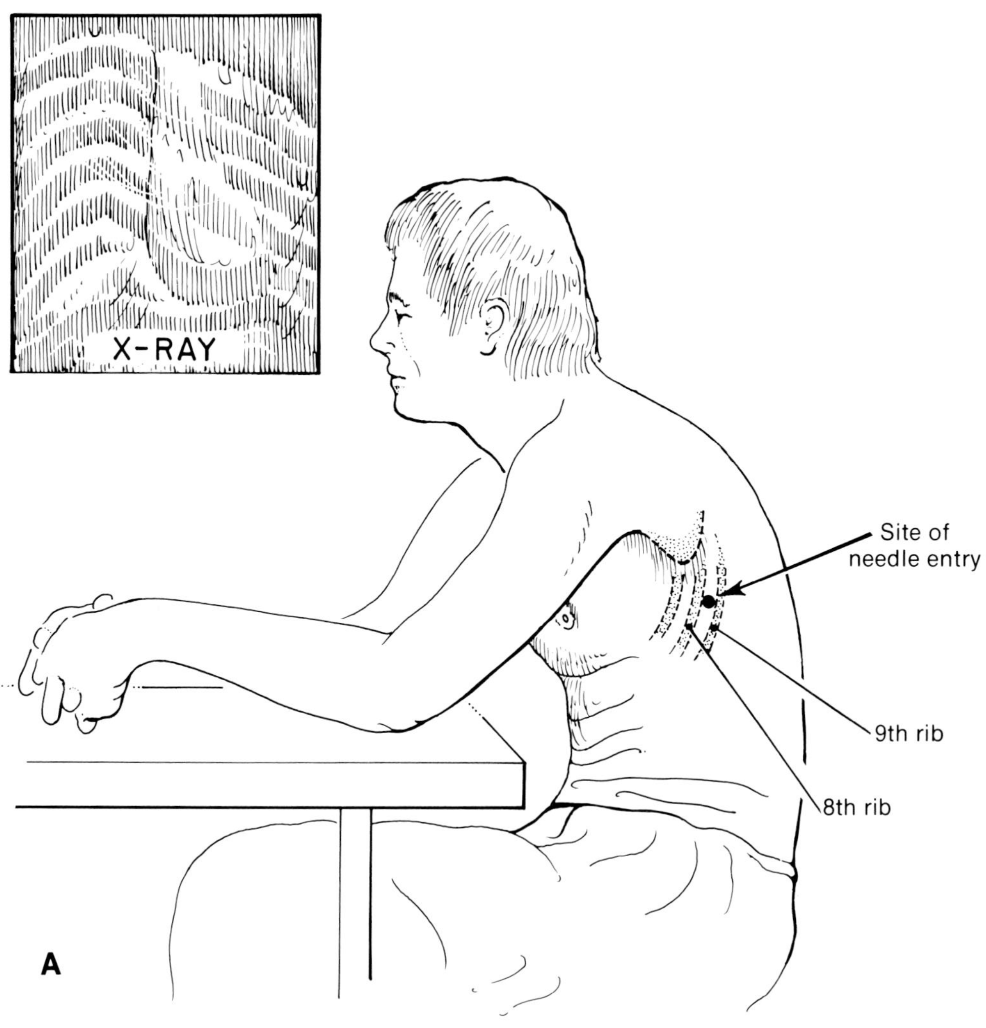

This technique of thoracentesis is offered as an alternative to that described in Chapter 32.

A, The patient is comfortably seated with arms held forward and forearms resting on a movable table. A chest x-ray film is at hand to permit identification of the proper side and rib level for aspiration. The site for entry is selected below the meniscus of fluid level and well above the diaphragm, and the skin and proposed track for the thoracentesis needle are infiltrated with 1% lidocaine (Xylocaine) without epinephrine.

B, The sterile no. 14 Intracath needle is inserted close to the lower rib (here shown as the 9th) to avoid laceration of the intercostal artery.

C, The needle is advanced so that the entire bevel is just within the parietal pleura. *D*, The catheter is then guided, within its plastic covering, through the needle into the pleural fluid. *E*, The needle is withdrawn, which minimizes the likelihood of laceration of the visceral pleura as fluid is aspirated and the lung expands. The collar of the catheter is attached to a three-way stopcock and 50-ml syringe for aspiration. A vacuum bottle of the type used for blood donation may be employed alternatively.

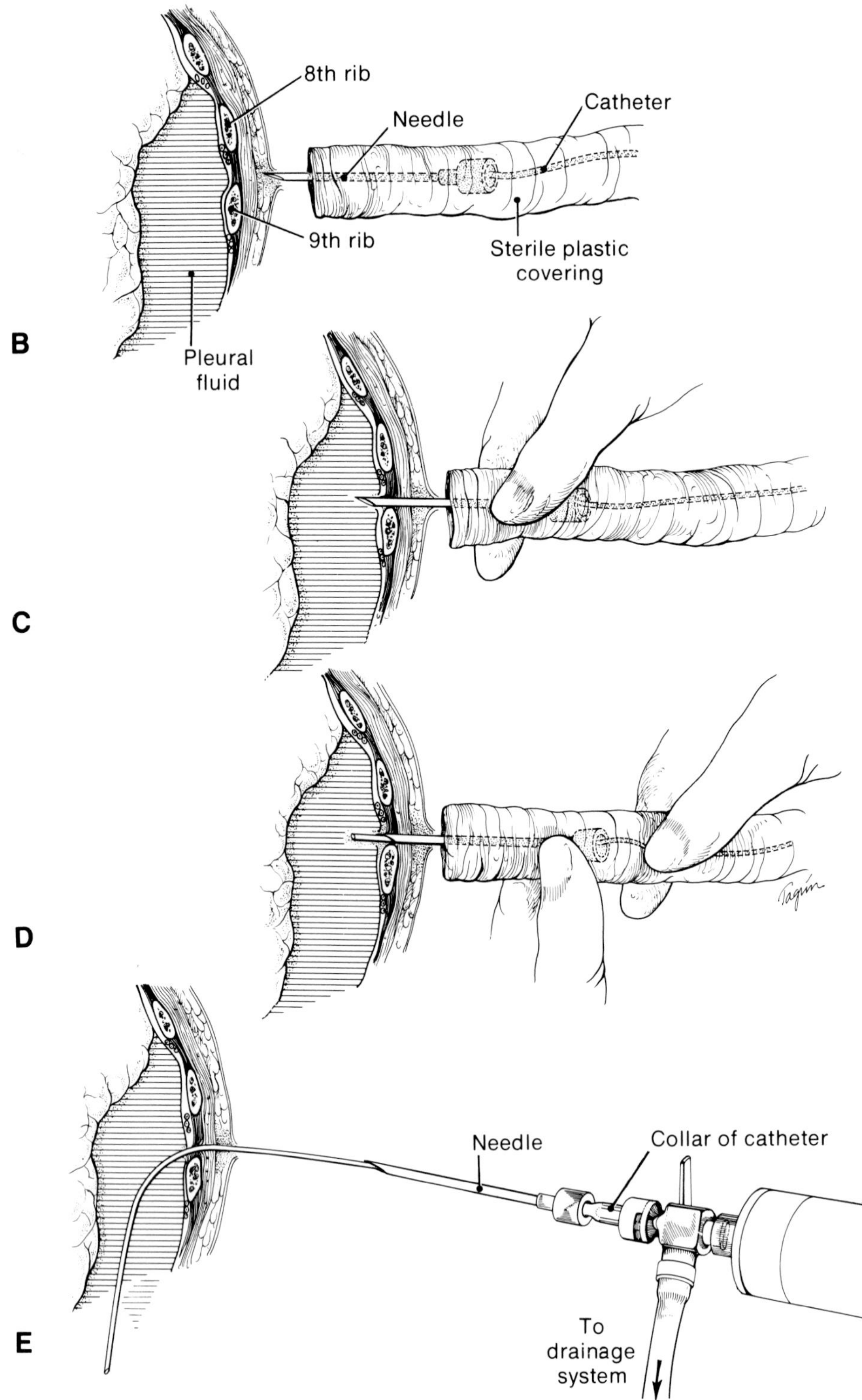
8th rib
Catheter
Needle
9th rib
Sterile plastic covering
Pleural fluid
B
C
D
Needle
Collar of catheter
To drainage system
E

13. CHEST TUBE INSERTION

CHARLES J. McCABE, M.D.

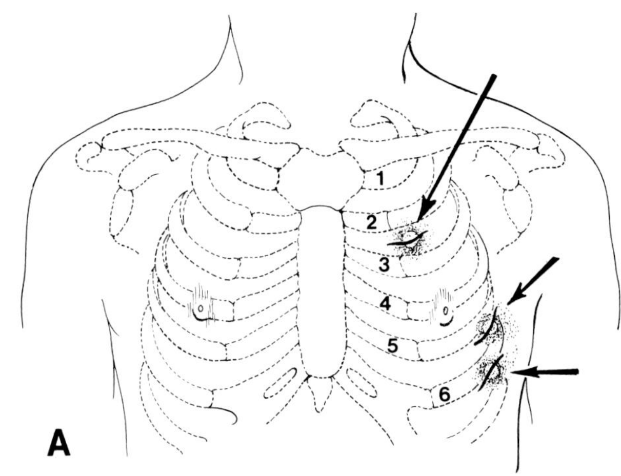

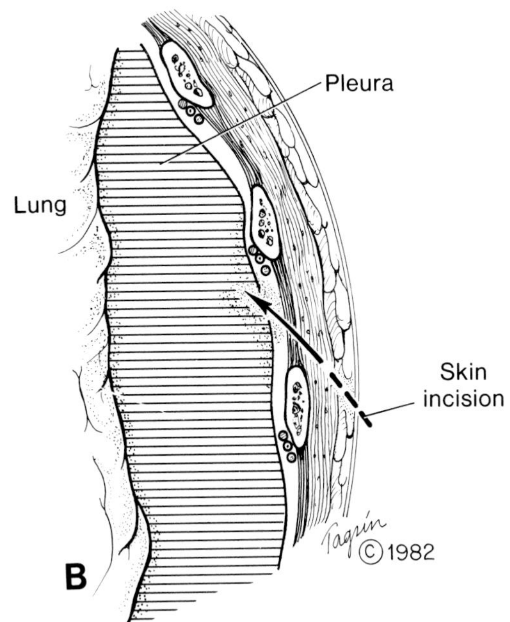

A, The site of insertion is usually the second intercostal space at the midclavicular line or the fifth or sixth interspace at the midaxillary line. A linear incision is made over the area of insertion after local anesthesia with 1% lidocaine (Xylocaine). Liberal use of lidocaine is recommended to provide anesthesia to the pleural level.

B, The skin incision is made 2–3 cm below the interspace through which the chest tube will be inserted. This allows for a skin and subcutaneous flap to develop with insertion. The neurovascular bundle that runs along the under surface of the rib is avoided.

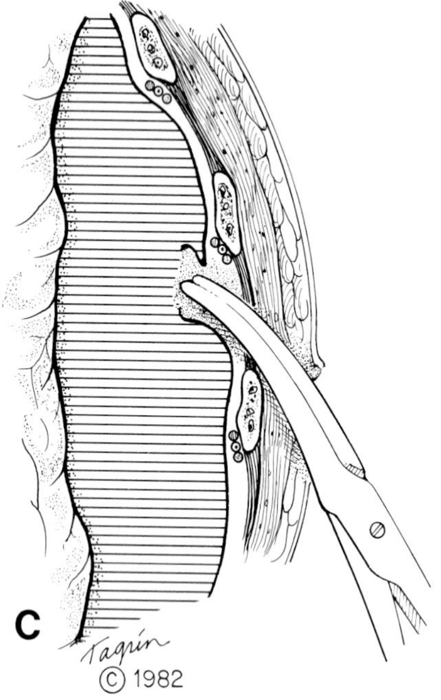

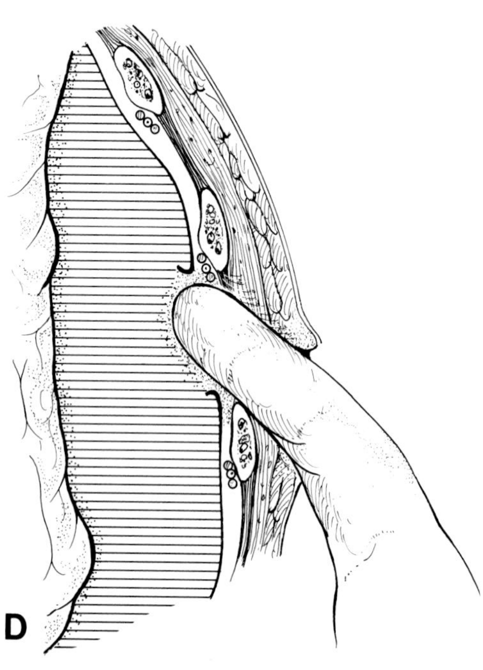

C, A Kelly clamp is used to spread the subcutaneous tissue and muscle fibers to allow penetration of the intercostal muscle.

D, Once the intercostal muscles have been spread, the digit is inserted through the intercostal space and muscle so that no damage to the underlying lung will occur. This allows digital exploration of a limited portion of the pleural space.

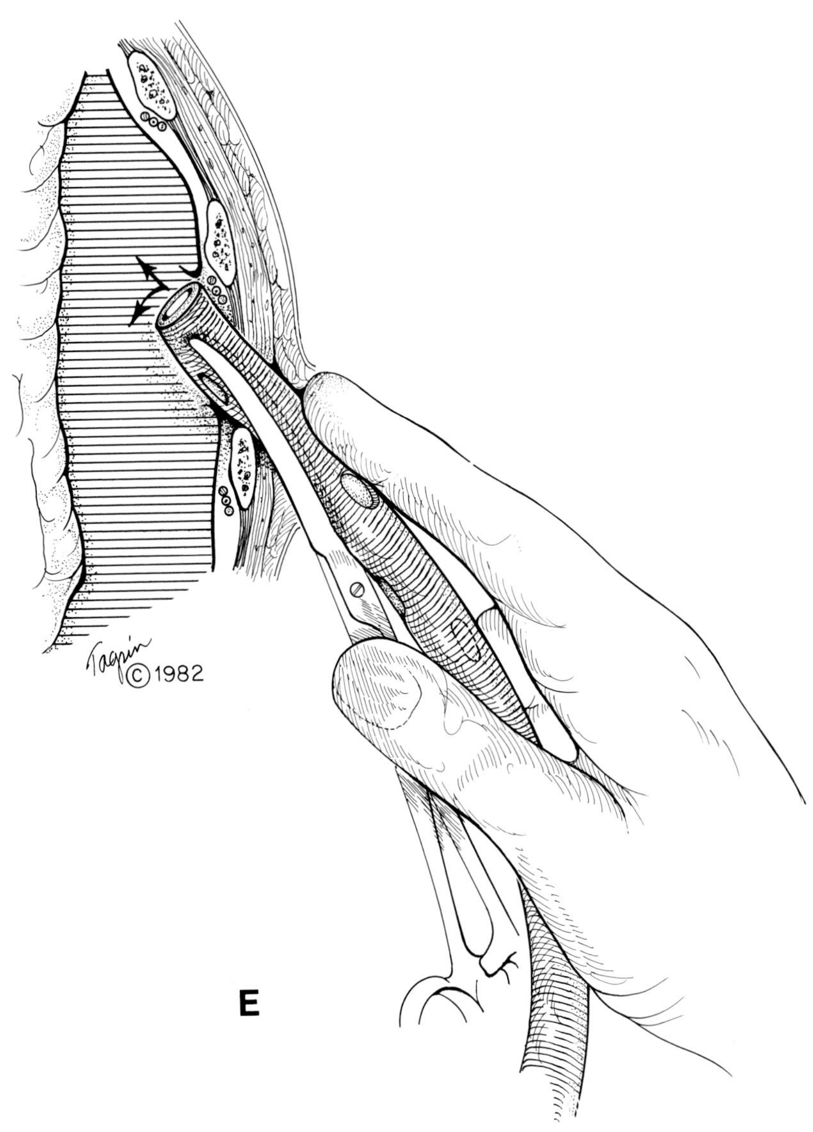

E, After an adequate tract is made using the digit, the chest tube is inserted through the created tract. The chest tube is threaded superiorly or inferiorly within the pleura. The chest tube should be inserted approximately 2–3 cm beyond the last (outer) hole in the catheter. The tube is secured to the chest wall with sutures and connected to the drainage device.

14. LUMBAR PUNCTURE

AMY A. PRUITT, M.D.

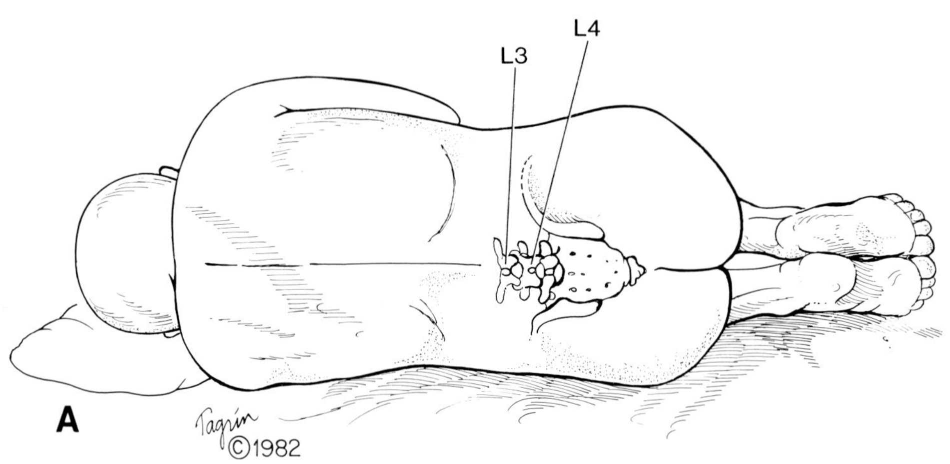

A–B, Positioning the patient. Whenever possible, place the patient on his/her side with the knees and hips flexed, the back perpendicular to the bed. For a right-handed physician, it is more convenient to have the patient on his/her left side, while for a left-handed physician, the patient is best positioned on the right side.

Place one hand on the iliac crest. A vertical line dropped from this landmark crosses the fourth lumbar vertebra. Use the other hand to feel the interspace just above this level. This is the L3–4 interspace. If this space cannot be used, L2–3 and L4–5 interspaces are acceptable.

Wash the patient's back with iodine-soaked sponges alternating with alcohol soaked-sponges, moving in concentric circles outward from the puncture site.

Put on sterile gloves and drape the patient with a sterile drape.

C, Introduction of the needle. Inject local anesthetic (1% lidocaine) into the skin at the proposed site. Raise a skin wheal with a slow intradermal injection of 0.2 ml followed by a further 0.5 ml into the deeper layers of the skin. There is no need to change needles for this procedure, nor to anesthetize deeper layers of muscle.

Introduce a 20-gauge lumbar puncture needle with a stylet in place. The needle should be directed

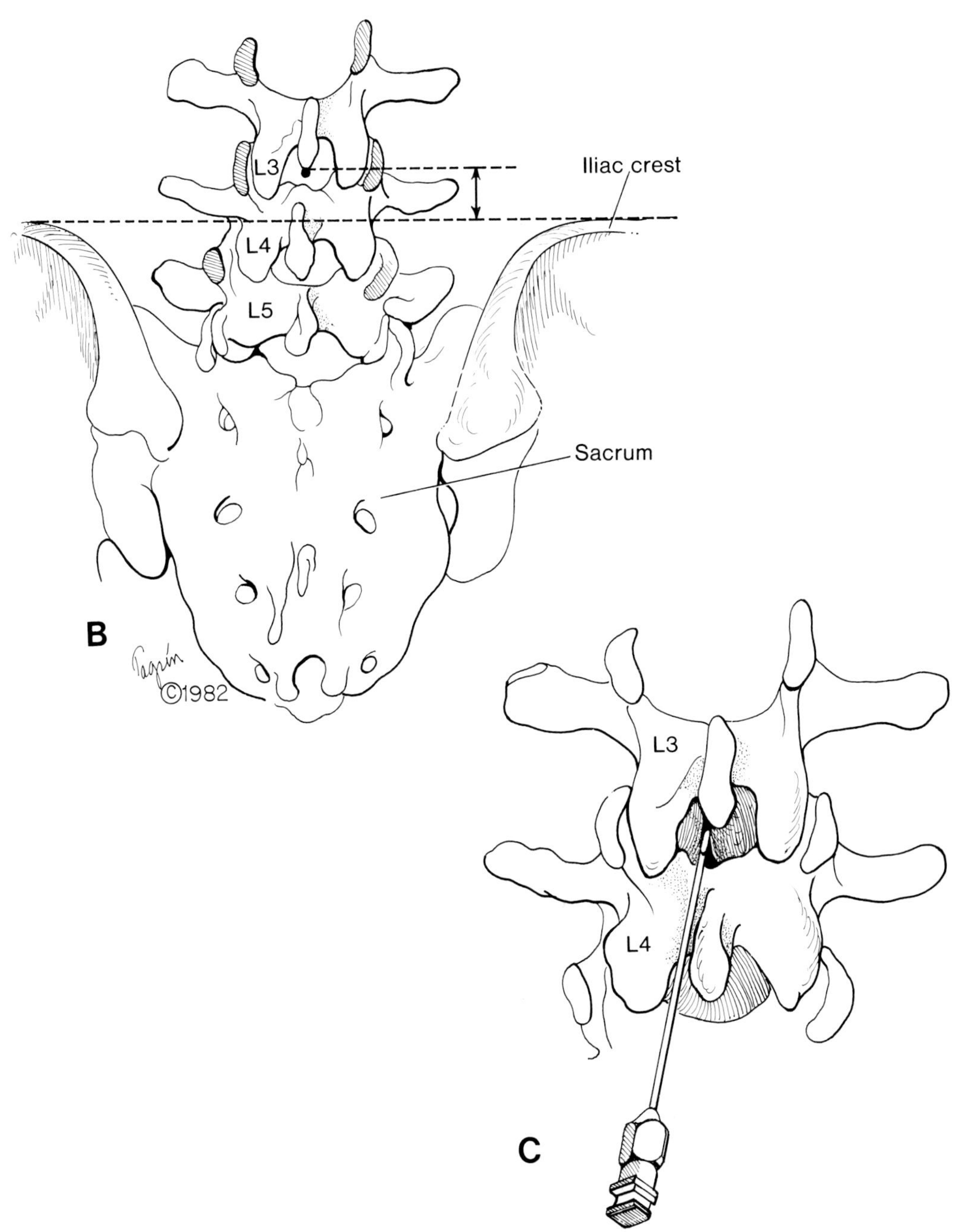

slightly cephalad (roughly toward the umbilicus) with the bevel parallel to the long axis of the patient's spine. The needle then spreads rather than cuts the fibers of the ligamentum flavum.

Advance the needle slowly until the "give" of the ligamentum flavum is felt as the needle enters the subdural space. At this point, advance the needle in 2-mm steps, removing the stylet between each step to check for cerebrospinal fluid (CSF) flow. If bone is encountered, withdraw the needle slowly and realign. Often, the give of the ligamentum flavum is not distinct. Therefore, the stylet should be removed frequently to check for CSF return.

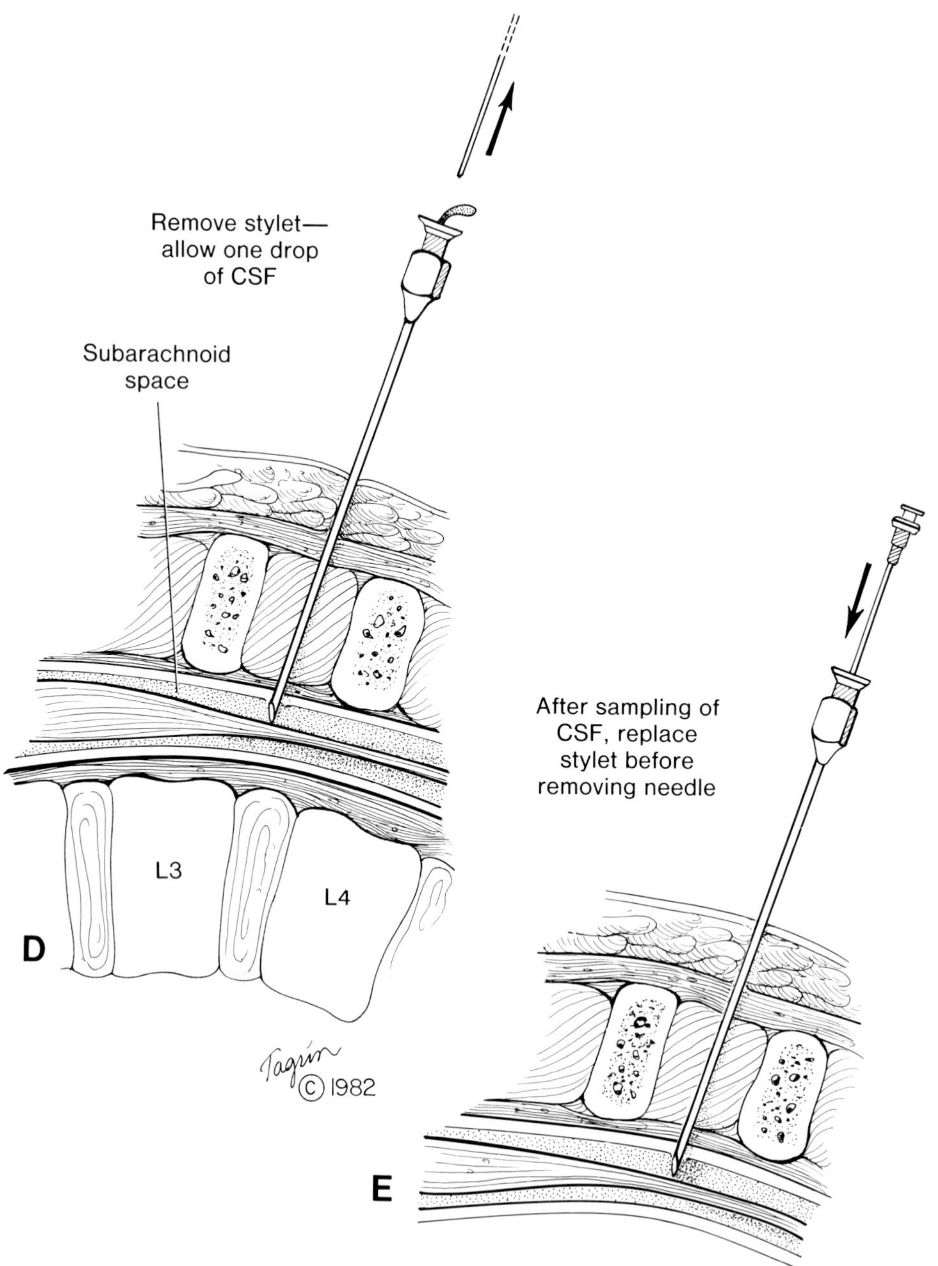

D, When the needle is in the subarachnoid space, one drop of CSF should be allowed to flow out. Then turn the bevel perpendicular to the long axis of the spine and replace the stylet.

Allow the patient to relax as much as possible, extending legs and hips slightly from the maximally flexed position. Remove the stylet, attach the manometer, and measure pressure. There should be good respiratory variation of the fluid level in the manometer.

Collect fluid in at least three sterile tubes. Tube #1 should be sent for protein and glucose (2–3 ml), tube #2 for culture and sensitivities (2 ml), and tube #3 for cell count (2 ml).

E, After all specimens are collected, replace stylet, and remove the needle. Press on the area of the puncture to prevent local bleeding, and put a small bandage over the site. The patient should be instructed to lie flat for 2–4 hours after the puncture.

15. PERITONEAL LAVAGE

ASHBY C. MONCURE, M.D.

After initial resuscitation, patients suspected of having blunt abdominal trauma who have equivocal physical findings or an altered state of consciousness may be more accurately evaluated by means of peritoneal lavage. If the patient has had a previous lower abdominal operation or disease process, peritoneal lavage is best managed by placing the catheter under direct vision through a small infraumbilical midline incision. If this is not the case, the catheter may be placed percutaneously.

If no blood is recovered, lavage with a balanced salt solution is then performed, the results being considered abnormal if frank blood is recovered in the lavage fluid, if the red blood cell count is more than 100,000/mm^3, if the white blood cell count is more than 500/mm^3, or if high concentrations of amylase, bile, or bacteria are present in the fluid.

A, The abdominal wall is prepared as a sterile field, and in the lower abdominal midline, one-third of the way between the umbilicus and the pubic bone, a small puncture wound is made with a no. 15 scalpel blade after infiltration with 1% lidocaine (Xylocaine). *B*, A peritoneal dialysis catheter with an indwelling stylet (Trocath, McGaw Laboratories) is placed through the puncture wound, and is advanced to the linea alba, where resistance is encountered.

C, The stylet tip is forced into the peritoneal cavity with a twisting motion; the depth of penetration is controlled by grasping the catheter with the thumb and index finger of the nondominant hand. *D*, The stylet is withdrawn. *E*, The catheter is advanced into the right or left pelvic gutter and is attached to an intravenous set with injection site for intravenous solution administration (McGaw Laboratories).

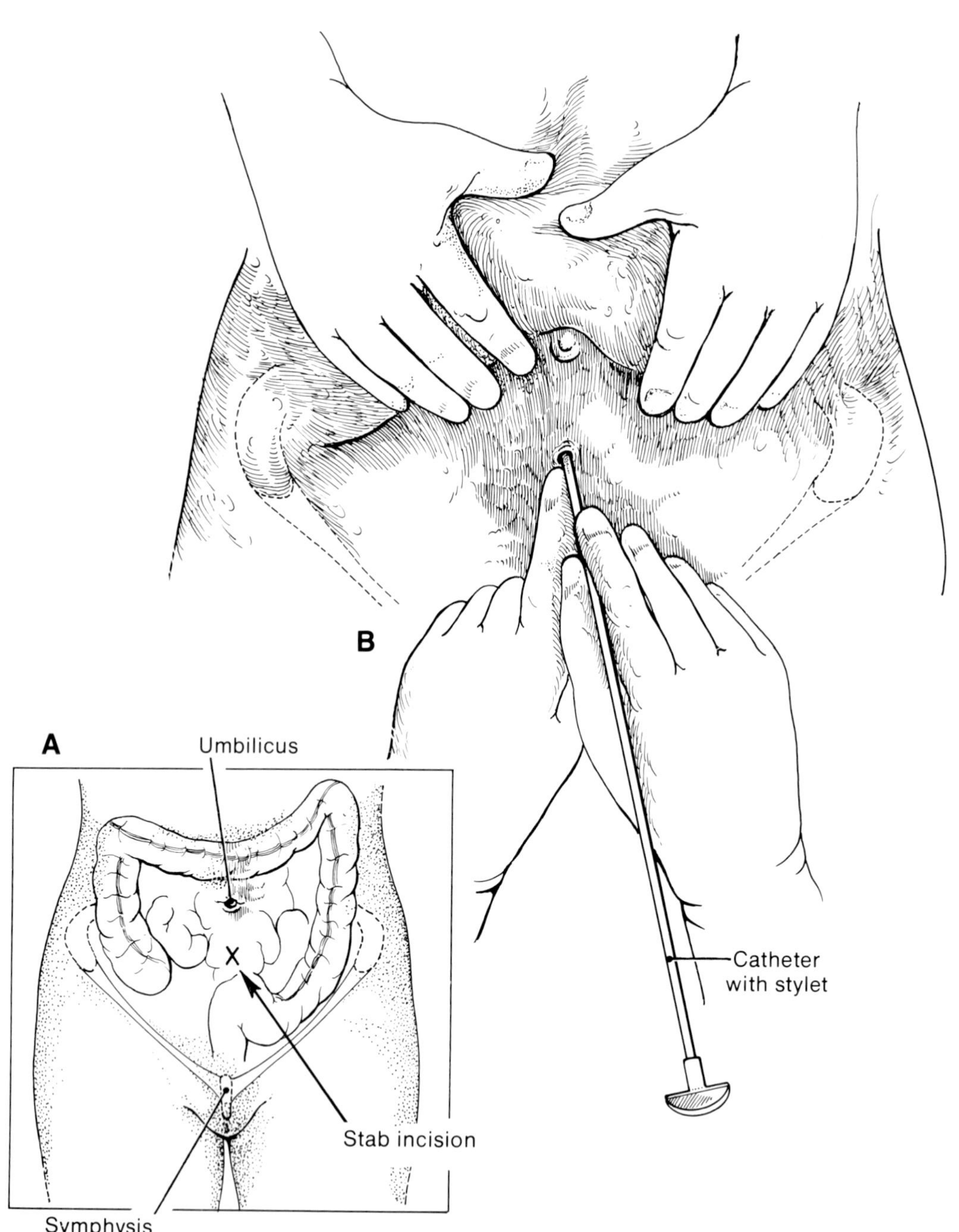
B
A
Umbilicus
Stab incision
Symphysis
Catheter with stylet

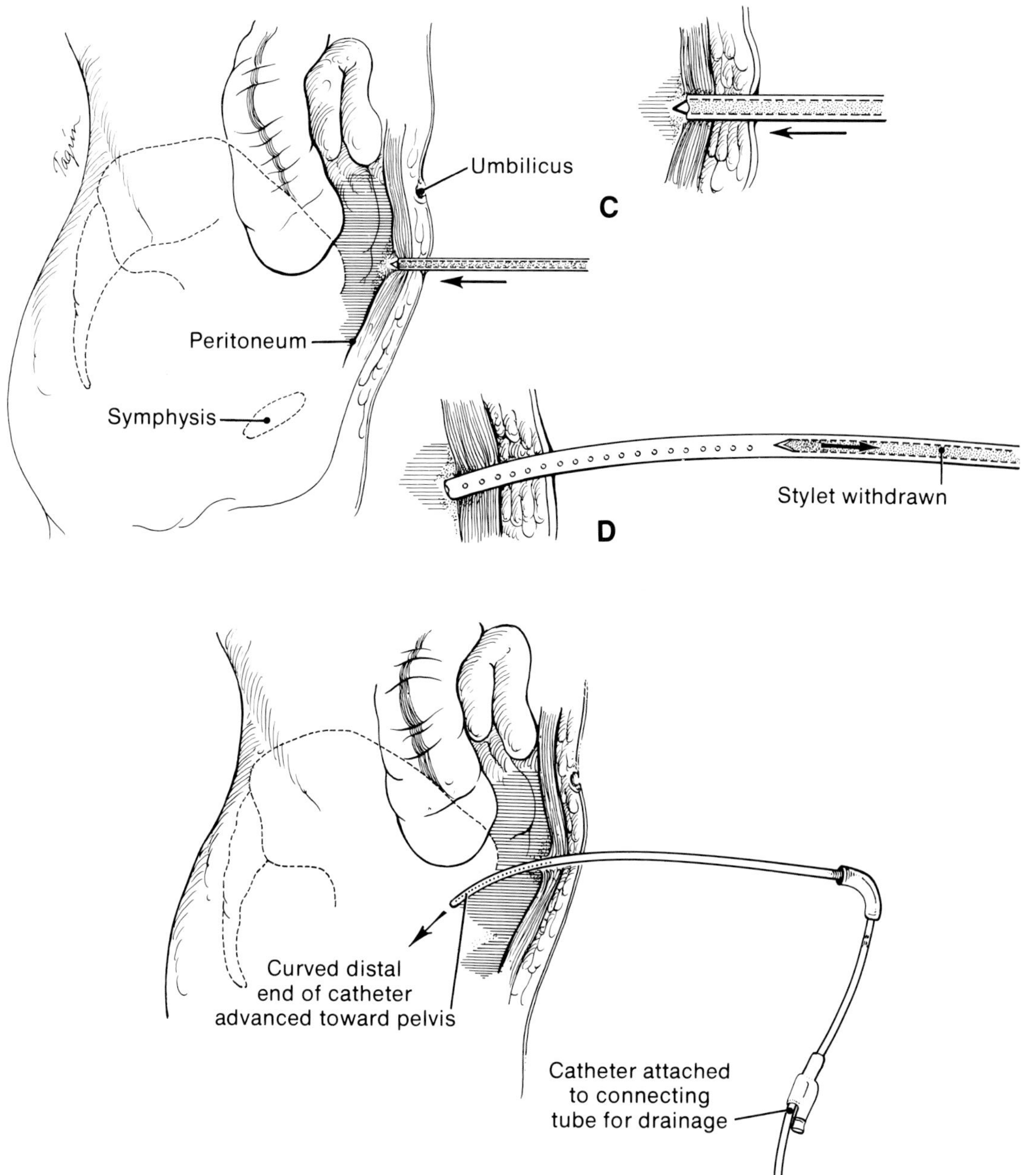
Umbilicus
C
Peritoneum
Symphysis
Stylet withdrawn
D
Curved distal end of catheter advanced toward pelvis
Catheter attached to connecting tube for drainage
E

16. PERCUTANEOUS SUPRAPUBIC CYSTOTOMY

ERIC J. SACKNOFF, M.D.

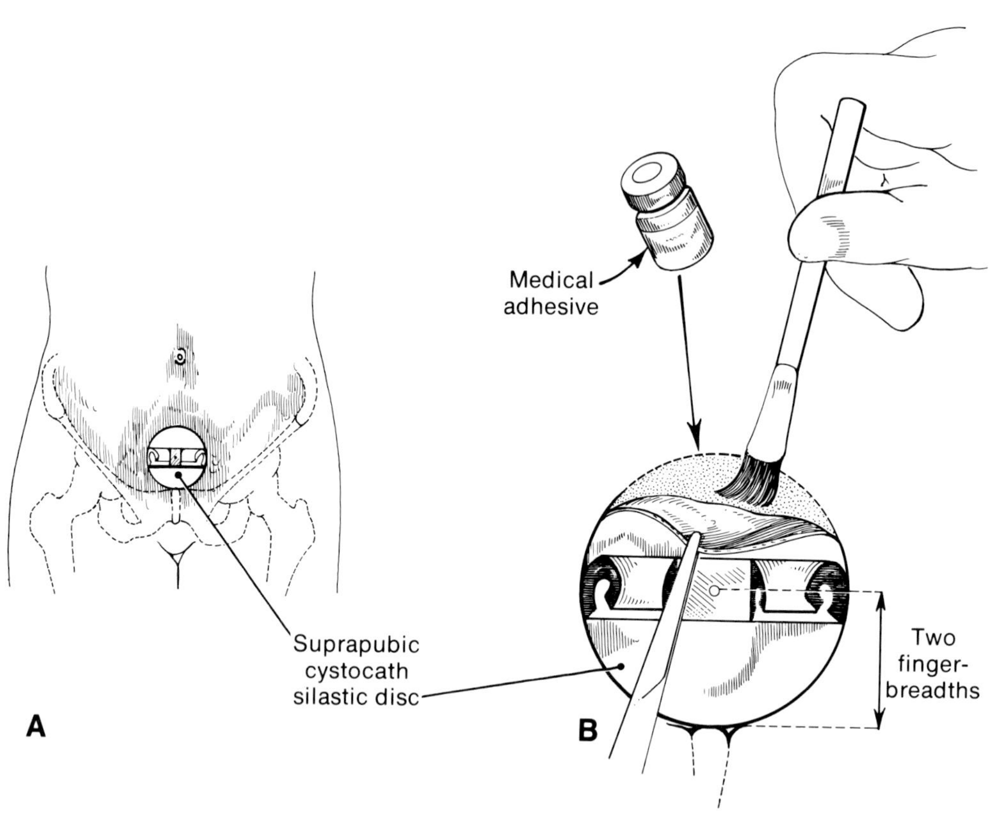

Indications

Acute epididymitis (severe)
Acute prostatitis (severe)
Acute urethritis (severe)
Urethral stricture
Urethral rupture
Urethral retention

Contraindications

Previous pelvic and lower abdominal bowel surgery
Bladder neoplasm
Previous transpubic vascular procedure
Previous pelvic radiation therapy
Pelvic sepsis

A, After the lower part of the abdomen is prepared with iodine and alcohol, the skin is anesthetized with 1% lidocaine (Xylocaine) in the midline two fingerbreadths above the pubic symphysis. The location where the Silastic disc will be affixed is shown.

B, The skin is brushed with medical adhesive provided in the Cystocath kit, and the Silastic disc is then applied in the midline.

C, Puncture of the skin surface with a no. 15 scalpel blade allows easy passage of the trocar and cannula through the skin and subcutaneous tissue.

D, At two fingerbreadths above the pubic symphysis in the midline, the trocar should be inserted in a direction slightly less than perpendicular to the skin so that the point is always directed inferiorly

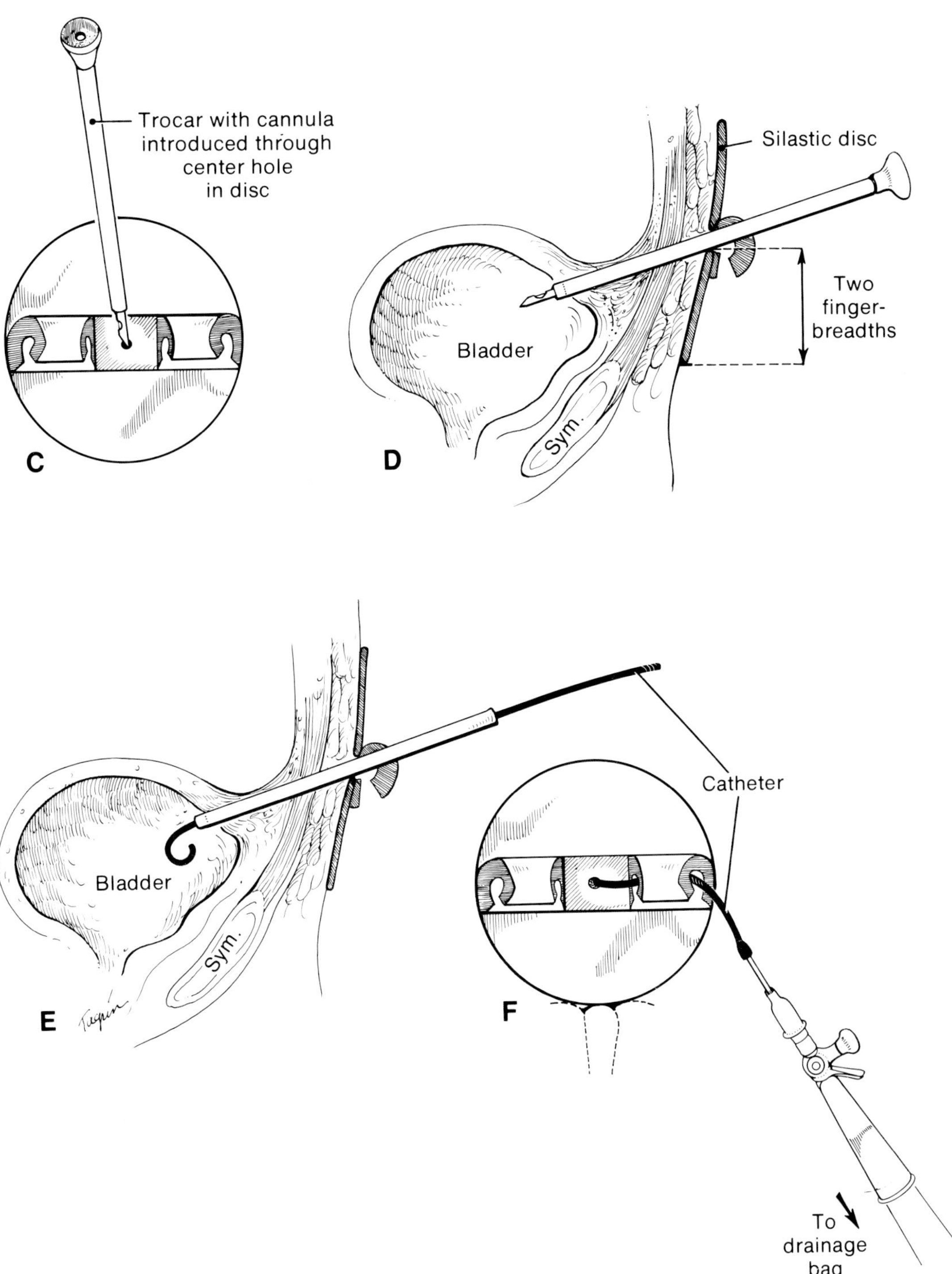

(*never* superiorly) to avoid entering the peritoneal cavity.

E, After the bladder is entered, the trocar is removed and a Silastic no. 8 French catheter is introduced through the cannula. *F*, Once the catheter is in the bladder, the cannula is removed. The catheter is then secured to the disc and attached to the three-way adapter and drainage system.

17. CULDOCENTESIS

DAVID S. CHAPIN, M.D.

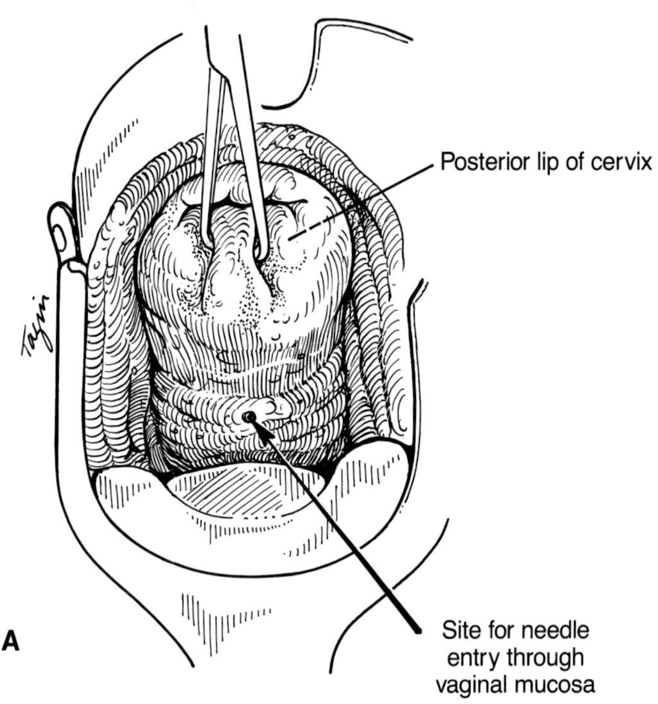

Indications

Suspected ectopic pregnancy
Suspected pelvic abscess

Contraindications

Markedly retroverted uterus
Obvious cul-de-sac obliteration

Instruments

Speculum
Tenaculum
5-ml syringe
20- or 22-gauge spinal needle

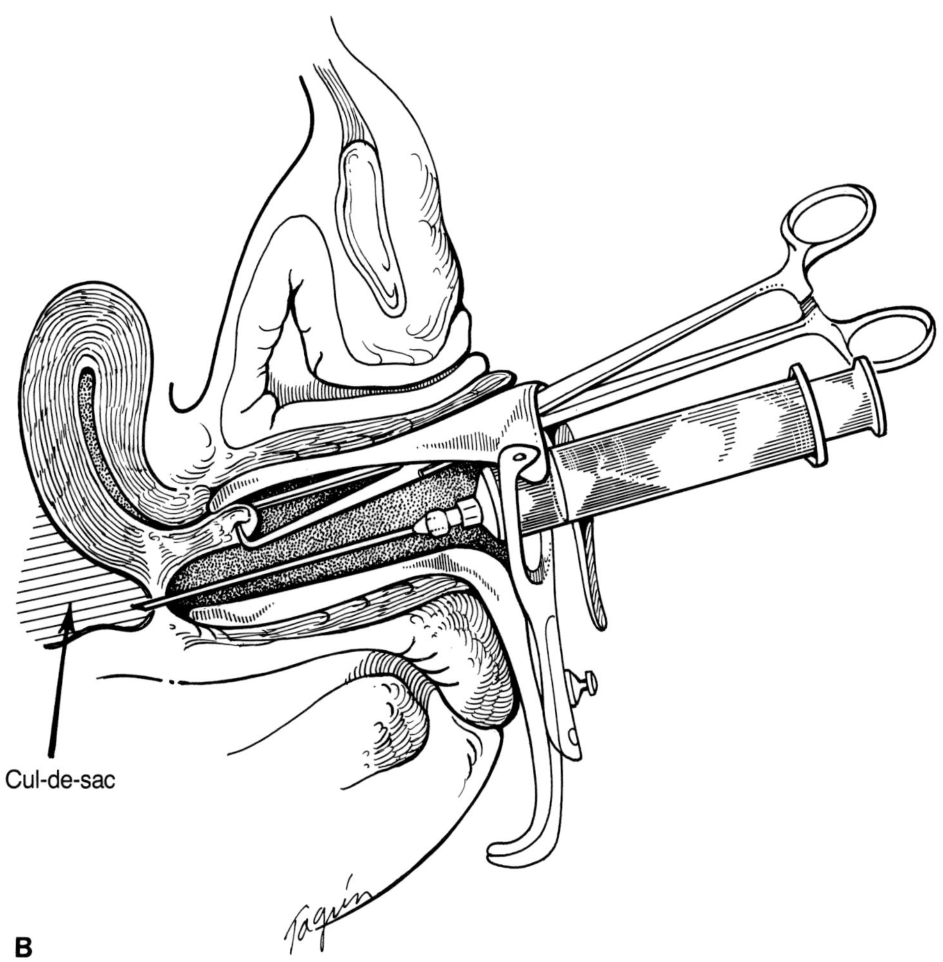

A–B, With the patient in the lithotomy position, the speculum is inserted, the cervix is visualized, and bulging of the cul-de-sac is noted. The vaginal apex is swabbed with antiseptic solution (Betadine). If desired, 1% lidocaine (Xylocaine) may be used to anesthetize the puncture site, although this step is usually unnecessary. The posterior lip of the cervix is grasped with the tenaculum and is elevated. The needle, mounted on the syringe, is inserted through the mucosa into the cul-de-sac. Withdrawal of pus or blood on aspiration suggests the presumptive diagnosis. If no fluid can be aspirated, the cul-de-sac is empty, but the presumptive diagnosis is not ruled out.

18. METACARPAL NERVE BLOCK

CHARLES J. McCABE, M.D.

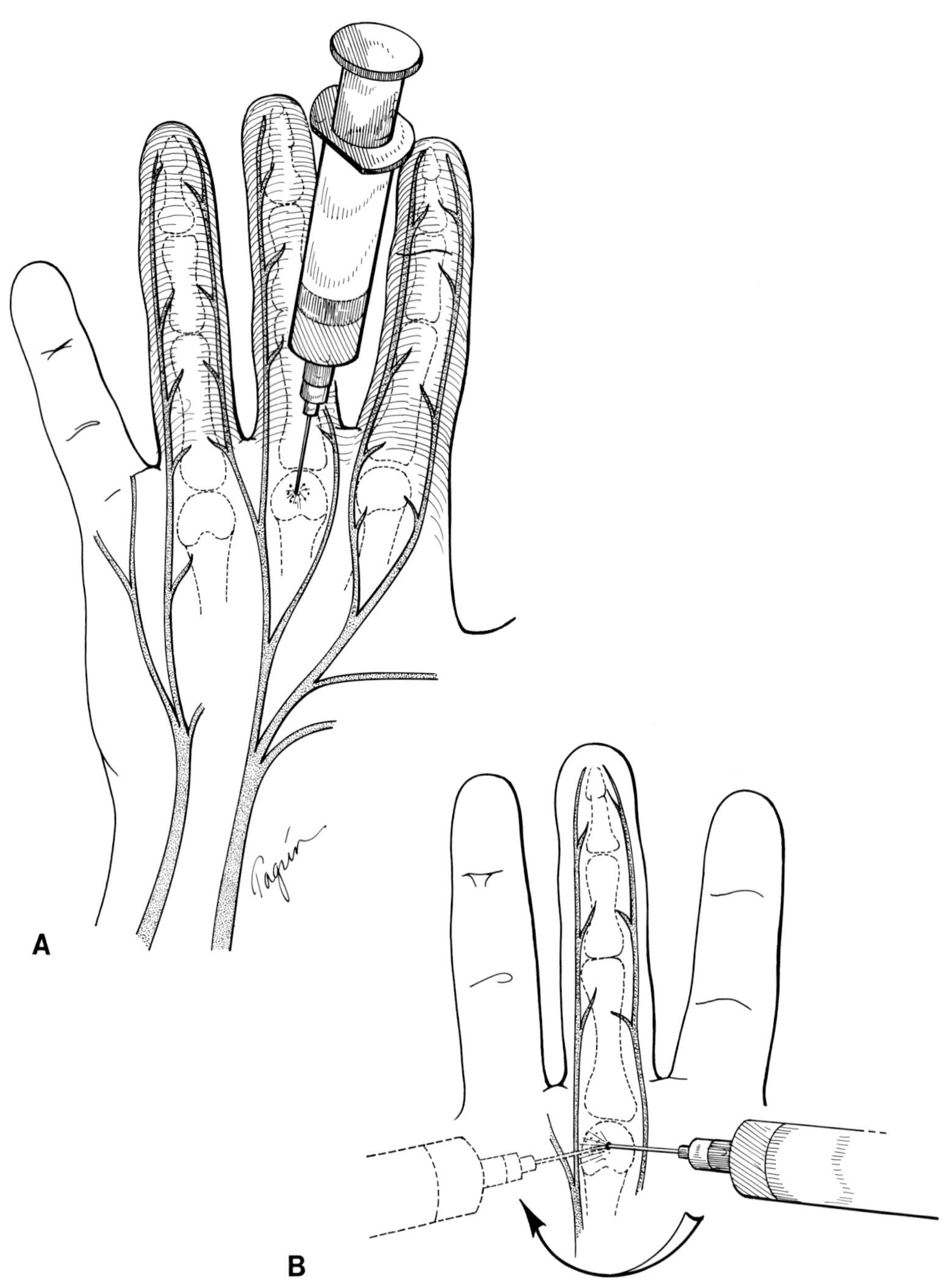

Equipment

1% lidocaine (Xylocaine) *without* epinephrine, 5 or 10-ml syringe, and 22-gauge needle

A, Palmar surface of the hand. Insert the needle directly to the metacarpal head of the digit involved.

B, Inject 1–2 ml of 1% lidocaine. Then gently direct the needle to the ulnar and to the radial side of the bone, injecting 2–3 ml lidocaine on each side.

19. DRAINAGE OF A PARONYCHIA

CHARLES J. McCABE, M.D.

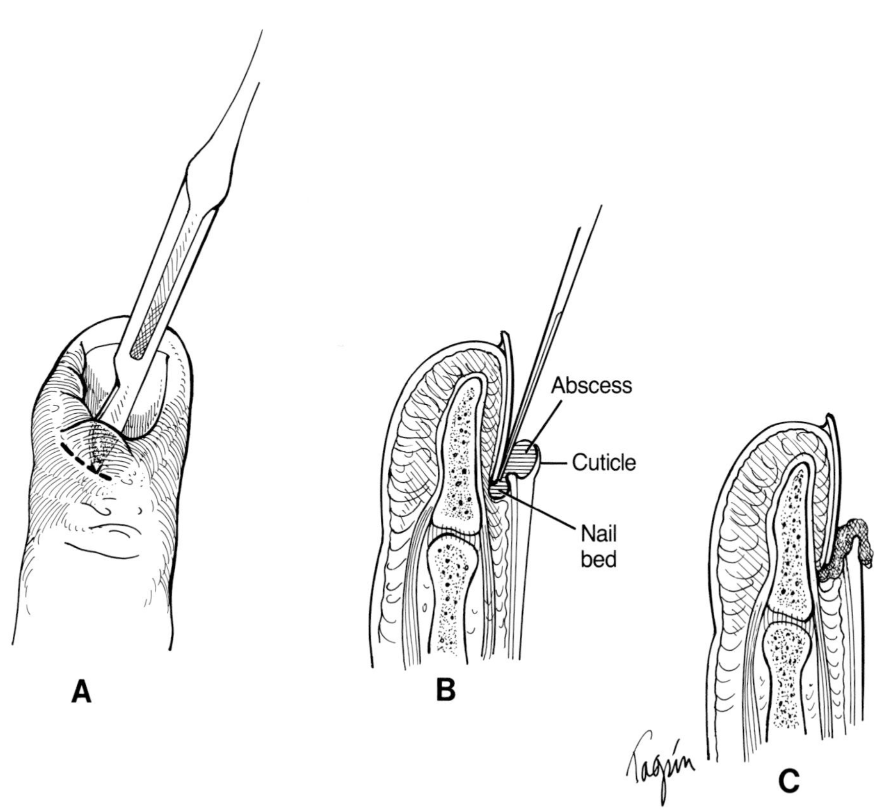

A paronychia is an infection at the base of the nail. Clinically, the area surrounding the nail base is red, swollen, tender, and fluctuant.

A digital block or metacarpal nerve block provides local anesthesia with 1% lidocaine (Xylocaine) without epinephrine.

A–C, An incision is made in the abscess between the nail and the overlying cuticle by sliding a knife

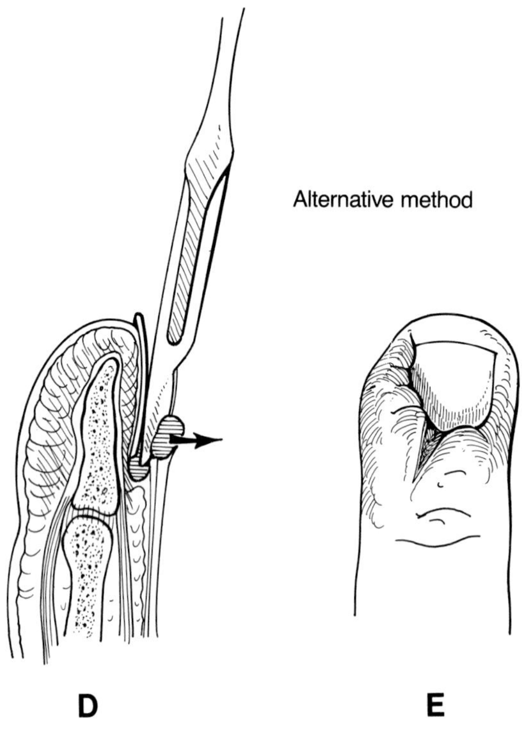

or the bevel of a needle between the cuticle and the base of the nail. This usually permits drainage of the abscess. A small Vaseline gauze wick may be placed in the wound for drainage for 24 hours.

D–E, The skin overlying the abscess may be incised by the technique diagrammed. The knife is used as in *B* and turned 90° so that the cutting edge faces the abscess.

20. DRAINAGE OF A FELON

CHARLES J. McCABE, M.D.

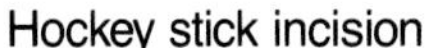

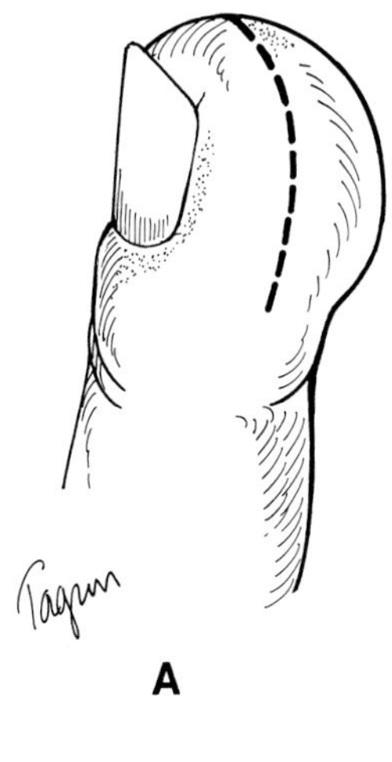

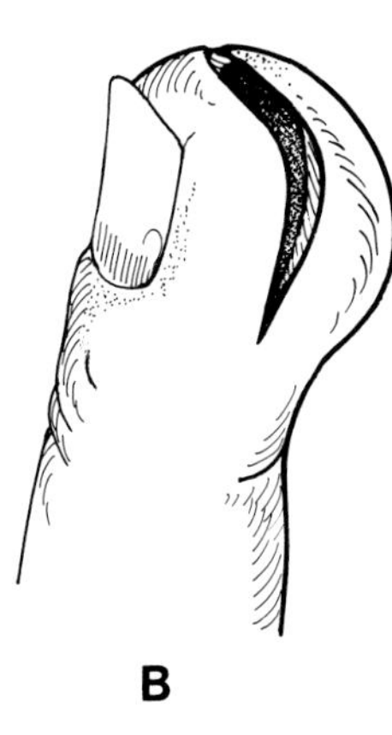

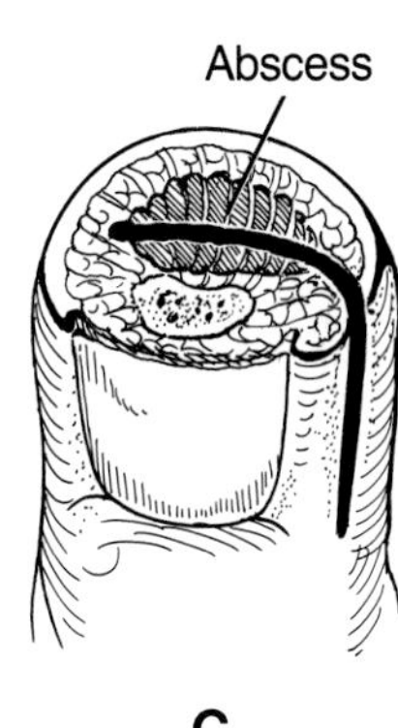

A felon is a collection of purulent material in the pulp of the palmar surface of the distal phalanx. In order to drain this purulent material, local anesthesia by metacarpal or digital nerve block is acceptable using 1% lidocaine (Xylocaine) without epinephrine.

A–B, To effect drainage, a hockey stick incision is made along the ulnar aspect of the distal phalanx extending onto the tip of the digit. This incision is begun in a plane opposite the volar aspect of the bony phalanx and extended onto the tip in the same line. All loculations are disrupted. A small Vaseline gauze or rubber wick drain is left in place for 24 hours. A dry, sterile dressing is applied.

C, This cross-sectional plane shows the abscess pocket in the pulp space volar to bone.

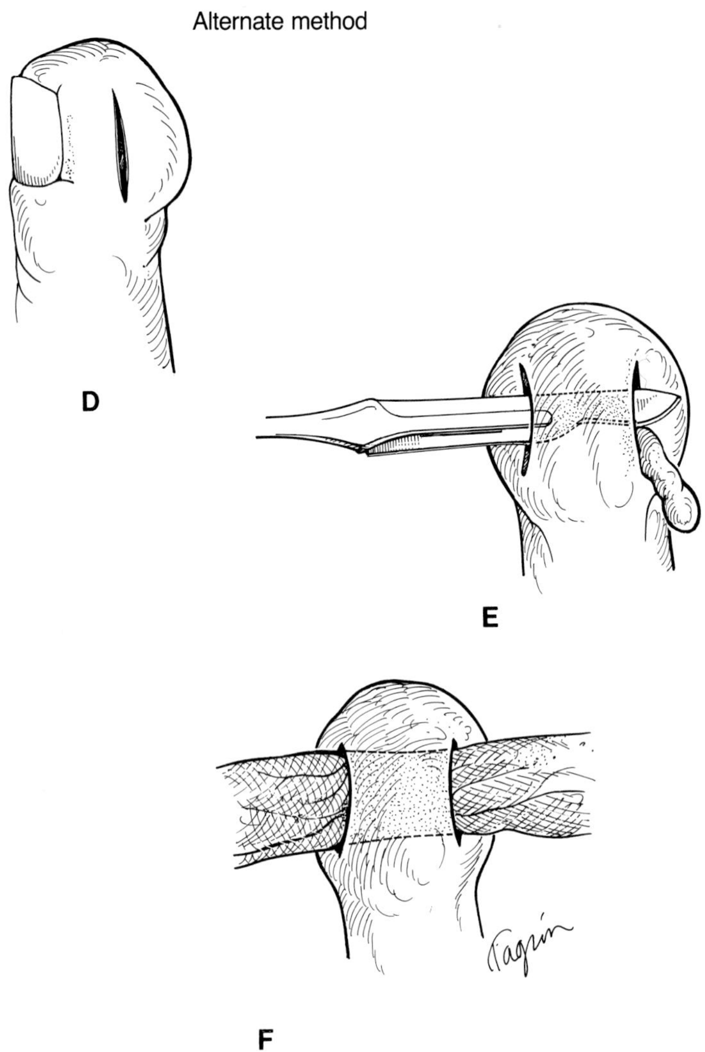

D–F, Alternative method. Drainage is accomplished by the through-and-through technique with incisions on the ulnar and radial surfaces of the distal phalanx. Care must be taken to open the entire pulp space. A drain is left in place.

21. EVACUATION OF A SUBUNGUAL HEMATOMA

CHARLES J. McCABE, M.D.

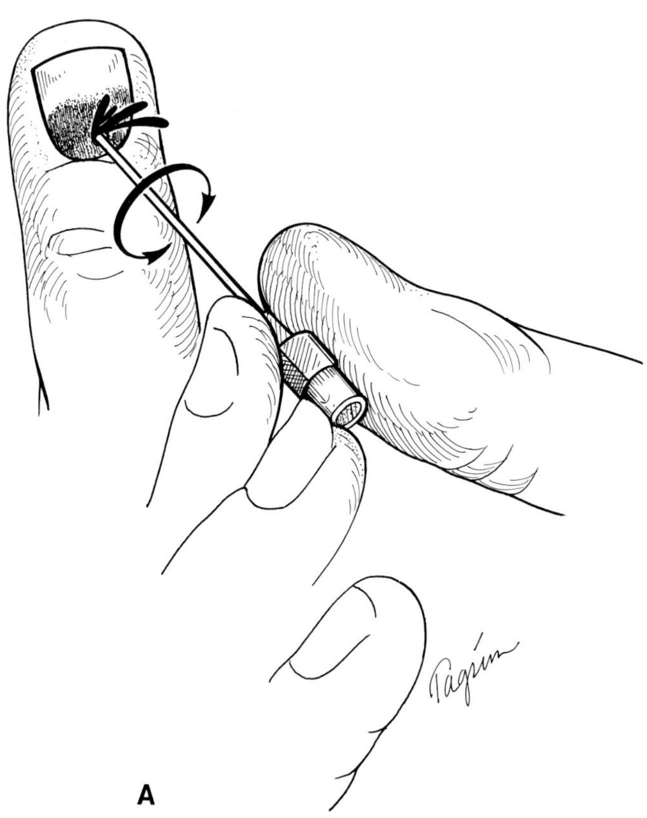

A

This lesion is often painful with blood under pressure beneath the fingernail. Therapy will depend on the extent of the hematoma. If the hematoma involves greater than one-half of the nail, the chances of a fracture of the distal phalanx through the nail bed is high.

Simple Hematoma (*A*)

This often does not require anesthesia, but occasionally a metacarpal or digital nerve block is helpful, using 1% lidocaine (Xylocaine) without epinephrine.

A small trephination is created directly over the area of hematoma (with a twisting motion of a no. 16–18 gauge needle.) A small amount of blood will "spurt" from the hole, and pain relief is usually immediate.

Complicated Hematoma (*B–F*)

B, If a distal fracture is present or if the hematoma involves more than 50% of the nail, an exploration of the nail bed should be undertaken. *C–D*, This is performed by elevating and removing the nail and identifying the nail bed defect using metacarpal or digital nerve block with 1% lidocaine (Xylocaine) without epinephrine. *E*, The nail bed is repaired by using 6-O absorbable suture. *F*, The nail is then returned to its normal location as a protective splint to promote comfort. A sterile dressing is then applied.

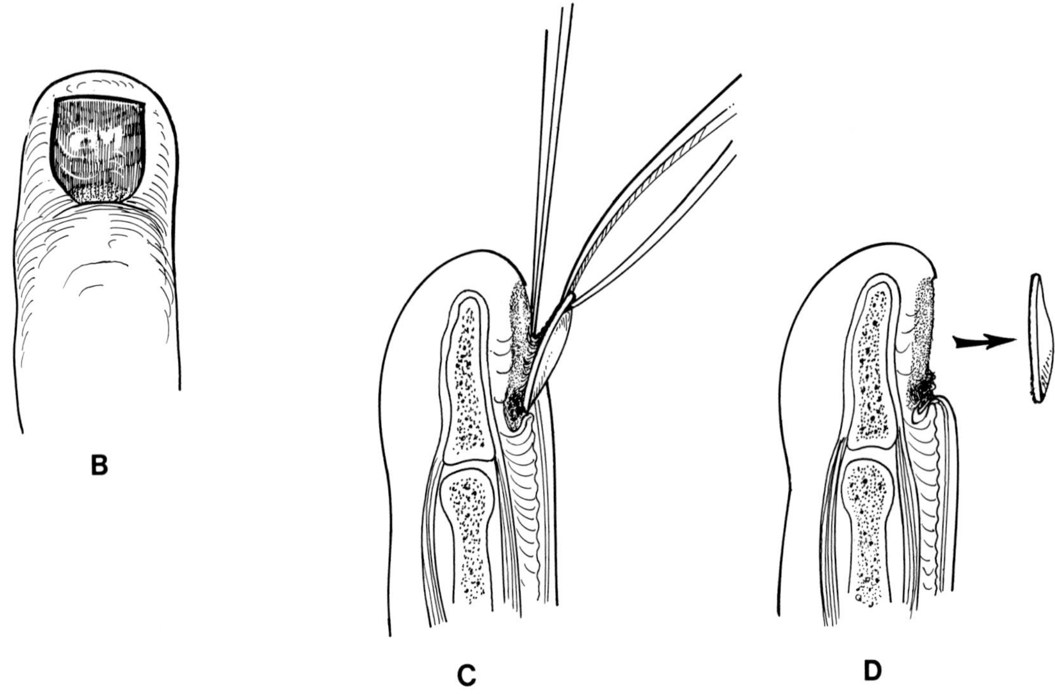
B
C
D

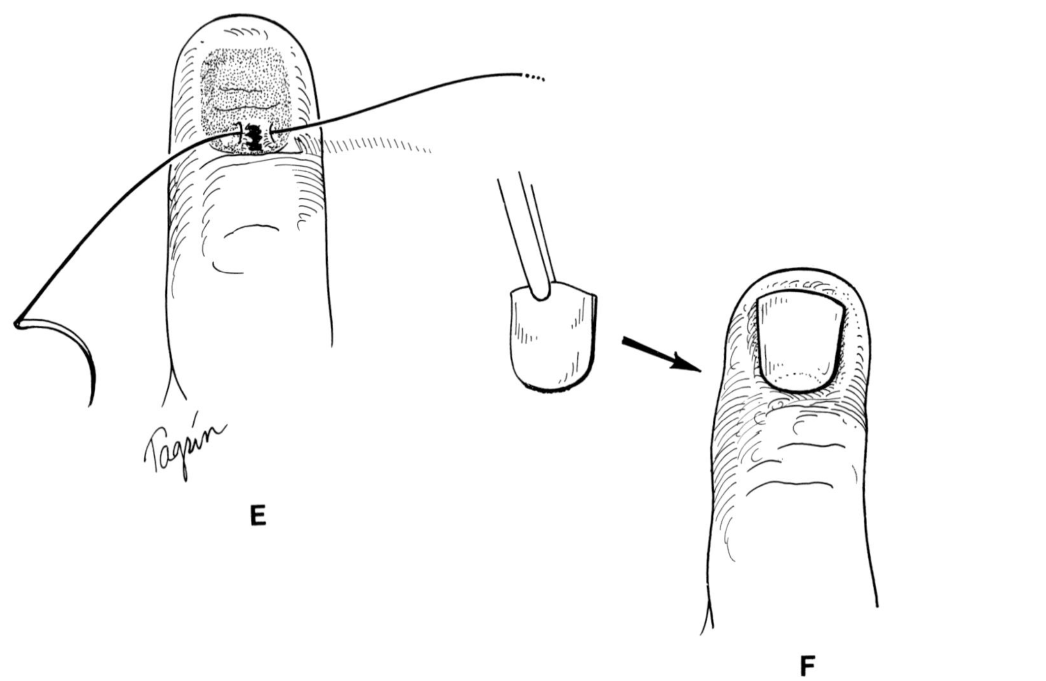
E
F

22. SUTURING TECHNIQUES

CHARLES J. McCABE, M.D.

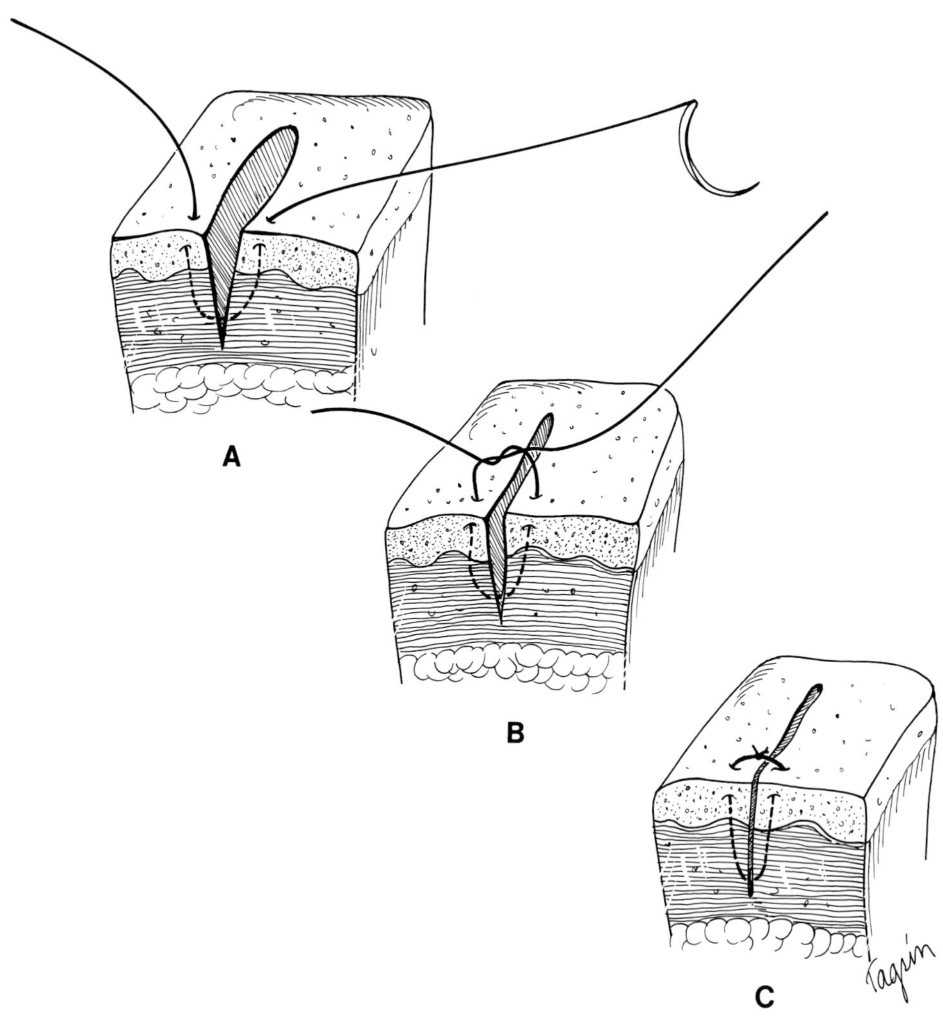

Isolate and sterilize the area to be sutured with saline irrigation and Betadine solution. If the laceration involves the wrist, hand, and/or fingers, or any anatomic area in proximity to major nerve or vascular structures, an examination should be performed before the area is anesthetized for neurologic function and circulation.

Locally anesthetize the area to be sutured with 1% lidocaine (Xylocaine) *without* epinephrine. A metacarpal or digital nerve block is useful for finger lacerations. After anesthesia is obtained, a more vigorous debridement and wound preparation is possible. Remove debris, foreign bodies, and obviously necrotic tissue.

Obtain hemostasis by suture ligature with no. 4-5-O chromic catgut.

The deep laceration may be closed in one (*A–C*) or two layers (*D, E*). The deeper layer is closed with fine absorbable suture. The skin is approximated using simple suturing techniques. Dividing the wound into progressive halves is the simplest means of setting the suture number and space intervals (*F*). The needle is grasped close to the point to avoid bending. The needle should enter the skin as far back from the edge as the anticipated space between stitches. The needle should be inserted perpendicularly to the skin surface, and the natural curve of the needle followed (*G*). The other hand manipulates the skin edge using atraumatic forceps in order to expose and stabilize the area to be sutured.

A dry sterile dressing is applied to provide occlusive covering of the area.

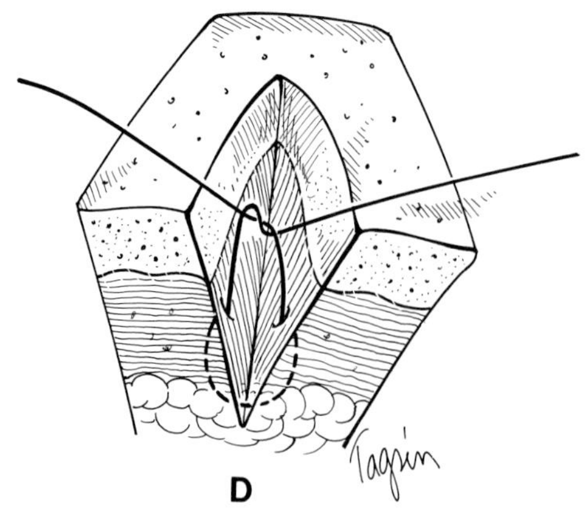

D

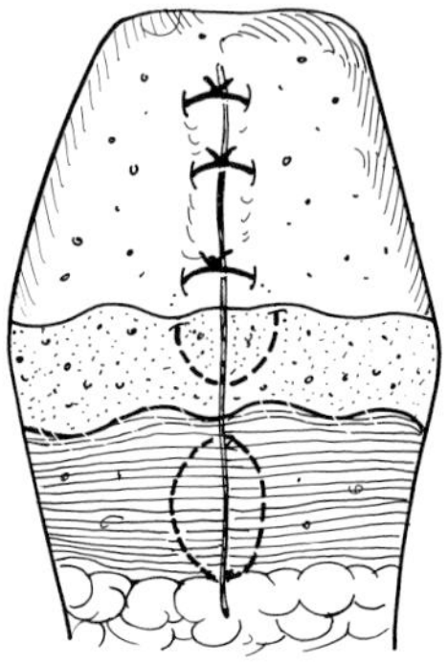

E

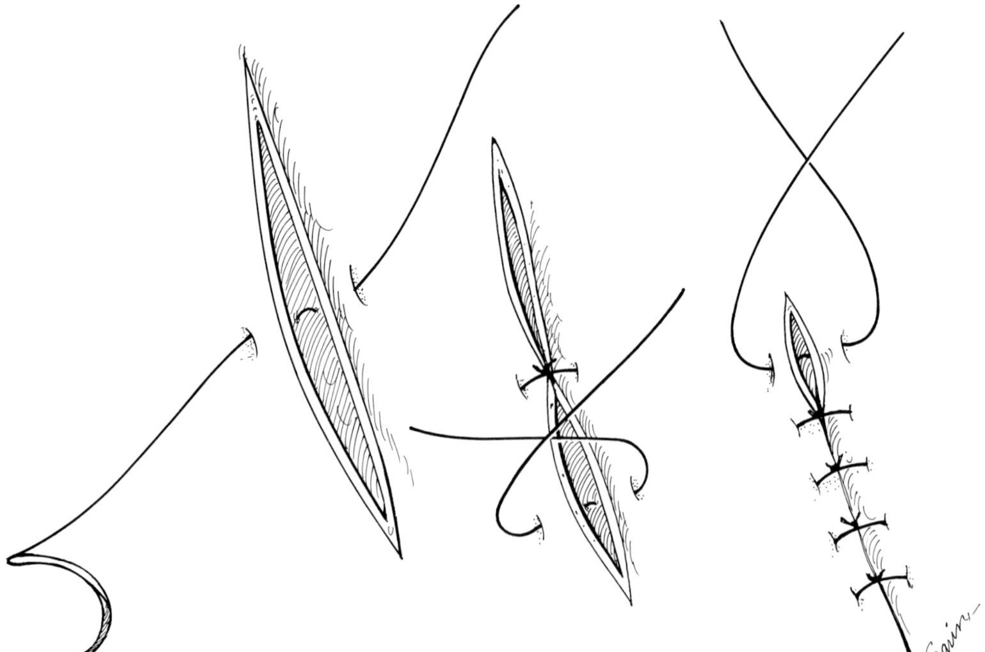

F

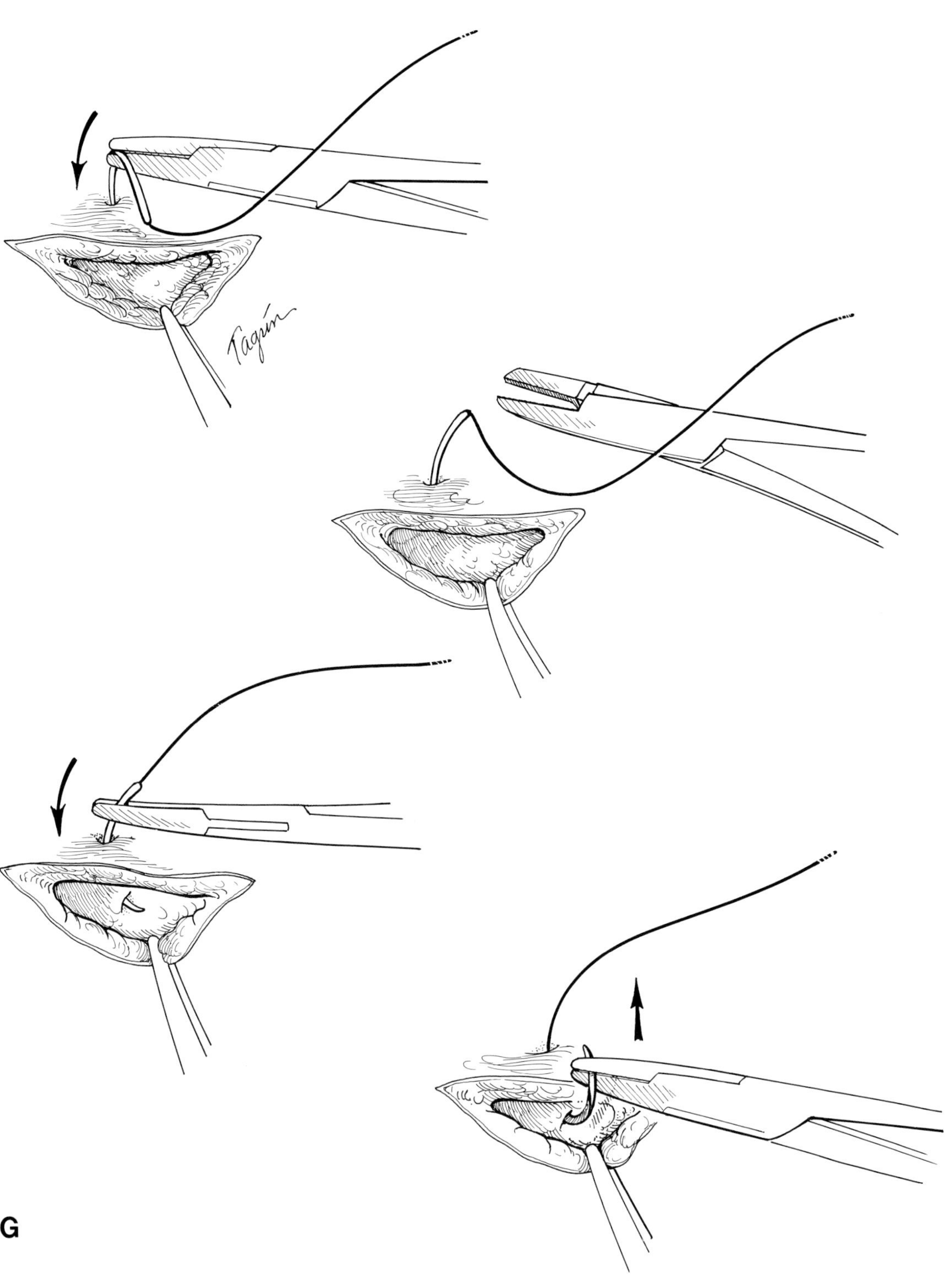
Fagún
G

23. INJECTION FOR BURSITIS—SHOULDER

BERTRAM ZARINS, M.D.
CARTER R. ROWE, M.D.

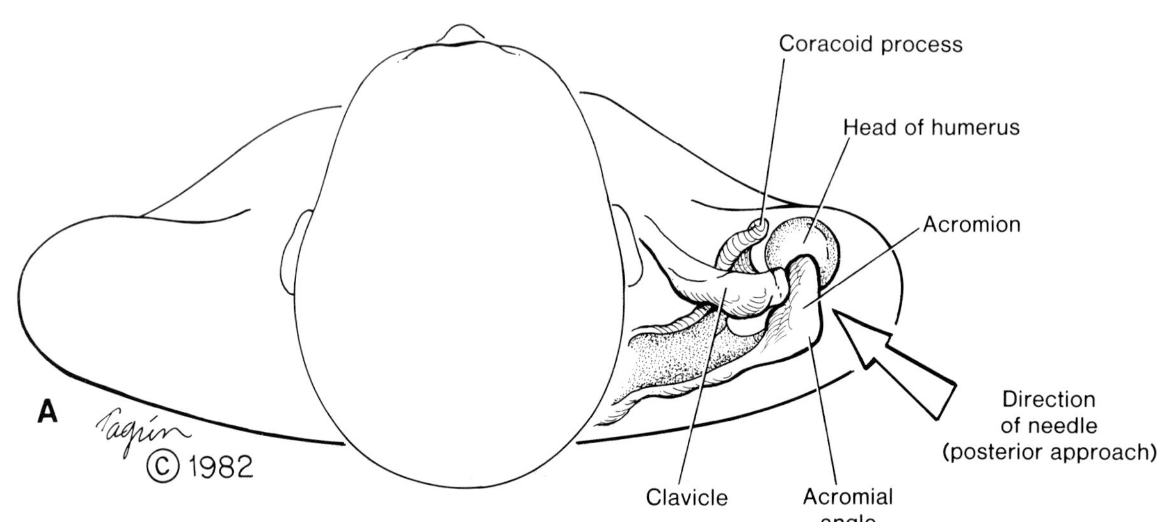

The most common cause of acute "bursitis" of the shoulder is calcific tendonitis involving the rotator cuff. If injected, steroid should be instilled into the overlying bursa rather than the tendon itself. Anteroposterior and axillary roentgenograms should be taken prior to steroid injection. Roentgenograms are evaluated for the presence of possible calcium deposition in the rotator cuff.

Injection into the subacromial bursa is carried out with the patient in a seated position and under sterile conditions. The posterolateral approach is the easiest and least painful (*A*). Palpate the spine of the scapula posteriorly, acromial angle, and acromion process; locate a "soft spot" 1 cm below the acromial angle and anesthetize the skin with local anesthesia using 1% lidocaine (Xylocaine). Instruct the patient to relax the muscles so that the humerus drops downward. Pass a 22-gauge needle underneath the acromion near the acromial angle into the space between the acromion and the rotator cuff (*B*). Instill 5–10 ml of 1% lidocaine into the bursa. When anesthesia has been achieved, puncture multiple holes into the bursa with the tip of the needle if this is not too painful. Leaving the needle in place, switch syringes to one containing a steroid solution, such as triamcinolone acetonide (Kenalog-40 Injection) 40 mg, and instill the solution into the bursa. Avoid infiltrating the skin or subcutaneous tissues with steroid solution.

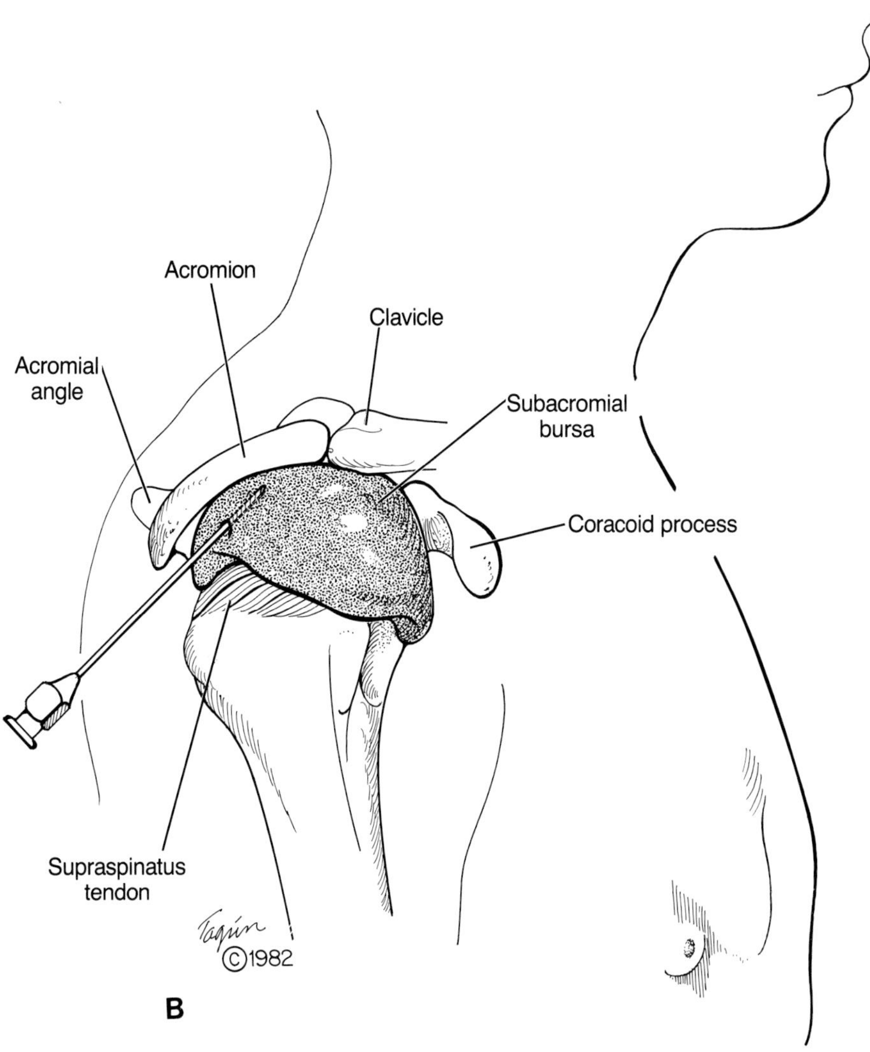
Acromion
Clavicle
Acromial angle
Subacromial bursa
Coracoid process
Supraspinatus tendon
©1982

B

24. ARTHROCENTESIS—KNEE

BERTRAM ZARINS, M.D.

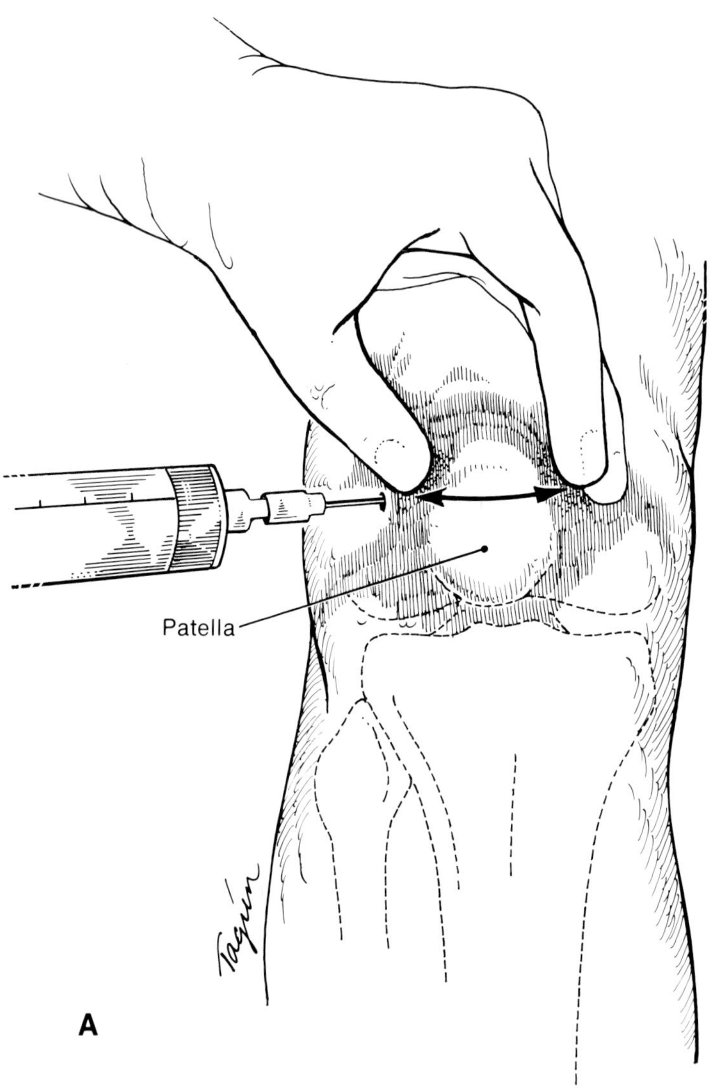

A, Arthrocentesis of the knee is performed with the patient's knee extended and the quadriceps muscles and patella relaxed so that the patella can be moved mediolaterally. With sterile technique and adequate local anesthesia using 1% lidocaine (Xylocaine), a large-bore needle (15- to 19-gauge) attached to a 50-ml syringe is introduced into the joint space at a point just lateral to the patella near its upper pole. The needle is inserted parallel to the posterior (articular) surface of the patella. A lateral approach is easier than a medial one, but both are satisfactory. *B*, Insertion of the needle just behind the patella avoids the suprapatellar and infrapatellar fat pads. If there is excess fluid in the knee, the needle can be inserted just above the patella into the suprapatellar bursa.

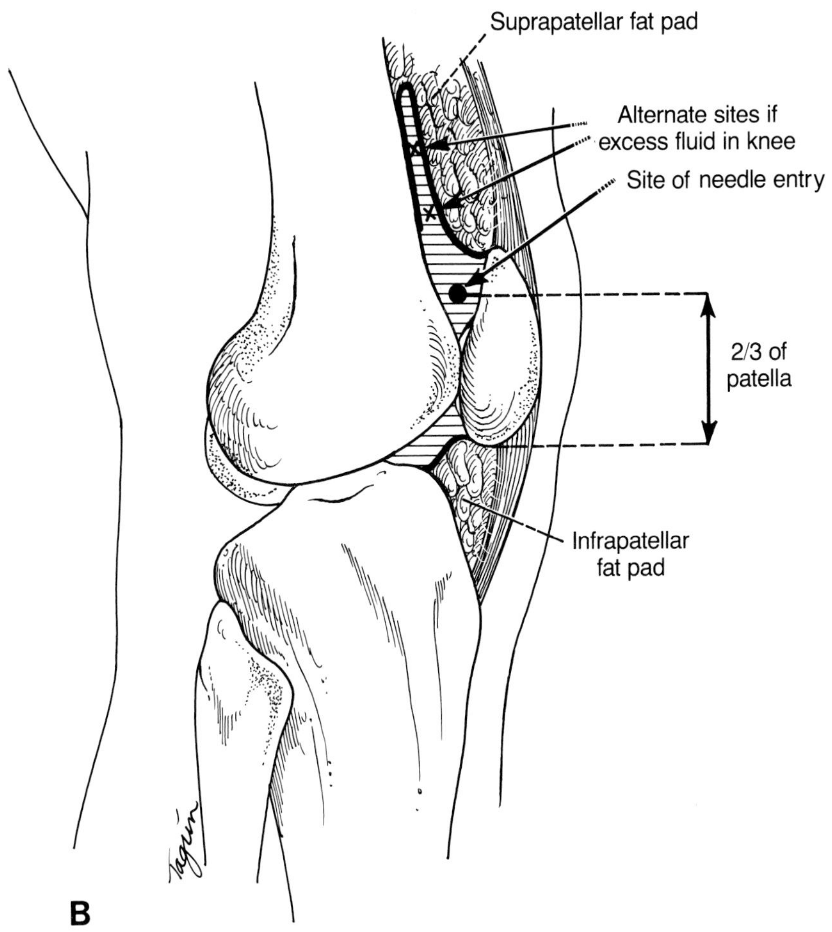
Suprapatellar fat pad
Alternate sites if excess fluid in knee
Site of needle entry
2/3 of patella
Infrapatellar fat pad
B

25. ARTHROCENTESIS—ANKLE

BERTRAM ZARINS, M.D.

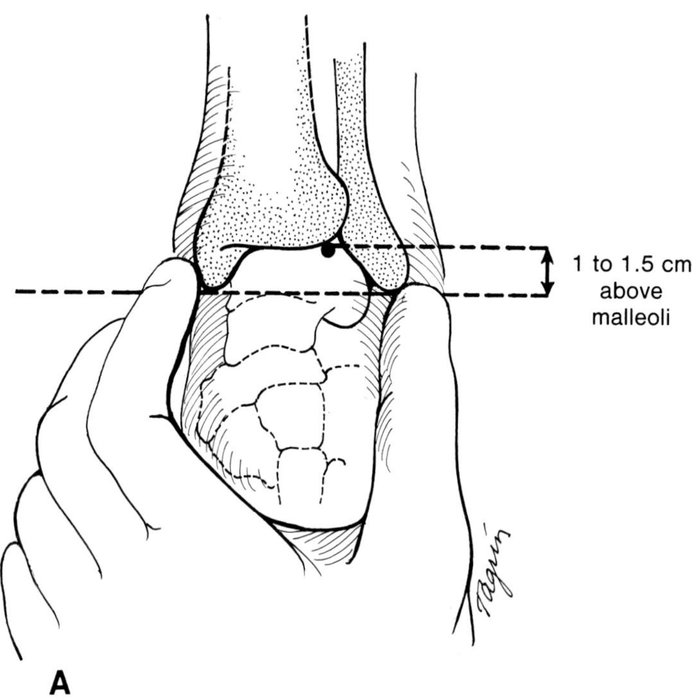

Arthrocentesis of the ankle is performed using sterile technique from the anterior approach. Local anesthesia is obtained with 1% lidocaine (Xylocaine). *A,* Palpate the medial and lateral malleoli with the thumb and index finger. The joint space is located 1–1½ cm above the line joining the tips of the malleoli. *B,* Palpate the dorsalis pedis artery and choose a puncture site anywhere on the anterior aspect of the ankle, avoiding the dorsalis pedis artery. *C,* The needle should enter the joint parallel to the articular surface of the distal tibia; this is at approximately a right angle to the shaft of the tibia.

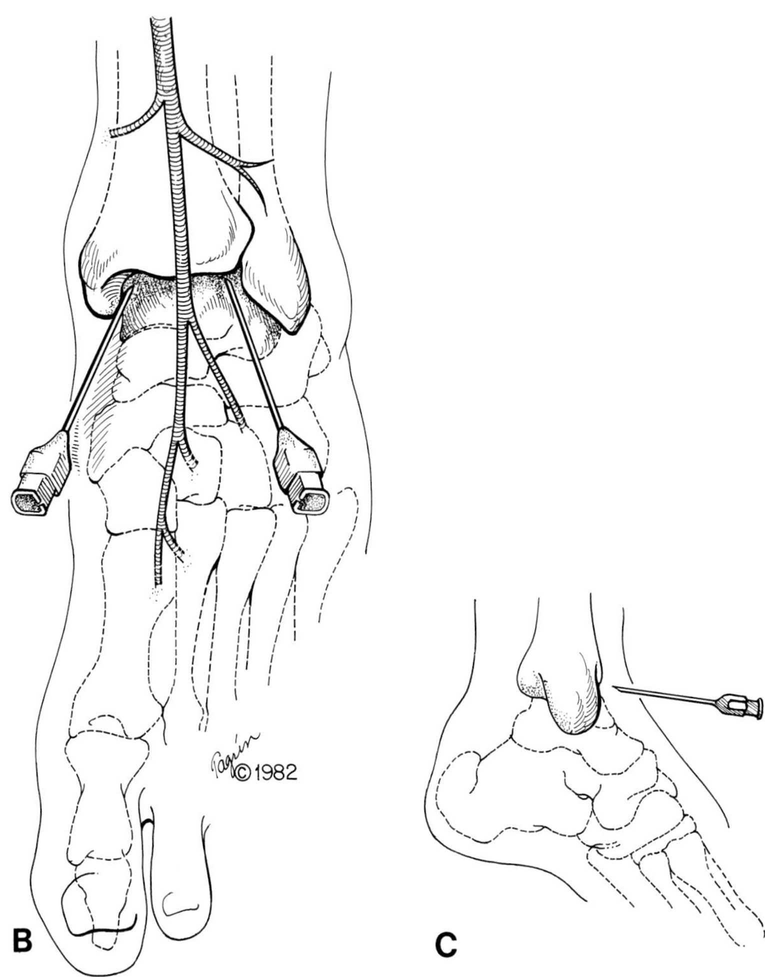
Pagán
©1982
B
C

26. EVACUATION OF A THROMBOSED HEMORRHOID

CHARLES J. McCABE, M.D.

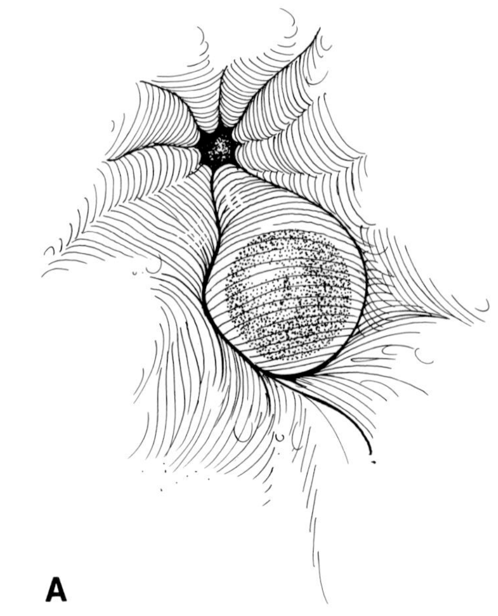

A

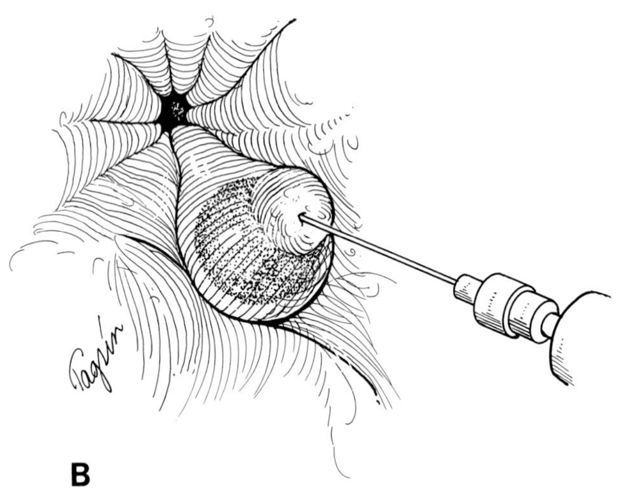

B

Editor's note: Under certain circumstances, the emergency physician may elect surgical consultation to consider primary excision of the thrombosed hemorrhoid.

Hemorrhoids rarely cause pain. When they do, it may indicate thrombosis. Evacuation of the thrombosed material is necessary to relieve pain.

The patient is placed in the same lateral position as for sigmoidoscopy, thighs flexed. Using wide tape, the buttocks can be separated in order to allow visualization of the perianal area.

A, The thrombosed hemorrhoid is visualized. The area is very tender, firm, and swollen. Rarely, there may be some inflammation surrounding the thrombosed hemorrhoid.

B, 1% lidocaine (Xylocaine) is used to anesthetize the skin immediately overlying the hemorrhoidal tissue.

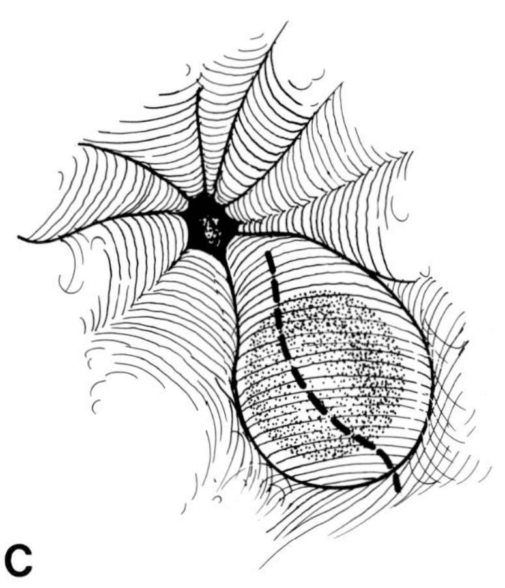

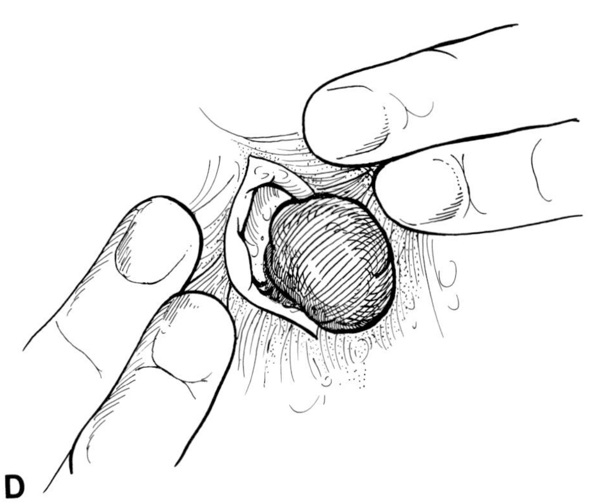

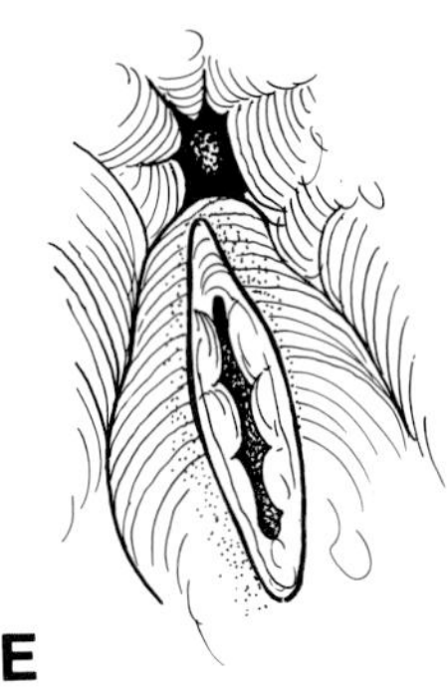

C, With a scalpel and no. 15 blade, an incision is made through the skin into the thrombosed hemorrhoid. It may spontaneously express itself, or with minimal digital pressure to the surrounding tissues, the clot can be evacuated (*D*). Any bleeding requires chromic catgut suture or Gelfoam packing of the empty hemorrhoidal space (*E*). A dry sterile dressing is maintained with a T-binder.

27. DRAINAGE OF A PERIANAL ABSCESS

CHARLES J. McCABE, M.D.

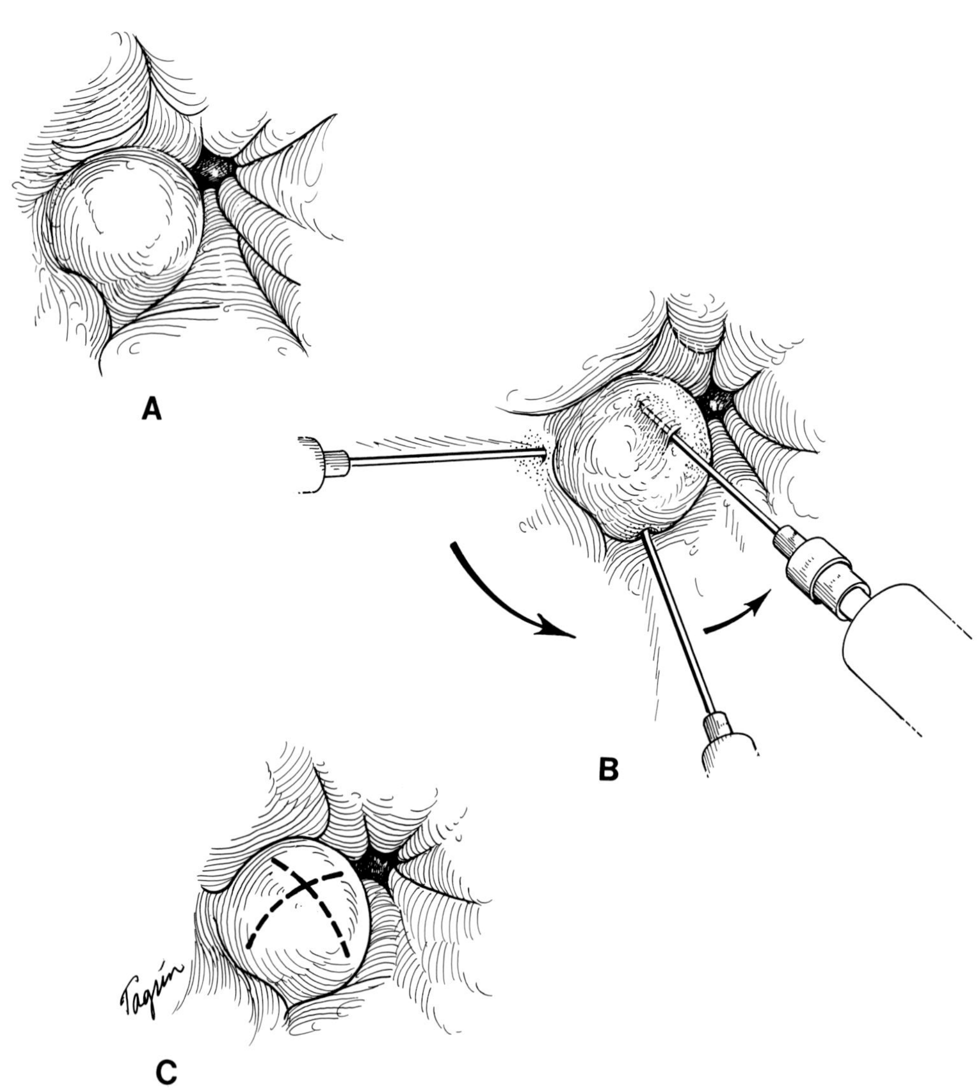

This technique is applicable to the drainage of any abscess, such as a Bartholin's gland abscess.

A, The area involved is prepared and draped.

B, 1% lidocaine (Xylocaine) is used to anesthetize the involved area. This is injected in the periabscess skin, as well as in the very superficial skin layer overlying the abscess. The abscess should not be penetrated with this needle. (Ethyl chloride spray may be used instead of the lidocaine injection.)

C, A cruciate incision is made directly over the area of maximal fluctuance. *D,* A curved hemostat or Kelly clamp is spread in the abscess cavity to ensure drainage of any loculations.

E–F, The abscess cavity is packed with gauze to provide hemostasis and allow continued drainage. A dry sterile dressing is applied.

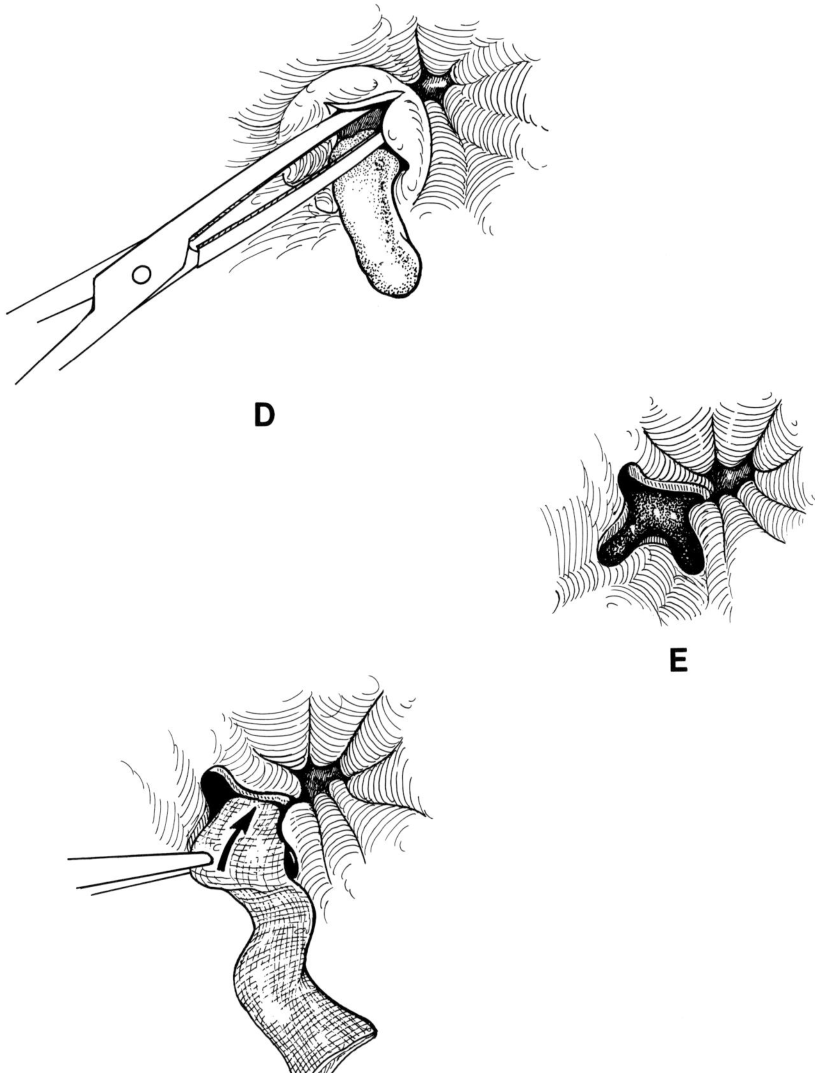
D
E
F

Drug Index

HAROLD DeMONACO, M.S., Director of Pharmacy
PAMELA MANWARING, R.Ph., Drug Information Coordinator
GLENN SIEGMANN, R.Ph., Assistant Director of Pharmacy
Massachusetts General Hospital, Boston, Massachusetts

DRUG LIST

Acetazolamide
Acetylcysteine
Activated charcoal
Acyclovir Sodium
Alteplase (TPA)
Amikacin Sulfate
Aminophylline
Amphotericin B
Ampicillin
Amrinone Lactate
Apomorphine
Atracurium
Atropine Sulfate
Bacitracin
Bretylium Tosylate
Bumetanide
Calcium Chloride Injection 10%
Carbenicillin
Cefotaxime
Ceftriaxone
Cefuroxime
Cephalothin
Chlordiazepoxide
Chlorothiazide
Chlorpheniramine Maleate
Chlorpromazine Hydrochloride
Cimetidine
Clindamycin
Crystalline Zinc Insulin (CZI)
Dantrolene
Desferoxamine
Desmopressin
Dexamethasone Sodium Phosphate
Dextran —40
Diazepam
Diazoxide
Digoxin
Diphenhydramine
Dobutamine
Dopamine Hydrochloride
Doxycycline
Edrophonium Chloride
Enalaprilat
Ephedrine Sulfate
Epinephrine
Erythromycin
Ethacrynic Acid
Furosemide
Gentamicin
Glucagon
Haloperidol (Lactate or Decanoate)
Heparin
Hetastarch
Hydralazine
Hydrocortisone Sodium Succinate
Imipenem
Indomethacin Sodium Trihydrate
Ipecac
Isoproterenol Hydrochloride
Labetalol Hydrochloride
Lactulose
Lidocaine Hydrochloride
Lorazepam
Mannitol
Methylene Blue
Methylprednisolone Sodium Succinate
Metoclopramide
Metoprolol
Metronidazole
Mithramycin (Plicamycin)
Morphine
Nafcillin
Naloxone
Neostigmine
Nitroglycerin
Norepinephrine Bitartrate
Oxacillin
Oxytocin
Pancuronium Bromide
Penicillin G (Potassium or Sodium)
Phenobarbital
Phenylephrine
Phenytoin Sodium
Physostigmine
Pralidoxime Chloride or 2-Pam
Procainamide
Prochlorperazine Edisylate
Propanolol
Pyridostigmine Bromide
Quinidine Gluconate
Ranitidine
Sodium Bicarbonate
Sodium Nitroprusside
Spectinomycin
Streptokinase
Succinylcholine Chloride
Terbutaline Sulfate
Tobramycin
Trimethaphan Camsylate
Trimethobenzamide Hydrochloride
Trimethoprim-Sulfamethoxazole
Urokinase
Vancomycin
Vasopressin
Vecuronium
Verapamil

Drug Monographs are organized as follows:

Generic Name: Listed are the generic name(s).
Trade Name: Common brand name(s) are listed.
Dosage Forms: Parenteral and oral dosage form(s) are listed.
Uses: Indications listed are primarily those encountered in an emergency setting.
Usual Dosages: Usual parenteral dosages or dosage ranges are listed for emergency indications. Refer to specialized references for dosages used in specific indications.
Precautions: Common precautions to be aware of during administration are listed.
Incompatibilities: Generalized physical incompatibilities are listed with specific drugs mentioned where applicable.

Editor's note: The drug list is not intended to be all-inclusive. A knowledge of generic names is required in above list. For further details it is suggested that one consult the Physicians Desk Reference (Medical Economics).

Generic Name: **Acetazolamide**
Trade Name: **Diamox**
Dosage Forms: Injection: 500 mg vial
Oral: 125 mg, 250 mg tablets and 500 mg extended release capsules
Uses: A carbonic anhydrase inhibitor used for the treatment of glaucoma, epilepsy and edema.
Usual Dosages: Adult: for open angle glaucoma: 250 mg orally 1–4 times daily.
Pediatric: 8–30 mg/kg/day orally given in divided doses every 6–8 hours.
Adult: for rapid lowering of intraocular pressure: 500 mg IV or IM, may repeat in 2–4 hours if needed.
Pediatric: 5–10 mg/kg IM or IV every 6 hours.
Adult: prophylactic management of epilepsy with other anticonvulsants: initial dose is 250 mg PO daily and maintenance doses range from 375 mg–1 g daily given in divided doses every 6 hours.
Pediatric: 8–30 mg/kg daily PO given in 1–4 divided doses.
Precautions: Contraindicated in patients with hepatic disease, low serum sodium or potassium, adrenocortical insufficiency, hyperchloremic acidosis, or severe renal disease. May cause hyperglycemia or glycosuria in diabetics. Caution in patients with respiratory acidosis or respiratory insufficiency. Painful when given by IM injection.
Adverse Reactions: Usually dose related; renal and metabolic effects, bone marrow depression, CNS disturbances and hepatic insufficiency.
Incompatibilities:

Generic Name: **Acetylcysteine**
Trade Name: **Mucomyst, Mucosol**
Dosage Forms: Solution for inhalation: 10% and 20% vials
Uses: Orally: an antidote for acetaminophen overdosage nebulized: as a mucolytic agent
Usual Dosages: Adults and adolescents: Acetaminophen overdose: determine plasma or serum concentration as soon as possible, but at least 4 hours after ingestion. The serum concentration is used along with a nomogram to determine potential hepatotoxicity and duration of therapy. Do not withhold therapy waiting for serum concentration. Administer a loading dose of 140 mg/kg orally, then 70 mg/kg orally every 4 hours times 17 doses. If the patient vomits within 1 hour of administration, repeat dose. Solution may be mixed in a 1:4 dilution in a carbonated beverage to mask taste.
Mucolytic agent: 3–5 ml of a 20% solution diluted with an equal portion of saline and give via a nebulizer every 4–6 hours.
Precautions: Use with caution in asthmatic patients and in patients with respiratory insufficiency. May cause bronchospasm.
Adverse Reactions: Stomatitis, nausea, vomiting, drowsiness, clamminess, fever, chills, severe rhinorrhea, chest tightness and bronchoconstriction.
Incompatibilities:

Generic Name: **Activated charcoal**
Trade Name: **Acta Char, Actidose, Arm-a-Char, Charcoaid, Charcolex and others**
Dosage Forms: Oral: 15, 30, 40, and 120 grams powder and suspensions in sorbitol
Uses: Treatment of drug or substance overdose, intentional or unintentional.
Usual Dosages: Adults and children: 30–100 grams. Repeated doses every 2–6 hours. If given every 2 hours, smaller dosages are used. Co-administer with a cathartic every other dose unless diarrhea develops.
Precautions: Use caution in patients who have an ileus or an absence of bowel sounds with co-administration of cathartics. Activated charcoal may cause vomiting which may be hazardous in caustic substances ingestion. Many inorganic acids and alkali are not significantly absorbed by charcoal. May impair visualization of gastroesophageal lesions by endoscopy.
Adverse Reactions: Black stools, vomiting, aspiration pneumonitis, and empyema.
Incompatibilities:

Generic Name: **Acyclovir Sodium**
Trade Name: **Zovirax**
Dosage Forms: Injection: 500 mg vial
Oral: 200 mg capsules
Uses: A synthetic antiviral used primarily in the treatment of herpes simplex in immunocompromised adults and children. Also used in the treatment of various herpes zoster infections.

Usual Dosages: Adult: 5 mg/kg intravenously every 8 hours.
Adult oral dose: 200 mg every 4 hours while awake
Pediatric: 250 mg/meter squared intravenously every 9 hours.
Precautions: Infuse each dose over a period of not less than one hour. Dosage adjustment is necessary with impaired renal function. Patient should be adequately hydrated during IV therapy.
Adverse Reactions: Local irritation at injection site. Transient increases in BUN and/or creatinine; incidence can be minimized with proper administration and hydration. Headache, nausea and vomiting common with oral administration.
Incompatibilities: Bacteriostatic water for injection containing parabens. Blood products and other colloidal products.

Generic Name: **Alteplase (tissue plasminogen activator)**
Trade Name: **Activase**
Dosage Forms: Injection: 50 mg, 20 mg vials
Uses: A thrombolytic agent used in the management of coronary artery thrombosis and acute myocardial infarction.
Usual Dosages: Adult: 6 mg by rapid intravenous injection followed by 54 mg/hour for the first hour and 20 mg/hour for the second and third hours
Pediatric dose: dose range not established.
Precautions: Use with caution in patients with pre-existing bleeding disorders or with a recent history of CVA or internal bleeding. EKG and blood pressure monitoring should be available during infusions, especially in patients treated for myocardial infarction. Use with caution in patients with a history of antiplatelet therapy.
Adverse Reactions: Hypotension, reperfusion arrhythmias and bleeding disorders
Incompatibilities: Do not add other medications to infusion solutions.

Generic Name: **Amikacin Sulfate**
Trade Name: **Amikin**
Dosage Forms: Injection: 500 mg
Uses: An aminoglycoside used in treatment of serious gram-negative infections caused by susceptible organisms such as Pseudomonas, Serratia and Proteus species.
Usual Dosages: Adults and children: 15 mg/kg daily divided equally every 8–12 hours IV or IM.
Pediatric: 7.5 mg/kg/dose given IV or IM every 8–24 hours depending on the age of the infant.
Precautions: Dosage adjustment is necessary with impaired renal function. Use with caution in patients with a previous history of sulfite allergy.
Adverse Reactions: Ototoxicity and nephrotoxicity
Incompatibilities: Heparin and some of the penicillins.

Generic Name: **Aminophylline**
Trade Name: **Aminophyllin**
Dosage Forms: Injection: 25 mg/ml vial
Oral: 100, 200 mg tablets
Uses: Acute bronchospasm and other pulmonary diseases.
Usual Dosages: Aminophylline should be carefully monitored and dosage based on lean body weight. Dosage varies significantly depending on patients age, concurrent disease state and social habits.
Adults: IV—6 mg/kg loading dose given over 20 minutes followed by 0.5 mg/kg/hr.
Pediatric: IV—0.2–1.0 mg/kg/hr depending on age.
Precautions: Avoid rapid IV injection. Sulfite allergic patients. Use with caution in patients with peptic ulcer, hyperthyroidism, glaucoma, diabetes, hypertension or with compromised cardiac or circulatory function.
Adverse Reactions: Rapid IV injection produces dizziness, faintness, lightheadedness, palpitation, syncope, flushing, profound bradycardia, PVC's, hypotension. Local pain with IM injection. GI irritation and CNS excitation.
Incompatibilities: Acidic solutions.

Generic Name: **Amphotericin B**
Trade Name: **Fungizone**
Dosage Forms: Injection: 50 mg vial
Uses: Treatment of severe systemic fungal infections and meningitis caused by susceptible fungi such as Candida, Aspergillus, Cryptococcus and Coccidioides species.

Usual Dosages: Adults: Two methods:
(1) After a test dose of 1 mg given over 2-4 hours; then 0.5-1 mg/kg daily given by slow IV infusion over 4-6 hours.
(2) A 1 mg test dose followed by 5-10 mg daily given by slow IV infusion, increase dose by 5 mg daily until a maximum of 1 mg/kg/day is reached.
—Alternatively drug can be given on an every other day basis at a dose of 1.5 mg/kg if desired.
Pediatric: A test dose of 0.1 mg/kg given by slow IV infusion followed by 0.25 mg/kg and increased to 0.5 mg/kg if tolerated.
—All doses are suspended in dextrose 5% in water at a concentration no greater than 1 mg/ml and given slowly over a 4-6 hour period.

Precautions: Fever, chills, headache, nausea and vomiting may occur and may be reduced by premedicating with acetaminophen, diphenhydramine and low dose steroids. Patients may become tolerant to these side effects in time.

Adverse Reactions: Nephrotoxicity and hypokalemia are common.

Incompatibilities: Electrolytes and most common medications with the exception of heparin and hydrocortisone in low doses.

Generic Name: **Ampicillin**

Trade Name: **Omnipen, Amcill, Principen, Polycillin and others**

Dosage Forms: Injection: 125 mg to 2 g vials
Oral: 250, 500 mg capsules and suspensions—various strengths

Uses: A semisynthetic penicillin used in the treatment of infections caused by susceptiple organisms such as H. influenza, Proteus mirabilis, E. coli and Salmonella. Also used in infections caused by S. pneumonia, Enterococcus, non-penicillinase producing Staphlococcus and Listeria.

Usual Dosages: Adults: Mild-moderate infections: 50-100 mg/kg/day in divided doses every 4-6 hours IV or IM.
Severe infections: 200-400 mg/kg/day in divided doses every 4-6 hours IV or IM.
Pediatric: Less than 7 days old: 50-100 mg/kg/day in divided doses every 12 hours IV or IM.
Greater than 7 days old: 75-200 mg/kg/day in divided doses every 6-8 hours IV or IM.

Precautions: Hypersensitivity to any penicillin-like drug.

Adverse Reactions: Rash, GI side effects (especially with oral administration), antibiotic-associated pseudomembranous colitis (<1%).

Incompatibilities: Stability decreases in dextrose containing solutions and at concentrations greater than 20 mg/ml. Incompatible with most aminoglycosides.

Generic Name: **Amrinone Lactate**

Trade Name: **Inocor**

Dosage Forms: Injection: 5 mg/ml ampoule

Uses: An inotropic agent used in short-term management of congestive heart failure.

Usual Dosages: Adult: Initial dose 0.75 mg/kg by direct IV injection given slowly over 1-2 minutes, followed by continuous infusion of 5-10 mcg/kg/min.
Pediatric: Dose not established

Precautions: Amrinone is a potent vasodilator. Hypotension should be watched for and anticipated. Adequate hemodynamic monitoring should be available during use of amrinone, with measurement of pulmonary artery wedge pressure, central venous pressure and cardiac output desirable. Amrinone should be used with caution in patients with a history of sensitivity to sulfites.

Adverse Reactions: Arrhythmias have been associated with use. Fever, chest pain, thrombocytopenia and pain at the site of injection have also been reported.

Incompatibilities: Do not mix in dextrose solutions, however it may be piggy-backed into these solutions. Furosemide.

Generic Name: **Apomorphine**

Trade Name: **Apomorphine**

Dosage Forms: Injection: 6 mg (soluble tablet)

Uses: To induce vomiting in acute poisonings or drug overdosages. Produces emesis by direct stimulation of the medullary chemoreceptor trigger zone.

Usual Dosages: Adults: 5-6 mg (0.07-1.0 mg/kg) given subcutaneously. Vomiting should occur within 15 minutes. Repeat dosing is not advised.
Pediatric: 0.07-0.1 mg/kg given subcutaneously.
—Emesis is facilitated with administration of 200-300 ml of water immediately following dose, use smaller volumes with children.

Precautions: Contraindicated in any person who lacks a gag reflex or is at risk of seizures, use with caution in debilitated and geriatric patients. Contraindicated in persons hypersensitive to other opiates.

Adverse Reactions: Causes CNS and respiratory depression.
Incompatibilities: Alkaline solutions, iodides, iron salts and oxidizing agents.

Generic Name: **Atracurium**
Trade Name: **Tracrium**
Dosage Forms: Injection: 10 mg/ml vial
Uses: A non-depolarizing skeletal muscle relaxant used to produce muscle relaxation during endotracheal intubation and surgery.
Usual Dosages: Adult: 30–35 mg IV push initially for endotracheal intubation.
Pediatric: Children 2 years and older: 0.4–0.5 mg/kg IV push initially for endotracheal intubation.
Precautions: Adequate facilities for intubation as well as oxygen administration and ventilatory support must be available prior to use. Reversal may be accomplished with intravenous administration of neostigmine, physostigmine or edrophonium and atropine.
Adverse Reactions: Respiratory depression.
Incompatibilities: Alkaline solutions.

Generic Name: **Atropine sulfate**
Trade Name: **Atropine sulfate**
Dosage Forms: Injection: 0.05 mg, 0.4 mg, 0.5 mg, 0.6 mg, 0.8 mg, 1.0 mg and 1.2 mg/ml vials; prefilled syringe 1 mg/10 ml
Uses: Sinus bradycardia, atrioventricular block (especially Wenckebach) and ventricular asystole.
Usual Dosages: Adult: Initially 0.5 mg–0.75 mg intravenously, repeated PRN up to a total dose of 2.5 mg or until a suitable heart rate is achieved (60 beats/min). Doses of less than 0.5 mg in adults may cause paradoxical slowing of heart rate.
—Dose may be administered via endotracheal tube.
Pediatric: Initially 0.01 mg–0.02 mg/kg intravenously, repeated as needed up to a total dose of 0.3 mg/kg or until a suitable heart rate is achieved.
Precautions: Administer rapidly to prevent paradoxical slowing of the heart rate. Use of atropine in the presence of myocardial infarction may worsen ischemia as heart rate increases.
Adverse Reactions: Ventricular tachycardia, ventricular fibrillation with excessive dose. Blurred vision, dry mouth, mydriasis, fever, "atropine flush", excitement, hallucinations. Elderly patients appear to be more prone to anticholinergic side effects which may last for several days after administration.
Incompatibilities: Sodium bicarbonate, levarterenol bitartrate, metaraminol bitartrate.

Generic Name: **Bacitracin**
Trade Name: **Bacitin, Baci-M**
Dosage Forms: Injection: 10,000 and 50,000 units
Uses: A polypeptide antibiotic that is active against many gram-positive organisms especially Staphylococcal species and Clostridia. Various strength topical solutions are used to irrigate wounds.
Usual Dosages: Adult: 10,000–25,000 units IM every 6 hours.
Pediatric: Less than 2.5 kg: 900 units/kg daily IM given in 2–3 doses.
Greater than 2.5 kg: 1000 units/kg daily IM given in 2–3 doses.
Precautions: Nephrotoxicity, especially tubular and glomerular necrosis; related to total daily dose and duration of therapy. Not to be administered IV because of severe thrombophlebitis.
Adverse Reactions: GI side effects, pain at the site of injection and anaphylactoid reactions.
Incompatibilities: Acidic and alkaline solutions.

Generic Name: **Bretylium Tosylate**
Trade Name: **Bretylol**
Dosage Forms: Injection: 50 mg/ml vials
For IV infusion: 1, 2, 4, 8 mg/ml in 5% dextrose
Uses: Ventricular arrhythmias, ventricular tachycardia and ventricular fibrillation.
Usual Dosages: Adult: ventricular tachycardias: 5–10 mg/kg given over 8–10 minutes, dose may be repeated every 1–2 hours or by continuous infusion of 1–2 mg/kg/minute.
Adult: ventricular fibrillation: 5–10 mg/kg given IV push rapidly over 1 minute, additional doses may be administered every 15-30 minutes.
Pediatric: not approved for use.
Precautions: Adequate patient monitoring including EKG and blood pressure measurement must be available. Use with caution in digitalized patients and only if arrhythmia is not digitalis induced.
—Safety and efficacy of use in children has not been established.

Adverse Reactions: Hypotension is frequently encountered especially when bretylium is given IV push, as is nausea and vomiting. Transient hypertension and increased heart rate due to initial release of norepinephrine.

Incompatibilities:

Generic Name: **Bumetanide**
Trade Name: **Bumex**
Dosage Forms: Injection: 0.25 mg/ml vials
Oral: 0.5, 1 and 2 mg tablets
Uses: A loop diuretic used in the treatment of hypertension and various edematous conditions such as pulmonary edema and congestive heart failure.
Usual Dosages: Adults: 0.5–2 mg initially (IV/IM). Repeated at 2–3 hour intervals as needed. Administer as a slow IV push over 1–2 minutes or as a small volume infusion.
Pediatric: not established however, 0.015–0.1 mg/kg daily has been used.
Precautions: Excessive use can cause profound fluid and electrolyte imbalances. Use extreme caution in patients allergic to furosemide.
Adverse Reactions: Ototoxicity and altered glucose metabolism.
Incompatibilities: Dobutamine.

Generic Name: **Calcium Chloride Injection 10%**
Trade Name: **Calcium Chloride**
Dosage Forms: Injection: for IV or intracardiac use: 10% (1 g/10 ml) in prefilled syringe or ampoules (1.36 meq calcium/ml)
Uses: Second line drug in the treatment of electromechanical dissociation, asystole and ventricular fibrillation refractory to countershock. Also used as a second line drug for the management of ineffective ventricular contractions where epinephrine and isoproterenol have failed. Antagonizes the cardiotoxicity of hyperkalemia (EKG shows broad QRS complexes or absent P waves).
Usual Dosages: Adult: initially 5–10 ml of a 10% solution (7–14 meq) injected slowly IV push.
Intracardiac dose: initially 2–5 ml of a 10% solution (3–6 meq).
Pediatric: initially 0.1–0.25 ml/kg of a 10% solution injected slowly IV push.
Precautions: Rapid injection may cause hypotension, bradycardia, vasodilatation, arrhythmias and cardiac arrest. Intramuscular or subcutaneous injection will cause tissue necrosis. May exacerbate toxicities related to digitalis glycosides.
Adverse Reactions: Hypercalcemia especially when given in large doses to patients with renal dysfunction.
Incompatibilities: Sodium bicarbonate, dobutamine, phosphate salts and magnesium salts.

Generic Name: **Carbenicillin**
Trade Name: **Geopen, Pyopen**
Dosage Forms: Injection: 1 to 5 gram vials
Uses: A beta-lactamase susceptible, extended spectrum penicillin used in the treatment of infections caused by susceptible gram-negative organisms such as Proteus, E. coli, Enterobacter and some strains of Pseudomonas.
Usual Dosages: Adult: 200–500 mg/kg/day given by IV infusion in divided doses every 4 hours. Maximum recommended daily dose is 40 grams.
—Can also be given by continuous infusion.
Pediatric: Neonates: 225–400 mg/kg/day given by IV infusion in divided doses every 6–8 hours.
Older than 1 month: 50–600 mg/kg/day given by IV infusion in divided doses every 4–6 hours.
—Can also be given by continuous infusion.
Precautions: Administer by slow IV intermittent infusion over 30 min.–1 hour. Each gram of carbenicillin contains 4.7 milliequivalents of sodium. Contraindicated in individuals allergic to penicillin-like drugs.
Adverse Reactions: Bleeding complications have occurred especially in patients with renal impairment. Hypokalemia has occurred with large dosages.
Incompatibilities: Aminoglycosides.

Generic Name: **Cefotaxime**
Trade Name: **Claforan**
Dosage Forms: Injection: 1 and 2 gram vials
Uses: A third generation cephalosporin used in the treatment of intra-abdominal, gynecologic, and respiratory infections caused by susceptible organisms such as E. coli, Proteus, Klebsiella, Enterobacter and some Bacteriodes species. Also used in the treatment of ampicillin resistant H. influenza meningitis in neonates and children.

Usual Dosages: Adults: moderate to severe: 1-2 g every 6-8 hours given IV or IM.
Severe to life-threatening: 2 g every 4 hours given IV or IM.
Uncomplicated gonorrhea: single 1 g intramuscular dose.
Neonates: less than 7 days old: 50-100 mg/kg/day in divided doses every 12 hours given IV or IM.
Infants and children: 150 mg/kg/day in divided doses every 6-8 hours given IV or IM.

Precautions: Hypersensitivity to cephalosporins and possible cross reactivity to patients allergic to penicillin-like drugs. Adjust dosage in patients with severe renal impariment.

Adverse Reactions: Elevated SGOT and eosinophilia. Local reactions at injection site.

Incompatibilities: Alkaline solutions.

Generic Name: **Ceftriaxone**

Trade Name: **Rocephine**

Dosage Forms: Injection: 250 mg, 500 mg, 1 and 2 gram vials

Uses: A third generation cephalosporin used in the treatment of intra-abdominal, lower respiratory tract, urinary tract and some CNS infections caused by susceptible organisms such as E. coli, Klebsiella, Serratia, Proteus and H. influenza. Used in treatment of uncomplicated gonorrhea and pelvic inflammatory disease caused by penicillinase producing Neisseria gonorrhoeae (PPNG).

Usual Dosages: Adult: 1-2 g/day given as a single dose or divided doses every 12 hours IV or IM.
—For PPNG: a single dose of 125-250 mg IM.
Pediatric: 50-75 mg/kg/day in divided doses every 12 hours given IV or IM.
—For meningitis: 100 mg/kg/day in divided doses every 12 hours given IV; may initiate therapy with a loading dose of 75 mg/kg.
—Children over 12 years old may receive adult dosage.

Precautions: Hypersensitivity to cephalosporins and other penicillin-like drugs.

Adverse Reactions: Rash, thrombocytosis and eosinophilia. A transient increase in SGOT and SGPT can occur. GI side effects.

Incompatibilities: Amikacin and clindamycin.

Generic Name: **Cefuroxime**

Trade Name: **Zinacef and Kefurox**

Dosage Forms: Injection: 750 mg and 1.5 gram vials

Uses: A second generation cephalosporin used in the treatment of lower respiratory tract, genitourinary tract and CNS infections caused by susceptible gram-negative organisms such as H. influenza, E. coli, Klebsiella and N. gonorrhoeae.

Usual Dosages: Adult: 750 mg-1.5 grams every 8 hours given IV or IM.
Pediatric: 50-100 mg/kg/day given in divided doses every 6-8 hours IV or IM.
For meningitis: 200-240 mg/kg/day given in divided doses every 6-8 hours.

Precautions: Dosage adjustment required in renal impairment. Hypersensitivity to cephalosporins and other penicillin-like drugs.

Adverse Reactions: Decreased hemoglobin concentration and eosinophilia. Transient increase in SGOT and SGPT.

Incompatibilities: Some aminoglycosides.

Generic Name: **Cephalothin**

Trade Name: **Keflin, Seffin**

Dosage Forms: Injection: 1, 2 and 4 gram vials

Uses: A first generation cephalosporin used in the treatment of infections caused by susceptible gram-positive aerobic cocci such as Streptococcus and Staphylococcus.

Usual Dosages: Adults: 0.5-2 grams IV every 4-6 hours.
Pediatric: 80-160 mg/kg/day given IV in divided doses every 4-6 hours.

Precautions: Hypersensitivity to cephalosporins and penicillin-like drugs.

Adverse Reactions: Thrombophlebitis, rash, fever and eosinophilia.

Incompatibilities: Aminophylline and some aminoglycosides.

Generic Name: **Chlordiazepoxide**

Trade Name: **Librium, Libritabs and others**

Dosage Forms: Injection: 100 mg ampoules
Oral: 5 mg, 10 mg, 25 mg capsules and tablets

Uses: A benzodiazepine used for management of anxiety disorders and agitation associated with alcohol withdrawal.

Usual Dosages: Adult: for acute to severe management of anxiety: 50–100 mg initially, then 25–50 mg 3–4 times daily as needed given IV or IM.
For agitation due to acute alcohol withdrawal: 50–100 mg initially IV or IM, may repeat in 2–4 hours if needed.
—IV dose usually should not exceed 300 mg in a 6 hour period.
—Usually 25–50 mg dosages are used in geriatric and debilitated patients and children 12–18 years of age.

Precautions: Administer by slow IV push, may cause hypotension and/or respiratory depression if administered too rapidly. Reconstitute immediately prior to use and discard any unused portion. Pain at site of IM injection.

Adverse Reactions: CNS and respiratory depression.

Incompatibilities: Most common medications.

Generic Name: **Chlorothiazide**

Trade Name: **Diuril, Diachlor**

Dosage Forms: Injection: 500 mg vial

Incompatibilities: Oral: 250 and 500 mg tablets and suspension

Uses: A thiazide diuretic used in the treatment of hypertension and a variety of edematous conditions.

Usual Dosages: Adults: 50 mg–2 grams IV push daily given in 1–2 divided doses.
Pediatric: 20–30 mg/kg/day given orally in 2 divided doses. IV route is generally not recommended.

Precautions: Avoid extravasation of this alkaline solution. Excessive use can cause fluid and electrolyte imbalances. Injection must not be given subcutaneously or intramuscularly. Use with caution in patients wiht severe renal disease.

Adverse Reactions: Impaired glucose metabolism, hyperuricemia, hypokalemia and alkalosis.

Incompatibilities: Acidic solutions and medications. Exceptions are cimetidine, lidocaine and nafcillin.

Generic Name: **Chlorpheniramine Maleate**

Trade Name: **Chlor-Trimeton, Chlor-Pro and others**

Dosage Forms: Injection: 10 mg/ml for IV use, 100 mg/ml (IM or SC only)
Oral: 2, 4 mg tablets and 6, 8 and 12 mg extended release capsules and tablets

Uses: An antihistamine used in the symptomatic management of allergic reactions.

Usual Dosages: For allergic reactions to blood or plasma: adults and children over 12 years old: 10–20 mg SC, IV or IM administered as a single dose. Maximum dose is 40 mg daily.
Pediatric: safety and efficacy of IV dosage form in children less than 12 years old has not been established.

Precautions: CNS disturbances such as drowsiness, confusion and dizziness may impair ability to perform activities requiring attention.

Adverse Reactions: Sedation and anticholinergic side effects such as dry mouth, mydriasis and blurred vision.

Incompatibilities: Calcium chloride, norepinephrine and pentobarbital.

Generic Name: **Chlorpromazine Hydrochloride**

Trade Name: **Thorazine, Promaz, Ormazine and others**

Dosage Forms: Injection: 25 mg/ml

Uses: A phenothiazine used in the symptomatic treatment of psychotic disorders. Also used in the prevention of nausea and vomiting as well as the management of tetanus and hiccups.

Usual Dosages: Adult: for the treatment of psychosis: 25 mg initially intramuscularly, repeated in 1–2 hours as needed.
—For nausea and vomiting: 25–50 mg every 3–4 hours IV or IM.
—For adjunctive treatment of tetanus: 25–50 mg every 6–8 hours IV or IM.
—For intractable hiccups: 25–50 mg given IM or by slow IV infusion.
Pediatric: 2 mg/kg/day given in divided doses every 6–8 hours IM or IV. Maximum dose for children between 6 months and 5 years old is 40 mg/day; between 5–12 years old is 75 mg/day.

Precautions: IV administration should be reserved for emergency use only. Dilute injection prior to direct IV injection. Give diluted injection slowly or by IV infusion. Alpha adrenergic blockade resulting in hypotension can occur. Extrapyramidal side effects are occasionally seen, especially in elderly patients. Should be used with caution in patients with a history of sulfite allergy.

Adverse Reactions: Dystonic reactions, akathisia, neuroleptic malignant syndrome, tardive dyskinesia, blurred vision, drowsiness, hypotension and hypothermia. Other reactions seen with long term use include blood dyscrasias, dermatologic lesions, ocular changes, galactorrhea, gynecomastia and cholestatic jaundice.

Incompatibilities: Should not be mixed with other drugs.

Generic Name: **Cimetidine**
Trade Name: **Tagamet**
Dosage Forms: Injection: 150 mg/ml vials
Oral: 200, 300, 400 and 800 mg tablets and solution
Uses: An H2-receptor antagonist used to decrease gastric acid secretion in the treatment of duodenal ulcer, gastroesophageal reflux and various hypersecretory syndromes such as Zollinger—Ellison syndrome.
Usual Dosages: Adult: 1.2 grams given in divided doses every 6 hours. Administered by intramuscular, slow intravenous injection or intermittent infusion.
—In hypersecretory conditions, higher doses may be required. Increases in dosage should be done by increasing the frequency of administration. Total dosage usually should not exceed 2.4 grams daily.
Pediatric: 20–40 mg/kg/day in divided doses every 6 hours. Administered by intramuscular, slow intravenous injection or intermittent infusion.
Precautions: Dosage adjustment required in renal and hepatic impairment. Dosage adjustment may be needed in geriatric and debilitated patients. Cimetidine may inhibit the metabolism of some drugs (ie. warfarin, phenytoin and theophylline) and dosage adjustments may be required.
Adverse Reactions: Gynecomastia; a dose-related and reversible CNS side effect, characterized by confusion and disorientation. Rare hematological side effects.
Aminophylline and barbiturates

Generic Name: **Clindamycin**
Trade Name: **Cleocin**
Dosage Forms: Injection: 300, 600 and 900 mg vials
Oral: 75 and 150 mg capsules and solution
Uses: A lincomycin derivative used in the treatment of serious respiratory tract and intra-abdominal infections including pelvic inflammatory disease caused by susceptible organisms such as aerobic gram-positive cocci and anaerobic gram-negative bacteria.
Usual Dosages: Adults: 150–600 mg given by IV infusion or IM every 8 hours.
Pediatric: 15–40 mg/kg/day given in divided doses every 6–8 hours by IV infusion or IM.
Precautions: Reduce dose in patients with severe hepatic and renal impairment. May enhance neuromuscular blockade produced by other medications.
Adverse Reactions: GI side effects including antibiotic-induced pseudomembranous colitis. A generalized morbilliform rash.
Incompatibilities: Aminophylline, ampicillin, barbiturates, phenytoin and magnesium sulfate.

Generic Name: **Crystalline Zinc Insulin (Regular)**
Trade Name: **Iletin**
Dosage Forms: Injection: 100 units/ml and 500 units/ml (usually used for insulin resistant patients)
Uses: Regular insulin is used in the treatment of hyperglycemia when rapid control of blood glucose is indicated. Because of its rapid onset and short duration of action, it is often used to supplement longer acting insulins or administered intravenously in the treatment of diabetic ketoacidosis.
Usual Dosages: Adults and children: dosage is highly individualized and based on blood or urine glucose levels.
IV infusions: loading dose of 0.1 mg/kg given as a bolus, followed by 0.1 mg/kg/hour as a constant infusion.
Precautions: Regular insulin is the *ONLY* insulin that can be given intravenously. Profound hypoglycemia from excessive use.
Adverse Reactions: Hyperglycemic rebound (Somogyi effect) and localized allergic reactions including atrophy or hypertrophy of subcutaneous tissue at the site of injection.
Incompatibilities: Alkaline solutions and medications.

Generic Name: **Dantrolene**
Trade Name: **Dantrium**
Dosage Forms: Injection: 20 mg
Oral: 25, 50 and 100 mg
Uses: A skeletal muscle relaxant used in the management of spasticity caused by upper motor neuron disorders and the treatment of malignant hyperthermia crisis. Has also been used experimentally in the treatment of malignant neuroleptic syndrome.

Usual Dosages: Management of malignant hyperthermia crisis: adults or children: 1 mg/kg given by rapid IV administration. Repeat as necessary until stable or a total maximum of 10 mg/kg is attained. Follow with oral doses of 4-8 mg/kg/day in 4 divided doses for up to 3 days following crisis.
Prevention of malignant hyperthermia crisis: adults and children: 4-8 mg/kg/day in 3-4 divided doses 1-2 days before surgery or 2.5 mg/kg as an IV infusion over 1 hour 1.25 hours before anesthesia.

Precautions: Each 20 mg vial contains 3 grams of mannitol. Malignant hyperthermia is a life threatening condition that requires immediate therapy.

Adverse Reactions: Difficulty swallowing, muscle weakness, drowsiness and dizziness may persist for 48 hours following IV therapy. Abnormal liver function test, hepatitis and severe hepatotoxicity can occur with oral administration.

Incompatibilities: Injection must be reconstituted with preservation-free sterile water for injection.

Generic Name: **Deferoxamine**
Trade Name: **Desferal**
Dosage Forms: Injection: 500 mg
Uses: A chelating agent used in the treatment of acute iron intoxication and chronic iron overload.

Usual Dosages: For acute iron intoxication: adults and children: 1 g intramuscularly or by *slow* IV infusion, then 500 mg at 4 hour intervals for 2 doses. An additional 500 mg dose may be given every 4-12 hours as needed.
Alternatively, children may be given 20 mg/kg initially intramuscularly or by *slow* IV infusion, then 10 mg/kg at 4 hour intervals for 2 doses. An additional dose of 10 mg/kg may be given every 4-12 hours as needed.
—Maximum dose of 6 g in adults and children over 24 hours.

Precautions: IV infusion must be administered slowly, a severe histamine release occurs with rapid IV administration causing hypotension, urticaria and possible shock. Contraindicated in patients with severe renal disease and pyelonephritis.

Adverse Reactions: Pain at site of injection, cataracts (primarily with long term therapy), and allergic type reactions.

Incompatibilities:

Generic Name: **Desmopressin**
Trade Name: **DDAVP**
Dosage Forms: Injection: 4 mcg/ml ampoule
Nasal solution: 100 mcg/ml (0.01%)

Uses: A synthetic polypeptide related to ADH used in the management of polyuria, polydipsia and dehydration in patients with diabetes insipidus. Also used to increase factor VII activity and control or prevent trauma induced hemorrhage in patients with hemophilia A and type I von Willebrand's disease. Desmopressin is used experimentally in uremic patients with prolonged bleeding times.

Usual Dosages: Adult: for diabetes insipidus:
Intranasal: 5-40 mcg (0.05-0.4 ml) of a 0.01% solution.
Intravenous or subcutaneously: 2-4 mcg daily given in divided doses twice daily.
Pediatric: for diabetes insipidus—children under 12 years:
Intranasal: 5-30 mcg (0.05-0.3 ml) of a 0.01% solution.
Intravenous or subcutaneously: dose range not established.
For bleeding disorders: adults and children over 3 months: 0.3 mcg/kg given as an IV infusion slowly over 15-20 minutes.

Precautions: Should not be used in patients with type II B von Willebrand's disease. Tachyphylaxis can develope when doses are repeated more frequently than every 48 hours. Water intoxication and hyponatremia can occur. Parenteral dose is usually 1/10 the maintenance intranasal dose.

Adverse Reactions: Hypersensitivity reactions. Tachycardia, flushing and hypotension with large doses.

Incompatibilities: Do not mix with other drugs.

Generic Name: **Dexamethasone Sodium Phosphate**
Trade Name: **Decadron**
Dosage Forms: Injection: 4, 10, 20 and 24 mg/ml
Uses: A synthetic glucocorticoid used in adrenal insufficiency and a variety of conditions including respiratory diseases, hematological disorders, gastrointestinal diseases and neoplastic disorders. Also used as an anti-inflammatory in the adjunctive treatment of allergic conditions, thyroditis, dermatological conditions and rheumatic disorders. Also it has been used to prevent emesis induced by chemotherapy administration.

Usual Dosages: Adult: ranges from 0.5 mg to 24 mg IV or IM daily, higher dosages are used in the treatment of shock.
Life-threatening shock: 1-6 mg/kg single IV injection or 40 mg IV every 2-6 hours.
Use in chemotherapy induced vomiting: 10-20 mg given IV before chemotherapy.
Pediatric: 6-40 mcg/kg/day IV or IM given in 1 or 2 divided doses.

Precautions: May increase susceptibility to infection or reactivate tuberculosis. Caution should be used in withdrawing patients with HPA-axis suppression (ie. high doses for a long period of time). May cause fetal damage when administered to pregnant women.

Adverse Reactions: Short term use, even in high dosages, usually does not produce harmful effects. When used in suppressive doses for longer than brief periods, may produce many effects such as adrenocortical atrophy, CNS disturbances, musculoskeletal conditions, gastrointestinal disorders and metabolic imbalances.

Incompatibilities:

Generic Name: **Dextran—40**
Trade Name: **Rheomacrodex**
Dosage Forms: Injection: 10% in 5% dextrose or 0.9% sodium chloride.
Uses: A polymer of glucose used for fluid replacement and as a volume expander in the adjunctive treatment of hypovolemic shock. Also used as rheologic agent to improve microcirculation and in the prophylactic management of thromboembolic complications due to certain surgical procedures.
Usual Dosages: Up to 1500 ml infused over 24 hours. Prior administration of promit (a dextran hapten) is advisable to limit both incidence and severity of allergic reactions.
Precautions: Severe anaphylactoid reactions have been reported. Close patient monitoring and resuscitative equipment should be available during infusion. Dextran 40 should be used with caution in patients with cardiac dysfunction.
Adverse Reactions: Anaphylactoid reactions.
Incompatibilities: Compatible with most intravenous fluids.

Generic Name: **Diazepam**
Trade Name: **Valium and others**
Dosage Forms: Injection: 5 mg/ml
Oral: 2, 5 and 10 mg tablets and solution.
Uses: A benzodiazepine used in the management of variety of anxiety disorders, agitated conditions, seizure disorders and for preoperative sedation. Also used as a skeletal muscle relaxant and antispasmodic for spasticity caused by upper motor neuron disorders.
Usual Dosages: Adults: for status epilepticus: 5-10 mg given IV push slowly. This does may be repeated at 5-10 minute intervals to a maximum of 30 mg. If necessary, the initial dose may be repeated in 2-4 hours. May be given by deep IM injection at the same dosage but absorption is slow and erratic.
For use as a skeletal muscle relaxant, sedative or anxiolytic: 2-10 mg given IV or IM every 3-4 hours as needed.
—Use lower doses of 2-5 mg in geriatric and debilitated patients, slowly increase if needed.
For acute alcohol withdrawal: 10-20 mg IV push initially, additional doses of 5-10 mg may be administered every 1-4 hours depending on patient response.
Pediatric: not recommended for use in neonates.
Children from 1 month to 5 years old: for status epilepticus: 0.2-0.5 mg IV push slowly over a 3 minute period. This may be repeated every 2-5 minutes to a maximum of 5 mg.
Children 5 years or older: 1 mg IV push initially. This may be repeated every 2-5 minutes until a maximum of 10 mg is given.
Children: for use as a skeletal muscle relaxant, sedative or anxiolytic: 0.04-0.025 mg/kg/dose, repeat if needed in 3-4 hours.
—Administer all pediatric doses slowly over a 3 minute period.
Precautions: Administer as an undiluted solution at a rate no greater than 5 mg/minute. Parenteral administration may cause hypotension and/or respiratory depression if administered IV too fast. Do not administer by intra-arterial injection. Use with caution in patients receiving other CNS depressants or patients with compromised pulmonary function. Patients with acute angle closure glaucoma or benzodiazipine sensitivity should not receive diazepam.
Adverse Reactions: Pain, swelling, and thrombophlebitis at the IV injection site. Apnea, bradycardia, cardiac arrest, arrythymias and a decreased gag reflex can occur.
Incompatibilities: Should not be mixed with other drugs or IV fluids.

Generic Name: **Diazoxide**
Trade Name: **Proglycem**
Dosage Forms: Injection: 15 mg/ml
Oral: 50 mg capsule and suspension
Uses: A hypotensive, hyperglycemic agent used in the treatment of hypertensive emergencies when resistant to other hypotensive agents. Also used in the treatment of hypoglycemia, however side effects associated with chronic use often limit therapy.
Usual Dosages: Adults: 1–3 mg/kg (up to 150 mg) every 5–15 minutes until adequate blood pressure reduction has been achieved. Administered undiluted as a rapid IV push over less than 30 seconds.
Pediatric: children: 3–5 mg/kg as a rapid IV push. May repeat in 30 minutes if needed.
Precautions: Sodium and water retention. Hyperglycemia occurs in the majority of patients. Monitor blood pressure closely for hypotension. Patients should remain in supine position for at least 1 hour after administration.
Adverse Reactions: Hypotension, nausea, vomiting, dizziness and generalized weakness primarily occur with bolus doses greater than 150 mg. Extrapyramidal side effects and hirsutism appear more with chronic oral therapy.
Incompatibilities:

Generic Name: **Digoxin**
Trade Name: **Lanoxin, Lanoxicaps and others**
Dosage Forms: Injection: 0.1 mg/ml and 0.25 mg/ml ampoules
Oral: 0.125 mg, 0.25 mg, 0.5 mg tablets and 0.05 mg, 0.1 mg and 0.2 mg liquid-filled capsules; and 0.05 mg/ml elixir
Uses: A digitalis glycoside used for prophylactic and therapeutic management of congestive heart failure and to control the ventricular response in supraventricular arrhythmias.
Usual Dosages: Adult: for "digitalization": 0.25–0.5 mg IV initially then 0.25 mg every 4–6 hours for 2–4 doses or 0.5–0.75 mg PO initially, then 0.25–0.5 mg every 6–8 hours until full digitalizing dose (0.5–1.0 mg/24 hours) is given.
Adult maintenance: 0.125–0.5 mg daily given IV or PO as a single dose. Dosage is dependent on renal function.
Pediatric: for oral digitalization:
Premature infants: 20–30 mcg/kg
Full term infants: 25–35 mcg/kg
1–24 months old: 35–60 mcg/kg
2–5 years old: 30–40 mcg/kg
5–10 years old: 20–35 mcg/kg
Older than 10 years: 10–15 mcg/kg
—Administered in divided doses every 6 hours with 50% of digitalizing dose administered as first dose.
—For intravenous digitalization, approximately 80% of oral dose is given in divided doses every 6 hours.
Pediatric maintenance:
Premature infants: 20–30% of the digitalizing dose.
All other age groups: 25–35% of the digitalizing dose.
Precautions: Digoxin has a narrow therapeutic index. Therapeutic blood levels should be used as a guideline only. Significant inter- and intra-patient variability exists and toxicity can occur even at "therapeutic" blood levels. Hypokalemia, hypercalcemia and hypomagnesemia may predispose patient to cardiac toxicity. Maintenance dose should be adjusted in patients with renal dysfunction. Renal and/or hepatic dysfunction may interfere with digoxin radioimmunassay to produce falsely elevated blood levels.
Adverse Reactions: Adverse reactions are usually confined to the cardiac, gastrointestinal and central nervous systems. Cardiac manifestations of toxicity include arrhythmias, AV block (partial or complete), bradycardia and ventricular irritability including fibrillation. Gatrointestinal symptoms include nausea, vomiting and anorexia. Central nervous system reactions most commonly include headache, fatigue, drowsiness, visual distrubances and generalized muscle weakness.
Incompatibilities: Acid and alkaline solutions; should not be mixed with most medications.

Generic Name: **Diphenhydramine**
Trade Name: **Benadryl and others**
Dosage Forms: Injection: 10 and 50 mg/ml
Oral: 25 and 50 mg capsules and various solutions and elixirs.

Uses: A antihistamine (ethanolamine deriviative) used as an adjunct in the management of allergic reactions. It is also used in the symptomatic treatment of extrapyramidal side effects in patients unable to tolerate more potent agents. It is used alone or in combination with other drugs as a sleep aide, antitussive.

Usual Dosages: Adult: 10–50 mg given IV or by deep IM injection every 6–8 hours, with a maximum daily dose of 400 mg.
Pediatric: not recommended in neonates.
Children: 5 mg/kg/day given IV or by deep IM injection in divided doses every 6 hours, with a maximum daily dose of 300 mg.

Precautions: CNS disturbances like drowsiness, confusion and dizziness may impair ability to perform activities requiring attention. Due to a strong anticholinergic activity, use may be contraindicated in patients with angle closure glaucoma, prostatic hypertrophy, stenosing peptic ulcer, pyloroduodenal closure, bladder neck obstruction and asthma. Some formulations of diphenhydramine contain sodium metabisulfite.

Adverse Reactions: Anticholinergic side effects, CNS depression and paradoxical excitement especially in children.

Incompatibilities: Furosemide, hydrocortisone, methylprednisolone and iodides.

Generic Name: **Dobutamine**
Trade Name: **Dobutrex**
Dosage Forms: Injection: 250 mg vial

Uses: A positive inotropic agent used in the short term management of congestive heart failure and cardiac decompensation.

Usual Dosages: Adult: given as a continuous IV infusion at rates of 2.5–10 mcg/kg/minute. Higher infusion rates have been used but are associated with an increased frequency of adverse effects such as tachycardia.
Pediatric: dosage range has not been established.

Precautions: May cause increase in heart rate including ventricular tachycardia and fibrillation. Hypovolemia should be corrected prior to use of dobutamine. Dobutamine is said to be contraindicated for use in patients with idiopathic hypertrophic subaortic stenosis. Dobutamine has no pressor effect and should be used with caution in patients with inadequate vascular resistance.

Adverse Reactions: Adverse effects are dose related and are usually seen with doses in excess of 20–25 mcg/kg/minute. Tachycardia, ventricular premature beats and fibrillation can occur.

Incompatibilities: Alkaline solutions such as sodium bicarbonate and aminophylline.

Generic Name: **Dopamine Hydrochloride**
Trade Name: **Intropin, Dopastat and others**
Dosage Forms: Injection: 200 and 400 mg vial; premixed solutions of 0.8, 1.6, 3.2 mg/ml for IV infusion

Uses: A sympathomimetic with dose dependent effects on cardiac function, renal and splanchnic blood flow and peripheral vascular resistance.

Usual Dosages: Adults: dosage must be adjusted to patient response as indicated by parameters such as heart rate, blood pressure, urine output and others. In general, at low doses (50–200 mcg/minute), renal blood flow increases with little demonstrable effect on peripheral vascular resistance or cardiac performance. At moderate doses (250–500 mcg/minute), cardiac effects predominate with increase in heart rate and stroke volume seen. At high doses, increase in peripheral vascular resistance is seen as the predominant clinical sign. Wide inter- and intra-patient variability exists to given dosage range and response.
Pediatric: safety and efficacy have not been established, but dosages of 2–10 mcg/kg/minute have been used.

Precautions: Patients should be monitored closely during dopamine therapy. Heart rate, blood pressure and urine output should be used to guide therapy. As with all pressor agents hypovolemia and acid-base disturbances should be corrected as soon as possible and preferably prior to initiation of therapy. Whenever possible, central venous access should be used for dopamine infusions. Use with caution in patients with a history of sulfite allergy.

Adverse Reactions: Adverse effects are dose related. Tachycardia and ventricular irritability can be seen at any dosage range. Effects of excessive vasoconstriction usually seen with high dose infusions. Hypotension due to excess vasodilatation is sometimes seen with low dose infusions.

Incompatibilities: Alkaline solutions and medications. A slight pink discoloration of dopamine solutions is indicative of oxidation with resulting loss of potency.

Generic Name: **Doxycycline**
Trade Name: **Vibramycin**
Dosage Forms: Injection: 100 and 200 mg vial
Oral: 50 and 100 mg tablets/capsules
Uses: A semisynthetic tetracycline derivative used in bacterial infections caused by uncommon gram-positive and gram-negative organisms. Also used in the treatment of rickettsial, chlamydial and mycoplasmal infections.
Usual Dosages: Adults: 100 mg every 12 hours times 1 day followed by 100 mg daily in 1–2 divided doses given intravenously.
Pediatric: do not use in children less than 8 years old. Children less than 45 kg can be given 4.4 mg/kg/day in 2 divided doses initially followed by 2.2 mg/kg/day in 1–2 divided doses given intravenously.
Precautions: Administer each IV dose slowly over a minimum of 1 hour. Avoid extravasation. Use with caution in hepatic and renal disease. Hypersensitivity to any tetracycline derivative. Protect from light.
Adverse Reactions: GI side effects particularly with oral administration. Photosensitivity and thrombophlebitis.
Incompatibilities: Alkaline solutions.

Generic Name: **Edrophonium Chloride**
Trade Name: **Tensi'on and Enlon**
Dosage Forms: Injection: 10 mg/ml
Uses: A parasympathomimetic agent used in the diagnosis of myasthenia gravis, also used for the treatment of supraventricular tachyarrhythmias such as paroxysmal atrial tachycardia when vagal stimulation is ineffective.
Usual Dosages: Adult: for SVT: 5–10 mg by slow intravenous injection, dose may be repeated in 15–20 minutes.
Pediatric: for SVT: 0.1–0.2 mg/kg/total dose; give 20% of dose slowly IV every 2 minutes as needed.
Precautions: Edrophonium is a potent cholinergic agent. Atropine sulfate injection should always be available as a specific antagonist. Should be used with caution in patients with a known sensitivity to sulfites. May cause uterine contractions and premature labor in pregnant women near term.
Adverse Reactions: Cholinergic excess with nausea, vomiting, diarrhea, blurred vision, increased salivation, bronchospasm, skeletal muscle spasm and bradycardia.
Incompatibilities:

Generic Name: **Enalaprilat**
Trade Name: **Vasotec**
Dosage Forms: Injection: 1.25 mg/ml vial
Uses: An angiotensin converting enzyme inhibitor used as an adjuvant in the management of hypertension when oral therapy is not practical.
Usual Dosages: Adult: 1.25 mg every 6 hours administered intravenously over a 5 minute period. An initial dose of 0.625 mg administered over a 5 minute period is used for patients on diuretic therapy.
Pediatric: dosage has not been established.
Precautions: Adequate hemodynamic monitoring should be available during use of enalaprilat, especially in the treatment of congestive heart failure. Use with caution in hypovolemic patients. Dosage adjustment is required with renal impairment.
Adverse Reactions: Enalaprilat is a potent antihypertensive. Hypotension should be watched for and anticipated. Renal function should be monitored closely during prolonged therapy.
Incompatibilities:

Generic Name: **Ephedrine Sulfate**
Trade Name: **Ephedrine Sulfate**
Dosage Forms: Injection: 5, 25 and 50 mg/ml solutions
Oral: 25 and 50 mg capsules
Nasal: 0.5 and 1% solutions
Uses: An indirect acting sympathomimetic used in the treatment of hypotension and shock; temporary support of the ventricular rate in the treatment of bradycardia and atrioventricular nodal block ("slow nodal rhythm") when accompanied by hemodynamic compromise.
Usual Dosages: Adult: 25–50 mg SC or IM initially and repeated as needed. 10–25 mg IV injected slowly, additional doses may be repeated as needed in 5–10 minutes.
Pediatric: 0.5–0.6 mg/kg by SC or slow IV injection.

Precautions: Hypovolemia and acid-base disturbances should be corrected as soon as possible or prior to the initiation of therapy. Hemodynamics must be monitored during therapy. Ephedrine may deplete norepinephrine stores with resulting tachyphylaxis.

Incompatibilities: Alkaline solutions and medications.

Generic Name: **Epinephrine**

Trade Name: **Epinephrine, Adrenalin, Susphrine**

Dosage Forms: Injection: 1 mg/ml (1:1000), 0.5 mg/ml (1:2000) and 0.1 mg/ml (1:10,000)
Suspension for SC injection: 5 mg/ml (1:200)
Inhalation: 1% and 2.25% (racemic) solution

Uses: An endogenous catecholamine used to increase myocardial contractility; convert fine ventricular fibrillation to coarse prior to electrical defibrillation and produce bronchodilatation and relieve bonchospasm. Also used in the treatment of severe acute anaphylactic reactions including shock.

Usual Dosages: Adult: for bronchospasm and sensitivity reactions: 0.1–0.5 mg (0.1–0.5 ml) of 1:1000 solution SC or IM, dose may be repeated every 15–20 minutes. For prolonged effect: 0.1–0.3 ml of a 1:200 suspension may be given SC and repeated every 4 hours.
For cardiac arrest: 0.1–0.5 mg (1–5 mls) of 1:10,000 solution administered IV or via an endotracheal tube or direct intracardiac injection.
Pediatric: for bronchospasm and sensitivity reactions: 0.01 mg/kg (0.01 ml/kg of 1:1000 injection) given SC, dose may be repeated every 15–20 minutes. For prolonged effect: 0.004–0.005 ml/kg of 1:200 suspension may be given SC and repeated every four hours.
For cardiac arrest: 0.01 mg/kg (0.01 ml/kg of 1:1000 injection) given IV.

Precautions: Caution should be exercised when administering epinephrine to patients with hypertension, hyperthyroidism, coronary artery disease, myocardial infarction, cardiac arrhythmias or a history of allergy to sulfites.

Adverse Reactions: Hypertension, tachycardia, myocardial ischemia, ventricular arrhythmias, anxiety, tremor and tissue necrosis if extravasated.

Incompatibilities: Alkaline solutions, sodium bicarbonate, aminophylline, calcium salts and oxidizing agents.

Generic Name: **Erythromycin**

Trade Name: **Erythrocin, Ilotycin and others**

Dosage Forms: Injection: 500 mg and 1 gram vials
Oral: 250–500 mg tablets and suspensions

Uses: A macrolide antibiotic used in the treatment of respiratory and soft tissue infections caused by susceptible organisms such as Staphylococcal, Streptococcal and Mycoplasmal species. Currently considered the drug of choice for legionella infections.

Usual Dosages: Adults: 2–4 grams daily given by IV infusion in divided doses every 6 hours.
Pediatric: 15–20 mg/kg/day given by continuous IV infusion or in 4 divided doses.

Precautions: Administer in dilute concentrations over a prolonged period of time. Avoid IM route of administration. Use with caution in liver disease.

Adverse Reactions: GI side effects, thrombophlebitis and a rare hepatotoxicity.

Incompatibilities: Acidic solutions; powder for injection should only be reconstituted with preservative free sterile water for injection.

Generic Name: **Ethacrynic Acid**

Trade Name: **Edecrin**

Dosage Forms: Injection: 50 mg vial
Oral: 25 and 50 mg tablets

Uses: A loop diuretic used in the treatment of hypertension and various edematous conditions such as pulmonary edema and congestive heart failure.

Usual Dosages: Adult: 50–100 mg given IV push slowly.
—Maximum single dose should not exceed 100 mg.
Pediatric: dosage has not been established, but 1 mg/kg doses given IV push slowly have been used.

Precautions: Use with caution in patients with severe renal impairment or in patients receiving other ototoxic drugs. Excessive use can cause fluid and electrolyte imbalances such as hypokalemia, hypocalcemia and alkalosis. Injection should not be administered by subcutaneous or intramuscular injection.

Adverse Reactions: Thrombophlebitis and ototoxicity.

Incompatibilities: Alkaline and acid solutions.

Generic Name:	**Furosemide**
Trade Name:	**Lasix**
Dosage Forms:	Injection: 10 mg/ml vials Oral: 20, 40 and 80 mg tablets
Uses:	A loop diuretic used in the treatment of hypertension and various edematous conditions such as pulmonary edema and congestive heart failure.
Usual Dosages:	Adults: 20–100 mg initially given as a slow IV push over 1–2 minutes. Repeat as needed every 2–4 hours. Pediatric: 1–2 mg/kg given as a slow IV push. —Doses may also be given intramuscularly.
Precautions:	Hypersensitivity to sulfa containing medications. Excessive use can cause fluid and electrolyte imbalances such as hypokalemia, hypocalcemia and alkalosis. Injection should not be administered by subcutaneous or intramuscular injection.
Adverse Reactions:	Ototoxicity.
Incompatibilities:	Acidic solutions.

Generic Name:	**Gentamicin**
Trade Name:	**Garamycin**
Dosage Forms:	Injection: 10 and 40 mg/ml vials Intrathecal: 2 mg/ml ampoule
Uses:	An aminoglycoside antibiotic used in the treatment of serious gram-negative infections caused by susceptible organisms such as Pseudomonas, Serratia and Proteus species.
Usual Dosages:	Adults: 3–5 mg/kg/day given in divided doses every 8 hours IM or IV. Intrathecal dose: 4 mg every 12 hours. Pediatric: 2.5–7.5 mg/kg/day given in divided doses IV or IM every 8–24 hours, depending on the age of the infant.
Precautions:	Dosage adjustment required in renal insufficiency.
Adverse Reactions:	Ototoxicity and nephrotoxicity.
Incompatibilities:	Heparin, ampicillin, carbenicillin and ticarcillin.

Generic Name:	**Glucagon**
Trade Name:	**Glucagon**
Dosage Forms:	Injection: 1 and 10 unit vials
Uses:	A hormone used for the treatment of severe hypoglycemia. Also used to relax smooth muscle of the gastrointestinal tract to aid in radiological examination.
Usual Dosages:	Adult: 0.5–1 unit given by subcutaneous, intramuscular or intravenous injection. Repeat dose in 20–30 minutes if no response. Pediatric: less than 10 kg: 0.1 mg/kg IM, up to 1 mg every 30 minutes. Greater than 10 kg: 1 mg/dose IM, every 30 minutes.
Precautions:	1 unit approximately equals 1 mg. Only effective if liver glycogen stores are not depleted. Use caution in patients with history of insulinoma or pheochromocytoma.
Adverse Reactions:	Hypersensitivity reactions could occur. Cardiostimulant in big doses. Nausea and vomiting most common.
Incompatibilities:	Use only diluent provided with glucagon to reconstitute powder for injection.

Generic Name:	**Haloperidol (Lactate or Decanoate)**
Trade Name:	**Haldol and others**
Dosage Forms:	Injection: 5 mg/ml of the lactate 50 mg/ml of the decanoate in oil.
Uses:	A butyrophenone derivative used in the symptomatic treatment of various psychotic disorders and agitated conditions. The decanoate form is a repository drug used for long term management, with 4 week duration of action. It also has been used in the prevention and control of severe nausea and vomiting.
Usual Dosages:	Adult: haloperidol decanoate: 10–15 times the previous daily oral dose (no greater than 100 mg) by deep IM injection. Adult: haloperidol lactate: based on severity of symptoms. Usual starting dose for acute psychosis: 2–5 mg IM, dose may be repeated every 30–60 minutes as needed. —Intravenous route has been used but is not currently an approved method of administration. Pediatric: dose range not established.
Precautions:	Extrapyramidal side effects are occasionally seen in elderly patients.
Adverse Reactions:	Dystonic reactions, akathisia, neuroleptic malignant syndrome, tardive dyskinesia, drowsiness, hypothermia and hyperpyrexia. Other reactions usually seen only with long term administration include galactorrhea, gynecomastia and other metabolic derangements.

Incompatibilities: Heparin and alkaline solutions and medications.

Generic Name: **Heparin**
Trade Name: **Liquaemin, Monoparin and others**
Dosage Forms: Injection: variety ranging from 10–40,000 units/ml.
Uses: A naturally occurring anticoagulant used for the prophylaxis and treatment of venous thrombosis, pulmonary embolism and many other conditions requiring anticoagulation. It has no effect on existing thrombi but works to prevent further thrombosis. It is the anticoagulant of choice when rapid anticoagulation therapy is indicated.
Usual Dosages: Dosage regimens vary depending on indications and patient response.
Adult: continuous IV infusion: 5,000–10,000 units IV bolus followed by 500–1200 units/hour, titrated to patient response.
IV intermittent: 10,000 unit IV bolus followed by 5,000–10,000 units in every 4 hours.
Subcutaneous: 5,000 unit IV bolus followed by 8,000–10,000 units every 8 hours or 15,000–20,000 units every 12 hours.
—Adjust clotting time to 20–30 minutes or partial thromboplastin time 1.5 to 2.5 times the control value.
Adult: low dose therapy: 5,000 units subcutaneously every 8–12 hours.
Pediatric: continuous IV infusion: 50 units/kg IV push followed by 10–25 units/kg/hour.
IV intermittent: 100 units/kg IV push initially followed by 50–100 units/kg every 4 hours.
Precautions: Monitor patient closely for bleeding complications during therapy. Screen patients carefully, and use caution in patients at risk of hemorrhage. Antidote is protamine sulfate. Use with caution in neonates; benzyl alcohol is used as a preservative in some preparations. Patients with antithrombin III deficiency may be resistant to heparin therapy.
Adverse Reactions: Hypersensitivity reactions. Most adverse reactions are due to excessive anticoagulation and resulting hemorrhage. Hematological side effects, especially thrombocytopenia and local reactions at site of injection.
Incompatibilities: Aminoglycosides, some penicillins, erythromycin, vancomycin, haloperidol, droperidol and diazepam.

Generic Name: **Hetastarch**
Trade Name: **Hespan**
Dosage Forms: Injection: 6% solution 500 ml
Uses: A synthetic polymer used as a plasma volume expander in the adjunctive treatment of certain types of shock.
Usual Dosages: Adult: 500–1000 ml administered by IV infusion depending on degree of volume depletion.
Pediatric: Dosage has not been established.
Precautions: Use with caution in patients with congestive heart failure, bleeding disorders and renal failure with oliguria or anuria. Blood pressure monitoring should be available during use of hetastarch, especially in the treatment of severe volume depletion.
Adverse Reactions: Allergic reactions, although rare, have been reported. Bleeding time may be altered in patients who receive large doses.
Incompatibilities:

Generic Name: **Hydralazine**
Trade Name: **Apresoline**
Dosage Forms: Injection: 20 mg/ml
Oral: 10, 25, 50, and 100 mg tablets
Uses: A vasodilator used in the management of moderate to severe hypertension. Currently, the first line agent in the treatment of hypertensive emergencies associated with pregnancy.
Usual Dosages: Adult: hypertensive emergency: 10–50 mg IM or IV initially and repeat as needed depending on response. Administer in small doses and increase dose gradually.
For hypertensive emergencies in pregnant women: 5 mg IV initially followed by 5–10 mg IV every 20 to 30 minutes as needed to reduce blood pressure.
Children: 0.1–0.5 mg/kg/dose IM or IV every 4–6 hours as needed.
Precautions: Adjust dosage in severe renal impairment. May cause systemic lupus-like syndrome. Slow acetylators and patients with decreased renal function have a higher risk of developing SLE. Use caution in sulfite sensitive patients.
Adverse Reactions: Headache, palpitations, tachycardia and SLE.
Incompatibilities: Physically incompatible with most drugs.

Generic Name: **Hydrocortisone Sodium Succinate**
Trade Name: **Solu-Cortef, A-Hydrocort and others**
Dosage Forms: Injection: 100, 250, 500 and 1000 mg vials.
Uses: A synthetic glucocorticoid used in adrenal insufficiency and a variety of conditions including respiratory diseases, hematological disorders, gastrointestinal diseases and neoplastic disorders. Also used as an anti-inflammatory in the adjunctive treatment of allergic conditions, thyroiditis, dermatological conditions and rheumatic disorders.
Usual Dosages: Adult: ranges from 100 mg to 8 grams daily, higher dosages are used in the treatment of shock.
Usual adult: 100–500 mg given IV or IM every 6 hours.
Life-threatening shock: 50 mg/kg given IV initially and repeated in 4 hours and/or every 24 hours if needed.
Usual pediatric: 0.16–1 mg/kg given IV or IM 1–2 times daily.
Precautions: Administer IV push doses over a 1 minute period. Hydrocortisone has significant mineralocorticoid activity and is more likely to cause electrolyte imbalances with prolonged use. May increase susceptibility to infection or reactivate tuberculosis. Caution should be used in withdrawing patients with HPA-axis suppression (ie. high doses for a long period of time). May cause fetal damage when administered to pregnant women.
Adverse Reactions: Short term use, even in high dosages, usually does not produce harmful effects. When used in suppressive doses for longer than brief periods, may produce many effects such as adrenocortical atrophy, CNS disturbances, musculoskeletal conditions, gastrointestinal disorders and metabolic imbalances.
Incompatibilities: Diphenhydramine, epinephrine, heparin, gentamicin and vancomycin.

Generic Name: **Imipenem**
Trade Name: **Primaxin**
Dosage Forms: Injection: 250 and 500 mg vials
Uses: A carbapenem antibiotic used in the treatment of serious respiratory tract, soft tissue, intra-abdominal and gynecological infections caused by gram-positive and gram-negative bacteria especially P. aeruginosa and mixed aerobic/anaerobic infections.
Usual Dosages: Adults: 0.5–1 gram given by IV infusion every 6–8 hours.
Pediatric: 50–100 mg/kg/day given in divided doses every 6–12 hours.
Precautions: Give each dose slowly over 30–60 minutes by intermittent infusion. Dosage adjustment required in renal insufficiency.
Adverse Reactions: GI side effects, eosinophilia, thrombophlebitis and transient increases in BUN and creatinine.
Incompatibilities: Acidic or alkaline solutions, most stable at a neutral pH.

Generic Name: **Indomethacin Sodium Trihydrate**
Trade Name: **Indocin**
Dosage Forms: Injection: 1 mg vial
Uses: A nonsteroidial anti-inflammatory used in the treatment of rheumatoid and osteoarthritis and a variety of inflammatory diseases. The injectable form is used exclusively for the treatment of patent ductus arteriosus (PDA) in neonates.
Usual Dosages: Closure of patient ductus arteriosus: 0.1–0.25 mg/kg/dose. Repeat at 12–24 hour intervals up to 3 doses.
Neonates less than 48 hours old: 0.2 mg/kg (first dose) followed by 0.1 mg/kg (second dose), then 0.1 mg/kg (third dose).
From 2–7 days old: 0.2 mg/kg (first dose) followed by 0.2 mg/kg (second dose), then 0.2 mg/kg (third dose).
Greater than 7 days old: 0.2 mg/kg (first dose) followed by 0.25 mg/kg (second dose), then 0.25 mg/kg (third dose).
Precautions: Care should be taken not to extravasate injection. Monitor hepatic and renal function. May impair platelet aggregation.
Adverse Reactions: Adverse effects are common and numerous with oral indomethacin use. The most frequent effect is nausea and dyspepsia. Renal and hepatic dysfunction has been reported.
Incompatibilities: Do not mix with other solutions or medications.

Generic Name: **Ipecac**
Trade Name: **Same**
Dosage Forms: Oral: 30 ml containers
Uses: An emetic used for acute poisoning. It produces emesis by stimulation of the medullary chemoreceptor trigger zone and by irritation of the gastric mucosa.

Usual Dosages: Adults and children over 12 years old: 30 ml
Children 1 to 12 years old: 15 ml
Infants 7 months to 1 year: 10 ml
Infants 6 months and younger: 5 ml
—Follow each dose with water or clear liquid, 100-200 ml in adults and smaller volumes in children, to facilitate emesis. Younger infants can be gently bounced to promote emesis.
—If emesis has not occurred within 30 minutes, may repeat the initial dose. If the second dose does not cause vomiting within 30 minutes, start alternative therapy (activated charcoal, gastric lavage).

Precautions: Ipecac syrup should not be used in volatile oils, caustic or corrosive ingestions. It should not be used in patients who are sedated, severely inebriated, in shock, seizing, or lacking a gag reflex.
—Do not administer concurrently with activated charcoal. Activated charcoal administration, when indicated, should follow ipecac therapy.
—Do not use ipecac fluid extract which is 14 times more potent than ipecac syrup.

Adverse Reactions: Gastrointestinal, CNS and myocardial effects are seen when used excessively or over a prolonged period of time. Protracted vomiting, diarrhea, lethargy and abdominal cramping are seen in doses used in emergencies.

Incompatibilities: Milk may delay the onset of effect of ipecac.

Generic Name: **Isoproterenol Hydrochloride**
Trade Name: **Isuprel**
Dosage Forms: Injection: 0.02 and 0.2 mg/ml ampoules
Uses: A beta adrenergic agonist used in the management of bronchospasm and ventricular arrhythmias due to A-V block. Also used in the management of bradycardia unresponsive to atropine.

Usual Dosages: Adult: 0.2-0.6 mg (1-3 ml) of hte 0.02 mg/ml solution by direct intravenous injection.
IV infusion: initial dose of 5 mcg/minute given as a continuous IV infusion with dose titration based on patient's response.
Pediatric: intravenous infusion; initial dose of 0.1 mcg/kg/minute with dose titration based on patient response.

Precautions: Isoproterenol should only be administered where adequate hemodynamic and EKG monitoring is available. Use with caution in patients with a history of sulfite allergies.

Adverse Reactions: Hypotension due to vasodilatation. Cardiac tacharrhythmias including ventricular tachycardia and fibrillation. CNS side effects such as nervousness, tremulousness and anxiety have been reported.

Incompatibilities: Alkaline solutions.

Generic Name: **Labetolol hydrochloride**
Trade Name: **Normodyne**
Dosage Forms: Injection: 50 mg/ml vial
Oral: 100, 200 and 300 mg tablets
Uses: An alpha and beta adrenergic blocking agent used in the management of hypertension and severe hypertensive emergencies. Also used to produce controlled hypotension during surgery.

Usual Dosages: Adult: 5-20 mg IV push initially, then additional doses ranging from 20-80 mg can be given every 10 minutes as needed depending on the patient's hemodynamic response.
Alternatively, it can be administered by continuous IV infusion; 5-20 mg as an initial bolus, followed by a continuous IV infusion of 20-160 mg/hour.
Pediatric: dosage range has not been established.

Precautions: EKG and blood pressure monitoring must be available during intravenous administration of labetolol. Use with caution in patients with cardiac conduction defects, bradycardia, chronic obstructive pulmonary disease and insulin dependent diabetes.

Adverse Reactions: Hypotension, A-V block and bronchospasm.
Incompatibilities: Alkaline solutions.

Generic Name: **Lactulose**
Trade Name: **Chronulac and Cephulac**
Dosage Forms: Oral and Rectal: 10 g/15 ml
Uses: A disaccharide sugar used as an adjunct to protein restriction and supportive therapy for the prevention and treatment of portal-systemic encephalopathy. Also used as a laxative in the treatment of chronic constipation in adults and geriatric patients.

Usual Dosages: Adult: for portal systemic encephalopathy: 20–30 g (30–45 ml) 3–4 times daily.
Rectal administration: dilute 200 g (300 ml) with 700 ml water or 0.9% sodium chloride solution. Administer via a rectal balloon catheter. May repeat every 4 to 6 hours as needed.
Pediatric: infants: 1.67–6.67 g (2.5–10 ml) daily in 3–4 divided doses orally.
Older children and adolescents: 27–60 g daily (40–90 ml) in 3–4 divided doses orally.
—Dosages should be adjusted to produce 2–3 soft stools daily.

Precautions: Monitor electrolytes with special attention to potassium. Caution in patients who require surgery and electrocautery procedures during proctoscopy or colonoscopy. Contains lactose and diabetics should be monitored for increased blood sugar. Cleansing enemas and alkaline solutions should not be administered concurrently with lactulose enemas.

Adverse Reactions: Gaseous distention, belching, flatulence, borborygmi and cramping when initiating therapy.

Incompatibilities:

Generic Name: **Lidocaine Hydrochloride**
Trade Name: **Xylocaine**
Dosage Forms: Injection: 2, 4, 8 mg/ml in dextrose 5% in water for IV infusion
For direct injection: 10, 20 mg/ml pre-filled syringes
For preparation of infusion: 1 and 2 gram vials

Uses: A local anesthetic which also is a class 1 antiarrhythmic agent used in the management of ventricular tachyarrhythmias.

Usual Dosages: Adult: Ventricular arrhythmias: 50–100 mg IV push followed by a continuous infusion of 1–4 mg/minute.
Pediatric: Dose range not established, however initial boluses of 0.5–1 mg/kg followed by IV infusions of 25–50 mcg/kg/minute have been used.

Precautions: Use with caution in patients with hepatic dysfunction and congestive heart failure. EKG monitoring should be available during lidocaine use.

Adverse Reactions: CNS disturbances including confusion, nervousness and convulsions. In large doses may cause significant cardiac dysfunction.

Incompatibilities: Compatible with most intravenous fluids and medications.

Generic Name: **Lorazepam**
Trade Name: **Ativan and Loraz**
Dosage Forms: Injection: 2 mg/ml
Oral: 0.5, 1 and 2 mg tablet

Uses: A benzodiazepine used in the management of variety of anxiety disorders, agitated conditions and for preoperative sedation.

Usual Dosages: Adult: For preoperative sedation: 0.05 mg/kg (maximum 4 mg) given in 2 hours before surgery or 0.04 mg/kg (up to 2 mg) given slow IV push 15–20 minutes before surgery.
—Use lower doses in geriatric and debilitated patients.
Pediatric: dose has not been established.

Precautions: Dilute injection prior to IV push administration, give slowly at a rate no greater than 2 mg/minute. Do not administer by intra-arterial injection. Generally, patients greater than 50 years old should not be given doses higher than 2 mg because excessive and prolonged sedation may occur. Use with caution in patients receiving other CNS depressants or patients with compromised pulmonary function. Patients with acute angle closure glaucoma or benzodiazipine sensitivity should not receive lorazepam.

Adverse Reactions: Sedation, possibly lasting 6–8 hours, and respiratory depression. Pain and thrombophlebitis locally at the site of injection.

Incompatibilities: Stable in most IV solutions.

Generic Name: **Mannitol**
Trade Name: **Osmitrol**
Dosage Forms: Injection: 5, 10, 15, 20 and 25% solutions.

Uses: An osmotic agent used as a diuretic to promote excretion of toxins alone or in combination with other diuretics and to promote diuresis during the oliguric phase of acute renal failure. Also used to decrease intracranial and intraocular pressure.

Usual Dosages: Adult: in acute renal failure: initially 0.2 mg/kg is given intravenously over 3-5 minutes; if effective, give 50-100 g as an IV infusion over 90 minutes to several hours.
To decrease intracranial or intraocular pressure: 1.5-2 g/kg administered as an IV infusion over a 30-60 minute period.
In the treatment of intoxications: 25 g IV push followed by an infusion to maintain urine output greater than 100 mg/hour.
Pediatric: in acute renal failure: 0.2 g/kg is given intravenously over 3-5 minutes.
To decrease intracranial or intraocular pressure: 0.2 g/kg is given as an IV infusion over 30-60 minutes.
In the treatment of intoxications: 0.2 g/kg IV push initially followed by an IV infusion to maintain proper urine output.
Precautions: May cause circulatory overload and electrolyte imbalances. Solutions greater than 20% can crystallize, use filter. Avoid extravasation. Do not use in anuric patients who do not respond to test dose.
Adverse Reactions: Metabolic imbalances, CNS and renal side effects.
Incompatibilities: Blood and strongly acidic or alkaline solutions.

Generic Name: **Methylene Blue**
Trade Name: **Methylene Blue**
Dosage Forms: Injection: 10 mg/ml
Oral: 65 mg tablets
Uses: A thiazine dye used in the treatment drug-induced methemoglobinemia and cyanide poisoning. Also used as an indication dye for the diagnosis of esophageal reflux.
Usual Dosages: Adults and children: 1-2 mg/kg given by slow IV injection over several minutes, may repeat in 1 hour if needed.
For maintenance of chronic methemoglobinemia: 100-300 mg PO daily.
Precautions: Should not be used alone in cyanide poisonings and in general is inferior to sodium nitrite for this indication. Methylene blue will not reverse methemoglobinemia in patients with glucose-6-phosphate dehydrogenase deficiency and may produce an acute hemolytic episode. If methylene blue is injected subcutaneously or extravasated, a necrotic abscess may form. Do not use doses greater than 7 mg/kg total in patients with renal impairment.
Adverse Reactions: Discolors skin, urine and feces. Anemia with chronic use. Nausea, vomiting, abdominal pain, precordial pain, dizziness, headache, hypertension, sweating and confusion can occur with intravenous use.
Incompatibilities:

Generic Name: **Methylprednisolone Sodium Succinate**
Trade Name: **Solu-Medrol and others**
Dosage Forms: Injection: 40 mg, 125 mg, 500 mg, 1 and 2 gram vials
Uses: A synthetic glucocorticoid used in adrenal insufficiency and a variety of conditions including respiratory diseases, hematological disorders, gastrointestinal diseases and neoplastic disorders. Also used as an anti-inflammatory in the adjunctive treatment of allergic conditions, thyroiditis, dermatological conditions and rheumatic disorders.
Usual Dosages: Adult: Ranges from 10 mg to 1.5 grams daily, higher dosages are used in the treatment of shock.
Usual adult: 10-250 mg/dose IM or IV up to 6 times daily.
Life-threatening shock: 30 mg/kg initially given by direct IV injection over 3-15 minutes period, repeat dose every 4-6 hours as needed or 100-250 mg initially, then repeated every 2-6 hours as needed.
Usual pediatric: 0.4-1.6 mg/kg/day given in divided doses IM or IV every 6-12 hours.
Precautions: May increase susceptibility to infection or reactivate tuberculosis. Caution should be used in withdrawing patients with HPA-axis suppression (ie. high doses for a long period of time). May cause fetal damage when administered to pregnant women.
Adverse Reactions: Short term use, even in high dosages, usually does not produce harmful effects. When used in suppressive doses for longer than brief periods, may produce many effects such as adrenocortical atrophy, CNS disturbances, musculoskeletal conditions, gastrointestinal disorders and metabolic imbalances.
Incompatibilities: Penicillins, diphenhydramine, calcium and magnesium salts.

Generic Name: **Metoclopramide**
Trade Name: **Reglan and others**
Dosage Forms: Injection: 5 mg/ml vials
Oral: 5 and 10 mg tablets and solution
Uses: A dopamine receptor antagonist used as an antiemetic and a stimulant of upper GI motility. Also used to facilitate intubation of the small intestine.

Usual Dosages: Adults and children: antiemetic for chemotherapy induced emesis: 1–2 mg/kg/dose given by IV infusion every 2 hours, starting 30 minutes before and continuing for 2 doses after chemotherapy.
—If extrapyramidal symptoms occur, 50 mg of diphenhydramine may be given.
For small intestine intubation:
Adults: 10 mg IV push
Children from 6 to 14 years old: 2.5–5 mg IV push
Children less than 6 years old: 0.1 mg/kg IV push

Precautions: Extrapyramidal reactions especially in pediatric patients. Use with caution in patients with allergies to sulfite or procainamide, or with pheochromocytoma or epilepsy.

Adverse Reactions: CNS side effects including restlessness, drowsiness, lassitude and fatigue.

Incompatibilities: Aminoglycosides, calcium salts and sodium bicarbonate.

Generic Name: **Metoprolol**
Trade Name: **Lopressor**
Dosage Forms: Injection: 1 mg/ml vial
Oral: 50 and 100 mg tablets

Uses: A beta-1 adrenergic blocking agent used in management of hypertension, tachycardia and as adjunctive treatment to lower mortality post-myocardial infarction.

Usual Dosages: Adult: hypertension/tachycardia: 5–20 mg by rapid intravenous injection, initial dose depending on degree of hypertension with repeat doses as needed.
Reduction of post-myocardial infarction mortality: 5 mg by rapid intravenous injection repeated every two minutes for a total of three doses, followed by an oral maintenance dose of 50 mg every 6 hours.
Pediatric: not established.

Precautions: Use with caution in patients with congestive heart failure, asthma and sinus node dysfunction. EKG and blood pressure monitoring should be available.

Adverse Reactions: Hypotension, bradycardia, congestive heart failure. Bronchospasm has been reported in susceptible patients.

Incompatibilities:

Generic Name: **Metronidazole**
Trade Name: **Flagyl**
Dosage Forms: Injection: 500 mg IV infusion vial
Oral: 250 and 500 mg tablets

Uses: A bactericidal antibiotic used in the treatment of infections caused by susceptible anaerobic bacteria such as Bacteriodes, Clostridia and Trichomonas species.

Usual Dosages: Adults: 2 grams daily given by IV infusion in divided doses every 6 hours.
Pediatric: 15 mg/kg loading dose followed by 7.5 mg/kg/dose given by IV infusion every 6–12 hours, depending on the age of the child.

Precautions: Reduce dosage in severe hepatic failure. Disulfuram-like reaction can occur rarely.

Adverse reactions: GI side effects, CNS side effects and thrombophlebitis.

Incompatibilities:

Generic Name: **Mithramycin (Plicamycin)**
Trade Name: **Mithracin**
Dosage Forms: Injection: 2.5 mg vial

Uses: An antineoplastic antibiotic used in the treatment of testicular cancer and hypercalcemia/hypercalciuria.

Usual Dosages: Adult: testicular cancer: 25–30 mcg/kg/day given as an IV infusion over 4–6 hours for 8–10 days.
Hypercalcemia: 25 mcg/kg/daily for 3 to 4 days given as an IV infusion over 4–6 hours; repeated every 7 days as needed.
Pediatric: dose has not been established.

Precautions: Give by slow IV infusion into a freely running IV line, care should be taken not to extravasate infusion. Use with caution and reduce dosage in patients with renal and hepatic insufficiency. Contraindicated in patients with existing bleeding disorders.

Adverse Reactions: GI side effects, bone marrow depression, hematologic side effects and abnormalities in liver function tests.

Incompatibilities: Strongly acidic solutions.

Generic Name: **Morphine**
Trade Name: **Morphine**
Dosage Forms: Injection: variety of strengths ranging from 1 to 15 mg/ml
Preservative-free injections: 0.5 and 1 mg/ml for epidural and intrathecal use.

Uses: An opiate agonist used in the treatment of severe pain. It is the drug of choice in relieving pain of myocardial infarction. It is also used in patients with acute pulmonary edema.

Usual Dosages: Adult: varies depending on route of administration.

Intramuscular or subcutaneous: 10 mg every 4 hours as needed, dosages range from 5–20 mg every 4 hours.

Intravenous: 2.5–15 mg diluted and given slowly over 4–5 minutes.

IV infusion: initially 1–10 mg/hour, then titrated as needed, dosages range from 20 to 150 mg/hour.

Pediatric: Intravenous, intramuscular or subcutaneous: 0.1–0.2 mg/kg every 4 hours, single dose not to exceed 15 mg.

IV infusion: 0.025–2.6 mg/kg/hour as a maintenance dose.

Precautions: CNS and respiratory depression effects may be abolished with naloxone. Histamine release with flushing, hypotension and urticaria can occur. Increase biliary tract pressure and decrease GI motility.

Adverse Reactions: Respiratory depression, urinary retention and constipation.

Incompatibilities: Alkaline solutions and medications.

Generic Name: **Nafcillin**

Trade Name: **Unipen, Nafcil and Nalpen**

Dosage Forms: Injection: 1 and 2 gram vials

Uses: A semisynthetic penicillinase-resistant penicillin used in the treatment of infections caused by gram-positive organisms such as the penicillinase-producing Staphyloccocci species.

Usual Dosages: Adults: 6–12 daily grams IV or IM given in divided doses every 4–6 hours.

Pediatric: Less than 7 days old: 40 mg/kg/day given in divided doses IV or IM every 12 hours.

Greater than 7 days old: 60 mg/kg/day given in divided doses IV or IM every 6–8 hours.

Older infants and children: 50–200 mg/kg/day given in divided doses every 4–6 hours.

Precautions: Administer each dose slowly over a minimum of 30 minutes. Hypersensitivity to penicillin-like drugs.

Adverse Reactions: Hematological, hepatic and GI side effects. Thrombophlebitis is common as well as pain at the site of IM injections. Hypokalemia has been associated with high dosages.

Incompatibilities: Hydrocortisone, methylprednisolone and aminoglycosides.

Generic Name: **Nalaxone**

Trade Name: **Narcan**

Dosage Forms: Injection: 0.02, 0.4 and 1 mg/ml ampoules

Uses: An opiate antagonist used in acute opiate overdose and opiate induced respiratory depression. It has been used experimentally as adjunctive therapy in the treatment of septic shock unresponsive to conventional therapy.

Usual Dosages: Adult: For opiate overdose and respiratory depression: 0.4–2 mg IV push given at 2–3 minute intervals. If no response is evident after 10 minutes, it is unlikely that the problem is due to opiates.

—When frequent administration is required to counteract effect of long acting opiates, a continuous infusion of naloxone can be given at a rate of 0.4 mg/hour after a loading dose of 0.4 mg.

Pediatric: Neonates: 0.01 mg/kg with repeat doses every 2–3 minutes according to neonates response.

Children: 0.01 mg/kg IV push initially, a subsequent dose of 0.1 mg/kg may be administered if no response is seen with initial dose.

Precautions: The reversal of opiate effects may produce severe withdrawal symptoms, hypertension, tachycardia, nausea and vomiting. Use with caution in patients with cardiovascular disease.

Adverse Reactions: Tremor, hyperventilation, cardiovascular effects, e.g. hypotension, hypertension, ventricular tachycardia and fibrillation.

Incompatibilities: Alkaline solutions and medications.

Generic Name: **Neostigmine**

Trade Name: **Prostigmine**

Dosage Forms: Injection: 0.25, 0.5 and 1 mg/ml vials

Oral: 15 mg tablets

Uses: An anticholinesterase used in the treatment and diagnosis of myasthenia gravis. Also used to reverse the effects of the nondepolarizing neuromuscular blocking agents.

Usual Dosages: Adult: Diagnosis of myasthenia gravis: stop all anticholinergics 8 hours before administering dose. 0.022 mg/kg neostigmine by IM injection, if test results are inconclusive, repeat test on another day.
—Administer atropine 0.011 mg/kg IV with neostigmine administration to prevent adverse muscarinic effects.
—Positive test shows a dramatic increase in muscle strength in response to neostigmine administration.
For reversal of nondepolarizing neuromuscular blockade: usually 0.5–2.5 mg given slowly IV push along with 0.6–1.2 mg of atropine to counteract muscarinic side effects.
Pediatric: Diagnosis of myasthenia gravis: 0.025–0.04 mg/kg IM injection as above.
For reversal of nondepolarizing neuromuscular blockade: 0.07–0.08 mg/kg given slowly IV push along with atropine to counteract muscarinic side effects.

Precautions: Use with caution in patients with epilepsy, bronchial asthma, coronary artery occlusion, vagotonia, hyperthyroidism, cardiac arrhythmias, peptic ulcer and GI motility disorders. Contraindicated in patients with peritonitis and mechanical obstruction of the intestinal or urinary tract.

Adverse Reactions: Primarily adverse effects are due to excessive parasympathetic stimulation.

Incompatibilities: Light sensitive.

Generic Name: **Nitroglycerin**
Trade Name: **Tridil, Nitro-Bid, Nitrostat, Nitrol and others**
Dosage Forms: Injection: 0.5, 0.8, 5 and 10 mg/ml ampoules
Sublingual: 0.15, 0.3, 0.4 and 0.6 mg tablets
Topical: 2% ointment and various transdermal systems

Uses: A vasodilating agent used in the management of hypertension, angina, congestive heart failure and myocardial ischemia.

Usual Dosages: Adult: Dosage based on hemodynamics of patient, usual starting dose of 25–50 mcg/minute by continuous intravenous infusion.
Pediatric: dose range not established.

Precautions: Use with caution in patients with myocardial ischemia and hypotension. EKG and blood pressure monitoring should be available during infusions, especially in patients treated for myocardial infarction. Nitroglycerin is adsorbed by plastic used in intravenous administration sets and intravenous solution containers. When special non-PVC tubing and containers are used, the dosage must be lowered accordingly. Tachyphylaxis is seen with prolonged sustained administration of nitrates.

Adverse Reactions: Headache, hypotension and methemoglobinemia with large doses.

Incompatibilities: Very alkaline or acidic solutions or medication. Manufacturer recommends that nitroglycerin not be mixed with other drugs. Nitroglycerin is compatible with normal saline and dextrose 5% in water.

Generic Name: **Norepinephrine Bitartrate**
Trade Name: **Levophed**
Dosage Forms: Injection: 1 mg/ml ampoule

Uses: A potent alpha and beta adrenergic stimulant used in the management of severe hypotension and shock. Norepinephrine is a potent vasoconstrictor and cardiac stimulant.

Usual Dosages: Adult: initially, 5–10 mcg/minute administered by continuous IV infusion with dose titrations based on the patient's hemodynamic response.
Pediatric: initially, 0.1 mcg/kg/minute with dose titrations based on the patient's hemodynamic response.

Precautions: Norepinephrine is a potent adrenergic agent. Adequate patient monitoring including EKG and blood pressure monitoring should be available during therapy. Norepinephrine should only be administered using a central indwelling intravenous line. Use with caution in patients with history of sulfite allergies.

Adverse Reactions: Hypertension. May cause severe peripheral vasoconstriction as well as decrease in perfusion to kidneys, liver and viscera. Can cause tissue necrosis if extravasated.

Incompatibilities: Alkaline solutions and oxidizing agents. Dextrose 5% in water is the preferred diluent.

Generic Name: **Oxacillin**
Trade Name: **Prostaphlin and Bactocill**
Dosage Forms: Injections: 500 mg, 1, 2 and 4 gram vials

Uses: A semisynthetic penicillinase-resistant penicillin used in the treatment of infections caused by gram-positive organisms such as the penicillinase-producing staphylococcal species.

Usual Dosages: Adults: mild to moderate infections: 2-4 grams daily given by IV infusion in divided doses every 4-6 hours.
Severe infections: 4-12 grams daily given by IV infusion in divided doses every 4-6 hours.
Pediatric: Use in neonates is controversial. Doses of 50-100 mg/kg/day given as a IV infusion in divided doses every 8-12 hours, depending on age, have been used.
Children: 50-200 mg/kg/day given in IV or IM in divided doses every 4-6 hours, depending on the weight of the child.

Precautions: Administer each dose slowly over a minimum of 30 minutes. Hypersensitivity to penicillin-like drugs.

Adverse Reactions: Hematological, hepatic and GI side effects. Thrombophlebitis is common as well as pain at the site of IM injections.

Incompatibilities: Aminoglycosides.

Generic Name: **Oxytocin**
Trade Name: **Syntocinon and Pitocin**
Dosage Forms: Injection: 10 units/ml
Nasal solution: 40 units/ml

Uses: A synthetic hormone used to induce labor at term by stimulating contractions during the first and second stages of labor. Postpartum it is used to reduce bleeding after the expulsion of the placenta. As a nasal solution it is used to promote milk ejection before breast feeding.

Usual Dosages: For induction of labor: start infusion at 1 milliunit/minute, increase the rate at 1 milliunit/minute increments at 15 minute intervals depending on response up to a maximum of 20 milliunits/minute.

Precautions: Dilute injection prior to use. Monitor uterine contractions, fetal and maternal heart rate and maternal blood pressure during administration. Do not use nasal spray during pregnancy.

Adverse Reactions: Hyperstimulation of the uterus. Increased uterine motility may cause fetal effects such as bradycardia, tachycardia, PVC's and CNS damage. Large doses may cause maternal hypotension, tachycardia and increased cardiac output, especially in patients with valvular heart disease or those with spinal and epidural anesthesia.

Incompatibilities: Sodium bisulfite and alkaline solutions.

Generic Name: **Pancuronium Bromide**
Trade Name: **Pavulon**
Dosage Forms: Injection: 1 and 2 mg/ml

Uses: A non-depolarizing skeletal muscle relaxant used to produce muscle relaxation during endotracheal intubation and surgery.

Usual Dosages: Adult: 4-8 mg IV push initially for endotracheal intubation.
Pediatric:
Neonates: use cautiously. 0.02 mg/kg initially then titrate to patient response.
Infants and children greater than 1 month: 0.04-0.1 mg/kg IV push initially.

Precautions: Facilities for intubation, oxygen administration and ventilatory support must be available prior to use. Duration of action can be prolonged in patients with renal and/or hepatic failure.

Adverse Reactions: Tachycardia and respiratory depression.

Incompatibilities: Alkaline solutions and medications.

Generic Name: **Penicillin G (Potassium or Sodium)**
Trade Name: **Pfizerpen, Pharmapen and others**
Dosage Forms: Injection: 1, 5, 10 and 20 million unit vials

Uses: A natural penicillin used in the treatment of infections caused by gram-positive organisms such as Staphylococcus, Streptococcus and Spirochetes.

Usual Dosages: Dosage depends on the severity of infection and the causative organism.
Adults: 4-20 million units daily as an IV infusion given in divided doses every 4 hours;
Pediatric: Less than 7 days old: 50,000-150,000 units/kg/day given in divided doses IV or IM every 6-8 hours.
Children: 25,000-500,000 units/kg/day in divided doses IV or IM every 4-6 hours.

Precautions: Hypersensitivity to penicillin-like drugs. When high doses are used, adjustments should be made for patients with renal failure.
—Penicillin G sodium contains sodium 2 meq/million units.
—Penicillin G potassium contains potassium 1.7 meq/million units.

Adverse Reactions: Hypersensitivity reactions including anaphylaxis and skin rashes. CNS side effects as well as electrolyte disturbances can occur with high dosages and patients with renal insufficiency.

Incompatibilities: Aminophylline, sodium bicarbonate and acidic solutions.

Generic Name: **Phenobarbital**
Trade Name: **Luminal**
Dosage Forms: Injection: 30, 60, 65 and 130 mg/ml vials.
Uses: A barbiturate derivative used as an anticonvulsant and as a sedative/hypnotic.
Usual Dosages: Adult: acute seizures and status epilepticus: 300–400 mg is given *slowly* IV with repeated doses of 100–200 mg every 2 hours until a total maximum dose of 800 mg has been reached.
—Give IV injection at a rate no greater than 60 mg/minute.
Pediatric: 15–25 mg/kg is given as an IV infusion at a rate no greater than 30 mg/minute.
Precautions: Respiratory depression can occur with rapid administration. Up to 30 minutes may be required for maximum anticonvulsant effect. Phenobarbital has a long duration of action, with a half-life of 2–6 days.
Adverse Reactions: Paradoxical reaction in children might cause CNS excitation. Skin rashes occur in 1–3% of patients.
Incompatibilities: Acidic solutions and most medications.

Generic Name: **Phenylephrine**
Trade Name: **Neosynephrine**
Dosage Forms: Injection: 10 mg/ml ampoule
Uses: A sympathomimetic amine used as a potent vasoconstrictor in the treatment of shock and hemodynamic instability. Phenylephrine acts primarily on the alpha adrenergic receptors to constrict resistance vessels with a reflex bradycardia.
Usual Dosages: Adults: 1–4 mcg/minute as an IV infusion, carefully titrating to the desired response.
Pediatric: 0.1–0.5 mcg/kg/minute as an IV infusion, carefully titrating to the desired response.
Precautions: Avoid extravasation, severe tissue necrosis and sloughing can occur. Proper hemodynamic and cardiac monitoring is required during administration. Severe vasoconstriction of peripheral and visceral vessels with reduced organ blood flow.
Adverse Reactions: Hypertension, severe bradycardia and decreased cardiac output. CNS excitation including restlessness, anxiety and tremor.
Incompatibilities: Alkaline solutions and medications.

Generic Name: **Phenytoin Sodium**
Trade Name: **Dilantin**
Dosage Forms: Injection: 50 mg/ml
Uses: A hydantoin derivative used as a primary agent in the management of tonic-clonic seizures and as a secondary agent in the acute management of ventricular arrhythmias and arrhythmias associated with digitalis intoxication.
Usual Dosages: Adult: loading dose: 750–1000 mg by slow intravenous injection (at a rate no greater than 50 mg/minute). Usual daily dose is 300–600 mg/day in 1–2 divided doses.
Pediatric: loading dose: 10–15 mg/kg given as described above. Usual daily dose is 4–7 mg/kg/day.
Precautions: Intramuscular route is not recommended because of erratic absorption. Intravenous injection rate should not exceed 50 mg/minute (25 mg/minute in elderly patients). Monitoring of blood pressure and EKG is essential during loading dose administration.
Adverse Reactions: Cardiovascular collapse especially with rapid intravenous injection. CNS dysfunction usually seen with large doses or serum levels in excess of 25 mcg/ml.
Incompatibilities: Phenytoin injection is incompatible with most drugs and intravenous fluids. Phenytoin injection should only be administered via a rapidly running intravenous fluid, preferably normal saline.

Generic Name: **Physostigmine**
Trade Name: **Antilirium**
Dosage Forms: Injection: 1 mg/ml ampoule
Uses: An anticholinesterase used to reverse effects produced from a serious overdose of an anticholinergic agent such as a tricyclic antidepressant, atropine or belladonna.

Usual Dosages: Adult: 0.5–2 mg given *slowly* IV push initially. May repeat every 20 minutes until response occurs. If initial doses are effective, additional doses may be given every 30–60 minutes as needed.
—Administer at a rate no greater than 1 mg/minute.
Pediatric: children in life threatening situations only: 0.02 mg/kg given *slowly* IV push initially. May repeat at 5–10 minute intervals as needed, until a total of 2 mg has been given.
—Administer at a rate no greater than 0.5 mg/minute.

Precautions: Do not administer IV injection rapidly. Atropine should always be available as an antidote. Use with caution in patients with epilepsy, bronchial asthma, coronary artery occlusion, vagotonia, hyperthyroidism, cardiac arrhythmias, ulcers and GI motility disorders. Contraindicated in patients with peritonitis and mechanical obstruction of the intestinal or urinary tract.

Adverse Reactions: Primarily adverse effects are due to excessive parasympathetic stimulation.

Incompatibilities: Alkaline solutions.

Generic Name: **Pralidoxime Chloride or 2-PAM**

Trade Name: **Protopam**

Dosage Forms: Injection: 1 g vial
Oral: 500 mg tablet

Uses: A cholinesterase reactivator used to reverse muscle paralysis associated with toxic exposure to organophosphate pesticides and chemicals with anticholinesterase activity.

Usual Dosages: For treatment of toxic exposure to organophosphate cholinesterase inhibitors: initiate at the same time as atropine.
Adults: 1–2 grams given by IV infusion, slow IV injection (over 10–15 minutes) or intramuscularly.
Administer atropine sulfate 2–6 mg IV or IM every 5–60 minutes in adults until muscarinic symptoms subside.
Pediatric: 20–40 mg/kg given as above.
—Repeat dose in 1 hour if muscle weakness is not relieved. Additional doses should be repeated cautiously if muscle weakness continues.

Precautions: Reduce dosage in patients with impaired renal function. May precipitate myasthenic crisis in patients with myasthenia gravis.

Adverse Reactions: Dizziness, blurred vision, diplopia, headache, drowsiness, nausea, tachycardia, hyperventilation, maculopapular rash and muscular weakness. Rapid IV injection has produced tachycardia, hypertension, laryngospasm, muscle rigidity, and transient neuromuscular blockage. Pain at the IM injection site.

Incompatibilities: Stable in 0.9% sodium chloride.

Generic Name: **Procainamide**

Trade Name: **Pronestyl, Procan-SR and Promine**

Dosage Forms: Injection: 100 and 500 mg/ml vials
Oral: 250, 375, 500 mg tablets and capsules; 250, 500, 750 and 1000 mg sustained release tablets

Uses: A class-1A antiarrhythmic agent used in management of supraventricular and ventricular arrhythmias.

Usual Dosages: Adult: 500–1000 mg IM every 4–8 hours or IV loading dose of 500 mg given as a diluted solution over 20–30 minutes followed by continuous infusion of 1–6 mg/minute.
Pediatric: 20–30 mg/kg IM given in divided doses every 6 hours or 3–6 mg/kg IV given slowly followed by a continuous infusion of 0.02–0.08 mg/kg/minute.

Precautions: Use with caution in patients with congestive heart failure and sinus node dysfunction. EKG signs such as excessive widening of the QRS complex and prolongation of the PR interval should be observed closely. Blood pressure monitoring should be available. Contraindicated in torsade de pointe. Use with caution in patients with known hypersensitivity to procaine.

Adverse Reactions: Hypotension, tachycardia and congestive heart failure. Systemic lupus erythematous-like syndrome.

Incompatibilities: Alkaline solutions.

Generic Name: **Prochlorperazine Edisylate**

Trade Name: **Compazine and others**

Dosage Forms: Injection: 5 mg/ml

Uses: A phenothiazine derivative used for the control of severe nausea and vomiting. Also used for the symptomatic management of psychotic disorders.

Usual Dosages: Adult: nausea and vomiting: 5–10 mg IM with repeat doses every 4–6 hours. Also can be given as a direct IV injection, once diluted to a 1 mg/ml concentration and given at a rate no greater than 5 mg/minute.
Moderate to severe symptoms of psychosis: 10–20 mg IM with repeat doses every 4–6 hours as needed.
Pediatric: children greater than 2 years old: 0.1–0.15 mg/kg IM with repeat doses every 6–8 hours as needed. Do not use IV route in children.

Precautions: Give slowly or by IV infusion. Alpha adrenergic blockade resulting in hypotension can occur. Extrapyramidal side effects are occasionally seen, especially in elderly patients. Should be used with caution in patients with a history of sulfite allergy.

Adverse Reactions: Dystonic reactions, akathisia, neuroleptic malignant syndrome, tardive dyskinesia, blurred vision, drowsiness, hypotension and hypothermia. Other reactions seen with long term use include blood dyscrasias, dermatologic lesions, ocular changes, galactorrhea, gynecomastia and cholestatic jaundice.

Incompatibilities: Should not be mixed with other drugs.

Generic Name: **Propranolol**
Trade Name: **Inderal**
Dosage Forms: Injection: 1 mg/ml ampoule
Oral: 10, 20, 40, 60, 80 mg tablets and 80, 120 and 160 mg sustained release capsules

Uses: A nonselective beta adrenergic blocker used as an antihypertensive agent and adjunct in the management of angina pectoris; also a class-1B antiarrhythmic agent used in management of supraventricular and ventricular arrhythmias.

Usual Dosages: Adults: rate related ischemia: 0.25–5 mg given slowly IV push every 5 minutes as needed.
Arrhythmias: 0.5–3 mg given slowly IV push and repeated as needed.
Pediatric: dose not well established. Initial doses of 10–20 mcg/kg IV have been used.

Precautions: Administer at a rate no greater than 1 mg/minute. Use with caution in patients with congestive heart failure, chronic obstructive pulmonary disease and sinus node dysfunction. EKG and blood pressure monitoring should be available.

Adverse Reactions: Hypotension, bradycardia and congestive heart failure.

Incompatibilities: Alkaline solutions.

Generic Name: **Pyridostigmine Bromide**
Trade Name: **Mestinon and Regonol**
Dosage Forms: Injection: 5 mg/ml
Oral: 60 and 180 mg tablets and solution

Uses: An anticholinesterase used in the treatment of myasthenia gravis. Also used to reverse the effects of the nondepolarizing neuromuscular blocking agents.

Usual Dosages: Adult: 2 mg or 1/30 of the oral dose IM or very slow IV injection every 2–3 hours.
Reversal of nondepolarizing neuromuscular blocking agents: 10–20 mg given slowly IV push.

Precautions: Large parenteral doses should have atropine administered at 0.6–1.2 mg IV or IM to avoid adverse muscarinic effects. Use with caution in patients with epilepsy, bronchial asthma, coronary artery occlusion, vagotonia, hyperthyroidism, cardiac arrhythmias, peptic ulcer and GI motility disorders. Contraindicated in patients with peritonitis and mechanical obstruction of the intestinal or urinary tract.

Adverse Reactions: Primarily adverse effects are due to excessive parasympathetic stimulation.

Incompatibilities: Alkaline solutions.

Generic Name: **Quinidine Gluconate**
Trade Name: **Quinaglute and Quinidine Gluconate**
Dosage Forms: Injection: 80 mg/ml quinidine gluconate equivalent to 50 mg/ml of quinidine base.
Oral: 324 mg sustained release tablets equivalent to 200 mg quinidine base.

Uses: A class-1A antiarrhythmic agent used in management of supraventricular and ventricular arrhythmias.

Usual Dosages: Dosage expressed in terms of quinidine gluconate
Adult: 600 mg IM followed by 400 mg every two hours as needed for suppression of atrial arrhythmias or a loading dose of 800 mg (10 ml) in 40 ml of 5% dextrose in water given over 30–45 minutes for acute management of life threatening arrhythmias.
Pediatric: dose range not established.

Precautions: Use with caution in patients with congestive heart failure and sinus node dysfunction. EKG and blood pressure monitoring should be available. Contraindicated in torsade de pointe. Widening of the QRS complex to greater than 125% of baseline may be indicator of drug toxicity.

Adverse Reactions: Hypotension, tachycardia with 1:1 atrial/ventricular response in atrial fibrillation and congestive heart failure.

Incompatibilities: Alkaline solutions.

Generic Name: **Ranitidine**

Trade Name: **Zantac**

Dosage Forms: Injection: 25 mg/ml
Oral: 150 and 300 mg tablets

Uses: A H2-receptor antagonist used to decrease gastric acid secretion in the treatment of duodenal ulcers, gastroesophageal reflux and various hypersecretory syndromes such as Zollinger-Ellison syndrome.

Usual Dosages: Adult: 50 mg every 6–8 hours administered by intramuscular, slow intravenous injection or IV intermittent infusion.
—In hypersecretory conditions, higher doses may be required. Increases in dosage should be done by increasing the frequency of administration. Total dosage usually should not exceed 400 mg daily.
Pediatric: 1–2 mg/kg/day administered by intramuscular, slow intravenous injection or IV intermittent infusion in divided doses every 6–8 hours.

Precautions: Dosage adjustment required with renal impairment.

Adverse Reactions: Gynecomastia; a dose-related and reversible CNS side effects and rare hematological side effects.

Incompatibilities: Hydroxyzine, diazepam and phenobarbital.

Generic Name: **Sodium Bicarbonate**

Trade Name: **Sodium Bicarbonate**

Dosage Forms: Injection: 4.2% (0.5 meq/ml) and 8.4% (1 meq/ml) prefilled syringes

Uses: An alkalizing agent used to correct metabolic acidosis.

Usual Dosages: Adult: 1 meq/kg intravenously initially, then 0.5 meq/kg at 10 minute intervals or until base deficit is corrected.
Pediatric: 1–2 meq/kg by slow intravenous injection (1–2 meq/kg/min) initially, then 0.5–1 meq/kg at 10 minute intervals or until base deficit is corrected.

Precautions: Rapid injection in children under the age of two may cause hypernatremia and possible intracranial hemorrhage. Overdosage with resultant metabolic alkalosis.

Adverse Reactions: Hypernatremia, metabolic alkalosis, decreased ionized calcium levels, hypokalemia, congestive heart failure. Intramuscular or subcutaneous injection may cause tissue necrosis.

Incompatibilities: Atropine sulfate, levarterenol bitartrate, isoproterenol, dopamine, tubocurarine, dobutamine and calcium salts.

Generic Name: **Sodium Nitroprusside**

Trade Name: **Nipride and Nitropress**

Dosage Forms: Injection: 50 mg vial

Uses: A vasodilating agent used in the management of hypertension, angina, congestive heart failure and myocardial ischemia.

Usual Dosages: Adult: usual starting dose of 25–50 mcg/minute by continuous intravenous infusion then titrated based on hemodynamic response of patient. Dosage range is from 0.5–10 mcg/kg/minute.
Pediatric: dose range not established.

Precautions: Use with caution in patients with myocardial ischemia and hypotension. EKG and blood pressure monitoring should be available during infusions especially in patients treated for myocardial infarction. Nitroprusside when used in high dose and for prolonged periods may cause cyanide toxicity.

Adverse Reactions: Headache, hypotension and increasing myocardial ischemia in susceptible patients.

Incompatibilities: Nitroprusside is only compatible with dextrose 5% in water; other diluents should not be used. Nitroprusside should not be mixed with other drugs and should be protected from light.

Generic Name: **Spectinomycin**

Trade Name: **Trobicin**

Dosage Forms: Injection: 2 and 4 gram vials for IM use

Uses: An aminocyclitol antibiotic used in the treatment of infections caused by penicillinase-producing N. gonorrhoeae or susceptible strains of N. gonorrhoeae in patients allergic to penicillins or cephalosporins.

Usual Dosages: Adults: 2 grams given intramuscularly as a single dose.
Pediatric: not recommended for neonates. Children: 40 mg/kg given intramuscularly as a single dose.
—Administer all dosages by deep IM injection.

Precautions: Spectinomycin is ineffective in treating syphilis and may mask signs of infection. Coexisting infections caused by chlamydial and mycoplasmal organisms are also insensitive to spectinomycin and may require combination therapy.

Adverse Reactions: Local pain at IM injection sites. Skin rash, vertigo, malaise, nausea and chills have been associated with administration.

Incompatibilities:

Generic Name: **Streptokinase**
Trade Name: **Streptase and Kabikinase**
Dosage Forms: Injection: 250,000, 600,000, 750,000 and 1,500,000 IU vials
Uses: A thrombolytic agent used in the management of coronary artery thrombosis and acute myocardial infarction, pulmonary embolism and deep vein thrombosis.

Usual Dosages: Adult: coronary artery thrombosis: 1,500,000 units over 60 minutes intravenously or 15,000–20,000 units by intracoronary injection over 1–2 minutes, followed by a continuous IV infusion of 2000 units/minute for 60 minutes.
Pulmonary embolism and deep vein thrombosis: 250,000 units intravenously over a 30 minute period followed by 100,000 units/hour by continuous IV infusion over 24–72 hours.
Pediatric: dose range not established.

Precautions: Use with caution in patients with pre-existing bleeding disorders or with a recent history of CVA or internal bleeding. EKG and blood pressure monitoring should be available during infusions especially in patients treated for myocardial infarction. Use with caution in patients with a history of antiplatelet therapy.

Adverse Reactions: Hypotension, reperfusion arrhythmias, bleeding disorders and allergic reactions, although rare have been reported.

Incompatibilities: Dextrose 5% and normal saline are preferred diluents. Diluent should be added slowly to powder during reconstitution and vial should not be shaken since flocculation will occur. Incompatible with dextran solutions.

Generic Name: **Succinylcholine Chloride**
Trade Name: **Anectine, Quelicin and Sucostrin**
Dosage Forms: Injection: 20, 50 and 100 mg/ml.
Uses: A depolarizing skeletal muscle relaxant used to produce muscle relaxation during endotracheal intubation and surgery.

Usual Dosages: Adult: 20–30 mg IV push initially for endotracheal intubation.
—Continuous IV infusion: 0.5–10 mg/minute carefully titrated to patient response for prolonged procedures.
Pediatric: 1–2 mg/kg IV push initially for endotracheal intubation.
—Continuous IV infusion is not recommended for children.

Precautions: Facilities for intubation, oxygen administration and ventilatory support must be available prior to use. May need to premedicate patient with atropine prior to administration to decrease secretions. Malignant hyperthermia has been associated with the use of succinylcholine. Contraindicated in patients with a familial history of malignant hyperthermia or myopathies associated with elevated serum creatine kinase levels. Use with caution in patients with extensive burns or history of pseudocholinesterase deficiency.

Adverse Reactions: Hyperkalemia, respiratory depression, fasciculations and malignant hyperthermia.
Incompatibilities: Alkaline solutions and medications.

Generic Name: **Terbutaline Sulfate**
Trade Name: **Brethine and Bricanyl**
Dosage Forms: Injection: 1 mg/ml ampoules
Oral: 2.5 and 5 mg tablets
Uses: A beta-adrenergic agonist used as a bronchodilator in the treatment of various bronchial disorders such as bronchial asthma, bronchospasm and emphysema. Has also been used to inhibit spontaneous uterine contractions during preterm labor.

Usual Dosages: Adults: 0.25 mg subcutaneously. Dose may be repeated once in 15–30 minutes if needed.
Pediatric: 5–10 mcg/kg (0.25 mg maximum) subcutaneously. Dose may be repeated once in 15–30 minutes if needed.

Precautions: Tolerance may develop with prolonged or excessive use. Use with caution in patients with a history of cardiac arrhythmias.

Adverse Reactions: CNS excitation, increased heart rate, headache, nausea and vomiting.

Incompatibilities: Alkaline solutions.

Generic Name: **Tobramycin**
Trade Name: **Nebcin**
Dosage Forms: Injection: 10 and 40 mg/ml vials
Uses: An aminoglycoside antibiotic used in the treatment of serious gram-negative infections caused by susceptible organisms such as Pseudomonas, Serratia and Proteus species.
Usual Dosages: Adults: 3–5 mg/kg/day given in divided doses every 8 hours IM or IV. Intrathecal dose: 4 mg every 12 hours.
Pediatric: 2.5–7.5 mg/kg/day given in divided doses IV or IM every 8–24 hours, depending on the age of the infant.
Precautions: Dosage adjustment required in renal insufficiency.
Adverse Reactions: Ototoxicity and nephrotoxicity.
Incompatibilities: Heparin, ampicillin, carbenicillin and ticarcillin.

Generic Name: **Trimethaphan Camsylate**
Trade Name: **Arfonad**
Dosage Forms: Injection: 50 mg/ml ampoule
Uses: A nondepolarizing ganglionic blocker used as a vasodilating agent in the management of severe hypertensive emergencies. Also used in controlled hypotensive anesthesia during surgery.
Usual Dosages: Adult: for severe hypertension: initial dose of 0.5–1 mg/minute with dose slowly increased as warranted by the patient's hemodynamic response.
Pediatric: not established
Precautions: Trimethaphan should only be used where adequate blood pressure monitoring is available. Hypotensive action is dependent on patient posture. Prolonged hypotension can occur with excessive dosages. Trimethaphan may cause mydriasis especially when used in high dose.
Adverse Reactions: Hypotension and other symptoms associated with a generalized autonomic blockade.
Incompatibilities: Alkaline solutions.

Generic Name: **Trimethobenzamide Hydrochloride**
Trade Name: **Tigan, Tebamide, Stemetic, Ticon and others**
Dosage Forms: Injection: 100 mg/ml
Oral: 100 and 250 mg capsules
Rectal: 100 and 200 mg suppositories
Uses: An antiemetic related to the antihistamines used for control of nausea and vomiting.
Usual Dosages: Adults: 200 mg given intramuscularly every 6–8 hours.
Rectally: 200 mg every 6–8 hours.
Orally: 250 mg every 6–8 hours.
Pediatric: Injectable form is not for use in children. Rectal form is not for use in neonates.
—Children less than 15 kg: 100 mg every 6–8 hours.
—Children between 15 and 40 kg: 100–200 mg every 6–8 hours.
Precautions: CNS disturbances such as drowsiness, confusion and dizziness may impair ability to perform activities requiring attention. Use with caution in patients sensitive to ester type local anesthetics (such as benzocaine). Trimethobenzamide has been associated with Reye's syndrome.
Adverse Reactions: Extrapyramidal side effects, Parkinsonism symptoms, hypersensitivity reactions and hypotension have occurred with injectable form. Local irritation at IM injection site and with rectal administration. Blood dyscrasias, blurred vision, disorientation, vertigo, dizziness, drowsiness and headache.
Incompatibilities:

Generic Name: **Trimethoprim-Sulfamethoxazole**
Trade Name: **Bactrim, Septra**
Dosage Forms: Injection: vials containing—sulfamethoxazole 80 mg/ml and trimethoprim 16 mg/ml.
Oral: tablets containing—400 mg/80 mg sulfamethoxazole/trimethoprim (single strength) and 800 mg/160 mg sulfamethozazole/trimethoprim (double strength) and suspensions
Uses: A combination of folate antagonist antibiotics used in the treatment of infections caused by a variety of gram-positive and gram-negative bacteria and Pneumocystis carinii.

Usual Dosages: Based on trimethoprim component—
Adults: 10–20 mg/kg/day given as an IV infusion in divided doses every 6 hours.
—For Pneumocystis carinii: 20 mg/kg/day given as an IV infusion in divided doses every 6 hours.
Pediatric: use of any sulfonamide in children less than 2 months old is not advised.
Children older than 2 months: 8–10 mg/kg/day given as an IV infusion in divided doses every 6–12 hours.
—For Pneumocystis carinii: 20 mg/kg/day given as an IV infusion in divided doses every 6 hours.

Precautions: Hypersensitivity to sulfonamides. Infusions should be diluted in dextrose 5% in water only. Each dose should be given over 60–90 minutes. Reduce dosage in patients with renal impairment. Adequate hydration should be maintained during therapy.

Adverse Reactions: Skin rashes and hematological reactions.

Incompatibilities: Most common medications.

Generic Name: **Urokinase**

Trade Name: **Abbokinase**

Dosage Forms: Injection: 5,000 and 250,000 IU vials

Uses: A thrombolytic agent used in the management of coronary artery thrombosis and acute myocardial infarction, pulmonary embolism and deep vein thrombosis.

Usual Dosages: Adult: Coronary artery thrombosis: 6,000 units/minute by intracoronary infusion for up to 2 hours.
Pulmonary embolism and deep vein thrombosis: 4,400 units/kg intravenously over a 10 minute period followed by 4,400 units/kg/hour by continuous IV infusion for 12 hours.
Pediatric: dose range not established.

Precautions: Use with caution in patients with pre-existing bleeding disorders or with a recent history of cerebrovascular accident or internal bleeding. EKG and blood pressure monitoring should be available during infusions, especially in patients treated for myocardial infarction. Use with caution in patients with a history of antiplatelet therapy.

Adverse Reactions: Hypotension, reperfusion arrhythmias and bleeding disorders.

Incompatibilities: Do not mix with other medications. Solutions should be prepared in 0.9% sodium chloride and dextrose 5% in water only.

Generic Name: **Vancomycin**

Trade Name: **Vancocin and Vancoled**

Dosage Forms: Injection: 500 mg and 1 gram vials
Oral: 125 and 250 mg capsules and solution

Uses: A narrow spectrum glycopeptide antibiotic used in the treatment of serious infections caused by a variety of susceptible gram-positive organisms such as Staphylococci, Streptococci, Enterococci, Corynebacterium and Clostridia.

Usual Dosages: Adults: 1–2 grams daily given as a slow IV infusion in divided doses every 6–12 hours.
Pediatrics: Neonates (0–7 days):
—Less than 1 kg: 10 mg/kg every 24 hours
—Between 1–2 kg: 10 mg/kg every 18 hours
—Greater than 2 kg: 10 mg/kg every 12 hours
Infants greater than 7 days: 30–45 mg/kg/day given as an IV infusion in divided doses every 8 hours (less in preterm infants).
—Oral preparations are used exclusively for the treatment of antibiotic-induced pseudomembraneous colitis caused by C. difficile because of little systemic absorption.

Precautions: Administer each dose slowly over at least 1 hour. Reduce dosage in patients with renal impairment. Do not administer intramuscularly and avoid extravasation.

Adverse Reactions: Hypotension which may be combined with a rash on the face, neck and chest (red man's syndrome) can occur and has been associated with rapid administration and large single doses. Ototoxicity and nephrotoxicity can occur, especially when given with other drugs causing similar adverse effects.

Incompatibilities: Heparin, aminophylline and various alkaline solutions and medications.

Generic Name: **Vasopressin**

Trade Name: **Pitresssin**

Dosage Forms: Injection: 20 units/ml (aqueous) and 5 units/ml (suspension) for IM or SC injection.

Uses: A polypeptide hormone (ADH) used in the treatment of diabetes insipidus and the acute treatment of GI hemorrhage.

Usual Dosages: Adult: GI hemorrhage—0.2–0.4 units/minute as a continuous IV infusion. The aqueous injection should be diluted to a concentration between 0.1–1 mg/ml prior to infusion.
—The aqueous solution is the *only* injection that can be given intravenously.

Precautions: May precipitate angina in patients with coronary artery disease. Vasopressin is a very potent vasoconstrictor and care should be taken not to extravasate the infusion; administer via central line if possible.

Adverse Reactions: Overhydration, abdominal cramps, sweating and headache. Hypersensitivity reactions have been reported.

Incompatibilities: Alkaline solutions.

Generic Name: **Vecuronium**
Trade Name: **Norcuron**
Dosage Forms: Injection: 10 mg vial
Uses: A non-depolarizing skeletal muscle relaxant used to produce muscle relaxation during endotracheal intubation and surgery.
Usual Dosages: Adult: 3–7 mg IV push initially for intubation.
Pediatric dose: 0.08–0.1 mg/kg IV push initially for intubation.
Precautions: Adequate facilities for intubation as well as oxygen administration and ventilatory support must be available prior to use. Reversal may be accomplished with intravenous administration of neostigmine, physostigmine or endrophonium and atropine.
Adverse Reactions: Respiratory depression.
Incompatibilities: Compatible with most intravenous fluids.

Generic Name: **Verapamil**
Trade Name: **Calan, Isoptin and others**
Dosage Forms: Injection: 2.5 mg/ml vial
Oral: 80 and 120 mg tablets and 240 mg sustained release tablets and capsules
Uses: A calcium channel blocking agent used in management of supraventricular arrhythmias, hypertension and angina.
Usual Dosages: Adult: 5–10 mg by direct IV injection, followed by repeated IV boluses every 4–6 hours or by a continuous IV infusion of 1.25–5.0 mg/hour.
Pediatric: dose range not established, however 0.1–0.3 mg/kg (up to 5 mg) have been used.
Precautions: Use with caution in patients with congestive heart failure and sinus node dysfunction. EKG and blood pressure monitoring should be available. Prolongation of the P-R interval may precede cardiac toxicity. Reduce dosage in renal severe impairment.
Adverse Reactions: Hypotension, congestive heart failure and conduction defects such as first degree AV block.
Incompatibilities: Alkaline solutions and medications.

Subject Index

Page numbers in *italics* denote figures; those followed by "t" denote tables.